Taylor's Clinical Nursing Skills

A Nursing Process Approach

Fourth Edition

Pamela Lynn, MSN, RN
Instructor
Gwynedd Mercy University
Frances M. Maguire School of Nursing and Health Professions
Gwynedd Valley, Pennsylvania

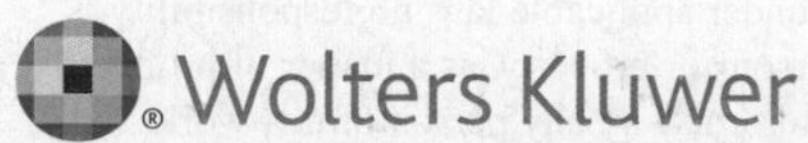

Philadelphia • Baltimore • New York • London
Buenos Aires • Hong Kong • Sydney • Tokyo

Publisher: Lisa McAllister
Executive Editor: Sherry Dickinson
Product Developmental Editor: Christine Abshire
Developmental Editor: Sarah Kyle
Editorial Assistant: Dan Reilly
Marketing Manager: Dean Karampelas
Production Project Manager: Cynthia Rudy
Design Coordinator: Holly Reid McLaughlin
Illustration Coordinator: Jennifer Clements
Manufacturing Coordinator: Karin Duffield
Prepress Vendor: Aptara, Inc.

4th Edition

9 8 7 6 5 4 3 2 1

Printed in China

Library of Congress Cataloging-in-Publication Data

Lynn, Pamela (Pamela Barbara), 1961- author.
Taylor's clinical nursing skills : a nursing process approach / Pamela Lynn. – Fourth edition.
p. ; cm.
Clinical nursing skills
Includes bibliographical references and index.
ISBN 978-1-4511-9271-1 (alk. paper)
I. Title. II. Title: Clinical nursing skills.
[DNLM: 1. Nursing Process. 2. Nursing Care–methods. WY 100]
RT51
610.73–dc23

2014021573

LWW.com

CCS0814

To past, present, and future nursing students and my family:

Each one of you helps me to continue learning and caring every day.

Contributors and Reviewers

Contributors to Previous Editions

Sheryl Kathleen Buckner, RN, MS, CM
Academic and Staff Developer, Case Manager, Clinical Instructor
University of Oklahoma, College of Nursing
Oklahoma City, Oklahoma
Unit III: Integrated Case Studies

Lynn Burbank, MSN, RN, CPNP
Learning Resource Coordinator
Dixon School of Nursing
Abington Memorial Hospital
Abington, Pennsylvania
Chapter 5: Medications

Pamela Evans-Smith, MSN, FNP
Clinical Nursing Instructor
University of Missouri
Columbia, Missouri

Mary Hermann, BSN, MSN, EdD
Professor
Gwynedd Mercy University
Gwynedd Valley, Pennsylvania
Chapter 3: Health Assessment
Chapter 6: Perioperative Nursing
Chapter 8: Skin Integrity and Wound Care
Chapter 11: Nutrition
Chapter 15: Fluid, Electrolyte, and Acid–Base Balance

Connie J. Hollen, RN, MS
Adjunct Instructor
University of Oklahoma, College of Nursing
Oklahoma City, Oklahoma
Unit III: Integrated Case Studies

Loren Nell Melton Stein, RNC, MSN
Adjunct Instructor
University of Oklahoma, College of Nursing
Oklahoma City, Oklahoma
Unit III: Integrated Case Studies

For a list of the contributors to the Student and Instructor Resources accompanying this book, please visit thePoint.

Reviewers

Esther Levine Brill, PhD, APRN-BC (ANP), RN
Professor
Long Island University
School of Nursing
Brooklyn, New York

Denise Doliveira, MSN, CMSRN
Professor of Nursing
Community College of Allegheny County, Boyce Campus
Monroeville, Pennsylvania

Jaime Huffman, PhD
Assistant Professor
Saginaw Valley State University
University Center, Michigan

Kathryn Konrad, MS, RNC-OB, LCCE, FACCE
Instructor, Nursing Academic Programs
The University of Oklahoma College of Nursing
Oklahoma City, Oklahoma

Catherine Leipold, MS, CCRN, APRN-BC
Clinical Instructor
University of Illinois–Urbana
Chicago, Illinois

Patricia Lisk, RN, MS, DACCE
Professor of Nursing
Dean of Nursing and Health Technologies
Germanna Community College
Locust Grove, Virginia

April Magoteaux, PhD, RN, CNS, NHA, AC
Associate Professor
Columbus State Community College
Columbus, Ohio

Marjorie Norquist, RN, MA, MPA, BSN
Professor
Community College of Rhode Island
Warwick, Rhode Island

Valinda Pearson, PhD, RN, CRRN, CNE
Professor of Nursing
St, Catherine University
Minneapolis, Minnesota

Janette Petro, RN, MSN, BSN
Professor
Community College of Allegheny County, Boyce Campus
Monroeville, Pennsylvania

Amy Ragnone, MSN, MA, RN
Professor
College of Southern Nevada
Las Vegas, Nevada

Pamela Santarlasci, PhD, RN, CRNP, CNE
Assistant Professor
Delaware County Community College
Media, Pennsylvania

Jeanine Speakman, MSN, BSN, ADN
Assistant Professor
Victor Valley College
Victorville, California

Donna Spivey, MSN, RN, CEN
Nursing Program Director
Lone Star College–Kingwood
Kingwood, Texas

Linda Tate, MSN, APRN-BC
Assistant Professor
Arkansas State University
Jonesboro, Arkansas

Robin Zachary, EdS, MSN, RN
Instructor of Nursing
Lincoln Memorial University
Harrogate, Tennessee

For a list of the reviewers of the Test Generator accompanying this book, please visit thePoint.

Preface

Taylor's Clinical Nursing Skills: A Nursing Process Approach aims to help nursing students or graduate nurses incorporate cognitive, technical, interpersonal, and ethical/legal skills into safe and effective patient care. This book is written to meet the needs of novice to advanced nurses. Many of the skills shown in this book may not be encountered by the student while in school, but may be encountered once the graduate nurse has entered the workforce.

Because it emphasizes the basic principles of patient care, we believe this book can easily be used with any Fundamentals text. However, this Skills book was specifically designed to accompany *Fundamentals of Nursing: The Art and Science of Person-Centered Nursing Care,* Eighth Edition, by Taylor, Lillis, and Lynn to provide a seamless learning experience. Some of the Skills and Guidelines for Nursing Care from the Taylor Fundamentals book may also be found in this book, but its content has been embellished here to:

- Highlight the nursing process
- Emphasize unexpected situations that the nurse may encounter, along with related interventions for how to respond to these unexpected situations
- Draw attention to critical actions within skills
- Illustrate specific actions within a skill through the use of nearly 1,000 four-color photographs and illustrations
- Highlight available best practice guidelines and/or research-based evidence to support the skills as available
- Reference appropriate case study or studies included at the end of the book, emphasizing which case studies utilize and enhance the content of each chapter

Additionally, this book contains numerous higher-level skills that are not addressed in the Taylor Fundamentals book.

LEARNING EXPERIENCE

This text and the entire Taylor Suite have been created with the student's experience in mind. Care has been taken to appeal to all learning styles. The student-friendly writing style ensures that students will comprehend and retain information. The extensive art program enhances understanding of important actions. Free video clips clearly demonstrate and reinforce important skill steps; as students watch and listen to the videos, comprehension increases. In addition, each element of the Taylor Suite, which is described later in the preface, coordinates to provide a consistent and cohesive learning experience.

ORGANIZATION

Taylor's Clinical Nursing Skills is organized into three units. Ideally, the text will be followed sequentially, but every effort has been made to respect the differing needs of diverse curricula and students. Thus, each chapter stands on its own merit and may be read independently of others.

Unit I, Actions Basic to Nursing Care

This unit introduces the foundational skills used by nurses: maintaining asepsis, measuring vital signs, assessing health, promoting safety, administering medication, and caring for surgical patients.

In Chapter 3, Health Assessment, revised physical assessment content reflects the practice needs of beginning and general nurses. Assessment procedures performed by advanced practice professionals are clearly identified. Assessments identified as advanced procedures and skills are available on thePoint.

Unit II, Promoting Healthy Physiologic Responses

This unit focuses on the physiologic needs of patients: hygiene; skin integrity and wound care; activity; comfort and pain management; nutrition; urinary elimination; bowel elimination; oxygenation; fluid, electrolyte, and acid–base balance; neurologic care; cardiovascular care; and specimen collection.

Unit III, Integrated Case Studies

Although nursing skills textbooks generally present content in a linear fashion for ease of understanding, in reality, many nursing skills are performed in combination for patients with complicated health needs. The integrated case studies in this unit are designed to challenge the reader to think critically and outside the norm, consider the multiple needs of patients, and prioritize care appropriately—ultimately preparing the student and graduate nurse for complex situations that may arise in everyday practice.

TEACHING/LEARNING PACKAGE

To facilitate mastery of this text's content, a comprehensive teaching/learning package has been developed to assist faculty and students.

Resources for Instructors

Tools to assist you with teaching your course are available upon adoption of this text on thePoint at http://thepoint.lww.com/Lynn4e.

- The **Test Generator** has over 500 NCLEX®-Style questions to help you put together exclusive new tests from a bank with questions spanning the book's topics, which will assist you in assessing your students' understanding of the material.

- **PowerPoint Presentations,** provided for each book chapter, enhance teaching by providing key visuals and reinforcing content. These provide an easy way for you to integrate the textbook with your students' learning experience, either via slide shows or handouts.
- **Skills Lab Teaching Plans** walk you through each chapter, objective by objective, and provide a lecture outline and teaching guidelines. In addition to one teaching plan for each chapter, there is one bonus teaching plan to assist with lab simulations.
- **A Master Checklist for Skills Competency** is provided to help you track your students' progress on all the skills in this book.
- A sample **Syllabus** is provided to help you organize your course.
- **Journal Articles** offer access to current research available in Wolters Kluwer journals.
- **WebCT/Blackboard-Ready Materials** can be accessed on thePoint, plus access to all Student Resources, including Watch & Learn video clips, Practice & Learn activities, and Concepts in Action Animations.
- The **Image Bank** provides free access to illustrations and photos from the textbook for use in PowerPoint presentations and handouts.

Resources for Students

Valuable learning tools for students are available on thePoint at http://thepoint.lww.com/Lynn4e.

- **NCLEX®-Style Review Questions** correspond with each book chapter for review of important concepts and to help practice for the NCLEX examination. Nearly 400 questions are included.
- **Watch & Learn** video clips, **Practice & Learn** activities, and **Concepts in Action Animations** demonstrate important concepts related to skills.
- **Journal Articles** offer access to current research available in Wolters Kluwer journals.
- A **Spanish–English Audio Glossary** provides helpful terms and phrases for communicating with patients who speak Spanish.
- **Dosage Calculation Quizzes** provide opportunities for students to practice math skills and calculate drug dosages.

Taylor Suite Resources

From traditional texts to video and interactive products, the Taylor Fundamentals/Skills suite is tailored to fit every learning style. This integrated suite of products offers students a seamless learning experience not found elsewhere. To learn more about any solution with the Taylor suite, please contact your local Wolters Kluwer representative.

- ***Fundamentals of Nursing: The Art and Science of Person-Centered Nursing Care,* 8th Edition,** by Carol Taylor, Carol Lillis and Pamela Lynn. This traditional Fundamentals text promotes nursing as an evolving art and science, directed to human health and well-being. It challenges students to focus on the four blended skills of nursing care, which prepare students to combine the highest level of scientific knowledge and technologic skill with responsible, caring practice. The text includes engaging features to promote critical thinking and comprehension.
- ***Taylor's Handbook of Clinical Nursing Skills,* 2nd Edition,** by Pamela Lynn. The second edition provides streamlined skills consistent with those in *Taylor's Clinical Nursing Skills,* Fourth Edition. Presented for quick reference or on-the-go review, skills are organized alphabetically by key word.
- ***Taylor's Video Guide to Clinical Nursing Skills,* 3rd Edition.** With more than 12 hours of video footage, this updated series follows nursing students and their instructors as they perform a range of essential nursing procedures. Institutions can purchase the videos on enhanced DVD or access them online.
- ***Skill Checklists for Taylor's Clinical Nursing Skills,* 4th Edition.** This collection of checklists with convenient perforated pages is designed to accompany the Skills textbook and promote proper technique while increasing students' confidence.

vSim for Nursing SIMULATION

vSim for Nursing* | *Fundamentals, a new virtual simulationplatform *(available via* thePoint). Co-developed by Laerdal Medical and Wolters Kluwer, *vSim for Nursing | Fundamentals* helps students develop clinical competence and decision-making skills as they interact with virtual patients in a safe, realistic environment. *vSim for Nursing* records and assesses student decisions throughout the simulation, then provides a personalized feedback log highlighting areas needing improvement.

Lippincott CoursePoint A COMPREHENSIVE, DIGITAL, INTEGRATED COURSE SOLUTION

Lippincott CoursePoint is the only integrated digital course solution for nursing education, combining the power of digital course content with interactive resources and virtual simulation. Pulling these resources together into one solution, the integrated product offers a seamless experience for learning, studying, applying, and remediating. Lippincott CoursePoint provides a personalized learning experience that is structured in the way students study. It drives students to immediate remediation in their text; digital course content and interactive course resources, such as case studies, videos, and journal articles, are also immediately available in the same digitally integrated course solution to help expand on concepts and bring them to life. The SmartSense links feature included throughout CoursePoint integrates all of the content, offering immediate remediation and additional learning resources at the click of a mouse. With Lippincott CoursePoint, instructors can collaborate with students at any time, identify common misunderstandings, evaluate student comprehension, and differentiate instruction as needed. And students can learn and retain course material in a personalized way. This unique offering creates an unparalleled learning experience for students. Contact your Wolters Kluwer sales representative for more information about the Lippincott CoursePoint solution.

Pamela Lynn, MSN, RN

How to Use *Taylor's Clinical Nursing Skills*

FOCUS ON PATIENT CARE!

Each chapter in Units I and II begins with a description of three real-world case scenarios that put the skills into context. These scenarios provide a framework for the chapter content to be covered.

GET READY TO LEARN!

Before reading the chapter content, read the **Learning Objectives.** These roadmaps help you understand what is important and why. Create your own learning outline or use them for self-testing.

Review the **Key Terms** lists to become familiar with new vocabulary presented throughout the narrative. Look for them in bold type throughout the chapter.

2 Vital Signs

FOCUSING ON PATIENT CARE

This chapter will explain some of the skills related to vital signs needed to care for the following patients:

TYRONE JEFFRIES, age 5, is in the emergency department with a temperature of 101.3°F (38.9°C).

TOBY WHITE, age 26, has a history of asthma and is now breathing 32 times per minute.

CARL GLATZ, age 58, has recently started taking medications to control his hypertension (high blood pressure).

Refer to Focusing on Patient Care: Developing Clinical Reasoning at the end of the chapter to apply what you learn.

LEARNING OBJECTIVES

After studying this chapter, you will be able to:

1. Assess body temperature via the oral, tympanic, temporal, axillary, and rectal routes.
2. Regulate an infant's temperature using an overhead radiant warmer.
3. Regulate temperature using a cooling blanket.
4. Assess peripheral pulses by palpation.
5. Assess an apical pulse by auscultation.
6. Assess peripheral pulses using Doppler ultrasound.
7. Assess respiration.
8. Assess blood pressure by auscultation or using an automatic electronic blood pressure monitor.
9. Assess systolic blood pressure using Doppler ultrasound.

KEY TERMS

apnea: absence of breathing
bell: (of stethoscope) hollowed, upright, curved portion used to auscultate low-pitched sounds, such as murmurs
blood pressure: force of blood against arterial walls
bradypnea: abnormally slow rate of breathing
diaphragm: (of stethoscope) large, flat disk on the stethoscope used to auscultate high-pitched sounds, such as respiratory sounds

35

DEVELOP CRITICAL THINKING AND CLINICAL REASONING!

Fundamentals Review. Because of the breadth and depth of nursing knowledge that must be absorbed, nursing students and graduate nurses can easily become overwhelmed. Thus, this book is designed to eliminate excessive content and redundancy and to better focus the reader's attention. To this end, each chapter in Units I and II includes several boxes, tables, or figures that summarize important concepts that should be understood before performing a skill. For a more in-depth study of these concepts, readers are encouraged to refer to their Fundamentals textbook.

FUNDAMENTALS REVIEW 2-2

TECHNIQUES FOR OBTAINING VITAL SIGNS OF INFANTS AND CHILDREN

- Due to the "fear factor" of blood pressure measurement, save the blood pressure measurement for last. Children and infants often begin to cry during blood pressure assessment, and this may affect the respiration and pulse rate assessment.
- Perform as many tasks as possible while the child is sitting on the parent's lap or in a chair next to the parent.
- Let the child see and touch the equipment before you begin to use it.
- Make measuring vital signs a game. For instance, if you are using a tympanic thermometer that makes a chirping sound, tell the child you are looking for "birdies" in the ear. While auscultating the pulse, tell the child you are listening for another type of animal.
- If the child has a doll or stuffed animal, pretend to take the doll's vital signs first.

Enhance Your Understanding, located at the end of each chapter, gives readers an opportunity to further their understanding and apply what they have learned. It includes three sections:

Focusing on Patient Care: Developing Clinical Reasoning asks readers to consider questions that reflect back to the opening scenarios for added cohesion throughout the chapters. Readers are challenged to apply the skills and use the new knowledge they have gained to "think through" learning exercises designed to show how critical thinking and clinical reasoning can result in a clinical judgment, leading to a possible change in outcomes and an impact on patient care.

Suggested Answers for Focusing on Patient Care: Developing Clinical Reasoning represent possible nursing care solutions to the problems. The answers can be found after the bibliography section at the end of the chapter.

Integrated Case Study Connection refers readers to the appropriate case study or studies discussion in Unit III, emphasizing which case studies utilize and enhance the content of that chapter.

ENHANCE YOUR UNDERSTANDING

FOCUSING ON PATIENT CARE: DEVELOPING CLINICAL REASONING

Consider the case scenarios at the beginning of the chapter as you answer the following questions to enhance your understanding and apply what you have learned.

QUESTIONS

1. While preparing the sterile table in the cardiac catheterization lab for Mr. Wilson, you realize that a sterile bowl is missing. How can you obtain a sterile bowl?
2. While you are putting on sterile gloves in preparation for an indwelling urinary catheter insertion, your patient, Sheri Lawrence, moves her leg. You do not *think* that Sheri's leg touched the glove, but you are not positive. What should you do?
3. Edgar Barowski's son is visiting and asks you why the masks that are outside Edgar's room are different from the ones that people wear in the operating room. What should you tell Edgar's son?

You can find suggested answers after the Bibliography at the end of this chapter.

INTEGRATED CASE STUDY CONNECTION

The case studies in the back of the book are designed to focus on integrating concepts. Refer to the following case studies to enhance your understanding of the concepts related to the skills in this chapter.

- Basic Case Studies: Tiffany Jones, page 1064; John Willis, page 1068.
- Intermediate Case Studies: Tula Stillwater, page 1081; Gwen Galloway, page 1089; George Patel, page 1091.

TAYLOR SUITE RESOURCES

Explore these additional resources to enhance learning for this chapter:

- NCLEX-Style Questions and other resources on thePoint, http://thePoint.lww.com/Lynn4e
- *Skill Checklists for Taylor's Clinical Nursing Skills,* 4e
- *Taylor's Video Guide to Clinical Nursing Skills:* Asepsis
- *Fundamentals of Nursing:* Chapter 23, Asepsis and Infection Control

New! Delegation Considerations assist students and graduate nurses in developing the critical decision-making skills necessary to transfer responsibility for the performance of an activity to another individual and to ensure safe and effective nursing care. Delegation decision-making information is provided in each skill and Appendix A, using delegation guidelines based on American Nurses Association (ANA) and National Council of State Boards of Nursing (NCSBN) principles and recommendations.

Updated and expanded in this edition, **Evidence for Practice** highlights available best practice guidelines and/or research-based evidence to support the skills as available.

EVIDENCE FOR PRACTICE ▶

PPE AND PREVENTION OF TRANSFER OF MICROORGANISMS

Prevention of health care–associated infections is a major challenge for health care providers. The removal of PPE after patient care may result in transfer of microorganisms to hands and clothing of health care workers. How can this risk of transfer be reduced?

Related Research

Casanova, L.M., Rutala, W.A., Weber, D.J., & Sobsey, M.D. (2012). Effect of single- versus double-gloving on virus transfer to healthcare workers' skin and clothing during removal of personal protective equipment. *American Journal of Infection Control, 40*(4), 369–374.

The focus of this study was to determine whether double-gloving reduces virus transfer to the hands and clothing of health care workers during removal of contaminated PPE. There was a double-gloving phase and a single-gloving phase of the experiment. Participants put on PPE, including a gown, N95 respirator, eye protection, and gloves. The gown, respirator, eye protection, and dominant glove were contaminated with bacteriophage. Participants then removed the PPE, and their hands, face, and clothing were sampled for virus. Transfer of virus to hands during PPE removal was significantly more frequent with single-gloving than with double-gloving. Significantly more virus was transferred to participants' hands after single-gloving than after double-gloving. Transfer to clothing was similar during single-gloving and double-gloving. The researchers concluded double-gloving can reduce the risk of viral contamination of the hands of health care workers during PPE removal.

Relevance for Nursing Practice

Nurses should continually strive to improve practice and be alert for interventions to help achieve better practice. The use of double gloves is an inexpensive and simple intervention. Incorporating the use of double-gloving with the use of full PPE may be an effective method to reduce the risk of transmission of microorganisms.

MASTER NURSING PROCESS!

The **nursing process** framework is used to integrate related nursing responsibilities for each of the five steps: Assessment, Nursing Diagnoses,* Outcome Identification and Planning, Implementation, and Evaluation, as well as Documentation.

Documentation Guidelines direct students and graduate nurses in accurate documentation of the skill and their findings. **Sample Documentation** demonstrates proper documentation.

SKILL 2-1 ASSESSING BODY TEMPERATURE continued

ACTION	RATIONALE
46. Dispose of the probe cover by holding the probe over an appropriate waste receptacle and pressing the release button.	Proper probe cover disposal reduces risk of microorganism transmission.
47. Using toilet tissue, wipe the anus of any feces or excess lubricant. Dispose of the toilet tissue. Remove gloves and discard them.	Wiping promotes cleanliness. Disposing of the toilet tissue avoids transmission of microorganisms.
48. Cover the patient and help him or her to a position of comfort.	Ensures patient comfort.
49. Place the bed in the lowest position; elevate rails as needed.	These actions provide for the patient's safety.
50. Return the thermometer to the charging unit.	The thermometer needs to be recharged for future use.

EVALUATION

The expected outcomes are met when the patient's temperature is assessed accurately without injury and the patient experiences minimal discomfort.

DOCUMENTATION

Guidelines

Record temperature on paper, flow sheet, or computerized record. Report abnormal findings to the appropriate person. Identify the site of assessment if other than oral.

Sample Documentation

10/20/15 Tympanic temperature assessed. Temperature 102.5°F. Patient states she has "a pounding" headache; denies chills, malaise. Physician notified. Received order to give 650 mg PO acetaminophen now. Incentive spirometer × 10 q 2 hours.

M. Evans, RN

UNEXPECTED SITUATIONS AND ASSOCIATED INTERVENTIONS

- *Temperature reading is higher or lower than expected based on your assessment:* Reassess temperature with a different thermometer. The thermometer may not be calibrated correctly. If using a tympanic thermometer, you will get lower readings if the probe is not inserted far enough into the ear.
- *During rectal temperature assessment, the patient reports feeling light-headed or passes out:* Remove the thermometer immediately. Quickly assess the patient's blood pressure and heart rate. Notify the physician. Do not attempt to take another rectal temperature on this patient.

SPECIAL CONSIDERATIONS

General Considerations

- Nonmercury glass thermometers used for oral readings commonly have long, thin bulbs. Those for rectal readings have a blunt bulb to prevent injury. See the accompanying Skill Variation for information on assessing temperature with a nonmercury glass thermometer.
- If the patient smoked, chewed gum, or consumed hot or cold food or fluids recently, wait 30 minutes before taking an oral temperature to allow the oral tissues to return to baseline temperature.
- Nasal oxygen is not thought to affect oral temperature readings. Do not assess oral temperatures in patients receiving oxygen by mask. Removal of the mask for the time period required for assessment could result in a serious drop in the patient's blood oxygen level.
- When using a tympanic thermometer, make sure to insert the probe into the ear canal sufficiently tightly to seal the opening to ensure an accurate reading.
- A dirty probe lens and cone on the temporal artery thermometer can cause a falsely low reading. If the lens is not shiny in appearance, clean the lens and cone with an alcohol preparation or swab moistened in alcohol.
- If the patient's axilla has been washed recently, wait 15 to 30 minutes before taking an axillary temperature to allow the skin to return to baseline temperature.
- Axillary temperatures are generally about one degree less than oral temperatures; rectal temperatures are generally about one degree higher.

*Material related to nursing diagnoses is from *Nursing Diagnoses–Definitions and Classification 2012–2014*. To make safe and effective judgments using NANDA-I nursing diagnoses it is essential that nurses refer to the definitions and defining characteristics of the diagnoses listed in this work.

DEVELOP THE NECESSARY SKILLS!

Step-by-Step Skills. Each chapter presents a host of related step-by-step skills. The skills are presented in a concise, straightforward, and simplified two-column format to facilitate competent performance of nursing skills.

Scientific Rationales accompany each nursing action to promote a deeper understanding of the basic principles supporting nursing care.

Nursing Alerts draw attention to crucial information.

Photo Atlas Approach. When learning a new skill, it is often overwhelming to only *read* how to perform a skill. With nearly 1,000 photographs, this book offers a pictorial guide to performing each skill. The skill will not only be learned but also remembered through the use of text with pictures.

SKILL 1-2 PERFORMING HAND HYGIENE USING SOAP AND WATER (HANDWASHING) continued

ACTION	RATIONALE
4. Wet the hands and wrist area. Keep hands lower than elbows to allow water to flow toward fingertips (Figure 3).	Water should flow from the cleaner area toward the more contaminated area. Hands are more contaminated than forearms.
5. Use about 1 teaspoon liquid soap from dispenser or rinse bar of soap and lather thoroughly (Figure 4). Cover all areas of hands with the soap product. Rinse soap bar again and return to soap rack without touching the rack.	Rinsing the soap before and after use removes the lather, which may contain microorganisms.

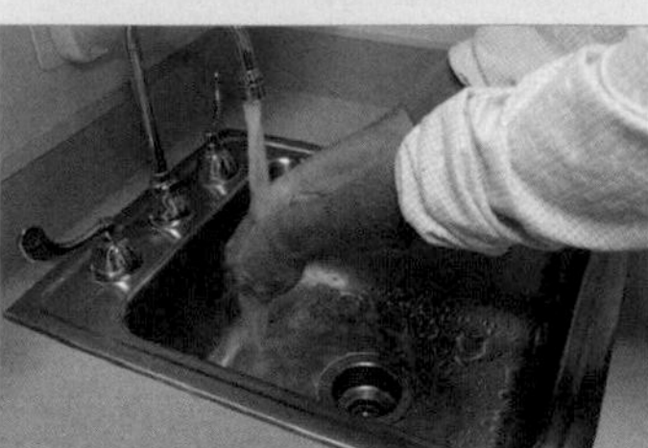

FIGURE 3 Wetting hands to the wrist.

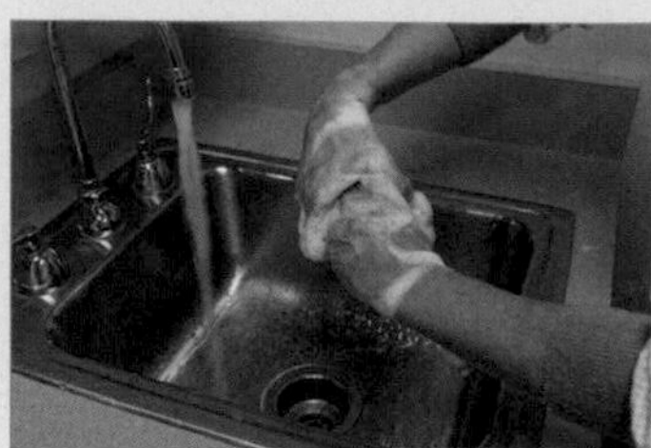

FIGURE 4 Lathering hands with soap and rubbing with firm circular motion.

ACTION	RATIONALE
6. With firm rubbing and circular motions, wash the palms and backs of the hands, each finger, the areas between the fingers (Figure 5), and the knuckles, wrists, and forearms. **Wash at least 1 inch above area of contamination.** If hands are not visibly soiled, wash to 1 inch above the wrists (Figure 6).	Friction caused by firm rubbing and circular motions helps to loosen dirt and organisms that can lodge between the fingers, in skin crevices of knuckles, on the palms and backs of the hands, and on the wrists and forearms. Cleaning less contaminated areas (forearms and wrists) after hands are clean prevents spreading microorganisms from the hands to the forearms and wrists.

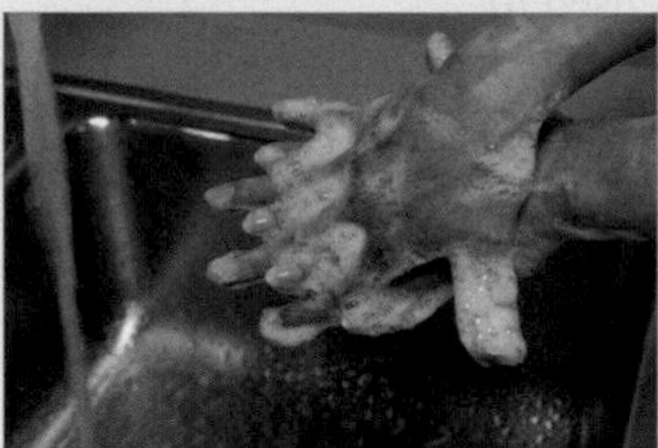

FIGURE 5 Washing areas between fingers.

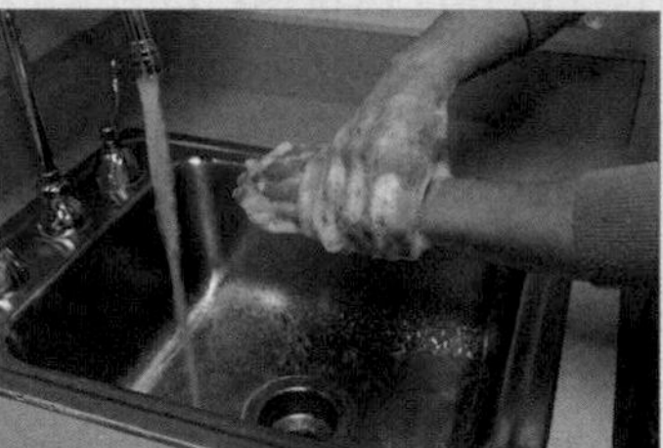

FIGURE 6 Washing to 1 inch above the wrist.

ACTION	RATIONALE
7. Continue this friction motion for at least 20 seconds.	Length of handwashing is determined by degree of contamination. Hands that are visibly soiled need a longer scrub.

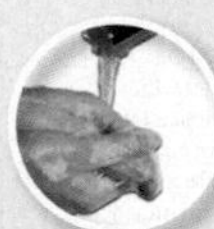

Hand Hygiene icons alert you to this crucial step that is the best way to prevent the spread of microorganisms. Important information related to this icon is included inside the back cover.

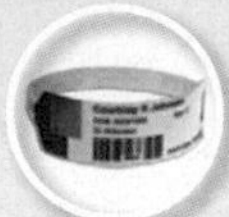

Patient Identification icons alert you to this critical step ensuring the right patient receives the intervention, to help prevent errors. Important information related to this icon is included inside the back cover.

Skill Variations provide clear, start-to-finish instructions for variations in equipment or technique.

Special Considerations, including **Infant, Child, Older Adult,** and **Home Care Considerations** (e.g., modifications and home care), appear throughout to explain the varying needs of patients across the lifespan and in various settings.

Unexpected Situations are provided after the explanation of normal outcomes. Each situation is followed by an explanation of how best to react, with rationales. This feature serves as a starting point for group discussion.

Many skills have free accompanying video clips, indicated by the **Watch & Learn** icon, or free accompanying activities, indicated by the **Practice & Learn** icon. All of these are available on thePoint website at http://thepoint.lww.com/Lynn4e.

Acknowledgments

This updated edition is the work of many talented people. I would like to acknowledge the hard work of all who have contributed to the completion of this project. Thanks to Carol Taylor, Carol Lillis, and Priscilla LeMone for offering generous support and encouragement. You have been excellent mentors.

The work of this revision was skillfully coordinated by my dedicated Product Developmental Editors in the Nursing Education division of Wolters Kluwer. I am grateful to each of you for your patience, support, unending encouragement, and total commitment. My thanks to Christine Abshire, Product Developmental Editor, for her insight and tireless work on this edition. My thanks to Sherry Dickinson, Executive Editor, for her hard work and guidance throughout most of the project; and to Cynthia Rudy, Production Project Manager; Holly Reid McLaughlin, Design Coordinator; and Jennifer Clements, Illustration Coordinator.

A special thanks to my colleagues at Gwynedd Mercy University, who offer unending support and professional guidance.

Finally, I would like to gratefully acknowledge my family, for their love, understanding, and encouragement. Their support was essential during the long hours of research and writing.

Pamela Lynn

Contents

UNIT I

Actions Basic to Nursing Care 1

UNIT III Integrated Case Studies

UNIT

I

Actions Basic to Nursing Care

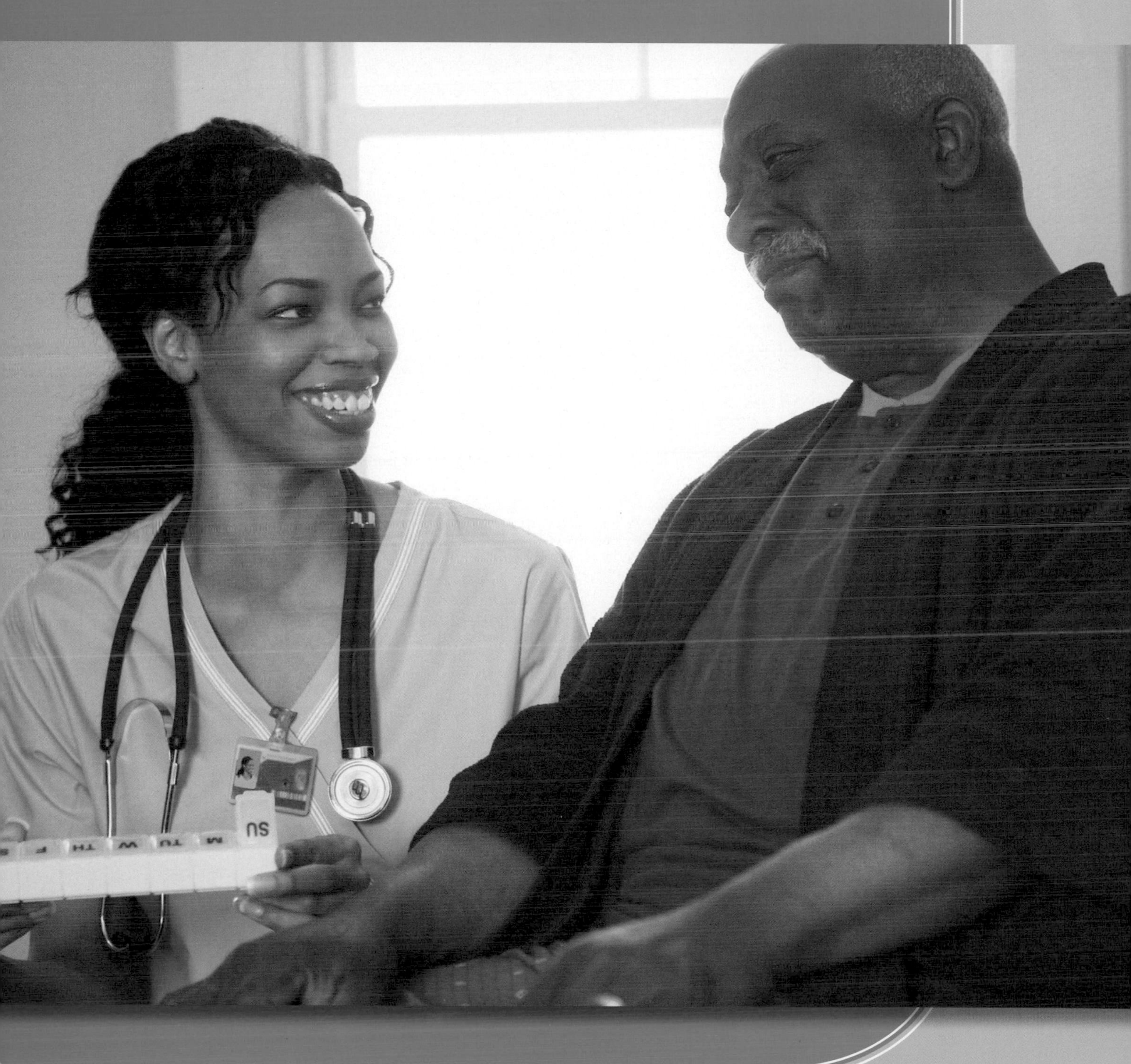

1 Asepsis and Infection Control

FOCUSING ON PATIENT CARE

This chapter will help you develop some of the skills related to asepsis and infection control necessary to care for the following patients:

JOE WILSON, is scheduled to undergo a cardiac catheterization later this morning.

SHERI LAWRENCE, has been ordered to have an indwelling urinary catheter inserted.

EDGAR BAROWSKI, is suspected of having tuberculosis and requires infection-control precautions.

Refer to Focusing on Patient Care: Developing Clinical Reasoning at the end of the chapter to apply what you learn.

LEARNING OBJECTIVES

After studying this chapter, you will be able to:

1. Perform hand hygiene using an alcohol-based handrub.
2. Perform hand hygiene using soap and water (handwashing).
3. Put on and remove personal protective equipment safely.
4. Prepare a sterile field.
5. Add sterile items to a sterile field.
6. Put on and remove sterile gloves.

KEY TERMS

health care–associated infection: infection not present on admission to a health care agency; acquired during the course of treatment for other conditions

medical asepsis: clean technique; involves procedures and practices that reduce the number and transfer of pathogens

personal protective equipment (PPE): equipment and supplies necessary to minimize or prevent exposure to infectious material, including gloves, gowns, masks, and protective eye gear

standard precautions: precautions used in the care of all hospitalized patients regardless of their diagnosis or possible infection status; these precautions apply to blood, all body fluids, secretions and excretions (except sweat), nonintact skin, and mucous membranes

surgical asepsis: sterile technique; involves practices used to render and keep objects and areas free from microorganisms

transmission-based precautions: precautions used in addition to *Standard Precautions* for patients in hospitals who are suspected of being infected with pathogens that can be transmitted by airborne, droplet, or contact routes; these precautions encompass all the diseases or conditions previously listed in the disease-specific or category-specific classifications

Nurses and other health care workers play a key role in reducing the spread of disease, minimizing complications, and reducing adverse outcomes for their patients. Prevention of health care–associated infections (HAIs) is a major challenge for health care providers. In the United States, HAIs account for tens of thousands of deaths and 28 to 33 billion dollars of additional health care costs annually (AHRQ, 2010). Limiting the spread of microorganisms is accomplished by breaking the chain of infection. The practice of asepsis includes all activities to prevent infection or break the chain of infection. **Medical asepsis**, or clean technique, involves procedures and practices that reduce the number and transfer of pathogens. Procedures incorporating medical asepsis include, for example, performing hand hygiene and wearing gloves. Refer to Fundamentals Review 1-1. **Surgical asepsis**, or sterile technique, includes practices used to render and keep objects and areas free from microorganisms. Procedures incorporating surgical asepsis include, for example, inserting an indwelling urinary catheter or inserting an intravenous catheter. Refer to Fundamentals Review 1-2.

This chapter focuses on nursing skills to assist in preventing the spread of infection. These skills include performing hand hygiene, using personal protective equipment (PPE), preparing a sterile field, adding sterile items to a sterile field, and putting on and removing sterile gloves.

Hand hygiene is the most effective way to help prevent the spread of infectious agents. The Joint Commission (TJC) has included a recommendation to use hand hygiene as part of the 2014 Patient Safety Goal to "prevent infection" (TJC, 2014). In addition, as part of their "Speak Up" program, TJC encourages consumers to insist on hand hygiene measures from all health care staff involved in their care (TJC, 2010). The World Health Organization (WHO, 2009) has defined the "Five Moments for Hand Hygiene." These include:

- Moment 1: Before touching a patient
- Moment 2: Before a clean or aseptic procedure
- Moment 3: After body fluid exposure risk
- Moment 4: After touching a patient
- Moment 5: After touching patient surroundings.

If the health care worker's hands are not visibly soiled, alcohol-based handrubs are recommended because they save time, are more accessible and easy to use, and reduce bacterial count on the hands (IHI, 2011). Refer to Fundamentals Review 1-3 for general guidelines regarding hand hygiene for health care workers.

The use of **Standard** and **Transmission-Based Precautions** is another important part of protecting patients and health care providers and preventing the spread of infection. Fundamentals Review 1-4 and Fundamentals Review 1-5 outline a summary of CDC recommended practices for *Standard* and *Transmission-Based Precautions.*

FUNDAMENTALS REVIEW 1-1

BASIC PRINCIPLES OF MEDICAL ASEPSIS IN PATIENT CARE

- Practice good hand hygiene techniques.
- Carry soiled items, including linens, equipment, and other used articles, away from the body to prevent them from touching the clothing.
- Do not place soiled bed linen or any other items on the floor, which is grossly contaminated. It increases contamination of both surfaces.
- Avoid allowing patients to cough, sneeze, or breathe directly on others. Provide patients with disposable tissues, and instruct them, as indicated, to cover their mouth and nose to prevent spread by airborne droplets.
- Move equipment away from you when brushing, dusting, or scrubbing articles. This helps prevent contaminated particles from settling on your hair, face, and uniform.
- Avoid raising dust. Use a specially treated or a dampened cloth. Do not shake linens. Dust and lint particles constitute a vehicle by which organisms can be transported from one area to another.
- Clean the least soiled areas first and then move to the more soiled ones. This helps prevent having the cleaner areas soiled by the dirtier areas.
- Dispose of soiled or used items directly into appropriate containers. Wrap items that are moist from body discharge or drainage in waterproof containers, such as plastic bags, before discarding into the refuse holder so that handlers will not come in contact with them.
- Pour liquids that are to be discarded, such as bath water, mouth rinse, and the like, directly into the drain to avoid splattering in the sink and onto you.
- Sterilize items that are suspected of containing pathogens. After sterilization, they can be managed as clean items if appropriate.
- Use personal grooming habits that help prevent spreading microorganisms. Shampoo your hair regularly; keep your fingernails short and free of broken cuticles and ragged edges; do not wear artificial nails; and do not wear rings with grooves and stones that might harbor microorganisms.
- Follow guidelines conscientiously for infection-control or barrier techniques as prescribed by your agency.

FUNDAMENTALS REVIEW 1-2

BASIC PRINCIPLES OF SURGICAL ASEPSIS IN PATIENT CARE

- Only a sterile object can touch another sterile object. Unsterile touching sterile means contamination has occurred.
- Open sterile packages so that the first edge of the wrapper is directed away from you to avoid the possibility of a sterile surface touching unsterile clothing. The outside of the sterile package is considered contaminated.
- Avoid spilling any solution on a cloth or paper used as a field for a sterile setup. The moisture penetrates the sterile cloth or paper and carries organisms by capillary action to contaminate the field. A wet field is considered contaminated if the surface immediately below it is not sterile.
- Hold sterile objects above waist level. This will ensure keeping the object within sight and preventing accidental contamination.
- Avoid talking, coughing, sneezing, or reaching over a sterile field or object. This helps to prevent contamination by droplets from the nose and the mouth or by particles dropping from your arm.
- Never walk away from or turn your back on a sterile field. This prevents possible contamination while the field is out of your view.
- All items brought into contact with broken skin, used to penetrate the skin to inject substances into the body, or used to enter normally sterile body cavities should be sterile. These items include dressings used to cover wounds and incisions, needles for injection, and tubes (catheters) used to drain urine from the bladder.
- Use dry, sterile forceps when necessary. Forceps soaked in disinfectant are not considered sterile.
- Consider the outer 1-inch edge of a sterile field to be contaminated.
- Consider an object contaminated if you have any doubt about its sterility.

FUNDAMENTALS REVIEW 1-3

HAND HYGIENE FOR HEALTH CARE WORKERS

HAND HYGIENE IS REQUIRED

- Before and after contact with each patient
- Before putting on gloves
- Before performing any invasive procedure, such as placement of a peripheral vascular catheter
- After accidental contact with body fluids or excretions, mucous membranes, nonintact skin, and wound dressings, even if hands are not visibly soiled
- When moving from a contaminated body site to a clean body site during patient care
- After contact with inanimate objects near the patient
- After removal of gloves

ADDITIONAL GUIDELINES

- The use of gloves does not eliminate the need for hand hygiene.
- The use of hand hygiene does not eliminate the need for gloves.
- Natural fingernails should be kept less than 1/4 inch long.
- Artificial fingernails or extenders should not be worn when having direct contact with patients at high risk.
- Gloves should be worn when contact with blood, infectious material, mucous membranes, and nonintact skin could occur.
- Hand lotions or creams are recommended to moisturize and protect skin related to the occurrence of irritant dermatitis associated with hand hygiene.

(Modified with permission from Centers for Disease Control and Prevention [2002]. Guidelines for hand hygiene in health-care settings. *Morbidity and Mortality Weekly Report, 51*(RR16), 1–45.)

FUNDAMENTALS REVIEW 1-4

STANDARD PRECAUTIONS

Standard Precautions are to be used for all patients receiving care in hospitals without regard to their diagnosis or presumed infection status. *Standard Precautions* apply to blood; all body fluids, secretions, and excretions except sweat, whether or not blood is present or visible; nonintact skin; and mucous membranes. *Standard Precautions* reduce the risk of transmission of microorganisms that cause infections in hospitals.

STANDARD PRECAUTIONS (TIER 1)

- Follow hand hygiene techniques.
- Wear clean nonsterile gloves when touching blood, body fluids, excretions, secretions, contaminated items, mucous membranes, and nonintact skin. Change gloves between tasks on the same patient, as necessary, and remove gloves promptly after use.
- Wear **personal protective equipment** such as mask, eye protection, face shield, or fluid-repellent gown during procedures and care activities that are likely to generate splashes or sprays of blood or body fluids. Use gown to protect skin and prevent soiling of clothing.
- Avoid recapping used needles. If you must recap, never use two hands. Use a needle-recapping device or the one-handed scoop technique. Place needles, sharps, and scalpels in appropriate puncture-resistant containers after use.
- Wear gloves to handle used patient-care equipment that is soiled with blood or identified body fluids, secretions, and excretions to prevent transfer of microorganisms. Clean and reprocess items appropriately if used for another patient.
- Follow Respiratory Hygiene/Cough Etiquette. These strategies are targeted at patients and accompanying family members and friends with undiagnosed transmissible respiratory infections. These strategies apply to any person entering a health care facility with signs of illness, including cough, congestion, rhinorrhea, or increased production of respiratory secretions. Educate patients and visitors to health care facilities to cover the mouth/nose with a tissue when coughing; to dispose of used tissues promptly; to use surgical masks on the coughing person when tolerated and appropriate; to use hand hygiene after contact with respiratory secretions; and to use spatial separation, ideally >3 feet, between people with respiratory infections in common waiting areas when possible. Health care personnel are advised to observe *Droplet Precautions* (i.e., wear a mask) and perform hand hygiene when examining and caring

FUNDAMENTALS REVIEW 1-4 continued

STANDARD PRECAUTIONS

for patients with signs and symptoms of a respiratory infection. Health care personnel who have a respiratory infection are advised to avoid direct patient contact, especially with high-risk patients. If this is not possible, then a mask should be worn while providing patient care.

- Use Safe Injection Practices: Use basic principles of aseptic technique for the preparation and administration of parenteral medications, including the use of a sterile, single-use, disposable needle and syringe for each injection given and prevention of contamination of injection equipment and medication. Whenever possible, use of single-dose vials is preferred over multiple-dose vials, especially when medications will be administered to multiple patients.
- Wear a face mask if placing a catheter or injecting material into the spinal or epidural space.

FUNDAMENTALS REVIEW 1-5

TRANSMISSION-BASED PRECAUTIONS

Transmission-Based Precautions are used in addition to *Standard Precautions* for patients with suspected infection with pathogens that can be transmitted by airborne, droplet, or contact routes. Any of the three types can be used in combination with the others. Equipment required for patient care, such as a thermometer, sphygmomanometer, and stethoscope, should be disposable, kept in the patient's room, and not used for other patients.

AIRBORNE PRECAUTIONS (TIER 2)

- Use *Airborne Precautions* for patients who have infections that spread through the air such as tuberculosis, varicella (chicken pox), rubeola (measles), and possibly severe acute respiratory syndrome (SARS).
- Place patient in a private room that has monitored negative air pressure in relation to surrounding areas, 6 to 12 air changes per hour, and appropriate discharge of air outside or monitored filtration if air is recirculated. Keep door closed and patient in room.
- Use respiratory protection when entering room of patient with known or suspected tuberculosis. If patient has known or suspected rubeola or varicella, respiratory protection should be worn unless the person entering the room is immune to these diseases.
- Transport patient out of room only when necessary and place a surgical mask on the patient if possible.
- Consult CDC Guidelines for additional prevention strategies for tuberculosis.

DROPLET PRECAUTIONS

- Use *Droplet Precautions* for patients with an infection that is spread by large-particle droplets, such as rubella, mumps, diphtheria, and the adenovirus infection in infants and young children.
- Use a private room, if available. Door may remain open.
- Wear PPE upon entry into the room for all interactions that may involve contact with the patient and potentially contaminated areas in the patient's environment.
- Transport patient out of the room only when necessary and place a surgical mask on the patient if possible.
- Keep visitors 3 feet away from the infected person.

CONTACT PRECAUTIONS

- *Contact Precautions* are intended to prevent transmission of infectious agents that are spread by direct or indirect contact with the patient or the patient's environment.
- Use *Contact Precautions* for patients who are infected or colonized by a multidrug-resistant organism (MDRO).
- Observe *Contact Precautions* in the presence of excessive wound drainage, fecal incontinence, or other discharges from the body that suggest an increased potential for extensive environmental contamination and risk of transmission.
- Place patient in a private room if available.
- Wear PPE whenever you enter the room for all interactions that may involve contact with the patient and potentially contaminated areas in the patient's environment. Change gloves after having contact with infective material. Remove PPE before leaving the patient environment, and wash hands with an antimicrobial or waterless antiseptic agent.
- Limit movement of the patient out of the room.
- Avoid sharing patient-care equipment.

(Adapted from Centers for Disease Control and Prevention (CDC). (2007d). *Guideline for isolation precautions: Preventing transmission of infectious agents in healthcare settings.* Available www.cdc.gov/hicpac/pdf/isolation. Isolation2007.pdf.)

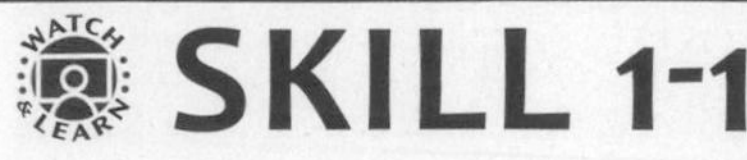

SKILL 1-1 PERFORMING HAND HYGIENE USING AN ALCOHOL-BASED HANDRUB

Alcohol-based handrubs can be used in the health care setting; they take less time to use than traditional handwashing. When using these products, check the product labeling for correct amount of product needed. Alcohol-based handrubs (CDC, 2002; IHI, 2011):

- May be used if hands are not visibly soiled or have not come in contact with blood or body fluids
- May be used before inserting urinary catheters, peripheral vascular catheters, or invasive devices that do not require surgical placement; before donning sterile gloves prior to an invasive procedure (e.g., inserting a central intravascular catheter); and if moving from a contaminated body site to a clean body site during patient care
- Should be used before and after each patient contact, or contact with surfaces in the patient's environment, and after removing gloves
- Significantly reduce the number of microorganisms on skin; alcohol-based handrubs are fast acting and cause less skin irritation

DELEGATION CONSIDERATIONS

The application and use of hand hygiene is appropriate for all health care providers.

EQUIPMENT

- Alcohol-based handrub
- Oil-free lotion (optional)

ASSESSMENT

Assess hands for any visible soiling or contact with blood or body fluids. Alcohol-based handrubs can be used if hands are not visibly soiled, or have not come in contact with blood or body fluids. Wash hands with soap and water before eating and after using the restroom. In addition, if hands are visibly soiled, proceed with washing the hands with soap and water. If hands have been in contact with blood or body fluids, even if there is no visible soiling, proceed with washing the hands with soap and water.

NURSING DIAGNOSIS

Determine the related factors for the nursing diagnosis based on the patient's current status. Appropriate nursing diagnoses may include Risk for Infection.

OUTCOME IDENTIFICATION AND PLANNING

The expected outcome to achieve when performing hand decontamination with alcohol-based rubs is that transient microorganisms will be eliminated from the hands. Other outcomes may be appropriate, depending on the specific nursing diagnosis identified for the patient.

IMPLEMENTATION

ACTION	RATIONALE
1. Remove jewelry, if possible, and secure in a safe place. A plain wedding band may remain in place.	Removal of jewelry facilitates proper cleansing. Microorganisms may accumulate in settings of jewelry. If jewelry was worn during patient care, it should be left on during handwashing.
2. Check the product labeling for correct amount of product needed (Figure 1).	Amount of product required to be effective varies from manufacturer to manufacturer, but is usually 1 to 3 mL.

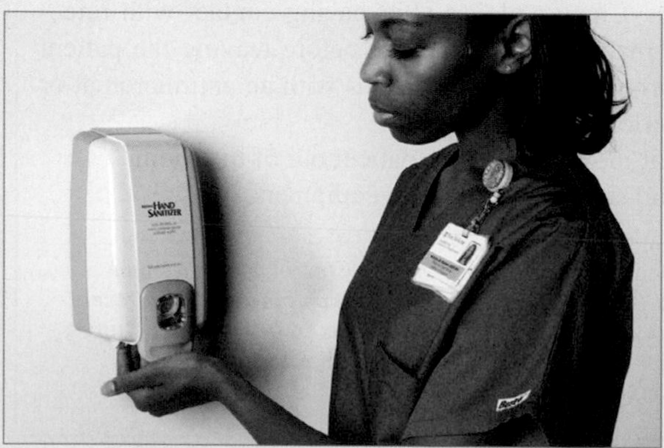

FIGURE 1 Checking product label for correct amount of product needed.

ACTION	RATIONALE
3. Apply the correct amount of product to the palm of one hand (Figure 2). Rub hands together, covering all surfaces of hands and fingers, and between fingers. Also clean the fingertips and the area beneath the fingernails.	Adequate amount of product is required to cover hand surfaces thoroughly. All surfaces must be treated to prevent disease transmission.
4. Rub hands together until they are dry (at least 15 seconds) (Figure 3).	Drying ensures antiseptic effect.

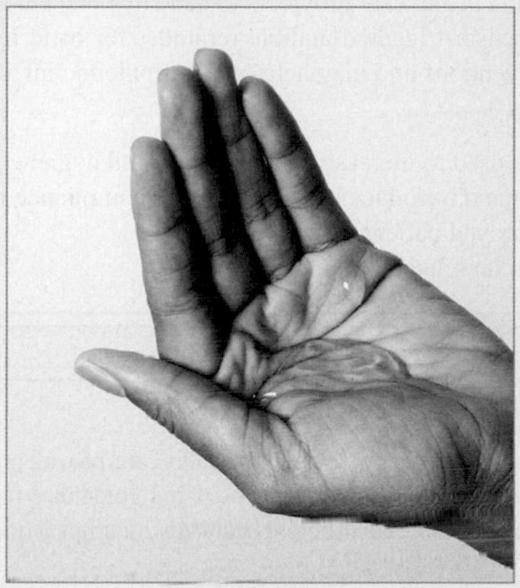

FIGURE 2 Applying the correct amount of product to the palm of one hand.

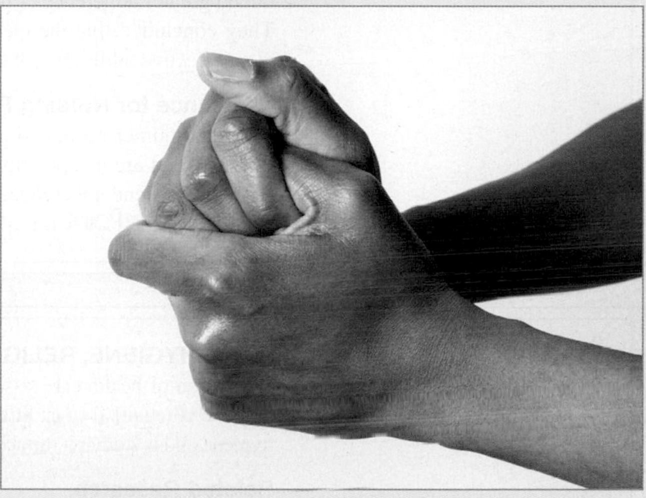

FIGURE 3 Rubbing hands together until dry.

ACTION	RATIONALE
5. Use oil-free lotion on hands, if desired.	Oil-free lotion helps to keep the skin soft and prevents chapping. It is best applied after patient care is complete and from a small, personal container. Oil-based lotions should be avoided because they can cause deterioration of gloves.

EVALUATION The expected outcome is met when transient microorganisms are eliminated from the hands.

DOCUMENTATION The performance of hand hygiene using an alcohol-based handrub is not generally documented.

SPECIAL CONSIDERATIONS

Home Care Considerations

- Proper hand hygiene, including the use of alcohol-based handrubs, is imperative before leaving a home and immediately upon entering another home (Kenneley, 2010; McGoldrick & Rhinehart, 2007).

EVIDENCE FOR PRACTICE ▶

IMPROVING THE USE OF HAND HYGIENE MEASURES

Prevention of health care–associated infections is a major challenge for health care providers. Hand hygiene is regarded as an effective preventive measure. What types of interventions can be used to increase adherence to hand hygiene guidelines by health care workers and visitors to health care institutions?

Fakhry, M., Hanna, G.B., Anderson, O., Holmes, A., & Nathwani, D. (2012). Effectiveness of an audible reminder on hand hygiene adherence. *American Journal of Infection Control, 40*(4), 320–323.

(continued)

SKILL 1-1 PERFORMING HAND HYGIENE USING AN ALCOHOL-BASED HANDRUB continued

An electronic motion sensor-triggered audible hand hygiene reminder was installed at the entrance of each patient unit at one hospital. The audible alert sounded the following message: "Please clean your hands with handrub from the dispensers when entering or exiting any clinical area." An 8-month preinterventional and postinterventional study was carried out to measure the adherence of hospital visitors and staff with hand hygiene guidelines. Researchers directly observed visitors and staff entering and exiting the units to measure use of alcohol-based handrub placed at each entrance. The authors reported an immediate and significantly improved and sustained greater adherence of hospital visitors and health care providers to hand hygiene guidelines. They concluded that the electronic motion sensor-triggered audible reminder for hand hygiene is an effective addition to hand hygiene interventions and may help control epidemic infections.

Relevance for Nursing Practice

There are numerous interventions that can be used to increase adherence to hand hygiene guidelines. Nurses are in a position to advocate for and introduce ideas to increase compliance related to hand hygiene adherence, resulting in improved patient care.

Refer to thePoint for additional research on related nursing topics.

EVIDENCE FOR PRACTICE ▶

HAND HYGIENE, RELIGION, AND CULTURE

Prevention of health care–associated infections is a major challenge for health care providers. Hand hygiene is regarded as an effective preventive measure. The WHO has prepared guidelines for hand hygiene and is studying the acceptability of these guidelines in different health care settings worldwide.

Related Research

Allegranzi, B., Memish, Z., Donaldson, L., et al. (2009). World Health Organization Global Patient Safety Challenge Task Force on Religious and Cultural Aspects of Hand Hygiene. Religion and culture: Potential undercurrents influencing hand hygiene promotion in health care. *American Journal of Infection Control, 37*(1), 28–34.

The authors conducted a literature search and consulted experts and religious authorities to investigate religious and cultural factors that may potentially influence hand hygiene promotion, offer possible solutions, and suggest areas for future research. Data were retrieved on specific indications for hand cleansing according to the seven main religions worldwide, interpretation of hand gestures, the concept of "visibly dirty" hands, and the use of alcohol-based handrubs and prohibition of alcohol use by some religions. They concluded that religious faith and culture can strongly influence hand hygiene behavior in health care workers and potentially affect compliance with best practices.

Relevance for Nursing Practice

Nurses need to consider the impact of religious faith and cultural specificities when implementing patient care and teaching related to hand hygiene.

Refer to thePoint for additional research on related nursing topics.

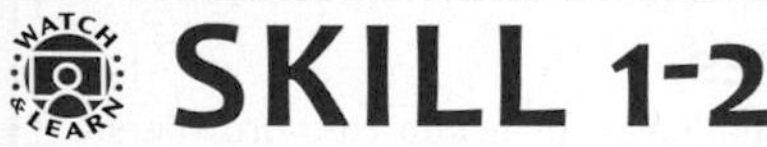

SKILL 1-2 PERFORMING HAND HYGIENE USING SOAP AND WATER (HANDWASHING)

Handwashing, as opposed to hand hygiene with an alcohol-based rub, is required (CDC, 2002):

- When hands are visibly dirty
- When hands are visibly soiled with (or in contact with) blood or other body fluids
- Before eating and after using the restroom
- If exposure to certain organisms, such as those causing anthrax or *Clostridium difficile,* is known or suspected. (Other agents, such as alcohol-based handrubs, have poor activity against these organisms.)

DELEGATION CONSIDERATIONS

The application and use of hand hygiene is appropriate for all health care providers.

EQUIPMENT

- Antimicrobial or nonantimicrobial soap (if in bar form, soap must be placed on a soap rack)
- Paper towels
- Oil-free lotion (optional)

ASSESSMENT

Assess for any of the above requirements for handwashing. If no requirements are fulfilled, the caregiver has the option of decontaminating hands with soap and water or using an alcohol-based handrub.

NURSING DIAGNOSIS

Determine the related factors for the nursing diagnosis based on the patient's current status. Appropriate nursing diagnoses may include Risk for Infection.

OUTCOME IDENTIFICATION AND PLANNING

The expected outcome to achieve when performing handwashing is that the hands will be free of visible soiling and transient microorganisms will be eliminated. Other outcomes may be appropriate, depending on the specific nursing diagnosis identified for the patient.

IMPLEMENTATION

ACTION	RATIONALE
1. Gather the necessary supplies. Stand in front of the sink. Do not allow your clothing to touch the sink during the washing procedure (Figure 1).	The sink is considered contaminated. Clothing may carry organisms from place to place.
2. Remove jewelry, if possible, and secure in a safe place. A plain wedding band may remain in place.	Removal of jewelry facilitates proper cleansing. Microorganisms may accumulate in settings of jewelry. If jewelry was worn during care, it should be left on during handwashing.
3. Turn on water and adjust force (Figure 2). Regulate the temperature until the water is warm.	Water splashed from the contaminated sink will contaminate clothing. Warm water is more comfortable and is less likely to open pores and remove oils from the skin. Organisms can lodge in roughened and broken areas of chapped skin.

FIGURE 1 Standing in front of sink.

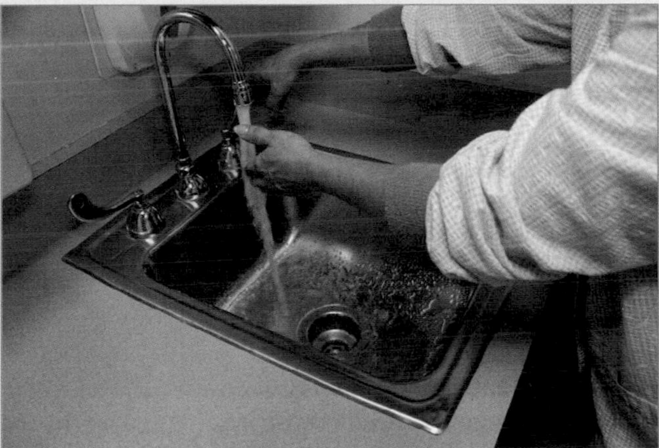

FIGURE 2 Turning on the water at the sink.

(*continued*)

SKILL 1-2 PERFORMING HAND HYGIENE USING SOAP AND WATER (HANDWASHING) continued

ACTION	RATIONALE
4. Wet the hands and wrist area. Keep hands lower than elbows to allow water to flow toward fingertips (Figure 3).	Water should flow from the cleaner area toward the more contaminated area. Hands are more contaminated than forearms.
5. Use about 1 teaspoon liquid soap from dispenser or rinse bar of soap and lather thoroughly (Figure 4). Cover all areas of hands with the soap product. Rinse soap bar again and return to soap rack without touching the rack.	Rinsing the soap before and after use removes the lather, which may contain microorganisms.

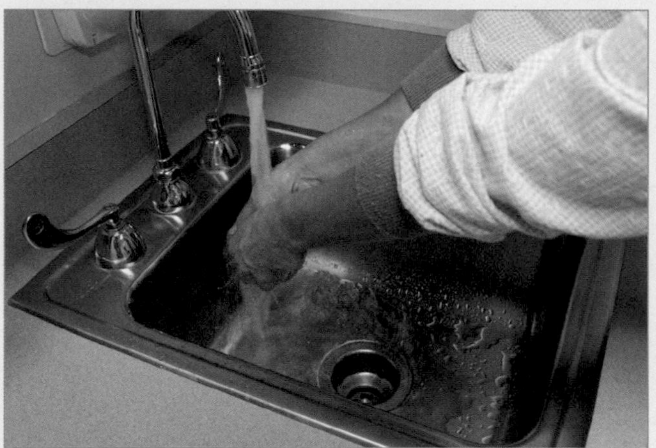

FIGURE 3 Wetting hands to the wrist.

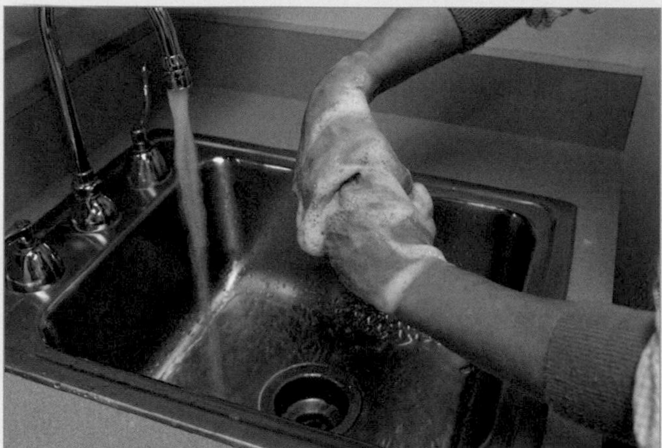

FIGURE 4 Lathering hands with soap and rubbing with firm circular motion.

ACTION	RATIONALE
6. With firm rubbing and circular motions, wash the palms and backs of the hands, each finger, the areas between the fingers (Figure 5), and the knuckles, wrists, and forearms. **Wash at least 1 inch above area of contamination.** If hands are not visibly soiled, wash to 1 inch above the wrists (Figure 6).	Friction caused by firm rubbing and circular motions helps to loosen dirt and organisms that can lodge between the fingers, in skin crevices of knuckles, on the palms and backs of the hands, and on the wrists and forearms. Cleaning less contaminated areas (forearms and wrists) after hands are clean prevents spreading microorganisms from the hands to the forearms and wrists.

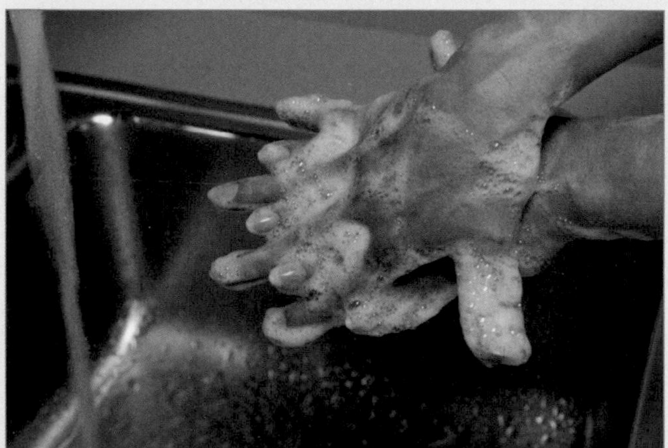

FIGURE 5 Washing areas between fingers.

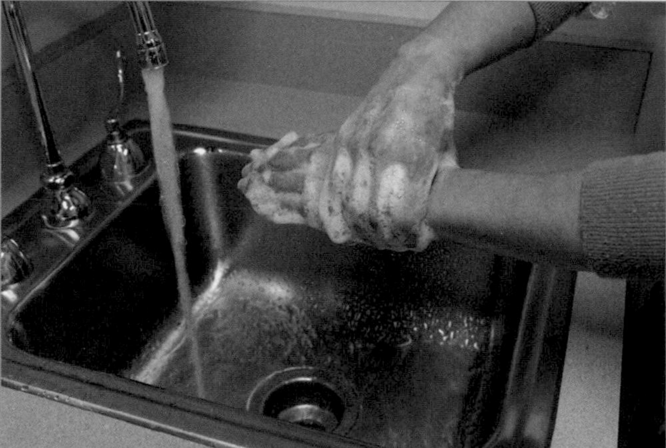

FIGURE 6 Washing to 1 inch above the wrist.

ACTION	RATIONALE
7. Continue this friction motion for at least 20 seconds.	Length of handwashing is determined by degree of contamination. Hands that are visibly soiled need a longer scrub.

ACTION	RATIONALE
8. Use fingernails of the opposite hand or a clean orangewood stick to clean under fingernails (Figure 7).	Area under nails has a high microorganism count, and organisms may remain under the nails, where they can grow and be spread to other persons.
9. Rinse thoroughly with water flowing toward fingertips (Figure 8).	Running water rinses microorganisms and dirt into the sink.

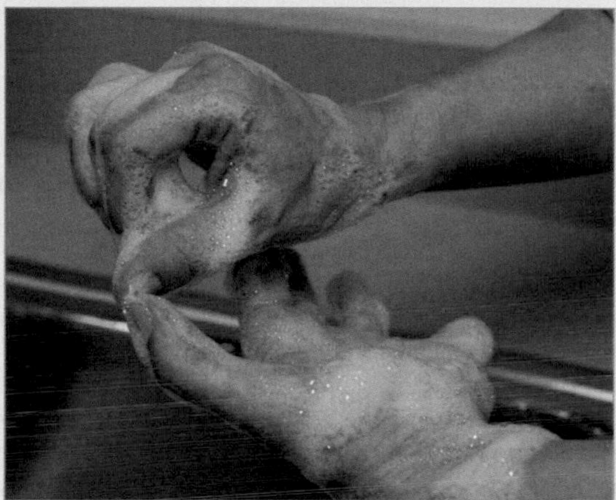

FIGURE 7 Using fingernails to clean under nails of opposite hand.

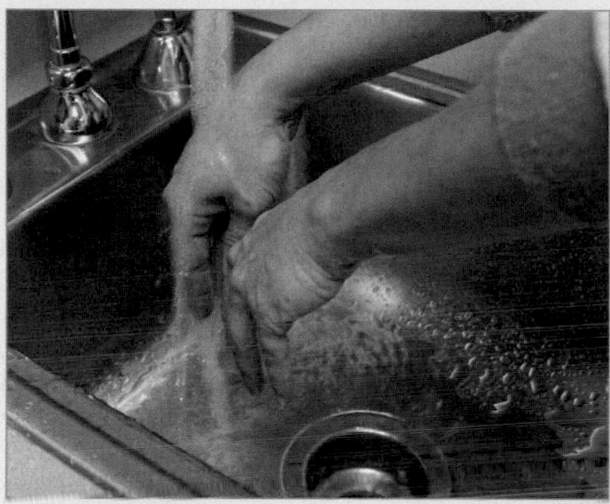

FIGURE 8 Rinsing hands under running water with water flowing toward fingertips.

ACTION	RATIONALE
10. Pat hands dry with a paper towel, beginning with the fingers and moving upward toward forearms, and discard it immediately. Use another clean towel to turn off the faucet. Discard towel immediately without touching other clean hand.	Patting the skin dry prevents chapping. Dry hands first because they are considered the cleanest and least contaminated area. Turning the faucet off with a clean paper towel protects the clean hands from contact with a soiled surface.
11. Use oil-free lotion on hands, if desired	Oil-free lotion helps to keep the skin soft and prevents chapping. It is best to apply after patient care is complete and from a small, personal container. Oil-based lotions should be avoided because they can cause deterioration of gloves.

EVALUATION

The expected outcome is met when the hands are free of visible soiling and transient microorganisms are eliminated.

DOCUMENTATION

The performance of handwashing is not generally documented.

SPECIAL CONSIDERATIONS

General Considerations

- Use of an antimicrobial soap product is recommended with handwashing before participating in an invasive procedure and after exposure to blood or body fluids. The length of the scrub will vary based on need.
- Liquid or bar soap, granules, or leaflets are all acceptable forms of nonantimicrobial soap.

Home Care Considerations

- Home care providers should consider bringing their own liquid soap and disposable paper towels into the home for washing and drying their hands instead of using potentially contaminated bar soap and towels in the patient's home (Grossman & DeBartolomeo, 2008).
- Proper hand hygiene before leaving a home and immediately upon entering another home is imperative (Kenneley, 2010; McGoldrick & Rhinehart, 2007).

(*continued*)

SKILL 1-2 PERFORMING HAND HYGIENE USING SOAP AND WATER (HANDWASHING) continued

EVIDENCE FOR PRACTICE ▶

IMPROVING THE USE OF HAND HYGIENE MEASURES

Prevention of **health care–associated infections** is a major challenge for health care providers. Hand hygiene is regarded as an effective preventive measure. This procedure is still not performed consistently in health care settings, however (The Joint Commission Center for Transforming Healthcare, 2012).

Related Research

Gould, D.J., Moralejo, D., Drey, N., & Chudleigh, J.H. (2011). Interventions to improve hand hygiene compliance in patient care. *Cochrane Database of Systematic Reviews*. Art. No.: CD005186. DOI: 10.1002/14651858.CD005186.pub3. Available http://summaries.cochrane.org/CD005186/methods-to-improve-healthcare-worker-hand-hygiene-to-decrease-infection-in-hospitals.

The objective of this literature review was to assess the short- and longer-term success of strategies to improve hand hygiene compliance and to determine whether sustained increase in hand hygiene compliance can reduce rates of health care–associated infection. Four studies met the criteria for review: two from the original review and two from the update. Two studies evaluated simple education initiatives, one using a randomized clinical trial design and the other a controlled before and after design. Both measured hand hygiene compliance by direct observation. The other two studies were both interrupted times series studies. One study presented three separate interventions within the same paper: simple substitutions of product and two multifaceted campaigns, one of which included involving practitioners in making decisions about choice of hand hygiene products and the components of the hand hygiene program. The other study also presented two separate multifaceted campaigns, one of which involved application of social marketing theory. In these two studies follow-up data collection continued beyond 12 months, and a proxy measure of hand hygiene compliance (product use) was recorded. Microbiological data were recorded in one study. Hand hygiene compliance increased for one of the studies where it was measured by direct observation, but the results from the other study were not conclusive. Product use increased in the two studies in which it was reported, with inconsistent results reported for one initiative. Methicillin-resistant *Staphylococcus aureus* (MRSA) incidence decreased in the one study reporting microbiological data. The authors concluded there is little robust evidence to influence the choice of interventions to improve hand hygiene. They identified a need to undertake methodologically robust research to explore the effectiveness of soundly designed interventions to increase hand hygiene compliance.

Relevance for Nursing Practice

Effective hand hygiene is a mandatory part of nursing care. Nurses should consider undertaking studies related to improving hand hygiene compliance to ensure safe patient care. Such studies would also add to the body of knowledge to support evidence-based nursing practice.

Refer to thePoint for additional research on related nursing topics.

EVIDENCE FOR PRACTICE ▶

HAND HYGIENE, RELIGION, AND CULTURE

Prevention of health care–associated infections is a major challenge for health care providers. Hand hygiene is regarded as an effective preventive measure. The WHO has prepared guidelines for hand hygiene and is studying the acceptability of these guidelines in different health care settings worldwide.

Allegranzi, B., Memish, Z., Donaldson, L., et al. (2009). World Health Organization Global Patient Safety Challenge Task Force on Religious and Cultural Aspects of Hand Hygiene. Religion and culture: Potential undercurrents influencing hand hygiene promotion in health care. *American Journal of Infection Control, 37*(1), 28–34.

Refer to Skill 1-1 for detailed information related to this research, and refer to thePoint for additional research on related nursing topics.

SKILL 1-3 USING PERSONAL PROTECTIVE EQUIPMENT

Personal protective equipment refers to specialized clothing or equipment worn by an employee for protection against infectious materials. PPE is used in health care settings to improve personnel safety in the health care environment through the appropriate use of PPE (CDC, 2004). This equipment includes clean (nonsterile) and sterile gloves, impervious gowns/aprons, surgical and high-efficiency particulate air (HEPA) masks, N95 disposable masks, face shields, and protective eyewear/goggles.

Understanding the potential contamination hazards related to the patient's diagnosis and condition and the institutional policies governing PPE is very important. The type of PPE used will vary based on the type of exposure anticipated and category of precautions: Standard Precautions and Transmission-Based Precautions, including Contact, Droplet, or Airborne Precautions. It is the nurse's responsibility to enforce the proper wearing of PPE during patient care for members of the health care team. Refer to Fundamentals Review 1-4 and Fundamentals Review 1-5 for a summary of CDC-recommended practices for Standard and Transmission-based Precautions. Box 1-1 provides Guidelines for Effective Use of PPE.

BOX 1-1 GUIDELINES FOR EFFECTIVE USE OF PPE

- Put on PPE before contact with the patient, preferably before entering the patient's room.
- Choose appropriate PPE based on the type of exposure anticipated and type of transmission-based precautions.
- When wearing gloves, work from "clean" areas to "dirty" areas.
- Touch as few surfaces and items with your PPE as possible.
- Avoid touching or adjusting other PPE.
- Keep gloved hands away from your face.
- If gloves become torn or heavily soiled, remove and replace. Perform hand hygiene before putting on the new gloves.
- Personal glasses are not a substitute for goggles.

(Adapted from Centers for Disease Control and Prevention (CDC). (2007e). (Updated 2012). Personal protective equipment for healthcare personnel. Excerpted from guideline for isolation precautions: Preventing transmission of infectious agents in healthcare settings. Available www.cdc.gov/hicpac/pdf/isolation/Isolation2007.pdf.)

DELEGATION CONSIDERATIONS

The application and use of PPE is appropriate for all health care providers.

EQUIPMENT

- Gloves
- Mask (surgical or particulate respirator)
- Impervious gown
- Protective eyewear (does not include eyeglasses)

Note: Equipment for PPE may vary depending on facility policy.

ASSESSMENT

Assess the situation to determine the necessity for PPE. In addition, check the patient's chart for information about a suspected or diagnosed infection or communicable disease. Determine the possibility of exposure to blood and body fluids and identify the necessary equipment to prevent exposure. Refer to the infection control manual provided by your facility.

NURSING DIAGNOSIS

Determine the related factors for the nursing diagnoses based on the patient's current status. Appropriate nursing diagnoses may include:

- Risk for Infection
- Ineffective Protection
- Diarrhea

OUTCOME IDENTIFICATION AND PLANNING

The expected outcome to achieve when using PPE is prevention of microorganism transmission. Other outcomes that may be appropriate include the following: Patient and staff remain free of exposure to potentially infectious microorganisms; and patient verbalizes information about the rationale for use of PPE.

(*continued*)

SKILL 1-3 USING PERSONAL PROTECTIVE EQUIPMENT continued

IMPLEMENTATION

ACTION	RATIONALE
1. Check medical record and nursing plan of care for type of precautions and review precautions in infection control manual.	Mode of transmission of organism determines type of precautions required.
2. Plan nursing activities before entering patient's room.	Organization facilitates performance of task and adherence to precautions.
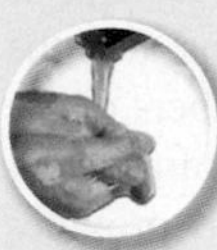 3. Perform hand hygiene.	Hand hygiene prevents the spread of microorganisms.
4. Provide instruction about precautions to patient, family members, and visitors.	Explanation encourages cooperation of patient and family and reduces apprehension about precaution procedures.
5. Put on gown, mask, protective eyewear, and gloves based on the type of exposure anticipated and category of isolation precautions.	Use of PPE interrupts chain of infection and protects patient and nurse. Gown should protect entire uniform. Gloves protect hands and wrists from microorganisms. Masks protect nurse or patient from droplet nuclei and large-particle aerosols. Eyewear protects mucous membranes in the eye from splashes.
a. Put on the gown, with the opening in the back. Tie gown securely at neck and waist (Figure 1).	Gown should fully cover the torso from the neck to knees, arms to the end of wrists, and wrap around the back.
b. Put on the mask or respirator over your nose, mouth, and chin (Figure 2). Secure ties or elastic bands at the middle of the head and neck. If respirator is used, perform a fit check. Inhale; the respirator should collapse. Exhale; air should not leak out.	Masks protect nurse or patient from droplet nuclei and large-particle aerosols. A mask must fit securely to provide protection.
c. Put on goggles (Figure 3). Place over eyes and adjust to fit. Alternately, a face shield could be used to take the place of the mask and goggles (Figure 4).	Eyewear protects mucous membranes in the eye from splashes. Must fit securely to provide protection.

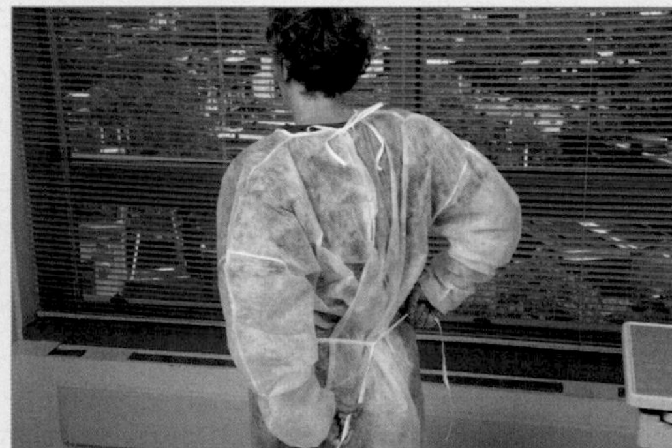

FIGURE 1 Tying gown at neck and waist.

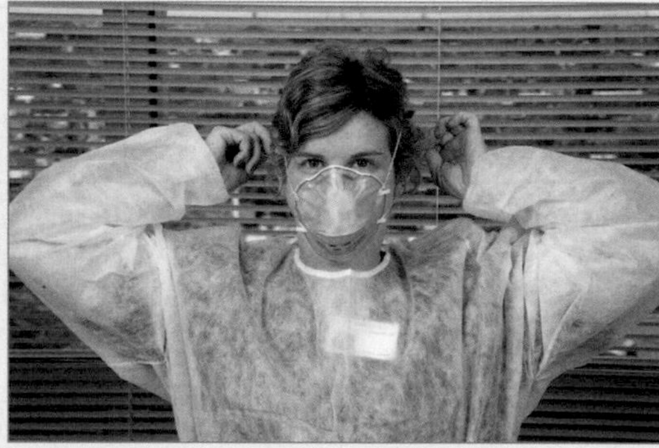

FIGURE 2 Applying mask over nose, mouth, and chin.

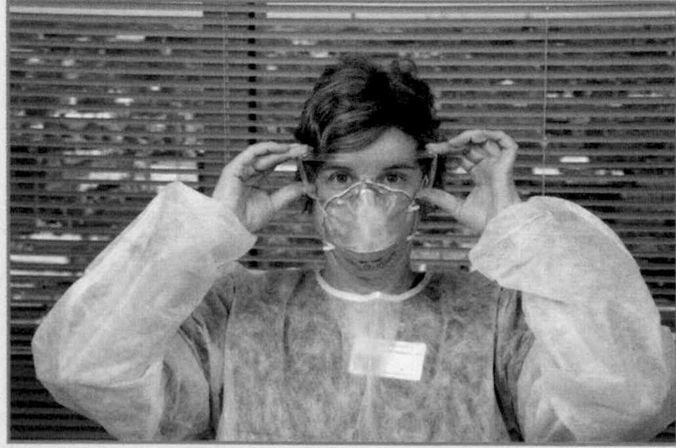

FIGURE 3 Putting on goggles.

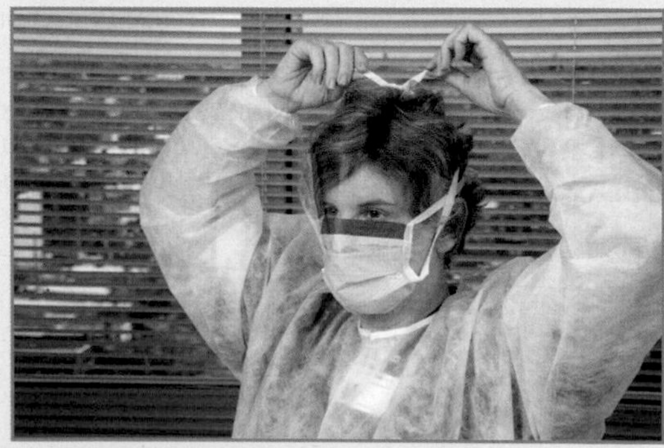

FIGURE 4 Putting on face shield.

ACTION	RATIONALE
d. Put on clean disposable gloves. Extend gloves to cover the cuffs of the gown (Figure 5).	Gloves protect hands and wrists from microorganisms.

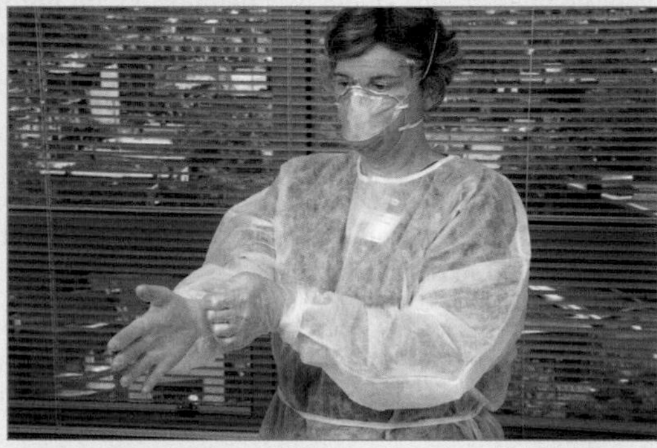

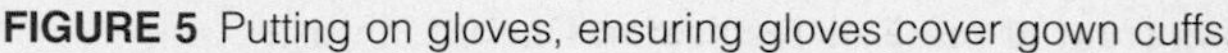

FIGURE 5 Putting on gloves, ensuring gloves cover gown cuffs.

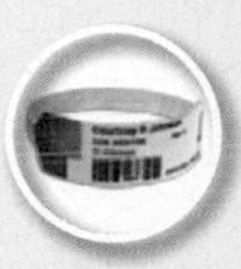

ACTION	RATIONALE
6. Identify the patient. Explain the procedure to the patient. Continue with patient care as appropriate.	Patient identification validates the correct patient and correct procedure. Discussion and explanation help allay anxiety and prepare the patient for what to expect.

Remove PPE

ACTION	RATIONALE
7. Remove PPE: Except for respirator, remove PPE at the doorway or in an anteroom. **Remove respirator after leaving the patient's room and closing the door.**	Proper removal prevents contact with and the spread of microorganisms. Removing respirator outside the patient's room prevents contact with airborne microorganisms.
a. If impervious gown has been tied in front of the body at the waistline, untie waist strings before removing gloves.	Outside front of equipment is considered contaminated. The inside, outside back, ties on head and back, are considered clean, which are areas of PPE that are not likely to have been in contact with infectious organisms. Front of gown, including waist strings, are contaminated. If tied in front of body, the ties must be untied before removing gloves.
b. Grasp the outside of one glove with the opposite gloved hand and peel off, turning the glove inside out as you pull it off (Figure 6). Hold the removed glove in the remaining gloved hand.	Outside of gloves are contaminated.
c. Slide fingers of ungloved hand under the remaining glove at the wrist, **taking care not to touch the outer surface of the glove** (Figure 7).	Ungloved hand is clean and should not touch contaminated areas.

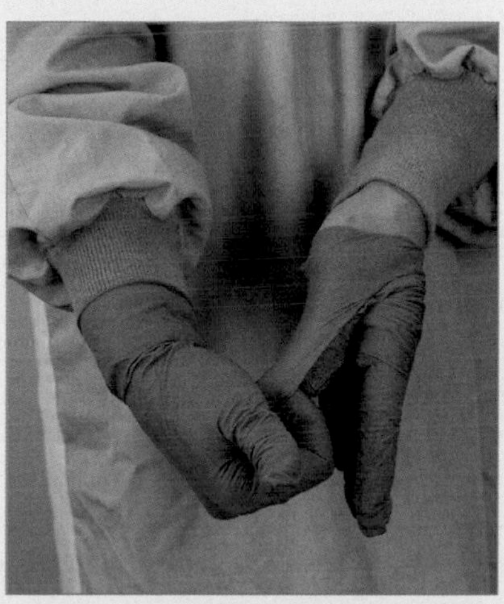

FIGURE 6 Grasping the outside of one glove and peeling off.

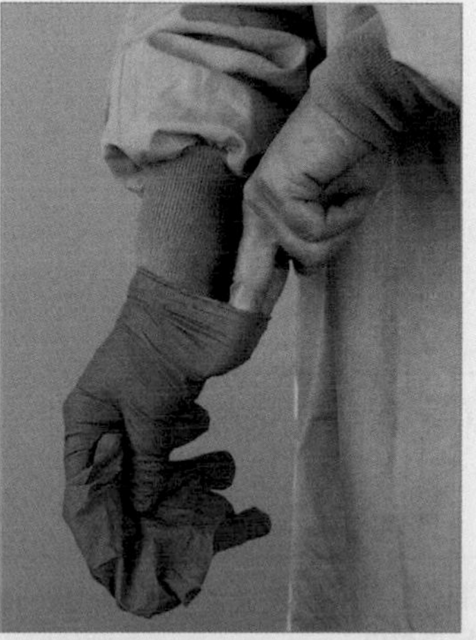

FIGURE 7 Sliding fingers of ungloved hand under the remaining glove at the wrist.

(continued)

SKILL 1-3 USING PERSONAL PROTECTIVE EQUIPMENT continued

ACTION	RATIONALE
d. Peel off the glove over the first glove, containing the one glove inside the other (Figure 8). Discard in appropriate container.	Proper disposal prevents transmission of microorganisms.
e. To remove the goggles or face shield: Handle by the headband or earpieces (Figure 9). Lift away from the face. Place in designated receptacle for reprocessing or in an appropriate waste container.	Outside of goggles or face shield is contaminated; **do not touch.** Handling by headband or earpieces and lifting away from face prevents transmission of microorganisms. Proper disposal prevents transmission of microorganisms.
f. To remove gown: Unfasten ties, if at the neck and back. Allow the gown to fall away from shoulders. **Touching only the inside of the gown,** pull away from the torso. Keeping hands on the inner surface of the gown, pull gown from arms. Turn gown inside out. Fold or roll into a bundle and discard.	Gown front and sleeves are contaminated. Touching only the inside of the gown and pulling it away from the torso prevents transmission of microorganisms. Proper disposal prevents transmission of microorganisms.
g. To remove mask or respirator: Grasp the neck ties or elastic, then top ties or elastic and remove. **Take care to avoid touching front of mask or respirator.** Discard in waste container. If using a respirator, save for future use in the designated area.	Front of mask or respirator is contaminated; **do not touch.** Not touching the front and proper disposal prevent transmission of microorganisms.

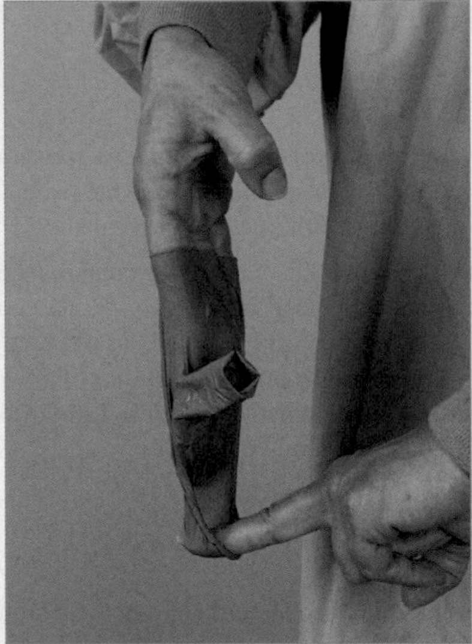

FIGURE 8 Pulling glove off the hand and over the other glove.

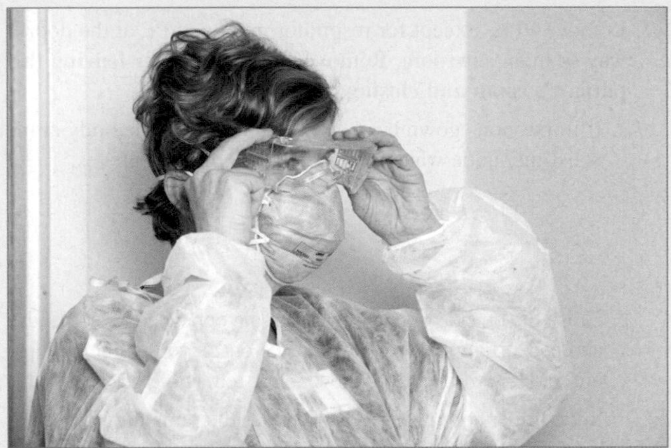

FIGURE 9 Removing goggles by grasping earpieces.

ACTION	RATIONALE
8. Perform hand hygiene immediately after removing all PPE.	Hand hygiene prevents spread of microorganisms.

EVALUATION

The expected outcome is met when the transmission of microorganisms is prevented; the patient and staff remain free from exposure to potentially infectious microorganisms; and the patient verbalizes an understanding about the rationale for use of PPE.

DOCUMENTATION

It is not usually necessary to document the use of specific articles of PPE or each application of PPE. However, document the implementation and continuation of specific transmission-based precautions as part of the patient's care.

UNEXPECTED SITUATIONS AND ASSOCIATED INTERVENTIONS

- *You did not realize the need for protective equipment at beginning of task:* Stop task and obtain appropriate protective wear.
- *You are accidentally exposed to blood and body fluids:* Stop task and immediately follow agency protocol for exposure, including reporting the exposure.

EVIDENCE FOR PRACTICE ▶

PPE AND PREVENTION OF TRANSFER OF MICROORGANISMS

Prevention of health care–associated infections is a major challenge for health care providers. The removal of PPE after patient care may result in transfer of microorganisms to hands and clothing of health care workers. How can this risk of transfer be reduced?

Related Research

Casanova, L.M., Rutala, W.A., Weber, D.J., & Sobsey, M.D. (2012). Effect of single- versus double-gloving on virus transfer to healthcare workers' skin and clothing during removal of personal protective equipment. *American Journal of Infection Control, 40*(4), 369–374.

The focus of this study was to determine whether double-gloving reduces virus transfer to the hands and clothing of health care workers during removal of contaminated PPE. There was a double-gloving phase and a single-gloving phase of the experiment. Participants put on PPE, including a gown, N95 respirator, eye protection, and gloves. The gown, respirator, eye protection, and dominant glove were contaminated with bacteriophage. Participants then removed the PPE, and their hands, face, and clothing were sampled for virus. Transfer of virus to hands during PPE removal was significantly more frequent with single-gloving than with double-gloving. Significantly more virus was transferred to participants' hands after single-gloving than after double-gloving. Transfer to clothing was similar during single-gloving and double-gloving. The researchers concluded double-gloving can reduce the risk of viral contamination of the hands of health care workers during PPE removal.

Relevance for Nursing Practice

Nurses should continually strive to improve practice and be alert for interventions to help achieve better practice. The use of double gloves is an inexpensive and simple intervention. Incorporating the use of double-gloving with the use of full PPE may be an effective method to reduce the risk of transmission of microorganisms.

Refer to thePoint for additional research on related nursing topics.

EVIDENCE FOR PRACTICE ▶

USING PPE CORRECTLY

The proper use of PPE is essential to reduce the risk of transfer of infectious microorganisms and diseases. Are health care workers using PPE properly?

Related Research

Beam, E.L., Gibbs, S.G., Boulter, K.C., Beckerdite, M.E., & Smith, P.W. (2011). A method for evaluating health care workers' personal protective equipment technique. *American Journal of Infection Control, 39*(5), 415–420.

This pilot study was conducted to examine the feasibility of using a simulated health care environment to assess the technique of health care workers when implementing standard airborne and contact isolation precautions. The participants were assigned patient care tasks based on their specific professional roles. The encounters were recorded during the application and removal of PPE, as well as during interactions with the simulated patient. Powdered fluorescent marker was used as a measure of contamination. The pilot data showed various inconsistencies in the health care workers' PPE technique. Each of the participants committed at least one breach of standard airborne and contact isolation precautions. The authors concluded an expanded research study of health care workers' behaviors is needed to properly examine possible contamination and exposure pathways. In addition, it was concluded training programs should be developed that emphasize the common errors in PPE technique. Infection control programs need to focus on both the policies for the use of PPE and the quality of the PPE techniques used while caring for patients to protect health care workers, patients, and the community.

Relevance for Nursing Practice

Nurses need continually to review infection control standards and guidelines for best practice. Nurses should be responsible practitioners. It is important to examine and reflect on individual practice to ensure appropriate use of infection control measures, including use of PPE, to provide safe and responsible nursing care.

Refer to thePoint for additional research on related nursing topics.

SKILL 1-4 PREPARING A STERILE FIELD USING A PACKAGED STERILE DRAPE

A sterile field is created to provide a surgically aseptic workspace. It should be considered a restricted area. A sterile drape may be used to establish a sterile field or to extend the sterile working area. The sterile drape should be waterproof on one side, with that side placed down on the work surface. After establishing the sterile field, add other sterile items, as needed, including solutions. Sterile items and sterile gloved hands are the only objects allowed in the sterile field. Refer to Fundamentals Review 1-2 to review basic principles of surgical asepsis.

DELEGATION CONSIDERATIONS

Procedures requiring the use of a sterile field and other sterile items are not delegated to nursing assistive personnel (NAP) or unlicensed assistive personnel (UAP). Depending on the state's nurse practice act and the organization's policies and procedures, these procedures may be delegated to licensed practical/vocational nurses (LPN/LVN). The decision to delegate must be based on careful analysis of the patient's needs and circumstances, as well as the qualifications of the person to whom the task is being delegated. Refer to the Delegation Guidelines in Appendix A.

EQUIPMENT

- Sterile wrapped drape
- Additional sterile supplies, such as dressings, containers, or solution, as needed
- PPE, as indicated

ASSESSMENT

Assess the situation to determine the necessity for creating a sterile field. Assess the area in which the sterile field is to be prepared. Move any unnecessary equipment out of the immediate vicinity.

NURSING DIAGNOSIS

Determine the related factors for the nursing diagnoses based on the patient's current status. Appropriate nursing diagnoses may include:

- Risk for Infection
- Ineffective Protection

OUTCOME IDENTIFICATION AND PLANNING

The expected outcome to achieve when preparing a sterile field is that the sterile field is created without contamination and the patient remains free of exposure to potential infection-causing microorganisms.

IMPLEMENTATION

ACTION	RATIONALE
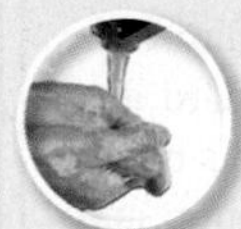 1. Perform hand hygiene and put on PPE, if indicated.	Hand hygiene and PPE prevent the spread of microorganisms. PPE is required based on transmission precautions.
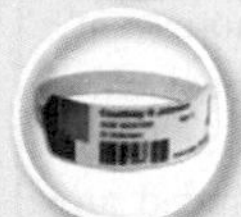 2. Identify the patient. Explain the procedure to the patient.	Patient identification validates the correct patient and correct procedure. Discussion and explanation help allay anxiety and prepare the patient for what to expect.
3. Check that packaged sterile drape is dry and unopened. Also note expiration date, making sure that the date is still valid.	Moisture contaminates a sterile package. Expiration date indicates period that package remains sterile.
4. Select a work area that is waist level or higher.	Work area is within sight. Bacteria tend to settle, so there is less contamination above the waist.
5. Open the outer covering of the drape. Remove sterile drape, lifting it carefully by its corners. Hold away from body and above the waist and work surface.	Outer 1 inch (2.5 cm) of drape is considered contaminated. Any item touching this area is also considered contaminated.

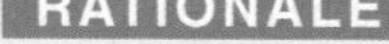

ACTION	RATIONALE
6. Continue to hold only by the corners. Allow the drape to unfold, away from your body and any other surface (Figure 1).	Touching the outer side of the wrapper maintains the sterile field. Contact with any surface would contaminate the field.
7. Position the drape on the work surface with the moisture-proof side down (Figure 2). This would be the shiny or blue side. Avoid touching any other surface or object with the drape. If any portion of the drape hangs off the work surface, that part of the drape is considered contaminated.	Moisture-proof side prevents contamination of the field if it becomes wet. The moisture penetrates the sterile cloth or paper and carries organisms by capillary action to contaminate the field. A wet field is considered contaminated if the surface immediately below it is not sterile.

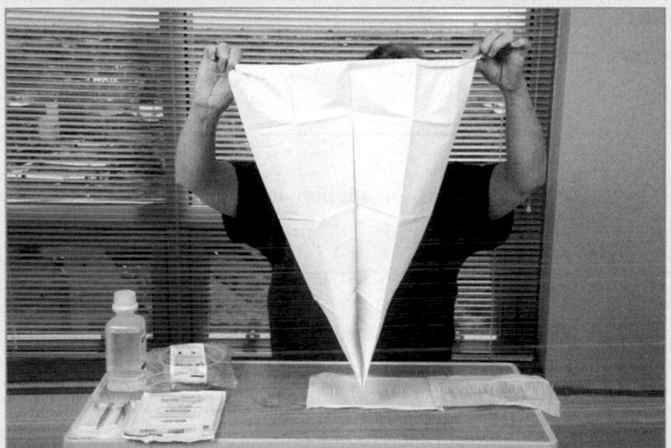

FIGURE 1 Holding drape by corners and allowing it to unfold away from body and surfaces.

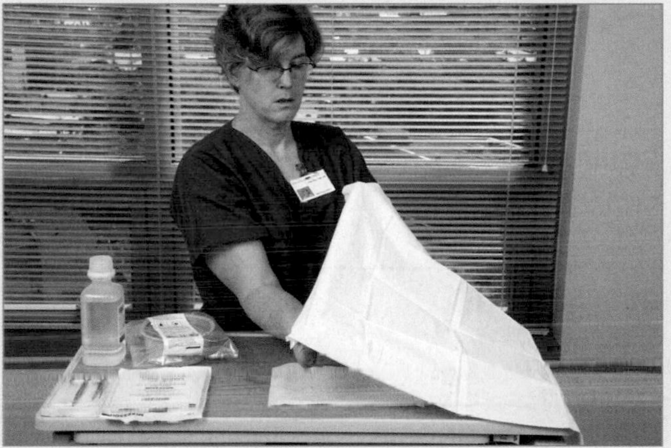

FIGURE 2 Positioning drape on work surface with the moisture-proof side down.

ACTION	RATIONALE
8. Place additional sterile items on field as needed. Refer to Skill 1-6. Continue with the procedure as indicated.	Sterility of the field is maintained.
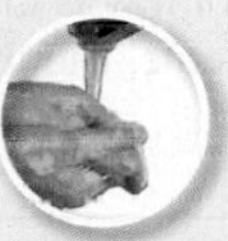 9. When procedure is completed, remove PPE, if used. Perform hand hygiene.	Removing PPE properly reduces the risk for infection transmission and contamination of other items. Hand hygiene prevents the spread of microorganisms.

EVALUATION

The expected outcome is met when the sterile field is prepared without contamination and the patient has remained free of exposure to potentially infectious microorganisms.

DOCUMENTATION

It is not usually necessary to document the preparation of a sterile field. However, document the use of sterile technique for any procedure performed using sterile technique.

UNEXPECTED SITUATIONS AND ASSOCIATED INTERVENTIONS

- *A part of the sterile field becomes contaminated:* When any portion of the sterile field becomes contaminated, discard all portions of the sterile field and start over.
- *The nurse realizes a supply is missing after setting up the sterile field:* Call for help. Do not leave the sterile field unattended. If the nurse is not able to visualize the sterile field at all times, it is considered contaminated.
- *The patient touches the sterile field:* If the patient touches the sterile field, discard the supplies and prepare a new sterile field. If the patient is confused, have someone assist by holding the patient's hands and/or reinforcing what is happening.

SKILL 1-5 PREPARING A STERILE FIELD USING A COMMERCIALLY PREPARED STERILE KIT OR TRAY

A sterile field is created to provide a surgically aseptic workspace. Consider it a restricted area. Commercially prepared sterile kits and trays are wrapped in a sterile wrapper that, once opened, becomes the sterile field. Sterile items and sterile gloved hands are the only objects allowed in the sterile field. If the area is breached, the entire sterile field is considered contaminated. Refer to Fundamentals Review 1-2 to review basic principles of surgical asepsis.

DELEGATION CONSIDERATIONS

Procedures requiring the use of a sterile field and other sterile items are not delegated to nursing assistive personnel (NAP) or unlicensed assistive personnel (UAP). Depending on the state's nurse practice act and the organization's policies and procedures, these procedures may be delegated to licensed practical/vocational nurses (LPN/LVN). The decision to delegate must be based on careful analysis of the patient's needs and circumstances, as well as the qualifications of the person to whom the task is being delegated. Refer to the Delegation Guidelines in Appendix A.

EQUIPMENT

- Commercially prepared sterile package
- Additional sterile supplies, such as dressings, containers, or solution, as needed
- PPE, as indicated

ASSESSMENT

Assess the situation to determine the necessity for creating a sterile field. Assess the area in which the sterile field is to be prepared. Move any unnecessary equipment out of the immediate vicinity.

NURSING DIAGNOSIS

Determine the related factors for the nursing diagnoses based on the patient's current status. Appropriate nursing diagnoses may include:

- Risk for Infection
- Ineffective Protection

OUTCOME IDENTIFICATION AND PLANNING

The expected outcome to achieve when opening a commercially packaged sterile kit or tray is that a sterile field is created without contamination, the contents of the package remain sterile, and the patient remains free of exposure to potential infection-causing microorganisms.

IMPLEMENTATION

ACTION	RATIONALE
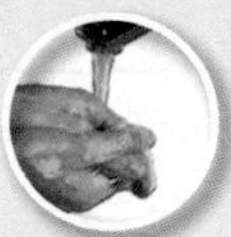 1. Perform hand hygiene and put on PPE, if indicated.	Hand hygiene and PPE prevent the spread of microorganisms. PPE is required based on transmission precautions.
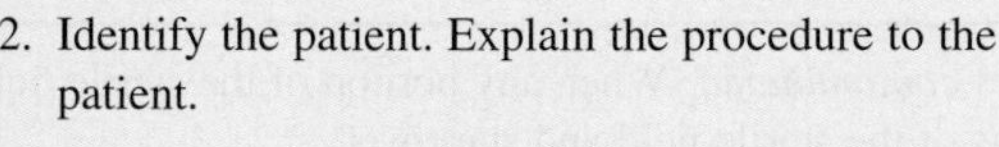 2. Identify the patient. Explain the procedure to the patient.	Patient identification validates the correct patient and correct procedure. Discussion and explanation help allay anxiety and prepare the patient for what to expect.
3. Check that the packaged kit or tray is dry and unopened. Also note expiration date, making sure that the date is still valid.	Moisture contaminates a sterile package. Expiration date indicates period that package remains sterile.
4. Select a work area that is waist level or higher.	Work area is within sight. Bacteria tend to settle, so there is less contamination above the waist.

ACTION	RATIONALE
5. Open the outside cover of the package and remove the kit or tray (Figure 1). Place in the center of the work surface, with the topmost flap positioned on the far side of the package. Discard outside cover.	This allows sufficient room for sterile field.
6. Reach around the package and grasp the outer surface of the end of the topmost flap, holding no more than 1 inch from the border of the flap. Pull open away from the body, keeping the arm outstretched and away from the inside of the wrapper (Figure 2). Allow the wrapper to lie flat on the work surface.	This maintains sterility of inside of wrapper, which is to become the sterile field. Outer surface of the wrapper is considered unsterile. Outer 1-inch border of the wrapper is considered contaminated.

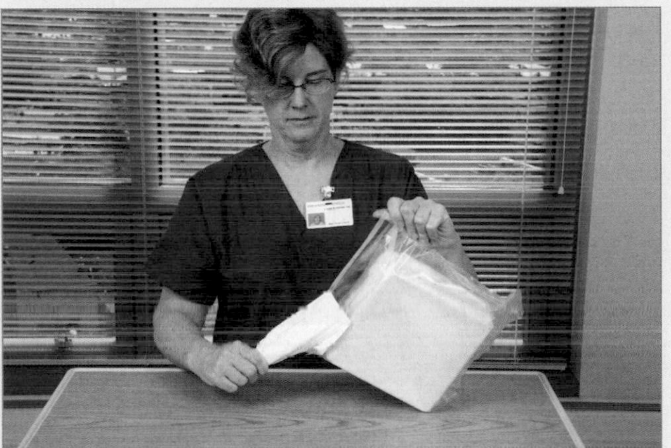

FIGURE 1 Opening outside cover of package.

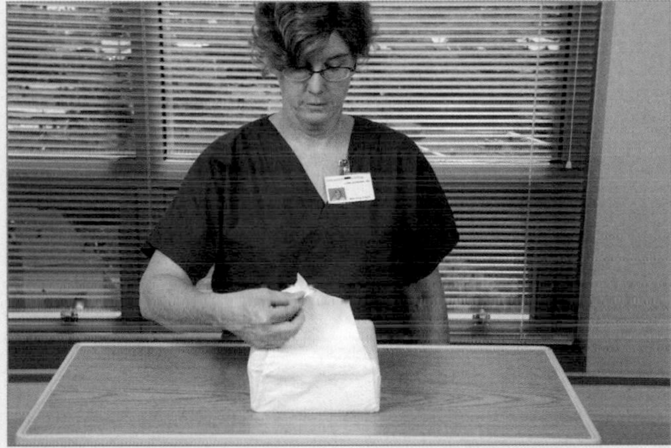

FIGURE 2 Pulling top flap open, away from body.

ACTION	RATIONALE
7. Reach around the package and grasp the outer surface of the first side flap, holding no more than 1 inch from the border of the flap. Pull open to the side of the package, keeping the arm outstretched and away from the inside of the wrapper (Figure 3). Allow the wrapper to lie flat on the work surface.	This maintains sterility of inside of wrapper, which is to become the sterile field. Outer surface of the wrapper is considered unsterile. Outer 1-inch border of the wrapper is considered contaminated.
8. Reach around the package and grasp the outer surface of the remaining side flap, holding no more than 1 inch from the border of the flap. Pull open to the side of the package, keeping the arm outstretched and away from the inside of the wrapper (Figure 4). Allow the wrapper to lie flat on the work surface.	This maintains sterility of inside of wrapper, which is to become the sterile field. Outer surface of the wrapper is considered unsterile. Outer 1 inch of border of the wrapper is considered contaminated.

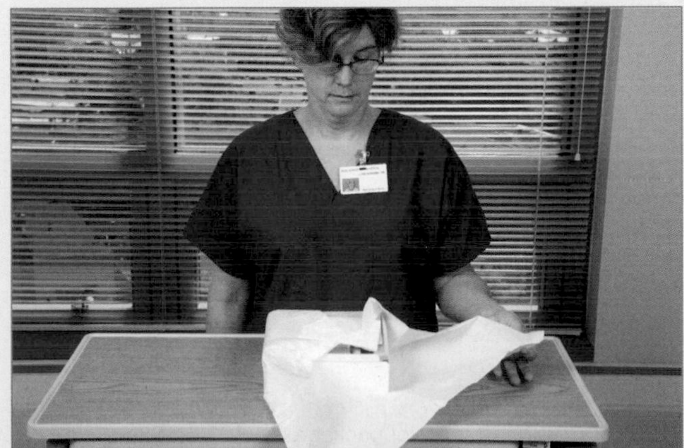

FIGURE 3 Pulling open the first side flap.

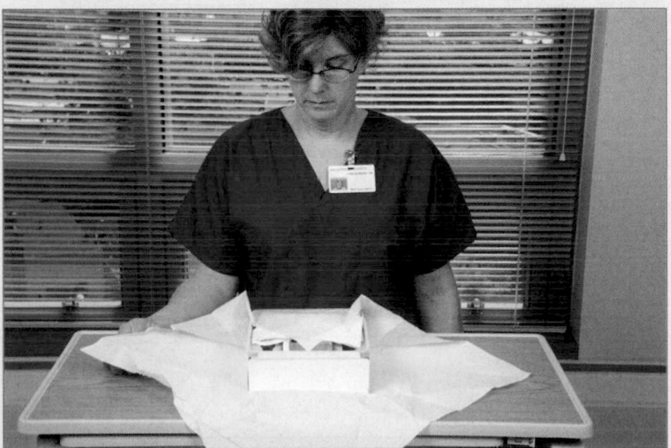

FIGURE 4 Pulling open the remaining side flap.

(continued)

SKILL 1-5 PREPARING A STERILE FIELD USING A COMMERCIALLY PREPARED STERILE KIT OR TRAY continued

ACTION	RATIONALE
9. Stand away from the package and work surface. Grasp the outer surface of the remaining flap closest to the body, holding not more than 1 inch from the border of the flap. Pull the flap back toward the body, keeping arm outstretched and away from the inside of the wrapper (Figure 5). Keep this hand in place. Use other hand to grasp the wrapper on the underside (the side that is down to the work surface). Position the wrapper so that when flat, edges are on the work surface, and do not hang down over sides of work surface (Figure 6). Allow the wrapper to lie flat on the work surface.	This maintains sterility of the inside of the wrapper, which is to become the sterile field. Outer surface of the wrapper is considered unsterile. Outer 1-inch border of the wrapper is considered contaminated.

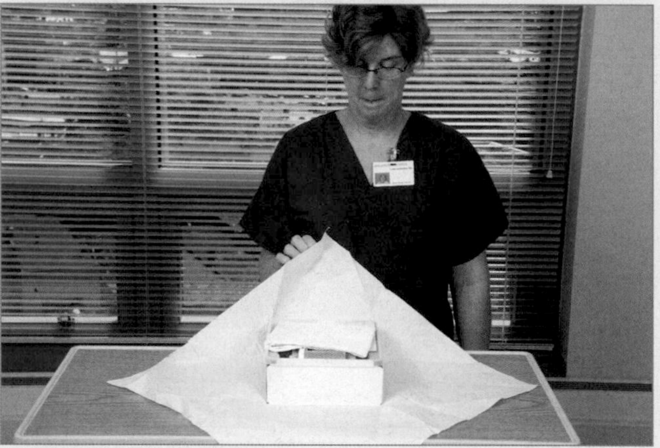

FIGURE 5 Pulling open flap closest to body.

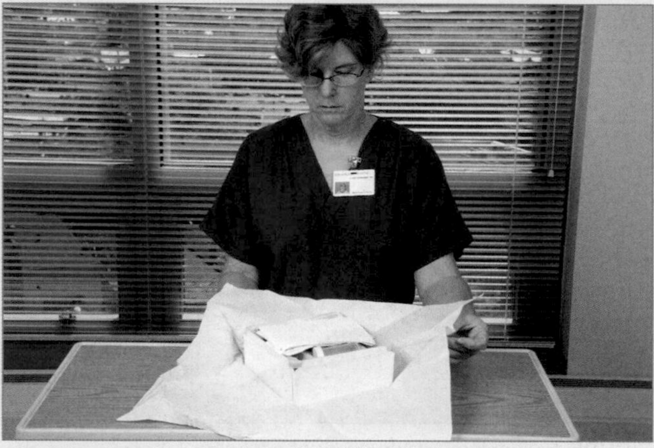

FIGURE 6 Positioning wrapper on work surface.

ACTION	RATIONALE
10. The outer wrapper of the package has become a sterile field with the packaged supplies in the center (Figure 7). Do not touch or reach over the sterile field. Place additional sterile items on field as needed. Refer to Skill 1-6. Continue with the procedure as indicated.	Sterility of the field and contents are maintained.
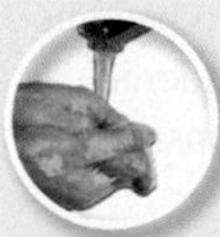 11. When procedure is completed, remove PPE, if used. Perform hand hygiene.	Removing PPE properly reduces the risk for infection transmission and contamination of other items. Hand hygiene prevents the spread of microorganisms.

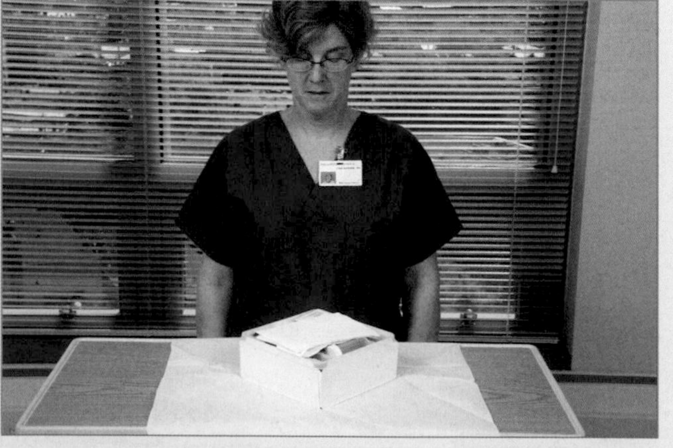

FIGURE 7 Outside wrapper of package is now sterile field.

EVALUATION

The expected outcome is met when the sterile field is prepared without contamination, the contents of the package remain sterile, and the patient remains free of exposure to potential infection-causing microorganisms.

DOCUMENTATION

It is not usually necessary to document the preparation of a sterile field. However, do document the use of sterile technique for any procedure performed using sterile technique.

UNEXPECTED SITUATIONS AND ASSOCIATED INTERVENTIONS

- *A part of the sterile field becomes contaminated:* When any portion of the sterile field becomes contaminated, discard all portions of the sterile field and start over.
- *You realize a supply is missing after setting up the sterile field:* Call for help. Do not leave the sterile field unattended. If you are unable to visualize the sterile field at all times, it is considered contaminated.
- *The patient touches the sterile field:* If the patient touches the sterile field, discard the supplies and prepare a new sterile field. If the patient is confused, have someone assist by holding the patient's hands and/or reinforcing what is happening.

SKILL 1-6 ADDING STERILE ITEMS TO A STERILE FIELD

A sterile field is created to provide a surgically aseptic workspace. It should be considered a restricted area. After establishing the sterile field, add other sterile items, including solutions, as needed. Items can be wrapped and sterilized within the agency or commercially prepared. Take care to ensure that nothing unsterile touches the field or other items in the field, including hands or clothes. Refer to Fundamentals Review 1-2 to review basic principles of surgical asepsis.

DELEGATION CONSIDERATIONS

Procedures requiring the use of a sterile field and other sterile items are not delegated to nursing assistive personnel (NAP) or unlicensed assistive personnel (UAP). Depending on the state's nurse practice act and the organization's policies and procedures, these procedures may be delegated to licensed practical/vocational nurses (LPN/LVN). The decision to delegate must be based on careful analysis of the patient's needs and circumstances, as well as the qualifications of the person to whom the task is being delegated. Refer to the Delegation Guidelines in Appendix A.

EQUIPMENT

- Sterile field
- Sterile gauze, forceps, dressings, containers, solutions, or other sterile supplies, as needed
- PPE, as indicated

ASSESSMENT

Assess the situation to determine the necessity for creating a sterile field. Assess the area in which the sterile field is to be prepared. Move any unnecessary equipment out of the immediate vicinity. Identify additional supplies needed for the procedure.

NURSING DIAGNOSIS

Determine the related factors for the nursing diagnoses based on the patient's current status. Appropriate nursing diagnoses may include:

- Risk for Infection
- Ineffective Protection

OUTCOME IDENTIFICATION AND PLANNING

The expected outcome to achieve when adding items to a sterile field is that the sterile field is created without contamination, the sterile supplies are not contaminated, and the patient remains free of exposure to potential infection-causing microorganisms.

(*continued*)

SKILL 1-6 ADDING STERILE ITEMS TO A STERILE FIELD continued

IMPLEMENTATION

ACTION	RATIONALE
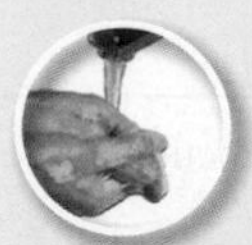 1. Perform hand hygiene and put on PPE, if indicated.	Hand hygiene and PPE prevent the spread of microorganisms. PPE is required based on transmission precautions.
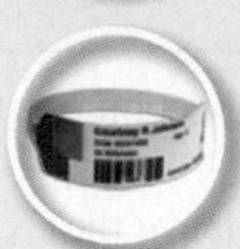 2. Identify the patient. Explain the procedure to the patient.	Patient identification validates the correct patient and correct procedure. Discussion and explanation help allay anxiety and prepare the patient for what to expect.
3. Check that the sterile, packaged drape and supplies are dry and unopened. Also note expiration date, making sure that the date is still valid.	Moisture contaminates a sterile package. Expiration date indicates period that package remains sterile.
4. Select a work area that is waist level or higher.	Work area is within sight. Bacteria tend to settle, so there is less contamination above the waist.
5. Prepare sterile field as described in Skill 1-4 or Skill 1-5.	Proper technique maintains sterility.
6. Add sterile item:	
To Add an Agency-Wrapped and Sterilized Item	
a. Hold agency-wrapped item in the dominant hand, with top flap opening away from the body. With other hand, reach around the package and unfold top flap and both sides.	Only sterile surface and item are exposed before dropping onto sterile field.
b. Keep a secure hold on the item through the wrapper with the dominant hand. Grasp the remaining flap of the wrapper closest to the body, taking care not to touch the inner surface of the wrapper or the item. Pull the flap back toward the wrist, so the wrapper covers the hand and wrist.	Only sterile surface and item are exposed before dropping onto sterile field.
c. Grasp all the corners of the wrapper together with the nondominant hand and pull back toward wrist, covering hand and wrist. Hold in place.	Only sterile surface and item are exposed before dropping onto sterile field.
d. Hold the item 6 inches above the surface of the sterile field and drop onto the field. Be careful to avoid touching the surface or other items or dropping any item onto the 1-inch border.	This prevents contamination of the field and inadvertent dropping of the sterile item too close to the edge or off the field. Any items landing on the 1-inch border are considered contaminated.
To Add a Commercially Wrapped and Sterilized Item	
a. Hold package in one hand. Pull back top cover with other hand. Alternately, carefully peel the edges apart using both hands (Figure 1).	Contents remain uncontaminated by hands.

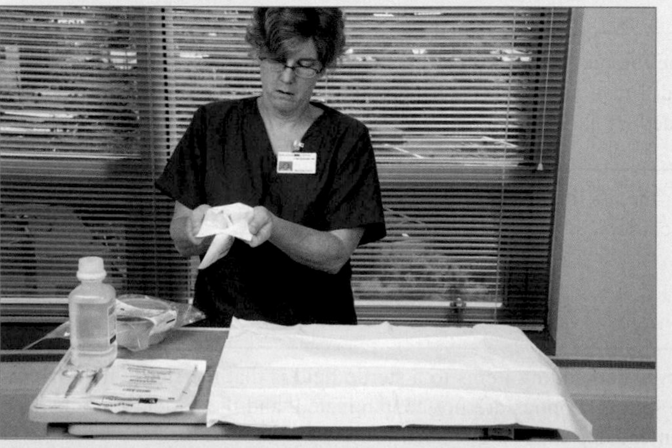

FIGURE 1 Carefully peeling edges apart.

ACTION	RATIONALE
b. After top cover or edges are partially separated, hold the item 6 inches above the surface of the sterile field. Continue opening the package and drop the item onto the field (Figure 2). **Be careful to avoid touching the surface or other items or dropping an item onto the 1-inch border.**	This prevents contamination of the field and inadvertent dropping of the sterile item too close to the edge or off the field. Any items landing on the 1-inch border are considered contaminated.
c. Discard wrapper.	A neat work area promotes proper technique and avoids inadvertent contamination of the field.

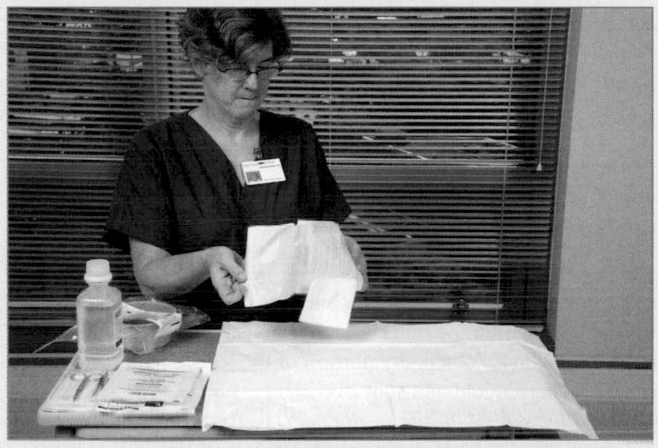

FIGURE 2 Dropping sterile item onto sterile field.

To Add a Sterile Solution

ACTION	RATIONALE
a. Obtain appropriate solution and check expiration date.	Once opened, label any bottles with date and time. Solution remains sterile for 24 hours once opened.
b. Open solution container according to directions and **place cap on table away from the field with edges up (Figure 3).**	Sterility of inside cap is maintained.
c. Hold bottle outside the edge of the sterile field with the label side facing the palm of your hand and prepare to pour from a height of 4 to 6 inches (10 to 15 cm). **Never touch the tip of the bottle to the sterile container or field.**	Label remains dry, and solution may be poured without reaching across sterile field. Minimal splashing occurs from that height. Accidentally touching the tip of the bottle to a container or dressing contaminates them both.
d. Pour required amount of solution steadily into sterile container previously added to the sterile field and positioned at side of sterile field or onto dressings (Figure 4). **Avoid splashing any liquid.**	A steady stream minimizes the risk of splashing; moisture contaminates sterile field.

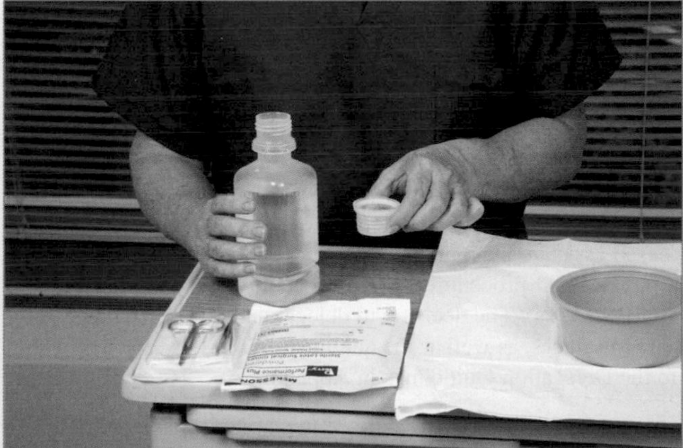

FIGURE 3 Opening bottle of sterile solution and placing cap on table with edges up.

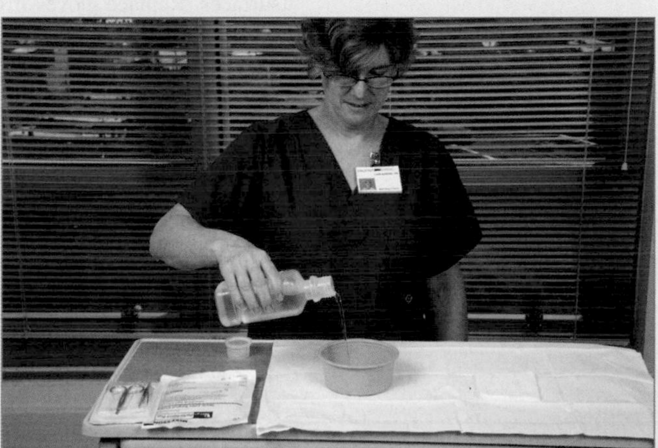

FIGURE 4 Pouring solution into sterile container.

(continued)

SKILL 1-6 ADDING STERILE ITEMS TO A STERILE FIELD continued

ACTION	RATIONALE
e. Touch only the outside of the lid when recapping. Label solution with date and time of opening.	Solution remains uncontaminated and available for future use.
7. Continue with procedure as indicated.	
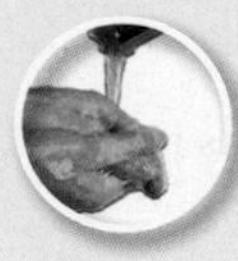 8. When procedure is completed, remove PPE, if used. Perform hand hygiene.	Removing PPE properly reduces the risk for infection transmission and contamination of other items. Hand hygiene prevents the spread of microorganisms.

EVALUATION

The expected outcome to achieve when adding items to a sterile field is that the sterile field is created without contamination, the sterile supplies are not contaminated, and the patient remains free of exposure to potential infection-causing microorganisms.

DOCUMENTATION

It is not usually necessary to document the addition of sterile items to a sterile field. However, document the use of performing sterile technique for any procedure.

UNEXPECTED SITUATIONS AND ASSOCIATED INTERVENTIONS

- *The item being added falls close to or on the edge of the field:* Consider the outer 1-inch edge of a sterile field to be contaminated. Any item within the outer 1-inch is considered contaminated.
- *A part of the sterile field becomes contaminated:* When any portion of the sterile field becomes contaminated, discard all portions of the sterile field and start over.
- *The nurse realizes a supply is missing after setting up the sterile field:* Call for help. Do not leave the sterile field unattended. If you are unable to visualize the sterile field at all times, it is considered contaminated.
- *The patient touches the sterile field:* If the patient touches the sterile field, discard the supplies and prepare a new sterile field. If the patient is confused, have someone assist by holding the patient's hands and/or reinforcing what is happening.

SKILL 1-7 PUTTING ON STERILE GLOVES AND REMOVING SOILED GLOVES

When applying and wearing sterile gloves, keep hands above waist level and away from nonsterile surfaces. Replace gloves if they develop an opening or tear; the integrity of the material becomes compromised; or the gloves come in contact with any nonsterile surface or nonsterile item. Refer to Fundamentals Review 1-2 for additional guidelines related to working with sterile gloves. It is a good idea to bring an extra pair of gloves with you when gathering supplies, according to facility policy. That way, if the first pair is contaminated in some way and needs to be replaced, you will not have to leave the procedure to get a new pair.

DELEGATION CONSIDERATIONS

Procedures requiring the use of sterile gloves and other sterile items are not delegated to nursing assistive personnel (NAP) or unlicensed assistive personnel (UAP). Depending on the state's nurse practice act and the organization's policies and procedures, these procedures may be delegated to licensed practical/vocational nurses (LPN/LVNs). The decision to delegate must be based on careful analysis of the patient's needs and circumstances, as well as the qualifications of the person to whom the task is being delegated. Refer to the Delegation Guidelines in Appendix A.

EQUIPMENT

- Sterile gloves of the appropriate size
- PPE, as indicated

ASSESSMENT

Assess the situation to determine the necessity for sterile gloves. In addition, check the patient's medical record for information about a possible latex allergy. Also, question the patient about any history of allergy, including latex allergy, or sensitivity and signs and symptoms that have occurred. If the patient has a latex allergy, anticipate the need for latex-free gloves.

NURSING DIAGNOSIS

Determine the related factors for the nursing diagnoses based on the patient's current status. Appropriate nursing diagnoses may include:

- Risk for Infection
- Ineffective Protection
- Risk for Latex Allergy Response

OUTCOME IDENTIFICATION AND PLANNING

The expected outcome to achieve when putting on and removing sterile gloves is that the gloves are applied and removed without contamination. Other outcomes that may be appropriate include the following: The patient remains free of exposure to infectious microorganisms, and the patient does not exhibit signs and symptoms of a latex allergy response.

IMPLEMENTATION

ACTION	RATIONALE
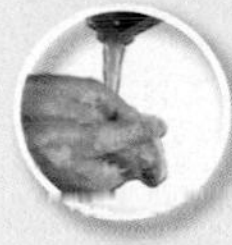 1. Perform hand hygiene and put on PPE, if indicated.	Hand hygiene and PPE prevent the spread of microorganisms. PPE is required based on transmission precautions.
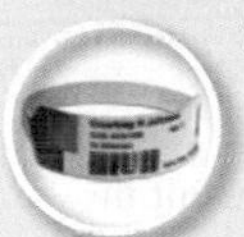 2. Identify the patient. Explain the procedure to the patient.	Patient identification validates the correct patient and correct procedure. Discussion and explanation help allay anxiety and prepare the patient for what to expect.
3. Check that the sterile glove package is dry and unopened. Also note expiration date, making sure that the date is still valid.	Moisture contaminates a sterile package. Expiration date indicates the period that the package remains sterile.
4. Place sterile glove package on clean, dry surface at or above your waist.	Moisture could contaminate the sterile gloves. Any sterile object held below the waist is considered contaminated.
5. Open the outside wrapper by carefully peeling the top layer back (Figure 1). Remove inner package, handling only the outside of it.	This maintains sterility of gloves in inner packet.
6. Place the inner package on the work surface with the side labeled "cuff end" closest to the body.	Allows for ease of glove application.
7. Carefully open the inner package. Fold open the top flap, then the bottom and sides (Figure 2). **Take care not to touch the inner surface of the package or the gloves.**	The inner surface of the package is considered sterile. The outer 1-inch border of the inner package is considered contaminated. The sterile gloves are exposed with the cuff end closest to the nurse.

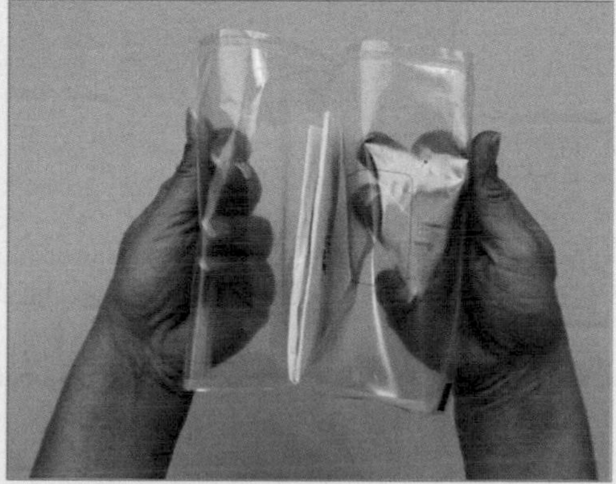

FIGURE 1 Pulling top layer of outside wrapper back.

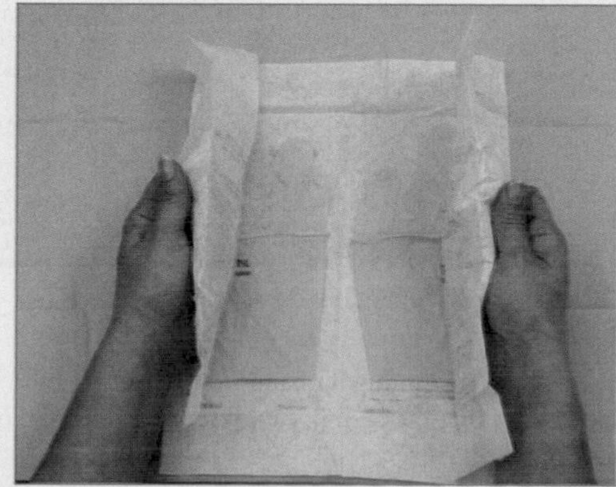

FIGURE 2 Folding back side flaps.

(*continued*)

SKILL 1-7 PUTTING ON STERILE GLOVES AND REMOVING SOILED GLOVES continued

ACTION	RATIONALE
8. With the thumb and forefinger of the nondominant hand, grasp the folded cuff of the glove for the dominant hand, touching only the exposed inside of the glove (Figure 3).	Unsterile hand touches only inside of glove. Outside remains sterile.
9. Keeping the hands above the waistline, lift and hold the glove up and off the inner package with fingers down (Figure 4). **Be careful that it does not touch any unsterile object.**	Glove is contaminated if it touches any unsterile objects.

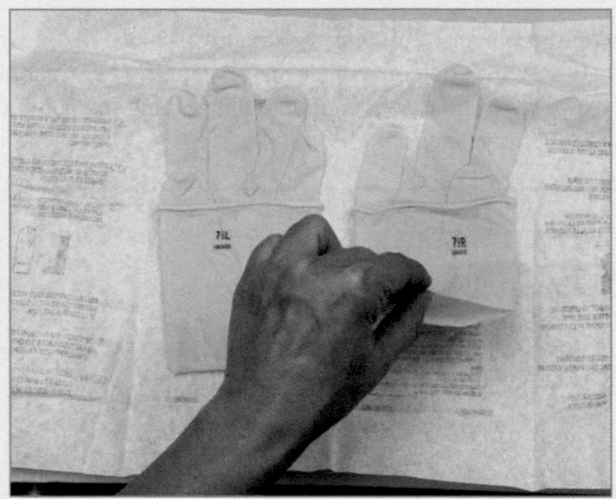

FIGURE 3 Grasping cuff of glove for dominant hand.

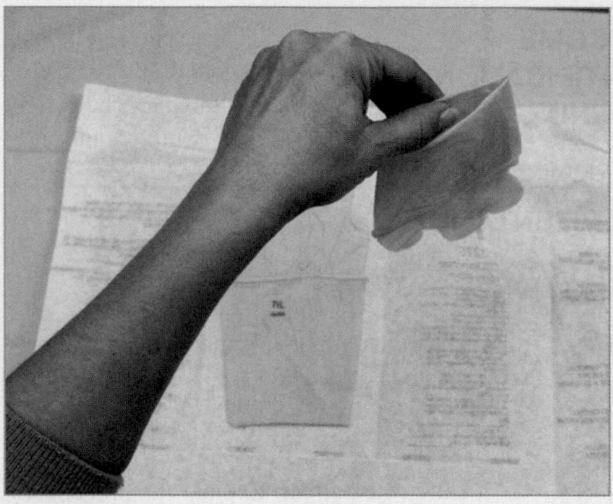

FIGURE 4 Lifting glove from package.

ACTION	RATIONALE
10. Carefully insert dominant hand palm up into glove (Figure 5) and pull glove on. Leave the cuff folded until the opposite hand is gloved.	Attempting to turn upward with unsterile hand may result in contamination of sterile glove.
11. Hold the thumb of the gloved hand outward. Place the fingers of the gloved hand inside the cuff of the remaining glove (Figure 6). Lift it from the wrapper, taking care not to touch anything with the gloves or hands.	Thumb is less likely to become contaminated if held outward. Sterile surface touching sterile surface prevents contamination.

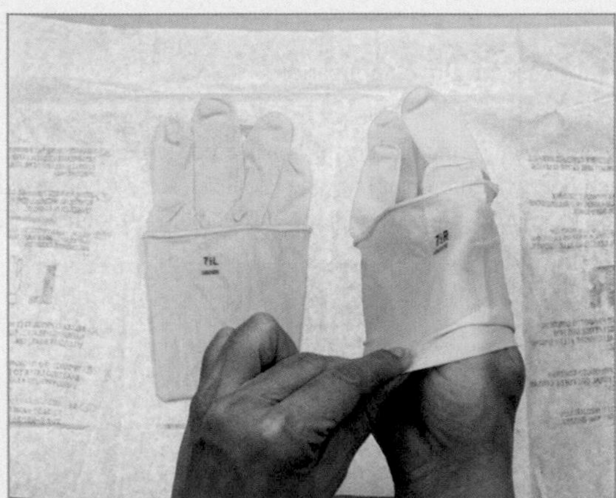

FIGURE 5 Inserting dominant hand into glove.

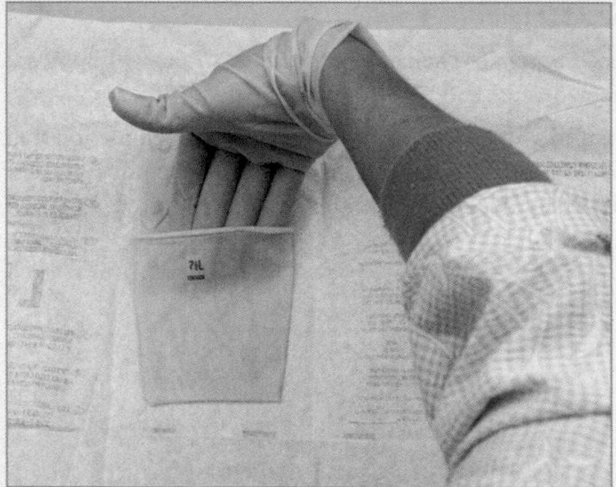

FIGURE 6 Sliding fingers under cuff of glove for nondominant hand.

ACTION	RATIONALE
12. Carefully insert nondominant hand into glove. Pull the glove on, taking care that the skin does not touch any of the outer surfaces of the gloves.	Sterile surface touching sterile surface prevents contamination.

ACTION	RATIONALE
13. **Slide the fingers of one hand under the cuff of the other and fully extend the cuff down the arm, touching only the sterile outside of the glove (Figure 7). Repeat for the remaining hand.**	Sterile surface touching sterile surface prevents contamination.
14. Adjust gloves on both hands if necessary, **touching only sterile areas with other sterile areas** (Figure 8).	Sterile surface touching sterile surface prevents contamination.
15. Continue with procedure as indicated.	

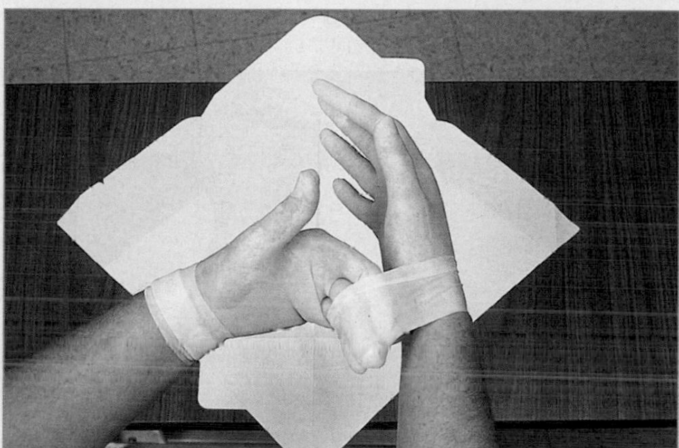

FIGURE 7 Sliding fingers of one hand under cuff of other hand and extending cuff down the arm.

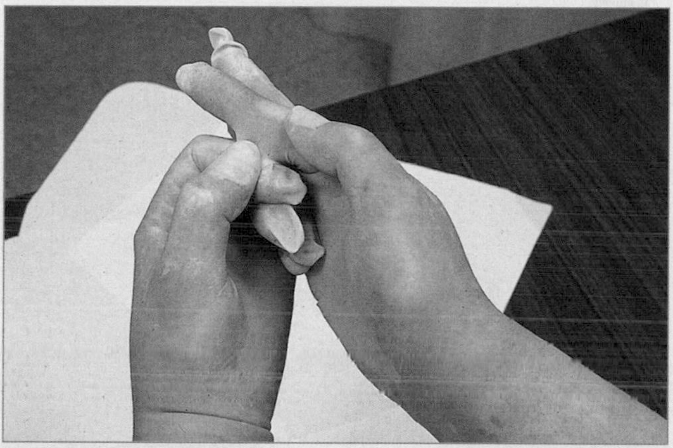

FIGURE 8 Adjusting gloves as necessary.

Removing Soiled Gloves

ACTION	RATIONALE
16. Use dominant hand to grasp the opposite glove **near cuff end on the outside exposed area.** Remove it by pulling it off, inverting it as it is pulled, keeping the contaminated area on the inside (Figure 9). Hold the removed glove in the remaining gloved hand.	Contaminated area does not come in contact with hands or wrists.

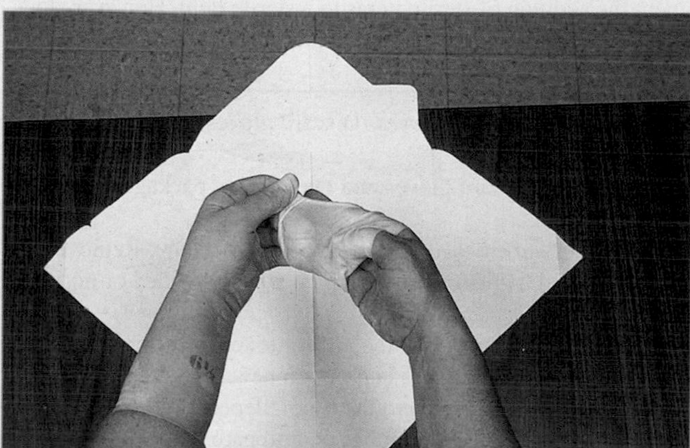

FIGURE 9 Inverting glove as it is removed.

(continued)

SKILL 1-7 PUTTING ON STERILE GLOVES AND REMOVING SOILED GLOVES continued

ACTION	RATIONALE
17. Slide fingers of ungloved hand between the remaining glove and the wrist (Figure 10). **Take care to avoid touching the outside surface of the glove.** Remove it by pulling it off, inverting it as it is pulled, keeping the contaminated area on the inside, and securing the first glove inside the second (Figure 11).	Contaminated area does not come in contact with hands or wrists.
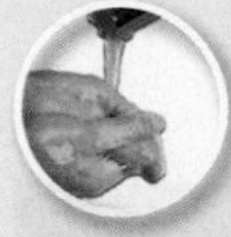 18. Discard gloves in appropriate container. Remove additional PPE, if used. Perform hand hygiene.	Proper disposal and removal of PPE reduces the risk for infection transmission and contamination of other items. Hand hygiene prevents the spread of microorganisms.

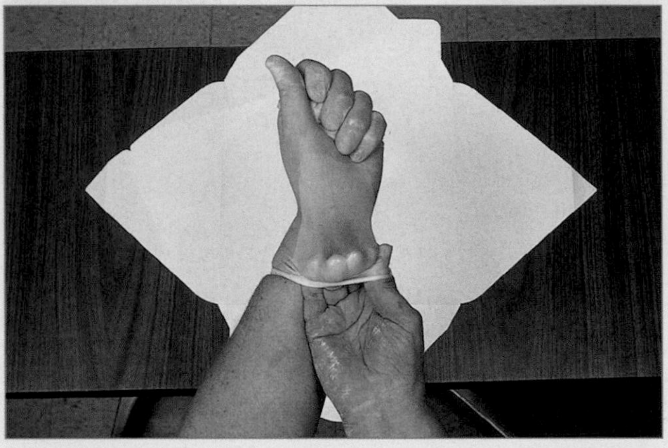

FIGURE 10 Sliding fingers of ungloved hand inside remaining glove.

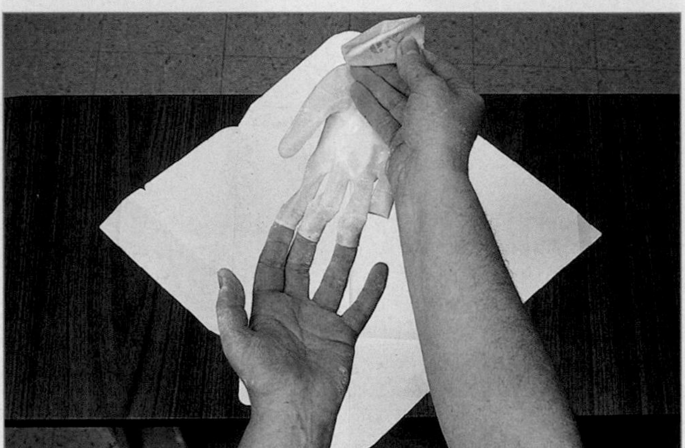

FIGURE 11 Inverting glove as it is removed; securing first glove inside it.

EVALUATION

The expected outcome is met when gloves are applied and removed without contamination. Other expected outcomes are met when the patient remains free of exposure to potential infection-causing microorganisms, and does not exhibit signs and symptoms of a latex-allergy response.

DOCUMENTATION

It is not usually necessary to document the addition of sterile items to a sterile field. However, document the use of sterile technique for any procedure performed using sterile technique.

UNEXPECTED SITUATIONS AND ASSOCIATED INTERVENTIONS

- *Contamination occurs during application of the sterile gloves:* Discard gloves and open new package of sterile gloves.
- *A hole or tear is noticed in one of the gloves:* Discard gloves and open a new package of sterile gloves.
- *A hole or tear is noticed in one of the gloves during the procedure:* Stop procedure. Remove damaged gloves. Wash hands or perform hand hygiene (depending on whether soiled or not) and put on new sterile gloves.
- *The patient touches the nurse's hands or the sterile field:* If the patient touches your hands and nothing else, you may remove the contaminated gloves and put on new, sterile gloves. It is always a good idea to bring two pairs of sterile gloves into the room, depending on facility policy. If the patient touches the sterile field, discard the supplies and prepare a new sterile field. If the patient is confused, have someone assist you by holding the patient's hands or reinforcing what is happening.
- *Patient has a latex allergy:* Obtain latex-free sterile gloves.

ENHANCE YOUR UNDERSTANDING

FOCUSING ON PATIENT CARE: DEVELOPING CLINICAL REASONING

Consider the case scenarios at the beginning of the chapter as you answer the following questions to enhance your understanding and apply what you have learned.

QUESTIONS

1. While preparing the sterile table in the cardiac catheterization lab for Mr. Wilson, you realize that a sterile bowl is missing. How can you obtain a sterile bowl?
2. While you are putting on sterile gloves in preparation for an indwelling urinary catheter insertion, your patient, Sheri Lawrence, moves her leg. You do not *think* that Sheri's leg touched the glove, but you are not positive. What should you do?
3. Edgar Barowski's son is visiting and asks you why the masks that are outside Edgar's room are different from the ones that people wear in the operating room. What should you tell Edgar's son?

You can find suggested answers after the Bibliography at the end of this chapter.

INTEGRATED CASE STUDY CONNECTION

The case studies in the back of the book are designed to focus on integrating concepts. Refer to the following case studies to enhance your understanding of the concepts related to the skills in this chapter.

- Basic Case Studies: Tiffany Jones, page 1064; John Willis, page 1068.
- Intermediate Case Studies: Tula Stillwater, page 1081; Gwen Galloway, page 1089; George Patel, page 1091.

TAYLOR SUITE RESOURCES

Explore these additional resources to enhance learning for this chapter:

- NCLEX-Style Questions and other resources on thePoint, http://thePoint.lww.com/Lynn4e
- *Skill Checklists for Taylor's Clinical Nursing Skills,* 4e
- *Taylor's Video Guide to Clinical Nursing Skills:* Asepsis
- *Fundamentals of Nursing:* Chapter 23, Asepsis and Infection Control

Bibliography

Agency for Healthcare Research and Quality (AHRQ). (2010). *AHRQ's efforts to prevent and reduce healthcare-associated infections.* Available at www .ahrq.gov/qual/haiflyer.pdf.

Ahmed-Lecheheb, D., Cunat, L., Hartemann, P., & Hautemanière, A. (2012). Prospective observational study to assess hand skin condition after application of alcohol-based hand rub solutions. *American Journal of Infection Control, 40*(2), 160–164.

Allegranzi, B., Memish, Z., Donaldson, L., et al. (2009). World Health Organization Global Patient Safety Challenge Task Force on Religious and Cultural Aspects of Hand Hygiene. Religion and culture: Potential undercurrents influencing hand hygiene promotion in health care. *American Journal of Infection Control, 37*(1), 28–34.

Association of Perioperative Registered Nurses (AORN). (2012). *Perioperative standards and recommended practices.* Denver, CO: AORN, Inc.

Association for Professionals in Infection Control and Epidemiology (APIC). (2010). *Guide to the elimination of methicillin-resistant Staphylococcus aureus (MRSA) Transmission in Hospital Settings,* (2nd ed.) Available at http://www.apic.org/Resource_/EliminationGuideForm/631fcd91-8773-4067-9f85-ab2a5b157eab/File/MRSA-elimination-guide-2010.pdf.

Association for Professionals in Infection Control and Epidemiology (APIC). (2005). *Hand hygiene for healthcare workers.* Available at http://www.apic.org/Resource_/EducationalBrochureForm/370c41f0-380f-4d4d-aa33-67ca4407f3ef/File/Hand-Hygiene-Health-care-Workers-Brochure.pdf

Beam, E.L., Gibbs, S.G., Boulter, K.C., Beckerdite, M.E., & Smith, P.W. (2011). A method for evaluating health care workers' personal protective equipment technique. *American Journal of Infection Control, 39*(5), 415–420.

Bulechek, G.M, Butcher, H.K., Dochterman, J.M., & Wagner, C.M. (Eds.). (2013). *Nursing interventions classification (NIC)* (6th ed.). St. Louis, MO: Mosby Elsevier.

Casanova, L.M., Rutala, W.A., Weber, D.J., & Sobsey, M.D. (2012). Effect of single- versus double-gloving on virus transfer to healthcare workers' skin and clothing during removal of personal protective equipment. *American Journal of Infection Control, 40*(4), 369–374.

Centers for Disease Control and Prevention. (2002). Guidelines for hand hygiene in health-care settings. *Morbidity and Mortality Weekly Report, 51*(RR16), 1–45.

Centers for Disease Control and Prevention (CDC). (2011). *Hand hygiene basics.* Available at www.cdc. gov/handhygiene/Basics.html.

Centers for Disease Control and Prevention. (2010). (Updated 2011). *Healthcare-associated infections (HAIs). Tools for protecting healthcare personnel. Sequence for donning and removing personal protective equipment (PPE).* Poster. Available at http://www.cdc. gov/HAI/prevent/ppe.html.

Centers for Disease Control and Prevention. (2004). *Guidance for the selection and use of personal protective equipment (PPE) in healthcare settings.* (Slide presentation). Available at http://www.cdc.gov/HAI/pdfs/ppe/PPEslides6-29-04.pdf.

Centers for Disease Control and Prevention (CDC). (2007a). (Updated 2012). *Airborne infection isolation precautions. Excerpted from guideline for isolation precautions: Preventing transmission of infectious agents in healthcare settings.* Available at www.cdc. gov/hicpac/pdf/isolation/Isolation2007.pdf.

Centers for Disease Control and Prevention (CDC). (2007b). (Updated 2012). *Contact precautions. Excerpted from guideline for isolation precautions: Preventing transmission of infectious agents in healthcare settings.* Available at www.cdc.gov/hicpac/pdf/ isolation/Isolation2007.pdf.

Centers for Disease Control and Prevention (CDC). (2007c). (Updated 2012). *Droplet precautions. Excerpted from guideline for isolation precautions: Preventing transmission of infectious agents in healthcare settings.* Available at www.cdc.gov/hicpac/pdf/ isolation/Isolation2007.pdf.

Centers for Disease Control and Prevention (CDC). (2007d). (Updated 2012). *Standard precautions. Excerpted from guideline for isolation precautions: Preventing transmission of infectious agents in healthcare settings.* Available at www.cdc.gov/hicpac/pdf/ isolation/Isolation2007.pdf.

Centers for Disease Control and Prevention (CDC). (2007e). (Updated 2012). *Personal protective equipment for healthcare personnel. Excerpted from guideline for isolation precautions: Preventing transmission of infectious agents in healthcare settings.* Available at www.cdc.gov/hicpac/pdf/isolation/Isolation2007.pdf.

Fakhry, M., Hanna, G.B., Anderson, O., Holmes, A., & Nathwani, D. (2012). Effectiveness of an audible reminder on hand hygiene adherence. *American Journal of Infection Control, 40*(4), 320–323.

Felembam, O, St. John, W. & Shaban, R. (2012). Hand hygiene practices of home visiting community nurses. *Home Healthcare Nurse, 30*(3), 152–160.

Gould, D.J., Moralejo, D., Drey, N., & Chudleigh, J.H. (2011). Interventions to improve hand hygiene compliance in patient care. *Cochrane Database of Systematic Reviews.* Art. No.: CD005186. DOI: 10.1002/14651858.CD005186.pub3. Available at http://summaries.cochrane.org/CD005186/methods-to-improve-healthcare-worker-hand-hygiene-to-decrease-infection-in-hospitals.

Grossman, S., & DeBartolomeo, D.M. (2008). Managing the threat of methicillin-resistant *staphylococcus aureus* in home care. *Home Healthcare Nurse,* 26(6), 356–366.

Grossman, S., & Porth, C.M. (2014). *Porth's pathophysiology: Concepts of altered health states.* (9th ed.). Philadelphia: Wolters Kluwer Health/Lippincott Williams & Wilkins.

Healthy People 2020. (2012). *Healthcare-associated infections.* Available at http:www.healthypeople.gov/2020/topicsobjectives2020/overview.aspx?topicid =17.

Hinkle, J.L., & Cheever, K.H. (2014). *Brunner & Suddarth's textbook of medical-surgical nursing* (13th ed.). Philadelphia: Wolters Kluwer Health/Lippincott Williams & Wilkins.

Institute for Healthcare Improvement (IHI). (2011). *How-to guide: Improving hand hygiene.* Available at http://www.IHI.org.

Jabbar, U., Leischner, J., Kasper, D., et al. (2010). Effectiveness of alcohol-based hand rubs for removal of *Clostridium difficile. Infection Control & Hospital Epidemiology, 30*(10), 565–570.

The Joint Commission. Center for Transforming Healthcare. (2012). *Facts about the hand hygiene project.* Available at http://www.centerfortransforminghealthcare.org/assets/4/6/CTH_HH_Fact_Sheet.pdf.

The Joint Commission (TJC). (2010). *Speak up: Five things you can do to prevent infection.* Available at http://www.jointcommission.org/speakup.aspx.

The Joint Commission (TJC). (2014). *National patient safety goals. Hospital: 2014 National patient safety goals.* Available at http://www.jointcommission.org/standards_information/npsgs.aspx.

Kenneley, I.L. (2010). Infection control and the home care environment. *Home Health Care Management & Practice, 22*(3), 195–201.

Kilpatrick, C., Murdoch, H., & Storr, J. (2012). Importance of hand hygiene during invasive procedures. *Nursing Standard, 26*(41), 42–46.

McGoldrick, M., & Rhinehart, E. (2007). Managing multidrug-resistant organisms in home care and hospice: Surveillance, prevention, and control. *Home Healthcare Nurse, 25*(9), 580–588.

Moorhead, S., Johnson, M., Maas, M.L., & Swanson, E. (Eds). (2013). *Nursing Outcomes Classification (NOC).* (5th ed.). St. Louis: Mosby Elsevier.

Mortell, M. (2012). Hand hygiene compliance: Is there a theory-practice-ethics gap? *British Journal of Nursing, 21*(17), 1011–1014.

NANDA International. (2012). *Nursing diagnoses: Definitions & classification 2012–2014.* West Sussex, UK: Wiley-Blackwell.

Pincock, T., Bernstein, P., Warthman, S., & Holst, E. (2012). Bundling hand hygiene interventions and measurement to decrease health care-associated infections. *American Journal of Infection Control, 40* (Supplement), S18–S27.

Taylor, C., Lillis, C., & Lynn, P. (2015). *Fundamentals of nursing.* (8th ed.). Philadelphia: Wolters Kluwer Health/Lippincott Williams & Wilkins.

Walker, B. (2007). New guidelines for fighting multidrug-resistant organisms. *Nursing, 37*(5), 20.

World Health Organization. (2009). *WHO guidelines on hand hygiene in health care.* Available at http://www.who.int/gpsc/5may/background/5moments/en/.

SUGGESTED ANSWERS FOR FOCUSING ON PATIENT CARE: DEVELOPING CLINICAL REASONING

1. You should call for or ask another staff member to obtain the bowl. Never walk away from or turn your back on a sterile field. This prevents possible contamination while the field is out of your view.
2. You should change gloves. Only a sterile object can touch another sterile object. Nonsterile touching sterile means contamination has occurred. Consider an object contaminated if you have any doubt about its sterility.
3. You should explain the rationale for transmission-based precautions, including specific information about airborne precautions. Airborne precautions are used for patients who have infections that spread through the air, such as tuberculosis, varicella (chicken pox), rubeola (measles), and possibly SARS. Place patient in a private room that has monitored negative air pressure in relation to surrounding areas, 6 to 12 air changes per hour, and appropriate discharge of air outside or monitored filtration if air is recirculated. Keep door closed and patient in room. Respiratory protection is used when entering the room of patient with known or suspected tuberculosis.

2 Vital Signs

FOCUSING ON PATIENT CARE

This chapter will explain some of the skills related to vital signs needed to care for the following patients:

TYRONE JEFFRIES, age 5, is in the emergency department with a temperature of 101.3°F (38.9°C).

TOBY WHITE, age 26, has a history of asthma and is now breathing 32 times per minute.

CARL GLATZ, age 58, has recently started taking medications to control his hypertension (high blood pressure).

Refer to Focusing on Patient Care: Developing Clinical Reasoning at the end of the chapter to apply what you learn.

LEARNING OBJECTIVES

After studying this chapter, you will be able to:

1. Assess body temperature via the oral, tympanic, temporal, axillary, and rectal routes.
2. Regulate an infant's temperature using an overhead radiant warmer.
3. Regulate temperature using a hypothermia blanket.
4. Assess peripheral pulses by palpation.
5. Assess an apical pulse by auscultation.
6. Assess peripheral pulses using Doppler ultrasound.
7. Assess respiration.
8. Assess blood pressure by auscultation or using an automatic electronic blood pressure monitor.
9. Assess systolic blood pressure using Doppler ultrasound.

KEY TERMS

apnea: absence of breathing

bell: (of stethoscope) hollowed, upright, curved portion used to auscultate low-pitched sounds, such as murmurs

blood pressure: force of blood against arterial walls

bradypnea: abnormally slow rate of breathing

diaphragm: (of stethoscope) large, flat disk on the stethoscope used to auscultate high-pitched sounds, such as respiratory sounds

diastolic pressure: least amount of pressure exerted on arterial walls, which occurs when the heart is at rest between ventricular contractions

expiration: act of breathing out; synonym is exhalation

febrile: a condition in which the body temperature is elevated

hypertension: blood pressure elevated above the upper limit of normal

hypotension: blood pressure below the lower limit of normal

hypothermia: body temperature below the lower limit of normal

inspiration: act of breathing in; synonym is inhalation

Korotkoff sounds: series of sounds that correspond to changes in blood flow through an artery as pressure is released

orthostatic hypotension: temporary fall in blood pressure associated with assuming an upright position; synonym for postural hypotension

respiration: act of breathing and using oxygen in body cells

systolic pressure: highest point of pressure on arterial walls when the ventricles contract

tachypnea: abnormally rapid rate of breathing

vital signs: body temperature, pulse, respiratory rates, and blood pressure; synonym for cardinal signs

Vital signs are a person's temperature, pulse, **respiration**, and **blood pressure**, abbreviated as T, P, R, and BP. Pain, often called the fifth vital sign, is discussed in Chapter 10, Comfort. Pulse oximetry, the noninvasive measurement of arterial oxyhemoglobin saturation of arterial blood, is also often included with the measurement of vital signs and is discussed in Chapter 14, Oxygenation. The health status of an individual is reflected in these indicators of body function. A change in vital signs may indicate a change in health.

Vital signs are assessed and compared with accepted normal values and the patient's usual patterns in a wide variety of instances. Examples of appropriate times to measure vital signs include, but are not limited to, screenings at health fairs and clinics, in the home, upon admission to a health care setting, when medications are given that may affect one of the vital signs, before and after invasive diagnostic and surgical procedures, and in emergency situations. Nurses take vital signs as often as the condition of a patient requires such assessment.

Careful attention to the details of vital sign procedures and accuracy in the interpretation of the findings are extremely important. Although vital sign assessment may be delegated to other health care personnel when the condition of the patient is stable, it is the nurse's responsibility to ensure the accuracy of the data, interpret vital sign findings, and report abnormal findings. Principles of delegation should be followed (see Appendix A). If a patient has abnormal or unusual physical signs or symptoms (e.g., chest pain or dizziness) or has unexpected changes in vital signs, the nurse should validate the findings and further assess the patient. Techniques for measuring each of the vital signs are presented in this chapter. Fundamentals Review 2-1 outlines age-related variations in normal vital signs. Fundamentals Review 2-2 provides guidelines for obtaining vital signs for infants and children.

FUNDAMENTALS REVIEW 2-1

AGE-RELATED VARIATIONS IN NORMAL VITAL SIGNS

Age	Temperature °C °F	Pulse beats/min	Respirations breaths/min	Blood pressure mm Hg
Newborn (axillary)	35.9–36.9 96.7–98.5	70–190	30–55	73/55
Infants (temporal)	37.1–38.1 98.7–100.5	80–150	20–40	85/37
Toddler (temporal)	37.1–38.1 98.7–100.5	70–120	20–30	89/46
Child (tympanic)	36.8–37.8 98.2–100	70–115	20–25	95/57
Preteen (oral)	35.8–37.5 96.4–99.5	65–110	18–26	102/61
Teen (oral)	35.8–37.5 96.4–99.5	55–105	12–22	112/64
Adult (oral)	35.8–37.5 96.4–99.5	60–100	12–20	120/80

Adapted from Jensen, S. (2011.) *Nursing health assessment. A best practice approach.* Philadelphia: Wolters Kluwer Health | Lippincott Williams & Wilkins; and Kyle, T., & Carman, S. (2013). *Essentials of pediatric nursing* (2nd ed.). Philadelphia: Wolters Kluwer Health | Lippincott Williams & Wilkins.

FUNDAMENTALS REVIEW 2-2

TECHNIQUES FOR OBTAINING VITAL SIGNS OF INFANTS AND CHILDREN

- Due to the "fear factor" of blood pressure measurement, save the blood pressure measurement for last. Children and infants often begin to cry during blood pressure assessment, and this may affect the respiration and pulse rate assessment.
- Perform as many tasks as possible while the child is sitting on the parent's lap or in a chair next to the parent.
- Let the child see and touch the equipment before you begin to use it.
- Make measuring vital signs a game. For instance, if you are using a tympanic thermometer that makes a chirping sound, tell the child you are looking for "birdies" in the ear. While auscultating the pulse, tell the child you are listening for another type of animal.
- If the child has a doll or stuffed animal, pretend to take the doll's vital signs first.

SKILL 2-1 ASSESSING BODY TEMPERATURE

Body temperature is the difference between the amount of heat produced by the body and the amount of heat lost to the environment measured in degrees. Heat is generated by metabolic processes in the core tissues of the body, transferred to the skin surface by the circulating blood, and then dissipated to the environment. Core body temperature (intracranial, intrathoracic, and intra-abdominal) is higher than surface body temperature. Normal body temperature is 35.9°C to 38°C (96.7°F to 100.5°F), depending on the route used for measurement (Jensen, 2011). There are individual variations of these temperatures as well as variations related to age, gender, physical activity, state of health, and environmental temperatures. Body temperature also varies during the day, with temperatures being lowest in the early morning and highest in the late afternoon (Grossman & Porth, 2014).

Health agency policies and procedures often specify the site to be used for assessing patients' temperatures. However, the nurse is expected to choose an alternate, appropriate site, and the correct equipment, based on the patient's condition, facility policy, and medical orders. Factors affecting the site selection include the patient's age, state of consciousness, amount of pain, and other care or treatments (e.g., oxygen administration) being provided.

Several types of equipment and different procedures might be used to measure body temperature. Different types of thermometers are illustrated in Figure 1. To obtain an accurate measurement, choose an appropriate site, the correct equipment, and the appropriate tool based on the patient's condition. If a temperature reading is obtained from a site other than the oral route, document the site used along with the measurement. If no site is listed with the documentation, it is generally assumed to be the oral route.

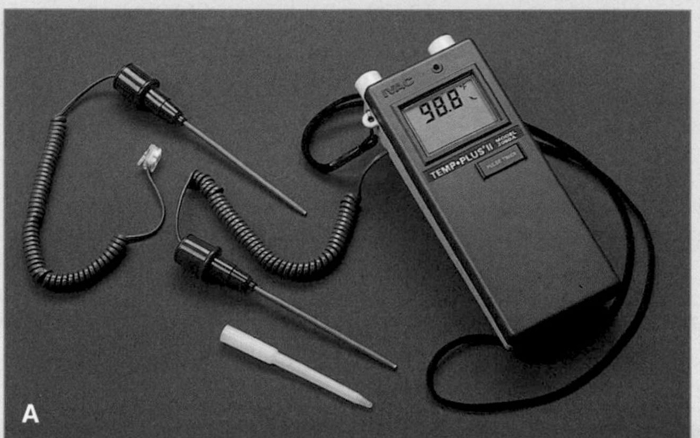

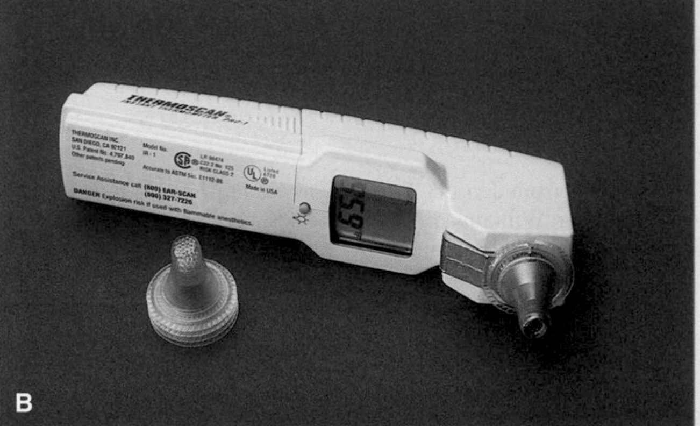

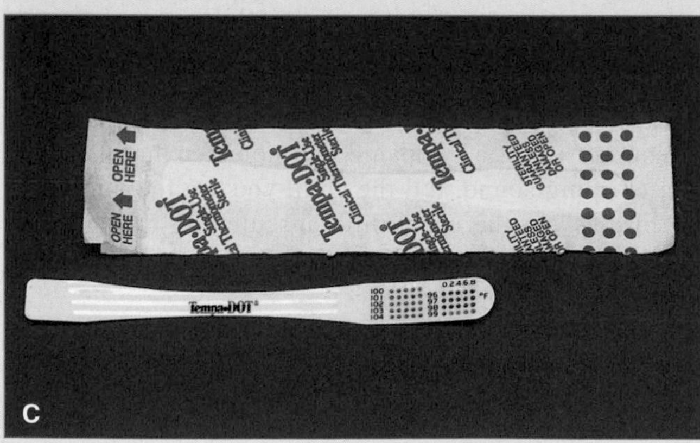

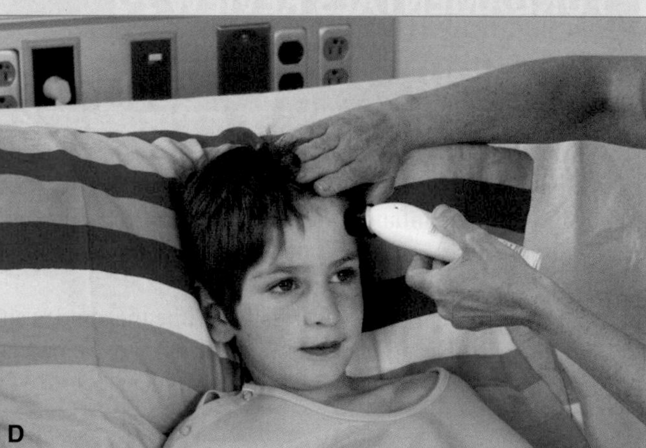

FIGURE 1 Types of thermometers. (**A**) Electronic thermometer. (**B**) Tympanic membrane thermometer. (**C**) Disposable thermometer for measuring oral temperature; the dots change color to indicate temperature. (**D**) Temporal artery thermometer.

Glass thermometers with mercury-filled bulbs have been used in the past for measuring body temperature. They are not used in health care institutions, based on federal safety recommendations (U.S. Environmental Protection Agency [EPA], 2012). However, patients may still have mercury thermometers at home and may be continuing to use them. Nurses should encourage patients to use alternative devices to measure body temperature and include patient teaching as part of nursing care.

Although bulb-type glass thermometers containing liquids other than mercury are available, they should never be used to measure the temperature of a person who is unconscious or irrational, or of infants and young children, because the glass could break.

DELEGATION CONSIDERATIONS

Assessment of body temperature may be delegated to nursing assistive personnel (NAP) or to unlicensed assistive personnel (UAP), as well as to licensed practical/vocational nurses (LPN/LVNs). The decision to delegate must be based on careful analysis of the patient's needs and circumstances, as well as the qualifications of the person to whom the task is being delegated. Refer to the Delegation Guidelines in Appendix A.

EQUIPMENT

- Digital, glass, or electronic thermometer, appropriate for site to be used
- Disposable probe covers
- Water-soluble lubricant for rectal temperature measurement
- Nonsterile gloves, if appropriate
- Additional personal protective equipment (PPE), as indicated
- Toilet tissue, if needed
- Pencil or pen, paper or flow sheet, computerized record

ASSESSMENT

Note baseline or previous temperature measurements. Assess the patient to ensure that his or her cognitive functioning is intact. Taking an oral temperature of a patient unable to follow directions can result in injury if the patient bites down on the thermometer. Assess whether the patient can close his or her lips around the thermometer. If the patient cannot, the oral method is not appropriate. Oral temperature measurement is contraindicated in patients with diseases of the oral cavity and in those who have had surgery of the nose or mouth. Ask the patient if he or she has recently smoked, has been chewing gum, or was eating and drinking immediately before having temperature assessed. If any of these have occurred, wait 30 minutes before taking an oral temperature because of the possible direct influence they may have had on the patient's temperature. **Tachypnea** and **bradypnea** may also influence results (Higgins, 2008; Quatrara, et al., 2007). The probe must remain in the sublingual pocket for the full period of measurement (Davie & Amoore, 2010).

If a patient has an earache, do not use the affected ear to take a tympanic temperature. The movement of the tragus may cause severe discomfort. Assess the patient for significant ear drainage or a scarred tympanic membrane. These conditions can provide inaccurate results and could cause problems for the patient. However, an ear infection or the presence of earwax in the canal will not significantly affect a tympanic thermometer reading. If the patient has been sleeping with the head turned to one side, take a tympanic temperature in the other ear. Heat may be increased on the side that was against the pillow, especially if it is a plastic-covered pillow. Otherwise, either ear can be used. Tympanic temperature readings are approximately equal to oral (Jensen, 2011).

When taking a temporal artery temperature, assess for head coverings. Anything covering the area, such as a hat, hair, wigs, or bandages, would insulate the area, resulting in falsely high readings. If a patient is lying on his or her side, measure only the side of the head exposed to the environment. Do not measure temporal artery temperature over scar tissue, open lesions, or abrasions. Move the thermometer across the forehead slowly and remain in contact with the skin to ensure accurate results. Temporal artery temperature readings are approximately equal to oral (Jensen, 2011).

When taking an axillary temperature, assess the patient's ability to hold the arm tight against his or her body. You may have to assist holding the arm firmly against the patient's body to ensure an accurate reading. Place the probe in the center of the axilla and ask the patient to hold his or her arm tightly by the side until the measurement is complete (Garner & Fendius, 2010). Axillary temperature readings are approximately 1 degree lower than oral (Jensen, 2011).

The rectal site should not be used in newborns, children with diarrhea, and in patients who have undergone rectal surgery or have a disease of the rectum. Because the insertion of the thermometer into the rectum can slow the heart rate by stimulating the vagus nerve, assessing a rectal temperature for patients with heart disease or after cardiac surgery may not be allowed in some institutions. In addition, assessing a rectal temperature is contraindicated in patients who are neutropenic (have low white blood cell counts, such as in leukemia) and in patients who have certain neurologic disorders (e.g., spinal cord injuries). Do not insert a rectal thermometer into a patient who has a low platelet count. The rectum is very vascular, and a thermometer could cause rectal bleeding. Rectal temperature readings are approximately 1 degree higher than oral (Jensen, 2011).

(*continued*)

SKILL 2-1 ASSESSING BODY TEMPERATURE continued

NURSING DIAGNOSIS

Determine related factors for the nursing diagnoses based on the patient's current status. Appropriate nursing diagnoses may include:

- Hyperthermia
- Hypothermia
- Risk for Imbalanced Body Temperature
- Ineffective Thermoregulation

OUTCOME IDENTIFICATION AND PLANNING

The expected outcomes to achieve when performing temperature assessment are that the patient's temperature is assessed accurately without injury and the patient experiences minimal discomfort. Other outcomes may be appropriate, depending on the patient's nursing diagnosis.

IMPLEMENTATION

ACTION	RATIONALE
1. Check the medical order or nursing care plan for frequency of measurement and route. More frequent temperature measurement may be appropriate based on nursing judgment.	Assessment and measurement of vital signs at appropriate intervals provide important data about the patient's health status.
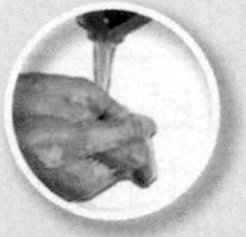 2. Perform hand hygiene and put on PPE, if indicated.	Hand hygiene and PPE prevent the spread of microorganisms. PPE is required based on transmission precautions.
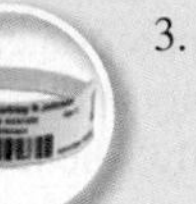 3. Identify the patient.	Identifying the patient ensures that the right patient receives the intervention and helps prevent errors.
4. Close the curtains around the bed and close the door to the room, if possible. Discuss the procedure with the patient and assess the patient's ability to assist with the procedure.	This ensures the patient's privacy. Explanation relieves anxiety and facilitates cooperation. Dialogue encourages patient participation and allows for individualized nursing care.
5. Assemble equipment on the overbed table within reach.	Organization facilitates performance of task.
6. Ensure that the electronic or digital thermometer is in working condition.	Improperly functioning thermometer may not give an accurate reading.
7. Put on gloves, if indicated.	Gloves prevent contact with blood and body fluids. Gloves are usually not required for an oral, axillary, or tympanic temperature measurement, unless contact with blood or body fluids is anticipated. Gloves should be worn for rectal temperature measurement.
8. Select the appropriate site based on previous assessment data.	This ensures safety and accuracy of measurement.
9. Follow the steps as outlined below for the appropriate type of thermometer.	
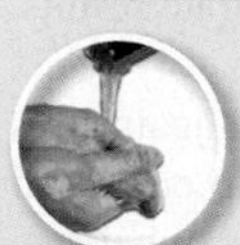 10. When measurement is completed, remove gloves, if worn. Remove additional PPE, if used. Perform hand hygiene.	Removing PPE properly reduces the risk for infection transmission and contamination of other items. Hand hygiene prevents the spread of microorganisms.

Measuring an Oral Temperature

ACTION	RATIONALE
11. Remove the electronic unit from the charging unit, and remove the probe from within the recording unit.	Electronic unit must be taken into the patient's room to assess the patient's temperature. On some models, by removing the probe the machine is already turned on.

ACTION	RATIONALE
12. Cover thermometer probe with disposable probe cover and slide it on until it snaps into place (Figure 2).	Using a cover prevents contamination of the thermometer probe.
13. **Place the probe beneath the patient's tongue in the posterior sublingual pocket (Figure 3). Ask the patient to close his or her lips around the probe.**	When the probe rests deep in the posterior sublingual pocket, it is in contact with blood vessels lying close to the surface.

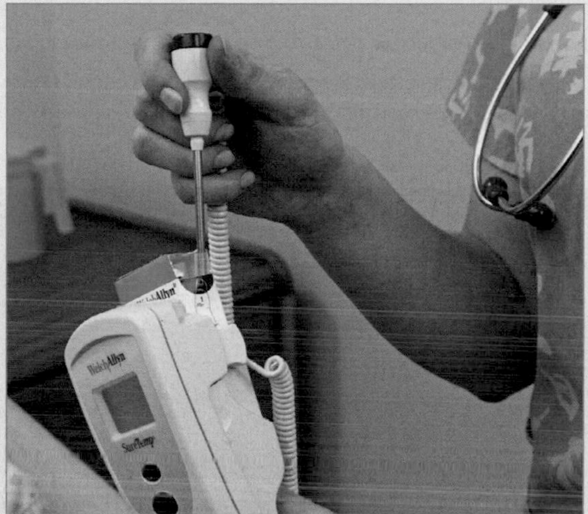

FIGURE 2 Putting probe cover on the thermometer.

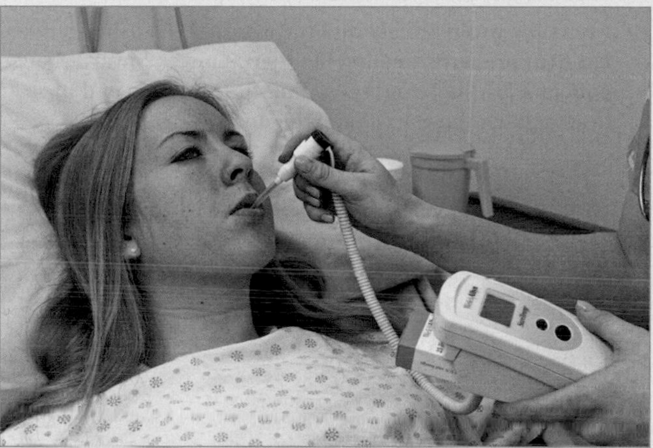

FIGURE 3 Inserting thermometer under the tongue in the posterior sublingual pocket.

ACTION	RATIONALE
14. Continue to hold the probe until you hear a beep (Figure 4). Note the temperature reading.	If left unsupported, the weight of the probe tends to pull it away from the correct location. The signal indicates that the measurement is completed. The electronic thermometer provides a digital display of the measured temperature.
15. Remove the probe from the patient's mouth. Dispose of the probe cover by holding the probe over an appropriate receptacle and pressing the probe release button (Figure 5).	Disposing of the probe cover ensures that it will not be reused accidentally on another patient. Proper disposal prevents spread of microorganisms.

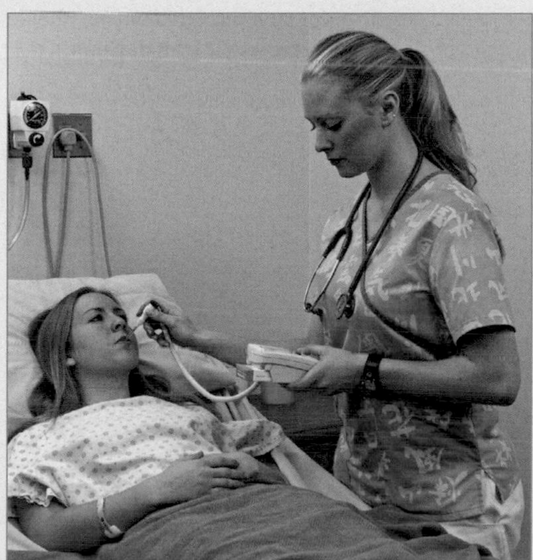

FIGURE 4 Holding probe in the patient's mouth.

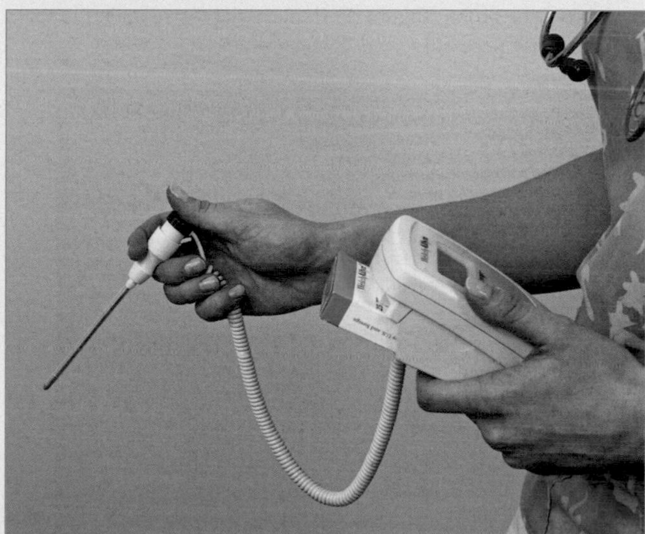

FIGURE 5 Pushing button to dispose of cover.

(continued)

SKILL 2-1 ASSESSING BODY TEMPERATURE continued

ACTION	RATIONALE
16. Return the thermometer probe to the storage place within the unit. Return the electronic unit to the charging unit, if appropriate.	The thermometer needs to be recharged for future use. If necessary, the thermometer should stay on the charger so that it is ready to use at all times.
Measuring a Tympanic Membrane Temperature	
17. If necessary, push the "ON" button and wait for the "ready" signal on the unit (Figure 6).	For proper function, the thermometer must be turned on and warmed up.
18. Slide the disposable cover onto the tympanic probe.	Use of a disposable cover deters the spread of microorganisms.
19. **Insert the probe snugly into the external ear using gentle but firm pressure, angling the thermometer toward the patient's jaw line (Figure 7). Pull the pinna up and back to straighten the ear canal in an adult.**	If the probe is not inserted correctly, the patient's temperature may be noted as lower than normal.

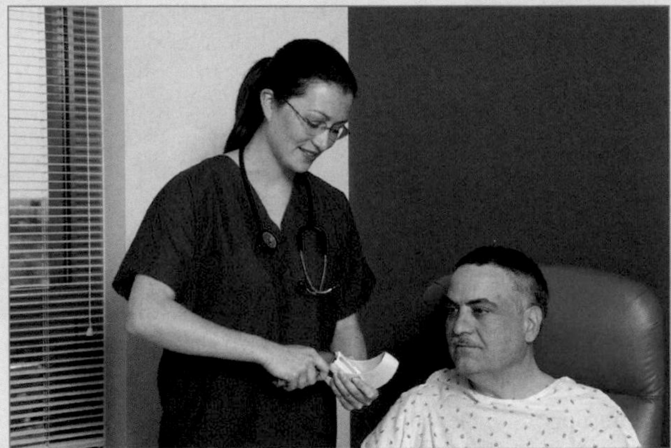

FIGURE 6 Turning unit on and awaiting the ready signal.

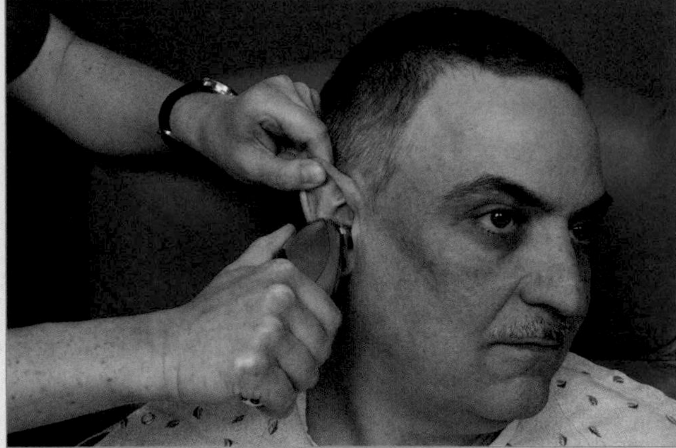

FIGURE 7 Thermometer in patient's ear canal with pinna pulled up and back.

ACTION	RATIONALE
20. Activate the unit by pushing the trigger button. The reading is immediate (usually within 2 seconds). Note the reading.	The digital thermometer must be activated to record the temperature.
21. Discard the probe cover in an appropriate receptacle by pushing the probe-release button or use the rim of cover to remove it from the probe (Figure 8). Replace the thermometer in its charger, if necessary.	Discarding the probe cover ensures that it will not be reused accidentally on another patient. Proper disposal prevents the spread of microorganisms. If necessary, the thermometer should stay on the charger so that it is ready to use at all times.

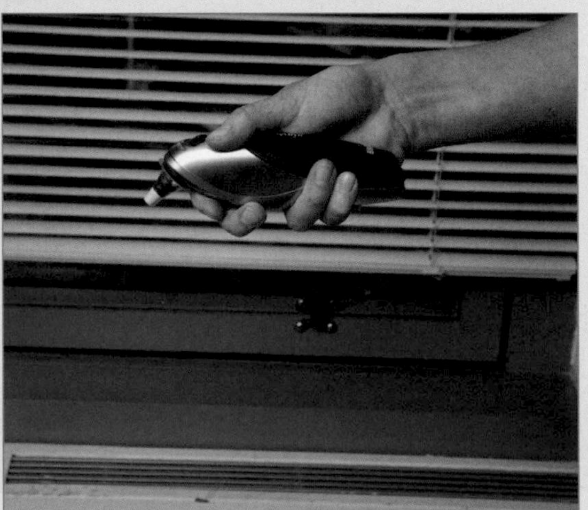

FIGURE 8 Disposing of probe cover.

ACTION

RATIONALE

Measuring Temporal Artery Temperature

22. Brush the patient's hair aside if it is covering the temporal artery area.

Anything covering the area—such as a hat, hair, wigs, or bandages—would insulate the area, resulting in falsely high readings. Measure only the side of the head exposed to the environment.

23. Apply a probe cover.

Using a cover prevents contamination of the thermometer probe.

24. Hold the thermometer like a remote control device, with your thumb on the red "ON" button. Place the probe flush on the center of the forehead, with the body of the instrument sideways (not straight up and down) so that it is not in the patient's face (Figure 9).

Allows for easy use of the device and reading of the display. Holding the instrument straight up and down could be intimidating for the patient, particularly young patients and/or those with alterations in mental status.

25. Depress the "ON" button. Keep the button depressed throughout the measurement.

26. Slowly slide the probe straight across the forehead, midline, to the hairline (Figure 10). The thermometer will click; fast clicking indicates a rise to a higher temperature, slow clicking indicates that the instrument is still scanning, but not finding any higher temperature.

Midline on the forehead, the temporal artery is less than 2 mm below the skin; whereas at the side of the face, the temporal artery is much deeper. Measuring there would result in falsely low readings.

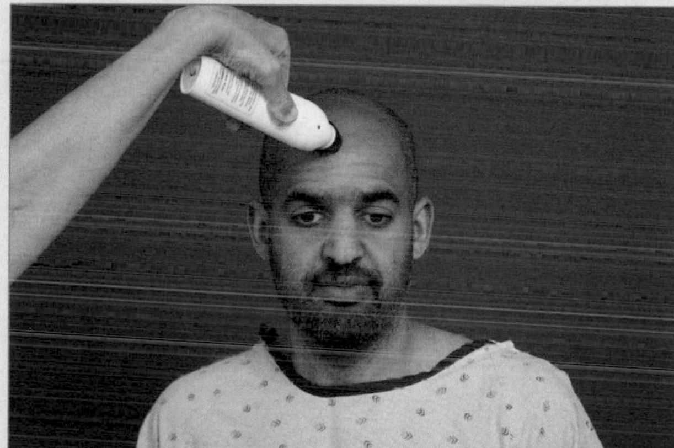

FIGURE 9 Placing the thermometer probe on the center of the forehead.

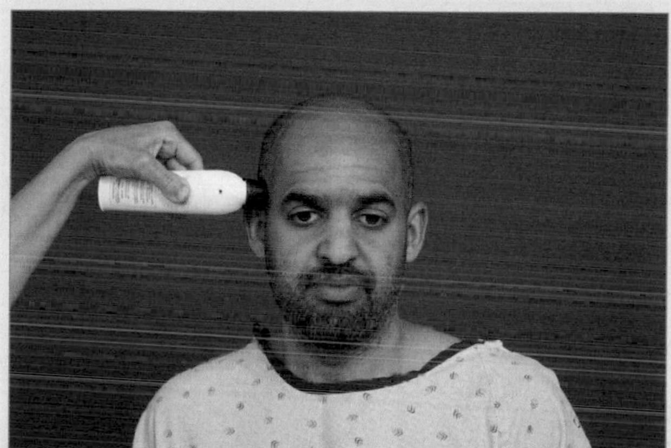

FIGURE 10 Sliding the probe across the forehead to the hairline.

27. Brush hair aside if it is covering the ear, exposing the area of the neck under the ear lobe. Lift the probe from the forehead and touch on the neck just behind the ear lobe, in the depression just below the mastoid (Figure 11).

Sweat causes evaporative cooling of the skin on the forehead, possibly leading to a falsely low reading. During diaphoresis, the area on the head behind the ear lobe exhibits high blood flow necessary for the arterial measurement; it is a double check for the thermometer (Exergen, 2007).

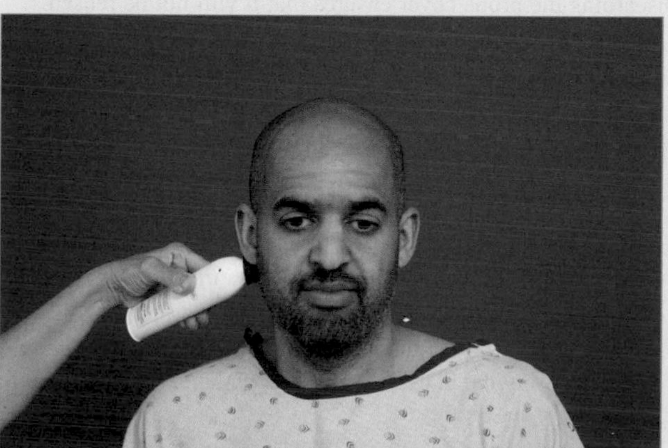

FIGURE 11 Touching the probe behind the ear.

(continued)

SKILL 2-1 ASSESSING BODY TEMPERATURE continued

ACTION	RATIONALE
28. Release the button and read the thermometer measurement.	
29. Hold the thermometer over a waste receptacle. Gently push the probe cover with your thumb against the proximal edge to dispose of the probe cover.	Discarding the probe cover ensures that it will not be reused accidentally on another patient.
30. The instrument will automatically turn off in 30 seconds, or press and release the power button.	Turns thermometer off.

Measuring Axillary Temperature

ACTION	RATIONALE
31. Move the patient's clothing to expose only the axilla (Figure 12).	The axilla must be exposed for placement of the thermometer. Exposing only the axilla keeps the patient warm and maintains his or her dignity.
32. Remove the probe from the recording unit of the electronic thermometer. Place a disposable probe cover on by sliding it on and snapping it securely.	Using a cover prevents contamination of the thermometer probe.
33. **Place the end of the probe in the center of the axilla (Figure 13). Have the patient bring the arm down and close to the body.**	The deepest area of the axilla provides the most accurate measurement; surrounding the bulb with skin surface provides a more reliable measurement.

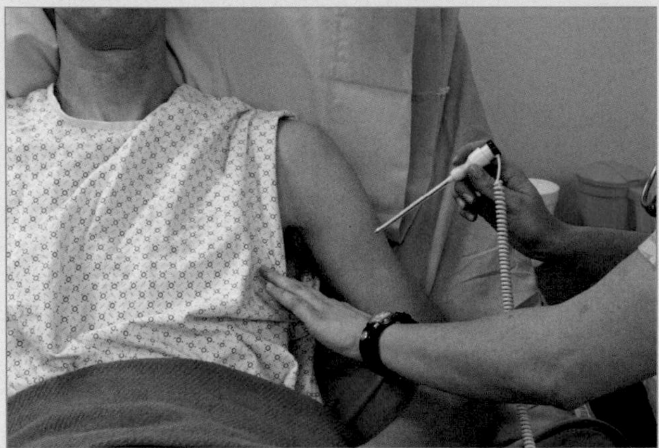

FIGURE 12 Exposing axilla to assess temperature.

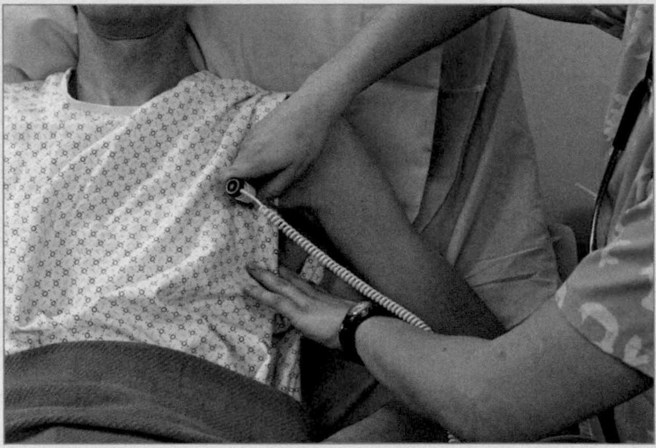

FIGURE 13 Placing thermometer in center of axilla.

ACTION	RATIONALE
34. Hold the probe in place until you hear a beep, and then carefully remove the probe. Note the temperature reading.	Axillary thermometers must be held in place to obtain an accurate temperature.
35. Cover the patient and help him or her to a position of comfort.	Ensures patient comfort.
36. Dispose of the probe cover by holding the probe over an appropriate waste receptacle and pushing the release button.	Discarding the probe cover ensures that it will not be reused accidentally on another patient.
37. Place the bed in the lowest position and elevate rails, as needed. Leave the patient clean and comfortable.	Low bed position and elevated side rails provide for patient safety.
38. Return the electronic thermometer to the charging unit.	Thermometer needs to be recharged for future use.

Measuring Rectal Temperature

ACTION	RATIONALE
39. Adjust the bed to a comfortable working height, usually elbow height of the care giver (VISN 8 Patient Safety Center, 2009). Put on nonsterile gloves.	Having the bed at the proper height prevents back and muscle strain. Gloves prevent contact with contaminants and body fluids.
40. Assist the patient to a side-lying position. Pull back the covers sufficiently to expose only the buttocks.	The side-lying position allows the nurse to visualize the buttocks. Exposing only the buttocks keeps the patient warm and maintains his or her dignity.

ACTION	RATIONALE
41. Remove the rectal probe from within the recording unit of the electronic thermometer. Cover the probe with a disposable probe cover and slide it until it snaps in place (Figure 14).	Using a cover prevents contamination of the thermometer.
42. **Lubricate about 1 inch of the probe with a water-soluble lubricant (Figure 15).**	Lubrication reduces friction and facilitates insertion, minimizing the risk of irritation or injury to the rectal mucous membranes.

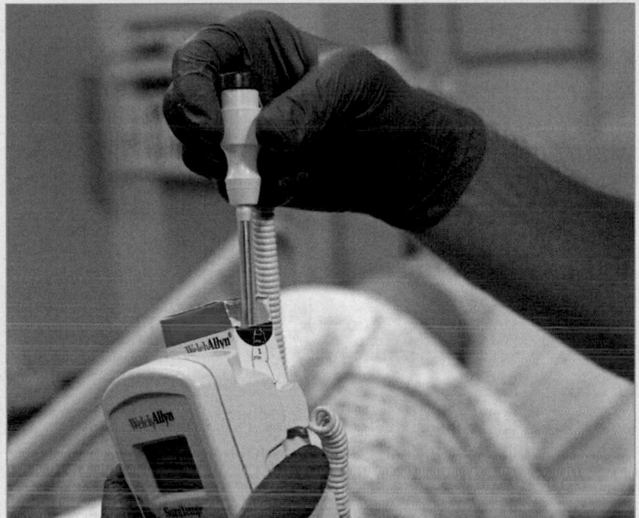

FIGURE 14 Removing appropriate probe and attaching disposable probe cover.

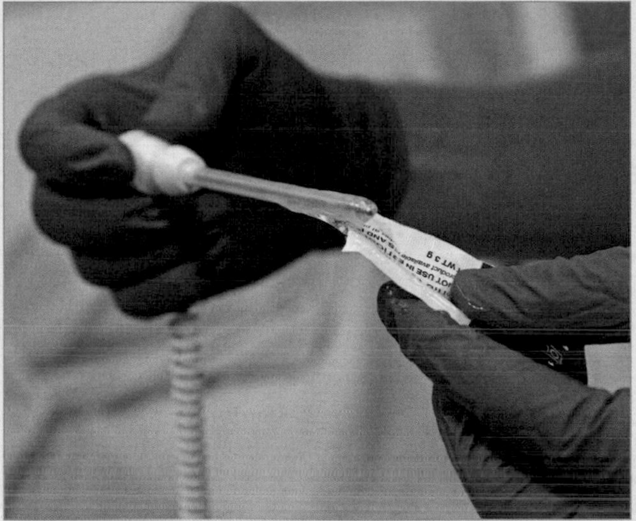

FIGURE 15 Lubricating thermometer tip.

ACTION	RATIONALE
43. Reassure the patient. Separate the buttocks until the anal sphincter is clearly visible.	If not placed directly into the anal opening, the thermometer probe may injure adjacent tissue or cause discomfort.
44. **Insert the thermometer probe into the anus about 1.5 inches in an adult or no more than 1 inch in a child (Figure 16).**	Depth of insertion must be adjusted based on the patient's age. Rectal temperatures are not normally taken in an infant, but may be indicated. Refer to the Special Considerations section at the end of the skill.

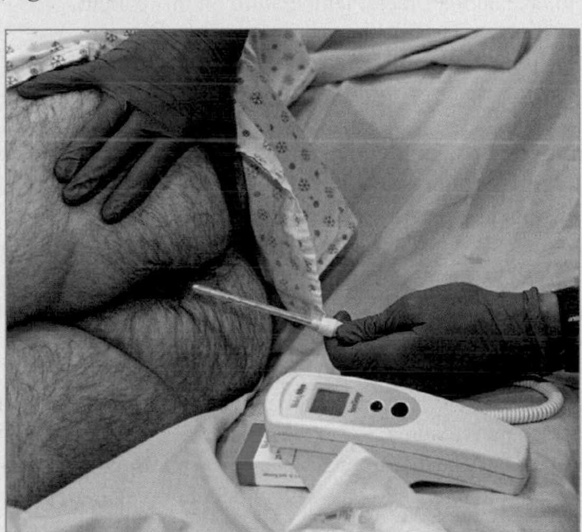

FIGURE 16 Inserting thermometer into the anus.

ACTION	RATIONALE
45. Hold the probe in place until you hear a beep, then carefully remove the probe. Note the temperature reading on the display.	If left unsupported, movement of the probe in the rectum could cause injury and/or discomfort. The signal indicates that the measurement is completed. The electronic thermometer provides a digital display of the measured temperature.

(continued)

SKILL 2-1 ASSESSING BODY TEMPERATURE continued

ACTION	RATIONALE
46. Dispose of the probe cover by holding the probe over an appropriate waste receptacle and pressing the release button.	Proper probe cover disposal reduces risk of microorganism transmission.
47. Using toilet tissue, wipe the anus of any feces or excess lubricant. Dispose of the toilet tissue. Remove gloves and discard them.	Wiping promotes cleanliness. Disposing of the toilet tissue avoids transmission of microorganisms.
48. Cover the patient and help him or her to a position of comfort.	Ensures patient comfort.
49. Place the bed in the lowest position; elevate rails as needed.	These actions provide for the patient's safety.
50. Return the thermometer to the charging unit.	The thermometer needs to be recharged for future use.

EVALUATION

The expected outcomes are met when the patient's temperature is assessed accurately without injury and the patient experiences minimal discomfort.

DOCUMENTATION

Guidelines

Record temperature on paper, flow sheet, or computerized record. Report abnormal findings to the appropriate person. Identify the site of assessment if other than oral.

Sample Documentation

Lippincott DocuCare Practice documenting body temperature and other vital signs in *Lippincott DocuCare.*

10/20/15 Tympanic temperature assessed. Temperature 102.5°F. Patient states she has "a pounding" headache; denies chills, malaise. Physician notified. Received order to give 650 mg PO acetaminophen now. Incentive spirometer × 10 q 2 hours.

—*M. Evans, RN*

UNEXPECTED SITUATIONS AND ASSOCIATED INTERVENTIONS

- *Temperature reading is higher or lower than expected based on your assessment:* Reassess temperature with a different thermometer. The thermometer may not be calibrated correctly. If using a tympanic thermometer, you will get lower readings if the probe is not inserted far enough into the ear.
- *During rectal temperature assessment, the patient reports feeling light-headed or passes out:* Remove the thermometer immediately. Quickly assess the patient's blood pressure and heart rate. Notify the physician. Do not attempt to take another rectal temperature on this patient.

SPECIAL CONSIDERATIONS

General Considerations

- Nonmercury glass thermometers used for oral readings commonly have long, thin bulbs. Those for rectal readings have a blunt bulb to prevent injury. See the accompanying Skill Variation for information on assessing temperature with a nonmercury glass thermometer.
- If the patient smoked, chewed gum, or consumed hot or cold food or fluids recently, wait 30 minutes before taking an oral temperature to allow the oral tissues to return to baseline temperature.
- Nasal oxygen is not thought to affect oral temperature readings. Do not assess oral temperatures in patients receiving oxygen by mask. Removal of the mask for the time period required for assessment could result in a serious drop in the patient's blood oxygen level.
- When using a tympanic thermometer, make sure to insert the probe into the ear canal sufficiently tightly to seal the opening to ensure an accurate reading.
- A dirty probe lens and cone on the temporal artery thermometer can cause a falsely low reading. If the lens is not shiny in appearance, clean the lens and cone with an alcohol preparation or swab moistened in alcohol.
- If the patient's axilla has been washed recently, wait 15 to 30 minutes before taking an axillary temperature to allow the skin to return to baseline temperature.
- Axillary temperatures are generally about one degree less than oral temperatures; rectal temperatures are generally about one degree higher.

Infant and Child Considerations

- Pull the pinna back and down when measuring tympanic temperature on a child younger than 3 years of age. For children older than 3 years of age, there is no need to manipulate the pinna (Kyle & Carman, 2013).
- Small children have a limited attention span and difficulty keeping their lips closed sufficiently long to obtain an accurate oral temperature reading. Based on an assessment of the child's ability to cooperate, it may be more appropriate to use the temporal or tympanic site.
- Chemical dot thermometers (liquid crystal skin contact thermometers) are sometimes used as alternatives in pediatric settings. These single-use, disposable, flexible thermometers have specific chemical mixtures in circles on the thermometer that change color to measure temperature increments of two tenths of a degree. Place the thermometer in the mouth with the dot side (sensor) down, into the posterior sublingual pocket. Keep this type of thermometer in the mouth for 1 minute, in the axilla 3 minutes, and in the rectum 3 minutes. Read the color change 10 to 15 seconds after removing the thermometer. Read away from any heat source. Wearable, continuous-use chemical dot thermometers are available. These are placed under the axilla and must remain in place at least 2 to 3 minutes before taking the first reading; continuously thereafter. Replace thermometer and assess the underlying skin every 48 hours (Higgins, 2008; Perry et al., 2010).
- The Society of Pediatric Nurses (SPN) recognizes that temporal artery thermometry is accurate for infants less than 90 days old without fever, as well as for all patients more than 90 days of age with or without fever, ill or well. The SPN recommends that the temporal artery method should not be used in infants 90 days or younger who are ill, have a fever, or have an ill diagnosis (Asher & Northington, 2008, p. 235). The rectal method should be used for these infants unless contraindicated by diagnosis, in which case the axillary method should be used. In addition, in children 6 months of age or older, the tympanic or oral methods may be used with correct positioning of the ear (tympanic) and if the patient can cooperate (oral) (Asher & Northington, 2008).

Home Care Considerations

- Teach patients who use electronic or digital thermometers to clean the probe after use to prevent transmission of microorganisms among family members. Clean according to manufacturer's directions.
- Teach patients using nonmercury glass thermometers to clean the thermometer after use in lukewarm soapy water and rinse in cool water. Store it in an appropriate place to prevent breakage and injury from the glass.
- Pacifier thermometers, which use the supralingual area, are available to screen for fever. These thermometers give an approximation to rectal temperature measurement in the home setting (Braun, 2006). Leave this thermometer in place for 3 to 6 minutes, based on the manufacturer's recommendations.

SKILL VARIATION Assessing Temperature with a Nonmercury Glass Thermometer

1. Check the medical order or nursing care plan for frequency of temperature assessment. More frequent temperature measurement may be appropriate based on nursing judgment.
2. Bring necessary equipment to the bedside stand or overbed table.
3. Perform hand hygiene and put on PPE, if indicated.
4. Identify the patient.
5. Close the curtains around the bed and close the door to the room, if possible.
6. If the thermometer is stored in a chemical solution, wipe the thermometer dry with a soft tissue, using a firm twisting motion. Wipe from the bulb toward the fingers.
7. Grasp the thermometer firmly with the thumb and the forefinger and, using strong wrist movements, shake it until the chemical line reaches at least 96°F.
8. Read the thermometer by holding it horizontally at eye level (Figure A). Rotate it between your fingers until you can see the chemical line. Verify the reading is less than or equal to 96°F.

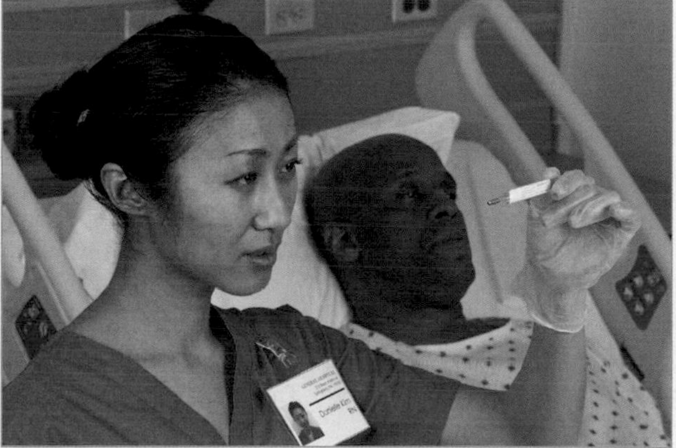

FIGURE A Reading thermometer. *(Photo by B. Proud.)*

(continued)

SKILL 2-1 ASSESSING BODY TEMPERATURE continued

SKILL VARIATION Assessing Temperature with a Nonmercury Glass Thermometer continued

9. Place a disposable cover on the thermometer.
10. **For oral use, place the bulb of the thermometer within the back of the right or left pocket under the patient's tongue and tell the patient to close the lips around the thermometer.**
11. **For rectal use, place the thermometer bulb in the rectum as described when using an electronic thermometer.**
12. **For axillary use, place the thermometer bulb in the center of the axilla. Move the patient's arm against the chest wall (Figure B).**
13. **Leave the thermometer in place for 3 minutes (for oral use); 2 to 3 minutes (for rectal use); and 10 minutes (for axillary use); or according to agency protocol.**
14. Remove the thermometer. Remove the disposable cover and place in a receptacle for contaminated items.
15. Read the thermometer to the nearest tenth of a degree.
16. Wash thermometer in lukewarm, soapy water. Rinse it in cool water. Dry and replace the thermometer in its container.

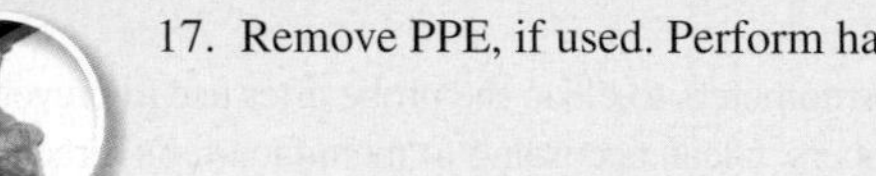

17. Remove PPE, if used. Perform hand hygiene.

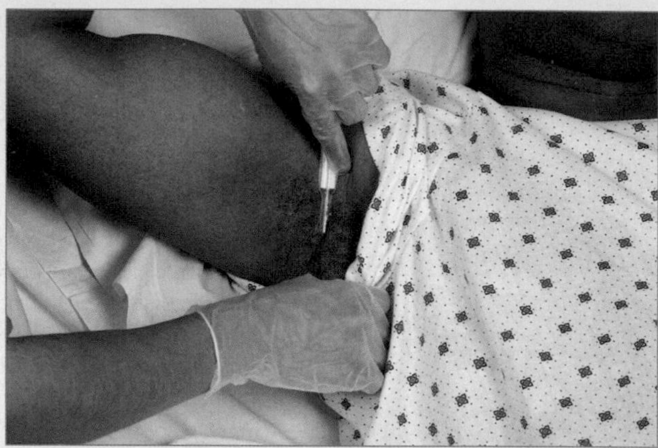

FIGURE B Place thermometer in the center of the axilla. *(Photo by B. Proud.)*

SKILL 2-2 REGULATING TEMPERATURE USING AN OVERHEAD RADIANT WARMER

Neonates, infants who are exposed to stressors or chilling (e.g., from undergoing numerous procedures), and infants who have an underlying condition that interferes with thermoregulation (e.g., prematurity) are highly susceptible to heat loss. Therefore, radiant warmers are used for infants who have trouble maintaining body temperature. In addition, use of a radiant warmer minimizes the oxygen and calories that the infant would expend to maintain body temperature, thereby minimizing the effects of body temperature changes on metabolic activity.

An overhead radiant warmer uses infrared light to warm the infant. The infant's skin is warmed, causing an increase in blood flow, which heats both the underlying blood and tissue surfaces. The warmed blood and tissue transfer this heat to the rest of the body (Dondelinger, 2010). The warmer is adjusted to maintain an anterior abdominal skin temperature of 36.5°C (97.7°F), but at least 36°C (96.8°F), using servo-control (automatic thermostat) (Dondelinger, 2010; Sinclair, 2002).

DELEGATION CONSIDERATIONS

The assessment of body temperature for an infant in a radiant warmer is not delegated to nursing assistive personnel (NAP) or to unlicensed assistive personnel (UAP). Depending on the state's nurse practice act and the organization's policies and procedures, the assessment of body temperature for an infant in a radiant warmer may be delegated to a licensed practical/vocational nurse (LPN/LVN). The decision to delegate must be based on careful analysis of the patient's needs and circumstances, as well as the qualifications of the person to whom the task is being delegated. Refer to the Delegation Guidelines in Appendix A.

EQUIPMENT

- Overhead warmer
- Temperature probe
- Aluminum foil probe cover
- Axillary or rectal thermometer, based on facility policy
- PPE, as indicated

ASSESSMENT

Assess the patient's temperature using the route specified in facility policy, and assess the patient's fluid intake and output.

NURSING DIAGNOSIS

Determine the related factors for the nursing diagnoses based on the patient's current status. Appropriate nursing diagnoses may include:

- Hyperthermia
- Hypothermia
- Risk for Imbalanced Body Temperature
- Ineffective Thermoregulation
- Risk for Deficient Fluid Volume

OUTCOME IDENTIFICATION AND PLANNING

The expected outcomes to achieve when using an overhead warmer are that the infant's temperature is maintained within normal limits without injury.

IMPLEMENTATION

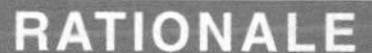

ACTION	RATIONALE
1. Check the medical order or nursing care plan for the use of a radiant warmer.	Provides for patient safety and appropriate care.
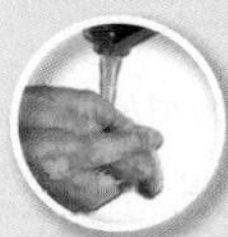 2. Perform hand hygiene and put on PPE, if indicated.	Hand hygiene and PPE prevent the spread of microorganisms. PPE is required based on transmission precautions.
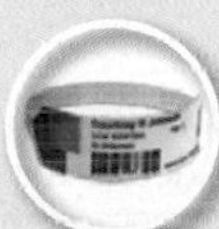 3. Identify the patient.	Identifying the patient ensures the right patient receives the intervention and helps prevent errors.
4. Close curtains around the bed and close the door to the room, if possible. Discuss the procedure with the patient's family.	This ensures the patient's privacy. Explanation reduces the family's apprehension and encourages family cooperation.
5. Plug in the warmer. Turn the warmer to the manual setting. Allow the blankets to warm before placing the infant under the warmer.	By allowing the blankets to warm before placing the infant under the warmer, you are preventing heat loss through conduction. By placing the warmer on the manual setting, you are keeping the warmer at a set temperature no matter how warm the blankets become.
6. Switch the warmer setting to automatic. Set the warmer to the desired abdominal skin temperature, usually 36.5°C (97.7°F).	The automatic setting ensures that the warmer will regulate the amount of radiant heat, depending on the temperature of the infant's skin. The temperature should be adjusted so that the infant does not become too warm or too cold.

(continued)

SKILL 2-2 REGULATING TEMPERATURE USING AN OVERHEAD RADIANT WARMER continued

ACTION	RATIONALE
7. Place the infant under the warmer. Attach the probe to the infant's abdominal skin at mid-epigastrium, halfway between the xiphoid and the umbilicus. Cover with a foil patch (Figure 1).	The foil patch prevents direct warming of the probe, allowing the probe to read only the infant's temperature.
8. When the abdominal skin temperature reaches the desired set point, check the patient's temperature using the route specified in facility policy to be sure it is within the normal range (Figure 2).	By monitoring the infant's temperature, you are watching for signs of hyperthermia or hypothermia.

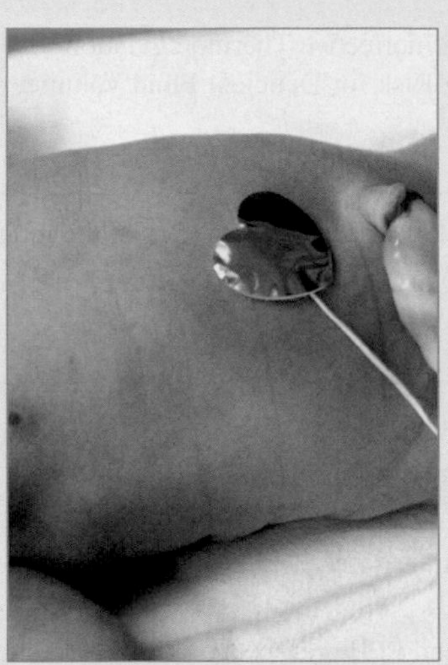

FIGURE 1 Probe in place with foil cover. *(Photo by Joe Mitchell.)*

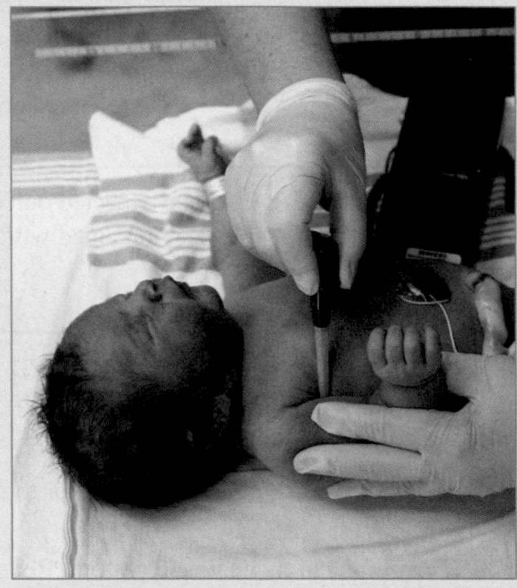

FIGURE 2 Taking infant's axillary temperature. *(Photo by Joe Mitchell.)*

ACTION	RATIONALE
9. Adjust the warmer's set point slightly, as needed, if the patient's temperature is abnormal. Do not change the set point if the temperature is normal.	By monitoring the infant's temperature, you are watching for signs of hyperthermia or hypothermia. This prevents the infant from becoming too warm or too cool.
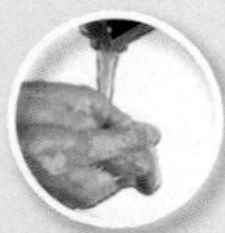 10. Remove additional PPE, if used. Perform hand hygiene.	Removing PPE properly reduces the risk for infection transmission and contamination of other items. Hand hygiene deters the spread of microorganisms.
11. Check frequently to be sure the probe maintains contact with the patient's skin. Continue to monitor temperature measurement and other vital signs.	Poor contact will cause overheating. Entrapment of the probe under the arm or between the infant and mattress will cause under-heating. Monitoring of vital signs assesses patient status.

EVALUATION

The expected outcomes are met when the infant is placed under the radiant warmer, the infant's temperature is well controlled, and the infant experiences no injury.

DOCUMENTATION

Guidelines

Document initial assessment of the infant, including body temperature; the placement of the infant under the radiant warmer; and the settings of the radiant warmer. Document incubator air temperatures, as well as subsequent skin and axillary or rectal temperatures, and other vital sign measurements.

Sample Documentation

10/13/15 1110 Infant placed under radiant warmer. Warmer on automatic setting 36.7°C (98°F), baby's skin temperature 36.8°C (98.2°F), rectal temperature 37°C (98.6°F), warmer air temperature 36.7°C (98°F).

—M. Evans, RN

UNEXPECTED SITUATIONS AND ASSOCIATED INTERVENTIONS

- *The infant becomes* ***febrile*** *under the radiant warmer:* Do not turn the warmer off and leave the infant naked. This could cause cold stress and even death. Leave the warmer on automatic and lower the set temperature. Notify the primary care provider.
- *The warmer's temperature is fluctuating constantly or is inaccurate:* Change the probe cover. If this does not improve the temperature variations, change the probe as well.

SPECIAL CONSIDERATIONS

General Considerations

- Sometimes, plastic surgeons order overhead radiant warmers to be used for patients who have undergone extremity or digit reattachment surgery. In this case, judge the heat by the probe's reading of the skin temperature.

Infant and Child Considerations

- Radiant warmers result in increased insensible water loss. This water loss needs to be taken into account when daily fluid requirements are calculated.

SKILL 2-3 REGULATING TEMPERATURE USING A HYPOTHERMIA BLANKET

A hypothermia blanket, or cooling pad, is a blanket sized aquathermia pad that conducts a cooled solution, usually distilled water, through coils in a plastic blanket or pad (Figure 1). Placing a patient on a hypothermia blanket or pad helps to lower body temperature. The nurse monitors the patient's body temperature and can reset the blanket setting accordingly. The blanket also can be preset to maintain a specific body temperature; the device continually monitors the patient's body temperature using a temperature probe (which is inserted rectally or in the esophagus, or placed on the skin) and adjusts the temperature of the circulating liquid accordingly.

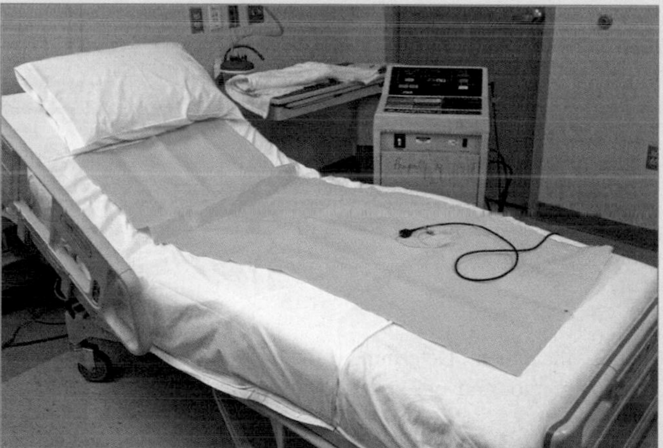

FIGURE 1 Hypothermia blanket.

DELEGATION CONSIDERATIONS

The application of a hypothermia pad is not delegated to nursing assistive personnel (NAP) or to unlicensed assistive personnel (UAP). The measurement of a patient's body temperature while a hypothermia pad is in use may be delegated to nursing assistive personnel (NAP) or unlicensed assistive personnel (UAP). Depending on the state's nurse practice act and the organization's policies and procedures, the application of a hypothermia pad may be delegated to a licensed practical/vocational nurse (LPN/LVN). The decision to delegate must be based on careful analysis of the patient's needs and circumstances, as well as the qualifications of the person to whom the task is being delegated. Refer to the Delegation Guidelines in Appendix A.

(continued)

SKILL 2-3 REGULATING TEMPERATURE USING A HYPOTHERMIA BLANKET continued

EQUIPMENT

- Disposable hypothermia blanket or pad
- Electronic control panel
- Distilled water to fill the device, if necessary
- Thermometer, if needed to monitor the patient's temperature
- Sphygmomanometer
- Stethoscope
- Temperature probe, if needed
- Thin blanket or sheet
- Towels
- Clean gloves
- Additional PPE, as indicated

ASSESSMENT

Assess the patient's condition, including current body temperature, to determine the need for the hypothermia blanket. Consider alternative measures to help lower the patient's body temperature before implementing the blanket. Also verify the medical order for the application of a hypothermia blanket. Assess the patient's vital signs, neurologic status, peripheral circulation, and skin integrity. Assess the equipment to be used, including the condition of cords, plugs, and cooling elements. Look for fluid leaks. Once the equipment is turned on, make sure there is a consistent distribution of cooling.

NURSING DIAGNOSIS

Determine the related factors for the nursing diagnoses based on the patient's current status. Appropriate nursing diagnoses may include:

- Risk for Injury
- Risk for Impaired Skin Integrity
- Hyperthermia
- Hypothermia
- Risk for Imbalanced Body Temperature
- Ineffective Thermoregulation

OUTCOME IDENTIFICATION AND PLANNING

The expected outcome to achieve when using a hypothermia blanket is that the patient maintains the desired body temperature. Other outcomes that may be appropriate include the patient does not experience shivering; the patient's vital signs are within normal limits; and the patient does not experience alterations in skin integrity, neurologic status, peripheral circulation, or fluid and electrolyte status and edema.

IMPLEMENTATION

ACTION	RATIONALE
1. Review the medical order for the application of the hypothermia blanket. Obtain consent for the therapy per facility policy.	Reviewing the order validates the correct patient and correct procedure.
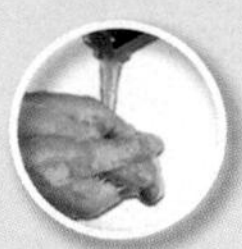 2. Perform hand hygiene and put on PPE, if indicated.	Hand hygiene and PPE prevent the spread of microorganisms. PPE is required based on transmission precautions.
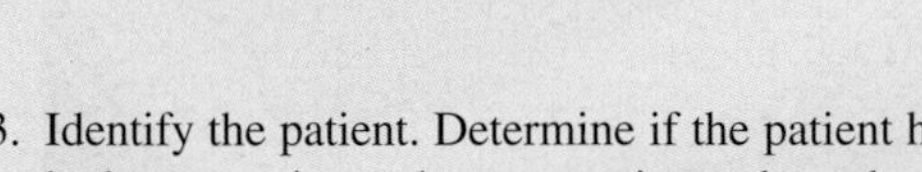 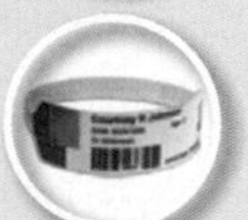 3. Identify the patient. Determine if the patient has had any previous adverse reaction to hypothermia therapy.	Identifying the patient ensures the right patient receives the intervention and helps prevent errors. Individual differences exist in tolerating specific therapies.
4. Assemble equipment on the overbed table within reach.	Organization facilitates performance of task.
5. Close curtains around the bed and close the door to the room, if possible. Explain what you are going to do and why you are going to do it to the patient.	This ensures the patient's privacy. Explanation relieves anxiety and facilitates cooperation.

ACTION	RATIONALE
6. Check that the water in the electronic unit is at the appropriate level. Fill the unit two thirds full with distilled water, or to the fill mark, if necessary. Check the temperature setting on the unit to ensure it is within the safe range.	Sufficient water in the unit is necessary to ensure proper function of the unit. Tap water leaves mineral deposits in the unit. Checking the temperature setting helps to prevent skin or tissue damage.
7. Assess the patient's vital signs, neurologic status, peripheral circulation, and skin integrity.	Assessment supplies baseline data for comparison during therapy and identifies conditions that may contraindicate the application.
8. Adjust bed to comfortable working height, usually elbow height of the care giver (VISN 8 Patient Safety Center, 2009).	Having the bed at the proper height prevents back and muscle strain.
9. Make sure the patient's gown has cloth ties, not snaps or pins.	Cloth ties minimize the risk of cold injury.
10. Apply lanolin or a mixture of lanolin and cold cream to the patient's skin where it will be in contact with the blanket.	These agents help protect the skin from cold.
11. Turn on the blanket and make sure the cooling light is on. Verify that the temperature limits are set within the desired safety range (Figure 2).	Turning on the blanket prepares it for use. Keeping temperature within the safety range prevents excessive cooling.
12. Cover the hypothermia blanket with a thin sheet or bath blanket.	A sheet or blanket protects the patient's skin from direct contact with the cooling surface, reducing the risk for injury.
13. Position the blanket under the patient so that the top edge of the pad is aligned with the patient's neck (Figure 3).	The blanket's rigid surface may be uncomfortable. The cold may lead to tissue breakdown.

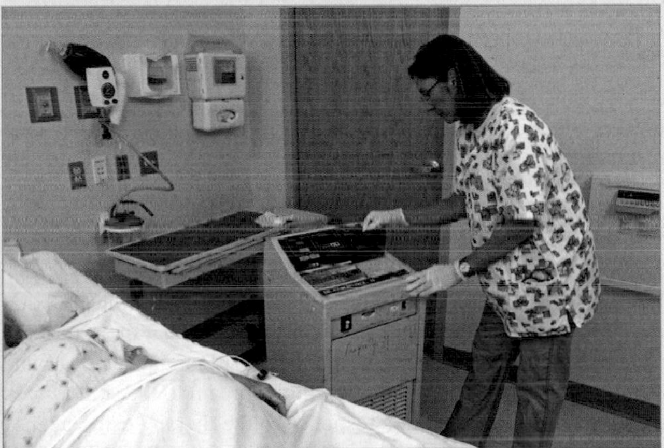

FIGURE 2 Checking the settings on the hypothermia blanket control unit and turning it on.

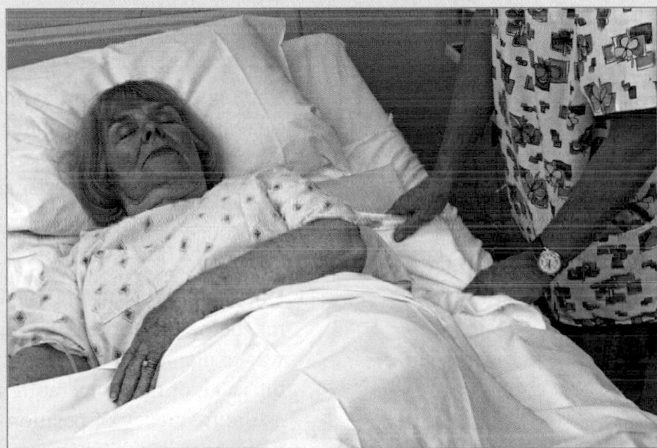

FIGURE 3 Aligning hypothermia blanket on bed.

ACTION	RATIONALE
14. Put on gloves. Lubricate the rectal probe and insert it into the patient's rectum unless contraindicated. Or tuck the skin probe deep into the patient's axilla and tape it in place. For patients who are comatose or anesthetized, use an esophageal probe. Remove gloves. Attach the probe to the control panel for the blanket.	The probe allows continuous monitoring of the patient's core body temperature. Rectal insertion may be contraindicated in patients with a low white blood cell or platelet count.
15. Wrap the patient's hands and feet in gauze if ordered, or if the patient desires. For male patients, elevate the scrotum off the hypothermia blanket with towels.	These actions minimize chilling, promote comfort, and protect sensitive tissues from direct contact with cold.
16. Place the patient in a comfortable position. Lower the bed. Dispose of any other supplies appropriately.	Repositioning promotes patient comfort and safety.
17. Recheck the thermometer and settings on the control panel.	Rechecking verifies that the blanket temperature is maintained at a safe level.

(continued)

SKILL 2-3 REGULATING TEMPERATURE USING A HYPOTHERMIA BLANKET continued

ACTION	RATIONALE
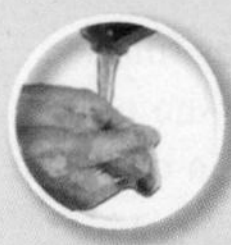 18. Remove any additional PPE, if used. Perform hand hygiene.	Removing PPE properly reduces the risk for infection transmission and contamination of other items. Hand hygiene prevents the spread of microorganisms.
19. **Turn and position the patient regularly (every 30 minutes to 1 hour).** Keep linens free from condensation. Reapply cream, as needed. Observe the patient's skin for change in color, changes in lips and nail beds, edema, pain, and sensory impairment.	Turning and repositioning prevent alterations in skin integrity and provide for assessment of potential skin injuries.
20. **Monitor vital signs and perform a neurologic assessment, per facility policy, usually every 15 minutes, until the body temperature is stable.** In addition, monitor the patient's fluid and electrolyte status.	Continuous monitoring provides evaluation of the patient's response to the therapy and permits early identification and intervention if adverse effects occur.
21. Observe for signs of shivering, including verbalized sensations, facial muscle twitching, hyperventilation, or twitching of extremities.	Shivering increases heat production, and is often controlled with medications.
22. Assess the patient's level of comfort.	Hypothermia therapy can cause discomfort. Prompt assessment and action can prevent injuries.
23. Turn off the blanket according to facility policy, usually when the patient's body temperature reaches 1 degree above the desired temperature. **Continue to monitor the patient's temperature until it stabilizes.**	Body temperature can continue to fall after this therapy.

EVALUATION

The expected outcome is met when the patient maintains the desired body temperature and other vital signs within acceptable parameters. In addition, the patient remains free from shivering; does not experience alterations in skin integrity, neurologic status, peripheral circulation, or fluid and electrolyte status, and edema.

DOCUMENTATION

Guidelines

Document assessments, such as vital signs, neurologic, peripheral circulation, and skin integrity status, before use of hypothermia blanket. Record verification of medical order and that the procedure was explained to the patient. Document the control settings, time of application and removal, and the route of the temperature monitoring. Include the application of lanolin cream to the skin as well as the frequency of position changes. Document the patient's response to the therapy using agency flow sheet, especially noting a decrease in temperature and discomfort assessment. Record the possible use of medication to reduce shivering or other discomforts. Include any pertinent patient and family teaching.

Sample Documentation

11/10/15 1800 Patient's temperature 106°F (41°C), pulse 122, respirations 24, BP 118/72. Dr. Fenter notified. Order received for application of hypothermia blanket. Procedure explained to patient. Lanolin applied to skin, bath sheet applied between blanket and patient, axillary probe applied, hypothermia blanket setting 99°F (37.2°C) per order. Vital signs, neurologic, neurovascular, and skin assessment every 30 minutes; see flow sheets. Patient without evidence of shivering.

—J. Lee, RN

11/10/15 1930 Patient reports chills and shivering. Temperature 100°F (37.8°C), pulse 104, respirations 20, BP 114/68. Dr. Fenter notified. Hypothermia blanket discontinued per order.

—J. Lee, RN

UNEXPECTED SITUATIONS AND ASSOCIATED INTERVENTIONS

- *The patient states he is cold and has chills. You observe shivering of his extremities:* Obtain vital signs. Assess for other symptoms. Increase the blanket temperature to a more comfortable range. If shivering persists or is excessive, discontinue the therapy. Notify the primary care provider of the findings and document the event in the patient's record.
- *When performing a skin assessment during therapy, you note increased pallor on pressure points and sluggish capillary refill. The patient reports alterations in sensation on these points:* Discontinue therapy, obtain vital signs, assess for other symptoms, notify the primary care provider, and document the event in the patient's record.

SPECIAL CONSIDERATIONS

General Considerations

- The patient may experience a secondary defense reaction, vasodilation, that causes body temperature to rebound, defeating the purpose of the therapy.

Older Adult Considerations

- Older adults are more at risk for skin and tissue damage because of their thin skin, loss of cold sensation, decreased subcutaneous tissue, and changes in the body's ability to regulate temperature. Check these patients more frequently during therapy.

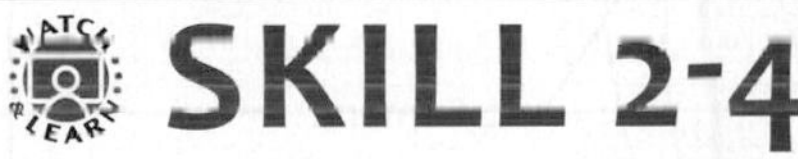

SKILL 2-4 ASSESSING A PERIPHERAL PULSE BY PALPATION

The pulse is a throbbing sensation that can be palpated over a peripheral artery, such as the radial artery or the carotid artery. Peripheral pulses result from a wave of blood being pumped into the arterial circulation by the contraction of the left ventricle. Each time the left ventricle contracts to eject blood into an already full aorta, the arterial walls in the cardiovascular system expand to compensate for the increase in pressure of the blood. Characteristics of the pulse, including rate, quality or amplitude, and rhythm, provide information about the effectiveness of the heart as a pump and the adequacy of peripheral blood flow.

Pulse rates are measured in beats per minute. The normal pulse rate for adolescents and adults ranges from 60 to 100 beats per minute. Pulse quality (amplitude) describes the quality of the pulse in terms of its fullness—strong or weak. It is assessed by the feel of the blood flow through the vessel. Pulse rhythm is the pattern of the pulsations and the pauses between them. Pulse rhythm is normally regular; the pulsations and the pauses between occur at regular intervals. An irregular pulse rhythm occurs when the pulsations and pauses between beats occur at unequal intervals.

Assess the pulse by palpating peripheral arteries, by auscultating the apical pulse with a stethoscope, or by using a portable Doppler ultrasound (see the accompanying Skill Variation). To assess the pulse accurately, you need to know which site to choose and what method is most appropriate for the patient.

The most commonly used sites to palpate peripheral pulses and a scale used to describe pulse amplitude are illustrated in Box 2-1. Place your fingers over the artery so that the ends of your fingers are flat against the patient's skin when palpating peripheral pulses. Do not press with the tip of the fingers only (refer to Figure 1, Step 8).

(*continued*)

SKILL 2-4 ASSESSING A PERIPHERAL PULSE BY PALPATION continued

Box 2-1 PULSE SITES AND PULSE AMPLITUDE

Pulse Sites

Arteries commonly used for assessing the pulse include the temporal, carotid, brachial, radial, femoral, popliteal, posterior tibial, and dorsalis pedis.

Pulse Amplitude

- 0: Absent, unable to palpate
- +1: Diminished, weaker than expected
- +2: Brisk, expected (normal)
- +3: Bounding

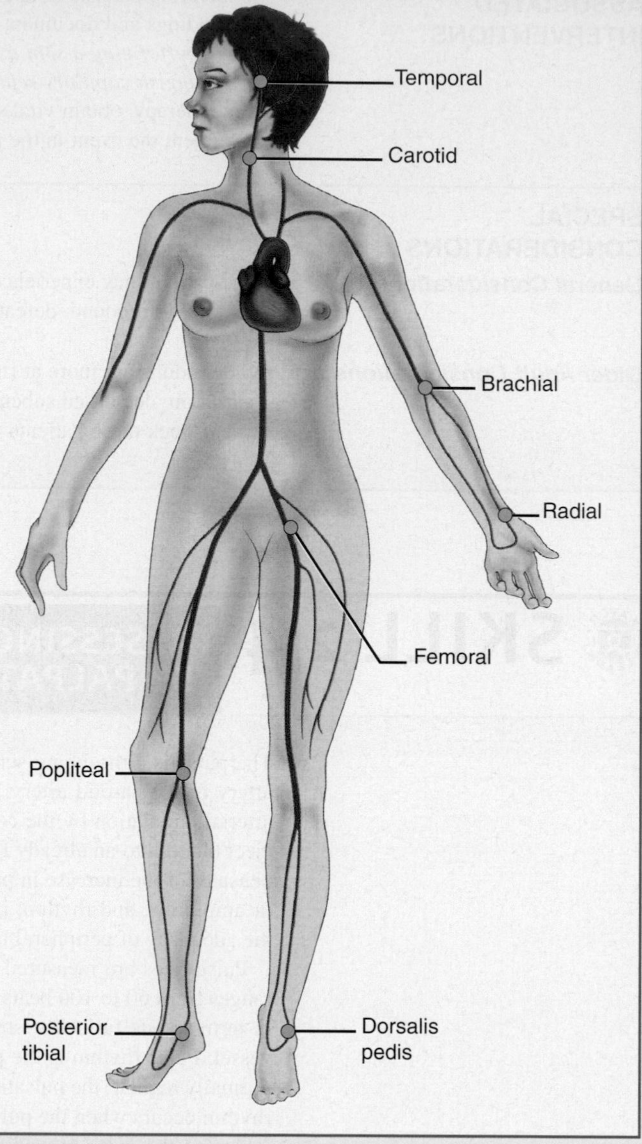

(Adapted from Hirsch, A.T., et al. (2006). ACC/AHA 2005 guidelines for the management of patients with peripheral arterial disease (lower extremity, renal, mesenteric, and abdominal aortic): Executive summary, a collaborative report from the American Association for Vascular Surgery/Society for Vascular Surgery, Society for Cardiovascular Angiography and Interventions, Society for Vascular Medicine and Biology, Society of Interventional Radiology, and the ACC/AHA Task Force on Practice Guidelines (Writing Committee to Develop Guidelines for the Management of Patients with Peripheral Arterial Disease). *Circulation, 113*(11), e463–e654.)

DELEGATION CONSIDERATIONS

The assessment of the radial and brachial peripheral pulses may be delegated to nursing assistive personnel (NAP) or to unlicensed assistive personnel (UAP). The assessment of peripheral pulses may be delegated to licensed practical/vocational nurses (LPN/LVN). The decision to delegate must be based on careful analysis of the patient's needs and circumstances, as well as the qualifications of the person to whom the task is being delegated. Refer to the Delegation Guidelines in Appendix A.

EQUIPMENT

- Watch with second hand or digital readout
- Pencil or pen, paper or flow sheet, computerized record
- Nonsterile gloves, if appropriate; additional PPE, as indicated

ASSESSMENT

Choose a site to assess the pulse. For an adult patient, adolescent, and older child, the most common site for obtaining a peripheral pulse is the radial pulse. Apical pulse measurement is the preferred method of pulse assessment for infants and children less than 2 years of age (Jarvis, 2012). (Refer to Skill 2-5.) Assess for factors that could affect pulse characteristics, such as the patient's age, amount of exercise, fluid balance, and medications. Note baseline or previous pulse measurements.

NURSING DIAGNOSIS

Determine the related factors for the nursing diagnoses based on the patient's current status. Appropriate nursing diagnoses may include:

- Decreased Cardiac Output
- Ineffective Peripheral Tissue Perfusion
- Acute Pain

OUTCOME IDENTIFICATION AND PLANNING

The expected outcomes to achieve when measuring a pulse rate are that the patient's pulse is assessed accurately without injury and that the patient experiences minimal discomfort. Other outcomes may be appropriate, depending on the patient's nursing diagnosis.

IMPLEMENTATION

ACTION	RATIONALE
1. Check medical order or nursing care plan for frequency of pulse assessment. More frequent pulse measurement may be appropriate based on nursing judgment.	Assessment and measurement of vital signs at appropriate intervals provide important data about the patient's health status.
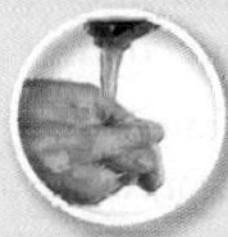 2. Perform hand hygiene and put on PPE, if indicated.	Hand hygiene and PPE prevent the spread of microorganisms. PPE is required based on transmission precautions.
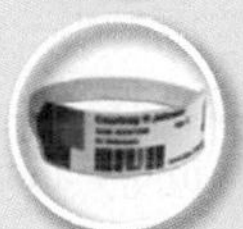 3. Identify the patient.	Identifying the patient ensures the right patient receives the intervention and helps prevent errors.
4. Close the curtains around the bed and close the door to the room, if possible. Discuss the procedure with the patient and assess the patient's ability to assist with the procedure.	This ensures the patient's privacy. Explanation relieves anxiety and facilitates cooperation.
5. Put on gloves, if indicated.	Gloves are not usually worn to obtain a pulse measurement unless contact with blood or body fluids is anticipated. Gloves prevent contact with blood and body fluids.
6. Select the appropriate peripheral site based on assessment data.	Ensures safety and accuracy of measurement.
7. Move the patient's clothing to expose only the site chosen.	The site must be exposed for pulse assessment. Exposing only the site keeps the patient warm and maintains his or her dignity.

(continued)

SKILL 2-4 ASSESSING A PERIPHERAL PULSE BY PALPATION continued

ACTION	RATIONALE
8. Place your first, second, and third fingers over the artery (Figure 1). **Lightly compress the artery so pulsations can be felt and counted.**	The sensitive fingertips can feel the pulsation of the artery.
9. Using a watch with a second hand, count the number of pulsations felt for 30 seconds (Figure 2). Multiply this number by 2 to calculate the rate for 1 minute. **If the rate, rhythm, or amplitude of the pulse is abnormal in any way, palpate and count the pulse for 1 minute.**	Ensures accuracy of measurement and assessment.

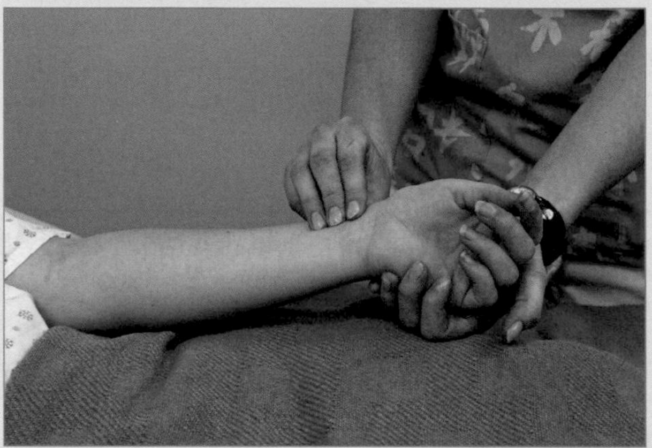

FIGURE 1 Palpating the radial pulse.

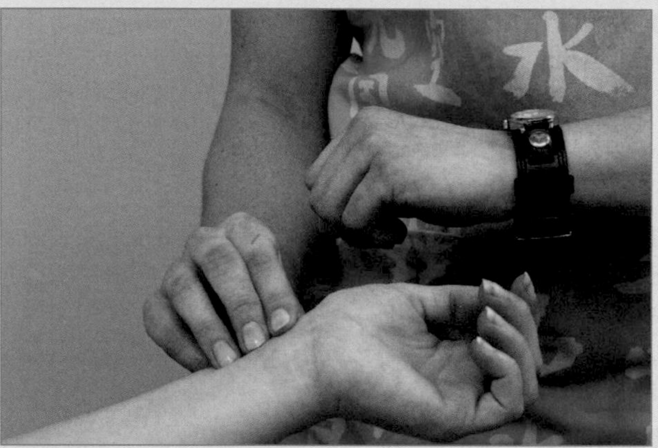

FIGURE 2 Counting the pulse.

ACTION	RATIONALE
10. Note the rhythm and amplitude of the pulse.	Provides additional assessment data regarding the patient's cardiovascular status.
11. When measurement is completed, remove gloves, if worn. Cover the patient and help him or her to a position of comfort.	Removing PPE properly reduces the risk for infection transmission and contamination of other items. Ensures patient comfort.
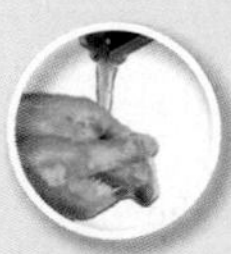 12. Remove additional PPE, if used. Perform hand hygiene.	Removing PPE properly reduces the risk for infection transmission and contamination of other items. Hand hygiene prevents the spread of microorganisms.

EVALUATION

The expected outcomes are met when the patient's pulse is assessed accurately without injury and the patient experiences minimal discomfort.

DOCUMENTATION

Guidelines

Record pulse rate, amplitude, and rhythm on paper, flow sheet, or computerized record. Identify site of assessment. Report abnormal findings to the primary care provider.

Sample Documentation

Lippincott DocuCare **Practice documenting pulse and other vital signs in *Lippincott DocuCare*.**

2/6/15 1000 Pulses 84, regular, 2+ and equal in radial, popliteal, and dorsalis pedis sites.
—*M. Evans, RN*

UNEXPECTED SITUATIONS AND ASSOCIATED INTERVENTIONS

- *The pulse is irregular:* Monitor the pulse for a full minute. If the pulse is difficult to assess, validate pulse measurement by taking the apical pulse for 1 minute. If this is a change for the patient, notify the primary care provider.
- *The pulse is palpated easily, but then disappears:* Apply only moderate pressure to the pulse. Applying too much pressure may obliterate the pulse.
- *You cannot palpate a pulse:* Use a portable Doppler ultrasound to assess the pulse. If this is a change in assessment or if you cannot find the pulse using a Doppler ultrasound, notify the primary care provider. If you can find the pulse using a Doppler ultrasound, place a small X over the spot where the pulse is located. This can make palpating the pulse easier because the exact location of the pulse is known.

SPECIAL CONSIDERATIONS

General Considerations

- The normal heart rate varies by age. Refer to Fundamentals Review 2-1.
- When palpating a carotid pulse, lightly press only one side of the neck at a time. Never attempt to palpate both carotid arteries at the same time. Bilateral palpation could result in reduced cerebral blood flow (Hogan-Quigley, et al., 2012).
- If a peripheral pulse is difficult to assess accurately because it is irregular, feeble, or extremely rapid, assess the apical rate.

Infant and Child Considerations

- For children younger than 10 years of age, the apical pulse measurement is the preferred method of pulse assessment (Jarvis, 2012) (see Skill 2-5). Do not measure the radial pulse in children younger than 2 years of age, because it is difficult to palpate accurately in this age group (Kyle & Carman, 2013). In older children, measure the radial pulse for a full minute.
- Measure the apical rate if the child has a cardiac problem or congenital heart defect (see Skill 2-5).

Home Care Considerations

- Teach the patient and family members how to take the patient's pulse, if appropriate.
- Inform the patient and family about digital pulse monitoring devices.
- Teach family members how to locate and monitor peripheral pulse sites, if appropriate.

SKILL VARIATION Assessing Peripheral Pulse Using a Portable Doppler Ultrasound

1. Check medical order or nursing care plan for frequency of pulse assessment. More frequent pulse measurement may be appropriate based on nursing judgment. Determine the need to use a Doppler ultrasound device for pulse assessment.
2. Bring necessary equipment to the bedside stand or overbed table.

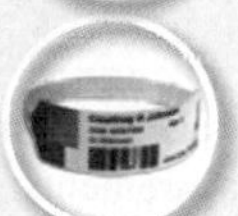

3. Perform hand hygiene and put on PPE, if indicated.
4. Identify the patient.
5. Close curtains around the bed and close the door to the room, if possible.
6. Explain the procedure to the patient.
7. Put on gloves, if indicated. Gloves are not usually worn to obtain a pulse measurement unless contact with blood or body fluids is anticipated.
8. Select the appropriate peripheral site based on assessment data.
9. Move the patient's clothing to expose only the site chosen.
10. Remove Doppler from charger and turn it on. Make sure that volume is set at low.
11. Apply conducting gel to the site where you are auscultating the pulse.
12. Hold the Doppler base in your nondominant hand. With your dominant hand, place the Doppler probe tip in the gel. Adjust the volume, as needed. Move the Doppler tip around until the pulse is heard (Figure A).
13. **Using a watch with a second hand, count the heartbeat for 1 minute.** Note the rhythm of the pulse.
14. Remove the Doppler tip and turn the Doppler off. Wipe excess gel off of the patient's skin with a tissue.

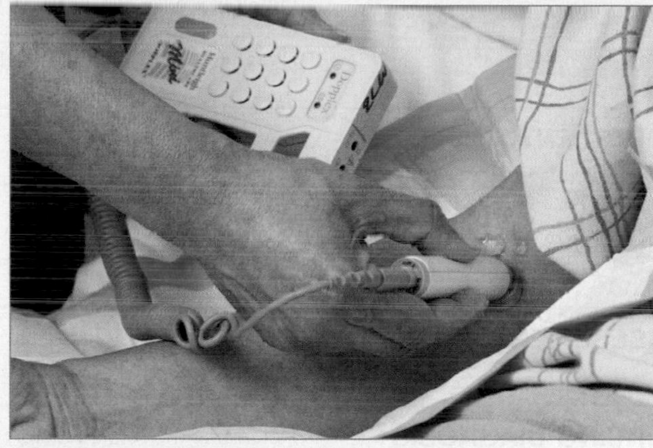

FIGURE A Moving the Doppler tip until pulse is heard.

15. Place a small X over the spot where the pulse is located with an indelible pen, depending on facility policy. Marking the site allows for easier future assessment. It can also make palpating the pulse easier because the exact location of the pulse is known.
16. Cover the patient and help him or her to a position of comfort.
17. Wipe any gel remaining on the Doppler probe off with a tissue. Clean the Doppler probe per facility policy or manufacturer's recommendations.

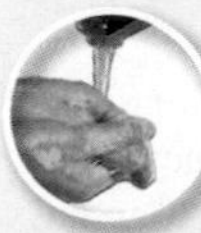

18. Remove PPE, if used. Perform hand hygiene.
19. Return the Doppler ultrasound device to the charge base.
20. Record pulse rate, rhythm, and site, and that it was obtained with a Doppler ultrasound device.

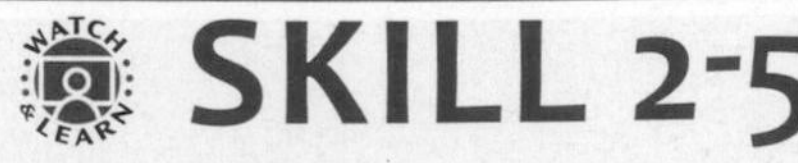

SKILL 2-5 ASSESSING THE APICAL PULSE BY AUSCULTATION

An apical pulse is auscultated (listened to) over the apex of the heart, as the heart beats. The heart is a cone-shaped, muscular pump, divided into four hollow chambers. The upper chambers, the atria (singular, atrium), receive blood from the veins (the superior and inferior vena cava and the left and right pulmonary veins). The lower chambers, the ventricles, force blood out of the heart through the arteries (the left and right pulmonary arteries and the aorta). One-way valves that direct blood flow through the heart are located at the entrance (tricuspid and mitral valves) and exit (pulmonic and aortic valves) of each ventricle. Heart sounds, which are produced by closure of the valves of the heart, are characterized as "lub-dub." The apical pulse is the result of closure of the mitral and tricuspid valves ("lub") and the aortic and pulmonic valves ("dub"). The combination of the two sounds is counted as one beat. Pulse rates are measured in beats per minute. The normal pulse rate for adolescents and adults ranges from 60 to 100 beats per minute. Pulse rhythm is also assessed. Pulse rhythm is the pattern of the beats and the pauses between them. Pulse rhythm is normally regular; the beats and the pauses between occur at regular intervals. An irregular pulse rhythm occurs when the beats and pauses between beats occur at unequal intervals.

An apical pulse is assessed when giving medications that alter heart rate and rhythm. In addition, if a peripheral pulse is difficult to assess accurately because it is irregular, feeble, or extremely rapid, assess the apical rate. In adults, the apical rate is counted for 1 full minute by listening with a stethoscope over the apex of the heart. Apical pulse measurement is also the preferred method of pulse assessment in children less than 10 years of age (Jarvis, 2012).

DELEGATION CONSIDERATIONS

The assessment of an apical pulse is not delegated to nursing assistive personnel (NAP) or to unlicensed assistive personnel (UAP). The assessment of an apical pulse may be delegated to a licensed practical/vocational nurse (LPN/LVN). The decision to delegate must be based on careful analysis of the patient's needs and circumstances, as well as the qualifications of the person to whom the task is being delegated. Refer to the Delegation Guidelines in Appendix A.

EQUIPMENT

- Watch with second hand or digital readout
- Stethoscope
- Alcohol swab
- Pencil or pen, paper or flow sheet, computerized record
- Nonsterile gloves, if appropriate; additional PPE, as indicated

ASSESSMENT

Assess for factors that could affect apical pulse rate and rhythm, such as the patient's age, amount of exercise, fluid balance, and medications. Note baseline or previous apical pulse measurements.

NURSING DIAGNOSIS

Determine the related factors for the nursing diagnoses based on the patient's current status. Appropriate nursing diagnoses may include:

- Decreased Cardiac Output
- Deficient Fluid Volume

OUTCOME IDENTIFICATION AND PLANNING

The expected outcomes to achieve when measuring an apical pulse rate are that the patient's pulse is assessed accurately without injury and the patient experiences minimal discomfort. Other outcomes may be appropriate, depending on the patient's nursing diagnosis.

IMPLEMENTATION

ACTION	RATIONALE
1. Check medical order or nursing care plan for frequency of pulse assessment. More frequent pulse measurement may be appropriate based on nursing judgment. Identify the need to obtain an apical pulse measurement.	Provides for patient safety and appropriate care.

ACTION	RATIONALE
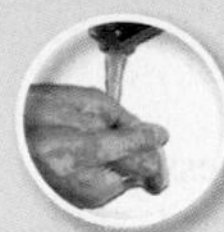 2. Perform hand hygiene and put on PPE, if indicated.	Hand hygiene and PPE prevent the spread of microorganisms. PPE is required based on transmission precautions.
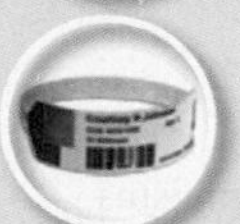 3. Identify the patient.	Identifying the patient ensures the right patient receives the intervention and helps prevent errors.
4. Close curtains around the bed and close the door to the room, if possible. Discuss the procedure with the patient and assess the patient's ability to assist with the procedure.	This ensures the patient's privacy. Explanation relieves anxiety and facilitates cooperation.
5. Put on gloves, if indicated.	Gloves are not usually worn to obtain a pulse measurement unless contact with blood or body fluids is anticipated. Gloves prevent contact with blood and body fluids.
6. Use an alcohol swab to clean the diaphragm of the stethoscope. Use another swab to clean the earpieces, if necessary.	Cleaning with alcohol deters transmission of microorganisms.
7. Assist the patient to a sitting or reclining position and expose the chest area.	This position facilitates identification of the site for stethoscope placement.
8. Move the patient's clothing to expose only the apical site.	The site must be exposed for pulse assessment. Exposing only the apical site keeps the patient warm and maintains his or her dignity.
9. Hold the stethoscope diaphragm against the palm of your hand for a few seconds.	Warming the diaphragm promotes patient comfort.
10. **Palpate the space between the fifth and sixth ribs (fifth intercostal space), and move to the left midclavicular line.** Place the stethoscope diaphragm over the apex of the heart (Figures 1 and 2).	Position the stethoscope over the apex of the heart, where the heartbeat is best heard.

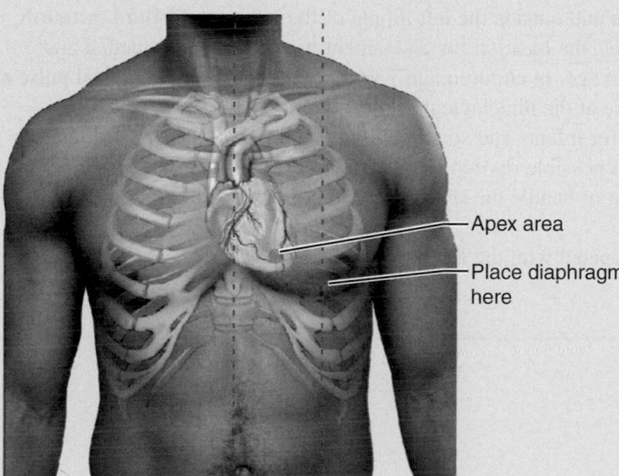

FIGURE 1 Locating the apical pulse: apex area.

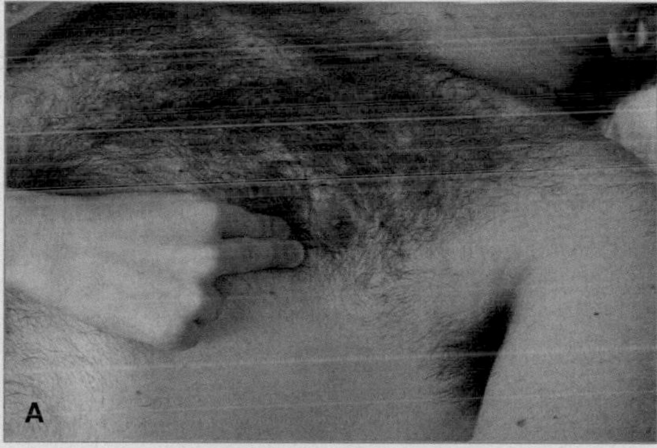

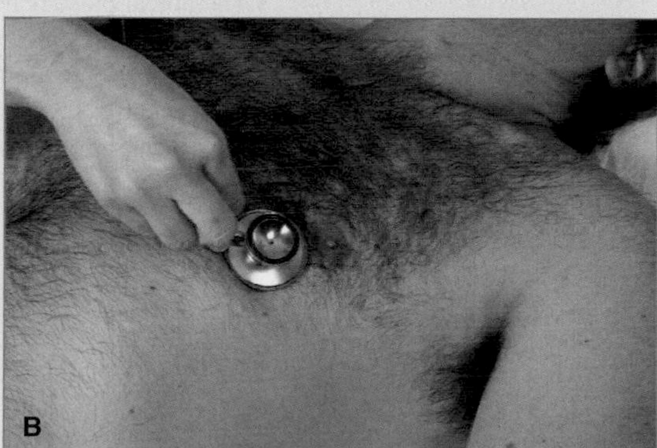

FIGURE 2 The apical pulse is usually found at (**A**) the fifth intercostal space just inside the midclavicular line and can be heard (**B**) over the apex of the heart.

(*continued*)

SKILL 2-5 ASSESSING THE APICAL PULSE BY AUSCULTATION continued

ACTION	RATIONALE
11. Listen for heart sounds ("lub-dub"). Each "lub-dub" counts as one beat.	These sounds occur as the heart valves close.
12. Using a watch with a second hand, count the heartbeat for 1 minute.	Counting for a full minute increases the accuracy of assessment.
13. When measurement is completed, cover the patient and help him or her to a position of comfort.	Ensures patient comfort.
14. Clean the diaphragm of the stethoscope with an alcohol swab.	Cleaning with alcohol deters transmission of microorganisms.
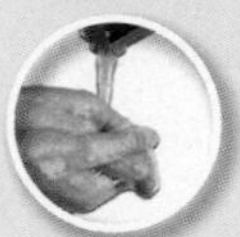 15. Remove gloves and additional PPE, if used. Perform hand hygiene.	Removing PPE properly reduces the risk for infection transmission and contamination of other items. Hand hygiene prevents the spread of microorganisms.

EVALUATION

The expected outcomes are met when the patient's apical pulse is assessed accurately without injury and the patient experiences minimal discomfort.

DOCUMENTATION

Guidelines

Record pulse rate and rhythm on paper, flow sheet, or computerized record. Report abnormal findings to the appropriate person. Identify site of assessment.

Sample Documentation

Lippincott DocuCare Practice documenting pulse and other vital signs in *Lippincott DocuCare*.

2/6/15 1000 Apical pulse 82 and regular. Digoxin 0.125 mg administered orally per order. Patient verbalized understanding of actions and untoward effects of medication.

—B. Clapp, RN

UNEXPECTED SITUATIONS AND ASSOCIATED INTERVENTIONS

- If the apical rate is irregular, assess the patient for other symptoms, such as light-headedness, dizziness, shortness of breath, or palpitations. Notify appropriate health care provider of findings.

SPECIAL CONSIDERATIONS

Infant and Child Considerations

- Assess the apical pulse just above and outside the left nipple of the infant at the third or fourth intercostal space. As the child ages, the location for assessment moves to a more medial and slightly lower area until 7 years of age. In children age 7 years or older, assess the apical pulse at the fourth or fifth intercostal space at the midclavicular line (Jensen, 2011).
- The apical pulse is most reliable for infants and small children. Count the rate for 1 full minute in infants and children because of possible rhythm irregularities (Perry et al., 2010).
- Allow the young child to examine or handle the stethoscope to become familiar with the equipment.
- Apical rate of infants is easily palpated with the fingertips.

SKILL 2-6 ASSESSING RESPIRATION

Under normal conditions, healthy adults breathe about 12 to 20 times per minute. Infants and children breathe more rapidly. Fundamentals Review 2-1 outlines respiratory rate ranges for different age groups. The depth of respirations varies normally from shallow to deep. The rhythm of respirations is normally regular, with each inhalation/exhalation and the pauses between occurring at regular intervals. An irregular respiratory rhythm occurs when the inhalation/exhalation cycle and the pauses between occur at unequal intervals. Table 2-1 outlines various respiratory patterns.

Assess respiratory rate, depth, and rhythm by inspection (observing and listening) or by listening with the stethoscope. Determine the rate by counting the number of breaths per minute. If respirations are very shallow and difficult to detect, observe the sternal notch, where respiration is more apparent. With an infant or young child, assess respirations before taking the temperature so that the child is not crying, which would alter the respiratory status.

Move immediately from the pulse assessment to counting the respiratory rate to avoid letting the patient know you are counting respirations. Patients should be unaware of the respiratory assessment because, if they are conscious of the procedure, they might alter their breathing patterns or rate.

Table 2-1 PATTERNS OF RESPIRATION

	DESCRIPTION	PATTERN	ASSOCIATED FEATURES
Normal	12–20 breaths/min; Regular		Normal pattern
Tachypnea	>24 breaths/min; Shallow		Fever, anxiety, exercise, respiratory disorders
Bradypnea	<10 breaths/min; Regular		Depression of the respiratory center by medications, brain damage
Hyperventilation	Increased rate and depth		Extreme exercise, fear, diabetic ketoacidosis (Kussmaul's respirations), overdose of aspirin
Hypoventilation	Decreased rate and depth; Irregular		Overdose of narcotics or anesthetics
Cheyne-Stokes respirations	Alternating periods of deep, rapid breathing followed by periods of **apnea**; Regular		Drug overdose, heart failure, increased intracranial pressure, renal failure
Biot's respirations	Varying depth and rate of breathing, followed by periods of apnea; Irregular		Meningitis, severe brain damage

DELEGATION CONSIDERATIONS

The assessment of respiration may be delegated to nursing assistive personnel (NAP) or to unlicensed assistive personnel (UAP), as well as to licensed practical/vocational nurses (LPN/LVN). The decision to delegate must be based on careful analysis of the patient's needs and circumstances, as well as the qualifications of the person to whom the task is being delegated. Refer to the Delegation Guidelines in Appendix A.

EQUIPMENT

- Watch with second hand or digital readout
- Pencil or pen, paper or flow sheet, computerized record
- PPE, as indicated

(continued)

SKILL 2-6 ASSESSING RESPIRATION continued

ASSESSMENT

Assess the patient for factors that could affect respirations, such as exercise, medications, smoking, chronic illness or conditions, neurologic injury, pain, and anxiety. Note baseline or previous respiratory measurements. Assess patient for any signs of respiratory distress, which include retractions, nasal flaring, grunting, **orthopnea**, or **tachypnea**. Note baseline or previous respiration measurements.

NURSING DIAGNOSIS

Determine the related factors for the nursing diagnoses based on the patient's current status. Appropriate nursing diagnoses may include:

- Ineffective Breathing Pattern
- Impaired Gas Exchange
- Risk for Activity Intolerance
- Ineffective Airway Clearance

OUTCOME IDENTIFICATION AND PLANNING

The expected outcomes to achieve when assessing respirations are that the patient's respirations are assessed accurately without injury and the patient experiences minimal discomfort. Other outcomes may be appropriate depending on the patient's nursing diagnosis.

IMPLEMENTATION

ACTION	RATIONALE
1. **While your fingers are still in place for the pulse measurement, after counting the pulse rate, observe the patient's respirations (Figure 1).**	The patient may alter the rate of respirations if he or she is aware they are being counted.

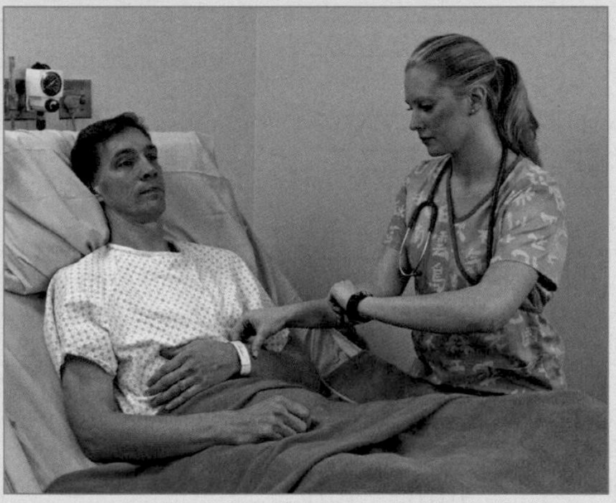

FIGURE 1 Assessing respirations.

ACTION	RATIONALE
2. Note the rise and fall of the patient's chest.	A complete cycle of an **inspiration** and an **expiration** composes one respiration.
3. Using a watch with a second hand, count the number of respirations for 30 seconds. Multiply this number by 2 to calculate the respiratory rate per minute.	Sufficient time is necessary to observe the rate, depth, and other characteristics.
4. **If respirations are abnormal in any way, count the respirations for at least 1 full minute.**	Increased time allows the detection of unequal timing between respirations.
5. Note the depth and rhythm of the respirations.	Provides additional assessment data regarding the patient's respiratory status.
6. When measurement is completed, remove gloves, if worn. Cover the patient and help him or her to a position of comfort.	Removing gloves properly reduces the risk for infection transmission and contamination of other items. Ensures patient comfort.
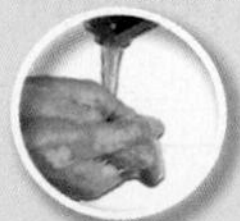 7. Remove additional PPE, if used. Perform hand hygiene.	Removing PPE properly reduces the risk for infection transmission and contamination of other items. Hand hygiene deters the spread of microorganisms.

EVALUATION

The expected outcome is met when the patient's respirations are assessed accurately without injury and the patient experiences minimal discomfort.

DOCUMENTATION

Guidelines

Document respiratory rate, depth, and rhythm on paper, flow sheet, or computerized record. Report any abnormal findings to the appropriate person.

Sample Documentation

Lippincott DocuCare Practice documenting respiration and other vital signs in *Lippincott DocuCare.*

10/23/15 0830 Patient breathing at a rate of 16 respirations per minute. Respirations regular and unlabored.

—*M. Evans, RN*

UNEXPECTED SITUATIONS AND ASSOCIATED INTERVENTIONS

- *The patient is breathing with such shallow respirations that you cannot count the rate:* Sometimes it is easier to count respirations by auscultating the lung sounds. Auscultate lung sounds and count respirations for 30 seconds. Multiply by 2 to calculate the respiratory rate per minute. If the respiratory rate is irregular, count for a full minute. Notify the physician of the respiratory rate and the shallowness of the respirations.

SPECIAL CONSIDERATIONS

General Considerations

- If respiratory rate is irregular, count respirations for 1 minute.

Infant and Child Considerations

- For infants, count respirations for 1 full minute due to a normally irregular rhythm.
- Assess respirations in infants and children when the child is resting or sitting quietly, because respiratory rate often changes when infants or young children cry, feed, or become more active. The most accurate respiratory rate is obtained before disturbing the infant or child (Kyle & Carman, 2013).
- Infants' respirations are primarily diaphragmatic; count abdominal movements to measure respiratory rate. After 1 year of age, count thoracic movements (Kyle & Carman, 2013).

EVIDENCE FOR PRACTICE ▶

EFFECTS OF MUSIC LISTENING IN POSTOPERATIVE PERIOD

Surgery and postoperative pain cause increased heart rate and blood pressure. Postoperative pain can alter respiratory function, and interfere with deep breathing, coughing, and moving. An important part of nursing care in the postoperative period includes nursing interventions to prevent complications from surgery. Listening to music can focus attention, facilitate breathing, and stimulate the relaxation response, aiding in pain control. Decreased pain allows patients to participate in important activities to prevent postoperative complications.

Related Research

Vaajoki, A., Kankkunen, P., Pietilä, A.M., & Vehviläinen-Julkunen, K. (2011). Music as a nursing intervention: Effects of music listening on blood pressure, heart rate, and respiratory rate in abdominal surgery patients. *Nursing and Health Sciences, 13*(4), 412–418.

The aim of this study was to evaluate the effects of music listening on blood pressure, heart rate, and respiratory rate on operation day, and on the first, second, and third postoperative days in patients having abdominal surgery. Those patients were assigned every second week to the music group (n = 83) or to the control group (n = 85) for 25 months. Patients in the music group chose their favorite music. In the music group, the respiratory rate was significantly lower after intervention on both the first and second postoperative days compared with the control group. A significant reduction in systolic blood pressure was demonstrated in the group that received music compared with the control group on both the first and second postoperative days. No differences were found between the two groups in diastolic blood pressure or heart rate.

Evaluation of the long-term effects of music on physiologic factors showed that the respiratory rate in the music group was significantly lower compared with the control group.

Relevance to Nursing Practice

Listening to music can significantly lower systolic blood pressure and respiratory rate in the postoperative period and was identified as a positive experience for patients. Nurses should strengthen their knowledge of the benefits of music listening as a nonpharmacologic intervention. Music can be used as part of the healing environment to support surgical patients during their recovery period, and can positively influence patient's experiences while in the hospital.

Refer to thePoint for additional research on related nursing topics.

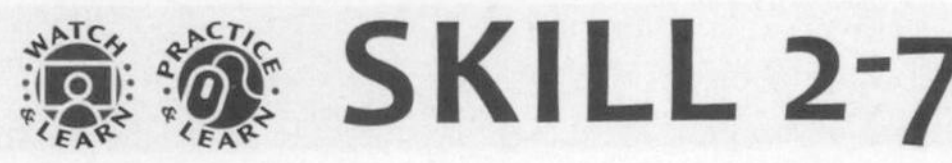

SKILL 2-7 ASSESSING BLOOD PRESSURE BY AUSCULTATION

Blood pressure refers to the force of the blood against arterial walls. **Systolic pressure** is the highest point of pressure on arterial walls when the ventricles contract and push blood through the arteries at the beginning of systole. When the heart rests between beats during diastole, the pressure drops. The lowest pressure present on arterial walls during diastole is the **diastolic pressure** (Taylor et al., 2015). Blood pressure, measured in millimeters of mercury (mm Hg), is recorded as a fraction. The numerator is the systolic pressure; the denominator is the diastolic pressure. The difference between the two is called the **pulse pressure.** For example, if the blood pressure is 120/80 mm Hg, 120 is the systolic pressure and 80 is the diastolic pressure. The pulse pressure, in this case, is 40. Table 2-2 outlines categories of blood pressure levels for adults.

Table 2-2 CATEGORIES FOR BLOOD PRESSURE LEVELS IN ADULTS (AGES 18 AND OLDER)

	BLOOD PRESSURE LEVEL (MM HG)		
CATEGORY	*Systolic*		*Diastolic*
Normal*	<120	AND	Less than 80
Prehypertension	120–139	OR	80–89
High Blood Pressure			
Stage 1	140–159	OR	90–99
Stage 2	≥160	OR	100 or higher

*In regard to risk of heart disease, optimal is defined as less than 120/80 mm Hg.
(Source: National Heart, Lung, and Blood Institute (NHLBI). National Institutes of Health (NIH). (2012). What is high blood pressure? Available http://www.nhlbi.nih.gov/health/health-topics/topics/hbp/)

To get an accurate assessment of blood pressure, you should know what equipment to use, which site to choose, and how to identify the sounds you hear. Take routine measurements after the patient has rested for a minimum of 5 minutes. In addition, make sure the patient does not have any caffeine or nicotine 30 minutes before measuring blood pressure. The American Heart Association recommends that blood pressure readings be measured on two or more subsequent occasions before determining if the blood pressure is outside acceptable parameters (AHA, 2012).

The series of sounds for which to listen when assessing blood pressure are called **Korotkoff sounds**. Table 2-3 describes and illustrates these sounds. Blood pressure can be assessed with different types of devices. Commonly, it is assessed by using a stethoscope and sphygmomanometer. Blood pressure can also be estimated with a Doppler ultrasound device, by palpation, and with electronic or automated devices. Auscultation is the preferred method of obtaining blood pressure readings in children older than one year (National Heart, Lung, and Blood Institute, 2005; Ogedegbe & Pickering, 2010). It is very important to use the correct technique and properly functioning equipment when assessing blood pressure to avoid errors in measurement. Use of a cuff of the correct size for the patient, correct limb placement, recommended deflation rate, and correct interpretation of the sounds heard are also necessary to ensure accurate blood pressure measurement (Hinkle & Cheever, 2014; Pickering et al., 2004). Table 2-4 outlines common errors in blood pressure measurement.

At times, it is necessary to assess a patient for **orthostatic hypotension** (postural hypotension). Orthostatic hypotension is a low blood pressure; it is defined as a decrease in systolic blood pressure of 20 mm Hg or a decrease in diastolic blood pressure of 10 mm Hg within 3 minutes of standing when compared with blood pressure from the sitting or supine position (Lanier et al., 2011). Box 2-2 outlines the procedure for blood pressure measurement to assess for orthostatic hypotension.

Table 2-3 KOROTKOFF SOUNDS

PHASE	DESCRIPTION	ILLUSTRATION
Phase I	Characterized by the first appearance of faint, but clear tapping sounds that gradually increase in intensity; the first tapping sound is the systolic pressure.	**FIGURE A** Blood flow interrupted by inflated cuff.
Phase II	Characterized by muffled or swishing sounds; these sounds may temporarily disappear, especially in hypertensive people; the disappearance of the sound during the latter part of phase I and during phase II is called the *auscultatory gap* and may cover a range of as much as 40 mm Hg; failing to recognize this gap may cause serious errors of underestimating systolic pressure or overestimating diastolic pressure	**FIGURE B** As the pressure in the cuff is released, blood starts flowing again and Korotkoff sounds are audible.
Phase III	Characterized by distinct, loud sounds as the blood flows relatively freely through an increasingly open artery.	
Phase IV	Characterized by a distinct, abrupt, muffling sound with a soft, blowing quality; in adults, the onset of this phase is considered to be the first diastolic pressure.	
Phase V	The last sound heard before a period of continuous silence; the pressure at which the last sound is heard is the second diastolic pressure.	**FIGURE C** Cuff is completely deflated after Phase V, restoring complete blood flow.

Various sites can be used to assess blood pressure. The brachial artery and the popliteal artery are used most commonly. This skill discusses using the brachial artery site to obtain a blood pressure measurement. The skill begins with the procedure for estimating systolic pressure. Estimation of systolic pressure prevents inaccurate readings in the presence of an auscultatory gap (a pause in the auscultated sounds). To identify the first Korotkoff sound accurately, the cuff must be inflated to a pressure above the point at which the pulse can no longer be felt.

(*continued*)

SKILL 2-7 ASSESSING BLOOD PRESSURE BY AUSCULTATION continued

Table 2-4 BLOOD PRESSURE ASSESSMENT ERRORS AND CONTRIBUTING CAUSES

ERROR	CONTRIBUTING CAUSES
Falsely low assessments	• Hearing deficit • Noise in the environment • Viewing the meniscus from above eye level • Applying too wide a cuff • Inserting ear tips of stethoscope incorrectly • Using cracked or kinked tubing • Releasing the valve rapidly • Misplacing the bell beyond the direct area of the artery • Failing to pump the cuff 20–30 mm Hg above the disappearance of the pulse
Falsely high assessments	• Using a manometer not calibrated at the zero mark • Assessing the blood pressure immediately after exercise • Viewing the meniscus from below eye level • Applying a cuff that is too narrow • Releasing the valve too slowly • Reinflating the bladder during auscultation

Box 2-2 BLOOD PRESSURE MEASUREMENT TO ASSESS FOR ORTHOSTATIC HYPOTENSION

Throughout the procedure, assess for signs and symptoms of **hypotension**, such as dizziness, light-headedness, pallor, diaphoresis, or syncope. If the patient is attached to a cardiac monitor, assess for arrhythmias. Immediately return the patient to a supine position if symptoms appear during the procedure. Do not have the patient stand if symptoms of hypotension occur when the patient is sitting. Use the following guidelines to assess for **orthostatic hypotension:**

- Lower the head of the bed. Place the bed in a low position.
- Ask the patient to lie in a supine position for 3 to 10 minutes. At the end of this time, take initial blood pressure and pulse measurements.
- Assist the patient to a sitting position on the side of the bed with the legs dangling. After 1 to 3 minutes, take the blood pressure and pulse measurements.
- Assist the patient to stand, unless standing is contraindicated. Wait 2 to 3 minutes, then take blood pressure and pulse measurements.
- Record the measurements for each position, noting the position with the readings. A decrease in systolic blood pressure of ≥20 mm Hg or a decrease in diastolic blood pressure of 10 mm Hg within 3 minutes of standing when compared with blood pressure from the sitting or supine position (Lanier et al., 2011).

(Adapted from Lanier, J.B., Mote, M.B., & Clay, E.C. (2011). Evaluation and management of orthostatic hypotension. *American Family Physician, 84*(5), 527–536; and Pickering, T., Hall, J., Appel, L., et al. (2004). American Heart Association Scientific Statement. Recommendations for blood pressure measurement in humans and experimental animals. Part 1: Blood pressure measurement in humans: A statement for professionals from the subcommittee of professional and public education of the American Heart Association Council on High Blood Pressure Research. Available at http://hyper.ahajournals.org/cgi/content/full/45/1/142.)

DELEGATION CONSIDERATIONS

The assessment of brachial artery blood pressure may be delegated to nursing assistive personnel (NAP) or unlicensed assistive personnel (UAP), as well as to licensed practical/vocational nurses (LPN/LVN). The decision to delegate must be based on careful analysis of the patient's needs and circumstances, as well as the qualifications of the person to whom the task is being delegated. Refer to the Delegation Guidelines in Appendix A.

EQUIPMENT

- Stethoscope
- Sphygmomanometer
- Blood pressure cuff of appropriate size
- Pencil or pen, paper, flow sheet, or computerized record
- Alcohol swab
- PPE, as indicated

ASSESSMENT

Assess the brachial pulse, or the pulse appropriate for the site being used. Assess for an intravenous infusion or breast or axilla surgery on the side of the body corresponding to the arm used. Assess for the presence of a cast, arteriovenous shunt, or injured or diseased limb. If any of these conditions are present, do not use the affected arm to monitor blood pressure. Assess the size of the limb so that the appropriate-sized blood pressure cuff can be used. The correct cuff should have a bladder length that is 80% of the arm circumference and a width that is at least 40% of the arm circumference: a length to width ratio of 2:1. Refer to Table 2-5 for recommended cuff sizes based on arm circumference. Assess for factors that could affect blood pressure reading, such as the patient's age, exercise, position, weight, fluid balance, smoking, and medications. Note baseline or previous blood pressure measurements. Assess the patient for pain. If the patient reports pain, give pain medication as ordered before assessing blood pressure. If the blood pressure is taken while the patient is in pain, make a notation concerning the pain if the blood pressure is elevated.

Table 2-5 RECOMMENDED BLOOD PRESSURE CUFF SIZES

CUFF SIZE	CUFF MEASUREMENTS	ARM CIRCUMFERENCE*
Newborn–premature infants	4 × 8 cm	
Infants	6 × 12 cm	
Older children	9 × 18 cm	
Small adult size	12 × 22 cm	22–26 cm
Adult size	16 × 30 cm	27–34 cm
Large adult size	16 × 36 cm	35–44 cm
Adult thigh size	16 × 42 cm	45–52 cm

*Select a blood pressure cuff that has a bladder width that is at least 40% of the arm circumference midway between the olecranon and the acromion. (Data from Pickering, T., Hall, J., Appel, L., et al. [2004]. American Heart Association Scientific Statement. Recommendations for blood pressure measurement in humans and experimental animals. Part 1: Blood pressure measurement in humans: A statement for professionals from the subcommittee of professional and public education of the American Heart Association Council on High Blood Pressure Research. Available at http://hyper.ahajournals.org/cgi/content/full/45/1/142.)

NURSING DIAGNOSIS

Determine the related factors for the nursing diagnoses based on the patient's current status. Appropriate nursing diagnoses may include:

- Decreased Cardiac Output
- Ineffective Health Maintenance
- Risk for Falls

OUTCOME IDENTIFICATION AND PLANNING

The expected outcome to achieve when measuring blood pressure is that the patient's blood pressure is measured accurately without injury. Other outcomes may be appropriate depending on the patient's nursing diagnosis.

(continued)

SKILL 2-7 ASSESSING BLOOD PRESSURE BY AUSCULTATION continued

IMPLEMENTATION

ACTION	RATIONALE
1. Check the medical order or nursing care plan for frequency of blood pressure measurement. More frequent measurement may be appropriate based on nursing judgment.	Provides for patient safety.
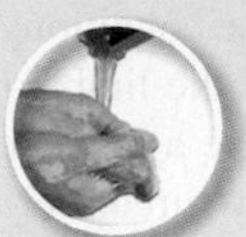 2. Perform hand hygiene and put on PPE, if indicated.	Hand hygiene and PPE prevent the spread of microorganisms. PPE is required based on transmission precautions.
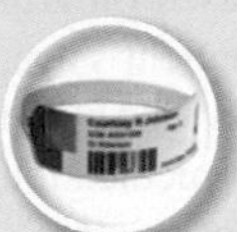 3. Identify the patient.	Identifying the patient ensures the right patient receives the intervention and helps prevent errors.
4. Close the curtains around the bed and close the door to the room, if possible. Discuss the procedure with the patient and assess patient's ability to assist with the procedure. Validate that the patient has relaxed for several minutes.	This ensures the patient's privacy. Explanation relieves anxiety and facilitates cooperation. Activity immediately before measurement can result in inaccurate results.
5. Put on gloves, if indicated.	Gloves prevent contact with blood and body fluids. Gloves are usually not required for measurement of blood pressure, unless contact with blood or body fluids is anticipated.
6. Select the appropriate arm for application of the cuff.	Measurement of blood pressure may temporarily impede circulation to the extremity.
7. Have the patient assume a comfortable lying or sitting position with the forearm supported at the level of the heart and the palm of the hand upward (Figure 1). If the measurement is taken in the supine position, support the arm with a pillow. In the sitting position, support the arm yourself or by using the bedside table. If the patient is sitting, have the patient sit back in the chair so that the chair supports his or her back. In addition, make sure the patient keeps the legs uncrossed.	The position of the arm can have a major influence when the blood pressure is measured; if the upper arm is below the level of the right atrium, the readings will be too high. If the arm is above the level of the heart, the readings will be too low (Pickering et al., 2004). If the back is not supported, the diastolic pressure may be elevated falsely; if the legs are crossed, the systolic pressure may be elevated falsely (Pickering et al., 2004). This position places the brachial artery on the inner aspect of the elbow so that the **bell** or diaphragm of the stethoscope can rest on it easily. This sitting position ensures accuracy.

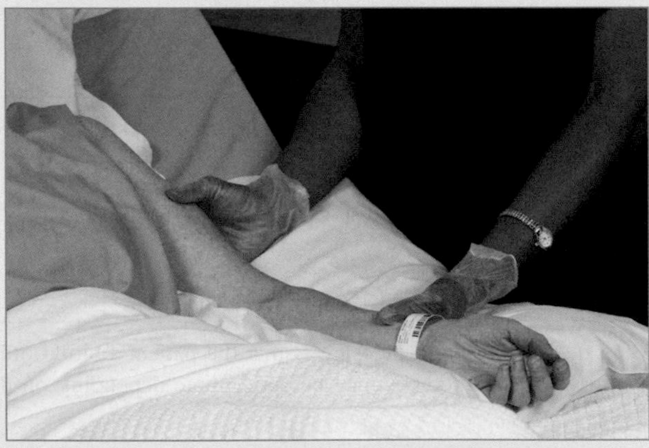

FIGURE 1 Proper positioning for blood pressure assessment using brachial artery. *(Photo by B. Proud.)*

ACTION	RATIONALE
8. Expose the brachial artery by removing garments or move a sleeve if it is not too tight, above the area where the cuff will be placed.	Clothing over the artery interferes with the ability to hear sounds and can cause inaccurate blood pressure readings. A tight sleeve would cause congestion of blood and possibly inaccurate readings.

ACTION

9. Palpate the location of the brachial artery. **Center the bladder of the cuff over the brachial artery, about midway on the arm, so that the lower edge of the cuff is about 2.5 to 5 cm (1 to 2 inches) above the inner aspect of the elbow. Line up the artery marking on the cuff with the patient's brachial artery.** The tubing should extend from the edge of the cuff nearer the patient's elbow (Figure 2).

RATIONALE

Pressure in the cuff applied directly to the artery provides the most accurate readings. If the cuff gets in the way of the stethoscope, readings are likely to be inaccurate. A cuff placed upside down with the tubing toward the patient's head may give a false reading.

10. Wrap the cuff around the arm smoothly and snugly, and fasten it. Do not allow any clothing to interfere with the proper placement of the cuff.

A smooth cuff and snug wrapping produce equal pressure and help promote an accurate measurement. A cuff wrapped too loosely results in an inaccurate reading.

11. Check that the needle on the aneroid gauge is within the zero mark (Figure 3). If using a mercury manometer, check to see that the manometer is in the vertical position and that the mercury is within the zero level with the gauge at eye level.

If the needle is not in the zero area, the blood pressure reading may not be accurate. Tilting a mercury manometer, inaccurate calibration, or improper height for reading the gauge can lead to errors in determining the pressure measurements.

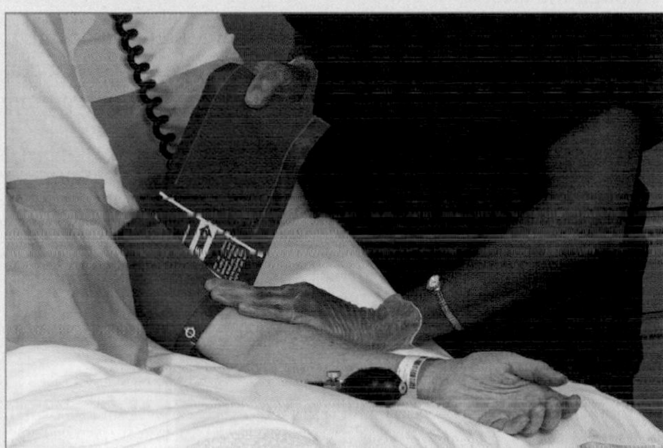

FIGURE 2 Placing the blood pressure cuff. *(Photo by B. Proud.)*

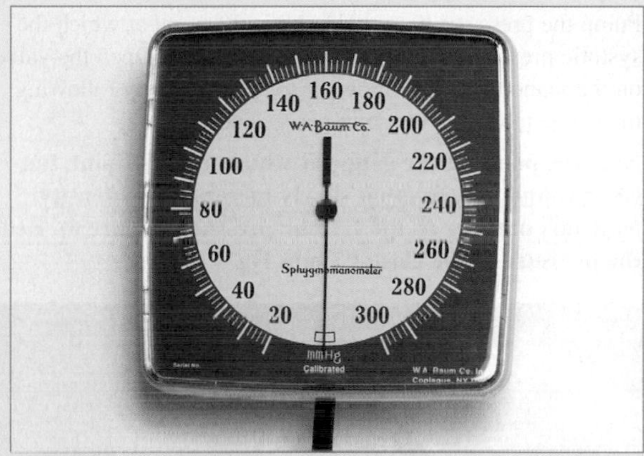

FIGURE 3 Ensuring gauge starts at zero. *(Photo by B. Proud.)*

Estimating Systolic Pressure

12. Palpate the pulse at the brachial or radial artery by pressing gently with the fingertips (Figure 4).

Palpation allows for measurement of the approximate systolic reading.

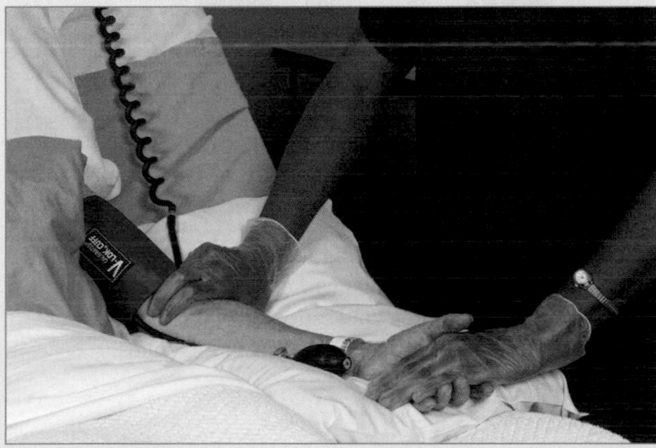

FIGURE 4 Palpating the brachial pulse. *(Photo by B. Proud.)*

13. Tighten the screw valve on the air pump.

The bladder within the cuff will not inflate with the valve open.

14. **Inflate the cuff while continuing to palpate the artery. Note the point on the gauge where the pulse disappears.**

The point where the pulse disappears provides an estimate of the systolic pressure. To identify the first Korotkoff sound accurately, the cuff must be inflated to a pressure above the point at which the pulse can no longer be felt.

(continued)

SKILL 2-7 ASSESSING BLOOD PRESSURE BY AUSCULTATION continued

ACTION	RATIONALE
15. Deflate the cuff and wait 1 minute.	Allowing a brief pause before continuing permits the blood to refill and circulate through the arm.
Obtaining Blood Pressure Measurement	
16. Assume a position that is no more than 3 feet away from the gauge.	A distance of more than about 3 feet can interfere with accurate reading of the numbers on the gauge.
17. Place the stethoscope earpieces in your ears. Direct the earpieces forward into the canal and not against the ear itself.	Proper placement blocks extraneous noise and allows sound to travel more clearly.
18. Place the bell or diaphragm of the stethoscope firmly but with as little pressure as possible over the brachial artery (Figure 5). Do not allow the stethoscope to touch clothing or the cuff.	Having the bell or diaphragm directly over the artery allows more accurate readings. Heavy pressure on the brachial artery distorts the shape of the artery and the sound. Placing the bell or diaphragm away from clothing and the cuff prevents noise, which would distract from the sounds made by blood flowing through the artery.
19. Pump the pressure 30 mm Hg above the point at which the systolic pressure was palpated and estimated. Open the valve on the manometer and allow air to escape slowly (allowing the gauge to drop 2 to 3 mm per second).	Increasing the pressure above the point where the pulse disappeared ensures a period before hearing the first sound that corresponds with the systolic pressure. It prevents misinterpreting phase II sounds as phase I sounds.
20. **Note the point on the gauge at which the first faint, but clear, sound appears that slowly increases in intensity. Note this number as the systolic pressure (Figure 6). Read the pressure to the closest 2 mm Hg.**	Systolic pressure is the point at which the blood in the artery is first able to force its way through the vessel at a similar pressure exerted by the air bladder in the cuff. The first sound is phase I of Korotkoff sounds.

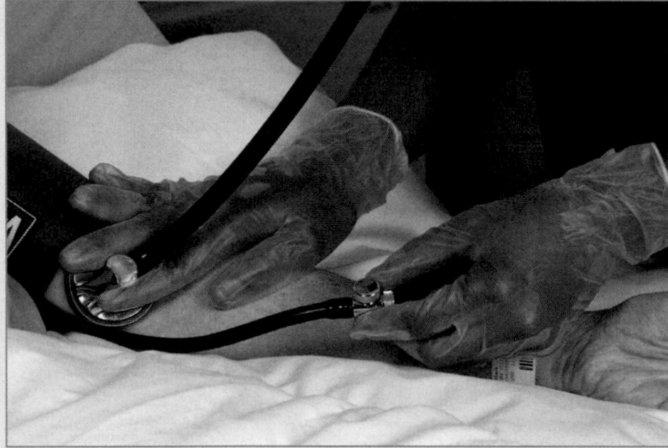

FIGURE 5 Proper placement of diaphragm of stethoscope. *(Photo by B. Proud.)*

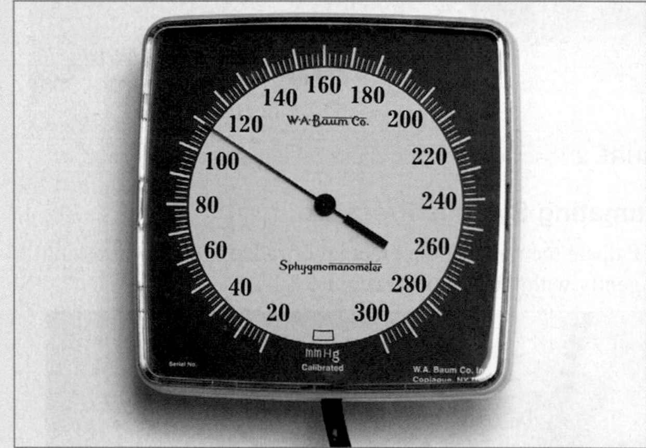

FIGURE 6 Measuring systolic blood pressure. *(Photo by B. Proud.)*

ACTION	RATIONALE
21. Do not reinflate the cuff once the air is being released to recheck the systolic pressure reading.	Reinflating the cuff while obtaining the blood pressure is uncomfortable for the patient and can cause an inaccurate reading. Reinflating the cuff causes congestion of blood in the lower arm, which lessens the loudness of Korotkoff sounds.

ACTION | **RATIONALE**

22. **Note the point at which the sound completely disappears. Note this number as the diastolic pressure (Figure 7). Read the pressure to the closest 2 mm Hg.**

The point at which the sound disappears corresponds to the beginning of phase V Korotkoff sounds and is generally considered the diastolic pressure reading (Pickering et al., 2004).

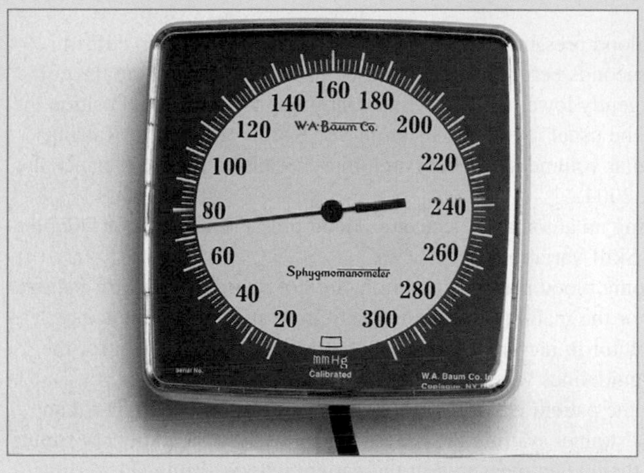

FIGURE 7 Measuring diastolic blood pressure. *(Photo by B. Proud.)*

23. Allow the remaining air to escape quickly. Repeat any suspicious reading, but wait at least 1 minute. Deflate the cuff completely between attempts to check the blood pressure.

False readings are likely to occur if there is congestion of blood in the limb while obtaining repeated readings.

24. When measurement is completed, remove the cuff. Remove gloves, if worn. Cover the patient and help him or her to a position of comfort.

Removing gloves properly reduces the risk for infection transmission and contamination of other items. Ensures patient comfort.

25. Clean the bell or diaphragm of the stethoscope with the alcohol wipe. Clean and store the sphygmomanometer, according to facility policy.

Appropriate cleaning deters the spread of microorganisms. Equipment should be left ready for use.

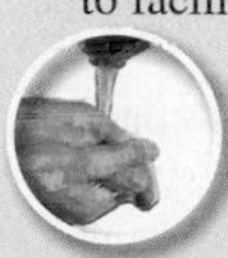

26. Remove additional PPE, if used. Perform hand hygiene.

Removing PPE properly reduces the risk for infection transmission and contamination of other items. Hand hygiene deters the spread of microorganisms.

EVALUATION

The expected outcome is met when the blood pressure is measured accurately without injury and with minimal patient discomfort.

DOCUMENTATION

Guidelines

Record the findings on paper, flow sheet, or computerized record. Report abnormal findings to the appropriate person. Identify arm used and site of assessment if other than brachial.

Sample Documentation

Lippincott DocuCare **Practice documenting blood pressure and other vital signs in *Lippincott DocuCare*.**

10/18/15 0945 Blood pressure taken in right arm 180/88. Physician notified. Ordered captopril 25 mg PO b.i.d. Blood pressure to be repeated 30 minutes after administering medication.

—*M. Evans, RN*

(continued)

SKILL 2-7 ASSESSING BLOOD PRESSURE BY AUSCULTATION continued

SPECIAL CONSIDERATIONS

General Considerations

- It is recommended that blood pressure measurements should be checked in both arms at the first examination. Most people have differences in blood pressure readings between arms. It is normal to have a 5- to 10-mm Hg difference in the systolic reading between arms. When there is a consistent inter-arm difference, use the arm with the higher pressure (Pickering et al., 2004).
- If you have difficulty hearing the blood pressure sounds, raise the patient's arm, with cuff in place, over his or her head for 30 seconds before rechecking the blood pressure. Inflate the cuff while the arm is elevated, and then gently lower the arm while continuing to support it. Position the stethoscope and deflate the cuff at the usual rate while listening for Korotkoff sounds. Raising the arm over the head reduces vascular volume in the limb and improves blood flow to enhance the Korotkoff sounds (Pickering et al., 2004).
- Blood pressure can be assessed using an automatic electronic blood pressure monitor or Doppler ultrasound (see the accompanying Skill Variation).
- Many versions of automatic electronic blood pressure monitors are not recommended for patients with irregular heart rates, tremors, or the inability to hold the extremity still. The presence of these conditions may cause the monitor to incorrectly overinflate the cuff, causing pain for the patient. Check the manufacturer's guidelines when considering use with these patients.
- Diastolic pressure measured while the patient is sitting is approximately 5 mm Hg higher than when measured while the patient is supine; systolic pressure measured while the patient is supine is approximately 8 mm Hg higher than when measured in the patient who is sitting (Pickering et al., 2004).
- Measuring blood pressure in the forearm by auscultating the radial artery for the Korotkoff sounds is becoming more common. Forearm measurements tend to be higher than the upper arm measurements (Domiano et al., 2008; Frese, et al., 2011). The accuracy of readings with forearm monitors is affected by the position of the wrist relative to the heart. This can be avoided if the wrist is always at heart level when the reading is taken (Pickering et al., 2004). This site for measurement has been suggested as an alternative for obtaining blood pressure readings in people who are obese. It is often difficult to obtain the appropriately sized cuff for the upper arm, given arm circumference and conical-shaped upper arms common in obesity. The conical shape of the upper arm makes it difficult to fit the cuff to the arm, increasing the likelihood of inaccurate blood pressure measurement (Palatini & Parati, 2011). Thus, measurement in the forearm can be a possible solution to this problem.
- When the patient's brachial artery is inaccessible and/or the use of the upper arm is contraindicated, you can assess the blood pressure using the popliteal artery in the leg. The systolic pressure is normally 10 to 40 mm Hg higher at this site, although the diastolic pressure is the same.

Infant and Child Considerations

- In infants and small children, the lower extremities are commonly used for blood pressure monitoring. The more common sites are the popliteal, dorsalis pedis, and posterior tibial. Blood pressures obtained in the lower extremities are generally higher than if taken in the upper extremities. In children over 1 year of age, the systolic pressure in the thigh tends to be 10 to 40 mm Hg higher than in the arm; the diastolic pressure remains the same (Kyle & Carman, 2013).
- Infants and children presenting with cardiac complaints may have blood pressures assessed in all four extremities. Large differences among blood pressure readings can indicate heart defects.
- The fifth Korotkoff sound corresponds to diastolic blood pressure in children. In some children, the Korotkoff sounds continue to 0 mm Hg. In this situation, document the reading as systolic pressure over "P" for pulse (Kyle & Carman, 2013).

Home Care Considerations

- Automated blood pressure devices in public locations are generally inaccurate and inconsistent. In addition, the cuffs on these devices are inadequate for persons with large arms (Pickering et al., 2004).
- Explain to the patient that it is important to use a cuff size appropriate for limb circumference. Inform the patient that cuff sizes range from a pediatric cuff to a large thigh cuff and that a poorly fitting cuff can result in an inaccurate measurement.
- Inform the patient about digital blood pressure monitoring equipment. Although more costly than manual cuffs, most provide an easy-to-read recording of systolic and diastolic measurements.
- Explain that three readings, at least 1 minute apart, should be taken while in a sitting position, both in the morning and at night. Measurement should occur after resting quietly in a chair for 3 to 5 minutes, with the upper arm at heart level. The readings should be recorded to show to the health care provider.
- Explain that home monitoring devices should be checked for accuracy every 1 to 2 years. Readings should be compared with auscultated measurement by a health care practitioner to ensure accuracy.

SKILL VARIATION Assessing Blood Pressure Using an Automatic Electronic Blood Pressure Monitor

Automatic, electronic equipment is often used to monitor blood pressure in acute care settings, during anesthesia, postoperatively, or any time frequent assessments are necessary (Figure A). This unit determines blood pressure by analyzing the sounds of blood flow or measuring oscillations. The machine can be set to take and record blood pressure readings at preset intervals. Irregular heart rates, excessive patient movement, and environmental noise can interfere with the readings. Because electronic equipment is more sensitive to outside interference, these readings are susceptible to error. The cuff is applied in the same manner as the auscultatory method, with the microphone or pressure sensor positioned directly over the artery. When using an automatic blood pressure device for serial readings, check the cuffed limb frequently. Incomplete deflation of the cuff between measurements can lead to inadequate arterial perfusion and venous drainage, compromising the circulation in the limb (Bern et al., 2007; Pickering et al., 2004).

1. Check the medical order or nursing care plan for frequency of blood pressure measurement. More frequent measurement may be appropriate based on nursing judgment.

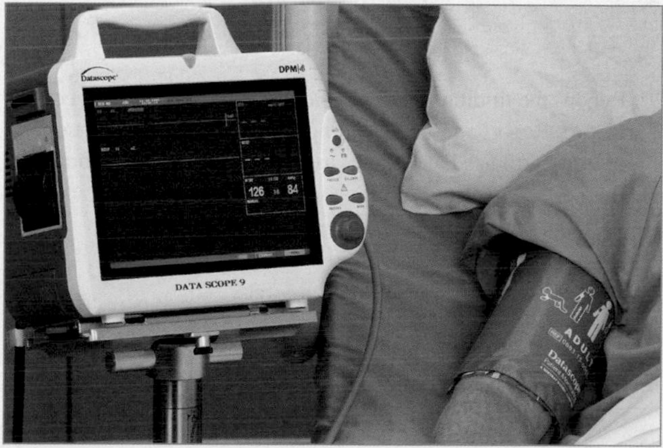

FIGURE A Electronic blood pressure device. *(Photo by B. Proud.)*

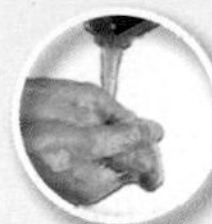

2. Perform hand hygiene and put on PPE, if indicated.

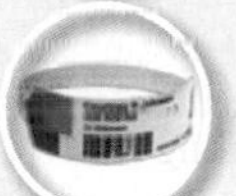

3. **Identify the patient.**
4. Close the curtains around the bed and close the door to the room, if possible.
5. Discuss the procedure with the patient and assess the patient's ability to assist with the procedure.
6. Validate that the patient has relaxed for several minutes.
7. Select the appropriate limb for application of cuff.
8. Have the patient assume a comfortable lying or sitting position with the limb exposed.
9. **Center the bladder of the cuff over the artery, lining up the artery mark on the cuff with the limb artery.**
10. Wrap the cuff around the limb smoothly and snugly, and fasten it. Do not allow any clothing to interfere with the proper placement of the cuff.
11. Turn on the machine. **If the machine has different settings for infants, children, and adults, select the appropriate setting.** Push the start button. Instruct the patient to hold the limb still.
12. Wait until the machine beeps and the blood pressure reading appears. Remove the cuff from the patient's limb and clean and store the equipment.

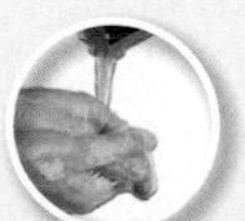

13. Remove PPE, if used. Perform hand hygiene.
14. Record the findings on paper, flow sheet, or computerized record. Report abnormal findings to the appropriate person. Identify arm used and site of assessment if other than brachial.

(continued)

SKILL 2-7 ASSESSING BLOOD PRESSURE BY AUSCULTATION continued

SKILL VARIATION Assessing Systolic Blood Pressure Using a Doppler Ultrasound

Blood pressure can be measured with a Doppler ultrasound device, which amplifies sound. It is especially useful if the sounds are indistinct or inaudible with a regular stethoscope. This method provides only an estimate of systolic blood pressure.

1. Check the medical order or nursing care plan for frequency of blood pressure measurement. More frequent measurement may be appropriate based on nursing judgment.
2. Perform hand hygiene and put on PPE, if indicated.
3. Identify the patient.

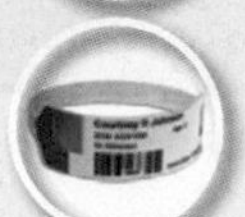

4. Explain the procedure to the patient.
5. Close the curtains around the bed and close the door to the room, if possible.
6. Select the appropriate limb for application of cuff.
7. Have the patient assume a comfortable lying or sitting position with the appropriate limb exposed.
8. **Center the bladder of the cuff over the artery, lining up the artery marker on the cuff with the artery.**
9. Wrap the cuff around the limb smoothly and snugly, and fasten it. Do not allow any clothing to interfere with the proper placement of the cuff.
10. Check that the needle on the aneroid gauge is within the zero mark. If using a mercury manometer, check to see that the manometer is in the vertical position and that the mercury is within the zero level with the gauge at eye level.
11. Place a small amount of conducting gel over the artery.
12. Hold the Doppler device in your nondominant hand. Using your dominant hand, place the Doppler tip in the gel. Adjust the volume as needed. Move the Doppler tip around until you hear the pulse.
13. Once the pulse is found using the Doppler device, close the valve to the sphygmomanometer. Tighten the screw valve on the air pump.

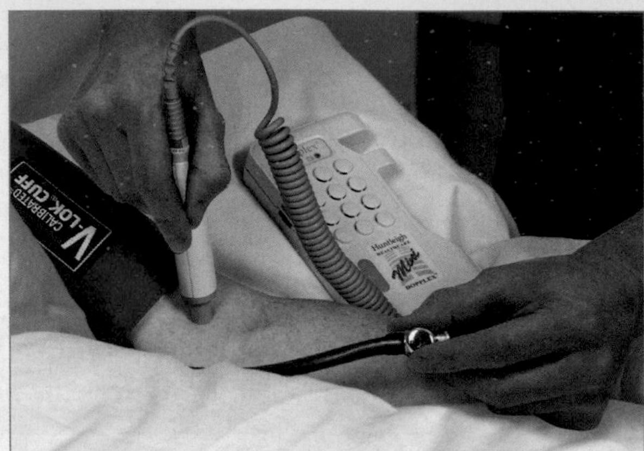

FIGURE B Inflating cuff while listening to artery pulsations. *(Photo by B. Proud.)*

14. **Inflate the cuff while continuing to use the Doppler device on the artery. Note the point on the gauge where the pulse disappears (Figure B).**
15. Open the valve on the manometer and allow air to escape quickly. Repeat any suspicious reading, but wait at least 1 minute between readings to allow normal circulation to return in the limb. Deflate the cuff completely between attempts to check the blood pressure.
16. Remove the Doppler tip and turn off the Doppler device. Wipe excess gel off the patient's skin with tissue. Remove the cuff.
17. Wipe any gel remaining on the Doppler probe off with a tissue. Clean the Doppler device according to facility policy or manufacturer's recommendations.
18. Return the Doppler device to the charge base.
19. Remove PPE, if used. Perform hand hygiene.

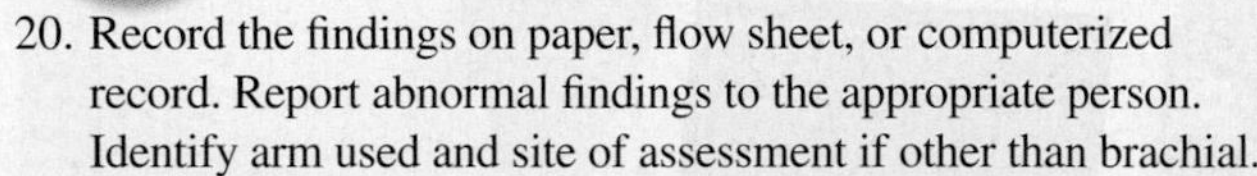

20. Record the findings on paper, flow sheet, or computerized record. Report abnormal findings to the appropriate person. Identify arm used and site of assessment if other than brachial.

EVIDENCE FOR PRACTICE ▶

AHA'S RECOMMENDATIONS FOR BLOOD PRESSURE MEASUREMENTS

Pickering, T., Hall, J., Appel, L., et al. (2004). American Heart Association Scientific Statement. Recommendations for blood pressure measurement in humans and experimental animals. Part 1: Blood pressure measurement in humans: A statement for professionals from the subcommittee of professional and public education of the American Heart Association Council on High Blood Pressure Research. Available at http://hyper.ahajournals.org/cgi/content/full/45/1/142.

The American Heart Association (AHA) has issued recommendations for blood pressure measurements. The new guidelines emphasize out-of-office blood pressure readings, proper cuff size, and more. When blood pressure is measured in a medical setting, the guidelines recommend that the cuff be placed on bare skin after the patient has relaxed for several minutes. Further recommendations call for the patient to be seated comfortably in a chair with the back and arm supported, legs uncrossed, and not talking. The first and fifth phases of the Korotkoff sounds are the preferred method for blood pressure measurement. Proper cuff size is critical to accurate measurement. When measuring blood pressure, the cuff should be inflated to 30 mm Hg above the point at which the radial pulse disappears. The sphygmomanometer pressure should then be reduced at 2 to 3 mm/second.

Refer to thePoint for additional research on related nursing topics.

EVIDENCE FOR PRACTICE ▶

HOME BLOOD PRESSURE MONITORING

Patients and/or their family members often need to check their own temperature, pulse, and/or blood pressure at home. Home blood pressure monitoring (HBPM) is being increasingly recommended (Parati et al., 2010; Pickering et al., 2008). Research has shown that readings at home are reliable; they are often lower than those taken in a health care provider setting, contribute to better adherence treatment, and provide multiple readings taken over prolonged periods, giving a better picture of the patient's status and response to treatment (Leblanc et al., 2011; Ogedegbe & Pickering, 2010).

Related Research

Leblanc, M.E., Cloutier, L., & Veiga, E.V. (2011). Knowledge and practice outcomes after home blood pressure measurement education programs. *Blood Pressure Monitoring*, *16*(6), 265–269.

This study investigated the outcomes of three home blood pressure measurement education programs on adult knowledge and practice. Adults were divided into three groups: individual training (A), group training (B), and self-learning (C), for education regarding home blood pressure measurement. Participants in groups A and B received interactive education led by a nurse. Participants in group C learned by themselves using an instruction booklet and a home blood pressure measurement device. Knowledge was assessed pretest and posttest and skills were evaluated by direct observation. While all groups demonstrated knowledge improvement, participants in groups A and B demonstrated significantly higher pretest to posttest improvements in scores. Adults attending an individual or group training program for home blood pressure measurement with a nurse retained the theoretic and practical principles better than those engaged in self-learning. The authors suggest these differences may be attributed to interaction with the nurse.

Relevance to Nursing Practice

Patient education is an important part of nursing care. Nurses can play an important role in assisting patients with hypertension to learn to measure their blood pressure accurately and in providing important information to give a better picture of the patient's status and response to treatment.

Refer to thePoint for additional research on related nursing topics.

ENHANCE YOUR UNDERSTANDING

FOCUSING ON PATIENT CARE: DEVELOPING CLINICAL REASONING

Consider the case scenarios at the beginning of the chapter as you answer the following questions to enhance your understanding and apply what you have learned.

QUESTIONS

1. Tyrone Jeffries, the 5-year-old with a fever of 101.3°F (38.5°C), is suspected of having a middle-ear infection. You need to obtain another set of vital signs for him. As you approach with the electronic thermometer, Tyrone begins to scream, saying, "Go away. I don't want it!" How would you respond?
2. Toby White, who is 26 years of age with a history of asthma, has a respiratory rate of 32 breaths per minute. What other assessments would be most important to make?
3. Carl Glatz, the 58-year-old man receiving medications for hypertension, asks you about how he should monitor his blood pressure at home. What information would you suggest?

You can find suggested answers after the Bibliography at the end of this chapter.

INTEGRATED CASE STUDY CONNECTION

The case studies in the back of the book are designed to focus on integrating concepts. Refer to the following case studies to enhance your understanding of the concepts related to the skills in this chapter.

- Basic Case Studies: Abigail Cantonelli, page 1063; James White, page 1066; Naomi Bell, page 1067; Joe LeRoy, page 1072.
- Intermediate Case Studies: Olivia Greenbaum, page 1077; Victoria Holly, page 1079; Lucille Howard, page 1086; Janice Romero, page 1088; Gwen Galloway, page 1089.
- Advanced Case Studies: Cole McKean, page 1093.

TAYLOR SUITE RESOURCES

Explore these additional resources to enhance learning for this chapter:

- NCLEX-Style Questions and other resources on thePoint, http://thePoint.lww.com/Lynn4e
- *Skill Checklists for Taylor's Clinical Nursing Skills,* 4e
- *Taylor's Video Guide to Clinical Nursing Skills:* Vital Signs
- *Fundamentals of Nursing:* Chapter 24, Vital Signs
- *Lippincott DocuCare* Fundamentals cases

Bibliography

Alexis, O. (2009). Providing best practice in manual blood pressure measurement. *British Journal of Nursing, 18*(7), 410–415.

Alexis, O. (2010). Providing best practice in manual pulse measurement. *British Journal of Nursing, 19*(4), 228–234.

American Heart Association. (2012). About high blood pressure. Available at http://www.heart.org/HEARTORG/Conditions/HighBloodPressure/AboutHighBloodPressure/About-High-Blood-Pressure_UCM_002050_Article.jsp.

Asher, C., & Northington, L. (2008). Society of Pediatric Nurses. Position statement for measurement of temperature/fever in children. *Journal of Pediatric Nursing, 23*(3), 234–326.

Bell, E. (2008). University of Iowa Children's Hospital. Department of Pediatrics. *Iowa neonatology handbook. Servocontrol: Incubator and radiant warmer.* Available at http://www.uihealthcare.com/depts/med/pediatrics/iowaneonatologyhandbook/temperature/servocontrol.html. Used with permission. Accessed August 24, 2012.

Bern, L., Brandt, M., Mbeiu, N., et al. (2007). Differences in blood pressure values obtained with automated and manual methods in medical inpatients. *MEDSURG Nursing, 16*(6), 356–361.

Boltz, M., Capezuti, E., Fulmer, T., & Zwicker, D. (eds.) (2012). *Evidence-based geriatric nursing protocols for best practice* (4th ed.). New York: Springer Publishing Company.

Braun, C. (2006). Accuracy of pacifier thermometers in young children. *Pediatric Nursing, 32*(5), 413–418.

Bulechek, G.M, Butcher, H.K., Dochterman, J.M., & Wagner, C.M. (Eds.). (2013). *Nursing interventions classification (NIC)* (6th ed.). St. Louis: Mosby Elsevier.

Carpenito-Moyet, L. (2008). *Nursing diagnosis: Application to clinical practice.* (12th ed.). Philadelphia: Wolters Kluwer Health|Lippincott Williams & Wilkins.

Carr, M.A., Wilmoth, M.L., Eliades, A.B., et al. (2011). Comparison of temporal artery to rectal temperature measurements in children up to 24 months. *Journal of Pediatric Nursing, 26*(3), 179–185.

Cunha, B.A. (2011). Fever myths and misconceptions: The beneficial effects of fever as a critical component of host defenses against infection. *Heart & Lung, 41*(1), 99–101.

Davie, A., & Amoore, J. (2010). Best practice in the measurement of body temperature. *Nursing Standard, 24*(42), 42–49.

Domiano, K.L., Hinck, S.M., Savinske, D.L., & Hope, K.L. (2008). Comparison of upper arm and forearm blood pressure. *Clinical Nursing Research, 17*(4), 241–250.

Dondelinger, R.M. (2010). The fundamentals of…Infant warmers. *Biomedical Instrumentation & Technology, 44*(6), 485–487.

Exergen. (2007). *Temporal scanner reference manual.* Watertown, MA: Author. Available at www.exergen.com/medical/TAT/TAT5000Manual5.pdf. Accessed October 29, 2008.

Flenady V, Woodgate PG. (2009). Radiant warmers versus incubators for regulating body temperature in newborn infants. *Cochrane Database of Systematic Reviews* 2003, Issue 4. Art. No.: CD000435. DOI: 10.1002/14651858.CD000435.

Frese, E.M., Fick, A., & Sadowsky, H.S. (2011). Blood pressure measurement guidelines for physical therapists. *Cardiopulmonary Physical Therapy Journal, 22*(2), 5–12.

Frommelt, T., Ott, C., & Hays, V. (2008). Accuracy of different devices to measure temperature. *MEDSURG Nursing, 17*(3), 171–182.

Garner, A., & Fendius, A. (2010). Temperature physiology, assessment, and control. *British Journal of Neuroscience Nursing, 6*(8), 397–400.

Gray-Miceli, D., Ratcliffe, S.J., Liu, S., et al. (2012). Orthostatic hypotension in older nursing home residents who fall: Are they dizzy? *Clinical Nursing Research, 211*, 64–78.

Grossman, S., & Porth, C.M. (2014). *Porth's pathophysiology: concepts of altered health states.* (9th ed.). Philadelphia: Wolters Kluwer Health/Lippincott Williams & Wilkins.

Higgins, D. (2008). Patient assessment Part 2: Measuring oral temperature. *Nursing Times, 104*(8), 24–25.

Hinkle, J.L. & Cheever, K.H. (2014). *Brunner & Suddarth's textbook of medical-surgical nursing.* (13th ed.). Philadelphia: Wolters Kluwer Health/Lippincott Williams & Wilkins.

Hirsch, A.T., Haskal, Z.J., Hertzer, N.R., et al. (2006). ACC/AHA 2005 guidelines for the management of patients with peripheral arterial disease (lower extremity, renal, mesenteric, and abdominal aortic): Executive summary a collaborative report from the American Association for Vascular Surgery/Society for Vascular Surgery, Society for Cardiovascular Angiography and Interventions, Society for Vascular Medicine and Biology, Society of Interventional Radiology, and the ACC/AHA Task Force on Practice Guidelines (Writing Committee to Develop Guidelines for the Management of Patients with Peripheral Arterial Disease). *Circulation, 113*(11), e463–e654.

Hogan-Quigley, B., Palm, M.L., & Bickley, L. (2012). *Bates' nursing guide to physical examination and history taking.* Philadelphia: Wolters Kluwer Health/Lippincott Williams & Wilkins.

Huether, S.E., & McCance, K.L. (2012.) *Understanding pathophysiology* (5th ed.). St. Louis: Elsevier.

Jarvis, C. (2012). *Physical examination & health assessment* (6th ed.). St. Louis: Saunders/Elsevier.

Jensen, S. (2011.) *Nursing health assessment. A best practice approach.* Philadelphia: Wolters Kluwer Health/Lippincott Williams & Wilkins.

Kyle, T., & Carman, S. (2013). *Essentials of pediatric nursing.* (2nd ed.). Philadelphia: Wolters Kluwer Health/Lippincott Williams & Wilkins.

Lanier, J.B., Mote, M.B., & Clay, E.C. (2011). Evaluation and management of orthostatic hypotension. *American Family Physician, 84*(5), 527–536.

Lawson, L., Bridges, E., Ballou, I., et al. (2007). Accuracy and precision of noninvasive temperature measurement in adult intensive care patients. *American Journal of Critical Care, 16*(5), 485–496.

Leblanc, M.E., Cloutier, L., & Veiga, E.V. (2011). Knowledge and practice outcomes after home blood pressure measurement education programs. *Blood Pressure Monitoring, 16*(6), 265–269.

Lee, G., Flannery-Bergey, D., Randall-Rollins, K., et al. (2011). Accuracy of temporal artery thermometry. *Advances in Neonatal Care, 11*(1), 62–70.

Lu, S.H., Leasure, A.R., & Dai, Y.T. (2009). A systematic review of body temperature variations in older people. *Journal of Clinical Nursing, 19*(1–2), 4–16.

Massey, D. (2010). Respiratory assessment 1: Why do it and how to do it? *British Journal of Cardiac Nursing, 5*(11), 537–41.

Moorhead, S., Johnson, M., Maas, M.L., & Swanson, E. (Eds). (2013). *Nursing Outcomes Classification (NOC).* (5th ed.). St. Louis: Mosby Elsevier.

NANDA International. (2012). *Nursing diagnoses: Definitions & classification 2012–2014.* West Sussex, UK: Wiley-Blackwell.

National Heart, Lung, and Blood Institute (NHLBI). National Institutes of Health (NIH). (2012). What is high blood pressure? Available at http://www.nhlbi.nih.gov/health/health-topics/topics/hbp/.

National Heart, Lung, and Blood Institute (NHLBI). National Institutes of Health (NIH). (2005). *The fourth report on the diagnosis, evaluation, and treatment of high blood pressure in children and adolescents.* (NIH Publication No. 05-5267). Washington, D.C.: U.S. Department of Health and Human Services.

Ogedegbe, G., & Pickering, T. (2010). Principles and techniques of blood pressure measurement. *Cardiology Clinics, 28*(4), 571–586.

Ogunlesi, TA. (2009). Radiant warmers versus incubators for regulating body temperature in newborn infants: RHL commentary. *The WHO Reproductive Health Library*; Geneva: World Health Organization. Available at http://apps.who.int/rhl/newborn/cd000435_ogunlesita_com/en/index.html#.

Palatini, P., & Parati, G. (2011). Blood pressure measurement in very obese patients: A challenging problem. *Journal of Hypertension, 29*(3), 425–429.

Parati, G., Krakoff, L.R., & Verdecchia, P. (2010). Methods of measurements: Home and ambulatory blood pressure monitoring. *Blood Pressure Monitoring, 15*(2), 100–105.

Parkes, R. (2011). Rate of respiration: The forgotten vital sign. *Emergency Nurse, 19*(2), 12–17.

Perry, S.E., Hockenberry, M.J., Lowdermilk, D.L., & Wilson, D. (2010). *Maternal child nursing care.* (4th ed.). Maryland Heights, MI: Mosby Elsevier.

Pickering, T., Miller, N., Ogedegbe, G., et al. (2008). Call to action on use and reimbursement for home health pressure monitoring: Executive summary. *Journal of Clinical Hypertension, 10*(6), 467–476.

Pickering, T., Hall, J., Appel, L., et al. (2004). American Heart Association Scientific Statement. Recommendations for blood pressure measurement in humans and experimental animals. Part 1: Blood pressure measurement in humans: A statement for professionals from the subcommittee of professional and public education of the American Heart Association Council on High Blood Pressure Research. Available at http://hyper.ahajournals.org/cgi/content/full/45/1/142.

Purssell, E., While, A., & Coomber, B. (2009). Tympanic thermometry–Normal temperature and reliability. *Paediatric Nursing 21*(6), 40–43.

Quatrara, B., Coffman, J., Kenkins, T., et al. (2007). The effects of respiratory rate and ingestion of hot and cold beverages on the accuracy of oral temperatures measured by electronic thermometers. *MEDSURG Nursing, 16*(2), 105–108, 100.

Sinclair, J. (2002). Servo-control for maintaining abdominal skin temperature at 36 C in low birth weight infants. *Cochrane Database of Systematic Reviews.* Issue 1. Article No.:CD001074. DOI 10.1002/14651858.CD0011074.

Skirton, H., Chamberlain, W., Lawson, C., Ryan, H., & Young, E. (2011). A systematic review of variability and reliability of manual and automated blood pressure readings. *Journal of Clinical Nursing, 20*(5/6), 602–613.

Smitz, S., Van de Winckel, A., & Smitz, M.F. (2009). Reliability of infrared ear thermometry in the prediction of rectal temperature in older inpatients. *Journal of Clinical Nursing, 18*(3), 451–456.

Sund-Levander, M., & Grodzinsky, E. (2009). Time for a change to assess and evaluate body temperature in clinical practice. *International Journal of Nursing Practice, 15*(4), 241–249.

Tabloski, P. (2010). *Gerontological nursing* (2nd ed.). Upper Saddle River, NJ: Pearson.

Taylor, C., Lillis, C., & Lynn, P. (2015). *Fundamentals of nursing: The art and science of nursing care.* (8th ed.). Philadelphia: Wolters Kluwer Health/Lippincott Williams & Wilkins.

Taylor, J.J., & Cohen, B.J. (2013). *Memmler's structure and function of the human body* (10th ed.). Philadelphia: Wolters Kluwer Health/Lippincott Williams & Wilkins.

U.S. Environmental Protection Agency (EPA). (2012). Mercury. Thermometers. Available at http://epa.gov/hg/thermometer-main.html. Accessed May 1, 2012.

Vaajoki, A., Kankkunen, P., Pietilä, A.M., & Vehviläinen-Julkunen, K. (2011). Music as a nursing intervention: Effects of music listening on blood pressure, heart rate, and respiratory rate in abdominal surgery patients. *Nursing and Health Sciences, 13*(4), 412–418.

VISN 8 Patient Safety Center. (2009). *Safe patient handling and movement algorithms.* Tampa, FL: Author. Available at http://www.visn8.va.gov/visn8/patientsafetycenter/safePtHandling/default.asp_

SUGGESTED ANSWERS FOR FOCUSING ON PATIENT CARE: DEVELOPING CLINICAL REASONING

1. First, assess the problem, talking with Tyrone and his mother, using age-appropriate communication with Tyrone. Because potentially he is thought to have an ear infection, he may be having pain in one or both ears. Assess his status and ability to cooperate and consider another route for temperature measurement. Temporal artery or axillary measurement may be indicated, based on your assessment and facility policy.
2. In addition to the respiratory rate, note the depth and rhythm of the respirations. Auscultate lung sounds. Measure the patient's oxygen saturation level with pulse oximetry. Ask the patient about recent activity and the presence of factors that may have caused an acute asthma attack, and for factors that could affect respirations, such as exercise, medications, smoking, chronic illness or conditions, neurologic injury, pain, and anxiety. Note baseline or previous respiratory measurements. Assess patient for any signs of respiratory distress, which include retractions, nasal flaring, grunting, and orthopnea (breathing more easily in an upright position).
3. Home monitoring of blood pressure for patients with hypertension is strongly recommended. Advise Mr. Glatz that automated blood pressure devices in public areas are generally inaccurate and inconsistent. Use a cuff size appropriate for limb circumference. Inform him that cuff sizes range from a pediatric cuff to a large thigh cuff and that a poorly fitting cuff can result in an inaccurate measurement. Discuss digital blood pressure monitoring equipment. Although more costly than manual cuffs, most provide an easy-to-read recording of systolic and diastolic measurements.

3 Health Assessment

FOCUSING ON PATIENT CARE

This chapter will help you develop some of the physical assessment skills related to health assessment necessary to care for the following patients:

WILLIAM LINCOLN, age 54, comes to the clinic for a routine checkup.

LOIS FELKER, age 30, has a history of type 1 diabetes. She is a patient in the hospital.

BOBBY WILLIAMS, a teenager brought to the emergency department by his parents, is suspected of having appendicitis.

Refer to Focusing on Patient Care: Developing Clinical Reasoning at the end of the chapter to apply what you learn.

LEARNING OBJECTIVES

After studying this chapter, you will be able to:

1. Describe the components of, and perform, a general survey.
2. Weigh the patient using a bed scale.
3. Use appropriate equipment while performing a head-to-toe physical assessment.
4. Assist in positioning the patient in the correct position to perform the head-to-toe physical assessment.
5. Verbalize the appropriate rationale for performing the specific head-to-toe assessment techniques.
6. Assess the skin, hair, and nails.
7. Assess the head and neck.
8. Assess the thorax, lungs, and breasts.
9. Assess the cardiovascular system.
10. Assess the abdomen.
11. Assess female genitalia.
12. Assess male genitalia.
13. Assess the neurologic, musculoskeletal, and peripheral vascular systems.

KEY TERMS

activities of daily living (ADLs): daily self-care activities within person's place of residence and/or in outdoor environments

adventitious breath sounds: sounds that are not normally heard in the lungs on auscultation

ascites: accumulation of serous fluid in the peritoneal cavity

auscultation: act of listening with a stethoscope to sounds produced within the body

body mass index (BMI): a ratio of weight (in kilograms) to height (in meters), used as an indicator of total body fat stores in the general population, and to estimate relative risk for diseases such as heart disease, diabetes, and hypertension

bruits: abnormal "swooshing" sounds heard on auscultation, indicating turbulent blood flow

cyanosis: bluish or grayish skin discoloration in response to inadequate oxygenation

ecchymosis: a collection of blood in the subcutaneous tissues, causing purplish discoloration

edema: excess fluid in the tissues, characterized by swelling

erythema: redness of the skin

general survey: overall impression of a person by the health care provider; includes physical appearance, body structure, mobility, and behavior

health history: a collection of subjective data that provides information about the patient's health status

inspection: process of performing deliberate, purposeful observations in a systematic manner

instrumental activities of daily living (IADLs): daily self-care activities needed for independent living; for example, housekeeping, meal preparation, management of finances, and transportation

jaundice: yellow color of the skin resulting from liver and gallbladder diseases, some types of anemia, and hemolysis

pallor: paleness of the skin

palpation: an assessment technique that uses the sense of touch

percussion: the act of striking one object against another to produce sound

petechiae: small hemorrhagic spots caused by capillary bleeding

physical assessment: a collection of objective data that provides information about changes in the patient's body systems

precordium: the area on the anterior chest corresponding to the aortic, pulmonic, tricuspid, and apical areas and Erb's point

turgor: fullness or elasticity of the skin

Health assessment involves gathering information about the health status of the patient. The information (data) is evaluated and synthesized. Based on these findings, the nurse plans appropriate nursing interventions and evaluates patient care outcomes to deliver the best possible care for each patient. A health assessment includes a health history and a physical assessment.

A **health history** is a collection of subjective data that provides information about the patient's health status. Components of the health history include biographical data; the reason the patient is seeking health care; present health concerns or history of those health concerns; health history; family history; functional health; psychosocial and lifestyle factors; and a review of systems. The nurse should adapt questions to the individual patient, omitting questions that do not apply and adding questions that seem pertinent, based on the setting, situation, the individual patient, and ongoing information as the health assessment proceeds. Be sure to use language the patient can understand; avoid using medical terms and jargon. Nurses use therapeutic communication skills, including interviewing techniques, during the health history to gather data to identify actual and potential health problems as well as sources of patient strength. Additionally, during the health history, the nurse begins to establish an effective nurse–patient relationship. Fundamentals Review 3-1 summarizes major components of a health history. Examples of health history questions related to each body system (review of systems) are included in the discussion of each region of the physical examination discussed in this chapter.

Generally, a physical assessment is performed after taking the health history. **Physical assessment** is a collection of objective data that provides information about changes in the patient's body systems. These data are obtained through direct observation or elicited through examination techniques, such as **inspection**, **palpation**, **percussion**, and **auscultation** (Fundamentals Review 3-2). The use of percussion and deep palpation are advanced physical assessment skills, usually performed by advanced practice professionals, health care providers with advanced education. *Percussion and deep palpation will not be discussed as part of physical assessment in this chapter. Refer to information on* thePoint *or a health assessment text for details of these advanced assessment skills.* To perform a physical examination, the nurse requires knowledge of anatomy and physiology, the equipment used for assessing body systems, and proper patient positioning and draping.

Nurses should be familiar with the general health beliefs and variances of various cultural and ethnic groups to improve the effectiveness of health care services and provide care within a cultural context (Ritter & Hoffman, 2010). Nurses should know risk factors for alterations in health that are based on racial inheritance and ethnic backgrounds, normal variations that occur within races, and then consider how religion and spirituality may impact health. In addition, laboratory and diagnostic tests provide crucial information about a patient's health. These results become a part of the total health assessment.

For a comprehensive assessment, the nurse integrates individual assessments following a systematic head-to-toe format. *However, not all assessments included in a comprehensive physical assessment are covered in this chapter.* Advanced practice professionals (health care providers with advanced education) typically perform some of the assessments included in a comprehensive or focused exam, such as an internal eye examination, a vaginal examination, or a rectal examination. *Refer to information on* thePoint *or a health assessment text for details of these advanced assessment skills.*

FUNDAMENTALS REVIEW 3-1

COMPONENTS OF A HEALTH HISTORY

BIOGRAPHIC DATA

Biographic information is often collected during admission to a health care facility or agency and documented on a specific form; it helps to identify the patient. Depending on the health care setting, some biographic data may be collected by people other than the nurse. Biographic data include:

- Name
- Address
- Billing and insurance information
- Gender
- Age and birth date
- Marital status
- Race
- Ethnicity
- Occupation
- Religious preference
- Advance directives/living will
- Health care financing
- Primary health care provider

REASON FOR SEEKING HEALTH CARE

The reason for seeking care is a statement in the patient's own words that describes the patient's reason for seeking care. This can help to focus the rest of the assessment. Ask an open-ended question, such as, "Tell me why you are here today." **Record whatever it is the person says; his or her description in exact words. Avoid paraphrasing or interpreting.**

For example, Nina Dunning comes into the clinic and states, "I'm having trouble sleeping. At night. I can't seem to stop my thoughts. All I do is worry."

- Incorrect documentation: Patient complains of insomnia and anxiety.
- Correct documentation: "I'm having trouble sleeping. At night, I can't seem to stop my thoughts. All I do is worry."

HISTORY OF PRESENT HEALTH CONCERN

When taking the patient's history of present health concern, be sure to explore the symptoms thoroughly.

FUNDAMENTALS REVIEW 3-1 continued

COMPONENTS OF A HEALTH HISTORY

Encourage the patient to describe and explain any symptoms. The description should include information regarding the onset of the problem; location; duration; intensity; quality/description; relieving/exacerbating factors; associated factors; past occurrences; any treatments; and how the problem has affected the patient. The mnemonic "PQRST," described below, is a helpful guide to analyze a patient's symptoms:

Provocative or palliative: What causes the symptom? What makes it better or worse?

- What were you doing when you first noticed it?
- What seems to trigger it? Stress? Position? Certain activities? An argument? (For a sign, such as an eye discharge: What seems to cause it or make it worse? For a psychological symptom, such as depression: Does the depression occur after specific events?)
- What relieves the symptom? Changing diet? Changing position? Taking medication? Being active?
- What makes the symptom worse? What makes the symptom better?

Quality or quantity: How does the symptom feel, look, or sound? How much of it are you experiencing now?

- How would you describe the symptom—how it feels, looks, or sounds?
- How much are you experiencing now? Is it so much that it prevents you from performing any activities? Is it more or less than you experienced at any other time?

Region or radiation: Where is the symptom located? Does it spread?

- Where does the symptom occur?
- In the case of pain, does it travel down your back or arms, up your neck, or down your legs?

Severity: How does the symptom rate on a scale of 1 to 10, with 10 being the most severe?

- How bad is the symptom at its worst? Does it force you to lie down, sit down, or slow down?
- Does the symptom seem to be getting better, getting worse, or staying about the same?

Timing: When did the symptom begin? Did it occur suddenly or gradually? How often does it occur?

- On what date and time did the symptom first occur?
- How did the symptom start? Suddenly? Gradually?
- How often do you experience the symptom? Hourly? Daily? Weekly? Monthly?
- When do you usually experience the symptom? During the day? At night? In the early morning? Does it awaken you? Does it occur before, during, or after meals? Does it occur seasonally?
- How long does an episode of the symptom last?

PAST MEDICAL HISTORY

A patient's past health history may provide insight to causes of current symptoms. It also alerts the nurse to certain risk factors. A past health history includes childhood and adult illnesses, chronic health problems and treatment, and previous surgeries or hospitalizations. This history should also include accidents or injuries, obstetric history, allergies, the date of most recent immunizations. Vaccine recommendations are updated each year by the Centers for Disease Control and Prevention (CDC). Current guidelines for different age groups can be found on the CDC's Web site at www.cdc.gov (CDC, 2012). Ask the patient about health maintenance screenings, including dates and results, as well as the use of safety measures. Ask the patient about prescribed and over-the-counter medications, including vitamins, supplements, and any home or herbal remedies. Include the name, dose, route, frequency, and purpose for each medication. Sample questions include:

- "Tell me about the childhood illnesses, such as measles or mumps, that you have had."
- "What are you allergic to?"
- "Describe any accidents, injuries, and surgeries you have had."
- "What prescribed or over-the counter medications do you use?"
- "Do you take any herbal or dietary supplements?"
- "What is the date of your most recent immunization for tetanus; pertussis; polio; measles; rubella; mumps; influenza; hepatitis A, B, and C; and pneumococcus?"
- "Tell me about your use of seat belts in cars."
- "Tell me about your family's use of sports helmets, padding, or other protective equipment."

FAMILY HISTORY

A person's family history will provide information about diseases and conditions for which a patient may be at increased risk. Certain disorders have genetic links. Information regarding contact with family members with communicable diseases or environmental hazards can provide clues to the patient's current health or risk factors for health issues. This information can also identify important topics for health teaching and counseling. Sample family history questions include:

- "How old are the members of your family?"
- "If any members of your family are not living, what caused their death?"
- "Is there any history of this health problem you have in other family members?"
- "Do any family members have long-term illnesses?"

(continued)

FUNDAMENTALS REVIEW 3-1 continued

COMPONENTS OF A HEALTH HISTORY

FUNCTIONAL HEALTH ASESSMENT

A functional health assessment focuses on the effects of health or illness on a patient's quality of life, including the strengths of the patient and areas that need to improve. Assess the patient's ability to perform **activities of daily living (ADLs)** or self-care activities. Eating, bathing, dressing, and toileting are examples of ADLs. Assess the patient's ability to perform **instrumental activities of daily living (IADLs)** or those needed for independent living. Housekeeping, meal preparation, management of finances, and transportation are examples of IADLs. Functional health may be further assessed using a formal tool, such as the Katz Index of Independence in Activities of Daily Living, which is used with older adults (Figure 1).

ACTIVITIES POINTS (1 OR 0)	**INDEPENDENCE:** (1 POINT) **NO** supervision, direction, or personal assistance	**DEPENDENCE:** (0 POINTS) **WITH** supervision, direction, personal assistance, or total care
BATHING POINTS:______	**(1 POINT)** Bathes self completely or needs help in bathing only a single part of the body such as the back, genital area, or disabled extremity.	**(0 POINTS)** Needs help with bathing more than one part of the body, getting in or out of the tub or shower. Requires total bathing.
DRESSING POINTS:______	**(1 POINT)** Gets clothes from closets and drawers and puts on clothes and outer garments complete with fasteners. May have help tying shoes.	**(0 POINTS)** Needs help with dressing self or needs to be completely dressed.
TOILETING POINTS:______	**(1 POINT)** Goes to toilet, gets on and off, arranges clothes, cleans genital area without help.	**(0 POINTS)** Needs help transferring to the toilet, cleaning self, or uses bedpan or commode.
TRANSFERRING POINTS:______	**(1 POINT)** Moves in and out of bed or chair unassisted. Mechanical transferring aides are acceptable.	**(0 POINTS)** Needs help in moving from bed to chair or requires a complete transfer.
CONTINENCE POINTS:______	**(1 POINT)** Exercises complete self-control over urination and defecation.	**(0 POINTS)** Is partially or totally incontinent of bowel or bladder.
FEEDING POINTS:______	**(1 POINT)** Gets food from plate into mouth without help. Preparation of food may be done by another person.	**(0 POINTS)** Needs partial or total help with feeding or requires parenteral feeding.

TOTAL POINTS = ______ 6 = High (*patient independent*) 0 = Low (*patient very dependent*)

FIGURE 1 Katz Index of Independence in Activities of Daily Living. (Slightly adapted from Katz, S., Down, T.D., Cash, H.R., & Grotz, R.C. (1970). Progress in the development of the index of ADL. *The Gerontologist*, *10*(1), 20–30. Copyright ©The Gerontological Society of America. Reproduced [Adapted] by permission of the publisher.)

FUNDAMENTALS REVIEW 3-1 continued

COMPONENTS OF A HEALTH HISTORY

Sample lifestyle questions include:

- "Do you have difficulty or require assistance with bathing or dressing?"
- "Do you have difficulty or require assistance with toileting or moving around?"
- "Do you have difficulty or require assistance with eating or preparing meals?"
- "Do you have difficulty or require assistance with shopping or administering your own medications?"
- "Tell me about your driving. Who provides transportation?"
- "Do you have difficulty or require assistance with housekeeping, finances, or laundry?"

PSYCHOSOCIAL AND LIFESTYLE FACTORS

A patient's lifestyle contributes to his or her overall health and well-being. Ask about the patient's social support and network of available assistance. Ask about confidants, skillful supporters and people who can help the patient cope with any health alteration, illness, or other change. Ask about the patient's level of activity and exercise; sleep and rest; and nutrition. Obtain information related to the patient's interpersonal relationships and resources; values, beliefs, and spiritual resources; self-esteem and self-concept; and coping and stress management. Question the patient regarding personal habits, including use of alcohol, illicit drugs, and/or tobacco; environmental and occupational hazards; intimate partner and family violence; sexual history and orientation; and mental health.

- "Do you smoke, drink, or use drugs? If so, what kind, for how long and how much?"
- "Describe the foods you eat during a typical day."
- "Tell me how well you sleep."
- "How much exercise do you get each day?"
- "Who in your family or community is available to help you with health problems if you need it?"
- "Does your religious faith or spirituality play an important part in your life?"
- "Tell me how you deal with stress."
- "Describe any changes that you have had in your mood or feelings."
- "Have you ever been treated for any problems with your mood or behavior?"

FUNDAMENTALS REVIEW 3-2

ASSESSMENT TECHNIQUES

Inspection is the process of performing deliberate, purposeful observations in a systematic manner. The nurse closely observes visually, but also uses hearing and smell to gather data throughout the assessment. The nurse assesses details of the patient's appearance, behavior, and movement. Inspection begins with the initial patient contact and continues through the entire assessment. Adequate natural or artificial lighting is essential for distinguishing the color, texture, and moisture of body surfaces. The nurse inspects each area of the body for size, color, shape, position, movement, and symmetry, noting normal findings and any deviations from normal.

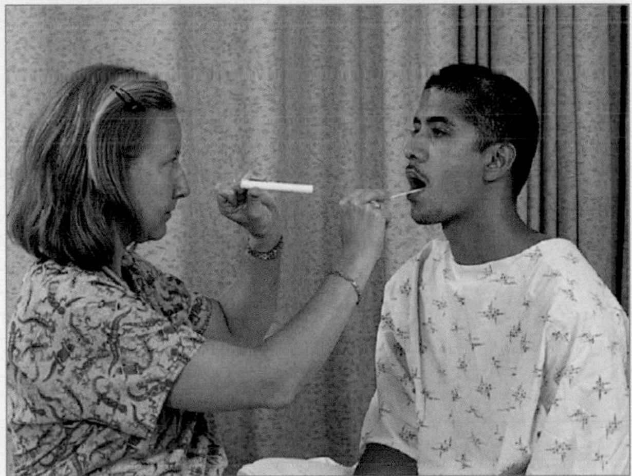

Inspection.

(*continued*)

FUNDAMENTALS REVIEW 3-2 continued

ASSESSMENT TECHNIQUES

Palpation uses the sense of touch. The hands and fingers are sensitive tools that can assess skin temperature, turgor, texture, and moisture, as well as vibrations within the body (e.g., the heart) and shape or structures within the body (e.g., the bones). Specific parts of the hand are more effective at assessing different qualities. The dorsum (back) surfaces of the hand and fingers are used for gross measure of temperature. The palmar (front) surfaces of the fingers and finger pads are used to assess firmness, contour, shape, tenderness, and consistency. The finger pads are best at fine discrimination. Use finger pads to locate pulses, lymph nodes and other small lumps, and to assess skin texture and edema. Vibration is palpated best with the ulnar, or outside, surface of the hand. For light palpation, apply light pressure with the dominant hand, using a circular motion to feel the surface structure; press down less than 1 cm (0.5 inch). *Advanced practitioners usually perform deep palpation. Refer to information on* thePoint *or a health assessment text for details of this advanced assessment skill.*

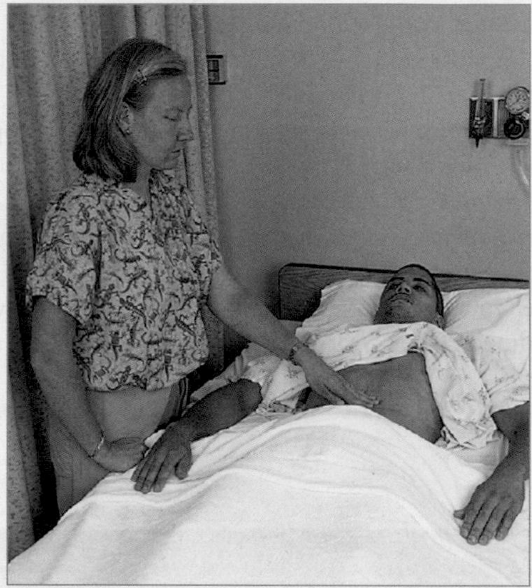
Light palpation.

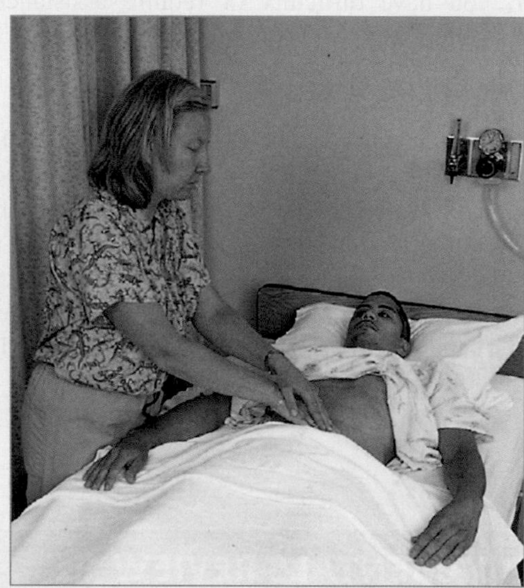
Deep palpation.

Percussion is the act of striking one object against another to produce sound. The fingertips are used to tap the body over body tissues to produce vibrations and sound waves. The characteristics of the sounds produced are used to assess the location, shape, size, and density of tissues. Abnormal sounds suggest alteration of tissues, such as an emphysematous lung, or the presence of a mass, such as an abdominal tumor. A quiet environment allows sounds to be heard. *Advanced practitioners usually perform percussion. Refer to information on* thePoint *or a health assessment text for details of this advanced assessment skill.*

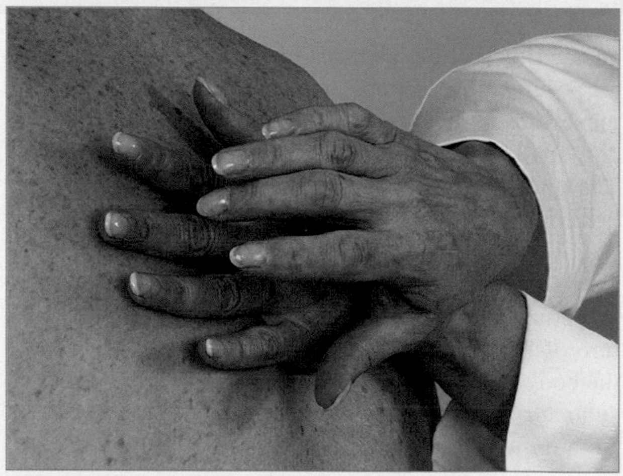
Percussion.

FUNDAMENTALS REVIEW 3-2 continued

ASSESSMENT TECHNIQUES

Auscultation is the act of listening with a stethoscope to sounds produced within the body. This technique is used to listen for blood pressure, and heart, lung, and bowel sounds. Four characteristics of sound are assessed by auscultation: (1) pitch (ranging from high to low); (2) loudness (ranging from soft to loud); (3) quality (e.g., gurgling or swishing); and (4) duration (short, medium, or long).

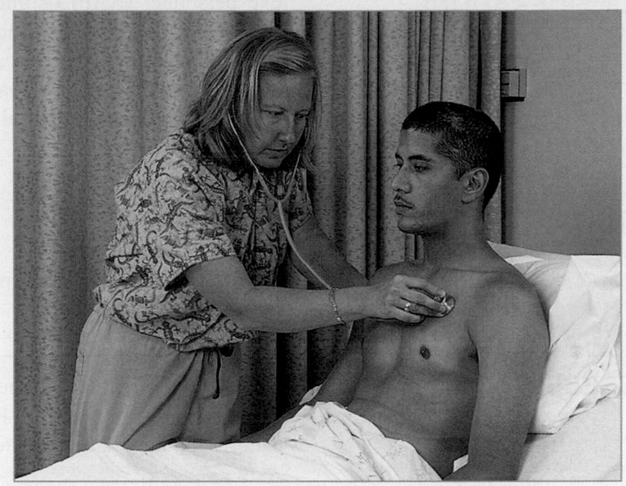

Auscultation. *(Photos by B. Proud.)*

SKILL 3-1 PERFORMING A GENERAL SURVEY

The general survey is the first component of the physical assessment, beginning with the first moment of patient contact and continuing throughout the nurse–patient relationship. The general survey contributes to the overall impression of the patient. It includes observing the patient's overall appearance and behavior; taking vital signs; measuring height, weight, and waist circumference; and calculating the BMI. Table 3-1 displays the relationship of the risks of obesity-associated diseases and conditions by BMI and waist circumference.

Table 3-1 RISK OF OBESITY-ASSOCIATED DISEASES AND CONDITIONS BY BMI AND WAIST CIRCUMFERENCE RELATIVE TO NORMAL WEIGHT AND WAIST CIRCUMFERENCE (DISEASE RISK FOR TYPE 2 DIABETES, HYPERTENSION, AND CARDIOVASCULAR DISEASE)

		WAIST CIRCUMFERENCE*	
	BMI (KG/M^2)	*Men ≤40 Inches (102 cm) Women ≤35 Inches (88 cm)*	*Men >40 Inches (102 cm) Women >35 Inches (88 cm)*
Underweight	<18.5	NA	NA
Normal	18.5–24.9	NA	NA
Overweight	25.0–29.9	Increased	High
Obesity, Class I	30.0–34.9	High	Very high
Obesity, Class II	35.0–39.9	Very high	Very high
Extreme Obesity	40.0+	Extremely high	Extremely high

*Increased waist circumference can also be a marker for increased risk even in persons of normal weight.
(National Institutes of Health, National Heart, Lung, and Blood Institute. [2000]. NHLBI Obesity Education Initiative. *The practical guide: Identification, evaluation, and treatment of overweight and obesity in adults.* NIH publication no. 00–4084. October 2000. Available at www.nhlbi.nih.gov/guidelines/obesity/prctgd_c.pdf.)

(continued)

SKILL 3-1 PERFORMING A GENERAL SURVEY continued

DELEGATION CONSIDERATIONS

Measurement of the patient's weight and height, and vital signs may be delegated to nursing assistive personnel (NAP) or unlicensed assistive personnel (UAP). Depending on the state's nurse practice act and the organization's policies and procedures, the licensed practical/vocational nurses (LPN/LVN) may perform some or all of the parts of the general survey. The decision to delegate must be based on careful analysis of the patient's needs and circumstances, as well as the qualifications of the person to whom the task is being delegated. Refer to the Delegation Guidelines in Appendix A.

EQUIPMENT

- Adequate lighting
- Tape measure
- A scale with height attachment; chair scale; or bed scale
- PPE, as indicated

ASSESSMENT

Develop an overall impression of the patient, focusing on overall appearance and behavior, vital signs, height, and weight. Ask the patient about any changes in weight, pain or discomfort, sleeping patterns, and any difficulty sleeping.

NURSING DIAGNOSIS

Determine the related factors for the nursing diagnosis based on the patient's current status. Appropriate nursing diagnoses may include:

- Self-Care Deficit (Toileting, Dressing, Bathing)
- Anxiety
- Ineffective Coping

OUTCOME IDENTIFICATION AND PLANNING

The expected outcome to achieve in performing a general survey is that the assessment is completed without the patient experiencing anxiety or discomfort, an overall impression of the patient is formulated, the findings are documented, and the appropriate referral is made to other health care professionals, as needed, for further evaluation. Other specific outcomes will depend on the identified nursing diagnosis.

IMPLEMENTATION

ACTION	RATIONALE
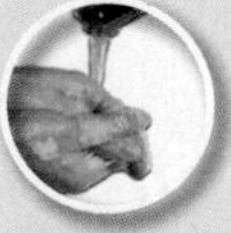 1. Perform hand hygiene and put on PPE, if indicated.	Hand hygiene and PPE prevent the spread of microorganisms. PPE is required based on transmission precautions.
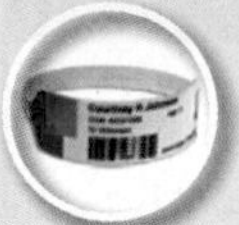 2. Identify the patient.	Identifying the patient ensures the right patient receives the intervention and helps prevent errors.
3. Close curtains around the bed and the door to the room, if possible. Explain the purpose of the health examination and what you are going to do. Answer any questions.	This ensures the patient's privacy. Explanation relieves anxiety and facilitates cooperation.
4. Assess the patient's physical appearance. Observe if the patient appears to be his or her stated age. Note the patient's mental status. Is the person alert and oriented, responsive to questions and responding appropriately? Are the facial features symmetric? Note any signs of acute distress, such as shortness of breath, pain, or anxiousness.	Appearance provides information about various aspects of the patient's health. Changes in cognitive processes, asymmetry, and signs of distress can be indicators of health abnormalities.

ACTION	RATIONALE
5. Assess the patient's body structure. Does the person's height appear within normal range for stated age and genetic heritage? Does the person's weight appear within normal range for height and body build? Note if body fat is evenly distributed. Do body parts appear equal bilaterally and relatively proportionate? Is the patient's posture erect and appropriate for age?	Height that is excessively short or tall, asymmetry, one-sided atrophy or hypertrophy, abnormal posture, and abnormal body proportion can be indicators of health problems.
6. Assess the patient's mobility. Is the patient's gait smooth, even, well-balanced, and coordinated? Is joint mobility smooth and coordinated with a general full range of motion (ROM)? Are involuntary movements evident?	Abnormalities in gait and ROM can indicate health concerns.
7. Assess the patient's behavior. Are facial expressions appropriate for the situation? Does the patient maintain eye contact, based on cultural norms? Does the person appear comfortable and relaxed with you? Is the patient's speech clear and understandable? Observe the person's hygiene and grooming. Is the clothing appropriate for climate, fit well, appear clean, and appropriate for the person's culture and age group? Does the person appear clean and well groomed, appropriate for age and culture?	Facial expressions, speech, eye contact, and other behaviors provide clues to mood and mental health. Deficits in hygiene and grooming may indicate alterations in health.
8. Assess for pain. (Refer to Chapter 10.)	Pain can indicate alterations in physical and psychological health.
9. Have the patient remove shoes and heavy outer clothing. Weigh the patient using a scale (Figure 1). Compare the measurement with previous weight measurements and recommended range for height.	Weight loss or gain may indicate health problems.
10. With shoes off, and standing erect, measure the patient's height using a wall-mounted measuring device or measuring pole (Figure 2).	Ratio of height and weight is a general assessment of overall health, hydration, and nutrition.

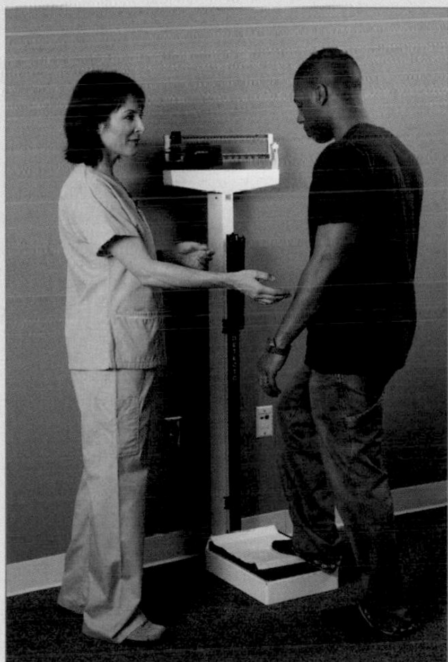

FIGURE 1 Weighing patient using scale. *(Photo by B. Proud.)*

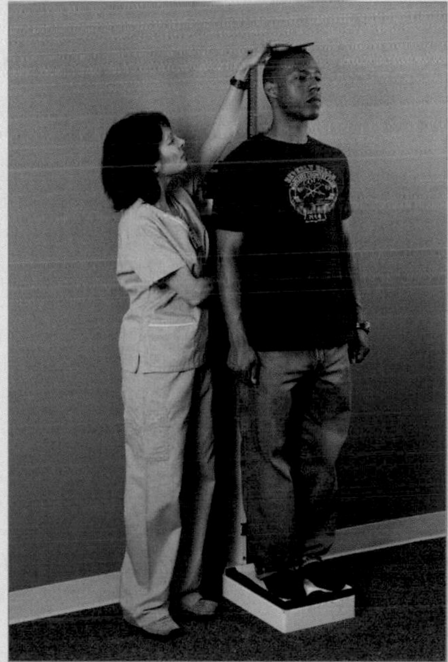

FIGURE 2 Measuring patient's height. *(Photo by B. Proud.)*

(continued)

SKILL 3-1 PERFORMING A GENERAL SURVEY continued

ACTION	RATIONALE
11. Use the patient's weight and height measurements to calculate the patient's BMI. $$\text{Body mass index} = \frac{\text{weight in kilograms}}{\text{height in meters}^2}$$	BMI, an indicator of total body fat stores in the general population, provides a more accurate weight calculation than weight measurement alone. In addition, it provides an estimation of risk for diseases, such as heart disease, diabetes, and hypertension. Refer to Table 3-1.
12. Using the tape measure, measure the patient's waist circumference. Place the tape measure snugly around the patient's waist at the level of the umbilicus.	Waist circumference is a good indicator of abdominal fat. It is thought to be an important and reliable indicator of risk for disease, such as type 2 diabetes, dyslipidemia, hypertension, and cardiovascular disease (Dudek, 2014).
13. Measure the patient's temperature, pulse, respirations, blood pressure, and oxygen saturation. (Refer to Chapter 2, and Chapter 14, for specific techniques.)	Vital signs and oxygen saturation are measured to establish a baseline for the database and to detect actual or potential health problems.
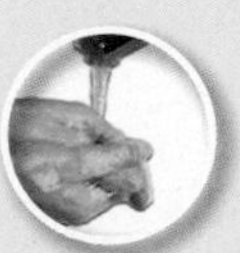 14. Remove PPE, if used. Clean equipment, based on facility policy. Perform hand hygiene. Continue with assessments of specific body systems as appropriate or indicated. Initiate appropriate referral to other health care practitioners for further evaluation as indicated.	Removing PPE properly reduces the risk for infection transmission and contamination of other items. Cleaning of equipment prevents transmission of microorganisms. Hand hygiene prevents the spread of microorganisms. Additional assessments should be completed, as indicated, to evaluate the patient's health status. Intervention by other health care providers may be indicated to evaluate and treat the patient's health status.

EVALUATION

The expected outcome is met when the assessment is completed without the patient experiencing anxiety or discomfort, an overall impression of the patient is formulated, the findings are documented, and the appropriate referral is made to other health care professionals, as needed, for further evaluation.

DOCUMENTATION

Guidelines

Document findings related to assessment of the patient's physical appearance, body structure, mobility, and behavior. Document the patient's height, weight, BMI, and waist circumference. Document the presence or absence of pain, as well as an initial pain assessment if present. Record the patient's temperature (T), pulse (P), respiration (R), and blood pressure (BP) measurements, as well as the oxygen saturation measurement. Note any referrals.

Sample Documentation

Lippincott DocuCare Practice documenting assessment techniques and findings in *Lippincott DocuCare.*

<u>1/26/15</u> 1015 Patient admitted to room 432. Patient is a 23-year-old Asian female graduate student at a local university, living in an apartment with three other female students. Appears well nourished, disheveled, clothing appropriate for age and season, and tired. Oriented, cooperative, with no signs of acute distress; patient denies pain at present. T 98.9°F, P 78, R 16, BP 114/58 mm Hg (left arm), sitting O_2 sat 96% on room air. Height 144 cm (5 ft). Weight 55 kg (121 lb). BMI 26.5. Waist circumference 32 inches. Information provided regarding use of call bell, lights, and phone, and location of bathroom. Patient verbalizes an understanding of information.

—*R. Robinson, RN*

UNEXPECTED SITUATIONS AND ASSOCIATED INTERVENTIONS

- *Patient is unable to tolerate standing for height or weight measurement:* Obtain a chair scale or bed scale to measure weight (see Skill 3-2). Obtain a measuring stick to measure height. Alternately, use tape to mark the patient's length in the bed with the patient supine, the head in the midline position, and the legs extended flat on the bed. Measure the resulting length.

SPECIAL CONSIDERATIONS

General Considerations

- BMI may not be accurate for people, such as athletes, with a large muscle mass; people with **edema** or dehydration; older adults and others who have lost muscle mass (NIH, 2012; Dudek, 2014).
- According to the most recent BMI guidelines published by the National Heart, Lung, and Blood Institute, an adult with a BMI below 18.5 is underweight; a BMI of 25 to 29.9 indicates that a person is overweight; a BMI of 30 or greater indicates obesity; and a BMI of 40 or greater indicates extreme obesity (NIH, 2012).
- Disease risk increases with a waist measurement of more than 40 inches in men and 35 inches in women (NIH, 2012).

Infant and Child Considerations

- Measure height in children up to 2 years of age in the recumbent position with legs fully extended.
- Weigh infants without clothing.
- Weigh children in their underwear.
- Overweight and obesity are defined differently for children and teens than for adults. Children are still growing, and boys and girls mature at different rates.
- BMIs for children and teens compare their heights and weights against growth charts that take age and sex into account. This is called BMI-for-age percentile. A child or teen's BMI-for-age percentile shows how his or her BMI compares with other boys and girls of the same age.
- Information about BMI-for-age and growth charts for children can be found at the Centers for Disease Control and Prevention's BMI-for-Age calculator (CDC, 2011).

SKILL 3-2 USING A BED SCALE

Obtaining a patient's weight is an important component of assessment. In addition to providing baseline information of the patient's overall status, weight is a valuable indicator of nutritional status and fluid balance. Changes in a patient's weight can provide clues to underlying problems, such as nutritional deficiencies or fluid excess or deficiency, or indicate the development of new problems, such as fluid overload. Weight also can be used to evaluate a patient's response to treatment. For example, if a patient is receiving nutritional supplementation, obtaining daily or biweekly weights is used to determine achievement of the expected outcome (i.e., weight gain).

Typically, the nurse will measure weight by having the patient stand on an upright scale. However, doing so requires that the patient is mobile and can maintain his or her balance. Chair scales are available for patient's who are unable to stand. For patients who are confined to the bed, have limited mobility, or cannot maintain a balanced upright or standing position for a short period of time, a bed scale can be used. With a bed scale, the nurse places the patient in a sling and raises the patient above the bed. To ensure safety, a second nurse should be on hand to assist with weighing the patient. Many facilities are providing beds for patient use with built-in scales. The following procedure explains how to weigh the patient with a portable bed scale.

DELEGATION CONSIDERATIONS

Measurement of body weight may be delegated to nursing assistive personnel (NAP) or unlicensed assistive personnel (UAP), as well as to licensed practical/vocational nurses (LPN/LVNs). The decision to delegate must be based on careful analysis of the patient's needs and circumstances, as well as the qualifications of the person to whom the task is being delegated. Refer to the Delegation Guidelines in Appendix A.

(continued)

SKILL 3-2 USING A BED SCALE continued

EQUIPMENT

- Bed scale with sling
- Cover for sling
- Sheet or bath blanket
- PPE, as indicated

ASSESSMENT

Assess the patient's ability to stand for a weight measurement. If the patient cannot stand, assess the patient's ability to sit in a chair or to lie still for a weight measurement. Assess the patient for pain. If necessary, give medication for pain or sedation before placing the patient on a bed scale. Assess for the presence of any material, such as tubes, drains, or IV tubing, which could become entangled in the scale or pulled during the weighing procedure.

NURSING DIAGNOSIS

Determine the related factors for the nursing diagnoses based on the patient's current status. Appropriate nursing diagnoses may include:

- Risk for Injury
- Impaired Physical Mobility
- Imbalanced Nutrition: Less Than Body Requirements
- Imbalanced Nutrition: More Than Body Requirements

OUTCOME IDENTIFICATION AND PLANNING

The expected outcomes to achieve when weighing a patient using a portable bed scale are that the patient's weight is assessed accurately, without injury, and the patient experiences minimal discomfort.

IMPLEMENTATION

ACTION	RATIONALE
1. Check the medical order or nursing plan of care for frequency of weight measurement. More frequent measurement of the patient's weight may be appropriate based on nursing judgment. Obtain the assistance of a second caregiver, based on the patient's mobility and ability to cooperate with the procedure.	This provides for patient safety and appropriate care.
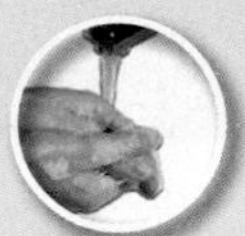 2. Perform hand hygiene and put on PPE, if indicated.	Hand hygiene and PPE prevent the spread of microorganisms. PPE is required based on transmission precautions.
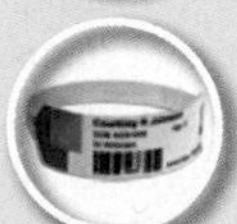 3. Identify the patient.	Identifying the patient ensures that the right patient receives the intervention and helps prevent errors.
4. Close the curtains around the bed and close the door to the room if possible. Discuss the procedure with the patient and assess the patient's ability to assist with the procedure.	This ensures the patient's privacy. Explanation relieves anxiety and facilitates cooperation.
5. Place a cover over the sling of the bed scale.	Using a cover deters the spread of microorganisms.
6. Attach the sling to the bed scale. Lay the sheet or bath blanket in the sling. Turn on the scale. **Balance the scale so that weight reads 0.0.**	Scale will add the sling into the weight unless it is zeroed with the sling, blanket, and cover.
7. Adjust the bed to a comfortable working position, usually elbow height of the caregiver (VISN 8, 2009). Position one caregiver on each side of the bed, if two caregivers are present. Raise side rail on the opposite side of the bed from where the scale is located, if not already in place. Cover the patient with the sheet or bath blanket. Remove other covers and any pillows.	Having the bed at the proper height prevents back and muscle strain. Having one caregiver on each side of the bed provides for patient safety and appropriate care. Side rail assists patient with movement. Blanket maintains patient's dignity and provides warmth.

ACTION	RATIONALE
8. Turn the patient onto his or her side facing the side rail, keeping his or her body covered with the sheet or blanket. Remove the sling from the scale. Place the cover on the sling. Roll cover and sling lengthwise. Place rolled sling under the patient, making sure the patient is centered in the sling.	Rolling the patient onto his or her side facilitates placing the patient onto the sling. Blanket maintains patient's dignity and provides warmth.
9. Roll the patient back over the sling and onto the other side. Pull the sling through, as if placing sheet under patient, unrolling the sling as it is pulled through.	This facilitates placing the patient onto the sling.
10. Roll the scale over the bed so that the arms of the scale are directly over the patient. **Spread the base of the scale.** Lower the arms of the scale and place the arm hooks into the holes on the sling.	By spreading the base, you are giving the scale a wider base, thus preventing the scale from toppling over with the patient. Hooking sling to scale provides secure attachment to the scale and prevents injury.
11. Once the scale arms are hooked onto the sling, gradually elevate the sling so that the patient is lifted up off of the bed (Figure 1). **Assess all tubes and drains, making sure that none have tension placed on them as the scale is lifted. Once the sling is no longer touching the bed, ensure that nothing else is hanging onto the sling (e.g., ventilator or IV tubing). If any tubing is connected to the patient, raise it up so that it is not adding any weight to the patient.**	The scale must be hanging free to obtain an accurate weight. Any tubing that is hanging off the scale will add weight to the patient.

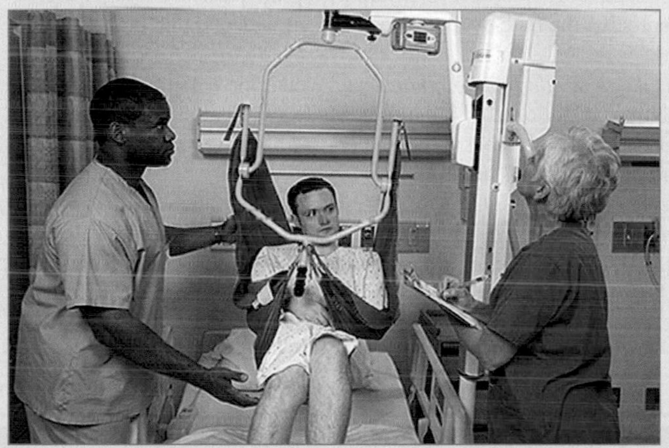

FIGURE 1 Using a bed scale.

ACTION	RATIONALE
12. Note the weight reading on the scale. Slowly and gently, lower the patient back onto the bed. Disconnect the scale arms from the sling. Close the base of the scale and pull it away from the bed.	Lowering the patient slowly does not alarm the patient. Closing the base of the scale facilitates moving the scale.
13. Raise the side rail. Turn the patient to the side rail. Roll the sling up against the patient's backside.	Raising the side rail is a safety measure.
14. Raise the other side rail. Roll the patient back over the sling and up facing the other side rail. Remove the sling from the bed. Remove gloves, if used. Raise the remaining side rail.	The patient needs to be removed from the sling before it can be removed from the bed.
15. Cover the patient and help him or her to a position of comfort. Place the bed in the lowest position.	Ensures patient comfort and safety.
16. Remove the disposable cover from the sling and discard in the appropriate receptacle.	Using a cover deters the spread of microorganisms.

(continued)

SKILL 3-2 USING A BED SCALE continued

ACTION	RATIONALE
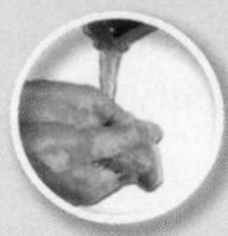 17. Remove additional PPE, if used. Clean equipment based on facility policy. Perform hand hygiene.	Removing PPE properly reduces the risk for infection transmission and contamination of other items. Cleaning equipment prevents transmission of microorganisms. Hand hygiene deters the spread of microorganisms.
18. Replace the scale and sling in the appropriate spot. Plug the scale into the electrical outlet.	Scale should be ready for use at any time.

EVALUATION

The expected outcome is met when the patient is weighed accurately without injury using the bed scale.

DOCUMENTATION

Guidelines

Document weight, unit of measurement, and scale used.

Sample Documentation

> <u>10/15/15</u> 0230 Patient reports pain in legs 5/10. Premedicated with Percocet 2 tabs po before obtaining weight per order. Patient weighed using bed scale, 75.2 kg.
>
> —M. Evans, RN

UNEXPECTED SITUATIONS AND ASSOCIATED INTERVENTIONS

- *As the patient is being lifted, the scale begins to tip over:* Stop lifting the patient. Slowly lower the patient back to the bed. Ensure that the base of the scale is spread wide enough before attempting to weigh the patient.
- *Weight differs from the previous day's weight by more than 1 kg:* Weigh the patient using the same scale at the same time each day. Check scale calibration. Make sure that the patient is wearing the same clothing. Make sure that no tubes or containers are hanging on the scale. If the patient is incontinent, make sure undergarments are clean and dry.
- *Patient becomes agitated as the sling is raised into the air:* Stop lifting the patient and reassure him or her. If the patient continues to be agitated, lower him or her back to the bed. Reevaluate necessity of obtaining weight at that exact time. If appropriate, obtain an order for sedation before attempting to obtain another weight measurement.

WATCH & LEARN SKILL 3-3 ASSESSING THE SKIN, HAIR, AND NAILS

The integumentary system includes the skin, hair, nails, sweat glands, and sebaceous glands. Assessment of the skin, hair, and nails provides information about the nutritional and hydration status and overall health of the patient. Additionally, this assessment can provide information associated with certain systemic diseases, infection, immobility, excessive sun exposure, and allergic reactions. Assessment often begins with an overall inspection of the skin's condition and skin assessment is integrated throughout the entire health assessment. Assessment of specific regions is usually integrated into specific body system assessments. Skin assessment is presented separately here for learning purposes in this text.

DELEGATION CONSIDERATIONS

The assessment of the patient's skin, hair, and nails should not be delegated to nursing assistive personnel (NAP) or unlicensed assistive personnel (UAP. However, the NAP or UAP may notice some items while providing care. The nurse must then validate, analyze, document, communicate, and act on these findings, as appropriate. Depending on the state's nurse practice act and the organization's policies and procedures, the licensed practical/vocational nurses (LPN/LVN) may perform some or all of the parts of assessment of the patient's skin, hair, and nails. The decision to delegate must be based on careful analysis of the patient's needs and circumstances, as well as the qualifications of the person to whom the task is being delegated. Refer to the Delegation Guidelines in Appendix A.

EQUIPMENT

- Gloves
- Additional PPE, as indicated
- Bath blanket or other drape
- Measuring tape or ruler
- Adequate light source

ASSESSMENT

Complete a health history, focusing on the integumentary system. Identify risk factors by asking about the following:

- History of rashes, lesions, change in color, or itching
- History of bruising or bleeding in the skin
- History of allergies to medications, plants, foods, or other substances
- History of bathing routines and products
- Exposure to the sun and sunburn history
- Presence of lesions (wounds, bruises, abrasions, or burns)
- Change in the color, size, or shape of a mole
- Recent chemotherapy or radiation therapy
- Exposure to chemicals that may be harmful to the skin, hair, or nails
- Degree of mobility
- Types of food eaten and liquids consumed each day
- Recent falls or injury
- Lifestyle choices: tattoos, body piercing
- Cultural practices related to skin

NURSING DIAGNOSIS

Determine the related factors for the nursing diagnoses based on the patient's current health status. Appropriate nursing diagnoses may include:

- Impaired Skin Integrity
- Disturbed Body Image
- Self-Mutilation

OUTCOME IDENTIFICATION AND PLANNING

The expected outcome to achieve in performing an integumentary assessment is that the assessment is completed without the patient experiencing anxiety or discomfort, the findings are documented, and the appropriate referral is made to the other health care professionals, as needed, for further evaluation. Other specific outcomes will be expected depending on the identified nursing diagnosis.

IMPLEMENTATION

ACTION	RATIONALE
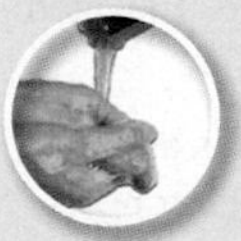 1. Perform hand hygiene and put on PPE, if indicated.	Hand hygiene and PPE prevent the spread of microorganisms. PPE is required based on transmission precautions.
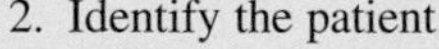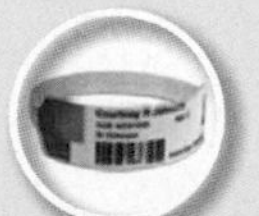 2. Identify the patient.	Identifying the patient ensures the right patient receives the intervention and helps prevent errors.
3. Close curtains around the bed and the door to room, if possible. Explain the purpose of the integumentary examination and what you are going to do. Answer any questions.	This ensures the patient's privacy. Explanation relieves anxiety and facilitates cooperation.
4. Ask the patient to remove all clothing and put on an examination gown (if appropriate). The patient remains in the sitting position for most of the examination, but will need to stand or lie on the side when the posterior part of the body is examined, exposing only the body part being examined.	Exposing only the body part being examined provides privacy for the patient. During the initial part of the examination, assess the skin areas that are exposed (e.g., face, arms, and hands). As the different assessments are completed, incorporate skin examination within these systems.

(continued)

SKILL 3-3 ASSESSING THE SKIN, HAIR, AND NAILS continued

ACTION	RATIONALE
5. Use the bath blanket or drape to cover any exposed area other than the one being assessed. Inspect the overall skin coloration (Figure 1).	Use of a bath blanket or drape provides for comfort and warmth. Overall coloration is a good indication of health status. Skin color varies among races and people; individual skin color should be relatively consistent across the body. Abnormal findings include **cyanosis**, **pallor**, **jaundice**, and **erythema**.
6. Inspect skin for vascularity, bleeding, or bruising.	These signs may relate to injury or cardiovascular, hematologic, or liver dysfunction.
7. Inspect the skin for lesions. Note bruises, scratches, cuts, insect bites, and wounds. (Refer to Wound Assessment [Fundamentals Review 8-3] in Chapter 8.) If present, note size, shape, color, exudates, and distribution/pattern, and presence of drainage or odor. Assess the location and condition of body piercings and/or tattoos.	Lesions can be normal variations, such as a macule or freckle, or an abnormal lesion, such as a melanoma.
8. Palpate skin using the backs of your hands to assess temperature. Wear gloves when palpating any potentially open area of the skin (Figure 2).	The back of the hand is more sensitive to temperature. Increase in skin temperature may indicate elevated body temperature.

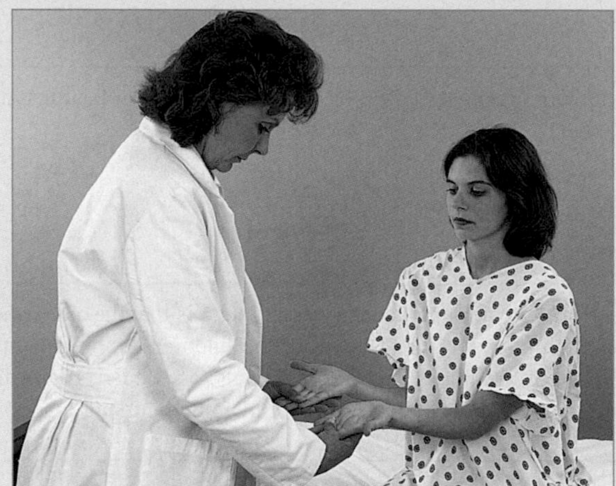

FIGURE 1 Inspecting overall skin coloration. *(Photo by B. Proud.)*

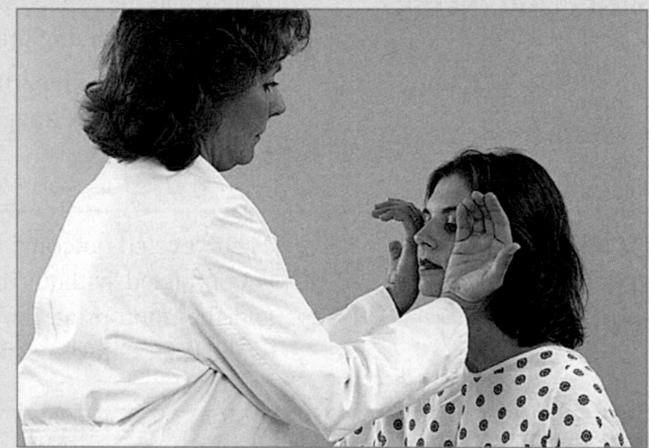

FIGURE 2 Assessing skin temperature. *(Photo by B. Proud.)*

ACTION	RATIONALE
9. Palpate for texture and moisture.	In a dehydrated patient, skin is dry, loose, and wrinkled. Elevated body temperature may result in increased perspiration.
10. Assess for skin turgor by gently pinching the skin under the clavicle (Figure 3).	Provides information about the patient's hydration status as well as skin mobility and elasticity. Decreased elasticity may be present in dehydrated patients.

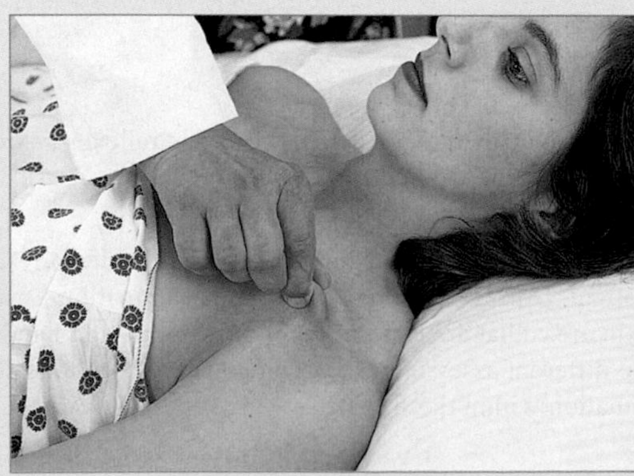

FIGURE 3 Palpating to assess turgor. *(Photo by B. Proud.)*

ACTION	RATIONALE
11. Palpate for edema, which is characterized by swelling, with taut and shiny skin over the edematous area.	Edema may be the result of overhydration, heart failure, kidney dysfunction, or peripheral vascular disease.
12. If lesions are present, put on gloves and palpate the lesion.	Palpation of lesions may result in drainage, which provides clues to the type or cause of the lesion. Gloves prevent contact with blood and body fluids.
13. Inspect the nail condition, including the shape, texture, and color as well as the nail angle; note if any clubbing is present.	Nail condition provides information about underlying illness and oxygenation status. Nails are normally convex and the cuticle is pink and intact. The angle of nail attachment is 160 degrees. Clubbing is present when the nail angle base exceeds 180 degrees.
14. Palpate nails for texture and capillary refill.	Normally, nails are firm and smooth and capillary refill should be brisk, less than 3 seconds.
15. Inspect the hair and scalp for color, texture, and distribution (Figure 4). Wear gloves for palpation if lesions or infestation is suspected or if hygiene is poor.	Hair condition provides information about nutritional and oxygenation status. Hair should be evenly distributed over the scalp. There are variations in hair color. Scalp should feel mobile and nontender.

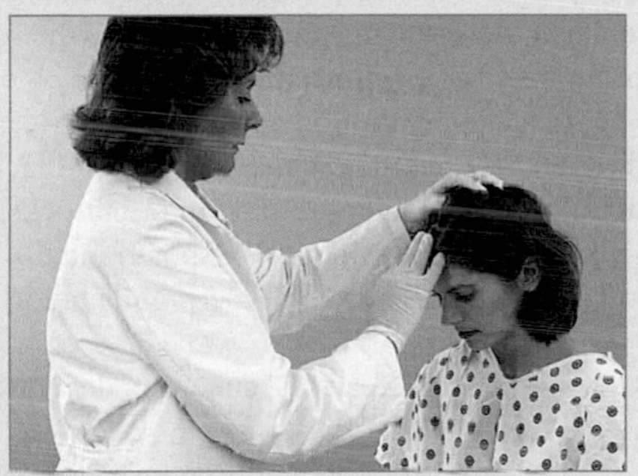

FIGURE 4 Inspecting the scalp and hair. *(Photo by B. Proud.)*

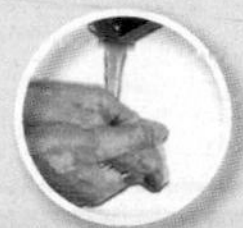

ACTION	RATIONALE
16. Remove gloves and any additional PPE, if used. Perform hand hygiene. Continue with assessments of specific body systems, as appropriate or indicated. Initiate appropriate referral to other health care practitioners for further evaluation, as indicated.	Removing PPE properly reduces the risk for infection transmission and contamination of other items. Hand hygiene prevents the spread of microorganisms. Additional assessments should be completed, as indicated, to evaluate the patient's health status. Intervention by other health care providers may be indicated to evaluate and treat the patient's health status.

EVALUATION

The expected outcome is met when the patient participates in the integumentary assessment, the patient verbalizes understanding of integumentary assessment techniques, as appropriate, the assessment is completed without the patient experiencing anxiety or discomfort, the findings are documented, and the appropriate referrals are made to the other health care professionals, as needed for further evaluation.

DOCUMENTATION

Guidelines

When documenting skin assessment, be sure to describe specific findings, including coloration, texture, moisture, temperature, turgor, capillary refill, and edema. Note hair distribution and texture. Describe the condition of nails, including any abnormal findings. If lesions are present, document specifics, describing type, size, shape (use tape measure if necessary), elevation, coloring, location, drainage, distribution, and patterns.

Sample Documentation

> 5/2/15 1030 Skin assessment performed. Patient reports history of atopic dermatitis. Uniform skin coloring (tan) with pink undertones. Skin on all areas, but the hands, is soft and warm. Skin returns to position when pinched. Multiple lesions, consistent with dermatitis, observed on the hands. Lesions are red, scaly, and dry. Brown hair, shiny and evenly distributed. Nails are firm and the cuticle is pink and intact and without ridging or pitting.
>
> —*B. Gentzler, RN*

(continued)

SKILL 3-3 ASSESSING THE SKIN, HAIR, AND NAILS continued

UNEXPECTED OUTCOMES AND ASSOCIATED INTERVENTIONS

- *While assessing the skin of a patient with dark skin tone, you are unsure if the change in coloration in a particular area of the body is normal or abnormal:* It is especially important when assessing people with dark skin tones to conduct the assessment with natural light rather than artificial lighting. When an abnormal condition is present, first examining an area of the skin that is not affected by the dermatologic disorder provides a comparison for identifying abnormal color conditions. Skin temperature becomes important to detect erythema in persons with dark skin tones; areas of erythema will feel warm compared with surrounding skin. Pallor in patients with dark skin tones is seen as an ashen gray or yellow tinge. Also, lesions that look red or brown on light skin may present as black or purple on dark skin.

SPECIAL CONSIDERATIONS

Older Adult Considerations

In the older adult patient expect to find overall thinning of the skin, reduced sweating and oil, and reduced skin turgor.

Cultural Considerations

- Pallor in people with dark skin tones appears as absence of the "glow" of brown or black skin, or may appear as ashen gray or yellow tinged. Lighter skin appears more yellowish-brown; darker skin looks ashen. Assess cyanosis in people with darker skin tones by examining the oral mucosa, the lips, nail beds, and the conjunctiva. Assess jaundice by observing the sclera of the eyes, the palms of the hands, and soles of the feet for a yellowish discoloration.
- Mongolian spot is a common variation of hyperpigmentation in newborns of African, African-American, Turkish, Asian, American Indian, and Hispanic heritage. It is a blue-black to purple macular area of hyperpigmentation that is usually located at the sacrum or buttocks, but sometimes occurs on the abdomen, thighs, shoulders, or arms. Mongolian spot gradually fades during the first year of life. It is important not to confuse these areas of hyperpigmentation with bruises (Jarvis, 2012).
- Asian patients may exhibit normal variations in physical features, such as a decrease in body hair and coarse head hair.

WATCH & LEARN SKILL 3-4 ASSESSING THE HEAD AND NECK

Examination of the head and neck region includes the assessment of multiple structures and body systems. The eyes, ears, nose, mouth, and throat are located within the facial structures. Anterior neck structures include the trachea, esophagus, and the thyroid gland, as well as the arteries, veins, and lymph nodes. Posterior neck areas involve the upper portion of the spine.

DELEGATION CONSIDERATIONS

Assessment of the patient's head and neck should not be delegated to nursing assistive personnel (NAP) or unlicensed assistive personnel (UAP). However, the NAP or UAP may notice some items while providing care. The nurse must then validate, analyze, document, communicate, and act on these findings, as appropriate. Depending on the state's nurse practice act and the organization's policies and procedures, the licensed practical/vocational nurses (LPN/LVNs) may perform some or all of the parts of assessment of the patient's head and neck. The decision to delegate must be based on careful analysis of the patient's needs and circumstances, as well as the qualifications of the person to whom the task is being delegated. Refer to the Delegation Guidelines in Appendix A.

EQUIPMENT

- Stethoscope
- Gloves
- Additional PPE, as indicated
- Bath blanket or other drape
- Lighting, including a penlight
- Tongue blades
- Visual acuity chart

ASSESSMENT

Complete a health history, focusing on the head and neck. Identify risk factors by asking about the following:

- Changes with aging in vision or hearing
- History of use of corrective lenses or hearing aids
- Loss of an eye (use of artificial eye)
- History of allergies
- History of disturbances in vision or hearing
- History of chronic illnesses, such as hypertension, diabetes mellitus, or thyroid disease
- Exposure to harmful substances or loud noises
- Exposure to ultraviolet light
- History of smoking, chewing tobacco, or cocaine use
- History of eye or ear infections
- History of head trauma
- Presence of body piercings and/or tattoos
- History of persistent hoarseness
- Oral and dental care practices

NURSING DIAGNOSIS

Determine the related factors for the nursing diagnoses based on the patient's current health status. Appropriate nursing diagnoses may include:

- Impaired Swallowing
- Impaired Dentition
- Impaired Oral Mucous Membrane

OUTCOME IDENTIFICATION AND PLANNING

The expected outcome to achieve in performing an examination of the structures in the head and neck region is that the assessment is completed without the patient experiencing anxiety or discomfort, the findings are documented, and the appropriate referral is made to the other health care professionals, as needed, for further evaluation. Other specific outcomes will be expected depending on the identified nursing diagnosis.

IMPLEMENTATION

ACTION	RATIONALE
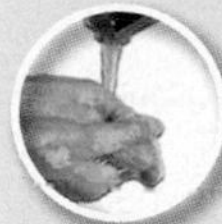 1. Perform hand hygiene and put on PPE, if indicated.	Hand hygiene and PPE prevent the spread of microorganisms. PPE is required based on transmission precautions.
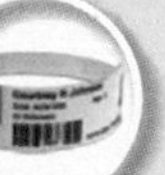 2. Identify the patient.	Identifying the patient ensures the right patient receives the intervention and helps prevent errors.
3. Close the curtains around the bed and close the door to the room, if possible. Explain the purpose of the head and neck examination and what you are going to do. Answer any questions.	This ensures the patient's privacy. Explanation relieves anxiety and facilitates cooperation.
4. Inspect the head for size and shape. Inspect the face for color, symmetry, lesions, and distribution of facial hair. Note facial expression. Palpate the skull.	Generally, the shape of the head is normocephalic and symmetric. Abnormal findings include a lack of symmetry or unusual size or contour of the head, which may be a result of trauma or disease. Facial expression is appropriate. Skull should be mobile and nontender.
5. Inspect the external eye structures (eyelids, eyelashes, eyeball, and eyebrows), cornea, conjunctiva, and sclera. Note color, edema, symmetry, and alignment.	Inspection detects abnormalities, such as ptosis, styes, conjunctivitis, or scleral color. Some abnormalities are associated with systemic disorders.

(continued)

SKILL 3-4 ASSESSING THE HEAD AND NECK continued

ACTION	RATIONALE
6. Examine the pupils for equality of size and shape (Figure 1). Examine the pupillary reaction to light: a. Darken the room. b. Ask the patient to look straight ahead. c. Bring the penlight from the side of the patient's face and briefly shine the light on the pupil (Figure 2). d. Observe the pupil's reaction; it normally constricts rapidly (direct response). Note pupil size. e. Repeat the procedure and observe the other eye; it too normally will constrict (consensual reflex). f. Repeat the procedure with the other eye.	Testing pupillary response to light and accommodation assesses cranial nerve III, the oculomotor nerve. The pupils are normally black, equal in size, round, and smooth. The normal and consensual pupillary response is constriction.

1 2 3 4 5 6 7

FIGURE 1 Pupillary gauge measures pupils in millimeters (mm).

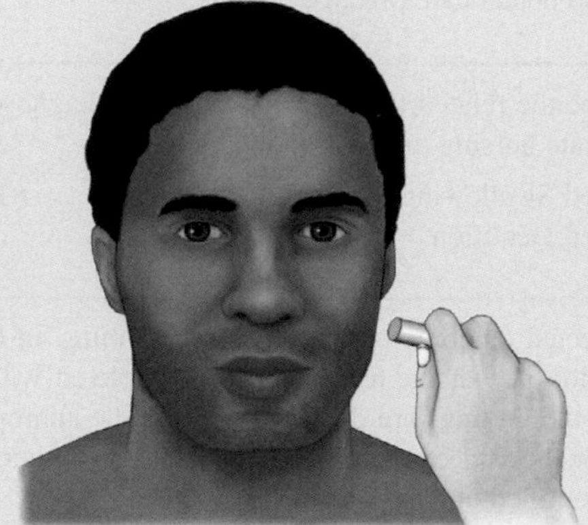

FIGURE 2 Assessing pupillary reaction to light.

ACTION	RATIONALE
7. Test for pupillary accommodation: a. Hold the forefinger, a pencil, or other straight object about 10 to 15 cm (4″ to 6″) from the bridge of the patient's nose. b. Ask the patient to first look at the object, then at a distant object, then back to the object being held. The pupil normally constricts when looking at a near object and dilates when looking at a distant object (Figure 3).	Testing pupillary response to light and accommodation assesses cranial nerve III, the oculomotor nerve. The normal pupillary response is constriction when focusing on a near object.

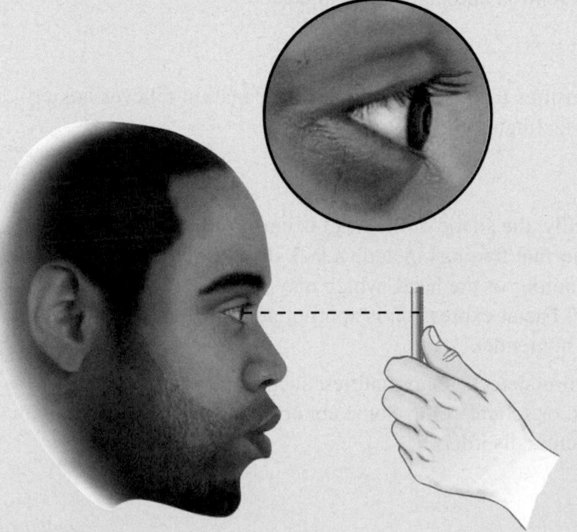

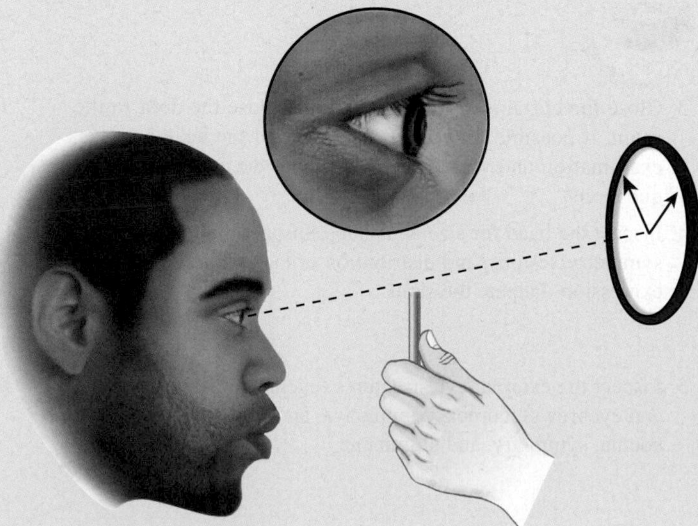

FIGURE 3 Accommodation.

ACTION

8. Assess extraocular movements.
   a. Ask the patient to hold the head still and follow the movement of your forefinger or a penlight with the eyes as you move the patient's eyes through the six cardinal positions of gaze.
   b. Keeping your finger or penlight about 1 foot from the patient's face, move it slowly through the cardinal positions: up and down, right and left, diagonally up and down to the left (Figure 4-A), diagonally up and down to the right (Figure 4-B).

RATIONALE

This evaluates the function of each of the six extraocular eye muscles (EOM) and tests cranial nerves III, IV, and VI (oculomotor, trochlear, and abducens nerves). Normally, both eyes move together, are coordinated, and are parallel.

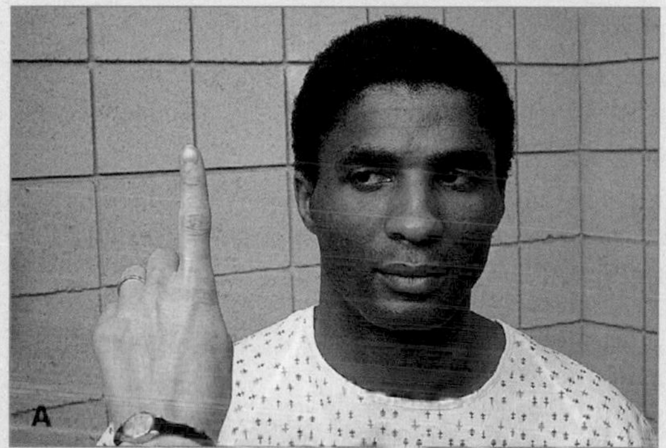

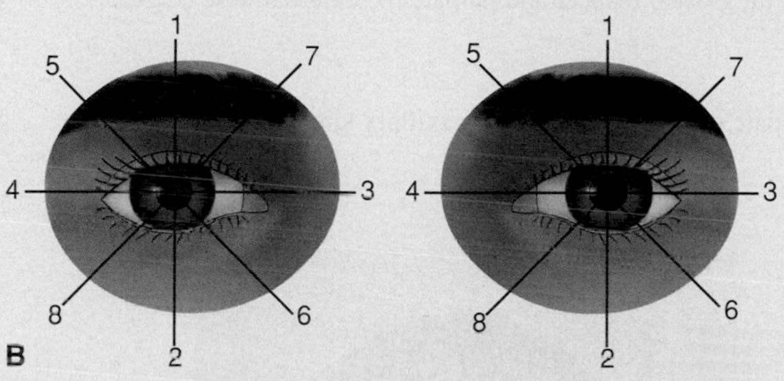

FIGURE 4 Six cardinal positions of gaze.

9. Test convergence:
   a. Hold your finger about 6″ to 8″ from the bridge of the patient's nose.
   b. Move your finger toward the patient's nose (Figure 5). The patient's eyes should normally converge (assume a cross-eyed appearance).

The patient's eyes should normally converge; converging eyes normally follow the object to within 5 cm of the nose (assume a cross-eyed appearance).

10. Test the patient's visual acuity with a Snellen chart. Have the patient stand 20 feet from the chart and ask the patient to read the smallest line of letters possible, first with both eyes and then with one eye at a time (with the opposite eye covered). Note whether the patient's vision is being tested with or without corrective lenses (Figure 6).

Evaluates the patient's distance vision and function of cranial nerve II (optic nerve). Additional tools are used to test for color perception.

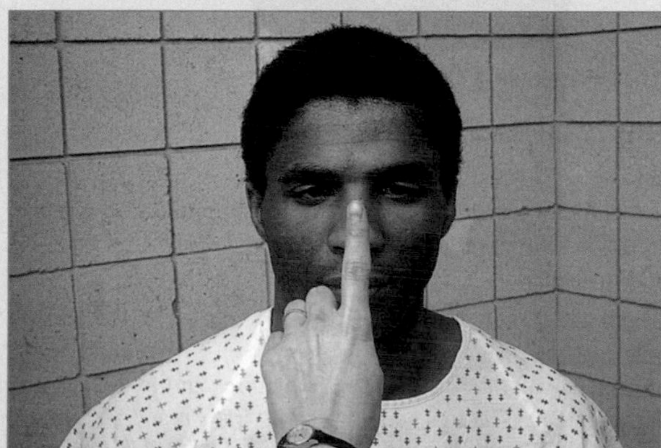

FIGURE 5 Convergence.

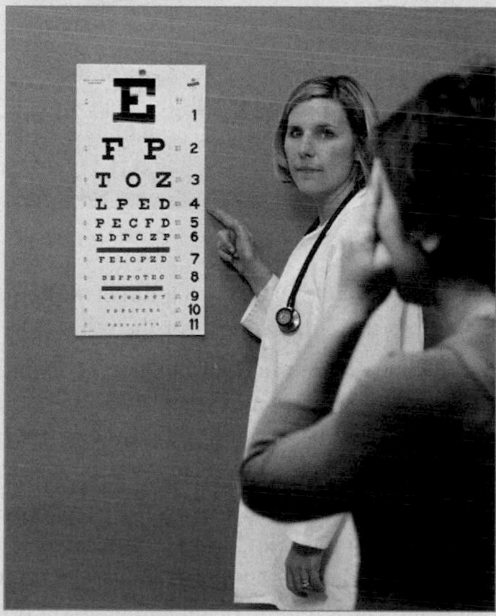

FIGURE 6 Testing visual acuity with a Snellen chart. (From Hogan-Quigley, B., Palm, M.L., & Bickley, L. (2012). *Bates' nursing guide to physical examination and history taking.* Philadelphia: Wolters Kluwer Health/Lippincott Williams & Wilkins, p. 221.)

(continued)

SKILL 3-4 ASSESSING THE HEAD AND NECK continued

ACTION	RATIONALE
11. Inspect the external ear bilaterally for shape, size, and lesions. Palpate the ear and mastoid process. Inspect the visible portion of the ear canal. Note cerumen (wax), edema, discharge, or foreign bodies.	Inspection may reveal abnormalities, such as uneven color, size, drainage, or lesions; inflammation (edema) or infection; nodules, lesions, or tenderness. Cerumen may normally be dark orange, brown, yellow, gray, or black and soft, moist, dry, or hard.
12. Use a whispered voice to test hearing. Stand about 1 to 2 feet away from the patient out of the patient's line of vision. Ask the patient to cover the ear not being tested. Determine whether the patient can hear a whispered sentence or group of numbers from a distance of 1 to 2 feet. Perform test on each ear.	Provides a gross assessment of cranial nerve VIII (acoustic nerve). The patient should repeat what has been said.
13. Put on gloves. Inspect and palpate the external nose (Figure 7).	Gloves prevent contact with blood and body fluids. These actions assess for the color, shape, consistency, and tenderness of the nose.
14. Palpate over the frontal and maxillary sinuses (Figure 8).	Sinus palpation is used to elicit tenderness, which may indicate sinus congestion or infection. Normally, the sinuses are not painful when palpated.

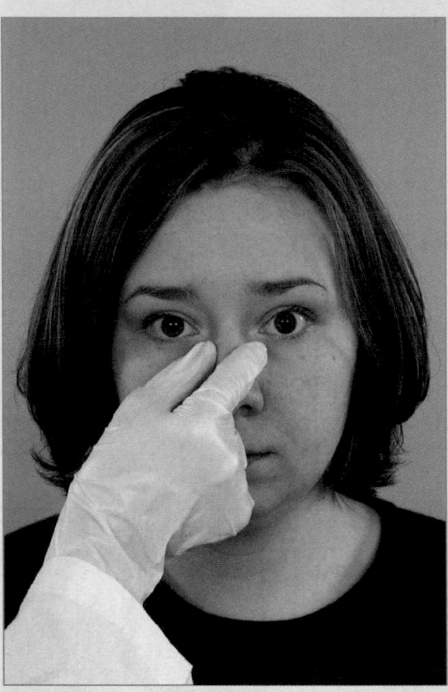

FIGURE 7 Palpating the nose. *(Photo by B. Proud.)*

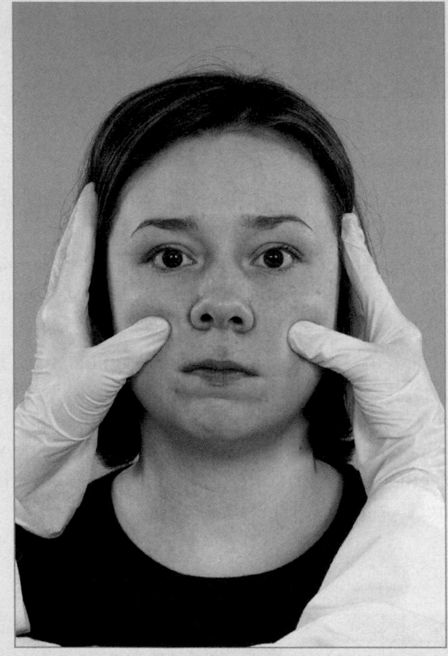

FIGURE 8 Palpating the sinuses. *(Photo by B. Proud.)*

ACTION	RATIONALE
15. Occlude one nostril externally with a finger while patient breathes through the other; repeat for the other side.	This technique checks the patency of the nasal passages.
16. Inspect each anterior nares and turbinates by tipping the patient's head back slightly and shining a light into the nares. Examine the mucous membranes for color and the presence of lesions, exudate, or growths. Also, inspect the nasal septum for intactness and deviation.	This technique can detect edema, inflammation, and excessive drainage. The nasal mucosa is moist and darker red than the oral mucosa.
17. Inspect the lips, oral mucosa, hard and soft palates, gingivae, teeth, and salivary gland openings. Ask the patient to open the mouth wide and use a tongue blade and penlight to visualize structures.	Evaluates the condition of the oral structures and hydration level of the patient. The lips should be pink, moist, and smooth. The gums should be pink and smooth. The teeth should be regular and free of cavities or have dental restoration. The tonsils, if present, are small, pink, and symmetric in size.

ACTION

18. Inspect the tongue. Ask the patient to stick out the tongue. Place a tongue blade at the side of the tongue while patient pushes it to the left and right with the tongue. Inspect the uvula by asking the patient to say "ahh" while sticking out the tongue (Figure 9). Palpate the tongue for muscle tone and tenderness. Remove gloves.

RATIONALE

Sticking out the tongue evaluates the function of cranial nerve XII (hypoglossal nerve). Saying "ahh" checks for movement of the uvula and soft palate.

The tongue and mucous membranes are normally pink, moist, and free of swelling or lesions. The uvula is normally centered and freely movable. Tongue should feel soft with positive muscle tone and be nontender.

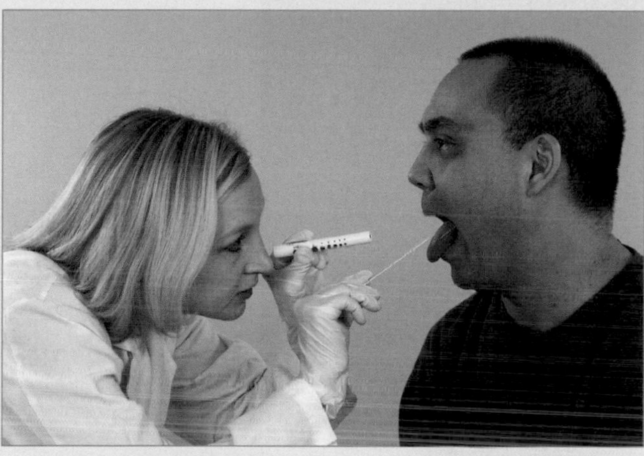

FIGURE 9 Inspecting the mouth using a tongue blade and penlight. *(Photo by B. Proud.)*

19. Inspect and palpate the lymph nodes (Figure 10) for enlargement, tenderness, and mobility, using the finger pads in a slow, circular motion (Figure 11).

Palpation can determine size, shape, mobility, consistency, and/or tenderness of enlarged lymph nodes.

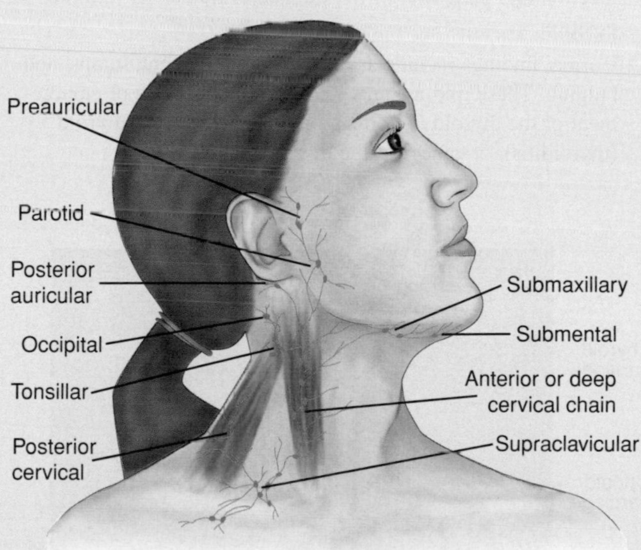

FIGURE 10 Location of lymph nodes in neck.

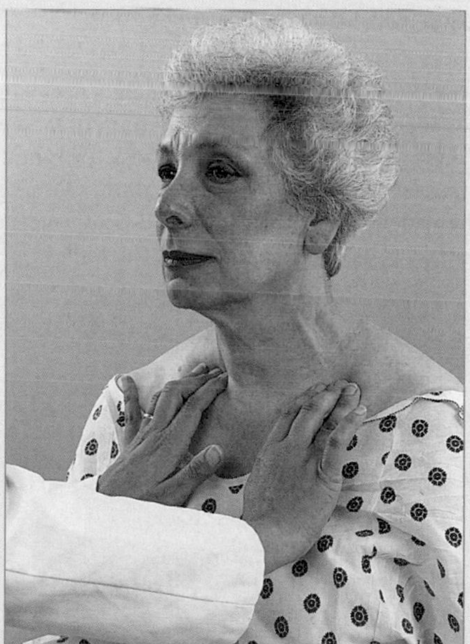

FIGURE 11 Palpating lymph nodes. *(Photo by B. Proud.)*

(continued)

SKILL 3-4 ASSESSING THE HEAD AND NECK continued

ACTION	RATIONALE
20. Inspect and palpate (Figure 12-A) the left and then the right carotid arteries. **Only palpate one carotid artery at a time.** Note the strength of the pulse and grade it as with peripheral pulses. Use the bell of the stethoscope to auscultate the arteries (Figure 12-B).	Palpation of this area evaluates circulation through the arteries. Palpating both arteries at once can reduce blood flow to the brain, potentially causing dizziness or loss of consciousness. Auscultation can detect a **bruit**, an abnormal "swooshing" sound heard on auscultation, indicating turbulent blood flow.

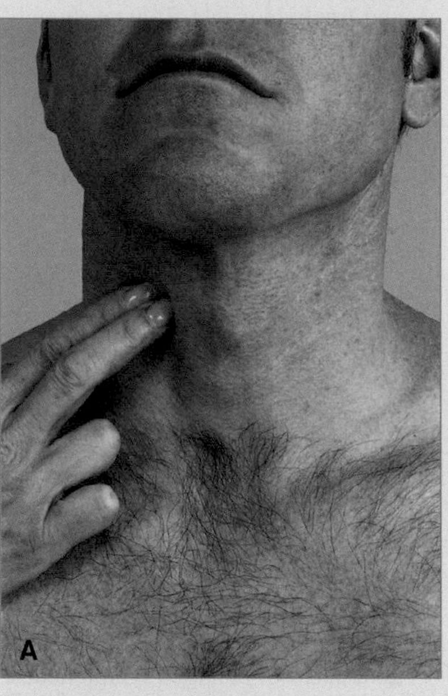

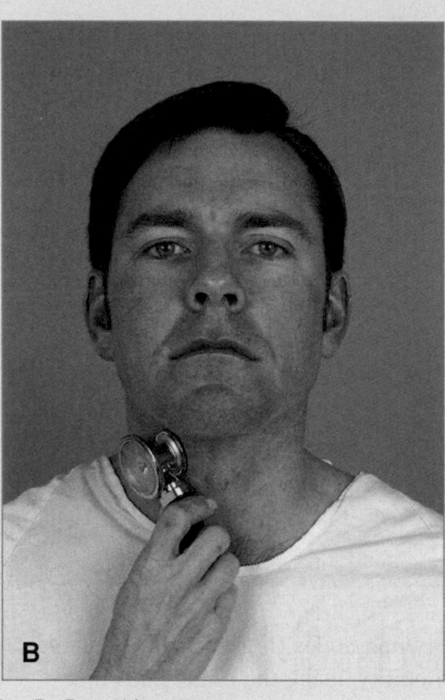

FIGURE 12 Palpating (**A**) and auscultating (**B**) carotid artery. *(Photos by B. Proud.)*

ACTION	RATIONALE
21. Inspect and palpate the trachea (Figure 13).	Inspection and palpation of the trachea evaluates its midline position.
22. Assess the thyroid gland with the patient's neck slightly hyperextended. Observe the lower portion of the neck overlying the thyroid gland (Figure 14). Assess for symmetry and visible masses. Ask the patient to swallow. Observe the area while the patient swallows. Offer a glass of water, if necessary, to make it easier for the patient to swallow.	Abnormal findings include asymmetry, enlargement, lumps, and bulging. These findings may indicate the presence of enlargement of the thyroid (a goiter), inflammation of the thyroid (thyroiditis), or cancer of the thyroid.

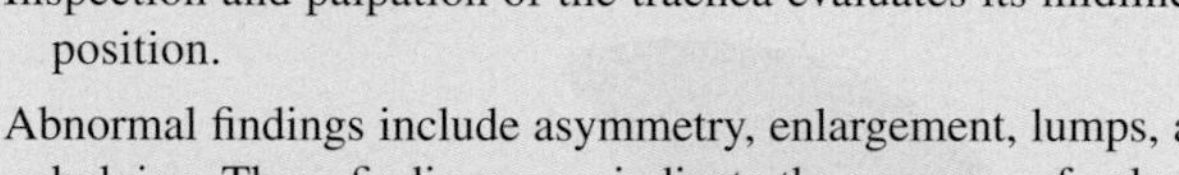

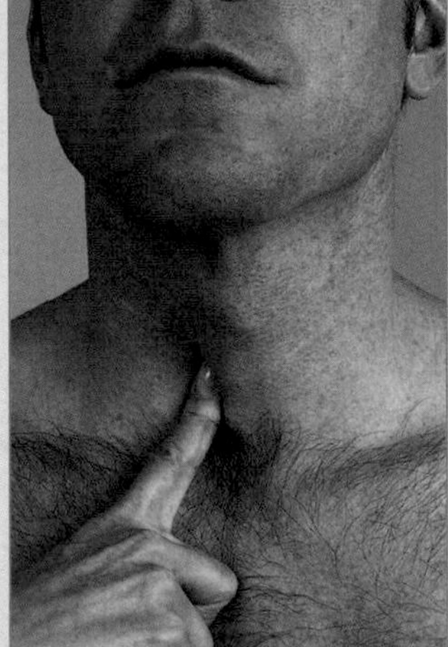

FIGURE 13 Palpating to determine position of trachea. *(Photo by B. Proud.)*

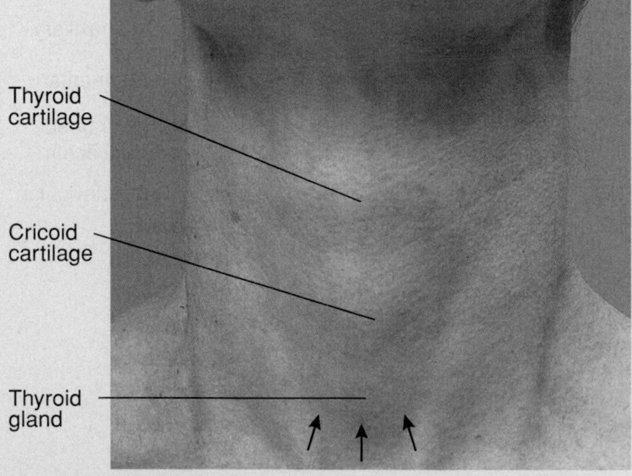

FIGURE 14 Assessing the thyroid gland. (From Hogan-Quigley, B., Palm, M.L., & Bickley, L. (2012). *Bates' nursing guide to physical examination and history taking.* Philadelphia: Wolters Kluwer Health/Lippincott Williams & Wilkins, p. 200.)

ACTION	RATIONALE
23. Inspect the ability of the patient to move the neck. Ask the patient to touch chin to chest and to each shoulder, each ear to the corresponding shoulder, and then tip the head back as far as possible.	These actions assess neck ROM, which is normally smooth and controlled.
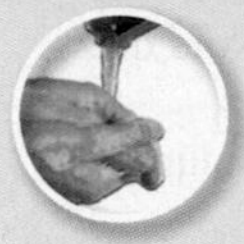 24. Remove any additional PPE, if used. Perform hand hygiene. Continue with assessments of specific body systems, as appropriate or indicated. Initiate appropriate referral to other health care practitioners for further evaluation, as indicated.	Removing PPE properly reduces the risk for infection transmission and contamination of other items. Hand hygiene prevents the spread of microorganisms. Additional assessments should be completed, as indicated, to evaluate the patient's health status. Intervention by other health care providers may be indicated to evaluate and treat the patient's health status.

EVALUATION

The expected outcome is met when the patient participates in head and neck assessment, the patient verbalizes understanding of these assessment techniques as appropriate, the assessment is completed without the patient experiencing anxiety or discomfort, the findings are documented, and the appropriate referrals are made to the other health care professionals, as needed, for further evaluation.

DOCUMENTATION

Guidelines

When documenting head and neck assessment, describe specific findings. For the head and face, document symmetry, coloration, and presence of lesions or edema. Note visual acuity, pupillary reaction, and condition of the external eye. Document results of tests for accommodation, convergence, and extraocular muscles. Describe condition of external and internal ear, noting any lesions or discharge. Document results of any hearing tests. Note condition of internal and external nose and sinuses. Describe condition of lips, gums, tongue, and buccal mucosa. Document quality of carotid pulse. Note position of trachea and any enlargement of the thyroid. Describe quality of any lymph nodes palpable. Note ROM of the neck. Document presence of pain or discomfort.

Sample Documentation

6/10/15 1545 Head and neck examination completed. Patient denies history of any sensory changes or sensory difficulties, but states, "I have some sores in my mouth." Overall skin coloring consistent, with pink undertones. Head symmetric and normal in size. Eyes are symmetric. No lesions or redness noted. Pupils equal and reactive to light; positive accommodation and convergence. Visual acuity 20/20 in both eyes. Eyes move smoothly through six fields of gaze. External ears and canal free of discharge, lesions, or tenderness. Whisper test negative for hearing loss. Nose and sinuses nontender. Minimal clear discharge present in the nostrils; nostrils patent. Lips free of lesions. Multiple white lesions approximately 1 cm in diameter noted on buccal mucosa and tongue. Uvula rise normal. No palpable lymph nodes. Carotid pulse strong bilaterally. No bruits auscultated. Trachea midline. Thyroid not enlarged.

—B. Gentzler, RN

UNEXPECTED SITUATIONS AND ASSOCIATED INTERVENTIONS

- *While you are testing a patient's visual acuity, the patient states that he can't see anything without his glasses:* Stop the test. Instruct the patient to put on his glasses, and then resume testing.
- *While performing an examination of the regional lymph nodes in the neck area, you palpate a lymph node that feels hard and fixed:* Ask the patient if he has felt this node before and, if so, for how long it has been present and if it is painful. Refer the patient to a primary care provider for follow-up care.

SPECIAL CONSIDERATIONS

General Considerations

- A patient who wears corrective lenses should have them on when visual acuity is being tested.
- A Snellen picture chart or Snellen E chart can be used to test vision in children and in patients who are unable to read English. The E chart uses the capital letter E in varying sizes pointing in different directions. The patient points his or her fingers in the direction the legs of the E are pointing.

(*continued*)

SKILL 3-4 ASSESSING THE HEAD AND NECK continued

- Near vision is tested with a handheld vision screen with varying sizes of print. A Jaeger card can be used for this measurement. The patient holds the card 14 inches from the eyes. Ask the patient to read the smallest line of letters possible, with one eye at a time (with the opposite eye covered), and corrective lenses in place, if used. The results are recorded as a fraction and written as 14 over the smallest line read by the patient. A normal result is 14/14.

Infant and Child Considerations

- When examining the neck of an infant or child, the preferred approach to assess ROM of the neck is to assess one movement at a time, rather than a full rotation of the neck, to avoid dizziness on movement.
- When examining the head of an infant, inspect and gently palpate the fontanels and sutures.
- Keep in mind that an infant's nose is usually slightly flattened.
- For a child under age 8 years, do not assess the frontal sinuses; they are usually too small to assess.
- Be aware that lymph nodes may be palpable in children under age 12 years, which is considered a normal variation.
- Note the number of teeth in a child; a child may have up to 20 temporary teeth.

Older Adult Considerations

- Look for a thin, grayish ring in the cornea (arcus senilis). This may be a normal finding in an older adult.
- When evaluating the neurologic system in the older adult patient, expect to find normal age-related sensory changes, such as a decrease in vision, hearing, olfaction, taste, proprioception, and touch.
- If the patient wears dentures, ask him or her to remove them for inspection of the gums and roof of the mouth.

Cultural Considerations

- Exophthalmos, protrusion of the eyeball, can be a normal finding in an African-American patient.

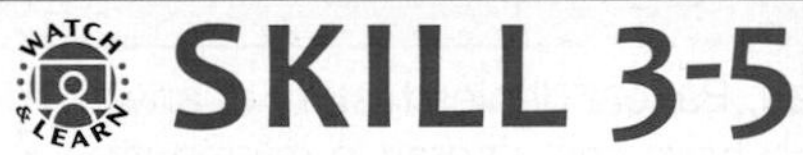

SKILL 3-5 ASSESSING THE THORAX, LUNGS, AND BREASTS

The thorax is composed of the lungs, rib cage, cartilage, and intercostal muscles. A thorough examination of the respiratory system is essential because the primary purpose of this system is to supply oxygen to, and remove carbon dioxide from, the body. Recognizing and identifying normal and abnormal breath sounds, a crucial component of lung assessment, takes practice (Tables 3-2 and 3-3). Assessment of the breasts and axillae is also included in this assessment.

Table 3-2 NORMAL BREATH SOUNDS

TYPE, DESCRIPTION, AND LOCATION	RATIO OF INSPIRATION TO EXPIRATION
Bronchial or Tubular	
Blowing, hollow sounds; auscultated over the larynx and trachea	Sound on expiration is longer, lower, and higher pitched than inspiration
Bronchovesicular	
Medium-pitched, medium intensity, blowing sounds; auscultated over the first and second intercostal spaces anteriorly and the scapula posteriorly	Inspiration and expiration sounds have similar pitch and duration
Vesicular	
Soft, low-pitched, whispering sounds; heard over most of the lung fields	Sound on inspiration is longer, louder, and higher pitched than expiration

Table 3-3 ADVENTITIOUS BREATH SOUNDS

TYPE AND CHARACTERISTICS	ILLUSTRATION
Wheeze (Sibilant) • Musical or squeaking • High-pitched, continuous sounds • Auscultated during inspiration and expiration • Air passing through narrowed airways	
Rhonchi (Sonorous Wheeze) • Sonorous or coarse; snoring quality • Low-pitched, continuous sounds • Auscultated during inspiration and expiration • Coughing may somewhat clear the sound • Air passing through or around secretions	Z Z Z Z Z Z
Crackles • Bubbling, crackling, popping • Low- to high-pitched, discontinuous sounds • Auscultated during inspiration and expiration • Opening of deflated small airways and alveoli; air passing through fluid in the airways	
Stridor • Harsh, loud, high-pitched • Auscultated on inspiration • Narrowing of upper airway (larynx or trachea); presence of foreign body in airway	
Friction Rub • Rubbing or grating • Loudest over lower lateral anterior surface • Auscultated during inspiration and expiration • Inflamed pleura rubbing against chest wall	

DELEGATION CONSIDERATIONS

Assessment of the patient's thorax, breasts, axillae, and lungs should not be delegated to nursing assistive personnel (NAP) or unlicensed assistive personnel (UAP). However, the NAP or UAP may notice some items while providing care. The nurse must then validate, analyze, document, communicate, and act on these findings, as appropriate. Depending on the state's nurse practice act and the organization's policies and procedures, the licensed practical/vocational nurses (LPN/LVNs) may perform some or all of the parts of assessment of the patient's thorax, breasts, axillae, and lungs. The decision to delegate must be based on careful analysis of the patient's needs and circumstances, as well as the qualifications of the person to whom the task is being delegated. Refer to the Delegation Guidelines in Appendix A.

EQUIPMENT

- Bath blanket or other drape
- Examination gown
- Light source
- Stethoscope
- PPE, as indicated

ASSESSMENT

Complete a health history, focusing on the thorax and lungs. Identify risk factors by asking about the following:

- History of trauma to the ribs or lung surgery
- Number of pillows used when sleeping
- History of chest pain with deep breathing
- History of persistent cough with or without producing sputum

(*continued*)

SKILL 3-5 ASSESSING THE THORAX, LUNGS, AND BREASTS continued

- History of allergies
- Environmental exposure to chemicals, asbestos, or smoke
- History of smoking (including pack-years)
- History of lung disease in family members or self
- History of frequent or chronic respiratory infections
- Breast discomfort, masses, or lumps, nipple discharge
- History of breast disease or surgeries
- History of breast disease in family members
- Use of breast self-examination
- Childbirth, use of oral contraceptives, breastfeeding

NURSING DIAGNOSIS

Determine the related factors for the nursing diagnoses based on the patient's current health status. Appropriate nursing diagnoses may include:

- Ineffective Airway Clearance
- Impaired Gas Exchange
- Disturbed Body Image

OUTCOME IDENTIFICATION AND PLANNING

The expected outcome to achieve in performing an examination of the thorax, lungs, breasts, and axillae is that the assessment is completed without the patient experiencing anxiety or discomfort, the findings are documented, and the appropriate referral is made to the other health care professionals, as needed, for further evaluation. Other specific outcomes will be expected, depending on the identified nursing diagnosis.

IMPLEMENTATION

ACTION	RATIONALE
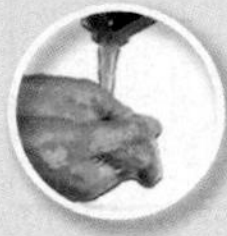 1. Perform hand hygiene and put on PPE, if indicated.	Hand hygiene and PPE prevent the spread of microorganisms. PPE is required based on transmission precautions.
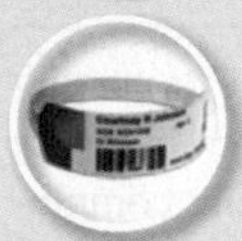 2. Identify the patient.	Identifying the patient ensures the right patient receives the intervention and helps prevent errors.
3. Close the curtains around the bed and close the door to the room, if possible. Explain the purpose of the thorax, lung, breast, and axillae examination and what you are going to do. Answer any questions.	This ensures the patient's privacy. Explanation relieves anxiety and facilitates cooperation.
4. Help the patient undress, if needed, and provide a patient gown. Assist the patient to a sitting position and expose the posterior thorax.	Having the patient wear a gown facilitates examination of the thorax while maintaining the patient's privacy.
5. Use the bath blanket to cover any exposed area other than the one being assessed.	Use of a bath blanket provides for comfort and warmth.
6. Inspect the posterior thorax. Examine the skin (Figure 1), bones, and muscles of the spine, shoulder blades, and back as well as symmetry of expansion and accessory muscle use during respirations.	Examination provides information about lung expansion and accessory muscle use during respiration. Inspection of skin reveals color, presence of lesions, rashes, or masses.
7. Assess the anteroposterior (AP) and lateral diameters of the thorax.	This assessment helps to detect deformities, such as a barrel chest. Normally, the AP is less than the transverse diameter (1:2 ratio).
8. Palpate over the spine and posterior thorax. Use the dorsal surface of the hand to palpate for temperature. Use the palmar surface of the hand to palpate for tenderness, muscle development, and masses (Figure 2).	Palpation may reveal abnormal findings, such as excessively dry or moist skin, muscle asymmetry, masses, tenderness, or vibrations.

ACTION | RATIONALE

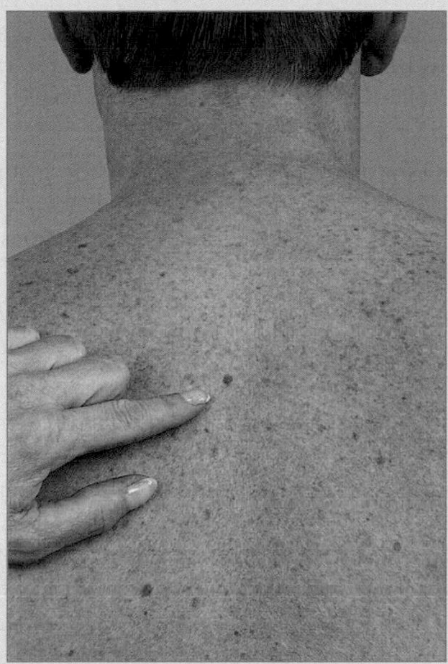

FIGURE 1 Inspecting the skin for abnormalities and variations. Any lesion or mole noted during inspection of the patient's back should be documented in the patient's medical record for follow-up evaluation. *(Photo by B. Proud.)*

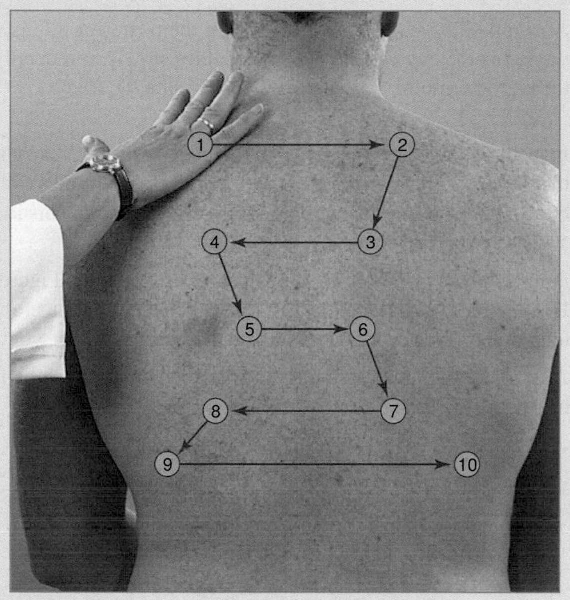

FIGURE 2 Palpating the posterior thorax and sequence for palpation.

9. Assess thoracic expansion by standing behind the patient and placing both thumbs on either side of the patient's spine at the level of T9 or T10 (Figure 3-A). Ask the patient to take a deep breath and note movement of your hands (Figure 3-B).

Movement should be symmetric bilaterally.

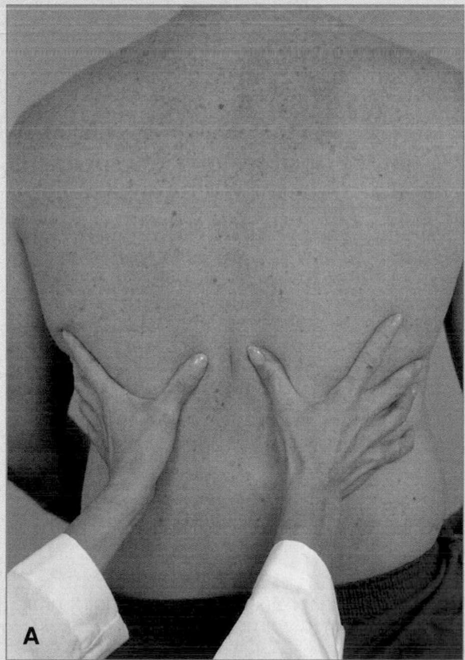

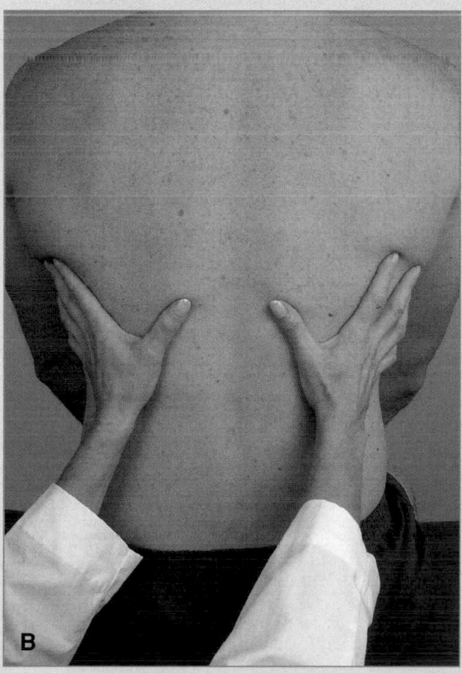

FIGURE 3 Palpating posterior thoracic excursion. **A.** The examiner's hands are placed symmetrically on the patient's back. **B.** As the patient inhales, the examiner's hands should move apart symmetrically. *(Photos by B. Proud.)*

(*continued*)

SKILL 3-5 ASSESSING THE THORAX, LUNGS, AND BREASTS continued

ACTION	RATIONALE
10. Auscultate the lungs across and down the posterior thorax to the bases of lungs as the patient breathes slowly and deeply through the mouth, comparing sides (Figure 4).	Lung auscultation assesses for normal breath sounds and for **adventitious breath sounds** (added, abnormal sounds). Abnormal breath sounds indicate respiratory compromise or diseases, such as asthma or bronchitis.
11. Inspect the anterior thorax. With the patient sitting, rearrange the gown so the anterior chest is exposed. Inspect the skin, bones, and muscles, as well as symmetry of lung expansion and accessory muscle use.	Examination of the anterior thorax provides information about lung expansion and accessory muscle use during respiration. Inspection of skin reveals color, presence of lesions, rashes, or masses.
12. Palpate the anterior thorax using the proper sequence (Figure 5). Use the palmar surface of the hand to palpate for temperature, tenderness, muscle development, and masses.	Palpation may reveal abnormal findings, such as excessively dry or moist skin, muscle asymmetry, masses, tenderness, or vibrations.
13. Auscultate the lungs through the anterior thorax as the patient breathes slowly and deeply through the mouth (Figure 6).	Lung auscultation assesses for normal breath and abnormal (adventitious) breath sounds. Abnormal breath sounds indicate respiratory compromise or diseases, such as asthma or bronchitis.

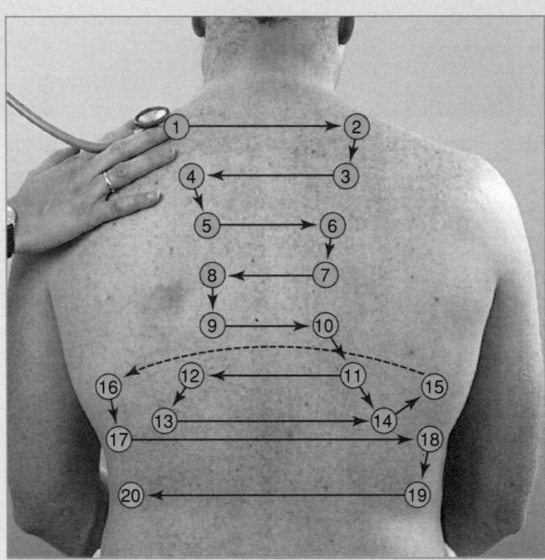

FIGURE 4 Sequence for auscultating posterior thorax.

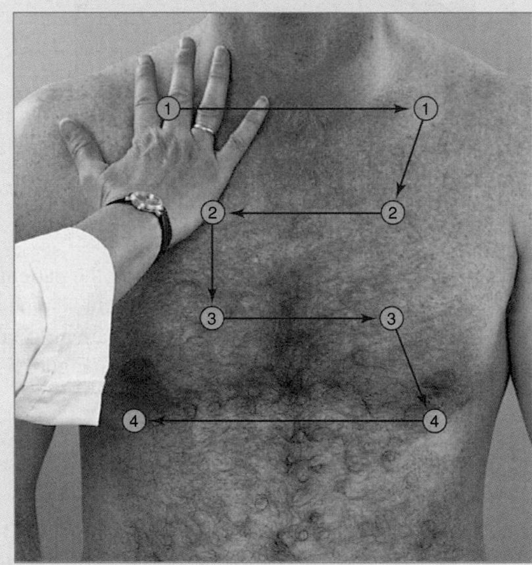

FIGURE 5 Sequence for palpating anterior thorax.

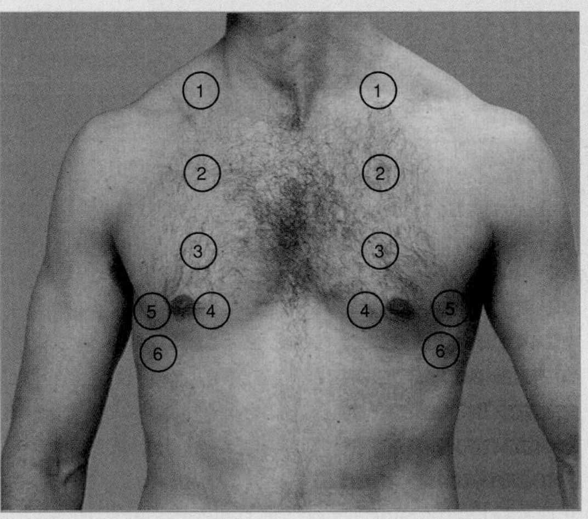

FIGURE 6 Sequence for auscultating anterior thorax. (From Hogan-Quigley, B., Palm, M.L., & Bickley, L. (2012). *Bates' nursing guide to physical examination and history taking.* Philadelphia: Wolters Kluwer Health/Lippincott Williams & Wilkins, p. 318.)

ACTION	RATIONALE
14. Inspect the breasts. Ask the patient to rest hands on both sides of the body, then on the hips and finally above the head. With the patient holding each position, inspect the breasts for size, shape, symmetry, color, texture, and skin lesions. Inspect the areola and nipples for size and shape and the nipples for discharge, crusting, and inversion.	This technique evaluates the general condition of the breasts and helps to identify any abnormalities.
15. Palpate the axillae with the patient's arms resting against the side of the body. If any nodes are palpable, assess their location, size, shape, consistency, tenderness, and mobility.	Palpating the axillae helps to detect nodular enlargement, tenderness, and other abnormalities.
16. Assist the patient into a supine position. Place a small pillow or towel under the patient's back and ask the patient to place a hand on the side being examined under the head, if possible.	Positioning facilitates the exam.
17. Wear gloves if there is any discharge from the nipples or if a lesion is present. Palpate each quadrant of each breast in a systematic method, using either the circular, wedge, or vertical strip technique (see Box 3-1). Palpate the nipple and areola and gently compress the nipple between the thumb and forefinger to assess for discharge.	Gloves prevent contact with blood and body fluids. Palpating the breasts evaluates the consistency and elasticity of breast tissue and nipples and for presence of lumps, masses, or discharge.
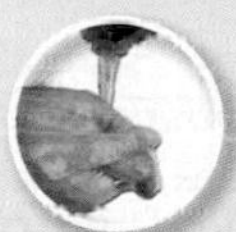 18. Assist the patient into a comfortable position and in replacing the gown. Remove gloves and any additional PPE, if used. Perform hand hygiene. Continue with assessments of specific body systems, as appropriate or indicated. Initiate appropriate referral to other health care practitioners for further evaluation, as indicated.	Replacing the gown ensures patient comfort. Removing PPE properly reduces the risk for infection transmission and contamination of other items. Hand hygiene prevents the spread of microorganisms. Additional assessments should be completed, as indicated, to evaluate the patient's health status. Intervention by other health care providers may be indicated to evaluate and treat the patient's health status.

BOX 3-1 METHODS FOR PALPATING THE BREASTS

Wedge Method

- Work in a clockwise direction and palpate from the periphery toward the areola (Figure 1).
- Use the pads of the first three fingers to gently compress the breast tissue against the chest wall.

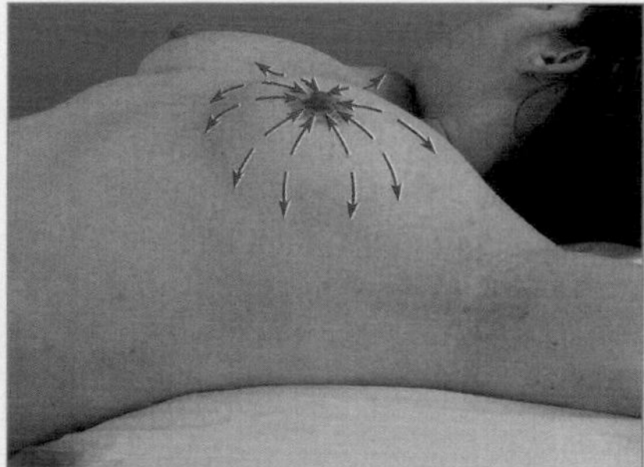

FIGURE 1 Wedge method of breast examination.

Circular Method

- Start at the tail of Spence and move in increasing smaller circles (Figure 2).
- Use the pads of the first three fingers to gently compress the breast tissue against the chest wall.

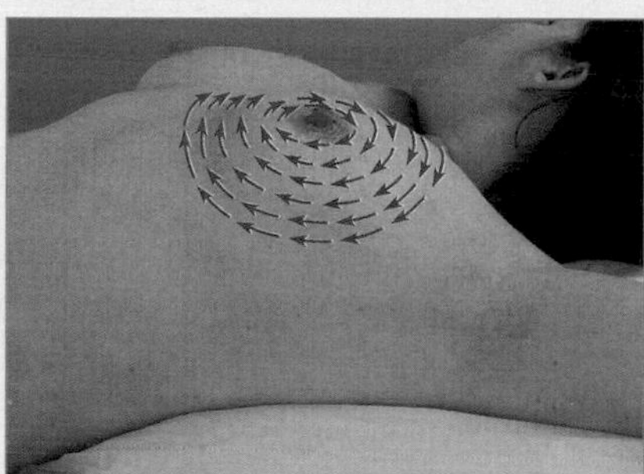

FIGURE 2 Circular method of breast examination.

Vertical Strip Method

- Start at the outer edge of the breast and palpate up and down the breast (Figure 3).
- Use the pads of the first three fingers to gently compress the breast tissue against the chest wall.

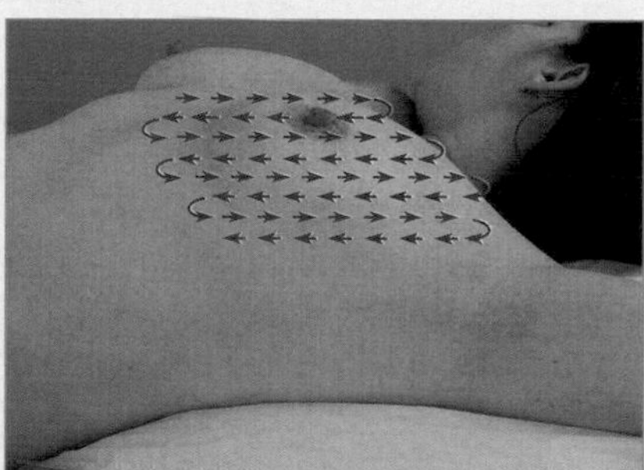

FIGURE 3 Vertical strip method of breast examination.

(continued)

SKILL 3-5 ASSESSING THE THORAX, LUNGS, AND BREASTS continued

EVALUATION

The expected outcome is met when the patient participates in the assessment of the thorax, lungs, breasts, and axillae; the patient verbalizes understanding of these assessment techniques as appropriate; the assessment is completed without the patient experiencing anxiety or discomfort; the findings are documented; and the appropriate referrals are made to the other health care professionals, as needed, for further evaluation.

DOCUMENTATION

Guidelines

When documenting the assessment of the thorax, lungs, breasts, and axillae, describe specific findings. Include specific findings for all assessment techniques performed. Note the location of elicited abnormalities. For breast assessment, clock position is often used to describe the location of findings.

Sample Documentation

Lippincott DocuCare Practice documenting assessment techniques and findings in *Lippincott DocuCare.*

6/10/15 2025 Patient states that she "has had a dry cough for the past week and feels weak." Skin pale. RR 30. Breathing effort moderately labored; right-sided intercostal retraction noted. Barrel-shaped chest. Vibrations palpated on right anterior and posterior chest. Rhonchi (sonorous wheezes) auscultated in RUL, RML, and RLL of lung fields. Breasts symmetric, skin smooth with even tone. Breasts and axillae without lumps, masses, dimpling, and discharge.

—*B. Gentzler, RN*

UNEXPECTED SITUATIONS AND ASSOCIATED INTERVENTIONS

- *When assessing a patient's lungs, you hear short, high-pitched popping sounds on inspiration:* Ask the patient to cough and auscultate again. If the sounds remain, suspect fine crackles and ask the patient if he or she is experiencing any difficulty in breathing or shortness of breath. Crackles may indicate disease such as pneumonia or heart failure. Document the findings. Continue to assess the patient and notify the primary care provider, as indicated.

SPECIAL CONSIDERATIONS

General Considerations

- Warm equipment, such as a stethoscope, before using it to prevent chilling the patient.
- Warm hands before palpating breasts to prevent chilling the patient and causing any discomfort.
- Attempt to reduce the noise level in the room while auscultating for breath sounds to ensure accuracy in listening. Also, the presence of chest hair may mimic the sound of crackles and bumping the stethoscope against clothing may distort the sound.
- Obtain the patient's subjective data as well as the physical examination findings. For example, the physical data may be normal; however, the patient may verbalize that he or she is having difficulty breathing. In this case, the patient needs to be monitored closely to assess for possible complications.

Infant and Child Considerations

- Auscultate a child's lungs before performing other assessment techniques that may cause crying.
- Expect to hear breath sounds that are harsher or more bronchial than those of an adult.

Older Adult Considerations

- In the older adult patient, expect to find a reduction in respiratory effort due to age-related changes. A common finding in the older adult is kyphoscoliosis, a skeletal deformity affecting the spinal column, which causes the AP diameter to increase and the thorax to shorten. Also, the alveoli of the lung tissue decreases, which reduces the amount of alveolar surface area available for gas exchange.

SKILL 3-6 ASSESSING THE CARDIOVASCULAR SYSTEM

The cardiovascular system transports oxygen, nutrients, and other substances to the body tissues and removes metabolic waste products to the kidneys and lungs. Careful assessment of this vital system is essential. In this skill, assessment data associated with the heart will be presented. The peripheral vascular system assessment is included in Skill 3-10, because peripheral vascular, neurologic, and musculoskeletal systems are usually combined when performing a head-to-toe assessment. While assessing the heart, careful auscultation is important. Identifying heart sounds takes practice; Box 3-2 provides a review of normal (and information about abnormal) heart sounds.

Box 3-2 HEART SOUNDS

Normal Heart Sounds

During auscultation, the first heart sound, S_1, is heard as the "lub" of "lub-dub." This sound occurs when the mitral and tricuspid valves close, and it corresponds to the onset of ventricular contraction. The sound, low-pitched and dull, is heard best at the apical area. The second heart sound, S_2, occurs at the termination of systole and corresponds to the onset of ventricular diastole. The "dub" of "lub-dub," it represents the closure of the aortic and pulmonic valves. The sound of S_2 is higher pitched and shorter than S_1. The two sounds occur within 1 second or less, depending on the heart rate.

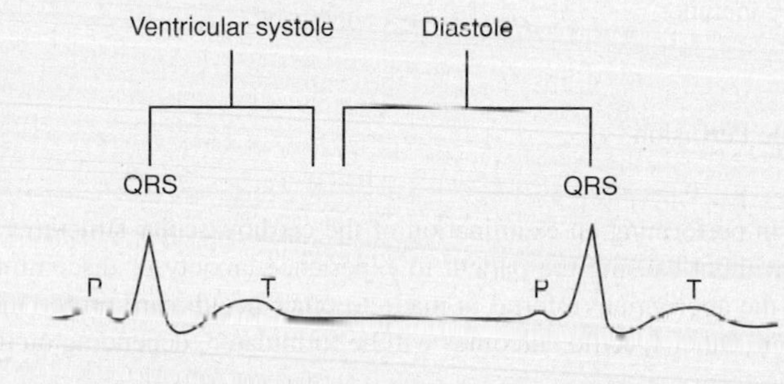

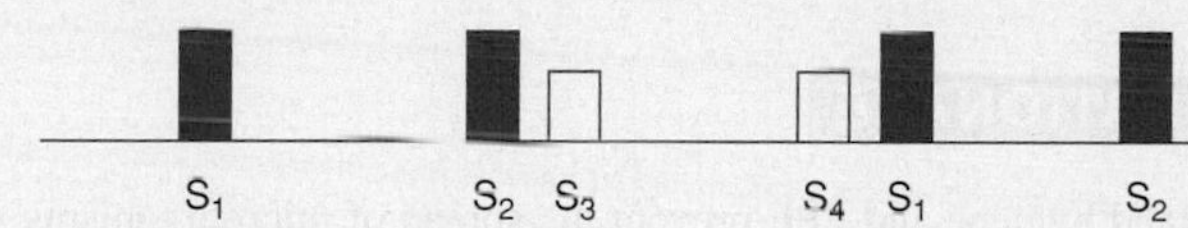

A. Electrocardiogram. **B.** Heart sounds. Heart sounds in relation to the cardiac cycle and an electrocardiogram.

Normal findings include S_1 that is louder at the tricuspid and apical areas, with S_2 louder at the aortic and pulmonic areas.

Heart sounds in relation to the cardiac cycle and an electrocardiogram.

Abnormal Heart Sounds

Abnormal findings include extra heart sounds at any of the cardiac landmarks and abnormal rate or rhythm. A wide variety of conditions may alter the normal heart rate or rhythm, including serious infections, anemia, diseases of the heart muscle or conducting system, dehydration or overhydration, endocrine disorders, respiratory disorders, and head trauma. Extra heart sounds may be S_3, S_4, murmurs, or bruits.

- S_3, known as the third heart sound, follows S_2, and is often represented by a "lub-dub-dee" pattern ("dee" being S_3). This sound is best heard with the stetho scope bell at the mitral area, with the patient lying on the left side. S_3 is considered normal in children and young adults and abnormal in middle-aged and older adults.
- S_4 is the fourth heart sound, occurring right before S_1, and is often represented by a "dee lub-dub" pattern ("dee" being S_4.) S_4 is considered normal in older adults but abnormal in children and adults.
- Heart murmurs are extra heart sounds caused by some disruption of blood flow through the heart. The characteristics of a murmur and grading depend on the adequacy of valve function, rate of blood flow, and size of the valve opening. Usually, nurses are more concerned with recognizing changes in murmurs rather than in diagnosing and labeling them (Jensen, 2011). Refer to information on thePoint or a health assessment text for grading details.

DELEGATION CONSIDERATIONS

Assessment of the patient's cardiovascular system should not be delegated to nursing assistive personnel (NAP) or unlicensed assistive personnel (UAP). However, the NAP or UAP may notice some items while providing care. The nurse must then validate, analyze, document, communicate, and act on these findings, as appropriate. Depending on the state's nurse practice act and the organization's policies and procedures, the licensed practical/vocational nurses (LPN/LVNs) may perform some or all of the parts of assessment of the patient's cardiovascular system. The decision to delegate must be based on careful analysis of the patient's needs and circumstances, as well as the qualifications of the person to whom the task is being delegated. Refer to the Delegation Guidelines in Appendix A.

(continued)

SKILL 3-6 ASSESSING THE CARDIOVASCULAR SYSTEM continued

EQUIPMENT

- Bath blanket or other drape
- Examination gown
- Stethoscope
- Centimeter ruler
- PPE, as indicated

ASSESSMENT

Complete a health history, focusing on the heart. Identify risk factors for altered health during the health history by asking about the following:

- History of chest pain, tightness, palpitations, dizziness, or fatigue
- Swelling in the ankles and feet
- Number of pillows used to sleep
- Type and amount of medications taken daily
- History of heart defect, rheumatic fever, or chest or heart surgery
- Family history of hypertension (high blood pressure), myocardial infarction (heart attack), coronary artery disease, high blood cholesterol levels, or diabetes mellitus
- History of smoking (including pack-years)
- History of alcohol use
- Type and amount of exercise
- Usual foods eaten each day

NURSING DIAGNOSIS

Determine the related factors for the nursing diagnoses based on the patient's current health status. Appropriate nursing diagnoses may include:

- Decreased Cardiac Output
- Impaired Gas Exchange
- Risk for Decreased Cardiac Tissue Perfusion

OUTCOME IDENTIFICATION AND PLANNING

The expected outcome to achieve in performing an examination of the cardiovascular structures is that the assessment is completed without causing the patient to experience anxiety or discomfort, the findings are documented, and the appropriate referral is made to other health care professionals, as needed, for further evaluation. Other specific outcomes will be formulated, depending on the identified nursing diagnosis.

IMPLEMENTATION

ACTION	RATIONALE
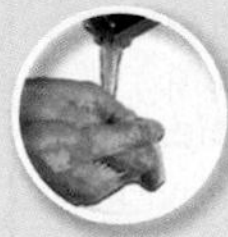 1. Perform hand hygiene and put on PPE, if indicated.	Hand hygiene and PPE prevent the spread of microorganisms. PPE is required based on transmission precautions.
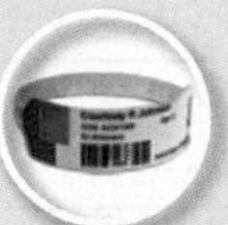 2. Identify the patient.	Identifying the patient ensures the right patient receives the intervention and helps prevent errors.
3. Close the curtains around the bed and close the door to the room, if possible. Explain the purpose of the cardiovascular examination and what you are going to do. Answer any questions.	This ensures the patient's privacy. Explanation relieves anxiety and facilitates cooperation.

ACTION	RATIONALE
4. Help the patient undress, if needed, and provide a patient gown. Assist the patient to a supine position with the head elevated about 30 to 45 degrees, if possible, and expose the anterior chest. Use the bath blanket to cover any exposed area other than the one being assessed.	Having the patient wear a gown facilitates examination of the cardiovascular system. Use of a bath blanket provides for comfort and warmth.
5. If not performed previously with the assessment of the head and neck, inspect and palpate the left and then the right carotid arteries. **Palpate only one carotid artery at a time.** Note the strength of the pulse and grade it as with peripheral pulses. Use the bell of the stethoscope to auscultate the arteries. Refer to Step 20, Skill 3-4.	Palpation of this area evaluates circulation through the arteries. Palpating both arteries at once can reduce blood flow to the brain, potentially causing dizziness or loss of consciousness. Auscultation can detect a bruit.
6. Inspect the neck for distention of the jugular veins.	Jugular venous distention (fullness) is associated with heart failure and fluid volume overload.
7. Inspect the **precordium** (the portion of the body over the heart and lower thorax, encompassing the aortic, pulmonic, tricuspid, and mitral (apical) areas, and Erb's point) for contour, pulsations, and heaves (Figure 1). Observe for the apical impulse at the fourth to fifth intercostal space (ICS) at the left midclavicular line.	Precordium inspection helps detect pulsations. There are normally no pulsations, except for the apical impulse.
8. Using the palmar surface with the four fingers held together, gently palpate the precordium for pulsations. Remember that hands should be warm. Palpation proceeds in a systematic manner, with assessment of specific cardiac landmarks—the aortic, pulmonic, tricuspid, and mitral areas and Erb's point. Palpate the apical impulse in the mitral area (Figure 2). Note size, duration, force, and location in relationship to the midclavicular line.	Normal findings include no pulsation palpable over the aortic and pulmonic areas, with a palpable apical impulse. Abnormal findings include precordial thrills, which are fine, palpable, rushing vibrations over the right or left second ICS, and any lifts or heaves, which involve a rise along the border of the sternum with each heartbeat.

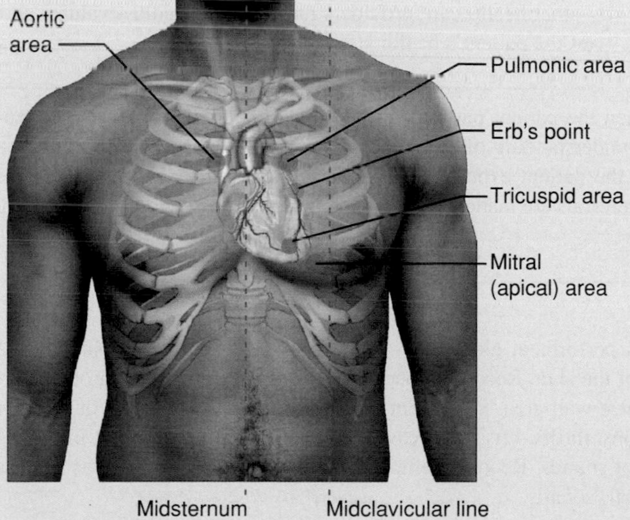

FIGURE 1 Cardiac landmarks.

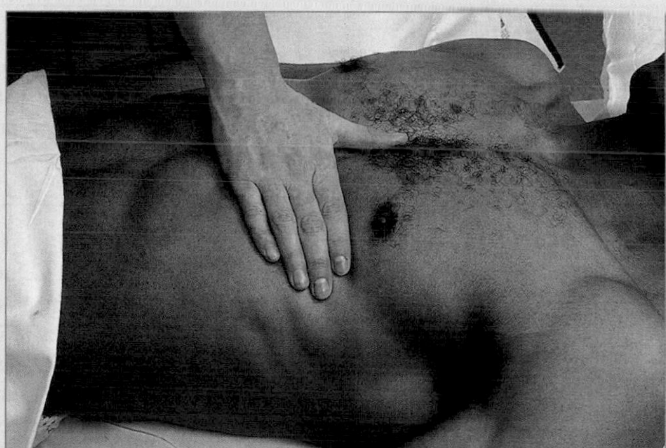

FIGURE 2 Palpating the apical impulse.

(continued)

SKILL 3-6 ASSESSING THE CARDIOVASCULAR SYSTEM continued

ACTION	RATIONALE
9. Auscultate heart sounds. Ask the patient to breathe normally. Use the diaphragm of the stethoscope first to listen to high-pitched sounds. Then use the bell to listen to low-pitched sounds. Focus on the overall rate and rhythm of the heart and the normal heart sounds (Box 3-2). Begin at the aortic area, move to the pulmonic area, then to Erb's point, then the tricuspid area, and finally listen at the mitral area (Figures 1 and 3).	Auscultation evaluates heart rate and rhythm and assesses for normal sounds (the lub, S_1; the dub, S_2) and abnormal heart sounds. The normal heart sounds (S_1 and S_2) are generated by the closing of the valves (the aortic, pulmonic, tricuspid, mitral). Extra heart sounds are often heard when the patient has anemia or heart disease. A wide variety of conditions may alter the normal heart rate or rhythm, including serious infections, diseases of the heart muscle or conducting system, dehydration or overhydration, endocrine disorders, respiratory disorders, and head trauma. Extra heart sounds may be S_3, S_4, murmurs, or bruits.

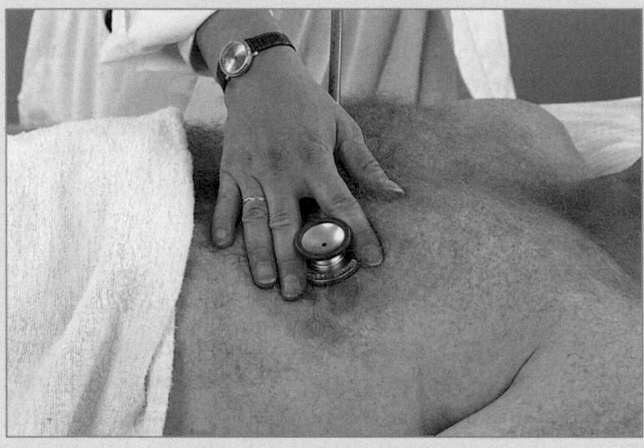

FIGURE 3 Auscultating the mitral area. *(Photo by B. Proud.)*

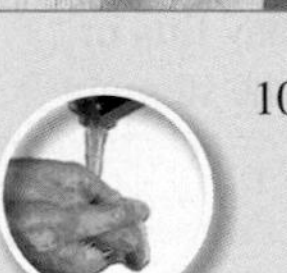

ACTION	RATIONALE
10. Assist the patient in replacing the gown. Remove PPE, if used. Perform hand hygiene. Continue with assessments of specific body systems as appropriate or indicated. Initiate appropriate referral to other health care practitioners for further evaluation, as indicated.	Replacing the gown ensures patient comfort. Removing PPE properly reduces the risk for infection transmission and contamination of other items. Hand hygiene prevents the spread of microorganisms. Additional assessments should be completed as indicated to evaluate the patient's health status. Intervention by other health care providers may be indicated to evaluate and treat the patient's health status.

EVALUATION

The expected outcome is met when the patient participates in the assessment of the cardiovascular system, the patient verbalizes understanding of these assessment techniques as appropriate, the assessment is completed without the patient experiencing anxiety or discomfort, the findings are documented, and the appropriate referrals are made to the other health care professionals, as needed, for further evaluation.

DOCUMENTATION

Guidelines

Document assessment techniques performed, along with specific findings. Note assessment data related to color and temperature of the skin. Record inspection findings related to the carotid arteries, jugular veins, and anterior chest wall area. Document findings related to palpation of anterior chest wall for presence of pulsations, thrills, lifts, and heaves. Note auscultation findings, including rate, rhythm, pitch, and location of sounds. Record the normal heart sounds (S_1 and S_2) as well as the presence of any extra (abnormal) sounds.

Sample Documentation

Lippincott DocuCare **Practice documenting assessment techniques and findings in *Lippincott DocuCare*.**

5/10/15 1015 Patient denies chest pain but states, "I have palpitations occurring about once a week." Skin pale, cool to touch, brisk capillary refill. Inspection and palpation of chest: no lifts, pulsations, or heaves were noted. Auscultation: S_1 loudest at the apex; S_2 loudest at the base; no extra sounds auscultated. Carotid pulse 88, regular rhythm, + 2, equal bilaterally. No carotid bruits auscultated.

—S. Moses, RN

SKILL 3-6 ASSESSING THE CARDIOVASCULAR SYSTEM continued

SPECIAL CONSIDERATIONS

General Considerations

- Warm equipment, such as a stethoscope, before using it to prevent chilling the patient.

Infant and Child Considerations

- The presence of abnormal heart sound S_3 is considered normal in children and young adults.
- The presence of abnormal heart sound S_4 is considered abnormal in children.

Older Adult Considerations

- The presence of abnormal heart sound S_3 is considered abnormal in middle-aged and older adults.
- The presence of abnormal heart sound S_4 is considered normal in older adults.

WATCH & LEARN SKILL 3-7 ASSESSING THE ABDOMEN

The abdominal cavity, the largest cavity in the body, contains the stomach, small intestine, large intestine, liver, gallbladder, pancreas, spleen, kidneys, urinary bladder, adrenal gland, and major blood vessels. In women, the uterus, fallopian tubes, and ovaries are also located in the abdomen. Not all of these organs can be assessed. For identification/documentation purposes, the abdomen can be divided into four quadrants (Figure 1).

The order of the techniques differs for the abdominal assessment from the other systems. Assessment of the abdomen starts with inspection, then auscultation, percussion, and palpation. The order of assessment differs for this system because palpation and percussion before auscultation may alter the sounds heard on auscultation. Advanced practice professionals perform percussion and deep palpation of the abdomen. Therefore, these techniques will not be discussed here. Before beginning the abdominal assessment, ask the patient to empty his/her bladder because a full bladder may cause discomfort during the examination.

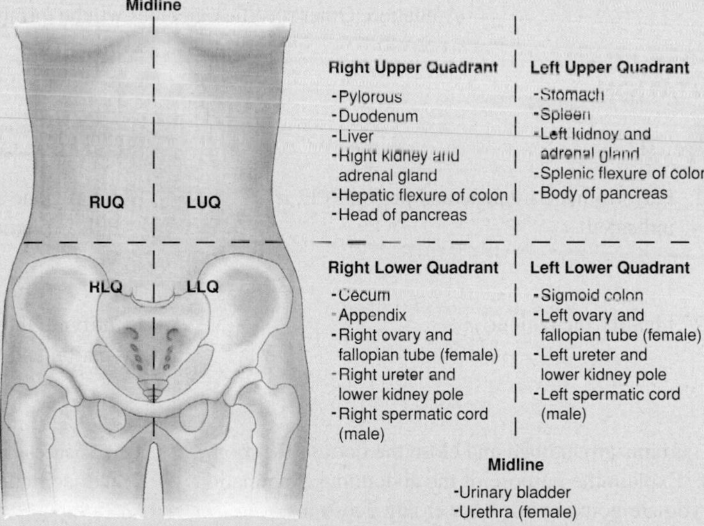

FIGURE 1 Diagram of abdominal quadrants and outline of underlying organs.

DELEGATION CONSIDERATIONS

Assessment of the patient's abdomen should not be delegated to nursing assistive personnel (NAP) or unlicensed assistive personnel (UAP). However, the NAP or UAP may notice some items while providing care. The nurse must then validate, analyze, document, communicate, and act on these findings, as appropriate. Depending on the state's nurse practice act and the organization's policies and procedures, the licensed practical/vocational nurses (LPN/LVNs) may perform some or all of the parts of assessment of the patient's abdomen. The decision to delegate must be based on careful analysis of the patient's needs and circumstances, as well as the qualifications of the person to whom the task is being delegated. Refer to the Delegation Guidelines in Appendix A.

(continued)

SKILL 3-7 ASSESSING THE ABDOMEN continued

EQUIPMENT

- PPE, as indicated
- Bath blanket or other drape
- Examination gown
- Stethoscope
- Penlight

ASSESSMENT

Complete a health history, focusing on the abdomen. Identify risk factors for altered health during the health history by asking about the following:

- History of abdominal pain
- History of indigestion, nausea or vomiting, constipation or diarrhea
- History of food allergies or lactose intolerance
- Appetite and usual food and fluid intake
- Usual bowel and bladder elimination patterns
- History of gastrointestinal disorders, such as peptic ulcer disease, bowel disease, gallbladder disease, liver disease, or appendicitis
- History of urinary tract disorders, such as infections, kidney stones, or kidney disease
- History of abdominal surgery or trauma
- Type and amount of prescribed and over-the-counter medications used
- Amount and type of alcohol ingestion
- For women, menstrual history

NURSING DIAGNOSIS

Determine the related factors for the nursing diagnoses based on the patient's current health status. Appropriate nursing diagnoses may include:

- Constipation
- Acute Pain
- Diarrhea

OUTCOME IDENTIFICATION AND PLANNING

The expected outcome to achieve in performing an examination of the abdomen is that the assessment is completed without causing the patient to experience anxiety or discomfort, the findings are documented, and the appropriate referral is made to other health care professionals, as needed, for further evaluation. Other specific outcomes will be formulated, depending on the identified nursing diagnosis.

IMPLEMENTATION

ACTION	RATIONALE
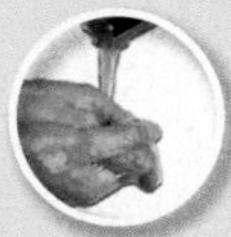 1. Perform hand hygiene and put on PPE, if indicated.	Hand hygiene and PPE prevent the spread of microorganisms. PPE is required based on transmission precautions.
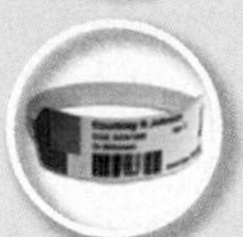 2. Identify the patient.	Identifying the patient ensures the right patient receives the intervention and helps prevent errors.
3. Close the curtains around bed and close the door to the room, if possible. Explain the purpose of the abdominal examination and what you are going to do. Answer any questions.	This ensures the patient's privacy. Explanation relieves anxiety and facilitates cooperation.
4. Help the patient undress, if needed, and provide a patient gown. Assist the patient to a supine position, if possible, and expose the abdomen. Use the bath blanket to cover any exposed area other than the one being assessed.	Having the patient wear a gown facilitates examination of the abdomen. Use of a bath blanket provides for comfort and warmth.
5. Inspect the abdomen for skin color, contour, pulsations, the umbilicus, and other surface characteristics (rashes, lesions, masses, scars).	The umbilicus should be centrally located and may be flat, rounded, or concave. The abdomen should be evenly rounded or symmetric, without visible peristalsis. In thin people, an upper midline pulsation may normally be visible. Abnormal findings include asymmetry (possibly from an enlarged organ or mass), distension (possibly indicating retained gas or air; obesity), swelling of the abdomen (possibly indicating **ascites**) and abdominal masses or unusual pulsations.

ACTION

RATIONALE

6. Ausculate all four quadrants of the abdomen (see Figure 1) for bowel sounds. Warm the stethoscope and, using light pressure, place the flat diaphragm on the right lower quadrant of the abdomen, then move to the right upper quadrant (Figure 2), left upper quadrant, and finally left lower quadrant. Listen carefully for bowel sounds (gurgles and clicks), and note their frequency and character.

Performing auscultation before percussion or palpation prevents percussion and palpation techniques from interfering with findings. Bowel sounds usually occur every 5 to 34 seconds. Before documenting bowel sounds as absent, listen for 2 minutes or longer in each abdominal quadrant. Abnormal findings include increased bowel sounds (often heard with diarrhea or in early bowel obstruction), decreased bowel sounds (heard after abdominal surgery or late bowel obstruction), or absent bowel sounds (indicating peritonitis or paralytic ileus). Bowel sounds of high-pitched tinkling or rushes of high-pitched sounds indicate a bowel obstruction.

7. Auscultate the abdomen for vascular sounds. Using the bell of the stethoscope, auscultate over the abdominal aorta, femoral arteries, and iliac arteries for bruits (Figure 3).

Bruits are abnormal sounds heard over a blood vessel, caused by blood that is swirling in the vessel, rather than normal smooth flow. A bruit may be heard in the presence of stenosis (narrowing) or occlusion of an artery. Bruits may also be caused by abnormal dilation of a vessel.

8. Palpate the abdomen lightly in all four quadrants The pads of the fingers are used to palpate with a light, gentle, dipping motion approximately 1 to 2 cm (Jensen, 2011). Watch the patient's face for nonverbal signs of pain during palpation. Palpate each quadrant in a systematic manner, noting muscular resistance, tenderness, enlargement of the organs, or masses. (Figure 4). **If the patient complains of pain or discomfort in a particular area of the abdomen, palpate that area last.**

Palpation provides information about the location, size, tenderness, and condition of the underlying structures. The abdomen should normally be soft, relaxed, and free of tenderness. Abnormal findings include involuntary rigidity, spasm, and pain (which may indicate trauma, peritonitis, infection, tumors, or enlarged or diseased abdominal organs, such as appendicitis).

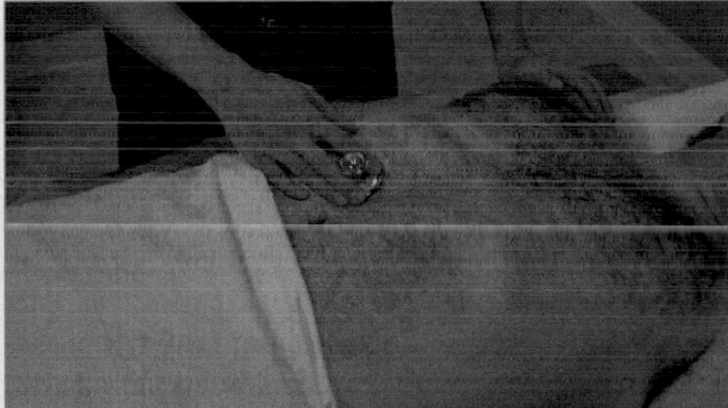

FIGURE 2 Auscultating the abdomen. (From Jensen, S. (2011). *Nursing health assessment. A best practice approach*. Philadelphia: Wolters Kluwer Health/Lippincott Williams & Wilkins, p. 606, Figure 22.6.)

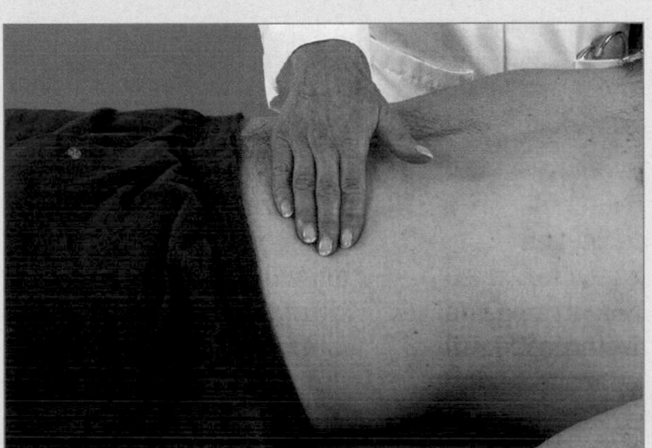

FIGURE 4 Palpating the abdomen lightly. *(Photo by B. Proud.)*

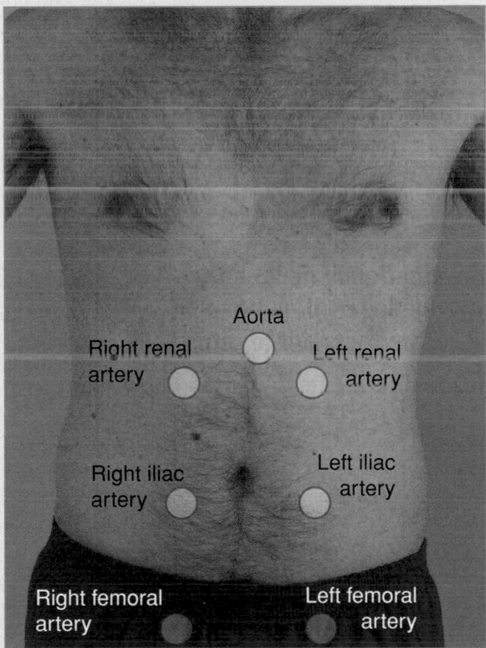

FIGURE 3 Locations to auscultate for bruits. *(Photo by B. Proud.)*

(continued)

SKILL 3-7 ASSESSING THE ABDOMEN continued

ACTION	RATIONALE
9. Palpate and then auscultate the femoral pulses in the groin. Note the strength of the pulse and grade it as with peripheral pulses (see Skill 3-10). Use the bell of the stethoscope to auscultate the arteries.	This is part of the assessment of the peripheral vascular system in Skill 3-10. However, some practitioners include this assessment here for organizational convenience and time management. This technique assesses flow of blood through the arteries. Auscultation can detect a bruit.
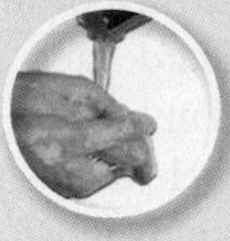 10. Assist the patient into a comfortable position and in replacing the gown. Remove PPE, if used. Perform hand hygiene. Continue with assessments of specific body systems, as appropriate, or indicated. Initiate appropriate referral to other health care practitioners for further evaluation, as indicated.	Replacing the gown ensures patient comfort. Removing PPE properly reduces the risk for infection transmission and contamination of other items. Hand hygiene prevents the spread of microorganisms. Additional assessments should be completed, as indicated, to evaluate the patient's health status. Intervention by other health care providers may be indicated to evaluate and treat the patient's health status.

EVALUATION

The expected outcome is met when the patient participates in the assessment of the abdomen, the patient verbalizes understanding of the assessment techniques as appropriate, the assessment is completed without the patient experiencing anxiety or discomfort, the findings are documented, and the appropriate referrals are made to the other health care professionals, as needed, for further evaluation.

DOCUMENTATION

Guidelines

Document assessment techniques performed, along with specific findings. For inspection, include a description of the color, presence of symmetry/asymmetry, distension, swelling, lesions, rashes, scars, or masses. For auscultation, note the character of the bowel sounds and if any bruits are present. For palpation, note the overall softness or hardness of the abdomen, presence of palpable masses, the presence of pain or tenderness, and unusual pulsations.

Sample Documentation

Lippincott DocuCare **Practice documenting assessment techniques and findings in *Lippincott DocuCare*.**

3/30/15 0930 Patient states, "I have been feeling sick to my stomach for the last 24 hours." Denies any abdominal pain. Abdomen symmetric; soft, slightly distended, umbilicus midline, no scars or pulsations, bowel sounds present in all four quadrants, but decreased.

—B. Gentzler, RN

SPECIAL CONSIDERATIONS

General Considerations

- Warm equipment, such as a stethoscope, before using it to prevent chilling the patient.

Infant and Child Considerations

- In infants, expect a large abdomen in relation to the pelvis.
- The abdomen of a child is normally protuberant.

SKILL 3-8 ASSESSING THE FEMALE GENITALIA

The external female genitalia consist of the mons pubis, labia majora and minora, clitoris, vestibular glands, vaginal vestibule, vaginal orifice, and urethral opening (Figure 1). During the physical assessment, examine the external genitalia by inspection and palpation. The internal pelvic examination is a skill most often performed by an advanced practice professional. Women from some cultures or those who practice certain religions (e.g., Islam) may agree to a physical examination of the genitalia only if it is performed by a female nurse or female practitioner.

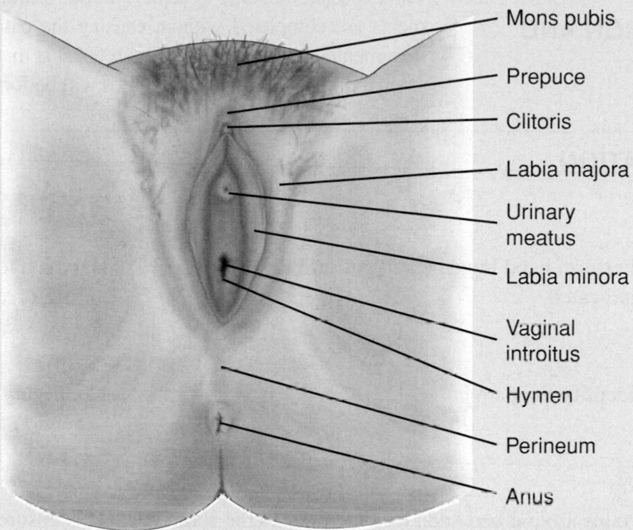

FIGURE 1 External female genitalia.

DELEGATION CONSIDERATIONS

Assessment of the patient's genitalia should not be delegated to nursing assistive personnel (NAP) or unlicensed assistive personnel (UAP). However, an NAP or UAP may notice some items while providing care. The nurse must then validate, analyze, document, communicate, and act on these findings, as appropriate. Depending on the state's nurse practice act and the organization's policies and procedures, the licensed practical/vocational nurses (LPN/LVNs) may perform some or all of the parts of assessment of the patient's genitalia. The decision to delegate must be based on careful analysis of the patient's needs and circumstances, as well as the qualifications of the person to whom the task is being delegated. Refer to the Delegation Guidelines in Appendix A.

EQUIPMENT

- PPE, as indicated
- Bath blanket or other drape
- Examination gown
- Gloves

ASSESSMENT

Complete a health history, focusing on the female genital system. Identify risk factors for altered health during the health history by asking about the following:

- Menstrual history (age of first and last period, length of flow, type of flow, pain)
- Sexual history (age at which sexual activity began, number and gender of partners)
- Pain with intercourse, difficulty achieving orgasm
- Number of pregnancies and live births
- History of sexually transmitted infection
- Use of contraceptives
- Frequency of pelvic examinations and Pap smears
- History of vaginal discharge, itching, or pain on urination
- Family history of reproductive or genital cancer
- Use of hormones and tobacco (how long, how much, how many packs/day)

(continued)

SKILL 3-8 ASSESSING THE FEMALE GENITALIA continued

NURSING DIAGNOSIS

Determine the related factors for the nursing diagnoses based on the patient's current health status. Appropriate nursing diagnoses may include:

- Ineffective Health Maintenance
- Risk for Infection
- Sexual Dysfunction

OUTCOME IDENTIFICATION AND PLANNING

The expected outcome to achieve in performing an examination of the female genitalia is that the assessments are completed without causing the patient to experience anxiety or discomfort, the findings are documented, and the appropriate referral is made to other health care professionals, as needed, for further evaluation. Other specific outcomes will be formulated, depending on the identified nursing diagnosis.

IMPLEMENTATION

ACTION	RATIONALE
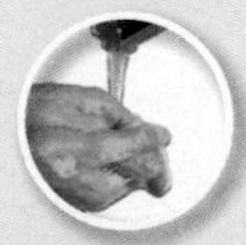 1. Perform hand hygiene and put on PPE, if indicated.	Hand hygiene and PPE prevent the spread of microorganisms. PPE is required based on transmission precautions.
 2. Identify the patient.	Identifying the patient ensures the right patient receives the intervention and helps prevent errors.
3. Close the curtains around bed and close the door to the room, if possible. Explain the purpose of the examination of genitalia and what you are going to do. Answer any questions.	This ensures the patient's privacy. Explanation relieves anxiety and facilitates cooperation.
4. Help the patient undress, if needed, and provide a patient gown. Assist the patient to a supine position, or lying on her side, if possible. Use the bath blanket to cover any exposed area other than the one being assessed.	Having the patient wear a gown facilitates examination of the genitalia. Use of a bath blanket provides for comfort and warmth.
5. Inspect the external genitalia for color, size of the labia majora and vaginal opening, lesions, and discharge.	The vulva normally has more pigmentation than other skin areas, and the mucous membranes are dark pink and moist. The skin and mucosa should be smooth, without lesions or swelling. The labia should be symmetric without lesions or swelling. Lesions may be the result of infections (e.g., herpes or syphilis). There may normally be a small amount of clear or whitish vaginal discharge.
6. Palpate the labia for masses.	The vulva should be without lumps or masses.
7. Assist the patient to a comfortable position.	This ensures the patient's comfort.
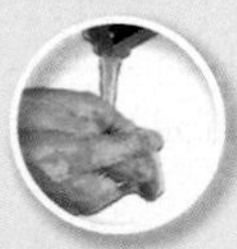 8. Remove PPE, if used. Perform hand hygiene. Continue with assessments of specific body systems, as appropriate, or indicated. Initiate appropriate referral to other health care practitioners for further evaluation, as indicated.	Removing PPE properly reduces the risk for infection transmission and contamination of other items. Hand hygiene prevents the spread of microorganisms. Additional assessments should be completed, as indicated, to evaluate the patient's health status. Intervention by other health care providers may be indicated to evaluate and treat the patient's health status.

EVALUATION

The expected outcome is met when the patient participates in the assessment of the genitalia; the patient verbalizes an understanding of the assessment techniques as appropriate; the assessment is completed without the patient experiencing anxiety or discomfort; the findings are documented; and the appropriate referrals are made to the other health care professionals as needed for further evaluation.

DOCUMENTATION

Guidelines

Document assessment techniques performed, along with specific findings. Note and record the color, size of the labia majora and vaginal opening, lesions, and presence of any discharge. Document any patient statements of pain and risk factors.

Sample Documentation

> 1/12/15 1645 Patient denies vaginal itching, pain, lumps, or discharge. Vulva with darker pigmentation than surrounding skin tone; mucous membranes are dark pink and moist. Skin and mucosa smooth, without lesions or swelling. Labia are symmetric without lesions or swelling. No discharge noted. Vulva are without lumps or masses.
>
> *—B. Holmes, RN*

SPECIAL CONSIDERATIONS

Infant and Child Considerations

- In newborns, enlargement of the labia and clitoris and breast enlargement occur, resulting from exposure to maternal hormones in utero and normally seen in the first week after birth, subsiding by the second week after birth.
- In children, loss of hymenal tissue between the 3 o'clock and 9 o'clock position indicates trauma (from digits, penis, or foreign objects).
- Pubic hair and breast development occur at puberty and follow a regular sequence of development.
- Menstruation begins about 2.5 years after puberty begins.
- Irregular menstrual cycle is common for first two years.

Older Adult Considerations

- Decreased size of labia and clitoris
- Decreased amount of pubic hair
- Decreased vaginal secretions
- Pale, thin, and dry vaginal mucosa

SKILL 3-9 ASSESSING MALE GENITALIA

The external male genitalia (Figure 1) include the penis and scrotum. In addition, the inguinal area may be assessed as part of this assessment. During the physical assessment, the nurse examines the external genitalia by inspection and palpation. Examination of the prostate gland is a skill performed by an advanced practice professional.

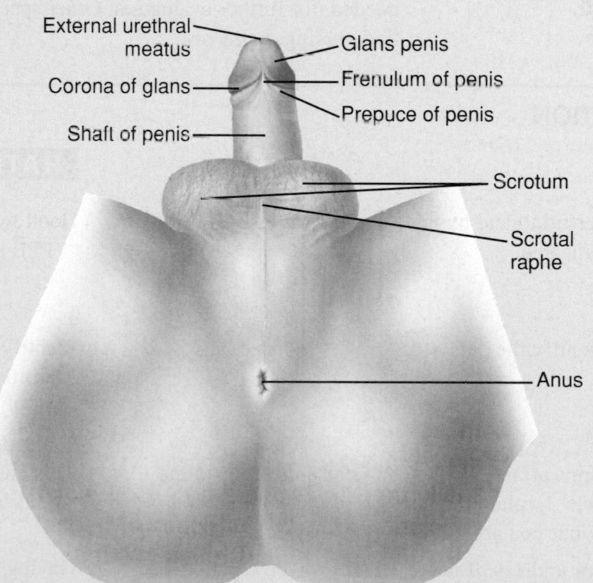

FIGURE 1 External male genitalia. (From Pansky, B., & Gest, T.R. (2013). *Lippincott's concise illustrated anatomy: Thorax, abdomen & pelvis*, Philadelphia: Wolters Kluwer Health/Lippincott Williams & Wilkins, p. 205, Figure 3.1F.)

(continued)

SKILL 3-9 ASSESSING MALE GENITALIA continued

DELEGATION CONSIDERATIONS

The assessment of the patient's genitalia should not be delegated to nursing assistive personnel (NAP) or unlicensed assistive personnel (UAP). However, the NAP or UAP may notice some items while providing care. The nurse must then validate, analyze, document, communicate, and act on these findings, as appropriate. Depending on the state's nurse practice act and the organization's policies and procedures, the licensed practical/vocational nurses (LPN/LVNs) may perform some or all of the parts of assessment of the patient's genitalia. The decision to delegate must be based on careful analysis of the patient's needs and circumstances, as well as the qualifications of the person to whom the task is being delegated. Refer to the Delegation Guidelines in Appendix A.

EQUIPMENT

- PPE, as indicated
- Bath blanket or other drape
- Examination gown
- Gloves

ASSESSMENT

Complete a health history, focusing on the male genitalia. Identify risk factors for altered health during the health history by asking about the following:

- Frequency of digital rectal examinations
- Frequency of testicular self-examination
- Use of contraceptives
- Occupational exposure to chemicals (tire and rubber manufacturing, farming, mechanics)
- History of sexually transmitted infection
- History of discharge from the penis
- Difficulty with urination (incontinence, hesitancy, frequency, voiding at night)
- History of erectile dysfunction

NURSING DIAGNOSIS

Determine the related factors for the nursing diagnoses based on the patient's current health status. Appropriate nursing diagnoses may include:

- Ineffective Health Maintenance
- Risk for Infection
- Sexual Dysfunction

OUTCOME IDENTIFICATION AND PLANNING

The expected outcome to achieve in performing an examination of the male genitalia is that the assessments are completed without causing the patient to experience anxiety or discomfort, the findings are documented, and the appropriate referral is made to other health care professionals, as needed, for further evaluation. Other specific outcomes will be formulated, depending on the identified nursing diagnosis.

IMPLEMENTATION

ACTION	RATIONALE
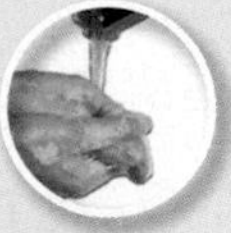 1. Perform hand hygiene and put on PPE, if indicated.	Hand hygiene and PPE prevent the spread of microorganisms. PPE is required based on transmission precautions.
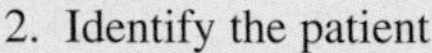 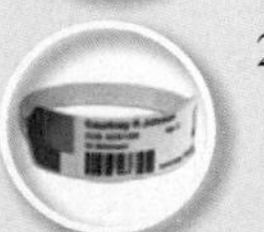 2. Identify the patient.	Identifying the patient ensures the right patient receives the intervention and helps prevent errors.
3. Close the curtains around the bed and close the door to the room, if possible. Explain the purpose of the examination of genitalia and what you are going to do. Answer any questions.	This ensures the patient's privacy. Explanation relieves anxiety and facilitates cooperation.
4. Help the patient undress, if needed, and provide a patient gown. Assist the patient to a supine or sitting position, if possible. Use a bath blanket to cover any exposed area other than the one being assessed.	Having the patient wear a gown facilitates examination of the genitalia. Use of a bath blanket provides for comfort and warmth.

ACTION	RATIONALE
5. Put on gloves. Inspect the external genitalia for size, placement, contour, appearance of the skin, redness, edema, and discharge. If the patient is uncircumcised, retract the foreskin for inspection of the glans penis. Assess the location of the urinary meatus. Inspect the scrotum for symmetry.	Gloves prevent contact with blood and body fluids. The size and shape of the scrotum should be similar bilaterally. It is not unusual for the left testicle to lie lower in the scrotal sac than the right testicle. Normal findings include skin that is free of lesions, and a foreskin (if present) that is intact, uniform in color, and easily retracted. The urinary meatus is normally located in the center of the glans penis and is free of discharge. Abnormal findings include lesions, redness, edema, discharge, and displacement of the urinary meatus or difficulties with voiding. Lesions may be the result of infections (e.g., herpes or syphilis). Edema, redness, or discharge may indicate an infection. Voiding difficulties may result from scarring caused by infections or prostate enlargement.
6. Palpate the scrotum for consistency, nodules, masses, and tenderness.	The consistency of the scrotal contents (i.e., testes) should be similar bilaterally. The scrotum and testes should be free of masses and nontender. Pain may indicate an infection.
7. Inspect the inguinal area. Ask the patient to bear down and look for bulging of the area.	Normally, the inguinal area is free of bulges.
8. Assist the patient to a comfortable position.	This ensures the patient's comfort.
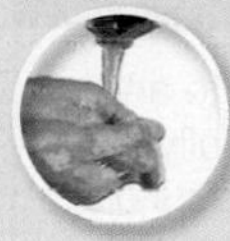 9. Remove PPE, if used. Perform hand hygiene. Continue with assessments of specific body systems, as appropriate, or indicated. Initiate appropriate referral to other health care practitioners for further evaluation, as indicated.	Removing PPE properly reduces the risk for infection transmission and contamination of other items. Hand hygiene prevents the spread of microorganisms. Additional assessments should be completed, as indicated, to evaluate the patient's health status. Intervention by other health care providers may be indicated to evaluate and treat the patient's health status.

EVALUATION

The expected outcome is met when the patient participates in the assessment of the genitalia; the patient verbalizes understanding of the assessment techniques as appropriate; the assessment is completed without the patient experiencing anxiety or discomfort; the findings are documented; and the appropriate referrals are made to the other health care professionals as needed for further evaluation.

DOCUMENTATION

Guidelines

Document assessment techniques performed, along with specific findings. Note and record the size, placement, contour, appearance of the skin, presence of foreskin, redness, edema, location of urinary meatus, and discharge. Document any patient statements of pain and risk factors.

Sample Documentation

09/23/15 1730 Patient denies pain and discharge from penis; denies lumps or changes in scrotum. Patient reports no difficulty with urination. Scrotum of equal size and shape. Skin without lesions, edema, redness; foreskin present and intact, uniform in color, and easily retracted. Urinary meatus located in the center of the glans penis and is free of discharge. Scrotum and testes free of masses and nontender. Inguinal area is free of bulges.

—*B. Holmes, RN*

SPECIAL CONSIDERATIONS

Infant and Child Considerations

- In newborns, breast enlargement occurs, resulting from exposure to maternal hormones in utero and normally seen in the first week after birth, subsiding by the second week after birth.
- Development of pubic hair and enlargement of the scrotum, testes, and penis occur at puberty and follow a regular sequence to adult configuration.
- Spontaneous nocturnal emission of seminal fluid occurs at puberty.

Older Adult Considerations

- Decreased penis size
- Decreased pubic hair
- Decreased size and firmness of testes

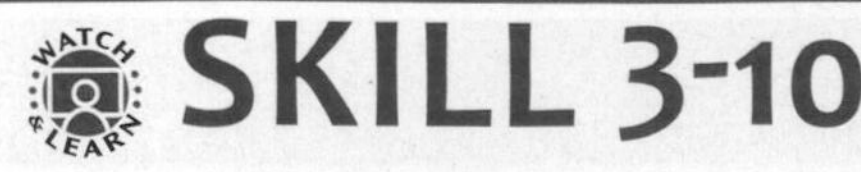

SKILL 3-10 ASSESSING THE NEUROLOGIC, MUSCULOSKELETAL, AND PERIPHERAL VASCULAR SYSTEMS

The focus of the following assessment is integration of the findings from the neurologic, musculoskeletal, and peripheral vascular systems. In assessing the neurologic system, ask the patient to respond to a series of questions that will enable you to obtain data related to overall cognitive function. In addition, evaluate sensation in different areas of the body as well as selected cranial nerves. Musculoskeletal examination will provide information concerning the condition and functioning of certain muscles and joints throughout the body. The peripheral vascular system assessment will identify the condition of the arteries and veins in the extremities as gained through inspection and palpation of the skin and peripheral pulses.

Musculoskeletal trauma, crush injuries, orthopedic surgery, and external pressure from a cast or tight-fitting bandage can cause damage to blood vessels and nerves. This damage causes localized inflammation and tissue edema, which can lead to significantly diminished perfusion and severe ischemia, with resulting severe and permanent dysfunction of the affected area and/or loss of a limb. Assessment of neurovascular status is an important nursing intervention leading to early identification of neurovascular impairment and timely intervention (Johnston-Walker & Hardcastle, 2011). A neurovascular assessment includes assessing for changes in circulation, oxygenation, and nerve function. Box 3-3 outlines the components of a neurovascular assessment.

Box 3-3 COMPONENTS OF A NEUROVASCULAR ASSESSMENT

- Pain: Extreme pain, especially on passive motion, is a significant sign of probable neurovascular impairment in an extremity. Subjective and objective assessments should be included. Opioid analgesia is unlikely to relieve the pain.
- Pallor (perfusion): Comparison between affected and unaffected limb is important. Color and temperature of the extremity: Pale skin, decreased tone, or white color may indicate poor arterial perfusion. Cyanosis may indicate venous stasis. Coolness or decreased temperature may indicate decreased arterial supply. Compare distal to proximal temperature variation in affected limb. Assess capillary refill. Using your thumb and forefinger, squeeze the patient's fingernail or toenail until it appears white. Release the pressure and observe the time it takes for normal color to return. Normally, color returns immediately, in less than 2 to 3 seconds.
- Peripheral pulses: Comparison between affected and unaffected limb is important. Assess the consistency of arterial blood flow (pulse presence, rate, quality) up to and past the affected area. Assess capillary refill, especially in patients whose pulses cannot be palpated due to casts or bandages (Judge, 2007, in Johnston-Walker & Hardcastle, 2001) and in nonverbal patients.
- Paraesthesia (sensation): May be first symptom of changes in sensory nerves to appear. Compare sensation to touch between affected and unaffected limb. Numbness, tingling, or 'pins and needles' sensations may be reported. Evaluate the areas above and below the affected area.
- Paralysis (movement): The ability of the patient to move the extremity distal to the injury. Paralysis of an extremity may be the result of prolonged nerve compression or irreversible muscle damage.
- Pressure: Comparison between affected and unaffected limb is important. Affected area may become taut and firm to the touch, with surrounding skin appearing shiny. The feeling of tightness or pressure may be present.

(Adapted from Hinkle, J.L., & Cheever, K.H. (2014). *Brunner & Suddarth's textbook of medical-surgical nursing* (13th ed.). Philadelphia: Wolters Kluwer Health/Lippincott Williams & Wilkins; and Johnston-Walker & Hardcastle, J. (2011). Neurovascular assessment in the critically ill patient. *Nursing in Critical Care, 16*(4), 170–177.)

DELEGATION CONSIDERATIONS

The assessment of the patient's neurologic, musculoskeletal, and peripheral vascular systems should not be delegated to nursing assistive personnel (NAP) or unlicensed assistive personnel (UAP). Some items may be noticed while providing care and noted by the NAP or UAP. The nurse must then validate, analyze, document, communicate, and act on these findings, as appropriate. Depending on the state's nurse practice act and the organization's policies and procedures, the licensed practical/vocational nurses (LPN/LVNs) may perform some or all of the parts of assessment of the patient's neurologic, musculoskeletal, and peripheral vascular systems. The decision to delegate must be based on careful analysis of the patient's needs and circumstances, as well as the qualifications of the person to whom the task is being delegated. Refer to the Delegation Guidelines in Appendix A.

EQUIPMENT

- PPE, as indicated
- Bath blanket or other drape
- Tongue depressor
- Examination gown
- Gloves
- Containers of odorous materials (e.g., coffee or chocolate) and substances for taste assessment (e.g., sugar, salt, vinegar)
- Miscellaneous items (e.g., coin, pin, cotton, key and paper clip)
- Cotton-tipped applicators

ASSESSMENT

Complete a health history, focusing on the neurologic, musculoskeletal, and peripheral vascular systems. Identify risk factors for altered health during the health history by asking about the following:

- History of numbness, tingling, or tremors
- History of seizures
- History of headaches
- History of dizziness
- History of trauma to the head or spine
- History of infections of the brain
- History of stroke
- Changes in the ability to hear, see, taste, or smell
- Loss of ability to control bladder and bowel
- History of smoking
- History of chronic alcohol use
- History of diabetes mellitus
- Use of prescription and over-the-counter medications
- Family history of Alzheimer's disease, epilepsy, cancer, Huntington's chorea, hypertension (high blood pressure), myocardial infarction (heart attack), coronary artery disease, high blood cholesterol levels, or diabetes mellitus
- Frequency of blood cholesterol tests and results
- Exposure to environmental hazards (e.g., lead, insecticides)
- History of trauma, arthritis, or neurologic disorder
- History of pain or swelling in the joints
- History of pain in the muscles
- Frequency and type of usual exercise
- Dietary intake of calcium
- Changes in color or temperature of the extremities
- History of pain in the legs when sleeping or pain that worsens by walking
- History of blood clots or sores on the legs that do not heal

NURSING DIAGNOSIS

Determine the related factors for the nursing diagnoses based on the patient's current health status. Appropriate nursing diagnoses may include:

- Risk for Falls
- Impaired Verbal Communication
- Risk for Peripheral Neurovascular Dysfunction
- Ineffective Peripheral Tissue Perfusion
- Impaired Physical Mobility

OUTCOME IDENTIFICATION AND PLANNING

The expected outcome to achieve in performing an examination of the neurologic, musculoskeletal, and peripheral vascular systems is that the assessments are completed without causing the patient to experience anxiety or discomfort, the findings are documented, and the appropriate referral is made to other health care professionals, as needed, for further evaluation. Other specific outcomes will be formulated, depending on the identified nursing diagnosis.

(*continued*)

SKILL 3-10 ASSESSING THE NEUROLOGIC, MUSCULOSKELETAL, AND PERIPHERAL VASCULAR SYSTEMS continued

IMPLEMENTATION

ACTION	RATIONALE
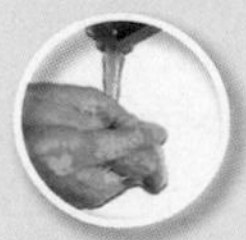 1. Perform hand hygiene and put on PPE, if indicated.	Hand hygiene and PPE prevent the spread of microorganisms. PPE is required based on transmission precautions.
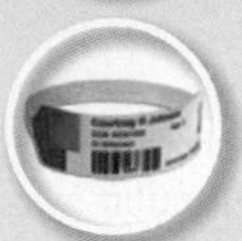 2. Identify the patient.	Identifying the patient ensures the right patient receives the intervention and helps prevent errors.
3. Close the curtains around the bed and close the door to the room, if possible. Explain the purpose of the neurologic, musculoskeletal, and peripheral vascular examinations and what you are going to do. Answer any questions.	This ensures the patient's privacy. Explanation relieves anxiety and facilitates cooperation.
4. Help the patient undress, if needed, and provide a patient gown. Assist the patient to a supine position, if possible. Use the bath blanket to cover any exposed area other than the one being assessed.	Having the patient wear a gown facilitates examination of the neurologic, musculoskeletal, and peripheral vascular systems. Use of a bath blanket provides for comfort and warmth.
5. Begin with a survey of the patient's overall hygiene and physical appearance.	This provides initial impressions of the patient. Hygiene and appearance can provide clues about the patient's mental state and comfort level.
6. Assess the patient's mental status.	
a. Evaluate the patient's orientation to person, place, and time.	This helps identify the patient's level of awareness.
b. Evaluate level of consciousness. Refer to Chapter 17 for standardized assessment tools to assess level of consciousness.	The patient should be awake and alert. Patients with altered level of consciousness may be lethargic, stuporous, or comatose.
c. Assess memory (immediate recall and past memory).	Memory problems may indicate neurologic impairment.
d. Assess abstract reasoning by asking the patient to explain a proverb, such as "The early bird catches the worm."	If intellectual ability is impaired, the patient usually gives a literal interpretation or repeats the phrase.
e. Evaluate the patient's ability to understand spoken and written word.	This helps assess for aphasia.
7. Test cranial nerve (CN) function.	
a. Ask the patient to close the eyes, occlude one nostril, and then identify the smell of different substances, such as coffee, chocolate, or alcohol. Repeat with other nostril.	This action tests the function of CN I (olfactory nerve).
b. Test visual acuity and pupillary constriction. Refer to previous discussion in the assessment of the head and neck.	This tests function of CN II and CN III (optic and oculomotor nerves).
c. Move the patient's eyes through the six cardinal positions of gaze. Refer to previous discussion in the assessment of the head and neck.	This testing evaluates the function of tests CN III, CN IV, and CN VI (oculomotor, trochlear, and abducens nerves).
d. Ask the patient to smile, frown, wrinkle the forehead, and puff out cheeks (Figure 1).	This maneuver evaluates the motor function of CN VII (facial nerve).
e. Ask the patient to protrude tongue and push against the cheek with the tongue.	This evaluates function of CN XII (hypoglossal nerve).
f. Palpate the jaw muscles. Ask the patient to open and clench jaws. Stroke the patient's face with a cotton ball.	This evaluates function of CN V (trigeminal nerve).
g. Test hearing with the whispered voice test. Refer to previous discussion in the assessment of the head and neck.	This evaluates function of CN VIII (acoustic nerve).

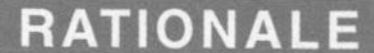

ACTION	RATIONALE
h. Put on gloves. Ask patient to open mouth. While observing soft palate, ask patient to say "ah"; observe upward movement of the soft palate. Test the gag reflex by touching the posterior pharynx with the tongue depressor. Explain to patient that this may be uncomfortable. Ask the patient to swallow. Remove gloves.	Gloves prevent contact with blood and body fluids. An intact gag reflex and swallowing indicates normal functioning of CN IX and X (glossopharyngeal and vagus nerves).
i. Place your hands on the patient's shoulders (Figure 2) while he or she shrugs against resistance. Then place your hand on the patient's left cheek, then the right cheek, and have the patient push against it.	These actions check CN XI (spinal accessory nerve) function and trapezius and sternocleidomastoid muscle strength.

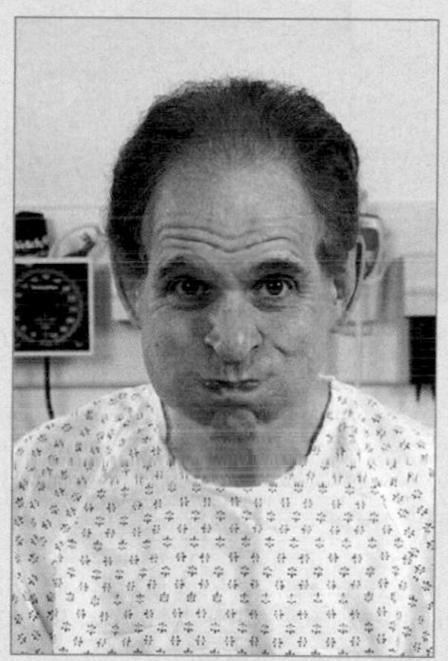

FIGURE 1 Putting out cheeks. (Weber, J.R., & Kelley, J.H. (2014). *Health assessment in nursing* (5th ed.). Philadelphia: Wolters Kluwer Health/Lippincott Williams & Wilkins.)

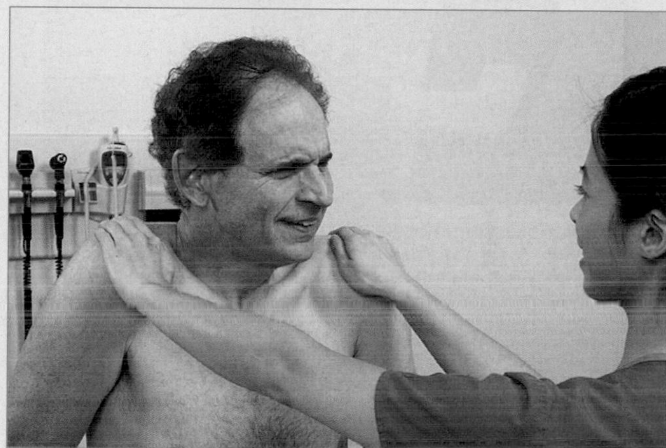

FIGURE 2 Assessing strength of the trapezius muscle. (Weber, J.R., & Kelley, J.H. (2014). *Health assessment in nursing* (5th ed.). Philadelphia: Wolters Kluwer Health/Lippincott Williams & Wilkins.)

ACTION	RATIONALE
8. Check the patient's ability to move his or her neck. Ask the patient to touch his or her chin to the chest and to each shoulder, then move each ear to the corresponding shoulder (Figure 3), and then tip the head back as far as possible.	These actions assess neck ROM, which is normally smooth and controlled.
9. Inspect the upper extremities. Observe for skin color, presence of lesions, rashes, and muscle mass. Palpate for skin temperature, texture, and presence of masses.	Examination of the upper extremities provides information about the circulatory, integumentary, and musculoskeletal systems.
10. Ask the patient to extend arms forward and then rapidly turn palms up and down.	This maneuver tests proprioception and cerebellar function.

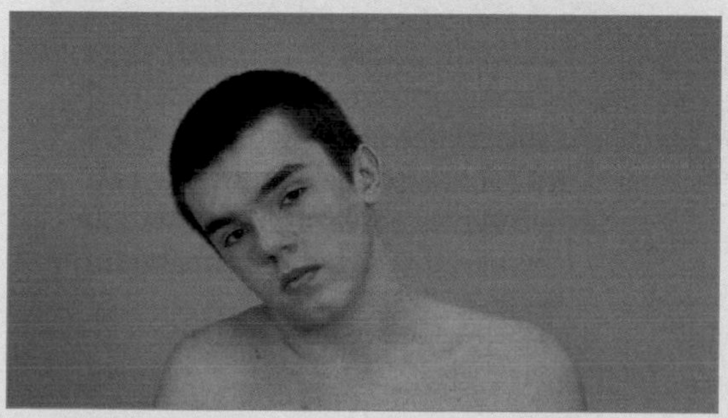

FIGURE 3 Moving each ear to the corresponding shoulder. (From Jensen, S. (2011). *Nursing health assessment. A best practice approach.* Philadelphia: Wolters Kluwer Health/Lippincott Williams & Wilkins, p. 654, Figure 23.16B.)

(*continued*)

SKILL 3-10 ASSESSING THE NEUROLOGIC, MUSCULOSKELETAL, AND PERIPHERAL VASCULAR SYSTEMS continued

ACTION	RATIONALE
11. Ask the patient to flex upper arm and to resist examiner's opposing force (Figure 4).	This technique assesses the muscle strength of the upper extremities.
12. Inspect and palpate the hands, fingers, wrists (Figure 5), and elbow joints.	Inspection and palpation provide information about abnormalities, tenderness, and ROM.

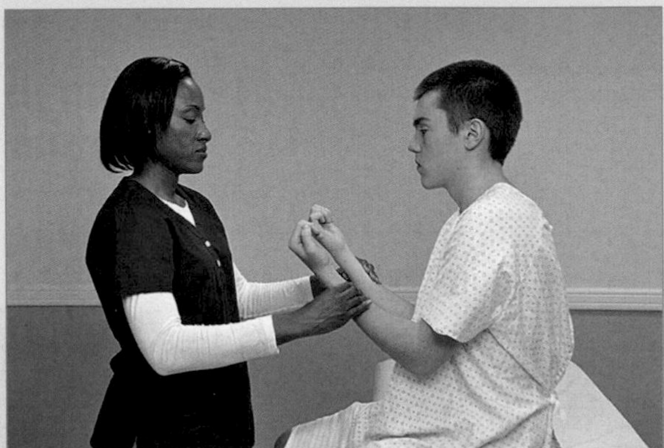

FIGURE 4 Assessing muscle strength of the upper extremities. (From Jensen, S. (2011). *Nursing health assessment. A best practice approach.* Philadelphia: Wolters Kluwer Health/Lippincott Williams & Wilkins, p. 658, Figure 23.20.)

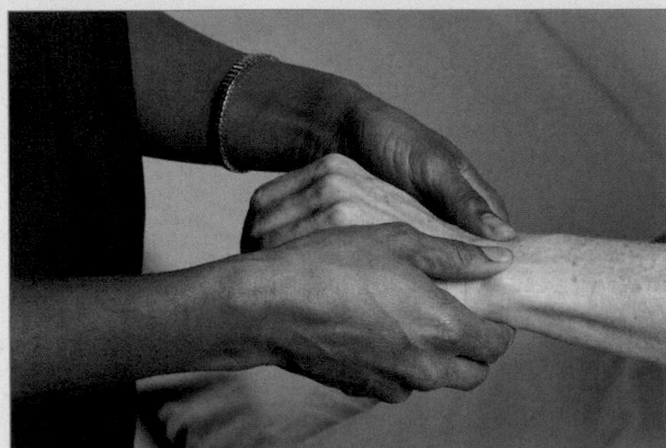

FIGURE 5 Palpating the wrist. *(Photo by B. Proud.)*

ACTION	RATIONALE
13. Ask the patient to bend and straighten the elbow, and flex and extend the wrists and hands.	Tests ROM of elbow joint and wrists.
14. Palpate the skin and the radial and brachial pulses. Assess the pulse rate, quality or amplitude, and rhythm. Test capillary refill (Refer to Box 3-2).	Pulse palpation and capillary refill evaluate the peripheral vascular status of the upper extremities.
15. Have the patient squeeze two of your fingers (Figure 6).	This maneuver tests the muscle strength of the hands.
16. Ask the patient to close his or her eyes. Using your finger or applicator, trace a one-digit number on the patient's palm and ask him or her to identify the number. Repeat on the other hand with a different number (Figure 7).	This test evaluates tactile discrimination, specifically graphesthesia.

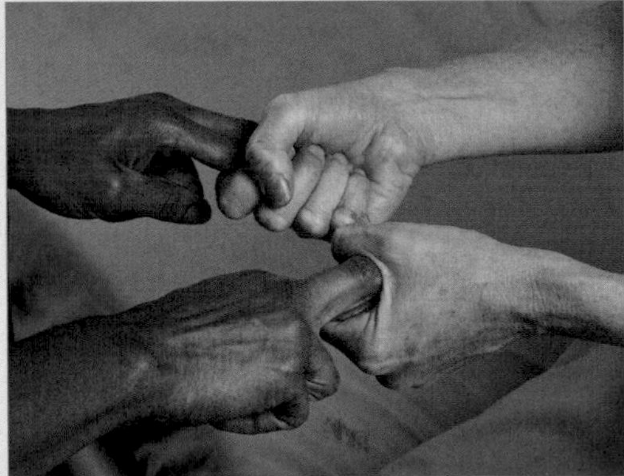

FIGURE 6 Testing grip. Patient squeezes nurse's index and middle fingers. *(Photo by B. Proud.)*

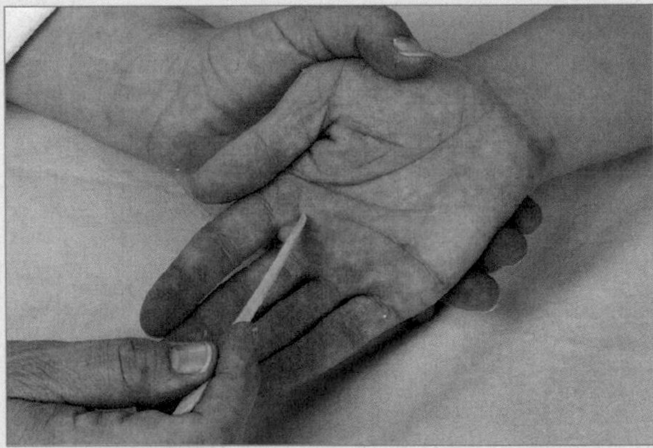

FIGURE 7 Testing tactile discrimination (graphesthesia). *(Photo by B. Proud.)*

ACTION	RATIONALE
17. Ask the patient to close his or her eyes. Place a familiar object, such as a key, in the patient's hand and ask him or her to identify the object. Repeat using another object for the other hand.	This test evaluates tactile discrimination, specifically stereognosis.

ACTION

RATIONALE

18. Assist the patient to a supine position. Palpate (Figure 8-A) and then use the bell of the stethoscope to auscultate the femoral pulses in the groin (Figure 8-B), if not done during assessment of the abdomen. Note the strength of the pulse and grade it as with peripheral pulses.

This technique assesses flow of blood through the arteries. Auscultation can detect a bruit.

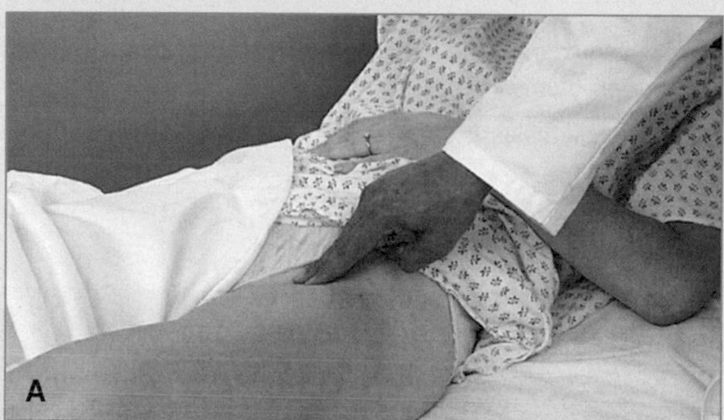

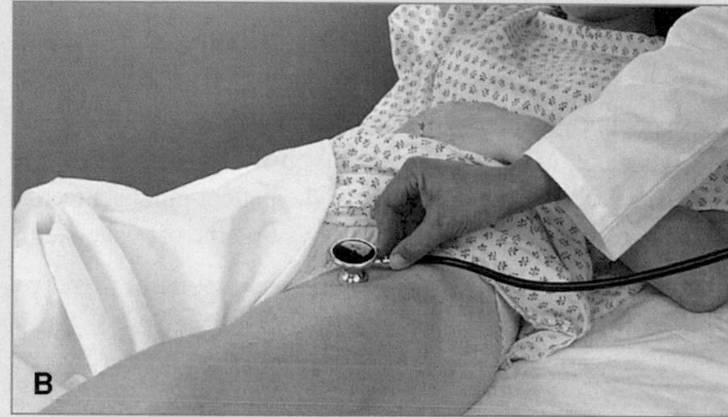

FIGURE 8 Palpating (**A**) and auscultating (**B**) the femoral pulses. *(Photos by B. Proud.)*

19. Examine the lower extremities. Inspect the legs and feet for color, lesions, varicosities, hair growth, nail growth, edema, and muscle mass.

Inspection provides information about peripheral vascular function.

20. Assess for pitting edema in the lower extremities by pressing fingers into the skin at the pretibial area and dorsum of the foot (Figure 9-A). If an indentation remains in the skin after the fingers have been lifted, pitting edema is present (Figure 9-B).

This technique reveals information about excess interstitial fluid. Refer to an edema scale in assessing the amount of edema: 1+ about 2 mm deep to 4+ about 8 mm deep.

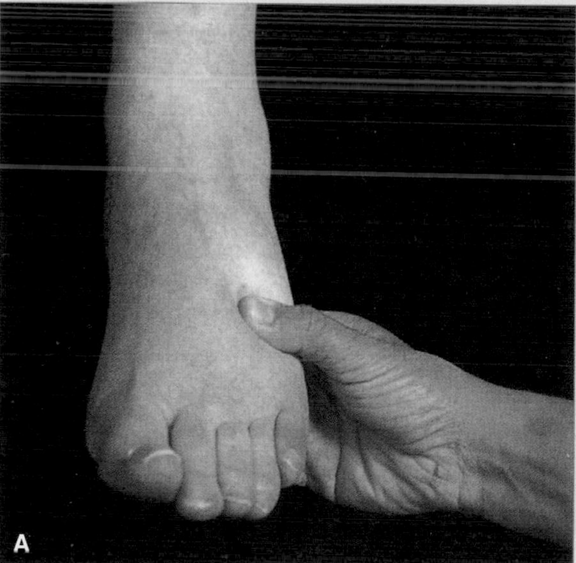

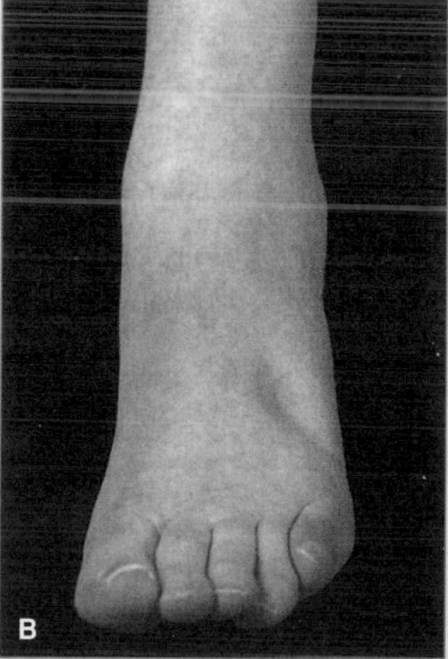

FIGURE 9 Assessing for pitting edema in lower extremities. (From Hogan-Quigley, B., Palm, M.L., & Bickley, L. (2012). *Bates' nursing guide to physical examination and history taking.* Philadelphia: Wolters Kluwer Health/Lippincott Williams & Wilkins, p. 412.)

(continued)

SKILL 3-10 ASSESSING THE NEUROLOGIC, MUSCULOSKELETAL, AND PERIPHERAL VASCULAR SYSTEMS continued

ACTION	RATIONALE
21. Palpate for pulses and skin temperature at the posterior tibial, dorsalis pedis, and popliteal areas. Assess the pulse rate, quality or amplitude, and rhythm. Test capillary refill (Refer to Box 3-2).	Pulses, skin temperature, and capillary refill provide information about the patient's peripheral vascular status.
22. Have the patient perform the straight leg test with one leg at a time (Figure 10).	This test checks for vertebral disk problems.
23. Ask the patient to move one leg laterally with the knee straight to test abduction and medially to test adduction of the hips.	This maneuver assesses ROM and provides information about joint problems.
24. Ask the patient to raise the thigh against the resistance of your hand (Figure 11); next have the patient push outward against the resistance of your hand; then have the patient pull backward against the resistance of your hand. Repeat on the opposite side.	These measures assess motor strength of the upper and lower legs.

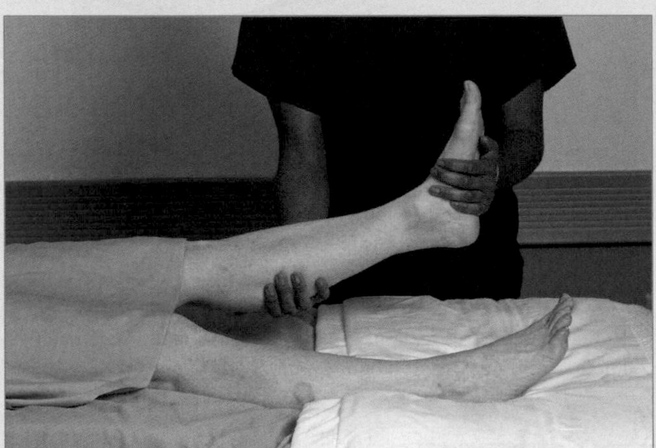

FIGURE 10 Performing straight leg test. *(Photo by B. Proud.)*

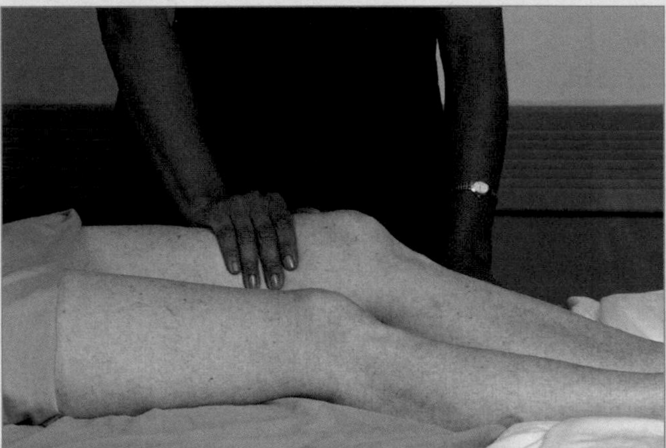

FIGURE 11 Testing motor strength of upper leg. Patient attempts to raise thigh against nurse's resistance. *(Photo by B. Proud.)*

ACTION	RATIONALE
25. Test plantar reflex. Stroke the sole of the patient's foot with the end of a hard object, such as the edge of a tongue depressor or a key. Begin at the heel and apply firm but gentle pressure to the lateral aspect of the foot. Continue to the base of the toes (Figure 12). Repeat on the other side.	Flexion of all the toes is considered a normal finding in an individual 18 months of age and older: a negative Babinski reflex.

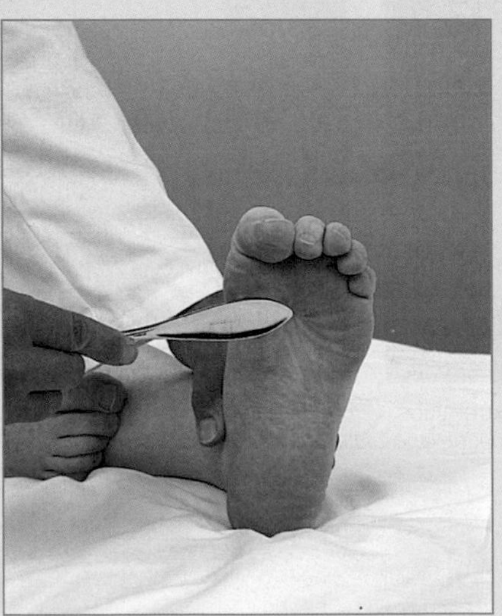

FIGURE 12 Eliciting plantar reflex.

ACTION	RATIONALE
26. Ask patient to dorsiflex and then plantarflex both feet against opposing resistance (Figure 13).	These measures test foot strength and ROM.

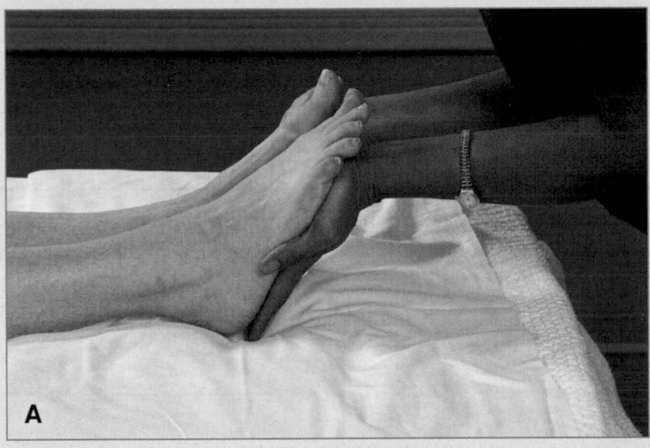

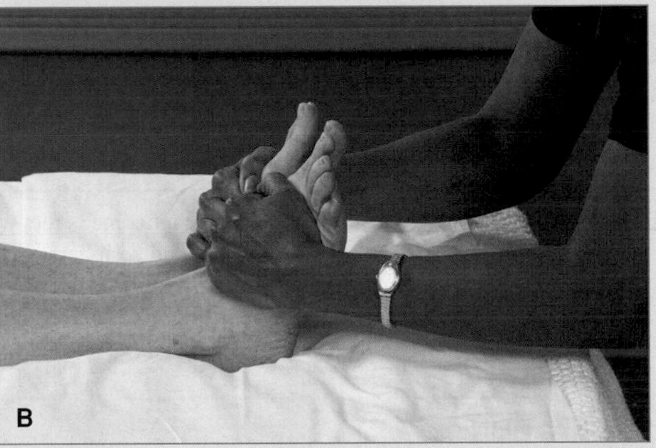

FIGURE 13 **A.** Testing ankle flexion and dorsiflexion. The patient first pushes the balls of the feet against resistance of the nurse's hands. **B.** Then attempts to pull against nurse's resistance. *(Photos by B. Proud.)*

ACTION	RATIONALE
27. As needed, assist the patient to a standing position. Observe the patient as he or she walks with a regular gait, on the toes, on the heels, and then heel to toe (Figure 14).	This procedure evaluates cerebellar and motor function.
28. Perform the Romberg test; ask the patient to stand straight with feet together, both eyes closed with arms at side (Figure 15). Wait 20 seconds and observe for patient swaying and ability to maintain balance. Be alert to prevent patient fall or injury related to losing balance during this assessment.	This test checks cerebellar functioning and evaluates balance, equilibrium, and coordination. Slight swaying is normal, but patient should be able to maintain balance.

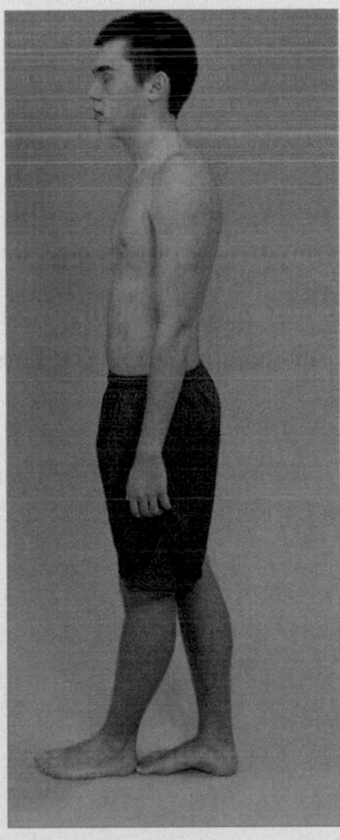

FIGURE 14 Testing heel to toe walking. (From Jensen, S. (2011). *Nursing health assessment. A best practice approach.* Philadelphia: Wolters Kluwer Health/Lippincott Williams & Wilkins, p. 707, Figure 24.13.)

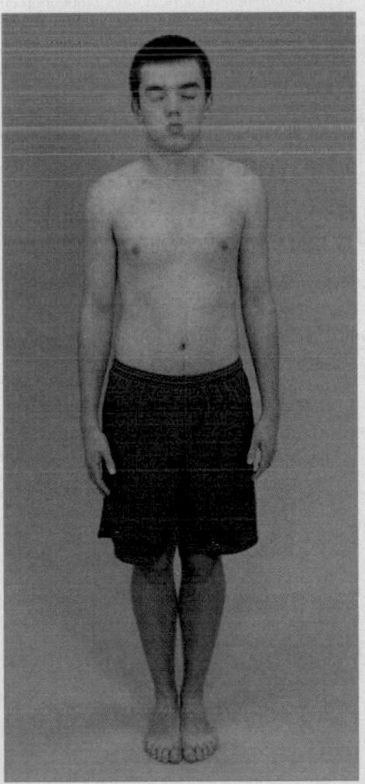

FIGURE 15 Positioning for the Romberg test. (From Jensen, S. (2011). *Nursing health assessment. A best practice approach.* Philadelphia: Wolters Kluwer Health/Lippincott Williams & Wilkins, p. 707, Figure 24.14.)

(*continued*)

SKILL 3-10 ASSESSING THE NEUROLOGIC, MUSCULOSKELETAL, AND PERIPHERAL VASCULAR SYSTEMS continued

ACTION	RATIONALE
29. Assist the patient to a comfortable position.	This ensures the patient's comfort.
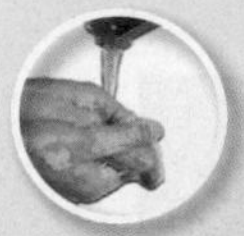 30. Remove PPE, if used. Perform hand hygiene. Continue with assessments of specific body systems, as appropriate, or indicated. Initiate appropriate referral to other health care practitioners for further evaluation, as indicated.	Removing PPE properly reduces the risk for infection transmission and contamination of other items. Hand hygiene prevents the spread of microorganisms. Additional assessments should be completed, as indicated, to evaluate the patient's health status. Intervention by other health care providers may be indicated to evaluate and treat the patient's health status.

EVALUATION

The expected outcome is met when the patient participates in the assessment of the neurologic, musculoskeletal, and peripheral vascular systems; the patient verbalizes understanding of the assessment techniques as appropriate; the assessment is completed without the patient experiencing anxiety or discomfort; the findings are documented; and the appropriate referrals are made to the other health care professionals as needed for further evaluation.

DOCUMENTATION

Guidelines

Document assessment techniques performed, along with specific findings. Note the cognitive responses of the patient, the tested cranial nerves, and sensation and motor responses. Document any patient statements of pain, muscle weakness, or joint abnormality. Record findings, including color, turgor, temperature, pulses, and capillary refill.

Sample Documentation

Lippincott DocuCare **Practice documenting assessment techniques and findings in *Lippincott DocuCare*.**

4/4/15 Patient alert, oriented, cognitively appropriate. Cranial nerves intact. Sensation intact. Full ROM of all joints. Muscles soft, firm, nontender, no atrophy. Patient states pain in right calf. Right calf skin paler tone and slightly cooler compared with left calf. Peripheral pulses 72, +2, regular rhythm, equal bilaterally; exception–right posterior tibial and dorsalis pedis pulses +1. Capillary refill right lower extremity sluggish, >3 seconds.

—*S. Moses, RN*

SPECIAL CONSIDERATIONS

General Considerations

- Before asking questions related to the mental status examination, inform the patient that some of the questions may seem unusual, but that you are attempting to evaluate overall cognitive function.

Infant and Child Considerations

- In an infant, jerky and brief twitching of the extremities may be noted and considered a normal finding.
- The Babinski sign is typically elicited in children age 18 months and younger.
- The infant's extremities move symmetrically through ROM, but lack full extension.
- Barlow-Ortolani's maneuver is used to assess hip abduction and adduction in an infant. (Refer to a pediatrics text for more information.)
- Before age 5 years, sensory function is normally not tested.
- Coordination of movement varies according to the developmental level of the young child.

Older Adult Considerations

- Be aware that short-term memory, such as recall of recent events, may diminish with age, as well as slowed reaction time.
- In the older adult patient, expect to find decreased musculoskeletal function, such as loss of muscle strength.
- Keep in mind that older adults may take longer to perform certain actions, such as completing activities for testing coordination.

ENHANCE YOUR UNDERSTANDING

FOCUSING ON PATIENT CARE: DEVELOPING CLINICAL REASONING

Consider the case scenarios at the beginning of the chapter as you answer the following questions to enhance your understanding and apply what you have learned.

QUESTIONS

1. When obtaining the history from Mr. Lincoln, he reports having a stuffed-up nose, postnasal drip, and a cough that sometimes produces mucus. He has smoked about one and a half packs of cigarettes a day for the past 20 years. Which areas of his physical examination would be most important?
2. Lois Felker, who has a history of type 1 diabetes mellitus, has arrived for her appointment with the physician. Due to this patient's diagnosis, what systems will be most important to include in the routine checkup?
3. Bobby Williams is suspected of having appendicitis. Which aspects of the physical examination would you use to help confirm this diagnosis?

You can find suggested answers after the Bibliography at the end of this chapter.

INTEGRATED CASE STUDY CONNECTION

The case studies in the back of the book are designed to focus on integrating concepts. Refer to the following case studies to enhance your understanding of the concepts related to the skills in this chapter.

- Basic Case Studies: Abigail Cantonelli, page 1063; James White, page 1066; Naomi Bell, page 1067; Joe LeRoy, page 1072; Kate Townsend, page 1073.
- Intermediate Case Studies: Olivia Greenbaum, page 1077; Victoria Holly, page 1079; Jason Brown, page 1083; Kent Clark, page 1085; Lucille Howard, page 1086; George Patel, page 1091.
- Advanced Case Studies: Cole McKean, page 1093; Dewayne Wallace, page 1095; Robert Espinoza, page 1097.

TAYLOR SUITE RESOURCES

Explore these additional resources to enhance learning for this chapter:

- NCLEX-Style Questions and other resources on thePoint, http://thePoint.lww.com/Lynn4e
- *Skill Checklists for Taylor's Clinical Nursing Skills,* 4e
- *Taylor's Video Guide to Clinical Nursing Skills:* Physical Assessment
- *Fundamentals of Nursing:* Chapter 25, Health Assessment
- *Lippincott DocuCare* Fundamentals cases

Bibliography

American Hearing Research Foundation. (2008). *Hearing testing.* Available at http://american-hearing.org/disorders/hearing-testing/. Accessed August 7, 2012.

Armstrong, J., & Mitchell, E. (2008). Comprehensive nursing assessment in the care of older people. *Nursing Older People, 1*(20), 36–40.

Bagai, A., Thavendiranathan, P., & Detsky, A.S. (2006). Does this patient have hearing impairment? *JAMA, 295*(4), 416–428.

Barker, E. (2008). *Neuroscience nursing* (3rd ed.). St. Louis: Mosby Elsevier.

Boltz, M., Capezuti, E., Fulmer, T., & Zwicker, D. (Eds.) (2012). *Evidence-based geriatric nursing protocols for best practice* (4th ed.). New York: Springer Publishing Company.

Centers for Disease Control and Prevention (CDC). (2012). *Immunization schedules.* Available at http://www.cdc.gov/vaccines/schedules/index.html. Accessed August 5, 2012.

Centers for Disease Control and Prevention. (2011). *BMI percentile calculator for child and teen.* Available at http://apps.nccd.cdc.gov/dnpabmi/. Accessed August 29, 2012.

Dudek, S. (2014). *Nutrition essentials for nursing practice.* (7th ed.). Philadelphia: Wolters Kluwer Health/Lippincott Williams & Wilkins.

Fennessey, A., & Wittmann-Price, R.A. (2011). Physical assessment: A continuing need for clarification. *Nursing Forum, 46*(1), 45–50.

Grossman, S., & Porth, C.M. (2014). *Porth's pathophysiology: concepts of altered health states.* (9th ed.). Philadelphia: Wolters Kluwer/Lippincott Williams & Wilkins.

Giddens, J. (2007). A survey of physical assessment techniques performed by RNs: Lessons for nursing education. *Journal of Nursing Education, 46*(2), 83–87.

Hassall, S., & Butler-Williams, C. (2010). Assessment of airway and breathing in adults. *British Journal of Neuroscience Nursing, 6*(6), 288–291.

Hinkle, J.L., & Cheever, K.H. (2014). *Brunner & Suddarth's textbook of medical-surgical nursing* (13th ed.). Philadelphia: Wolters Kluwer Health/Lippincott Williams & Wilkins.

Hogan-Quigley, B., Palm, M.L., & Bickley, L. (2012). *Bates' nursing guide to physical examination and history taking.* Philadelphia: Wolters Kluwer Health/Lippincott Williams & Wilkins.

Hotta, T. (2011). The basics of a health assessment. *Plastic Surgical Nursing, 31*,(3), 100–104.

Jarvis, C. (2012). *Physical examination & health assessment* (6th ed.). St. Louis: Saunders/Elsevier.

Jensen, S. (2011). *Nursing health assessment. A best practice approach.* Philadelphia: Wolters Kluwer Health/Lippincott Williams & Wilkins.

Johnston-Walker, E., & Hardcastle, J. (2011). Neurovascular assessment in the critically ill patient. *Nursing in Critical Care, 16*(4), 170–177.

Kyle, T., & Carman, S. (2013). *Essentials of pediatric nursing* (2nd ed.). Philadelphia: Wolters Kluwer Health/Lippincott Williams & Wilkins.

Massey, D. (2010). Respiratory assessment 1: Why do it and how to do it? *British Journal of Cardiac Nursing, 6*(11), 537–541.

Meredith, T., & Massey, D. (2011). Respiratory assessment 2: More key skills to improve care. *British Journal of Cardiac Nursing, 6*(2), 63–68.

National Institutes of Health (NIH). National Heart, Lung, and Blood Institute. (2012). *How are overweight and obesity diagnosed?* Available at http://www.nhlbi.nih.gov/health/health-topics/topics/obe/diagnosis.html. Accessed August 29, 2012.

National Institutes of Health, National Heart, Lung, and Blood Institute. (2000). NHLBI Obesity Education Initiative. *The practical guide: Identification, evaluation, and treatment of overweight and obesity in adults.* NIH publication no. 00-4084. October 2000. Available at www.nhlbi.nih.gov/guidelines/obesity/prctgd_c.pdf.

NANDA International. (2012). *Nursing diagnoses: Definitions & classification 2012–2014.* West Sussex, UK: Wiley-Blackwell.

Parkes, R. (2011). Rate of respiration: The forgotten vital sign. *Emergency Nurse, 19*(2), 12–17.

Perry, S.E., Hockenberry, M.J., Lowdermilk, D.L., & Wilson, D. (2010). *Maternal child nursing care* (4th ed.). Maryland Heights, MO: Mosby/Elsevier.

Ritter, L.A., & Hoffman, N.A. (2010). *Multicultural health.* Boston: Jones and Bartlett.

Spector, R.E. (2009). *Cultural diversity in health and illness* (7th ed.). Upper Saddle River, NJ: Pearson/Prentice Hall.

Tabloski, P. (2010). *Gerontological nursing* (2nd ed.). Upper Saddle River, NJ: Pearson.

Taylor, C.R, Lillis, C., & Lynn, P. (2015). *Fundamentals of nursing.* (8th ed.). Philadelphia: Wolters Kluwer Health/Lippincott Williams & Wilkins.

VISN8 Patient Safety Center. (2009). *Safe patient handling and movement algorithms.* Tampa, FL: Author. Available at http://www.visn8.va.gov/visn8/patientsafetycenter/safePtHandling/default.asp.

SUGGESTED ANSWERS FOR FOCUSING ON PATIENT CARE: DEVELOPING CLINICAL REASONING

1. Assessment of the patient's head and neck, as well as his thorax and lungs, would be most important. Examination of his head and neck will provide additional information related to his nasal symptoms, as well as his cough. Assessment of his thorax and lungs will provide additional information related to his cough and possible effects of smoking.
2. Assessment of integumentary, neurologic, and peripheral vascular systems would be important to include when caring for a patient with diabetes. Major complications of diabetes include retinopathy, nephropathy, and neuropathy. Assessment of these systems would aid in identifying possible complications from diabetes that should be addressed.
3. Assessment of the patient's abdomen would be important to aid in confirming a diagnosis of appendicitis. In particular, you should assess for tenderness, which can indicate peritoneal irritation, such as from appendicitis.

4 Safety

FOCUSING ON PATIENT CARE

This chapter will help you develop some of the skills related to safety issues for monitoring and interventions that may be necessary to care for the following patients:

MEGAN LEWIS, an 18-month-old who has an IV access in her left forearm.

KEVIN MALLORY, a 35-year-old professional body builder admitted with a severe closed head injury. He is intubated and is constantly reaching for his endotracheal tube.

JOHN FRAWLEY, a 72-year-old diagnosed with Alzheimer's disease who continues to try to get out of bed after falling and breaking a hip.

Refer to Focusing on Patient Care: Developing Clinical Reasoning at the end of the chapter to apply what you learn.

LEARNING OBJECTIVES

After studying this chapter, you will be able to:

1. Implement nursing interventions related to fall prevention.
2. Implement nursing interventions to be used as alternatives to restraints.
3. Identify guidelines for the use of physical restraints.
4. Apply an extremity restraint correctly and safely.
5. Apply a waist restraint correctly and safely.
6. Apply an elbow restraint correctly and safely.
7. Apply a mummy restraint correctly and safely.

KEY TERMS

restraint: any manual method, physical or mechanical device, material, or equipment that immobilizes or reduces the ability of a patient to move or access to his or her body freely; a drug or medication when it is used as a restriction to manage the patient's behavior or restrict the patient's freedom of movement and is not a standard treatment or dosage for the patient's condition (CMS, 2006, p. 71427).

safety event report: documentation that describes any occurrence that results in injury or has the potential to result in injury, to a patient, employee, or visitor; also called a variance, occurrence, or incident report

Safety and security are basic human needs. Safety is a paramount concern that underlies all nursing care, and patient safety is a responsibility of all healthcare providers. It is a focus in all healthcare facilities as well as in the home, workplace, and community. Nursing strategies that identify potential hazards and promote wellness evolve from an awareness of factors that affect safety in the environment. Fundamentals Review 4-1 outlines patient safety risks related to developmental stage, as well as patient teaching to promote patient safety. Guidelines to promote patient safety are provided by The Joint Commission (TJC). The purpose of the National Patient Safety Goals is to improve patient safety. These Safety Goals focus on problems in healthcare safety and how to solve them. They are updated yearly and can be found on The Joint Commission website at: http://www.jointcommission.org/PatientSafety/NationalPatientSafetyGoals.

This chapter covers the skills nurses will need when working with patients to monitor for safety, prevent injury, and to intervene when there are issues involving safety. The first two skills discuss fall prevention and utilizing alternatives to the use of restraints. The remaining skills address how to use several types of physical restraints safely and correctly. A physical restraint is any manual method, physical or mechanical device, material, or equipment that the person cannot remove easily, which immobilizes or reduces the person's freedom of movement or normal access to one's body (CMS, 2006). **Physical restraints should be considered as a last resort after other care alternatives have been unsuccessful.**

Whether or not a specific device is considered a restraint is determined by several factors:

- Intended use of a device, such as physical restriction
- Its involuntary application
- Identified patient need

For example, if a bed rail is used to facilitate mobility in and out of bed, it is not a restraint. If side rails could potentially restrict a patient's freedom to leave the bed, the rails would be a restraint. If a patient can release or remove a device, it is not a restraint.

When it is necessary to apply a restraint, the nurse should use the least restrictive method and should remove it at the earliest possible time. Consider the laws regulating the use of restraints and facility regulations and policies. Ensure compliance with ordering, assessment, and maintenance procedures. Fundamentals Review 4-2 provides general guidelines for restraint use and Fundamentals Review 4-3 defines the R-E-S-T-R-A-I-N-T acronym aimed at promoting effective use of restraints. Always treat patients with respect and protect their dignity.

FUNDAMENTALS REVIEW 4-1

PREVENTING ACCIDENTS AND PROMOTING SAFETY AT VARYING DEVELOPMENTAL STAGES

Developmental Stage/ Safety Risks	Teaching Tip	Why Is This Important
Fetus Abnormal growth & development	• Abstain from alcohol and caffeine while pregnant. • Stop smoking or reduce the number of cigarettes smoked per day. • Avoid all drugs, including OTC drugs, unless prescribed by a physician, midwife, or other licensed independent practitioner. • Avoid exposure to pesticides and certain environmental chemicals. • Avoid exposure to radiation.	Any factors, chemical or physical, can adversely affect the fertilized ovum, embryo, and developing fetus. A fetus is extremely vulnerable to environmental hazards.

FUNDAMENTALS REVIEW 4-1 continued

PREVENTING ACCIDENTS AND PROMOTING SAFETY AT VARYING DEVELOPMENTAL STAGES

Developmental Stage/ Safety Risks	Teaching Tip	Why Is This Important
Neonate (first 28 days of life) Infection Falls SIDS	• Wash hands frequently. • Never leave infant unsupervised on a raised surface without side rails. • Use appropriate infant car seat that is secured in the backseat facing the rear of the car. • Handle infant securely while supporting the head. • Place infant on back to sleep.	Physical care for the newborn includes maintaining a patent airway, protecting the baby from infection and injury, and providing optimal nutrition.
Infant Falls Injuries from toys Burns Suffocation or drowning Inhalation or ingestion of foreign bodies	• Supervise child closely to prevent injury. • Select toys appropriate for developmental level. • Use appropriate safety equipment in the home (e.g., locks for cabinets, gates, electrical outlet covers). • Never leave child alone in the bathtub. • Childproof the entire house.	Infants progress from rolling over to sitting, crawling, and pulling up to stand. They are very curious and will explore everything in their environment that they can.
Toddler Falls Cuts from sharp objects Burns Suffocation or drowning Inhalation or ingestion of foreign bodies/poisons	• Have poison control center phone number in readily accessible location. • Use appropriate car seat for toddler. • Supervise child closely to prevent injury. • Childproof house to ensure that poisonous products, drugs, and small objects are out of toddler's reach. • Never leave child alone and unsupervised outside. • Keep all hot items on stove out of child's reach.	Toddlers accomplish a wide variety of developmental tasks and progress to walking and talking. They become more independent and continue to explore their environment.
Preschooler Falls Cuts Burns Drowning Inhalation or ingestion Guns and weapons	• Teach child to wear proper safety equipment when riding bicycles or scooters. • Ensure that playing areas are safe. • Begin to teach safety measures to child. • Do not leave child alone in the bathtub or near water. • Practice emergency evacuation measures. • Teach about fire safety.	Though more independent, preschoolers still have an immature understanding of dangerous behavior. They may strive to imitate adults and thus attempt dangerous behavior.
School-aged child Burns Drowning Broken bones Concussions (TBI) Inhalation or ingestion Guns and weapons Substance abuse	• Teach accident prevention at school and home. • Teach child to wear safety equipment when playing sports. • Reinforce teaching about symptoms that require immediate medical attention. • Continue immunizations as scheduled. • Provide drug, alcohol, and sexuality education. • Reinforce use of seat belts and pedestrian safety.	School-aged children have developed more refined muscular coordination, but increasing involvement in sports and play activities increases their risk for injury. TBI can cause disruption in brain function and death. Cognitive maturity improves their ability to understand safety instructions.

(continued)

FUNDAMENTALS REVIEW 4-1 continued

PREVENTING ACCIDENTS AND PROMOTING SAFETY AT VARYING DEVELOPMENTAL STAGES

Developmental Stage/ Safety Risks	Teaching Tip	Why Is This Important
Adolescent Motor vehicle accidents Drowning Guns and weapons Inhalation and ingestion	• Teach responsibilities of new freedoms that accompany being a teenager. • Enroll teen in safety courses (driver education, water safety, emergency care measures). • Emphasize gun safety. • Get physical examination before participating in sports. • Make time to listen to and talk with your adolescent (helps with stress reduction). • Follow healthy lifestyle (nutrition, rest, etc.). • Teach about sexuality, sexually transmitted infections, and birth control. • Encourage child to report any sexual harassment or abuse of any kind.	Adolescence is a critical period in growth and development. The adolescent needs increasing freedom and responsibility to prepare for adulthood. During this time, the mind has a great ability to acquire and use knowledge. The teen's peer group is a greater influence than parents during this stage.
Adult Stress Domestic violence Motor vehicle accidents Industrial accidents Drug and alcohol abuse	• Practice stress reduction techniques (e.g., meditation, exercise). • Enroll in a defensive driving course. • Evaluate the workplace for safety hazards and utilize safety equipment as prescribed. • Practice moderation when consuming alcohol. • Avoid use of illegal drugs. • Provide options and referrals to domestic violence victims.	As people progress through the adult years, visible signs of aging become apparent. Lifestyle behaviors and situational or family crises can also impact an adult's overall health and cause stress. Preventive health practices help adults improve the quality and duration of life.
Older Adult Falls Motor vehicle accidents Elder abuse Sensorimotor changes Fires	• Identify safety hazards in the environment. • Modify the environment as necessary. • Attend defensive driving courses on courses designed for elderly drivers. • Encourage regular vision and hearing tests. • Ensure that prescribed eyeglasses and hearing aids are available and functioning. • Wear appropriate footwear. • Have operational smoke detectors in place. • Objectively document and report any signs of neglect and abuse.	Accidental injuries occur more frequently in older adults because of decreased sensory abilities, slower reflexes and reaction times, changes in hearing and vision, and loss of strength and mobility. Collaboration between family and healthcare providers can ensure a safe, comfortable environment and promote healthy aging.

FUNDAMENTALS REVIEW 4-2

GENERAL GUIDELINES FOR RESTRAINT USE

- The patient has the right to be free from restraints that are not medically necessary. Restraints *must not* be used for the convenience of staff or to punish a patient.
- The patient's family must be involved in the plan of care. They must be consulted when the decision is made to use restraints. The family must be instructed regarding the facility's restraint policy and alternatives to restraints that are available.
- Physical restraints should be considered only after assessment of the patient, environment, and the situation; interventions to relieve discomforting behaviors have been used, precipitating factors have been identified and eliminated, if possible; and consultation with other healthcare professionals has occurred (Park & Tang, 2007).
- **Alternatives to restraints and less-restrictive interventions must have been implemented and failed. All alternatives used must be documented.**
- Contradictions to physical restraints should be assessed.
- The benefit gained from using a restraint must outweigh the known risks for that patient.
- The restraints must be ordered by a physician or other licensed independent practitioner who is responsible for the care of the patient. The order can never be for use on an 'as needed' basis.
- Once in place, the patient must be monitored and reassessed frequently. The patient's vital signs must be assessed and the medical patient must be visually observed every hour or according to facility policy.
- A physician or licensed independent practitioner must reevaluate and assess the patient every 24 hours (in the medical–surgical setting).
- Personal needs must be met. Provide fluids, nutrition, and toileting assistance every 2 hours.
- Skin integrity must be assessed and range-of-motion exercises provided every 2 hours.
- Documentation regarding why, how, where, and for how long the restraints were placed, and patient monitoring is vital.

(Modified from Centers for Medicare & Medicaid Services [CMS]. [2006]. Department of Health and Human Services. 42 CFR Part 482. Conditions of Participation: Patients' Rights. Final Rule; Lane, C., & Harrington, A. (2011). The factors that influence nurses' use of physical restraint: A thematic literature review. *International Journal of Nursing Practice, 17*(2), 195–204; and Park, M., & Tang, J. [2007]. Evidence-based guideline. Changing the practice of physical restraint use in acute care. *Journal of Gerontological Nursing, 33*[2], 9–16.)

FUNDAMENTALS REVIEW 4-3

R-E-S-T-R-A-I-N-T ACRONYM

The following R-E-S-T-R-A-I-N-T acronym prompts effective use of restraints (DiBartolo, 1998).

- **R**espond to the present, not the past. The patient's current condition, not his or her past history, must determine the need for restraints. This includes assessment of physical condition and mental and behavior status.
- **E**valuate the potential for injury. Determine whether the patient is at increased risk for harming self or others.
- **S**peak with family members or caregivers. Ask them for insights into the patient's behavior, and enlist their help in making a decision.
- **T**ry alternative measures first. Also, investigate the patient's medication regimen and attempt to discuss options with the patient.
- **R**eassess the patient to determine whether alternatives are successful. Agency policy dictates the frequency of assessments and documentation.
- **A**lert the primary care provider and the patient's family if restraints are indicated. Agency policy, The Joint Commission, and state and federal guidelines require an order from a physician or other healthcare professional licensed to prescribe in the state. The order should include the type of restraint, justification, criteria for removal, and intended duration of use.
- **I**ndividualize restraint use. Choose the least-restrictive device.
- **N**ote important information on the chart. Document the date and time the restraint is applied, the type of restraint, alternatives that were attempted and their results, and notification of the patient's family and physician. Include frequency of assessment, your findings, regular intervals when the restraint is removed, and nursing interventions.
- **T**ime-limit the use of restraints. Release the patient from the restraint as soon as he or she is no longer a risk to self or others. Restraints should be used no longer than 24 hours on nonpsychiatric patients. After 24 hours, a new order is required.

(Modified from DiBartolo, V. [1998]. 9 steps to effective restraint use. *RN, 61*[12], 23–24.)

SKILL 4-1 FALL PREVENTION

Falls are associated with physical and psychological trauma, especially in older adults. Fall-related injuries are often serious and can be fatal. Falls are caused by and associated with multiple factors. Primary causes of falls include:

- Change in balance or gait disturbance
- Muscle weakness
- Dizziness, syncope, and vertigo
- Cardiovascular changes, such as postural hypotension
- Change in vision or vision impairment
- Physical environment/environmental hazards
- Acute illness
- Neurologic disease, such as dementia or depression
- Language disorders that impair communication
- Polypharmacy

Many of these causes are within the realm of nursing responsibility. Identifying at-risk patients is crucial to planning appropriate interventions to prevent a fall. The combination of an assessment tool with a care/intervention plan sets the stage for best practice (AGS, 2012b; AGS & BGS, 2010; Gray-Micelli, 2012; and Hendrich, 2007). Accurate assessment and use of appropriate multifactorial fall interventions lead to maximum prevention (Degelau, et al., 2012). Table 4-1 identifies examples

Table 4-1 RECOMMENDED FALL-PREVENTION STRATEGIES BY FALL RISK LEVEL

LOW FALL RISK	MODERATE FALL RISK	HIGH FALL RISK
Fall Risk Score: 0–5 Points Maintain safe unit environment, including: • Remove excess equipment/supplies/ furniture from rooms and hallways. • Coil and secure excess electrical and telephone wires. • Clean all spills in patient room or in hallway immediately. Place signage to indicate wet floor danger. • Restrict window openings. The following are examples of basic safety interventions: • Orient patient to surroundings, including bathroom location, use of bed, and location of call bell. • Keep bed in lowest position during use unless impractical (as in ICU nursing or specialty beds). • Keep top two side rails up (excludes box beds). In ICU, keep all side rails up. • Secure locks on beds, stretchers, and wheelchairs. • Keep floors clutter/obstacle free (with attention to path between bed and bathroom/ commode). • Place call bell and frequently needed objects within patient reach. Answer call bell promptly. • Encourage patients/families to call for assistance when needed. • Display special instructions for vision and hearing. • Ensure adequate lighting, especially at night. • Use properly fitting nonskid footwear.	*Fall Risk Score: 6–10 Points* *Color Code: Yellow* • Institute flagging system: yellow card outside room and yellow sticker on medical record. Hill ROM flag (if available), assignment board/electronic board. In addition to measures listed under low fall risk: • Monitor and assist patient in following daily schedules. • Supervise and/or assist bedside sitting, personal hygiene, and toileting, as appropriate. • Reorient confused patients, as necessary. • Establish elimination schedule, including use of bedside commode, if appropriate. • PT (physical therapy) consult if patient has a history of fall and/or mobility impairment Evaluate need for: • OT (occupational therapy) consult • Slip-resistant chair mat (do *not* use in shower chair) • Use of seat belt, when in wheelchair	*Fall Risk Score: >10 Points* *Color Code: Red* • Institute flagging system: red card outside room and red sticker on medical record, assignment board/ electronic board: nurse call system flag, if available. In addition to measures listed under moderate and low fall risk: • Remain with patient while toileting. • Observe every 60 minutes unless patient is on activated bed/chair alarm. • If patient requires an air overlay, remove mattress (unless contraindicated by overlay type) or use side rail protectors. • When necessary, transport throughout hospital with assistance of staff or trained caregivers. Consider alternatives, for example, bedside procedure. Notify receiving area of high fall risk. Evaluate need for the following, starting with less restrictive to more restrictive measures in the listed order: • Moving patient to room with best visual access to nursing station • Bed/chair alarm • Specialty fall-prevention bed • 24-hour supervision/sitter • Physical restraint/enclosed bed (only if less-restrictive alternatives have been considered and found to be ineffective)

(Recommended fall-prevention strategies by fall risk level. Reprinted with permission. ©2003, The Johns Hopkins Hospital.)

of fall-prevention strategies based on fall risk assessment. Fall risk assessment is discussed in the following assessment section. Providing patient education and a safer patient environment can reduce the incidence and severity of falls. The ultimate goal is to reduce the physical and psychological trauma experienced by patients and their significant others.

DELEGATION CONSIDERATIONS

After assessment of fall risk by the RN, activities related to the prevention of falls may be delegated to nursing assistive personnel (NAP) or unlicensed assistive personnel (UAP), as well as to licensed practical/vocational nurses (LPN/LVN). The decision to delegate must be based on careful analysis of the patient's needs and circumstances, as well as the qualifications of the person to whom the task is being delegated. Refer to the Delegation Guidelines in Appendix A.

EQUIPMENT

- Fall-risk assessment tool, if available
- PPE, as indicated
- Additional intervention tools, as appropriate, (refer to sample intervention equipment in this skill)

ASSESSMENT

At a minimum, fall-risk assessment needs to occur on admission to the facility, following a change in the patient's condition, after a fall, and when the patient is transferred. If it is determined that the patient is at risk for falling, regular assessment must continue. Assess the patient and the medical record for factors that increase the patient's risk for falling. The use of an objective, systematic fall assessment is made easier by the use of a fall assessment tool. Figure 1 provides an

Fall risk factor category* **(NA If comatose, complete paralysis, or completely immobilized)**	Points
Age • 70–79 y (2 points) • ≥80 y (3 points)	
Fall history • Fall within 3 months before admission (5 points) • Fall during this hospitalization (11 points)	
Mobility • Ambulates or transfers with unsteady gait and **NO** assistance or assistive devices (2 points) • Ambulates or transfers with assistance or assistive device (2 points) • Visual or auditory impairment affecting mobility (4 points)	
Elimination • Urgency/nocturia (2 points) • Incontinence (5 points)	
Mental status changes • Affecting awareness of environment (2 points) • Affecting awareness of one's physical limitations (4 points)	
Medications: One present (3 points); 2 or more present; or sedated procedure within the past 24 h (5 points) Psychotropics (antidepressants, hypnotics, antipsychotics, sedatives, benzodiazepines, some antiemetics) Anticonvulsants Diuretics/cathartics PCS/narcotics/opiates Antihypertensives	
Patient care equipment: One present (1 point); ≥ 2 present (2 points) (IV, chest tube, indwelling catheter, SCDs, etc)	
Total points	

***Moderate risk = 6–10 Total points, High risk > 10 Total points**

FIGURE 1 Johns Hopkins Fall Risk Assessment Tool. (Reprinted with permission. ©2003, The Johns Hopkins Hospital.)

(continued)

SKILL 4-1 FALL PREVENTION continued

example of a fall assessment tool. The Hendrich II Fall Risk Model, another tool to evaluate fall risk factors, can be viewed on thePoint. Assess for a history of falls. If the patient has experienced a previous fall, assess the circumstances surrounding the fall and any associated symptoms. Review the patient's medication history and medication record for medications that may increase the risk for falls. Assess for the following additional risk factors for falls (AGS & BGS, 2010; Gray-Micelli, 2012; Hendrich, 2007; Titler, et al., 2011):

- Lower extremity muscle weakness
- Gait or balance deficit
- Restraint use
- Use of an assistive device
- Presence of intravenous therapy
- Impaired activities of daily living
- Age older than 75 years
- Altered elimination
- History of falls
- Administration of high-risk drugs, such as narcotic analgesics, antiepileptics, benzodiazepines, and drugs with anticholinergic effects
- Use of four or more medications
- Depression
- Visual deficit
- Arthritis
- History of cerebrovascular accident
- Cognitive impairment
- Secondary diagnosis/chronic disease

NURSING DIAGNOSIS

Determine the related factors for nursing diagnoses based on the patient's current status. Appropriate nursing diagnoses may include:

- Risk for Falls
- Risk for Injury
- Impaired Physical Mobility

OUTCOME IDENTIFICATION AND PLANNING

The expected outcome to achieve is that the patient does not experience a fall and remains free of injury. Other outcomes that may be appropriate include the following: the patient's environment is free from hazards; patient and/or caregiver demonstrates an understanding of appropriate interventions to prevent falls; the patient uses assistive devices correctly; the patient uses safe transfer procedures; and appropriate precautions are implemented related to the use of medications that increase the risk for falls.

IMPLEMENTATION

ACTION	RATIONALE
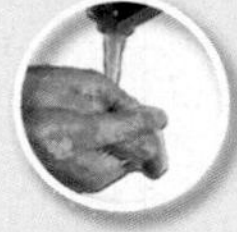 1. Perform hand hygiene and put on PPE, if indicated.	Hand hygiene and PPE prevent the spread of microorganisms. PPE is required based on transmission precautions.
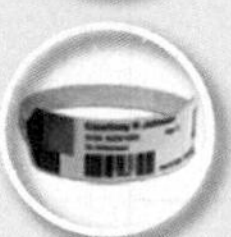 2. Identify the patient. Assess fall risk as outlined above.	Identifying the patient ensures the right patient receives the intervention and helps prevent errors. Fall-risk assessment aids in providing appropriate fall-prevention interventions for the individual patient.
3. Explain the rationale for fall prevention interventions to the patient and family/significant others.	Explanation helps reduce anxiety and promotes compliance and understanding.

ACTION	RATIONALE
4. Include the patient's family and/or significant others in the plan of care.	This promotes continuity of care and cooperation.
5. Provide adequate lighting. Use a night light during sleeping hours.	Good lighting reduces accidental tripping over and bumping into objects that may not be seen. Night light provides illumination in an unfamiliar environment.
6. Remove excess equipment, supplies, furniture, and other objects from rooms and walkways. Pay particular attention to high traffic areas and the route to the bathroom.	All are possible hazards.
7. Orient patient and significant others to new surroundings, including use of the telephone, call bell, patient bed, and room illumination. Indicate the location of the patient's bathroom.	Knowledge of proper use of equipment relieves anxiety and promotes compliance.
8. Provide a 'low bed' to replace regular hospital bed.	To be considered a 'low hospital bed' the frame of the bed must be lower so that the height of the mattress deck off the floor is between 6.5″ and 10.5″. This low height, as determined by the FDA, reduces the risk of fall-related injuries from bed.
9. Use floor mats if patient is at risk for serious injury (Figure 2).	Floor mats cushion falls and may prevent serious injury in patients at risk, such as those with osteoporosis (Gray-Micelli, 2012).
10. Provide nonskid footwear and/or walking shoes (Figure 3).	Nonskid footwear prevents slipping and walking shoes improve balance when ambulating or transferring.

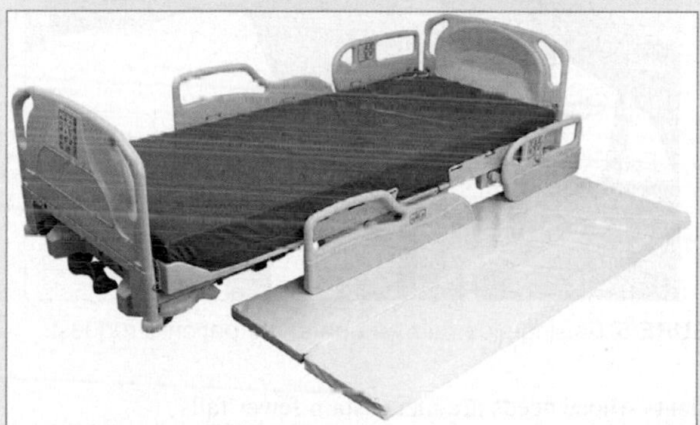

FIGURE 2 Low bed with floor mats. (Reprinted with permission from CHG Hospital Beds, London, ON.)

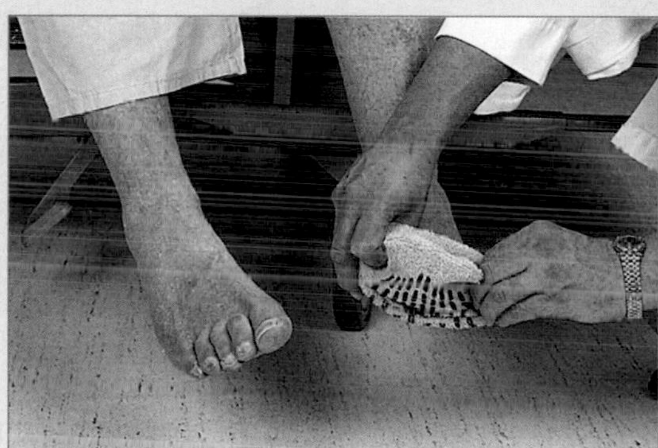

FIGURE 3 Providing nonskid footwear.

ACTION	RATIONALE
11. Institute a toileting regimen and/or continence program, if appropriate.	Toileting on a regular basis decreases risk for falls.
12. Provide a bedside commode and/or urinal/bedpan, if appropriate. Ensure that it is near the bed at all times.	This prevents falls related to incontinence or trying to get to the bathroom.
13. Ensure that the call bell, bedside table, telephone, and other personal items are within the patient's reach at all times.	This prevents the patient from having to overreach for a device or items, and/or possibly attempt ambulation or transfer unassisted.
14. Confer with primary care provider regarding appropriate exercise and physical therapy.	Exercise programs, such as muscle strengthening, balance training, and walking plans, decrease falls and fall-related injuries (AGS & BGS, 2010).
15. Confer with primary care provider regarding appropriate mobility aids, such as a cane or walker.	Mobility aids can help improve balance and steady the patient's gait.

(continued)

SKILL 4-1 FALL PREVENTION continued

ACTION	RATIONALE
16. Confer with primary care provider regarding the use of bone-strengthening medications, such as calcium, vitamin D, and drugs to prevent/treat osteoporosis.	Bone strengthening has been suggested to reduce fracture rates with falls (AGS & BGS, 2010).
17. Encourage the patient to rise or change position slowly and sit for several minutes before standing.	Gradual position changes reduce the risk of falls related to orthostatic hypotension.
18. Evaluate the appropriateness of elastic stockings for lower extremities.	Elastic stockings minimize venous pooling and promote venous return.
19. Review medications for potential hazards.	Certain medications and combinations of medications have been associated with increased risk for falls.
20. Keep the bed in the lowest position. If elevated to provide care (to reduce caregiver strain), ensure that it is lowered when care is completed.	Keeping bed in lowest position reduces the risk of a fall-related injury.
21. Make sure locks on the bed or wheelchair are secured at all times (Figure 4).	Locking prevents the bed or wheelchair from moving out from under the patient.
22. Use bed rails according to facility policy, when appropriate (Figure 5).	Inappropriate bed-rail use has been associated with patient injury and increased fall risk. Side rails may be considered a restraint when used to prevent an ambulatory patient from getting out of bed.

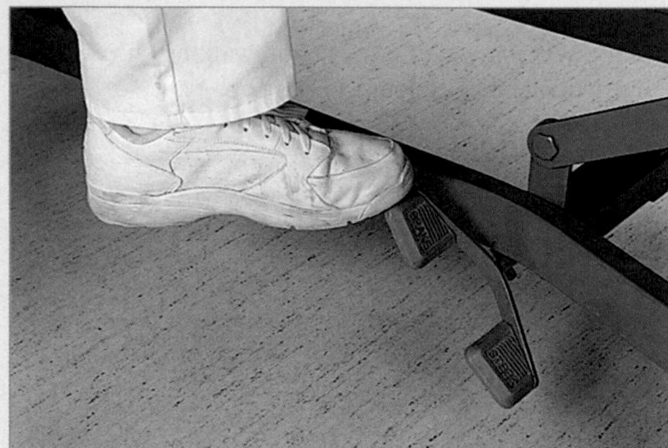

FIGURE 4 Engaging bed locks.

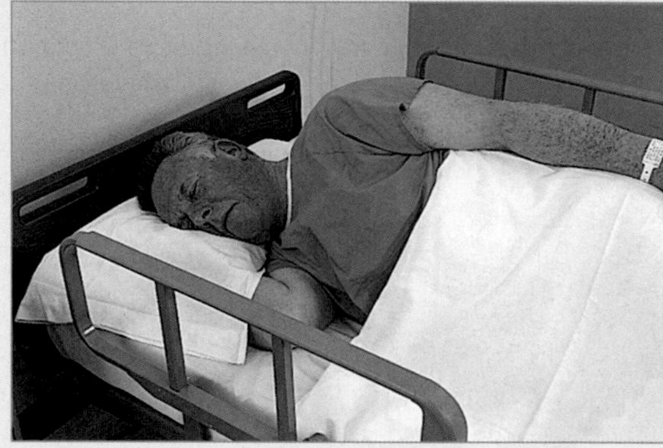

FIGURE 5 Raising side rails on bed at the patient's request.

ACTION	RATIONALE
23. Anticipate patient needs and provide assistance with activities instead of waiting for the patient to ask.	Patients whose needs are met sustain fewer falls.
24. Consider the use of an electronic personal alarm or pressure sensor alarm for the bed or chair (Figure 6).	The alarm helps alert staff to unassisted changes in position by the patient.

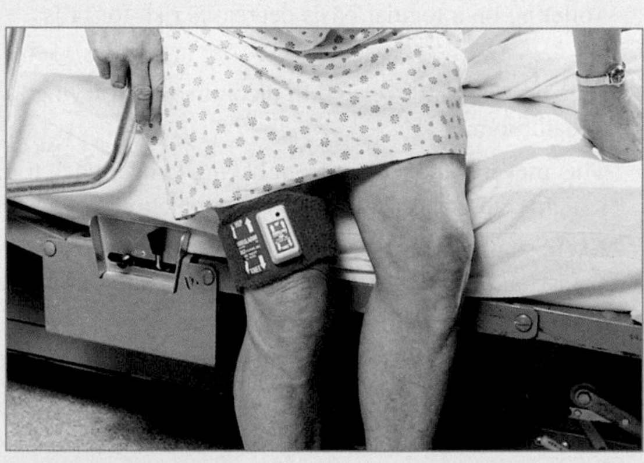

FIGURE 6 Patient wearing a personal alarm device.

ACTION	RATIONALE
25. Discuss the possibility of appropriate family member(s) staying with patient.	The presence of a family member provides familiarity and companionship.
26. Consider the use of patient attendant or sitter.	Attendant or sitter can provide companionship and supervision.
27. Increase the frequency of patient observation and surveillance. Utilize 1- or 2-hour nursing rounds, including pain assessment, toileting assistance, patient comfort, making sure personal items are in reach, and meeting patient needs.	Patient care rounds/nursing rounds can reduce patient falls (Kessler, et al., 2012; Olrich, et al., 2012; Meade, et al., 2006; Weisgram & Raymond, 2008).
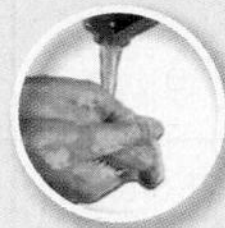 28. Remove PPE, if used. Perform hand hygiene.	Removing PPE properly reduces the risk for infection transmission and contamination of other items. Hand hygiene prevents transmission of microorganisms.

EVALUATION

The expected outcomes are met when the patient remains free of falls, and injury interventions to minimize risk factors that might precipitate a fall are implemented; patient's environment is free from hazards; patient and/or caregiver demonstrates an understanding of appropriate interventions to prevent falls; the patient uses assistive devices correctly; the patient uses safe transfer procedures; and appropriate precautions are implemented related to use of medications that increase the risk for falls.

DOCUMENTATION

Guidelines

Document patient fall-risk assessment. Include appropriate interventions to reduce fall risk in nursing care plan. Document patient and family teaching relative to fall-risk reduction. Document interventions included in care.

Sample Documentation

<u>11/1/15</u> 1730 Patient admitted to room 650W; oriented to room. Fall assessment low risk (5 pts). Basic safety interventions in place per facility Fall Prevention Guidelines. Will continue to monitor and reevaluate.

—B. Clapp, RN

UNEXPECTED SITUATIONS AND ASSOCIATED INTERVENTIONS

- *Patient experiences a fall:* Immediately assess the patient's condition. Provide care and interventions appropriate for status/injuries. Notify the patient's primary caregiver of the incident and your assessment of the patient. Ensure prompt follow-through for any orders for diagnostic tests, such as x-rays or CT scans, as ordered. Evaluate circumstances of the fall and the patient's environment and institute appropriate measures to prevent further incidents. Document incident, assessments, and interventions in the patient's medical record. Complete a **safety event report** per facility policy.

SPECIAL CONSIDERATIONS

Home Care Considerations

- Patients are at risk for falls in their home. Assess for risk factors in the home and assess the home environment. Include patient teaching regarding falls as part of the nursing plan of care. See Box 4-1 for possible interventions for the home setting.

(continued)

SKILL 4-1 FALL PREVENTION continued

BOX 4-1 PATIENT EDUCATION FOR PREVENTING FALLS IN THE HOME

- Talk with your doctor about a plan for an exercise program. Regular exercise helps maintain strength and flexibility, and can help slow bone loss.
- Have regular hearing and vision testing. Always wear glasses and hearing aids, if prescribed. Even small changes in sight and hearing can affect stability.
- Wear low-heeled, rubber-soled shoes. Avoid wearing only socks or shoes with smooth soles.
- Have hand rails on both sides of stairs and make use of them when using the stairs. Try not to carry things when using the steps. When necessary, hold item in one hand and use the hand rail with the other hand.
- Avoid using chairs and tables as ladders to reach items that are too high to reach.
- Keep electrical and telephone cords against the wall and out of walkways.
- Consider rails next to the toilet and in the shower or tub and raised toilet seats.
- Know the possible side effects of medications used. Some can affect coordination and balance.
- Use a cane, walking stick, or walker to help improve stability.
- Keep home temperature at a moderate level. Temperatures too hot or too cold can contribute to dizziness.
- Stand up slowly after eating, lying down, or resting. Standing too quickly can cause fainting or dizziness.
- Make sure there is good lighting, particularly at the stairs.
- Use a night light.
- Remove clutter from walkways inside and outside the house.
- Carpets should be fixed firmly to the floor to prevent slipping. Use no-slip strips on uncarpeted surfaces.
- Use nonskid mats, strips, or carpet on surfaces that get wet.
- Check all medications, including prescriptions, and over-the-counter drugs, herbs, and vitamins, with your health-care provider and/or pharmacist to find out if any put you at risk for falling.

(Adapted from American Geriatrics Society (AGS). [2012a]. *Tips for preventing serious falls.* Available at http://www.healthinaging.org/files/documents/tipsheets/falls_prevention.pdf; American Geriatrics Society (AGS). [2012b]. *Aging & health A to Z.* Available at http://www.healthinaging.org/aging-and-health-a-to-z/topic:falls; Bandos, J. [2008]. Protection in the home. Tips on safety for older adults. *Advance for Nurses, 10*[22], 40; and National Institute on Aging. [2012]. *Age page: Falls and fractures.* Available at http://www.nia.nih.gov/health/publication/falls-and-fractures.)

EVIDENCE FOR PRACTICE ▶

HOURLY PATIENT ROUNDS

Many factors increase a patient's risk for falling, including cognitive impairments, impaired ability to perform activities of daily living (ADLs), and impaired elimination. Can nursing interventions that focus on proactive, protective strategies, and patient comfort reduce the risk for falls?

Related Research

Olrich, T., Kalman, M., & Nigolian, C. (2012). Hourly rounding: A replication study. *MEDSURG Nursing, 21*(1), 23–36.

The purpose of this study was to determine the effect of hourly rounding on fall rates, call light usage, and patient satisfaction in an inpatient medical–surgical patient population. Data were collected for patient falls, patient satisfaction, and call-light use prior to the implementation of nurse rounding. Unlicensed assistive personnel (UAP) on the experimental unit attended a CNS-led educational session about performance of hourly rounding. The round process involved patient–nurse interaction (or patient–designee interaction), including evaluations of pain, toileting needs, and positioning, as well as a check of the patient's environment, including access to call bell, telephone, bedside table, tissues, water, television, and trash can. The nursing rounds were associated with reduction in patient use of the call bell, as well as a reduction of patient falls and increased patient satisfaction.

Relevance for Nursing Practice

Nursing rounds are a simple, easy-to-implement intervention. A protocol that incorporates hourly or once every 2-hour rounds can reduce the frequency of patients' call bell use, increase patient satisfaction with nursing care, and reduce falls, leading to more effective patient-care management and improved patient satisfaction, and safety.

Refer to thePoint for additional research on related nursing topics.

SKILL 4-2 IMPLEMENTING ALTERNATIVES TO THE USE OF RESTRAINTS

Physical restraints increase the possibility of serious injury due to a fall. They do not prevent falls. The adverse health consequences associated with restraint use actually result in the need for additional staff because the condition of residents in long-term care facilities can deteriorate when restraints are employed. Additional negative outcomes of restraint use include skin breakdown and contractures, incontinence, depression, delirium, anxiety, aspiration and respiratory difficulties, and even death (Taylor, et al., 2015). The American Nurses Association (ANA) has approved a position statement defining the nurses' role in reducing restraint use in healthcare. Their recommendations are included in Box 4-2. **Restraints should be used only after less-restrictive methods have failed.** The following skill outlines possible alternatives to restraint use.

Box 4-2 ANA BOARD OF DIRECTORS POSITION STATEMENT: REDUCTION OF PATIENT RESTRAINT AND SECLUSION IN HEALTH CARE SETTINGS

Recommendations: To ensure safe, quality care for all patients in the least restrictive environment, ANA supports nursing efforts to:

1. Educate nurses, nursing students, unlicensed personnel, other members of the interdisciplinary team, and family caregivers on the appropriate use of restraint and seclusion, and on the alternatives to these restrictive interventions;
2. Ensure sufficient nursing staff to monitor and individualize care with the goal of only using restraint when no other viable option is available;
3. Ensure policies and environment support services are in place to provide feasible alternatives to physical and chemical restraints;
4. Move progressively toward a restraint-free environment while providing a therapeutic sanctuary for all;
5. Enforce documentation requirements and education about what should be documented;
6. Explore the ethical implications of restraining patients with nursing students and discuss the need for institutional policy that clarifies when, where, and how patients are to be restrained and monitored while restrained;
7. Be aware of all implications of allowing the application of restraints in healthcare settings. The nurse administrator should make consultation available to nurses, including ethical consultation about decisions to restrain; and
8. Develop clear policies based on accepted national standards to guide decision-making regarding restraints.

(ANA Position Statement: *Reduction of patient restraint and seclusion in health care settings.* [2012]. p. 10–11. Available at http://www.nursingworld.org/restraintposition.

DELEGATION CONSIDERATIONS

After assessment by the RN, activities related to the use of alternatives to restraints may be delegated to nursing assistive personnel (NAP) or unlicensed assistive personnel (UAP), as well as to licensed practical/vocational nurses (LPN/LVN). The decision to delegate must be based on careful analysis of the patient's needs and circumstances, as well as the qualifications of the person to whom the task is being delegated. Refer to the Delegation Guidelines in Appendix A.

EQUIPMENT

- PPE, as indicated
- Additional intervention tools, as appropriate (refer to sample intervention equipment in this skill)

ASSESSMENT

Assess the patient's status. Determine whether the patient's pattern of behavior (wandering, fall risk, interfering with medical devices, resistive to care, danger to self or others) exists that increases the need for restraint use. Assess to determine the meaning of the behavior and its cause. Assess for pain. Assess respiratory status, vital signs, blood glucose level, fluid and electrolyte issues, and medications. Assess the patient's functional, mental, and psychological status. Evaluate the patient's environment, including noise level, lighting, floor surfaces, design/suitability of equipment and furniture, visual cues, barriers to mobility, space for privacy, and clothing. Assess and evaluate the effectiveness of restraint alternatives.

NURSING DIAGNOSIS

Determine the related factors for the nursing diagnosis based on the patient's current status. Appropriate nursing diagnoses may include:

- Acute Confusion
- Risk for Injury
- Risk for Other-Directed Violence

(continued)

SKILL 4-2 IMPLEMENTING ALTERNATIVES TO THE USE OF RESTRAINTS continued

OUTCOME IDENTIFICATION AND PLANNING

The expected outcome to be met when implementing alternatives to restraints is that the use of restraints is avoided and the patient and others remain free from harm.

IMPLEMENTATION

ACTION	RATIONALE
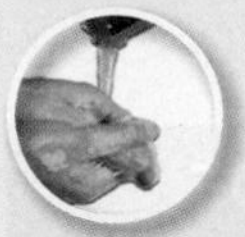 1. Perform hand hygiene and put on PPE, if indicated.	Hand hygiene and PPE prevent the spread of microorganisms. PPE is required based on transmission precautions.
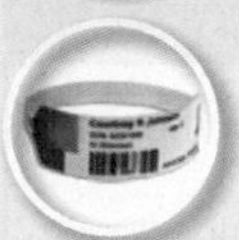 2. Identify the patient.	Identifying the patient ensures the right patient receives the intervention and helps prevent errors.
3. Explain the rationale for interventions to the patient and family/significant others.	Explanation helps reduce anxiety and promotes compliance and understanding.
4. Include the patient's family and/or significant others in the plan of care.	This promotes continuity of care and cooperation.
5. Identify behavior(s) that place the patient at risk for restraint use. Assess the patient's status and environment, as outlined above.	Behaviors, such as interference with therapy or treatment, risk for falls, agitation/restlessness, resistance to care, wandering, and/or cognitive impairment, put the patient at risk for restraint use. Assessment and interpretation of patient behavior identifies unmet physiologic or psychosocial needs, acute changes in mental or physical status, provides for appropriate environments and individualized care, and respects patient's needs and rights.
6. Identify triggers or contributing factors to patient behaviors. Evaluate medication usage for medications that can contribute to cognitive and movement dysfunction and to increased risk for falls.	Removal of contributing factors and/or triggers can decrease need for restraint use. Possible changes in prescribed medications can be addressed to decrease adverse effects and decrease the need for restraint use.
7. Assess the patient's functional, mental, and psychological status and the environment, as outlined above.	Assessment provides a better understanding of the reason for the behavior, leading to individualized interventions that can eliminate restraint use and provide for patient safety.
8. Provide adequate lighting. Use a night light during sleeping hours.	Appropriate lighting can reduce disruptive behavior related to fear in an unfamiliar environment.
9. Consult with primary care provider and other appropriate healthcare providers regarding the continued need for treatments/therapies and the use of the least invasive method to deliver care.	Exploring the possibility of administering treatment in a less intrusive manner or discontinuing treatment no longer needed can remove the stimulus for behavior that increases risk for use of restraints.
10. Assess the patient for pain and discomfort. Provide appropriate pharmacologic and nonpharmacologic interventions. (Refer to Chapter 10)	Unrelieved pain can contribute to behaviors that increase the risk for the use of restraints.
11. Ask a family member or significant other to stay with the patient.	Having someone stay with the patient provides companionship and familiarity.
12. Reduce unnecessary environmental stimulation and noise.	Increased stimulation can contribute to behaviors that increase the risk for use of restraints.
13. Provide simple, clear, and direct explanations for treatments and care. Repeat to reinforce, as needed.	Explanation helps reduce anxiety and promotes compliance and understanding.
14. Distract and redirect using a calm voice.	Distraction and redirection can reduce or remove behaviors that increase risk for use of restraints.

ACTION	RATIONALE
15. Increase the frequency of patient observation and surveillance; 1- or 2-hour nursing rounds, including pain assessment, toileting assistance, patient comfort, keeping personal items in reach, and meeting patient needs.	Patient care rounds/nursing rounds improve identification of unmet needs, which can decrease behaviors that increase risk for use of restraints.
16. Implement fall precaution interventions. Refer to Skill 4-1.	Behaviors that increase risk for use of restraints also increase risk for falls.
17. Camouflage tube and other treatment sites with clothing, elastic sleeves, or bandaging.	Camouflaging tubes and other treatment sites removes stimulus that can trigger behaviors that increase risk for use of restraints.
18. Ensure the use of glasses and hearing aids, if necessary.	Glasses and hearing aids allow for correct interpretation of the environment and activities to reduce confusion.
19. Consider relocation to a room close to the nursing station.	Relocation close to the nursing station provides the opportunity for increased frequency of observation.
20. Encourage daily exercise/provide exercise and activities or relaxation techniques.	Activity provides an outlet for energy and stimulation, decreasing behaviors associated with increased risk for use of restraints.
21. Make the environment as homelike as possible; provide familiar objects.	Familiarity provides reassurance and comfort, decreasing apprehension and reducing behaviors associated with increased risk for use of restraints.
22. Allow restless patient to walk after ensuring that environment is safe. Use a large plant or piece of furniture as a barrier to limit wandering from the designated area.	Activity provides an outlet for energy and stimulation, decreasing behaviors associated with increased risk for use of restraints.
23. Consider the use of patient attendant or sitter.	An attendant or sitter provides companionship and supervision.
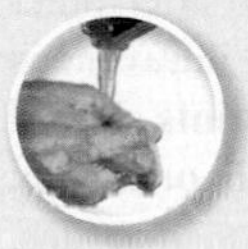 24. Remove PPE, if used. Perform hand hygiene.	Removing PPE properly reduces the risk for infection transmission and contamination of other items. Hand hygiene prevents transmission of microorganisms.

EVALUATION

The expected outcomes are met when use of restraints is avoided and the patient and others remain free from harm.

DOCUMENTATION

Guidelines

Document patient assessment. Include appropriate interventions to reduce need for restraints in nursing plan of care. Document patient and family teaching relative to use of interventions. Document interventions included in care.

Sample Documentation

1/1/15 2330 Patient pulling IV tubing and attempting to remove dressing at insertion site left antecubital. NPO status; IV necessary for hydration and medication. Explanation regarding IV access reinforced with patient and wife. IV site covered with gauze and tubing placed under top bed linen to minimize appearance. Wife provided CD of favorite music and a puzzle. Rounding increased to every 30 minutes when family not present.

—*B. Clapp, RN*

UNEXPECTED SITUATIONS AND ASSOCIATED INTERVENTIONS

- *Interventions to distract no longer effective. Patient continues to pull at IV site and tubing:* Reevaluate need for IV fluid infusion. Consult with primary care provider regarding possibility of converting to intermittent access. Reevaluate patient and environment; attempt additional/different interventions as outlined above.

(continued)

SKILL 4-2 IMPLEMENTING ALTERNATIVES TO THE USE OF RESTRAINTS continued

EVIDENCE FOR PRACTICE ▶

MINIMIZING RESTRAINT USE

These resources summarize current best evidence on the topic of interventions to be used as alternatives to the use of restraints, as well as minimizing and eliminating the use of restraints.

- Rutledge, D.N., & March, P.D. (2011). *Evidence-based care sheet. Restraint: Minimizing use in acute, nonpsychiatric care.* Glendale, CA: Cinahl Information Systems.
- Rutledge, D.N., & March, P.D. (2011). *Evidence-based care sheet. Restraint: Minimizing usage in skilled nursing facilities.* Glendale, CA: Cinahl Information Systems.
- Centers for Medicare & Medicaid Services (CMS). (2006). Department of Health and Human Services. 42 CFR Part 482. *Conditions of participation: Patients' rights. Final rule.* Available http://www.cms.gov/Regulations-and-Guidance/Legislation/CFCsAndCoPs/downloads/finalpatientrightsrule.pdf.
- Park, M., & Tang, J. (2007). Evidence-based guideline. Changing the practice of physical restraint use in acute care. *Journal of Gerontological Nursing, 33*(2), 9–16.

Refer to thePoint for additional research on related nursing topics.

SKILL 4-3 APPLYING AN EXTREMITY RESTRAINT

Cloth extremity restraints immobilize one or more extremities. They may be indicated after other measures have failed to prevent a patient from removing therapeutic devices, such as intravenous (IV) access devices, endotracheal tubes, oxygen, or other treatment interventions. **Restraints should be used only after less-restrictive methods have failed. Ensure compliance with ordering, assessment, and maintenance procedures.** Restraints can be applied to the hands, wrists, or ankles. Review the general guidelines for using restraints in the chapter introduction and in Fundamentals Review 4-2 and 4-3, as well as in Box 4-2 in Skill 4-2. See also Evidence for Practice after Skill 4-2 for best evidence on the topic of interventions to be used as alternatives to the use of restraints, as well as minimizing and eliminating the use of restraints.

DELEGATION CONSIDERATIONS

After assessment of the patient by the RN, the application of an extremity restraint may be delegated to nursing assistive personnel (NAP) or unlicensed assistive personnel (UAP), as well as to licensed practical/vocational nurses (LPN/LVNs). The decision to delegate must be based on careful analysis of the patient's needs and circumstances, as well as the qualifications of the person to whom the task is being delegated. Refer to the Delegation Guidelines in Appendix A.

EQUIPMENT

- Appropriate cloth restraint for the extremity that is to be immobilized
- Padding, if necessary, for bony prominences
- PPE, as indicated

ASSESSMENT

Assess both the patient's physical condition and the potential for injury to self or others. A confused patient who might remove devices needed to sustain life is considered at risk for injury to self and may require the use of restraints. Assess the patient's behavior, including the presence of confusion, agitation, and combativeness, as well as the patient's ability to understand and follow directions. Evaluate the appropriateness of the least restrictive restraint device. For example, if the patient has had a stroke and cannot move the left arm, a restraint may be needed only on the right arm. Inspect the extremity where the restraint will be applied. Establish baseline skin condition for comparison at future assessments while the restraint is in place. Consider using another form of restraint if the restraint may cause further injury at the site. Before application, assess for adequate circulation in the extremity to which the restraint is to be applied, including capillary refill and proximal pulses.

NURSING DIAGNOSIS

Determine the related factors for nursing diagnoses based on the patient's current status. Appropriate nursing diagnoses may include:

- Risk for Injury
- Risk for Impaired Skin Integrity
- Acute Confusion

OUTCOME IDENTIFICATION AND PLANNING

The expected outcome to achieve is that the patient is constrained by the restraint, remains free from injury, and the restraint does not interfere with therapeutic devices. Other outcomes that may be appropriate include the following: the patient does not experience impaired skin integrity; the patient does not injure himself or herself due to the restraints; and the patient's family will demonstrate an understanding about the use of the restraint and their role in the patient's care.

IMPLEMENTATION

ACTION	RATIONALE
1. Determine need for restraints. Assess patient's physical condition, behavior, and mental status. (Refer to Fundamentals Review 4-2 and 4-3 at the beginning of the chapter and Box 4-2 in Skill 4-2.)	Restraints should be used only as a last resort when alternative measures have failed and the patient is at increased risk for harming self or others.
2. Confirm agency policy for application of restraints. **Secure an order from the primary care provider, or validate that the order has been obtained within the required time frame.**	Policy protects the patient and the nurse and specifies guidelines for application as well as type of restraint and duration. **Each order for restraint or seclusion used for the management of violent or self-destructive behavior that jeopardizes the immediate physical safety of the patient, a staff member, or others may only be renewed in accordance with the following limits for up to a total of 24 hours: (A) 4 hours for adults 18 years of age or older; (B) 2 hours for children and adolescents 9 to 17 years of age; or (C) 1 hour for children under 9 years of age. After 24 hours, before writing a new order for the use of restraint or seclusion for the management of violent or self-destructive behavior, a physician or other licensed independent practitioner who is responsible for the care of the patient must see and assess the patient** (CMS, 2006).
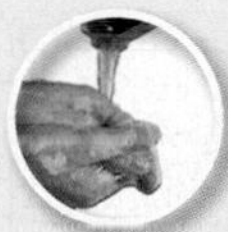 3. Perform hand hygiene and put on PPE, if indicated.	Hand hygiene and PPE prevent the spread of microorganisms. PPE is required based on transmission precautions.
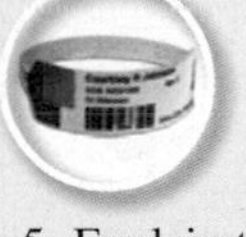 4. Identify the patient.	Identifying the patient ensures the right patient receives the intervention and helps prevent errors.
5. Explain the reason for restraint use to patient and family. Clarify how care will be given and how needs will be met. Explain that restraint is a temporary measure.	Explanation to patient and family may lessen confusion and anger and provide reassurance. A clearly stated agency policy on application of restraints should be available for patient and family to read. In a long-term care facility, the family must give consent before a restraint is applied.
6. Include the patient's family and/or significant others in the plan of care.	This promotes continuity of care and cooperation.
7. Apply restraint according to manufacturer's directions:	Proper application prevents injury.
a. Choose the least restrictive type of device that allows the greatest possible degree of mobility.	This provides minimal restriction.
b. Pad bony prominences.	Padding helps prevent skin injury.

(continued)

SKILL 4-3 APPLYING AN EXTREMITY RESTRAINT continued

ACTION	RATIONALE
c. Wrap the restraint around the extremity with the soft part in contact with the skin (Figure 1). If a hand mitt is being used, pull over the hand with cushion to the palmar aspect of hand (Figure 2).	This prevents excess pressure on the extremity.

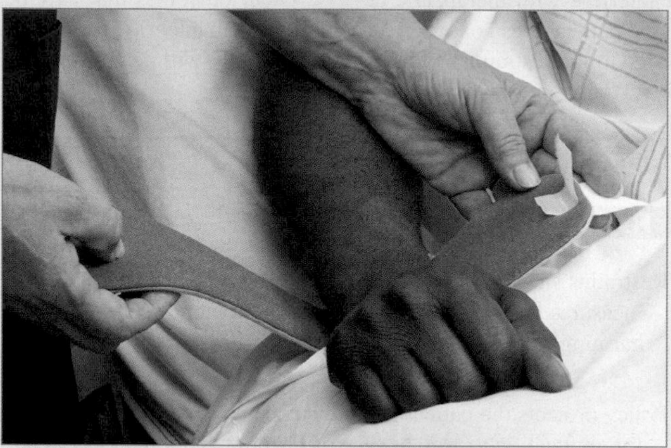

FIGURE 1 Wrapping the restraint around the extremity with the soft part in contact with the skin. (From Craven, C. F., & Hirnle, C. J., (2013). *Fundamentals of nursing* (7th ed). Philadelphia: Wolters Kluwer Health/Lippincott Williams & Wilkins, p. 596, Figure 1.)

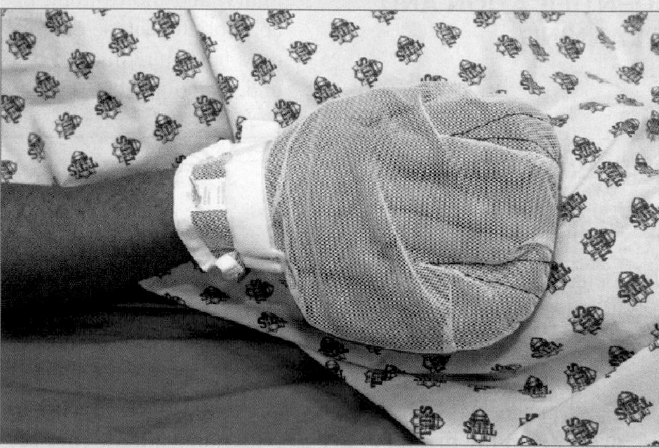

FIGURE 2 Using a hand mitt. (From Craven, C. F., & Hirnle, C. J., (2013). *Fundamentals of nursing* (7th ed). Philadelphia: Wolters Kluwer Health/Lippincott Williams & Wilkins, p. 597, Figure 4.)

ACTION	RATIONALE
8. Secure in place with the Velcro straps or other mechanism, depending on specific restraint device (Figure 3). Depending on characteristics of specific restraint, it may be necessary to tie a knot in the restraint ties, to ensure the restraint remains secure on the extremity.	Proper application secures restraint and ensures that there is no interference with patient's circulation and potential alteration in neurovascular status.
9. **Ensure that two fingers can be inserted between the restraint and patient's extremity (Figure 4).**	Proper application ensures that nothing interferes with patient's circulation and potential alteration in neurovascular status.

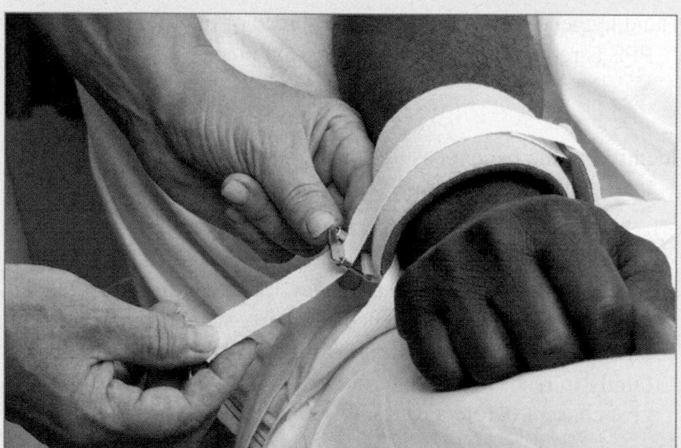

FIGURE 3 Securing restraint on extremity. (From Craven, C. F., & Hirnle, C. J., (2013). *Fundamentals of nursing* (7th ed). Philadelphia: Wolters Kluwer Health/Lippincott Williams & Wilkins, p. 597, Figure 2.)

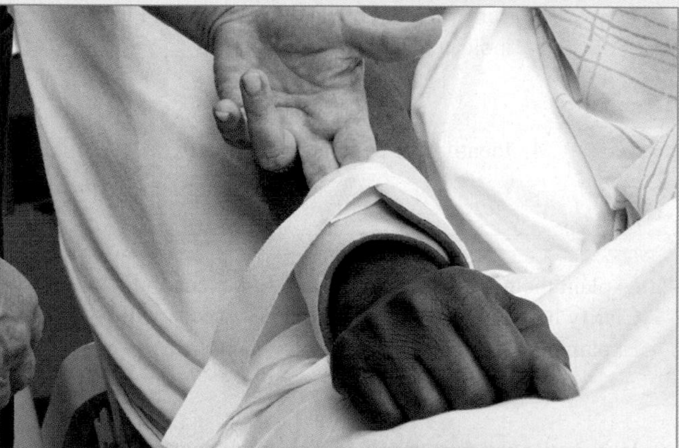

FIGURE 4 Ensuring that two fingers can be inserted between the restraint and the patient's extremity. (From Craven, C. F., & Hirnle, C. J., (2013). *Fundamentals of nursing* (7th ed). Philadelphia: Wolters Kluwer Health/Lippincott Williams & Wilkins, p. 597, Figure 3.)

ACTION	RATIONALE
10. Maintain restrained extremity in normal anatomic position. **Use a quick-release knot to tie the restraint to the bed frame, not side rail (Figure 5).** The restraint may also be attached to a chair frame. The site should not be readily accessible to the patient.	Maintaining a normal position lessens possibility of injury. A quick-release knot ensures that the restraint will not tighten when pulled and can be removed quickly in an emergency. Securing the restraint to a side rail may injure the patient when the side rail is lowered. Tying the restraint out of the patient's reach promotes security.

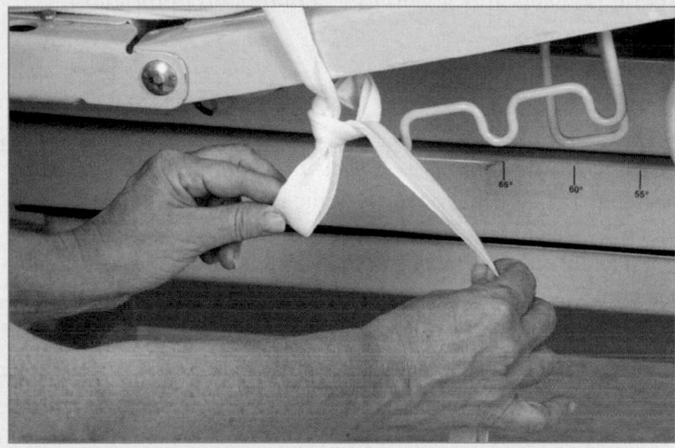

FIGURE 5 Securing restraint to bed frame. (From Craven, C. F., & Hirnle, C. J., (2009). *Fundamentals of nursing* (6th ed). Philadelphia: Wolters Kluwer Health/Lippincott Williams & Wilkins, p. 680, Figure 4.)

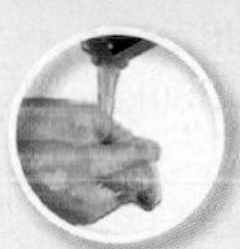

ACTION	RATIONALE
11. Remove PPE, if used. Perform hand hygiene.	Removing PPE properly reduces the risk for infection transmission and contamination of other items. Hand hygiene prevents transmission of microorganisms.
12. Assess the patient at least every hour or according to facility policy. Assessment should include the placement of the restraint, neurovascular assessment of the affected extremity, and skin integrity. In addition, assess for signs of sensory deprivation, such as increased sleeping, daydreaming, anxiety, panic, and hallucinations.	Improperly applied restraints may cause skin tears, abrasions, or bruises. Decreased circulation may result in paleness, coolness, decreased sensation, tingling, numbness, or pain in extremity. Use of restraints may decrease environmental stimulation and result in sensory deprivation.
13. **Remove restraint at least every 2 hours, or according to agency policy and patient need.** Perform range-of-motion exercises.	Removal allows you to assess the patient and re-evaluate need for restraint. It also allows interventions for toileting, provision of nutrition and liquids, exercise, and change of position. Exercise increases circulation in the restrained extremity.
14. Evaluate patient for continued need of restraint. Reapply restraint only if continued need is evident and order is still valid.	Continued need must be documented for reapplication.
15. Reassure patient at regular intervals. Provide continued explanation of rationale for interventions, reorientation if necessary, and plan of care. **Keep call bell within patient's easy reach.**	Reassurance demonstrates caring and provides an opportunity for sensory stimulation as well as ongoing assessment and evaluation. Patient can use call bell to summon assistance quickly.

EVALUATION

The expected outcomes are met when the patient remains free of injury to self or others, circulation to extremity remains adequate, skin integrity is not impaired under the restraint, and patient and family are aware of rationale for restraints.

DOCUMENTATION

Guidelines

Document alternative measures attempted before applying restraint. Document patient assessment before application. Record patient and family education and understanding regarding restraint use. Document family consent, if necessary, according to facility policy. Document reason for restraining patient, date and time of application, type of restraint, times when removed, and result and frequency of nursing assessment.

(continued)

SKILL 4-3 APPLYING AN EXTREMITY RESTRAINT continued

Sample Documentation

7/10/15 0830 Patient disoriented and combative. Attempting to remove tracheostomy and indwelling urinary catheter. Sitting at bedside, patient continued to tug at catheter and pull on tracheostomy. Family unwilling to sit with patient. Wrist restraints applied bilaterally as ordered.

—K. Urhahn, RN

7/10/15 1030 Patient continues to be disoriented and combative. Wrist restraints removed for 30 minutes during patient's bath; skin intact, hands warm, even skin tone, + radial pulses, + movement; passive and active range of motion completed. Wrist restraints reapplied.

—K. Urhahn, RN

UNEXPECTED SITUATIONS AND ASSOCIATED INTERVENTIONS

- *Patient has an IV catheter in the right wrist and is trying to remove the drain from the wound:* The left wrist may have a cloth restraint applied. Due to the IV in the right wrist, alternative forms of restraints should be tried, such as a cloth mitt or an elbow restraint.
- *Patient cannot move left arm:* Do not apply restraint to an extremity that is immobile. If patient cannot move the extremity, there is no need to apply a restraint. Restraint may be applied to right arm after obtaining an order from the primary care provider.

SPECIAL CONSIDERATIONS

- Do not position patient with wrist restraints flat in a supine position. If patient vomits, aspiration may occur.
- Check restraint for correct size before applying. Extremity restraints are available in different sizes. If restraint is too large, patient may free the extremity. If restraint is too small, circulation may be affected.
- Consider keeping a pair of scissors with emergency supplies in case the restraints cannot be untied quickly.

EVIDENCE FOR PRACTICE ▶

MINIMIZING RESTRAINT USE

Several resources summarize current best evidence on the topic of interventions to be used as alternatives to the use of restraints, as well as minimizing and eliminating the use of restraints. Refer to the Evidence for Practice placed after Skill 4-2, and refer to thePoint for additional research on related nursing topics.

SKILL 4-4 APPLYING A WAIST RESTRAINT

Waist restraints are a form of restraint that is applied to the patient's torso. It is applied over the patient's clothes, gown, or pajamas. When using a waist restraint, patients can move their extremities, but cannot get out of the chair or bed. **Restraints should be used only after less-restrictive methods have failed. Ensure compliance with ordering, assessment, and maintenance procedures. Historically, vest or jacket restraints were used to prevent similar patient movement, but their use has significantly decreased due to concerns for the potential risk for asphyxiation with these devices. However, research suggests that waist restraints pose the same potential risk for asphyxial death as vest restraints (Capezuti, et al., 2008).** Healthcare providers need to be aware of the potential outcome of using this device and weigh it against possible benefit from its use. Review the general guidelines for using restraints in the chapter introduction and Fundamentals Review 4-2 and 4-3, as well as in Box 4-2 in Skill 4-2. See also Evidence for Practice in Skill 4-2 for best evidence on the topic of interventions to be used as alternatives to the use of restraints, as well as minimizing and eliminating the use of restraints.

DELEGATION CONSIDERATIONS

After assessment of the patient by the RN, the application of a waist restraint may be delegated to nursing assistive personnel (NAP) or unlicensed assistive personnel (UAP), as well as to licensed practical/vocational nurses (LPN/LVNs). The decision to delegate must be based on careful analysis of the patient's needs and circumstances, as well as the qualifications of the person to whom the task is being delegated. Refer to the Delegation Guidelines in Appendix A.

EQUIPMENT

- Waist restraint
- Additional padding as needed
- PPE, as indicated

ASSESSMENT

Assess the patient's physical condition and for the potential for injury to self or others. A confused patient who is being treated with devices needed to sustain life, such as pulmonary intubation, might attempt to ambulate and is considered at risk for injury to self, and may require the use of restraints. Assess the patient's behavior, including the presence of confusion, agitation, combativeness, and ability to understand and follow directions. Evaluate the appropriateness of the least restrictive restraint device.

Inspect the patient's torso for any wounds or therapeutic devices that may be affected by the waist restraint. Consider using another form of restraint if the restraint may cause further injury at the site. Assess the patient's respiratory effort. If applied incorrectly, the waist restraint can restrict the patient's ability to breathe.

NURSING DIAGNOSIS

Determine the related factors for nursing diagnoses based on the patient's current status. Appropriate nursing diagnoses may include:

- Risk for Injury
- Wandering
- Acute Confusion

OUTCOME IDENTIFICATION AND PLANNING

The expected outcome to achieve is that the patient is constrained by the restraint, remains free from injury, and the restraint does not interfere with therapeutic devices. Other outcomes that may be appropriate include the following: the patient does not experience impaired skin integrity; the patient does not injure himself or herself due to the restraints; and the patient's family will demonstrate an understanding about the use of the restraint and their role in the patient's care.

IMPLEMENTATION

ACTION	RATIONALE
1. Determine need for restraints. Assess patient's physical condition, behavior, and mental status. (Refer to Fundamentals Review 4-2 and 4-3 at the beginning of the chapter and Box 4-2 in Skill 4-2.)	Restraints should be used only as a last resort when alternative measures have failed and the patient is at increased risk for harming self or others.
2. Confirm agency policy for application of restraints. **Secure an order from the primary care provider, or validate that the order has been obtained within the required time frame.**	Policy protects the patient and the nurse and specifies guidelines for application as well as type of restraint and duration. **Each order for restraint or seclusion used for the management of violent or self-destructive behavior that jeopardizes the immediate physical safety of the patient, a staff member, or others may only be renewed in accordance with the following limits for up to a total of 24 hours: (A) 4 hours for adults 18 years of age or older; (B) 2 hours for children and adolescents 9 to 17 years of age; or (C) 1 hour for children under 9 years of age. After 24 hours, before writing a new order for the use of restraint or seclusion for the management of violent or self-destructive behavior, a physician or other licensed independent practitioner who is responsible for the care of the patient must see and assess the patient** (CMS, 2006).

(continued)

SKILL 4-4 APPLYING A WAIST RESTRAINT continued

ACTION	RATIONALE
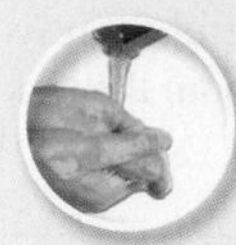 3. Perform hand hygiene and put on PPE, if indicated.	Hand hygiene and PPE prevent the spread of microorganisms. PPE is required based on transmission precautions.
 4. Identify the patient.	Identifying the patient ensures the right patient receives the intervention and helps prevent errors.
5. Explain reason for use of restraint to patient and family. Clarify how care will be given and how needs will be met. Explain that restraint is a temporary measure.	Explanation to patient and family may lessen confusion and anger and provide reassurance. A clearly stated agency policy on application of restraints should be available for patient and family to read. In a long-term care facility, the family must give consent before a restraint is applied.
6. Include the patient's family and/or significant others in the plan of care.	This promotes continuity of care and cooperation.
7. Apply restraint according to manufacturer's directions:	Proper application prevents injury. Proper application ensures that there is no interference with patient's respiration.
a. Choose the correct size of the least restrictive type of device that allows the greatest possible degree of mobility.	This provides minimal restriction.
b. Pad bony prominences that may be affected by the waist restraint.	Padding helps prevent injury.
c. Assist patient to a sitting position, if not contraindicated.	This will assist you in helping the patient into the waist restraint.
d. Place waist restraint on patient over gown. Bring ties through slots in restraint. Position slots at patient's back (Figure 1).	Placing the waist restraint over the gown protects the patient's skin. Positioning the slots with the ties at the back keeps them out of the patient's vision.
e. Pull the ties secure. **Ensure that the restraint is not too tight and has no wrinkles.**	Securing too tightly could impede breathing. Wrinkles in the restraint may lead to skin impairment.
f. **Insert fist between restraint and patient to ensure that breathing is not constricted. Assess respirations after restraint is applied.**	This prevents impaired respirations.
8. **Use a quick-release knot to tie the restraint to the bed frame, not side rail.** If patient is in a wheelchair, lock the wheels and place the ties under the arm rests and tie behind the chair (Figure 2). Site should not be readily accessible to the patient.	A quick-release knot ensures that the restraint will not tighten when pulled and can be removed quickly in an emergency. Securing the restraint to a side rail may injure the patient when the side rail is lowered. Tying the restraint out of patient's reach promotes security.
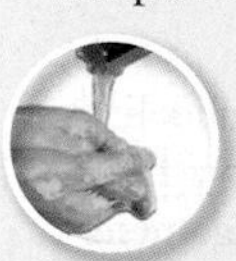 9. Remove PPE, if used. Perform hand hygiene.	Removing PPE properly reduces the risk for infection transmission and contamination of other items. Hand hygiene prevents transmission of microorganisms.

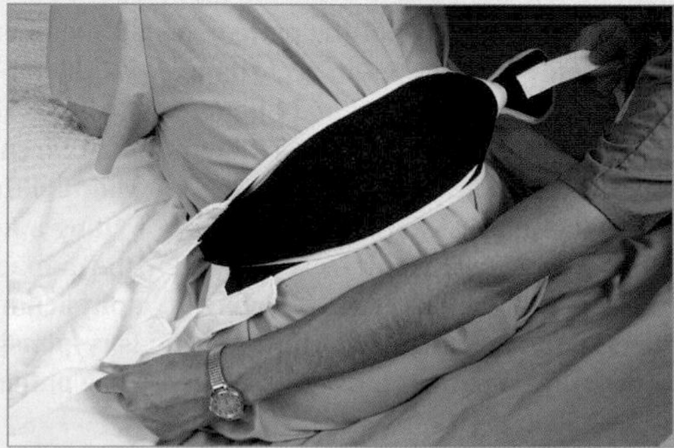

FIGURE 1 Waist restraint in place.

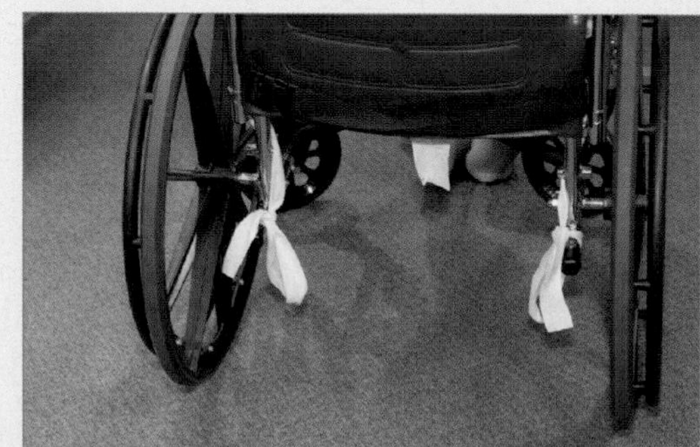

FIGURE 2 Restraint secured behind chair, out of the patient's reach.

ACTION	RATIONALE
10. Assess the patient at least every hour or according to facility policy. An assessment should include the placement of the restraint, respirations, and skin integrity. Assess for signs of sensory deprivation, such as increased sleeping, daydreaming, anxiety, panic, and hallucinations.	Improperly applied restraints may cause difficulty breathing, skin tears, abrasions, or bruises. Decreased circulation can result in impaired skin integrity. Use of restraints may decrease environmental stimulation and result in sensory deprivation.
11. **Remove restraint at least every 2 hours or according to agency policy and patient need.** Perform ROM exercises.	Removal allows you to assess patient and reevaluate need for restraint. Allows interventions for toileting, provision of nutrition and liquids, exercise, and change of position. Exercise increases circulation in restrained extremity.
12. Evaluate patient for continued need of restraint. Reapply restraint only if continued need is evident and order is still valid.	Continued need must be documented for reapplication.
13. Reassure patient at regular intervals. Provide continued explanation of rationale for interventions, reorientation if necessary, and plan of care. **Keep call bell within easy reach of patient.**	Reassurance demonstrates caring and provides an opportunity for sensory situation as well as ongoing assessment and evaluation. Patient can use call bell to summon assistance quickly.

EVALUATION

The expected outcomes are met when the patient remains free of injury; the restraints prevent injury to the patient or others; respirations are easy and effortless; skin integrity is maintained under the restraint; and the patient and family demonstrate understanding of the rationale for using the restraints.

DOCUMENTATION

Guidelines

Document alternative measures attempted before applying restraint. Document patient assessment before application. Record patient and family education and understanding regarding restraint use. Document family consent, if necessary, according to facility policy. Document reason for restraining patient, date and time of application, type of restraint, times when removed, and result and frequency of nursing assessment.

Sample Documentation

9/30/15 2130 Patient continues to attempt to get out of bed without assistance. Waist restraint applied at night, as ordered, when family leaves. Bed height low; side rails up × 2.

—B. Clapp, RN

9/30/15 2300 Waist restraint removed; skin intact, patient ambulated to restroom with assistance. Patient requested to ambulate to kitchen for snack; patient assisted to kitchen; graham crackers and milk obtained. Patient returned to bed and waist restraint reapplied after snack.

—B. Clapp, RN

UNEXPECTED SITUATIONS AND ASSOCIATED INTERVENTIONS

- *Patient slides down and neck is caught in restraint:* Immediately release restraint. Determine alternate methods for restraining.
- *Patient slides down and out of restraint:* Immediately release restraint. Ensure restraint is properly applied. Determine alternate methods for restraining.
- *Patient is exhibiting signs of respiratory distress:* Release restraint. Restraint may be applied too tightly and cause difficulty with chest expansion.

SPECIAL CONSIDERATIONS

- Consider keeping a pair of scissors with emergency supplies in case the restraints cannot be untied quickly.

EVIDENCE FOR PRACTICE ▶

MINIMIZING RESTRAINT USE

Several resources summarize current best evidence on the topic of interventions to be used as alternatives to the use of restraints, as well as minimizing and eliminating the use of restraints. Refer to the Evidence for Practice after Skill 4-2, and refer to thePoint for additional research on related nursing topics.

SKILL 4-5 APPLYING AN ELBOW RESTRAINT

Elbow restraints are generally used on infants and children, but may be used with adults. They prevent the patient from bending the elbows and reaching incisions or therapeutic devices. The patient can move all joints and extremities except the elbow. **Restraints should be used only after less-restrictive methods have failed.** Ensure compliance with ordering, assessment, and maintenance procedures. Review the general guidelines for using restraints in the chapter introduction and Fundamentals Review 4-2 and 4-3, as well as in Box 4-2 in Skill 4-2. See also Evidence for Practice in Skill 4-2 for best evidence on the topic of interventions to be used as alternatives to the use of restraints, as well as minimizing and eliminating the use of restraints.

DELEGATION CONSIDERATIONS

After assessment of the patient by the RN, the application of an elbow restraint may be delegated to nursing assistive personnel (NAP) or unlicensed assistive personnel (UAP), as well as to licensed practical/vocational nurses (LPN/LVNs). The decision to delegate must be based on careful analysis of the patient's needs and circumstances, as well as the qualifications of the person to whom the task is being delegated. Refer to the Delegation Guidelines in Appendix A.

EQUIPMENT

- Elbow restraint
- Padding, as necessary
- PPE, as indicated

ASSESSMENT

Assess the patient's physical condition and for the potential for injury to self or others. A confused patient who might remove devices needed to sustain life is considered at risk for injury to self and may require the use of restraints. Assess the patient's behavior, including the presence of confusion, agitation, combativeness, and ability to understand and follow directions. Evaluate the appropriateness of the least restrictive restraint device. Inspect the arm where the restraint will be applied. Baseline skin condition should be established for comparison at future assessments while the restraint is in place. Consider using another form of restraint if the restraint may cause further injury at the site. Assess capillary refill and proximal pulses in the arm to which the restraint is to be applied. This helps to determine the circulation in the extremity before applying the restraint. The restraint should not interfere with circulation. Measure the distance from the patient's shoulder to wrist to determine the appropriate size of elbow restraint to apply.

NURSING DIAGNOSIS

Determine the related factors for nursing diagnoses based on the patient's current status. Appropriate nursing diagnoses may include:

- Risk for Injury
- Acute Confusion
- Risk for Impaired Skin Integrity

OUTCOME IDENTIFICATION AND PLANNING

The expected outcome to achieve when applying an elbow restraint is that the patient is constrained by the restraint, remains free from injury, and the restraint does not interfere with therapeutic devices. Other outcomes that may be appropriate include the following: the patient does not experience impaired skin integrity; the patient does not injure self due to the restraints; and the patient's family demonstrates an understanding about the use of the restraint and its role in the patient's care.

IMPLEMENTATION

ACTION	RATIONALE
1. Determine need for restraints. Assess the patient's physical condition, behavior, and mental status. (Refer to Fundamentals Review 4-2 and 4-3 at the beginning of the chapter and Box 4-2 in Skill 4-2.)	Restraints should be used only as a last resort when alternative measures have failed and the patient is at increased risk for harming self or others.

ACTION	RATIONALE
2. Confirm agency policy for application of restraints. **Secure an order from the primary care provider, or validate that the order has been obtained within the required time frame.**	Policy protects the patient and the nurse and specifies guidelines for application as well as type of restraint and duration of use. **Each order for restraint or seclusion used for the management of violent or self-destructive behavior that jeopardizes the immediate physical safety of the patient, a staff member, or others may only be renewed in accordance with the following limits for up to a total of 24 hours: (A) 4 hours for adults 18 years of age or older; (B) 2 hours for children and adolescents 9 to 17 years of age; or (C) 1 hour for children under 9 years of age. After 24 hours, before writing a new order for the use of restraint or seclusion for the management of violent or self-destructive behavior, a physician or other licensed independent practitioner who is responsible for the care of the patient must see and assess the patient** (CMS, 2006).
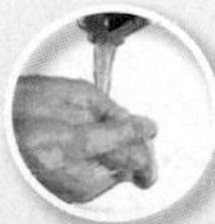 3. Perform hand hygiene and put on PPE, if indicated.	Hand hygiene and PPE prevent the spread of microorganisms. PPE is required based on transmission precautions.
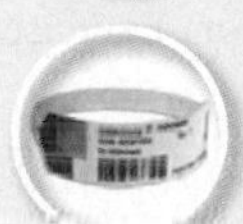 4. Identify the patient.	Identifying the patient ensures the right patient receives the intervention and helps prevent errors.
5. Explain the reason for use to the patient and family. Clarify how care will be given and how needs will be met. Explain that restraint is a temporary measure.	Explanation to patient and family may lessen confusion and anger and provide reassurance. A clearly stated agency policy on application of restraints should be available for patient and family to read. In a long-term care facility, the family must give consent before a restraint is applied.
6. Apply restraint according to manufacturer's directions:	Proper application prevents injury. Proper application ensures that there is no interference with patient's circulation.
a. Choose the correct size of the least restrictive type of device that allows the greatest possible degree of mobility.	This provides minimal restriction.
b. Pad bony prominences that may be affected by the restraint.	Padding helps prevent injury.
c. Spread elbow restraint out flat. Place middle of elbow restraint behind patient's elbow. **The restraint should not extend below the wrist or place pressure on the axilla.**	Elbow restraint should be placed in the middle of the arm to ensure that the patient cannot bend the elbow. Patient should be able to move the wrist. Pressure on the axilla may lead to skin impairment.
d. **Wrap restraint snugly around patient's arm, but make sure that two fingers can easily fit under the restraint.**	Wrapping snugly ensures that the patient will not be able to remove the device. Being able to insert two fingers helps to prevent impaired circulation and potential alterations in neurovascular status.
e. Secure Velcro straps around the restraint (Figure 1).	Velcro straps will hold the restraint in place and prevent removal of the restraint.

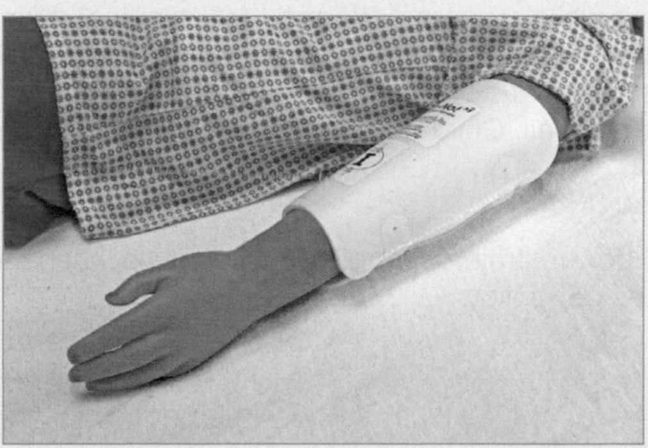

FIGURE 1 Child with elbow restraint in place.

(continued)

SKILL 4-5 APPLYING AN ELBOW RESTRAINT continued

ACTION	RATIONALE
f. Apply the restraint to the opposite arm if the patient can move arm.	Bilateral elbow restraints are needed if the patient can move both arms.
g. Thread Velcro strap from one elbow restraint across the back and into the loop on the opposite elbow restraint.	Strap across the back prevents the patient from wiggling out of elbow restraints.
7. **Assess circulation to fingers and hand.**	Circulation should not be impaired by the elbow restraint.
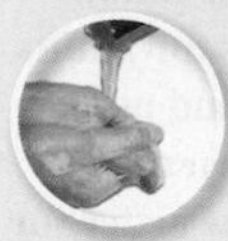 8. Remove PPE, if used. Perform hand hygiene.	Removing PPE properly reduces the risk for infection transmission and contamination of other items. Hand hygiene prevents transmission of microorganisms.
9. Assess the patient at least every hour or according to facility policy. An assessment should include the placement of the restraint, neurovascular assessment, and skin integrity. Assess for signs of sensory deprivation, such as increased sleeping, daydreaming, anxiety, inconsolable crying, and panic.	Improperly applied restraints may cause alterations in circulation, skin tears, abrasions, or bruises. Decreased circulation may result in impaired skin integrity. Use of restraints may decrease environmental stimulation and result in sensory deprivation.
10. **Remove restraint at least every 2 hours or according to agency policy and patient need. Remove restraint at least every 2 hours for children ages 9 to 17 years and at least every 1 hour for children under age 9, or according to agency policy and patient need.** Perform ROM exercises.	Removal allows you to assess patient and reevaluate need for restraint. Allows interventions for toileting; provision of nutrition and liquids, and exercise; and change of position. Exercise increases circulation in restrained extremity.
11. Evaluate patient for continued need of restraint. Reapply restraint only if continued need is evident.	Continued need must be documented for reapplication.
12. Reassure patient at regular intervals. **Keep call bell within easy reach of patient.**	Reassurance demonstrates caring and provides opportunity for sensory situation as well as ongoing assessment and evaluation. Parent or child old enough to use call bell can use it to summon assistance quickly.

EVALUATION

The expected outcome is met when the restraint prevents injury to self or others. In addition, the patient cannot bend the elbow; skin integrity is maintained under the restraint; and the family demonstrates an understanding of the rationale for the elbow restraint.

DOCUMENTATION

Guidelines

Document alternative measures attempted before applying restraint. Document patient assessment before application. Record patient and family education regarding restraint use and their understanding. Document family consent, if necessary, according to facility policy. Document reason for restraining patient, date and time of application, type of restraint, times when removed, and result and frequency of nursing assessment.

Sample Documentation

<u>9/1/15</u> 0800 Elbow restraints removed while AM care performed (45 minutes). Skin warm, dry, even tone; + radial and brachial pulses, equal bilaterally, capillary refill < 3 seconds. Patient moving arms appropriately. Continues to pick at colostomy bag. Distraction techniques used to no avail. Child removes abdominal binder when applied.

—B. Clapp, RN

<u>9/1/12</u> 0855 Skin intact and warm. Elbow restraints reapplied. Will remove when family arrives at bedside or every 2 hours as per policy.

—B. Clapp, RN

UNEXPECTED SITUATIONS AND ASSOCIATED INTERVENTIONS

- *Skin breakdown is noted on elbows:* Ensure that restraints are being removed routinely for at least 30 minutes and a skin inspection is done. If restraints are still needed, a padded dressing should be applied under the elbow restraint.
- *Patient reports discomfort and pain or cries when elbow is moved:* Restraints need to be removed more frequently, with active and/or passive ROM. If elbow is not moved, it will become stiff and painful.
- *Application of elbow restraint does not control the patient's body movement to allow for needed examination or treatment:* Reassess situation and consider more restrictive type of restraint.

EVIDENCE FOR PRACTICE ▶

MINIMIZING RESTRAINT USE

Several resources summarize current best evidence on the topic of interventions to be used as alternatives to the use of restraints, as well as minimizing and eliminating the use of restraints. Refer to the Evidence for Practice after Skill 4-2, and refer to thePoint for additional research on related nursing topics.

SKILL 4-6 APPLYING A MUMMY RESTRAINT

A mummy restraint is appropriate for short-term restraint of an infant or small child to control the child's movements during examination or to provide care for the head and neck. **Restraints should be used only after less-restrictive methods have failed.** Ensure compliance with ordering, assessment, and maintenance procedures. Review the general guidelines for using restraints in the chapter introduction and Fundamentals Review 4-2 and 4-3, as well as in Box 4-2 in Skill 4-2. See also Evidence for Practice after Skill 4-2 for best evidence on the topic of interventions to be used as alternatives to the use of restraints, as well as minimizing and eliminating the use of restraints.

DELEGATION CONSIDERATIONS

After assessment of the patient by the RN, the application of a mummy restraint may be delegated to nursing assistive personnel (NAP) or unlicensed assistive personnel (UAP), as well as to licensed practical/vocational nurses (LPN/LVNs). The decision to delegate must be based on careful analysis of the patient's needs and circumstances, as well as the qualifications of the person to whom the task is being delegated. Refer to the Delegation Guidelines in Appendix A.

EQUIPMENT

- Small blanket or sheet
- PPE, as indicated

ASSESSMENT

Assess patient's behavior and need for restraint. Assess for wounds or therapeutic devices that may be affected by the restraint. Evaluate the appropriateness of the least restrictive restraint device. Another form of restraint may be more appropriate to prevent injury.

NURSING DIAGNOSIS

Determine the related factors for nursing diagnoses based on the patient's current status. Appropriate nursing diagnoses may include:

- Risk for Injury
- Anxiety
- Impaired Physical Mobility

OUTCOME IDENTIFICATION AND PLANNING

The expected outcome to achieve is that the patient is constrained by the restraint, remains free from injury, and that the restraint does not interfere with therapeutic devices. Other outcomes that may be appropriate include the following: examination and/or treatment is provided without incident and the patient's family will demonstrate an understanding about the use of the restraint and its role in the patient's care.

(continued)

SKILL 4-6 APPLYING A MUMMY RESTRAINT continued

ACTION	RATIONALE
1. Determine need for restraints. Assess patient's physical condition, behavior, and mental status. (Refer to Fundamentals Review 4-2 and 4-3 at the beginning of the chapter and Box 4-2 in Skill 4-2.)	Restraints should be used only as a last resort when alternative measures have failed, and the patient is at increased risk for harming self or others.
2. Confirm agency policy for application of restraints. **Secure an order from the primary care provider, or validate that the order has been obtained within the required time frame.**	Policy protects the patient and the nurse and specifies guidelines for application as well as type of restraint and duration. **Each order for restraint or seclusion used for the management of violent or self-destructive behavior that jeopardizes the immediate physical safety of the patient, a staff member, or others may only be renewed in accordance with the following limits for up to a total of 24 hours: (A) 4 hours for adults 18 years of age or older; (B) 2 hours for children and adolescents 9 to 17 years of age; or (C) 1 hour for children under 9 years of age. After 24 hours, before writing a new order for the use of restraint or seclusion for the management of violent or self-destructive behavior, a physician or other licensed independent practitioner who is responsible for the care of the patient must see and assess the patient** (CMS, 2006).
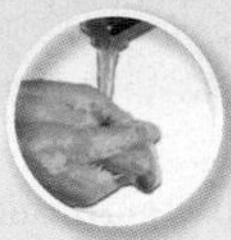 3. Perform hand hygiene and put on PPE, if indicated.	Hand hygiene and PPE prevent the spread of microorganisms. PPE is required based on transmission precautions.
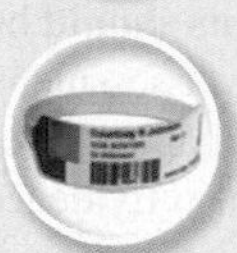 4. Identify the patient.	Identifying the patient ensures the right patient receives the intervention and helps prevent errors.
5. Explain the reason for use to the patient and family. Clarify how care will be given and how needs will be met. Explain that restraint is a temporary measure.	Explanation to patient and family may lessen confusion and anger and provide reassurance. A clearly stated agency policy on application of restraints should be available for patient and family to read. In a long-term care facility, the family must give consent before a restraint is applied.
6. Open the blanket or sheet. Place the child on the blanket, with the edge of the blanket at or above neck level.	This positions the child correctly on the blanket.
7. Position the child's right arm alongside the child's body. Left arm should not be constrained at this time. Pull the right side of the blanket tightly over the child's right shoulder and chest. Secure under the left side of the child's body (Figure 1).	Wrapping snugly ensures that child will not be able to wiggle out.

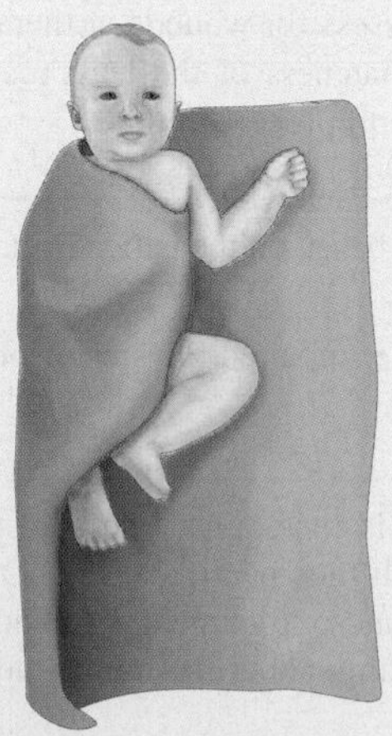

FIGURE 1 Pulling blanket over right shoulder and chest and securing under patient's left side.

ACTION | RATIONALE

8. Position the left arm alongside the child's body. Pull the left side of the blanket tightly over the child's left shoulder and chest. Secure under the right side of the child's body (Figure 2).

   Wrapping snugly ensures that child will not be able to wiggle out.

9. Fold the lower part of blanket up and pull over the child's body. Secure under the child's body on each side or with safety pins (Figure 3).

   This ensures that child will not be able to wiggle out.

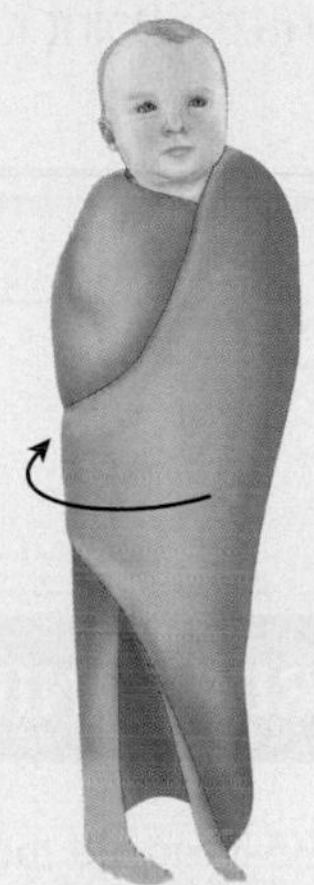

FIGURE 2 Securing blanket under right side of body

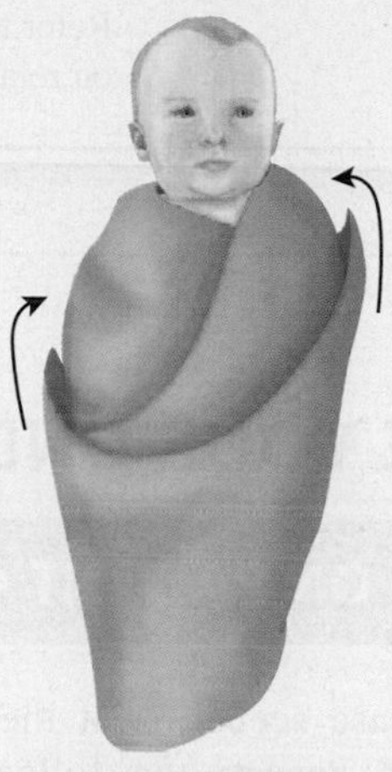

FIGURE 3 Securing lower corner of blanket under each side of patient's body.

10. Stay with child while the mummy wrap is in place. Reassure the child and parents at regular intervals. Once examination or treatment is completed, unwrap the child.

    Remaining with the child prevents injury. Reassurance demonstrates caring and provides opportunity for ongoing assessment and evaluation.

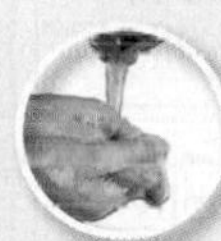

11. Remove PPE, if used. Perform hand hygiene.

    Removing PPE properly reduces the risk for infection transmission and contamination of other items. Hand hygiene prevents transmission of microorganisms.

EVALUATION

The expected outcome is met when the restraint prevents injury to self or others. In addition, the examination or treatment is provided without incident; and the family demonstrates an understanding of the rationale for the mummy restraint.

DOCUMENTATION

Guidelines

Document alternative measures attempted before applying restraint. Document patient assessment before application. Record patient and family education and understanding regarding restraint use. Document family consent, if necessary, according to facility policy. Document reason for restraining patient, date and time of application, type of restraint, times when removed, and result and frequency of nursing assessment.

Sample Documentation

6/9/15 0230 Patient requires suturing of forehead. Parent attempted to hold child for procedure without success. Need to restrain child explained to parents. Mummy restraint applied with parents' consent. Restraint removed after 20 minutes; sutures intact. Wound care instructions (verbal and written) provided to parents; parents verbalize understanding.

—*D. Dunn, RN*

(continued)

SKILL 4-6 APPLYING A MUMMY RESTRAINT continued

UNEXPECTED SITUATIONS AND ASSOCIATED INTERVENTIONS

- *Application of mummy wrap does not control the infant's or child's body movement to allow for needed examination or treatment:* Reassess situation and consider more restrictive type of restraint.

EVIDENCE FOR PRACTICE ▶

MINIMIZING RESTRAINT USE

Several resources summarize current best evidence on the topic of interventions to be used as alternatives to the use of restraints, as well as minimizing and eliminating the use of restraints. Refer to the Evidence for Practice after Skill 4-2, and refer to thePoint for additional research on related nursing topics.

ENHANCE YOUR UNDERSTANDING

FOCUSING ON PATIENT CARE: DEVELOPING CLINICAL REASONING

Consider the case scenarios at the beginning of the chapter as you answer the following questions to enhance your understanding and apply what you have learned.

QUESTIONS

1. Megan Lewis, an 18-month-old with an IV access in her left forearm, is continually picking at the IV and dressing. What interventions would be appropriate as alternatives to restraints? If unsuccessful, what restraints would be appropriate for Megan?
2. Kevin Mallory, a 35-year-old body builder with a closed head injury, is extremely strong. The fear is that he will rip the cloth restraints and extubate himself. What other type of restraints could be tried?
3. John Frawley, a 72-year-old patient with Alzheimer's disease, continually tries to get out of bed without assistance. He has an unsteady gait and has one broken hip due to a fall. What are the appropriate interventions to try with Mr. Frawley?

You can find suggested answers after the Bibliography at the end of this chapter.

INTEGRATED CASE STUDY CONNECTION

The case studies in the back of the book are designed to focus on integrating concepts. Refer to the following case studies to enhance your understanding of the concepts related to the skills in this chapter.

- Basic Case Studies: Abigail Cantonelli, page 1063; Claudia Tran, page 1070.
- Intermediate Case Studies: Olivia Greenbaum, page 1077; Kent Clark, page 1085.

TAYLOR SUITE RESOURCES

Explore these additional resources to enhance learning for this chapter:

- NCLEX-Style Questions and other resources on thePoint, http://thePoint.lww.com/Lynn4e
- *Skill Checklists for Taylor's Clinical Nursing Skills,* 4e
- *Fundamentals of Nursing:* Chapter 26, Safety, Security, and Emergency Preparedness

Bibliography

Ackley, B.J., & Ladwig, G.B. (2011). *Nursing diagnosis handbook* (9th ed.). St. Louis: Mosby/Elsevier.

American Geriatrics Society (AGS). (2012a). *Tips for preventing serious falls.* Available at http://www.healthinaging.org/files/documents/tipsheets/falls_prevention.pdf.

American Geriatrics Society (AGS). (2012b). *Aging & health A to Z.* Available at http://www.healthinaging.org/aging-and-health-a-to-z/topic:falls/.

American Geriatrics Society and British Geriatrics Society. (2010). *AGS/BGS Clinical practice guideline: Prevention of falls in older persons.* Available at http://www.medcats.com/FALLS/frameset.htm.

American Nurses Association (ANA). (2012). *Reduction of patient restraint and seclusion in health care settings.* Available at http://www.nursingworld.org/restraintposition.

Ang, E., Mordiffi, S.Z., & Wong, H.B. (2011). Evaluating the use of a targeted multiple intervention strategy in reducing patient falls in an acute care hospital: A randomized controlled trial. *Journal of Advanced Nursing, 67*(9), 1984–1992.

Bandos, J. (2008). Protection in the home. Tips on safety for older adults. *Advance for Nurses, 10*(22), 40.

Barnsteiner, J. (2011). Teaching the culture of safety. *Online Journal of Issues in Nursing, 16*(3). Available at http://www.medscape.com/viewarticle/758853_1.

Benike, L., Cognetta-Rieke, C., Dahlby, M., & Disch, J. (2012). Quality and safety in home and ambulatory settings. *Nursing Clinics of North America, 47*(3), 323–331.

Boltz, M., Capezuti, E., Fulmer, T., & Zwicker, D. (Eds.) (2012). *Evidence-based geriatric nursing protocols for best practice* (4th ed.). New York: Springer Publishing Company.

Bulechek, G.M, Butcher, H.K., Dochterman, J.M., & Wagner, C.M. (Eds.). (2013). *Nursing interventions classification (NIC)* (6th ed.). St. Louis: Mosby Elsevier.

Capezuti, E., Brush, B., Won, R., et al. (2008). Least restrictive or least understood? Waist restraints, provider practices, and risk of harm. *Journal of Aging & Social Policy, 20*(3), 305–322.

Centers for Disease Control and Prevention (CDC). (2012c). *Costs of falls among older adults.* Available at http://www.cdc.gov/HomeandRecreationalSafety/Falls/fallcost.html

Centers for Disease Control and Prevention (CDC). (2012d). *Health alert network (HAN).* Available at http://www.bt.cdc.gov/HAN/

Centers for Medicare & Medicaid Services (CMS). (2006). Department of Health and Human Services. Federal Register. 42 CFR Part 482. *Conditions of participation: Patients' rights. Final rule.* Available at http://www.cms.gov/Regulations-and-Guidance/Legislation/CFCsAndCoPs/downloads/finalpatientrightsrule.pdf.

Choi, Y.S., Lawler, E., Boenecke, C.A., Ponatoski, E.R., & Zimring, C.M. (2011). Developing a multi-systemic fall prevention model, incorporating the physical environment, the care process and technology: a systematic review. *Journal of Advanced Nursing, 67*(12), 2501–2524.

Davies, K. (2010). Hourly patient rounding. *Advance for Nurses, 12*(13), 13–15.

Degelau, J., Belz, M., Bungum, L., et al. (2012). *Institute for Clinical Systems Improvement (ICSI). Prevention of falls (acute care). Health care protocol.* Bloomington, MN: Institute for Clinical Systems Improvement (ICSI). Agency for Healthcare Research and Quality (AHRQ). Available at http://guideline.gov/content.aspx?id=36906#Section420.

DiBartolo, V. (1998). 9 steps to effective restraint use. *RN, 61*(12), 23–24.

Dickinson, A., Machen, I., Horton, K., et al. (2011). Fall prevention in the community: What older people say they need. *British Journal of Community Nursing, 16*(4), 174–180.

Dykes, P., Carroll, D., Hurley, A., et al. (2010). *Fall prevention in acute care hospitals.* Available at http://www.ncbi.nlm.nih.gov/pmc/articles/PMC3107709/

Evans, L., & Cotter, V. (2008). Avoiding restraints in patients with dementia: Understanding, prevention, and management are the keys. *American Journal of Nursing, 108*(3), 40–49.

Ferris, M. (2008). Protecting hospitalized elders from falling. *Topics in Advanced Practice Nursing eJournal, 8*(4). Available at www.medscape.com/viewarticle/585961.

Ford, B.M. (2010). Hourly rounding: A strategy to improve patient satisfaction scores. *MEDSURGNursing, 19*(3), 188–191.

Graham, B.C. (2012). Examining evidence-based interventions to prevent inpatient falls. *MEDSURGNursing, 21*(5), 267–270.

Gray-Micelli, D. (2012). Hartford Institute for Geriatric Nursing. FALLS. *Nursing standard of practice protocol: Fall prevention.* Available at www.consultgerirn.org/topics/falls/want_to_know_more.

Gulpers, M.J.M., Bleijlevens, M.H.C., Ambergen, T., et al. (2011). Belt restraint reduction in nursing homes: Effects of a multicomponent intervention program. *Journal of the American Geriatrics Society, 59*(11), 2029–2036.

Hendrich, A. (2007). Predicting patient falls. *American Journal of Nursing, 107*(11), 50–58.

Henneman, E.A., Gawlinski, A., & Giuliano, K.K. (2012). Surveillance: A strategy for improving patient safety in acute and critical care units. *Critical Care Nurse, 32*(2), e9–e18.

Hinkle, J.L., & Cheever, K.H. (2014). *Brunner & Suddarth's textbook of medical-surgical nursing* (13th ed.). Philadelphia: Wolters Kluwer Health/Lippincott Williams & Wilkins.

The Joint Commission (TJC). (2014). *National patient safety goals. Hospital: 2014.* Available at http://www.jointcommission.org/standards_information/npsgs.aspx.

The Joint Commission Center for Transforming Healthcare. (2012). *Facts about the preventing falls with injury project.* Available at http://www.centerfortransforminghealthcare.org/assets/4/6/CTH_PFWI_Fact_Sheet.pdf

Jorgensen, J. (2011). Reducing patient falls: A call to action. (pp. 2–5). In *Best practices for falls reduction: A practical guide.* Special supplement to *The American Nurse Today,* March 2011.

Kessler, B., Claude-Gutekunst, M., Donchez, A.M., Dries, R.F., & Snyder, M.M. (2012). The merry-go-round of patient rounding: Assure your patients get the brass ring. *MEDSURGNursing, 21*(4), 240–245.

Kibayashi, K., Shimada, R., & Nakao, K. (2011). Accidental deaths occurring in bed: Review of cases and proposal of preventive strategies. *Journal of Forensic Nursing, 7*(3), 130–136.

Koczy, P., Becker, C., Rapp, K., et al. (2011). Effectiveness of a multifactorial intervention to reduce physical restraints in nursing home residents. *Journal of the American Geriatrics Society, 59*(2), 333–339.

Kulik, C. (2011). Components of a comprehensive fall-risk assessment. (pp. 4–5). In *Best practices for falls reduction: A practical guide.* Special supplement to *The American Nurse Today,* March 2011.

Kyle, T., & Carman, S. (2013). *Essentials of pediatric nursing.* (2nd ed.). Philadelphia: Wolters Kluwer Health/Lippincott Williams & Wilkins.

Lach, H.W. (2012). The Hartford Institute for Geriatric Nursing. *Try this: Best practices in nursing care to older adults with dementia. Home safety inventory for older adults with dementia.* Available at http://consultgerirn.org/uploads/File/trythis/try_this_d12.pdf.

Lane, C., & Harrington, A. (2011). The factors that influence nurses' use of physical restraint: A thematic literature review. *International Journal of Nursing Practice, 17*(2), 195–204.

Lowe, L., & Hodgson, G. (2012). Hourly rounding in a high dependency unit. *Nursing Standard, 27*(8), 35–40.

McNamara, S.A. (2011). Reducing fall risk for surgical patients. *AORN Journal, 93*(3), 390–394.

McPhall, K. (2011). Safe at home. *Advances for Nurses, 13*(12), 17–18.

Meade, C., Bursell, A., & Ketelsen, L. (2006). Effects of nursing rounds on patients' call light use, satisfaction and safety. *American Journal of Nursing, 106*(9), 58–71.

Moorhead, S., Johnson, M., Maas, M.L., & Swanson, E. (Eds). (2013). *Nursing Outcomes Classification (NOC).* (5th ed.). St. Louis: Mosby Elsevier.

National Institute on Aging. (2012). *Age page: Falls and fractures.* Available at http://www.nia.nih.gov/health/publication/falls-and-fractures.

NANDA-I International. (2012). *Nursing diagnoses: Definitions & classification 2012–2014.* West Sussex, UK: Wiley-Blackwell.

Nowicki, T., Fulbrook, P., & Burns, C. (2010). Bed safety off the rails. *Australian Nursing Journal, 18*(1), 31–34.

Olrich, T., Kalman, M., & Nigolian, C. (2012). Hourly rounding: A replication study. *MEDSURG Nursing, 21*(1), 23–36.

Park, M., & Tang, J. (2007). Evidence-based guideline. Changing the practice of physical restraint use in acute care. *Journal of Gerontological Nursing, 33*(2), 9–16.

Pellfolk, T.J.E., Gustafson, Y., Bucht, G., & Karlsson, S. (2010). Effects of a restraint minimization program on staff knowledge, attitudes, and practice: A cluster randomized trial. *Journal of the American Geriatrics Society, 58*(1), 62–69.

Perry, S.E., Hockenberry, M.J., Lowdermilk, D.L., & Wilson, D. (2012). *Maternal child nursing care.* (4th ed.). Maryland Heights, MI: Mosby Elsevier.

Ponce, M. (2012). *How to prevent falls among older adults in outpatient settings.* Available at http://www.americannursetoday.com/Popups/ArticlePrint.aspx?id=10854.

Quigley, P. & Goff, L. (2011). Current and emerging innovations to keep patients safe. (pp. 14–17). In *Best practices for falls reduction: A practical guide.* Special supplement to *The American Nurse Today,* March 2011.

Restraint use cut in half. (2010). *Nursing, 40*(10), 20.

Rutledge, D.N., & March, P.D. (2011). Evidence-based care sheet. *Restraint: Minimizing use in acute, nonpsychiatric care.* Glendale, CA: Cinahl Information Systems.

Rutledge, D.N., & March, P.D. (2011). Evidence based care sheet. *Restraint: Minimizing usage in skilled nursing facilities.* Glendale, CA: Cinahl Information Systems.

Sherrington, C., Whitney, J., Lord, S., et al. (2008). Effective exercise for the prevention of falls: A systematic review and meta-analysis. *Journal of the American Geriatrics Society, 56*(12), 2234–2243.

Tabloski, P. (2010). *Gerontological nursing* (2nd ed.). Upper Saddle River, NJ: Pearson.

Taylor, C., Lillis, C., & Lynn P. (2015). *Fundamentals of nursing.* (8th ed.). Philadelphia: Wolters Kluwer Health/Lippincott Williams & Wilkins.

Titler, M.G., Shever, L.L., Kanak, M.F., Picone, D.M., & Qin, R. (2011), Factors associated with falls during hospitalization in an older adult population. *Research and Theory for Nursing Practice: An International Journal, 25*(2), 127–152.

Tzeng, H., Yin, C., & Grunawalt, J. (2008). Effective assessment of use of sitters by nurses in inpatient care settings. *Journal of Advanced Nursing, 64*(2), 176–184.

U.S. Food and Drug Administration (FDA). (2010). Medical devices. *A guide to bed safety bed rails in hospitals, nursing homes, and home health care: The facts.* Available at http://www.fda.gov/MedicalDevices/ProductsandMedicalProcedures/GeneralHospitalDevicesandSupplies/HospitalBeds/ucm123676.htm.

Weisgram, B., & Raymond, S. (2008). Using evidence-based nursing rounds to improve patient outcomes. *MEDSURG Nursing, 17*(6), 429–430.

SUGGESTED ANSWERS FOR FOCUSING ON PATIENT CARE: DEVELOPING CLINICAL REASONING

1. Nursing interventions for Megan should include the use of distraction, such as play, toys, music, games, and so forth. (Refer to Skill 4-2.) Megan's parent should be encouraged to stay with her to provide supervision and distraction, also. Cover the IV access site with a dressing and gauze, or other cover, such as the I.V. House® dressing. If all other alternatives to restraints are attempted, and it is necessary to maintain the IV infusion, an elbow restraint (Skill 4-5) or hand mitt (Skill 4-3) would be the least restrictive restraints to prevent dislodgement of Megan's IV access.
2. You must implement as many alternatives to restraints as possible for Mr. Mallory. Refer to Skill 4-2. In addition, consult with the primary care provider to discuss a possible time frame for extubation. Increase frequency of monitoring, repeat explanations, and provide distraction as part of the nursing plan of care for this patient. Elbow restraints (Skill 4-5) would be a possible solution if it is determined that restraints are required.
3. Fall prevention is best achieved through the implementation of multiple strategies. Begin by assessing the patient's motivation for attempting activity unassisted. Provide reassurance and explanations related to care. If possible, Mr. Frawley could be moved to a room closer to the nursing station to allow increased monitoring. Additional nursing interventions to try could include asking family members to stay with Mr. Frawley, providing distraction based on information from the family regarding favorite activities, more frequent rounding to ensure that his toileting needs are met, as well as need for hydration. Provide a low bed for the patient, as well as floor mats, to reduce the risk for serious injury if Mr. Frawley should fall. Refer to Skill 4-1 for additional intervention suggestions.

5 Medication Administration

FOCUSING ON PATIENT CARE

This chapter will help you develop the skills needed to administer medications safely to the following patients:

COOPER JACKSON, age 2 years, does not want to take his ordered oral antibiotic.

ERIKA JENKINS, age 20, is extremely afraid of needles and is at the clinic for her birth-control injection.

JONAH DINERMAN, age 63, was recently diagnosed with diabetes and needs to be taught how to give himself insulin injections.

Refer to Focusing on Patient Care: Developing Clinical Reasoning at the end of the chapter to apply what you learn.

LEARNING OBJECTIVES

After studying this chapter, you will be able to:

1. Prepare medications for administration in a safe manner.
2. Administer oral medications.
3. Administer medications via a gastric tube.
4. Remove medication from an ampule.
5. Remove medication from a vial.
6. Mix medications from two vials in one syringe.
7. Identify appropriate needle size and angle of insertion for intradermal, subcutaneous, and intramuscular injections.
8. Locate appropriate sites for intradermal injection.
9. Administer an intradermal injection.
10. Locate appropriate sites for a subcutaneous injection.
11. Administer a subcutaneous injection.
12. Locate appropriate sites for an intramuscular injection.
13. Administer an intramuscular injection.
14. Apply an insulin pump.
15. Administer medications by intravenous bolus or push through an intravenous infusion.
16. Administer a piggyback, intermittent, intravenous infusion of medication.
17. Administer an intermittent intravenous infusion of medication via a volume-control administration set.
18. Introduce drugs through a medication or drug-infusion lock using the saline flush.

19. Apply a transdermal patch.
20. Instill eye drops.
21. Administer eye irrigation.
22. Instill ear drops.
23. Administer ear irrigation.
24. Administer a nasal spray.
25. Administer a vaginal cream.
26. Administer a rectal suppository.
27. Administer medication via a metered-dose inhaler.
28. Administer medication via a dry-powder inhaler.
29. Administer medication via a small-volume nebulizer.

KEY TERMS

adverse drug effect: undesirable effect other than the intended therapeutic effect of a drug

ampule: a glass flask that contains a single dose of medication for parenteral administration

inhalation: route to administer medications directly into the lungs or airway passages

intradermal injection: injection placed just below the epidermis; sites commonly used are the inner surface of the forearm, the dorsal aspect of the upper arm, and the upper back

intramuscular injection: injection placed into muscular tissue; sites commonly used are the ventrogluteal, vastus lateralis, and deltoid muscles

intravenous (IV) route: route to administer medications directly into the vein or venous system; the most dangerous route of medication administration

metered-dose inhaler (MDI): device to deliver a controlled dose of medication for inhalation

nebulizer: instrument that produces a fine spray or mist; in this case, passing air through a liquid medication to produce fine particles for inhalation

needle gauge: measurement of the diameter of a needle

subcutaneous injection: injection placed between the epidermis and muscle, into the subcutaneous tissue; sites commonly used are the outer aspect of the upper arm, the abdomen, the anterior aspects of the thigh, the upper back, and the upper ventral or dorsogluteal area

suppository: oval or cone-shaped substance that is inserted into a body cavity; it melts at body temperature

vial: a glass bottle with a self-sealing stopper through which medication is removed

Medication administration is a basic nursing function that involves skillful technique and consideration of the patient's development, health status, and safety. The nurse administering medications needs a knowledge base about drugs, including drug names, preparations, classifications, adverse effects, and physiologic factors that affect drug action (Fundamentals Review 5-1).

Use of the three checks and the rights of medication administration when administering medications can assist with safe administration of medications. Check the label on the medication package or container three times during medication preparation and administration (Fundamentals Review 5-2). The rights of medication administration (Fundamentals Review 5-3) can help to ensure accuracy when administering medications. However, the Institute for Safe Medication Practices (2007) states, "They (rights of medication administration) are merely broadly stated goals or desired outcomes of safe medication practices." The rights themselves do not ensure medication safety. The nurse assumes individual accountability for safe drug administration by engaging in behavior that follows standards of practice and behaviors prescribed by the institution to achieve the goals of the rights (Aschenbrenner & Venable, 2012). Suggested rights of administration vary slightly between references. However, in general, eight to ten rights of medication administration seem to be common in the literature (Elliott & Liu, 2012; Macdonald, 2010; Kee, et al., 2012).

Nursing responsibilities for drug administration are summarized in Fundamentals Review 5-4. This chapter covers skills that the nurse needs to administer medications safely via multiple routes. Proper use of equipment and proper technique are imperative. Fundamentals Review 5-5 and Figure 5-1 review important guidelines related to administering parenteral medications. Nurses should be aware of the higher risk of making an error when their workflow is disrupted from either a distraction or interruption; (Popescu, et al., 2011). As a result, it is important to prepare medications in a relatively quiet location. The nurse who is preparing drugs should work alone. This practice helps to avoid distractions and interruptions, which may lead to errors (Klejka, 2012; Popescu, et al., 2011).

When administering medication, consider factors that may affect drug action, such as age considerations. Older adults are more sensitive to medications because their bodies have experienced physiologic changes associated with the aging process, including decreased gastric motility, muscle mass, acid production, and blood flow, which affect drug absorption. They may also be more susceptible to certain drug side effects. The physiologic changes in older adults that increase drug susceptibility are summarized in Fundamentals Review 5-6. Drug interactions in older adults are a very real and dangerous problem because older adults are more likely to be prescribed more than one drug (Lorenz, 2010; Tabloski, 2010).

FUNDAMENTALS REVIEW 5-1

KNOW YOUR MEDICATIONS

Before administering any unfamiliar medications, know the following:

- Mode of action and purpose of medication (making sure that this medication is appropriate for the patient's diagnosis)
- Side effects of, and contraindications for, medication
- Antagonist of medication (as appropriate)
- Safe dosage range for medication
- Interactions with other medications
- Precautions to take before administration
- Proper administration technique

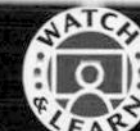

FUNDAMENTALS REVIEW 5-2

THE THREE CHECKS

"Three Checks" denotes that the label on the medication package or container should be checked three times during medication preparation and administration.

1. Read the Computer-generated Medication Administration Record (CMAR) or Medication Administration Record (MAR) and select the proper medication from the patient's medication drawer or unit stock. This is the *first check* of the medication label.
2. After retrieving the medication from the drawer, compare the medication label with the CMAR/MAR. Note: Compare with the CMAR/MAR immediately before pouring from a multidose container. This is the *second check* of the medication label.
3. The *third check* can be performed in one of two ways, depending on facility policy:
   - When all medications for one patient have been prepared, recheck the labels with the CMAR/MAR before taking the medication to the patient.
   - At the bedside, recheck the labels with the CMAR/MAR after identifying the patient and before administration.

FUNDAMENTALS REVIEW 5-3

RIGHTS OF MEDICATION ADMINISTRATION

The "Rights of Medication Administration" can help to ensure accuracy when administering medications. To prevent medication errors, always ensure that the:

1. **Right medication** is given to the
2. **Right patient** in the
3. **Right dosage** (in the right form) through the
4. **Right route** at the
5. **Right time** for the
6. **Right reason** based on the
7. **Right (appropriate) assessment** data using the
8. **Right documentation** and monitoring for the
9. **Right response** by the patient.

Additional rights have been suggested to include (10) the **right to education**, ensuring patients receive accurate and thorough information about the medication, and (11) the **right to refuse**, acknowledging that patients can and do refuse to take a medication.

FUNDAMENTALS REVIEW 5-4

NURSING RESPONSIBILITIES FOR ADMINISTERING DRUGS

- Assessing the patient and understanding clearly why the patient is receiving a particular medication
- Preparing the medication to be administered (checking labels, preparing injections, observing proper asepsis techniques with needles and syringes)
- Calculating accurate dosages
- Validating medication calculations with another nurse
- Administering the medication (e.g., proper injection techniques, aids to help swallowing, topical methods, and so on)
- Documenting the medications given
- Monitoring the patient's reaction and evaluating the patient's response
- Educating the patient regarding his or her medications and medication regimen

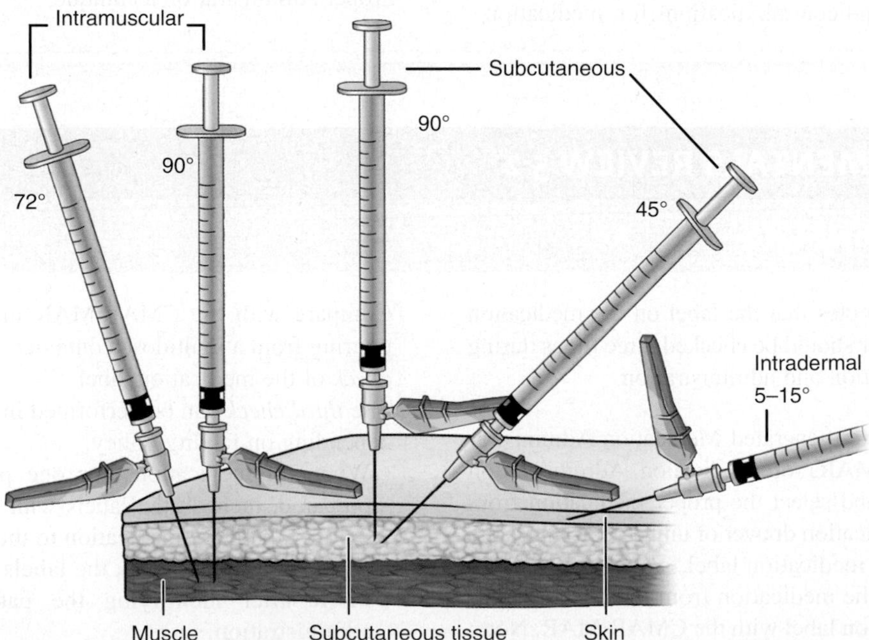

FIGURE 5-1 Comparison of insertion angles for intramuscular, subcutaneous, and intradermal injections.

FUNDAMENTALS REVIEW 5-5

NEEDLE/SYRINGE SELECTION

- When looking at a needle package, the first number is the gauge or diameter of the needle (e.g., 18, 20) and the second number is the length in inches (e.g., 1, 1.5).
- As the gauge number becomes larger, the size of the needle becomes smaller; for instance, a 24-gauge needle is smaller than an 18-gauge needle.
- When giving an injection, the viscosity of the medication directs the choice of gauge (diameter). A thicker medication, such as a hormone, is given through a needle with a larger gauge, such as a 20-gauge. A thinner-consistency medication, such as morphine, is given through a needle with a smaller gauge, such as a 24-gauge.
- The size of the syringe is directed by the amount of medication to be given. If the amount is less than 1 mL, use a 1-mL syringe to administer the medication. In a 1-mL syringe, the amount of medication may be rounded to the 100th decimal place. In syringes larger than 1 mL, the amount is rounded to the 10th decimal place. If the amount of medication to be administered is less than 3 mL, use a 3-mL syringe. If the amount of medication is equal to the size of the syringe (e.g., 1 mL and using a 1-mL syringe), you may go up to the next size syringe to prevent awkward movements when deploying the plunger.

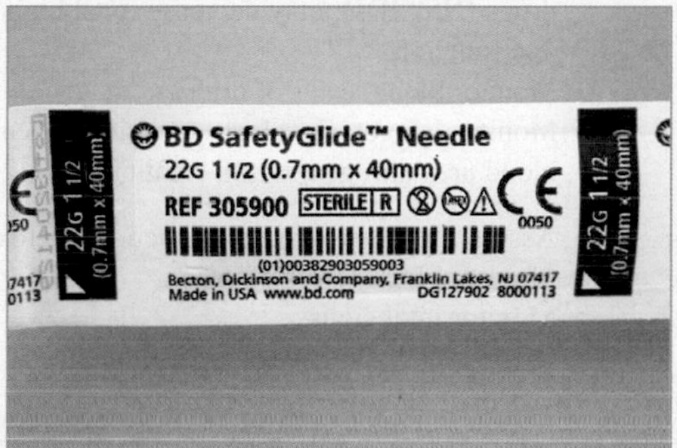

Needle package showing first number (gauge or diameter of the needle) and second number (length of the needle in inches).

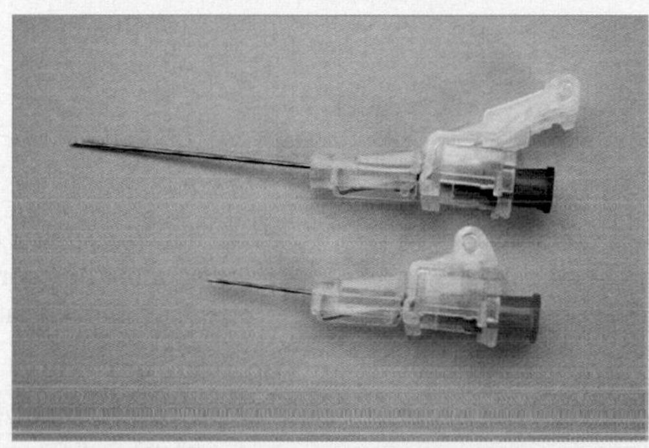

Different needle sizes. An 18-gauge needle (*top*) and a 24-gauge needle (*bottom*).

FUNDAMENTALS REVIEW 5-6

ALTERED DRUG RESPONSE IN OLDER PEOPLE

Age-Related Changes	Implication or Response	Nursing Interventions
Decreased gastric motility; increased gastric pH	Stomach irritation; nausea; vomiting; gastric ulceration	• Assess for symptoms of gastrointestinal discomfort. • Assess stools for blood.
Decreased lean body mass; decreased total body water	Decreased distribution of water-soluble drugs and higher plasma concentrations, leading to an increased possibility of drug toxicity	• Assess for signs of drug interactions or toxicity. • Monitor blood levels of drugs. • Monitor fluid balance; intake and output.
Increased adipose tissue	Accumulation of fat-soluble drugs; delay in elimination from, and accumulation of, drug in the body, leading to prolonged action and increased possibility of toxicity	• Assess for signs of drug interactions or toxicity. • Monitor blood levels of drugs.

(*continued*)

FUNDAMENTALS REVIEW 5-6 continued

ALTERED DRUG RESPONSE IN OLDER PEOPLE

Age-Related Changes	Implication or Response	Nursing Interventions
Decreased number of protein-binding sites	Higher drug plasma concentrations, leading to increased possibility of drug toxicity	• Assess for signs of drug interactions or toxicity. • Monitor blood levels of drugs. • Monitor laboratory values—albumin and prealbumin.
Decreased liver function; decreased enzyme production for drug metabolism; decreased hepatic perfusion	Decreased rate of drug metabolism; higher drug plasma concentrations, leading to prolonged action and increased possibility of drug toxicity	• Assess for signs of drug interactions or toxicity. • Monitor blood levels of drugs. • Monitor laboratory values—hepatic enzymes.
Decreased kidney function, renal mass, and blood flow	Decreased excretion of drugs, leading to possible increased serum levels/toxicity	• Assess for signs of drug interactions or toxicity. • Monitor use of non-steroidal anti-inflammatory drugs (NSAIDs); may decrease renal blood flow and function. • Monitor blood levels of drugs. • Monitor laboratory values—creatinine clearance, blood urea nitrogen, serum creatinine.
Alterations in normal homeostatic responses; altered peripheral venous tone	Exacerbated response to cardiovascular drugs; more pronounced hypotensive effects from medications	• Assess for signs of drug interactions or toxicity. • Monitor blood levels of drugs. • Monitor vital signs. • Orthostatic hypotension precautions
Alterations in blood–brain barrier	Enhanced central nervous system penetration of fat-soluble drugs; increased possibility for alterations in mental status, dizziness, gait disturbances	• Assess for signs of drug interactions or toxicity. • Assess for dizziness and light-headedness. • Institute fall safety precautions.
Decreased central nervous system efficiency	Prolonged effect of drugs on the central nervous system; exacerbated response to analgesics and sedatives	• Assess for signs of drug interactions or toxicity. • Assess for alterations in neurologic status. • Monitor vital signs and pulse oximetry.
Decreased production of oral secretions; dry mouth	Difficulty swallowing oral medications	• Monitor ability to swallow medications, especially tablets and capsules. • Discuss changing medications to forms that can be crushed and/or liquid forms with prescribing practitioner.
Decreased lipid content in skin	Possible decrease in absorption of transdermal medications	• Monitor effectiveness of transdermal preparations.

(Adapted from Aschenbrenner, D., & Venable, S. (2012). *Drug therapy in nursing* (3rd ed.). Philadelphia: Wolters Kluwer Health/Lippincott Williams & Wilkins; Hinkle, J.L., & Cheever, K.H. (2014). *Brunner & Suddarth's textbook of medical-surgical nursing* (13th ed.). Philadelphia: Wolters Kluwer Health/Lippincott Williams & Wilkins; Tabloski, P. (2010). *Gerontological nursing* (2nd ed.). Upper Saddle River, NJ: Pearson Prentice Hall; Grossman, S., & Porth, C.M. (2014). *Porth's pathophysiology: concepts of altered health states.* (9th ed.). Philadelphia: Wolters Kluwer Health/Lippincott Williams & Wilkins.)

SKILL 5-1 ADMINISTERING ORAL MEDICATIONS

Drugs given orally are intended for absorption in the stomach and small intestine. The oral route is the most commonly used route of administration. It is usually the most convenient and comfortable route for the patient. After oral administration, drug action has a slower onset and a more prolonged, but less potent, effect than other routes.

DELEGATION CONSIDERATIONS

The administration of oral medications is not delegated to nursing assistive personnel (NAP) or to unlicensed assistive personnel (UAP) in the acute care setting. The administration of specified oral medications to stable patients in some long-term care settings may be delegated to nursing assistive personnel (NAP) or unlicensed assistive personnel (UAP) who have received appropriate training. Depending on the state's nurse practice act and the organization's policies and procedures, the administration of oral medications may be delegated to licensed practical/vocational nurses (LPN/LVNs). The decision to delegate must be based on careful analysis of the patient's needs and circumstances, as well as the qualifications of the person to whom the task is being delegated. Refer to the Delegation Guidelines in Appendix A.

EQUIPMENT

- Medication in disposable cup or oral syringe
- Liquid (e.g., water, juice) with straw, if not contraindicated
- Medication cart or tray
- Computer-generated Medication Administration Record (CMAR) or Medication Administration Record (MAR)
- PPE, as indicated

ASSESSMENT

Assess the appropriateness of the drug for the patient. Review medical history, allergy, assessment, and laboratory data that may influence drug administration. Assess the patient's ability to swallow medications; check the gag reflex, if indicated. If the patient cannot swallow, is NPO, does not have gag reflex, or is experiencing nausea or vomiting, withhold the medication, notify the primary care provider, and complete proper documentation. Assess the patient's knowledge of the medication. If the patient has a knowledge deficit about the medication, this may be the appropriate time to begin education about the medication. If the medication may affect the patient's vital signs, assess them before administration. If the medication is for pain relief, assess the patient's pain level before and after administration. Verify the patient name, dose, route, and time of administration.

NURSING DIAGNOSIS

Determine related factors for the nursing diagnoses based on the patient's current status. Appropriate nursing diagnoses may include:

- Impaired Swallowing
- Deficient Knowledge
- Risk for Aspiration

OUTCOME IDENTIFICATION AND PLANNING

The expected outcome to achieve when administering an oral medication is that the patient will swallow the medication. Other outcomes that may be appropriate include the following: the patient will experience the desired effect from the medication; the patient will not aspirate; the patient experiences decreased anxiety; the patient does not experience adverse effects; and the patient understands and complies with the medication regimen.

IMPLEMENTATION

ACTION	RATIONALE
1. Gather equipment. Check each medication order against the original in the medical record, according to facility policy. Clarify any inconsistencies. Check the patient's medical record for allergies.	This comparison helps to identify errors that may have occurred when orders were transcribed. The primary care provider's order is the legal record of medication orders for each facility.
2. Know the actions, special nursing considerations, safe dose ranges, purpose of administration, and adverse effects of the medications to be administered. Consider the appropriateness of the medication for this patient.	This knowledge aids the nurse in evaluating the therapeutic effect of the medication in relation to the patient's disorder and can also be used to educate the patient about the medication.

(continued)

SKILL 5-1 ADMINISTERING ORAL MEDICATIONS continued

ACTION	RATIONALE
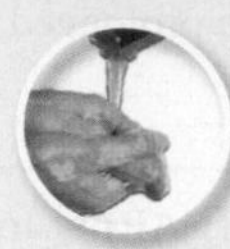 3. Perform hand hygiene.	Hand hygiene prevents the spread of microorganisms.
4. Move the medication cart to the outside of the patient's room or prepare for administration in the medication area.	Organization facilitates error-free administration and saves time.
5. Unlock the medication cart or drawer. Enter pass code into the computer and scan employee identification, if required.	Locking the cart or drawer safeguards each patient's medication supply. Hospital accrediting organizations require medication carts to be locked when not in use. Entering pass code and scanning ID allows only authorized users into the computer system and identifies the user for documentation by the computer.
6. **Prepare medications for one patient at a time.**	This prevents errors in medication administration.
7. Read the CMAR/MAR and select the proper medication from the unit stock or patient's medication drawer.	This is the *first* check of the medication label.
8. Compare the medication label with the CMAR/MAR (Figure 1). Check expiration dates and perform calculations, if necessary. Scan the bar code on the package, if required.	This is the *second* check of the label. Verify calculations with another nurse to ensure safety, if necessary.
9. Prepare the required medications:	
a. *Unit dose packages:* Place unit dose-packaged medications in a disposable cup. **Do not open the wrapper until at the bedside.** Keep opioids and medications that require special nursing assessments in a separate container.	Wrapper is kept intact because the label is needed for an additional safety check. Special assessments may be required before giving certain medications. These may include assessing vital signs and checking laboratory test results.
b. *Multidose containers:* When removing tablets or capsules from a multidose bottle, pour the necessary number into the bottle cap and then place the tablets or capsules in a medication cup. Break only scored tablets, if necessary, to obtain the proper dosage. Do not touch tablets or capsules with hands.	Pouring medication into the cap allows for easy return of excess medication to the bottle. Pouring tablets or capsules into your hand is unsanitary.
c. *Liquid medication in multidose bottle:* When pouring liquid medications out of a multidose bottle, hold the bottle so the label is against the palm. Use the appropriate measuring device when pouring liquids, and read the amount of medication at the bottom of the meniscus at eye level (Figure 2). Wipe the lip of the bottle with a paper towel.	Liquid that may drip onto the label makes the label difficult to read. Accuracy is possible when the appropriate measuring device is used and then read accurately.

FIGURE 1 Comparing medication label with CMAR.

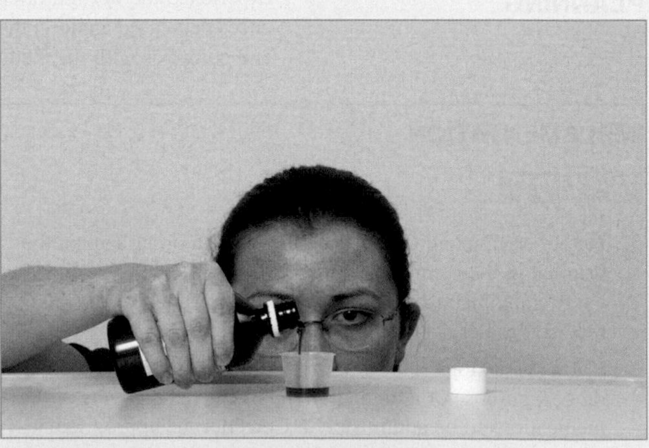

FIGURE 2 Measuring at eye level. *(Photo by B. Proud.)*

ACTION	RATIONALE
10. **Depending on facility policy, the third check of the label may occur at this point. If so, when all medications for one patient have been prepared, recheck the labels with the CMAR/MAR before taking the medications to the patient.**	This *third* check ensures accuracy and helps to prevent errors. *Note:* Many facilities require the third check to occur at the bedside, after identifying the patient and before administration.
11. Replace any multidose containers in the patient's drawer or unit stock. **Lock the medication cart before leaving it.**	Locking the cart or drawer safeguards the patient's medication supply. Hospital accrediting organizations require medication carts to be locked when not in use.
12. Transport medications to the patient's bedside carefully, and keep the medications in sight at all times.	Careful handling and close observation prevent accidental or deliberate disarrangement of medications.
13. **Ensure that the patient receives the medications at the correct time.**	Check agency policy, which may allow for administration within a period of 30 minutes before or 30 minutes after the designated time.
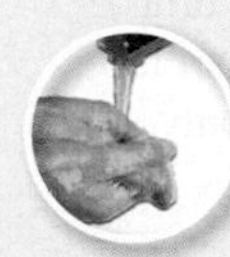 14. Perform hand hygiene and put on PPE, if indicated.	Hand hygiene and PPE prevent the spread of microorganisms. PPE is required based on transmission precautions.
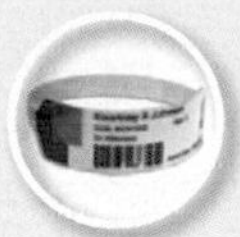 15. **Identify the patient. Compare the information with the CMAR/MAR. The patient should be identified using at least two methods** (The Joint Commission, 2013):	Identifying the patient ensures the right patient receives the medications and helps prevent errors. The patient's room number or physical location is not used as an identifier (The Joint Commission, 2013). Replace the identification band if it is missing or inaccurate in any way.
a. Check the name on the patient's identification band (Figure 3).	
b. Check the identification number on the patient's identification band.	
c. Check the birth date on the patient's identification band.	
d. Ask the patient to state his or her name and birth date, based on facility policy.	This requires a response from the patient, but illness and strange surroundings often cause patients to be confused.
16. **Complete necessary assessments before administering medications. Check the patient's allergy bracelet or ask the patient about allergies. Explain the purpose and action of each medication to the patient.**	Assessment is a prerequisite to administration of medications.
17. Scan the patient's bar code on the identification band, if required (Figure 4).	The bar code provides an additional check to ensure that the medication is given to the right patient.

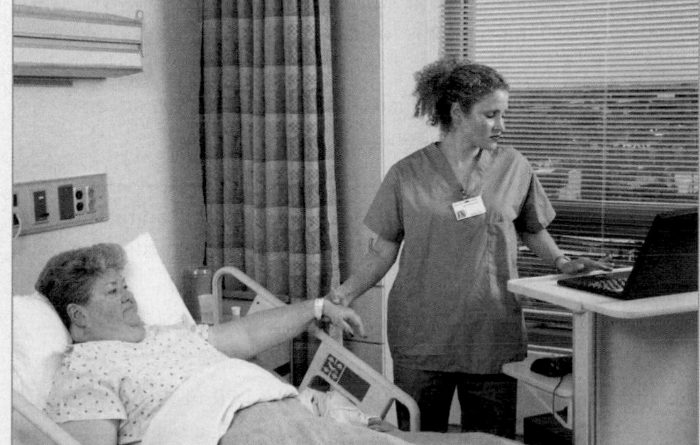

FIGURE 3 Comparing patient's name and identification number with CMAR.

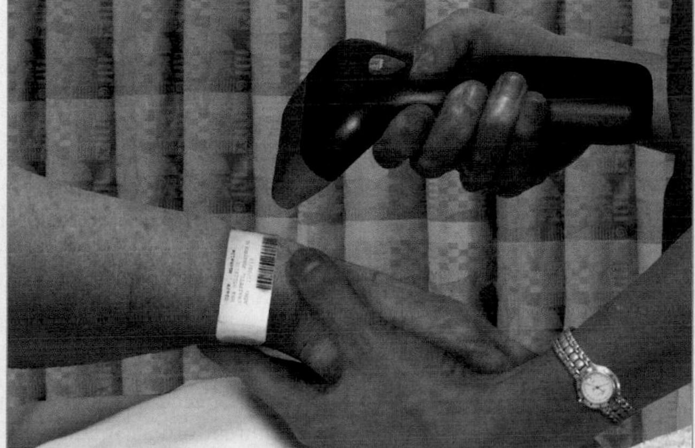

FIGURE 4 Scanning bar code on patient's identification bracelet. *(Photo by B. Proud.)*

(continued)

SKILL 5-1 ADMINISTERING ORAL MEDICATIONS continued

ACTION	RATIONALE
18. **Based on facility policy, the third check of the medication label may occur at this point. If so, recheck the label with the CMAR/MAR before administering the medications to the patient.**	Many facilities require the *third* check to occur at the bedside, after identifying the patient and before administration. If facility policy directs the *third* check at this time, this *third* check ensures accuracy and helps prevent errors.
19. Assist the patient to an upright or lateral (side-lying) position.	Swallowing is facilitated by proper positioning. An upright or side-lying position protects the patient from aspiration.
20. Administer medications:	
a. Offer water or other permitted fluids with pills, capsules, tablets, and some liquid medications.	Liquids facilitate swallowing of solid drugs. Some liquid drugs are intended to adhere to the pharyngeal area, in which case liquid is not offered with the medication.
b. Ask whether the patient prefers to take the medications by hand or in a cup.	This encourages the patient's participation in taking the medications.
21. **Remain with the patient until each medication is swallowed. Never leave medication at the patient's bedside** (Figure 5).	Unless you have seen the patient swallow the drug, the drug cannot be recorded as administered. The patient's chart is a legal record. Medications can be left at the bedside only with a prescriber's order.

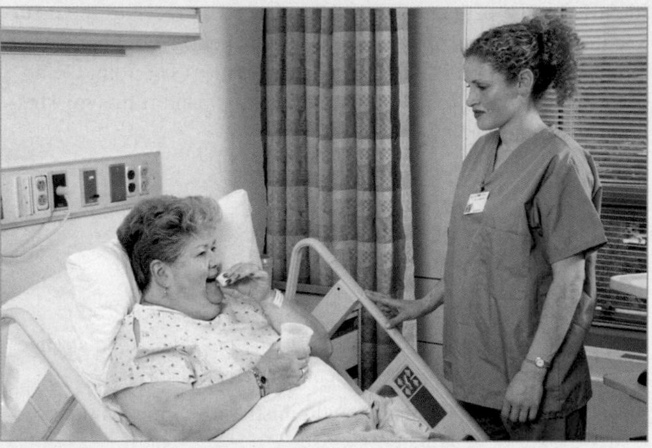

FIGURE 5 Remaining with patient until each medication is swallowed.

ACTION	RATIONALE
22. Assist the patient to a comfortable position. Remove PPE, if used. Perform hand hygiene.	Promotes patient comfort. Proper removal of PPE prevents transmission of microorganisms. Hand hygiene deters the spread of microorganisms.
23. Document the administration of the medication immediately after administration. See Documentation section below.	Timely documentation helps to ensure patient safety.
24. Evaluate the patient's response to the medication within the appropriate time frame.	The patient needs to be evaluated for therapeutic and adverse effects from the medication.

EVALUATION

The expected outcomes are met when the patient swallows the medication, does not aspirate, verbalizes an understanding of the medication, experiences the desired effect from the medication, and does not experience adverse effects.

DOCUMENTATION

Guidelines

Record each medication immediately after it is administered on the CMAR/MAR or record using the required format. Include the date and time of administration (Figure 6). If using a bar-code system, medication administration is automatically recorded when the bar code is scanned. PRN medications require documentation of the reason for administration. Prompt recording avoids the possibility of accidentally repeating the administration of the drug. If the drug was refused or omitted, record this in the appropriate area on the medication record and notify the primary care provider. This verifies the reason medication was omitted and ensures that the primary care provider is aware of the patient's condition. Recording administration of an opioid may require additional documentation on a controlled-substance record, stating drug count and other specific information. A record of fluid intake and output measurement is required.

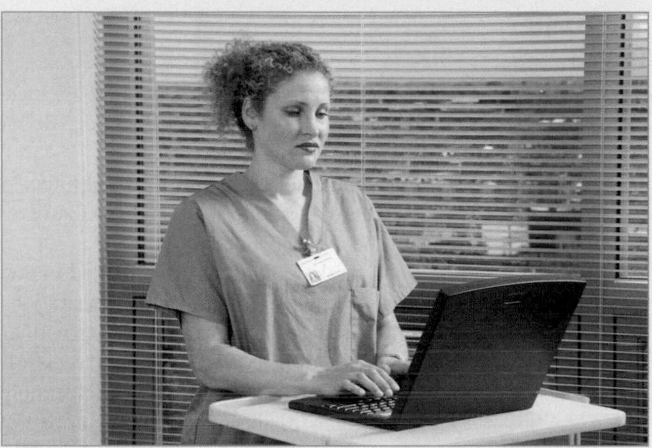

FIGURE 6 Recording each medication administered on CMAR.

Sample Documentation

DocuCare Practice documenting medication administration in *Lippincott DocuCare*.

8/6/15 0835 Patient states he is having constant stabbing leg pains. Rates pain as an 8/10. Percocet 2 tabs administered.

—*K. Sanders, RN*

8/6/15 0905 Patient resting comfortably. Rates leg pain as a 1/10

—*K. Sanders, RN*

8/6/15 1300 Patient states he does not want pain medication, despite return of leg pain. States, "It made me feel woozy last time." Feelings discussed with patient. Patient agrees to take Percocet 1 tab at this time.

—*K. Sanders, RN*

8/6/15 1320 Percocet, 1 tablet given PO.

—*K. Sanders, RN*

UNEXPECTED SITUATIONS AND ASSOCIATED INTERVENTIONS

- *Patient states that it feels like medication is lodged in throat:* Offer patient more fluids to drink. If allowed, offer the patient bread or crackers to help move the medication to the stomach.
- *It is unclear whether the patient swallowed the medication:* Check in the patient's mouth, under tongue, and between cheek and gum. Patients with altered mental status may not be aware that the medication was not swallowed. Also, patients may "cheek" medications to avoid taking the medication or to save it for later use. Watch patients requiring suicide precautions closely to ensure that they are not "cheeking" the medication or hiding it in the mouth. These patients may be trying to accumulate a large amount of medication to take all at once in a suicide attempt. Substance abusers may cheek medication to accumulate a large amount to take all at once so that they may feel a high from medication.
- *Patient vomits immediately or shortly after receiving oral medication:* Assess vomit, looking for pills or fragments. Do not re-administer medication without notifying primary care provider. If a whole pill is seen and can be identified, the primary care provider may ask that the medication be administered again. If a pill is not seen or medications cannot be identified, do not re-administer the medication in order to prevent the patient from receiving too large a dose.
- *Child refuses to take oral medications:* Some medications may be mixed in a small amount of food, such as pudding or ice cream. Do not add the medication to liquids because the medication may alter the taste of liquids; if child then refuses to drink the rest of the liquid, you will not know how much of the medication was ingested. Use creativity when devising ways to administer medications to a child. See the section below, Infant and Child Considerations, for suggestions.

(continued)

SKILL 5-1 ADMINISTERING ORAL MEDICATIONS continued

- *Capsule or tablet falls to the floor during administration:* Discard and obtain a new dose for administration. This prevents contamination and transmission of microorganisms.
- *Patient refuses medication:* Explore the reason for the patient's refusal. Review the rationale for using the drug and any other information that may be appropriate. If you are unable to administer the medication despite education and discussion, document the omission according to facility policy and notify the primary care provider.

SPECIAL CONSIDERATIONS

General Considerations

- Some liquid medication preparations, such as suspensions, require agitation to ensure even distribution of medication in the solution. Be familiar with the specific requirements for medications you are administering.
- Place medications intended for sublingual absorption under the patient's tongue. Instruct the patient to allow the medication to dissolve completely. Reinforce the importance of not swallowing the medication tablet.
- Some oral medications are provided in powdered forms. Verify the correct liquid in which to dissolve the medication for administration. This information is usually included on the package. Verify any unclear instructions with a pharmacist or medication reference. If there is more than one possible liquid in which to dissolve the medication, include the patient in the decision process; patients may find one choice more palatable than another.
- Ongoing assessment is an important part of nursing care for both evaluation of patient response to administered medications and early detection of adverse effects. If an adverse effect is suspected, withhold further medication doses and notify the patient's primary care provider. Additional intervention is based on type of reaction and patient assessment.
- If the patient questions a medication order or states the medication is different from the usual dose, always recheck and clarify with the original order and/or primary care provider before giving the medication.
- If the patient's level of consciousness is altered or his or her swallowing is impaired, check with the primary care provider to clarify the route of administration or alternative forms of medication. This may also be a solution for a pediatric or a confused patient who is refusing to take a medication.
- Patients with poor vision can request large-type labels on medication containers. A magnifying lens also may be helpful.
- Provide written medication information to reinforce discussion and education in the appropriate language, if the patient is literate. If the patient is unable to read, provide written information to family or significant other, if appropriate. Written information should be at a 5th-grade level to ensure ease of understanding.
- If the patient has difficulty swallowing tablets, it may be appropriate to crush the medication to facilitate administration. However, not all medications can be crushed or altered; long-acting and slow-release drugs are examples of medications that cannot be crushed. Therefore, it is important to consult a medication reference and/or pharmacist. If the medication can be crushed, use a pill-crusher or mortar and pestle to grind the tablet into a powder. Crush each pill one at a time. Dissolve the powder with water or other recommended liquid in a liquid medication cup, keeping each medication separate from the others. Keep the package label with the medication cup for future comparison of information. Combine the crushed medication with a small amount of soft food, such as applesauce or pudding, to facilitate administration.

Infant and Child Considerations

- Special devices, such as oral syringes and calibrated nipples, are available in a pharmacy to ensure accurate dose calculations for young children and infants.
- Some creative ways to administer medications to children include the following: have a "tea party" with medicine cups; place oral syringe (without needle) or dropper in the space between the cheek and gum and slowly administer the medication; save a special treat for after the medication administration (e.g., movie, playroom time, or a special food, if allowed).
- The Institute for Safe Medication Practices (ISMP) and the U.S. Food and Drug Administration (FDA) have received reports of infants choking on the plastic caps that fit on the end of syringes when used to administer oral medications. They recommend the following: Remove and dispose of caps before giving syringes to patients or families, caution family caregivers to dispose of caps on syringes they buy over the counter, and report any problems with syringe caps to the FDA. Companies manufacture syringes labeled "oral use" without the caps on them (ISMP, 2012b; FDA, 2012d).

Older Adult Considerations

- Older patients with arthritis may have difficulty opening childproof caps. On request, the pharmacist can substitute a cap that is easier to open. A rubber band twisted around the cap may provide a more secure grip for older patients.
- Consider large-print written medication information, when appropriate.
- Physiologic changes associated with the aging process, including decreased gastric motility, muscle mass, acid production, and blood flow, can affect patient's response to medication, including drug absorption and increased risk of adverse effects. Older adults are more likely to take multiple drugs, so drug interactions in the older adult are a very real and dangerous problem. Refer to Fundamentals Review 5-6.

Home Care Considerations

- Encourage the patient to discard expired prescription medications based on label instructions or community guidelines.
- Discuss safe storage of medications when there are children and pets in the home environment.
- Discuss with parents the difference in over-the-counter medications made for infants and medications made for children. Many times parents do not realize that there are different strengths to the actual medications, leading to under- or overdosing.
- Encourage patients to carry a card listing all medications they take, including dosage and frequency, in case of an emergency.
- Discuss the importance of using an appropriate measuring device for liquid medications. Caution patients not to use eating utensils for measuring medications; use a liquid medication cup, oral syringe, or measuring spoon to provide accurate dosing.

EVIDENCE FOR PRACTICE ▶

MEDICATION ERRORS

Medication errors occur frequently and are a serious problem in health care. Medication errors may have serious consequences. Health care providers, including nurses, have a responsibility to prevent medication errors. What nursing practices may help improve the medication administration process?

Related Research

Murphy, M., & While, A. (2012). Medication administration practices among children's nurses: A survey. *British Journal of Nursing, 21*(15), 928–933.

This study investigated the medication administration practices of children's nurses to identify practices that may improve the medication administration process. Clinical staff working in all areas in a children's hospital were surveyed about medication errors and medication administration practices. Nurses identified interruptions in the medication process, a heavy workload, and fatigue as contributing factors to medication errors. In addition, the authors identified inadequate knowledge and skills and a failure to comply with hospital policy as additional contributing factors. The authors concluded that a lack of adherence to hospital policy and the frequency of interruptions in the medication administration process are important practices that require change.

Relevance to Nursing Practice

Medication administration is an important nursing responsibility. Nurses need to be aware of the factors that contribute to medication errors and work to reduce these factors in their practice. Nurses have a responsibility to be familiar with, and conform to, facility policies, as well as to maintain professional competency in regard to current and best practice guidelines. In addition, nurses should strive to work with facilities to ensure the provision of correct environment where interruptions and distractions can be kept to a minimum during all stages of the medication administration process.

Refer to thePoint for additional research on related nursing topics.

(continued)

SKILL 5-1 ADMINISTERING ORAL MEDICATIONS continued

EVIDENCE FOR PRACTICE ▶

MEDICATION MANAGEMENT IN OLDER ADULTS

Older adults are often prescribed multiple medications. Low health literacy can affect the understanding of complex medication regimens by older adults. What nursing interventions can be used to address low health literacy and improve medication use among older adults?

Related Research

Martin, D., Kripalani, S., & DuRapau, J.J. (2012). Improving medication management among at-risk older adults. *Journal of Gerontological Nursing*, *38*(6), 24–34.

Community-dwelling older adults in this study were enrolled at an inner-city adult day center. Participants completed a baseline measure of health literacy, medication self-efficacy, and medication adherence. They were provided with a personalized, illustrated daily medication schedule. Six weeks later, their medication self-efficacy and adherence were assessed. Among the 20 participants in this pilot study, 70% had high likelihood of limited health literacy and took an average of 13.2 prescription medications. Both self-efficacy and medication adherence increased significantly after provision of the personalized illustrated daily medication schedule. All participants rated the schedules as very helpful in terms of helping them remember the medication's purpose and dosing. The authors concluded that illustrated daily medication schedules improve medication self-efficacy and adherence among at-risk community-dwelling older adults.

Relevance to Nursing Practice

Patient education is an important nursing responsibility. Nurses need to be creative and diligent in their approach to meeting the needs of their patients. Simple interventions, such as illustrated written schedules, along with explanation, can improve patient understanding and compliance.

Refer to thePoint for additional research on related nursing topics.

SKILL 5-2 ADMINISTERING MEDICATIONS VIA A GASTRIC TUBE

Patients with a gastrointestinal tube (nasogastric, nasointestinal, percutaneous endoscopic gastrostomy [PEG], or jejunostomy [J] tube) often receive medication through the tube. Care of the patient with an enteral feeding tube is described in Chapter 11. Use liquid medications, when possible, because they are readily absorbed and less likely to cause tube occlusions. Certain solid dosage medications can be crushed and combined with liquid. Crush each pill, one at a time, to a fine powder and mix with 15 to 30 mL of water before delivery through the tube, keeping each medication separate from the others. Also, certain capsules may be opened, emptied into liquid, and administered through the tube (Toedter Williams, 2008). **Not all medications can be crushed or altered; long-acting and slow-release drugs are examples of medications that cannot be crushed.** Check manufacturer's recommendations and/or with a pharmacist to verify. Keep the package label with the medication cup for future comparison of information.

DELEGATION CONSIDERATIONS

The administration of medications via a gastric tube is not delegated to nursing assistive personnel (NAP) or to unlicensed assistive personnel (UAP). Depending on the state's nurse practice act and the organization's policies and procedures, the administration of medications via a gastric tube may be delegated to licensed practical/vocational nurses (LPN/LVNs). The decision to delegate must be based on careful analysis of the patient's needs and circumstances, as well as the qualifications of the person to whom the task is being delegated. Refer to the Delegation Guidelines in Appendix A.

EQUIPMENT	• Irrigation set (60-mL syringe and irrigation container) • Medications • Water (gastrostomy tubes) or sterile water (nasogastric [NG] tubes), according to facility policy	• Gloves • Additional PPE, as indicated

ASSESSMENT

Research each medication to be given, especially for mode of action, side effects, nursing implications, ability to be crushed, and whether the medication should be given with or without food. Verify patient name, dose, route, and time of administration. Also assess patient's knowledge of the medication and the reason for its administration. Auscultate the abdomen for evidence of bowel sounds. Palpate the abdomen for tenderness and distention. Ascertain the time of the patient's last bowel movement and measure abdominal girth, if appropriate.

NURSING DIAGNOSIS

Determine the related factors for the nursing diagnoses based on the patient's current status. Possible nursing diagnoses may include:

- Deficient Knowledge
- Risk for Injury
- Impaired Swallowing

OUTCOME IDENTIFICATION AND PLANNING

The expected outcome to achieve is that the patient receives the medication via the tube and experiences the intended effect of the medication. In addition, the patient verbalizes knowledge of the medications given; the patient remains free from adverse effects and injury; and the gastrointestinal tube remains patent.

IMPLEMENTATION

ACTION	RATIONALE
1. Gather equipment. Check each medication order against the original in the medical record, according to facility policy. Clarify any inconsistencies. Check the patient's chart for allergies.	This comparison helps to identify errors that may have occurred when orders were transcribed. The primary care provider's order is the legal record of medication orders for each facility.
2. Know the actions, special nursing considerations, safe dose ranges, purpose of administration, and adverse effects of the medications to be administered. Consider the appropriateness of the medication for this patient.	This knowledge aids the nurse in evaluating the therapeutic effect of the medication in relation to the patient's disorder and can also be used to educate the patient about the medication.
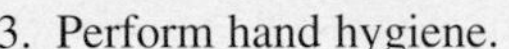 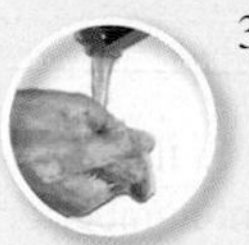 3. Perform hand hygiene.	Hand hygiene prevents the spread of microorganisms.
4. Move the medication cart to the outside of the patient's room or prepare for administration in the medication area.	Organization facilitates error-free administration and saves time.
5. Unlock the medication cart or drawer. Enter pass code into the computer and scan employee identification, if required.	Locking the cart or drawer safeguards each patient's medication supply. Hospital accrediting organizations require medication carts to be locked when not in use. Entering pass code and scanning ID allows only authorized users into the computer system and identifies the user for documentation by the computer.
6. **Prepare medications for one patient at a time.**	This prevents errors in medication administration.
7. Read the CMAR/MAR and select the proper medication from the unit stock or patient's medication drawer.	This is the *first* check of the label.
8. Compare the label with the CMAR/MAR. Check expiration dates and perform calculations, if necessary. Scan the bar code on the package, if required.	This is the *second* check of the label. Verify calculations with another nurse to ensure safety, if necessary.

(continued)

SKILL 5-2 ADMINISTERING MEDICATIONS VIA A GASTRIC TUBE continued

ACTION	RATIONALE
9. Check to see if medications to be administered come in a liquid form. **If pills or capsules are to be given, check with pharmacy or drug reference to verify the ability to crush tablets or open capsules.**	To prevent the tube from becoming clogged, all medications should be given in liquid form whenever possible. Medications in extended-release formulations should not be crushed before administration.
10. Prepare medication. *Pills:* Using a pill crusher, crush each pill one at a time. Dissolve the powder with water or other recommended liquid in a liquid medication cup, keeping each medication separate from the others. Keep the package label with the medication cup, for future comparison of information. *Liquid:* When pouring liquid medications from a multidose bottle, hold the bottle with the label against the palm. Use the appropriate measuring device when pouring liquids, and read the amount of medication at the bottom of the meniscus at eye level. Wipe the lip of the bottle with a paper towel.	Some medications require dissolution in liquid other than water. The label is needed for an additional safety check. Some medications require pre-administration assessments. Liquid that may drip onto the label makes the label difficult to read. Accuracy is possible when the appropriate measuring device is used and then read accurately.
11. **Depending on facility policy, the third check of the label may occur at this point. If so, when all medications for one patient have been prepared, recheck the labels with the CMAR/MAR before taking the medications to the patient.**	This *third* check ensures accuracy and helps to prevent errors. *Note:* Many facilities require the *third* check to occur at the bedside, after identifying the patient and before administration.
12. Replace any multidose containers in the patient's drawer or unit stock.	Proper storage safeguards medications.
13. **Lock the medication cart before leaving it.**	Locking the cart or drawer safeguards the patient's medication supply. Hospital accrediting organizations require medication carts to be locked when not in use.
14. Transport medications to the patient's bedside carefully, and keep the medications in sight at all times.	Careful handling and close observation prevent accidental or deliberate disarrangement of medications.
15. **Ensure that the patient receives the medications at the correct time.**	Check agency policy, which may allow for administration within a period of 30 minutes before or 30 minutes after the designated time.
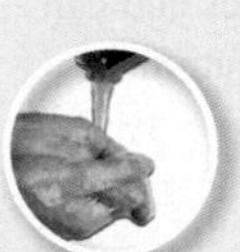 16. Perform hand hygiene and put on PPE, if indicated.	Hand hygiene and PPE prevent the spread of microorganisms. PPE is required based on transmission precautions.
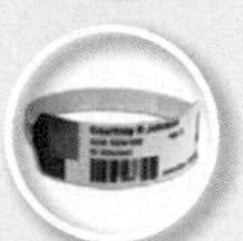 17. **Identify the patient. Compare the information with the CMAR/MAR. The patient should be identified using at least two methods** (The Joint Commission, 2013):	Identifying the patient ensures the right patient receives the medications and helps prevent errors. The patient's room number or physical location is not used as an identifier (The Joint Commission, 2013). Replace the identification band if it is missing or inaccurate in any way.
a. Check the name on the patient's identification band. b. Check the identification number on the patient's identification band. c. Check the birth date on the patient's identification band.	
d. Ask the patient to state his or her name and birth date, based on facility policy.	This requires a response from the patient, but illness and strange surroundings often cause patients to be confused.
18. **Complete necessary assessments before administering medications. Check the patient's allergy bracelet or ask the patient about allergies. Explain what you are going to do, and the reason for doing it, to the patient.**	Assessment is a prerequisite to administration of medications. Explanation relieves anxiety and facilitates cooperation.

ACTION	RATIONALE
19. Scan the patient's bar code on the identification band, if required (Figure 1).	This provides an additional check to ensure that the medication is given to the right patient.
20. **Based on facility policy, the third check of the label may occur at this point. If so, recheck the labels with the CMAR/MAR before administering the medications to the patient.**	Many facilities require the *third* check to occur at the bedside, after identifying the patient and before administration. If facility policy directs the *third* check at this time, this *third* check ensures accuracy and helps to prevent errors.
21. Assist the patient to the high Fowler's position, unless contraindicated.	This reduces the risk of aspiration.
22. Put on gloves.	Gloves prevent contact with mucous membranes and body fluids.
23. If patient is receiving continuous tube feedings, pause the tube-feeding pump (Figure 2).	If the pump is not stopped, tube feeding will flow out of the tube and onto the patient.

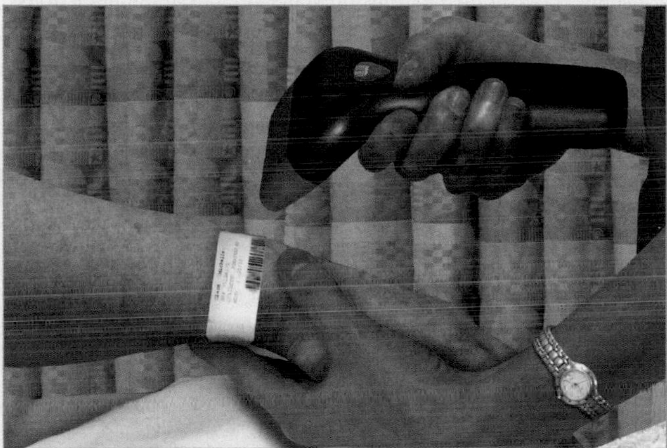

FIGURE 1 Scanning bar code on the patient's identification bracelet. *(Photo by B. Proud.)*

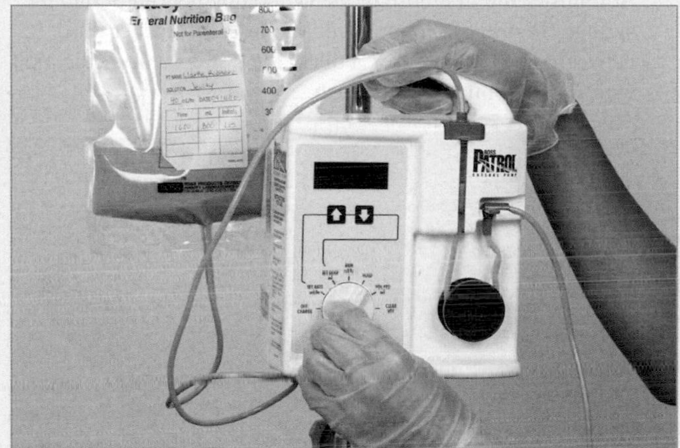

FIGURE 2 Pausing feeding pump. *(Photo by B. Proud.)*

ACTION	RATIONALE
24. Pour the water into the irrigation container. Measure 30 mL of water. Apply clamp on feeding tube, if present. Alternately, pinch gastric tube below port with fingers, or position stopcock to correct direction. Open port on gastric tube delegated to medication administration (Figure 3) or disconnect tubing for feeding from gastric tube and place cap on end of feeding tubing.	Fluid is ready for flushing of the tube. Applying clamp, folding the tube over, and clamping, or the correct positioning of the stopcock prevents any backflow of gastric drainage. Covering end of feeding tubing prevents contamination.
25. **Check tube placement, depending on type of tube and facility policy.** (Refer to Chapter 11.)	Tube placement must be confirmed before administering anything through the tube to avoid inadvertent instillation in the respiratory tract.

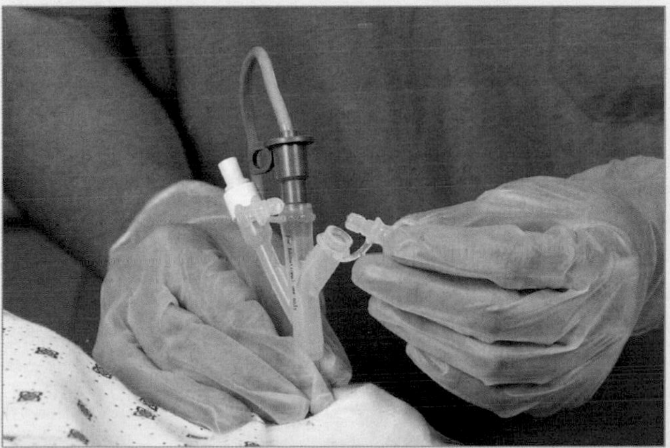

FIGURE 3 Pinching gastric tubing to prevent backflow of gastric drainage and opening medication administration port. *(Photo by B. Proud.)*

(continued)

SKILL 5-2 ADMINISTERING MEDICATIONS VIA A GASTRIC TUBE continued

ACTION	RATIONALE
26. Note the amount of any residual. Refer to Chapter 11. Replace residual back into stomach, based on facility policy.	Research findings are inconclusive on the benefit of returning gastric volumes to the stomach or intestine to avoid fluid or electrolyte imbalance, which has been accepted practice. Consult agency policy concerning this practice (Bourgault, et al., 2007; Keithley & Swanson, 2004; Metheny, 2008).
27. Apply clamp on feeding tube, if present. Alternately, pinch the gastric tube below port with fingers, or position stop-cock to correct direction. Remove 60-mL syringe from gastric tube. Remove the plunger of the syringe. Reinsert the syringe in the gastric tube without the plunger. Pour 30 mL of water into the syringe (Figure 4). **Unclamp the tube and allow the water to enter the stomach via gravity infusion.**	Clamping prevents backflow of gastric drainage. Flushing the tube ensures that all the residual is cleared from the tube.
28. Administer the first dose of medication by pouring it into the syringe (Figure 5). Follow with a 5- to 10-mL water flush between medication doses. Follow the last dose of medication with 30 to 60 mL of water flush.	Flushing between medications prevents any possible interactions between the medications. Flushing at the end maintains tube patency, prevents blockage by medication particles, and ensures all doses enter the stomach.

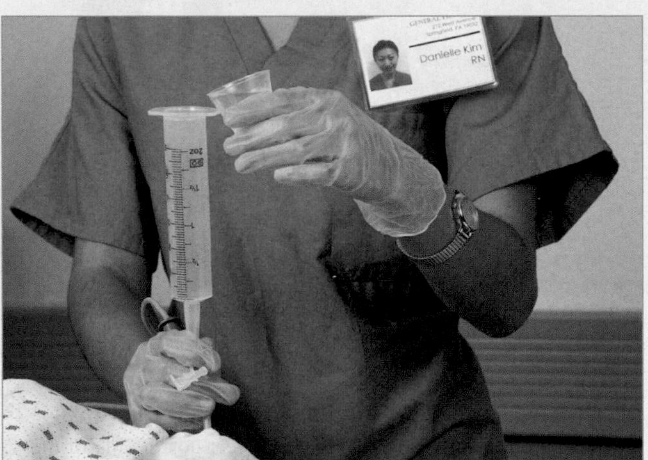

FIGURE 4 Pouring water into syringe inserted in gastric tube. *(Photo by B. Proud.)*

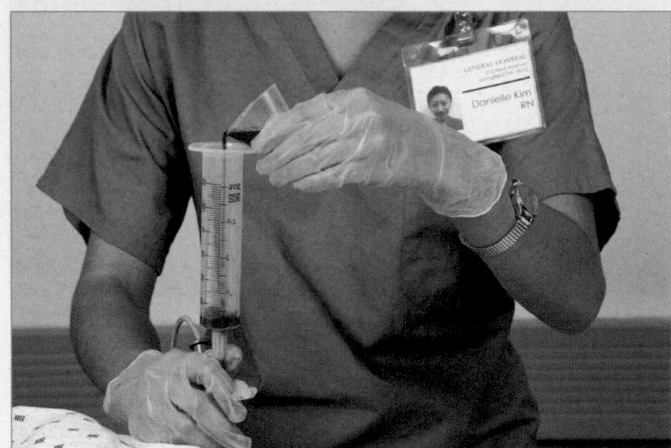

FIGURE 5 Pouring medication into syringe inserted in gastric tube. *(Photo by B. Proud.)*

ACTION	RATIONALE
29. Clamp the tube, remove the syringe, and replace the feeding tubing. If a stopcock is used, position it to correct direction. If a tube medication port was used, cap the port. Unclamp the gastric tube and restart tube feeding, if appropriate for medications administered.	Some medications require the holding of the tube feeding for a certain period of time after administration. Consult a drug reference or a pharmacist.
30. Remove gloves. Assist the patient to a comfortable position. If receiving a tube feeding, the head of the bed must remain elevated at least 30 degrees.	Ensures patient comfort. Keeping the head of the bed elevated helps prevent aspiration.
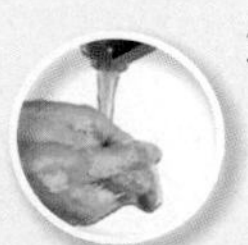 31. Remove additional PPE, if used. Perform hand hygiene.	Removing PPE properly reduces the risk for infection transmission and contamination of other items. Hand hygiene prevents the spread of microorganisms.
32. Document the administration of the medication immediately after administration. See Documentation section below.	Timely documentation helps to ensure patient safety.
33. Evaluate the patient's response to the medication within the appropriate time frame.	The patient needs to be evaluated for therapeutic and adverse effects from the medication.

EVALUATION

The expected outcome is met when the patient receives the prescribed medications and experiences the intended effects of the medications administered. In addition, the patient demonstrates a patent and functioning gastric tube, verbalizes knowledge of the medications given, and remains free from adverse effects and injury.

DOCUMENTATION

Guidelines

Document the administration of the medication immediately after administration, including date, time, dose, and route of administration on the CMAR/MAR or record using the required format. If using a bar-code system, medication administration is automatically recorded when the bar code is scanned. PRN medications require documentation of the reason for administration. Prompt recording avoids the possibility of accidentally repeating the administration of the drug. Record the amount of gastric residual, if appropriate. Record the amount of liquid given on the intake and output record. If the drug was refused or omitted, record this in the appropriate area on the medication record and notify the primary care provider. This verifies the reason medication was omitted and ensures that the primary care provider is aware of the patient's condition.

UNEXPECTED SITUATIONS AND ASSOCIATED INTERVENTIONS

- *Medication enters tube and then tube becomes clogged:* Attach a 10-mL syringe onto end of tube. Pull back and then lightly apply pressure to plunger in a repetitive motion. This may dislodge the medication. If the medication does not move through the tube, notify the primary care provider. The tube may have to be replaced.

SPECIAL CONSIDERATIONS

- If medications are being administered via an NG tube that is attached to suction, the tube should remain clamped, off suction, for a period of time after medication administration. This allows for medication absorption before returning to suction. Check facility policy and drug reference for specific drug requirements.
- If necessary to use plunger in irrigation syringe to administer medications, instill gently and slowly. Gravity administration is considered best to avoid excess pressure.
- Give medications separately and flush with water between each drug. Some medications may interact with each other or become less effective if mixed with other drugs.
- If the patient is receiving tube feedings, review information about the drugs to be administered. Absorption of some drugs, such as phenytoin (Dilantin), is affected by tube feeding formulas. Discontinue a continuous tube feeding and leave the tube clamped for the required period of time before and after the medication has been given, according to the reference and facility protocol.
- Ongoing assessment is an important part of nursing care for both evaluation of patient response to administered medications and early detection of adverse effects. If an adverse effect is suspected, withhold further medication doses and notify the patient's primary care provider. Additional intervention is based on type of reaction and patient assessment.

SKILL 5-3 REMOVING MEDICATION FROM AN AMPULE

An **ampule** is a glass flask that contains a single dose of medication for parenteral administration. Because there is no way to prevent contamination of any unused portion of medication after the ampule is opened, discard any remaining medication if not all the medication is used for the prescribed dose. You must break the thin neck of the ampule to remove the medication.

DELEGATION CONSIDERATIONS

The preparation of medication from an ampule is not delegated to nursing assistive personnel (NAP) or to unlicensed assistive personnel (UAP). Depending on the state's nurse practice act and the organization's policies and procedures, the preparation of medication from an ampule may be delegated to a licensed practical/vocational nurse (LPN/LVN). The decision to delegate must be based on careful analysis of the patient's needs and circumstances, as well as the qualifications of the person to whom the task is being delegated. Refer to the Delegation Guidelines in Appendix A.

(continued)

SKILL 5-3 REMOVING MEDICATION FROM AN AMPULE continued

EQUIPMENT

- Sterile syringe and filter needle
- Ampule of medication
- Small gauze pad
- Computer-generated Medication Administration Record (CMAR) or Medication Administration Record (MAR)

ASSESSMENT

Assess the medication in the ampule for any particles or discoloration. Assess the ampule for any cracks or chips. Check expiration date before administering the medication. Verify patient name, dose, route, and time of administration. Assess the appropriateness of the drug for the patient. Review assessment and laboratory data that may influence drug administration.

NURSING DIAGNOSIS

Determine related factors for the nursing diagnoses based on the patient's current status. Appropriate nursing diagnoses may include:

- Risk for Infection
- Risk for Injury
- Deficient Knowledge

OUTCOME IDENTIFICATION AND PLANNING

The expected outcome to achieve when removing medication from an ampule is that the medication will be removed in a sterile manner; it will be free from glass shards and the proper dose prepared.

IMPLEMENTATION

ACTION	RATIONALE
1. Gather equipment. Check the medication order against the original order in the medical record, according to facility policy. Clarify any inconsistencies. Check the patient's chart for allergies.	This comparison helps to identify errors that may have occurred when orders were transcribed. The primary care provider's order is the legal record of medication orders for each facility.
2. Know the actions, special nursing considerations, safe dose ranges, purpose of administration, and adverse effects of the medications to be administered. Consider the appropriateness of the medication for this patient.	This knowledge aids the nurse in evaluating the therapeutic effect of the medication in relation to the patient's disorder and can also be used to educate the patient about the medication.
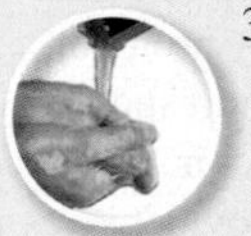 3. Perform hand hygiene.	Hand hygiene prevents the spread of microorganisms.
4. Move the medication cart to the outside of the patient's room or prepare for administration in the medication area.	Organization facilitates error-free administration and saves time.
5. Unlock the medication cart or drawer. Enter pass code and scan employee identification, if required.	Locking the cart or drawer safeguards each patient's medication supply. Hospital accrediting organizations require medication carts to be locked when not in use. Entering pass code and scanning ID allows only authorized users into the computer system and identifies the user for documentation by the computer.
6. **Prepare medications for one patient at a time.**	This prevents errors in medication administration.
7. Read the CMAR/MAR and select the proper medication from unit stock or the patient's medication drawer.	This is the *first* check of the label.
8. Compare the label with the CMAR/MAR. Check expiration dates and perform calculations, if necessary. Scan the bar code on the package, if required.	This is the *second* check of the label. Verify calculations with another nurse to ensure safety, if necessary.

ACTION	RATIONALE
9. Tap the stem of the ampule (Figure 1) or twist your wrist quickly (Figure 2) while holding the ampule vertically.	This facilitates movement of medication in the stem to the body of the ampule.
10. Wrap a small gauze pad around the neck of the ampule.	This will protect your fingers from the glass as the ampule is broken.

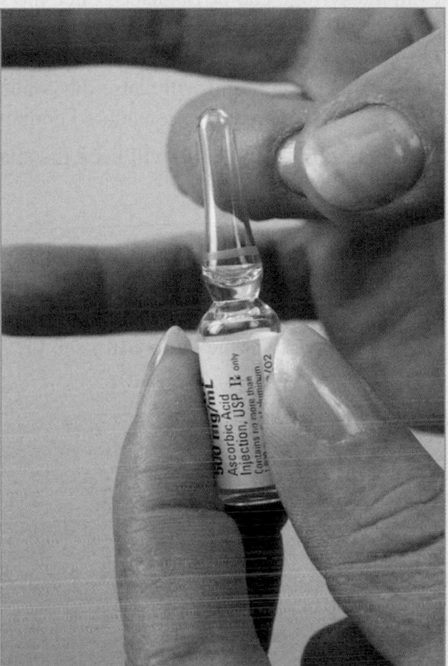

FIGURE 1 Tapping stem of the ampule.

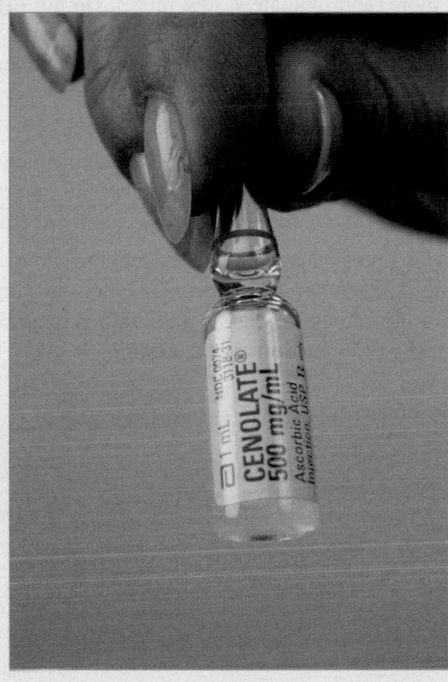

FIGURE 2 Twisting wrist quickly while holding ampule vertically.

ACTION	RATIONALE
11. Use a snapping motion to break off the top of the ampule along the scored line at its neck (Figure 3). **Always break away from your body.**	This protects your face and fingers from any shattered glass fragments.

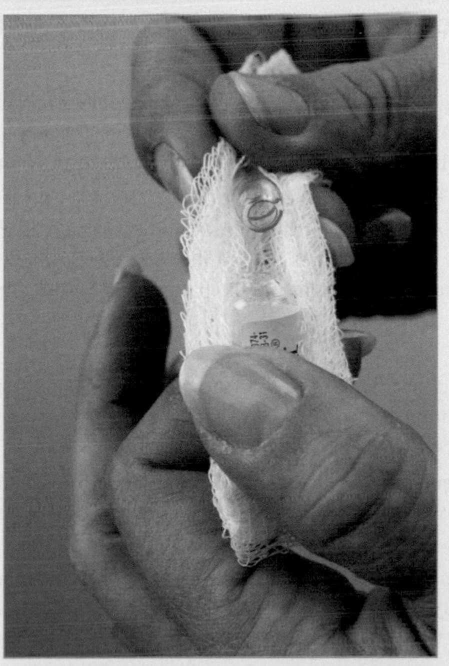
FIGURE 3 Using a snapping motion to break top of ampule.

(continued)

SKILL 5-3 REMOVING MEDICATION FROM AN AMPULE continued

ACTION	RATIONALE
12. Attach filter needle to syringe. Remove the cap from the filter needle by pulling it straight off.	Use of a filter needle prevents the accidental withdrawing of small glass particles with the medication. Pulling the cap off in a straight manner prevents accidental needlestick.
13. Withdraw medication in the amount ordered plus a small amount more (approximately 30% more). **Do not inject air into the solution. While inserting the filter needle into the ampule, be careful not to touch the rim.** Use either of the following methods to withdraw the medication:	By withdrawing an additional small amount of medication, any air bubbles in the syringe can be displaced once the syringe is removed while allowing ample medication to remain in the syringe. The contents of the ampule are not under pressure; therefore, air is unnecessary and will cause the contents to overflow. The rim of the ampule is considered contaminated.
a. Insert the tip of the needle into the ampule, which is upright on a flat surface, and withdraw fluid into the syringe (Figure 4). **Touch the plunger only at the knob.**	Handling the plunger only at the knob will keep the shaft of the plunger sterile.
b. Insert the tip of the needle into the ampule and invert the ampule. Keep the needle centered and not touching the sides of the ampule. Withdraw fluid into syringe (Figure 5). **Touch the plunger only at the knob.**	Surface tension holds the fluids in the ampule when inverted. If the needle touches the sides or is removed and then reinserted into the ampule, surface tension is broken, and fluid runs out. Handling the plunger only at the knob will keep the shaft of the plunger sterile.

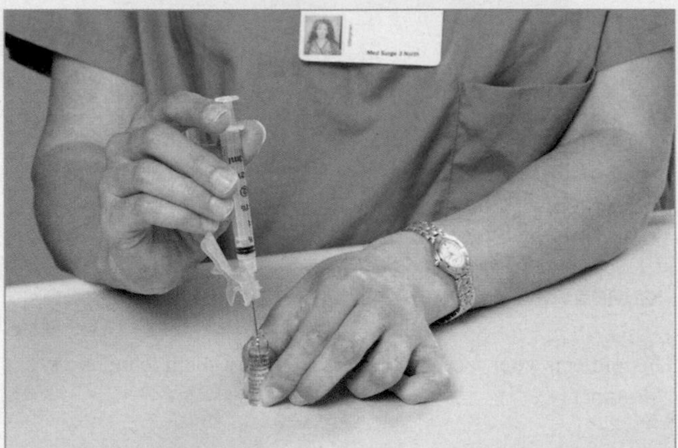

FIGURE 4 Withdrawing medication from upright ampule. *(Photo by B. Proud.)*

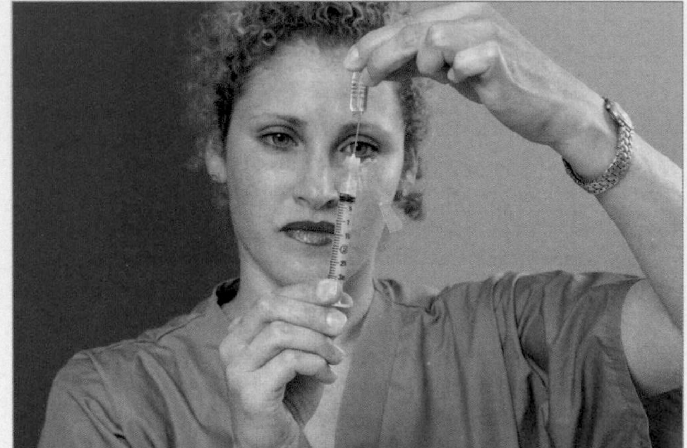

FIGURE 5 Withdrawing medication from inverted ampule. *(Photo by B. Proud.)*

ACTION	RATIONALE
14. Wait until the needle has been withdrawn to tap the syringe and expel the air carefully by pushing on the plunger. **Check the amount of medication in the syringe with the medication dose and discard any surplus, according to facility policy.**	Ejecting air into the solution increases pressure in the ampule and can force the medication to spill out over the ampule. Ampules may have overfill. Careful measurement ensures that the correct dose is withdrawn.
15. **Depending on facility policy, the third check of the label may occur at this point. If so, when all medications for one patient have been prepared, recheck the labels with the CMAR/MAR before taking the medications to the patient.**	This *third* check ensures accuracy and helps to prevent errors. *Note:* Many facilities require the *third* check to occur at the bedside, after identifying the patient and before administration.
16. **Engage safety guard on filter needle and remove the needle. Discard the filter needle in a suitable container. Attach appropriate administration device to syringe.**	The filter needle used to draw up medication should not be used to administer the medication. This will prevent any glass shards from entering the patient during administration.
17. Discard the ampule in a suitable container.	Any medication that has not been removed from the ampule must be discarded because sterility of contents cannot be maintained in an opened ampule.
18. Lock the medication cart before leaving it.	Locking the cart or drawer safeguards the patient's medication supply. Hospital accrediting organizations require medication carts to be locked when not in use.

ACTION	RATIONALE
19. Perform hand hygiene.	Hand hygiene deters the spread of microorganisms.
20. Proceed with administration, based on prescribed route.	See appropriate skill for prescribed route.

EVALUATION

The expected outcome is met when the medication is removed from the ampule in a sterile manner, is free from glass shards, and the proper dose is prepared.

DOCUMENTATION

Guidelines

It is not necessary to record the removal of the medication from the ampule. Prompt recording of administration of the medication is required immediately after it is administered.

UNEXPECTED SITUATIONS AND ASSOCIATED INTERVENTIONS

- *You cut yourself while trying to open the ampule:* Discard ampule in case contamination has occurred. Clean and bandage the wound and obtain a new ampule. Report according to facility policy.
- *All of medication was not removed from the stem and insufficient medication remains in body of ampule for dose:* Discard ampule and drawn medication. Obtain a new ampule and start over. Medication in original ampule stem is considered contaminated once neck of ampule has been placed on a nonsterile surface.
- *You inject air into inverted ampule, spraying medication:* Wash hands to remove any medication. If any medication has gotten into eyes, perform eye irrigation. Obtain a new ampule for medication dose. Report injury, if appropriate, according to facility policy.
- *Medication is drawn up without using a filter needle:* Replace needle with a filter needle. Inject the medication through the filter needle into a new syringe and then administer to patient.
- *Plunger becomes contaminated before inserted into ampule:* Discard needle and syringe and start over. If plunger is contaminated after medication is drawn into the syringe, it is not necessary to discard and start over. The contaminated plunger will enter the barrel of the syringe when pushing the medication out and will not contaminate the medication.

SKILL 5-4 REMOVING MEDICATION FROM A VIAL

A vial is a glass bottle with a self-sealing stopper through which medication is removed. For safety in transporting and storing, the vial top is usually covered with a soft metal cap that can be removed easily. The self-sealing stopper that is then exposed is the means of entrance into the vial. Single-dose vials are used once, and then discarded, regardless of the amount of the drug that is used from the vial. Multi-dose vials contain several doses of medication and can be used multiple times. The Centers for Disease Control and Prevention (CDC) recommends that medications packaged as multiuse vials be assigned to a single patient whenever possible (CDC, 2011). In addition, it is recommended that the top of the vial be cleaned before each entry, and that a new sterile needle and syringe are used for each entry. The medication contained in a vial can be in liquid or powder form. Powdered forms must be dissolved in an appropriate diluent before administration. The following skill reviews removing liquid medication from a vial. Refer to the accompanying Skill Variation for steps to reconstitute powdered medication.

DELEGATION CONSIDERATIONS

The preparation of medication from a vial is not delegated to nursing assistive personnel (NAP) or to unlicensed assistive personnel (UAP). Depending on the state's nurse practice act and the organization's policies and procedures, the preparation of medication from a vial may be delegated to licensed practical/vocational nurses (LPN/LVNs). The decision to delegate must be based on careful analysis of the patient's needs and circumstances, as well as the qualifications of the person to whom the task is being delegated. Refer to the Delegation Guidelines in Appendix A.

(continued)

SKILL 5-4 REMOVING MEDICATION FROM A VIAL continued

EQUIPMENT

- Sterile syringe and needle or blunt cannula (size depends on medication being administered)
- Vial of medication
- Antimicrobial swab
- Second needle (optional)
- Filter needle (optional)
- Computer-generated Medication Administration Record (CMAR) or Medication Administration Record (MAR)

ASSESSMENT

Assess the medication in the vial for any discoloration or particles. Check expiration date before administering medication. Verify patient name, dose, route, and time of administration. Assess the appropriateness of the drug for the patient. Review assessment and laboratory data that may influence drug administration.

NURSING DIAGNOSIS

Determine related factors for the nursing diagnoses based on the patient's current status. Appropriate nursing diagnoses include:

- Risk for Infection
- Deficient Knowledge
- Risk for Injury

OUTCOME IDENTIFICATION AND PLANNING

The expected outcome to achieve when removing medication from a vial is withdrawal of the medication into a syringe in a sterile manner and preparation of the proper dose.

IMPLEMENTATION

ACTION	RATIONALE
1. Gather equipment. Check the medication order against the original order in the medical record, according to facility policy. Clarify any inconsistencies. Check the patient's chart for allergies.	This comparison helps to identify errors that may have occurred when orders were transcribed. The primary care provider's order is the legal record of medication orders for each facility.
2. Know the actions, special nursing considerations, safe dose ranges, purpose of administration, and adverse effects of the medications to be administered. Consider the appropriateness of the medication for this patient.	This knowledge aids the nurse in evaluating the therapeutic effect of the medication in relation to the patient's disorder and can also be used to educate the patient about the medication.
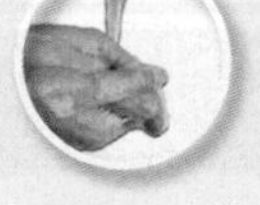 3. Perform hand hygiene.	Hand hygiene deters the spread of microorganisms.
4. Move the medication cart to the outside of the patient's room or prepare for administration in the medication area.	Organization facilitates error-free administration and saves time.
5. Unlock the medication cart or drawer. Enter pass code and scan employee identification, if required.	Locking the cart or drawer safeguards each patient's medication supply. Hospital accrediting organizations require medication carts to be locked when not in use. Entering pass code and scanning ID allows only authorized users into the system and identifies the user for documentation by the computer.
6. **Prepare medications for one patient at a time.**	This prevents errors in medication administration.
7. Read the CMAR/MAR and select the proper medication from unit stock or the patient's medication drawer.	This is the *first* check of the label.
8. Compare the label with the CMAR/MAR. Check expiration dates and perform calculations, if necessary. Scan the bar code on the package, if required.	This is the *second* check of the label. Verify calculations with another nurse to ensure safety, if necessary.
9. Remove the metal or plastic cap on the vial that protects the rubber stopper.	Cap needs to be removed to access medication in the vial.

ACTION	RATIONALE
10. **Swab the rubber top with the antimicrobial swab and allow to dry.**	Antimicrobial swab removes surface bacterial contamination. Allowing the alcohol to dry prevents it from entering the vial on the needle.
11. Remove the cap from the needle or blunt cannula by pulling it straight off. Touch the plunger only at the knob. Draw back an amount of air into the syringe that is equal to the specific dose of medication to be withdrawn. Some facilities require use of a filter needle when withdrawing premixed medication from multidose vials.	Pulling the cap off in a straight manner prevents accidental needlestick injury. Handling the plunger only at the knob will keep the shaft of the plunger sterile. Because a vial is a sealed container, injection of an equal amount of air (before fluid is removed) is required to prevent the formation of a partial vacuum. If not enough air is injected, the negative pressure makes it difficult to withdraw the medication. Using a filter needle prevents any solid material from being withdrawn through the needle.
12. Hold the vial on a flat surface. Pierce the rubber stopper in the center with the needle tip and inject the measured air into the space above the solution (Figure 1). Do not inject air into the solution.	Air bubbled through the solution could result in withdrawal of an inaccurate amount of medication.
13. Invert the vial. **Keep the tip of the needle or blunt cannula below the fluid level (Figure 2).**	This prevents air from being aspirated into the syringe.
14. Hold the vial in one hand and use the other to withdraw the medication. **Touch the plunger only at the knob. Draw up the prescribed amount of medication while holding the syringe vertically and at eye level (Figure 3).**	Handling the plunger only at the knob will keep the shaft of the plunger sterile. Holding the syringe at eye level facilitates accurate reading, and the vertical position makes removal of air bubbles from the syringe easy.

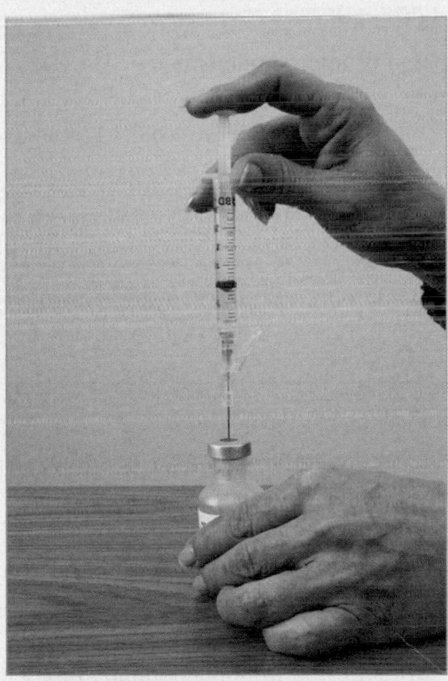

FIGURE 1 Injecting air with vial upright.

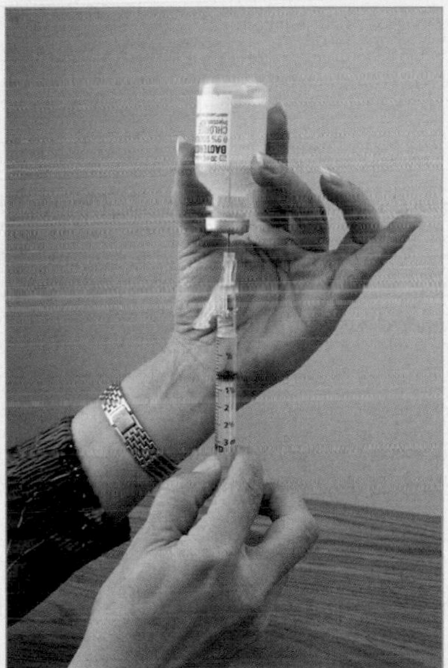

FIGURE 2 Positioning needle tip in solution.

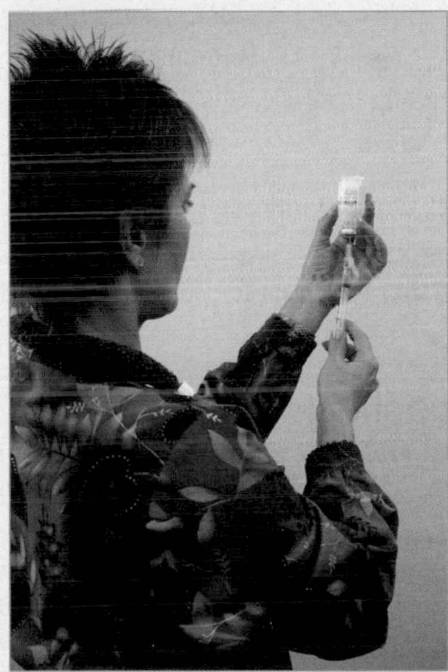

FIGURE 3 Withdrawing medication at eye level.

ACTION	RATIONALE
15. If any air bubbles accumulate in the syringe, tap the barrel of the syringe sharply and move the needle past the fluid into the air space to re-inject the air bubble into the vial. Return the needle tip to the solution and continue withdrawal of the medication.	Removal of air bubbles is necessary to ensure an accurate dose of medication.

(*continued*)

SKILL 5-4 REMOVING MEDICATION FROM A VIAL continued

ACTION	RATIONALE
16. After the correct dose is withdrawn, remove the needle from the vial and carefully replace the cap over the needle. **If a filter needle has been used to draw up the medication, remove it and attach the appropriate administration device.** Some facilities require changing the needle, if one was used to withdraw the medication, before administering the medication.	This prevents contamination of the needle and protects against accidental needlesticks. A one-handed recap method may be used as long as care is taken not to contaminate the needle during the process. A filter needle used to draw up medication should not be used to administer the medication to prevent any solid material from entering the patient. Changing the needle may be necessary because passing the needle through the stopper on the vial may dull the needle. In addition, it ensures the tip of the needle is free from medication residue, significantly reducing pain intensity associated with the injection (Ağaç & Güneş, 2010).
17. **Check the amount of medication in the syringe with the medication dose and discard any surplus.**	Careful measurement ensures that the correct dose is withdrawn.
18. **Depending on facility policy, the third check of the label may occur at this point. If so, when all medications for one patient have been prepared, recheck the labels with the CMAR/MAR before taking the medications to the patient.**	This *third* check ensures accuracy and helps to prevent errors. *Note:* Many facilities require the *third* check to occur at the bedside, after identifying the patient and before administration.
19. **If a multidose vial is being used, label the vial with the date and time opened, and store the vial containing the remaining medication according to facility policy.**	Because the vial is sealed, the medication inside remains sterile and can be used for future injections. Labeling the opened vials with a date and time limits its use after a specific time period.
20. Lock the medication cart before leaving it.	Locking the cart or drawer safeguards the patient's medication supply. Hospital accrediting organizations require medication carts to be locked when not in use.
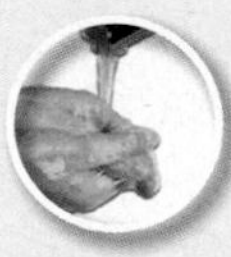 21. Perform hand hygiene.	Hand hygiene deters the spread of microorganisms.
22. Proceed with administration, based on prescribed route.	See appropriate skill for prescribed route.

EVALUATION

The expected outcome is met when the medication is withdrawn into the syringe in a sterile manner and the proper dose is prepared.

DOCUMENTATION

Guidelines

It is not necessary to record the removal of the medication from the ampule. Prompt recording of administration of the medication is required immediately after it is administered.

UNEXPECTED SITUATIONS AND ASSOCIATED INTERVENTIONS

- *A piece of rubber stopper is noticed floating in the medication in the syringe:* Discard the syringe, needle, and vial. Obtain a new vial, syringe, and needle and prepare dose as ordered.
- *As needle attached to syringe filled with air is inserted into vial, the plunger is immediately pulled down:* If possible to withdraw medication, continue steps as explained above. If such a vacuum has formed that this is impossible, remove syringe and inject more air into the vial. This is caused by previous withdrawal of medication without the addition of air into the vial.
- *Plunger is contaminated before injecting air into vial:* Discard needle and syringe and start over.
- *Plunger is contaminated after medication is drawn into syringe:* It is not necessary to discard needle and syringe and start over. The contaminated plunger will enter the barrel of the syringe when pushing the medication out and will not contaminate the medication.

SKILL VARIATION Reconstituting Powdered Medication in a Vial

Drugs that are unstable in liquid form are often provided in a dry powder form. The powder must be mixed with the correct amount of appropriate solution to prepare the medication for administration. Verify the correct amount and correct solution type for the specific medication prescribed. This information is found on the vial label, package insert, in a drug reference, an on-line pharmacy source, or from the pharmacist. To reconstitute powdered medication:

1. Gather equipment. Check the medication order against the original order in the medical record, according to agency policy.
2. Know the actions, special nursing considerations, safe dose ranges, purpose of administration, and adverse effects of the medications to be administered. Consider the appropriateness of the medication for this patient.
3. Perform hand hygiene.

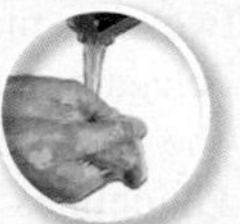

4. Move the medication cart to the outside of the patient's room or prepare for administration in the medication area.
5. Unlock the medication cart or drawer. Enter pass code and scan employee identification, if required.
6. **Prepare medications for one patient at a time.**
7. Read the CMAR/MAR and select the proper medication and diluent from unit stock or from the patient's medication drawer. This is the *first* check of the medication label.
8. Compare the labels with the CMAR/MAR. This is the *second* check of the medication label. Check expiration dates and perform calculations, check medication calculation with another nurse. Scan the bar code on the package, if required.
9. Remove the metal or plastic cap on the medication vial and diluent vial that protects the self-sealing stoppers.
10. Swab the self-sealing tops with the antimicrobial swab and allow to dry.
11. **Draw up the appropriate amount of diluent into the syringe.**
12. Insert the needle or blunt cannula through the center of the self-sealing stopper on the powdered medication vial.
13. Inject the diluent into the powdered medication vial.
14. Remove the needle or blunt cannula from the vial and replace cap.
15. **Gently agitate the vial to mix the powdered medication and the diluent completely. Do not shake the vial.**
16. **Draw up the prescribed amount of medication while holding the syringe vertically and at eye level.**
17. After the correct dose is withdrawn, remove the needle from the vial and carefully replace the cap over the needle. **If a filter needle has been used to draw up the medication, remove it and attach the appropriate administration device.** Some facilities require changing the needle, if one was used to withdraw the medication, before administering the medication.
18. **Check the amount of medication in the syringe with the medication dose and discard any surplus.**
19. **Depending on facility policy, the third check of the label may occur at this point. If so, recheck the label with the CMAR/MAR before taking the medications to the patient.**
20. Lock the medication cart before leaving it.
21. Perform hand hygiene.

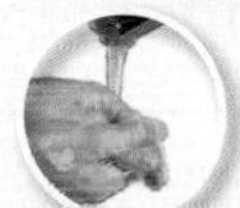

22. Proceed with administration, based on prescribed route.

SKILL 5-5 MIXING MEDICATIONS FROM TWO VIALS IN ONE SYRINGE

Preparation of medications in one syringe depends on how the medication is supplied. When using a single-dose vial and a multidose vial, air is injected into both vials and the medication in the multidose vial is drawn into the syringe first. This prevents the contents of the multidose vial from being contaminated with the medication in the single-dose vial. The CDC recommends that medications packaged as multiuse vials be assigned to a single patient whenever possible (CDC, 2011). In addition, it is recommended that the top of the vial be cleaned before each entry, and that a new sterile needle and syringe are used before each entry.

When considering mixing two medications in one syringe, you must ensure that the two drugs are compatible. Be aware of drug incompatibilities when preparing medications in one syringe. Certain medications, such as diazepam (Valium), are incompatible with other drugs in the same syringe. Incompatible drugs may become cloudy or form a precipitate in the syringe. Such medications are discarded and prepared again in separate syringes. Other drugs have limited compatibility and should be administered within 15 minutes of preparation. Mixing more than two drugs in one

(continued)

SKILL 5-5 MIXING MEDICATIONS FROM TWO VIALS IN ONE SYRINGE continued

syringe is not recommended. If it must be done, contact the pharmacist to determine the compatibility of the three drugs, as well as the compatibility of their pH values and the preservatives that may be present in each drug. A drug-compatibility table should be available to nurses who are preparing medications.

Insulin, with many types available for use, is an example of a medication that may be combined together in one syringe for injection. Insulins vary in their onset and duration of action and are classified as rapid acting, short acting, intermediate acting, and long acting. Before administering any insulin, be aware of the onset time, peak, and duration of effects, and ensure that proper food is available. Be aware that some insulins, such as Lantus and Levemir, cannot be mixed with other insulins. Refer to a drug reference for a listing of the different types of insulin and action specific to each type. Insulin dosages are calculated in units. The scale commonly used is U100, which is based on 100 units of insulin contained in 1 mL of solution.

DELEGATION CONSIDERATIONS

The preparation of medication from two vials is not delegated to nursing assistive personnel (NAP) or to unlicensed assistive personnel (UAP). Depending on the state's nurse practice act and the organization's policies and procedures, the preparation of medication from two vials may be delegated to licensed practical/vocational nurses (LPN/LVNs). The decision to delegate must be based on careful analysis of the patient's needs and circumstances, as well as the qualifications of the person to whom the task is being delegated. Refer to the Delegation Guidelines in Appendix A.

EQUIPMENT

The preparation of two types of insulin in one syringe is used as the example in the following procedure.

- Two vials of medication (insulin in this example)
- Sterile syringe (insulin syringe in this example)
- Antimicrobial swabs
- Computer-generated Medication Administration Record (CMAR) or Medication Administration Record (MAR)

ASSESSMENT

Determine the compatibility of the two medications. Not all insulin can be mixed together. For example, Lantus and Levemir cannot be mixed with another insulin.

Assess the contents of each vial of insulin. It is very important to be familiar with the particular drug's properties to be able to assess the quality of the medication in the vial before withdrawal. Unmodified preparations of insulin typically appear as clear substances, so they should be without particles or foreign matter. Modified preparations of insulin are typically suspensions, so they do not appear as clear substances.

Check the expiration date before administering the medication. Assess the appropriateness of the drug for the patient. Review the assessment and laboratory data that may influence drug administration. Check the patient's blood glucose level, if appropriate, before administering the insulin. Verify patient name, dose, route, and time of administration.

NURSING DIAGNOSIS

Determine related factors for the nursing diagnoses based on the patient's current status. Appropriate nursing diagnoses include:

- Risk for Infection
- Deficient Knowledge
- Risk for Injury

OUTCOME IDENTIFICATION AND PLANNING

The expected outcome to achieve when mixing two different types of medication in one syringe is the accurate withdrawal of the medication into a syringe in a sterile manner and that the proper dose is prepared.

IMPLEMENTATION

ACTION	RATIONALE
1. Gather equipment. Check medication order against the original order in the medical record, according to facility policy.	This comparison helps to identify errors that may have occurred when orders were transcribed. The primary care provider's order is the legal record of medication orders for each facility.
2. Know the actions, special nursing considerations, safe dose ranges, purpose of administration, and adverse effects of the medications to be administered. Consider the appropriateness of the medication for this patient.	This knowledge aids the nurse in evaluating the therapeutic effect of the medication in relation to the patient's disorder and can also be used to educate the patient about the medication.
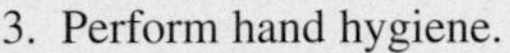 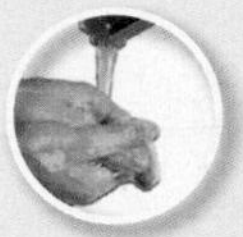 3. Perform hand hygiene.	Hand hygiene prevents the spread of microorganisms.
4. Move the medication cart to the outside of the patient's room or prepare for administration in the medication area.	Organization facilitates error-free administration and saves time.
5. Unlock the medication cart or drawer. Enter pass code and scan employee identification, if required.	Locking the cart or drawer safeguards each patient's medication supply. Hospital accrediting organizations require medication carts to be locked when not in use. Entering pass code and scanning ID allows only authorized users into the system and identifies the user for documentation by the computer.
6. **Prepare medications for one patient at a time.**	This prevents errors in medication administration.
7. Read the CMAR/MAR and select the proper medications from unit stock or the patient's medication drawer.	This is the *first* check of the label.
8. Compare the labels with the CMAR/MAR. Check expiration dates and perform dosage calculations, if necessary. Scan the bar code on the package, if required.	This is the *second* check of the labels. Verify calculations with another nurse to ensure safety, if necessary.
9. If necessary, remove the cap that protects the rubber stopper on each vial.	The cap protects the rubber top.
10. **If medication is a suspension (e.g., a modified insulin, such as NPH insulin), roll and agitate the vial to mix it well.**	There is controversy regarding how to mix insulin in suspension. Some sources advise rolling the vial; others advise shaking the vial. Consult facility policy. Regardless of the method used, it is essential that the suspension be mixed well to avoid administering an inconsistent dose.
11. **Cleanse the rubber tops with antimicrobial swabs.** Allow the top to dry.	Antimicrobial swab removes surface bacterial contamination. Allowing the alcohol to dry prevents it from entering the vial on the needle.
12. Remove cap from needle by pulling it straight off. Touch the plunger only at the knob. Draw back an amount of air into the syringe that is equal to the dose of modified insulin to be withdrawn.	Pulling the cap off in a straight manner prevents accidental needlestick. Handling the plunger only by the knob ensures sterility of the shaft of the plunger. Before fluid is removed, injection of an equal amount of air is required to prevent the formation of a partial vacuum, because a vial is a sealed container. If not enough air is injected, the negative pressure makes it difficult to withdraw the medication.
13. Hold the modified vial on a flat surface. Pierce the rubber stopper in the center with the needle tip and inject the measured air into the space above the solution (Figure 1). Do not inject air into the solution. Withdraw the needle.	Unmodified insulin should never be contaminated with modified insulin. Placing air in the modified insulin first without allowing the needle to contact the insulin ensures that the second vial-entered (unmodified) insulin is not contaminated by the medication in the other vial. Air bubbled through the solution could result in withdrawal of an inaccurate amount of medication.

(*continued*)

SKILL 5-5 MIXING MEDICATIONS FROM TWO VIALS IN ONE SYRINGE continued

ACTION	RATIONALE
14. Draw back an amount of air into the syringe that is equal to the dose of unmodified insulin to be withdrawn.	A vial is a sealed container. Therefore, injection of an equal amount of air (before fluid is removed) is required to prevent the formation of a partial vacuum. If not enough air is injected, the negative pressure makes it difficult to withdraw the medication.
15. Hold the unmodified vial on a flat surface. Pierce the rubber stopper in the center with the needle tip and inject the measured air into the space above the solution (Figure 2). Do not inject air into the solution. Keep the needle in the vial.	Air bubbled through the solution could result in withdrawal of an inaccurate amount of medication.

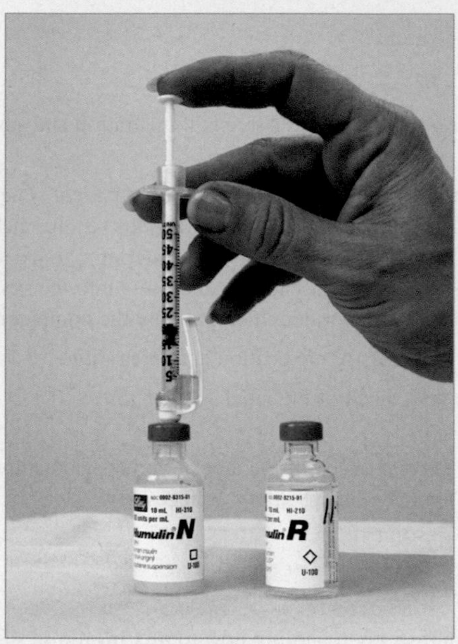

FIGURE 1 Injecting air into modified insulin preparation.

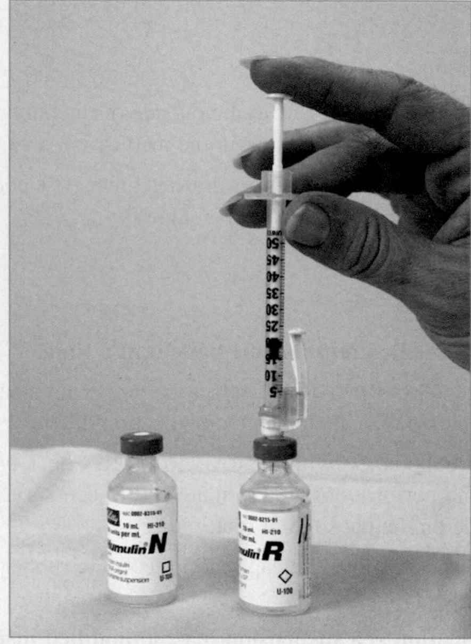

FIGURE 2 Injecting air into unmodified insulin vial.

ACTION	RATIONALE
16. Invert the vial of unmodified insulin. Hold the vial in one hand and use the other to withdraw the medication. **Touch the plunger only at the knob. Draw up the prescribed amount of medication while holding the syringe at eye level and vertically (Figure 3).** Turn the vial over and then remove the needle from the vial.	Holding the syringe at eye level facilitates accurate reading, and the vertical position allows easy removal of air bubbles from the syringe. First dose is prepared and is not contaminated by insulin that contains modifiers.
17. Check that there are no air bubbles in the syringe.	The presence of air in the syringe would result in an inaccurate dose of medication.
18. **Check the amount of medication in the syringe with the medication dose and discard any surplus.**	Careful measurement ensures that correct dose is withdrawn.
19. **Recheck the vial label with the CMAR/MAR.**	This is the *third* check to ensure accuracy and to prevent errors. It must be checked now for the first medication in the syringe, as it is not possible to ensure accuracy once a second drug is in the syringe.
20. Calculate the endpoint on the syringe for the combined insulin amount by adding the number of units for each dose together.	Allows for accurate withdrawal of the second dose.

ACTION	RATIONALE
21. Insert the needle into the modified vial and invert it, taking care not to push the plunger and inject medication from the syringe into the vial. Invert vial of modified insulin. Hold the vial in one hand and use the other to withdraw the medication. **Touch the plunger only at the knob. Draw up the prescribed amount of medication while holding the syringe at eye level and vertically (Figure 4). Take care to withdraw only the prescribed amount.** Turn the vial over and then remove the needle from the vial. Carefully recap the needle. Carefully replace the cap over the needle.	Previous addition of air eliminates need to create positive pressure. Holding the syringe at eye level facilitates accurate reading. Capping the needle prevents contamination and protects the nurse against accidental needlesticks. A one-handed recap method may be used as long as care is taken to ensure that the needle remains sterile.

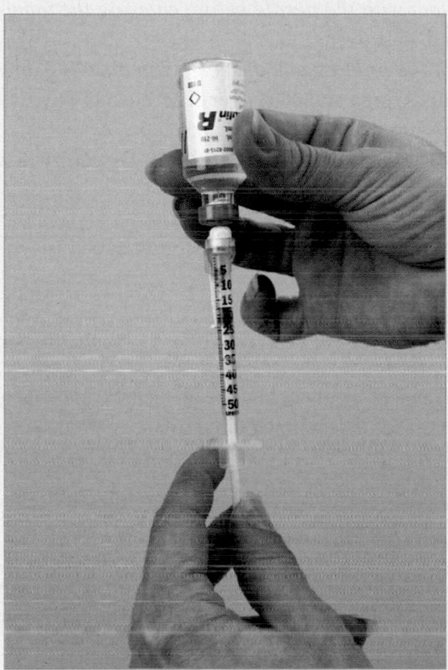

FIGURE 3 Withdrawing prescribed amount of unmodified insulin.

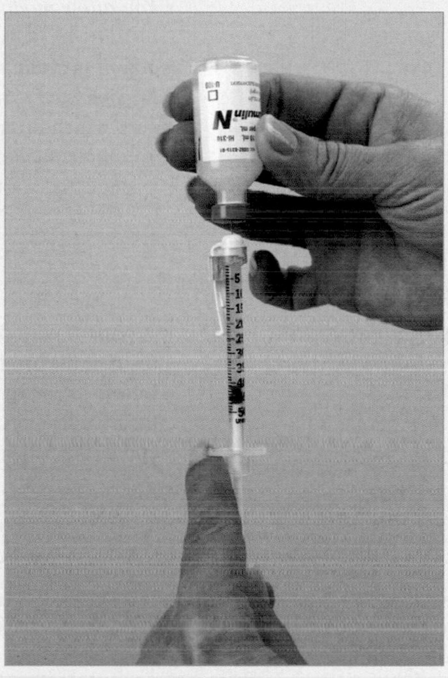

FIGURE 4 Withdrawing modified insulin.

ACTION	RATIONALE
22. **Check the amount of medication in the syringe with the medication dose.**	Careful measurement ensures that correct dose is withdrawn.
23. **Depending on facility policy, the third check of the label may occur at this point. If so, recheck the label with the MAR before taking the medications to the patient.**	This *third* check ensures accuracy and helps to prevent errors. *Note:* Many facilities require the *third* check to occur at the bedside, after identifying the patient and before administration.
24. **Label the vials with the date and time opened, and store the vials containing the remaining medication, according to facility policy.**	Because the vial is sealed, the medication inside remains sterile and can be used for future injections. Labeling the opened vials with a date and time limits its use after a specific time period. The CDC recommends that medications packaged as multiuse vials be assigned to a single patient whenever possible (CDC, 2011).
25. Lock medication cart before leaving it.	Locking the cart or drawer safeguards the patient's medication supply. Hospital accrediting organizations require medication carts to be locked when not in use.
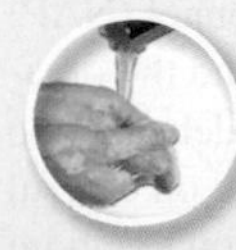 26. Perform hand hygiene.	Hand hygiene deters the spread of microorganisms.
27. Proceed with administration, based on prescribed route.	See appropriate skill for prescribed route.

(continued)

SKILL 5-5 MIXING MEDICATIONS FROM TWO VIALS IN ONE SYRINGE continued

EVALUATION

The expected outcome is met when the medication is withdrawn into a syringe in a sterile manner, and the proper dose is prepared.

DOCUMENTATION

Guidelines

It is not necessary to record the removal of the medication from the ampule. Prompt recording of administration of the medication is required immediately after it is administered.

UNEXPECTED SITUATIONS AND ASSOCIATED INTERVENTIONS

- *You contaminate the plunger before injecting air into the insulin vial:* Discard the needle and syringe and start over. *If plunger is contaminated after medication is drawn into the syringe,* it is not necessary to discard and start over. The contaminated plunger will enter the barrel of the syringe when pushing the medication out and will not contaminate the medication.
- *You allow modified insulin to come in contact with the needle before entering the unmodified insulin vial:* Discard needle and syringe and start over.
- *You notice that the combined amount is not the ordered amount (e.g., you have less or more units in combined syringe than ordered):* Discard syringe and start over. There is no way to know for sure which dosage is wrong or which medication should be expelled.
- *You inject medication from the first vial (in syringe) into the second vial:* Discard vial and syringe and start over.

SPECIAL CONSIDERATIONS

General Considerations

- A patient with diabetes who is visually impaired may find it helpful to use a magnifying apparatus that fits around the syringe.
- Before attempting to explain or demonstrate devices that help low-vision diabetic patients to prepare their medication, attempt to use the device yourself under similar circumstances. To detect any difficulties the patient may experience, practice using the aid with your eyes closed or in a poorly lit room.

Infant and Child Considerations

School-age children are generally able to prepare and administer their own injections, such as insulin, with supervision (Kyle & Carman, 2013). Parents/significant others and the child should be involved in teaching.

SKILL 5-6 ADMINISTERING AN INTRADERMAL INJECTION

Intradermal injections are administered into the dermis, just below the epidermis. The intradermal route has the longest absorption time of all parenteral routes. For this reason, intradermal injections are used for sensitivity tests, such as tuberculin and allergy tests, and local anesthesia. The advantage of the intradermal route for these tests is that the body's reaction to substances is easily visible, and degrees of reaction are discernible by comparative study.

Sites commonly used are the inner surface of the forearm and the upper back, under the scapula. Equipment used for an intradermal injection includes a tuberculin syringe calibrated in tenths and hundredths of a milliliter and a 0.25- to 0.5-inch, 25- or 27-gauge needle. The dosage given intradermally is small, usually less than 0.5 mL. The angle of administration for an intradermal injection is 5 to 15 degrees (see Figure 5-1 in the chapter opener).

DELEGATION CONSIDERATIONS

The administration of an intradermal injection is not delegated to nursing assistive personnel (NAP) or to unlicensed assistive personnel (UAP). Depending on the state's nurse practice act and the organization's policies and procedures, the administration of an intradermal injection may be delegated to licensed practical/vocational nurses (LPN/LVNs). The decision to delegate must be based on careful analysis of the patient's needs and circumstances, as well as the qualifications of the person to whom the task is being delegated. Refer to the Delegation Guidelines in Appendix A.

EQUIPMENT

- Prescribed medication
- Sterile syringe, usually a tuberculin syringe calibrated in tenths and hundredths, and a needle, ¼- to ½-inch, 25- or 27-gauge
- Antimicrobial swab
- Disposable gloves
- Small gauze square
- Computer-generated Medication Administration Record (CMAR) or Medication Administration Record (MAR)
- PPE, as indicated

ASSESSMENT

Assess the patient for any allergies. Check expiration date before administering medication. Assess the appropriateness of the drug for the patient. Review assessment and laboratory data that may influence drug administration. Assess the site on the patient where the injection is to be given. Avoid areas of broken or open skin. Avoid areas that are highly pigmented, and those that have lesions, bruises, or scars and are hairy. Assess the patient's knowledge of the medication. This may provide an opportune time for patient education. Verify the patient's name, dose, route, and time of administration.

NURSING DIAGNOSIS

Determine related factors for the nursing diagnoses based on the patient's current status. Appropriate nursing diagnoses may include:

- Deficient Knowledge
- Risk for Infection
- Risk for Injury

OUTCOME IDENTIFICATION AND PLANNING

The expected outcome to achieve when administering an intradermal injection is the appearance of a wheal at the injection site. Other outcomes that may be appropriate include the following: the patient refrains from rubbing the site; the patient's anxiety is decreased; the patient does not experience adverse effects; and the patient understands and complies with the medication regimen.

IMPLEMENTATION

ACTION	RATIONALE
1. Gather equipment. Check each medication order against the original order in the medical record according to facility policy. Clarify any inconsistencies. Check the patient's chart for allergies.	This comparison helps to identify errors that may have occurred when orders were transcribed. The primary care provider's order is the legal record of medication orders for each facility.
2. Know the actions, special nursing considerations, safe dose ranges, purpose of administration, and adverse effects of the medications to be administered. Consider the appropriateness of the medication for this patient.	This knowledge aids the nurse in evaluating the therapeutic effect of the medication in relation to the patient's disorder and can also be used to educate the patient about the medication.
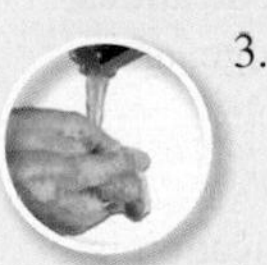 3. Perform hand hygiene.	Hand hygiene deters the spread of microorganisms.
4. Move the medication cart to the outside of the patient's room or prepare for administration in the medication area.	Organization facilitates error-free administration and saves time.
5. Unlock the medication cart or drawer. Enter pass code and scan employee identification, if required.	Locking the cart or drawer safeguards each patient's medication supply. Hospital accrediting organizations require medication carts to be locked when not in use. Entering pass code and scanning ID allows only authorized users into the system and identifies the user for documentation by the computer.
6. **Prepare medications for one patient at a time.**	This prevents errors in medication administration.
7. Read the CMAR/MAR and select the proper medication from unit stock or the patient's medication drawer.	This is the *first* check of the label.

(continued)

SKILL 5-6 ADMINISTERING AN INTRADERMAL INJECTION continued

ACTION	RATIONALE
8. Compare the label with the CMAR/MAR. Check expiration dates and perform calculations, if necessary. Scan the bar code on the package, if required.	This is the *second* check of the label. Verify calculations with another nurse to ensure safety.
9. If necessary, withdraw the medication from an ampule or vial as described in Skills 5-3 and 5-4.	
10. **Depending on facility policy, the third check of the label may occur at this point. If so, when all medications for one patient have been prepared, recheck the labels with the CMAR/MAR before taking the medications to the patient.**	This *third* check ensures accuracy and helps to prevent errors. *Note:* Many facilities require the *third* check to occur at the bedside, after identifying the patient and before administration.
11. Lock the medication cart before leaving it.	Locking the cart or drawer safeguards the patient's medication supply. Hospital accrediting organizations require medication carts to be locked when not in use.
12. Transport medications to the patient's bedside carefully, and keep the medications in sight at all times.	Careful handling and close observation prevent accidental or deliberate disarrangement of medications.
13. **Ensure that the patient receives the medications at the correct time.**	Check agency policy, which may allow for administration within a period of 30 minutes before or 30 minutes after the designated time.
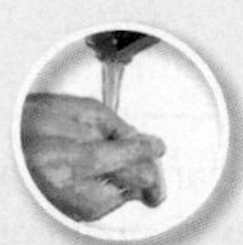 14. Perform hand hygiene and put on PPE, if indicated.	Hand hygiene and PPE prevent the spread of microorganisms. PPE is required based on transmission precautions.
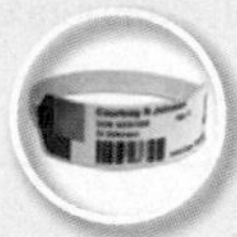 15. **Identify the patient. Compare the information with the CMAR/MAR. The patient should be identified using at least two methods** (The Joint Commission, 2013):	Identifying the patient ensures the right patient receives the medications and helps prevent errors. The patient's room number or physical location is not used as an identifier (The Joint Commission, 2013). Replace the identification band if it is missing or inaccurate in any way.
a. Check the name on the patient's identification band.	
b. Check the identification number on the patient's identification band.	
c. Check the birth date on the patient's identification band.	
d. Ask the patient to state his or her name and birth date, based on facility policy.	This requires a response from the patient, but illness and strange surroundings often cause patients to be confused.
16. Close the door to the room or pull the bedside curtain.	This provides patient privacy.
17. **Complete necessary assessments before administering medications. Check allergy bracelet or ask the patient about allergies. Explain the purpose and action of the medication to the patient.**	Assessment is a prerequisite to administration of medications. Explanation provides rationale, increases knowledge, and reduces anxiety.
18. Scan the patient's bar code on the identification band, if required.	Provides an additional check to ensure that the medication is given to the right patient.
19. **Based on facility policy, the third check of the label may occur at this point. If so, recheck the labels with the CMAR/MAR before administering the medications to the patient.**	Many facilities require the *third* check to occur at the bedside, after identifying the patient and before administration. If facility policy directs the *third* check at this time, this *third* check ensures accuracy and helps to prevent errors.
20. Put on clean gloves.	Gloves help prevent exposure to contaminants.
21. Select an appropriate administration site. Assist the patient to the appropriate position for the site chosen. Drape, as needed, to expose only site area to be used.	Appropriate site prevents injury and allows for accurate reading of the test site at the appropriate time. Draping provides privacy and warmth.
22. Cleanse the site with an antimicrobial swab while wiping with a firm, circular motion and moving outward from the injection site. Allow the skin to dry.	Pathogens on the skin can be forced into the tissues by the needle. Moving from the center outward prevents contamination of the site. Allowing skin to dry prevents introducing alcohol into the tissue, which can be irritating and uncomfortable.

ACTION	RATIONALE
23. Remove the needle cap with the nondominant hand by pulling it straight off.	This technique lessens the risk of an accidental needlestick.
24. Use the nondominant hand to spread the skin taut over the injection site (Figure 1).	Taut skin provides an easy entrance into intradermal tissue.
25. Hold the syringe in the dominant hand, between the thumb and forefinger with the bevel of the needle up.	Using the dominant hand allows for easy, appropriate handling of the syringe. Having the bevel up allows for smooth piercing of the skin and introduction of medication into the dermis.
26. Hold the syringe at a 5- to 15-degree angle from the site. Place the needle almost flat against the patient's skin (Figure 2), bevel side up, and insert the needle into the skin. Insert the needle only about 1/8 inch with entire bevel under the skin.	The dermis is entered when the needle is held as nearly parallel to the skin as possible and is inserted about 1/8 inch.

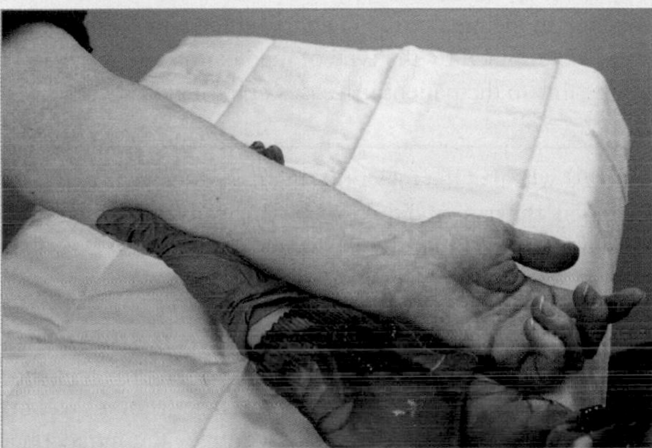
FIGURE 1 Spreading skin taut over injection site.

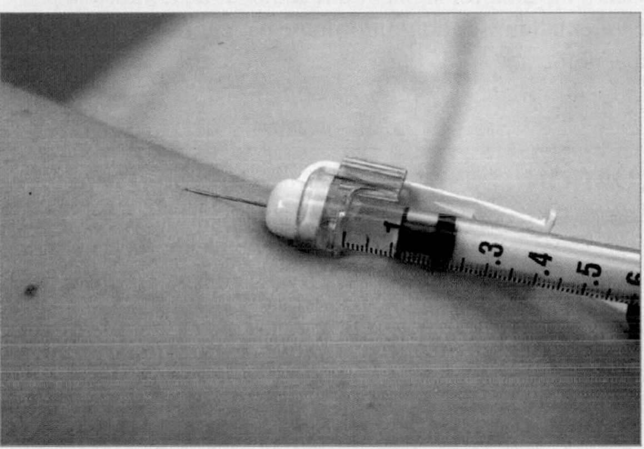

FIGURE 2 Inserting needle almost level with skin.

ACTION	RATIONALE
27. Once the needle is in place, steady the lower end of the syringe. Slide your dominant hand to the end of the plunger.	Prevents injury and inadvertent advancement or withdrawal of needle.
28. Slowly inject the agent while watching for a small wheal or blister to appear (Figure 3).	The appearance of a wheal indicates the medication is in the dermis.

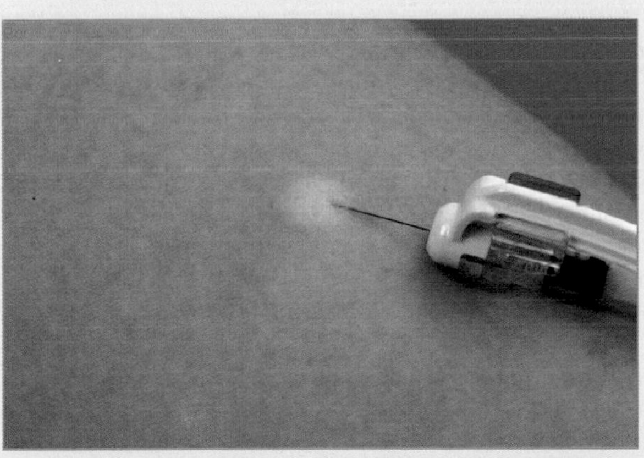
FIGURE 3 Observing for wheal while injecting medication.

ACTION	RATIONALE
29. Withdraw the needle quickly at the same angle that it was inserted. Do not recap the used needle. Engage the safety shield or needle guard.	Withdrawing the needle quickly and at the angle at which it entered the skin minimizes tissue damage and discomfort for the patient. Safety shield or needle guard prevents accidental needlestick injury.
30. **Do not massage the area after removing needle. Tell the patient not to rub or scratch the site. If necessary, gently blot the site with a dry gauze square. Do not apply pressure or rub the site.**	Massaging the area where an intradermal injection is given may spread the medication to underlying subcutaneous tissue.

(continued)

SKILL 5-6 ADMINISTERING AN INTRADERMAL INJECTION continued

ACTION	RATIONALE
31. Assist the patient to a position of comfort.	This provides for the well-being of the patient.
32. Discard the needle and syringe in the appropriate receptacle.	Proper disposal of the needle prevents injury.
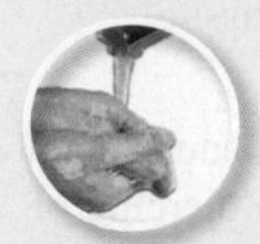 33. Remove gloves and additional PPE, if used. Perform hand hygiene.	Removing PPE properly reduces the risk for infection transmission and contamination of other items. Hand hygiene prevents the spread of microorganisms.
34. Document the administration of the medication immediately after administration. See Documentation section below.	Timely documentation helps to ensure patient safety.
35. Evaluate the patient's response to the medication within the appropriate time frame.	The patient needs to be evaluated for therapeutic and adverse effects from the medication.
36. Observe the area for signs of a reaction at determined intervals after administration. Inform the patient of the need for inspection.	With many intradermal injections, you need to look for a localized reaction in the area of the injection at the appropriate interval(s) determined by the type of medication and purpose. Explaining this to the patient increases compliance.

EVALUATION

The expected outcomes are met when you note a wheal at the injection site; the patient refrains from rubbing the site; the patient's anxiety is decreased; the patient did not experience adverse effects; and the patient verbalizes an understanding of, and complies with, the medication regimen.

DOCUMENTATION

Guidelines

Record each medication administered on the CMAR/MAR or record using the required format, including date, time, and the site of administration, immediately after administration. Some facilities recommend circling the injection site with ink. Circling the injection site easily identifies the intradermal injection site and allows for future careful observation of the exact area. If using a bar-code system, medication administration is automatically recorded when the bar code is scanned. PRN medications require documentation of the reason for administration. Prompt recording avoids the possibility of accidentally repeating the administration of the drug. If the drug was refused or omitted, record this in the appropriate area on the medication record and notify the primary care provider. This verifies the reason medication was omitted and ensures that the primary care provider is aware of the patient's condition.

UNEXPECTED SITUATIONS AND ASSOCIATED INTERVENTIONS

- *You do not note a wheal or blister at the injection site:* Medication has been injected subcutaneously. Document according to facility policy and inform the primary care provider. You may need to obtain an order to repeat the procedure.
- *Medication leaks out of the injection site before the needle is withdrawn:* Needle was inserted less than ⅛ inch. Document according to facility policy and inform the primary care provider. You may need to obtain an order to repeat the procedure.
- *You stick yourself with the needle before injection:* Discard needle and syringe appropriately. Follow facility policy regarding needlestick injury. Prepare new syringe with medication and administer to patient. Complete appropriate paperwork and follow facility's policy regarding accidental needlestick injuries.
- *You stick yourself with the needle after injection:* Discard needle and syringe appropriately. Follow facility policy regarding needlestick injury. Complete appropriate paperwork and follow facility's policy regarding accidental needlesticks.

SPECIAL CONSIDERATIONS

- Ongoing assessment is an important part of nursing care for both evaluation of patient response to administered medications and early detection of adverse effects. If an adverse effect is suspected, withhold further medication doses and notify the patient's primary care provider. Additional intervention is based on type of reaction and patient assessment.
- Aspiration, pulling back on the plunger after insertion and before administration, is not recommended for an intradermal injection. The dermis does not contain large blood vessels.
- Some agencies recommend administering intradermal injections with the bevel down instead of the bevel up. Check facility policy.

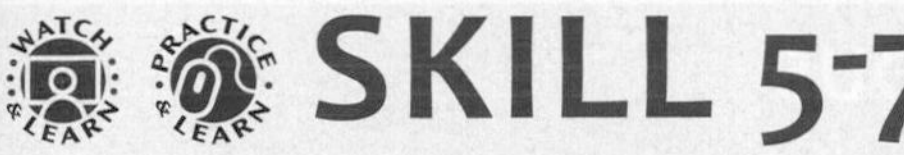

SKILL 5-7 ADMINISTERING A SUBCUTANEOUS INJECTION

Subcutaneous injections are administered into the adipose tissue layer just below the epidermis and dermis. This tissue has few blood vessels, so drugs administered here have a slow, sustained rate of absorption into the capillaries.

It is important to choose the right equipment to ensure depositing the medication into the intended tissue layer and not the underlying muscle. Equipment used for a subcutaneous injection includes a syringe of appropriate volume for the amount of drug being administered. An insulin injection pen may be used for subcutaneous injection of insulin (see the accompanying Skill Variation for technique). A 25- to 30-gauge, ⅜- to 1-inch needle can be used; ⅜- and ⅝-inch needles are most commonly used for subcutaneous injections. Choose the needle length based on the amount of subcutaneous tissue present, which is based on the patient's body weight and build (Annersten & Willman, 2005). Some medications are packaged in prefilled cartridges with a needle attached. Confirm that the provided needle is appropriate for the patient before use. If not, the medication will have to be transferred to another syringe and the appropriate needle attached.

Review the specifics of the particular medication before administrating it to the patient. Various sites may be used for subcutaneous injections, including the outer aspect of the upper arm, the abdomen (from below the costal margin to the iliac crests), the anterior aspects of the thigh, the upper back, and the upper ventral gluteal area. Figure 1 displays the sites on the body where subcutaneous injections can be given. Absorption rates differ at different sites. Injections in the abdomen are absorbed most rapidly; ones in the arms are absorbed somewhat more slowly; those in the thighs, even more slowly; and those in the upper ventral or dorsogluteal areas have the slowest absorption (American Diabetes Association [ADA], 2004).

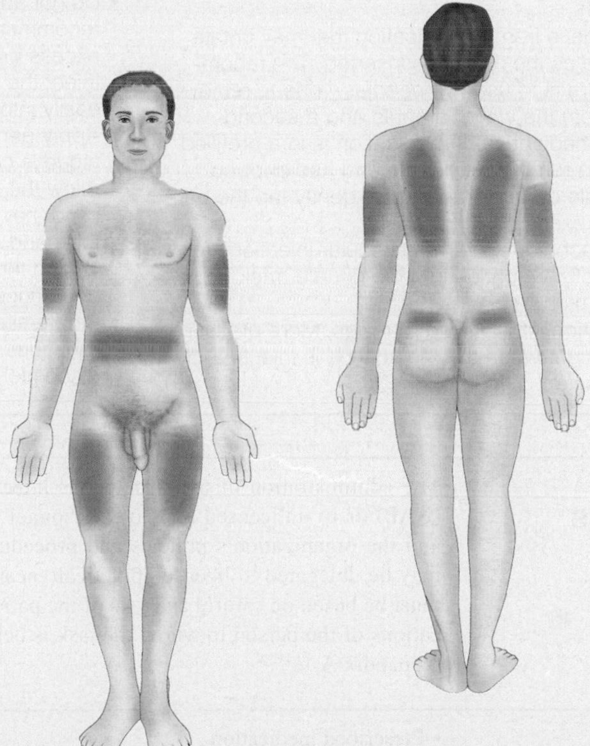

FIGURE 1 Body sites where subcutaneous injections can be given.

Subcutaneous injections are administered at a 45- to 90-degree angle. Choose the angle of needle insertion based on the amount of subcutaneous tissue present and the length of the needle. Generally, insert the shorter, ⅜-inch needle, at a 90-degree angle and the longer, ⅝-inch needle, at a 45-degree angle. Figure 5-1 in the chapter opener shows the angles of insertion for subcutaneous injections.

Recommendations differ regarding pinching or bunching a skin fold for administration. Pinching is advised for thinner patients and when a longer needle is used, to lift the adipose tissue away from underlying muscle and tissue. If pinching is used, once the needle is inserted, release the skin to avoid injecting into the compressed tissue.

(continued)

SKILL 5-7 ADMINISTERING A SUBCUTANEOUS INJECTION continued

Aspiration, or pulling back on the plunger to check that a blood vessel has been entered, is not necessary and has not proved to be a reliable indicator of needle placement. The likelihood of injecting into a blood vessel is small (Crawford & Johnson, 2012). The American Diabetes Association (2004) has stated that routine aspiration is not necessary when injecting insulin. **Aspiration is definitely contraindicated with administration of heparin because this action can result in hematoma formation.**

Usually, no more than 1 mL of solution is given subcutaneously. Giving larger amounts adds to the patient's discomfort and may predispose to poor absorption. It is necessary to rotate sites or areas for injection if the patient is to receive frequent injections. This helps to prevent buildup of fibrous tissue and permits complete absorption of the medication.

Box 5-1 discusses techniques for reducing discomfort when injecting medications subcutaneously or intramuscularly.

Box 5-1 REDUCING DISCOMFORT IN SUBCUTANEOUS AND INTRAMUSCULAR ADMINISTRATIONS

The following are recommended techniques for reducing discomfort when injecting medications subcutaneously or intramuscularly:

- Select a needle of the smallest gauge that is appropriate for the site and solution to be injected, and select the correct needle length.
- Be sure the needle is free of medication that may irritate superficial tissues as the needle is inserted. The recommended procedure is to use two needles—one to remove the medication from the vial or ampule and a second one to inject the medication. If medication is in a prefilled syringe with a non-removable needle and has dripped back on the needle during preparation, gently tap the barrel to remove the excess solution.
- Use the Z-track technique for intramuscular injections to prevent leakage of medication into the needle track, thus minimizing discomfort.
- Inject the medication into relaxed muscles. More pressure and discomfort occur when the medication is injected into a contracted muscle.
- Do not inject areas that feel hard on palpation or tender to the patient.
- Insert the needle with a dart-like motion without hesitation, and remove it quickly at the same angle at which it was inserted. These techniques reduce discomfort and tissue irritation.
- Do not administer more solution in one injection than is recommended for the site. Injecting more solution creates excess pressure in the area and increases discomfort.
- Inject the solution slowly so that it may be dispersed more easily into the surrounding tissue (10 seconds per 1 mL).
- Apply gentle pressure after injection, unless this technique is contraindicated.
- Allow the patient who is fearful of injections to talk about his or her fears. Answer the patient's questions truthfully, and explain the nature and purpose of the injection. Taking the time to offer support often allays fears and decreases discomfort.
- Rotate sites when the patient is to receive repeated injections. Injections in the same site may cause undue discomfort, irritation, or abscesses in tissues.

DELEGATION CONSIDERATIONS

The administration of a subcutaneous injection is not delegated to nursing assistive personnel (NAP) or to unlicensed assistive personnel (UAP). Depending on the state's nurse practice act and the organization's policies and procedures, the administration of a subcutaneous injection may be delegated to licensed practical/vocational nurses (LPN/LVNs). The decision to delegate must be based on careful analysis of the patient's needs and circumstances, as well as the qualifications of the person to whom the task is being delegated. Refer to the Delegation Guidelines in Appendix A.

EQUIPMENT

- Prescribed medication
- Sterile syringe and needle. Needle size depends on the medication to be administered and patient body type (see previous discussion).
- Antimicrobial swab
- Non-latex, disposable gloves
- Small gauze square
- Computer-generated Medication Administration Record (CMAR) or Medication Administration Record (MAR)
- PPE, as indicated

ASSESSMENT

Assess the patient for any allergies. Check expiration date before administering medication. Assess the appropriateness of the drug for the patient. Verify patient name, dose, route, and time of administration. Review assessment and laboratory data that may influence drug administration. Assess the site on the patient where the injection is to be given. Avoid sites that are bruised, tender, hard, swollen, inflamed, or scarred. These conditions could affect absorption or cause discomfort and injury (Hunter, 2008). Assess the patient's knowledge of the medication. If the patient has deficient knowledge about the medication, this may be the appropriate time to begin education about it. If the medication may affect the patient's vital signs, assess them before administration. If the medication is for pain relief, assess the patient's pain before and after administration.

NURSING DIAGNOSIS

Determine related factors for the nursing diagnoses based on the patient's current status. Appropriate nursing diagnoses may include:

- Deficient Knowledge
- Risk for Injury
- Acute Pain

OUTCOME IDENTIFICATION AND PLANNING

The expected outcome is that the patient receives the medication via the subcutaneous route. Other outcomes that may be appropriate include the following: the patient's anxiety is decreased; the patient does not experience adverse effects; and the patient understands and complies with the medication regimen.

IMPLEMENTATION

ACTION	RATIONALE
1. Gather equipment. Check each medication order against the original order in the medical record, according to facility policy. Clarify any inconsistencies. Check the patient's chart for allergies.	This comparison helps to identify errors that may have occurred when orders were transcribed. The primary care provider's order is the legal record of medication orders for each facility.
2. Know the actions, special nursing considerations, safe dose ranges, purpose of administration, and adverse effects of the medications to be administered. Consider the appropriateness of the medication for this patient.	This knowledge aids the nurse in evaluating the therapeutic effect of the medication in relation to the patient's disorder and can also be used to educate the patient about the medication.
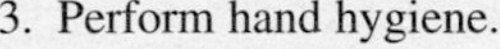 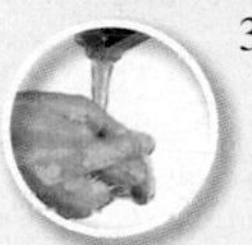 3. Perform hand hygiene.	Hand hygiene prevents the spread of microorganisms.
4. Move the medication cart to the outside of the patient's room or prepare for administration in the medication area.	Organization facilitates error-free administration and saves time.
5. Unlock the medication cart or drawer. Enter pass code and scan employee identification, if required.	Locking the cart or drawer safeguards each patient's medication supply. Hospital accrediting organizations require medication carts to be locked when not in use. Entering pass code and scanning ID allows only authorized users into the computer system and identifies the user for documentation by the computer.
6. **Prepare medications for one patient at a time.**	This prevents errors in medication administration.
7. Read the CMAR/MAR and select the proper medication from unit stock or the patient's medication drawer.	This is the *first* check of the label.
8. Compare the label with the CMAR/MAR. Check expiration dates and perform calculations, if necessary. Scan the bar code on the package, if required.	This is the *second* check of the label. Verify calculations with another nurse to ensure safety, if necessary.
9. If necessary, withdraw medication from an ampule or vial as described in Skills 5-3 and 5-4.	

(continued)

SKILL 5-7 ADMINISTERING A SUBCUTANEOUS INJECTION continued

ACTION	RATIONALE
10. **Depending on facility policy, the third check of the label may occur at this point. If so, when all medications for one patient have been prepared, recheck the labels with the CMAR/MAR before taking the medications to the patient.**	This *third* check ensures accuracy and helps to prevent errors. *Note:* Many facilities require the *third* check to occur at the bedside, after identifying the patient and before administration.
11. Lock the medication cart before leaving it.	Locking the cart or drawer safeguards the patient's medication supply. Hospital accrediting organizations require medication carts to be locked when not in use.
12. Transport medications to the patient's bedside carefully, and keep the medications in sight at all times.	Careful handling and close observation prevent accidental or deliberate disarrangement of medications.
13. **Ensure that the patient receives the medications at the correct time.**	Check agency policy, which may allow for administration within a period of 30 minutes before or 30 minutes after the designated time.
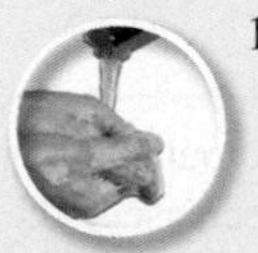 14. Perform hand hygiene and put on PPE, if indicated.	Hand hygiene and PPE prevent the spread of microorganisms. PPE is required based on transmission precautions.
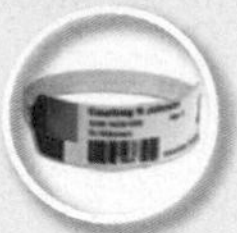 15. **Identify the patient. Compare the information with the CMAR/MAR. The patient should be identified using at least two methods** (The Joint Commission, 2013):	Identifying the patient ensures the right patient receives the medications and helps prevent errors. The patient's room number or physical location is not used as an identifier (The Joint Commission, 2013). Replace the identification band if it is missing or inaccurate in any way.
a. Check the name on the patient's identification band.	
b. Check the identification number on the patient's identification band.	
c. Check the birth date on the patient's identification band.	
d. Ask the patient to state his or her name and birth date, based on facility policy.	This requires a response from the patient, but illness and strange surroundings often cause patients to be confused.
16. Close the door to the room or pull the bedside curtain.	This provides patient privacy.
17. **Complete necessary assessments before administering medications. Check the patient's allergy bracelet or ask the patient about allergies. Explain the purpose and action of the medication to the patient.**	Assessment is a prerequisite to administration of medications. Explanation provides rationale, increases knowledge, and reduces anxiety.
18. Scan the patient's bar code on the identification band, if required (Figure 2).	Scanning provides an additional check to ensure that the medication is given to the right patient.

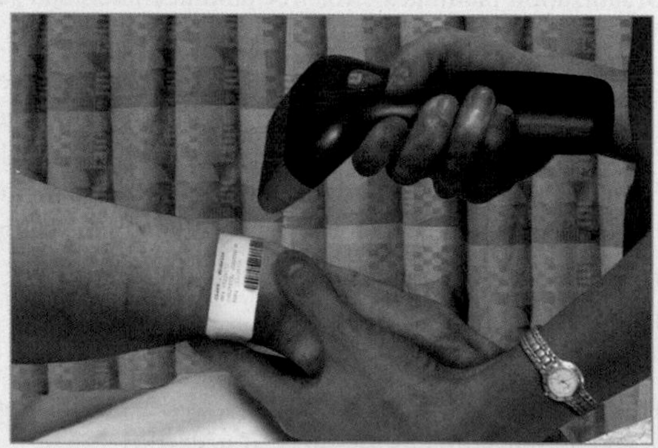

FIGURE 2 Scanning bar code on the patient's identification bracelet. *(Photo by B. Proud.)*

ACTION	RATIONALE
19. **Based on facility policy, the third check of the label may occur at this point. If so, recheck the labels with the CMAR/MAR before administering the medications to the patient.**	Many facilities require the *third* check to occur at the bedside, after identifying the patient and before administration. If facility policy directs the *third* check at this time, this *third* check ensures accuracy and helps to prevent errors.

ACTION	RATIONALE
20. Put on clean gloves.	Gloves help prevent exposure to contaminants.
21. Select an appropriate administration site.	Appropriate site prevents injury and allows for accurate reading of the test site at the appropriate time.
22. Assist the patient to the appropriate position for the site chosen. Drape, as needed, to expose only site area to be used.	Appropriate site prevents injury. Draping helps maintain the patient's privacy.
23. Identify the appropriate landmarks for the site chosen.	Good visualization is necessary to establish the correct site location and to avoid tissue damage.
24. Cleanse the area around the injection site with an antimicrobial swab. Use a firm, circular motion while moving outward from the injection site (Figure 3). Allow the area to dry.	Pathogens on the skin can be forced into the tissues by the needle. Moving from the center outward prevents contamination of the site. Allowing skin to dry prevents introducing alcohol into the tissue, which can be irritating and uncomfortable.
25. Remove the needle cap with the nondominant hand, pulling it straight off.	The cap protects the needle from contact with microorganisms. This technique lessens the risk of an accidental needlestick.
26. Grasp and bunch the area surrounding the injection site or spread the skin taut at the site (Figure 4).	Decision to create a skin fold is based on the nurse's assessment of the patient and needle length used. Pinching is advised for thinner patients and when a longer needle is used, to lift the adipose tissue away from underlying muscle and tissue. If pinching is used, once the needle is inserted, release the skin to avoid injecting into compressed tissue. If skin is pulled taut, it provides easy, less painful entry into the subcutaneous tissue.

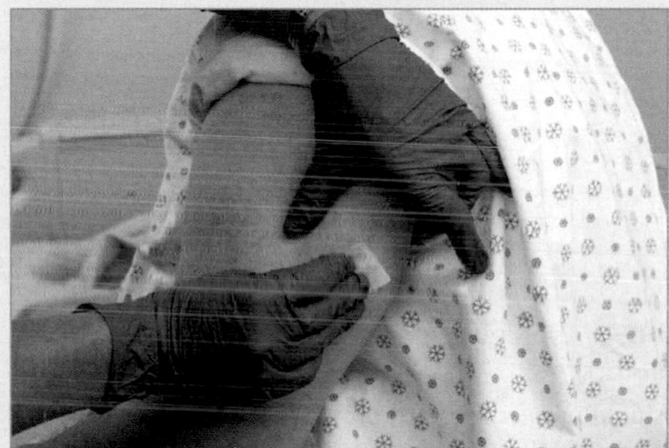

FIGURE 3 Cleaning injection site.

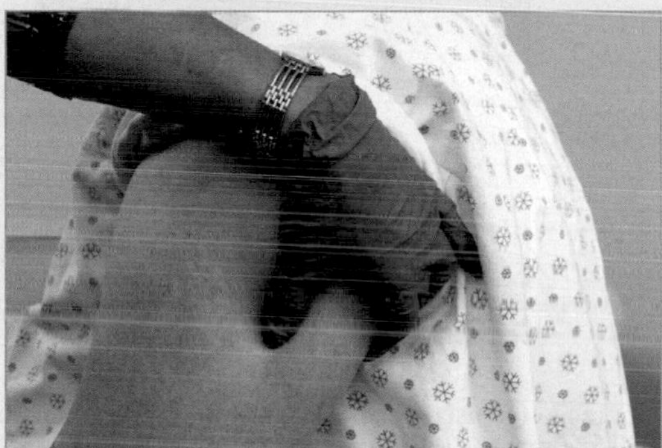

FIGURE 4 Bunching tissue at injection site.

ACTION	RATIONALE
27. Hold the syringe in the dominant hand between the thumb and forefinger. Inject the needle quickly at a 45- to 90-degree angle (Figure 5).	Inserting the needle quickly causes less pain to the patient. Subcutaneous tissue is abundant in well-nourished, well-hydrated people and spare in emaciated, dehydrated, or very thin persons. For a person with little subcutaneous tissue, it is best to insert the needle at a 45-degree angle.

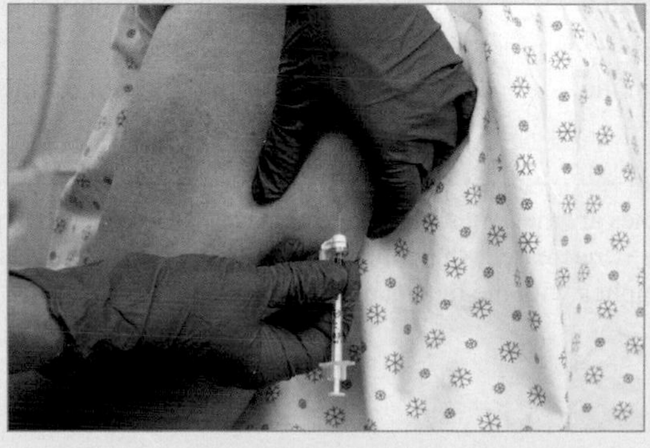

FIGURE 5 Inserting needle.

(continued)

SKILL 5-7 ADMINISTERING A SUBCUTANEOUS INJECTION continued

ACTION	RATIONALE
28. After the needle is in place, release the tissue. If you have a large skin fold pinched up, ensure that the needle stays in place as the skin is released. Immediately move your nondominant hand to steady the lower end of the syringe. Slide your dominant hand to the end of the plunger. Avoid moving the syringe.	Injecting the solution into compressed tissues results in pressure against nerve fibers and creates discomfort. If there is a large skin fold, the skin may retract away from the needle. The nondominant hand secures the syringe. Moving the syringe could cause damage to the tissues and inadvertent administration into an incorrect area.
29. Inject the medication slowly (at a rate of 10 sec/mL).	Rapid injection of the solution creates pressure in the tissues, resulting in discomfort.
30. Withdraw the needle quickly at the same angle at which it was inserted, while supporting the surrounding tissue with your nondominant hand.	Slow withdrawal of the needle pulls the tissues and causes discomfort. Applying counter traction around the injection site helps to prevent pulling on the tissue as the needle is withdrawn. Removing the needle at the same angle at which it was inserted minimizes tissue damage and discomfort for the patient.
31. Using a gauze square, apply gentle pressure to the site after the needle is withdrawn (Figure 6). **Do not massage the site.**	Massaging the site can damage underlying tissue and increase the absorption of the medication. Massaging after heparin administration can contribute to hematoma formation. Massaging after an insulin injection may contribute to unpredictable absorption of the medication.

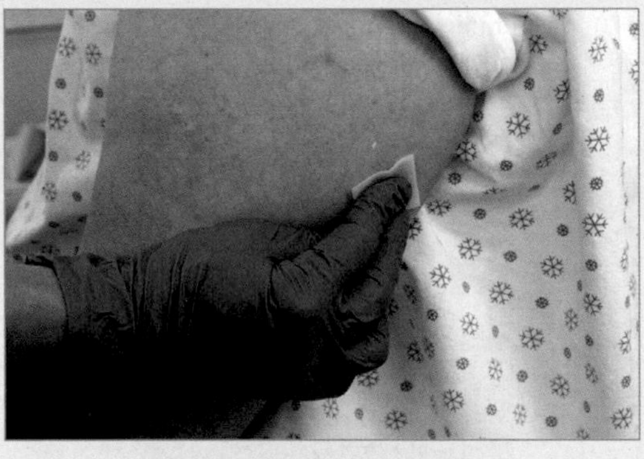

FIGURE 6 Applying pressure to injection site.

ACTION	RATIONALE
32. Do not recap the used needle. Engage the safety shield or needle guard. Discard the needle and syringe in the appropriate receptacle.	Safety shield or needle guard prevents accidental needlestick. Proper disposal of the needle prevents injury.
33. Assist the patient to a position of comfort.	This provides for the well-being of the patient.
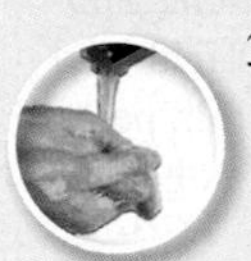 34. Remove gloves and additional PPE, if used. Perform hand hygiene.	Removing PPE properly reduces the risk for infection transmission and contamination of other items. Hand hygiene prevents the spread of microorganisms.
35. Document the administration of the medication immediately after administration. See Documentation section on page 211.	Timely documentation helps to ensure patient safety.
36. Evaluate the patient's response to the medication within the appropriate time frame for the particular medication.	The patient needs to be evaluated for therapeutic and adverse effects from the medication.

EVALUATION

The expected outcomes are met when the patient receives the medication via the subcutaneous route; the patient's anxiety is decreased; the patient does not experience adverse effects; and the patient understands and complies with the medication regimen.

DOCUMENTATION

Guidelines

Record each medication given on the CMAR/MAR or record using the required format, including date, dose, time, and the site of administration, immediately after administration. If using a bar-code system, medication administration is automatically recorded when the bar code is scanned. PRN medications require documentation of the reason for administration. Prompt recording avoids the possibility of accidentally repeating the administration of the drug. If the drug was refused or omitted, record this in the appropriate area on the medication record and notify the primary care provider. This verifies the reason medication was omitted and ensures that the primary care provider is aware of the patient's condition.

UNEXPECTED SITUATIONS AND ASSOCIATED INTERVENTIONS

- *When skin fold is released, needle pulls out of skin:* Engage safety shield or needle guard. Appropriately discard needle. Attach new needle to syringe and administer injection.
- *Patient refuses to let you administer medication in a different location:* Explain the rationale behind rotating injection sites. Discuss other available injection sites with the patient. If the patient will still not allow injection in another area, administer medication to patient, document patient's refusal of rotation of injection site and discussion, and notify primary care provider.
- *You stick yourself with the needle before injection:* Discard needle and syringe appropriately. Follow facility policy regarding needlestick injury. Prepare new syringe with medication and administer to patient. Complete appropriate paperwork and follow facility's policy regarding accidental needlestick injuries.
- *You stick yourself with the needle after injection:* Discard needle and syringe appropriately. Complete appropriate paperwork and follow facility's policy regarding accidental needlestick injuries.
- *During injection, patient pulls away from the needle before the medication is delivered fully:* Remove and appropriately discard needle. Attach a new needle to syringe and administer remaining medication at a different site. Document events and interventions according to facility policy.

SPECIAL CONSIDERATIONS

General Considerations

- Ongoing assessment is an important part of nursing care for both evaluation of patient response to administered medications and early detection of adverse effects. If an adverse effect is suspected, withhold further medication doses and notify the patient's primary care provider. Additional intervention is based on type of reaction and patient assessment.
- Heparin is administered subcutaneously. The abdomen is the most commonly used administration site. Avoid the area 2 inches around the umbilicus and the belt line. The manufacturer's directions for subcutaneous administration of low–molecular-weight heparin preparations, such as enoxaparin (Lovenox), include specific instructions regarding administration site and technique (Sanofi Aventis, 2012). Administer enoxaparin in an area on the abdomen between the left or right anterolateral and left or right posterolateral abdominal wall (Figure 7). To administer the medication, pinch the tissue gently and insert the needle at a 90-degree angle. In addition, enoxaparin is packaged in a prefilled syringe with an air bubble. Do not expel the air bubble before administration.

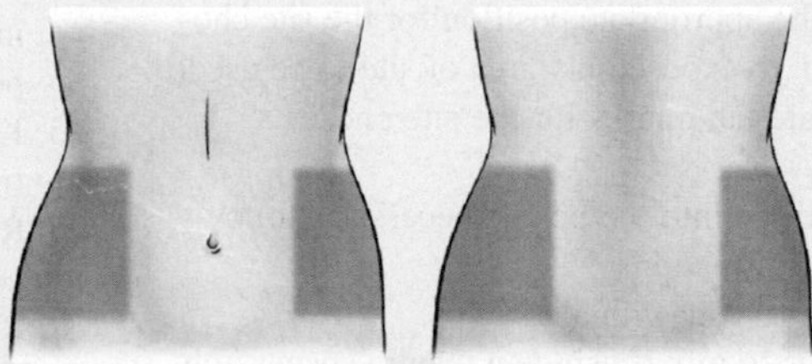

FIGURE 7 Sites for administration of enoxaparin.

Infant and Child Considerations

- Do not tell a child that an injection will not hurt. Describe the feel of the injection as a pinch or a sting. A child who believes you have been dishonest with him/her is less likely to cooperate with future procedures.

Older Adult Considerations

- Many older patients have less adipose tissue. Adjust the needle length and insertion angle accordingly. (Refer to discussion earlier in Skill.) You do not want to inadvertently give a subcutaneous medication intramuscularly.

(continued)

SKILL 5-7 ADMINISTERING A SUBCUTANEOUS INJECTION continued

Home Care Considerations

- Reuse of syringes in the home setting is not recommended.
- Because absorption rates vary from site to site, it is recommended that patients administering their own insulin use the same area of the body at the same time every day to ensure more consistent absorption and prevent tissue changes from repeated use of the same site (Ashenbrenner & Veneble, 2012; ADA, 2004). Rotate injection sites within the area of the body being used.
- Changes and improvements to insulin syringes to make injections painless have resulted in thinner, shorter, sharper, and better lubricated needles. As a result, after one injection the tip of the fine needles can bend and form a hook that can tear tissue if reused. In addition, these fine needles can break and leave fragments in the skin and tissue if reused. Reuse results in more painful injections related to a reduction in needle lubricant and tip damage. Therefore, teach patients to use a new needle and syringe for each injection.
- Encourage patients to consult the policies of their local government regarding contaminated and sharps waste disposal. Teach patients to dispose of needles and syringes in a hard, plastic container. Liquid detergent or liquid fabric softener containers are good choices. Never use glass containers.

SKILL VARIATION Using an Insulin Injection Pen to Administer Insulin via the Subcutaneous Route

Prepare medication as outlined in steps 1–13 above (Skill 5-7).

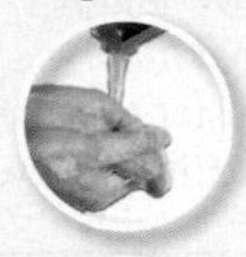

1. Perform hand hygiene and put on PPE, as indicated.

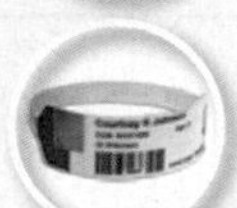

2. Identify the patient.
3. Explain the procedure to patient.
4. Close the door to the room or pull the bedside curtain.
5. **Complete necessary assessments before administering medications. Check the patient's allergy bracelet or ask the patient about allergies. Explain the purpose and action of the medication to the patient.**
6. Scan the patient's bar code on the identification band, if required.
7. **Based on facility policy, the third check of the label may occur at this point. If so, recheck the labels with the CMAR/MAR before administering the medications to the patient.**
8. Select an appropriate administration site.
9. Assist the patient to the appropriate position for the site chosen. Drape, as needed, to expose only area of site to be used.
10. Identify the appropriate landmarks for the site chosen.
11. Remove the pen cap.
12. Insert an insulin cartridge into the pen, if necessary, following the manufacturer's directions.
13. Clean the tip of the reservoir with alcohol.
14. Invert the pen 20 times to mix if using an insulin suspension.
15. Remove the protective tab from the needle.
16. Screw the needle onto the reservoir.
17. Remove the outer and inner needle caps.
18. Hold the pen upright and tap to force any air bubbles to the top.
19. Dial the dose selector to 2 units to perform an "air shot" to get rid of bubbles.
20. Hold the pen upright and press the plunger firmly. Watch for a drop of insulin at the needle tip.

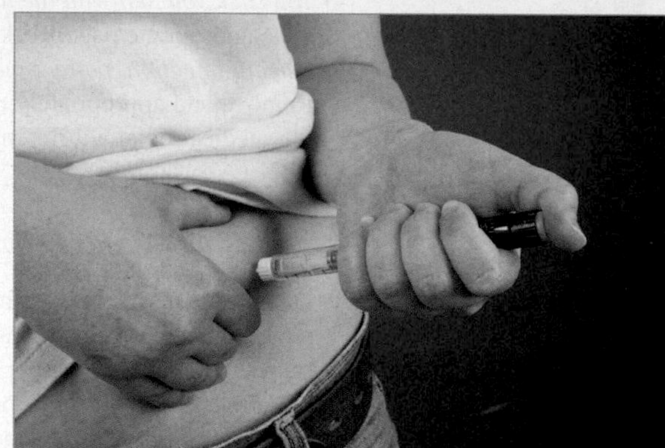

FIGURE A Patient using insulin pen. *(Photo by B. Proud.)*

21. Check the drug reservoir to make sure sufficient insulin is available for the dose.
22. Check that the dose selector is at "0," then dial the units of insulin for the dose.
23. Put on gloves.
24. Clean the injection site and administer the subcutaneous injection, holding the pen like a dart. Push the button on the pen all the way in (Figure A).
25. Keep the button depressed and count to 6 before removing from the skin.
26. Remove the needle from the pen and dispose in a sharps container.
27. Remove gloves and additional PPE, if used.

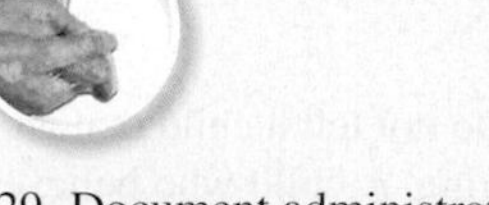

28. Perform hand hygiene.
29. Document administration on the CMAR/MAR, including the injection site.

(Adapted from Moshang, J. (2005). Making a point about insulin pens. *Nursing, 35*(2), 46–47.)

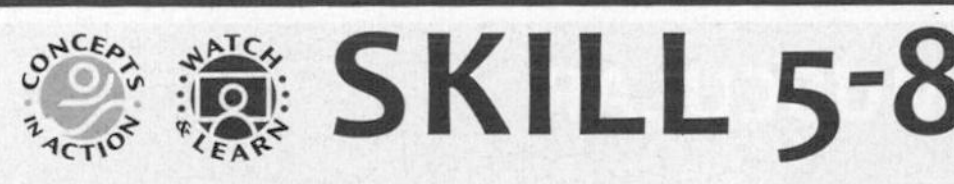

SKILL 5-8 ADMINISTERING AN INTRAMUSCULAR INJECTION

Intramuscular injections deliver medication through the skin and subcutaneous tissues into certain muscles. Muscles have a larger and a greater number of blood vessels than subcutaneous tissue, allowing faster onset of action than with subcutaneous injections. An intramuscular injection is chosen when a reasonably rapid systemic uptake of the drug is needed by the body and when a relatively prolonged action is required. Some medications administered intramuscularly are formulated to have a longer duration of effect. The deposit of medication creates a depot at the injection site, designed to deliver slow, sustained release over hours, days, or weeks.

To administer an intramuscular injection correctly and effectively, choose the right equipment, select the appropriate location, use the correct technique, and deliver the correct dose. Inject the medication into the denser part of the muscle fascia below the subcutaneous tissues. This is ideal because skeletal muscles have fewer pain-sensing nerves than subcutaneous tissue and can absorb larger volumes of solution because of the rapid uptake of the drug into the bloodstream via the muscle fibers (Hunter, 2008).

It is important to choose the right needle length for a particular intramuscular injection. Needle length should be based on the site for injection and the patient's age. (See Table 5-1 for intramuscular needle length recommendations.) Patients who are obese may require a longer needle, and emaciated patients may require a shorter needle. Appropriate gauge is determined by the medication being administered. Generally, biologic agents and medications in aqueous solutions should be administered with a 20- to 25-gauge needle. Medications in oil-based solutions should be administered with an 18- to 25-gauge needle. Many medications come in prefilled syringe units. If a needle is provided on the prefilled unit, ensure that the needle on the unit is the appropriate length for the patient and situation.

Table 5-1 INTRAMUSCULAR INJECTION NEEDLE LENGTH

SITE/AGE	NEEDLE LENGTH
Vastus lateralis	5⁄8″ to 1¼″
Deltoid (children)	5⁄8″ to 1¼″
Deltoid (adults)	1″ to 1½″
Ventrogluteal (adults)	1½″

Note: Patients who are obese may require a longer needle (Zaybak et al., 2007) and those who are emaciated may require a shorter needle. (Adapted from Centers for Disease Control and Prevention (CDC). (2012). *The pink book: Appendices. Epidemiology and prevention of vaccine preventable diseases* (11th ed.). Appendix D. Vaccine administration. Vaccine administration guidelines. Available www.cdc.gov/vaccines/pubs/pinkbook/pinkappendx.htm#appd; Centers for Disease Control and Prevention (CDC). (2008). *Needle length and injection site of intramuscular injections.* Available http://www.cdc.gov/vaccines/ed/encounter08/Downloads/Table7.pdf; and Nicoll, L., & Hesby, A. (2002). Intramuscular injection: An integrative research review and guideline for evidence-based practice. *Applied Nursing Research, 16*(2), 149–162.)

To avoid complications, be able to identify anatomic landmarks and site boundaries. See Figure 1 for a depiction of anatomic landmarks and site boundaries for potential intramuscular injection sites. Consider the age of the patient, medication type, and medication volume when selecting an intramuscular injection site. (See Table 5-2 on page 215 for information related to intramuscular site selection.) Rotate the sites used to administer intramuscular medications when therapy requires repeated injections. Whatever pattern of rotating sites is used, a description of it should appear in the patient's plan of nursing care. Depending on the site selected, it may be necessary to reposition the patient (see Table 5-3 on page 215).

Use accurate, careful technique when administering intramuscular injections. If care is not taken, possible complications include abscesses; cellulites; injury to blood vessels, bones, and nerves; lingering pain; tissue necrosis; and periostitis (inflammation of the membrane covering a bone). Administer the intramuscular injection so that the needle is perpendicular to the patient's body. This ensures it is given using an injection angle between 72 and 90 degrees (Katsma & Katsma, 2000). Figure 5-1 in the chapter opener shows the angles of insertion for intramuscular injections.

(*continued*)

SKILL 5-8 ADMINISTERING AN INTRAMUSCULAR INJECTION continued

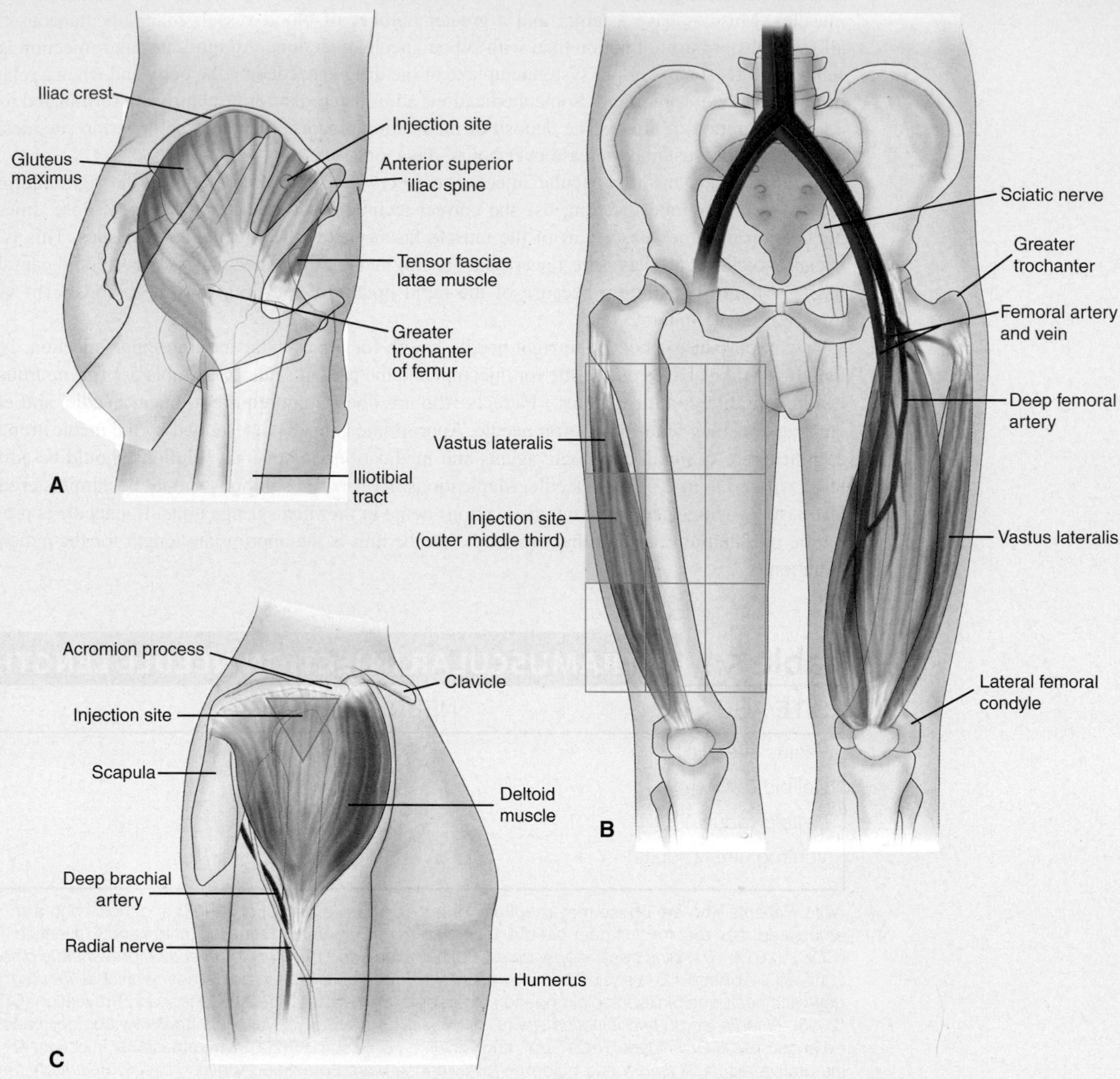

FIGURE 1 Sites for intramuscular injections.Descriptions for locating sites are given in the text. (**A**) Ventrogluteal site is located by placing palm on greater trochanter and index finger toward the anterosuperior iliac spine. (**B**) Vastus lateralis site is identified by dividing the thigh into thirds, horizontally and vertically. (**C**) Deltoid muscle site is located by palpating lower edge of acromion process.

The medication volume that can be administered intramuscularly varies based on the intended site. Generally, 1 to 4 mL is the accepted volume range, with no more than 1 to 2 mL given at the deltoid site. The less-developed muscles of children and older people limit the intramuscular injection to 1 to 2 mL.

According to the CDC (2012) and current review of evidence (Crawford & Johnson, 2012), aspiration is not required for intramuscular injections. Some literature suggests aspiration *may* be indicated when administering large molecule medications such as penicillin (Crawford & Johnson, 2012). Consult facility policy and manufacturer recommendations to ensure safe administration.

Refer to Box 5-1 in Skill 5-7 for techniques for reducing discomfort when injecting medications subcutaneously or intramuscularly.

Table 5-2 INTRAMUSCULAR SITE SELECTION

AGE OF PATIENT	RECOMMENDED SITE
Infants	Vastus lateralis
Toddlers (1–2 years)	Vastus lateralis (preferred) or deltoid
Child/Adolescent (3–18 years)	Deltoid (preferred) or vastus lateralis
Adults	Deltoid or ventrogluteal
MEDICATION TYPE	**RECOMMENDED SITE**
Biologicals (infants and young children)	Vastus lateralis
Biologicals (older children and adults)	Deltoid
Hepatitis B/Rabies	Deltoid
Medications that are known to be irritating, viscous, or oily solutions	Ventrogluteal

(Adapted from Centers for Disease Control and Prevention (CDC). (2012). *The pink book: Appendices. Epidemiology and prevention of vaccine preventable diseases* (11th ed.). Appendix D. Vaccine administration. Vaccine administration guidelines. Available www.cdc.gov/vaccines/pubs/pinkbook/pinkappendx.htm#appd; Centers for Disease Control and Prevention (CDC). (2008). *Needle length and injection site of intramuscular injections.* Available http://www.cdc.gov/vaccines/ed/encounter08/Downloads/Table7.pdf; and Nicoll, L., & Hesby, A. (2002). Intramuscular injection: An integrative research review and guideline for evidence-based practice. *Applied Nursing Research, 16*(2), 149–162.)

Table 5-3 PATIENT POSITIONING

INJECTION SITE	PATIENT POSITION
Deltoid	Patient may sit or stand. A child may be held in an adult's lap.
Ventrogluteal	Patient may stand, sit, lie laterally, and lie supine.
Vastus lateralis	Patient may sit or lie supine. Infants and young children may lie supine or be held in an adult's lap.

(Adapted from Centers for Disease Control and Prevention (CDC). (2012). *The pink book: Appendices. Epidemiology and prevention of vaccine preventable diseases* (11th ed.). Appendix D. Vaccine administration. Vaccine administration guidelines. Available www.cdc.gov/vaccines/pubs/pinkbook/pinkappendx.htm#appd)

DELEGATION CONSIDERATIONS

The administration of an intramuscular injection is not delegated to nursing assistive personnel (NAP) or to unlicensed assistive personnel (UAP). Depending on the state's nurse practice act and the organization's policies and procedures, the administration of an intramuscular injection may be delegated to licensed practical/vocational nurses (LPN/LVNs). The decision to delegate must be based on careful analysis of the patient's needs and circumstances, as well as the qualifications of the person to whom the task is being delegated. Refer to the Delegation Guidelines in Appendix A.

EQUIPMENT

- Gloves
- Additional PPE, as indicated
- Medication
- Sterile syringe and needle of appropriate size and gauge
- Antimicrobial swab
- Small gauze square
- Computer-generated Medication Administration Record (CMAR) or Medication Administration Record (MAR)

ASSESSMENT

Assess the patient for any allergies. Check the expiration date before administering the medication. Assess the appropriateness of the drug for the patient. Verify patient name, dose, route, and time of administration. Review assessment and laboratory data that may influence drug administration. Assess the site on the patient where the injection is to be given. Avoid any site that is bruised, tender, hard, swollen, inflamed, or scarred.

(continued)

SKILL 5-8 ADMINISTERING AN INTRAMUSCULAR INJECTION continued

Assess the patient's knowledge of the medication. If the patient has deficient knowledge about the medication, this may be the appropriate time to begin education about it. If the medication may affect the patient's vital signs, assess them before administration. If the medication is intended for pain relief, assess the patient's pain before and after administration.

NURSING DIAGNOSIS

Determine related factors for the nursing diagnoses based on the patient's current status. Appropriate diagnoses may include:

- Acute Pain
- Risk for Injury
- Anxiety

OUTCOME IDENTIFICATION AND PLANNING

The expected outcome to achieve when administering an intramuscular injection is that the patient receives the medication via the intramuscular route. Other outcomes that may be appropriate include the following: the patient's anxiety is decreased; the patient does not experience adverse effects; and the patient understands and complies with the medication regimen.

IMPLEMENTATION

ACTION	RATIONALE
1. Gather equipment. Check each medication order against the original order in the medical record according to facility policy. Clarify any inconsistencies. Check the patient's chart for allergies.	This comparison helps to identify errors that may have occurred when orders were transcribed. The primary care provider's order is the legal record of medication orders for each facility.
2. Know the actions, special nursing considerations, safe dose ranges, purpose of administration, and adverse effects of the medications to be administered. Consider the appropriateness of the medication for this patient.	This knowledge aids the nurse in evaluating the therapeutic effect of the medication in relation to the patient's disorder and can also be used to educate the patient about the medication.
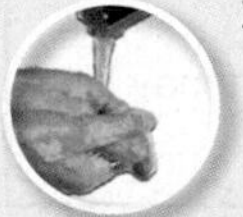 3. Perform hand hygiene.	Hand hygiene prevents the spread of microorganisms.
4. Move the medication cart to the outside of the patient's room or prepare for administration in the medication area.	Organization facilitates error-free administration and saves time.
5. Unlock the medication cart or drawer. Enter pass code and scan employee identification, if required.	Locking the cart or drawer safeguards each patient's medication supply. Hospital accrediting organizations require medication carts to be locked when not in use. Entering pass code and scanning ID allows only authorized users into the system and identifies the user for documentation by the computer.
6. **Prepare medications for one patient at a time.**	This prevents errors in medication administration.
7. Read the CMAR/MAR and select the proper medication from unit stock or the patient's medication drawer.	This is the *first* check of the label.
8. Compare the label with the CMAR/MAR. Check expiration dates and perform calculations, if necessary. Scan the bar code on the package, if required.	This is the *second* check of the label. Verify calculations with another nurse to ensure safety, if necessary.
9. If necessary, withdraw medication from an ampule or vial as described in Skills 5-3 and 5-4.	
10. **Depending on facility policy, the third check of the label may occur at this point. If so, when all medications for one patient have been prepared, recheck the labels with the CMAR/MAR before taking the medications to the patient.**	This *third* check ensures accuracy and helps to prevent errors. *Note:* Many facilities require the *third* check to occur at the bedside, after identifying the patient and before administration.

ACTION	RATIONALE
11. Lock the medication cart before leaving it.	Locking the cart or drawer safeguards the patient's medication supply. Hospital accrediting organizations require medication carts to be locked when not in use.
12. Transport medications to the patient's bedside carefully, and keep the medications in sight at all times.	Careful handling and close observation prevent accidental or deliberate disarrangement of medications.
13. **Ensure that the patient receives the medications at the correct time.**	Check agency policy, which may allow for administration within a period of 30 minutes before or 30 minutes after the designated time.
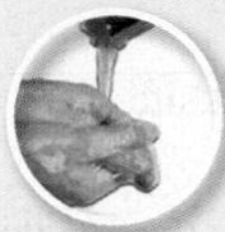 14. Perform hand hygiene and put on PPE, if indicated.	Hand hygiene and PPE prevent the spread of microorganisms. PPE is required based on transmission precautions.
 15. **Identify the patient. Compare the information with the CMAR/MAR. The patient should be identified using at least two methods** (The Joint Commission, 2013):	Identifying the patient ensures the right patient receives the medications and helps prevent errors. The patient's room number or physical location is not used as an identifier (The Joint Commission, 2013). Replace the identification band if it is missing or inaccurate in any way.
a. Check the name on the patient's identification band.	
b. Check the identification number on the patient's identification band.	
c. Check the birth date on the patient's identification band.	
d. Ask the patient to state his or her name and birth date, based on facility policy.	This requires a response from the patient, but illness and strange surroundings often cause patients to be confused.
16. Close the door to the room or pull the bedside curtain.	This provides patient privacy.
17. **Complete necessary assessments before administering medications. Check the patient's allergy bracelet or ask the patient about allergies. Explain the purpose and action of the medication to the patient.**	Assessment is a prerequisite to administration of medications. Explanation provides rationale, increases knowledge, and reduces anxiety.
18. Scan the patient's bar code on the identification band, if required (Figure 2).	Provides an additional check to ensure that the medication is given to the right patient.

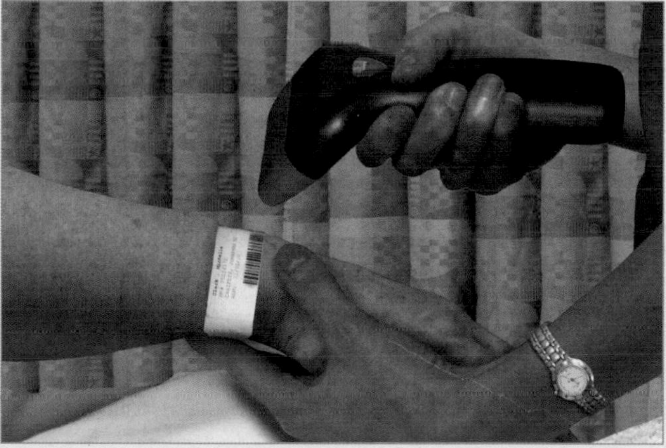

FIGURE 2 Scanning bar code on the patient's identification bracelet. *(Photo by B. Proud.)*

(continued)

SKILL 5-8 ADMINISTERING AN INTRAMUSCULAR INJECTION continued

ACTION	RATIONALE
19. **Based on facility policy, the third check of the label may occur at this point. If so, recheck the labels with the CMAR/MAR before administering the medications to the patient.**	Many facilities require the *third* check to occur at the bedside, after identifying the patient and before administration. If facility policy directs the *third* check at this time, this *third* check ensures accuracy and helps to prevent errors.
20. Put on clean gloves.	Gloves help prevent exposure to contaminants.
21. Select an appropriate administration site.	Selecting the appropriate site prevents injury.
22. Assist the patient to the appropriate position for the site chosen. See Table 5-3. Drape, as needed, to expose only the site area being used.	Appropriate positioning for the site chosen prevents injury. Draping helps maintain the patient's privacy.
23. Identify the appropriate landmarks for the site chosen.	Good visualization is necessary to establish the correct site location and to avoid tissue damage.
24. Cleanse the area around the injection site with an antimicrobial swab. Use a firm, circular motion while moving outward from the injection site. Allow the area to dry.	Pathogens on the skin can be forced into the tissues by the needle. Moving from the center outward prevents contamination of the site. Allowing skin to dry prevents introducing alcohol into the tissue, which can be irritating and uncomfortable.
25. Remove the needle cap by pulling it straight off. Hold the syringe in your dominant hand between the thumb and forefinger.	This technique lessens the risk of an accidental needlestick and also prevents inadvertently unscrewing the needle from the barrel of the syringe.
26. Displace the skin in a Z-track manner. Pull the skin down or to one side about 1 inch (2.5 cm) with your nondominant hand and hold the skin and tissue in this position (Figure 3). (See the accompanying Skill Variation for information on administering an intramuscular injection without using the Z-track technique.)	Z-track technique is recommended for all intramuscular injections to ensure medication does not leak back along the needle track and into the subcutaneous tissue (Nicoll & Hesby, 2002; Zimmerman, 2010). This technique reduces pain and discomfort, particularly for patients receiving injections over an extended period. The Z-track method is also suggested for older patients who have decreased muscle mass. Some agents, such as iron, are best given via the Z-track method due to the irritation and discoloration associated with this agent.

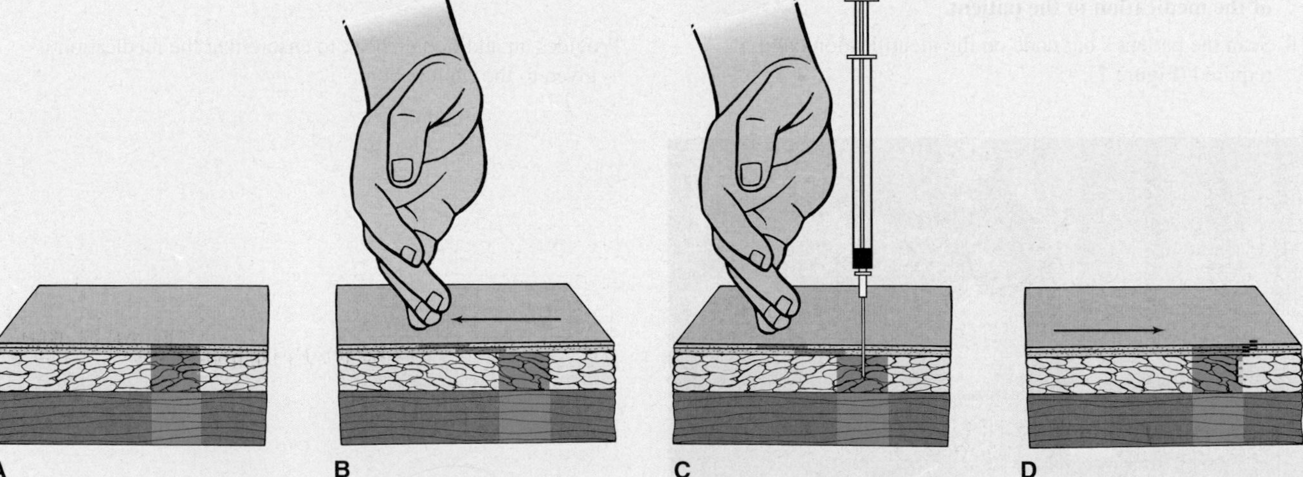

FIGURE 3 Z-track or zigzag technique is recommended for intramuscular injections. (**A**) Normal skin and tissues. (**B**) Moving skin to one side. (**C**) Needle is inserted at a 90-degree angle. (**D**) Once needle is withdrawn, displaced tissue is allowed to return to its normal position, preventing solution from escaping from muscle tissue.

ACTION	RATIONALE
27. Quickly dart the needle into the tissue so that the needle is perpendicular to the patient's body (Figure 4). This should ensure that the medication is administered using an injection angle between 72 and 90 degrees.	A quick injection is less painful. Inserting the needle at a 72- to 90-degree angle facilitates entry into muscle tissue.
28. As soon as the needle is in place, use the thumb and forefinger of your nondominant hand to hold the lower end of the syringe. Slide your dominant hand to the end of the plunger. Inject the solution slowly (10 sec/mL of medication).	Moving the syringe could cause damage to the tissues and inadvertent administration into an incorrect area. Rapid injection of the solution creates pressure in the tissues, resulting in discomfort. According to the CDC (2012) and current review of evidence (Crawford & Johnson, 2012), aspiration is not required for intramuscular injections. Some literature suggests aspiration *may* be indicated when administering large molecule medications such as penicillin (Crawford & Johnson, 2012). Consult facility policy and manufacturer recommendations to ensure safe administration.
29. Once the medication has been instilled, wait 10 seconds before withdrawing the needle.	Allows medication to begin to diffuse into the surrounding muscle tissue (Nicoll & Hesby, 2002).
30. Withdraw the needle smoothly and steadily at the same angle at which it was inserted, supporting tissue around the injection site with your nondominant hand.	Slow withdrawal of the needle pulls the tissues and causes discomfort. Applying counter traction around the injection site helps to prevent pulling on the tissue as the needle is withdrawn. Removing the needle at the same angle at which it was inserted minimizes tissue damage and discomfort for the patient.
31. Apply gentle pressure at the site with a dry gauze (Figure 5). **Do not massage the site.**	Light pressure causes less trauma and irritation to the tissues. Massaging can force medication into subcutaneous tissues.

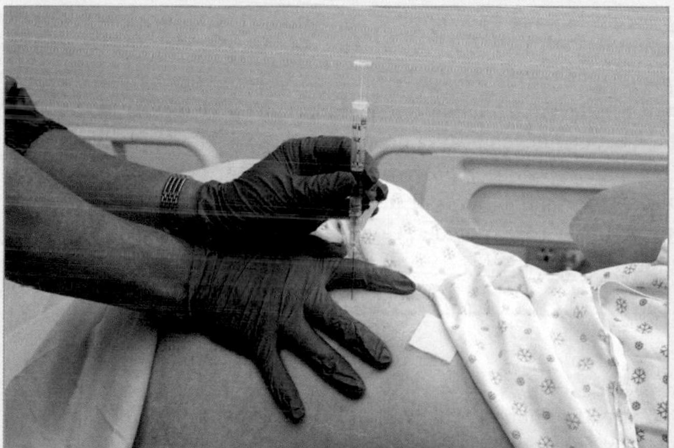

FIGURE 4 Darting needle into tissue.

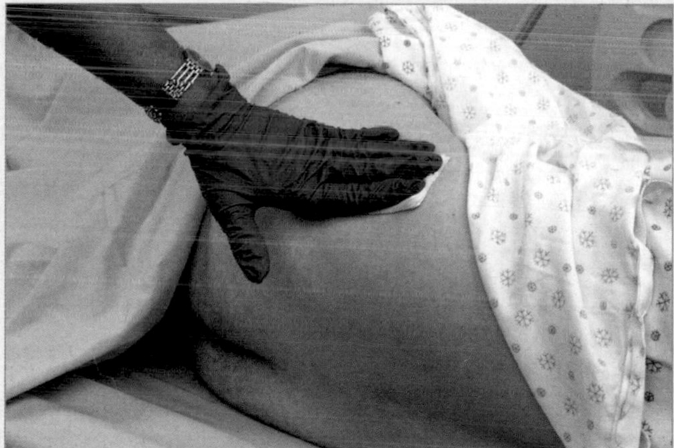

FIGURE 5 Applying pressure at injection site.

ACTION	RATIONALE
32. Do not recap the used needle. Engage the safety shield or needle guard, if present. Discard the needle and syringe in the appropriate receptacle.	Proper disposal of the needle prevents injury.
33. Assist the patient to a position of comfort.	This provides for the well-being of the patient.
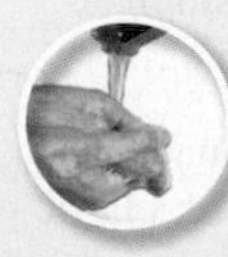 34. Remove gloves and additional PPE, if used. Perform hand hygiene.	Removing PPE properly reduces the risk for infection transmission and contamination of other items. Hand hygiene prevents the spread of microorganisms.

(continued)

SKILL 5-8 ADMINISTERING AN INTRAMUSCULAR INJECTION continued

ACTION	RATIONALE
35. Document the administration of the medication immediately after administration. See Documentation section below.	Timely documentation helps to ensure patient safety.
36. Evaluate the patient's response to the medication within the appropriate time frame. Assess site, if possible, within 2 to 4 hours after administration.	The patient needs to be evaluated for therapeutic and adverse effects from the medication. Visualization of the site allows for assessment of any untoward effects.

EVALUATION

The expected outcomes are met when the patient receives the medication via the intramuscular route; the patient's anxiety is decreased; the patient does not experience adverse effects or injury; and the patient understands and complies with the medication regimen.

DOCUMENTATION

Guidelines

Record each medication given on the CMAR/MAR or record using the required format, including date, time, and the site of administration, immediately after administration. If using a bar-code system, medication administration is automatically recorded when the bar code is scanned. PRN medications require documentation of the reason for administration. Prompt recording avoids the possibility of accidentally repeating the administration of the drug. If the drug was refused or omitted, record this in the appropriate area on the medication record and notify the primary care provider. This verifies the reason medication was omitted and ensures that the primary care provider is aware of the patient's condition.

UNEXPECTED SITUATIONS AND ASSOCIATED INTERVENTIONS

- *You stick yourself with the needle before injection:* Discard needle and syringe appropriately. Follow agency policy regarding needlestick injury. Prepare new syringe with medication and administer to patient. Complete appropriate paperwork and follow facility's policy regarding accidental needlesticks.
- *You stick yourself with the needle after injection:* Discard needle and syringe appropriately. Follow agency policy regarding needlestick injury. Complete appropriate paperwork and follow facility's policy regarding accidental needlesticks.
- *During injection, the patient pulls away from the needle before the medication is delivered fully:* Remove and appropriately discard needle. Attach a new needle to syringe and administer remaining medication at a different site. Document events and interventions, according to facility policy.
- *While injecting the needle into the patient, you hit patient's bone:* Withdraw and discard the needle. Apply a new needle to the syringe and administer in an alternate site. Document incident in patient's medical record. Notify primary care provider. Complete appropriate paperwork related to special events, according to facility policy.

SPECIAL CONSIDERATIONS

General Considerations

- Ongoing assessment is an important part of nursing care for both evaluation of patient response to administered medications and early detection of adverse effects. If an adverse effect is suspected, withhold further medication doses and notify the patient's primary care provider. Additional intervention is based on the type of reaction and patient assessment.

Infant and Child Considerations

- The vastus lateralis is the preferred site for intramuscular injections in infants.

Older Adult Considerations

- Muscle mass atrophies as a person ages. Take care to evaluate the patient's muscle mass and body composition. Use appropriate needle length and gauge for patient's body composition. Choose appropriate site based on the patient's body composition.

Home Care Considerations

- Encourage patients to consult the policies of their local government regarding contaminated and sharps waste disposal. Explain that needles and syringes should be disposed of in a hard, plastic container. Liquid detergent or liquid fabric softener containers are good choices. Glass containers should not be used.
- Reuse of syringes in the home setting is not recommended.

SKILL VARIATION Administering an Intramuscular Injection Without Using the Z-Track Technique

The Z-track technique is recommended for all intramuscular injections to ensure medication does not leak back along the needle track and into the subcutaneous tissue (Nicoll & Hesby, 2002; Zimmerman, 2010). This technique reduces pain and discomfort, particularly for patients receiving injections over an extended period. The Z-track method is also suggested for older patients who have decreased muscle mass. Some agents, such as iron, are best given via the Z-track method due to the irritation and discoloration associated with this agent. If the nurse chooses not to use the Z-Track technique, the skin should be stretched flat between two fingers and held taut for needle insertion. Prepare medication as outlined in steps 1–13 above (Skill 5–8). To administer the injection:

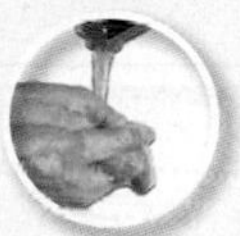

1. Perform hand hygiene and put on PPE, as indicated.

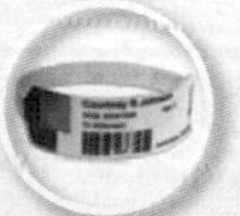

2. Identify the patient.
3. Explain the procedure to the patient.
4. Close the door to the room or pull the bedside curtain.
5. **Complete necessary assessments before administering medications. Check the patient's allergy bracelet or ask the patient about allergies. Explain the purpose and action of the medication to the patient.**
6. Scan the patient's bar code on the identification band, if required.
7. **Based on facility policy, the third check of the label may occur at this point. If so, recheck the labels with the CMAR/MAR before administering the medications to the patient.**
8. Put on clean gloves.
9. Select an appropriate administration site.
10. Assist the patient to the appropriate position for the site chosen. Drape, as needed, to expose only site area to be used.
11. Identify the appropriate landmarks for the site chosen with your nondominant hand.
12. Clean the area around the injection site with an antimicrobial swab. Use a firm, circular motion while moving outward from the injection site. Allow the area to dry.
13. Remove the needle cap by pulling it straight off. Hold the syringe in your dominant hand between the thumb and forefinger.
14. Stretch the skin flat between two fingers and hold taut for needle insertion.
15. Quickly dart the needle into the tissue so that the needle is perpendicular to the patient's body. This should ensure that it is given using an injection angle between 72 and 90 degrees.
16. As soon as the needle is in place, use your thumb and forefinger of your nondominant hand to hold the lower end of the syringe. Slide your dominant hand to the end of the plunger.
17. Inject the solution slowly (10 sec/mL of medication).
18. Withdraw the needle smoothly and steadily at the same angle at which it was inserted, supporting tissue around the injection site with your nondominant hand.
19. Apply gentle pressure at the site with a dry gauze.
20. Do not recap the used needle. Engage the safety shield or needle guard. Discard the needle and syringe in the appropriate receptacle.
21. Assist the patient to a position of comfort.
22. Remove gloves and additional PPE, if used. Perform hand hygiene.
23. Document administration of the medication on the CMAR/MAR immediately after performing the procedure.
24. Evaluate the patient's response to the medication within the appropriate time frame. Assess site, if possible, within 2 to 4 hours after administration.

EVIDENCE FOR PRACTICE ▶

INTRAMUSCULAR INJECTIONS AND ADMINISTRATION SITE CHOICE

Safe medication administration, including the administration of intramuscular (IM) injections, is an expected competency for nurses. The focus of evidence-based practice and recommendation in the recent nursing literature advocate use of the ventrogluteal site over the dorsogluteal site, to avoid damage to the sciatic nerve. Are nurses incorporating current best practice into their delivery of nursing care?

Related Research

Walsh, L., & Brophy, K. (2010). Staff nurses' sites of choice for administering intramuscular injections to adult patients in the acute care setting. *Journal of Advanced Nursing*, *67*(5), 1034–1040.

(*continued*)

SKILL 5-8 ADMINISTERING AN INTRAMUSCULAR INJECTION continued

A convenience sample of nurses employed in acute care settings was accessed through a database at a professional association. A questionnaire was sent to 652 nurses; 264 questionnaires were returned, a response rate of 42.2%. Nurses responding to the survey preferentially used the dorsogluteal site over the ventrogluteal site. Only 15.2% of nurses based site selection on recommendations in the nursing literature. Site selection varied significantly with age, level of preparation, years in nursing, and knowledge of nerve injury as a complication with the selected site. The authors concluded nurses are not using the ventrogluteal site for IM injections in adults as recommended in the nursing literature.

Relevance for Nursing Practice

Nurses have a responsibility to provide professional and safe nursing care. This involves maintaining current knowledge and incorporating evidenced-based guidelines and best practices into care provided to patients. Nurses must take responsibility for keeping abreast of current practice guidelines and maintaining involvement in the decision-making process for health care facilities' policies and procedures to ensure safe patient care. In addition, there is a need to explore why nurses are not using current guidelines as recommended in the nursing literature.

Refer to thePoint for additional research on related nursing topics.

SKILL 5-9 ADMINISTERING A CONTINUOUS SUBCUTANEOUS INFUSION: APPLYING AN INSULIN PUMP

Some medications, such as insulin and morphine, may be administered continuously via the subcutaneous route. Continuous subcutaneous insulin infusion (CSII or insulin pump) allows for multiple preset rates of insulin delivery. This system uses a small, computerized reservoir that delivers insulin via tubing through a small plastic cannula or needle inserted into the subcutaneous tissue. The pump is programmed to deliver multiple preset rates of insulin. The settings can be adjusted for exercise and illness, and bolus dose delivery can be timed in relation to meals. It is recommended that the site is changed every 2 to 3 days to prevent tissue damage or absorption problems (American Association of Diabetes Educators, 2008). Advantages of continuous subcutaneous medication infusion include the longer rate of absorption via the subcutaneous route and convenience for the patient. There are many different manufacturers of insulin pumps. Nurses need to be familiar with the particular pump in use by their patient and to refer to the specific manufacturer's recommendations for use.

DELEGATION CONSIDERATIONS

The administration of a continuous subcutaneous infusion using an insulin pump is not delegated to nursing assistive personnel (NAP) or to unlicensed assistive personnel (UAP). Depending on the state's nurse practice act and the organization's policies and procedures, the management of an insulin pump in some settings may be delegated to licensed practical/vocational nurses (LPN/LVNs) who have received appropriate training. The decision to delegate must be based on careful analysis of the patient's needs and circumstances, as well as the qualifications of the person to whom the task is being delegated. Refer to the Delegation Guidelines in Appendix A.

EQUIPMENT

- Insulin pump
- Pump syringe and vial of insulin or prefilled cartridge, as ordered
- Sterile infusion set
- Insertion (triggering) device
- Needle (24- or 22-gauge, or blunt-ended needle)
- Antimicrobial swabs
- Sterile non-occlusive dressing

- Computer-generated Medication Administration Record (CMAR) or Medication Administration Record (MAR)
- Disposable gloves
- Additional PPE, as indicated

ASSESSMENT

Assess the patient for any allergies. Check the expiration date before administering the medication. Assess the appropriateness of the drug for the patient. Review assessment and laboratory data that may influence drug administration. Verify patient name, dose, route, and time of administration. Assess the infusion site. Typical infusion sites include those areas used for subcutaneous insulin injection. Assess the area where the pump is to be applied. Do not place the pump on skin that is irritated or broken down.

Assess the patient's knowledge of the medication. If the patient has a knowledge deficit about the medication, this may be the appropriate time to begin education about it. Assess the patient's blood glucose level as appropriate or as ordered.

NURSING DIAGNOSIS

Determine related factors for the nursing diagnoses based on the patient's current status. Appropriate nursing diagnoses may include:

- Deficient Knowledge
- Risk for Unstable Blood Glucose Level
- Risk for Infection

OUTCOME IDENTIFICATION AND PLANNING

The expected outcome is that the device is applied successfully and medication is administered correctly. Other outcomes that may be appropriate include the following: the patient understands the rationale for the pump use and mechanism of action; the patient experiences no allergy response; the patient's skin remains intact; pump is applied using aseptic technique; and the patient does not experience unstable blood glucose levels or adverse effect.

IMPLEMENTATION

ACTION	RATIONALE
1. Gather equipment. Check each medication order against the original order in the medical record, according to facility policy. Clarify any inconsistencies. Check the patient's chart for allergies.	This comparison helps to identify errors that may have occurred when orders were transcribed. The primary care provider's order is the legal record of medication orders for each facility.
2. Know the actions, special nursing considerations, safe dose ranges, purpose of administration, and adverse effects of the medications to be administered. Consider the appropriateness of the medication for this patient.	This knowledge aids the nurse in evaluating the therapeutic effect of the medication in relation to the patient's disorder and can also be used to educate the patient about the medication.
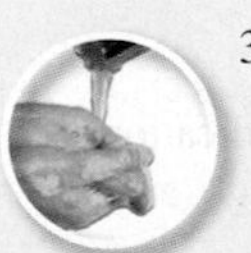 3. Perform hand hygiene.	Hand hygiene prevents the spread of microorganisms.
4. Move the medication cart to the outside of the patient's room or prepare for administration in the medication area.	Organization facilitates error-free administration and saves time.
5. Unlock the medication cart or drawer. Enter pass code and scan employee identification, if required.	Locking the cart or drawer safeguards each patient's medication supply. Hospital accrediting organizations require medication carts to be locked when not in use. Entering pass code and scanning ID allows only authorized users into the system and identifies the user for documentation by the computer.
6. **Prepare medications for one patient at a time.**	This prevents errors in medication administration.
7. Read the CMAR/MAR and select the proper medication from unit stock or the patient's medication drawer.	This is the *first* check of the label.

(continued)

SKILL 5-9 ADMINISTERING A CONTINUOUS SUBCUTANEOUS INFUSION: APPLYING AN INSULIN PUMP continued

ACTION	RATIONALE
8. Compare the label with the CMAR/MAR. Check expiration dates and perform calculations, if necessary. Scan the bar code on the package, if required.	This is the *second* check of the label. Verify calculations with another nurse to ensure safety, if necessary.
9. Attach a blunt-ended needle or a small-gauge needle to a syringe. Follow Skill 5–4 to prepare insulin from a vial, if necessary. Prepare enough insulin to last the patient 2 to 3 days, plus 30 units for priming tubing. If using a prepackaged insulin syringe or cartridge, remove from packaging.	Patient will wear pump for up to 3 days without changing syringe or tubing.
10. **Depending on facility policy, the third check of the label may occur at this point. If so, when all medications for one patient have been prepared, recheck the labels with the CMAR/MAR before taking the medications to the patient.**	This *third* check ensures accuracy and helps to prevent errors. *Note:* Many facilities require the *third* check to occur at the bedside, after identifying the patient and before administration.
11. Lock the medication cart before leaving it.	Locking the cart or drawer safeguards the patient's medication supply. Hospital accrediting organizations require medication carts to be locked when not in use.
12. Transport medications to the patient's bedside carefully, and keep the medications in sight at all times.	Careful handling and close observation prevent accidental or deliberate disarrangement of medications.
13. **Ensure that the patient receives the medications at the correct time.**	Check agency policy, which may allow for administration within a period of 30 minutes before or 30 minutes after the designated time.
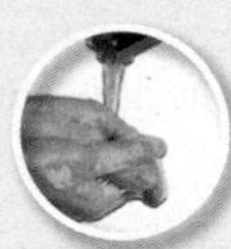 14. Perform hand hygiene and put on PPE, if indicated.	Hand hygiene and PPE prevent the spread of microorganisms. PPE is required based on transmission precautions.
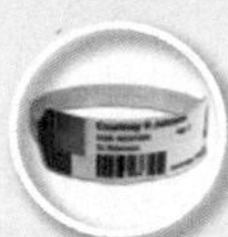 15. **Identify the patient. Compare the information with the CMAR/MAR. The patient should be identified using at least two methods** (The Joint Commission, 2013):	Identifying the patient ensures the right patient receives the medications and helps prevent errors. The patient's room number or physical location is not used as an identifier (The Joint Commission, 2013). Replace the identification band if it is missing or inaccurate in any way.
a. Check the name on the patient's identification band.	
b. Check the identification number on the patient's identification band.	
c. Check the birth date on the patient's identification band.	
d. Ask the patient to state his or her name and birth date, based on facility policy.	This requires a response from the patient, but illness and strange surroundings often cause patients to be confused.
16. Close the door to the room or pull the bedside curtain.	This provides patient privacy.
17. **Complete necessary assessments before administering medications. Check the patient's allergy bracelet or ask the patient about allergies. Explain the purpose and action of the medication to the patient.**	Assessment is a prerequisite to administration of medications. Explanation provides rationale, increases knowledge, and reduces anxiety.
18. Scan the patient's bar code on the identification band, if required (Figure 1).	Provides an additional check to ensure that the medication is given to the right patient.
19. **Based on facility policy, the third check of the label may occur at this point. If so, recheck the labels with the CMAR/MAR before administering the medications to the patient.**	Many facilities require the *third* check to occur at the bedside, after identifying the patient and before administration. If facility policy directs the *third* check at this time, this *third* check ensures accuracy and helps to prevent errors.
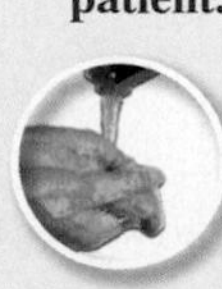 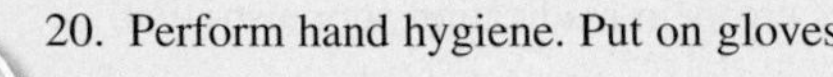 20. Perform hand hygiene. Put on gloves.	Hand hygiene prevents the spread of microorganisms. Gloves prevent contact with blood and body fluids.

ACTION	RATIONALE
21. Remove the cap from the syringe or insulin cartridge (Figure 2). Attach sterile tubing to the syringe or insulin cartridge. Open the pump and place the syringe or cartridge in compartment according to manufacturer's directions (Figure 3). Close the pump.	Tubing must be attached correctly and syringe must be placed in pump correctly for insulin delivery.

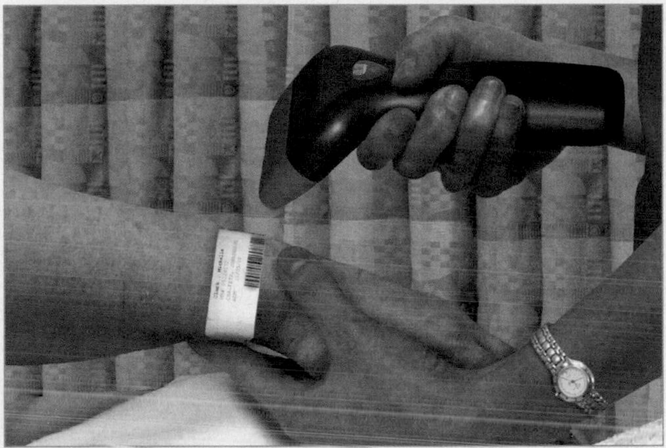

FIGURE 1 Scanning bar code on patient's identification bracelet. *(Photo by B. Proud.)*

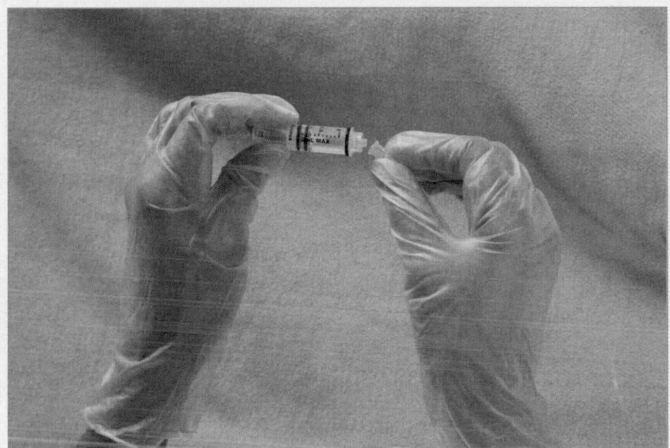

FIGURE 2 Removing cap from syringe or insulin cartridge.

ACTION	RATIONALE
22. Initiate priming of the tubing, according to manufacturer's directions. Program the pump according to manufacturer's recommendations following primary care provider's orders (Figure 4). **Check for any bubbles in the tubing.**	Removing all the air from the tubing and correct programming of pump ensures the patient receives the correct dose of insulin.

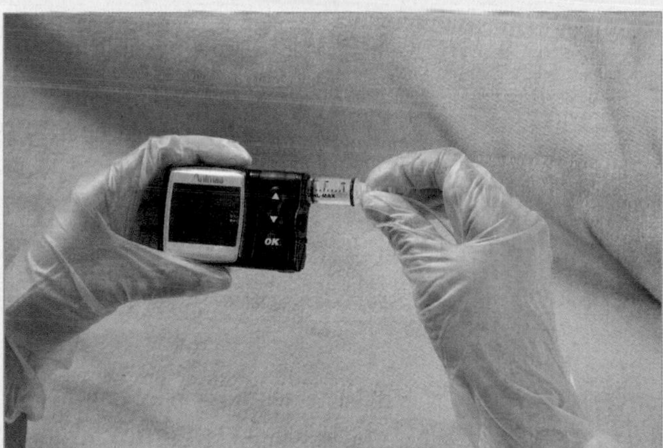

FIGURE 3 Placing syringe or cartridge in compartment according to manufacturer's directions.

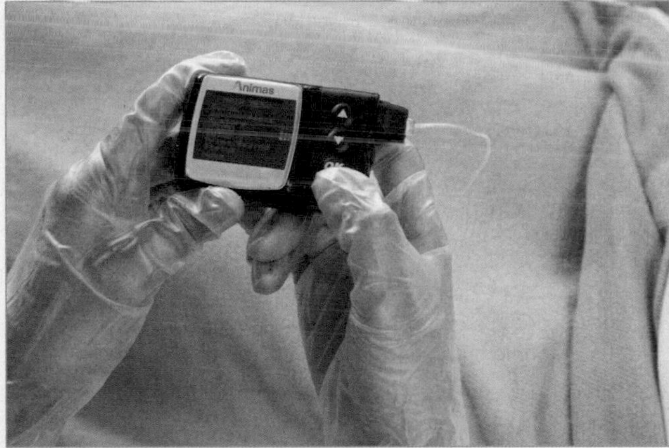

FIGURE 4 Programming pump according to manufacturer's recommendations following primary care provider's orders.

ACTION	RATIONALE
23. Activate the delivery device. Place the needle between prongs of the insertion device with the sharp edge facing out. Push insertion set down until a click is heard.	To ensure correct placement of insulin pump needle, an insertion device must be used.
24. Select an appropriate administration site.	Appropriate site prevents injury.
25. Assist the patient to the appropriate position for the site chosen. Drape, as needed, to expose only site area to be used.	Appropriate site prevents injury. Draping maintains privacy and warmth.

(continued)

SKILL 5-9 ADMINISTERING A CONTINUOUS SUBCUTANEOUS INFUSION: APPLYING AN INSULIN PUMP continued

ACTION	RATIONALE
26. Identify the appropriate landmarks for the site chosen.	Good visualization is necessary to establish the correct site location and to avoid tissue damage.
27. Cleanse area around injection site with antimicrobial swab (Figure 5). Use a firm, circular motion while moving outward from insertion site. Allow antiseptic to dry.	Pathogens on the skin can be forced into the tissues by the needle. Moving from the center outward prevents contamination of the site. Allowing skin to dry prevents introducing alcohol into the tissue, which can be irritating and uncomfortable.
28. Remove paper from adhesive backing. Remove the needle guard. Pinch skin at insertion site, press insertion device on site, and press release button to insert needle. Remove triggering device.	To ensure delivery of insulin into subcutaneous tissue, a skin fold is made with a pinch *before* insertion of the medication.
29. Apply sterile occlusive dressing over the insertion site, if not part of the insertion device. Attach the pump to patient's clothing, as desired (Figure 6).	Dressing prevents contamination of site. Pump can be dislodged easily if not attached securely to patient.

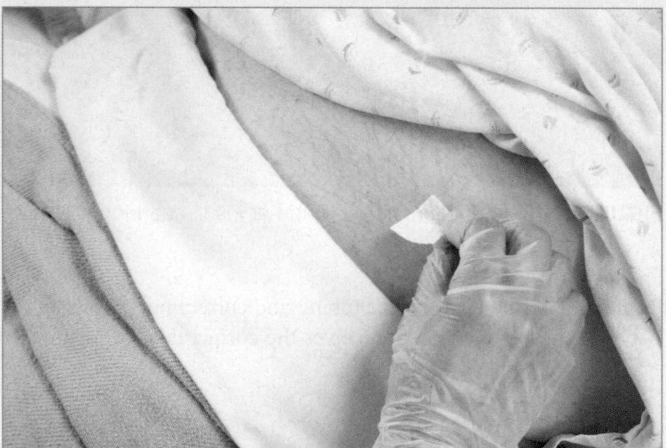

FIGURE 5 Cleansing area around injection site with antimicrobial swab.

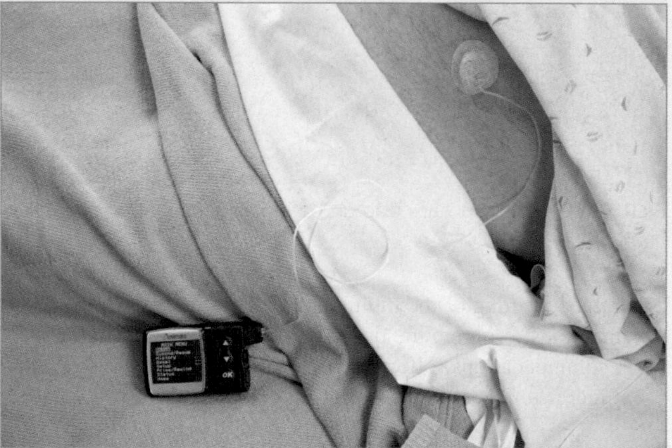

FIGURE 6 Insulin pump in place.

ACTION	RATIONALE
30. Assist the patient to a position of comfort.	This provides for the well-being of the patient.
31. Discard the needle and syringe in the appropriate receptacle.	Proper disposal of the needle prevents injury.
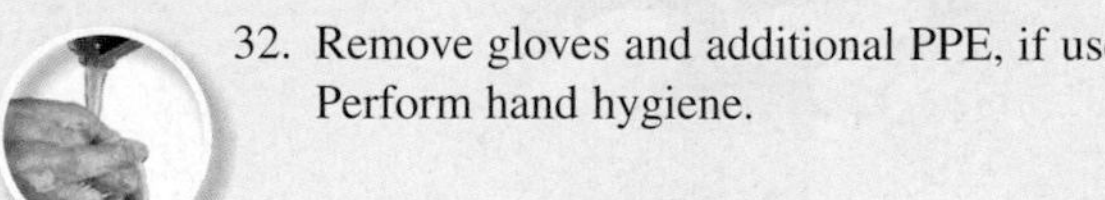 32. Remove gloves and additional PPE, if used. Perform hand hygiene.	Removing PPE properly reduces the risk for infection transmission and contamination of other items. Hand hygiene prevents the spread of microorganisms.
33. Document the administration of the medication immediately after administration. See Documentation section below.	Timely documentation helps to ensure patient safety.
34. Evaluate the patient's response to the medication within the appropriate time frame. Monitor the patient's blood glucose levels, as appropriate, or as ordered.	Patient needs to be evaluated to ensure that the pump is delivering the drug appropriately. The patient needs to be evaluated for therapeutic and adverse effects from the medication.

EVALUATION

The expected outcomes are met when the patient receives insulin from the attached pump successfully without hypo- or hyperglycemic effects noted; the patient understands the rationale for the pump attachment; the patient experiences no allergy response; the patient's skin remains intact; the patient remains infection free; and the patient experiences no or minimal pain.

DOCUMENTATION

Guidelines

Document the application of the pump, the type of insulin used, pump settings, insertion site, and any teaching done with the patient on the CMAR/MAR or record using the required format, including date, time, and the site of administration, immediately after administration. If using a bar-code system, medication administration is automatically recorded when the bar code is scanned. PRN medications require documentation of the reason for administration. Prompt recording avoids the possibility of accidentally repeating the administration of the drug. If the drug was refused or omitted, record this in the appropriate area on the medication record and notify the primary care provider. This verifies the reason medication was omitted and ensures that the primary care provider is aware of the patient's condition.

Sample Documentation

9/22/15 1000 Insulin pump inserted by patient on left upper quadrant of abdomen with minimal assistance. Pump filled with 300 units (3 mL) of lispro insulin. Rate set at 1 unit per hour. Patient verbalizes desire to apply pump without assistance when site next changed.

—B. Clapp, RN

UNEXPECTED SITUATIONS AND ASSOCIATED INTERVENTIONS

- *After the pump is attached to the patient, a large amount of air is noted in tubing:* Remove the pump from patient. Obtain new sterile tubing with insertion needle. Prime the tubing and reinsert.

SPECIAL CONSIDERATIONS

General Considerations

- *Patient must rotate site more frequently than every 2 to 3 days due to insulin usage:* Check manufacturer's recommendations. Most pumps are initially set in a smaller mode but can be changed for a larger amount of insulin delivery.
- *Patient is refusing to rotate site at least every 3 days:* Inform the patient that absorption of medication decreases after 3 days, which may increase his or her need for insulin. Rotating sites prevents this decrease in absorption from developing. In addition, sit rotation reduces risk of infection at the site.
- *You note that the insertion site is now erythematous:* Remove the stylet, obtain a new pump setup, and insert at a different site at least 1 inch from old site.
- *Occlusive dressing will not stick due to perspiration:* Apply deodorant around insertion site but not over insertion site. Alternately, apply skin barrier around insertion site but not over insertion site.
- Assess infusion site areas routinely for inflammation, allergic reactions, infection, and lipodystrophy.
- Good hygiene and frequent catheter site changes reduce the risk of site complications. Change catheter site every 2 to 3 days.
- Contact dermatitis is sometimes a problem at the catheter site area. The primary care provider may order topical antibiotics, aloe, vitamin E, or corticosteroids to treat a contact dermatitis.
- Insulin self-administered by the patient through the insulin pump should be communicated to the nurse at the time of administration. This allows for accurate documentation of insulin requirements.
- Ongoing assessment is an important part of nursing care for both evaluation of patient response to administered medications and early detection of adverse effects. If an adverse effect is suspected, withhold further medication doses and notify the patient's primary care provider. Additional intervention is based on type of reaction and patient assessment.

Home Care Considerations

- Encourage patients to consult the policies of their local government regarding contaminated and sharps waste disposal. Explain that needles and other sharps should be disposed of in a hard, plastic container. Liquid detergent or liquid fabric softener containers are good choices. Glass containers should not be used.

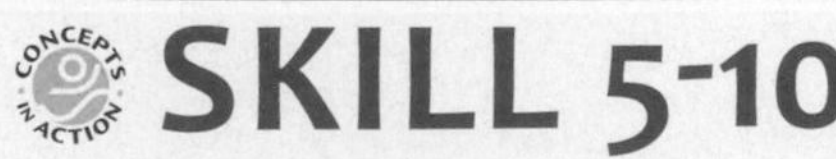

SKILL 5-10 ADMINISTERING MEDICATIONS BY INTRAVENOUS BOLUS OR PUSH THROUGH AN INTRAVENOUS INFUSION

A medication can be administered via the **intravenous (IV) route** as an IV bolus or push. This involves a single injection of a concentrated solution directly into an IV line. Drugs given by IV push are used for intermittent dosing or to treat emergencies. The drug is administered very slowly over at least 1 minute. This can be done manually or by using a syringe pump. Confirm exact administration times by consulting a pharmacist or drug reference. Needleless devices prevent needlesticks and provide access to the intravenous line. Either a blunt-ended cannula or a recessed connection port may be used to administer the medication.

DELEGATION CONSIDERATIONS

The administration of medications by intravenous bolus is not delegated to nursing assistive personnel (NAP) or to unlicensed assistive personnel (UAP). Depending on the state's nurse practice act and the organization's policies and procedures, the administration of specified intravenous medications in some settings may be delegated to licensed practical/vocational nurses (LPN/LVNs) who have received appropriate training. The decision to delegate must be based on careful analysis of the patient's needs and circumstances, as well as the qualifications of the person to whom the task is being delegated. Refer to the Delegation Guidelines in Appendix A.

EQUIPMENT

- Antimicrobial swab
- Watch with second hand, or stopwatch
- Disposable gloves
- Additional PPE, as indicated
- Prescribed medication
- Syringe with a needleless device or 23- to 25-gauge, 1-inch needle (follow facility policy)
- Syringe pump, if necessary
- Computer-generated Medication Administration Record (CMAR) or Medication Administration Record (MAR)

ASSESSMENT

Assess the patient for any allergies. Check the expiration date before administering the medication. Assess the appropriateness of the drug for the patient. Assess the compatibility of the ordered medication and the IV fluid. Review assessment and laboratory data that may influence drug administration. Verify the patient's name, dose, route, and time of administration. Assess the patient's IV site, noting any swelling, coolness, leakage of fluid from the IV site, or pain. Assess the patient's knowledge of the medication.

If the patient has a knowledge deficit about the medication, this may be the appropriate time to begin education about the medication. If the medication may affect the patient's vital signs, assess them before administration. If the medication is for pain relief, assess the patient's pain before and after administration.

NURSING DIAGNOSIS

Determine related factors for the nursing diagnoses based on the patient's current status. Appropriate nursing diagnoses may include:

- Risk for Injury
- Risk for Allergy Response
- Risk for Infection

OUTCOME IDENTIFICATION AND PLANNING

The expected outcome to achieve is that the medication is given safely via the IV route. Other outcomes that may be appropriate include the following: the patient experiences no adverse effects; the patient experiences no allergy response; the patient is knowledgeable about medication being added by bolus IV; the patient remains infection free; and the patient has no, or decreased, anxiety.

IMPLEMENTATION

ACTION	RATIONALE
1. Gather equipment. Check medication order against the original order in the medical record, according to facility policy. Clarify any inconsistencies. Check the patient's chart for allergies. Verify the compatibility of the medication and IV fluid. Check a drug resource to clarify whether the medication needs to be diluted before administration. Check the administration rate.	This comparison helps to identify errors that may have occurred when orders were transcribed. The primary care provider's order is the legal record of medication orders for each facility. Compatibility of medication and solution prevents complications. Delivers the correct dose of medication as prescribed.
2. Know the actions, special nursing considerations, safe dose ranges, purpose of administration, and adverse effects of the medications to be administered. Consider the appropriateness of the medication for this patient.	This knowledge aids the nurse in evaluating the therapeutic effect of the medication in relation to the patient's disorder and can also be used to educate the patient about the medication.
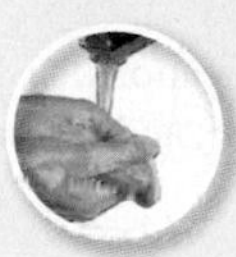 3. Perform hand hygiene.	Hand hygiene prevents the spread of microorganisms.
4. Move the medication cart to the outside of the patient's room or prepare for administration in the medication area.	Organization facilitates error-free administration and saves time.
5. Unlock the medication cart or drawer. Enter pass code and scan employee identification, if required.	Locking the cart or drawer safeguards each patient's medication supply. Hospital accrediting organizations require medication carts to be locked when not in use. Entering pass code and scanning ID allows only authorized users into the system and identifies the user for documentation by the computer.
6. **Prepare medication for one patient at a time.**	This prevents errors in medication administration.
7. Read the CMAR/MAR and select the proper medication from unit stock or the patient's medication drawer.	This is the *first* check of the label.
8. Compare the label with the CMAR/MAR. Check expiration dates and perform calculations, if necessary. Scan the bar code on the package, if required.	This is the *second* check of the label. Verify calculations with another nurse to ensure safety, if necessary.
9. If necessary, withdraw medication from an ampule or vial as described in Skills 5-3 and 5-4.	
10. **Depending on facility policy, the third check of the label may occur at this point. If so, when all medications for one patient have been prepared, recheck the labels with the CMAR/MAR before taking the medications to the patient.**	This *third* check ensures accuracy and helps to prevent errors. *Note:* Many facilities require the *third* check to occur at the bedside, after identifying the patient and before administration.
11. Lock the medication cart before leaving it.	Locking the cart or drawer safeguards the patient's medication supply. Hospital accrediting organizations require medication carts to be locked when not in use.
12. Transport medications and equipment to the patient's bedside carefully, and keep the medications in sight at all times.	Careful handling and close observation prevent accidental or deliberate disarrangement of medications. Having equipment available saves time and facilitates performance of the task.
13. **Ensure that the patient receives the medications at the correct time.**	Check agency policy, which may allow for administration within a period of 30 minutes before or 30 minutes after the designated time.
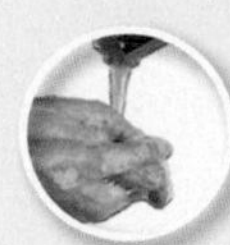 14. Perform hand hygiene and put on PPE, if indicated.	Hand hygiene and PPE prevent the spread of microorganisms. PPE is required based on transmission precautions.

(continued)

SKILL 5-10 ADMINISTERING MEDICATIONS BY INTRAVENOUS BOLUS OR PUSH THROUGH AN INTRAVENOUS INFUSION continued

ACTION	RATIONALE
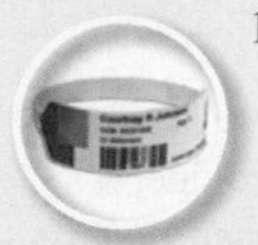 15. **Identify the patient. Compare the information with the CMAR/MAR. The patient should be identified using at least two methods** (The Joint Commission, 2013):	Identifying the patient ensures the right patient receives the medications and helps prevent errors. The patient's room number or physical location is not used as an identifier (The Joint Commission, 2013). Replace the identification band if it is missing or inaccurate in any way.
a. Check the name on the patient's identification band.	
b. Check the identification number on the patient's identification band.	
c. Check the birth date on the patient's identification band.	
d. Ask the patient to state his or her name and birth date, based on facility policy.	This requires a response from the patient, but illness and strange surroundings often cause patients to be confused.
16. Close the door to the room or pull the bedside curtain.	This provides patient privacy.
17. Complete necessary assessments before administering medications. Check the patient's allergy bracelet or ask the patient about allergies. Explain the purpose and action of the medication to the patient.	Assessment is a prerequisite to administration of medications. Explanation provides rationale, increases knowledge, and reduces anxiety.
18. Scan the patient's bar code on the identification band, if required.	Provides an additional check to ensure that the medication is given to the right patient.
19. **Based on facility policy, the third check of the label may occur at this point. If so, recheck the label with the CMAR/MAR before administering the medications to the patient.**	Many facilities require the *third* check to occur at the bedside, after identifying the patient and before administration. If facility policy directs the *third* check at this time, this *third* check ensures accuracy and helps to prevent errors.
20. **Assess IV site for presence of inflammation or infiltration.**	IV medication must be given directly into a vein for safe administration.
21. If IV infusion is being administered via an infusion pump, pause the pump.	Pausing prevents infusion of fluid during bolus administration and activation of pump occlusion alarms.
22. Put on clean gloves.	Gloves prevent contact with blood and body fluids.
23. Select injection port on tubing that is closest to venipuncture site. Clean port with antimicrobial swab.	Using port closest to the needle insertion site minimizes dilution of medication. Cleaning deters entry of microorganisms when port is punctured.
24. Uncap syringe. Steady port with your nondominant hand while inserting syringe into center of port.	This supports the injection port and lessens the risk for accidentally dislodging the IV or entering the port incorrectly.
25. Move your nondominant hand to the section of IV tubing just above the injection port. Fold the tubing between your fingers.	This temporarily stops flow of gravity IV infusion and prevents medication from backing up tubing.
26. Pull back slightly on plunger just until blood appears in tubing.	This ensures injection of medication into the bloodstream.
27. **Inject the medication at the recommended rate** (see Special Considerations on page 231) (Figure 1).	This delivers the correct amount of medication at the proper interval according to manufacturer's directions.

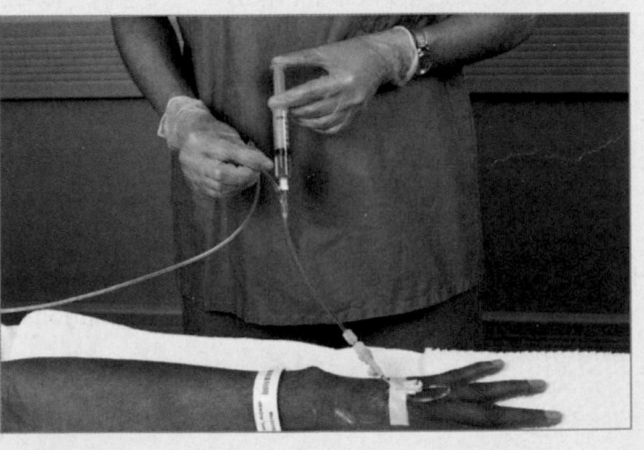

FIGURE 1 Injecting medication while interrupting IV flow. *(Photo by B. Proud.)*

ACTION	RATIONALE
28. Release the tubing. Remove the syringe. Do not recap the used needle, if used. Engage the safety shield or needle guard, if present. Release the tubing and allow the IV fluid to flow. Discard the needle and syringe in the appropriate receptacle.	Proper disposal of the needle prevents injury.
29. Check IV fluid infusion rate. Restart infusion pump, if appropriate.	Injection of bolus may alter fluid infusion rate, if infusing by gravity.
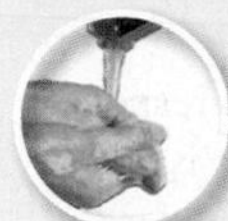 30. Remove gloves and additional PPE, if used. Perform hand hygiene.	Removing PPE properly reduces the risk for infection transmission and contamination of other items. Hand hygiene prevents the spread of microorganisms.
31. Document the administration of the medication immediately after administration. See Documentation section below.	Timely documentation helps to ensure patient safety.
32. Evaluate the patient's response to the medication within the appropriate time frame.	The patient needs to be evaluated for therapeutic and adverse effects from the medication.

EVALUATION

The expected outcomes are met when the medication is safely administered via IV bolus; the patient's anxiety is decreased; the patient does not experience adverse effects; and the patient understands and complies with the medication regimen.

DOCUMENTATION

Guidelines

Document the administration of the medication immediately after administration, including date, time, dose, route of administration, site of administration, and rate of administration on the CMAR/MAR or record using the required format. If using a bar-code system, medication administration is automatically recorded when the bar code is scanned. PRN medications require documentation of the reason for administration. Prompt recording avoids the possibility of accidentally repeating the administration of the drug. If the drug was refused or omitted, record this in the appropriate area on the medication record and notify the primary care provider. This verifies the reason medication was omitted and ensures that the primary care provider is aware of the patient's condition.

UNEXPECTED SITUATIONS AND ASSOCIATED INTERVENTIONS

- *Upon assessing the IV site before administering medication, no blood return is aspirated:* If IV appears patent, without signs of infiltration, and IV fluid infuses without difficulty, proceed with administration. Observe closely for signs and symptoms of infiltration during and after administration.
- *Upon assessing the patient's IV site before administering medication, you note that IV has infiltrated:* Stop IV fluid and remove IV from extremity. Restart IV in a different location. Continue to monitor new IV site as medication is administered.
- *While administering medication, you note a cloudy, white substance forming in the IV tubing:* Stop the IV from flowing and stop administering medication. Clamp IV at the site nearest to the patient. Change administration tubing and restart infusion. Check literature or consult pharmacist regarding compatibility of medication and IV fluid.
- *While you are administering the medication, the patient begins to complain of pain at the IV site:* Stop medication. Assess IV site for any signs of infiltration or phlebitis. Flush the IV with normal saline to check for patency. If the IV site appears within normal limits, resume medication administration at a slower rate.

SPECIAL CONSIDERATIONS

- Facility policy may recommend the following variations when injecting a bolus IV medication:
  - Release folded tubing after each increment of the drug has been administered at the prescribed rate to facilitate delivery of medication.
  - Use a syringe with 1 mL normal saline to flush tubing after an IV bolus is delivered to ensure that residual medication in tubing is not delivered too rapidly.

(continued)

SKILL 5-10 ADMINISTERING MEDICATIONS BY INTRAVENOUS BOLUS OR PUSH THROUGH AN INTRAVENOUS INFUSION continued

- Consider how fast IV fluid is flowing to determine whether a flush of normal saline is in order after administering the medication. If IV fluid is flowing less than 50 mL per hour, it may take up to 30 minutes for the medication to reach the patient. This depends on what type of tubing is being used in the agency.
- If the IV is a small gauge (22- to 24-gauge) placed in a small vein, a blood return may not occur even if IV is intact. Also, the patient may complain of stinging and pain at the site while medication is being administered due to irritation of vein. Placing a warm pack over the vein or slowing the rate may relieve discomfort.
- If the medication and IV solution are incompatible, a bolus may be given by flushing the tubing with normal saline before and after the medication bolus. Consult facility policy.
- Ongoing assessment is an important part of nursing care for both evaluation of patient response to administered medications and early detection of adverse effects. If an adverse effect is suspected, withhold further medication doses and notify the patient's primary care provider. Additional intervention is based on type of reaction and patient assessment.

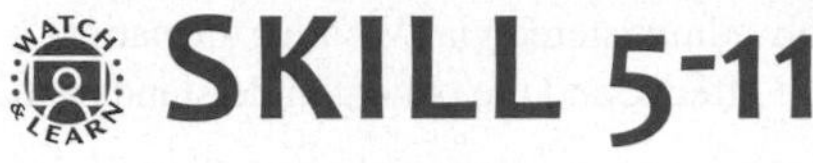

SKILL 5-11 ADMINISTERING A PIGGYBACK INTERMITTENT INTRAVENOUS INFUSION OF MEDICATION

With intermittent IV infusion, the drug is mixed with a small amount of the IV solution, such as 50 to 100 mL, and administered over a short period at the prescribed interval (e.g., every 4 hours). The administration is most often performed using an IV infusion pump, which requires the nurse to program the infusion rate into the pump. "Smart (computerized) pumps" are being used by many facilities for IV infusions, including intermittent infusions. Smart pumps also require programming of infusion rates by the nurse, but also are able to identify dosing limits and practice guidelines to aid in safe administration. Administration may also be achieved by gravity infusion, which requires the nurse to calculate the infusion rate in drops per minute. The best practice, however, is to use an IV infusion pump.

The IV piggyback delivery system requires the intermittent or additive solution to be placed higher than the primary solution container. An extension hook provided by the manufacturer provides for easy lowering of the main IV container. The port on the primary IV line has a back-check valve that automatically stops the flow of the primary solution, allowing the secondary or piggyback solution to flow when connected. Because manufacturers' designs vary, it is important to check the directions carefully for the systems used in the facility. The nurse is responsible for calculating and regulating the infusion with an infusion pump or manually adjusting the flow rate of the IV intermittent infusion. Needleless devices (recommended by the CDC and the Occupational Safety and Health Administration [OSHA]) prevent needlesticks and provide access to the primary venous line. Either a blunt-ended cannula or a recessed connection port may be used to connect intermittent IV infusions.

DELEGATION CONSIDERATIONS

The administration of medications by intermittent IV infusion is not delegated to nursing assistive personnel (NAP) or to unlicensed assistive personnel (UAP). Depending on the state's nurse practice act and the organization's policies and procedures, the administration of specified IV medications in some settings may be delegated to licensed practical/vocational nurses (LPN/LVNs) who have received appropriate training. The decision to delegate must be based on careful analysis of the patient's needs and circumstances, as well as the qualifications of the person to whom the task is being delegated. Refer to the Delegation Guidelines in Appendix A.

EQUIPMENT

- Medication prepared in labeled small-volume bag
- Short secondary infusion tubing (microdrip or macrodrip)
- IV pump
- Needleless connector, if required, based on facility system
- Antimicrobial swab
- Metal or plastic hook
- IV pole
- Date label for tubing
- Computer-generated Medication Administration Record (CMAR) or Medication Administration Record (MAR)
- PPE, as indicated

ASSESSMENT

Assess the patient for any allergies. Check the expiration date before administering the medication. Assess the appropriateness of the drug for the patient. Assess the compatibility of the ordered medication, diluent, and the infusing IV fluid. Review assessment and laboratory data that may influence drug administration. Verify patient name, dose, route, and time of administration. Assess the patient's knowledge of the medication. If the patient has a knowledge deficit about the medication, this may be the appropriate time to begin education about the medication. If the medication may affect the patient's vital signs, assess them before administration. Assess the IV insertion site, noting any swelling, coolness, leakage of fluid at site, redness, or pain.

NURSING DIAGNOSIS

Determine related factors for the nursing diagnoses based on the patient's current status. Appropriate nursing diagnoses include:

- Risk for Allergy Response
- Risk for Infection
- Risk for Injury

OUTCOME IDENTIFICATION AND PLANNING

The expected outcome to achieve is that the medication is delivered via the intravenous route using sterile technique. Other outcomes that may be appropriate include the following: medication is delivered to the patient in a safe manner and at the appropriate infusion rate; the patient experiences no allergy response; the patient remains infection free; and the patient understands and complies with the medication regimen.

IMPLEMENTATION

ACTION	RATIONALE
1. Gather equipment. Check each medication order against the original order in the medical record, according to facility policy. Clarify any inconsistencies. Check the patient's chart for allergies.	This comparison helps to identify errors that may have occurred when orders were transcribed. The primary care provider order is the legal record of medication orders for each facility.
2. Know the actions, special nursing considerations, safe dose ranges, purpose of administration, and adverse effects of the medications to be administered. Consider the appropriateness of the medication for this patient.	This knowledge aids the nurse in evaluating the therapeutic effect of the medication in relation to the patient's disorder and can also be used to educate the patient about the medication.
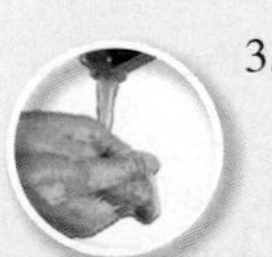 3. Perform hand hygiene.	Hand hygiene prevents the spread of microorganisms.
4. Move the medication cart to the outside of the patient's room or prepare for administration in the medication area.	Organization facilitates error-free administration and saves time.
5. Unlock the medication cart or drawer. Enter pass code and scan employee identification, if required.	Locking the cart or drawer safeguards each patient's medication supply. Hospital accrediting organizations require medication carts to be locked when not in use. Entering pass code and scanning ID allows only authorized users into the system and identifies the user for documentation by the computer.
6. **Prepare medications for one patient at a time.**	This prevents errors in medication administration.
7. Read the CMAR/MAR and select the proper medication from unit stock or the patient's medication drawer.	This is the *first* check of the label.

(continued)

SKILL 5-11 ADMINISTERING A PIGGYBACK INTERMITTENT INTRAVENOUS INFUSION OF MEDICATION continued

ACTION	RATIONALE
8. Compare the label with the CMAR/MAR. Check expiration dates. Confirm the prescribed or appropriate infusion rate. Calculate the drip rate if using a gravity system. Scan the bar code on the package, if required.	This is the *second* check of the label. Verify calculations with another nurse to ensure safety, if necessary. Infusing medication at an appropriate rate prevents injury.
9. **Depending on facility policy, the third check of the label may occur at this point. If so, when all medications for one patient have been prepared, recheck the labels with the CMAR/MAR before taking the medications to the patient.**	This *third* check ensures accuracy and helps to prevent errors. *Note:* Many facilities require the *third* check to occur at the bedside, after identifying the patient and before administration.
10. Lock the medication cart before leaving it.	Locking the cart or drawer safeguards the patient's medication supply. Hospital accrediting organizations require medication carts to be locked when not in use.
11. Transport medications to the patient's bedside carefully, and keep the medications in sight at all times.	Careful handling and close observation prevent accidental or deliberate disarrangement of medications.
12. **Ensure that the patient receives the medications at the correct time.**	Check facility policy, which may allow for administration within a period of 30 minutes before or 30 minutes after the designated time.
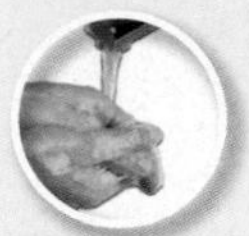 13. Perform hand hygiene and put on PPE, if indicated.	Hand hygiene and PPE prevent the spread of microorganisms. PPE is required based on transmission precautions.
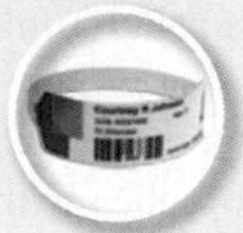 14. **Identify the patient. Compare the information with the CMAR/MAR. The patient should be identified using at least two methods** (The Joint Commission, 2013):	Identifying the patient ensures the right patient receives the medications and helps prevent errors. The patient's room number or physical location is not used as an identifier (The Joint Commission, 2013). Replace the identification band if it is missing or inaccurate in any way.
a. Check the name on the patient's identification band.	
b. Check the identification number on the patient's identification band.	
c. Check the birth date on the patient's identification band.	
d. Ask the patient to state his or her name and birth date, based on facility policy.	This requires a response from the patient, but illness and strange surroundings often cause patients to be confused.
15. Close the door to the room or pull the bedside curtain.	This provides patient privacy.
16. **Complete necessary assessments before administering medications. Check the patient's allergy bracelet or ask the patient about allergies. Explain the purpose and action of the medication to the patient.**	Assessment is a prerequisite to administration of medications. Explanation provides rationale, increases knowledge, and reduces anxiety.
17. Scan the patient's bar code on the identification band, if required.	Scanning provides an additional check to ensure that the medication is given to the right patient.
18. **Based on facility policy, the third check of the label may occur at this point. If so, recheck the labels with the CMAR/MAR before administering the medications to the patient.**	Many facilities require the *third* check to occur at the bedside, after identifying the patient and before administration. If facility policy directs the *third* check at this time, this *third* check ensures accuracy and helps to prevent errors.
19. Assess the IV site for the presence of inflammation or infiltration.	IV medication must be given directly into a vein for safe administration.
20. Close the clamp on the short secondary infusion tubing. Using aseptic technique, remove the cap on the tubing spike and the cap on the port of the medication container, taking care to avoid contaminating either end.	Closing the clamp prevents fluid from entering the system until the nurse is ready. Maintaining sterility of the tubing and the medication port prevents contamination.

ACTION	RATIONALE
21. Attach infusion tubing to the medication container by inserting the tubing spike into the port with a firm push and twisting motion, taking care to avoid contaminating either end.	Maintaining sterility of tubing and medication port prevents contamination.
22. Hang piggyback container on IV pole, positioning it higher than primary IV according to manufacturer's recommendations (Figure 1). Use metal or plastic hook to lower primary IV fluid container. (See the accompanying Skill Variation for information on administering an intermittent IV medication using a tandem piggyback setup.)	Position of containers influences the flow of IV fluid into the primary setup.
23. Place label on tubing with appropriate date.	Tubing for piggyback setup may be used for 48 to 96 hours, depending on agency policy. Label allows for tracking of the next date to change the medication.
24. Squeeze drip chamber on tubing and release. Fill to the line or about half full. Open clamp and prime tubing. Close clamp. Place needleless connector on the end of the tubing, using sterile technique, if required.	This removes air from tubing and preserves the sterility of the setup.
25. Use an antimicrobial swab to clean the access port or stopcock above the roller clamp on the primary IV infusion tubing (Figure 2).	This deters entry of microorganisms when the piggyback setup is connected to the port. Backflow valve in the primary line secondary port stops flow of primary infusion while piggyback solution is infusing. Once completed, backflow valves open and flow of primary solution resumes.
26. Connect piggyback setup to the access port or stopcock (Figure 3). If using, turn the stopcock to the open position.	Needleless systems and stopcock setup eliminate the need for a needle and are recommended by the CDC.

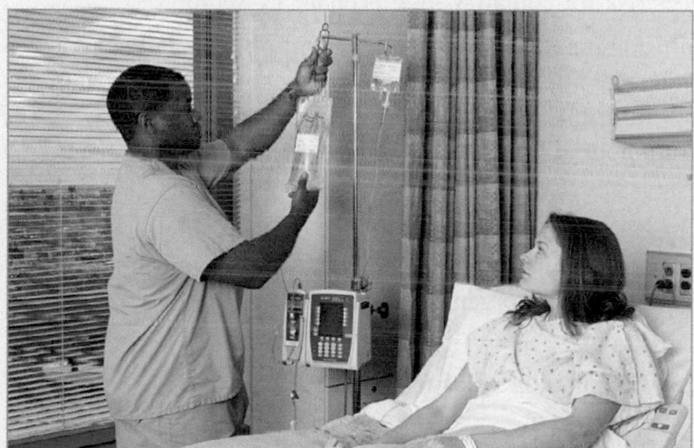

FIGURE 1 Positioning piggyback container on IV pole. *(Photo by B. Proud.)*

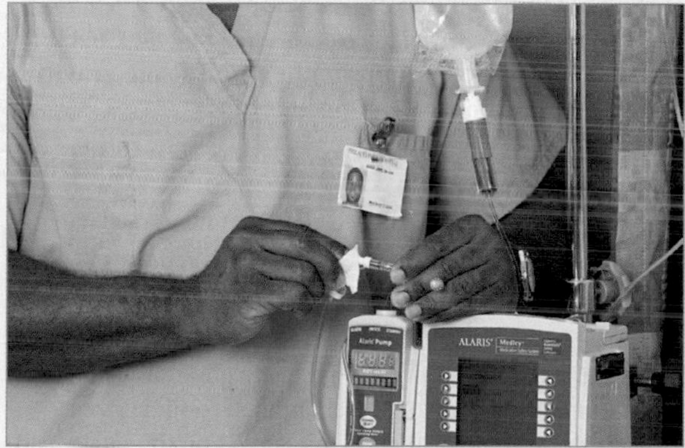

FIGURE 2 Cleaning access port. *(Photo by B. Proud.)*

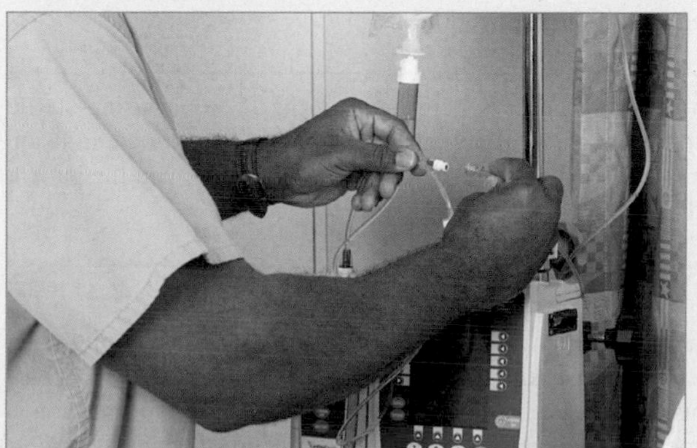

FIGURE 3 Connecting piggyback setup to access port. *(Photo by B. Proud.)*

(continued)

SKILL 5-11 ADMINISTERING A PIGGYBACK INTERMITTENT INTRAVENOUS INFUSION OF MEDICATION continued

ACTION	RATIONALE
27. Open clamp on the secondary tubing. Set rate for secondary infusion on infusion pump and begin infusion (Figure 4). If using gravity infusion, use the roller clamp on the primary infusion tubing to regulate the flow at the prescribed delivery rate (Figure 5). Monitor medication infusion at periodic intervals.	Backflow valve in the primary line secondary port stops flow of primary infusion while piggyback solution is infusing. Once completed, backflow valves open and flow of primary solution resumes. It is important to verify the safe administration rate for each drug to prevent adverse effects.

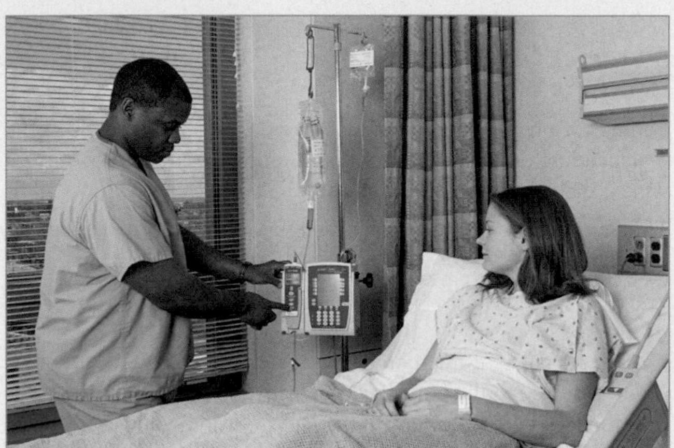

FIGURE 4 Setting rate on infusion pump. *(Photo by B. Proud.)*

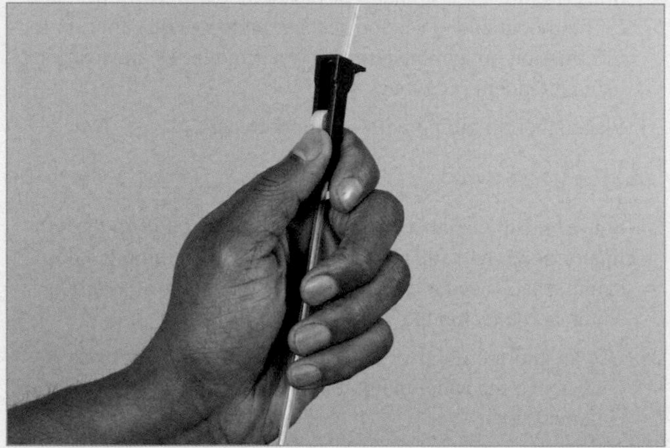

FIGURE 5 Using roller clamp on primary infusion tubing to regulate gravity flow. *(Photo by B. Proud.)*

ACTION	RATIONALE
28. Clamp tubing on piggyback set when solution is infused. Follow facility policy regarding disposal of equipment.	Most facilities allow the reuse of tubing for 48 to 96 hours. This reduces risk for contaminating primary IV setup.
29. Raise primary IV fluid container to original height. **Check primary infusion rate on infusion pump. If using gravity infusion, readjust flow rate of primary IV.**	Most infusion pumps automatically restart primary infusion at previous rate after secondary infusion is completed. If using gravity infusion, piggyback medication administration may interrupt normal flow rate of primary IV. Rate readjustment may be necessary.
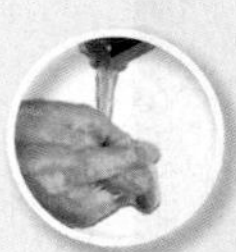 30. Remove PPE, if used. Perform hand hygiene.	Removing PPE properly reduces the risk for infection transmission and contamination of other items. Hand hygiene prevents the spread of microorganisms.
31. Document the administration of the medication immediately after administration. See Documentation section below. Document the volume of fluid administered on the intake and output record, if necessary.	Timely documentation helps to ensure patient safety.
32. Evaluate the patient's response to the medication within an appropriate time frame. Monitor IV site at periodic intervals.	The patient needs to be evaluated for therapeutic and adverse effects from the medication.

EVALUATION

The expected outcomes are met when the medication is delivered via the IV route using sterile technique; the medication is delivered to the patient in a safe manner and at the appropriate infusion rate; the patient experiences no allergy response; the patient remains infection free; and the patient understands and complies with the medication regimen.

DOCUMENTATION

Guidelines

Document the administration of the medication immediately after administration, including date, time, dose, route of administration, site of administration, and rate of administration on the CMAR/MAR or record using the required format. If using a bar-code system, medication administration is automatically recorded when the bar code is scanned. PRN medications require documentation of the reason for administration. Prompt recording avoids the possibility of accidentally repeating the administration of the drug. If the drug was refused or omitted, record this in the appropriate area on the medication record and notify the primary care provider. This verifies the reason medication was omitted and ensures that the primary care provider is aware of the patient's condition. Document the volume of fluid administered on the intake and output record, if necessary.

UNEXPECTED SITUATIONS AND ASSOCIATED INTERVENTIONS

- *Upon assessing the IV site before administering medication, you note that the IV has infiltrated:* Stop IV fluid and remove the IV from the extremity. Restart the IV in a different location. Continue to monitor the new IV site as medication is administered.
- *While administering medication, you note a cloudy, white substance forming in the IV tubing:* Stop the IV from flowing and stop administering the medication to prevent precipitate from entering the patient's circulation. Clamp the IV at the site nearest to the patient. Replace tubing on primary and secondary infusions. Check the literature regarding incompatibilities of medications before administering. Medication infusion may require a second IV site or flushing of tubing before and after administration, using the tandem system.
- *While you are administering medication, the patient begins to complain of pain at the IV site:* Stop the medication. Assess the IV site for any signs of infiltration or phlebitis. Flush the IV with normal saline to check for patency. If the IV site appears within normal limits, resume medication administration at a slower rate.

SPECIAL CONSIDERATIONS

General Considerations

- An alternate way to prime the secondary tubing, particularly if administration set is in place from a previous infusion, is to "backfill" the secondary tubing. Attach the medication bag to the secondary infusion tubing. Lower the medication bag below the main IV solution container and open the clamp on the secondary infusion tubing. This allows the primary IV solution to flow up the secondary tubing to the drip chamber, "backfilling" the tubing. Allow the solution to enter the drip chamber until the drip chamber is half full. Close the clamp on the secondary tubing and hang the medication container on the IV pole. Proceed with administration by lowering the primary IV container, as described above. This "backfill" method keeps the infusion system intact, preventing both introduction of microorganisms and loss of medication when the tubing is primed. Check facility policy regarding the use of "backfilling."
- Ongoing assessment is an important part of nursing care for both evaluation of patient response to administered medications and early detection of adverse effects. If an adverse effect is suspected, withhold further medication doses and notify the patient's primary care provider. Additional intervention is based on type of reaction and patient assessment.

Infant and Child Considerations

- Infants and small children with fluid restrictions may not tolerate the added IV fluid needed for administration with piggyback or volume-control systems. For these children, consider using the mini-infusion pump (see Skill 5-12).

SKILL VARIATION Tandem Piggyback Setup

A tandem delivery setup allows for simultaneous infusion of the primary and secondary IV solutions. Both solution containers are hung at the same height. Tubing for the secondary infusion is attached to an access port below the roller clamp on the primary tubing. There is no back-check valve at the secondary port on the primary line. This type of setup is used infrequently because the solution from the primary IV line will back up into the tandem line if this intermittent infusion is not clamped immediately after it is infused. It requires a second IV infusion pump to control the rate of the secondary infusion (or the use of primary tubing, if using gravity infusion).

Prepare medication as outlined in steps 1–12 above (Skill 5-11).

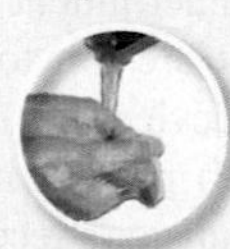

1. Perform hand hygiene and put on PPE, if indicated.

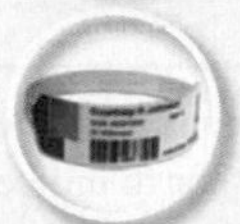

2. Identify the patient. The patient should be identified using two methods.
3. Close the door to the room or pull the bedside curtain.

(continued)

SKILL 5-11 ADMINISTERING A PIGGYBACK INTERMITTENT INTRAVENOUS INFUSION OF MEDICATION continued

SKILL VARIATION Tandem Piggyback Setup continued

4. **Complete necessary assessments before administering medications. Check the patient's allergy bracelet or ask the patient about allergies. Explain the purpose and action of the medication to the patient.**
5. Scan the patient's bar code on the identification band, if required.
6. **Based on facility policy, the third check of the label may occur at this point. If so, recheck the labels with the CMAR/MAR before administering the medications to the patient.**
7. Assess the IV site for the presence of inflammation or infiltration.
8. Close the clamp on the secondary infusion tubing. Using aseptic technique, remove the cap on the tubing spike and the cap on the port of the medication container, taking care not to contaminate either end.
9. Attach infusion tubing to the medication container by inserting the tubing spike into the port with a firm push and twisting motion, taking care not to contaminate either end.
10. Hang the secondary container on the IV pole, positioning it at the same height as the primary IV.
11. Place label on tubing with appropriate date.
12. Squeeze drip chamber and release. Fill to the line or about half full. Open clamp and prime tubing. Close clamp. Place needleless connector on the end of the tubing using sterile technique, if required. Insert tubing into infusion pump, according to manufacturer's directions.
13. Use an antimicrobial swab to clean the access port or stopcock below the roller clamp on the primary IV infusion tubing, usually the port closest to the IV insertion site.
14. Connect the secondary setup to the access port or stopcock. If using, turn the stopcock to the open position.
15. Open the clamp on the secondary tubing. Set rate for secondary infusion on infusion pump. If using gravity infusion, use the roller clamp on the primary infusion tubing to regulate the flow at the prescribed delivery rate. Monitor medication infusion at periodic intervals.
16. Turn off secondary infusion pump. Clamp tubing on secondary set when solution is infused. Remove secondary tubing from access port and cap, or replace connector with a new, capped one, if reusing. Follow facility policy regarding disposal of equipment.
17. Check primary infusion rate.

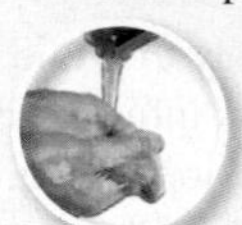

18. Remove PPE, if used. Perform hand hygiene.
19. Evaluate the patient's response to the medication within an appropriate time frame. Monitor the IV site at periodic intervals.

SKILL 5-12 ADMINISTERING AN INTERMITTENT INTRAVENOUS INFUSION OF MEDICATION VIA A MINI-INFUSION PUMP

With intermittent IV infusion, the drug is mixed with a small amount of the IV solution, and administered over a short period at the prescribed interval (e.g., every 4 hours). The mini-infusion pump (syringe pump) for intermittent infusion is battery or electrical operated and allows medication mixed in a syringe to be connected to the primary line and delivered by mechanical pressure applied to the syringe plunger. "Smart (computerized) pumps" are being used by many facilities for IV infusions, including intermittent infusions. Smart pumps also require programming of infusion rates by the nurse, but also are able to identify dosing limits and practice guidelines to aid in safe administration. Needleless devices (recommended by the CDC and the Occupational Safety and Health Administration [OSHA]) prevent needlesticks and provide access to the primary venous line. Either a blunt-ended cannula or a recessed connection port may be used to connect intermittent IV infusions.

DELEGATION CONSIDERATIONS

The administration of medications by intermittent IV infusion is not delegated to nursing assistive personnel (NAP) or to unlicensed assistive personnel (UAP). Depending on the state's nurse practice act and the organization's policies and procedures, the administration of specified IV medications in some settings may be delegated to licensed practical/vocational nurses (LPN/LVNs) who have received appropriate training. The decision to delegate must be based on careful analysis of the patient's needs and circumstances, as well as the qualifications of the person to whom the task is being delegated. Refer to the Delegation Guidelines in Appendix A.

EQUIPMENT

- Medication prepared in labeled syringe
- Mini-infusion pump and tubing
- Needleless connector, if required, based on facility system
- Antimicrobial swab
- Date label for tubing
- Computer-generated Medication Administration Record (CMAR) or Medication Administration Record (MAR)
- PPE, as indicated

ASSESSMENT

Assess the patient for any allergies. Check the expiration date before administering medication. Assess the appropriateness of the drug for the patient. Assess the compatibility of the ordered medication, diluent, and the infusing IV fluid. Review assessment and laboratory data that may influence drug administration. Verify patient name, dose, route, and time of administration. Assess the patient's knowledge of the medication. If the patient has a knowledge deficit about the medication, this may be the appropriate time to begin education about the medication. If the medication may affect the patient's vital signs, assess them before administration. Assess the IV insertion site, noting any swelling, coolness, leakage of fluid at site, redness, or pain.

NURSING DIAGNOSIS

Determine related factors for the nursing diagnoses based on the patient's current status. Appropriate nursing diagnoses include:

- Risk for Allergy Response
- Risk for Injury
- Risk for Infection

OUTCOME IDENTIFICATION AND PLANNING

The expected outcome is that the medication is delivered via the IV route using sterile technique. Other outcomes that may be appropriate include the following: medication is delivered to the patient in a safe manner and at the appropriate infusion rate; the patient experiences no allergy response; the patient remains infection free; and the patient understands and complies with the medication regimen.

IMPLEMENTATION

ACTION	RATIONALE
1. Gather equipment. Check each medication order against the original order in the medical record according to facility policy. Clarify any inconsistencies. Check the patient's chart for allergies.	This comparison helps to identify errors that may have occurred when orders were transcribed. The primary care provider's order is the legal record of medication orders for each facility. Compatibility of medication and solution prevents complications.
2. Know the actions, special nursing considerations, safe dose ranges, purpose of administration, and adverse effects of the medications to be administered. Consider the appropriateness of the medication for this patient.	This knowledge aids the nurse in evaluating the therapeutic effect of the medication in relation to the patient's disorder and can also be used to educate the patient about the medication.
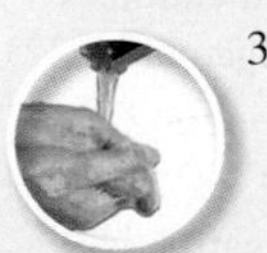 3. Perform hand hygiene.	Hand hygiene prevents the spread of microorganisms.
4. Move the medication cart to the outside of the patient's room or prepare for administration in the medication area.	Organization facilitates error-free administration and saves time.
5. Unlock the medication cart or drawer. Enter pass code and scan employee identification, if required.	Locking the cart or drawer safeguards each patient's medication supply. Hospital accrediting organizations require medication carts to be locked when not in use. Entering pass code and scanning ID allows only authorized users into the system and identifies the user for documentation by the computer.

(continued)

SKILL 5-12 ADMINISTERING AN INTERMITTENT INTRAVENOUS INFUSION OF MEDICATION VIA A MINI-INFUSION PUMP continued

ACTION	RATIONALE
6. **Prepare medications for one patient at a time.**	This prevents errors in medication administration.
7. Read the CMAR/MAR and select the proper medication from unit stock or the patient's medication drawer.	This is the *first* check of the label.
8. Compare the label with the CMAR/MAR. Check expiration dates. Confirm the prescribed or appropriate infusion rate. Scan the bar code on the package, if required.	This is the *second* check of the label. Verify calculations with another nurse to ensure safety, if necessary. Infusing medication at appropriate rate prevents injury.
9. **Depending on facility policy, the third check of the label may occur at this point. If so, when all medications for one patient have been prepared, recheck the labels with the CMAR/MAR before taking the medications to the patient.**	This *third* check ensures accuracy and helps to prevent errors. *Note:* Many facilities require the *third* check to occur at the bedside, after identifying the patient and before administration.
10. Lock the medication cart before leaving it.	Locking the cart or drawer safeguards the patient's medication supply. Hospital accrediting organizations require medication carts to be locked when not in use.
11. Transport medications to the patient's bedside carefully, and keep the medications in sight at all times.	Careful handling and close observation prevent accidental or deliberate disarrangement of medications.
12. **Ensure that the patient receives the medications at the correct time.**	Check agency policy, which may allow for administration within a period of 30 minutes before or 30 minutes after the designated time.
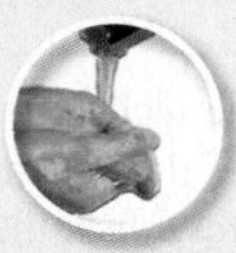 13. Perform hand hygiene and put on PPE, if indicated.	Hand hygiene and PPE prevent the spread of microorganisms. PPE is required based on transmission precautions.
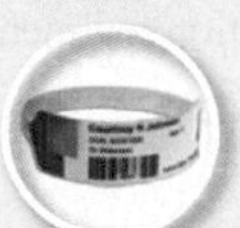 14. **Identify the patient. Compare the information with the CMAR/MAR. The patient should be identified using at least two methods** (The Joint Commission, 2013):	Identifying the patient ensures the right patient receives the medications and helps prevent errors. The patient's room number or physical location is not used as an identifier (The Joint Commission, 2013). Replace the identification band if it is missing or inaccurate in any way.
a. Check the name on the patient's identification band.	
b. Check the identification number on the patient's identification band.	
c. Check the birth date on the patient's identification band.	
d. Ask the patient to state his or her name and birth date, based on facility policy.	This requires a response from the patient, but illness and strange surroundings often cause patients to be confused.
15. Close the door to the room or pull the bedside curtain.	Provides patient privacy.
16. **Complete necessary assessments before administering medications. Check the patient's allergy bracelet or ask the patient about allergies. Explain the purpose and action of the medication to the patient.**	Assessment is a prerequisite to administration of medications. Explanation provides rationale, increases knowledge, and reduces anxiety.
17. Scan the patient's bar code on the identification band, if required.	Provides an additional check to ensure that the medication is given to the right patient.
18. **Based on facility policy, the third check of the label may occur at this point. If so, recheck the labels with the CMAR/MAR before administering the medications to the patient.**	Many facilities require the *third* check to occur at the bedside, after identifying the patient and before administration. If facility policy directs the *third* check at this time, this *third* check ensures accuracy and helps to prevent errors.
19. Assess the IV site for the presence of inflammation or infiltration.	IV medication must be given directly into a vein for safe administration.
20. Using aseptic technique, remove the cap on the tubing and the cap on the syringe, taking care not to contaminate either end.	Maintaining sterility of tubing and medication port prevents contamination.

ACTION	RATIONALE
21. Attach infusion tubing to the syringe, taking care not to contaminate either end.	Maintaining sterility of tubing and medication port prevents contamination.
22. Place label on tubing with appropriate date.	Tubing for piggyback setup may be used for 48 to 96 hours, depending on facility policy. Label allows for tracking of the next date to change.
23. Fill tubing with medication by applying gentle pressure to syringe plunger. Place needleless connector on the end of the tubing, using sterile technique, if required.	This removes air from tubing and maintains sterility.
24. Insert syringe into mini-infusion pump according to manufacturer's directions (Figure 1).	Syringe must fit securely in pump apparatus for proper operation.
25. Use antimicrobial swab to clean the access port or stopcock below the roller clamp on the primary IV infusion tubing, usually the port closest to the IV insertion site (Figure 2).	This deters entry of microorganisms when the piggyback setup is connected to the port. Proper connection allows IV medication to flow into the primary line.
26. Connect the secondary infusion to the primary infusion at the cleansed port (Figure 3).	Allows for delivery of medication.
27. Program the pump to the appropriate rate and begin infusion (Figure 4). Set the alarm if recommended by the manufacturer.	Pump delivers medication at a controlled rate. Alarm is recommended for use with IV lock apparatus.

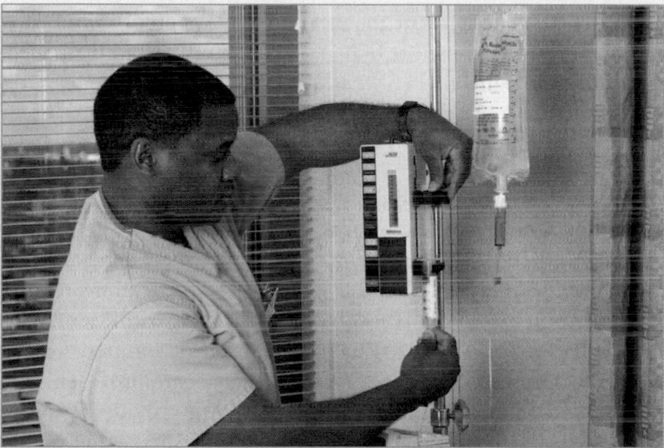
FIGURE 1 Inserting syringe into mini-infusion pump.

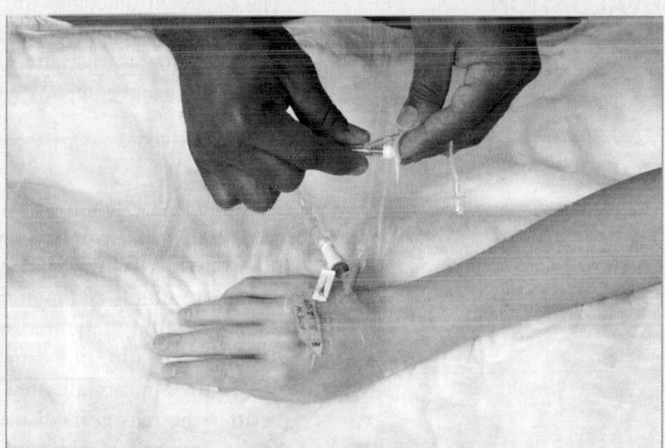
FIGURE 2 Cleaning access port closest to IV insertion site.

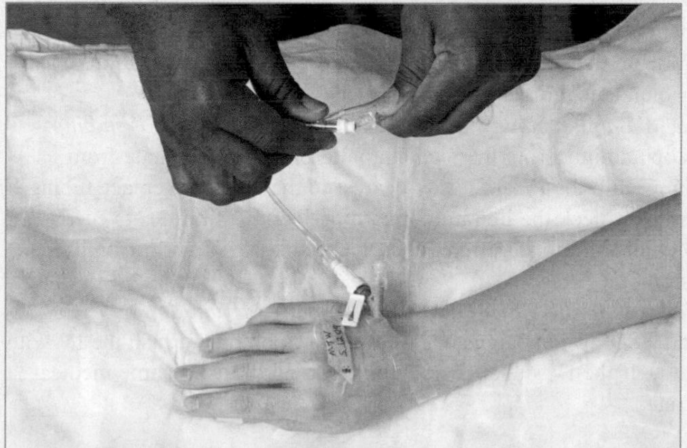
FIGURE 3 Connecting secondary infusion tubing to primary infusion.

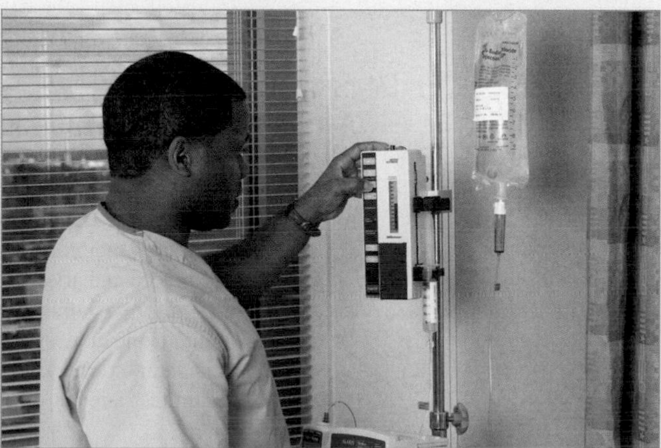
FIGURE 4 Programming mini-infusion pump.

(*continued*)

SKILL 5-12 ADMINISTERING AN INTERMITTENT INTRAVENOUS INFUSION OF MEDICATION VIA A MINI-INFUSION PUMP continued

ACTION	RATIONALE
28. Clamp tubing on secondary set when solution is infused. Remove secondary tubing from access port and cap, or replace connector with a new, capped one, if reusing. Follow facility policy regarding disposal of equipment.	Many facilities allow reuse of tubing for 48 to 96 hours. Replacing connector or needle with a new, capped one maintains system sterility.
29. Check rate of primary infusion.	Administration of secondary infusion may interfere with primary infusion rate.
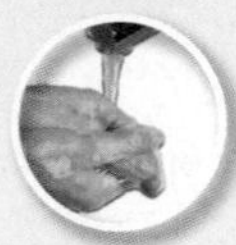 30. Remove PPE, if used. Perform hand hygiene.	Removing PPE properly reduces the risk for infection transmission and contamination of other items. Hand hygiene prevents the spread of microorganisms.
31. Document the administration of the medication immediately after administration. See Documentation section below. Document the volume of fluid administered on the intake and output record, if necessary.	Timely documentation helps to ensure patient safety.
32. Evaluate the patient's response to the medication within appropriate time frame. Monitor IV site at periodic intervals.	The patient needs to be evaluated for therapeutic and adverse effects from the medication.

EVALUATION

The expected outcomes are met when the medication is delivered via the IV route using sterile technique; the medication is delivered to the patient in a safe manner and at the appropriate infusion rate; the patient experiences no allergy response; the patient remains infection free; and the patient understands and complies with the medication regimen.

DOCUMENTATION

Guidelines

Document the administration of the medication immediately after administration, including date, time, dose, route of administration, site of administration, and rate of administration on the CMAR/MAR or record using the required format. If using a bar-code system, medication administration is automatically recorded when the bar code is scanned. PRN medications require documentation of the reason for administration. Prompt recording avoids the possibility of accidentally repeating the administration of the drug. If the drug was refused or omitted, record this in the appropriate area on the medication record and notify the primary care provider. This verifies the reason medication was omitted and ensures that the primary care provider is aware of the patient's condition. Document the volume of fluid administered on the intake and output record, if necessary.

UNEXPECTED SITUATIONS AND ASSOCIATED INTERVENTIONS

- *Upon assessing the IV site before administering medication, you note that the IV has infiltrated:* Stop IV fluid and remove the IV from the extremity. Restart the IV in a different location. Continue to monitor the new IV site as medication is administered.
- *While administering medication, you note a cloudy, white substance forming in the IV tubing:* Stop the IV from flowing and stop administering the medication to prevent precipitate from entering the patient's circulation. Clamp the IV at the site nearest to the patient. Replace tubing on primary and secondary infusions. Check the literature regarding incompatibilities of medications before administering. Medication infusion may require a second IV site or flushing of tubing before and after administration.
- *While you are administering medication, the patient begins to complain of pain at the IV site:* Stop the medication. Assess the IV site for any signs of infiltration or phlebitis. Flush the IV with normal saline to check for patency. If the IV site appears within normal limits, resume medication administration at a slower rate.

SPECIAL CONSIDERATIONS

General Considerations

- Ongoing assessment is an important part of nursing care for both evaluation of patient response to administered medications and early detection of adverse effects. If an adverse effect is suspected, withhold further medication doses and notify the patient's primary care provider. Additional intervention is based on type of reaction and patient assessment.

Infant and Child Considerations

- Infants and small children with fluid restrictions may not tolerate the added IV fluid needed for administration with piggyback or volume-control systems. For these children, consider using the mini-infusion pump.

SKILL 5-13 ADMINISTERING AN INTERMITTENT INTRAVENOUS INFUSION OF MEDICATION VIA A VOLUME-CONTROL ADMINISTRATION SET

With intermittent IV infusion, the drug is mixed with a small amount of the IV solution (e.g., 50 to 100 mL) and administered over a short period at the prescribed interval (e.g., every 4 hours). The administration is most often performed using an IV infusion pump, which requires the nurse to program the infusion rate into the pump. "Smart (computerized) pumps" are being used by many facilities for IV infusions, including intermittent infusions. Smart pumps also require programming of infusion rates by the nurse, but also are able to identify dosing limits and practice guidelines to aid in safe administration. Administration may also be achieved by gravity infusion, which requires the nurse to calculate the infusion rate in drops per minute. The best practice, however, is to use an intravenous infusion pump.

This skill discusses using a volume-control administration set for intermittent IV infusion. The medication is diluted with a small amount of solution and administered through the patient's IV line. This type of equipment may be used for infusing solutions into children, critically ill patients, and older patients when the fluid volume to be infused is a concern. Needleless devices (recommended by the CDC and the Occupational Safety and Health Administration [OSHA]) prevent needlesticks and provide access to the primary venous line. Either a blunt-ended cannula or a recessed connection port may be used to connect intermittent IV infusions.

DELEGATION CONSIDERATIONS

The administration of medications by intermittent IV infusion is not delegated to nursing assistive personnel (NAP) or to unlicensed assistive personnel (UAP). Depending on the state's nurse practice act and the organization's policies and procedures, the administration of specified IV medications in some settings may be delegated to licensed practical/vocational nurses (LPN/LVNs) who have received appropriate training. The decision to delegate must be based on careful analysis of the patient's needs and circumstances, as well as the qualifications of the person to whom the task is being delegated. Refer to the Delegation Guidelines in Appendix A.

EQUIPMENT

- Prescribed medication
- Syringe with a needless device or blunt needle, if required, based on facility system
- Volume-control set (Volutrol, Buretrol, Burette)
- Needleless connector or stopcock, if required
- Infusion pump, if needed
- Antimicrobial swab
- Date label for tubing
- Medication label

(continued)

SKILL 5-13 ADMINISTERING AN INTERMITTENT INTRAVENOUS INFUSION OF MEDICATION VIA A VOLUME-CONTROL ADMINISTRATION SET continued

- Computer-generated Medication Administration Record (CMAR) or Medication Administration Record (MAR)
- PPE, as indicated

ASSESSMENT

Assess the patient for any allergies. Check the expiration date before administering the medication. Assess the appropriateness of the drug for the patient. Assess the compatibility of the ordered medication, diluent, and the infusing IV fluid. Review assessment and laboratory data that may influence drug administration. Assess the patient's knowledge of the medication. If the patient has a knowledge deficit about the medication, this may be the appropriate time to begin education about the medication. If the medication may affect the patient's vital signs, assess them before administration. Assess the IV insertion site, noting any swelling, coolness, leakage of fluid at site, redness, or pain.

NURSING DIAGNOSIS

Determine related factors for the nursing diagnoses based on the patient's current status. Appropriate nursing diagnoses include:

- Risk for Allergy Response
- Risk for Injury
- Risk for Infection

OUTCOME IDENTIFICATION AND PLANNING

The expected outcome to achieve when administering an intermittent IV infusion of medication via a volume-control set is that the medication is delivered via the IV route using sterile technique. Other outcomes that may be appropriate include the following: medication is delivered to the patient in a safe manner and at the appropriate infusion rate; the patient experiences no allergy response; the patient remains infection free; and the patient understands and complies with the medication regimen.

IMPLEMENTATION

ACTION	RATIONALE
1. Gather equipment. Check the medication order against the original order in the medical record according to facility policy. Clarify any inconsistencies. Check the patient's chart for allergies. Verify the compatibility of the medication and IV fluid.	This comparison helps to identify errors that may have occurred when orders were transcribed. The primary care provider's order is the legal record of medication orders for each facility.
2. Know the actions, special nursing considerations, safe dose ranges, purpose of administration, and adverse effects of the medications to be administered. Consider the appropriateness of the medication for this patient.	This knowledge aids the nurse in evaluating the therapeutic effect of the medication in relation to the patient's disorder and can also be used to educate the patient about the medication.
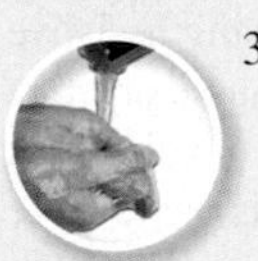 3. Perform hand hygiene.	Hand hygiene prevents the spread of microorganisms.
4. Move the medication cart to the outside of the patient's room or prepare for administration in the medication area.	Organization facilitates error-free administration and saves time.
5. Unlock the medication cart or drawer. Enter pass code and scan employee identification, if required.	Locking the cart or drawer safeguards each patient's medication supply. Hospital accrediting organizations require medication carts to be locked when not in use. Entering pass code and scanning ID allows only authorized users into the computer system and identifies the user for documentation by the computer.
6. **Prepare medication for one patient at a time.**	This prevents errors in medication administration.
7. Read the CMAR/MAR and select the proper medication from unit stock or the patient's medication drawer.	This is the *first* check of the label.

ACTION	RATIONALE
8. Compare the label with the CMAR/MAR. Check expiration dates and perform calculations, if necessary. Confirm the prescribed or appropriate infusion rate. Calculate the drip rate if using a gravity system. Scan the bar code on the package, if required. Check the infusion rate.	This is the *second* check of the label. Verify calculations with another nurse to ensure safety, if necessary. Delivers the correct dose of medication as prescribed.
9. If necessary, withdraw medication from an ampule or vial as described in Skills 5-3 and 5-4. Attach needleless connector or blunt needle to end of syringe, if necessary.	Allows for entry into the volume-control administration set chamber.
10. **Depending on facility policy, the third check of the label may occur at this point. If so, when all medications for one patient have been prepared, recheck the label with the CMAR/MAR before taking the medications to the patient.**	This *third* check ensures accuracy and helps to prevent errors. *Note:* Many facilities require the *third* check to occur at the bedside, after identifying the patient and before administration.
11. Prepare medication label, including name of medication, dose, total volume, including diluent, and time of administration.	Allows for accurate identification of medication.
12. Lock the medication cart before leaving it.	Locking the cart or drawer safeguards the patient's medication supply. Hospital accrediting organizations require medication carts to be locked when not in use.
13. Transport medications and equipment to the patient's bedside carefully, and keep the medications in sight at all times.	Careful handling and close observation prevent accidental or deliberate disarrangement of medications. Having equipment available saves time and facilitates performance of the task.
14. **Ensure that the patient receives the medications at the correct time.**	Check facility policy, which may allow for administration within a period of 30 minutes before or 30 minutes after the designated time.
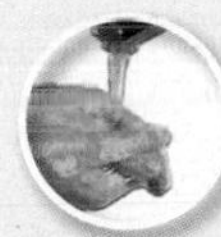 15. Perform hand hygiene and put on PPE, if indicated.	Hand hygiene and PPE prevent the spread of microorganisms. PPE is required based on transmission precautions.
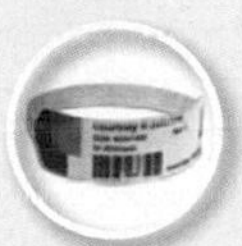 16. **Identify the patient. Compare the information with the CMAR/MAR. The patient should be identified using at least two methods** (The Joint Commission, 2013):	Identifying the patient ensures the right patient receives the medications and helps prevent errors. The patient's room number or physical location is not used as an identifier (The Joint Commission, 2013). Replace the identification band if it is missing or inaccurate in any way.
a. Check the name on the patient's identification band.	
b. Check the identification number on the patient's identification band.	
c. Check the birth date on the patient's identification band.	
d. Ask the patient to state his or her name and birth date, based on facility policy.	This requires a response from the patient, but illness and strange surroundings often cause patients to be confused.
17. Close the door to the room or pull the bedside curtain.	This provides patient privacy.
18. **Complete necessary assessments before administering medications. Check the patient's allergy bracelet or ask the patient about allergies. Explain the purpose and action of the medication to the patient.**	Assessment is a prerequisite to administration of medications. Explanation provides rationale, increases knowledge, and reduces anxiety.

(*continued*)

SKILL 5-13 ADMINISTERING AN INTERMITTENT INTRAVENOUS INFUSION OF MEDICATION VIA A VOLUME-CONTROL ADMINISTRATION SET continued

ACTION	RATIONALE
19. Scan the patient's bar code on the identification band, if required (Figure 1).	Provides an additional check to ensure that the medication is given to the right patient.
20. **Based on facility policy, the third check of the label may occur at this point. If so, recheck the labels with the CMAR/MAR before administering the medications to the patient.**	Many facilities require the *third* check to occur at the bedside, after identifying the patient and before administration. If facility policy directs the *third* check at this time, this *third* check ensures accuracy and helps to prevent errors.
21. Assess IV site for presence of inflammation or infiltration.	IV medication must be given directly into a vein for safe administration.
22. Fill the volume-control administration set (Figure 2) with the prescribed amount of IV fluid by opening the clamp between IV solution and the volume-control administration set. Follow manufacturer's instructions and fill with prescribed amount of IV solution (Figure 3). Close clamp.	This dilutes the medication in a minimal amount of solution. Reclamping prevents the continued addition of fluid to the volume to be mixed with the medication.

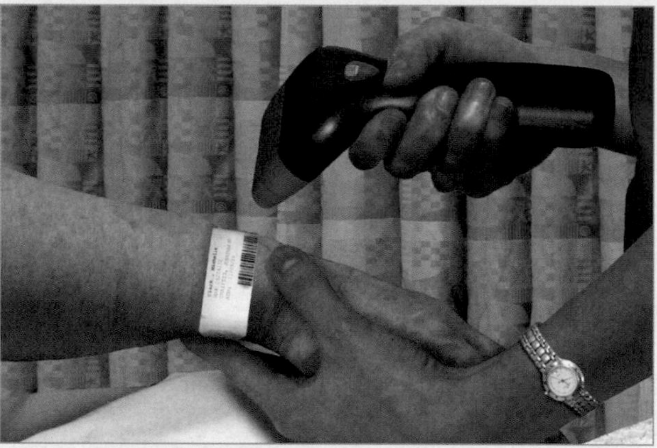

FIGURE 1 Scanning bar code on the patient's identification bracelet. *(Photo by B. Proud.)*

FIGURE 2 Volume-control administration set and IV solution for dilution of medication. *(Photo by B. Proud.)*

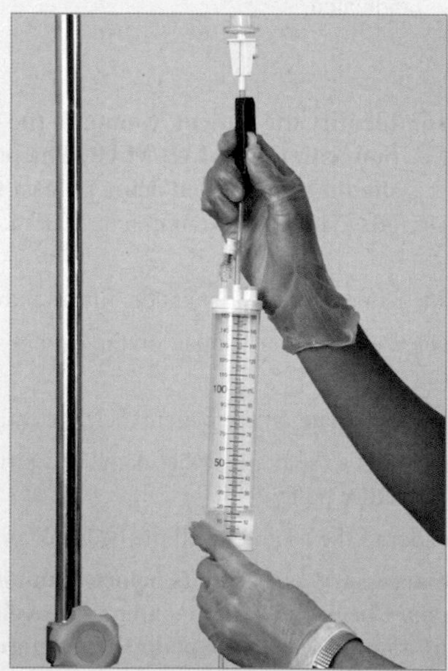

FIGURE 3 Opening clamp between IV solution and volume-control administration set to fill chamber with prescribed amount of solution. *(Photo by B. Proud.)*

ACTION	RATIONALE
23. Check to ensure the air vent on the volume-control administration set chamber is open.	Air vent allows fluid in the chamber to flow at a regular rate.
24. Use an antimicrobial swab to clean the access port on the volume-control administration set chamber (Figure 4).	This deters entry of microorganisms when the syringe enters the chamber.
25. Attach the syringe with a twisting motion into the access port while holding the syringe steady (Figure 5). Alternately, insert the needleless device or blunt needle into the port. Inject the medication into the chamber (Figure 6). Gently rotate the chamber.	This ensures that medication is evenly mixed with the solution.

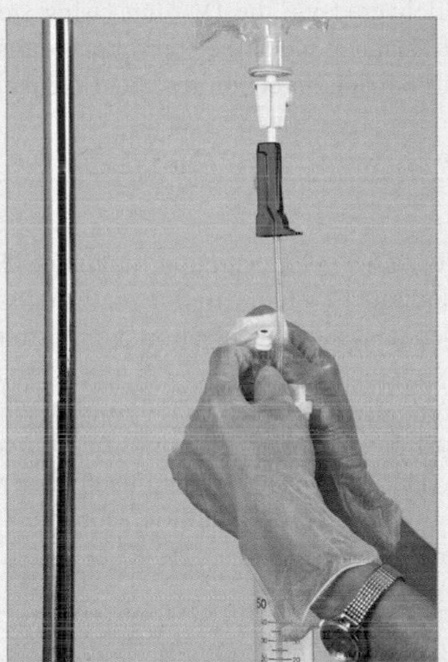

FIGURE 4 Cleaning access port. *(Photo by B. Proud.)*

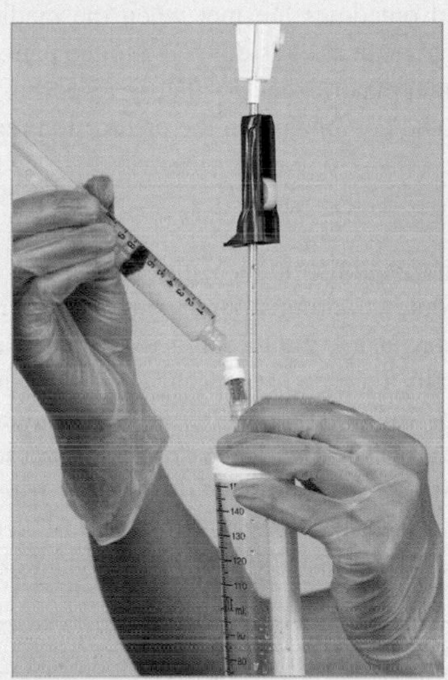

FIGURE 5 Attaching syringe to access port. *(Photo by B. Proud.)*

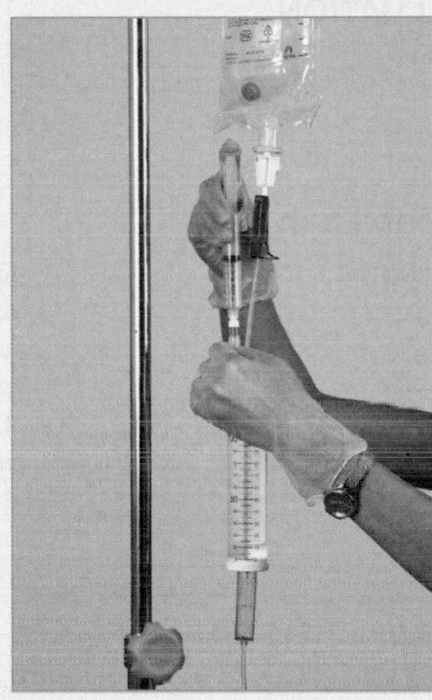

FIGURE 6 Injecting medication into chamber. *(Photo by B. Proud.)*

ACTION	RATIONALE
26. Attach the medication label to the volume-control device.	This identifies contents of the set and prevents medication error.
27. Use an antimicrobial swab to clean the access port or stopcock below the roller clamp on the primary IV infusion tubing, usually the port closest to the IV insertion site.	This deters entry of microorganisms when the piggyback setup is connected to the port. Proper connection allows IV medication to flow into primary line.
28. Connect the secondary infusion to the primary infusion at the cleansed port.	This allows for delivery of medication.
29. The volume-control administration set may be placed on an infusion pump with the appropriate dose programmed into the pump. Alternately, use the roller clamp on the volume-control administration set tubing to adjust the infusion to the prescribed rate.	Delivery over a 30- to 60-minute interval is a safe method of administering IV medication.
30. Discard the syringe in the appropriate receptacle.	Proper disposal prevents injury.
31. Clamp tubing on secondary set when solution is infused. Remove secondary tubing from access port and cap or replace connector with a new, capped one, if reusing. Follow facility policy regarding disposal of equipment.	Many facilities allow reuse of tubing for 48 to 96 hours. Replacing connector or needle with a new, capped one maintains sterility of system.
32. Check rate of primary infusion.	Administration of a secondary infusion may interfere with the primary infusion rate.
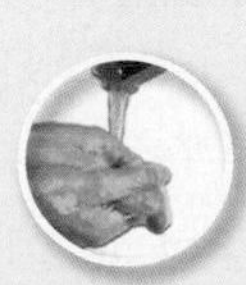 33. Remove PPE, if used. Perform hand hygiene.	Removing PPE properly reduces the risk for infection transmission and contamination of other items. Hand hygiene prevents the spread of microorganisms.

(continued)

SKILL 5-13 ADMINISTERING AN INTERMITTENT INTRAVENOUS INFUSION OF MEDICATION VIA A VOLUME-CONTROL ADMINISTRATION SET continued

ACTION	RATIONALE
34. Document the administration of the medication immediately after administration. See Documentation section below. Document the volume of fluid administered on the intake and output record, if necessary.	Timely documentation helps to ensure patient safety.
35. Evaluate the patient's response to the medication within appropriate time frame. Monitor IV site at periodic intervals.	The patient needs to be evaluated for therapeutic and adverse effects from the medication. Visualization of the site also allows for assessment of any untoward effects.

EVALUATION

The expected outcomes are met when the medication is delivered via the IV route using sterile technique; the medication is delivered to the patient in a safe manner and at the appropriate infusion rate; the patient experiences no allergy response; the patient remains infection free; and the patient understands and complies with the medication regimen.

DOCUMENTATION

Guidelines

Document the administration of the medication immediately after administration, including date, time, dose, route of administration, site of administration, and rate of administration on the CMAR/MAR or record using the required format. If using a bar-code system, medication administration is automatically recorded when bar code is scanned. PRN medications require documentation of the reason for administration. Prompt recording avoids the possibility of accidentally repeating the administration of the drug. If the drug was refused or omitted, record this in the appropriate area on the medication record and notify the primary care provider. This verifies the reason medication was omitted and ensures that the primary care provider is aware of the patient's condition. Document the volume of fluid administered on the intake and output record, if necessary.

UNEXPECTED SITUATIONS AND ASSOCIATED INTERVENTIONS

- *Upon assessing the IV site before administering the medication, you note that the IV has infiltrated:* Stop IV fluid and remove the IV from the extremity. Restart the IV in a different location. Continue to monitor the new IV site as medication is administered.
- *While administering the medication, you note a cloudy, white substance forming in the IV tubing:* Stop the IV from flowing and stop administering the medication to prevent precipitate from entering the patient's circulation. Clamp the IV at the site nearest to the patient. Replace tubing on primary and secondary infusions. Check the literature regarding incompatibilities of medications before administering. Medication infusion may require a second IV site or flushing of tubing before and after administration.
- *While you are administering the medication, the patient begins to complain of pain at the IV site:* Stop the medication. Assess the IV site for any signs of infiltration or phlebitis. Flush the IV with normal saline to check for patency. If the IV site appears within normal limits, resume medication administration at a slower rate.

SPECIAL CONSIDERATIONS

General Considerations

- Ongoing assessment is an important part of nursing care for both evaluation of patient response to administered medications and early detection of adverse effects. If an adverse effect is suspected, withhold further medication doses and notify the patient's primary care provider. Additional intervention is based on type of reaction and patient assessment.

Infant and Child Considerations

- Infants and small children with fluid restrictions may not tolerate the added IV fluid needed for administration with piggyback or volume-control systems. For these children, consider using a mini-infusion pump (Skill 5-12).

SKILL 5-14 INTRODUCING DRUGS THROUGH A MEDICATION OR DRUG-INFUSION LOCK (INTERMITTENT PERIPHERAL VENOUS ACCESS DEVICE) USING THE SALINE FLUSH

A medication or drug-infusion lock, also known as an intermittent peripheral venous access device, is used for patients who require intermittent IV medication, but not a continuous IV infusion. This device consists of a needle or catheter connected to a short length of tubing capped with a sealed injection port. After the catheter is in place in the patient's vein, the catheter and tubing are anchored to the patient's arm so that the catheter remains in place until the patient no longer requires the repeated medication intravenously.

The device is kept patent (working) by flushing with small amounts of saline pushed through the device on a routine basis. Using saline eliminates any possible systemic effects on coagulation, development of a heparin allergy, and drug incompatibility, which may occur when a heparin solution is used. The nurse must confirm IV placement before administration of medication. It is important to flush the drug-infusion lock before and after the medication is administered to clear the vein of any medication and to prevent clot formation in the device. If infiltration or phlebitis occurs, the lock is removed and replaced in a new site.

DELEGATION CONSIDERATIONS

The administration of medications through an intermittent peripheral venous access device is not delegated to nursing assistive personnel (NAP) or to unlicensed assistive personnel (UAP). Depending on the state's nurse practice act and the organization's policies and procedures, the administration of specified IV medications in some settings may be delegated to licensed practical/vocational nurses (LPN/LVNs) who have received appropriate training. The decision to delegate must be based on careful analysis of the patient's needs and circumstances, as well as the qualifications of the person to whom the task is being delegated. Refer to the Delegation Guidelines in Appendix A.

EQUIPMENT

- Medication
- Saline flushes (2), volume according to facility policy, usually 2 to 3 mL
- Antimicrobial swabs
- Watch with second hand or stopwatch feature
- Disposable gloves
- Computer-generated Medication Administration Record (CMAR) or Medication Administration Record (MAR)

ASSESSMENT

Assess the patient for any allergies. Check the expiration date before administering the medication. Assess the appropriateness of the drug for the patient. Review assessment and laboratory data that may influence drug administration. Assess the patient's IV site, noting any swelling, coolness, leakage of fluid from IV site, or pain. Assess the patient's knowledge of the medication. If the patient has a knowledge deficit about the medication, this may be the appropriate time to begin education about the medication. If the medication may affect the patient's vital signs, assess them before administration. If the medication is for pain relief, assess the patient's pain before and after administration.

NURSING DIAGNOSIS

Determine related factors for the nursing diagnoses based on the patient's current status. Appropriate nursing diagnoses may include:

- Risk for Allergy Response
- Risk for Infection
- Deficient Knowledge

OUTCOME IDENTIFICATION AND PLANNING

The expected outcome to achieve when administering medication via a medication or drug-infusion lock is that the medication is delivered via the IV route using sterile technique. Other outcomes that may be appropriate include the following: medication is delivered to the patient in a safe manner and at the appropriate infusion rate; the patient experiences no adverse effect; and the patient understands and complies with the medication regimen.

(continued)

SKILL 5-14 INTRODUCING DRUGS THROUGH A MEDICATION OR DRUG-INFUSION LOCK (INTERMITTENT PERIPHERAL VENOUS ACCESS DEVICE) USING THE SALINE FLUSH continued

IMPLEMENTATION

ACTION	RATIONALE
1. Gather equipment. Check the medication order against the original order in the medical record, according to agency policy. Clarify any inconsistencies. Check the patient's chart for allergies. Check a drug resource to clarify whether medication needs to be diluted before administration. Verify the recommended administration rate.	This comparison helps to identify errors that may have occurred when orders were transcribed. The primary care provider's order is the legal record of medication orders for each facility. Compatibility of medication and solution prevents complications. Recommended infusion rate delivers the correct dose of medication as prescribed.
2. Know the actions, special nursing considerations, safe dose ranges, purpose of administration, and adverse effects of the medications to be administered. Consider the appropriateness of the medication for this patient.	This knowledge aids the nurse in evaluating the therapeutic effect of the medication in relation to the patient's disorder and can also be used to educate the patient about the medication.
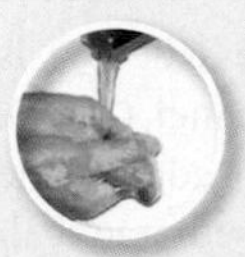 3. Perform hand hygiene.	Hand hygiene prevents the spread of microorganisms.
4. Move the medication cart to the outside of the patient's room or prepare for administration in the medication area.	Organization facilitates error-free administration and saves time.
5. Unlock the medication cart or drawer. Enter pass code and scan employee identification, if required.	Locking the cart or drawer safeguards each patient's medication supply. Hospital accrediting organizations require medication carts to be locked when not in use. Entering pass code and scanning ID allows only authorized users into the system and identifies the user for documentation by the computer.
6. **Prepare medication for one patient at a time.**	This prevents errors in medication administration.
7. Read the CMAR/MAR and select the proper medication from unit stock or the patient's medication drawer.	This is the *first* check of the label.
8. Compare the label with the CMAR/MAR. Check expiration dates and perform calculations, if necessary. Scan the bar code on the package, if required.	This is the *second* check of the label. Verify calculations with another nurse to ensure safety, if necessary.
9. If necessary, withdraw medication from an ampule or vial as described in Skills 5-3 and 5-4.	Allows administration of medication.
10. **Depending on facility policy, the third check of the label may occur at this point. If so, when all medications for one patient have been prepared, recheck the labels with the CMAR/MAR before taking the medications to the patient.**	This *third* check ensures accuracy and helps to prevent errors. *Note:* Many facilities require the *third* check to occur at the bedside, after identifying the patient and before administration.
11. Lock the medication cart before leaving it.	Locking the cart or drawer safeguards the patient's medication supply. Hospital accrediting organizations require medication carts to be locked when not in use.
12. Transport medications and equipment to the patient's bedside carefully, and keep the medications in sight at all times.	Careful handling and close observation prevent accidental or deliberate disarrangement of medications. Having equipment available saves time and facilitates performance of the task.
13. **Ensure that the patient receives the medications at the correct time.**	Check facility policy, which may allow for administration within a period of 30 minutes before or 30 minutes after the designated time.

ACTION | RATIONALE

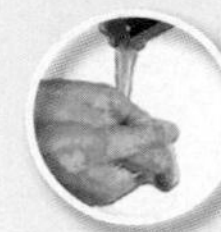

14. Perform hand hygiene and put on PPE, if indicated.

Hand hygiene and PPE prevent the spread of microorganisms. PPE is required based on transmission precautions.

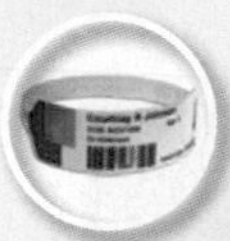

15. **Identify the patient. Compare the information with the CMAR/MAR. The patient should be identified using at least two methods** (The Joint Commission, 2013):

Identifying the patient ensures the right patient receives the medications and helps prevent errors. The patient's room number or physical location is not used as an identifier (The Joint Commission, 2013). Replace the identification band if it is missing or inaccurate in any way.

a. Check the name on the patient's identification band.

b. Check the identification number on the patient's identification band.

c. Check the birth date on the patient's identification band.

d. Ask the patient to state his or her name and birth date, based on facility policy.

This requires a response from the patient, but illness and strange surroundings often cause patients to be confused.

16. Close the door to the room or pull the bedside curtain.

This provides patient privacy.

17. **Complete necessary assessments before administering medications. Check the patient's allergy bracelet or ask the patient about allergies. Explain the purpose and action of the medication to the patient.**

Assessment is a prerequisite to administration of medications. Explanation provides rationale, increases knowledge, and reduces anxiety.

18. Scan the patient's bar code on the identification band, if required (Figure 1).

Scanning provides an additional check to ensure that the medication is given to the right patient.

19. **Based on facility policy, the third check of the label may occur at this point. If so, recheck the labels with the CMAR/MAR before administering the medications to the patient.**

Many facilities require the *third* check to occur at the bedside, after identifying the patient and before administration. If facility policy directs the *third* check at this time, this *third* check ensures accuracy and helps to prevent errors.

20. Assess IV site for presence of inflammation or infiltration.

IV medication must be given directly into a vein for safe administration.

21. Put on clean gloves.

Gloves protect the nurse's hands from contact with the patient's blood.

22. Clean the access port of the medication lock with antimicrobial swab (Figure 2).

Cleaning removes surface contaminants at the lock entry site.

FIGURE 1 Scanning bar code on patient's identification bracelet.

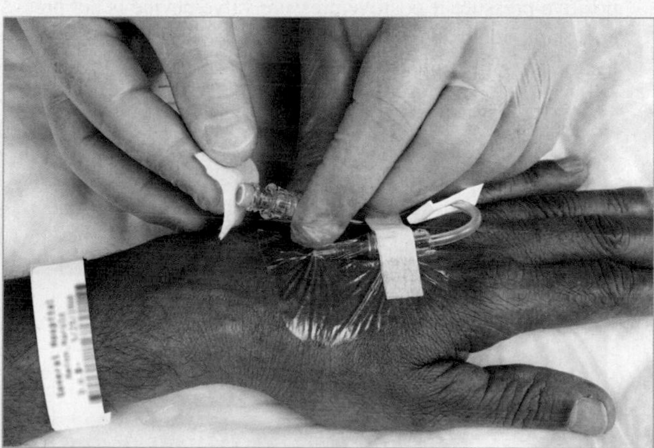

FIGURE 2 Cleaning access port.

(continued)

SKILL 5-14 INTRODUCING DRUGS THROUGH A MEDICATION OR DRUG-INFUSION LOCK (INTERMITTENT PERIPHERAL VENOUS ACCESS DEVICE) USING THE SALINE FLUSH continued

ACTION	RATIONALE
23. Stabilize the port with your nondominant hand and insert the syringe, or needleless access device, of normal saline into the access port (Figure 3).	This allows for careful insertion into the center circle of the lock.
24. Release the clamp on the extension tubing of the medication lock. Aspirate gently and check for blood return (Figure 4).	This ensures the catheter of the medication lock is in a vein.

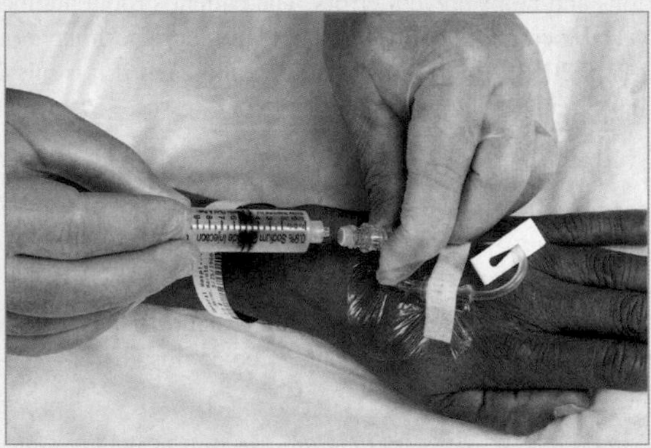

FIGURE 3 Inserting syringe into access port.

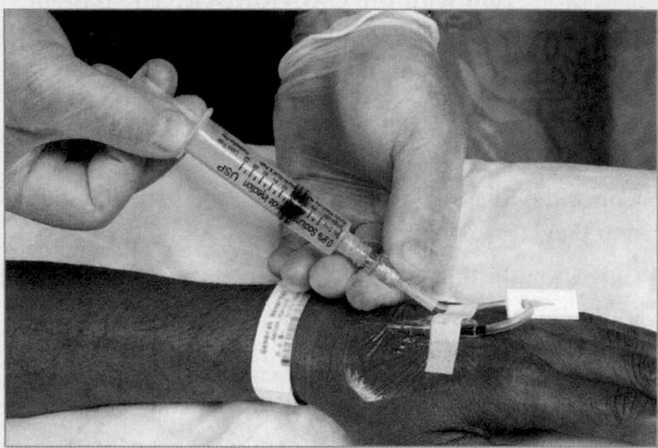

FIGURE 4 Aspirating for blood return.

ACTION	RATIONALE
25. Gently flush with normal saline by pushing slowly on the syringe plunger. Observe the insertion site while inserting the saline. Remove syringe.	Saline flush ensures that the IV line is patent. Puffiness or swelling as the site is flushed could indicate infiltration of the catheter.
26. Insert syringe, or needleless access device, with medication into the port and gently inject medication, using a watch to verify correct administration rate. **Do not force the injection if resistance is felt.**	Easy installation of medication usually indicates that the lock is still patent and in the vein. If force is used against resistance, a clot may break away and cause a blockage elsewhere in the body.
27. Remove the medication syringe from the port. Stabilize the port with your nondominant hand and insert the syringe, or needleless access device, of normal saline into the port. Gently flush with normal saline by pushing slowly on the syringe plunger (Figure 5). If the medication lock is capped with positive pressure valve/device, remove syringe, and then clamp the extension tubing (Figure 6). Alternately, to gain positive pressure if positive pressure valve/device is not present, clamp the extension tubing as you are still flushing the last of the saline into the medication lock. Remove syringe.	Positive pressure prevents blood from backing into the catheter and causing the medication lock to clot off.

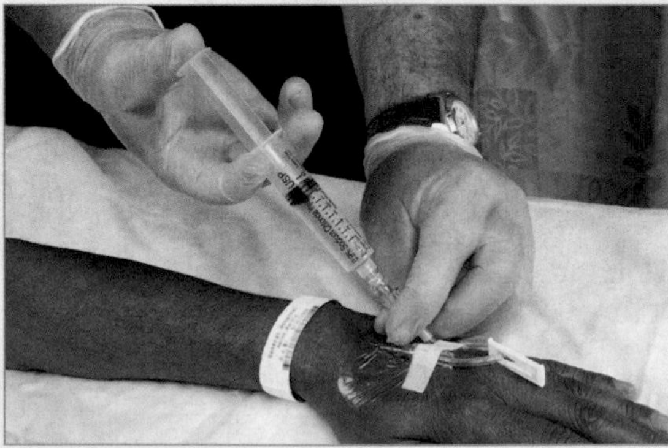

FIGURE 5 Flushing port with normal saline.

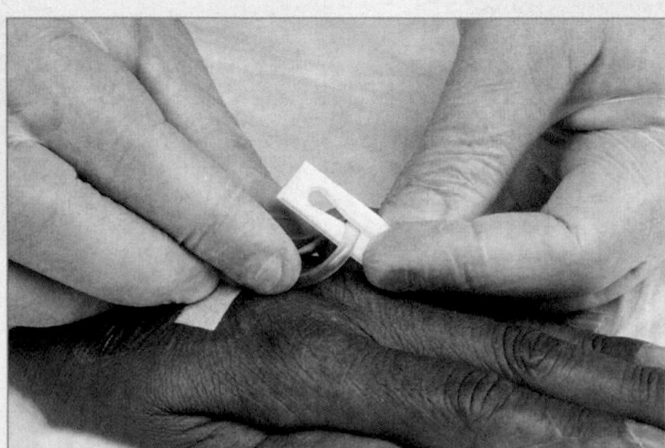

FIGURE 6 Clamping access port.

ACTION	RATIONALE
28. Discard the syringe in the appropriate receptacle.	Proper disposal prevents injury.
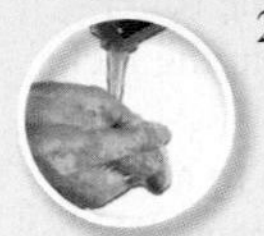 29. Remove PPE, if used. Perform hand hygiene.	Removing PPE properly reduces the risk for infection transmission and contamination of other items. Hand hygiene prevents the spread of microorganisms.
30. Document the administration of the medication immediately after administration. See Documentation section below.	Timely documentation helps to ensure patient safety.
31. Evaluate the patient's response to the medication within an appropriate time frame.	The patient needs to be evaluated for therapeutic and adverse effects from the medication.
32. Check the medication lock site at least every 8 hours or according to facility policy.	This ensures patency of system.

EVALUATION

The expected outcomes are met when the medication is delivered via the IV route using sterile technique; the medication is delivered to the patient in a safe manner and at the appropriate infusion rate; the patient experiences no adverse effect; the intermittent peripheral venous access device remains patent; and the patient understands and complies with the medication regimen.

DOCUMENTATION

Guidelines

Document the administration of the medication and saline flush, including date, time, dose, route of administration, site of administration, and rate of administration on the CMAR/MAR or record using the required format, immediately after administration. If using a bar-code system, medication administration is automatically recorded when the bar code is scanned. PRN medications require documentation of the reason for administration. Prompt recording avoids the possibility of accidentally repeating the administration of the drug. If the drug was refused or omitted, record this in the appropriate area on the medication record and notify the primary care provider. This verifies the reason medication was omitted and ensures that the primary care provider is aware of the patient's condition.

UNEXPECTED SITUATIONS AND ASSOCIATED INTERVENTIONS

- *Upon assessing the medication lock site before administering the medication, you note that the medication lock has infiltrated:* Remove the medication lock from the extremity. Restart peripheral venous access in a different location. Continue to monitor the new site as medication is administered.
- *While you are administering medication, the patient begins to complain of pain at the site:* Stop the medication. Assess the medication lock site for signs of infiltration and phlebitis. Flush the medication lock with normal saline again to recheck patency. If the IV site appears within normal limits, resume medication administration at a slower rate. If pain persists, stop, remove medication lock and restart in a different location.
- *As you are attempting to access the lock, the syringe tip touches the patient's arm:* Discard syringe. Prepare a new dose for administration.
- *No blood return is noted upon aspiration:* If the medication lock appears patent, without signs of infiltration, and normal saline fluid infuses without difficulty, proceed with administration. Observe closely for signs and symptoms of infiltration during and after administration.

SPECIAL CONSIDERATIONS

General Considerations

- If a medication lock is not used, flush with saline every 8 to 12 hours to maintain patency, according to facility policy.
- Routinely change the medication lock site every 72 to 96 hours, according to facility policy. This reduces the risk of infection and emboli in the bloodstream.

(continued)

SKILL 5-14 INTRODUCING DRUGS THROUGH A MEDICATION OR DRUG-INFUSION LOCK (INTERMITTENT PERIPHERAL VENOUS ACCESS DEVICE) USING THE SALINE FLUSH continued

- Intermittent infusions of small-volume IV medications can also be administered through the medication lock. Attach IV medication container to infusion tubing and prime. After flushing the medication lock with saline as outlined above, attach the infusion tubing to the medication lock. Set the infusion rate in the infusion pump. Alternately, adjust the infusion rate with the roller clamp on the gravity infusion tubing. After infusion is completed, remove tubing from the lock and flush with saline as outlined above.
- Ongoing assessment is an important part of nursing care to evaluate patient response to administered medications and early detection of adverse effects. If an adverse effect is suspected, withhold further medication doses and notify the patient's primary care provider. Additional intervention is based on type of reaction and patient assessment.

Infant and Child Considerations

- If the volume of medication being administered is small (less than 1.0 mL), always include the amount of flush solution as part of the total amount to be injected and take this into account when determining how fast to push a medication. For example, if the medication is to be injected at a rate of 1.0 mL per minute and the total amount of solution to be injected is 2.25 mL (0.25 mL medication volume plus 2.0 mL saline flush solution volume equals 2.25 mL), then the medication would be injected over a period of 2 minutes 15 seconds.

SKILL 5-15 APPLYING A TRANSDERMAL PATCH

The transdermal route is being used more frequently to deliver medication. A disk or patch that contains medication intended for daily use or longer is applied to the patient's skin. Transdermal patches are commonly used to deliver hormones, opioid analgesics, cardiac medications, and nicotine. Medication errors have occurred when patients apply multiple patches at once or fail to remove the overlay on the patch that exposes the skin to the medication. Opioid analgesic patches are associated with the most **adverse drug effects**. Clear patches have a cosmetic advantage, but they can be difficult to find on the patient's skin when they need to be removed or replaced.

DELEGATION CONSIDERATIONS

The administration of medication via a transdermal patch is not delegated to nursing assistive personnel (NAP) or to unlicensed assistive personnel (UAP). Depending on the state's nurse practice act and the organization's policies and procedures, the administration of a transdermal patch may be delegated to licensed practical/vocational nurses (LPN/LVNs). The decision to delegate must be based on careful analysis of the patient's needs and circumstances, as well as the qualifications of the person to whom the task is being delegated. Refer to the Delegation Guidelines in Appendix A.

EQUIPMENT

- Medication patch
- Disposable gloves
- Scissors (optional)
- Washcloth, soap, and water
- Computer-generated Medication Administration Record (CMAR) or Medication Administration Record (MAR)
- Additional PPE, as indicated

ASSESSMENT

Assess the patient for any allergies. Check the expiration date before administering the medication. Assess the appropriateness of the drug for the patient. Review assessment and laboratory data that may influence drug administration. Verify patient name, dose, route, and time of administration. Assess the skin at the location where the patch will be applied. Many patches have different and specific instructions for where the patch is to be placed. For example, transdermal patches that contain estrogen cannot be placed on breast tissue. Check the manufacturer's instructions for the appropriate location for the patch. The site should be clean, dry, and free of hair. Do not place transdermal patches on irritated or broken skin. Assess the patient for any old patches. Do not place a new transdermal patch until old patches have been removed. Verify the application frequency for the specific medication. Assess the patient's knowledge of the medication. If the patient has a knowledge deficit about the medication, this may be the appropriate time to begin education about the medication. If the medication may affect the patient's vital signs, assess them before administration. If the medication is for pain relief, assess the patient's pain before and after administration.

NURSING DIAGNOSIS

Determine related factors for the nursing diagnoses based on the patient's current status. Appropriate nursing diagnoses may include:

- Risk for Allergy Response
- Risk for Impaired Skin Integrity
- Deficient Knowledge

OUTCOME IDENTIFICATION AND PLANNING

The expected outcome is that the medication is delivered via the transdermal route. Other outcomes that may be appropriate include the following: the patient experiences no adverse effect; the patient's skin remains free from injury; and the patient understands and complies with the medication regimen.

IMPLEMENTATION

ACTION	RATIONALE
1. Gather equipment. Check medication order against the original order in the medical record, according to facility policy. Clarify any inconsistencies. Check the patient's chart for allergies.	This comparison helps to identify errors that may have occurred when orders were transcribed. The primary care provider's order is the legal record of medication orders for each facility.
2. Know the actions, special nursing considerations, safe dose ranges, purpose of administration, and adverse effects of the medications to be administered. Consider the appropriateness of the medication for this patient.	This knowledge aids the nurse in evaluating the therapeutic effect of the medication in relation to the patient's disorder and can also be used to educate the patient about the medication.
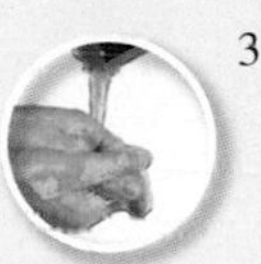 3. Perform hand hygiene.	Hand hygiene prevents the spread of microorganisms.
4. Move the medication cart to the outside of the patient's room or prepare for administration in the medication area.	Organization facilitates error-free administration and saves time.
5. Unlock the medication cart or drawer. Enter pass code and scan employee identification, if required.	Locking the cart or drawer safeguards each patient's medication supply. Hospital accrediting organizations require medication carts to be locked when not in use. Entering pass code and scanning ID allows only authorized users into the system and identifies the user for documentation by the computer.
6. **Prepare medications for one patient at a time.**	This prevents errors in medication administration.
7. Read the CMAR/MAR and select the proper medication from unit stock or the patient's medication drawer.	This is the *first* check of the label.
8. Compare the label with the CMAR/MAR. Check expiration dates and perform calculations, if necessary. Scan the bar code on the package, if required.	This is the *second* check of the label. Verify calculations with another nurse to ensure safety, if necessary.
9. **Depending on facility policy, the third check of the label may occur at this point. If so, when all medications for one patient have been prepared, recheck the labels with the CMAR/MAR before taking the medications to the patient.**	This *third* check ensures accuracy and helps to prevent errors. *Note:* Many facilities require the *third* check to occur at the bedside, after identifying the patient and before administration.

(*continued*)

SKILL 5-15 APPLYING A TRANSDERMAL PATCH continued

ACTION	RATIONALE
10. Lock the medication cart before leaving it.	Locking the cart or drawer safeguards the patient's medication supply. Hospital accrediting organizations require medication carts to be locked when not in use.
11. Transport medications to the patient's bedside carefully, and keep the medications in sight at all times.	Careful handling and close observation prevent accidental or deliberate disarrangement of medications.
12. **Ensure that the patient receives the medications at the correct time.**	Check agency policy, which may allow for administration within a period of 30 minutes before or 30 minutes after the designated time.
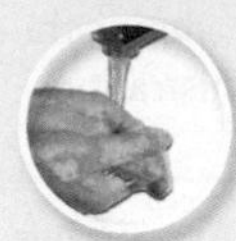 13. Perform hand hygiene and put on PPE, if indicated.	Hand hygiene and PPE prevent the spread of microorganisms. PPE is required based on transmission precautions.
 14. **Identify the patient. Compare the information with the CMAR/MAR. The patient should be identified using at least two methods** (The Joint Commission, 2013):	Identifying the patient ensures the right patient receives the medications and helps prevent errors. The patient's room number or physical location is not used as an identifier (The Joint Commission, 2013). Replace the identification band if it is missing or inaccurate in any way.
a. Check the name on the patient's identification band.	
b. Check the identification number on the patient's identification band.	
c. Check the birth date on the patient's identification band.	
d. Ask the patient to state his or her name and birth date, based on facility policy.	This requires a response from the patient, but illness and strange surroundings often cause patients to be confused.
15. **Complete necessary assessments before administering medications. Check the patient's allergy bracelet or ask the patient about allergies. Explain the purpose and action of each medication to the patient.**	Assessment is a prerequisite to administration of medications.
16. Scan the patient's bar code on the identification band, if required (Figure 1).	This provides an additional check to ensure that the medication is given to the right patient.

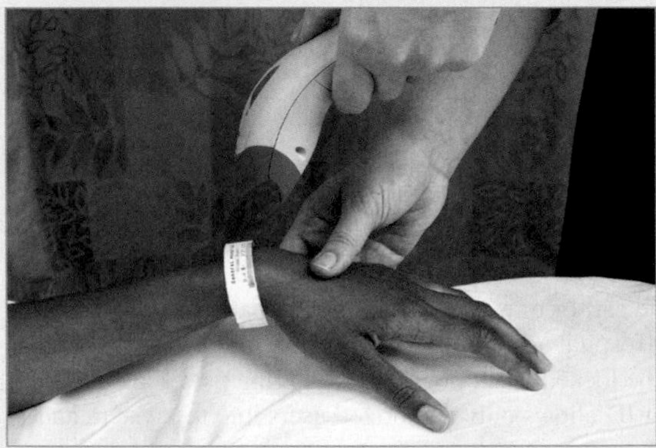

FIGURE 1 Scanning bar code on patient's identification bracelet.

ACTION	RATIONALE
17. **Based on facility policy, the third check of the label may occur at this point. If so, recheck the labels with the CMAR/MAR before administering the medications to the patient.**	Many facilities require the *third* check to occur at the bedside, after identifying the patient and before administration. If facility policy directs the *third* check at this time, this *third* check ensures accuracy and helps to prevent errors.
18. Put on gloves.	Gloves protect the nurse when handling the medication on the transdermal patch.
19. Assess the patient's skin where patch is to be placed, looking for any signs of irritation or breakdown. Site should be clean, dry, and free of hair. Rotate application sites.	Transdermal patches should not be placed on skin that is irritated or broken down. Hair can prevent the patch from sticking to the skin. Rotating sites reduces risk for skin irritation.

ACTION	RATIONALE
20. **Remove any old transdermal patches from the patient's skin.** Fold the old patch in half with the adhesive sides sticking together and discard according to facility policy. Gently wash the area where the old patch was with soap and water.	Leaving old patches on a patient while applying new ones may lead to delivery of a toxic level of the drug. Folding sides together prevents accidental contact with remaining medication. Washing area with soap and water removes all traces of medication in that area.
21. Remove the patch from its protective covering. Remove the covering on the patch without touching the medication surface (Figure 2). Apply the patch to the patient's skin (Figure 3). Use the palm of your hand to press firmly for about 10 seconds. Do not massage.	Touching the adhesive side may alter the amount of medication left on the patch. Pressing firmly for 10 seconds ensures that the patch stays on the patient's skin. Massaging the site may increase absorption of the medication.

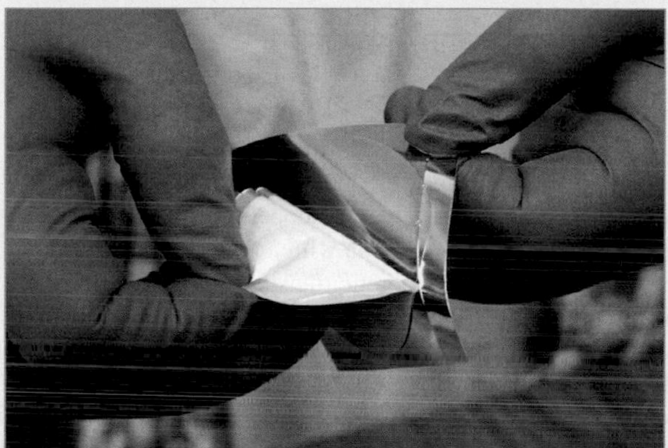

FIGURE 2 Removing covering on patch.

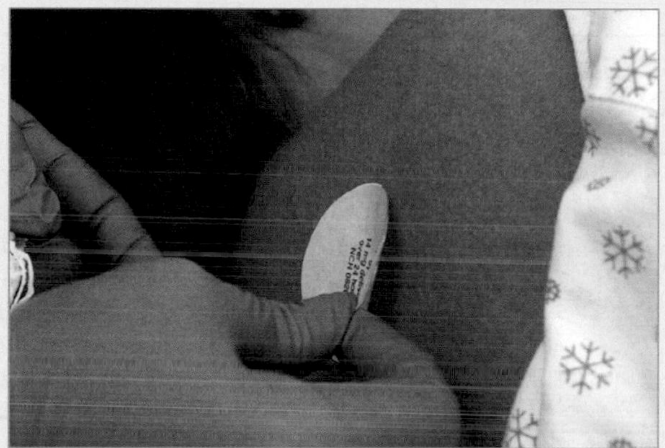

FIGURE 3 Applying patch to patient's skin.

ACTION	RATIONALE
22. Depending on facility policy, initial and write the date and time of administration on a piece of medical tape. Apply the tape to the patient's skin in close proximity to the patch. **Do not write directly on the medication patch.**	Most manufacturers recommend against writing on patches due to insufficient data on the practice. Writing on the patch could damage or tear it. Moreover, if ink is used, it may leach through and come into contact with the medication, and it is not known whether ink might interact with a given medication or impede its delivery.
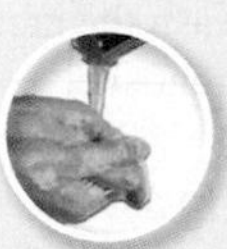 23. Remove gloves and additional PPE, if used. Perform hand hygiene.	Removing PPE properly reduces the risk for infection transmission and contamination of other items. Hand hygiene prevents the spread of microorganisms.
24. Document the administration of the medication immediately after administration. See Documentation section below.	Timely documentation helps to ensure patient safety.
25. Evaluate the patient's response to the medication within the appropriate time frame.	The patient needs to be evaluated for therapeutic and adverse effects from the medication.

EVALUATION

The expected outcomes are met when the medication is delivered via the transdermal route; the patient experiences no adverse effect; the patient's skin remains free from injury; and the patient understands and complies with the medication regimen.

DOCUMENTATION

Guidelines

Document the administration of the medication immediately after administration, including date, time, dose, route of administration, and site of administration on the CMAR/MAR or record using the required format. If using a bar-code system, medication administration is automatically recorded when the bar code is scanned. PRN medications require documentation of the reason for administration. Prompt recording avoids the possibility of accidentally repeating the administration of the drug. If the drug was refused or omitted, record this in the appropriate area on the medication record and notify the primary care provider. This verifies the reason the medication was omitted and ensures that the primary care provider is aware of the patient's condition.

(continued)

SKILL 5-15 APPLYING A TRANSDERMAL PATCH continued

UNEXPECTED SITUATIONS AND ASSOCIATED INTERVENTIONS

- *You did not wear gloves while applying the transdermal patch:* Immediately perform good hand hygiene using soap and water to remove any medication that may be on the skin. You may feel the effects of the medication if any came into contact with your skin.
- *You find more than one old transdermal patch while applying a new transdermal patch:* Remove all old patches of the same kind; remember that more than one medication may be delivered via a transdermal patch. Check orders in the medical record to ensure that the patient is still receiving medication. Failure to remove old transdermal patches is considered a medication error and special event. Notify the primary care provider of potential medication overdose. Follow facility policy regarding documentation for special events.
- *When removing an old transdermal patch, you note the skin underneath is erythematosus and swollen:* Wash skin with soap and water and assess the patient for any latex or adhesive allergies. Discuss with the patient whether the patch site has been rotated. Notify the primary care provider before applying a new patch.

SPECIAL CONSIDERATIONS

General Considerations

- Transdermal drug products have specific application sites, application intervals, and considerations. It is important to be knowledgeable about the specific drug administered. For example, fentanyl (Duragesic) may be applied to the chest, back, flank, and upper arm; it is reapplied every 3 days; and patients may experience increased absorption with a temperature elevation higher than 102°F (Ball & Smith, 2008). Fentanyl iontophoretic transdermal system (Ionsys) may be applied to the chest or upper outer arm; it is reapplied every 24 hours or after 80 doses have been delivered; it contains metal parts, so it should be removed before MRI, cardioversion, or defibrillation (Ball & Smith, 2008). Nitroglycerin (Minitran) may be placed on any hairless surface, except on extremities below the knees or elbows, with the chest being the preferred site. It is reapplied every 12 to 14 hours, and patients should have a nitrate-free interval each day of 10 to 12 hours to ensure tolerance does not develop (Ball & Smith, 2008).
- Apply the patch at the same time of the day, according to the order and medication specifications.
- Check for dislodgement of the patch if the patient is active. Read information about the patch or consult with the pharmacist to determine reapplication schedule and procedure.
- Aluminum backing on a patch necessitates precautions if defibrillation is required. Burns and smoke may result. In addition, these patches should be removed before an MRI is performed to avoid burning of the skin.
- Assess for any skin irritation at the application site. If necessary, remove the patch, wash the area carefully with soap and water, and allow skin to air dry. Apply a new patch at a different site. Assess the potential for adverse reaction.
- Ongoing assessment is an important part of nursing care to evaluate patient response to administered medications and early detection of adverse effects. If an adverse effect is suspected, withhold further medication doses and notify the patient's primary care provider. Additional intervention is based on type of reaction and patient assessment.

Home Care Considerations

- Some manufacturers recommend that patients wearing patches avoid external heat sources (e.g., heating pads, electric blankets, heat lamps, saunas, hot tubs, sunlight), as heat may promote drug absorption through the skin. Consult specific information from the manufacturer related to a particular medication.
- Caregivers and patients should be sure to remove an old transdermal medication before applying a new one, as many patches have residual drug content even after the recommended application time.
- Instruct patients and caregivers to rotate application sites to decrease the risk of skin irritation.
- Instruct patients and caregivers to wash their hands thoroughly after the application of a transdermal medication to avoid inadvertent eye contact.
- Instruct patients and caregivers to discard used transdermal medications according to manufacturer's instructions and out of reach of children, to avoid inadvertent exposure by children and pets (Durand, et al., 2012).

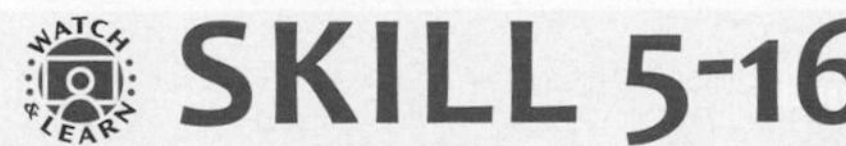

SKILL 5-16 INSTILLING EYE DROPS

Eye drops are instilled for their local effects, such as for pupil dilation or constriction when examining the eye, for infection treatment, or for controlling intraocular pressure (for patients with glaucoma). The type and amount of solution administered depends on the purpose of the instillation.

The eye is a delicate organ, highly susceptible to infection and injury. Although the eye is never free of microorganisms, the secretions of the conjunctiva protect against many pathogens. For maximal safety for the patient, the equipment, solutions, and ointments introduced into the conjunctival sac should be sterile. If this is not possible, follow careful guidelines for medical asepsis.

Refer to the accompanying Skill Variation for the steps to administer eye ointment.

DELEGATION CONSIDERATIONS

The administration of medication via drops in the eye is not delegated to nursing assistive personnel (NAP) or to unlicensed assistive personnel (UAP). Depending on the state's nurse practice act and the organization's policies and procedures, the administration of eye drops may be delegated to licensed practical/vocational nurses (LPN/LVNs). The decision to delegate must be based on careful analysis of the patient's needs and circumstances, as well as the qualifications of the person to whom the task is being delegated. Refer to the Delegation Guidelines in Appendix A.

EQUIPMENT

- Gloves
- Additional PPE, as indicated
- Medication
- Tissues
- Normal saline solution
- Washcloth, cotton balls, or gauze squares
- Computer-generated Medication Administration Record (CMAR) or Medication Administration Record (MAR)

ASSESSMENT

Assess the patient for any allergies. Check the expiration date before administering the medication. Assess the appropriateness of the drug for the patient. Review assessment and laboratory data that may influence drug administration. Verify patient name, dose, route, and time of administration. Assess the affected eye for any drainage, erythema, or swelling. Assess the patient's knowledge of the medication. If the patient has a knowledge deficit about the medication, this may be the appropriate time to begin education about the medication. If the medication may affect the patient's vital signs, assess them before administration.

NURSING DIAGNOSIS

Determine related factors for the nursing diagnoses based on the patient's current status. Appropriate nursing diagnoses may include:

- Risk for Allergy Response
- Deficient Knowledge
- Risk for Injury

OUTCOME IDENTIFICATION AND PLANNING

The expected outcome to achieve when administering eye drops is that the medication is delivered successfully into the eye. Other outcomes that may be appropriate include the following: the patient experiences no allergy response; the patient does not exhibit systemic effects of the medication; the patient's eye remains free from injury; and patient understands the rationale for medication administration.

IMPLEMENTATION

ACTION	RATIONALE
1. Gather equipment. Check medication order against the original order in the medical record, according to facility policy. Clarify any inconsistencies. Check the patient's chart for allergies.	This comparison helps to identify errors that may have occurred when orders were transcribed. The primary care provider's order is the legal record of medication orders for each facility.
2. Know the actions, special nursing considerations, safe dose ranges, purpose of administration, and adverse effects of the medications to be administered. Consider the appropriateness of the medication for this patient.	This knowledge aids the nurse in evaluating the therapeutic effect of the medication in relation to the patient's disorder and can also be used to educate the patient about the medication.

(continued)

SKILL 5-16 INSTILLING EYE DROPS continued

ACTION	RATIONALE
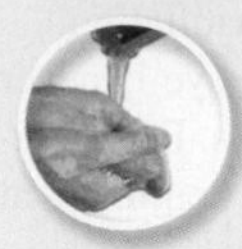 3. Perform hand hygiene.	Hand hygiene prevents the spread of microorganisms.
4. Move the medication cart to the outside of the patient's room or prepare for administration in the medication area.	Organization facilitates error-free administration and saves time.
5. Unlock the medication cart or drawer. Enter pass code and scan employee identification, if required.	Locking the cart or drawer safeguards each patient's medication supply. Hospital accrediting organizations require medication carts to be locked when not in use. Entering pass code and scanning ID allows only authorized users into the system and identifies the user for documentation by the computer.
6. **Prepare medications for one patient at a time.**	This prevents errors in medication administration.
7. Read the CMAR/MAR and select the proper medication from the patient's medication drawer or unit stock.	This is the *first* check of the label.
8. Compare the label with the CMAR/MAR. Check expiration dates and perform calculations, if necessary. Scan the bar code on the package, if required.	This is the *second* check of the label. Verify calculations with another nurse to ensure safety, if necessary.
9. **Depending on facility policy, the third check of the label may occur at this point. If so, when all medications for one patient have been prepared, recheck the labels with the CMAR/MAR before taking the medications to the patient.**	This *third* check ensures accuracy and helps to prevent errors. *Note:* Many facilities require the *third* check to occur at the bedside, after identifying the patient and before administration.
10. Lock the medication cart before leaving it.	Locking the cart or drawer safeguards the patient's medication supply. Hospital accrediting organizations require medication carts to be locked when not in use.
11. Transport medications to the patient's bedside carefully, and keep the medications in sight at all times.	Careful handling and close observation prevent accidental or deliberate disarrangement of medications.
12. **Ensure that the patient receives the medications at the correct time.**	Check agency policy, which may allow for administration within a period of 30 minutes before or 30 minutes after the designated time.
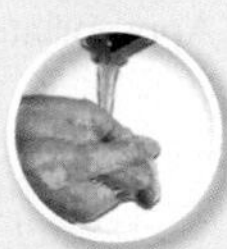 13. Perform hand hygiene and put on PPE, if indicated.	Hand hygiene and PPE prevent the spread of microorganisms. PPE is required based on transmission precautions.
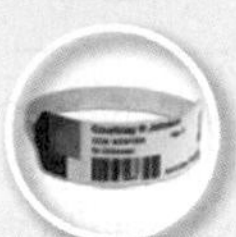 14. **Identify the patient. Compare the information with the CMAR/MAR. The patient should be identified using at least two methods** (The Joint Commission, 2013):	Identifying the patient ensures the right patient receives the medications and helps prevent errors. The patient's room number or physical location is not used as an identifier (The Joint Commission, 2013). Replace the identification band if it is missing or inaccurate in any way.
a. Check the name on the patient's identification band.	
b. Check the identification number on the patient's identification band.	
c. Check the birth date on the patient's identification band.	
d. Ask the patient to state his or her name and birth date, based on facility policy.	This requires a response from the patient, but illness and strange surroundings often cause patients to be confused.
15. **Complete necessary assessments before administering medications. Check the patient's allergy bracelet or ask the patient about allergies. Explain the purpose and action of each medication to the patient.**	Assessment is a prerequisite to administration of medications.

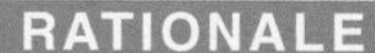

ACTION	RATIONALE
16. Scan the patient's bar code on the identification band, if required (Figure 1).	Provides an additional check to ensure that the medication is given to the right patient.
17. **Based on facility policy, the third check of the label may occur at this point. If so, recheck the labels with the CMAR/MAR before administering the medications to the patient.**	Many facilities require the *third* check to occur at the bedside, after identifying the patient and before administration. If facility policy directs the *third* check at this time, this *third* check ensures accuracy and helps to prevent errors.
18. Put on gloves.	Gloves protect the nurse from potential contact with mucous membranes and body fluids.
19. Offer tissue to patient.	Solution and tears may spill from the eye during the procedure.
20. Cleanse the eyelids and eyelashes of any drainage with a washcloth, cotton balls, or gauze squares moistened with normal saline solution. Use each area of the cleaning surface once, moving from the inner toward the outer canthus (Figure 2).	Debris can be carried into the eye when the conjunctival sac is exposed. Using each area of the gauze once and moving from the inner canthus to the outer canthus prevents carrying debris to the lacrimal ducts.

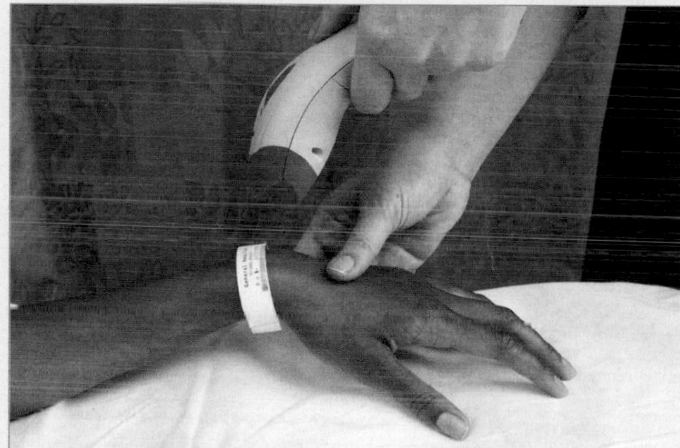

FIGURE 1 Scanning bar code on patient's identification bracelet.

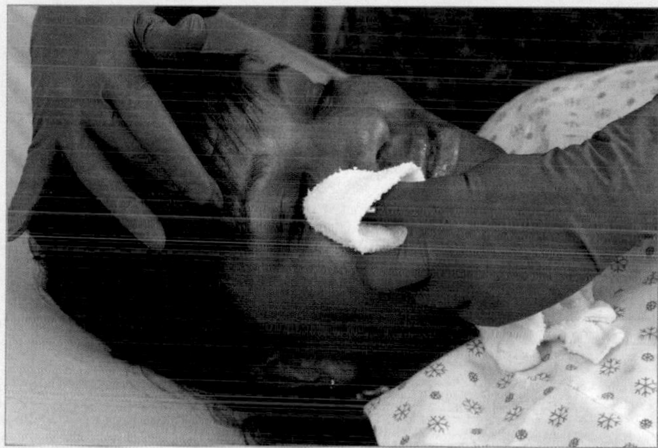

FIGURE 2 Cleaning lids and lashes from inside of eye to outside.

ACTION	RATIONALE
21. Tilt the patient's head back slightly if sitting, or place the patient's head over a pillow if lying down. **Tilting the patient's head should be avoided if the patient has a cervical spine injury.** The head may be turned slightly to the affected side to prevent solution or tears from flowing toward the opposite eye (Figure 3).	Tilting the patient's head back slightly makes it easier to reach the conjunctival sac. Turning the head to the affected side helps to prevent solution or tears from flowing toward the opposite eye.

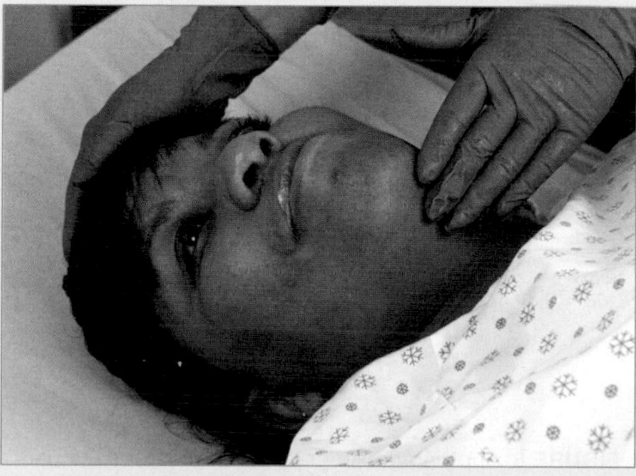

FIGURE 3 Turning head slightly to affected side.

(continued)

SKILL 5-16 INSTILLING EYE DROPS continued

ACTION	RATIONALE
22. Remove the cap from the medication bottle, being careful not to touch the inner side of the cap. (See the accompanying Skill Variation for administering ointment.)	Touching the inner side of the cap may contaminate the bottle of medication.
23. Invert the monodrip plastic container that is commonly used to instill eye drops. Have the patient look up and focus on something on the ceiling.	By having the patient look up and focus on something else, the procedure is less traumatic and keeps the eye still.
24. Place thumb or two fingers near margin of lower eyelid immediately below eyelashes, and exert pressure downward over bony cheek prominence. The lower conjunctival sac is exposed as the lower lid is pulled down (Figure 4).	The eye drop should be placed in the conjunctival sac, not directly on the eyeball.
25. **Hold the dropper close to the eye, but avoid touching eyelids or lashes.** Squeeze container and allow prescribed number of drops to fall in lower conjunctival sac (Figure 5).	Touching the eye, eyelids, or lashes can contaminate the medication in the bottle; startle the patient, causing blinking; or injure the eye. Do not allow medication to fall onto the cornea. This may injure the cornea or cause the patient to have an unpleasant sensation.

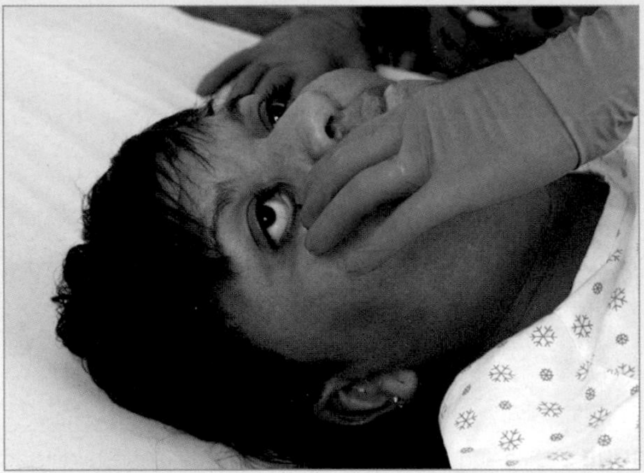

FIGURE 4 Exerting pressure downward to expose lower conjunctival sac.

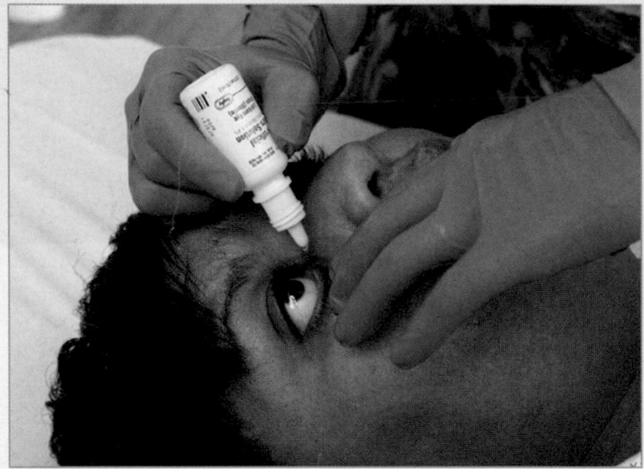

FIGURE 5 Administering drops into conjunctival sac.

ACTION	RATIONALE
26. Release lower lid after eye drops are instilled. Ask patient to close eyes gently.	This allows the medication to be distributed over the entire eye.
27. Apply gentle pressure over inner canthus to prevent eye drops from flowing into tear duct (Figure 6).	This minimizes the risk of systemic effects from the medication.

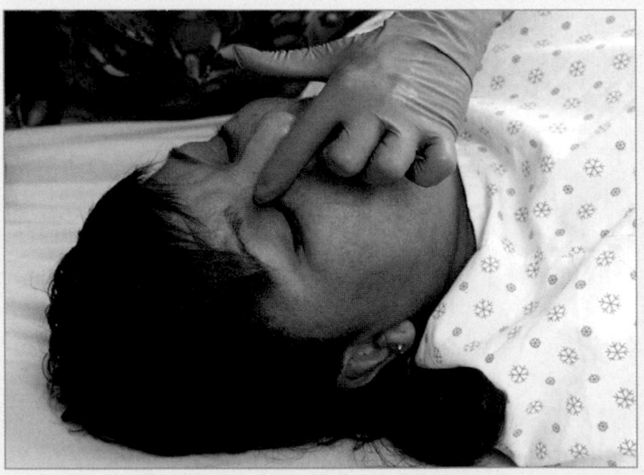

FIGURE 6 Applying gentle pressure over inner canthus.

ACTION	RATIONALE
28. Instruct patient not to rub affected eye.	This prevents injury and irritation to the eye.
29. Remove gloves. Assist the patient to a comfortable position.	This ensures patient comfort.
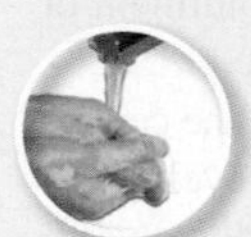 30. Remove additional PPE, if used. Perform hand hygiene.	Removing PPE properly reduces the risk for infection transmission and contamination of other items. Hand hygiene prevents the spread of microorganisms.
31. Document the administration of the medication immediately after administration. See Documentation section below.	Timely documentation helps to ensure patient safety.
32. Evaluate the patient's response to the medication within an appropriate time frame.	The patient needs to be evaluated for therapeutic and adverse effects from the medication.

EVALUATION

The expected outcomes are met when the patient receives the eye drops; experiences no adverse effects, including allergy response, systemic effect, or injury; and understands the rationale for the medication administration.

DOCUMENTATION

Guidelines

Document the administration of the medication immediately after administration, including date, time, dose, route of administration, and site of administration, specifically right, left, or both eyes, on the CMAR/MAR or record using the required format. If using a bar-code system, medication administration is automatically recorded when the bar code is scanned. PRN medications require documentation of the reason for administration. Prompt recording avoids the possibility of accidentally repeating the administration of the drug. If the drug was refused or omitted, record this in the appropriate area on the medication record and notify the primary care provider. This verifies the reason medication was omitted and ensures that the primary care provider is aware of the patient's condition.

UNEXPECTED SITUATIONS AND ASSOCIATED INTERVENTIONS

- *Drop is placed on eyelid or outer margin of eyelid due to patient blinking or moving:* Do not count this drop in total number of drops administered. Allow the patient to regain composure and proceed with application of medication. Consider approaching the patient from below the line of sight.
- *You cannot open eyelids due to dried crust and matting of eyelids:* Place a warm, wet washcloth over the eye and allow it to remain there for approximately 3 minutes. Cleanse eye as described previously. You may need to repeat this procedure if there is a large amount of matting.
- *Bottle or tube of medication comes in contact with the eyeball when applying medication:* Bottle is contaminated; discard appropriately. Notify pharmacy or retrieve a new bottle for the oncoming shift.

SPECIAL CONSIDERATIONS

General Considerations

- Ongoing assessment is an important part of nursing care to evaluate patient response to administered medications and early detection of adverse effects. If an adverse effect is suspected, withhold further medication doses and notify the patient's primary care provider. Additional intervention is based on type of reaction and patient assessment.

Infant and Child Considerations

- To apply eye drops in a small child, two or more people may be needed to restrain the child. Make sure the child does not reach up to the eye, causing the nurse to jab the medication bottle into the eye.

(continued)

SKILL 5-16 INSTILLING EYE DROPS continued

SKILL VARIATION Administering Eye Ointment

Prepare medication as outlined in steps 1–12 above (Skill 5-16).

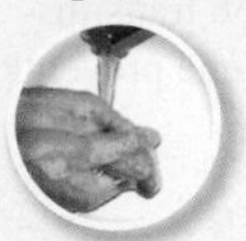

1. Perform hand hygiene and put on PPE, if indicated.

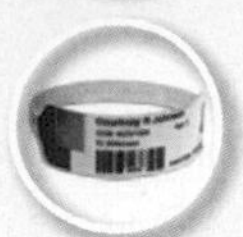

2. Identify the patient. The patient should be identified using two methods.
3. Close the door to the room or pull the bedside curtain.
4. Complete necessary assessments before administering medications. Check allergy bracelet or ask patient about allergies. Explain the purpose and action of the medication to the patient.
5. Scan the patient's bar code on the identification band, if required.
6. Based on facility policy, the *third check* of the label may occur at this point. If so, recheck the labels with the CMAR/MAR before administering the medications to the patient.
7. Put on gloves. Offer the patient a tissue.
8. Cleanse the eyelids and eyelashes of any drainage with cotton balls or gauze squares moistened with normal saline solution. Use each area of the gauze square once, moving from the inner toward the outer canthus of the eye.
9. Tilt the patient's head back slightly if sitting, or place the patient's head over a pillow if lying down. The head may be turned slightly to the affected side to prevent ointment or tears from flowing toward the opposite eye.
10. Have the patient look up and focus on something on the ceiling.
11. Place thumb or two fingers near margin of lower eyelid immediately below eyelashes and exert pressure downward over bony cheek prominence. Lower conjunctival sac is exposed as lower lid is pulled down.
12. Hold the ointment tube close to eye, but avoid touching eyelids or lashes. Squeeze container and apply about 0.5 inch of ointment from the tube along the exposed sac. Apply the medication, moving from the inner canthus to the outer canthus. Twist tube to break off ribbon of ointment. Do not touch the tip to the eye.
13. Release lower lid after ointment is instilled. Ask the patient to close eyes gently.
14. The warmth helps to liquefy the ointment. Instruct the patient to move the eye, because this helps to spread the ointment under the lids and over the surface of the eyeball.
15. Assist the patient to a comfortable position. Explain that the ointment may temporarily blur vision; encourage the patient not to rub the eye.
16. Remove gloves and additional PPE, if used. Perform hand hygiene.
17. Document administration of the medication on the CMAR/MAR immediately after administering the medication.
18. Evaluate the patient's response to the medication within an appropriate time frame.

SKILL 5-17 ADMINISTERING AN EYE IRRIGATION

Eye irrigation is performed to remove secretions or foreign bodies or to cleanse and soothe the eye. When irrigating one eye, take care that the overflowing irrigation fluid does not contaminate the other eye.

DELEGATION CONSIDERATIONS

The administration of an eye irrigation is not delegated to nursing assistive personnel (NAP) or to unlicensed assistive personnel (UAP). Depending on the state's nurse practice act and the organization's policies and procedures, the administration of an eye irrigation may be delegated to licensed practical/vocational nurses (LPN/LVNs). The decision to delegate must be based on careful analysis of the patient's needs and circumstances, as well as the qualifications of the person to whom the task is being delegated. Refer to the Delegation Guidelines in Appendix A.

EQUIPMENT

- Sterile irrigation solution (warmed to 37°C [98.6°F])
- Sterile irrigation set (sterile container and irrigating or bulb syringe)
- Emesis basin or irrigation basin
- Washcloth
- Waterproof pad
- Towel
- Gloves
- Additional PPE, as indicated

ASSESSMENT

Assess the patient's eyes for redness, erythema, edema, drainage, or tenderness. Assess the patient for allergies. Verify patient name, dose, route, and time of administration. Assess the patient's knowledge of the procedure. If the patient has a knowledge deficit about the procedure, this may be an appropriate time to begin patient education. Assess the patient's ability to cooperate with the procedure.

NURSING DIAGNOSIS

Determine related factors for the nursing diagnoses based on the patient's current status. Appropriate nursing diagnoses may include:

- Deficient Knowledge
- Acute Pain
- Risk for Injury

OUTCOME IDENTIFICATION AND PLANNING

The expected outcome to achieve is that the eye is cleansed successfully. Other outcomes that may be appropriate include the following: the patient understands the rationale for the procedure and is able to participate; the patient's eye remains free from injury; and the patient remains free from pain.

IMPLEMENTATION

ACTION / 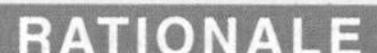

ACTION	RATIONALE
1. Gather equipment. Check the original order in the medical record for the irrigation, according to facility policy. Clarify any inconsistencies. Check the patient's chart for allergies.	This comparison helps to identify errors that may have occurred when orders were transcribed. The primary care provider's order is the legal record of medication orders for each facility.
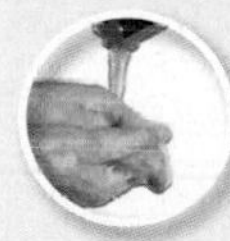 2. Perform hand hygiene and put on PPE, if indicated.	Hand hygiene and PPE prevent the spread of microorganisms. PPE is required based on transmission precautions.
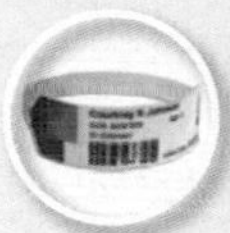 3. **Identify the patient. Compare the information with the CMAR/MAR. The patient should be identified using at least two methods** (The Joint Commission, 2013):	Identifying the patient ensures the right patient receives the medications and helps prevent errors. The patient's room number or physical location is not used as an identifier (The Joint Commission, 2013). Replace the identification band if it is missing or inaccurate in any way.
a. Check the name on the patient's identification band.	
b. Check the identification number on the patient's identification band.	
c. Check the birth date on the patient's identification band.	
d. Ask the patient to state his or her name and birth date, based on facility policy.	This requires a response from the patient, but illness and strange surroundings often cause patients to be confused.
4. Explain the procedure to the patient.	Explanation facilitates cooperation and reassures the patient.
5. Scan the patient's bar code on the identification band, if required.	Provides an additional check to ensure that the medication is given to the right patient.
6. Assemble equipment at the patient's bedside.	This provides for an organized approach to the task.
7. Have the patient sit or lie with head tilted toward side of affected eye (Figure 1). Protect the patient and bed with a waterproof pad.	Gravity aids flow of the solution away from the unaffected eye and from the inner canthus of the affected eye toward the outer canthus.

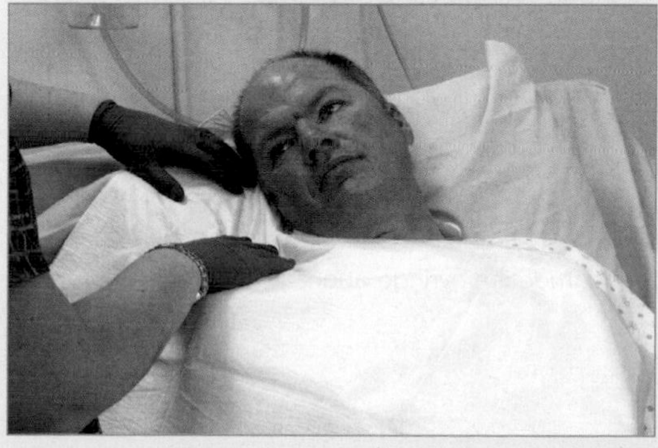

FIGURE 1 Tilting head toward affected eye.

(continued)

SKILL 5-17 ADMINISTERING AN EYE IRRIGATION continued

ACTION	RATIONALE
8. Put on gloves. Clean lids and lashes with washcloth moistened with normal saline or the solution ordered for the irrigation. Wipe from inner canthus to outer canthus (Figure 2). Use a different corner of washcloth with each wipe.	Gloves protect the nurse from contact with mucous membranes, body fluids, and contaminants. Materials lodged on lids or in lashes may be washed into the eye. Wiping from the inner to outer canthus protects the nasolacrimal duct and the other eye. Use of a different part of the washcloth prevents transmission of bacteria.
9. Place curved basin at cheek on the side of the affected eye to receive irrigating solution (Figure 3). If patient is able, ask him/her to support the basin.	Gravity aids flow of solution.
10. Expose lower conjunctival sac and hold upper lid open with your nondominant hand (Figure 4).	Solution is directed only into lower conjunctival sac because the cornea is sensitive and easily injured. This also prevents reflex blinking.
11. Fill the irrigation syringe with the prescribed fluid. **Hold irrigation syringe about 2.5 cm (1 inch) from eye (Figure 5). Direct flow of solution from inner to outer canthus along the conjunctival sac.**	This minimizes the risk for injury to the cornea. Directing solution toward the outer canthus helps to prevent the spread of contamination from the eye to the lacrimal sac, the lacrimal duct, and the nose.

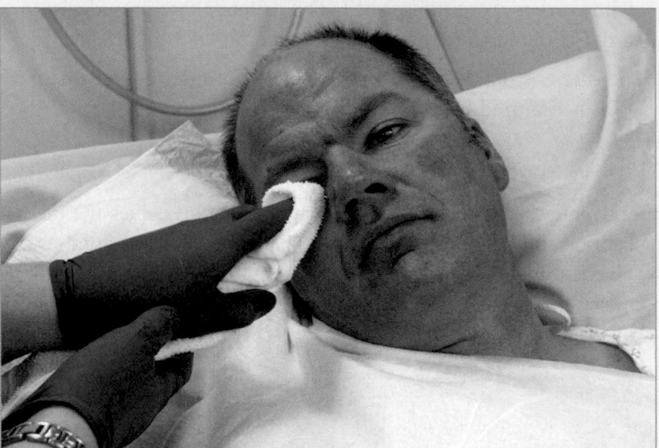

FIGURE 2 Cleaning lids and lashes from inside of eye to outside.

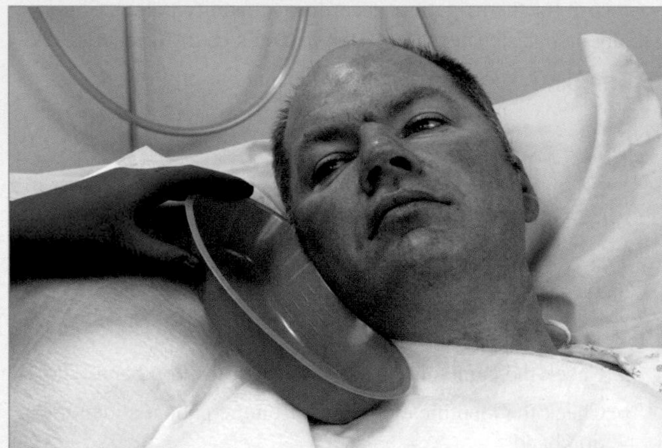

FIGURE 3 Placing basin to catch irrigating fluid.

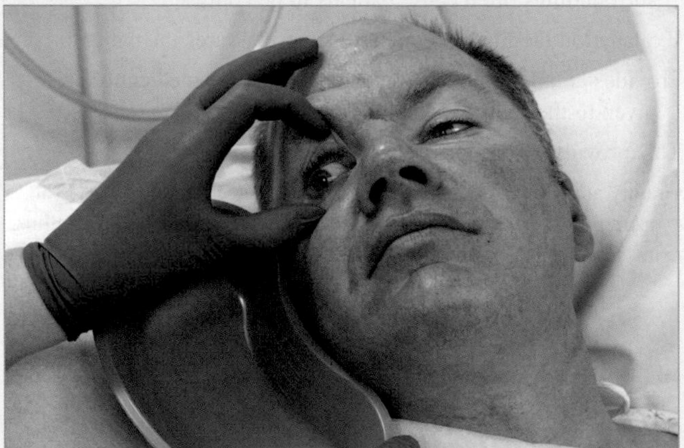

FIGURE 4 Holding eyelid in position.

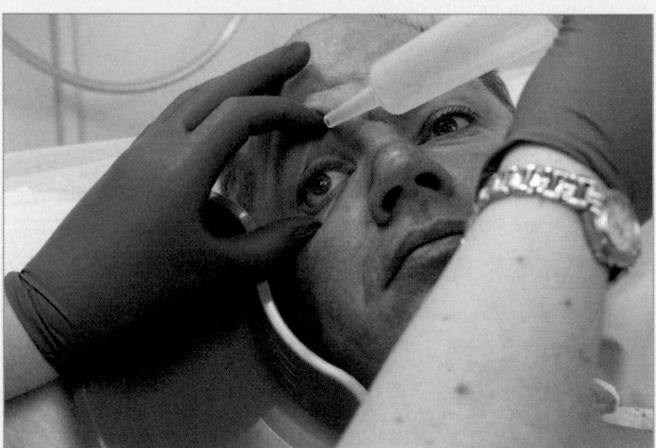

FIGURE 5 Holding irrigation syringe about 1 inch from eye.

ACTION	RATIONALE
12. Irrigate until the solution is clear or all the solution has been used. **Use only enough force to remove secretions gently from the conjunctiva. Avoid touching any part of the eye with the irrigating tip.**	Directing solutions with force may cause injury to the tissues of the eye as well as to the conjunctiva. Touching the eye is uncomfortable for the patient and may cause damage to the cornea.
13. Pause the irrigation and have the patient close the eye periodically during the procedure.	Movement of the eye when the lids are closed helps to move secretions from the upper to the lower conjunctival sac.
14. Dry the periorbital area after irrigation with gauze sponge. Offer a towel to the patient if face and neck are wet.	Leaving the skin moist after irrigation is uncomfortable for the patient.
15. Remove gloves. Assist the patient to a comfortable position.	This ensures patient comfort.
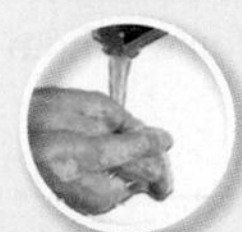 16. Remove additional PPE, if used. Perform hand hygiene.	Removing PPE properly reduces the risk for infection transmission and contamination of other items. Hand hygiene prevents the spread of microorganisms.
17. Evaluate the patient's response to the medication within an appropriate time frame.	The patient needs to be evaluated for therapeutic and adverse effects from the medication.

EVALUATION

The expected outcomes are met when the eye has been irrigated successfully; the patient understands the rationale for the procedure and is able to comply with the procedure; the eye is not injured; and the patient experiences minimal discomfort.

DOCUMENTATION

Guidelines

Document the procedure, site, the type of solution and volume used, length of time irrigation performed, pre- and post-procedure assessments, characteristics of any drainage, and the patient's response to the treatment.

Sample Documentation

8/26/15 1820 Sclera of left eye reddened, with periorbital edema and erythema. Thick, yellow liquid draining from left eye. Irrigation of left eye performed using 500 mL of sterile saline. Patient's sclera remains reddened, with slight periorbital edema and erythema. No drainage noted from left eye after irrigation. Patient tolerated procedure with minimal discomfort. Denies need for pain medication at this time. Patient rates pain at present as 1/10.

—*B. Clapp, RN*

UNEXPECTED SITUATIONS AND ASSOCIATED INTERVENTIONS

- *Patient complains of significant pain during the procedure:* Stop the procedure and notify the primary care provider. Primary care provider may need to check for any foreign objects, such as glass, before proceeding with irrigation.
- *Patient cannot keep the eye open during the procedure:* You may need assistance to help the patient keep the eye open.

SPECIAL CONSIDERATIONS

- Ongoing assessment is an important part of nursing care to evaluate patient response to administered treatments and early detection of adverse effects. If an adverse effect is suspected, notify the patient's primary care provider. Provide additional intervention based on type of reaction and patient assessment.

SKILL 5-18 INSTILLING EAR DROPS

Drugs are instilled into the auditory canal for their local effect. They are used to soften wax, relieve pain, apply local anesthesia, and treat infections.

The tympanic membrane separates the external ear from the middle ear. Normally, it is intact and closes the entrance to the middle ear completely. If it is ruptured or has been opened by surgical intervention, the middle ear and the inner ear have a direct passage to the external ear. When this occurs, perform instillations with the greatest of care to prevent forcing materials from the outer ear into the middle ear and the inner ear. Use sterile technique to prevent infection.

DELEGATION CONSIDERATIONS

The administration of medication via drops in the ear is not delegated to nursing assistive personnel (NAP) or to unlicensed assistive personnel (UAP). Depending on the state's nurse practice act and the organization's policies and procedures, the administration of ear drop may be delegated to licensed practical/vocational nurses (LPN/LVNs). The decision to delegate must be based on careful analysis of the patient's needs and circumstances, as well as the qualifications of the person to whom the task is being delegated. Refer to the Delegation Guidelines in Appendix A.

EQUIPMENT

- Medication (warmed to 37°C [98.6°F])
- Dropper
- Tissue
- Cotton balls (optional)
- Gloves
- Additional PPE, as indicated
- Washcloth (optional)
- Normal saline solution
- Computer-generated Medication Administration Record (CMAR) or Medication Administration Record (MAR)

ASSESSMENT

Assess the affected ear for redness, erythema, edema, drainage, or tenderness. Assess the patient for allergies. Verify patient name, dose, route, and time of administration. Assess the patient's knowledge of medication and procedure. If the patient has a knowledge deficit about the medication, this may be an appropriate time to begin education about the medication. Assess the patient's ability to cooperate with the procedure.

NURSING DIAGNOSIS

Determine related factors for the nursing diagnoses based on the patient's current status. Appropriate nursing diagnoses may include:

- Anxiety
- Risk for Injury
- Acute Pain

OUTCOME IDENTIFICATION AND PLANNING

The expected outcome to achieve is that drops are administered successfully. Other outcomes that may be appropriate include the following: the patient understands the rationale for the ear drop instillation and has decreased anxiety; the patient remains free from pain; and the patient experiences no allergy response or injury.

IMPLEMENTATION

ACTION	RATIONALE
1. Gather equipment. Check medication order against the original order in the medical record, according to facility policy. Clarify any inconsistencies. Check the patient's chart for allergies.	This comparison helps to identify errors that may have occurred when orders were transcribed. The primary care provider's order is the legal record of medication orders for each facility.
2. Know the actions, special nursing considerations, safe dose ranges, purpose of administration, and adverse effects of the medication to be administered. Consider the appropriateness of the medication for this patient.	This knowledge aids the nurse in evaluating the therapeutic effect of the medication in relation to the patient's disorder and can also be used to educate the patient about the medication.

ACTION	RATIONALE
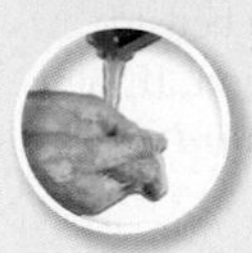 3. Perform hand hygiene.	Hand hygiene prevents the spread of microorganisms.
4. Move the medication cart to the outside of the patient's room or prepare for administration in the medication area.	Organization facilitates error-free administration and saves time.
5. Unlock the medication cart or drawer. Enter pass code and scan employee identification, if required.	Locking the cart or drawer safeguards each patient's medication supply. Hospital accrediting organizations require medication carts to be locked when not in use. Entering pass code and scanning ID allows only authorized users into the system and identifies the user for documentation by the computer.
6. **Prepare medications for one patient at a time.**	This prevents errors in medication administration.
7. Read the CMAR/MAR and select the proper medication from the patient's medication drawer or unit stock.	This is the *first* check of the label.
8. Compare the label with the CMAR/MAR. Check expiration dates and perform calculations, if necessary. Scan the bar code on the package, if required.	This is the *second* check of the label. Verify calculations with another nurse to ensure safety, if necessary.
9. **Depending on facility policy, the third check of the label may occur at this point. If so, when all medications for one patient have been prepared, recheck the labels with the CMAR/MAR before taking the medications to the patient.**	This *third* check ensures accuracy and helps to prevent errors. *Note:* Many facilities require the *third* check to occur at the bedside, after identifying the patient and before administration.
10. Lock the medication cart before leaving it.	Locking the cart or drawer safeguards the patient's medication supply. Hospital accrediting organizations require medication carts to be locked when not in use.
11. Transport medications to the patient's bedside carefully, and keep the medications in sight at all times.	Careful handling and close observation prevent accidental or deliberate disarrangement of medications.
12. **Ensure that the patient receives the medications at the correct time.**	Check agency policy, which may allow for administration within a period of 30 minutes before or 30 minutes after the designated time.
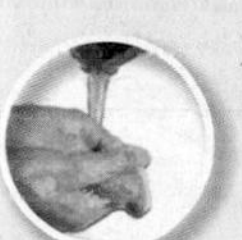 13. Perform hand hygiene and put on PPE, if indicated.	Hand hygiene and PPE prevent the spread of microorganisms. PPE is required based on transmission precautions.
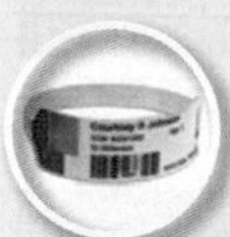 14. **Identify the patient. Compare the information with the CMAR/MAR. The patient should be identified using at least two methods** (The Joint Commission, 2013):	Identifying the patient ensures the right patient receives the medications and helps prevent errors. The patient's room number or physical location is not used as an identifier (The Joint Commission, 2013). Replace the identification band if it is missing or inaccurate in any way.
a. Check the name on the patient's identification band.	
b. Check the identification number on the patient's identification band.	
c. Check the birth date on the patient's identification band.	
d. Ask the patient to state his or her name and birth date, based on facility policy.	This requires a response from the patient, but illness and strange surroundings often cause patients to be confused.
15. **Complete necessary assessments before administering medications. Check the patient's allergy bracelet or ask the patient about allergies. Explain the purpose and action of each medication to the patient.**	Assessment is a prerequisite to administration of medications.
16. Scan the patient's bar code on the identification band, if required.	Provides an additional check to ensure that the medication is given to the right patient.

(continued)

SKILL 5-18 INSTILLING EAR DROPS continued

ACTION	RATIONALE
17. **Based on facility policy, the third check of the label may occur at this point. If so, recheck the labels with the CMAR/MAR before administering the medications to the patient.**	Many facilities require the *third* check to occur at the bedside, after identifying the patient and before administration. If facility policy directs the *third* check at this time, this *third* check ensures accuracy and helps to prevent errors.
18. Put on gloves.	Gloves protect the nurse from potential contact with mucous membranes and body fluids.
19. Cleanse external ear of any drainage with cotton ball or washcloth moistened with normal saline (Figure 1).	Debris and drainage may prevent some of the medication from entering the ear canal.
20. Place patient on his or her unaffected side in bed, or, if ambulatory, have patient sit with head well tilted to the side so that the affected ear is uppermost (Figure 2).	This positioning prevents the drops from escaping from the ear.
21. Draw up the amount of solution needed in the dropper. Do not return excess medication to stock bottle. A prepackaged, monodrip plastic container may also be used (Figure 3).	Risk for contamination is increased when medication is returned to the stock bottle.
22. Straighten auditory canal by pulling cartilaginous portion of pinna up and back for an adult. (See Infant and Child Considerations for correct positioning for this age group.)	Pulling on the pinna as described helps to straighten the canal properly for ear drop instillation.
23. Hold dropper in the ear with its tip above the auditory canal (Figure 4). Do not touch the dropper to the ear. For an infant or an irrational or confused patient, protect the dropper with a piece of soft tubing to help prevent injury to the ear.	By holding the dropper in the ear, most of the medication will enter the ear canal. Touching the dropper to the ear contaminates the dropper and medication. The hard tip of the dropper can damage the tympanic membrane if it is jabbed into the ear.

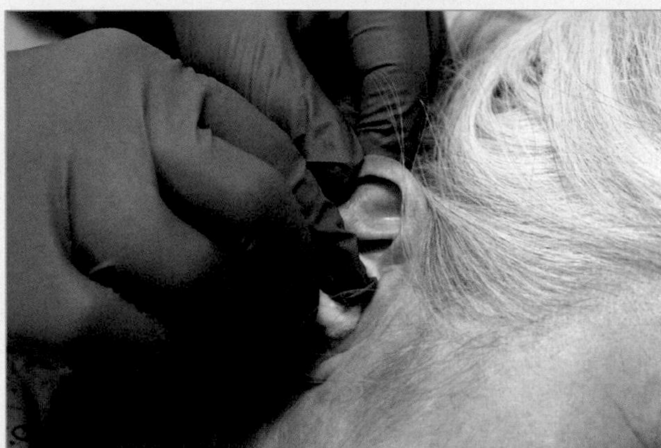
FIGURE 1 Cleaning external ear.

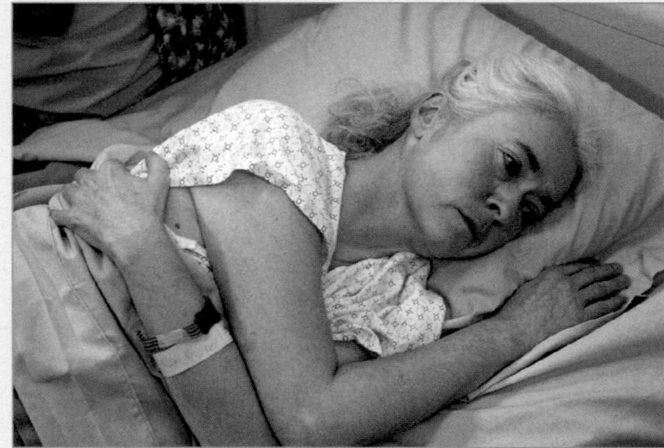
FIGURE 2 Positioning patient on unaffected side.

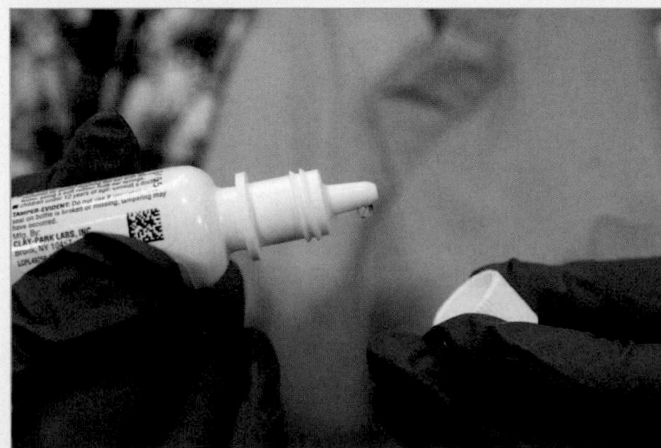
FIGURE 3 Prepackaged ear drop solution.

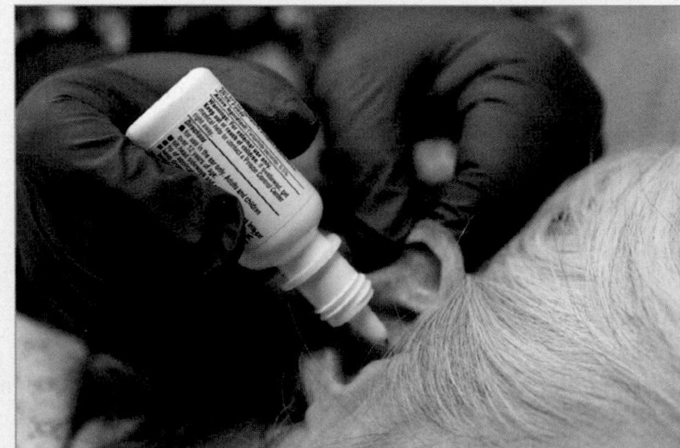
FIGURE 4 Pulling the pinna up and back and placing dropper tip above auditory canal.

ACTION	RATIONALE
24. **Allow drops to fall on the side of the canal. Avoid instilling in the middle of the canal, to avoid instilling directly onto the tympanic membrane.**	It is uncomfortable for the patient if the drops fall directly onto the tympanic membrane.
25. Release pinna after instilling drops, and have patient maintain the head position to prevent escape of medication.	Medication should remain in ear canal for at least 5 minutes.
26. Gently press on the tragus a few times (Figure 5).	Pressing on the tragus causes medication from the canal to move toward the tympanic membrane.
27. If ordered, loosely insert a cotton ball into the ear canal (Figure 6).	A cotton ball can help prevent medication from leaking out of the ear canal.

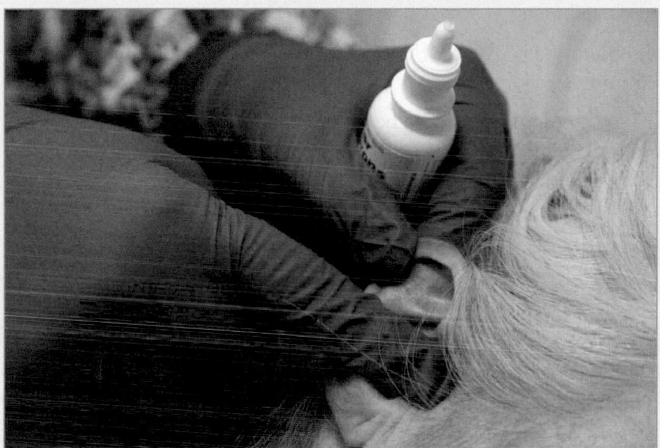
FIGURE 5 Applying pressure to tragus.

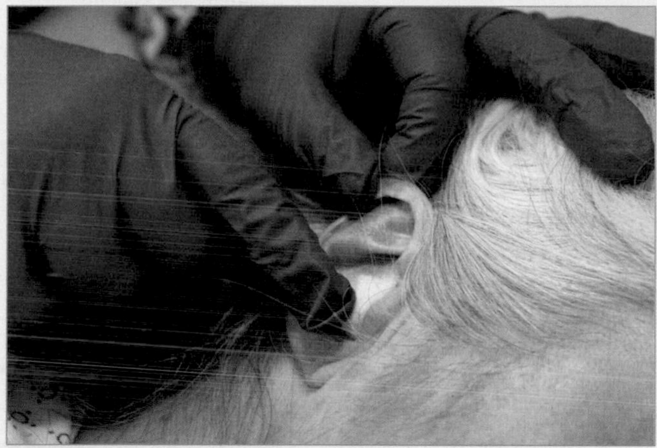
FIGURE 6 Inserting cotton ball into ear canal.

ACTION	RATIONALE
28. Remove gloves. Assist the patient to a comfortable position.	This ensures patient comfort.
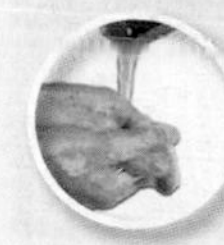 29. Remove additional PPE, if used. Perform hand hygiene.	Removing PPE properly reduces the risk for infection transmission and contamination of other items. Hand hygiene prevents the spread of microorganisms.
30. Document the administration of the medication immediately after administration. See Documentation section below.	Timely documentation helps to ensure patient safety.
31. Evaluate the patient's response to medication within an appropriate time frame.	The patient needs to be evaluated for therapeutic and adverse effects from the medication.

EVALUATION

The expected outcomes are met when the patient receives the ear drops successfully; the patient understands the rationale for ear drop instillation and exhibits no or decreased anxiety; the patient experiences no or minimal pain and no allergy response or injury.

DOCUMENTATION

Guidelines

Document the administration of the medication immediately after administration, including date, time, dose, route of administration, and site of administration, specifically right, left, or both ears, on the CMAR/MAR or record using the required format. If using a bar-code system, medication administration is automatically recorded when the bar code is scanned. PRN medications require documentation of the reason for administration. Prompt recording avoids the possibility of accidentally repeating the administration of the drug. Document pre- and post-administration assessments, characteristics of any drainage, and the patient's response to the treatment, if appropriate. If the drug was refused or omitted, record this in the appropriate area on the medication record and notify the primary care provider. This verifies the reason medication was omitted and ensures that the primary care provider is aware of the patient's condition.

(continued)

SKILL 5-18 INSTILLING EAR DROPS continued

UNEXPECTED SITUATIONS AND ASSOCIATED INTERVENTIONS

- *Medication runs from ear into eye:* Notify primary care provider and check with the pharmacy. Eye irrigation may need to be performed.
- *Patient complains of extreme pain when you press on the tragus:* Allow patient to press on tragus. If pressure causes too much pain, this part may be deferred.

SPECIAL CONSIDERATIONS

General Considerations

- If both ears are to be treated, wait 5 minutes before instilling drops into the second ear.
- Ongoing assessment is an important part of nursing care to evaluate patient response to administered treatments and early detection of adverse effects. If an adverse effect is suspected, notify the patient's primary care provider. Additional intervention is based on type of reaction and patient assessment.

Infant and Child Considerations

- Pull pinna straight back for a child older than 3 years (Figure 7) and down and back for an infant or a child younger than 3 years (Figure 8).
- Distraction techniques, such as TV or a quiet toy, may be helpful when attempting to keep a child quiet for 5 minutes. Reading to the child may not be appropriate because the child's hearing may be compromised during medication administration.

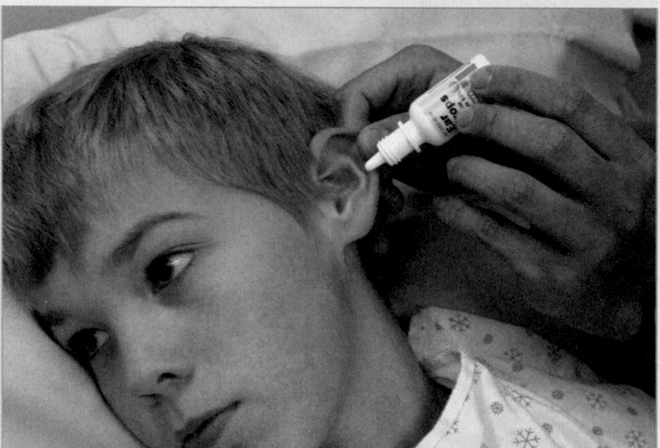

FIGURE 7 Pulling pinna straight back for child older than 3 years.

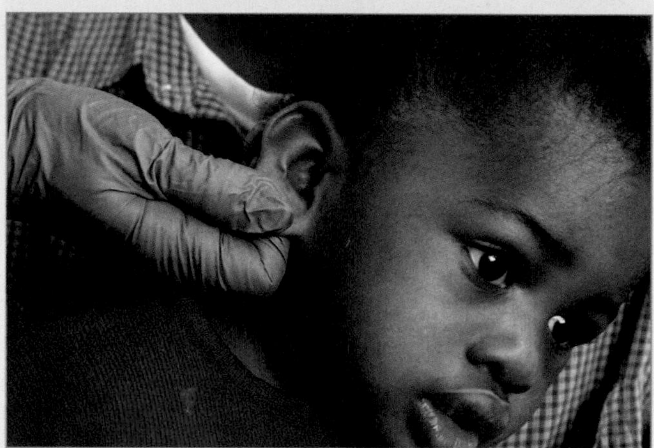

FIGURE 8 Pulling pinna down and back for an infant or child younger than 3 years.

SKILL 5-19 ADMINISTERING AN EAR IRRIGATION

Irrigations of the external auditory canal are ordinarily performed for cleaning purposes or for applying heat to the area. Typically, a normal saline solution is used, although an antiseptic solution may be indicated for local action. To prevent pain, make sure the irrigation solution is at least room temperature. Usually, an irrigation syringe is used. However, an irrigating container with tubing and an ear tip may also be used, especially if the purpose of the irrigation is to apply heat to the area.

DELEGATION CONSIDERATIONS

The administration of an irrigation of the ear is not delegated to nursing assistive personnel (NAP) or to unlicensed assistive personnel (UAP). Depending on the state's nurse practice act and the organization's policies and procedures, the irrigation of the ear may be delegated to licensed practical/vocational nurses (LPN/LVNs). The decision to delegate must be based on careful analysis of the patient's needs and circumstances, as well as the qualifications of the person to whom the task is being delegated. Refer to the Delegation Guidelines in Appendix A.

EQUIPMENT

- Prescribed irrigating solution (warmed to 37°C [98.6°F])
- Irrigation set (container and irrigating or bulb syringe)
- Waterproof pad
- Emesis basin
- Cotton-tipped applicators
- Gloves
- Additional PPE, as indicated
- Cotton balls
- Computer-generated Medication Administration Record (CMAR) or Medication Administration Record (MAR)

ASSESSMENT

Assess the affected ear for redness, erythema, edema, drainage, or tenderness. Assess the patient's ability to hear. Assess the patient for allergies. Verify patient name, dose, route, and time of administration. Assess the patient's knowledge of medication and procedure. If the patient has a knowledge deficit about the medication, this may be an appropriate time to begin education about the medication. Assess the patient's ability to cooperate with the procedure.

NURSING DIAGNOSIS

Determine related factors for the nursing diagnoses based on the patient's current status. Appropriate nursing diagnoses may include:

- Acute Pain
- Deficient Knowledge
- Risk for Injury

OUTCOME IDENTIFICATION AND PLANNING

The expected outcome to achieve is that the irrigation is administered successfully. Other outcomes that may be appropriate include the following: the patient remains free from pain and injury; the patient will experience improved hearing; and the patient understands the rationale for the procedure.

IMPLEMENTATION

ACTION	RATIONALE
1. Gather equipment. Check medication order against the original order in the medical record, according to facility policy. Clarify any inconsistencies. Check the patient's chart for allergies.	This comparison helps to identify errors that may have occurred when orders were transcribed. The primary care provider's order is the legal record of medication orders for each facility.
2. Know the actions, special nursing considerations, safe dose ranges, purpose of administration, and adverse effects of the medication to be administered. Consider the appropriateness of the medication for this patient.	This knowledge aids the nurse in evaluating the therapeutic effect of the medication in relation to the patient's disorder and can also be used to educate the patient about the medication.
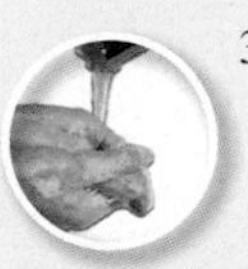 3. Perform hand hygiene.	Hand hygiene prevents the spread of microorganisms.
4. Move the medication cart to the outside of the patient's room or prepare for administration in the medication area.	Organization facilitates error-free administration and saves time.
5. Unlock the medication cart or drawer. Enter pass code and scan employee identification, if required.	Locking the cart or drawer safeguards each patient's medication supply. Hospital accrediting organizations require medication carts to be locked when not in use. Entering pass code and scanning ID allows only authorized users into the computer system and identifies the user for documentation by the computer.
6. **Prepare medications for one patient at a time.**	This prevents errors in medication administration.
7. Read the CMAR/MAR and select the proper medication from unit stock or the patient's medication drawer.	This is the *first* check of the label.
8. Compare the label with the CMAR/MAR. Check expiration dates and perform calculations, if necessary. Scan the bar code on the package, if required.	This is the *second* check of the label. Verify calculations with another nurse to ensure safety, if necessary.

(continued)

SKILL 5-19 ADMINISTERING AN EAR IRRIGATION continued

ACTION	RATIONALE
9. **Depending on facility policy, the third check of the label may occur at this point. If so, when all medications for one patient have been prepared, recheck the labels with the CMAR/MAR before taking the medications to the patient.**	This *third* check ensures accuracy and helps to prevent errors. *Note:* Many facilities require the *third* check to occur at the bedside, after identifying the patient and before administration.
10. Lock the medication cart before leaving it.	Locking the cart or drawer safeguards the patient's medication supply. Hospital accrediting organizations require medication carts to be locked when not in use.
11. Transport medications to the patient's bedside carefully, and keep the medications in sight at all times.	Careful handling and close observation prevent accidental or deliberate disarrangement of medications.
12. **Ensure that the patient receives the medications at the correct time.**	Check agency policy, which may allow for administration within a period of 30 minutes before or 30 minutes after the designated time.
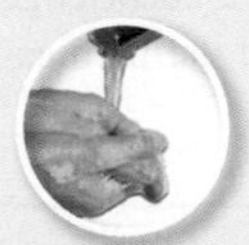 13. Perform hand hygiene and put on PPE, if indicated.	Hand hygiene and PPE prevent the spread of microorganisms. PPE is required based on transmission precautions.
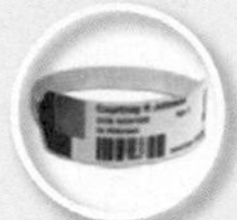 14. **Identify the patient. Compare the information with the CMAR/MAR. The patient should be identified using at least two methods** (The Joint Commission, 2013):	Identifying the patient ensures the right patient receives the medications and helps prevent errors. The patient's room number or physical location is not used as an identifier (The Joint Commission, 2013). Replace the identification band if it is missing or inaccurate in any way.
a. Check the name on the patient's identification band.	
b. Check the identification number on the patient's identification band.	
c. Check the birth date on the patient's identification band.	
d. Ask the patient to state his or her name and birth date, based on facility policy.	This requires a response from the patient, but illness and strange surroundings often cause patients to be confused.
15. Explain the procedure to the patient.	Explanation facilitates cooperation and reassures the patient.
16. Scan the patient's bar code on the identification band, if required.	Provides an additional check to ensure that the medication is given to the right patient.
17. Assemble equipment at patient's bedside.	This provides for an organized approach to the task.
18. Put on gloves.	Gloves protect the nurse from potential contact with contaminants and body fluids.
19. Have the patient sit up or lie with head tilted toward side of the affected ear. Protect the patient and bed with a waterproof pad. Have the patient support the basin under the ear to receive the irrigating solution (Figure 1).	Gravity causes the irrigating solution to flow from the ear to the basin.

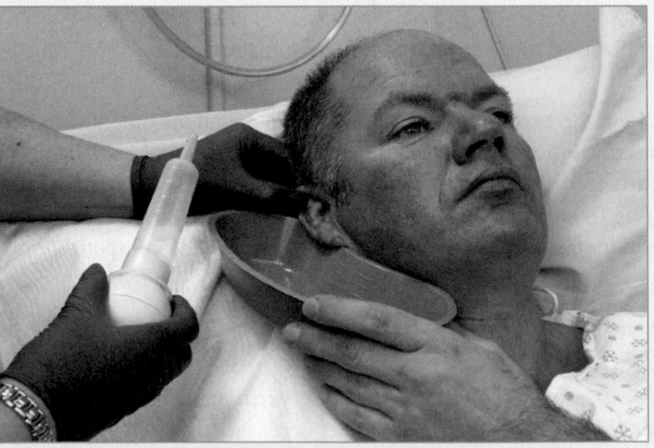

FIGURE 1 Positioning for ear irrigation.

ACTION	RATIONALE
20. Clean pinna and meatus of auditory canal, as necessary, with moistened cotton-tipped applicators dipped in warm tap water or the irrigating solution.	Materials lodged on the pinna and at the meatus may be washed into the ear.
21. Fill bulb syringe with warm solution. If an irrigating container is used, prime the tubing.	Priming the tubing allows air to escape from the tubing. Air forced into the ear canal is noisy and therefore unpleasant for the patient.
22. Straighten the auditory canal by pulling the cartilaginous portion of pinna up and back for an adult (Figure 2). (See Infant and Child Considerations for correct positioning for this age group.)	Straightening the ear canal allows solution to reach all areas of the canal easily.
23. **Direct a steady, slow stream of solution against the roof of the auditory canal, using only enough force to remove secretions (Figure 3). Do not occlude the auditory canal with the irrigating nozzle. Allow solution to flow out unimpeded.**	Directing the solution at the roof of the canal helps prevent injury to the tympanic membrane. Continuous in-and-out flow of the irrigating solution helps to prevent pressure in the canal.
24. When irrigation is complete, place a cotton ball loosely in the auditory meatus (Figure 4) and have the patient lie on side of affected ear on a towel or absorbent pad.	The cotton ball absorbs excess fluid, and gravity allows the remaining solution in the canal to escape from the ear.

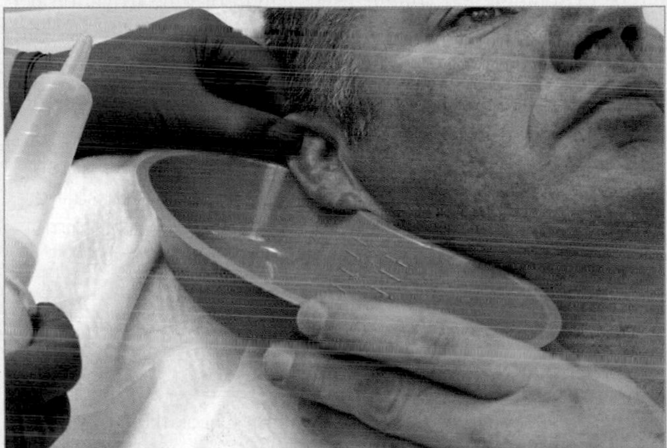

FIGURE 2 Straightening ear canal for irrigation.

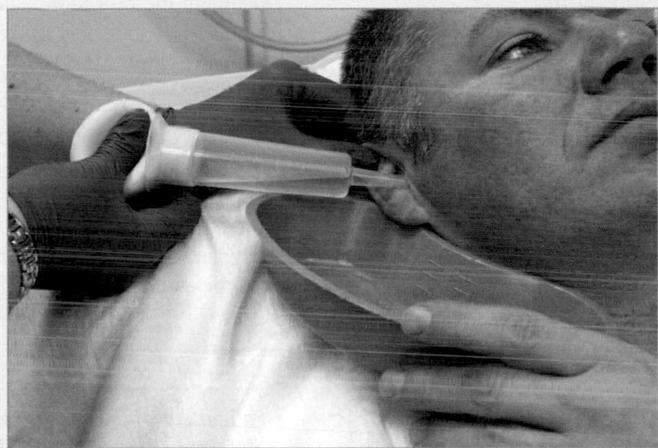

FIGURE 3 Instilling irrigation fluid.

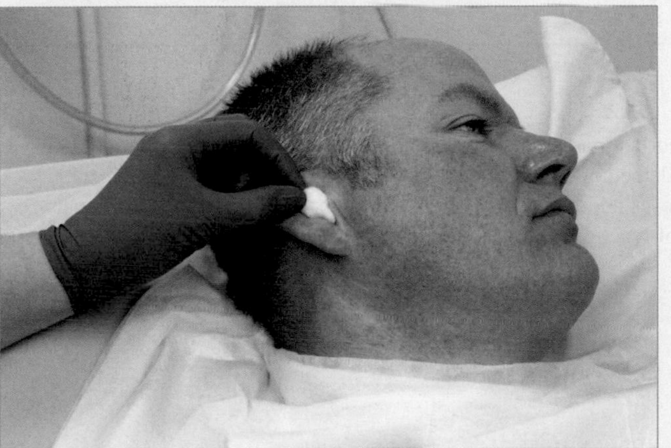

FIGURE 4 Placing cotton ball in ear.

(continued)

SKILL 5-19 ADMINISTERING AN EAR IRRIGATION continued

ACTION	RATIONALE
25. Remove gloves. Assist the patient to a comfortable position.	This ensures patient comfort.
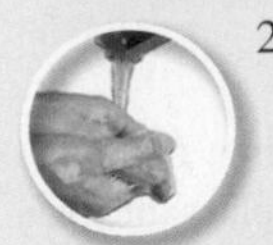 26. Remove additional PPE, if used. Perform hand hygiene.	Removing PPE properly reduces the risk for infection transmission and contamination of other items. Hand hygiene prevents the spread of microorganisms.
27. Document the administration of the medication immediately after administration. See Documentation section below.	Timely documentation helps to ensure patient safety.
28. Evaluate the patient's response to the procedure. Return in 10 to 15 minutes and remove cotton ball and assess drainage. Evaluate the patient's response to the medication within an appropriate time frame.	The patient needs to be evaluated for any adverse effects from the procedure. Drainage or pain may indicate injury to the tympanic membrane. The patient needs to be evaluated for therapeutic and adverse effects from the medication.

EVALUATION

The expected outcomes are met when the ear canal is irrigated successfully; the patient experiences no or minimal pain or discomfort; the patient's hearing is improved; and the patient understands the rationale for the ear irrigation procedure.

DOCUMENTATION

Guidelines

Document the procedure, site, the type of solution and volume used, length of time irrigation performed, pre- and post-procedure assessments, characteristics of any drainage, and the patient's response to the treatment.

Sample Documentation

7/6/15 1830 Right ear noted to be without external edema and redness. No drainage noted. Patient reports slightly decreased hearing in right ear. Slight tenderness noted on palpation. Irrigation of right ear performed using 100 mL of warmed normal saline. Clear return with particles of cerumen noted. Patient tolerated procedure with minimal discomfort. Patient reports no change in hearing in right ear. Denies need for pain medication at this time. Patient rates pain at present as 1/10.

—B. Clapp, RN

UNEXPECTED SITUATIONS AND ASSOCIATED INTERVENTIONS

- *Patient complains of significant pain during irrigation:* Stop the irrigation. Check the temperature of the solution. If the solution has cooled, rewarm it and try again. If the patient still complains of pain, stop the irrigation and notify the primary care provider.

SPECIAL CONSIDERATIONS

General Considerations

- Ongoing assessment is an important part of nursing care to evaluate patient response to administered medications and early detection of adverse effects. If an adverse effect is suspected, withhold further medication doses and notify the patient's primary care provider. Additional intervention is based on type of reaction and patient assessment.

Infant and Child Considerations

- Pull pinna straight back for a child older than 3 years (Figure 5) and down and back for an infant or a child younger than 3 years (Figure 6).

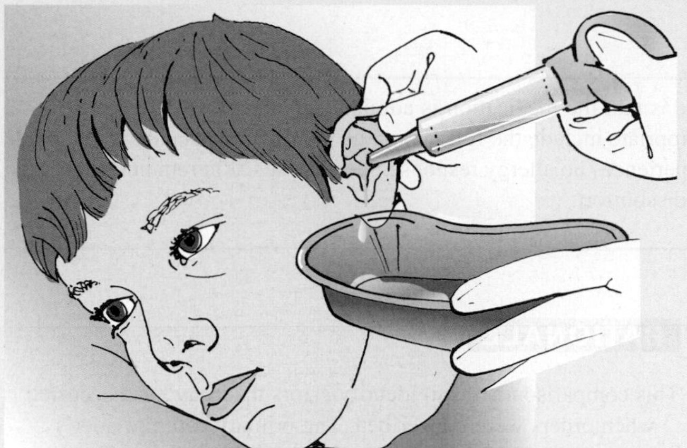

FIGURE 5 Pulling pinna straight back for child older than 3 years.

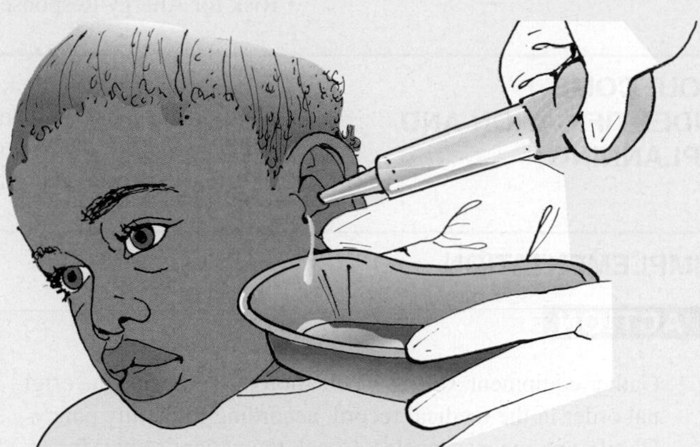

FIGURE 6 Pulling pinna down and back for an infant or child younger than 3 years.

SKILL 5-20 ADMINISTERING A NASAL SPRAY

Nasal instillations are used to treat allergies, sinus infections, and nasal congestion. Medications with a systemic effect, such as vasopressin, may also be prepared as a nasal instillation. The nose is normally not a sterile cavity, but because of its connection with the sinuses, it is important to observe medical asepsis carefully when using nasal instillations.

The following skill describes the steps to administer a nasal spray. Refer to the accompanying Skill Variation for guidelines to administer medication via nasal drops.

DELEGATION CONSIDERATIONS

The administration of medication using a nasal spray is not delegated to nursing assistive personnel (NAP) or to unlicensed assistive personnel (UAP). Depending on the state's nurse practice act and the organization's policies and procedures, administration of a nasal spray may be delegated to licensed practical/vocational nurses (LPN/LVNs). The decision to delegate must be based on careful analysis of the patient's needs and circumstances, as well as the qualifications of the person to whom the task is being delegated. Refer to the Delegation Guidelines in Appendix A.

EQUIPMENT

- Medication in nasal spray bottle
- Gloves
- Additional PPE, as indicated
- Tissue
- Computer-generated Medication Administration Record (CMAR) or Medication Administration Record (MAR)

ASSESSMENT

Assess the nares for redness, erythema, edema, drainage, or tenderness. Assess the patient for allergies. Verify patient name, dose, route, and time of administration. Assess the patient's knowledge of medication and the procedure. If the patient has a knowledge deficit about the medication, this may be an appropriate time to begin education about the procedure. Assess the patient's ability to cooperate with the procedure.

(continued)

SKILL 5-20 ADMINISTERING A NASAL SPRAY continued

NURSING DIAGNOSIS

Determine related factors for the nursing diagnoses based on the patient's current status. Appropriate nursing diagnoses may include:

- Deficient Knowledge
- Risk for Allergy Response

OUTCOME IDENTIFICATION AND PLANNING

The expected outcome to achieve is that the medication is administered successfully into the nose. Other outcomes that may be appropriate include the following: the patient understands the rationale for the nose spray; the patient experiences no allergy response; the patient's skin remains intact; and the patient experiences minimal discomfort.

IMPLEMENTATION

ACTION	RATIONALE
1. Gather equipment. Check medication order against the original order in the medical record, according to facility policy. Clarify any inconsistencies. Check the patient's chart for allergies.	This comparison helps to identify errors that may have occurred when orders were transcribed. The primary care provider's order is the legal record of medication orders for each facility.
2. Know the actions, special nursing considerations, safe dose ranges, purpose of administration, and adverse effects of the medication to be administered. Consider the appropriateness of the medication for this patient.	This knowledge aids the nurse in evaluating the therapeutic effect of the medication in relation to the patient's disorder and can also be used to educate the patient about the medication.
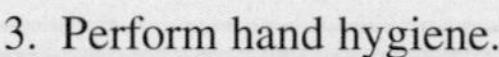 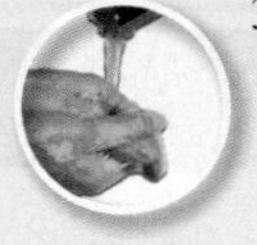 3. Perform hand hygiene.	Hand hygiene prevents the spread of microorganisms.
4. Move the medication cart to the outside of the patient's room or prepare for administration in the medication area.	Organization facilitates error-free administration and saves time.
5. Unlock the medication cart or drawer. Enter pass code and scan employee identification, if required.	Locking the cart or drawer safeguards each patient's medication supply. Hospital accrediting organizations require medication carts to be locked when not in use. Entering pass code and scanning ID allows only authorized users into the system and identifies the user for documentation by the computer.
6. **Prepare medications for one patient at a time.**	This prevents errors in medication administration.
7. Read the CMAR/MAR and select the proper medication from the patient's medication drawer or unit stock.	This is the *first* check of the label.
8. Compare the label with the CMAR/MAR. Check expiration dates and perform calculations, if necessary. Scan the bar code on the package, if required.	This is the *second* check of the label. Verify calculations with another nurse to ensure safety, if necessary.
9. **Depending on facility policy, the third check of the label may occur at this point. If so, when all medications for one patient have been prepared, recheck the labels with the CMAR/MAR before taking the medications to the patient.**	This *third* check ensures accuracy and helps to prevent errors. *Note:* Many facilities require the *third* check to occur at the bedside, after identifying the patient and before administration.
10. Lock the medication cart before leaving it.	Locking the cart or drawer safeguards the patient's medication supply. Hospital accrediting organizations require medication carts to be locked when not in use.
11. Transport medications to the patient's bedside carefully, and keep the medications in sight at all times.	Careful handling and close observation prevent accidental or deliberate disarrangement of medications.
12. **Ensure that the patient receives the medications at the correct time.**	Check agency policy, which may allow for administration within a period of 30 minutes before or 30 minutes after the designated time.

ACTION	RATIONALE
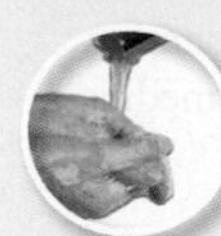 13. Perform hand hygiene and put on PPE, if indicated.	Hand hygiene and PPE prevent the spread of microorganisms. PPE is required based on transmission precautions.
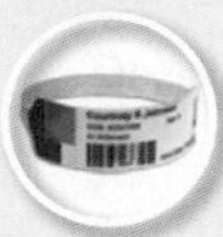 14. **Identify the patient. Compare the information with the CMAR/MAR. The patient should be identified using at least two methods** (The Joint Commission, 2013):	Identifying the patient ensures the right patient receives the medications and helps prevent errors. The patient's room number or physical location is not used as an identifier (The Joint Commission, 2013). Replace the identification band if it is missing or inaccurate in any way.
a. Check the name on the patient's identification band.	
b. Check the identification number on the patient's identification band.	
c. Check the birth date on the patient's identification band.	
d. Ask the patient to state his or her name and birth date, based on facility policy.	This requires a response from the patient, but illness and strange surroundings often cause patients to be confused.
15. **Complete necessary assessments before administering medications. Check the patient's allergy bracelet or ask the patient about allergies. Explain the purpose and action of each medication to the patient.**	Assessment is a prerequisite to administration of medications.
16. Scan the patient's bar code on the identification band, if required (Figure 1).	Provides an additional check to ensure that the medication is given to the right patient.

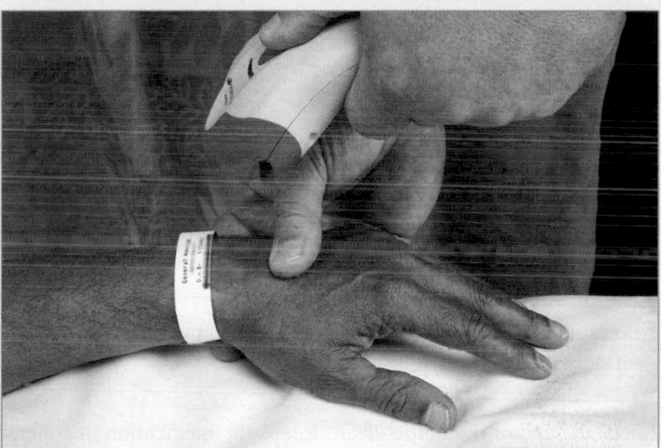

FIGURE 1 Scanning bar code on the patient's identification bracelet.

ACTION	RATIONALE
17. **Based on facility policy, the third check of the label may occur at this point. If so, recheck the labels with the CMAR/MAR before administering the medications to the patient.**	Many facilities require the *third* check to occur at the bedside, after identifying the patient and before administration. If facility policy directs the *third* check at this time, this *third* check ensures accuracy and helps to prevent errors.
18. Put on gloves.	Gloves protect the nurse from potential contact with contaminants and body fluids.
19. Provide patient with paper tissues and ask the patient to blow his or her nose.	Blowing the nose clears the nasal mucosa prior to medication administration.
20. Have the patient sit up with head tilted back. **Tilting the patient's head should be avoided if the patient has a cervical spine injury.**	Allows the spray to flow into the nares. Tilting the head is contraindicated with cervical spine injury.

(*continued*)

SKILL 5-20 ADMINISTERING A NASAL SPRAY continued

ACTION	RATIONALE
21. Instruct the patient to inhale gently through the nose as the spray is being administered or not to inhale gently as the spray is being administered. Your instruction to the patient will depend on the medication being administered. Consult the manufacturer's instructions for each medication.	Inhalation helps to distribute the spray in the nares. Inhalation during administration is not recommended for some medications.
22. Agitate the bottle gently, if required for specific medication. Insert the tip of the nosepiece of the bottle into one nostril (Figure 2). Close the opposite nostril with a finger. Instruct the patient to breathe in gently through the nostril, if required. Compress or activate the bottle to release one spray at the same time the patient breathes in.	Mixes medication thoroughly to ensure a consistent dose of medication.

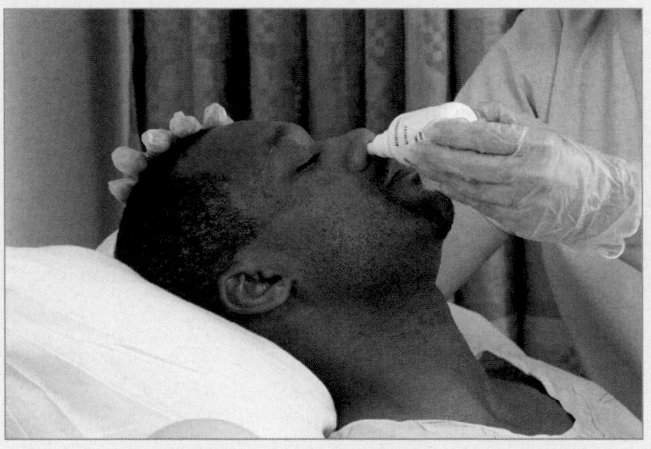

FIGURE 2 Inserting tip of bottle into one nostril. (From Craven & Hirnle, (2013). *Fundamentals of nursing* (7th ed). Philadelphia: Wolters Kluwer Health/Lippincott Williams & Wilkins, p. 425, Figure 19-8.)

ACTION	RATIONALE
23. Keep the medication container compressed and remove it from the nostril. Release the container from the compressed state. Do not allow the container to return to its original position until it is removed from the patient's nose.	Prevents contamination of the contents of the container.
24. Have the patient hold his or her breath for a few seconds, and then breathe out slowly through the mouth. Repeat in the other nostril, as prescribed or indicated.	Allows medication to remain in contact with mucous membranes of nose.
25. Wipe the outside of the bottle nose piece with a clean, dry tissue or cloth and replace the cap. Instruct the patient to avoid blowing his or her nose for 5 to 10 minutes, depending on the medication.	Keeps the end of the bottle clean. Keeps the medication in contact with the mucous membranes of the nose.
26. Remove gloves. Assist the patient to a comfortable position.	This ensures patient comfort.
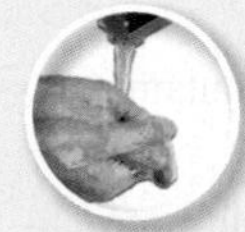 27. Remove additional PPE, if used. Perform hand hygiene.	Removing PPE properly reduces the risk for infection transmission and contamination of other items. Hand hygiene prevents the spread of microorganisms.
28. Document the administration of the medication immediately after administration. See Documentation section below.	Timely documentation helps to ensure patient safety.
29. Evaluate the patient's response to the procedure and medication within an appropriate time frame.	The patient needs to be evaluated for therapeutic and adverse effects from the medication.

EVALUATION

The expected outcomes are met when the patient receives the nose spray successfully; the patient understands the rationale for nose spray; the patient experiences no allergy response; the patient's skin remains intact; and the patient experiences minimal discomfort.

DOCUMENTATION

Guidelines

Document the administration of the medication, including date, time, dose, route of administration, and site of administration, specifically right, left, or both nares, on the CMAR/MAR or record using the required format. If using a bar-code system, medication administration is automatically recorded when the bar code is scanned. PRN medications require documentation of the reason for administration. Prompt recording avoids the possibility of accidentally repeating the administration of the drug. Document pre- and post-administration assessments, characteristics of any drainage, and the patient's response to the treatment, if appropriate. If the drug was refused or omitted, record this in the appropriate area on the medication record and notify the primary care provider. This verifies the reason medication was omitted and ensures that the primary care provider is aware of the patient's condition.

UNEXPECTED SITUATIONS AND ASSOCIATED INTERVENTIONS

- *Patient sneezes immediately after receiving nose spray:* Do not repeat the dosage, because you cannot determine how much medication was actually absorbed.

SPECIAL CONSIDERATIONS

- Ongoing assessment is an important part of nursing care to evaluate patient response to administered medications and early detection of adverse effects. If an adverse effect is suspected, withhold further medication doses and notify the patient's primary care provider. Additional intervention is based on type of reaction and patient assessment.

SKILL VARIATION Administering Medication via Nasal Drops

Prepare medication as outlined in steps 1–12 above (Skill 5-20).

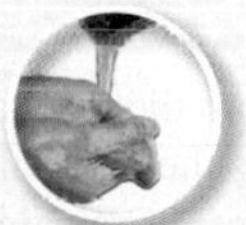

1. Perform hand hygiene and put on PPE, if indicated.

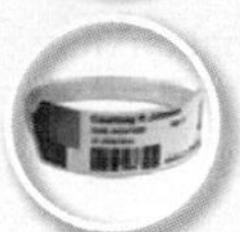

2. Identify the patient. The patient should be identified using two methods.
3. Close the door to the room or pull the bedside curtain.
4. **Complete necessary assessments before administering medications. Check allergy bracelet or ask patient about allergies. Explain the purpose and action of the medication to the patient.**
5. Scan the patient's bar code on the identification band, if required.
6. **Based on facility policy, the third check of the label may occur at this point. If so, recheck the labels with the CMAR/MAR before administering the medications to the patient.**
7. Put on gloves. Assist the patient to an upright position with the head tilted back.
8. Draw sufficient solution into the dropper for both nares. Do not return excess solution to the bottle to avoid contamination.
9. Have the patient breathe through the mouth. Hold tip of nose up and place dropper just above naris, about 1/3 inch. Instill the prescribed number of drops in one naris and then into the other. Avoid touching naris with dropper.
10. Have patient remain in position with head tilted back for a few minutes to prevent the escape of the medication.
11. Remove gloves. Assist the patient to a comfortable position.
12. Remove additional PPE, if used. Perform hand hygiene.
13. Document administration of the medication on the CMAR/MAR immediately after administering the medication. Document the site, if only one nostril is used.
14. Evaluate the patient's response to the medication within an appropriate time frame.

SKILL 5-21 ADMINISTERING A VAGINAL CREAM

Creams, foams, and tablets can be applied intravaginally using a narrow, tubular applicator with an attached plunger. Suppositories that melt when exposed to body heat are also administered by vaginal insertion (see Skill Variation 5-21). Refrigerate suppositories for storage. Time administration to allow the patient to lie down afterward to retain the medication.

DELEGATION CONSIDERATIONS

The administration of medication as a vaginal cream is not delegated to nursing assistive personnel (NAP) or to unlicensed assistive personnel (UAP). Depending on the state's nurse practice act and the organization's policies and procedures, administration of a vaginal cream may be delegated to licensed practical/vocational nurses (LPN/LVNs). The decision to delegate must be based on careful analysis of the patient's needs and circumstances, as well as the qualifications of the person to whom the task is being delegated. Refer to the Delegation Guidelines in Appendix A.

EQUIPMENT

- Medication with applicator, if appropriate
- Water-soluble lubricant
- Perineal pad
- Washcloth, skin cleanser, and warm water
- Gloves
- Additional PPE, as indicated
- Computer-generated Medication Administration Record (CMAR) or Medication Administration Record (MAR)

ASSESSMENT

Assess the external genitalia and vaginal canal for redness, erythema, edema, drainage, or tenderness. Assess the patient for allergies. Verify patient name, dose, route, and time of administration. Assess the patient's knowledge of medication and procedure. If the patient has a knowledge deficit about the medication, this may be an appropriate time to begin education about the medication. Assess the patient's ability to cooperate with the procedure.

NURSING DIAGNOSIS

Determine related factors for the nursing diagnoses based on the patient's current status. Appropriate nursing diagnoses may include:

- Deficient Knowledge
- Risk for Allergy Response
- Anxiety

OUTCOME IDENTIFICATION AND PLANNING

The expected outcome to achieve is that the medication is administered successfully into the vagina. Other outcomes that may be appropriate include the following: the patient understands the rationale for the vaginal instillation; the patient experiences no allergy response; the patient's skin remains intact; the patient experiences no, or minimal, pain; and the patient experiences minimal anxiety.

IMPLEMENTATION

ACTION	RATIONALE
1. Gather equipment. Check medication order against the original order in the medical record, according to facility policy. Clarify any inconsistencies. Check the patient's chart for allergies.	This comparison helps to identify errors that may have occurred when orders were transcribed. The primary care provider's order is the legal record of medication orders for each facility.
2. Know the actions, special nursing considerations, safe dose ranges, purpose of administration, and adverse effects of the medication to be administered. Consider the appropriateness of the medication for this patient.	This knowledge aids the nurse in evaluating the therapeutic effect of the medication in relation to the patient's disorder and can also be used to educate the patient about the medication.
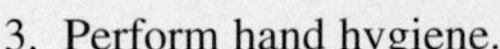 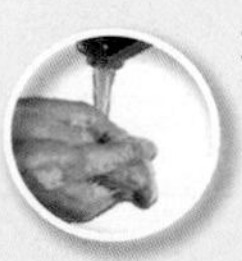 3. Perform hand hygiene.	Hand hygiene prevents the spread of microorganisms.

ACTION	RATIONALE
4. Move the medication cart to the outside of the patient's room or prepare for administration in the medication area.	Organization facilitates error-free administration and saves time.
5. Unlock the medication cart or drawer. Enter pass code and scan employee identification, if required.	Locking of the cart or drawer safeguards each patient's medication supply. Hospital accrediting organizations require medication carts to be locked when not in use. Entering pass code and scanning ID allows only authorized users into the system and identifies the user for documentation by the computer.
6. **Prepare medications for one patient at a time.**	This prevents errors in medication administration.
7. Read the CMAR/MAR and select the proper medication from unit stock or the patient's medication drawer.	This is the *first* check of the label.
8. Compare the label with the CMAR/MAR. Check expiration dates and perform calculations, if necessary. Scan the bar code on the package, if required.	This is the *second* check of the label. Verify calculations with another nurse to ensure safety, if necessary.
9. **Depending on facility policy, the third check of the label may occur at this point. If so, when all medications for one patient have been prepared, recheck the labels with the CMAR/MAR before taking the medications to the patient.**	This *third* check ensures accuracy and helps to prevent errors. *Note:* Many facilities require the *third* check to occur at the bedside, after identifying the patient and before administration.
10. Lock the medication cart before leaving it.	Locking the cart or drawer safeguards the patient's medication supply. Hospital accrediting organizations require medication carts to be locked when not in use.
11. Transport medications to the patient's bedside carefully, and keep the medications in sight at all times.	Careful handling and close observation prevent accidental or deliberate disarrangement of medications.
12. **Ensure that the patient receives the medications at the correct time.**	Check agency policy, which may allow for administration within a period of 30 minutes before or 30 minutes after the designated time.
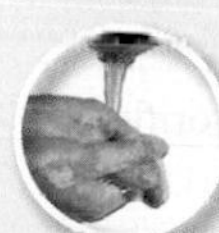 13. Perform hand hygiene and put on PPE, if indicated.	Hand hygiene and PPE prevent the spread of microorganisms. PPE is required based on transmission precautions.
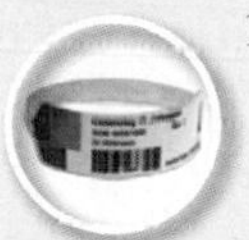 14. **Identify the patient. Compare the information with the CMAR/MAR. The patient should be identified using at least two methods** (The Joint Commission, 2013):	Identifying the patient ensures the right patient receives the medications and helps prevent errors. The patient's room number or physical location is not used as an identifier (The Joint Commission, 2013). Replace the identification band if it is missing or inaccurate in any way.
a. Check the name on the patient's identification band.	
b. Check the identification number on the patient's identification band.	
c. Check the birth date on the patient's identification band.	
d. Ask the patient to state his or her name and birth date, based on facility policy.	This requires a response from the patient, but illness and strange surroundings often cause patients to be confused.
15. **Complete necessary assessments before administering medications. Check the patient's allergy bracelet or ask the patient about allergies. Explain the purpose and action of each medication to the patient.**	Assessment is a prerequisite to administration of medications.

(continued)

SKILL 5-21 ADMINISTERING A VAGINAL CREAM continued

ACTION | **RATIONALE**

16. Scan the patient's bar code on the identification band, if required (Figure 1).

Provides an additional check to ensure that the medication is given to the right patient.

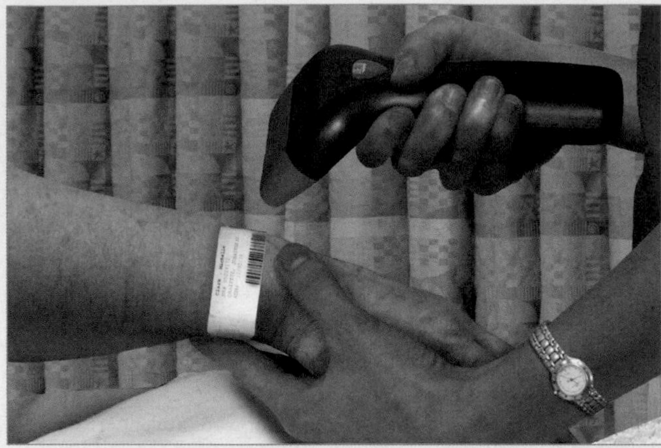

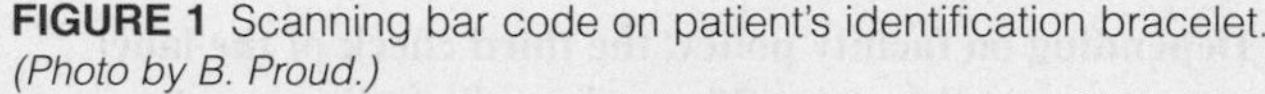

FIGURE 1 Scanning bar code on patient's identification bracelet. *(Photo by B. Proud.)*

17. **Based on facility policy, the third check of the label may occur at this point. If so, recheck the labels with the CMAR/MAR before administering the medications to the patient.**

Many facilities require the *third* check to occur at the bedside, after identifying the patient and before administration. If facility policy directs the *third* check at this time, this *third* check ensures accuracy and helps to prevent errors.

18. Ask the patient to void before inserting the medication.

Empties the bladder and helps to minimize pressure and discomfort during administration.

19. Put on gloves.

Gloves protect the nurse from potential contact with contaminants and body fluids.

20. Position the patient so that she is lying on her back with the knees flexed. Maintain privacy with draping. Provide adequate light to visualize the vaginal opening.

Position provides access to vaginal canal and helps to retain medication in the canal. Draping limits exposure of the patient and promotes warmth and privacy. Adequate light facilitates ease of administration.

21. Spread labia with fingers, and cleanse area at vaginal orifice with washcloth and warm water, using a different corner of the washcloth with each stroke. Wipe from above the vaginal orifice downward toward the sacrum (front to back) (Figure 2).

These techniques prevent contamination of the vaginal orifice with debris surrounding the anus.

22. Remove gloves and put on new gloves.

Prevents spread of microorganisms.

23. Fill vaginal applicator with prescribed amount of cream (Figure 3). (See the accompanying Skill Variation for administering a vaginal suppository.)

This ensures the correct dosage of medication will be administered.

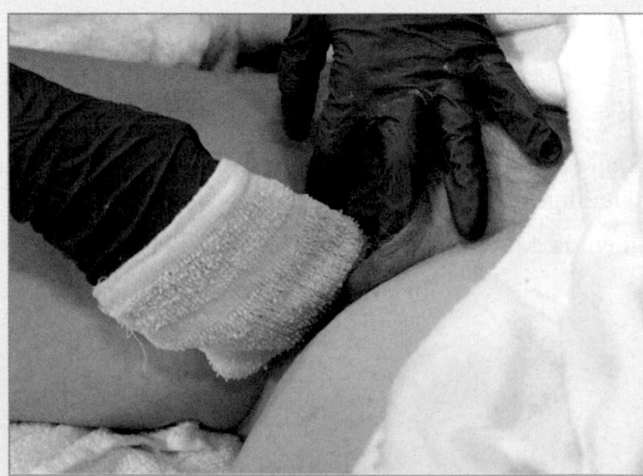

FIGURE 2 Performing perineal care.

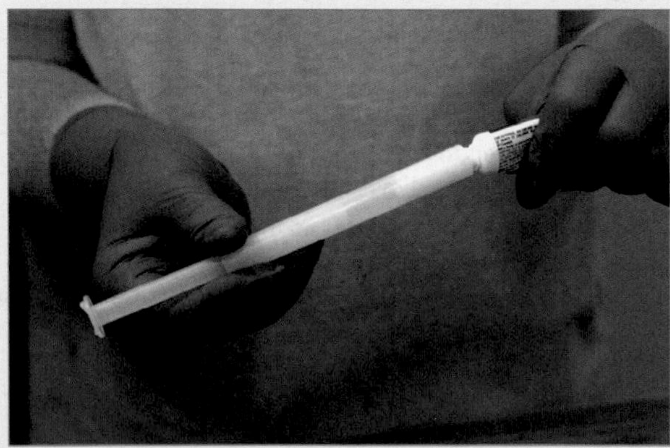

FIGURE 3 Filling vaginal applicator with cream.

ACTION	RATIONALE
24. Lubricate applicator with the lubricant, as necessary.	Ordinarily, lubrication is unnecessary, but it may be used to reduce friction while inserting the applicator.
25. Spread the labia with your nondominant hand and gently introduce the applicator with your dominant hand, in a rolling manner, while directing it downward and backward.	This follows the normal contour of the vagina for its full length.
26. After the applicator is properly positioned (Figure 4), labia may be allowed to fall in place if necessary to free the hand for manipulating the plunger. Push the plunger to its full length and then gently remove applicator with plunger depressed.	Pushing the plunger will gently deploy the cream into the vaginal orifice.

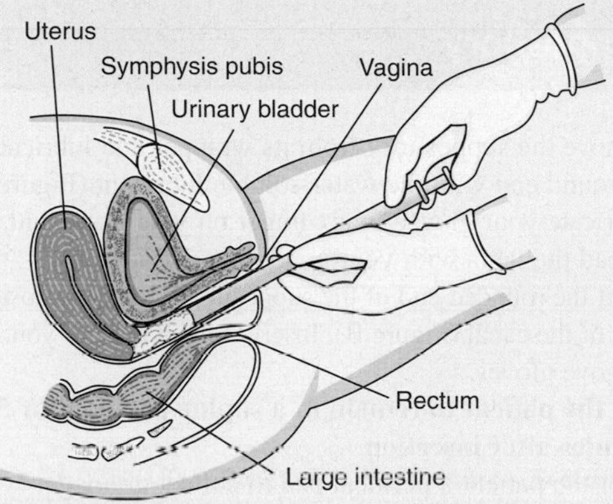

FIGURE 4 Positioning applicator in vagina for administration of medication.

ACTION	RATIONALE
27. **Ask the patient to remain in the supine position for 5 to 10 minutes after insertion.** Offer the patient a perineal pad to collect drainage.	This gives the medication time to be absorbed in the vaginal cavity. As medication heats up, some medication may leak from the vaginal orifice.
28. Dispose of the applicator in an appropriate receptacle or clean the nondisposable applicator according to manufacturer's directions.	Disposal prevents transmission of microorganisms. Cleaning prepares the applicator for future use by same patient for continuing treatment.
29. Remove gloves and additional PPE, if used. Perform hand hygiene.	Removing PPE properly reduces the risk for infection transmission and contamination of other items. Hand hygiene prevents the spread of microorganisms.
30. Document the administration of the medication immediately after administration. See Documentation section below.	Timely documentation helps to ensure patient safety.
31. Evaluate the patient's response to the medication within an appropriate time frame.	The patient needs to be evaluated for therapeutic and adverse effects from the medication.

EVALUATION

The expected outcomes are met when the patient receives the medication via the vagina; the patient understands the rationale for the medication administration; the patient experiences no allergy response; the patient experiences no or minimal discomfort; and the patient experiences no or minimal anxiety.

DOCUMENTATION

Guidelines

Document the administration of the medication immediately after administration, including date, time, dose, and route of administration on the CMAR/MAR or record using the required format. Prompt recording avoids the possibility of accidentally repeating the administration of the drug. If using a bar-code system, medication administration is automatically recorded when the bar code is scanned. PRN medications require documentation of the reason for administration. Document assessment, characteristics of any drainage, and the patient's response to the treatment, if appropriate. If the drug was refused or omitted, record this in the appropriate area on the medication record and notify the primary care provider. This verifies the reason medication was omitted and ensures that the primary care provider is aware of the patient's condition.

(continued)

SKILL 5-21 ADMINISTERING A VAGINAL CREAM continued

Sample Documentation

7/23/15 2300 Monistat vaginal cream administered as ordered. Small amount of curd-like, white discharge noted from vagina. Perineal skin remains erythematous. Patient states, "It doesn't itch as much."

—*K. Sanders, RN*

SPECIAL CONSIDERATIONS

- Ongoing assessment is an important part of nursing care to evaluate patient response to administered medications and early detection of adverse effects. If an adverse effect is suspected, withhold further medication doses and notify the patient's primary care provider. Additional intervention is based on type of reaction and patient assessment.

SKILL VARIATION Administering a Vaginal Suppository

Prepare medication as outlined in steps 1–12 above (Skill 5-21).

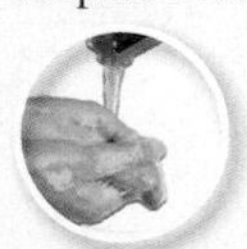

1. Perform hand hygiene and put on PPE, if indicated.

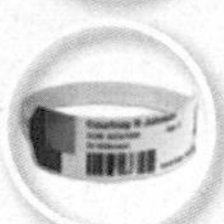

2. Identify the patient. The patient should be identified using two methods.
3. Close the door to the room or pull the bedside curtain.
4. **Complete necessary assessments before administering medications. Check allergy bracelet or ask patient about allergies. Explain the purpose and action of the medication to the patient.**
5. Scan the patient's bar code on the identification band, if required.
6. Ask the patient to void before inserting the medication.
7. **Based on facility policy, the third check of the label may occur at this point. If so, recheck the labels with the CMAR/MAR before administering the medications to the patient.**
8. Put on gloves. Position the patient so that she is lying on her back with the knees flexed. Maintain privacy with draping. Adequate light should be available to visualize the vaginal opening.
9. Spread labia with fingers, and clean area at vaginal orifice with washcloth and warm water, using a different corner of the washcloth with each stroke. Wipe from above orifice downward toward sacrum (front to back).
10. Remove gloves and put on new gloves.
11. Remove the suppository from its wrapper and lubricate the round end with the water-soluble lubricant (Figure A). Lubricate your gloved index finger on your dominant hand.
12. Spread the labia with your nondominant hand.
13. Insert the rounded end of the suppository along the posterior wall of the canal (Figure B). Insert to the length of your finger.
14. Remove gloves.
15. **Ask the patient to remain in a supine position for 5 to 10 minutes after insertion.**
16. Offer the patient a perineal pad to collect drainage.

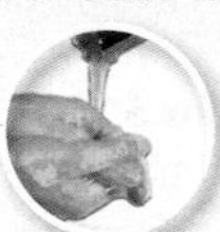

17. Remove additional PPE, if used. Perform hand hygiene.
18. Document administration of the medication on the CMAR/MAR immediately after administering the medication.
19. Evaluate the patient's response to the medication within an appropriate time frame.
20. Assist the patient to a comfortable position after the required 5 to 10 minutes in the supine position.

Unexpected Situations and Associated Interventions

- *Upon assessing the patient after administering a vaginal suppository, you note the suppository is not in the vagina but instead is between the labia:* Put on gloves and reinsert the suppository, ensuring that it is inserted fully.

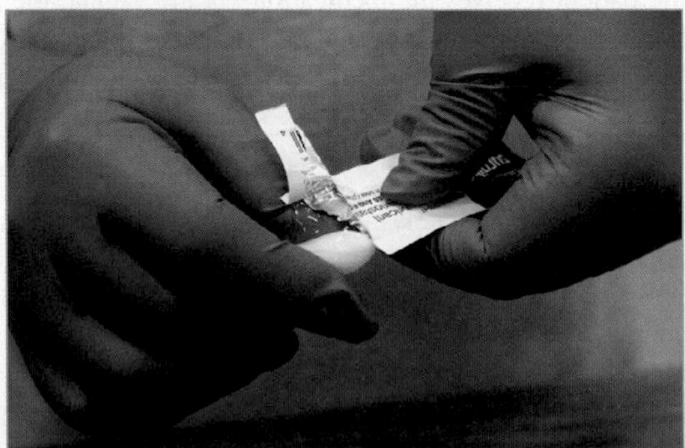

FIGURE A Lubricating suppository.

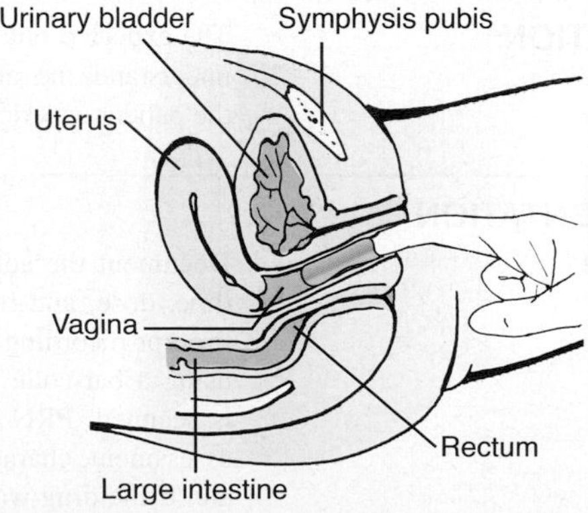

FIGURE B Inserting suppository into vagina.

SKILL 5-22 ADMINISTERING A RECTAL SUPPOSITORY

Rectal suppositories are used primarily for their local action, such as laxatives and fecal softeners. Systemic effects are also achieved with rectal suppositories. It is important to ensure the suppository is placed past the internal anal sphincter and against the rectal mucosa.

DELEGATION CONSIDERATIONS

The administration of medication as a rectal suppository is not delegated to nursing assistive personnel (NAP) or to unlicensed assistive personnel (UAP). Depending on the state's nurse practice act and the organization's policies and procedures, administration of a vaginal cream may be delegated to licensed practical/vocational nurses (LPN/LVNs). The decision to delegate must be based on careful analysis of the patient's needs and circumstances, as well as the qualifications of the person to whom the task is being delegated. Refer to the Delegation Guidelines in Appendix A.

EQUIPMENT

- Suppository (rectal)
- Water-soluble lubricant
- Nonlatex, disposable gloves
- Computer-generated Medication Administration Record (CMAR) or Medication Administration Record (MAR)
- Additional PPE, as indicated

ASSESSMENT

Assess the rectal area for any alterations in integrity. Do not administer suppositories to patients who have had recent rectal or prostate surgery. Assess recent laboratory values, particularly the patient's white blood cell and platelet counts. Patients who are thrombocytopenic or neutropenic should not receive rectal suppositories. Do not administer rectal suppositories to patients at risk for cardiac arrhythmias. Assess relevant body systems for the particular medication being administered. Assess the patient for allergies. Verify patient name, dose, route, and time of administration. Assess the patient's knowledge of the medication and procedure. If the patient has a knowledge deficit about the medication, this may be an appropriate time to begin education about the medication. Assess the patient's ability to cooperate with the procedure.

NURSING DIAGNOSIS

Determine the related factors for the nursing diagnoses based on the patient's current status. Possible nursing diagnoses may include:

- Anxiety
- Risk for Injury
- Constipation

OUTCOME IDENTIFICATION AND PLANNING

The expected outcome is that the medication is administered successfully into the rectum. Other outcomes that may be appropriate include the following: the patient understands the rationale for the rectal instillation; the patient experiences no allergy response; the patient's mucosa and skin remains intact; the patient experiences no, or minimal, pain; and the patient experiences minimal anxiety.

IMPLEMENTATION

ACTION	RATIONALE
1. Gather equipment. Check medication order against the original order in the medical record, according to facility policy. Clarify any inconsistencies. Check the patient's chart for allergies.	This comparison helps to identify errors that may have occurred when orders were transcribed. The primary care provider's order is the legal record of medication orders for each facility.
2. Know the actions, special nursing considerations, safe dose ranges, purpose of administration, and adverse effects of the medication to be administered. Consider the appropriateness of the medication for this patient.	This knowledge aids the nurse in evaluating the therapeutic effect of the medication in relation to the patient's mucosa and disorder and can also be used to educate the patient about the medication.
3. Perform hand hygiene.	Hand hygiene prevents the spread of microorganisms.

(continued)

SKILL 5-22 ADMINISTERING A RECTAL SUPPOSITORY continued

ACTION	RATIONALE
4. Move the medication cart to the outside of the patient's room or prepare for administration in the medication area.	Organization facilitates error-free administration and saves time.
5. Unlock the medication cart or drawer. Enter pass code and scan employee identification, if required.	Locking the cart or drawer safeguards each patient's medication supply. Hospital accrediting organizations require medication carts to be locked when not in use. Entering pass code and scanning ID allows only authorized users into the system and identifies the user for documentation by the computer.
6. **Prepare medications for one patient at a time.**	This prevents errors in medication administration.
7. Read the CMAR/MAR and select the proper medication from unit stock or the patient's medication drawer.	This is the *first* check of the label.
8. Compare the label with the CMAR/MAR. Check expiration dates and perform calculations, if necessary. Scan the bar code on the package, if required.	This is the *second* check of the label. Verify calculations with another nurse to ensure safety, if necessary.
9. **Depending on facility policy, the third check of the label may occur at this point. If so, when all medications for one patient have been prepared, recheck the labels with the CMAR/MAR before taking the medications to the patient.**	This *third* check ensures accuracy and helps to prevent errors. *Note:* Many facilities require the *third* check to occur at the bedside, after identifying the patient and before administration.
10. Lock the medication cart before leaving it.	Locking the cart or drawer safeguards the patient's medication supply. Hospital accrediting organizations require medication carts to be locked when not in use.
11. Transport medications to the patient's bedside carefully, and keep the medications in sight at all times.	Careful handling and close observation prevent accidental or deliberate disarrangement of medications.
12. **Ensure that the patient receives the medications at the correct time.**	Check agency policy, which may allow for administration within a period of 30 minutes before or 30 minutes after the designated time.
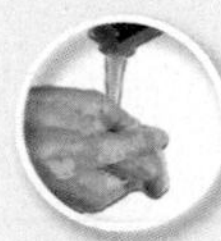 13. Perform hand hygiene and put on PPE, if indicated.	Hand hygiene and PPE prevent the spread of microorganisms. PPE is required based on transmission precautions.
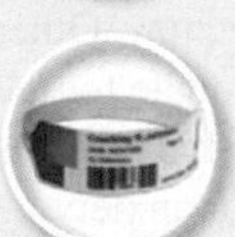 14. **Identify the patient. Compare the information with the CMAR/MAR. The patient should be identified using at least two methods** (The Joint Commission, 2013):	Identifying the patient ensures the right patient receives the medications and helps prevent errors. The patient's room number or physical location is not used as an identifier (The Joint Commission, 2013). Replace the identification band if it is missing or inaccurate in any way.
a. Check the name on the patient's identification band.	
b. Check the identification number on the patient's identification band.	
c. Check the birth date on the patient's identification band.	
d. Ask the patient to state his or her name and birth date, based on facility policy.	This requires a response from the patient, but illness and strange surroundings often cause patients to be confused.
15. **Complete necessary assessments before administering medications. Check the patient's allergy bracelet or ask the patient about allergies. Explain the purpose and action of each medication to the patient.**	Assessment is a prerequisite to administration of medications.

ACTION	RATIONALE
16. Scan the patient's bar code on the identification band, if required (Figure 1).	Provides an additional check to ensure that the medication is given to the right patient.
17. **Based on facility policy, the third check of the label may occur at this point. If so, recheck the labels with the CMAR/MAR before administering the medications to the patient.**	Many facilities require the *third* check to occur at the bedside, after identifying the patient and before administration. If facility policy directs the *third* check at this time, this *third* check ensures accuracy and helps to prevent errors.
18. Put on gloves.	Gloves protect the nurse from potential contact with contaminants and body fluids.
19. Assist the patient to his or her left side in a Sims' position. Drape accordingly to expose only the buttocks.	Sims' positioning allows for easy access to the anal area. Left side decreases chance of expulsion of the suppository. Proper draping maintains privacy.
20. Remove the suppository from its wrapper. Apply lubricant to the rounded end (Figure 2). Lubricate the index finger of your dominant hand.	Lubricant reduces friction on administration and increases patient comfort.

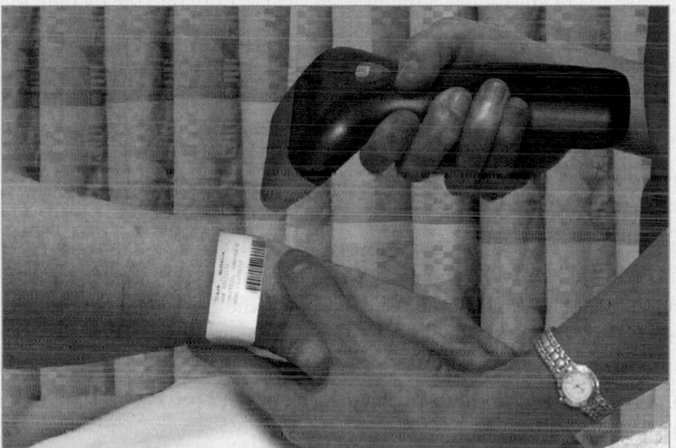

FIGURE 1 Scanning bar code on patient's identification bracelet. *(Photo by B. Proud.)*

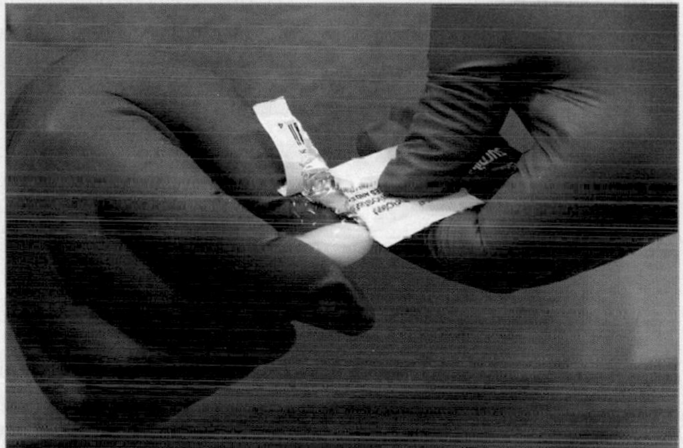

FIGURE 2 Applying lubricant to rounded end of suppository.

ACTION	RATIONALE
21. Separate the buttocks with your nondominant hand and instruct the patient to breathe slowly and deeply through his or her mouth while the suppository is being inserted.	Slow, deep breaths help to relax the anal sphincter and reduce discomfort.
22. Using your index finger, insert the suppository, round end first, along the rectal wall. Insert about 3 to 4 inches (Figure 3).	Suppository must make contact with the rectal mucosa for absorption to occur.

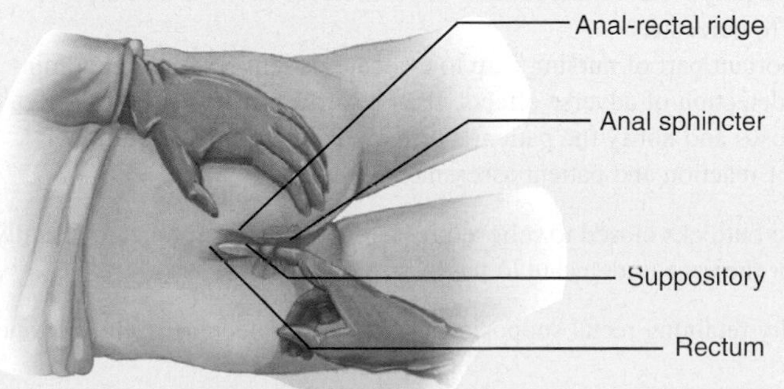

FIGURE 3 Inserting suppository round end first along rectal wall.

(continued)

SKILL 5-22 ADMINISTERING A RECTAL SUPPOSITORY continued

ACTION	RATIONALE
23. Use toilet tissue to clean any stool or lubricant from around the anus. Release the buttocks. Encourage the patient to remain on his or her side for at least 5 minutes and retain the suppository for the appropriate amount of time for the specific medication.	Prevents skin irritation. Prevents accidental expulsion of suppository and ensures absorption of the medication.
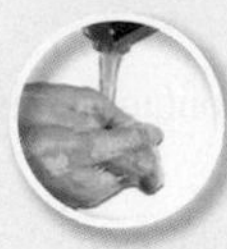 24. Remove additional PPE, if used. Perform hand hygiene.	Removing PPE properly reduces the risk for infection transmission and contamination of other items. Hand hygiene prevents the spread of microorganisms.
25. Document the administration of the medication immediately after administration. See Documentation section below.	Timely documentation helps to ensure patient safety.
26. Evaluate the patient's response to the medication within an appropriate time frame.	The patient needs to be evaluated for therapeutic and adverse effects from the medication.

EVALUATION

The expected outcome is achieved when the medication is administered successfully into the rectum; the patient understood the rationale for the rectal instillation; the patient did not experience adverse effects; the patient's mucosa and skin remains intact; and the patient experiences minimal anxiety.

DOCUMENTATION

Guidelines

Document the administration of the medication immediately after administration, including date, time, dose, and route of administration on the CMAR/MAR or record using the required format. If using a bar-code system, medication administration is automatically recorded when the bar code is scanned. PRN medications require documentation of the reason for administration. Prompt recording avoids the possibility of accidentally repeating the administration of the drug. Document your assessments, and the patient's response to the treatment, if appropriate. If the drug was refused or omitted, record this in the appropriate area on the medication record and notify the primary care provider. This verifies the reason medication was omitted and ensures that the primary care provider is aware of the patient's condition.

UNEXPECTED SITUATIONS AND ASSOCIATED INTERVENTIONS

- *Patient expels the suppository before it is absorbed:* Put on gloves and apply additional lubricant to the suppository. Reinsert past the internal sphincter. If the suppository has warmed and become too soft, discard the suppository and notify the primary care provider. An additional dose may be ordered.

SPECIAL CONSIDERATIONS

General Considerations

- If the suppository is for laxative purposes, it must remain in position for 35 to 45 minutes, or until the patient feels the urge to defecate.
- Ongoing assessment is an important part of nursing care to evaluate patient response to administered medications and early detection of adverse effects. If an adverse effect is suspected, withhold further medication doses and notify the patient's primary care provider. Additional intervention is based on type of reaction and patient assessment.

Infant and Child Considerations

- It may be necessary to hold the buttocks closed to relieve pressure on the anal sphincter. Usually, 5 to 10 minutes is sufficient for the urge to defecate to pass.

Older Adult Considerations

- Older adults may have difficulty retaining rectal suppositories because of decreased muscle tone and loss of sphincter control.

SKILL 5-23 ADMINISTERING MEDICATION VIA A METERED-DOSE INHALER (MDI)

Many medications for respiratory problems are delivered via the respiratory system. A **metered-dose inhaler (MDI)** is a handheld inhaler that uses an aerosol spray or mist to deliver a controlled dose of medication with each compression of the canister. The medication is then absorbed rapidly through the lung tissue, resulting in local and systemic effects.

DELEGATION CONSIDERATIONS

The administration of medication via a metered-dose inhaler is not delegated to nursing assistive personnel (NAP) or to unlicensed assistive personnel (UAP). Depending on the state's nurse practice act and the organization's policies and procedures, administration of a metered-dose inhaler may be delegated to licensed practical/vocational nurses (LPN/LVNs). The decision to delegate must be based on careful analysis of the patient's needs and circumstances, as well as the qualifications of the person to whom the task is being delegated. Refer to the Delegation Guidelines in Appendix A.

EQUIPMENT

- Stethoscope
- Medication in an MDI
- Spacer or holding chamber (optional, but recommended for many medications)
- Computerized-generated Medication Administration Record (CMAR) or Medication Administration Record (MAR)
- PPE, as indicated

ASSESSMENT

Assess respiratory rate, rhythm, and depth to establish a baseline. Assess lung sounds before and after use to establish a baseline and determine the effectiveness of the medication. Frequently, patients will have wheezes or coarse lung sounds before medication administration. If ordered, assess oxygen saturation level before medication administration. The oxygenation level usually increases after the medication is administered. Verify patient name, dose, route, and time of administration. Assess the patient's ability to manage an MDI; young and older patients may have dexterity problems. Assess the patient's knowledge and understanding of the medication's purpose and action.

NURSING DIAGNOSIS

Determine related factors for the nursing diagnoses based on the patient's current status. Appropriate nursing diagnoses may include:

- Ineffective Airway Clearance
- Impaired Gas Exchange
- Deficient Knowledge

OUTCOME IDENTIFICATION AND PLANNING

The expected outcome to achieve when using an MDI is that the patient receives the medication. Other outcomes that may be appropriate include the following: the patient demonstrates improved lung expansion and breath sounds; respiratory status is within acceptable parameters; the patient verbalizes an understanding of medication purpose and action; and the patient demonstrates correct use of an MDI.

IMPLEMENTATION

ACTION	RATIONALE
1. Gather equipment. Check each medication order against the original order in the medical record, according to facility policy. Clarify any inconsistencies. Check the patient's chart for allergies.	This comparison helps to identify errors that may have occurred when orders were transcribed. The primary care provider's order is the legal record of medication orders for each facility.
2. Know the actions, special nursing considerations, safe dose ranges, purpose of administration, and adverse effects of the medications to be administered. Consider the appropriateness of the medication for this patient.	This knowledge aids the nurse in evaluating the therapeutic effect of the medication in relation to the patient's disorder and can also be used to educate the patient about the medication.

(continued)

SKILL 5-23 ADMINISTERING MEDICATION VIA A METERED-DOSE INHALER (MDI) continued

ACTION	RATIONALE
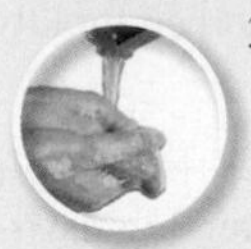 3. Perform hand hygiene.	Hand hygiene prevents the spread of microorganisms.
4. Move the medication cart to the outside of the patient's room or prepare for administration in the medication area.	Organization facilitates error-free administration and saves time.
5. Unlock the medication cart or drawer. Enter pass code and scan employee identification, if required.	Locking the cart or drawer safeguards each patient's medication supply. Hospital accrediting organizations require medication carts to be locked when not in use. Entering pass code and scanning ID allows only authorized users into the computer system and identifies the user for documentation by the computer.
6. **Prepare medications for one patient at a time.**	This prevents errors in medication administration.
7. Read the CMAR/MAR and select the proper medication from the patient's medication drawer or unit stock.	This is the *first* check of the label.
8. Compare the label with the CMAR/MAR. Check expiration dates and perform calculations, if necessary. Scan the bar code on the package, if required.	This is the *second* check of the label. Verify calculations with another nurse to ensure safety, if necessary.
9. **Depending on facility policy, the third check of the label may occur at this point. If so, when all medications for one patient have been prepared, recheck the labels with the CMAR/MAR before taking the medications to the patient.**	This *third* check ensures accuracy and helps to prevent errors. *Note:* Many facilities require the *third* check to occur at the bedside, after identifying the patient and before administration.
10. Lock the medication cart before leaving it.	Locking the cart or drawer safeguards the patient's medication supply. Hospital accrediting organizations require medication carts to be locked when not in use.
11. Transport medications to the patient's bedside carefully, and keep the medications in sight at all times.	Careful handling and close observation prevent accidental or deliberate disarrangement of medications.
12. **Ensure that the patient receives the medications at the correct time.**	Check agency policy, which may allow for administration within a period of 30 minutes before or 30 minutes after the designated time.
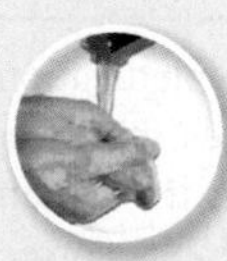 13. Perform hand hygiene and put on PPE, if indicated.	Hand hygiene and PPE prevent the spread of microorganisms. PPE is required based on transmission precautions.
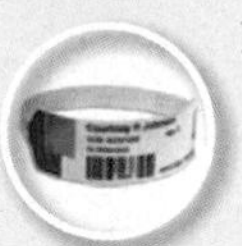 14. **Identify the patient. Compare the information with the CMAR/MAR. The patient should be identified using at least two methods** (The Joint Commission, 2013):	Identifying the patient ensures the right patient receives the medications and helps prevent errors. The patient's room number or physical location is not used as an identifier (The Joint Commission, 2013). Replace the identification band if it is missing or inaccurate in any way.
a. Check the name on the patient's identification band.	
b. Check the identification number on the patient's identification band.	
c. Check the birth date on the patient's identification band.	
d. Ask the patient to state his or her name and birth date, based on facility policy.	This requires a response from the patient, but illness and strange surroundings often cause patients to be confused.
15. **Complete necessary assessments before administering medications. Check the patient's allergy bracelet or ask the patient about allergies. Explain what you are going to do and the reason for doing it to the patient.**	Assessment is a prerequisite to administration of medications. Explanation relieves anxiety and facilitates cooperation.

ACTION	RATIONALE
16. Scan the patient's bar code on the identification band, if required (Figure 1).	Provides an additional check to ensure that the medication is given to the right patient.
17. **Based on facility policy, the third check of the label may occur at this point. If so, recheck the labels with the CMAR/MAR before administering the medications to the patient.**	Many facilities require the *third* check to occur at the bedside, after identifying the patient and before administration. If facility policy directs the *third* check at this time, this *third* check ensures accuracy and helps to prevent errors.
18. Remove the mouthpiece cover from the MDI and the spacer. Attach the MDI to the spacer. (See accompanying Skill Variation for using an MDI without a spacer.)	The use of a spacer is preferred because it traps the medication and aids in delivery of the correct dose.
19. Shake the inhaler and spacer well.	The medication and propellant may separate when the canister is not in use. Shaking well ensures that the patient is receiving the correct dosage of medication.
20. Have patient place the spacer's mouthpiece into mouth, grasping securely with teeth and lips (Figure 2). Have patient breathe normally through the spacer.	Medication should not leak out around the mouthpiece.

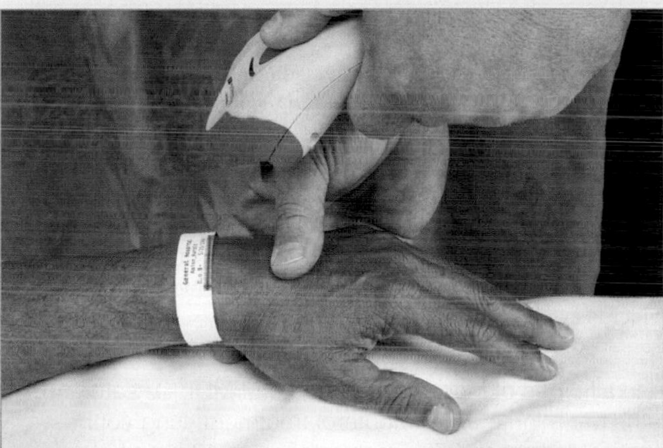
FIGURE 1 Scanning bar code on patient's identification bracelet.

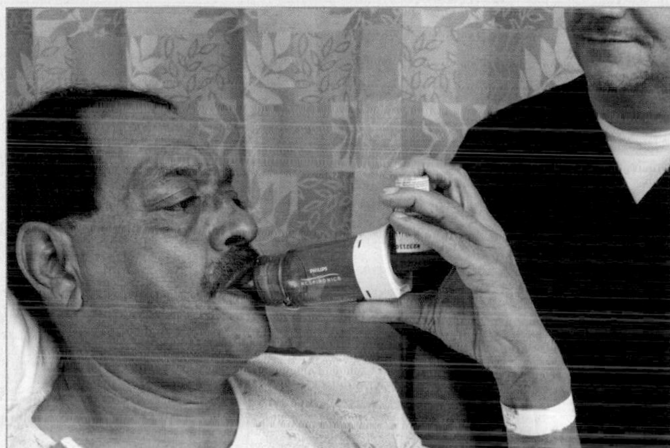
FIGURE 2 Using an MDI with a spacer.

ACTION	RATIONALE
21. Patient should depress the canister, releasing one puff into the spacer, then inhale slowly and deeply through the mouth.	The spacer will hold the medication in suspension for a short period so that the patient can receive more of the prescribed medication than if it had been projected into the air. Breathing slowly and deeply distributes the medication deep into the airways.
22. **Instruct patient to hold his or her breath for 5 to 10 seconds, or as long as possible, and then to exhale slowly through pursed lips.**	This allows better distribution and longer absorption time for the medication.
23. **Wait 1 to 5 minutes, as prescribed, before administering the next puff, as prescribed.**	This ensures that both puffs are absorbed as much as possible. Bronchodilation after the first puff allows for deeper penetration by subsequent puffs.
24. After the prescribed number of puffs has been administered, have the patient remove the MDI from the spacer and replace the caps on both MDI and spacer.	By replacing the caps, the patient is preventing any dust or dirt from entering and being propelled into the bronchioles with later doses.
25. Have the patient gargle and rinse with tap water after using an MDI, as necessary. Clean the MDI according to the manufacturer's directions.	Rinsing removes medication residue from the mouth. Rinsing is necessary when using inhaled steroids because oral fungal infections can occur. The buildup of medication in the device can attract bacteria and affect how the medication is delivered.

(continued)

SKILL 5-23 ADMINISTERING MEDICATION VIA A METERED-DOSE INHALER (MDI) continued

ACTION	RATIONALE
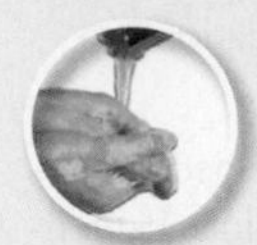 26. Remove gloves and additional PPE, if used. Perform hand hygiene.	Removing PPE properly reduces the risk for infection transmission and contamination of other items. Hand hygiene prevents the spread of microorganisms.
27. Document the administration of the medication immediately after administration. See Documentation section below.	Timely documentation helps to ensure patient safety.
28. Evaluate the patient's response to the medication within an appropriate time frame. **Reassess lung sounds, oxygen saturation level, and respirations.**	The patient needs to be evaluated for therapeutic and adverse effects from the medication. Lung sounds and oxygen saturation level may improve after MDI use. Respiratory rate may decrease after MDI use.

EVALUATION

The expected outcome is met when the medication is administered successfully using the MDI; the patient demonstrates improved lung sounds and ease of breathing; the patient demonstrates correct use of the MDI; and the patient verbalizes correct information about medication therapy associated with MDI use.

DOCUMENTATION

Guidelines

Document the administration of the medication immediately after administration, including date, time, dose, and route of administration on the CMAR/MAR or record using the required format. If using a bar-code system, medication administration is recorded automatically when the bar code is scanned. PRN medications require documentation of the reason for administration. Prompt recording avoids the possibility of accidentally repeating the administration of the drug. Document respiratory rate, oxygen saturation, if applicable, lung assessment, and the patient's response to the treatment, if appropriate. If the drug was refused or omitted, record this in the appropriate area on the medication record and notify the primary care provider. This verifies the reason medication was omitted and ensures that the primary care provider is aware of the patient's condition.

Sample Documentation

9/29/15 0820 Wheezes noted in all lobes of lungs before albuterol MDI, O_2 saturation 92%, respiratory rate 24 breaths per minute. After albuterol treatment, lung sounds are clear and equal in all lobes, O_2 saturation 97%, respiratory rate 18 breaths per minute. Patient able to demonstrate accurately the use of an MDI and spacer and verbalizes understanding of medication purpose and action.

—*C. Bausler, RN*

UNEXPECTED SITUATIONS AND ASSOCIATED INTERVENTIONS

- *Patient uses MDI, but symptoms are not relieved:* Check to make sure that the inhaler still contains medication. The patient may have received only propellant, without medication.
- *Patient is unable to use MDI:* Many companies have adaptive devices that allow patients to use MDIs.
- *Patient reports that relief of symptoms has decreased, even with increased number of puffs:* Have patient demonstrate the technique that he or she is using. Many patients develop poor habits over time. Poor administration technique can lead to a decrease in effectiveness and a need for an increased dosage of medication.

SPECIAL CONSIDERATIONS

General Considerations

- Spacers and inhalers should be cleaned at least weekly with warm water or soaked in a vinegar solution (1 pint of water to 2 oz. white vinegar) for 20 minutes. Rinse with clean water and allow to air dry.
- If the medication being administered is a steroid, the patient should rinse the mouth with water after administration to prevent irritation and secondary infection to the oral mucosa (Kee, et al., 2012).

- Ongoing assessment is an important part of nursing care to evaluate patient response to administered medications and early detection of adverse effects. If an adverse effect is suspected, withhold further medication doses and notify the patient's primary care provider. Additional intervention is based on type of reaction and patient assessment.

Infant and Child Considerations

- Young children usually require a spacer to use an MDI. Spacers with masks are available for young children; consider using these for children under 5 years of age to aid in the delivery of the medication. The mask must fit securely over both the nose and the mouth to ensure a good seal and prevent medication from escaping.
- Children must be able to seal their lips around the mouthpiece in order to use a spacer without a mask.
- Many medications can also be administered as a nebulizer (see Skill 5-25).

Home Care Considerations

- It is important for patients to know how to tell when medication levels are getting low. The most reliable method is to look on the canister and see how many puffs the canister contains. Divide this number by the number of puffs used daily to ascertain how many days the MDI will last. For instance, if the MDI contains 200 puffs and the patient takes 6 puffs per day, the MDI should last for 33 days. Keep a diary or record of inhaler use and discard the inhaler on reaching the labeled number of doses. This method may be cumbersome and impractical for some patients, but it is a reliable way to determine how much medication remains in an MDI. Another accurate way to know when the canister is depleted is to use a dose counter, which counts down each time the canister is activated (Rubin, 2010). **Floating the canister in water is not reliable and is contraindicated. Immersion in water can cause valve obstruction and threatens product integrity (Rubin, 2010).**

SKILL VARIATION Using an MDI Without a Spacer

Prepare medication as outlined in steps 1–12 above (Skill 5-23).

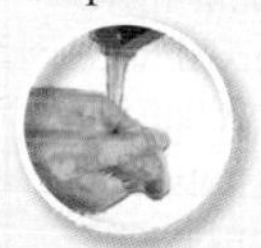

1. Perform hand hygiene and put on PPE, if indicated.

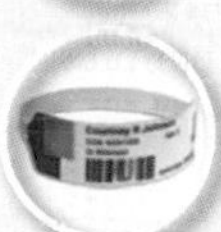

2. Identify the patient. The patient should be identified using two methods.
3. Close the door to the room or pull the bedside curtain.
4. **Complete necessary assessments before administering medications. Check allergy bracelet or ask patient about allergies. Explain the purpose and action of the medication to the patient.**
5. Scan the patient's bar code on the identification band, if required.
6. **Based on facility policy, the third check of the label may occur at this point. If so, recheck the labels with the CMAR/MAR before administering the medications to the patient.**
7. Remove the cap from the MDI. Shake the inhaler well.
8. Have the patient take a deep breath and exhale.
9. Have the patient hold the inhaler 1 to 2 inches away from the mouth (Figure A). Have the patient begin to inhale slowly and deeply, depress the medication canister, and continue to inhale for a full breath.
10. Instruct the patient to hold the breath for 5 to 10 seconds, or as long as possible, and then to exhale slowly through pursed lips.

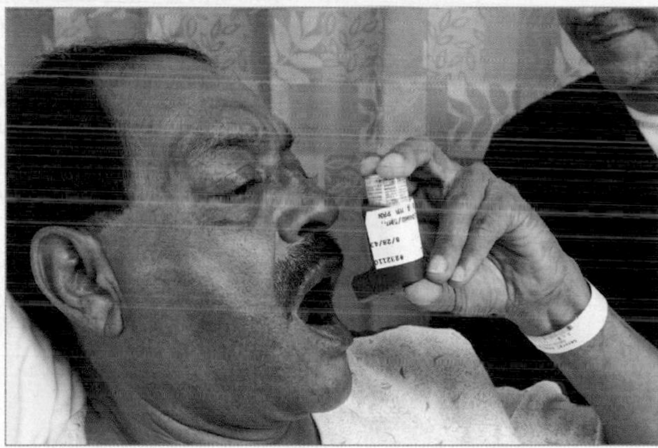

FIGURE A Preparing to use an MDI without spacer.

11. Wait 1 to 5 minutes, as prescribed, before administering the next puff.
12. After the prescribed number of puffs has been administered, have the patient replace the cap on the MDI.
13. Remove additional PPE, if used. Perform hand hygiene.
14. Document administration of the medication on the CMAR/MAR immediately after administering the medication.
15. Evaluate the patient's response to the medication within an appropriate time frame. Reassess lung sounds, oxygen saturation level, if ordered, and respirations.

(continued)

SKILL 5-23 ADMINISTERING MEDICATION VIA A METERED-DOSE INHALER (MDI) continued

EVIDENCE FOR PRACTICE ▶

INHALED MEDICATIONS

Correct use of a metered-dose inhaler is critical to ensure accurate dosing of medication. Patients who are prescribed medications delivered with an MDI must have accurate knowledge and demonstrate appropriate technique regarding use to ensure accurate medication delivery.

Related Research

Batterink, J., Dahri, K., Aulakh, A., & Rempel, C. (2012). Evaluation of the use of inhaled medications by hospital inpatients with chronic obstructive pulmonary disease. *Canadian Journal of Hospital Pharmacy*, *65*(2), 111–118.

The goal of this study was to evaluate the inhaler technique of patients with chronic obstructive pulmonary disease (COPD) and identify baseline patient characteristics and/or inhaler devices associated with poor inhaler technique. After giving informed consent, 37 patients admitted to a tertiary care hospital demonstrated their inhaler technique. The patients' technique was evaluated with standardized checklists. Errors in technique were categorized as noncritical or critical. Critical errors were defined as those resulting in little or no medication reaching the lungs. Of participants, 59% made critical errors while demonstrating their inhaler technique. Patients using metered-dose inhalers (93%) were more likely to make critical errors compared with patients using other inhalers (39%). Of the steps for using an inhaler, 26% were performed incorrectly. Sixty-two percent (62%) of patients reported having received previous counseling on inhaler technique, but only 57% of these patients had received such counseling in the previous 6 months. The authors concluded that more than half of the patients misused their inhaler devices, and many made critical errors that would result in inadequate amounts of drug reaching the lungs. Many of the patients were not receiving regular counseling on appropriate inhaler technique.

Relevance to Nursing Practice

This was a study with a small number of participants. However, over half of the patients in the study did not use their inhalers correctly. Accurate dosing of inhaled medications, and therefore control of symptoms and disease treatment, depends on correct use of the delivery device. Patient education is an important nursing responsibility. Providing patient education related to self-administration of medications, leading to accurate medication dosing, is a very important nursing intervention. Nurses need to be aware that poor inhaler technique is a problem. Nurses should routinely evaluate their patients' inhaler technique and provide counseling and reinforcement as necessary.

Refer to thePoint for additional research on related nursing topics.

SKILL 5-24 ADMINISTERING MEDICATION VIA A DRY POWDER INHALER

Dry powder inhalers (DPIs) are another type of delivery method for inhaled medications. The medication is supplied in a powder form, either in a small capsule or disk inserted into the DPI, or in a compartment inside the DPI. DPIs are breath activated. A quick breath by the patient activates the flow of medication, eliminating the need to coordinate activating the inhaler (spraying the medicine) while inhaling the medicine. However, the drug output and size distribution of the aerosol from a DPI is more or less dependent on the flow rate through the device, so the patient must be able to take a powerful, deep inspiration (Rubin, 2010). Many types of DPIs are available, with distinctive operating instructions. Some have to be loaded with a dose of medication each time they are used and some hold a number of preloaded doses. It is important to understand the particular instructions both for the medication and for the particular delivery device being used.

DELEGATION CONSIDERATIONS

The administration of medication via a dry powder inhaler is not delegated to nursing assistive personnel (NAP) or to unlicensed assistive personnel (UAP). Depending on the state's nurse practice act and the organization's policies and procedures, administration of medication using a dry powder inhaler may be delegated to licensed practical/vocational nurses (LPN/LVNs). The decision to delegate must be based on careful analysis of the patient's needs and circumstances, as well as the qualifications of the person to whom the task is being delegated. Refer to the Delegation Guidelines in Appendix A.

EQUIPMENT

- Stethoscope
- DPI and appropriate medication
- Computer-generated Medication Administration Record (CMAR) or Medication Administration Record (MAR)
- PPE, as indicated

ASSESSMENT

Assess respiratory rate, rhythm, and depth to establish a baseline. Assess lung sounds before and after use to establish a baseline and determine the effectiveness of the medication. If appropriate, assess oxygen saturation level before medication administration. Assess the patient's ability to manage the DPI. Verify patient name, dose, route, and time of administration. Assess the patient's knowledge and understanding of the medication's purpose and action.

NURSING DIAGNOSIS

Determine related factors for the nursing diagnoses based on the patient's current status. Appropriate nursing diagnoses may include:

- Deficient Knowledge
- Risk for Activity Intolerance
- Ineffective Breathing Pattern

OUTCOME IDENTIFICATION AND PLANNING

The expected outcome to achieve is that the patient receives the medication. Other outcomes that may be appropriate include the following: the patient demonstrates improved lung expansion and breath sounds; respiratory status is within acceptable parameters; the patient verbalizes an understanding of medication purpose and action; and the patient demonstrates correct use of the DPI.

IMPLEMENTATION

ACTION	RATIONALE
1. Gather equipment. Check each medication order against the original order in the medical record, according to facility policy. Clarify any inconsistencies. Check the patient's chart for allergies.	This comparison helps to identify errors that may have occurred when orders were transcribed. The primary care provider's order is the legal record of medication orders for each facility.
2. Know the actions, special nursing considerations, safe dose ranges, purpose of administration, and adverse effects of the medications to be administered. Consider the appropriateness of the medication for this patient.	This knowledge aids the nurse in evaluating the therapeutic effect of the medication in relation to the patient's disorder and can also be used to educate the patient about the medication.
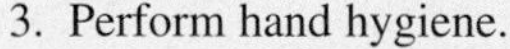 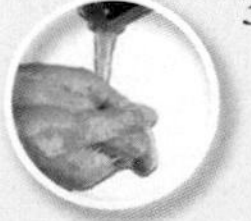 3. Perform hand hygiene.	Hand hygiene prevents the spread of microorganisms.
4. Move the medication cart to the outside of the patient's room or prepare for administration in the medication area.	Organization facilitates error-free administration and saves time.
5. Unlock the medication cart or drawer. Enter pass code and scan employee identification, if required.	Locking the cart or drawer safeguards each patient's medication supply. Hospital accrediting organizations require medication carts to be locked when not in use. Entering pass code and scanning ID allows only authorized users into the system and identifies the user for documentation by the computer.
6. **Prepare medications for one patient at a time.**	This prevents errors in medication administration.

(continued)

SKILL 5-24 ADMINISTERING MEDICATION VIA A DRY POWDER INHALER continued

ACTION	RATIONALE
7. Read the CMAR/MAR and select the proper medication from the patient's medication drawer or unit stock.	This is the *first* check of the label.
8. Compare the label with the CMAR/MAR. Check expiration dates and perform calculations, if necessary. Scan the bar code on the package, if required.	This is the *second* check of the label. Verify calculations with another nurse to ensure safety, if necessary.
9. **Depending on facility policy, the third check of the label may occur at this point. If so, when all medications for one patient have been prepared, recheck the labels with the CMAR/MAR before taking the medications to the patient.**	This *third* check ensures accuracy and helps to prevent errors. *Note:* Many facilities require the *third* check to occur at the bedside, after identifying the patient and before administration.
10. Lock the medication cart before leaving it.	Locking the cart or drawer safeguards the patient's medication supply. Hospital accrediting organizations require medication carts to be locked when not in use.
11. Transport medications to the patient's bedside carefully, and keep the medications in sight at all times.	Careful handling and close observation prevent accidental or deliberate disarrangement of medications.
12. **Ensure that the patient receives the medications at the correct time.**	Check agency policy, which may allow for administration within a period of 30 minutes before or 30 minutes after the designated time.
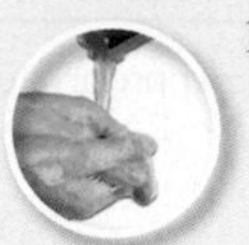 13. Perform hand hygiene and put on PPE, if indicated.	Hand hygiene and PPE prevent the spread of microorganisms. PPE is required based on transmission precautions.
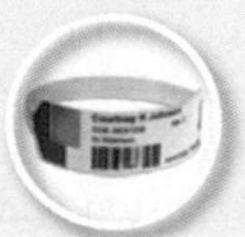 14. **Identify the patient. Compare the information with the CMAR/MAR. The patient should be identified using at least two methods** (The Joint Commission, 2013):	Identifying the patient ensures the right patient receives the medications and helps prevent errors. The patient's room number or physical location is not used as an identifier (The Joint Commission, 2013). Replace the identification band if it is missing or inaccurate in any way.
a. Check the name on the patient's identification band.	
b. Check the identification number on the patient's identification band.	
c. Check the birth date on the patient's identification band.	
d. Ask the patient to state his or her name and birth date, based on facility policy.	This requires a response from the patient, but illness and strange surroundings often cause patients to be confused.
15. **Complete necessary assessments before administering medications. Check the patient's allergy bracelet or ask the patient about allergies. Explain what you are going to do, and the reason for doing it, to the patient.**	Assessment is a prerequisite to administration of medications.
16. Scan the patient's bar code on the identification band, if required (Figure 1).	Provides an additional check to ensure that the medication is given to the right patient.

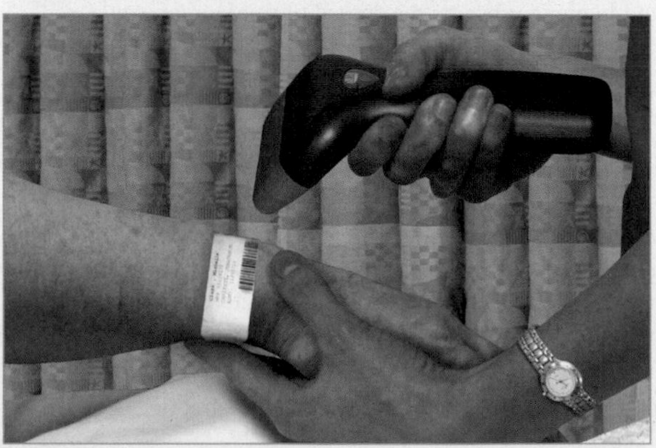

FIGURE 1 Scanning bar code on patient's identification bracelet. *(Photo by B. Proud.)*

ACTION	RATIONALE
17. **Based on facility policy, the third check of the label may occur at this point. If so, recheck the labels with the CMAR/MAR before administering the medications to the patient.**	Many facilities require the *third* check to occur at the bedside, after identifying the patient and before administration. If facility policy directs the *third* check at this time, this *third* check ensures accuracy and helps to prevent errors.
18. Remove the mouthpiece cover or remove the device from storage container. Load a dose into the device as directed by the manufacturer, if necessary. Alternately, activate the inhaler, if necessary, according to manufacturer's directions.	This is necessary to deliver the medication.
19. Have the patient breathe out slowly and completely, without breathing into the DPI.	This allows for deeper inhalation with the medication dose. Moisture from the patient's breath can clog the inhaler.
20. **Instruct the patient to place teeth over, and seal lips around, the mouthpiece. Do not block the opening with the tongue or teeth (Figure 2).**	Prevents medication from escaping and allows for a tight seal, ensuring maximal dosing of medication. Blocking of opening interferes with medication delivery.

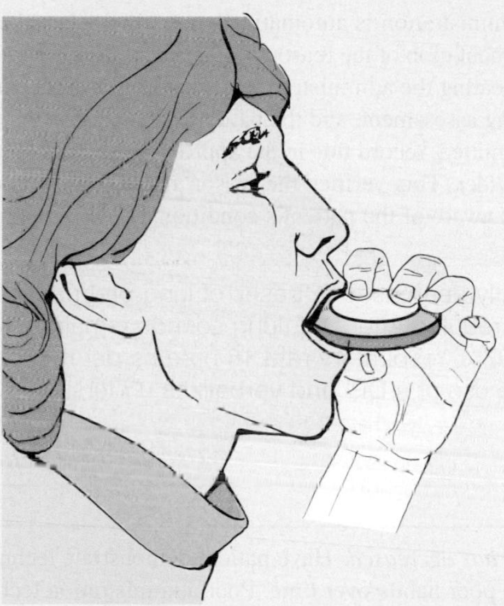

FIGURE 2 Patient with teeth and lips around mouthpiece of a dry powder inhalcr.

ACTION	RATIONALE
21. **Instruct patient to breathe in quickly and deeply through the mouth, for longer than 2 to 3 seconds.**	Activates the flow of medication. Deep inhalation allows for maximal distribution of medication to lung tissue.
22. Remove inhaler from mouth. Instruct patient to hold the breath for 5 to 10 seconds, or as long as possible, and then to exhale slowly through pursed lips.	This allows better distribution and longer absorption time for the medication.
23. Wait 1 to 5 minutes, as prescribed, before administering the next puff.	This ensures that both puffs are absorbed as much as possible. Bronchodilation after the first puff allows for deeper penetration by subsequent puffs.
24. After the prescribed number of puffs has been administered, have the patient replace the cap or storage container.	By replacing the cap, the patient is preventing any dust or dirt from entering the inhaler and being propelled into the bronchioles with later doses or from clogging the inhaler.
25. Have the patient gargle and rinse with tap water after using DPI, as necessary. Clean the DPI according to the manufacturer's directions.	Rinsing is necessary when using inhaled steroids, because oral fungal infections can occur. Rinsing removes medication residue from the mouth. Medication buildup in the device can affect how the medication is delivered, as well as attract bacteria.
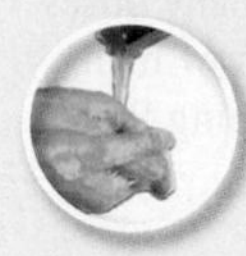 26. Remove gloves and additional PPE, if used. Perform hand hygiene.	Removing PPE properly reduces the risk for infection transmission and contamination of other items. Hand hygiene prevents the spread of microorganisms.

(continued)

SKILL 5-24 ADMINISTERING MEDICATION VIA A DRY POWDER INHALER continued

ACTION	RATIONALE
27. Document the administration of the medication immediately after administration. See Documentation section below.	Timely documentation helps to ensure patient safety.
28. Evaluate patient's response to the medication within an appropriate time frame. **Reassess lung sounds, oxygen saturation level, and respirations.**	The patient needs to be evaluated for therapeutic and adverse effects from the medication. Lung sounds and oxygen saturation level may improve after DPI use. Respirations may decrease after DPI use.

EVALUATION

The expected outcome is met when the patient demonstrates improved lung sounds and ease of breathing. In addition, the patient demonstrates correct use of the DPI and verbalizes correct information about medication therapy associated with DPI use.

DOCUMENTATION

Guidelines

Document the administration of the medication immediately after administration, including date, time, dose, and route of administration on the CMAR/MAR or record using the required format. If using a bar-code system, medication administration is automatically recorded when the bar code is scanned. PRN medications require documentation of the reason for administration. Prompt recording avoids the possibility of accidentally repeating the administration of the drug. Document respiratory rate, oxygen saturation, if applicable, lung assessment, and the patient's response to the treatment, if appropriate. If the drug was refused or omitted, record this in the appropriate area on the medication record and notify the primary care provider. This verifies the reason medication was omitted and ensures that the primary care provider is aware of the patient's condition.

Sample Documentation

12/22/15 1715 Breath sounds slightly decreased in bases of lung pretreatment, respirations 18 breaths per minute and regular. After DPI, lung sounds remain diminished bilaterally in bases, O_2 saturation 97%, respiratory rate 16 breaths per minute. Patient able to demonstrate accurately the use of a DPI and verbalizes understanding of medication purpose and action.

—C. Bausler, RN

UNEXPECTED SITUATIONS AND ASSOCIATED INTERVENTIONS

- *Patient reports that relief of symptoms has decreased:* Have patient demonstrate technique that he or she is using. Many patients develop poor habits over time. Poor administration technique can lead to a decrease in effectiveness.

SPECIAL CONSIDERATIONS

General Considerations

- Instruct the patient never to exhale into the mouthpiece.
- If mist can be seen from the mouth or nose, the DPI is being used incorrectly.
- Follow the manufacturer's directions to clean the DPI.
- Store inhaler, capsules, and disks away from moisture.
- Ongoing assessment is an important part of nursing care to evaluate patient response to administered medications and early detection of adverse effects. If an adverse effect is suspected, withhold further medication doses and notify the patient's primary care provider. Additional intervention is based on type of reaction and patient assessment.

Home Care Considerations

- Many DPIs have dosage counters to keep track of remaining doses.
- If a particular DPI does not have a dose counter, teach patients how to tell when medication levels are getting low. The most reliable method is to look on the package and see how many doses the DPI contains. Divide this number by the number of doses used daily to ascertain how many days the DPI will last. Keep a diary or record of DPI use and discard the DPI on reaching the labeled number of doses.

SKILL 5-25 ADMINISTERING MEDICATION VIA A SMALL-VOLUME NEBULIZER

Many medications prescribed for respiratory problems may be delivered via the respiratory system using a small-volume **nebulizer.** Nebulizers disperse fine particles of liquid medication into the deeper passages of the respiratory tract, where absorption occurs. The treatment continues until all the medication in the nebulizer cup has been inhaled.

DELEGATION CONSIDERATIONS

The administration of medication via a nebulizer is not delegated to nursing assistive personnel (NAP) or to unlicensed assistive personnel (UAP). Depending on the state's nurse practice act and the organization's policies and procedures, administration of medication using a nebulizer may be delegated to licensed practical/vocational nurses (LPN/LVNs). The decision to delegate must be based on careful analysis of the patient's needs and circumstances, as well as the qualifications of the person to whom the task is being delegated. Refer to the Delegation Guidelines in Appendix A.

EQUIPMENT

- Stethoscope
- Medication
- Nebulizer tubing and chamber
- Air compressor or oxygen hookup
- Sterile saline (if not premeasured)
- Computer-generated Medication Administration Record (CMAR) or Medication Administration Record (MAR)
- PPE, as indicated

ASSESSMENT

Assess respiratory rate, rhythm, and depth to establish a baseline. Assess lung sounds before and after use to establish a baseline and determine the effectiveness of the medication. Often, patients have wheezes or coarse lung sounds before medication administration. If ordered, assess patient's oxygen saturation level before medication administration. The oxygen saturation level may increase after the medication has been administered. Verify patient name, dose, route, and time of administration. Assess the patient's knowledge and understanding of the medication's purpose and action.

NURSING DIAGNOSIS

Determine related factors for the nursing diagnoses based on the patient's current status. Appropriate nursing diagnoses may include:

- Ineffective Airway Clearance
- Impaired Gas Exchange
- Ineffective Breathing Pattern

OUTCOME IDENTIFICATION AND PLANNING

The expected outcome to achieve is that the patient receives the medication. Other outcomes that may be appropriate include the following: the patient exhibits improved lung sounds and respiratory effort; and the patient demonstrates the steps for nebulizer use and verbalizes an understanding of the medication's purpose and action.

IMPLEMENTATION

ACTION	RATIONALE
1. Gather equipment. Check each medication order against the original order in the medical record, according to facility policy. Clarify any inconsistencies. Check the patient's chart for allergies.	This comparison helps to identify errors that may have occurred when orders were transcribed. The primary care provider's order is the legal record of medication orders for each facility.
2. Know the actions, special nursing considerations, safe dose ranges, purpose of administration, and adverse effects of the medications to be administered. Consider the appropriateness of the medication for this patient.	This knowledge aids the nurse in evaluating the therapeutic effect of the medication in relation to the patient's disorder and can also be used to educate the patient about the medication.

(continued)

SKILL 5-25 ADMINISTERING MEDICATION VIA A SMALL-VOLUME NEBULIZER continued

ACTION	RATIONALE
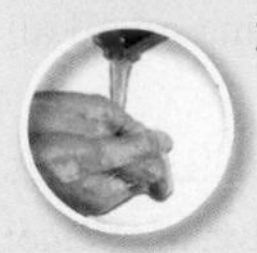 3. Perform hand hygiene.	Hand hygiene prevents the spread of microorganisms.
4. Move the medication cart to the outside of the patient's room or prepare for administration in the medication area.	Organization facilitates error-free administration and saves time.
5. Unlock the medication cart or drawer. Enter pass code and scan employee identification, if required.	Locking the cart or drawer safeguards each patient's medication supply. Hospital accrediting organizations require medication carts to be locked when not in use. Entering pass code and scanning ID allows only authorized users into the system and identifies the user for documentation by the computer.
6. **Prepare medications for one patient at a time.**	This prevents errors in medication administration.
7. Read the CMAR/MAR and select the proper medication from unit stock or the patient's medication drawer.	This is the *first* check of the label.
8. Compare the label with the CMAR/MAR. Check expiration dates and perform calculations, if necessary. Scan the bar code on the package, if required.	This is the *second* check of the label. Verify calculations with another nurse to ensure safety, if necessary.
9. **Depending on facility policy, the third check of the label may occur at this point. If so, when all medications for one patient have been prepared, recheck the labels with the CMAR/MAR before taking the medications to the patient.**	This *third* check ensures accuracy and helps to prevent errors. *Note:* Many facilities require the *third* check to occur at the bedside, after identifying the patient and before administration.
10. Lock the medication cart before leaving it.	Locking the cart or drawer safeguards the patient's medication supply. Hospital accrediting organizations require medication carts to be locked when not in use.
11. Transport medications to the patient's bedside carefully, and keep the medications in sight at all times.	Careful handling and close observation prevent accidental or deliberate disarrangement of medications.
12. **Ensure that the patient receives the medications at the correct time.**	Check agency policy, which may allow for administration within a period of 30 minutes before or 30 minutes after the designated time.
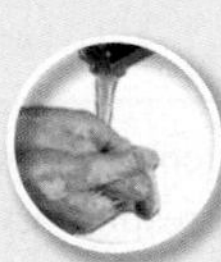 13. Perform hand hygiene and put on PPE, if indicated.	Hand hygiene and PPE prevent the spread of microorganisms. PPE is required based on transmission precautions.
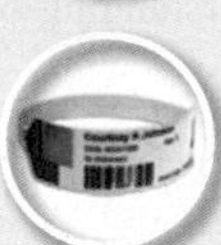 14. **Identify the patient. Compare the information with the CMAR/MAR. The patient should be identified using at least two methods** (The Joint Commission, 2013):	Identifying the patient ensures the right patient receives the medications and helps prevent errors. The patient's room number or physical location is not used as an identifier (The Joint Commission, 2013). Replace the identification band if it is missing or inaccurate in any way.
a. Check the name on the patient's identification band.	
b. Check the identification number on the patient's identification band.	
c. Check the birth date on the patient's identification band.	
d. Ask the patient to state his or her name and birth date, based on facility policy.	This requires a response from the patient, but illness and strange surroundings often cause patients to be confused.
15. **Complete necessary assessments before administering medications. Check the patient's allergy bracelet or ask the patient about allergies. Explain what you are going to do, and the reason for doing it, to the patient.**	Assessment is a prerequisite to administration of medications. Explanation relieves anxiety and facilitates cooperation.

ACTION	RATIONALE
16. Scan the patient's bar code on the identification band, if required.	Scanning provides an additional check to ensure that the medication is given to the right patient.
17. **Based on facility policy, the third check of the label may occur at this point. If so, recheck the labels with the CMAR/MAR before administering the medications to the patient.**	Many facilities require the *third* check to occur at the bedside, after identifying the patient and before administration. If facility policy directs the *third* check at this time, this *third* check ensures accuracy and helps to prevent errors.
18. Remove the nebulizer cup from the device and open it. Place premeasured unit-dose medication in the bottom section of the cup or use a dropper to place a concentrated dose of medication in the cup (Figure 1). Add prescribed diluent, if required.	To get enough volume to make a fine mist, normal saline may need to be added to the concentrated medication.
19. Screw the top portion of the nebulizer cup back in place and attach the cup to the nebulizer. Attach one end of tubing to the stem on the bottom of the nebulizer cuff and the other end to the air compressor or oxygen source.	Air or oxygen must be forced through the nebulizer to form a fine mist.
20. Turn on the air compressor or oxygen. Check that a fine medication mist is produced by opening the valve. Have the patient place the mouthpiece into the mouth and grasp securely with teeth and lips.	If there is no fine mist, make sure that medication has been added to the cup and that the tubing is connected to the air compressor or oxygen outlet. Adjust flow meter if necessary.
21. **Instruct the patient to inhale slowly and deeply through the mouth (Figure 2). A nose clip may be necessary if the patient is also breathing through the nose. Hold each breath for a slight pause, before exhaling.**	While the patient inhales and holds the breath, the medication comes in contact with the respiratory tissue and is absorbed. The longer the breath is held, the more medication can be absorbed.

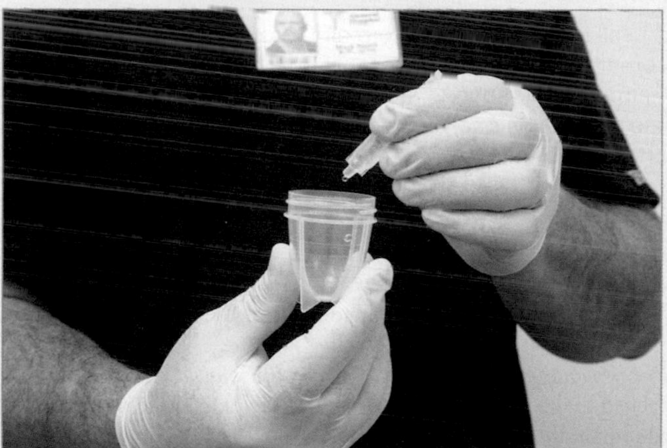

FIGURE 1 Putting medication into nebulizer chamber.

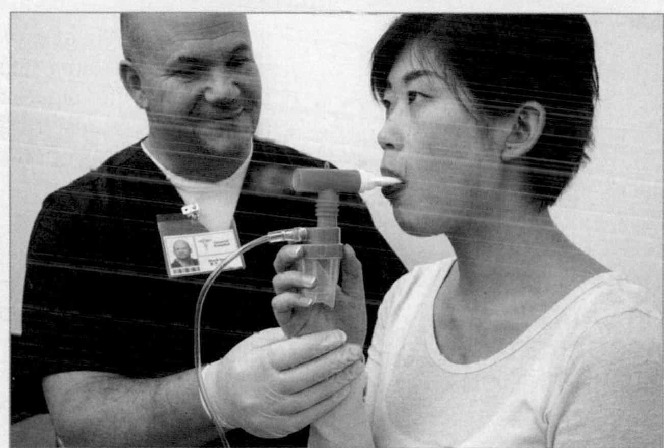

FIGURE 2 Using nebulizer for treatment.

ACTION	RATIONALE
22. Continue this inhalation technique until all medication in the nebulizer cup has been aerosolized (usually about 15 minutes). Once the fine mist decreases in amount, gently flick the sides of the nebulizer cup.	Once the fine mist stops, the medication is no longer being aerosolized. By gently flicking the cup sides, any medication that is stuck to the sides is knocked into the bottom of the cup, where it can become aerosolized.
23. Have the patient gargle and rinse with tap water after using the nebulizer, as necessary. Clean the nebulizer according to the manufacturer's directions.	Rinsing is necessary when using inhaled steroids, because oral fungal infections can occur. Rinsing removes medication residue from the mouth. The buildup of medication in the device can affect how the medication is delivered, as well as attract bacteria.
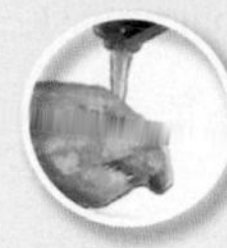 24. Remove gloves and additional PPE, if used. Perform hand hygiene.	Removing PPE properly reduces the risk for infection transmission and contamination of other items. Hand hygiene prevents the spread of microorganisms.

(continued)

SKILL 5-25 ADMINISTERING MEDICATION VIA A SMALL-VOLUME NEBULIZER continued

ACTION	RATIONALE
25. Document the administration of the medication immediately after administration. See Documentation section below.	Timely documentation helps to ensure patient safety.
26. Evaluate patient's response to the medication within an appropriate time frame. **Reassess lung sounds, oxygen saturation level, and respirations.**	The patient needs to be evaluated for therapeutic and adverse effects from the medication. Lung sounds and oxygen saturation level may improve after nebulizer use. Respirations may decrease after nebulizer use.

EVALUATION

The expected outcome is met when the patient receives the medication and exhibits improved lung sounds and respiratory effort. In addition, the patient demonstrates correct steps for use, and verbalizes an understanding, of the need for the medication.

DOCUMENTATION

Guidelines

Document the administration of the medication immediately after administration, including date, time, dose, and route of administration on the CMAR/MAR or record using the required format. If using a bar-code system, medication administration is automatically recorded when the bar code is scanned. PRN medications require documentation of the reason for administration. Prompt recording avoids the possibility of accidentally repeating the administration of the drug. Document respiratory rate, oxygen saturation, if applicable, lung assessment, and the patient's response to the treatment, if appropriate. If the drug was refused or omitted, record this in the appropriate area on the medication record and notify the primary care provider. This verifies the reason medication was omitted and ensures that the primary care provider is aware of the patient's condition.

Sample Documentation

9/29/13 2300 Wheezes noted in all lobes of lungs before albuterol nebulizer, O_2 saturation 92%, respiratory rate 24 breaths per minute, patient reports "feeling like I can't get my breath." After albuterol treatment, lung sounds are clear and equal in all lobes, O_2 saturation 97%, respiratory rate 18 breaths per minute unlabored. Patient verbalizes relief of shortness of breath and an understanding of medication purpose and action.

—C. Bausler, RN

UNEXPECTED SITUATIONS AND ASSOCIATED INTERVENTIONS

- *Patient reports that the nebulizer "doesn't smell or taste the way it usually does":* Double-check to make sure that medication was added to the nebulizer cup and that it is the appropriate medication.
- *Patient is unable to hold nebulizer in mouth and/or is unable to keep lips closed around device:* A plain oxygen mask can be attached to the nebulizer device and used to deliver the nebulized medication, eliminating the need to hold the device in the mouth.

SPECIAL CONSIDERATIONS

General Considerations

- Ongoing assessment is an important part of nursing care to evaluate patient response to administered medications and early detection of adverse effects. If an adverse effect is suspected, withhold further medication doses and notify the patient's primary care provider. Additional intervention is based on type of reaction and patient assessment.

Infant and Child Considerations

- A small child may use a mask instead of a mouthpiece. Mask must fit securely over both the nose and the mouth to ensure a good seal and prevent medication escaping.
- Children must be able to seal their lips around the mouthpiece to use a nebulizer without a mask.

ENHANCE YOUR UNDERSTANDING

FOCUSING ON PATIENT CARE: DEVELOPING CLINICAL REASONING

Consider the case scenarios at the beginning of the chapter as you answer the following questions to enhance your understanding and apply what you have learned.

QUESTIONS

1. When entering Cooper Jackson's room with the antibiotic, Cooper becomes visibly upset and runs to his mother. What is the best technique to administer liquid medication to an uncooperative 2-year-old? Thirty minutes after receiving an oral medication, Cooper vomits. Should the nurse re-administer the medication?
2. What are some ways that the nurse can make Erika Jenkins feel more relaxed about receiving her injection?
3. What are some priority points that the nurse needs to discuss with Jonah Dinerman, the patient with type 1 diabetes, if the education needs to be completed in a short time?

You can find suggested answers after the Bibliography at the end of this chapter.

INTEGRATED CASE STUDY CONNECTION

The case studies in the back of the book are designed to focus on integrating concepts. Refer to the following case studies to enhance your understanding of the concepts related to the skills in this chapter.

- Basic Case Studies: Naomi Bell, page 1067; Claudia Tran, page 1070; Tula Stillwater, page 1075.
- Intermediate Case Studies: Tula Stillwater, page 1081; Jason Brown, page 1083; Kent Clark, page 1085.
- Advanced Case Studies: Dewayne Wallace, page 1095; Robert Espinoza, page 1097.

TAYLOR SUITE RESOURCES

Explore these additional resources to enhance learning for this chapter:

- NCLEX-Style Questions and other resources on thePoint, http://thePoint.lww.com/Lynn4e
- *Skill Checklists for Taylor's Clinical Nursing Skills,* 4e
- *Taylor's Video Guide to Clinical Nursing Skills:* Oral and Topical Medications, Injectable Medications, and Intravenous Medications
- *Fundamentals of Nursing:* Chapter 28, Medications
- *Lippincott DocuCare* Fundamentals cases

Bibliography

Ackley, B.J., & Ladwig, G.B. (2011). *Nursing diagnosis handbook* (9th ed.). St. Louis: Mosby/Elsevier.

Ağaç, E., & Güneş, Ü.Y. (2010). Effect on pain of changing the needle prior to administering medicine intramuscularly: A randomized controlled trial. *Journal of Advanced Nursing, 67*(3), 563–568.

Alsaleh, F.M., Smith, F.J., Keady, S., & Taylor, K.M.G. (2010). Insulin pumps: From inception to the present and toward the future. *Journal of Clinical Pharmacy and Therapeutics, 35*(2), 127–138.

American Association of Diabetes Educators. (2008). *Insulin pump therapy: Guidelines for successful outcomes.* Available at http://www.diabeteseducator.org/export/sites/aade/_resources/pdf/ Insulin_Pump_White_Paper.pdf.

American Diabetes Association. (2004). Insulin administration: Position statement. *Diabetes Care, 27* (Suppl. 1), S106–S109.

American Society of Health-System Pharmacists (ASHP). (2009). ASHP statement on bar-code-enabled medication administration technology. *American Journal of Health-System Pharmacy, 66*(6), 588–590.

Annersten, M., & Willman, A. (2005). Performing subcutaneous injections: A literature review. *Worldviews on Evidence-Based Nursing, 2*(3), 122–130.

Arunthari, V., Bruinsma, R.S., Lee, A.S., Johnson, M.M. (2012). A prospective, comparative trial of standard and breath-actuated nebulizer: Efficacy, safety, and satisfaction. *Respiratory Care, 57*(8), 1242–1247.

Aschenbrenner, D., & Venable, S. (2012). *Drug therapy in nursing* (4th ed.). Philadelphia: Wolters Kluwer Health/Lippincott Williams & Wilkins.

Aziz, A.M. (2012). Subcutaneous injections: Preventing needle stick injuries in the community *British Journal of Community Nursing, 17*(6), 258–264.

Ball, A., & Smith, K. (2008). Optimizing transdermal drug therapy. *American Journal of Health-System Pharmacy, 65*(14), 1337–1346.

Batterink, J., Dahri, K., Aulakh, A., & Rempel, C. (2012). Evaluation of the use of inhaled medications by hospital inpatients with chronic obstructive pulmonary disease. *Canadian Journal of Hospital Pharmacy, 65*(2), 111–118.

Best, C., & Wilson, N. (2011). Advice on safe administration of medications via enteral feeding tubes. *Nutrition,* Supplement, S6–S8.

Boltz, M., Capezuti, E, Fulmer, T., & Zwicker, D. (Eds.). (2012). *Evidence-based geriatric nursing protocols for best practice* (4th ed.). New York. Springer Publishing Company.

Bourgault, A., Ipe, L., Weaver, J., et al. (2007). Development of evidence-based guidelines and critical care nurses' knowledge of enteral feeding. *Critical Care Nurse, 27*(4), 17–29.

Bulechek, G.M., Butcher, H.K., Dochterman, J.M., & Wagner, C.M. (Eds.). *Nursing interventions classification (NIC).* (6th ed.). St. Louis: Mosby Elsevier.

Burke, K. (2005). Executive summary: The state of the science on safe medication administration symposium. *American Journal of Nursing, 105*(3 Suppl.), 4–9.

Carter-Templeton, H., & McCoy, T. (2008). Are we on the same page? A comparison of intramuscular injection explanations in nursing fundamental texts. *MEDSURG Nursing, 17*(4), 237–240.

Centers for Disease Control and Prevention (CDC). (2011). Injection safety. Safe injection practices to prevent transmission of infections to patients. Available at www.cdc.gov/injectionsafety/IP07_standardPrecaution.html.

Centers for Disease Control and Prevention (CDC). (2012). *The pink book: Appendices. Epidemiology and prevention of vaccine preventable diseases* (11th ed.). Appendix D. Vaccine administration. Vaccine administration guidelines. Available at www.cdc.gov/vaccines/pubs/pinkbook/pink-appendx.htm#appd.

Choo, J., Hutchinson, A., & Bucknall, T. (2010). Nurses' role in medication safety. *Journal of Nursing Management, 18*(7), 853–861.

Chung, J.W., Ng, W.M., & Wong, T.K. (2002). An experimental study on the use of manual pressure to reduce pain in intramuscular injections. *Journal of Clinical Nursing, 11*(4), 457–461.

Cocoman, A., & Murray, J. (2010). Recognizing the evidence and changing practice on injection sites. *British Journal of Nursing, 19*(18), 1170–1174.

Cohen, M.R. (2012). Medication errors. *Nursing, 42*(9), 17.

Cranwell-Bruce, L. (2009). Update in diabetes management. *MEDSURG Nursing, 18*(1), 51–54.

Crawford, C.L., & Johnson, J.A. (2012). To aspirate or not: An integrative review of the evidence. *Nursing, 42*(3), 20–25.

Crawford, D. (2012). Maintaining good practice in the administration of medicines to children. *Nursing Children & Young People, 24*(4), 29–35.

Dasqupta, A., Sansgiry, S.S., Jacob, S.M., Frost, C.P., Dwibedi, N., & Tipton, J. (2011). Descriptive analysis of workflow variables associated with barcode-based approach to medication administration. *Journal of Nursing Care Quality, 26*(4), 377–384.

Deithley, J., & Swanson, B. (2004). Enteral nutrition: An update on practice recommendations. *MEDSURG Nursing, 13*(2), 131.

Dougherty, L., Sque, M., & Crouch, R. (2012). Decision-making processes used by nurses during intravenous drug preparation and administration. *Journal of Advanced Nursing, 68*(6), 1302–1311.

Dudek, S. (2014). *Nutrition essentials for nursing practice* (7th ed.). Philadelphia: Wolters Kluwer Health/Lippincott Williams & Wilkins.

Durand, C., Alhammad, A., & Willett, K.C. (2012). Practical considerations for optimal transdermal drug delivery. *American Journal of Health-System Pharmacy, 69*(2), 116–124.

Dychter, S.S., Gold, D.A., & Haller, M.F. (2012). Subcutaneous drug delivery. A route to increased safety, patient satisfaction, and reduced costs. *Journal of Infusion Nursing, 35*(3), 154–160.

Elliott, M., & Liu, Y. (2010). The nine rights of medication administration: An overview. *British Journal of Nursing, 19*(5), 300–305.

Flynn, L., Liang, Y., Dickson, G.L., Xie, M., & Suh, D.C. (2012). Nurses' practice environments, error interception practices, and inpatient medication errors. *Journal of Nursing Scholarship, 44*(2), 2nd Quarter: 180–186.

Gibney, M.A., Arce, C.H., Byron, K.J., & Hirsch, L.J. (2010). Skin and subcutaneous adipose layer thickness in adults with diabetes at sites used for insulin injections: Implications for needle length recommendations. *Current Medical Research & Opinion, 26*(6), 1519–1530.

Greenway, K. (2004). Using the ventrogluteal site for intramuscular injection. *Nursing Standard, 18*(25), 39–42.

Grossman, S., & Porth, C.M. (2014). *Porth's pathophysiology: concepts of altered health states.* (9th ed.). Philadelphia: Wolters Kluwer Health/Lippincott Williams & Wilkins.

Hess, D.R., MacIntyre, N.R., Mishoe, S.C., Galvin, W.F., & Adams, A.B. (2012). *Respiratory care. Principles and practice* (2nd ed.). Sudbury, MA: Jones & Bartlett Learning.

Hinkle, J.L., & Cheever, K.H. (2014). *Brunner & Suddarth's textbook of medical-surgical nursing* (13th ed.). Philadelphia: Wolters Kluwer Health/Lippincott Williams & Wilkins.

Hughes, L. (2012). Assessing a patient with an insulin pump. *Nursing, 42*(9), 62–64.

Hughes, R., & Ortiz, E. (2005). Medication errors. *American Journal of Nursing, 105*(3 Suppl.), 14–24.

Hunter, J. (2008). Subcutaneous injection technique. *Nursing Standard, 22*(21), 41–44.

Hunter, J., & Clark, G. (2008). Intramuscular injection technique. *Nursing Standard, 22*(24), 35–40.

Infusion Nurses Society. (2006). Infusion nursing standards of practice. *Journal of Infusion Nursing, 29*(1–S), S1–S92.

The Institute for Safe Medication Practices (ISMP). (2012a). ISMP and FDA campaign to eliminate use of error-prone abbreviations. Available at www.ismp.org/tools/abbreviations/.

The Institute for Safe Medication Practices (ISMP). (2012b). *ISMP medication safety alert. Preventing tragedies caused by syringe tip caps.* Available at http://www.ismp.org/Newsletters/acutecare/articles/19990310.asp

The Institute for Safe Medication Practices (ISMP). (2007). *The five rights: A destination without a map.* Available at http://www.ismp.org/newsletters/acutecare/articles/20070125.asp.

The Joint Commission (TJC). (2014). *National patient safety goals.* Available at http://www.jointcommission.org/standards_information/npsgs.aspx.

Katsma, D.L., & Katsma, R.P.E. (2000). The myth of the 90°-angle intramuscular injection. *Nurse Educator, 25*(1), 34–37.

Kee, J.L., Hayes, E.R., McCuistion, L.E. (2012). *Pharmacology. A nursing process approach* (7th ed.). St. Louis: Elsevier/Saunders.

Kelly. J. & Wright, D. (2010). Administering medication to adult patients with dysphagia: Part 2. *Nursing Standard, 24*(26), 61–68.

Kenny, D.J., & Goodman, P. (2010). Care of the patient with enteral tube feeding. An evidence-based practice protocol. *Nursing Research, 59*(1S), S22–S31.

Klejka, D.E. (2012). Shhh! Conducting a quiet zone pilot study for medication safety. *Nursing, 42*(9), 18–21.

Kyle, T., & Carman, S. (2013). *Essentials of pediatric nursing* (2nd ed.). Philadelphia: Wolters Kluwer Health/Lippincott Williams & Wilkins.

Lareau, S.C., & Hodder, R. (2012). Teaching inhaler use in chronic obstructive pulmonary disease patients. *Journal of the American Academy of Nurse Practitioners, 24*(2), 113–120.

Lavery, I. (2011). Intravenous therapy: Preparation and administration of IV medicines. *British Journal of Nursing, 20* (Intravenous Supplement), S28–S34.

Lemoine, J.B., & Hurst, H.M. (2012). Using smart pumps to reduce medication errors in the NICU. *Nursing for Women's Health, 16*(2), 151–158.

Leyshon, J. (2011). Improving inhaler technique in patients with asthma. *Nursing Standard, 26*(9), 49–56.

Love, G. (2006). Administering an intradermal injection. *Nursing, 36*(6), 20.

Lorenz, J.M. (2010). Polypharmacy in the elderly: Increased use of medications raises risk of drug interactions, side effects and adverse reactions. *Advance for Nurses, 7*(12), 11–14, 17.

Macdonald, M. (2010). Patient safety. Examining the adequacy of the 5 rights of medication administration. *Clinical Nurse Specialist, 24*(4), 196–201.

Mandrack, M., Cohen, M.R., Featherling, J., Gellner, L., Judd, K., Kienle, P.C., & Vanderveen, T. (2012). Nursing best practices using automated dispensing cabinets: Nurses' key role in improving medication safety. *MEDSURG Nursing, 21*(3), 134–144.

Marik, P.E. & Flemmer, M. (2012). Do dietary supplements have beneficial health effects in industrialized nations: What is the evidence? *Journal of Parenteral & Enteral Nutrition, 36*(2), 159–168.

Martin, D., Kripalani, S., & DuRapau, V.J. (2012). Improving medication management among at-risk older adults. *Journal of Gerontological Nursing, 38*(6), 24–34.

McRoberts, S. (2005). The use of bar code technology in medication administration. *Clinical Nurse Specialist, 19*(2), 55–56.

Meetoo, D., McAllister, G., West, A., & Turnbull, M. (2012). In pursuit of excellence in diabetes care: Trends in insulin delivery. *British Journal of Nursing, 21*(10), 588–595.

Metheny, N. (2008). Residual volume measurement should be retained in enteral feeding protocols. *American Journal of Critical Care, 17*(1), 62–64.

Mishra, P., & Stringer, M.D. (2010). Sciatic nerve injury from intramuscular injection: A persistent and global problem. *International Journal of Clinical Practice, 64*(11), 1573–1579.

Moorhead, S., Johnson, M., Maase, M.L., & Swanson, E. (Eds.). (2008). *Nursing outcomes classification (NOC).* (5th ed.). St. Louis: Mosby Elsevier.

Moshang, J. (2005). Making a point about insulin pens. *Nursing, 35*(2), 46–47.

Muñoz, C., & Hilgenberg, C. (2005). Ethnopharmacology. *American Journal of Nursing, 105*(8), 4047.

Murphy, M., & While, A. (2012). Medication administration practices among children's nurses: A survey. *British Journal of Nursing, 21*(15), 928–933.

NANDA International. (2012). *Nursing diagnoses: Definitions & classification 2012–2014.* West Sussex, UK: Wiley-Blackwell.

Nicoll, L., & Hesby, A. (2002). Intramuscular injection: An integrative research review and guideline for evidence-based practice. *Applied Nursing Research, 16*(2), 149–162.

Perry, S.E., Hockenberry, M.J., Lowdermilk, D.L., & Wilson, D. (2010). *Maternal child nursing care* (4th ed.). Maryland Heights, MO: Mosby/Elsevier.

Pezzotti, W., & Freuler, M. (2012). Using anticoagulants to steer clear of clots. *Nursing, 42*(2), 26–35.

Popescu, A., Currey, J., & Botti, M. (2011). Multifactorial influences on and deviations from medication administration safety and quality in the acute medical/surgical context. *Worldviews on Evidence-Based Nursing, 8*(1), 15–24.

Rack, L., Dudjak, L.A., & Wolf, G.A. (2012). Study of nurse workarounds in a hospital using bar code medication administration system. *Journal of Nursing Care Quality, 27*(3), 232–239.

Ritter, L.A., & Hoffman, N.A. (2010). *Multicultural health.* Boston: Jones and Bartlett.

Rubin, B.K. (2010). Air and soul: The science and application of aerosol therapy. *Respiratory Care, 55*(7), 911–921.

Rubin, B., & Durotoye, L. (2004). How do patients determine that their metered-dose inhaler is empty? *Chest, 126*(4), 1134–1137.

Sander, N., Fusco-Walker, S., Harder, J., et al. (2006). Dose counting and the use of pressurized metered-dose inhalers: Running on empty. *Annals of Allergy, Asthma & Immunology, 97*(1), 34–38.

Sanofi Aventis. (2012). *How to self-inject Lovenox®.* Available at http://www.lovenox.com/consumer/prescribed-lovenox/self-inject/inject-lovenox.aspx.

Shane, R. (2009). Current status of administration of medications. *American Journal of Health-System Pharmacy, 66*(3 Suppl), S42–S47.

Simmons, D., Graves, K., & Flynn, E. (2009). Threading needles in the dark. The effect of the physical work environment on nursing practice. *Critical Care Nursing Quarterly, 32*(2), 70–74.

Small, S. (2004). Preventing sciatic nerve injury from intramuscular injections: Literature review. *Journal of Advanced Nursing, 47*(3), 287–296.

Spector, R.E. (2009). *Cultural diversity in health and illness* (7th ed.). Upper Saddle River, NJ: Pearson/Prentice Hall.

Spollett, G.R. (2012). Improved disposable insulin pen devices provide an alternative to vials and syringes for insulin administration. *Diabetes Spectrum, 25*(2), 117–122.

Swanland, S., Scherck, K., Metcalf, S., & Jesek-Hale, S. (2008). Keys to successful self-management of medications. *Nursing Science Quarterly, 21*(3), 238–246.

Tabloski, P. (2010). *Gerontological nursing* (2nd ed.). Upper Saddle River, NJ: Pearson.

U.S. Food and Drug Administration (FDA). (2012a). *Drugs. Information for consumers.* Available at http://www.fda.gov/Drugs/ResourcesForYou/Consumers/default.htm.

U.S. Food and Drug Administration (FDA). (2012b). *Drugs. Medication errors.* Available at www.fda.gov/Drugs/DrugSafety/MedicationErrors/default.htm#abbreviations.

U.S. Food and Drug Administration (FDA). (2012c). *Safety. MedWatch: The FDA safety information, and adverse event reporting program.* Available at www.fda.gov/Safety/MedWatch/default.htm.

U.S. Food and Drug Administration (FDA). (2012d). *Preventing medical errors. Headline: Article on preventing asphyxiation from aspirated syringe tip caps.* Available at http://www.accessdata.fda.gov/psn/transcript.cfm?show=3.

Walsh, L., & Brophy, K. (2010). Staff nurses' sites of choice for administering intramuscular injections to adult patients in the acute care setting. *Journal of Advanced Nursing, 67*(5), 1034–1040.

Ward, H. (1988). *My friends' beliefs.* New York: Walker and Company.

Williams, N.T. (2008). Medication administration through enteral feeding tubes. *American Journal of Health-System Pharmacy, 65*(24), 2347–2357.

Wright, D., & Kelly, J. (2012). Reducing drug administration errors in patients with dysphagia. *Nurse Prescribing, 10*(7), 357–360.

Zaybak, A., Gunes, U., Tamsel, S., et al. (2007). Does obesity prevent the needle from reaching muscle in intramuscular injections? *Journal of Advanced Nursing, 58*(6), 552–556.

Zimmerman, P.G. (2010). Revisiting IM injections. *American Journal of Nursing, 110*(2), 60–61.

SUGGESTED ANSWERS FOR FOCUSING ON PATIENT CARE: DEVELOPING CLINICAL REASONING

1. Discuss routines and rituals typically used at home with Cooper's mother. Incorporating these routines and rituals if they are safe and positive can provide a positive way to administer medication. Offer simple choices to Cooper, such as allowing him the choice of having the nurse or his mother administer the medication. A toddler may enjoy using an oral syringe to squirt the medicine into his own mouth. The nurse could also allow Cooper to act out medication administration with a favorite toy, pretending to administer liquid medication to the toy.
2. Explore Erika's feelings related to injections and assess her knowledge of the procedure. Allow patients who are fearful of injections to talk about his or her fears. Answer the patient's questions truthfully, and explain the nature and purpose of the injection. Taking the time to offer support often allays fears and decreases discomfort. Explain to Erika how the injection will be given. Discuss possible injection sites and allow Erika to have a say in the location used for the injection, if possible. It is very important that the nurse selects the appropriate needle length and gauge for the medication and patient criteria, including site location, patient's body size, and age. The nurse must use the correct technique to administer the injection and minimize pain. The injection should be administered using the Z-track technique to reduce pain and discomfort.
3. Diabetes is a chronic illness that requires life-long self-management behaviors. However, it is important that, initially, Jonah learns the "survival skills." "Survival skills" are basic information that patients must know to survive. Jonah should have a basic understanding of the definition of diabetes, normal blood glucose ranges and target levels; the effect of insulin and exercise; the effect of food and stress; basic treatment approaches; administration of prescribed medications, including subcutaneous insulin and oral antidiabetes medications; and meal planning. Jonah must also have an understanding of how to recognize, treat, and prevent hypoglycemia and hyperglycemia before discharge. The nurse should include information related to the importance of continued diabetes education, once the basic skills are mastered and information understood. Patient knowledge and compliance with treatment are crucial to preventing complications related to diabetes.

6 Perioperative Nursing

FOCUSING ON PATIENT CARE

This chapter will help you develop the skills related to safe perioperative nursing care for the following patients:

JOSIE MCKEOWN, a 2-day-old girl who needs surgery to correct a heart defect.

TATUM KELLY, a 28-year-old woman having outpatient surgery for breast reduction.

DOROTHY GIBBS, an 81-year-old woman having surgery to remove a bowel obstruction.

Refer to Focusing on Patient Care: Developing Clinical Reasoning at the end of the chapter to apply what you learn.

LEARNING OBJECTIVES

After studying this chapter, you will be able to:

1. Provide patient teaching regarding deep breathing exercises, coughing, and splinting of an incision.
2. Provide patient teaching regarding leg exercises.
3. Provide safe and effective care for the preoperative patient.
4. Provide safe and effective care for the postoperative patient.
5. Apply a forced-warm air device.

KEY TERMS

anesthetic: medication that produces such states as loss of consciousness, analgesia, relaxation, and loss of reflexes

atelectasis: incomplete expansion or collapse of a part of the lungs

conscious sedation/analgesia: type of anesthesia used for short procedures; the intravenous administration of sedatives and analgesics raises the pain threshold and produces an altered mood and some degree of amnesia, but the patient maintains cardiopulmonary function and can respond to verbal commands

deep vein thrombosis: the presence of a blood clot (thrombus) in one or more of the deep veins in the body, most commonly in the lower legs

elective surgery: surgery that is recommended, but can be omitted or delayed without a negative effect

embolus: foreign body or air in the circulatory system

hemorrhage: excessive blood loss due to the escape of blood from blood vessels

hypothermia: core body temperature below 36°C (96°F); can lead to complications of poor wound healing, surgical site infection, hemodynamic stress, cardiac disturbances, coagulopathy, delayed emergence from anesthesia, and shivering and its associated discomfort (AORN, 2011a).

hypovolemic shock: shock due to a decrease in blood volume

perioperative nursing: wide variety of nursing activities carried out before, during, and after surgery

perioperative phase: time frame consisting of the preoperative phase (starts with decision that surgery is necessary and lasting until the patient is transferred to the operating room (OR) or procedural bed); the intraoperative phase (starts from the arrival in the OR until transfer to the postanesthesia care unit [PACU]); and the postoperative phase (begins with admission to the PACU or other recovery area and lasts until complete recovery from surgery and last follow-up physician visit)

postanesthesia care unit (PACU): an area often adjacent to the surgical suite designed to provide care for patients recovering from anesthesia or moderate sedation/analgesia.

thrombophlebitis: inflammation in a vein associated with thrombus formation

A wide range of illnesses and injuries may require treatment that includes some type of surgical intervention. Nursing care provided for the patient before, during, and after surgery is called **perioperative nursing**. Perioperative nursing involves three phases: *preoperative, intraoperative,* and *postoperative.*

Surgical procedures may be inpatient, performed in a hospital; or ambulatory or outpatient, performed in a hospital-based surgical center, a freestanding surgical center, or a physician's office. In an ambulatory or outpatient center, the patient goes to the surgical area the day of surgery and returns home on the same day. Whether the surgery is performed in the inpatient or outpatient setting, consistent written policies and procedures for perioperative care grounded in evidence-based practice and agency policy must be followed to ensure patient safety. The nurse follows specific criteria and guidelines while conducting the preadmission assessment and preparation. This preadmission assessment can be accomplished through a telephone call or a face-to face interview with the patient. A preoperative teaching plan should include preoperative instructions and patient preparation. This teaching should include both the patient and the patient's family members or guardian. For certain types of **elective surgery**, such as joint replacements, patients participate in a group patient teaching session before their admission to the hospital. Refer to Fundamentals Review 6-1, 6-2, and 6-3.

The postoperative care of the patient begins immediately after the surgical procedure is completed. This involves a short stay in the postanesthesia care unit (PACU) for about 1 to 2 hours, depending on the type of surgery and the patient's condition. After this time period and when the patient's condition is stabilized, the patient may be transferred either to the intensive care unit (ICU) if more in-depth monitoring and nursing care is required, or to the surgical floor in the hospital. If the surgery was ambulatory, the patient will be discharged to home. Nursing care throughout the postoperative period includes ongoing assessments, monitoring for complications, implementing specific nursing interventions, and patient and family teaching, as needed. Before discharge from either the hospital or the ambulatory care unit, all patients will receive both oral and written discharge instructions and information regarding a follow-up appointment with the surgeon. In addition, to ensure early identification of complications and address any patient concerns, the patient may receive a follow-up telephone call the next day after discharge.

With an increasing trend toward short-stay or same-day surgical treatment, the nursing interventions in each phase of perioperative nursing care may vary somewhat, but they remain basically the same. While caring for the surgical patient, the nurse should keep in mind that a surgical procedure of any extent is a stressor that requires physical and psychosocial adaptations for both the patient and the family (Fundamentals Review 6-4). This chapter will cover the skills the nurse needs to provide safe perioperative nursing care in the preoperative and postoperative phases.

FUNDAMENTALS REVIEW 6-1

NURSING ASSESSMENT AND INTERVENTION BEFORE SURGERY

The nurse assesses for the following during preadmission or upon admission:

- Baseline physical status
- Baseline mental status
- Allergies and sensitivities
- Signs of abuse or neglect
- Cultural, emotional, and socioeconomic factors
- Pain (comprehensive assessment)
- Medication history, including nonprescription medications and supplements
- Previous surgeries, complications, and implants
- Anesthetic history
- Results of radiologic examinations and other preoperative testing
- Referrals
- Physical alterations that require additional equipment or supplies

The nurse also:

- Provides preoperative patient teaching
- Determines informed consent and/or knowledge of planned procedure
- Asks about advance directive
- Develops a plan of care
- Documents and communicates all information per facility policy

(From Taylor, C.R., Lillis, C., & Lynn, P. [2015]. *Fundamentals of nursing.* [8th ed.]. Philadelphia: Wolters Kluwer Health/Lippincott Williams & Wilkins; and Association of periOperative Registered Nurses [AORN]. [2013]. Recommended practices for perioperative nursing. In: Conner, R., Blanchard, J., Burlingame, B., et al. [Eds.]. *2013 AORN perioperative standards and recommended practices.* Denver, CO: AORN, Inc.)

FUNDAMENTALS REVIEW 6-2

PREOPERATIVE INFORMATION FOR OUTPATIENT/SAME DAY SURGERY

Provide verbal and written instructions, in simple language the patient can understand, for patients having ambulatory surgery.

Ask the patient to:

- List all medications routinely taken, and ask the physician which should be taken or omitted the morning of surgery.
- Notify the surgeon's office if a cold or infection develops before surgery.
- List all allergies, and be sure the operating staff is aware of these.
- Follow all instructions from your surgeon regarding bathing or showering with a special soap solution.
- Remove nail polish and do not wear makeup on the day of the procedure.
- Leave all jewelry and valuables at home.
- Wear clothing that buttons in front; short-sleeved garments are better for surgery on the hands.
- Have someone available for transportation home after recovery from anesthesia.

Inform patient of:

- Limitations on eating or drinking before surgery, with a specific time to begin the limitations.
- When and where to arrive for the procedure, as well as the estimated time when the procedure will be performed.

FUNDAMENTALS REVIEW 6-3

SAMPLE PREOPERATIVE TEACHING: ACTIVITIES AND EVENTS FOR IN-HOSPITAL SURGERY PREOPERATIVE PHASE

- Exercises and physical activities:
  - Deep breathing exercises
  - Coughing
  - Incentive spirometry
  - Turning
  - Leg exercises
  - Pneumatic compression stockings
- Pain management:
  - Meaning of PRN orders for medications
  - Patient-controlled analgesia (PCA), as appropriate
  - Timing for best effect of medications
  - Splinting incision
  - Nonpharmacologic pain management options
- Visit by anesthesiologist
- Physical preparation:
  - NPO
  - Sleeping medication the night before
  - Preoperative checklist (review items)
- Visitors and waiting room
- Transport to operating room by stretcher

INTRAOPERATIVE PHASE

- Holding area:
  - Skin preparation
  - Intravenous lines and fluids
  - Medications
- Operating room:
  - Operating room bed
  - Lights and common equipment (e.g., cardiac monitor, pulse oximeter, warming device)
  - Safety belt
  - Sensations
  - Staff

POSTOPERATIVE PHASE

- Postanesthesia care unit:
  - Frequent vital signs, assessments (e.g., orientation, movement of extremities, strength of grasp)
  - Dressings, drains, tubes, catheters
  - Intravenous lines
  - Pain medications, comfort measures
  - Family notification
  - Sensations
  - Airway, oxygen therapy, pulse oximetry
  - Staff
- Transfer to unit (on stretcher):
  - Frequent vital signs
  - Sensations
  - Pain medications, nonpharmacologic strategies
  - Nothing by mouth (NPO), diet progression
  - Exercises
  - Early ambulation
  - Family visits

FUNDAMENTALS REVIEW 6-4

NURSING INTERVENTIONS TO MEET PSYCHOLOGICAL NEEDS OF PATIENTS HAVING SURGERY

- Establish and maintain a therapeutic relationship, allowing the patient to verbalize fears and concerns.
- Use active listening skills to identify and validate verbal and nonverbal messages revealing anxiety and fear.
- Use touch, as appropriate, to demonstrate genuine empathy and caring.
- Be prepared to respond to common patient questions about surgery:
  - Will I lose control of my body functions while I'm having surgery?
  - How long will I be in the operating room and PACU?
  - Where will my family be?
  - Will I have pain when I wake up?
  - Will the anesthetic make me sick?
  - Will I need a blood transfusion?
  - How long will it be before I can eat?
  - What kind of scar will I have?
  - When will I be able to be sexually active?
  - When can I go back to work?

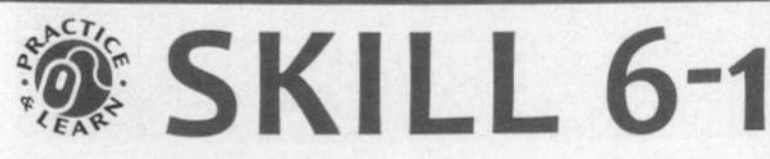

SKILL 6-1 TEACHING DEEP BREATHING EXERCISES, COUGHING, AND SPLINTING

During surgery, the cough reflex is suppressed, mucus accumulates in the tracheobronchial passages, and the lungs do not ventilate fully. After surgery, respirations are often less effective as a result of anesthesia, pain medication, and pain from the incision, particularly thoracic and high abdominal incisions. Alveoli do not inflate and may collapse. Along with retained secretions, this increases the risk for **atelectasis** and respiratory infection.

Deep breathing exercises hyperventilate the alveoli and prevent them from collapsing again, improve lung expansion and volume, help to expel anesthetic gases and mucus, and facilitate tissue oxygenation. Coughing, which helps to remove mucus from the respiratory tract, usually is taught in conjunction with deep breathing. Because coughing is often painful for the patient with a thoracic or abdominal incision, it is important to teach the patient how to splint the incision when coughing. This technique provides support to the incision and helps reduce pain during coughing and movement.

DELEGATION CONSIDERATIONS

Preoperative assessment and teaching is not delegated to nursing assistive personnel (NAP) or to unlicensed assistive personnel (UAP). Depending on the state's nurse practice act and the organization's policies and procedures, preoperative teaching may be delegated to licensed practical/vocational nurses (LPN/LVNs) after an assessment of education needs by the registered nurse. The decision to delegate must be based on careful analysis of the patient's needs and circumstances, as well as the qualifications of the person to whom the task is being delegated. Refer to the Delegation Guidelines in Appendix A.

EQUIPMENT

- Small pillow or folded bath blanket
- PPE, as indicated

ASSESSMENT

It is important for the nurse to identify patients who are considered at greater risk for respiratory complications after surgery, such as the very young and very old; obese or malnourished patients; patients with fluid and electrolyte imbalances; patients with chronic disease; patients who have underlying lung or cardiac disease; patients who have decreased mobility; and patients who are at risk for decreased compliance with postoperative activities, such as those with alterations in cognitive function. Depending on the particular at-risk patient, specific assessments and interventions may be warranted. Assess the patient's current level of knowledge regarding deep breathing, coughing, and splinting.

NURSING DIAGNOSIS

Determine related factors for the nursing diagnoses based on the patient's current status. Appropriate nursing diagnoses may include:

- Deficient Knowledge
- Risk for Infection
- Impaired Physical Mobility

OUTCOME IDENTIFICATION AND PLANNING

The expected outcome to achieve when teaching deep breathing, coughing, and splinting of an incision is that the patient and/or significant other verbalizes an understanding of the instructions and is able to demonstrate the activities.

IMPLEMENTATION

ACTION	RATIONALE
1. Check the patient's medical record for the type of surgery and review the medical orders. Gather the necessary supplies.	This check ensures that the care will be provided for the right patient and any specific teaching based on the type of surgery will be addressed. Preparation promotes efficient time management and an organized approach to the task.
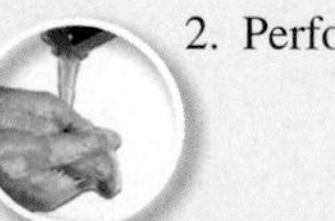 2. Perform hand hygiene and put on PPE, if indicated.	Hand hygiene and PPE prevent the spread of microorganisms. PPE is required based on transmission precautions.
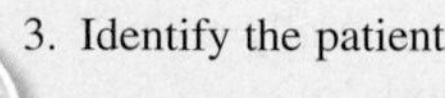 3. Identify the patient.	Identifying the patient ensures the right patient receives the intervention and helps prevent errors.

ACTION	RATIONALE
4. Close curtains around the bed and close the door to the room, if possible. Explain what you are going to do and why you are going to do it to the patient. Place necessary supplies on the bedside stand or overbed table, within easy reach.	This ensures the patient's privacy. Explanation relieves anxiety and facilitates cooperation. Bringing everything to the bedside conserves time and energy. Arranging items nearby is convenient, saves time, and avoids unnecessary stretching and twisting of muscles on the part of the nurse.
5. Identify the patient's learning needs and the patient's level of knowledge regarding deep breathing exercises, coughing, and splinting of the incision. If the patient has had surgery before, ask about this experience.	Identification of baseline knowledge contributes to individualized teaching. Previous surgical experience may impact preoperative/postoperative care positively or negatively, depending on this experience.
6. Explain the rationale for performing deep breathing exercises, coughing, and splinting of the incision.	Explanation facilitates patient cooperation. An understanding of the rationale may contribute to increased compliance.
7. Teach the patient how to perform deep breathing exercises and explain their importance.	Deep breathing exercises improve lung expansion and volume, help expel anesthetic gases and mucus from the airway, and facilitate the oxygenation of body tissues.
a. Assist or ask the patient to sit up (semi- or high-Fowler's position) (Figure 1), with the neck and shoulders supported. Ask the patient to place the palms of both hands along the lower anterior rib cage.	The upright position promotes chest expansion and lessens exertion of the abdominal muscles. Positioning the hands on the rib cage allows the patient to feel the chest rise and the lungs expand as the diaphragm descends.
b. Ask the patient to exhale gently and completely.	
c. Instruct the patient to breathe in through the nose as deeply as possible and hold breath for 3 to 5 seconds.	Deep inhalation promotes lung expansion.
d. Instruct the patient to exhale through the mouth, pursing the lips like when whistling.	
e. Have the patient practice the breathing exercise three times. Instruct the patient that this exercise should be performed every 1 to 2 hours for the first 24 hours after surgery, and as necessary thereafter, depending on risk factors and pulmonary status.	Return demonstration ensures that the patient is able to perform the exercises properly. Practice promotes effectiveness and compliance.
8. Provide teaching regarding coughing and splinting.	Coughing helps remove retained mucus from the respiratory tract. Splinting minimizes pain while coughing or moving.
a. Ask the patient to sit up (semi-Fowler's position), leaning forward. Apply a folded bath blanket or pillow against the part of the body where the incision will be (e.g., abdomen or chest) (Figure 2).	These interventions aim to decrease discomfort while coughing.

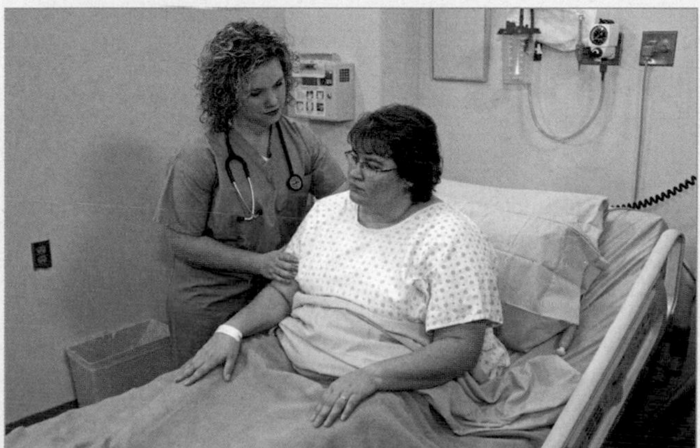

FIGURE 1 Assisting patient to semi- or high-Fowler's position.

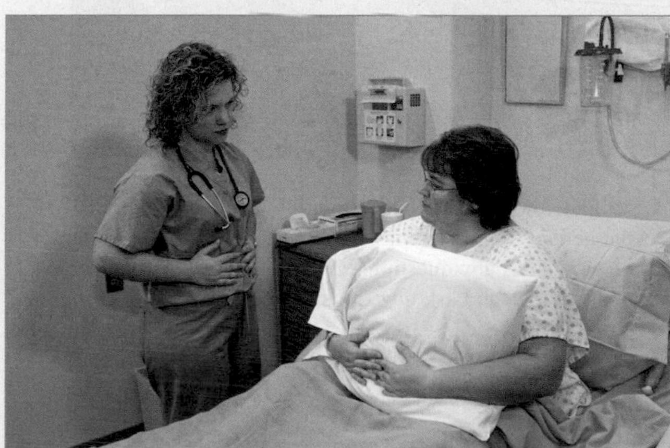

FIGURE 2 Having patient splint chest or abdominal incision by holding a folded bath blanket or pillow against the incision.

(continued)

SKILL 6-1 TEACHING DEEP BREATHING EXERCISES, COUGHING, AND SPLINTING continued

ACTION	RATIONALE
b. Ask the patient to inhale and exhale deeply and slowly through the nose three times.	
c. Ask the patient to take a deep breath and hold it for 3 seconds (Figure 3) and then cough out three short times (Figure 4).	
d. Ask the patient to take a quick breath through the mouth and strongly and deeply cough again one or two times (Figure 5).	
e. Ask the patient to take another deep breath.	
f. Instruct the patient that he or she should perform these actions every 2 hours when awake after surgery.	

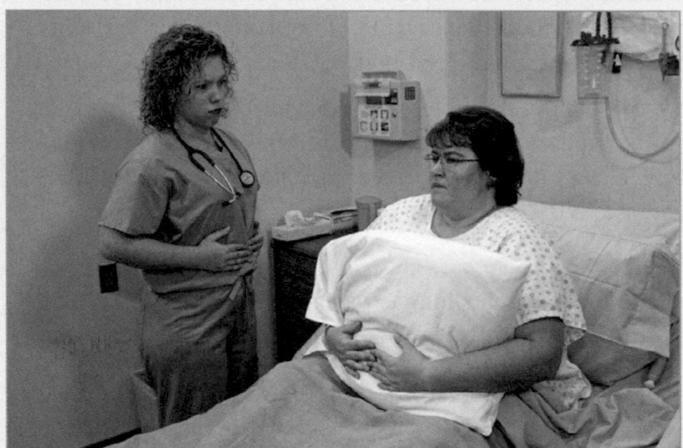

FIGURE 3 Telling patient to take a deep breath and hold for 3 seconds.

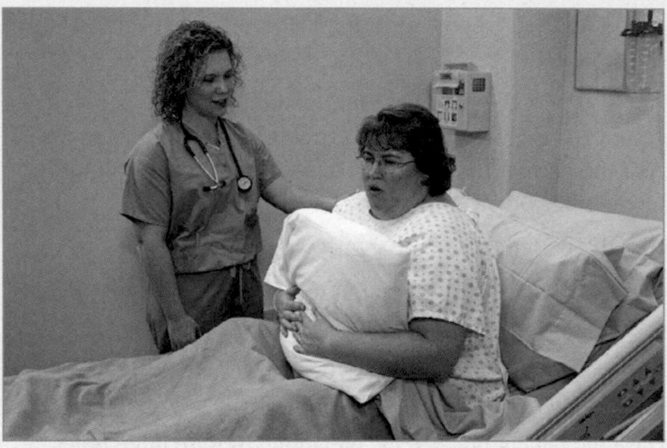

FIGURE 4 Encouraging patient to cough out three short times after holding breath.

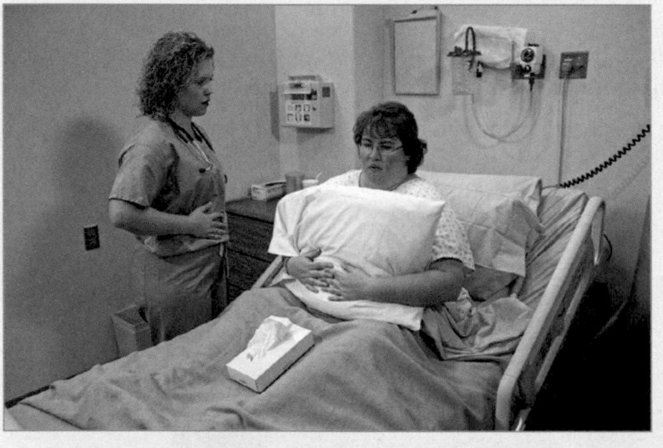

FIGURE 5 Encouraging patient to take another deep breath and cough strongly two times.

ACTION	RATIONALE
9. Validate the patient's understanding of the information. Ask the patient to give a return demonstration. Ask the patient if he or she has any questions. Encourage the patient to practice the activities and ask questions, if necessary.	Validation facilitates patient's understanding of information and performance of activities.
10. Remove PPE, if used. Perform hand hygiene.	Removing PPE properly reduces the risk for infection transmission and contamination of other items. Hand hygiene prevents the spread of microorganisms.

EVALUATION The expected outcome is met when the patient and/or significant other verbalizes an understanding of the instructions related to deep breathing, coughing, and splinting, and is able to demonstrate the activities.

DOCUMENTATION

Guidelines

Document the components of teaching related to deep breathing exercises, coughing, and splinting that were reviewed with the patient and family, if present. Record the patient's ability to demonstrate deep breathing exercises, coughing, and splinting and his or her response to the teaching; note if any follow-up instruction needs to be performed.

Sample Documentation

4/2/15 1030 Perioperative teaching points related to deep breathing, coughing, and splinting reviewed with patient and his wife, including the rationale for each of these points. Patient verbalized an understanding of the rationale for the activities. Patient demonstrated proper technique for deep breathing, coughing, and splinting. Patient stated that he was anxious about the surgery because this will be his first time to the OR. Emotional support and reassurance was provided.

—J. Lance, RN

UNEXPECTED SITUATIONS AND ASSOCIATED INTERVENTIONS

- *The patient verbalizes concern about being able to remember steps for deep breathing and coughing:* Discuss with the patient why he or she feels this way. Offer encouragement and support. Reinforce that nurses will assist the patient with postoperative activities and reinforce the required actions. Provide written instructions as necessary to reinforce material.

SPECIAL CONSIDERATIONS

General Considerations

- Respiratory disorders, such as pneumonia, and chronic obstructive pulmonary diseases increase the risk for respiratory depression from anesthesia as well as postoperative pneumonia and atelectasis.

Infant and Child Considerations

- Deep breathing and coughing can be accomplished through play to enhance a child's participation (Kyle & Carman, 2013).

EVIDENCE FOR PRACTICE ▶

POSTOPERATIVE INTERVENTIONS TO PREVENT PULMONARY COMPLICATIONS

The most important and serious postoperative pulmonary complications include atelectasis, pneumonia, respiratory failure, and the exacerbation of underlying lung disease. Pulmonary complications can be reduced by optimizing pulmonary function, intensive pulmonary hygiene, and early ambulation.

Related Research

Restrepo, R.D., Wettstein, R., Wittnebel, L., et al. (2011). AARC clinical practice guideline. Incentive spirometry: 2011. *Respiratory Care, 56*(10), 1600–1604.

This updated clinical practice guideline is the result of a review of 54 clinical trials and systematic reviews related to incentive spirometry and other postoperative interventions to prevent postoperative pulmonary complications. Based on this review, it is recommended that incentive spirometry, deep breathing techniques, directed coughing, early mobilization, and optimal analgesia be implemented to prevent postoperative pulmonary complications. In addition, the guideline suggests deep breathing exercises provide the same benefit as incentive spirometry in the preoperative and postoperative setting to prevent postoperative pulmonary complications.

Relevance for Nursing Practice

Patient teaching is an important part of nursing care. Nurses need to ensure that patients undergoing surgery, particularly those at increased risk of complications, understand and implement appropriate postoperative activities to help decrease these risks. Both preoperative and postoperative nursing care should include appropriate teaching related to appropriate patient activities, including the use of deep breathing exercises.

Refer to thePoint for additional research on related nursing topics.

SKILL 6-2 TEACHING LEG EXERCISES

During surgery, venous blood return from the legs slows. In addition, some patient positions used during surgery decrease venous return. **Thrombophlebitis**, **deep vein thrombosis (DVT)**, and the risk for emboli are potential complications from circulatory stasis in the legs. Leg exercises increase venous return through flexion and contraction of the quadriceps and gastrocnemius muscles. It is important to individualize leg exercises to patient needs, physical condition, primary care provider preference, and facility protocol.

DELEGATION CONSIDERATIONS

Preoperative assessment and teaching is not delegated to nursing assistive personnel (NAP) or to unlicensed assistive personnel (UAP). Depending on the state's nurse practice act and the organization's policies and procedures, preoperative teaching may be delegated to licensed practical/vocational nurses (LPN/LVNs) after an assessment of education needs by the registered nurse. The decision to delegate must be based on careful analysis of the patient's needs and circumstances, as well as the qualifications of the person to whom the task is being delegated. Refer to the Delegation Guidelines in Appendix A.

EQUIPMENT

• PPE, as indicated

ASSESSMENT

It is important to identify patients who are considered at greater risk, such as those with chronic disease; patients who are obese or have underlying cardiovascular disease; patients who have decreased mobility; and patients who are at risk for decreased compliance with postoperative activities, such as those with alterations in cognitive function.

Depending on the particular at-risk patient, specific assessments and interventions may be warranted. Assess the patient's current level of knowledge regarding leg exercises.

NURSING DIAGNOSIS

Determine related factors for the nursing diagnoses based on the patient's current status. Appropriate nursing diagnoses may include:

- Deficient Knowledge
- Impaired Physical Mobility
- Risk for Ineffective Cerebral Tissue Perfusion

OUTCOME IDENTIFICATION AND PLANNING

The expected outcome to achieve when teaching leg exercises is that the patient and/or significant other verbalizes an understanding of the instructions and is able to demonstrate the activity.

IMPLEMENTATION

ACTION	RATIONALE
1. Check the patient's medical record for the type of surgery and review the medical orders. Gather the necessary supplies.	This check ensures that the care will be provided for the right patient and any specific teaching based on the type of surgery will be addressed. Preparation promotes efficient time management and an organized approach to the task.
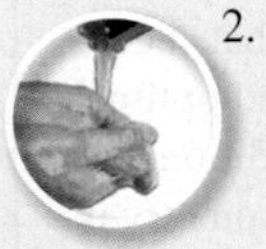 2. Perform hand hygiene and put on PPE, if indicated.	Hand hygiene and PPE prevent the spread of microorganisms. PPE is required based on transmission precautions.
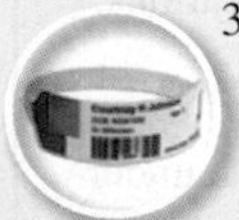 3. Identify the patient.	Identifying the patient ensures the right patient receives the intervention and helps prevent errors.

ACTION	RATIONALE
4. Close the curtains around the bed and close the door to the room, if possible. Explain what you are going to do and why you are going to do it to the patient. Place necessary supplies on the bedside stand or overbed table, within easy reach.	This ensures the patient's privacy. Explanation relieves anxiety and facilitates cooperation. Bringing everything to the bedside conserves time and energy. Arranging items nearby is convenient, saves time, and avoids unnecessary stretching and twisting of muscles on the part of the nurse.
5. Identify the patient's learning needs. Identify the patient's level of knowledge regarding leg exercises. If the patient has had surgery before, ask about this experience.	Identification of baseline knowledge contributes to individualized teaching. Previous surgical experience may impact preoperative/postoperative care positively or negatively, depending on this experience.
6. Explain the rationale for performing leg exercises.	Explanation facilitates patient cooperation. An understanding of rationale may contribute to increased compliance.
7. Teach leg exercises and explain their purpose.	Leg exercises assist in preventing muscle weakness, promote venous return, and decrease complications related to venous stasis.
a. Assist or ask the patient to sit up (semi-Fowler's position) (Figure 1) and explain to the patient that you will first demonstrate, and then coach him/her to exercise one leg at a time.	
b. Straighten the patient's knee, raise the foot (Figure 2), extend the lower leg, and hold this position for a few seconds (Figure 3). Lower the entire leg (Figure 4). Practice this exercise with the other leg.	

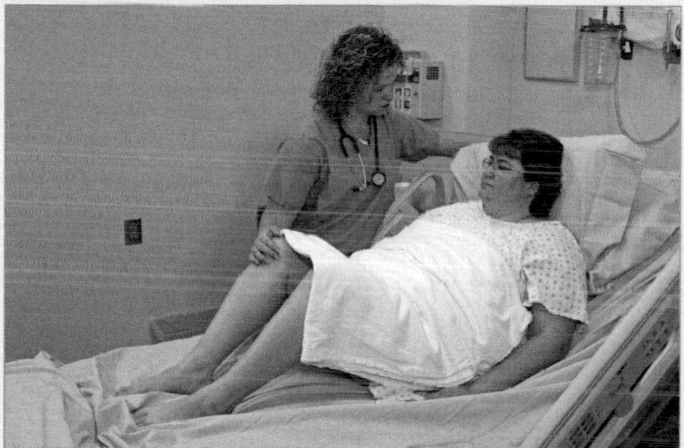

FIGURE 1 Assisting patient to semi-Fowler's position.

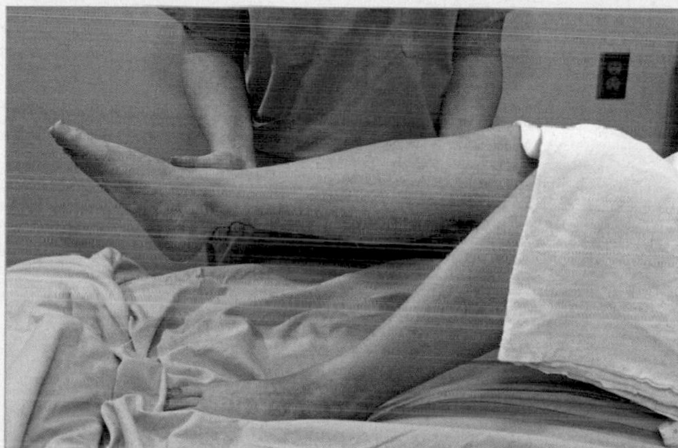

FIGURE 2 Raising patient's foot with knee straight.

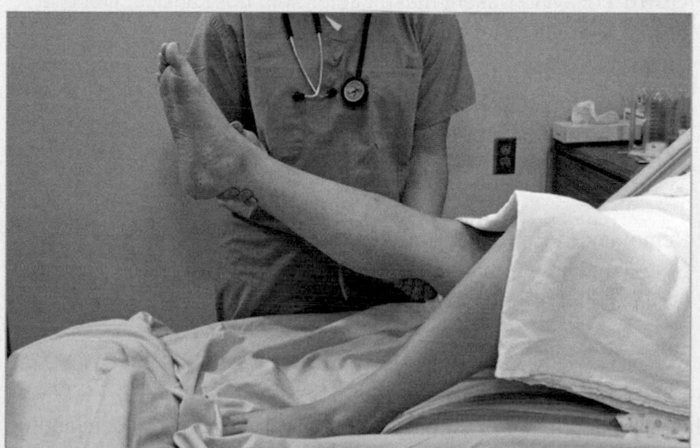

FIGURE 3 Extending lower portion of the leg and holding for a few seconds.

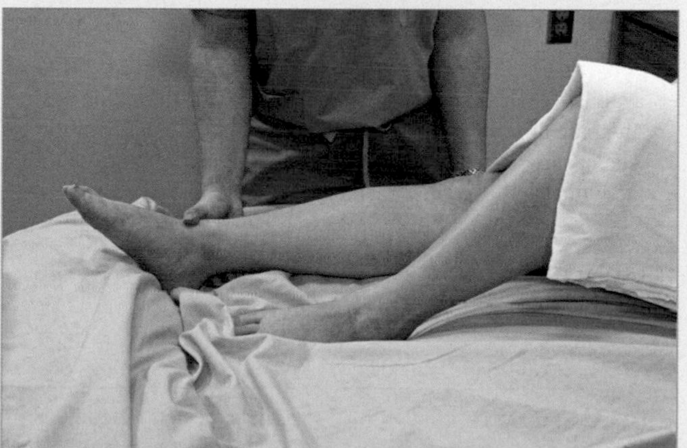

FIGURE 4 Lowering entire leg to bed.

(continued)

SKILL 6-2 TEACHING LEG EXERCISES continued

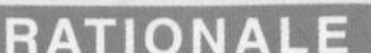

ACTION	RATIONALE
c. Assist or ask the patient to point the toes of both legs toward the foot of the bed, then relax them (Figure 5). Next, flex or pull the toes toward the chin (Figure 6).	
d. Assist or ask the patient to keep legs extended and to make circles with both ankles, first circling to the left and then to the right (Figure 7). Instruct the patient to repeat these exercises three times. Instruct the patient to perform leg exercises every 2 to 4 hours when awake after surgery.	

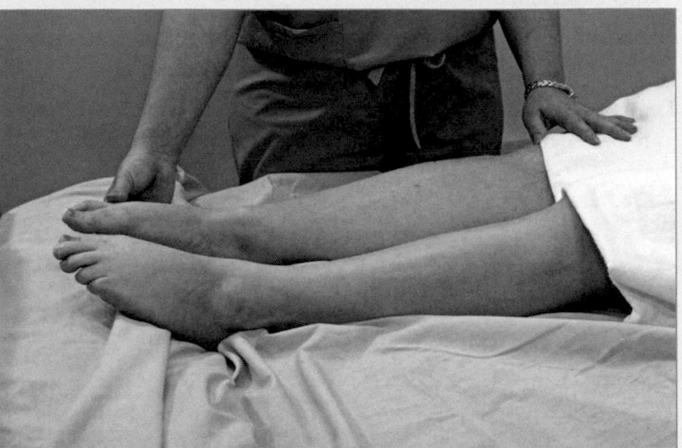

FIGURE 5 Pointing toes of both feet toward foot of bed.

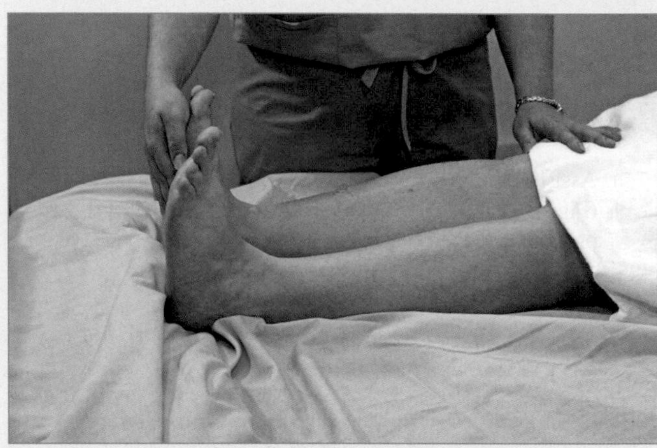

FIGURE 6 Pulling toes toward chin.

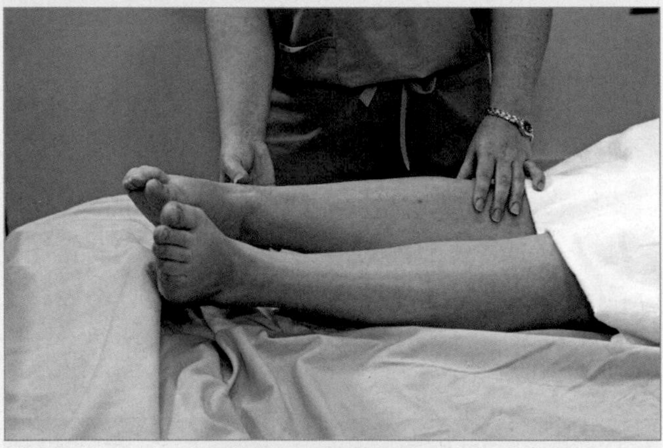

FIGURE 7 Having patient make circles with both ankles, first one way and then the other.

ACTION	RATIONALE
8. Validate the patient's understanding of the information. Ask the patient for a return demonstration. Ask the patient if he or she has any questions. Encourage the patient to practice the activities and ask questions, if necessary.	Validation facilitates the patient's understanding of information and performance of activities.
9. Remove PPE, if used. Perform hand hygiene.	Removing PPE properly reduces the risk for infection transmission and contamination of other items. Hand hygiene prevents the spread of microorganisms.

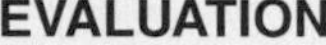

EVALUATION

The expected outcome is met when the patient and/or significant other verbalizes an understanding of the instructions related to leg exercises and is able to demonstrate the activities.

DOCUMENTATION

Guidelines

Document the components of teaching related to leg exercises that were reviewed with the patient and family, if present. Record the patient's ability to demonstrate the leg exercises and response to the teaching; note if any follow-up instruction needs to be performed.

Sample Documentation

> 11/2/15 2230 Perioperative teaching points related to leg exercises reviewed with patient and her husband, including the rationale for each of these points. Patient verbalized an understanding of the rationale for the activities. Patient demonstrated proper technique for leg exercises and asked appropriate questions. Patient stated that she was anxious about the surgery because this will be her first surgical experience. Emotional support and reassurance were provided.
>
> —J. Lynn, RN

UNEXPECTED SITUATIONS AND ASSOCIATED INTERVENTIONS

- *Patient unable to complete full range of motion of lower extremities due to pain from arthritis or other health issue:* Modify exercises based on patient's abilities. Encourage patient to perform to the best of his or her abilities. Document patient's ROM and limitations related to exercises.

SPECIAL CONSIDERATIONS

- Cardiovascular disorders, such as thrombocytopenia, hemophilia, myocardial infarction or cardiac surgery, and dysrhythmias, increase the risk for venous stasis and thrombophlebitis.
- Certain types of surgeries are associated with a higher risk of deep vein thrombosis and pulmonary embolism, including major orthopedic surgery, major cardiothoracic, vascular, and neurosurgery.

SKILL 6-3 PROVIDING PREOPERATIVE PATIENT CARE: HOSPITALIZED PATIENT

The preoperative phase consists of the time from when it is decided that surgery is needed until the patient is transferred to the OR or procedural bed. During this time the nurse will perform physical, emotional, and cultural assessments of the patient. In addition, the nurse will provide patient and family teaching. The nurse provides emotional support and allays anxiety, as appropriate, throughout the preoperative period.

DELEGATION CONSIDERATIONS

Preoperative assessment and teaching are not delegated to nursing assistive personnel (NAP) or to unlicensed assistive personnel (UAP). Depending on the state's nurse practice act and the organization's policies and procedures, preoperative teaching may be delegated to licensed practical/vocational nurses (LPN/LVNs) after an assessment of education needs by the registered nurse. The decision to delegate must be based on careful analysis of the patient's needs and circumstances, as well as the qualifications of the person to whom the task is being delegated. Refer to the Delegation Guidelines in Appendix A.

EQUIPMENT (varies, depending on the type of surgery)

- Blood pressure cuffs
- Electronic blood pressure monitor
- Pulse oximeter sensors
- IV pump
- Graduated compression stockings
- Pneumatic compression device
- Tubes, drains, vascular access tubing
- Incentive spirometer
- Small pillow
- PPE, as indicated

(continued)

SKILL 6-3 PROVIDING PREOPERATIVE PATIENT CARE: HOSPITALIZED PATIENT continued

ASSESSMENT

The preoperative nursing assessment, which includes a complete baseline health assessment, is completed upon admission to the surgical facility. This assessment can begin in various settings, such as the surgeon's office or an inpatient unit. Interview the patient to determine the medical and surgical history, including allergies, as well as any emotional, socioeconomic, cultural, and spiritual factors that may influence the patient's care. Ask about and review all medications the patient is taking, including nonprescription drugs, herbs, and supplements, as well as illicit drugs. Also explore any relevant preoperative needs of the patient or family. If the patient has a preferred speaking language other than English, it is essential to note this in the patient's record.

Perform physical assessments of skin, respiratory, cardiovascular, abdominal, neurologic, and musculoskeletal function. Take the patient's vital signs. Communicate any assessment abnormalities or areas of concern to the primary care provider. It is important for the nurse to identify patients who are considered at greater risk, such as the very young and very old; obese or malnourished patients; patients with fluid and electrolyte imbalances; patients with chronic disease; patients taking certain medications (e.g., anticoagulants or analgesics); and patients who are extremely anxious. Depending on the particular at-risk patient, specific assessments and interventions may be warranted.

NURSING DIAGNOSIS

Determine related factors for the nursing diagnoses based on the patient's current status. Appropriate nursing diagnoses may include:

- Anxiety
- Risk for Imbalanced Fluid Volume
- Deficient Knowledge
- Risk for Infection
- Hypothermia

OUTCOME IDENTIFICATION AND PLANNING

The expected outcome to achieve when providing preoperative patient care for the hospitalized patient is that the patient will proceed to surgery. Other outcomes that may be appropriate include the following: the patient will be free from anxiety and fear, and the patient will demonstrate an understanding of the need for surgery and the measures to minimize the postoperative risks associated with surgery.

IMPLEMENTATION

ACTION	RATIONALE
1. Check the patient's medical record for the type of surgery and review the medical orders. Review the nursing database, history, and physical examination. Check that the baseline data are recorded; report those that are abnormal.	These checks ensure that the care will be provided for the right patient and any specific teaching based on the type of surgery will be addressed. Also, this review helps to identify patients who are at increased surgical risk.
2. **Check that all diagnostic testing has been completed and results are available; identify and report abnormal results.** Gather the necessary supplies.	This check may influence the type of surgery performed and **anesthetic** used, as well as the timing of surgery or the need for additional consultation. Preparation promotes efficient time management and an organized approach to the task.
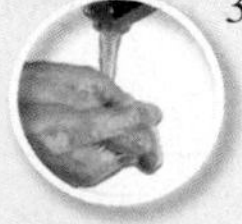 3. Perform hand hygiene and put on PPE, if indicated.	Hand hygiene and PPE prevent the spread of microorganisms. PPE is required based on transmission precautions.
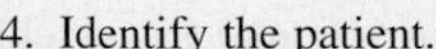 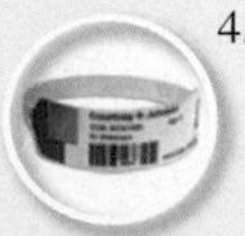 4. Identify the patient.	Identifying the patient ensures the right patient receives the intervention and helps prevent errors.

ACTION	RATIONALE
5. Close the curtains around the bed and close the door to the room, if possible. Explain what you are going to do and why you are going to do it to the patient and significant other. Place necessary supplies on the bedside stand or overbed table, within easy reach.	This ensures the patient's privacy. Explanation relieves anxiety and facilitates cooperation. Bringing everything to the bedside conserves time and energy. Arranging items nearby is convenient, saves time, and avoids unnecessary stretching and twisting of muscles on the part of the nurse.
6. Explore the psychological needs of the patient and family related to the surgery.	Meeting the psychological needs of the patient and family before surgery can have a beneficial effect on the postoperative course.
a. Establish a therapeutic relationship, encouraging the patient to verbalize concerns or fears.	
b. Use active listening skills, answering questions and clarifying any misinformation.	
c. Use touch, as appropriate, to convey genuine empathy.	
d. Offer to contact spiritual counselor (e.g., priest, minister, rabbi) to meet spiritual needs.	Spiritual beliefs for some patients and family can provide a source of support over the perioperative course.
7. **Identify learning needs of patient and family.** Ensure that the informed consent of the patient for the surgery has been signed, timed, dated, and witnessed. Inquire if the patient has any questions regarding the surgical procedure (Figure 1). Check the patient's record to determine if an advance directive has been completed. If an advance directive has not been completed, discuss with the patient the possibility of completing it, as appropriate. If patient has had surgery before, ask about this experience.	This enhances surgical recovery and allays anxiety by preparing the patient for postoperative convalescence, discharge plans, and self-care. The surgeon is responsible for explaining the details of the surgical procedure and potential risks and complications. The nurse is responsible for clarifying what the surgeon has explained to the patient and contacting the surgeon if the patient does not understand or has further questions. An advance directive provides written communication of the patient's wishes to the health care team related to the patient's desire for extraordinary life-sustaining treatments if the patient's condition is deemed unsalvageable. Previous surgical experience may impact preoperative care positively or negatively, depending on the patient's experience.
8. Teach deep breathing exercises. Refer to Skill 6-1.	Deep breathing exercises improve lung expansion and volume, help expel anesthetic gases and mucus from the airway, and facilitate the oxygenation of body tissues.
9. Teach coughing and splinting. Refer to Skill 6-1.	Coughing helps remove retained mucus from the respiratory tract. Splinting minimizes pain while coughing or moving.
10. Teach use of incentive spirometer (Figure 2). (Refer to Skill 14-2, Chapter 14, for specific information.)	Incentive spirometry improves lung expansion, helps expel anesthetic gases and mucus from the airway, and facilitates oxygenation of body tissues.

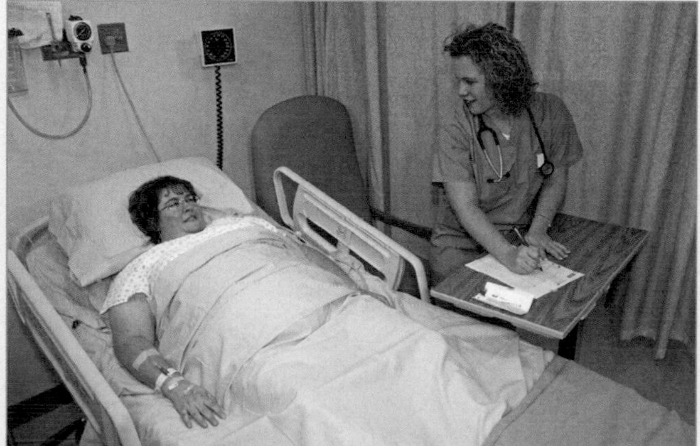

FIGURE 1 Identifying needs of patient and answering questions.

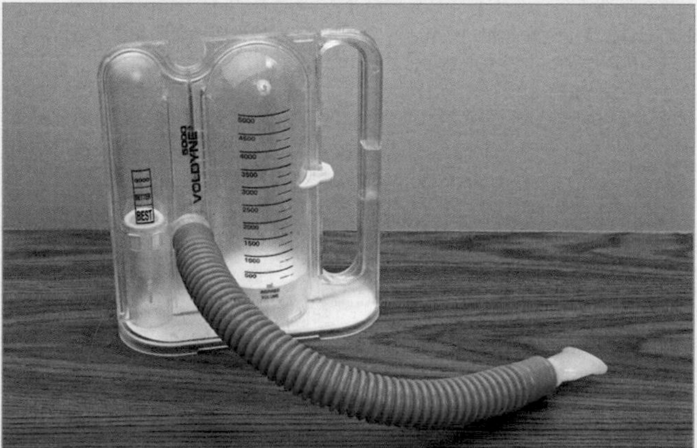

FIGURE 2 An incentive spirometer helps increase lung volume and promotes inflation of the alveoli.

(continued)

SKILL 6-3 PROVIDING PREOPERATIVE PATIENT CARE: HOSPITALIZED PATIENT continued

ACTION	RATIONALE
11. Teach leg exercises, as appropriate. Refer to Skill 6-2.	Leg exercises assist in preventing muscle weakness, promote venous return, and decrease complications related to venous stasis. Leg exercises may be contraindicated for patients with certain conditions, such as lower extremity fractures.
12. Assist the patient in putting on graduated compression stockings. (Refer to Skill 9-11, Chapter 9, for specific information.) and demonstrate how the pneumatic compression device operates. (Refer to Skill 9-12, Chapter 9, for specific information.)	Graduated compression stockings and pneumatic compression devices are used postoperatively for patients who are at risk for a deep vein thrombosis (DVT) and pulmonary embolism.
13. Teach about turning in the bed.	Turning and repositioning of the patient is important to prevent postoperative complications and to minimize pain.
a. Instruct the patient to use a pillow or bath blanket to splint where the incision will be. Ask the patient to raise his or her left knee and reach across to grasp the right side rail of the bed when turning toward his or her right side (Figure 3). If the patient is turning to the left side, he or she will bend the right knee and grasp the left side rail.	
b. When turning the patient onto the right side, ask the patient to push with bent left leg and pull on the right side rail (Figure 4). Explain to the patient that you will place a pillow behind his/her back to provide support, and that the call bell will be placed within easy reach (Figure 5).	
c. Explain to the patient that position change is recommended every 2 hours.	

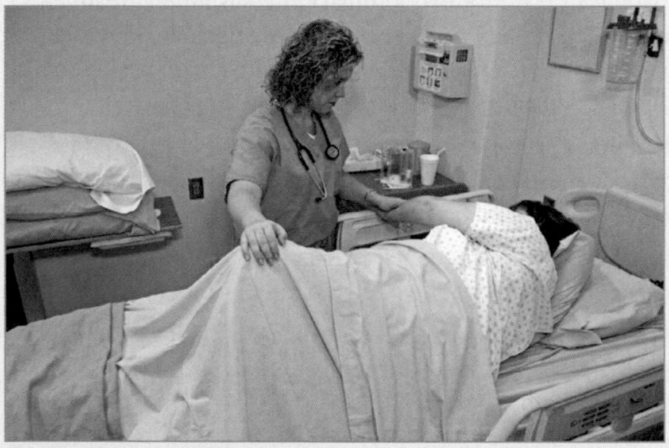

FIGURE 3 Instructing patient to raise left knee and reach across to grasp right side rail toward which she will be turning.

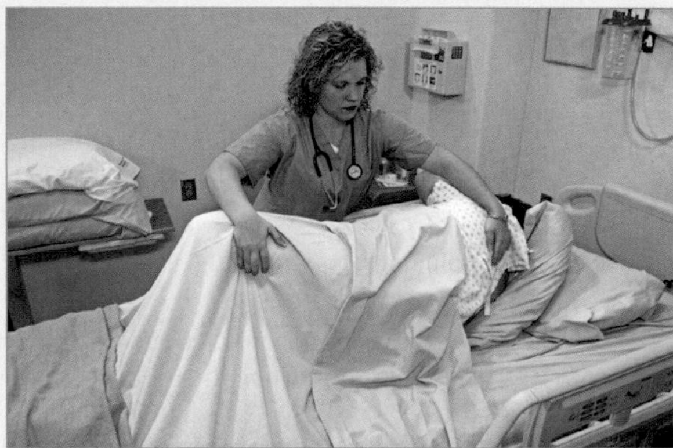

FIGURE 4 Helping patient to roll over to her right side while she pushes with left bent leg and pulls on the side rail.

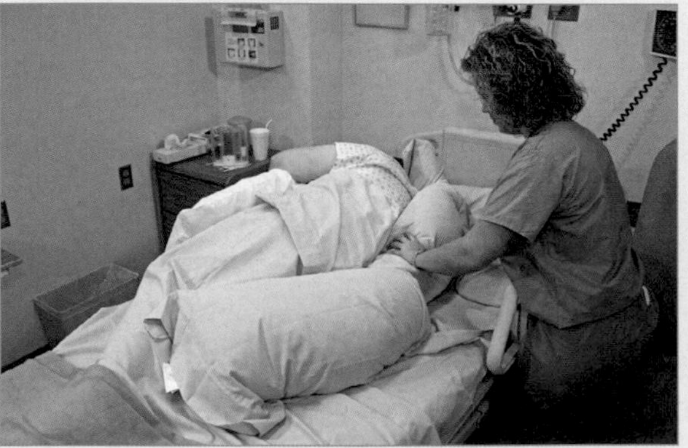

FIGURE 5 After patient is turned, provide support with pillows behind patient's back.

ACTION	RATIONALE
14. Teach about pain management.	Using prescribed analgesics to minimize pain helps prevent postoperative complications.
a. Discuss past experiences with pain and interventions that the patient has used to reduce pain.	Past experiences with pain can impact the patient's ability to manage surgical pain. Pain is a subjective experience and the interventions effective in reducing pain vary from patient to patient.
b. Discuss the availability of analgesic medication postoperatively.	Depending on the medical order, the patient may need to request analgesic medication, as needed, or a patient-controlled analgesia (PCA) or epidural analgesia may be ordered, for which the patient will need specific instruction on how to use. (See Chapter 10 for more information.)
c. Discuss the use of PCA, as appropriate. Refer to Skill 10-4, Chapter 10.	Patient understanding of the use of PCA is crucial for effective, safe administration.
d. Explore the use of other alternative and nonpharmacologic methods to reduce pain, such as position change, massage, relaxation/diversion, guided imagery, and meditation. Refer to Skills 10-1 and 10-2, Chapter 10.	These measures may reduce anxiety and may decrease the amount of pain medication that is needed. Analgesic therapy should involve a multimodal approach influenced by age, weight, and comorbidity.
15. Review equipment that may be used after surgery.	
a. Show the patient various equipment, such as IV pumps, electronic blood pressure cuff, tubes, and surgical drains.	Knowledge can reduce anxiety about equipment. The patient may need an indwelling urinary (Foley) catheter during and after surgery to keep the bladder empty and to monitor urinary output. Drains are frequently used to remove excess fluid around the surgical incision.
16. Provide skin preparation. a. **Ask the patient to bathe or shower with the antiseptic solution. Remind the patient to clean the surgical site.**	An antiseptic shower, bath, or cleansing with antimicrobial-impregnated wipes may be ordered the evening before surgery and repeated the morning of surgery to begin the process of preparing the skin before surgery and to prevent infection. Evidence-based practice advises against hair removal at the surgical site due to increased potential for infection. The Centers for Disease Control and Prevention (CDC) recommends that if shaving is necessary, it should be performed immediately before the surgery, using disposable supplies and aseptic technique. Follow facility policy regarding skin preparation of the surgical patient. In addition, immediately before the surgical procedure, the skin of the patient's operative site will be cleansed with a product that is compatible with the antiseptic used for showering.
17. Provide teaching about and follow dietary/fluid restrictions. **Explain to the patient that both food and fluid will be restricted before surgery to ensure that the stomach contains a minimal amount of gastric secretions. This restriction is important to reduce the risk of aspiration. Emphasize to the patient the importance of avoiding food and fluids during the prescribed time period, because failure to adhere may necessitate cancellation of the surgery.**	Ensure that fluid and dietary restrictions (NPO), as ordered by the primary care provider or in facility protocol, have been followed. These restrictions assist in preventing regurgitation and aspiration.

(continued)

SKILL 6-3 PROVIDING PREOPERATIVE PATIENT CARE: HOSPITALIZED PATIENT continued

ACTION	RATIONALE
18. Provide intestinal preparation, as appropriate. In certain situations, the bowel will need to be prepared by administering enemas or laxatives to evacuate the bowel and to reduce the intestinal bacteria.	This preparation will be needed when major abdominal, perineal, perianal, or pelvic surgery is planned.
a. As needed, explain the purpose of enemas or laxatives before surgery. If patient will be administering an enema, clarify the steps as needed.	Enemas can be stressful, especially when repeated enemas are required to obtain a clear fluid return. Repeated enemas may cause fluid and electrolyte imbalance, orthostatic hypotension, and weakness. Follow safety precautions to guard against patient falls. Anesthetic agents and abdominal surgery can interfere with normal elimination during the initial postoperative period. (Refer to Chapter 13 to review skill for enema administration.)
19. **Check administration of regularly scheduled medications.** Review with the patient routine medications, over-the-counter medications, and herbal supplements that are taken regularly. Check the medical orders and review with the patient which medications he or she will be permitted to take the day of surgery.	Many patients take medications for a variety of chronic medical conditions. Adjustments in taking these medications may be needed before surgery. Certain medications, such as aspirin, are stopped days before surgery due to their anticoagulant effect. Certain cardiac and respiratory drugs may be taken the day of surgery per medical order. If the patient is diabetic and takes insulin, the insulin dosage may be reduced.
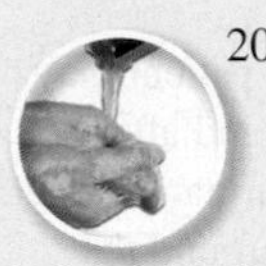 20. Remove PPE, if used. Perform hand hygiene.	Removing PPE properly reduces the risk for infection transmission and contamination of other items. Hand hygiene prevents the spread of microorganisms.

EVALUATION

The expected outcome is met when the patient prepares for surgery free from excessive anxiety and fear and demonstrates an understanding of the perioperative instructions.

DOCUMENTATION

Guidelines

Document that the patient's records were reviewed, including the history, physical assessment, and any laboratory values and diagnostic studies. Record that the surgeon was notified of any abnormal values. Document the components of perioperative teaching that were reviewed with the patient and family, if present, such as use of the incentive spirometer, deep breathing exercises, splinting, leg exercises, graduated compression stockings, and pneumatic compression devices. Record the patient's ability to demonstrate the skills and response to the teaching, and note if any follow-up instruction needs to be performed. Document other preoperative teaching, including pain management, intestinal preparation, medications, and preoperative skin preparation. Record any patient concerns about the surgery and whether the surgeon was contacted to provide any further explanations. Document the emotional support that was offered to the patient and if a spiritual counselor was notified per request of patient.

Sample Documentation

4/2/15 1030 Patient's records were reviewed and no abnormal results were identified. Perioperative teaching points reviewed with patient and his wife, including the rationale for each of these points. Patient demonstrated proper use of incentive spirometry, deep breathing, splinting while coughing, and leg exercises. Reviewed pain management, intestinal preparation, medications, and preoperative skin preparation. Patient stated that he was anxious about the surgery because this will be his first time to the OR. Emotional support and reassurance were provided.

—J. Grabes, RN

UNEXPECTED SITUATIONS AND ASSOCIATED INTERVENTIONS

- *Patient's laboratory results are noted to be abnormal:* Notify primary care provider. Some abnormalities, such as an elevated international normalized ratio (INR) or abnormalities in the complete blood count (CBC), may postpone the surgery.
- *A patient says to you, "I'm not sure I really want this surgery:"* Discuss with the patient why he or she feels this way. Notify primary care provider. Patients should not undergo surgery until they are sure that surgery is what they want.

SPECIAL CONSIDERATIONS

General Considerations

- Obese patients are at greater risk of surgical complications and death compared with optimal-weight patients. In taking an obese patient's history, be alert for other medical conditions, such as diabetes, hypertension, and sleep apnea.

Infant and Child Considerations

- Children have special needs related to their overall health, age, and size. Easing preoperative anxiety of the child is crucial and includes using simple and concrete terms when providing information.
- The nurse needs to be sensitive to the anxiety level of the parent and provide support, explanations, and patient teaching, as needed.
- Accurate weights are essential for correct medication dosages.
- Developmentally appropriate pain assessment and therapy needs to be initiated to ensure adequate pain management.

Older Adult Considerations

- Age-related changes and pre-existing chronic conditions can affect the postoperative course of the older adult patient.
- It is important to present preoperative teaching information slowly with reinforcement, because processing of information can be slower.
- Pain assessment and therapy may be suboptimal due to communication barriers and any comorbidity present in many older adult patients. These patients may respond differently to pain medication; therefore, careful and individualized attention is required.

EVIDENCE FOR PRACTICE ▶

PREVENTING POSTOPERATIVE SURGICAL SITE INFECTION

Surgical site infections occur as a result of microbial contamination of the surgical site and are a potential complication with any surgery. What is the best method to prevent postoperative surgical site infection?

Related Research

Kamel, C., McGahan, L., Polisena, J., et al. (2012). Preoperative skin antiseptic preparations for preventing surgical site infections: A systematic review. *Infection Control and Hospital Epidemiology, 33*(6), 608–617.

This article reports a systematic review of the literature related to interventions to prevent postoperative surgical site infections. The data sources consisted of a MEDLINE and EMBASE literature search, as well as other databases, for the period January 2001, through June 2011. Studies included in the review were randomized and non-randomized trials of preoperative skin antisepsis preparations and application techniques. Data were collected using standardized tables developed before the study and included study methods, quality, and clinical findings. The authors concluded that the evidence suggests that presurgical antiseptic showering is effective for reducing skin flora and may reduce surgical site infection rates. The authors could not conclude if one antiseptic is more effective than another at reducing surgical site infections.

Relevance for Nursing Practice

Patient teaching is an important part of nursing care. Nurses need to ensure patients undergoing surgery understand and implement appropriate activities to help decrease the risk of postoperative complications, including infections. Preoperative nursing should include appropriate teaching related to skin antisepsis.

Refer to thePoint for additional research on related nursing topics.

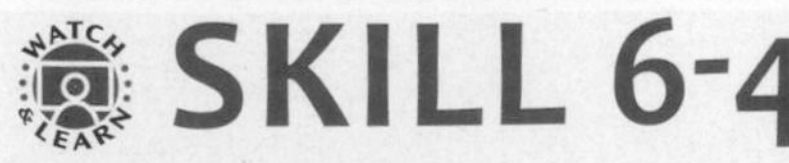

SKILL 6-4 PROVIDING PREOPERATIVE PATIENT CARE: HOSPITALIZED PATIENT (DAY OF SURGERY)

Due to the variety of outpatient and inpatient settings where elective surgery is performed, the day before surgery may be spent at home or in the hospital. If the patient will be arriving the morning of surgery to the surgical setting, he or she will receive a phone call the day before from a health care professional reminding the patient of the scheduled surgery, and key points, such as showering with an antiseptic cleansing agent, NPO restrictions, and any other pertinent information related to the particular procedure. Additionally, the nurse will clarify any questions that the patient may have. If the patient is a hospitalized patient, the nurse will review the same information, clarify any concerns, and reinforce any perioperative instructions, as needed.

DELEGATION CONSIDERATIONS

Preoperative measurement of vital signs may be delegated to nursing assistive personnel (NAP) or to unlicensed assistive personnel (UAP), as well as to licensed practical/vocational nurses (LPN/LVNs). Preoperative assessment and teaching is not delegated to NAP or to UAP. Depending on the state's nurse practice act and the organization's policies and procedures, preoperative teaching may be delegated to LPN/LVNs after an assessment of education needs by the registered nurse. The decision to delegate must be based on careful analysis of the patient's needs and circumstances, as well as the qualifications of the person to whom the task is being delegated. Refer to the Delegation Guidelines in Appendix A.

EQUIPMENT

- Blood pressure cuff
- Electronic blood pressure monitor
- Thermometer
- Pulse oximeter sensors
- IV pump, IV solution, vascular access tubing
- Graduated compression stockings (as ordered)
- Pneumatic compression device (as ordered)
- Incentive spirometer
- PPE, as indicated

ASSESSMENT

Immediately prior to the surgery, assess the patient's vital signs and report any abnormalities in vital signs, as well as any abnormalities in laboratory and diagnostic results to the surgeon. Also, review and complete the preoperative checklist and inquire if the patient or family members have any questions. Provide clarification as needed.

NURSING DIAGNOSIS

Determine related factors for the nursing diagnoses based on the patient's current status. Appropriate nursing diagnoses may include:

- Anxiety
- Deficient Knowledge
- Risk for Aspiration

OUTCOME IDENTIFICATION AND PLANNING

The expected outcome to achieve when providing preoperative patient care for the hospitalized patient is that the patient will proceed to surgery. Other outcomes that may be appropriate include the following: the patient will be free from anxiety; the patient will be free from fear; and the patient will demonstrate an understanding of the need for surgery and the measures to minimize the postoperative risks associated with surgery.

IMPLEMENTATION

ACTION	RATIONALE
1. Check the patient's medical record for the type of surgery and review the medical orders. Review the nursing database, history, and physical examination. Check that the baseline data are recorded; report those that are abnormal. Gather the necessary supplies.	A review of the medical record ensures that the care will be provided for the right patient and any specific teaching based on the type of surgery will be addressed. Also, review identifies patients who are surgical risks. Preparation promotes efficient time management and an organized approach to the task.
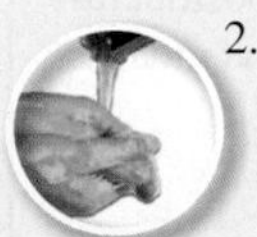 2. Perform hand hygiene and put on PPE, if indicated.	Hand hygiene and PPE prevent the spread of microorganisms. PPE is required based on transmission precautions.

ACTION	RATIONALE
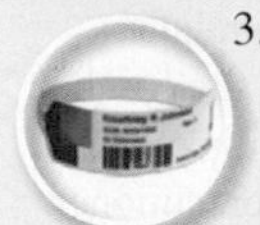 3. Identify the patient.	Identifying the patient ensures the right patient receives the intervention and helps prevent errors.
4. Close the curtains around the bed and close the door to the room, if possible. Explain what you are going to do and why you are going to do it to the patient and significant other. Place necessary supplies on the bedside stand or overbed table, within easy reach.	This ensures the patient's privacy. Explanation relieves anxiety and facilitates cooperation. Bringing everything to the bedside conserves time and energy. Arranging items nearby is convenient, saves time, and avoids unnecessary stretching and twisting of muscles on the part of the nurse.
5. Check that preoperative consent forms are signed, witnessed, and correct; that advance directives are in the medical record (as applicable); and that the patient's medical record is in order.	This fulfills legal requirements related to informed consent and educates the patient regarding advance directives.
6. Measure vital signs (Figure 1). Notify the primary care provider and surgeon of any pertinent changes (e.g., rise or drop in blood pressure, elevated temperature, cough, symptoms of infection).	This provides baseline data for comparison. Significant findings may require interventions and/or result in postponement of surgery.

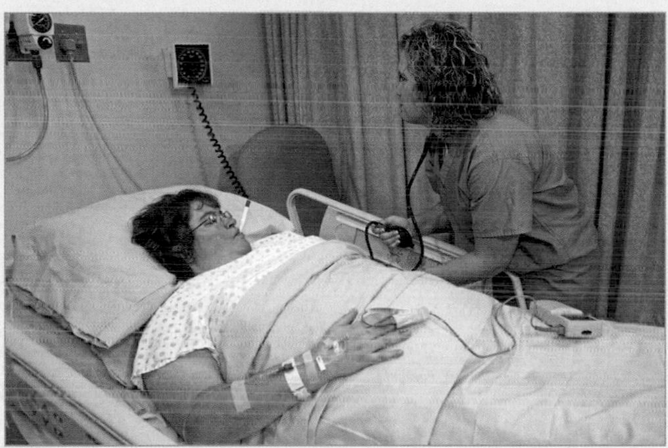

FIGURE 1 Obtaining preoperative vital signs.

ACTION	RATIONALE
7. Provide hygiene and oral care. Assess for loose teeth and caps. Remind the patient of food and fluid restrictions before surgery.	This promotes comfort and prevents intraoperative complications during anesthesia induction.
8. Instruct the patient to remove all personal clothing, including underwear, and to put on a hospital gown.	This permits access to the operative area and ease of assessment during the operative period.
9. Ask the patient to remove cosmetics, jewelry including body-piercing, nail polish, and prostheses (e.g., contact lenses, false eyelashes, dentures, and so forth). Some facilities allow a wedding band to be left in place depending on the type of surgery, provided it is secured to the finger with tape.	These interfere with assessment during surgery. Some hospital policies advise having the patient wear eyeglasses and leave hearing aids in place, if needed. Notify the postanesthesia care unit (PACU) nurse if the patient wears hearing aids.
10. If possible, give valuables to a family member or place them in an appropriate area, such as the hospital safe, if this is not possible. They should not be placed in the narcotics drawer.	This ensures safety of valuables and personal possessions. Document where valuables have been secured.
11. Have patient empty bladder and bowel before surgery.	An empty bladder and bowel minimizes risk for injury or complications during and after surgery.
12. Attend to any special preoperative orders, such as starting an IV line.	This prepares the patient for the operative procedure.
13. Complete preoperative checklist and record of patient's preoperative preparation.	This ensures accurate documentation and communication with the perioperative nurse caring for patient.

(*continued*)

SKILL 6-4 PROVIDING PREOPERATIVE PATIENT CARE: HOSPITALIZED PATIENT (DAY OF SURGERY) continued

ACTION	RATIONALE
14. Question patient regarding the location of the operative site. Document the location in the medical record according to facility policy. The actual site will be marked on the patient when the patient arrives in the preoperative holding area by the licensed independent practitioner who will be directly involved in the procedure (The Joint Commission, 2014b).	The Universal Protocol (National Patient Safety Goals) requires marking and documentation to validate the intended site for the procedure. The site will be marked before the patient is moved into the surgical location by a licensed independent practitioner who will be involved directly in the procedure and will be present at the time the procedure is performed (The Joint Commission, 2014b).
15. Administer preoperative medication as prescribed.	Medication reduces anxiety, provides sedation, and diminishes salivary and bronchial secretions. Preoperative medications may be given "on call" (when the OR nurse calls to tell the nurse to give the medication) or at a scheduled time. Certain patients undergoing specific cardiac, colorectal, gynecologic, ophthalmologic, and urinary surgical procedures also may be given antibiotic prophylaxis before surgery.
16. Raise side rails of bed, based on facility policy; place bed in lowest position. Instruct the patient to remain in bed or on stretcher. If necessary, use a safety belt.	These actions ensure the patient's safety once the preoperative medication has been given.
17. Help move the patient from the bed to the transport stretcher, if necessary. Reconfirm patient identification and ensure that all preoperative events and measures are documented.	Helping the patient move prevents injury. Reconfirming the patient identity helps to ensure that the correct patient is being transported to surgery.
18. Tell the patient's family where the patient will be taken after surgery and the location of the waiting area where the surgeon will come to explain the outcome of the surgery. If possible, take the family to the waiting area.	Informing the family members of what to expect helps allay anxiety and avoid confusion.
19. After the patient leaves for the OR, prepare the room and make a postoperative bed for the patient (Figure 2). Anticipate any necessary equipment based on the type of surgery and the patient's history.	Preparing for the patient's return helps to promote efficient care in the postoperative period.

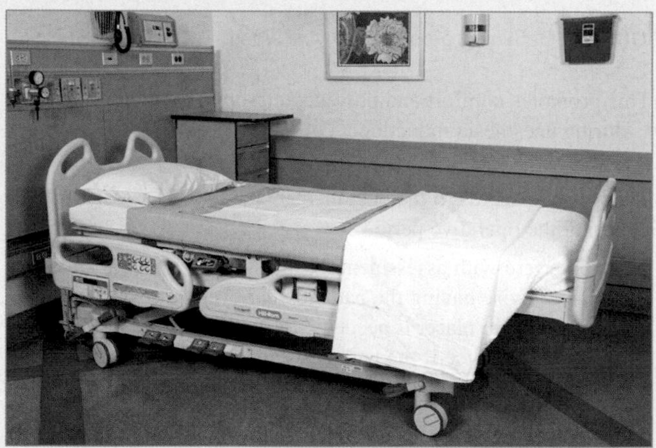

FIGURE 2 Postoperative bed, ready for patient's return.

ACTION	RATIONALE
20. Remove PPE, if used. Perform hand hygiene.	Removing PPE properly reduces the risk for infection transmission and contamination of other items. Hand hygiene prevents transmission of microorganisms.

EVALUATION

The expected outcome is met when the patient proceeds to surgery, is prepared for surgery so that he or she is free from anxiety and fear, and demonstrates understanding of the importance of pre- and postoperative instructions. Family members exhibit knowledge of what to expect over the remainder of the preoperative course.

DOCUMENTATION

Guidelines

Document that the preoperative checklist was completed, time of patient's last void, preoperative medications administered, intended procedure site, and any special interventions that were ordered before sending the patient to the OR. Record if there were any abnormal results that were communicated to the surgeon or OR nurse. Note if the patient's valuables were given to a family member. Document that the patient was safely transferred onto the stretcher and escorted to the OR without incident. Record that the patient's family members were instructed as to where to wait to meet the surgeon after the surgery is performed.

Sample Documentation

4/3/15 1045 Preoperative checklist completed with no abnormalities noted, patient voided, operative permit signed. Patient states surgical site is left knee. Maintained NPO status throughout night. IV started into right forearm, #18-gauge needle inserted without difficulty. IV solution of 1,000 mL of D5.45 sodium chloride at 80/mL/hour initiated. No preoperative medications ordered. Patient verbalized that he will be glad when the surgery is over. Patient assisted onto stretcher for transfer to OR without difficulty. Family also accompanied and instructed to wait in surgical waiting lounge.

—A. Lynn, RN

UNEXPECTED SITUATIONS AND ASSOCIATED INTERVENTIONS

- *A patient admits he ate "just a little bit" this morning upon waking from sleep:* Notify the surgeon. The patient's surgery may have to be postponed for a few hours to prevent aspiration during surgery.
- *Identification band is not in place:* Ensure identity of patient and obtain new identification band. Patient cannot proceed to surgery without an identification band. Two patient identifiers are required to meet current patient safety goals.
- *Consent form is not signed:* Notify the surgeon. It is the physician's responsibility to obtain consent for surgery and anesthesia. Preoperative medications cannot be given until the consent form is signed. The patient should not proceed to surgery without a signed consent form (unless it is an emergency).
- *Patient does not want to remove dentures before surgery, saying, "I never take my dentures out":* Discuss with surgeon or anesthesia provider. Patient may be allowed to go to the preoperative area with dentures and remove the dentures before entering the OR.
- *Patient refuses to take preoperative medication:* Notify surgeon and anesthesiologist before patient goes to the OR. Many medications are necessary to protect the patient pre- or postoperatively.

SPECIAL CONSIDERATIONS

General Considerations

- Appropriately sized equipment, such as blood pressure cuffs, wide stretchers, and lift devices, need to be available for obese patients.

Infant and Child Considerations

- In many institutions, the parents are allowed to enter the preoperative area with the child. This has been shown to decrease the child's and the parents' anxiety.
- The breastfed infant may be allowed to nurse closer to the time of surgery than a bottle-fed infant would be allowed to have a bottle of formula. Breast milk is easier for the stomach to digest, so the clearance time is shorter than for formula.
- Children have special needs related to their overall health, age, and size. Appropriately sized blood pressure cuffs are essential.

Older Adult Considerations

- Due to the prevalence of hearing and vision loss in this age group, the necessity of wearing eyeglasses and hearing aids is essential for processing preoperative teaching and throughout the postoperative course. The patient who requires glasses and hearing aids to understand and/or read instructions should be sent to the preoperative area with the glasses and/or hearing aid in place and then remove them before entering the OR.

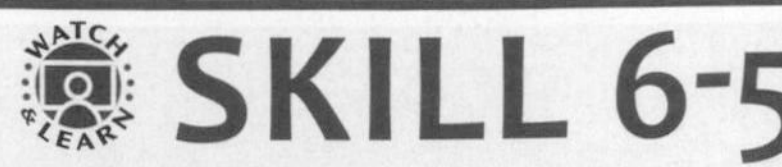

SKILL 6-5 PROVIDING POSTOPERATIVE CARE WHEN PATIENT RETURNS TO ROOM

Postoperative care facilitates recovery from surgery and supports the patient in coping with physical changes or alterations. Nursing interventions promote physical and psychological health, prevent complications, and teach self-care skills for the patient to use after the hospital stay. After surgery, patients spend time on the PACU. From the PACU, they are transferred back to their rooms. At this time, nursing care focuses on accurate assessments and associated interventions. Ongoing assessments are crucial for early identification of postoperative complications.

DELEGATION CONSIDERATIONS

Postoperative measurement of vital signs may be delegated to nursing assistive personnel (NAP) or to unlicensed assistive personnel (UAP), as well as to licensed practical/vocational nurses (LPN/LVNs). Postoperative assessment and teaching is not delegated to NAP or to UAP. Depending on the state's nurse practice act and the organization's policies and procedures, postoperative teaching may be delegated to LPN/LVNs after an assessment of education needs by the registered nurse. The decision to delegate must be based on careful analysis of the patient's needs and circumstances, as well as the qualifications of the person to whom the task is being delegated. Refer to the Delegation Guidelines in Appendix A.

EQUIPMENT (varies, depending on the surgery)

- Electronic blood pressure monitor
- Blood pressure cuff
- Electronic thermometer
- Pulse oximeter
- Stethoscope
- IV pump, IV solutions
- Graduated compression stockings
- Pneumatic compression devices
- Tubes, drains, vascular access tubing
- Incentive spirometer
- PPE, as indicated
- Blankets, as needed

ASSESSMENT

Assess the patient's mental status, positioning, and vital signs. Assess the patient's oxygen saturation level, skin color, respiratory status, and cardiovascular status. Assess the patient's neurovascular status, depending on the type of surgery. Assess the operative site, drains/tubes, and IV site(s). Perform a pain assessment. A wide variety of factors increase the risk for postoperative complications. Ongoing postoperative assessments and interventions are used to decrease the risk for postoperative complications. Assessment of the patient's and family's learning needs is also important.

NURSING DIAGNOSIS

Determine the related factors for the nursing diagnoses based on the patient's current status. Appropriate nursing diagnoses may include the following:

- Acute Pain
- Risk for Imbalanced Fluid Volume
- Impaired Gas Exchange
- Hypothermia
- Impaired Skin Integrity
- Risk for Aspiration

OUTCOME IDENTIFICATION AND PLANNING

The expected outcome to achieve when providing postoperative care to a patient is that the patient will recover from the surgery. Other outcomes that may be appropriate include the following: patient is free from anxiety; patient's temperature remains between 36.5°C and 37.5°C (97.7°F and 99.5°F); patient's vital signs remain stable; patient will remain free from infection; patient will not experience any skin breakdown; patient will regain mobility; patient will have pain managed appropriately; and patient is comfortable with body image. Specific expected outcomes are individualized based on risk factors, the surgical procedure, and the patient's unique needs.

IMPLEMENTATION

ACTION	RATIONALE
Immediate Care	
1. When patient returns from the PACU, participate in hand-off report from the PACU nurse and review the OR and PACU data. Gather the necessary supplies.	Obtaining a hand-off report ensures accurate communication and promotes continuity of care. Preparation promotes efficient time management and an organized approach to the task.

ACTION	RATIONALE
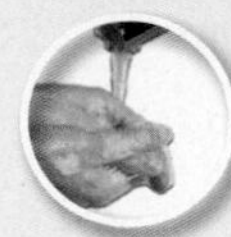 2. Perform hand hygiene and put on PPE, if indicated.	Hand hygiene and PPE prevent the spread of microorganisms. PPE is required based on transmission precautions.
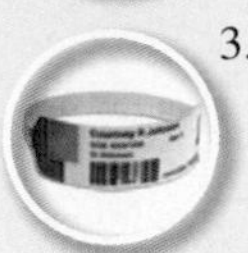 3. Identify the patient.	Identifying the patient ensures the right patient receives the intervention and helps prevent errors.
4. Close the curtains around the bed and close the door to the room, if possible. Explain what you are going to do and why you are going to do it to the patient or significant other. Place necessary supplies on the bedside stand or overbed table, within easy reach.	This ensures the patient's privacy. Explanation relieves anxiety and facilitates cooperation. Bringing everything to the bedside conserves time and energy. Arranging items nearby is convenient, saves time, and avoids unnecessary stretching and twisting of muscles on the part of the nurse.
5. **Place patient in safe position (semi- or high Fowler's or side-lying). Note level of consciousness.**	A sitting position (head of bed [HOB] elevated) facilitates deep breathing; the side-lying position with neck slightly extended prevents aspiration and airway obstruction. Alternate positions may be appropriate based on the type of surgery.
6. **Obtain vital signs. Monitor and record vital signs frequently.** Assessment order may vary, but usual frequency includes taking vital signs every 15 minutes the first hour, every 30 minutes the next 2 hours, every hour for 4 hours, and finally every 4 hours.	Comparison with baseline preoperative vital signs may indicate impending shock or **hemorrhage**. Some institutions use a paper or computer flow sheet to record initial postoperative data.
7. Assess the patient's respiratory status. (Refer to Skill 3-5, Chapter 3.) Measure the patient's oxygen saturation level (Figure 1).	Comparison with baseline preoperative respiratory assessment may indicate impending respiratory complications.
8. Assess the patient's cardiovascular status. (Refer to Skills 3-6 and 3-10, Chapter 3.)	Comparison with baseline preoperative cardiovascular assessment may indicate impending cardiovascular complications.
9. Assess the patient's neurovascular status, based on the type of surgery performed. (Refer to Skill 3-10, Chapter 3.)	Comparison with baseline preoperative neurovascular assessment may indicate impending neurovascular complications.
10. Provide for warmth, using heated or extra blankets, as necessary (Figure 2). Refer to Skill 6-6. Assess skin color and condition.	The OR is a cold environment. Hypothermia is uncomfortable and may lead to cardiac arrhythmias and impaired wound healing.

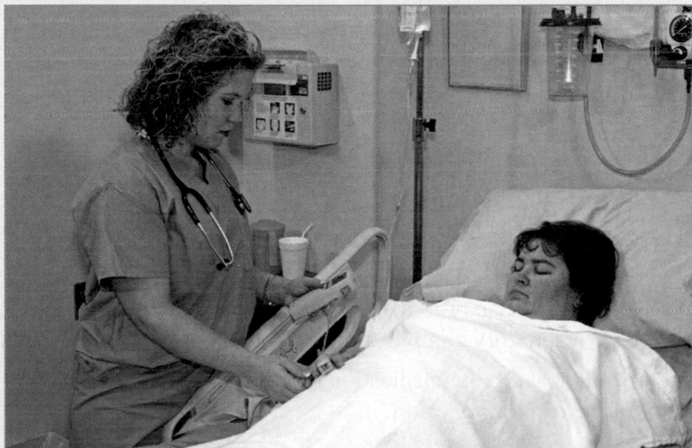

FIGURE 1 Obtaining postoperative oxygen saturation level.

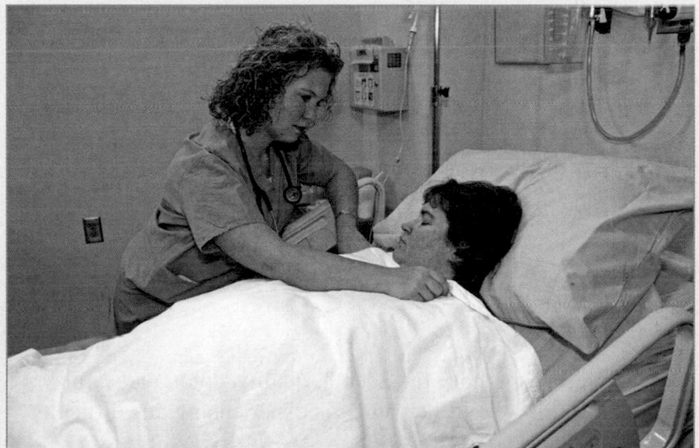

FIGURE 2 Providing extra blankets for warmth.

(continued)

SKILL 6-5 PROVIDING POSTOPERATIVE CARE WHEN PATIENT RETURNS TO ROOM continued

ACTION	RATIONALE
11. Check dressings for color, odor, presence of drains, and amount of drainage (Figure 3). Mark the drainage on the dressing by circling the amount, and include the time. Turn the patient to assess visually under the patient for bleeding from the surgical site.	Hemorrhage and shock are life-threatening complications of surgery and early recognition is essential.

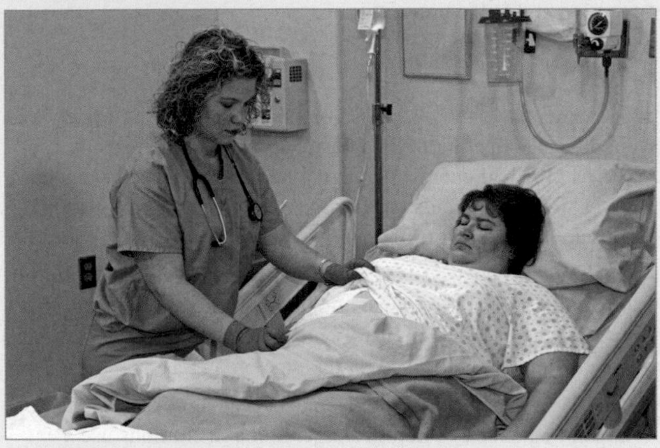

FIGURE 3 Checking dressings for color, odor, and amount of drainage.

ACTION	RATIONALE
12. Verify that all tubes and drains are patent and the equipment is working; note amount of drainage in collection device. If an indwelling urinary (Foley) catheter is in place, note urinary output.	This ensures function of drainage devices.
13. Verify and maintain IV infusion at prescribed rate.	This replaces fluid loss and prevents dehydration and electrolyte imbalances.
14. Assess for pain and relieve it by administering medications ordered by the primary care provider. If the patient has been instructed in the use of PCA for pain management, review its use. Check record to verify if analgesic medication was administered in the PACU.	Use a facility-approved pain scale. Observe for nonverbal behavior that may indicate pain, such as grimacing, crying, and restlessness. Analgesics and other nonpharmacologic pain strategies are used for relief of postoperative pain.
15. Provide for a safe environment. Keep bed in low position with side rails up, based on facility policy. Have call bell within patient's reach.	This prevents accidental injury. Easy access to call bell permits patient to call for nurse when necessary.
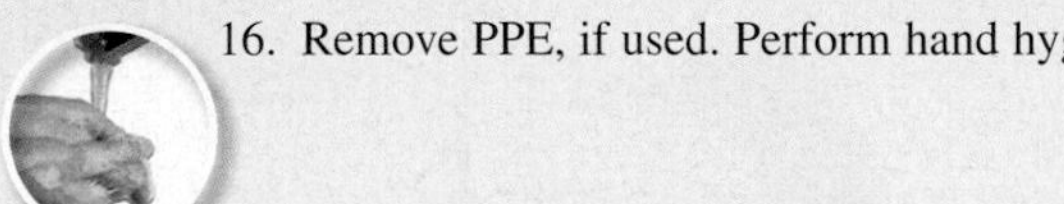 16. Remove PPE, if used. Perform hand hygiene.	Removing PPE properly reduces the risk for infection transmission and contamination of other items. Hand hygiene prevents transmission of microorganisms.

Ongoing Care

ACTION	RATIONALE
17. Promote optimal respiratory function.	Anesthetic agents may depress respiratory function. Patients who have existing respiratory or cardiovascular disease, have abdominal or chest incisions, who are obese, older (Shippee-Rice, et al., 2012), or in a poor state of nutrition are at greater risk for respiratory complications.
a. Assess respiratory rate, depth, quality, color, and capillary refill. Ask if the patient is experiencing any difficulty breathing.	Postoperative analgesic medication can reduce the rate and quality of the respiratory effort.
b. Assist with coughing and deep breathing exercises. (Refer to Skill 6-1.)	
c. Assist with incentive spirometry. (Refer to Skill 14-2, Chapter 14.)	

ACTION	RATIONALE
d. Assist with early ambulation.	
e. Provide frequent position changes.	
f. Administer oxygen, as ordered.	
g. Monitor pulse oximetry. (Refer to Skill 14-1, Chapter 14.)	
18. Promote optimal cardiovascular function:	Preventive measures can improve venous return and circulatory status.
a. Assess apical rate, rhythm, and quality and compare with peripheral pulses, color, and blood pressure. Ask if the patient has any chest pains or shortness of breath.	
b. Provide frequent position changes.	
c. Assist with early ambulation.	
d. Apply graduated compression stockings or pneumatic compression devices, if ordered and not in place. If in place, assess for integrity.	
e. Provide leg and range-of-motion exercises if not contraindicated. (Refer to Skill 6-2.)	
19. Promote optimal neurologic function:	
a. Assess level of consciousness, movement, and sensation.	Anesthetic and pain management agents can alter neurologic function.
b. Determine the level of orientation to person, place, and time.	Older patients may take longer to return to their level of orientation before surgery. Drug and anesthetics will delay this return (Shippee-Rice, et al., 2012).
c. Test motor ability by asking the patient to move each extremity.	Anesthesia alters motor and sensory function.
d. Evaluate sensation by asking the patient if he or she can feel your touch on an extremity.	
20. Promote optimal renal and urinary function and fluid and electrolyte status. Assess intake and output, evaluate for urinary retention and monitor serum electrolyte levels.	Anesthetic agents and surgical manipulation in the area may temporarily depress bladder tone and response causing urinary retention.
a. Promote voiding by offering bedpan at regular intervals, noting the frequency, amount, and if any burning or urgency symptoms.	Frequency, burning, or urgency may indicate possible urinary tract abnormality.
b. Monitor urinary catheter drainage if present.	The primary care provider needs to be notified if the urinary output is less than 30 mL/hour or 240 mL/8-hour period.
c. Measure intake and output.	Intake and output are good indicators of fluid balance.
21. Promote optimal gastrointestinal function and meet nutritional needs:	Anesthetic agents and narcotics depress peristalsis and normal functioning of the gastrointestinal tract. Flatus indicates return of peristalsis.
a. Assess abdomen for distention and firmness. Ask if patient feels nauseated, any vomiting, and if passing flatus.	
b. Auscultate for bowel sounds.	Presence of bowel sounds indicates return of peristalsis.
c. Assist with diet progression; encourage fluid intake; monitor intake.	Patients may experience nausea after surgery and are encouraged to resume diet slowly, starting with clear liquids and advancing as tolerated.
d. Medicate for nausea and vomiting, as ordered.	Antiemetics are frequently ordered to alleviate postoperative nausea.

(*continued*)

SKILL 6-5 PROVIDING POSTOPERATIVE CARE WHEN PATIENT RETURNS TO ROOM continued

ACTION	RATIONALE
22. Promote optimal wound healing.	Alterations in nutritional, circulatory, and metabolic status may predispose the patient to infection and delayed healing.
a. Assess condition of wound for presence of drains and any drainage.	
b. Use surgical asepsis for dressing changes and drain care. Refer to Skills 8-1, 8-2, 8-7, 8-8, 8-9, and 8-10, Chapter 8.	Surgical asepsis reduces the risk of infection.
c. Inspect all skin surfaces for beginning signs of pressure ulcer development and use pressure-relieving supports to minimize potential skin breakdown.	Lying on the OR table in the same position can predispose some patients to pressure ulcer formation, especially in patients who have undergone lengthy procedures.
23. Promote optimal comfort and relief from pain.	This shortens recovery period and facilitates return to normal function.
a. Assess for pain (location and intensity using pain scale).	Control of postoperative pain promotes patient comfort and recovery.
b. Provide for rest and comfort; provide extra blankets, as needed, for warmth.	Patients may experience chills in the postoperative period.
c. Administer pain medications, as needed, and/or initiate nonpharmacologic methods, as appropriate.	
24. Promote optimal meeting of psychosocial needs:	This facilitates individualized care, anxiety reduction, and patient's return to normal health.
a. Provide emotional support to patient and family, as needed.	
b. Explain procedures and offer explanations regarding post-operative recovery, as needed, to both patient and family members.	

EVALUATION

The expected outcome is met when the patient recovers from surgery; patient is free from anxiety; patient's temperature remains between 36.5°C and 37.5°C (97.7°F and 99.5°F); patient's vital signs remain stable; patient remains free from infection; patient does not experience skin breakdown; patient regains mobility; patient experiences adequate pain control; and patient is comfortable with body image. Specific expected outcomes are individualized based on risk factors, the surgical procedure, and the patient's unique needs.

DOCUMENTATION

Guidelines

Document the time that the patient returns from PACU to the surgical unit. Record the patient's level of consciousness, vital signs, all assessments, and condition of dressing. If patient has oxygen running, an IV, or any other equipment, record this information. Document pain assessment, interventions that were instituted to alleviate pain, and the patient's response to the interventions. Document any patient teaching that is reviewed with the patient, such as use of incentive spirometer.

Sample Documentation

4/10/15 1330 Patient returned to room at 1315, drowsy but easily aroused; answers to name. Patient's temperature 98.8°F, pulse 78, BP 122/84, O_2 sat 96% on O_2 2 L/min. Right lower abdominal dressing dry and intact. Rates pain at a "4" on scale of 1–10, was medicated in PACU with 10 mg morphine sulfate IV at 1030. Incentive spirometry completed × 10 cycles, 750 mL each. Patient deep breathing and coughing without production and turned to right side with HOB elevated. See flow sheet for additional system assessments.

—J. Grabbs, RN

UNEXPECTED SITUATIONS AND ASSOCIATED INTERVENTIONS

- *Vital signs are progressively increasing or decreasing from baseline:* Notify primary care provider. A continued decrease in blood pressure or an increase in heart rate could indicate internal bleeding.
- *Dressing was clean before but now has large amount of fresh blood:* Do not remove dressing. Reinforce dressing with more bandages. Removing the bandage could dislodge any clot that is forming and lead to further blood loss. Notify primary care provider.
- *Patient reports pain that is not relieved by ordered medication:* After fully assessing pain (location, description, alleviating factors, aggravating factors), notify primary care provider. Pain can be a clue to other problems, such as hemorrhage.
- *Patient is febrile within 12 hours of surgery:* Assist patient with coughing and deep breathing. If ordered, begin incentive spirometry. Continue to monitor vital signs and laboratory values such as complete blood count (CBC).
- *Adult patient has a urine output of less than 30 mL/hour:* Unless this is expected, notify primary care provider. Urine output is a good indicator of tissue perfusion. Patient may need more fluid or may need medication to increase blood pressure if it is low.

SPECIAL CONSIDERATIONS

General Considerations

- Be aware of baseline sensory deficits. Ensure appropriate aids are in place, such as glasses or hearing aids. Lack of appropriate aids may impact postoperative assessments, such as level of consciousness.
- For patients undergoing throat surgery, such as a tonsillectomy, evaluate swallowing pattern. A patient who has had throat surgery and swallows frequently may be bleeding from the incision site.
- In the obese patient, medications may not perform as expected related to the lack of serum proteins that are needed to bind with the drugs to support their effectiveness. Additionally, due to the larger kidney mass of the obese patient, renal elimination rates of certain drugs are increased, reducing the effectiveness of these drugs.
- Check to make sure that the mattress for the obese patient is of high quality, because this patient is at greater risk for skin breakdown due to the poor vascular supply of adipose tissue.
- Ensure that written postoperative instructions specific to the patient and follow-up appointments with the surgeon or other health care professionals are provided to each patient upon discharge from the hospital or outpatient center. Information, such as signs and symptoms to report to the primary care provider, as well as restrictions in activity and diet, are addressed. In addition, patients discharged the same day as their surgery are required to have a responsible individual accompany them home, and a contact telephone number is to be provided in case of emergency. The patient should be alert and oriented, or mental status should be at the patient's baseline. The vital signs of the patient should be stable. Have the patient "teach back" important information/instructions in their own words.

Infant and Child Considerations

- Postoperative complications are often related to the respiratory system in this age group. After receiving general anesthesia, premature infants are at greater risk for apnea.
- Infants and children are at great risk for temperature-related complications because their body temperature can change rapidly. It is essential to have warmed blankets and other warming equipment available to avoid this complication.

Older Adult Considerations

- In the older adult patient, postoperative pneumonia can be a very serious complication resulting in death. Therefore, it is especially important to encourage and assist the patient in using the incentive spirometer and with deep breathing exercises (see Skill 14-2 in Chapter 14 and Skill 6-1 above).
- Older patients may take longer to return to normothermia and their level of orientation before surgery. Drugs and anesthetics will delay this return.

(continued)

SKILL 6-5 PROVIDING POSTOPERATIVE CARE WHEN PATIENT RETURNS TO ROOM continued

EVIDENCE FOR PRACTICE ▶

PAIN MANAGEMENT IN THE PERIOPERATIVE PERIOD

American Society of Anesthesiologists Task Force on Acute Pain Management. (2012). Practice guidelines for acute pain management in the perioperative setting: An updated report by the American Society of Anesthesiologists Task Force on Acute Pain Management. *Anesthesiology, 116*(2), 248–273.

This practice guideline provides basic recommendations that are supported by a synthesis and analysis of the current literature, expert and practitioner opinion, open forum commentary, and clinical feasibility data. This document updates the "Practice Guidelines for Acute Pain Management in the Perioperative Setting: An Updated Report by the American Society of Anesthesiologists (ASA) Task Force on Acute Pain Management," adopted by the ASA in 2003 and published in 2004. These recommendations are intended to facilitate the safety and effectiveness of acute pain management in the perioperative setting and reduce the risk of adverse outcomes related to pain management. In addition, this guideline discusses recommendations to maintain the patient's ability to function and enhance the quality of life for patients with acute pain in the perioperative period.

Refer to thePoint for additional research on related nursing topics.

SKILL 6-6 APPLYING A FORCED-WARM AIR DEVICE

Patients returning from surgery are often hypothermic. The application of a forced-air warming device is a more effective way of rewarming the patient compared to using warm blankets. This device circulates warm air around the patient.

DELEGATION CONSIDERATIONS

Application of a forced-warm air device is not delegated to nursing assistive personnel (NAP) or to unlicensed assistive personnel (UAP). Application of a forced-warm air device may be delegated to licensed practical/vocational nurses (LPN/LVNs). The decision to delegate must be based on careful analysis of the patient's needs and circumstances, as well as the qualifications of the person to whom the task is being delegated. Refer to the Delegation Guidelines in Appendix A.

EQUIPMENT

- Forced-warm air device
- Forced-air blanket
- Electronic thermometer
- PPE, as indicated

ASSESSMENT

Assess patient's temperature and skin color and perfusion. Patients who are hypothermic are generally pale to dusky and cool to the touch and have decreased peripheral perfusion. Inspect nail beds and mucous membranes of patients with darker skin tones for signs of decreased perfusion.

NURSING DIAGNOSIS

Determine the related factors for the nursing diagnoses based on the patient's current status. Appropriate nursing diagnoses may include the following:

- Risk for Imbalanced Body Temperature
- Hypothermia

OUTCOME IDENTIFICATION AND PLANNING

The expected outcome to achieve when applying a forced-air warming device is that the patient will return to and maintain a temperature of 97.7°F to 99.5°F (36.5°C to 37.5°C). Other outcomes that may be appropriate include the following: skin will become warm, capillary refill will be less than 2 to 3 seconds, and the patient will not experience shivering.

IMPLEMENTATION

ACTION	RATIONALE
1. Check the patient's medical record for the order for the use of a forced-air warming device. Gather the necessary supplies.	Reviewing the order validates the correct patient and correct procedure. Organization facilitates performance of the task. Preparation promotes efficient time management and an organized approach to the task.
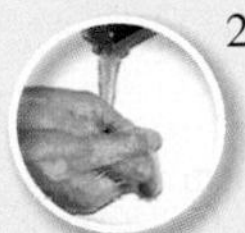 2. Perform hand hygiene and put on PPE, if indicated.	Hand hygiene and PPE prevent the spread of microorganisms. PPE is required based on transmission precautions.
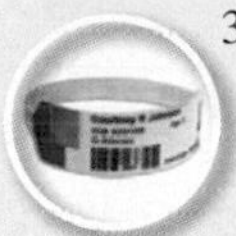 3. Identify the patient.	Identifying the patient ensures the right patient receives the intervention and helps prevent errors.
4. Close the curtains around the bed and close the door to the room, if possible. Explain what you are going to do and why you are going to do it to the patient or significant other. Place necessary supplies on the bedside stand or overbed table, within easy reach.	This ensures the patient's privacy. Explanation relieves anxiety and facilitates cooperation. Bringing everything to the bedside conserves time and energy. Arranging items nearby is convenient, saves time, and avoids unnecessary stretching and twisting of muscles on the part of the nurse.
5. **Assess the patient's temperature.**	Baseline temperature validates the need for use of the device and provides baseline information for future comparison.
6. Plug forced-air warming device into electrical outlet. Place forced-air blanket over patient, with plastic side up (Figure 1). Keep air-hose inlet at foot of bed.	Blanket should always be used with the device. To avoid causing burns, *do not* place air hose under cotton blankets with airflow blanket.

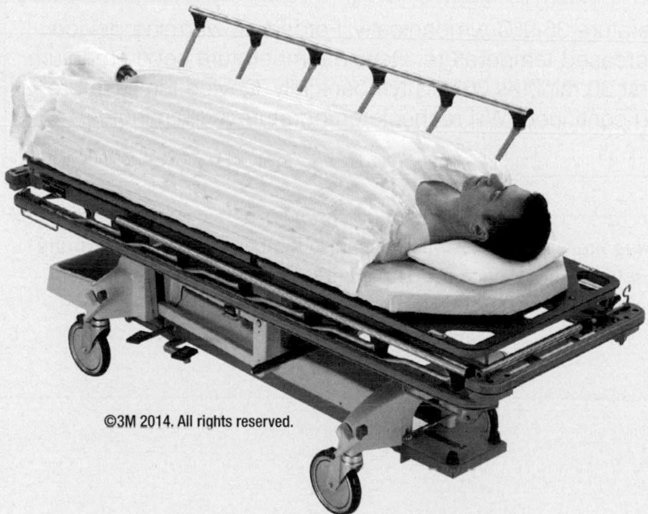

FIGURE 1 Forced-air blanket on patient, plastic side up, with air hose inlet at foot of bed. (The photograph is reproduced herein with permission. © 3M 2014. All rights reserved.)

(continued)

SKILL 6-6 APPLYING A FORCED-WARM AIR DEVICE continued

ACTION	RATIONALE
7. Securely insert air hose into inlet. Place a lightweight fabric blanket over the forced-air blanket, according to manufacturer's instructions. Turn the machine on and adjust temperature of air to desired effect.	Air hose must be properly inserted to ensure that it will not fall out. Blanket will help keep warmed air near the patient. Adjust air temperature, depending on desired patient temperature. If blanket is being used to maintain an already stable temperature, it may be turned down lower than if needed to raise patient's temperature.
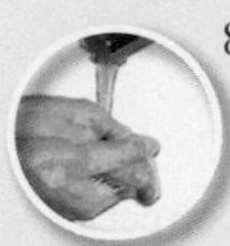 8. Remove PPE, if used. Perform hand hygiene.	Removing PPE properly reduces the risk for infection transmission and contamination of other items. Hand hygiene prevents transmission of microorganisms.
9. **Monitor the patient's temperature at least every 30 minutes while using the forced-air device. If rewarming a patient with hypothermia, do not raise the temperature more than 1°C/hour to prevent a rapid vasodilation effect.**	Monitoring the patient's temperature ensures that the patient does not experience too rapid a rise in body temperature, resulting in vasodilation.
10. Discontinue use of the forced-air device once patient's temperature is adequate and the patient can maintain the temperature without assistance.	Forced-air device is not needed once the patient is warm and stable enough to maintain temperature.
11. Remove device and clean according to agency policy and manufacturer's instructions.	Proper care of equipment helps to maintain function of the device.

EVALUATION

The expected outcome is met when the patient's temperature returns to the normal range of 97.7°F to 99.5°F (36.5°C to 37.5°C) and the patient is able to maintain this temperature; skin is warm; and patient is free from shivering.

DOCUMENTATION

Guidelines

Document the patient's temperature and the route used for measurement. Record that the forced-air warming device was applied to the patient. Document appearance of the skin and that the patient did not experience any adverse effects from the warming device. Record that the patient's temperature was monitored every 30 minutes, as well as the actual temperature after 30 minutes.

Sample Documentation

<u>4/23/15</u> 1440 Patient's temperature 35.9°C tympanically. Forced-air warming device applied to patient due to decreased temperature. Device temperature set on medium. Patient's temperature after first 30 minutes 36.4°C tympanically. Device temperature setting decreased to low and continued. Will recheck temperature in 30 minutes.

—*J. Grabbs, RN*

UNEXPECTED SITUATIONS AND ASSOCIATED INTERVENTIONS

- *Patient's temperature is increasing more than 1°C/hour:* Decrease temperature of air-warming device. If air is down to lowest setting, turn device off. If patient's temperature increases too rapidly, it can lead to a vasodilation effect that will cause the patient to become hypotensive.

ENHANCE YOUR UNDERSTANDING

FOCUSING ON PATIENT CARE: DEVELOPING CLINICAL REASONING

Consider the case scenarios at the beginning of the chapter as you answer the following questions to enhance your understanding and apply what you have learned.

QUESTIONS

1. In Josie's medical record there is an order for a prophylactic antibiotic to be given "on call to the OR," which means the nurse is to administer the prescribed medication after receiving the phone call to send Josie to the OR. However, the phone call comes during a busy period, and the nurse realizes that Josie has been transported down to the preoperative holding area without receiving her dose of prophylactic antibiotics. What should the nurse do?
2. After her surgery, Ms. Kelly rates her pain as 8 of 10. The nurse administers the ordered pain medication. Fifteen minutes later, Ms. Kelly is now rating her pain as 9 of 10 and is beginning to writhe with pain. She has no more ordered pain medication for another hour. What should the nurse do?
3. Dorothy Gibbs returns from surgery with a core temperature of 95.4°F (35.2°C), blood pressure of 128/72 mm Hg, and pulse of 60 beats per minute. Her skin is pale and cool to the touch. A forced-air warming device is placed on Ms. Gibbs, and the nurse turns the warmer to the highest heat setting. An hour later, the nurse takes Ms. Gibbs' vital signs. Her tympanic temperature is 37.8°C (100.0°F), her blood pressure is 82/48 mm Hg, and her pulse is 100 beats per minute. What should the nurse do?

You can find suggested answers after the Bibliography at the end of this chapter.

INTEGRATED CASE STUDY CONNECTION

The case studies in the back of the book are designed to focus on integrating concepts. Refer to the following case studies to enhance your understanding of the concepts related to the skills in this chapter.

- Basic Case Studies: Tiffany Jones, page 1064; Kate Townsend, page 1073; Tula Stillwater, page 1075.
- Intermediate Case Studies: Jason Brown, page 1083.
- Advanced Case Studies: Robert Espinoza, page 1097.

TAYLOR SUITE RESOURCES

Explore these additional resources to enhance learning for this chapter:

- NCLEX-Style Questions and other resources on thePoint, http://thePoint.lww.com/Lynn4e
- *Skill Checklists for Taylor's Clinical Nursing Skills,* 4e
- *Taylor's Video Guide to Clinical Nursing Skills:* Perioperative Nursing
- *Fundamentals of Nursing:* Chapter 29, Perioperative Nursing

Bibliography

Ackley, B.J., & Ladwig, G.B. (2011). *Nursing diagnosis handbook* (9th ed.). St. Louis: Mosby/Elsevier.

Alexander-Magalee, M. (2013). Mechanical and pharmacologic prophylaxis for DVT. *OR Nurse 7*(1), 45–47. American College of Surgeons (ACS) Annual Clinical Congress, 2012. *New respiratory care program suggests promise in decreasing pulmonary complications in surgical patients.* Available at http://www.facs.org/clincon2012/press/mcaneny.html.

American Society of Anesthesiologists Task Force on Acute Pain Management. (2012). Practice guidelines for acute pain management in the perioperative setting: An updated report by the American Society of Anesthesiologists Task Force on Acute Pain Management. *Anesthesiology, 116*(2), 248–273.

American Society of Anesthesiologists Task Force on Postanesthetic Care. (2013). Practice guidelines for postanesthetic care: A report by the American Society of Anesthesiologists Task Force on Postanesthetic Care. *Anesthesiology, 118*(2), 291–307.

American Society of Anesthesiologists. (2011). Practice guidelines for preoperative fasting and the use of pharmacologic agents to reduce the risk of pulmonary aspiration: Application to healthy patients undergoing elective procedures: An updated report by the American Society of Anesthesiologists Committee on Standards and Practice Parameters. *Anesthesiology, 114*(3), 495–511.

Association of periOperative Registered Nurses (AORN). (2011a). Recommended practices for perioperative nursing. In: Conner, R., Retzlaff, K., Brusco, J., et al. (Eds.). *2011 AORN perioperative standards and recommended practices.* Denver, CO: AORN, Inc.

Association of Perioperative Registered Nurses (AORN). (2011b). Recommended practices for perioperative nursing. Preoperative patient skin antisepsis. In: Conner, R., Retzlaff, K., Brusco, J., et al. (Eds.). *2011 AORN perioperative standards and recommended practices.* Denver, CO: AORN, Inc., p. 361–379.

Association of Perioperative Registered Nurses (AORN). (2011c). AORN guidance statement: Preoperative patient care in the ambulatory surgery setting. In: Conner, R., Retzlaff, K., Brusco, J., et al. (Eds.). *2011 AORN perioperative standards and recommended practices.* Denver, CO: AORN, Inc., p. 599–604.

Association of Perioperative Registered Nurses (AORN). (2011d). AORN guidance statement: Postoperative patient care in the ambulatory surgery setting. In: Conner, R., Retzlaff, K., Brusco, J., et al. (Eds.). *2011 AORN perioperative standards and recommended practices.* Denver, CO: AORN, Inc., p. 592–598.

Boltz, M., Capezuti, E., Fulmer, T., et al. (Eds.) (2012). *Evidence-based geriatric nursing protocols for best practice* (4th ed.). New York: Springer Publishing Company.

Bulechek, G.M, Butcher, H.K., Dochterman, J.M., et al. (Eds.). (2013). *Nursing interventions classification (NIC)* (6th ed.). St. Louis: Mosby Elsevier.

Carlson, D.S., & Pfadt, E. (2012). Preventing deep vein thrombosis in perioperative patients. *OR Nurse, 6*(5), 14–21.

Franson, H.E. (2010). Postoperative patient-controlled analgesia in the pediatric population: A literature review. *American Association of Nurse Anesthetists Journal, 78*(5), 374–378.

Grossman, S., & Porth, C.M. (2014). *Porth's pathophysiology: concepts of altered health states.* (9th ed.). Philadelphia: Wolters Kluwer Health/Lippincott Williams & Wilkins.

Herr, K., Coyne, P., Key, T., et al. (2006). Pain assessment in the nonverbal patient: Position statement with clinical practice recommendations. *Pain Management Nursing, 7*(2), 44–52.

Hicks, R.W., Hernandez, J., & Wanzer, L.J. (2012). Perioperative pharmacology: Patient-controlled analgesia. *AORN Journal, 95*(2), 255–262.

Hinkle, J.L., & Cheever, K.H. (2014). *Brunner & Suddarth's textbook of medical-surgical nursing* (13th ed.). Philadelphia: Wolters Kluwer Health/Lippincott Williams & Wilkins.

Hogan-Quigley, B., Palm, M.L., & Bickley, L. (2012). *Bates' nursing guide to physical examination and history taking.* Philadelphia: Wolters Kluwer Health/Lippincott Williams & Wilkins.

Jarvis, C. (2012). *Physical examination & health assessment.* (6th ed.). St. Louis: Saunders/Elsevier.

The Joint Commission. (2014a). *National patient safety goals.* Available at http://www.jointcommission.org/standards_information/npsgs.aspx.

The Joint Commission. (2014b). *Universal protocol for preventing wrong site, wrong procedure, wrong person surgery.* Available at http://www.jointcommission.org/standards_information/up.aspx.

Kamel, C., McGahan, L., Polisena, J., et al. (2012). Preoperative skin antiseptic preparations for preventing surgical site infections: A systematic review. *Infection Control and Hospital Epidemiology, 33*(6), 608–617.

Kyle, T., & Carman, S. (2013). *Essentials of pediatric nursing* (2nd ed.). Philadelphia: Wolters Kluwer Health/Lippincott Williams & Wilkins.

Lawrence, V., Cornell, J., & Smetana, G. (2006). Strategies to reduce postoperative pulmonary complications after noncardiothoracic surgery: Systematic review for the American College of Physicians. *Annals of Internal Medicine, 144*(8), 596–608.

Lipke, V.L., & Hyott, A.S. (2010). Reducing surgical site infections by bundling multiple risk reduction strategies and active surveillance. *AORN Journal, 92*(3), 288–296.

Massey, R. (2012). Return of bowel sounds indicating an end of postoperative ileus: Is it time to cease this long-standing nursing tradition? *MEDSURGNursing, 21*(3), 146–150.

Moorhead, S., Johnson, M., Maas, M.L., et al. (Eds.). (2013). *Nursing outcomes classification (NOC).* (5th ed.). St. Louis: Mosby Elsevier.

NANDA-I International. (2012). *Nursing diagnoses: Definitions & classification 2012–2014.* West Sussex, UK: Wiley-Blackwell.

Perry, S.E., Hockenberry, M.J., Lowdermilk, D.L., et al. (2010). *Maternal child nursing care* (4th ed.). Maryland Heights, MO: Mosby/Elsevier.

Restrepo, R.D., Wettstein, R., Wittnebel, L., et al. (2011). AARC clinical practice guideline. Incentive spirometry: 2011. *Respiratory Care, 56*(10), 1600–1604.

Rothrock, J. (2011). *Alexander's care of the patient in surgery* (14th ed.). St. Louis: Mosby Elsevier.

Sajid, M.S., Desai, M., Morris, R.W., et al. (2012). Knee length versus thigh length graduated compression stockings for prevention of deep vein thrombosis in postoperative surgical patients. *Cochrane Database of Systematic Reviews,* Issue 5. Art. No.: CD007162. DOI: 10.1002/14651858.CD007162.pub2.

Shippee-Rice, R.V., Fetzer, S.J., Long J.V. (2012). *Gerioperative nursing care.* New York: Springer.

Smith Collins, A. (2011). Postoperative nausea and vomiting in adults: Implications for critical care. *Critical Care Nurse, 31*(6), 36–45.

Sullivan, J.M. (2011). Caring for older adults after surgery. *Nursing, 41*(4), 48–51.

Tabloski, P. (2010). *Gerontological nursing* (2nd ed.). Upper Saddle River, NJ: Pearson.

Taylor, C., Lillis, C., & Lynn, P. (2015). *Fundamentals of nursing.* (8th ed.). Philadelphia: Wolters Kluwer Health/Lippincott Williams & Wilkins.

Tinsley, M.H., & Barone, C.P. (2012). Preventing postoperative nausea and vomiting. *OR Nurse, 6*(3), 18–26.

Topolovec-Vranic, J., Canzian, S., Innis, J., et al. (2010). Patient satisfaction and documentation of pain assessments and management after implementing the Adult Nonverbal Pain Scale. *American Journal of Critical Care, 19*(4), 345–354.

Ward, C.W. (2012). Fast track program to prevent postoperative ileus. *NEDSURGNursing, 21*(4), 214–232.

SUGGESTED ANSWERS FOR FOCUSING ON PATIENT CARE: DEVELOPING CLINICAL REASONING

1. Preoperative medications may be ordered for administration before transfer to the preoperative holding area or for administration in the preoperative holding area. The nurse needs to call the nursing staff in the preoperative holding area. The nurse should explain the circumstances, identify the ordered medication, and state that the medication was not administered. The nurse should also notify the primary care provider, in this case the surgeon, of the missed medication dose. It is important that the appropriate health care personnel are aware of the missing dose of medication, so that appropriate action can be taken to ensure the patient receives the required medication to prevent intraoperative or postoperative complications.
2. The nurse needs to consider the onset of action and peak effect of the administered medication. If the appropriate time has not lapsed for the medication to take effect, the nurse should provide further explanation and reassurance to the patient. The nurse should initiate additional nonpharmacologic interventions to aid in pain management (refer to Chapter 10, Comfort). If the pain persists, the nurse should perform a complete pain assessment (refer to Chapter 10, Comfort). In addition, the nurse should assess for other postoperative complications. Pain can be a clue to other problems, such as hemorrhage. The nurse should notify the primary care provider of the initial assessment findings, information regarding analgesics administered, nonpharmacologic interventions, and the patient's response to interventions. In addition, some patients do not obtain adequate relief from the initial analgesic prescribed and require a change in analgesics to achieve adequate pain management.
3. Monitor the patient's temperature at least every 30 minutes while using the forced-air device. If rewarming a patient with hypothermia, do not raise temperature more than 1°C/hour to prevent a rapid vasodilation effect. The nurse should not have waited 60 minutes to recheck the patient's temperature. Ms. Gibbs is experiencing the effects of rapid vasodilation, resulting in lowered blood pressure and increased heart rate. The nurse should discontinue the forced-air warming device. Assess the patient's cardiovascular and respiratory status. Notify the primary care provider of the assessment findings. Provide for the patient's safety; make sure the call bell is within reach and instruct the patient to remain in bed, to avoid a fall or other injury related to hypotension. Monitor the patient's vital signs at least every 30 minutes. Be prepared to reapply the forced-air heating device if the patient's temperature drops below prescribed limits.

UNIT

II

Promoting Healthy Physiologic Responses

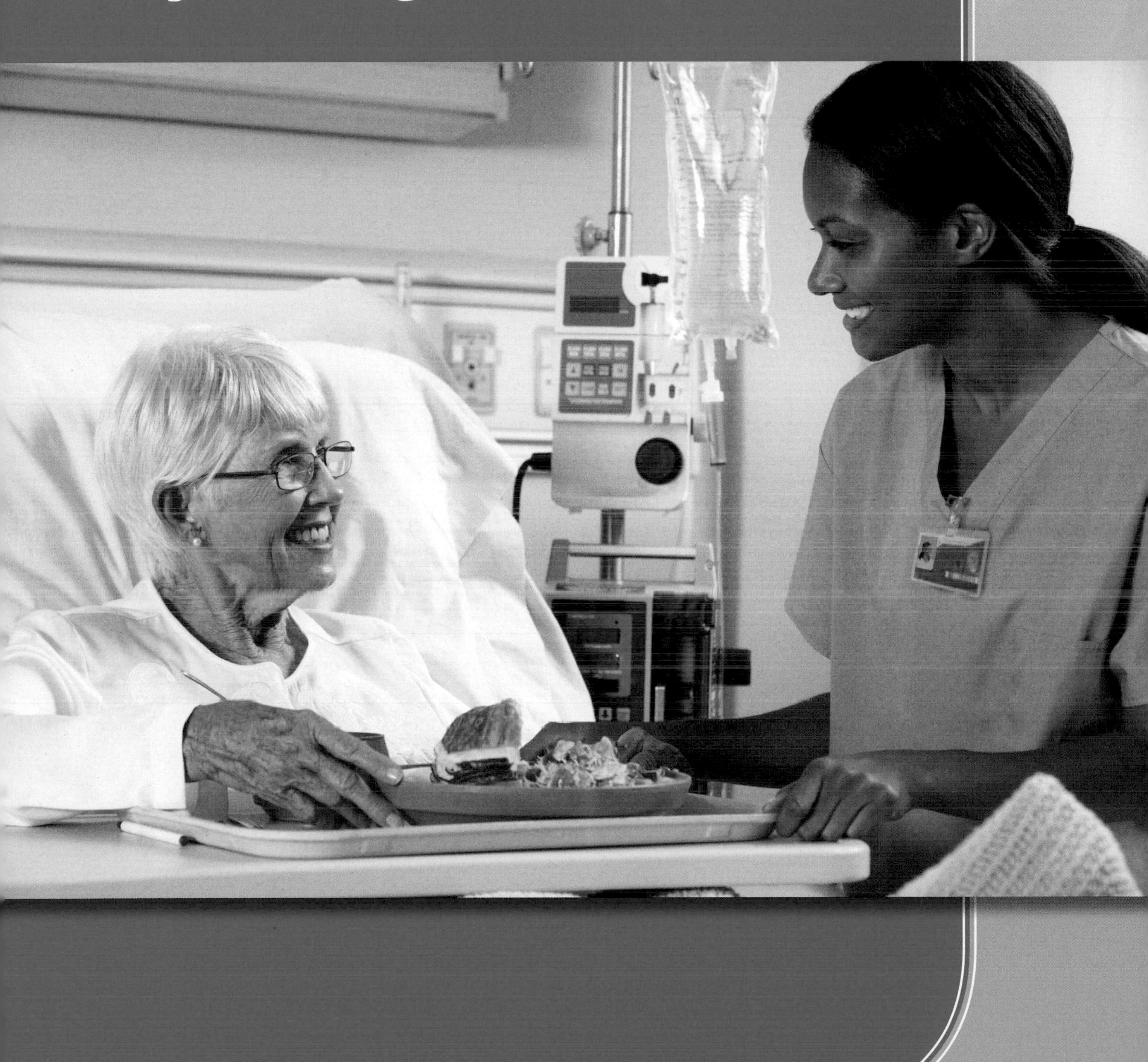

7 Hygiene

FOCUSING ON PATIENT CARE

This chapter will help you develop some of the skills related to hygiene necessary to care for the following patients:

DENASIA KERR, a 6-year-old who is on bed rest after surgery and needs her hair washed.

CINDY VORTEX, age 34, who is in a coma after a car accident and needs her contact lenses removed.

CARL SHEEN, age 76, who needs help cleaning his dentures.

Refer to Focusing on Patient Care: Developing Clinical Reasoning at the end of the chapter to apply what you learn.

LEARNING OBJECTIVES

After studying this chapter, you will be able to:

1. Assist with a shower or tub bath.
2. Provide a bed bath.
3. Assist with oral care.
4. Provide oral care for a dependent patient.
5. Provide denture care.
6. Remove contact lenses.
7. Shampoo a patient's hair in bed.
8. Assist with shaving.
9. Provide nail care.
10. Make an unoccupied bed.
11. Make an occupied bed.

KEY TERMS

caries: cavities of the teeth
dysphagia: inability to swallow or difficulty in swallowing
gingivitis: inflammation of the gingivae (gums)
halitosis: offensive breath
integument: skin
pediculosis: infestation with lice
plaque: transparent, adhesive coating on teeth consisting of mucin, carbohydrate, and bacteria
pyorrhea: extensive inflammation of the gums and alveolar tissues; synonym for periodontitis
tartar: hard deposit on the teeth near the gum line formed by plaque buildup and dead bacteria

Personal hygiene involves measures people take for personal cleanliness and grooming that promote physical and psychological well-being. Personal hygiene practices vary widely among people. The time of day one bathes and how often a person shampoos his or her hair or changes the bed linens are very individualized choices. It is important that the nurse carry out personal care for each patient conveniently and frequently enough to promote personal hygiene and wellness.

People who are well ordinarily are responsible for their own hygiene. In some cases, the nurse may provide teaching to assist a well person to develop personal hygiene habits he or she may lack. Acute and chronic illness, hospitalization, and institutionalization generally require modifications in hygiene practices. In these situations, the nurse helps the patient to continue sound hygiene practices and can teach the patient and family members, when necessary, about hygiene. When assisting with basic hygiene, it is important to respect individual patient preferences and give only the care that patients cannot, or should not, provide for themselves. This chapter covers skills that the nurse needs to promote hygiene, including bathing, skin care, oral care, removing dentures and contact lenses, shampooing hair, shaving, and changing bed linens. Fundamentals Review 7-1 outlines general skin care principles. Fundamentals Review 7-2 shows an example of a patient care flow sheet. Flow sheets are documentation tools used to record routine aspects of nursing care, and are often used to document hygiene-related interventions.

FUNDAMENTALS REVIEW 7-1

GENERAL SKIN CARE PRINCIPLES

- Assess the patient's skin daily.
- Cleanse the skin, when indicated, such as when soiled, using a no-rinse, pH-balanced cleanser.
- Avoid using soap and hot water; avoid excessive friction and scrubbing.
- Minimize skin exposure to moisture (incontinence, wound leakage); use a skin barrier product, as necessary.
- Use emollients.

(Adapted from Voegeli, D. (2010). Care or harm: Exploring essential components in skin care regimens. *British Journal of Nursing, 19*(13), 812, 814, 816, 818–819; Wound Ostomy and Continence Nurses Society, 2003, as cited in Voegeli, 2010.)

FUNDAMENTALS REVIEW 7-2

PATIENT CARE FLOW SHEET

Esposito, Tomas Gender: **Male**, DOB: **1/16/1967 (46y)** Height: **72 in** Weight: **185 lb** MRN: **984521** Allergies: Penicillin
Primary Adm Dx: Pneumonia Location: Mercy Hospital Rm: 412 Contact Precaution: Standard
Adm Provider: Tom Rankle, Admitting Adm On: 11/29/2013 14:45 (3 day(s)) Adv Directive: Full Code

Patient Information | Assessment | ADLs | Notes | Nursing Dx | Orders | MAR | I/O | Vital Signs | Diagnostics | Flowsheet

Monday, December 2, 2013 15:56:35

Back To Current Assessment

Charted at 12/2/2013 14:45 By: Tom Rankle, Admitting

ADL Assessment

- ✓ Bed mobility
  Description of assessment activity: Limited assistance
- ✓ Transfer
  Description of assessment activity: Limited assistance
- ✓ Walking
  Description of assessment activity: Supervision needed
- ✓ Dressing
  Description of assessment activity: Extensive assistance
- ✓ Eating
  Description of assessment activity: Limited assistance
- ✓ Toilet use
  Description of assessment activity: Extensive assistance
- ✓ Personal hygiene
  Description of assessment activity: Limited assistance
- ✓ Bathing
  Description of assessment activity: Total dependence

Diet Consumption

- 25%
- 50%
- ✓ 75%
- 100%

Diet Assessment

- ☐ Increased appetite
- ✓ Decreased appetite
- ☐ Aspiration risk
- ☐ Difficulty chewing
- ☐ Dysphagia
- ☐ Weight gain
- ☐ Weight loss

Communication

- ✓ Short-term memory intact
- ✓ Long-term memory intact
- ✓ Has ability to understand
- ✓ Has ability to make self-understood

Speech Assessment

- ☐ Rate
- ☐ Rhythm
- ✓ Content

Speech clear and appropriate.

- ☐ Loudness
- ☐ Fluency
- ☐ Quantity
- ☐ Articulation
- ☐ Pattern

Mood and Behavior

- ☐ Verbal expression of distress
- ☐ Loss of interest
- ☐ Sleep pattern disturbance
- ☐ Apathetic
- ☐ Anxious
- ☐ Sad appearance
- ✓ Appropriate for patient

Notes:

How does the resident make decisions about ADLs

Patient requires direction to complete personal hygiene ADLs.

SKILL 7-1 ASSISTING WITH A SHOWER OR TUB BATH

A shower may be the preferred method of bathing for patients who are ambulatory and able to tolerate the activity. Tub baths may be an option, particularly in long-term care or other community-based settings, depending on facility policy. Make any necessary adaptations for individual patients. For example, if the patient is confused and becomes agitated as a result of overstimulation when bathing, reduce the stimuli. Turn down the lights and play soft music and/or warm the room before taking the patient into it (Johnson, 2011). Box 7-1 outlines possible measures to implement to meet the bathing needs of patients with dementia.

Bathing is performed in a matter-of-fact and dignified manner. If this approach is followed, patients generally do not find care by a person of the opposite gender to be offensive or embarrassing.

Box 7-1 MEETING THE BATHING NEEDS OF PATIENTS WITH DEMENTIA

- Shift the focus of the interaction from the "task of bathing" to the needs and abilities of the patient. Focus on comfort, safety, autonomy, and self-esteem, in addition to cleanliness.
- Individualize patient care. Consult the patient, the patient's record, family members, and other caregivers to determine patient preferences.
- Consider what can be learned from the behaviors associated with dementia about the needs and preferences of the patient. A patient's behavior may be an expression of unmet needs; unwillingness to participate may be a response to uncomfortable water temperatures or levels of sound or light in the room.
- Ensure privacy and warmth.
- Consider other methods for bathing. Showers and tub baths are not the only options in bathing. Towel baths, washing under clothes, and bathing "body sections" one day at a time are other possible options.
- Maintain a relaxed demeanor. Use calming language. Use one-step commands. Try to determine phrases and terms the patient understands in relation to bathing and make use of them. Offer frequent reassurance.
- Encourage independence. Using hand-over-hand or a guided hand technique to cue the person regarding the purpose of the interaction can allow patients to perform some activities for themselves.
- Explore the need for routine analgesia before bathing. Move limbs carefully and be aware of signs of discomfort during bathing.
- Wash the face and hair at the end of the bath or at a separate time. Water dripping in the face and having a wet head are often the most upsetting parts of the bathing process for people with dementia.

(Adapted from Jablonski, R.A., Therrien, B., & Kolanowski, A. (2011). No more fighting and biting during mouth care: Applying the theoretical constructs of threat perception to clinical practice. *Research and Theory for Nursing Practice: An International Journal, 25*(3), 163–175; Johnson, R.H. (2011). Practical care: Creative strategies for bathing. *Nursing & Residential Care, 13*(8), 392–394; Keefe, S. (2010). Bath safety and dementia. *Advance for Long-term Care Management*. Available http://long-term-care.advanceweb.com/Features/Articles/Bath-Safety-and-Dementia.aspx; Papa, K.S. (2011). A dignified bathing experience. *Advance for Long-Term Care Management, 14*(6), 16.)

DELEGATION CONSIDERATIONS

The implementation of a shower or tub bath may be delegated to nursing assistive personnel (NAP) or unlicensed assistive personnel (UAP), as well as to licensed practical/vocational nurses (LPN/LVNs). The decision to delegate must be based on careful analysis of the patient's needs and circumstances, as well as the qualifications of the person to whom the task is being delegated. Refer to the Delegation Guidelines in Appendix A.

EQUIPMENT

- Personal hygiene supplies (deodorant, lotion, and others)
- Skin-cleaning agent
- Emollient and skin barrier, as indicated
- Towels and washcloths
- Robe and slippers or nonskid socks
- Gown or pajamas, or clothing
- Laundry bag
- Shower or tub chair, as needed
- Nonsterile gloves, as indicated
- Additional PPE, as indicated

ASSESSMENT

Assess the patient's knowledge of hygiene practices and bathing preferences: frequency, time of day, and type of hygiene products. Assess for any physical-activity limitations. Assess the patient's ability to bathe him- or herself. Assess the patient's skin for dryness, redness, or areas of breakdown, and gather any other appropriate supplies that may be needed as a result of the assessment.

NURSING DIAGNOSIS

Determine the related factors for the nursing diagnoses based on the patient's current status. Appropriate nursing diagnoses may include:

- Bathing Self-Care Deficit
- Risk for Infection
- Risk for Impaired Skin Integrity
- Deficient Knowledge

OUTCOME IDENTIFICATION AND PLANNING

The expected outcome to achieve when assisting with a shower or tub bath is that the patient will be clean and fresh, and without injury. Other outcomes that may be appropriate include the following: patient regains feelings of control by assisting with the bath; patient verbalizes positive body image; and patient demonstrates understanding about the need for cleanliness.

IMPLEMENTATION

ACTION	RATIONALE
1. Review the patient's health record for any limitations in physical activity. Check presence of medical order for clearing the patient to shower, if required by facility policy.	Identifying limitations prevents patient discomfort and injury. In some settings, a medical order is required for showering.
2. Check to see that the bathroom is available, clean, and safe. Make sure showers and tubs have mats or nonskid strips to prevent patients from falling. Place a mat or towel on floor in front of shower or tub. Put a shower or tub chair in place, as appropriate. Place 'occupied' sign on door of room.	A clean bathroom prevents transmission of microorganisms. Mats and nonskid materials prevent patients from slipping and falling. Having a place for a weak or physically disabled patient to sit in a shower prevents falls; warm water could cause vasodilation and pooling of blood in lower extremities, contributing to lightheadedness or dizziness. Use of sign allows others to be aware of use of room and ensures patient privacy.
3. Gather necessary hygienic and toiletry items, and linens. Place within easy reach of shower or tub.	Bringing everything to the bathing location conserves time and energy. Arranging items nearby is convenient, saves time, and avoids unnecessary reaching and possible falls.
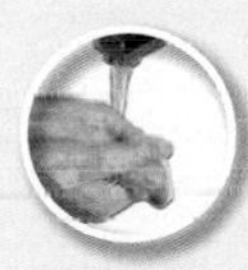 4. Perform hand hygiene.	Hand hygiene prevents the spread of microorganisms.
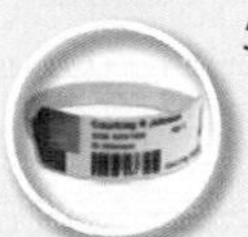 5. Identify the patient. Discuss the procedure with the patient and assess the patient's ability to assist in the bathing process, as well as personal hygiene preferences.	Identifying the patient ensures the right patient receives the intervention and helps prevent errors. Discussion promotes reassurance and provides knowledge about the procedure. Dialogue encourages patient participation and allows for individualized nursing care.
6. Assist patient to bathroom to void or defecate, if appropriate.	Voiding or defecating before the bath lessens the likelihood that the bath will be interrupted, because warm bath water may stimulate the urge to void.
7. Assist the patient to put on a robe and slippers or nonskid socks. Cover IV access site(s) according to facility policy.	This ensures the patient's privacy, prevents chilling, and decreases the risk for slipping and fallings. Coverage of IV site prevents loosening of dressings from exposure to moisture, and maintains integrity of IV access.
8. Assist the patient to the shower or tub.	This prevents accidental falls.
9. Close the curtains around the shower or tub, as appropriate, and close the door to the bathroom. Adjust the room temperature, if necessary. Shower: Turn shower on. Check to see that the water temperature is safe and comfortable. Tub: Fill tub halfway with water. Check to see that the water temperature is safe and comfortable. **Water temperature should be 100°F to less than 120°F to 125 °F.**	This ensures the patient's privacy and lessens the risk for loss of body heat during the bath. Adjusting the water temperature to 100°F to less than 120°F to 125°F decreases risk of burns and drying of the skin. The lower temperature is recommended for children and adults over 65 years of age (Burn Foundation, 2012). Warm water is relaxing, stimulates circulation, and provides for more effective cleansing.
10. Explain the use of the call device and ensure that it is within reach of the shower or tub.	Use of the call device allows the patient to call for help if necessary.

(continued)

SKILL 7-1 ASSISTING WITH A SHOWER OR TUB BATH continued

ACTION	RATIONALE
11. Put on gloves, as indicated. Help the patient get in and out of the shower or tub, as necessary. Use safety bars. For a tub: Have the patient grasp the handrails at the side of the tub, or place a chair at the side of the tub. The patient sits on the chair and eases to the edge of the tub. After putting both feet into the tub, have the patient reach to the opposite side and ease down into the tub. The patient may kneel first in the tub and then sit in it.	Gloves are required if contact with blood or body fluids is anticipated. Gloves prevent the transmission of microorganisms. This prevents slipping and falling.
12. If necessary, use a hydraulic lift, when available, to lower patients who are unable to maneuver safely or completely bear their own weight. Some community-based settings have walk-in tubs available.	This prevents slipping and falling and prevents strain and injury to patients and nurses.
13. Adjust water temperature, if appropriate, based on patient preference (Figure 1). Keep room door unlocked. Remain in room with patient to offer assistance, as appropriate. If assistance is needed with bathing, put on gloves. Otherwise, check on patient every 5 minutes. **Never leave young children or confused patients alone in the bathroom.**	These actions promote safety. Health personnel should be able to enter with ease if the patient needs help. Gloves are required if contact with blood or body fluids is anticipated. Gloves prevent the transmission of microorganisms.
14. Assist patient out of shower or tub when bathing is complete. Obtain the assistance of additional personnel, as appropriate. Use safety bars. For a tub: Drain the water from the tub. Have the patient grasp the handrails at the side of the tub. Assist the patient to the edge of the tub. Have the patient ease to a chair placed at the side of the tub, then remove feet out of tub. The patient may kneel first in the tub and then move to the side of the tub.	This prevents slipping and falling. Use of additional personnel prevents strain and injury to patients and nurses.
15. If necessary, use a hydraulic lift, when available, to raise patients who are unable to maneuver safely or completely bear their own weight.	This prevents slipping and falling and prevents strain and injury to patients and nurses.
16. Put on gloves, as indicated. Assist the patient with drying, application of emollients, and dressing, as appropriate or necessary. Remove cover from IV access site.	Gloves are required if contact with blood or body fluids is anticipated. Gloves prevent the transmission of microorganisms. Prevents chilling and promotes patient comfort. Use of emollients is recommended to restore and maintain skin integrity (Voegeli, 2010).
17. Remove gloves, if used. Assist patient to room (Figure 2) and into a position of comfort.	Removing gloves properly reduces risk for infection transmission and contamination of other items. Promotes patient comfort and safety.

FIGURE 1 Adjusting water temperature, based on patient preference.

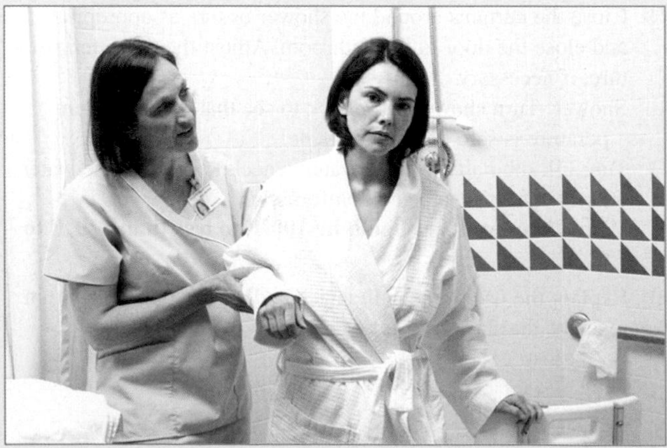

FIGURE 2 Assisting patient to room.

ACTION	RATIONALE
18. Clean shower or tub according to facility policy. Dispose of soiled linens according to facility policy. Remove 'occupied' sign from door of bathroom.	Reduces risk for infection transmission and contamination of other items. Allows others to make use of room.
19. Perform hand hygiene.	Hand hygiene prevents the spread of microorganisms.

EVALUATION

The expected outcomes are met when the patient is clean; demonstrates some feeling of control in his or her care; verbalizes an improved body image; and verbalizes the importance of cleanliness.

DOCUMENTATION

Guidelines

Record any significant observations and communication. Document the condition of the patient's skin. Record the procedure, amount of assistance given, and patient participation. Document the application of skin care products, such as an emollient.

Sample Documentation

<u>7/14/15</u> 1030 Shower provided with minimal assistance. Skin intact. Patient states improved sense of cleanliness and increased comfort.

—*C. Stone, RN*

UNEXPECTED SITUATIONS AND ASSOCIATED INTERVENTIONS

- *Patient becomes chilled during bath:* If the room temperature is adjustable, increase temperature. Provide additional assistance to dry and dress quickly, to decrease chilling.
- *The patient becomes excessively fatigued during the bath process:* Allow for rest period sitting down after walking to bathing room and/or completion of bath, before returning to room. Assist patient to and from bath in wheelchair, to conserve energy. Schedule bath after rest period or nap.

SPECIAL CONSIDERATIONS

General Considerations

- Incontinent patients require special attention to perineal care. Patients with urinary or fecal incontinence are at risk for perineal skin damage. This damage is related to moisture, changes in the pH of the skin, overgrowth of bacteria and infection of the skin, and erosion of perineal skin from friction on moist skin. Skin care for these patients should include measures to reduce overhydration (excess exposure to moisture), reduce contact with ammonia and bacteria, and reduce friction. Remove soil and irritants from the skin during routine hygiene, as well as cleansing, when the skin becomes exposed to irritants. Avoid using soap and excessive force for cleaning. The use of perineal skin cleansers, moisturizers, and moisture barriers is recommended for skin care for the incontinent patient. These products help promote healing and prevent further skin damage.

Infant and Child Considerations

- When bathing an infant or young child, have supplies within easy reach, and support or hold the child securely at all times to ensure safety.
- Never leave the child alone.

Older Adult Considerations

- Check the temperature of the water carefully before bathing an older patient, because sensitivity to temperature may be impaired in older people.
- An older, continent patient may not require a bath every day. If dry skin is a problem, water and skin lotion or bath oil may be used on alternate days. Do not use bath oil in tub water, as it can cause tub surfaces to become slippery.

Home Care Considerations

- Evaluate the safety of the bathing area in the home. Tub mats, adhesive strips, grab bars, and shower stools can help prevent falls.
- Instruct patients to apply emollients, lotions, or oils after leaving tub or shower to prevent slipping and falling.

(continued)

SKILL 7-1 ASSISTING WITH A SHOWER OR TUB BATH continued

EVIDENCE FOR PRACTICE ▶

BATHING PEOPLE WITH DEMENTIA

Bathing patients with dementia can be challenging. People with dementia often respond negatively to bathing and develop resistive behaviors related to bathing. This patient population is increasing in size with the aging of society. There is a need to ensure care providers are able to meet the needs and preserve the dignity of patients who have lost the ability to initiate and complete activities of daily living (ADLs), including hygiene-related activities.

Related Research

Gaspard, G., & Cox. L. (2012). Bathing people with dementia: When education is not enough. *Journal of Gerontological Nursing, 38*(9), 43–51.

This qualitative study describes health care assistants' (HCA) perceptions and experiences related to bathing people with dementia in residential care settings. Data were collected from three focus groups with 18 HCA participants from 12 different residential care facilities. HCAs constructed two definitions of a successful bath, which informed their choice of bathing strategies. Three themes emerged from the data analysis in regard to their bathing strategies: I Know You, I Am All Alone, and I Am Not Prepared. These data were used in the development of a framework to guide gerontologic nurses in creating and supporting the opportunity for successful bathing.

Relevance for Nursing Practice

This study suggests that successful bathing is not solely reliant on the skills and abilities of the HCA, but also includes the need for a supportive system. Nurses ought to engage in the deliberate practice of sharing a person-centered vision, providing both professional and emotional support, as well as enhancing HCAs' knowledge. A significant role exists for gerontologic nurses at all levels in the health care system to improve bathing experiences of people with dementia and their care providers.

Refer to thePoint for additional research on related nursing topics.

WATCH & LEARN SKILL 7-2 PROVIDING A BED BATH

Some patients must remain in bed as a part of their therapeutic regimen, but can still bathe themselves. Other patients are not on bed rest, but require total or partial assistance with bathing in bed due to physical limitations, such as fatigue or limited range of motion. A bed bath may be considered a partial bed bath if the patient is well enough to perform most of the bath, and the nurse needs to assist with washing areas that the patient cannot reach easily. A partial bath may also refer to bathing only those body parts that absolutely have to be cleaned, such as the perineal area, and any soiled body parts. Many of the bedside skin-cleaning products available today do not require rinsing. After cleaning the body part, dry it thoroughly. See Table 7-1 for a summary of common cleaning products. Perform bathing in a matter-of-fact and dignified manner. If this approach is followed, patients generally do not find care by a person of the opposite gender to be offensive or embarrassing. This skill reviews providing a bed bath using water and cleanser. Refer to the Skill Variation at the end of the skill for guidelines to use a disposable bathing system. Giving a Bath Using a Disposable Self-contained Bathing System.

Make any necessary adaptations for individual patients. For example, if the patient is confused and becomes agitated as a result of overstimulation when bathing, reduce the stimuli. Turn down the lights and play soft music and/or warm the room before giving the patient a bath (Johnson, 2011). Box 7-1 in Skill 7-1 outlines possible measures to implement to meet the bathing needs of patients with dementia.

Table 7-1 BEDSIDE CLEANING AND SKIN-CARE PRODUCTS

PRODUCT	DESCRIPTION
Bathing cloths	Premoistened, pH-balanced, microwaveable, disposable cloths for rinse-free skin cleaning and moisturizing. Each package provides one complete bath using 8 to 10 cloths.
Bathing wipes	Packaged dry cloths. Adding water to the cloths causes them to foam, providing rinse-free skin pH-balanced cleaning. Cloths are in a resealable package for multiple uses.
No-rinse body wash and shampoo	No-rinse, concentrated skin cleanser and moisturizer. Mix with water, apply with a cloth, lather, and dry.
Body foam	Foam cleanser and moisturizer to be used as a body wash, no-rinse shampoo, and perineal cleanser. Pump bottle dispenses foam to be applied with a cloth.
Chlorhexidine gluconate	Reduces colonization of skin with pathogens. Chlorhexidine can be added to bath water, but is also available, and easier to use, in prepackaged impregnated cloths. Bathing with chlorhexidine may be used to reduce the incidence of hospital-acquired infections, such as central line-associated bloodstream infections and surgical site infections, as well as to reduce the acquisition of or decolonization with multidrug-resistant organisms (Ritz, et al., 2012; Sievert, et al., 2011).

DELEGATION CONSIDERATIONS

The implementation of a shower or tub bath may be delegated to nursing assistive personnel (NAP) or to unlicensed assistive personnel (UAP), as well as to licensed practical/vocational nurses (LPN/LVNs). The decision to delegate must be based on careful analysis of the patient's needs and circumstances, as well as the qualifications of the person to whom the task is being delegated. Refer to the Delegation Guidelines in Appendix A.

EQUIPMENT

- Washbasin and warm water
- Personal hygiene supplies (deodorant, lotion, and others)
- Skin-cleaning agent
- Emollient and skin barrier, as indicated
- Towels (2)
- Washcloths (2)
- Bath blanket
- Gown or pajamas
- Bedpan or urinal
- Laundry bag
- Nonsterile gloves; other PPE, as indicated

ASSESSMENT

Assess the patient's knowledge of hygiene practices and bathing preferences: frequency, time of day, and type of hygiene products. Assess for any physical activity limitations. Assess the patient's ability to bathe him- or herself. Allow the patient to do any part of the bath that he or she can do. For example, the patient may be able to wash the face, while the nurse does the rest. Assess the patient's skin for dryness, redness, or areas of breakdown, and gather any other appropriate supplies that may be needed as a result of the assessment.

NURSING DIAGNOSIS

Determine the related factors for the nursing diagnoses based on the patient's current status. Appropriate nursing diagnoses may include:

- Bathing Self Care Deficit
- Impaired Skin Integrity
- Risk for Infection
- Risk for Impaired Skin Integrity

OUTCOME IDENTIFICATION AND PLANNING

The expected outcome to achieve when giving a bed bath is that the patient will be clean and fresh. Other outcomes that may be appropriate include the following: patient regains feelings of control by assisting with the bath; patient verbalizes positive body image; and patient demonstrates understanding about the need for cleanliness.

(continued)

SKILL 7-2 PROVIDING A BED BATH continued

IMPLEMENTATION

ACTION	RATIONALE
1. Review the patient's health record for any limitations in physical activity.	Identifying limitations prevents patient discomfort and injury.
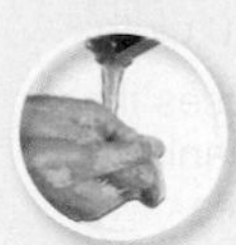 2. Perform hand hygiene and put on gloves and/or other PPE, if indicated.	Hand hygiene and PPE prevent the spread of microorganisms. PPE is required based on transmission precautions.
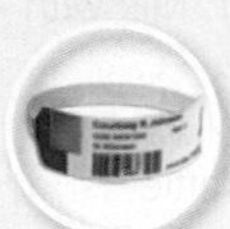 3. Identify the patient. Discuss the procedure with the patient and assess the patient's ability to assist in the bathing process, as well as personal hygiene preferences.	Identifying the patient ensures the right patient receives the intervention and helps prevent errors. Discussion promotes reassurance and provides knowledge about the procedure. Dialogue encourages patient participation and allows for individualized nursing care.
4. Assemble equipment on overbed table within reach.	Organization facilitates performance of the task.
5. Close the curtains around the bed and close the door to the room, if possible. Adjust the room temperature, if necessary.	This ensures the patient's privacy and lessens the risk for loss of body heat during the bath.
6. Adjust the bed to a comfortable working height; usually elbow height of the caregiver (VISN 8 Patient Safety Center, 2009).	Having the bed at the proper height prevents back and muscle strain.
7. Remove sequential compression devices and antiembolism stockings from lower extremities according to agency protocol.	Most manufacturers and agencies recommend removal of these devices before the bath to allow for assessment.
8. Put on gloves. Offer patient bedpan or urinal.	Gloves are necessary for potential contact with blood or body fluids. Voiding or defecating before the bath lessens the likelihood that the bath will be interrupted, because warm bath water may stimulate the urge to void.
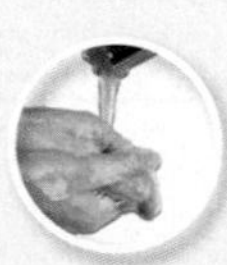 9. Remove gloves and perform hand hygiene.	Hand hygiene deters the spread of microorganisms.
10. Put on a clean pair of gloves. Lower side rail nearest to you and assist patient to side of bed where you will work. Have patient lie on his or her back.	Gloves prevent transmission of microorganisms. Having the patient positioned near the nurse and lowering the side rail prevent unnecessary stretching and twisting of muscles on the part of the nurse.
11. Loosen top covers and remove all except the top sheet. Place bath blanket over patient and then remove top sheet while patient holds bath blanket in place. If linen is to be reused, fold it over a chair. Place soiled linen in laundry bag. Take care to prevent linen from coming in contact with your clothing.	The patient is not exposed unnecessarily, and warmth is maintained. If a bath blanket is unavailable, the top sheet may be used in its place.
12. Remove patient's gown and keep bath blanket in place. If patient has an IV line and is not wearing a gown with snap sleeves, remove gown from other arm first. Lower the IV container and pass gown over the tubing and the container. **Rehang the container and check the drip rate.**	This provides uncluttered access during the bath and maintains warmth of the patient. IV fluids must be maintained at the prescribed rate.

ACTION	RATIONALE
13. **Raise side rails.** Fill basin with a sufficient amount of comfortably warm water (100°F to 120°F to 125°F). Add the skin cleanser, if appropriate, according to manufacturer's directions. Change, as necessary, throughout the bath. Lower side rail nearest to you when you return to the bedside to begin the bath.	Side rails maintain patient safety. Adjusting the water temperature to 100°F to less than 120°F to 125°F decreases risk of burns and drying of the skin. The lower temperature is recommended for children and adults over 65 years of age (Burn Foundation, 2012). Warm water is comfortable and relaxing for the patient. It also stimulates circulation and provides for more effective cleansing.
14. Put on gloves, if necessary. If desired, fold the washcloth like a mitt on your hand so that there are no loose ends (Figure 1, Figure 2, Figure 3).	Gloves are necessary if there is potential contact with blood or body fluids. Having loose ends of cloth drag across the patient's skin is uncomfortable. Loose ends cool quickly and feel cold to the patient.
15. Lay a towel across the patient's chest and on top of bath blanket.	This prevents chilling and keeps the bath blanket dry.
16. **With no cleanser on the washcloth, wipe one eye from the inner part of the eye, near the nose, to the outer part (Figure 4). Rinse or turn the cloth before washing the other eye.**	Soap is irritating to the eyes. Moving from the inner to the outer aspect of the eye prevents carrying debris toward the nasolacrimal duct. Rinsing or turning the washcloth prevents spreading organisms from one eye to the other.

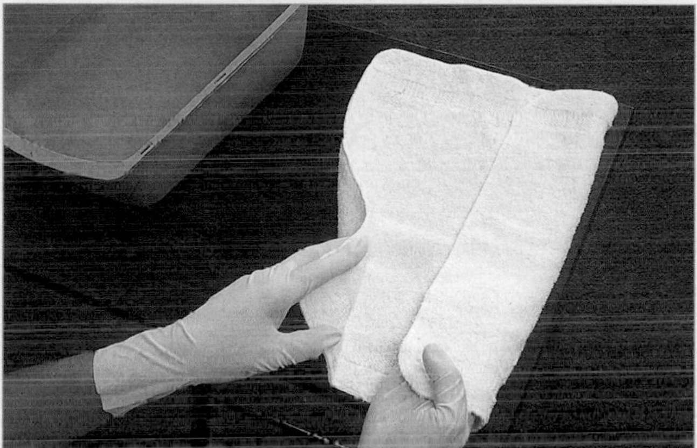

FIGURE 1 Folding washcloth in thirds around hand to make a bath mitt.

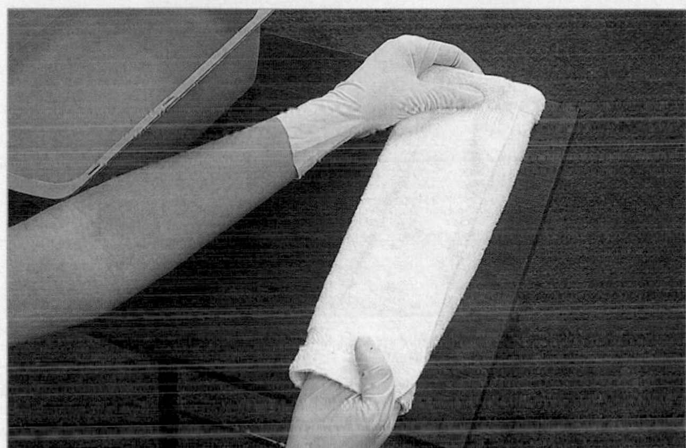

FIGURE 2 Straightening washcloth before folding into mitt.

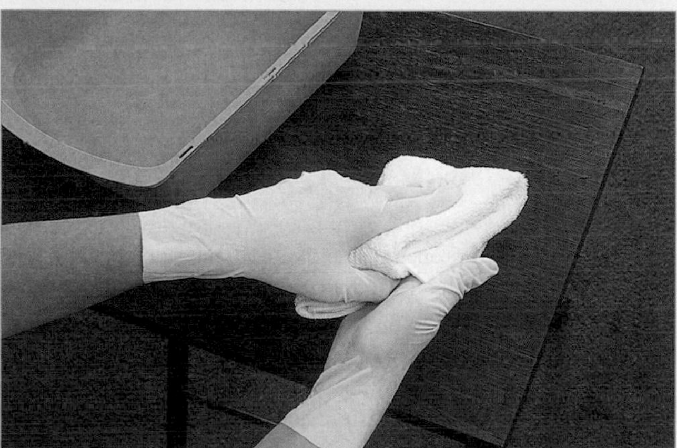

FIGURE 3 Folding ends over and tucking ends under folded washcloth over palm.

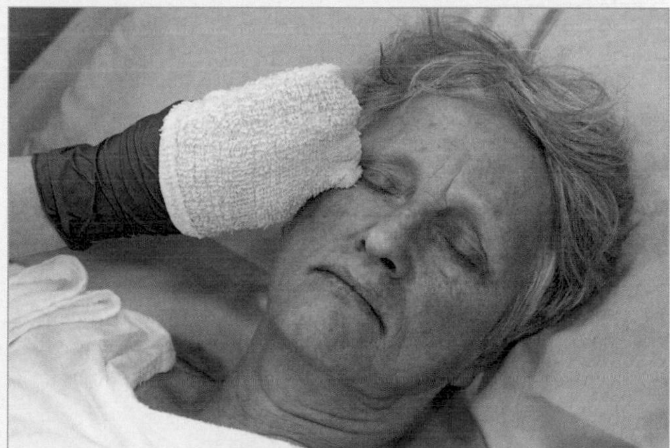

FIGURE 4 Washing from the inner corner of the eye outward.

ACTION	RATIONALE
17. Bathe patient's face, neck, and ears. Apply appropriate emollient.	Use of emollients is recommended to restore and maintain skin integrity (Voegeli, 2010).

(*continued*)

SKILL 7-2 PROVIDING A BED BATH continued

ACTION	RATIONALE
18. Expose patient's far arm and place towel lengthwise under it. Using firm strokes, wash hand, arm, and axilla, lifting the arm as necessary to access axillary region (Figure 5). Rinse, if necessary, and dry. Apply appropriate emollient.	The towel helps to keep the bed dry. Washing the far side first eliminates contaminating a clean area once it is washed. Gentle friction stimulates circulation and muscles and helps remove dirt, oil, and organisms. Long, firm strokes are relaxing and more comfortable than short, uneven strokes. Rinsing is necessary when using some cleansing products. Use of emollients is recommended to restore and maintain skin integrity (Voegeli, 2010).
19. Place a folded towel on the bed next to the patient's hand and put basin on it. Soak the patient's hand in basin (Figure 6). Wash, rinse if necessary, and dry hand. Apply appropriate emollient.	Placing the hand in the basin of water is an additional comfort measure for the patient. It facilitates thorough washing of the hands and between the fingers and aids in removing debris from under the nails. Use of emollients is recommended to restore and maintain skin integrity (Voegeli, 2010).

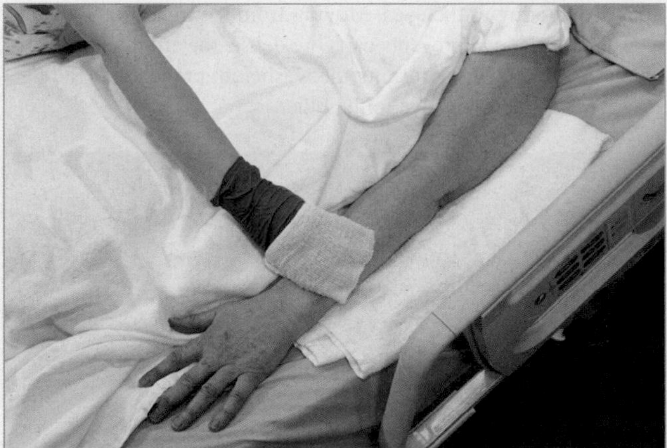

FIGURE 5 Exposing the far arm and washing it.

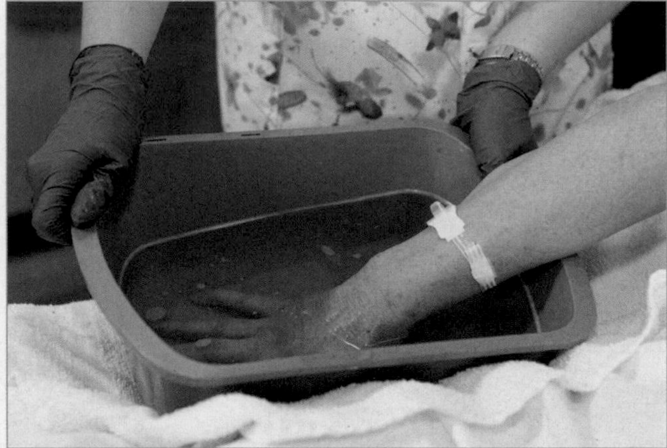

FIGURE 6 Soaking hand in basin.

ACTION	RATIONALE
20. Repeat Actions 18 and 19 for the arm nearest you. An option for the nurse who is shorter or susceptible to back strain might be to bathe one side of the patient first and then move to the other side of the bed to complete the bath.	
21. Spread a towel across patient's chest. Lower bath blanket to patient's umbilical area. Wash, rinse, if necessary, and dry chest. Keep chest covered with towel between the wash and rinse. Pay special attention to the folds of skin under the breasts. Apply appropriate emollient.	Exposing, washing, rinsing, and drying one part of the body at a time avoids unnecessary exposure and chilling. Areas of skin folds may be sources of odor and skin breakdown if not cleaned and dried properly. Use of emollients is recommended to restore and maintain skin integrity (Voegeli, 2010).
22. Lower bath blanket to the perineal area. Place a towel over patient's chest.	Keeping the bath blanket and towel in place avoids exposure and chilling.
23. Wash, rinse, if necessary, and dry abdomen (Figure 7). Carefully inspect and clean umbilical area and any abdominal folds or creases. Apply appropriate emollient.	Skin-fold areas may be sources of odor and skin breakdown if not cleaned and dried properly. Use of emollients is recommended to restore and maintain skin integrity (Voegeli, 2010).
24. Return bath blanket to original position and expose far leg. Place towel under far leg. Using firm strokes, wash, rinse, if necessary, and dry leg from ankle to knee and knee to groin (Figure 8). Apply appropriate emollient.	The towel protects linens and prevents the patient from feeling uncomfortable from a damp or wet bed. Washing from ankle to groin with firm strokes promotes venous return. Use of emollients is recommended to restore and maintain skin integrity (Voegeli, 2010).
25. Wash, rinse if necessary, and dry the foot. Pay particular attention to the areas between toes. Apply appropriate emollient.	Drying of the feet is important to prevent irritation, possible skin breakdown, and infections (National Institute on Aging, 2012). Use of emollients is recommended to restore and maintain skin integrity (Voegeli, 2010).

ACTION | RATIONALE

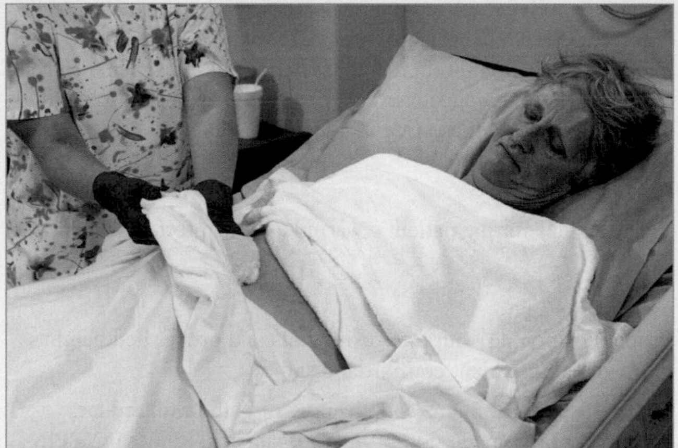

FIGURE 7 Washing the abdomen, with perineal and chest areas covered.

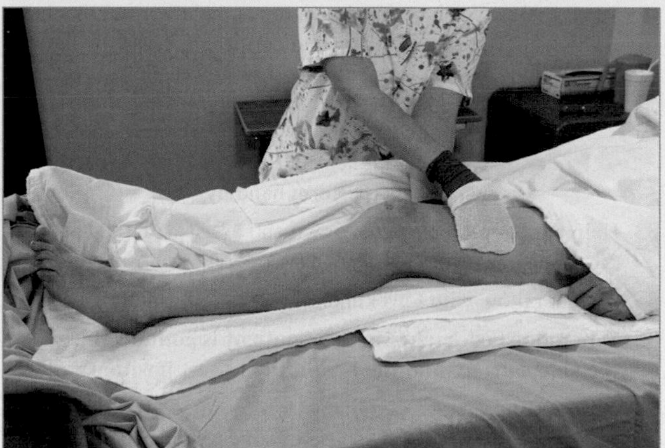

FIGURE 8 Washing and drying far leg, keeping the other leg covered.

26. Repeat Actions 24 and 25 for the other leg and foot.

27. Make sure patient is covered with bath blanket. Change water and washcloth at this point or earlier, if necessary.

The bath blanket maintains warmth and privacy. Clean, warm water prevents chilling and maintains patient comfort.

28. Assist patient to a prone or side-lying position. Put on gloves, if not applied earlier. Position bath blanket and towel to expose only the back and buttocks.

Positioning the towel and bath blanket protects the patient's privacy and provides warmth. Gloves prevent contact with body fluids.

29. Wash, rinse, if necessary, and dry back and buttocks area (Figure 9). **Pay particular attention to cleansing between gluteal folds, and observe for any redness or skin breakdown in the sacral area.**

Fecal material near the anus may be a source of microorganisms. Prolonged pressure on the sacral area or other bony prominences may compromise circulation and lead to development of decubitus ulcer.

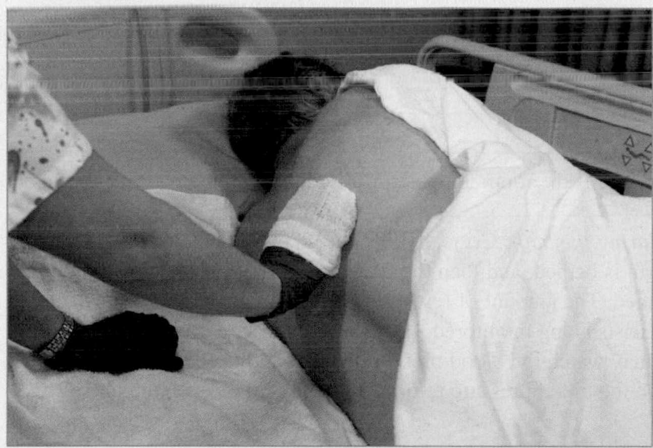

FIGURE 9 Washing the upper back.

30. If not contraindicated, give patient a backrub, as described in Skill 10-2, Chapter 10. Alternatively, back massage may be given after perineal care. Apply appropriate emollient and/or skin barrier product.

A backrub improves circulation to the tissues and is an aid to relaxation. A backrub may be contraindicated in patients with cardiovascular disease or musculoskeletal injuries. Use of emollients is recommended to restore and maintain skin integrity (Voegeli, 2010). Skin barriers protect the skin from damage caused by excessive exposure to water and irritants, such as urine and feces.

31. Raise the side rail. Refill basin with clean water. Discard washcloth and towel. Remove gloves and put on clean gloves.

The washcloth, towel, and water are contaminated after washing the patient's gluteal area. Changing to clean supplies decreases the spread of organisms from the anal area to the genitals.

(*continued*)

SKILL 7-2 PROVIDING A BED BATH continued

ACTION	RATIONALE
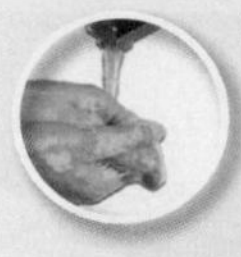 32. Clean perineal area or set patient up so that he or she can complete perineal self-care. If the patient is unable to do so, lower the side rail and complete perineal care. Follow the guidelines in the accompanying Skill Variation. Apply skin barrier, as indicated. Raise side rail, remove gloves, and perform hand hygiene.	Providing perineal self-care may decrease embarrassment for the patient. Effective perineal care reduces odor and decreases the risk for infection through contamination. Skin barriers protect the skin from damage caused by excessive exposure to water and irritants, such as urine and feces.
33. Help patient put on a clean gown and assist with the use of other personal toiletries, such as deodorant or cosmetics.	This provides for the patient's warmth and comfort.
34. Protect pillow with towel and groom patient's hair.	
35. **When finished, make sure the patient is comfortable, with the side rails up and the bed in the lowest position.**	Proper positioning with raised side rails and proper bed height provides for patient comfort and safety.
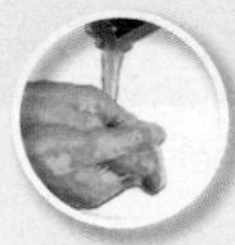 36. Change bed linens, as described in Skills 7-10 and 7-11. Dispose of soiled linens according to facility policy. Clean bath basin according to facility policy before returning to storage at bedside. Remove gloves and any other PPE, if used. Perform hand hygiene.	Proper disposal of linens and cleaning of bath basin reduce the risk for transmission of microorganisms. Removing PPE properly reduces the risk for infection transmission and contamination of other items. Hand hygiene prevents the spread of microorganisms.

EVALUATION

The expected outcomes are met when the patient is clean; demonstrates some feeling of control in his or her care; verbalizes an improved body image; and verbalizes the importance of cleanliness.

DOCUMENTATION

Guidelines

Record any significant observations and communication. Document the condition of the patient's skin. Record the procedure, amount of assistance given, and patient participation. Document the application of skin care products, such as a skin barrier.

Sample Documentation

7/14/15 2130 Bath provided with complete assistance; reddened area (3 cm × 3 cm) noted on patient's sacral area; skin-care team consultation made.

—C. Stone, RN

UNEXPECTED SITUATIONS AND ASSOCIATED INTERVENTIONS

- *Patient becomes chilled during bath:* If the room temperature is adjustable, increase it. Another bath blanket may be needed.
- *The patient becomes unstable during the bath:* Critically ill patients often need to be bathed in stages. For instance, the right arm is bathed, and then the patient is allowed to rest for a short period before the left arm is bathed. The amount of rest time needed depends on how unstable the patient is and which parameter is being monitored. If the blood pressure drops when the patient is stimulated, the nurse may watch the blood pressure while bathing the patient and stop when it begins to decrease. Once the blood pressure returns to the previous level, the nurse can begin to bathe the patient again.

SPECIAL CONSIDERATIONS

General Considerations

- To remove the gown from a patient with an IV line, take the gown off the uninvolved arm first and then thread the IV tubing and bottle or bag through the arm of the gown. To replace the gown, place the clean gown on the unaffected arm first and thread the IV tubing and bottle or bag from inside the arm of the gown on the involved side. Never disconnect IV tubing to change a gown, because this causes a break in a sterile system and could introduce infection.

- Lying flat in bed during the bed bath may be contraindicated for certain patients. The position may have to be modified to accommodate their needs.
- Incontinent patients require special attention to perineal care. Patients with urinary or fecal incontinence are at risk for perineal skin damage. This damage is related to moisture, changes in skin pH, overgrowth of bacteria and skin infection, and erosion of perineal skin from friction on moist skin. Skin care for these patients should include measures to reduce overhydration (excess exposure to moisture), reduce contact with ammonia and bacteria, and reduce friction. Remove soil and irritants from the skin during routine hygiene, as well as cleansing when the skin becomes exposed to irritants. Avoid using soap and excessive force for cleaning. The use of perineal skin cleansers, moisturizers, and moisture barriers is recommended for skin care for the incontinent patient. These products help promote healing and prevent further skin damage.
- If the patient has an indwelling catheter, use mild soap and water or a perineal cleanser to clean the perineal area; rinse the area well. Do not use powders and lotions after cleaning. Do not use antibiotic or other antimicrobial cleaners or betadine at the urethral meatus (Herter & Wallace Kazer, 2010; Society of Urologic Nurses and Associates [SUNA], 2010). Facility policy may recommend use of an antiseptic cleaning agent or plain soap and water to clean the actual catheter. Put on clean gloves before cleaning the catheter. Clean 6 to 8 inches of the catheter, moving from the meatus downward. Be careful not to pull or tug on the catheter during the cleaning motion. Inspect the meatus for drainage and note the characteristics of the urine.
- The use of chlorhexidine gluconate for bathing has been shown to reduce colonization of skin with pathogens and is becoming part of personal hygiene policies in some facilities. Chlorhexidine can be added to bath water, but is also available, and easier to use, in prepackaged impregnated cloths. Bathing with chlorhexidine may be used to reduce the incidence of hospital-acquired infections, such as central line-associated bloodstream infections and surgical site infections, as well as to reduce the acquisition of or decolonization with multidrug-resistant organisms (Ritz, et al., 2012; Sievert, et al., 2011).
- If applying lotion, warm the lotion in your hands before applying it to the patient to prevent chilling.

Infant and Child Considerations

- When bathing an infant or young child, have supplies within easy reach, and support or hold the child securely at all times to ensure safety.
- Never leave the child alone.

Older Adult Considerations

- Check the temperature of the water carefully before bathing an older patient, because sensitivity to temperature may be impaired in older adults.
- An older, continent patient may not require a full bed bath with soap and water every day. If dry skin is a problem, water and skin lotion or bath oil may be used on alternate days.

Home Care Considerations

- Evaluate the safety of the bathing area in the home. Tub mats, adhesive strips, grab bars, and shower stools can help prevent falls.
- Use plastic trash bags or a plastic shower-curtain liner to protect the mattress when bathing or shampooing a patient in bed. Disposable washcloths may also be an option to consider. A large plastic container or baby bathtub can effectively serve as a shampoo basin.
- If linens are soiled with blood or body fluids, instruct family members to wear gloves when handling them. They should be rinsed first in cold water and then washed separately from other household wash, using hot water, laundry detergent, and bleach.
- Teach a family member or caregiver how to perform comfort measures, such as a backrub.
- If patients are home with an indwelling catheter, instruct them or their caregivers to wash the urinary meatus and perineal area twice daily with mild soap and water or a perineal cleanser.
- Teach patients to clean the anal area after each bowel movement. Careful handwashing is imperative.

(*continued*)

SKILL 7-2 PROVIDING A BED BATH continued

SKILL VARIATION Performing Perineal Cleansing

Perineal care may be carried out while the patient remains in bed. Perform perineal cleaning in a matter-of-fact and dignified manner. If this approach is followed, patients generally do not find care by a person of the opposite gender to be offensive or embarrassing. When performing perineal care, follow these guidelines:

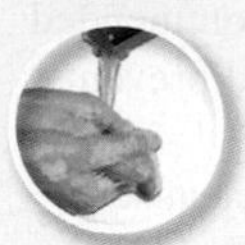

1. Perform hand hygiene and put on PPE, if indicated.

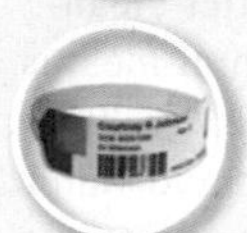

2. Identify the patient.
3. Explain what you are going to do and the reason for doing it to the patient.
4. Assemble necessary equipment on the bedside stand or overbed table.
5. Close curtains around the bed and close the door to the room, if possible.
6. Put on gloves. Cover the patient with a bath blanket and remove top linens to expose only the perineal area. Wash and rinse the groin area (both male and female patients):
   - **For a female patient,** spread the labia and move the washcloth from the pubic area toward the anal area to prevent carrying organisms from the anal area back over the genital area (Figure A). Always proceed from the least contaminated area to the most contaminated area. Use a clean portion of the washcloth for each stroke. Rinse the washed areas well with plain water.
   - **For a male patient,** clean the tip of the penis first, moving the washcloth in a circular motion from the meatus outward. Wash the shaft of the penis using downward strokes toward the pubic area (Figure B). Always proceed from the least contaminated area to the most contaminated area. Rinse the washed areas well with plain water.

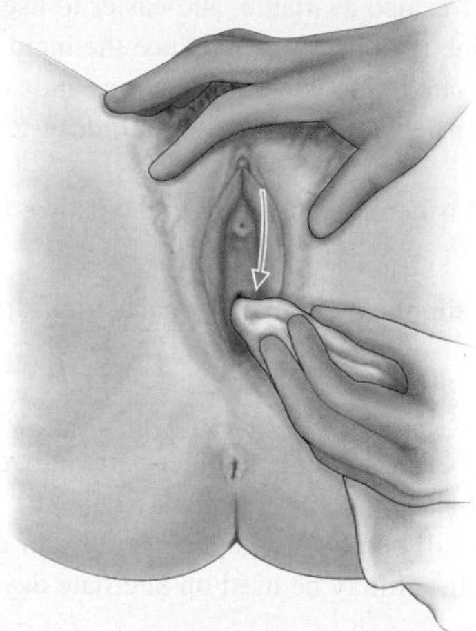

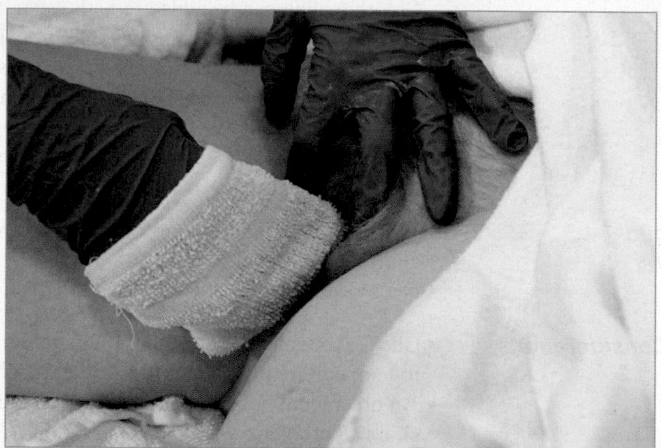

FIGURE A Performing female perineal care.

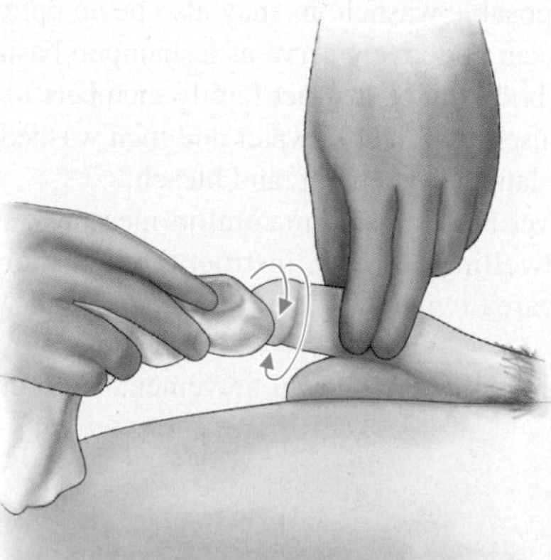

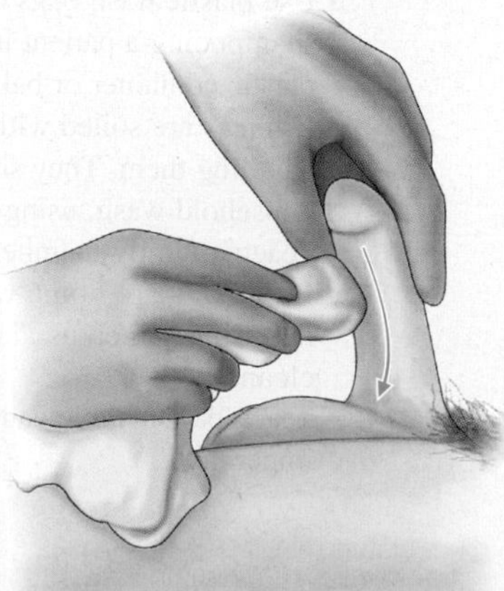

FIGURE B Performing male perineal care.

(continued)

SKILL VARIATION Performing Perineal Cleansing continued

In an *uncircumcised male patient* (teenage or older), retract the foreskin (prepuce) while washing the penis. **It is not recommended to retract the foreskin for cleaning during infancy and childhood, because injury and scarring could occur (MedlinePlus, 2012).** Pull the *uncircumcised male patient's* foreskin back into place over the glans penis to prevent constriction of the penis, which may result in edema and tissue injury. Wash and rinse the male patient's scrotum. Handle the scrotum, which houses the testicles, with care because the area is sensitive.

7. Dry the cleaned areas and apply an emollient, as indicated. Apply skin barrier (protectant) to area, as indicated. Avoid the use of powder. Powder may become a medium for bacteria growth.
8. Turn the patient on his or her side and continue cleansing the anal area. Continue in the direction of least contaminated to most contaminated area. In the female, cleanse from the vagina toward the anus. In both female and male patients, change the washcloth with each stroke until the area is clean. Rinse and dry the area. Apply skin barrier (protectant) to area, as indicated.

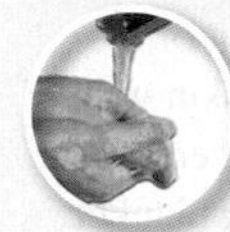

9. Remove gloves and perform hand hygiene. Continue with additional care as necessary.

SKILL VARIATION Giving a Bath Using a Disposable Self-contained Bathing System

A disposable bathing system is packaged with 8 to 10 premoistened disposable washcloths. If more than 8 cloths are available in the package, use a separate cloth for hands and feet. When giving a bath with a disposable system, follow these guidelines:

1. Warm the unopened package in the microwave, according to manufacturer's directions or remove package from storage warmer (Figure A).

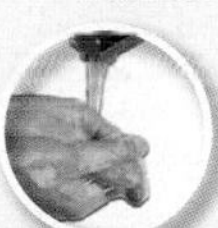

2. Perform hand hygiene and put on PPE, if indicated.

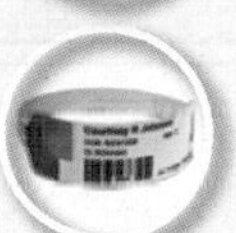

3. Identify the patient.
4. Explain what you are going to do and the reason for doing it to the patient.
5. Assemble necessary equipment on the bedside stand or overbed table.
6. Close the curtains around the bed and close the door to the room, if possible.
7. Put on gloves. Cover the patient with a bath blanket and remove top linens. Remove patient's gown and keep the bath blanket in place.
8. Remove first cloth from the package. Wipe one eye from the inner part of the eye, near the nose, to the outer part. Use a different part of the cloth for the other eye.
9. Bathe the face, neck, and ears. Allow the skin to air dry for approximately 30 seconds, according to manufacturer's directions. Air drying allows the emollient ingredient of the

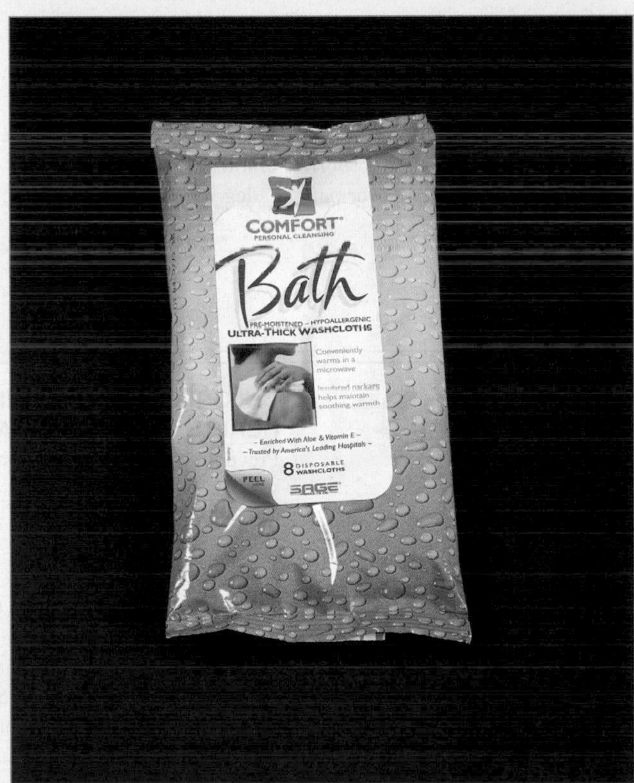

FIGURE A Commercial self-contained bathing system. *(Photo by B. Proud.)*

(continued)

SKILL 7-2 PROVIDING A BED BATH continued

SKILL VARIATION Giving a Bath Using a Disposable Self-contained Bathing System continued

cleanser to remain on the skin. Alternately, dry the skin with a towel, based on the product used. Apply appropriate emollient. Dispose of cloth in trash receptacle.

10. Expose the patient's far arm. Remove another cloth. Using firm strokes, wash hand, arm, and axilla. Allow the skin to air dry for approximately 30 seconds, according to manufacturer's directions. Air drying allows the emollient ingredient of the cleanser to remain on the skin. Alternately, dry the skin with a towel, based on the product used. Apply appropriate emollient. Dispose of cloth in trash receptacle. Cover arm with blanket.
11. Repeat for nearer arm with a new cloth. Cover arm with blanket.
12. Expose the patient's chest. Remove new cloth and cleanse chest. Allow the skin to air dry for approximately 30 seconds, according to manufacturer's directions. Cover chest with a towel. Expose patient's abdomen. Cleanse abdomen. Allow the skin to air dry for approximately 30 seconds, according to manufacturer's directions. Air drying allows the emollient ingredient of the cleanser to remain on the skin. Alternately, dry the skin with a towel, based on the product used. Apply appropriate emollient. Dispose of cloth in trash receptacle. Cover patient's body with blanket.
13. Expose far leg. Remove new cloth and cleanse leg and foot. Allow the skin to air dry for approximately 30 seconds, according to manufacturer's directions. Air drying allows the emollient ingredient of the cleanser to remain on the skin. Alternately, dry the skin with a towel, based on the product used. Apply appropriate emollient. Dispose of cloth in trash receptacle. Cover patient's leg with blanket.
14. Repeat for nearer leg with a new cloth. Cover leg with blanket.
15. Assist patient to prone or side-lying position. Put on gloves, if not applied earlier. Position blanket to expose back and buttocks. Remove a new cloth and cleanse back and buttocks area. Allow the skin to air dry for approximately 30 seconds, according to manufacturer's directions. Air drying allows the emollient ingredient of the cleanser to remain on the skin. Alternately, dry the skin with a towel, based on the product used. Apply appropriate emollient. Dispose of cloth in trash receptacle. If not contraindicated, give the patient a back massage. Apply skin barrier, as indicated. Cover patient with blanket.
16. Remove gloves and put on clean gloves. Remove last cloth and cleanse the perineal area. Refer to the guidelines in the previous Skill Variation. Dispose of cloth in trash receptacle. Apply skin barrier, as indicated.

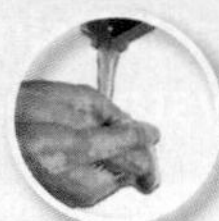

17. Remove gloves. Assist the patient to put on a clean gown. Perform hand hygiene. Assist with the use of other personal toiletries.
18. Change bed linens as described in Skills 7-10 and 7-11. Dispose of soiled linens according to facility policy.

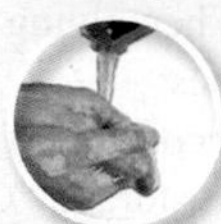

19. Remove gloves and additional PPE, if used. Perform hand hygiene.

EVIDENCE FOR PRACTICE ▶

CHLORHEXIDINE BATHING AND PREVENTION OF HEALTH CARE-ASSOCIATED INFECTIONS (HAIs)

Prevention of health care-associated infections (HAIs) is a major challenge for health care providers. Health care agencies constantly strive to implement evidence-based practices to reduce the risk of HAIs for patients and promote patient health.

Related Research

Ritz, J., Pashnik, B., Padula, C., et al. (2012). Effectiveness of 2 methods of chlorhexidine bathing. *Journal of Nursing Care Quality, 27*(2), 171–175.

This study examined the impact of chlorhexidine gluconate (CHG) bathing on the transmission of methicillin-resistant *Staphylococcus aureus* (MRSA) *and* vancomycin-resistant *Enterococcus* (VRE) on an inpatient oncology unit, using a convenience sample of 405 patients, over a six-month period. The study also compared the cost of two chlorhexidine bath delivery methods, and evaluated nursing time and satisfaction related to bath administration. Specific protocols were developed for each type of bath, based on a review of the literature. Patients received a daily bath using two ounces of 4% CHG solution added to the bathing water or were bathed daily with prepackaged 2% CHG impregnated cloths. MRSA and VRE transmission rates decreased from those during the previous years. Costs associated with bathing increased, but the time to administer the bath decreased with the chlorhexidine cloths. The nursing staff reported satisfaction with the use of the chlorhexidine cloths; all of the 32 nursing staff reported that the product was easier to use, took less time, and required fewer supplies. Most (94%) of the staff preferred the cloth bathing method.

Relevance for Nursing Practice

This study suggests that the implementation of a relatively simple procedure, daily bathing with a consistent dose of CHG, along with a continued emphasis on hand hygiene and transmission-based precautions, can reduce the risk of transmission of MRSA and VRE. These results can be useful to other facilities in decreasing HAIs. Nurses and nursing staff are the primary providers of bathing activities in many health care settings and should consider the implementation of interventions to break the chain of infection, improve patient health, and decrease health care costs.

Refer to thePoint for additional research on related nursing topics.

SKILL 7-3 ASSISTING THE PATIENT WITH ORAL CARE

Adequate oral hygiene care is imperative to promote the patient's sense of well-being and prevent deterioration of the oral cavity. Poor oral hygiene is reported to lead to the colonization of the oropharyngeal secretions by respiratory pathogens. Diligent oral hygiene care can improve oral health and limit the growth of pathogens in oropharyngeal secretions, decreasing the incidence of aspiration pneumonia, community-acquired pneumonia, ventilator-associated pneumonia, and other systemic diseases, such as diabetes, heart disease, and stroke (Tada & Miura, 2012; CDC, 2011a; Durgunde & Cocks, 2011; AACN, 2010). The mouth requires care even during illness, but sometimes care must be modified to meet a patient's needs. If the patient can assist with mouth care, provide the necessary materials. Oral care is important not only to prevent dental **gingivitis** and **caries**, but also to improve the patient's self-image. Teeth should be brushed and flossed twice a day; the mouth should be rinsed after meals. If the patient is unable to perform oral hygiene, make certain that the mouth receives care as often as necessary to keep it clean and moist, as often as every 1 or 2 hours if necessary. This is especially important for patients who cannot drink or are not permitted fluids by mouth. Refer to Box 7-2 for suggestions to meet the oral hygiene needs for patients with cognitive impairments.

Box 7-2 MEETING THE ORAL HYGIENE NEEDS OF PATIENTS WITH COGNITIVE IMPAIRMENTS

- Choose a time of day when the patient is most calm and accepting of care.
- Enlist the aid of a family member or significant other.
- Break the task into small steps.
- Provide distraction, such as playing favorite music, while providing care.
- Allow the patient to participate. The nurse can put a hand over the patient's to guide the activity.
- The nurse can start the activity, show the patient what to do, then let the patient take over.
- If the patient strongly refuses care, withdraw and reapproach later.
- Effective and ineffective interventions should be documented to provide appropriate information for staff to give consistent, effective care.

(Adapted from Tabloski, P.A. [2010]. *Gerontological nursing* (2nd ed.). Upper Saddle River, NJ: Pearson.)

(*continued*)

SKILL 7-3 ASSISTING THE PATIENT WITH ORAL CARE continued

DELEGATION CONSIDERATIONS

The implementation of oral care may be delegated to nursing assistive personnel (NAP) or to unlicensed assistive personnel (UAP), as well as to licensed practical/vocational nurses (LPN/LVNs). The decision to delegate must be based on careful analysis of the patient's needs and circumstances, as well as the qualifications of the person to whom the task is being delegated. Refer to the Delegation Guidelines in Appendix A.

EQUIPMENT

- Toothbrush
- Toothpaste
- Emesis basin
- Glass with cool water
- Disposable gloves
- Additional PPE, as indicated
- Towel
- Mouthwash (optional)
- Washcloth or paper towel
- Lip lubricant (optional)
- Dental floss

ASSESSMENT

Assess the patient's oral hygiene preferences: frequency, time of day, and type of hygiene products. Assess for any physical activity limitations. An oral assessment tool can assist with assessment of the status of the oral cavity, as well as help to determine the frequency and procedure for oral care. Assess the patient's oral cavity and dentition. Look for any inflammation or bleeding of the gums. Look for ulcers, lesions, and yellow or white patches. The yellow or white patches may indicate a fungal infection called thrush. Assess for signs of dehydration (dry mucosa) and dental decay. Look at the lips for dryness or cracking. Ask the patient if he or she is having pain, dryness, soreness, or difficulty chewing or swallowing. Assess the patient's ability to perform own care.

NURSING DIAGNOSIS

Determine the related factors for the nursing diagnoses based on the patient's current status. Possible nursing diagnoses may include:

- Risk for Aspiration
- Impaired Oral Mucous Membrane
- Deficient Knowledge

OUTCOME IDENTIFICATION AND PLANNING

The expected outcome is that the patient's mouth and teeth will be clean; the patient will exhibit a positive body image; and the patient will verbalize the importance of oral care.

IMPLEMENTATION

ACTION	RATIONALE
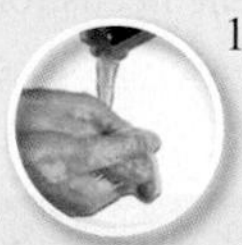 1. Perform hand hygiene and put on gloves if assisting with oral care, and/or other PPE, if indicated.	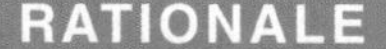 Hand hygiene and PPE prevent the spread of microorganisms. PPE is required based on transmission precautions.
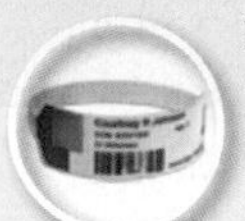 2. Identify the patient. Explain the procedure to the patient.	Identifying the patient ensures the right patient receives the intervention and helps prevent errors. Explanation facilitates cooperation.
3. Assemble equipment on overbed table within patient's reach.	Organization facilitates performance of the task.
4. Close the room door or curtains. Place the bed at an appropriate and comfortable working height; usually elbow height of the caregiver (VISN 8 Patient Safety Center, 2009).	Closing the door or curtains provides privacy. Proper bed height helps reduce back strain while performing the procedure.
5. Lower side rail and assist the patient to a sitting position, if permitted, or turn the patient onto side. Place towel across the patient's chest.	The sitting or side-lying position prevents aspiration of fluids into the lungs. The towel protects the patient from dampness.

ACTION	RATIONALE
6. Encourage the patient to brush own teeth according to the following guidelines. Assist, if necessary.	
a. Moisten toothbrush and apply toothpaste to bristles.	Water softens the bristles.
b. Place brush at a 45-degree angle to gum line (Figure 1) and brush from gum line to crown of each tooth (Figure 2). Brush outer and inner surfaces. Brush back and forth across biting surface of each tooth.	Facilitates removal of **plaque** and **tartar**. The 45-degree angle of brushing permits cleansing of all tooth surface areas.
c. Brush tongue gently with toothbrush (Figure 3).	Removes coating on the tongue. Gentle motion does not stimulate gag reflex.
d. Have patient rinse vigorously with water and spit into emesis basin (Figure 4). Repeat until clear. Suction may be used as an alternative for removal of fluid and secretions from the mouth.	The vigorous swishing motion helps to remove debris. Suction is appropriate if the patient is unable to expectorate well.

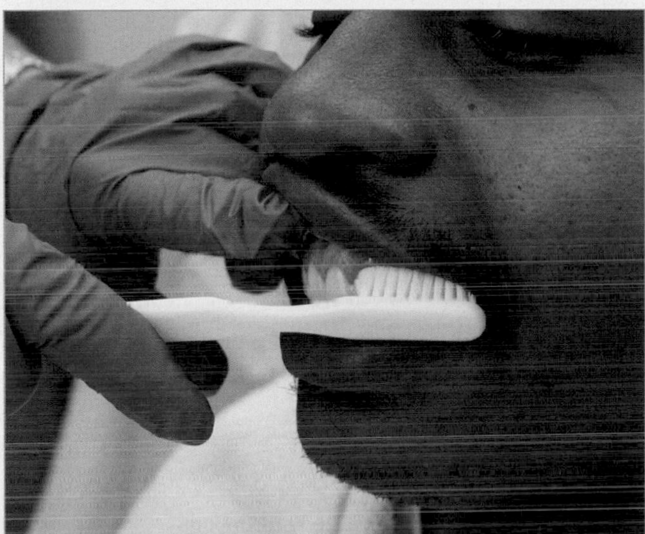

FIGURE 1 Placing brush at a 45 degree angle to gum line.

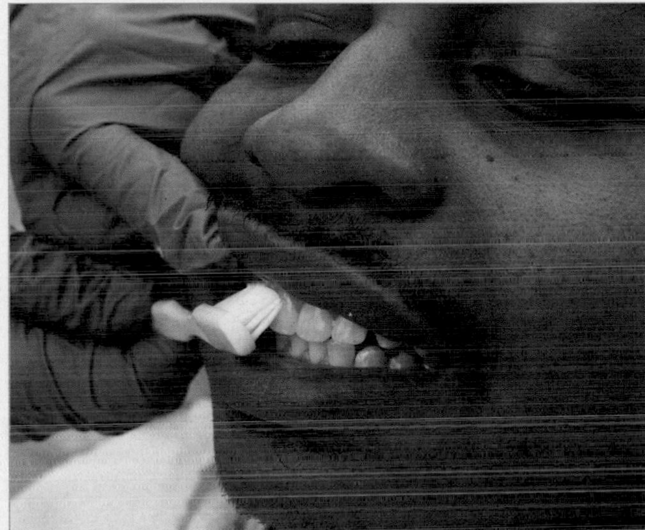

FIGURE 2 Brushing from gum line to the crown of each tooth.

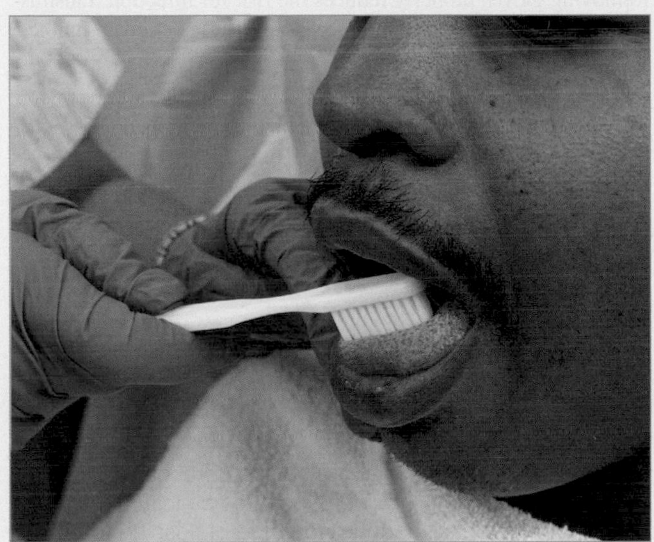

FIGURE 3 Brushing tongue.

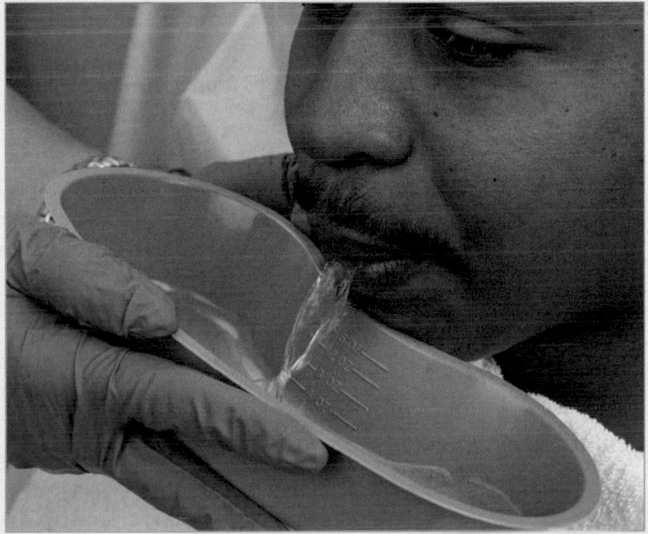

FIGURE 4 Holding emesis basin for patient to rinse and spit.

(continued)

SKILL 7-3 ASSISTING THE PATIENT WITH ORAL CARE continued

ACTION	RATIONALE
7. Assist patient to floss teeth, if appropriate:	Flossing aids in removal of plaque and promotes healthy gum tissue.
a. Remove approximately 6 inches of dental floss from container or use a plastic floss holder. Wrap the floss around the index fingers, keeping about 1 to 1.5 inches of floss taut between the fingers.	The floss must be held taut to get between the teeth.
b. Insert floss gently between teeth, moving it back and forth downward to the gums.	Trauma to the gums can occur if floss is forced between teeth.
c. Move the floss up and down, first on one side of a tooth and then on the side of the other tooth, until the surfaces are clean (Figure 5). Repeat in the spaces between all teeth.	This ensures that the sides of both teeth are cleaned.
d. Instruct patient to rinse mouth well with water after flossing.	Vigorous rinsing helps to remove food particles and plaque that have been loosened by flossing.

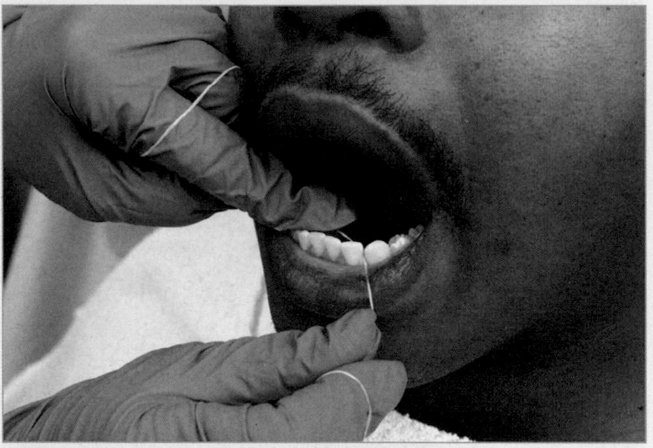

FIGURE 5 Flossing teeth.

ACTION	RATIONALE
8. Offer mouthwash if patient prefers.	Mouthwash leaves a pleasant taste in the mouth.
9. Offer lip balm or petroleum jelly.	Lip balm lubricates lips and prevents drying.
10. Remove equipment. Remove gloves and discard. Raise side rail and lower bed. Assist patient to a position of comfort.	Removing gloves properly reduces the risk for infection transmission and contamination of other items. These actions promote patient comfort and safety.
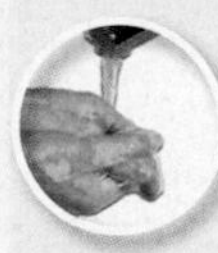 11. Remove any other PPE, if used. Perform hand hygiene.	Removing PPE properly reduces the risk for infection transmission and contamination of other items. Hand hygiene prevents the spread of microorganisms.

EVALUATION

The expected outcomes are met when the patient receives oral care, experiences little to no discomfort, states mouth feels refreshed, and demonstrates understanding the reasons for proper oral care.

DOCUMENTATION

Guidelines

Record oral assessment, significant observations, and unusual findings, such as bleeding or inflammation. Document any teaching done. Document procedure and patient response.

Sample Documentation

10/20/15 0930 Patient performed oral care with minimal assistance. Oral cavity mucosa pink and moist. No evidence of bleeding or ulceration. Lips slightly dry; lip moisturizer applied. Reinforcement provided related to importance of flossing teeth every day. Patient demonstrates appropriate flossing technique.

—L. Schneider, RN

UNEXPECTED SITUATIONS AND ASSOCIATED INTERVENTIONS

- *While cleaning the teeth, you notice a large amount of bleeding from the gum line:* Stop brushing. Allow patient to gently rinse mouth with water and spit into emesis basin. Before brushing again, check most recent platelet level. Consider the use of a softer toothbrush to provide oral hygiene.
- *Patient has braces on teeth:* Brush extra thoroughly. Braces collect food particles.

SPECIAL CONSIDERATIONS

General Considerations

- Use a soft bristled toothbrush with a small head even when the patient has no or few teeth. It is the only effective way to remove plaque and debris from the teeth, gums, and tongue.
- A patient receiving chemotherapy medication may have bleeding gums and extremely sensitive mucous membranes. Use a soft sponge toothette for cleaning, and a saltwater rinse (half teaspoon salt in 1 cup of warm water) (Polovich, et al., 2009).
- Automatic toothbrushes, electric or battery operated, are simple to use and are as good as manual brushes for removing debris and plaque. These devices are very useful for patients with arthritis or other conditions that make it difficult to brush effectively (Mayo Foundation for Medical Education and Research, 2011d).
- The use of chlorhexidine gluconate as part of oral hygiene has been integrated into oral hygiene regimens and is available in an oral spray and dental gel (Ames, et al., 2011; Kelly, et al., 2010). The use of CHG as part of protocols for systematic oral care for critically ill patients has been shown to reduce the incidence of health care-associated pneumonia (Ames, et al., 2011).

Infant and Child Considerations

- When assisting small children with oral care, do not use toothpaste that contains fluoride if the child cannot spit out excess. Excessive amounts of ingested fluoride can lead to a discoloration of the teeth.
- Oral hygiene should begin as soon as an infant's teeth erupt. Clean teeth and gums by wiping with a damp cloth. As the infant gets more teeth, introduce a small toothbrush. Use water to clean an infant's teeth, not toothpaste.

EVIDENCE FOR PRACTICE ▶

ORAL HYGIENE AND DYSPHAGIA

Oral care is an essential component of quality nursing care. Diligent oral hygiene care can improve oral health and decrease the incidence of aspiration pneumonia, community-acquired pneumonia, ventilator-associated pneumonia, and other systemic diseases. What is nurses' knowledge regarding appropriate oral hygiene for patients with **dysphagia**?

Related Research

Durgude, Y., & Cocks, N. (2011). Nurse's knowledge of the provision of oral care for patients with dysphagia. *British Journal of Community Nursing, 16*(12), 604–610.

This study surveyed nurses' knowledge and practices concerning oral care for patients with dysphagia. Participants reported limited knowledge of medical conditions secondary to poor oral care, and a lack of knowledge related to medications associated with poor oral hygiene. Only 3% of participants correctly associated poor oral hygiene as a risk factor for pneumonia. RNs in the study did report that they gave mouth care to patients with dysphagia more frequently than to patients without dysphagia, but some of the practices, such as the use of mouthwash, were actually dangerous for patients with dysphagia. The study authors suggest that these differences between knowledge and practice suggest that the RNs may have been instructed to provide frequent oral care to patients with dysphagia, but were not aware of why they were doing this.

Relevance for Nursing Practice

Nurses should maintain up-to-date knowledge regarding appropriate interventions to provide oral care. Frequent educational updates and evidence-based training are needed to improve nursing care related to oral health, particularly in relation to patients with dysphagia. Nurses should investigate the use of appropriate tools to aid in improved oral care practice, and work to ensure adequate supplies are on hand to provide appropriate oral care for patients.

Refer to thePoint for additional research on related nursing topics.

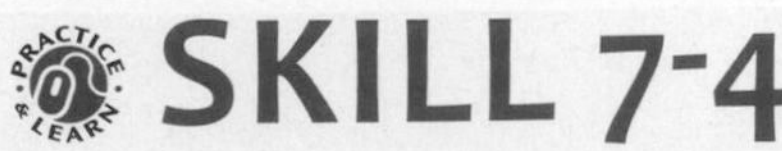

SKILL 7-4 PROVIDING ORAL CARE FOR THE DEPENDENT PATIENT

Physical limitations, such as those associated with aging, often lead to less than adequate oral hygiene. The dexterity required for adequate brushing and flossing may decrease with age, or illness. Older patients may be dependent on caregivers for oral hygiene. Patients with cognitive impairment, such as dementia, are also at risk for inadequate oral hygiene (Jablonski, et al., 2011). Refer to Box 7-2 in Skill 7-3 for suggestions to meet the oral hygiene needs for patients with cognitive impairments.

Teeth should be brushed and flossed twice a day; the mouth should be rinsed after meals. If the patient is unable to perform oral hygiene, make certain that the mouth receives care as often as necessary to keep it clean and moist, as often as every 1 or 2 hours, if necessary. This is especially important for patients who cannot drink or are not permitted fluids by mouth. Moisten the mouth with water, if allowed, and lubricate the lips often enough to keep the membranes well moistened.

DELEGATION CONSIDERATIONS

The implementation of oral care for a dependent patient may be delegated to nursing assistive personnel (NAP) or to unlicensed assistive personnel (UAP) after assessment by the registered nurse, as well as to licensed practical/vocational nurses (LPN/LVNs). The decision to delegate must be based on careful analysis of the patient's needs and circumstances, as well as the qualifications of the person to whom the task is being delegated. Refer to the Delegation Guidelines in Appendix A.

EQUIPMENT

- Toothbrush
- Toothpaste
- Emesis basin
- Glass with cool water
- Disposable gloves
- Additional PPE, as indicated
- Towel
- Mouthwash (optional)
- Dental floss (optional)
- Denture-cleaning equipment (if necessary)
- Denture cup
- Denture cleaner
- 4 × 4 gauze
- Washcloth or paper towel
- Lip lubricant (optional)
- Sponge toothette
- Irrigating syringe with rubber tip (optional)
- Suction catheter with suction apparatus (optional)

ASSESSMENT

Assess the patient's oral hygiene preferences: frequency, time of day, and type of hygiene products. Assess for any physical activity limitations. Assess the patient's level of consciousness and overall ability to assist with oral care and respond to directions. Assess the patient's risk for oral hygiene problems. Alterations in cognitive function and/or consciousness increase the risk for alterations in oral tissue and structure integrity. Assess the patient's gag reflex. Decreased or absent gag reflex increases the risk for aspiration. An oral assessment tool can assist with assessment of the status of the oral cavity, as well as help to determine the frequency and procedure for oral care. Assess patient's oral cavity and dentition. Look for any inflammation or bleeding of the gums. Look for ulcers, lesions, and yellow or white patches. The yellow or white patches may indicate a fungal infection called thrush. Assess for signs of dehydration (dry mucosa) and dental decay. Look at the lips for dryness or cracking. If the patient is conscious and/or cognitively able to respond, ask the patient if he or she is having pain, dryness, soreness, or difficulty chewing or swallowing.

NURSING DIAGNOSIS

Determine the related factors for the nursing diagnoses based on the patient's current status. Possible nursing diagnoses may include:

- Impaired Oral Mucous Membrane
- Deficient Knowledge
- Risk for Aspiration

OUTCOME IDENTIFICATION AND PLANNING

The expected outcome to achieve when performing oral care is that the patient's mouth and teeth will be clean; the patient will not experience impaired oral mucous membranes; the patient will demonstrate improvement in body image; and the patient will verbalize, if able, an understanding about the importance of oral care.

IMPLEMENTATION

ACTION	RATIONALE
1. Perform hand hygiene and put on PPE, if indicated.	Hand hygiene and PPE prevent the spread of microorganisms. PPE is required based on transmission precautions.

ACTION	RATIONALE
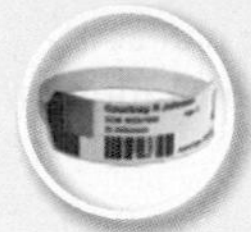 2. Identify the patient. Explain the procedure to the patient.	Identifying the patient ensures the right patient receives the intervention and helps prevent errors. Explanation facilitates cooperation.
3. Assemble equipment on overbed table within reach.	Organization facilitates performance of task.
4. Close the room door or curtains. Place the bed at an appropriate and comfortable working height, usually elbow height of the caregiver (VISN 8 Patient Safety Center, 2009). Lower one side rail and position the patient on the side, with head tilted forward. Place towel across the patient's chest and emesis basin in position under chin. Put on gloves.	Cleaning another person's mouth is invasive and may be embarrassing (Holman, et al., 2005). Closing the door or curtains provides privacy. Proper bed height helps reduce back strain while performing the procedure. The side-lying position with head forward prevents aspiration of fluid into lungs. Towel and emesis basin protects the patient from dampness. Gloves prevent the spread of microorganisms.
5. Gently open the patient's mouth by applying pressure to the lower jaw at the front of the mouth. Remove dentures, if present. (Refer to Skill 7-5.) Brush the teeth and gums carefully with toothbrush and paste (Figure 1). Lightly brush the tongue.	Toothbrush provides friction necessary to clean areas where plaque and tartar accumulate.
6. Use toothette dipped in water to rinse the oral cavity. If desired, insert the rubber tip of the irrigating syringe into patient's mouth and rinse gently with a small amount of water (Figure 2). **Position patient's head to allow for return of water or use suction apparatus to remove the water from oral cavity** (Figure 3).	Rinsing helps clean debris from the mouth. Forceful irrigation may cause aspiration.

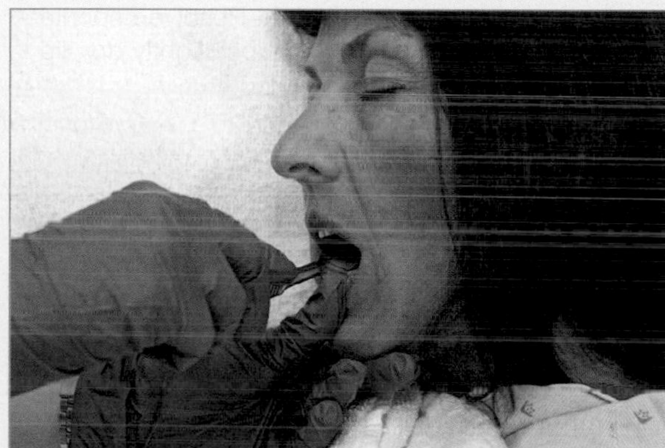

FIGURE 1 Carefully brushing patient's teeth.

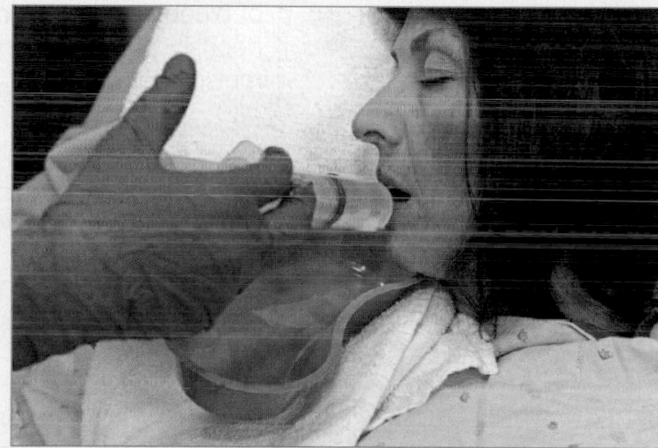

FIGURE 2 Using irrigating syringe and a small amount of water to rinse mouth.

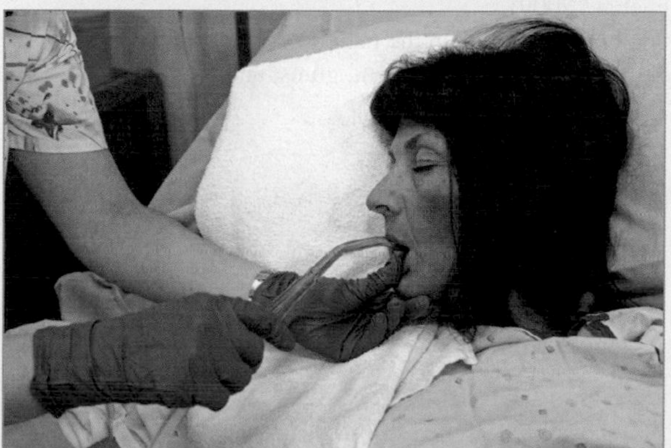

FIGURE 3 Using suction to remove excess fluid.

(continued)

SKILL 7-4 PROVIDING ORAL CARE FOR THE DEPENDENT PATIENT continued

ACTION	RATIONALE
7. Clean the dentures before replacing. (See Skill 7-5.)	Cleaning maintains dentures and oral hygiene. Plaque can accumulate on dentures and promote oropharyngeal colonization of pathogens.
8. Apply lubricant to patient's lips.	This prevents drying and cracking of lips.
9. Remove equipment and return patient to a position of comfort. Remove your gloves. Raise side rail and lower bed.	Promotes patient comfort and safety. Removing gloves properly reduces the risk for infection transmission and contamination of other items.
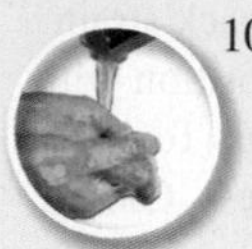 10. Remove additional PPE, if used. Perform hand hygiene.	Removing PPE properly reduces the risk for infection transmission and contamination of other items. Hand hygiene prevents the spread of microorganisms.

EVALUATION

The expected outcomes are met when the patient's oral cavity is clean and free from complications, and the patient states or demonstrates improved body image. In addition, if the patient is able, he or she verbalizes a basic understanding of the need for oral care.

DOCUMENTATION

Guidelines

Record oral assessment, significant observations, and unusual findings, such as bleeding or inflammation. Document any teaching done. Document procedure and patient response.

Sample Documentation

7/10/15 0945 Oral care performed. Oral cavity mucosa pink and moist. Small amount of bleeding noted from gums after using soft-bristled toothbrush. Resolved spontaneously when brushing completed. No evidence of ulceration. Lips slightly dry; lip moisturizer applied.

—C. Stone, RN

UNEXPECTED SITUATIONS AND ASSOCIATED INTERVENTIONS

- *Patient begins to bite the toothbrush:* Do not jerk the toothbrush out. Wait for patient to relax mouth before removing the toothbrush and continuing with care.
- *Mouth is extremely dry with crusts that remain after oral care provided:* Increase frequency of oral hygiene. Apply mouth moisturizer to oral mucosa.

SPECIAL CONSIDERATIONS

- Suction toothbrushes may be used with patients with dysphagia (Figure 4).
- A patient receiving chemotherapy medication may have bleeding gums and extremely sensitive mucous membranes. Use a soft sponge toothette for cleaning, and a saltwater rinse (half teaspoon salt in 1 cup of warm water) (Polovich, et al., 2009).
- Use a soft bristled toothbrush with a small head even when the patient has no or few teeth. It is the only effective way to remove plaque and debris from the teeth, gums, and tongue.

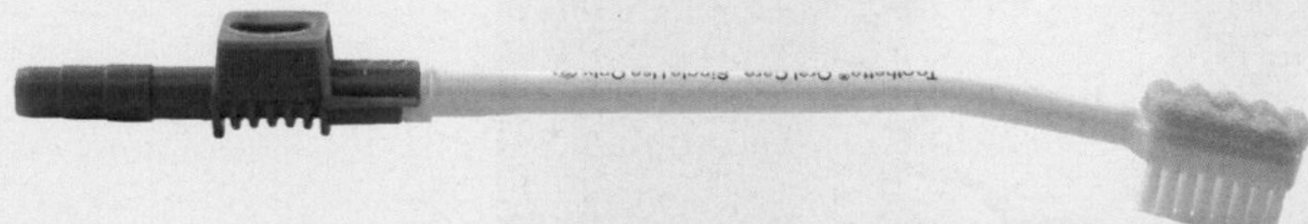

FIGURE 4 Example of a suction toothbrush. (From Sage Products, Suction Toothbrush Kit, http://www.sageproducts.com/.)

EVIDENCE FOR PRACTICE ▶

ORAL HYGIENE AND DYSPHAGIA

Oral care is an essential component of quality nursing care. Diligent oral hygiene care can improve oral health and decrease the incidence of aspiration pneumonia, community-acquired pneumonia, ventilator-associated pneumonia, and other systemic diseases. What is nurses' knowledge regarding appropriate oral hygiene for patients with dysphagia?

Related Research

Durgude, Y., & Cocks, N. (2011). Nurses' knowledge of the provision of oral care for patients with dysphagia. *British Journal of Community Nursing, 16*(12), 604–610.

For detailed information see the Evidence for Practice in Skill 7-3, and refer to thePoint for additional research on related nursing topics.

SKILL 7-5 PROVIDING DENTURE CARE

Plaque, which can accumulate on dentures, can promote oropharyngeal colonization of pathogens. Diligent oral hygiene care can improve oral health and decrease the incidence of aspiration pneumonia, community-acquired pneumonia, ventilator-associated pneumonia, and other systemic diseases. It is important to brush dentures twice a day and to remove and rinse dentures and mouth after meals. Dentures may be cleaned more often, based on need and the patient's personal preference. Dentures are often removed at night. Handle dentures with care to prevent breakage.

Refer to Box 7-2 in Skill 7-3 for suggestions to meet the oral hygiene needs for patients with cognitive impairments.

DELEGATION CONSIDERATIONS

The implementation of denture care may be delegated to nursing assistive personnel (NAP) or to unlicensed assistive personnel (UAP), as well as to licensed practical/vocational nurses (LPN/LVNs). The decision to delegate must be based on careful analysis of the patient's needs and circumstances, as well as the qualifications of the person to whom the task is being delegated. Refer to the Delegation Guidelines in Appendix A.

EQUIPMENT

- Soft toothbrush or denture brush
- Toothpaste
- Denture cleaner (optional)
- Denture adhesive (optional)
- Glass of cool water
- Emesis basin
- Denture cup (optional)
- Nonsterile gloves
- Additional PPE, as indicated
- Towel
- Mouthwash (optional)
- Washcloth or paper towel
- Lip lubricant (optional)
- Gauze

ASSESSMENT

Assess the patient's oral hygiene preferences: frequency, time of day, and type of hygiene products. Assess for any physical activity limitations. Assess for difficulty chewing, pain, tenderness, and discomfort. An oral assessment tool can assist with assessment of the status of the oral cavity, as well as help to determine the frequency and procedure for oral care. Assess patient's oral cavity. Look for inflammation, edema, lesions, bleeding, or yellow/white patches. The patches may indicate a fungal infection called thrush. Assess patient's ability to perform own care.

NURSING DIAGNOSIS

Determine the related factors for the nursing diagnoses based on the patient's current status. Possible nursing diagnoses may include:

- Ineffective Health Maintenance
- Impaired Oral Mucous Membrane
- Disturbed Body Image

(continued)

SKILL 7-5 PROVIDING DENTURE CARE continued

OUTCOME IDENTIFICATION AND PLANNING

The expected outcome to achieve is that the patient's mouth and dentures will be clean; the patient will exhibit a positive body image; and the patient will verbalize the importance of oral care.

IMPLEMENTATION

ACTION	RATIONALE
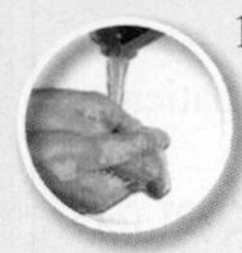 1. Perform hand hygiene and put on PPE, if indicated.	Hand hygiene and PPE prevent the spread of microorganisms. PPE is required based on transmission precautions.
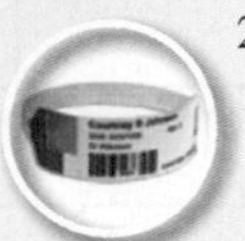 2. Identify patient. Explain the procedure to patient.	Identifying the patient ensures the right patient receives the intervention and helps prevent errors. Explanation facilitates cooperation.
3. Assemble equipment on overbed table within reach.	Organization facilitates performance of task.
4. Provide privacy for the patient.	Cleaning another person's mouth is invasive and may be embarrassing (Holman, et al., 2005). Patient may be embarrassed by removal of dentures.
5. Lower side rail and assist patient to sitting position, if permitted, or turn patient onto side. Place towel across patient's chest. Raise bed to a comfortable working position, usually elbow height of the caregiver (VISN 8 Patient Safety Center, 2009). Put on gloves.	The sitting or side-lying position prevents aspiration of fluids into the lungs. The towel protects the patient from dampness. Proper bed height helps reduce back strain while performing the procedure. Gloves prevent the spread of microorganisms.
6. Apply gentle pressure with 4 × 4 gauze to grasp upper denture plate and remove it (Figure 1). Place it immediately in denture cup. Lift lower dentures with gauze, using slight rocking motion. Remove, and place in denture cup.	Rocking motion breaks suction between denture and gum. Using 4 × 4 gauze prevents slippage and discourages spread of microorganisms.
7. Place paper towels or washcloth in sink while brushing. Using the toothbrush and paste, brush all denture surfaces gently but thoroughly (Figure 2). If patient prefers, add denture cleaner to cup with water and follow directions on preparation.	Putting paper towels or a washcloth in the sink protects against breakage. Dentures collect food and microorganisms and require daily cleaning.

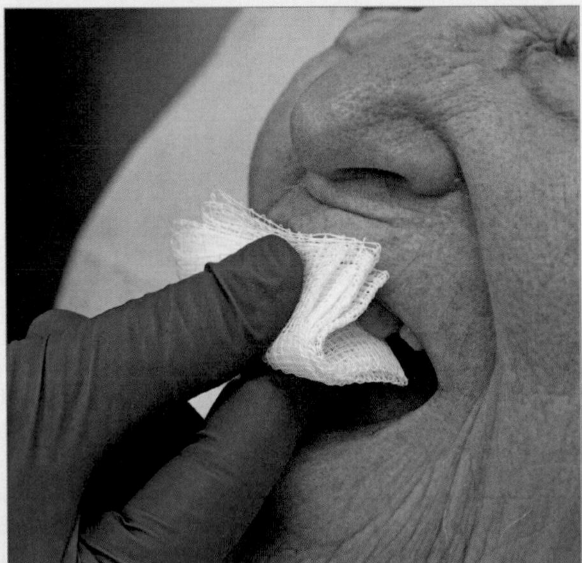

FIGURE 1 Removing dentures with a gauze sponge.

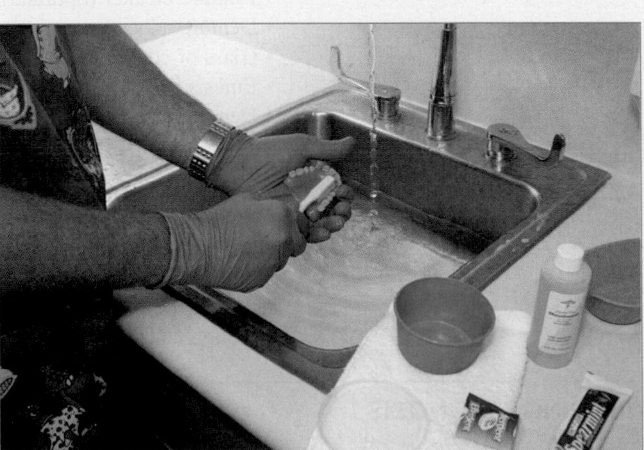

FIGURE 2 Cleaning dentures at sink.

ACTION	RATIONALE
8. Rinse thoroughly with water. Apply denture adhesive, if appropriate.	Water aids in removal of debris and acts as a cleaning agent.
9. Use a toothbrush and paste to gently clean gums, mucous membranes, and tongue. Offer water and/or mouthwash so patient can rinse mouth before replacing dentures.	Cleaning removes food particles and plaque, permitting proper fit and preventing infection. Mouthwash leaves a pleasant taste in the mouth.
10. Insert upper denture in mouth and press firmly. Insert lower denture. Check that the dentures are securely in place and comfortable.	This ensures patient comfort.
11. If the patient desires, dentures can be stored in the denture cup in cold water, instead of returning to the mouth. Label the cup and place it in the patient's bedside table.	Storing in water prevents warping of dentures. Proper storage prevents loss and damage.
12. Remove equipment and return the patient to a position of comfort. Remove your gloves. Raise side rail and lower bed.	Promotes patient comfort and safety. Removing gloves properly reduces the risk for infection transmission and contamination of other items.
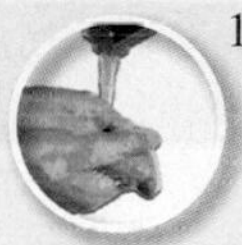 13. Remove additional PPE, if used. Perform hand hygiene.	Removing PPE properly reduces the risk for infection transmission and contamination of other items. Hand hygiene prevents transmission of microorganisms.

EVALUATION

The expected outcomes are met when the patient's oral cavity and dentures are clean, free from complications, and the patient states or demonstrates improved body image. In addition, the patient verbalizes a basic understanding of the need for oral care.

DOCUMENTATION

Guidelines

Record oral assessment, significant observations and unusual findings, such as bleeding or inflammation. Document any teaching done. Document procedure and patient response.

Sample Documentation

> 7/10/15 0945 Oral care performed. Oral cavity mucosa pink and moist. Denture and oral care given. No evidence of bleeding, ulceration, or inflammation.
>
> —*C. Stone, RN*

UNEXPECTED SITUATIONS AND ASSOCIATED INTERVENTIONS

- *Food or other material does not come off denture with brushing:* Place denture in cup with cool water and soak. After soaking, use toothbrush and toothpaste to clean again. If necessary, use commercial denture cleaner added to water in cup to soak, then brush clean.

SPECIAL CONSIDERATIONS

- Encourage the patient to wear his or her dentures, if not contraindicated. Dentures enhance appearance, assist in eating, facilitate speech, and maintain the gum line. Denture fit may be altered with long periods of nonuse.
- Encourage the patient to refrain from wrapping the denture in paper towels or napkins because they could be mistaken for trash.
- Encourage the patient to refrain from placing the dentures in the bedclothes because they can be lost in the laundry.
- Store dentures in cold water when not in the patient's mouth. Leaving dentures dry can cause warping, leading to discomfort when worn.

(continued)

SKILL 7-5 PROVIDING DENTURE CARE continued

EVIDENCE FOR PRACTICE ▶

ORAL HYGIENE AND DYSPHAGIA

Oral care is an essential component of quality nursing care. Diligent oral hygiene care can improve oral health and decrease the incidence of aspiration pneumonia, community-acquired pneumonia, ventilator-associated pneumonia, and other systemic diseases. What is nurses' knowledge regarding appropriate oral hygiene for patients with dysphagia?

Related Research

Durgude, Y., & Cocks, N. (2011). see the Evidence for Practice in Skill 7-3. Nurse's knowledge of the provision of oral care for patients with dysphagia. *British Journal of Community Nursing, 16*(12), 604–610.

For detailed information see the Evidence for Practice in Skill 7-3, and refer to thePoint for additional research on related nursing topics.

SKILL 7-6 REMOVING CONTACT LENSES

If a patient wears contact lenses but cannot remove them, the nurse is responsible for removing them. This may occur, for example, when the nurse is caring for an unconscious patient. Whenever an unconscious patient is admitted without any family present, always assess the patient to determine whether he or she wears contact lenses. Leaving contact lenses in place for long periods could result in permanent eye damage. Before removing lenses, use gentle pressure to center the lens on the cornea. Once removed, be sure to identify the lenses as being for the right or left eye, because the two lenses are not necessarily identical. If an eye injury is present, do not try to remove lenses because of the danger of causing an additional injury.

DELEGATION CONSIDERATIONS

The removal of contact lenses may be delegated to nursing assistive personnel (NAP) or to unlicensed assistive personnel (UAP), as well as to licensed practical/vocational nurses (LPN/LVNs). The decision to delegate must be based on careful analysis of the patient's needs and circumstances, as well as the qualifications of the person to whom the task is being delegated. Refer to the Delegation Guidelines in Appendix A.

EQUIPMENT

- Disposable gloves
- Additional PPE, if indicated
- Container for contact lenses (if unavailable, two small sterile containers marked "L" and "R" will suffice)
- Sterile normal saline solution
- Rubber pincer, if available (for removal of soft lenses)
- Suction-cup remover, if available (for removal of rigid lenses)

ASSESSMENT

Assess both eyes for contact lenses; some people wear them in only one eye. Assess eyes for any redness or drainage, which may indicate an eye infection or an allergic response. Assess for any eye injury. If an injury is present, notify the primary care provider about the presence of the contact lens. Do not try to remove the contact lens in this situation due to the risk for additional eye injury.

NURSING DIAGNOSIS

Determine the related factors for the nursing diagnoses based on the patient's current status. Appropriate nursing diagnoses may include:

- Risk for Injury
- Deficient Knowledge

OUTCOME IDENTIFICATION AND PLANNING

The expected outcome to achieve when removing contact lenses is that the lenses are removed without trauma to the eye and stored safely.

IMPLEMENTATION

ACTION	RATIONALE
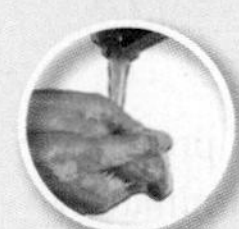 1. Perform hand hygiene and put on PPE, if indicated.	Hand hygiene and PPE prevent the spread of microorganisms. PPE is required based on transmission precautions.
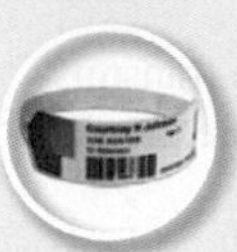 2. Identify the patient. Explain the procedure to the patient.	Patient identification validates the correct patient and correct procedure. Discussion and explanation help allay anxiety and prepare the patient for what to expect.
3. Assemble equipment on overbed table within reach.	Organization facilitates performance of task.
4. Close the curtains around the bed and close the door to the room, if possible.	This ensures the patient's privacy.
5. Assist the patient to a supine position. Raise the bed to a comfortable working position, usually elbow height of the caregiver (VISN 8 Patient Safety Center, 2009). Lower side rail closest to you.	Supine position with the bed raised and the side rail down is the least stressful position for removing a contact lens. Proper bed height helps reduce back strain while performing the procedure.
6. If containers are not already labeled, do so now. Place 5 mL of normal saline in each container.	Many patients have different prescription strengths for each eye. The saline will prevent the contact from drying out.
7. Put on gloves. Remove soft contact lens:	Gloves prevent the spread of microorganisms.
a. Have the patient look forward. Retract the lower lid with one hand. Using the pad of the index finger of the other hand, move the lens down to the sclera (Figure 1).	
b. Using the pads of the thumb and index finger, grasp the lens with a gentle pinching motion and remove it (Figure 2).	
See the accompanying Skill Variation figures for other techniques for removing both rigid and soft lenses.	
8. Place the first lens in its designated cup in the storage case before removing the second lens (Figure 3).	Lenses may be different for each eye. Avoids mixing them up.

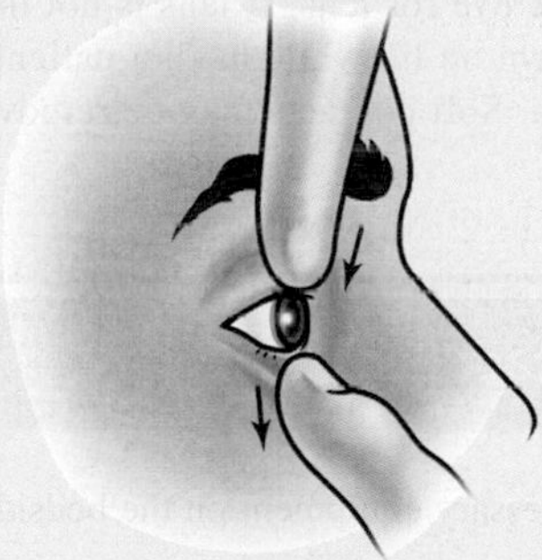

FIGURE 1 Retracting lower lid with one hand and using pad of index finger of other hand to move lens down to the sclera.

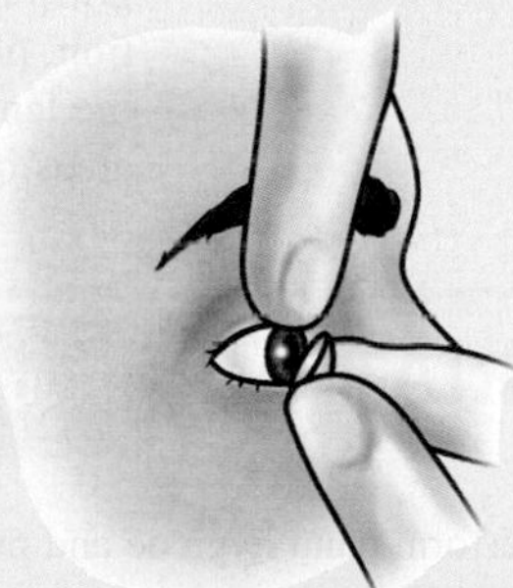

FIGURE 2 Using the pads of thumb and index finger to grasp lens with a gentle pinching motion to remove it.

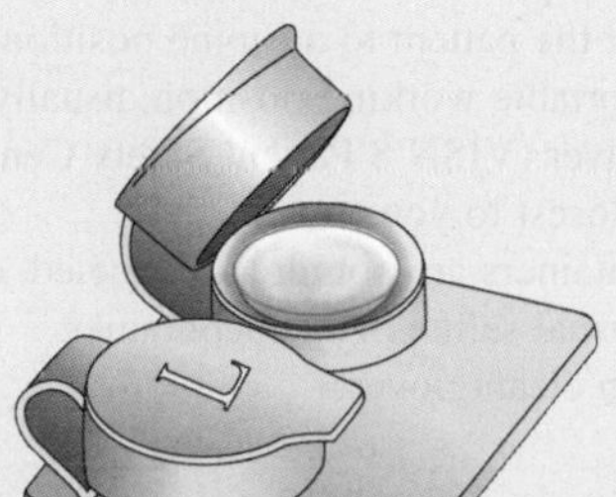

FIGURE 3 Storage cases are marked L and R, designating left and right lenses. Placing first lens in its designated cup before removing second lens avoids mixing them up.

(continued)

SKILL 7-6 REMOVING CONTACT LENSES continued

ACTION	RATIONALE
9. Repeat actions to remove other contact lens.	
10. If patient is awake and has glasses at bedside, offer patient glasses.	Not being able to see clearly creates anxiety.
11. Remove equipment and return the patient to a position of comfort. Remove your gloves. Raise side rail and lower bed.	Promotes patient comfort and safety. Removing gloves properly reduces the risk for infection transmission and contamination of other items.
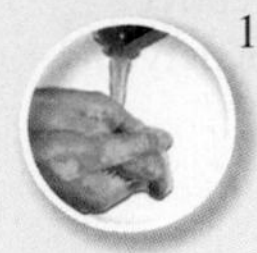 12. Remove additional PPE, if used. Perform hand hygiene.	Removing PPE properly reduces the risk for infection transmission and contamination of other items. Hand hygiene prevents transmission of microorganisms.

EVALUATION

The expected outcome is met when the patient remains free of injury as the contact lenses are removed. Eye exhibits no signs and symptoms of trauma, irritation, or redness.

DOCUMENTATION

Guidelines

Record your assessment, significant observations, and unusual findings, such as drainage or pain. Document any teaching done. Document the removal of the contact lenses, their storage, and patient response.

Sample Documentation

7/15/15 1045 Soft contacts removed from eyes without trauma. Stored in patient's lens case in normal saline. Sclera white with no drainage from eye. Glasses placed at bedside.

—*C. Stone, RN*

UNEXPECTED SITUATIONS AND ASSOCIATED INTERVENTIONS

- *The contact lens cannot be removed:* Use tool to remove lens. For hard lenses, the tool has a small suction cup that is placed over the contact lens. For soft lenses, the tool is a small pair of rubber grippers that can be placed over the contact lens to aid in removal.
- *Hard contact is not over the cornea:* Place a cotton-tipped applicator over upper eyelid and grasp lid, inverting lid over applicator. Examine eye for lens. If lens is not in the upper portion, place finger below eye and gently pull down on lid while having patient look up. When the lens is found, gently slide it over the cornea. Soft contacts may be removed from other areas of the eye.

SKILL VARIATION Removing Different Types of Contact Lens

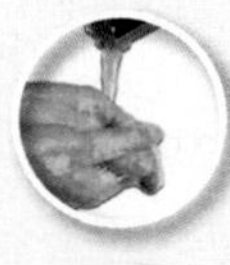

1. Perform hand hygiene and put on PPE, if indicated.

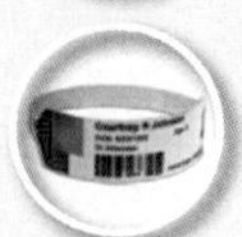

2. Identify the patient.
3. Explain what you are going to do and the reason for doing it to the patient.
4. Assemble necessary equipment on the bedside stand or overbed table.
5. Close the curtains around the bed and close the door to the room, if possible.
6. Assist the patient to a supine position. Raise bed to a comfortable working position, usually elbow height of the caregiver (VISN 8 Patient Safety Center, 2009). Lower side rail closest to you.
7. If containers are not already labeled, do so now. Place 5 mL of normal saline in each container.
8. Put on clean gloves.

SKILL VARIATION Removing Different Types of Contact Lens continued

To Remove Hard Contact Lenses—Patient is Able to Blink

a. If the lens is not centered over the cornea, apply gentle pressure on the lower eyelid to center the lens (Figure A).
b. Gently pull the outer corner of the eye toward the ear (Figure B).
c. Position the other hand below the lens to catch it and ask patient to blink (Figure C).

To Remove Hard Contact Lenses—Patient is Unable to Blink

a. Gently spread the eyelids beyond the top and bottom edges of the lens (Figure D).
b. Gently press the lower eyelid up against the bottom of the lens (Figure E).
c. After the lens is tipped slightly, move the eyelids toward one another to cause the lens to slide out between the eyelids (Figure F).

To Remove Hard Contact Lenses with a Suction Cup—Patient is Unable to Blink

a. Ensure that contact lens is centered on the cornea. Place a drop of sterile saline on the suction cup.
b. Place the suction cup in the center of the contact lens and gently pull the contact lens off the eye.
c. To remove the suction cup from the lens, slide the lens off sideways.

To Remove Soft Contact Lenses with a Rubber Pincer

a. Locate the contact lens and place the rubber pincers in the center of the lens.
b. Gently squeeze the pincers and remove the lens from the eye.

9. Place the first lens in its designated cup in the storage case before removing the second lens.
10. Repeat actions to remove other contact lens. Remove gloves.
11. If patient is awake and has glasses at bedside, offer patient glasses. Lower bed. Assist patient to a comfortable position.
12. Remove additional PPE, if used. Perform hand hygiene.

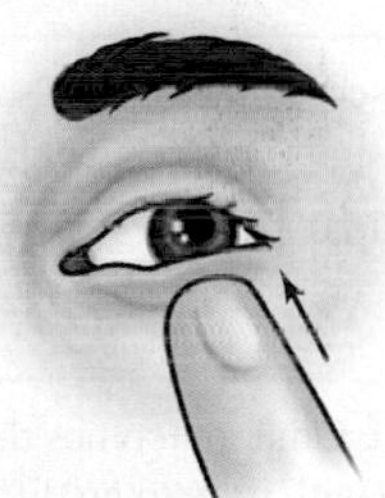
FIGURE A Centering lens.

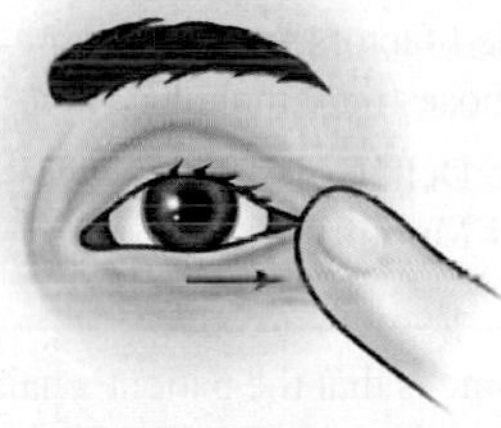
FIGURE B Gently pulling outer corner of eye toward ear.

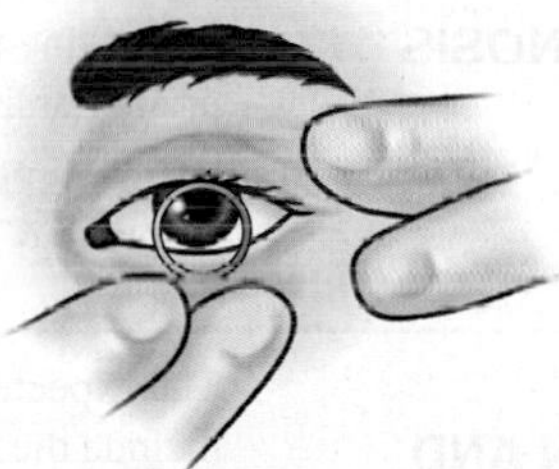
FIGURE C Receiving lens as patient blinks.

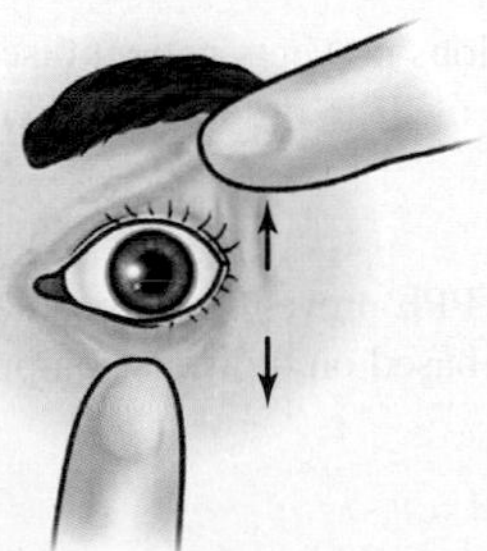
FIGURE D Spreading eyelids.

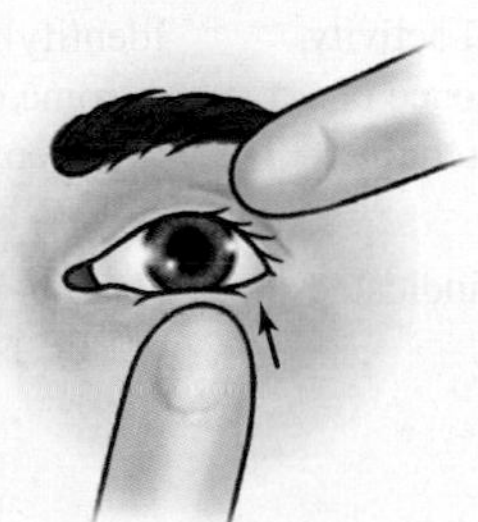
FIGURE E Pressing lower lid up against bottom of lens.

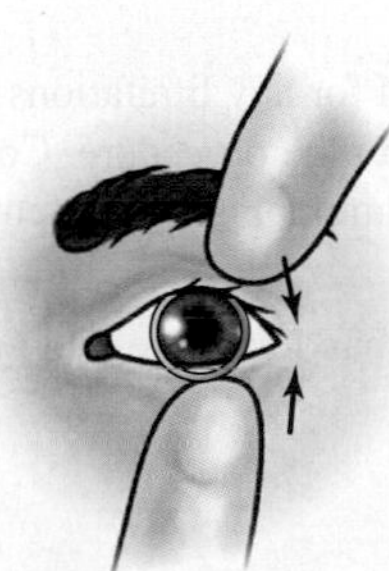
FIGURE F Sliding lens out between lids.

SKILL 7-7 SHAMPOOING A PATIENT'S HAIR IN BED

The easiest way to wash a patient's hair is to assist him or her in the shower, but not all patients can take showers. If the patient's hair needs to be washed but the patient is unable or not allowed to get out of bed, a bed shampoo can be performed. Shampoo caps are available, and are being used with increasing frequency. These commercially prepared, disposable caps contain a rinseless shampoo product. See the accompanying Skill Variation.

DELEGATION CONSIDERATIONS

The shampooing of a patient's hair may be delegated to nursing assistive personnel (NAP) or to unlicensed assistive personnel (UAP), as well as to licensed practical/vocational nurses (LPN/LVNs). The decision to delegate must be based on careful analysis of the patient's needs and circumstances, as well as the qualifications of the person to whom the task is being delegated. Refer to the Delegation Guidelines in Appendix A.

EQUIPMENT

- Water pitcher
- Warm water
- Shampoo
- Conditioner (optional)
- Disposable gloves
- Additional PPE, as indicated
- Protective pad for bed
- Shampoo board
- Bucket
- Towels
- Gown
- Comb or brush
- Blow dryer (optional)

ASSESSMENT

Assess the patient's hygiene preferences: frequency, time of day, and type of hygiene products. Assess for any physical activity limitations. Assess the patient's ability to get out of bed to have his or her hair washed. If the medical orders allow it and patient is physically able to wash his or her hair in the shower, the patient may prefer to do so. If the patient cannot tolerate being out of bed or is not allowed to do so, perform a bed shampoo. Assess for any activity or positioning limitations. Inspect the patient's scalp for any cuts, lesions, or bumps. Note any flaking, drying, or excessive oiliness, or evidence of problems, such as **pediculosis**.

NURSING DIAGNOSIS

Determine the related factors for the nursing diagnoses based on the patient's current status. Appropriate nursing diagnoses may include:

- Bathing Self-Care Deficit
- Impaired Physical Mobility
- Impaired Transfer Ability

OUTCOME IDENTIFICATION AND PLANNING

The expected outcome is that the patient's hair will be clean. Other outcomes that may be appropriate include the following: the patient will tolerate the shampoo with little to no difficulty, the patient will demonstrate an improved body image, and the patient will verbalize an increase in comfort.

IMPLEMENTATION

ACTION	RATIONALE
1. Review health record for any limitations in physical activity, or contraindications to the procedure. Confirm presence of medical order for shampooing the patient's hair, if required by facility policy.	Identifying limitations prevents patient discomfort and injury. In some settings, a medical order is required for shampooing a patient's hair.
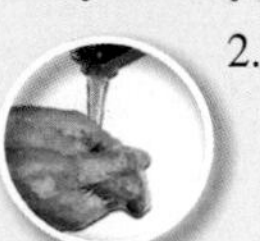 2. Perform hand hygiene. Put on PPE, as indicated.	Hand hygiene and PPE prevent the spread of microorganisms. PPE is required based on transmission precautions.
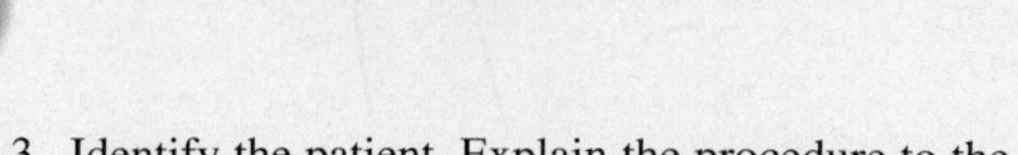	
 3. Identify the patient. Explain the procedure to the patient.	Patient identification validates the correct patient and correct procedure. Discussion and explanation help allay anxiety and prepare the patient for what to expect.

ACTION	RATIONALE
4. Assemble equipment on overbed table within reach.	Organization facilitates performance of task.
5. Close the curtains around the bed and close the door to the room, if possible.	Provides for patient privacy.
6. Lower the head of the bed. Raise bed to a comfortable working position, usually elbow height of the caregiver (VISN 8 Patient Safety Center, 2009). Lower side rail. Remove pillow and place protective pad under patient's head and shoulders (Figure 1).	Proper bed height helps reduce back strain while performing the procedure. A protective pad keeps the sheets from getting wet.
7. **Fill the pitcher with comfortably warm water (100°F to less than 120°F to 125°F).** Position the patient at the top of the bed, in a supine position. Have the patient lift his or her head and place the shampoo board underneath patient's head (Figure 2). If necessary, pad the edge of the board with a small towel.	Warm water is comfortable and relaxing for the patient. It also stimulates circulation and provides for more effective cleaning. Adjusting the water temperature to 100°F to less than 120°F to 125°F decreases risk of burns and drying of the skin. The lower temperature is recommended for children and adults over 65 years of age (Burn Foundation, 2012). Padding the edge of the shampoo board may help increase patient comfort.
8. Place a drain container underneath the drain of the shampoo board (Figure 3).	The container will catch the runoff water, preventing a mess on the floor.

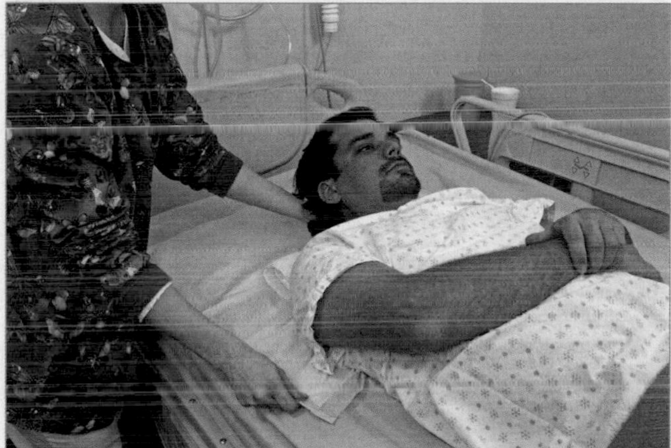

FIGURE 1 Placing protective pad under patient's head.

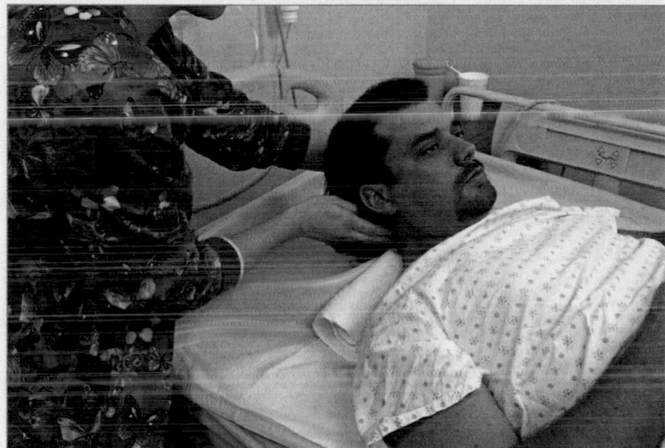

FIGURE 2 Placing patient's head on shampoo board.

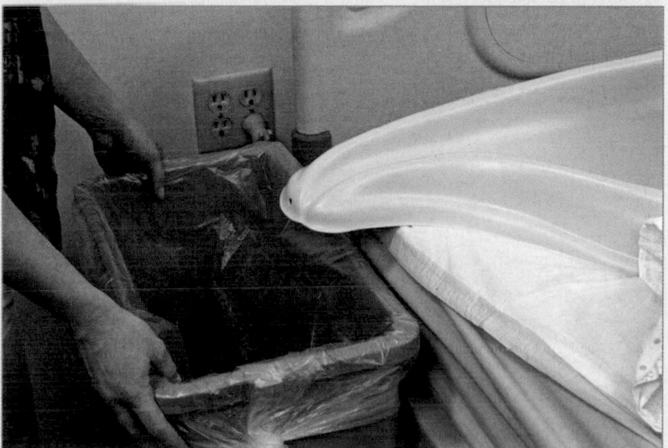

FIGURE 3 Positioning drain container for shampoo board.

(continued)

SKILL 7-7 SHAMPOOING A PATIENT'S HAIR IN BED continued

ACTION	RATIONALE
9. Put on gloves. If the patient is able, have him or her hold a folded washcloth at the forehead. Pour a pitcher of warm water slowly over the patient's head, making sure that all hair is saturated (Figure 4). Refill pitcher, if needed.	Gloves prevent the spread of microorganisms. A washcloth prevents water from running into the patient's eyes. By pouring slowly, more hair will become wet, and it is more soothing for the patient.
10. Apply a small amount of shampoo to patient's hair. Lather shampoo (Figure 5). Massage deep into the scalp, avoiding any cuts, lesions, or sore spots.	Shampoo will help to remove dirt or oil.
11. Rinse with comfortably warm water until all shampoo is out of hair (Figure 6). Repeat shampoo, if necessary.	Shampoo left in hair may cause pruritus. If hair is still dirty, another shampoo treatment may be needed.
12. If patient has thick hair or requests it, apply a small amount of conditioner to hair and massage throughout. Avoid any cuts, lesions, or sore spots.	Conditioner eases tangles and moisturizes hair and scalp.
13. If drain container is small, empty before rinsing hair. Rinse with comfortably warm water until all conditioner is out of hair.	Container may overflow if not emptied. Conditioner left in hair may cause pruritus.
14. Remove shampoo board (Figure 7). Place towel around patient's hair.	This prevents the patient from getting cold.

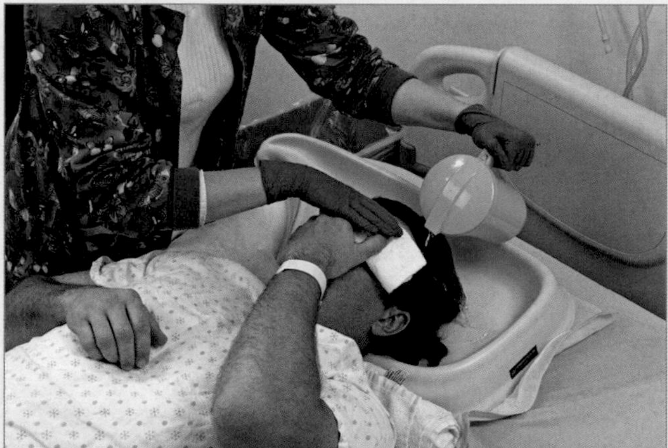

FIGURE 4 Pouring warm water over patient's head.

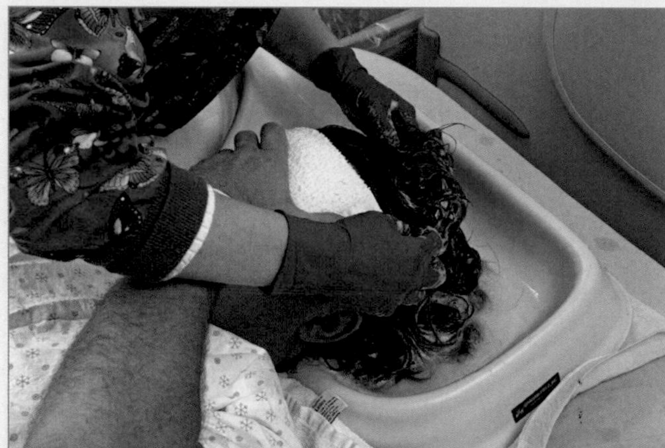

FIGURE 5 Lathering shampoo.

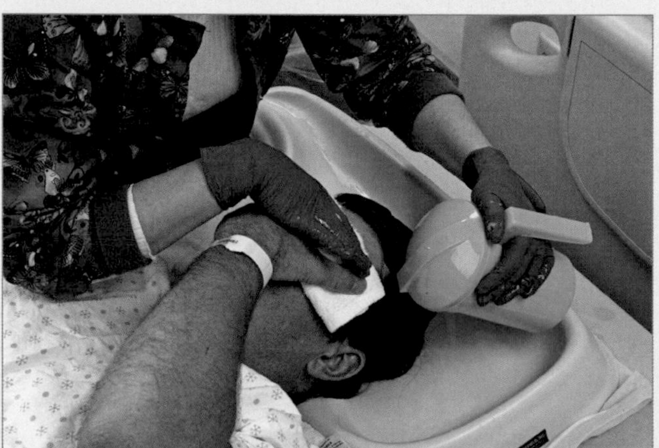

FIGURE 6 Rinsing shampoo from patient's head.

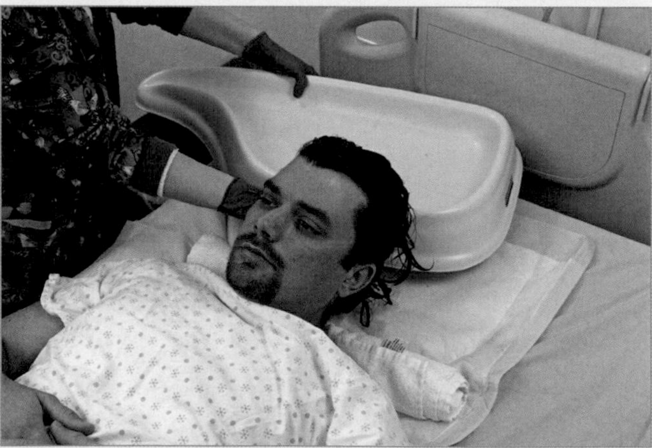

FIGURE 7 Removing shampoo board.

ACTION	RATIONALE
15. Pat hair dry, avoiding any cuts, lesions, or sore spots (Figure 8). Remove protective padding, but keep one dry protective pad under patient's hair (Figure 9).	Patting dry removes any excess water without damaging hair or scalp.

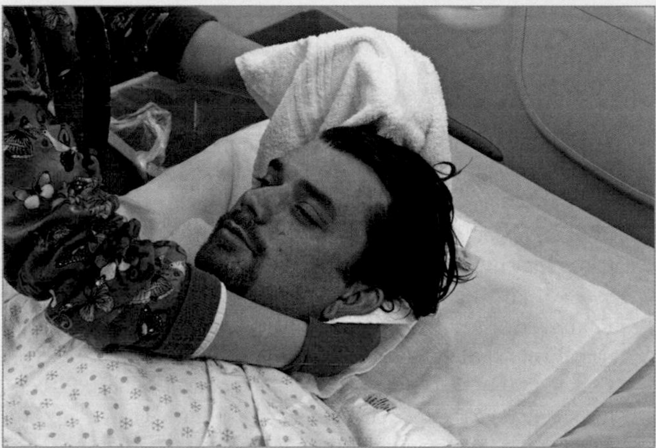

FIGURE 8 Patting patient's hair dry.

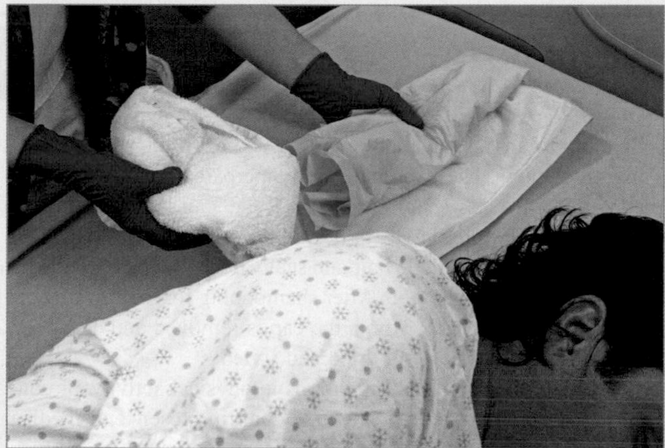

FIGURE 9 Removing wet protective padding.

ACTION	RATIONALE
16. Gently brush hair, removing tangles, as needed.	Removing tangles helps hair to dry faster. Brushing hair improves patient's self-image.
17. Blow-dry hair on a cool setting, if allowed and if patient wishes. If not, consider covering the patient's head with a dry towel, until hair is dry.	Blow-drying hair helps hair to dry faster and prevents patient from becoming chilled. Keeping the head covered prevents chilling while hair is drying.
18. Change patient's gown and remove protective pad. Replace pillow.	If patient's gown is damp, patient will become chilled. Protective pad is no longer needed once hair is dry.
19. Remove equipment and return patient to a position of comfort. Remove your gloves. Raise side rail and lower bed.	Promotes patient comfort and safety. Removing gloves properly reduces the risk for infection transmission and contamination of other items.
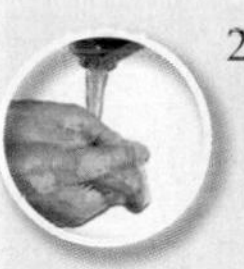 20. Remove additional PPE, if used. Perform hand hygiene.	Removing PPE properly reduces the risk for infection transmission and contamination of other items. Hand hygiene deters spread of microorganisms.

EVALUATION

The expected outcomes are met when the patient's hair is clean, the patient verbalizes a positive body image, and the patient reports an increase in comfort level.

DOCUMENTATION

Guidelines

Record your assessment, significant observations, and unusual findings, such as bleeding or inflammation. Document any teaching done. Document procedure and patient response.

Sample Documentation

7/4/15 1130 Hair washed. Moderate amount of dried blood in hair noted. A 3-cm laceration noted over left parietal area. Edges well approximated, slight redness of wound, surrounding skin consistent with rest of skin tone, sutures intact, and no drainage noted.

—*C. Stone, RN*

UNEXPECTED SITUATIONS AND ASSOCIATED INTERVENTIONS

- *Glass is found in hair:* Carefully comb through hair before washing to remove as much glass as possible. Discard glass in appropriate container. When massaging the scalp, be alert to signs of pain from the patient; glass could be cutting the patient's head.

(*continued*)

SKILL 7-7 SHAMPOOING A PATIENT'S HAIR IN BED continued

SPECIAL CONSIDERATIONS

- If the patient has a spinal cord or neck injury, use of the shampoo board may be contraindicated. In this case, a makeshift protection area can be created to wash the patient's hair without using the board. Place a protective pad underneath the patient's head and shoulders. Roll a towel into the bottom of the protective pad and direct the roll into one area so that water will drain into the container.

SKILL VARIATION Shampooing a Patient's Hair with a Shampoo Cap

Shampoo caps are available and are being used with increasing frequency. These commercially prepared, disposable caps contain a rinseless shampoo product. The cap is warmed in the microwave or stored in a warmer until use. The cap is placed on the patient's head and the hair and scalp are massaged through the cap, to lather the shampoo. After shampooing for the manufacturer's suggested length of time, the cap is removed and discarded. The patient's hair is towel dried and styled.

1. Review chart for any limitations in physical activity, or contraindications to the procedure. Confirm presence of medical order for shampooing patient's hair, if required by facility policy.
2. Warm the cap in the microwave, according to the manufacturer's directions, or remove it from the storage warmer.

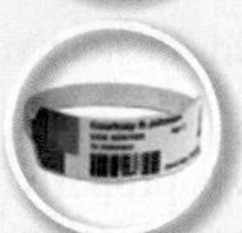

3. Perform hand hygiene and put on PPE, if indicated.
4. Identify the patient.
5. Explain what you are going to do and the reason for doing it to the patient.
6. Assemble necessary equipment on the bedside stand or overbed table.
7. Close the curtains around the bed and close the door to the room, if possible.
8. Put on gloves. Raise bed to a comfortable working position, usually elbow height of the caregiver (VISN 8 Patient Safety Center, 2009). Place a towel across the patient's chest. Place the shampoo cap on the patient's head (Figure A).
9. Massage the scalp and hair through the cap to lather the shampoo. Continue to massage according to the time frame specified by the manufacturer's directions (Figure B).
10. Remove and discard the shampoo cap.
11. Dry the patient's hair with a towel.
12. Remove the towel from the patient's chest.
13. Comb and style the hair.
14. Remove gloves. Lower bed. Assist the patient to a comfortable position.

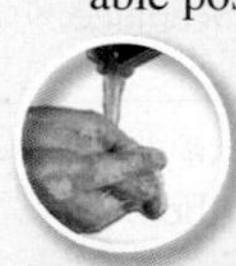

15. Remove additional PPE, if used. Perform hand hygiene.

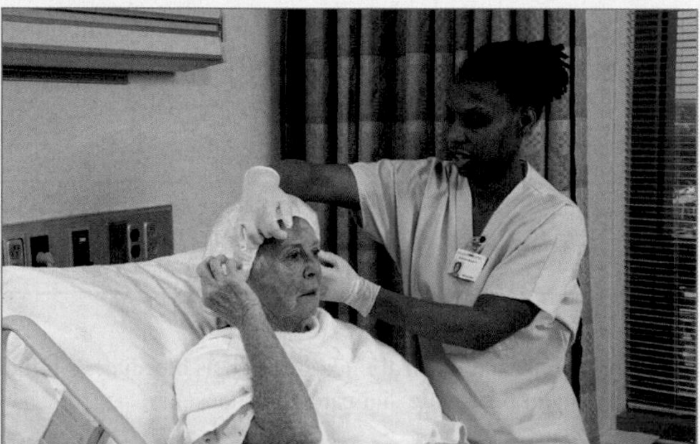

FIGURE A Placing warmed shampoo cap on the patient's head.

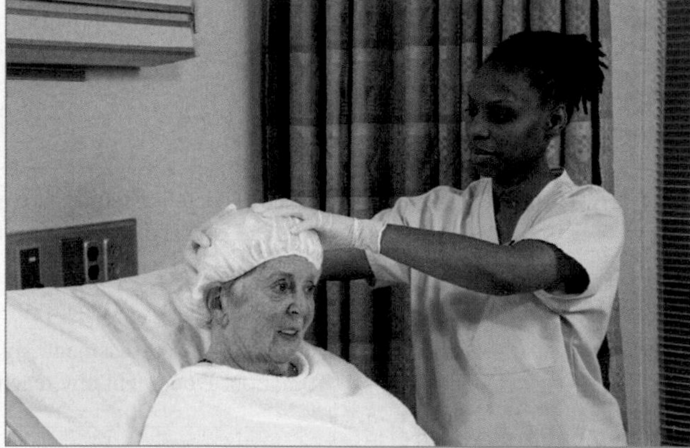

FIGURE B Massaging the hair and scalp.

SKILL 7-8 ASSISTING THE PATIENT TO SHAVE

For many patients shaving is a daily hygiene ritual. They may feel disheveled and unclean without shaving. Some patients may need help with shaving when using a regular blade or may require that the nurse perform the shaving procedure for them completely. Patients with beards or mustaches may require nursing assistance to keep the beard and mustache clean. However, never trim or shave a patient's beard or mustache without the patient's consent. Female patients may require assistance with shaving underarm and leg hair, depending on the patient's personal preference and abilities. If available and permitted by the facility, electric shavers are usually recommended when the patient is receiving anticoagulant therapy or has a bleeding disorder. Electric shavers are especially convenient for ill and bedridden patients.

DELEGATION CONSIDERATIONS

The shaving of a patient's hair may be delegated to nursing assistive personnel (NAP) or to unlicensed assistive personnel (UAP) after assessment by the registered nurse, as well as to licensed practical/vocational nurses (LPN/LVNs). The decision to delegate must be based on careful analysis of the patient's needs and circumstances, as well as the qualifications of the person to whom the task is being delegated. Refer to the Delegation Guidelines Appendix A.

EQUIPMENT

- Shaving cream
- Safety razor
- Towel
- Washcloth
- Bath basin
- Disposable gloves
- Additional PPE, as indicated
- Waterproof pad
- Aftershave or lotion (optional)

ASSESSMENT

Assess the patient's shaving preferences: frequency, time of day, and type of shaving products. Assess for any physical activity limitations. Assess patient for any bleeding problems. If patient is receiving any anticoagulant, such as heparin or warfarin (Coumadin), has received an antithrombolytic agent, or has a low platelet count, consider using an electric razor. Inspect the area to be shaved for any lesions or weeping areas. Assess the patient's ability to shave himself or assist with the procedure.

NURSING DIAGNOSIS

Determine related factors for the nursing diagnoses based on the patient's current status. Appropriate nursing diagnoses may include:

- Risk for Injury
- Bathing Self-Care Deficit
- Impaired Physical Mobility

OUTCOME IDENTIFICATION AND PLANNING

The expected outcome to achieve when assisting the patient with shaving is that the patient will be clean, without evidence of hair growth or trauma to the skin. Other outcomes that may be appropriate include the following: the patient tolerates shaving with minimal to no difficulty, and the patient verbalizes feelings of improved self-esteem.

IMPLEMENTATION

ACTION	RATIONALE
1. Review health record for any limitations in physical activity, or contraindications to the procedure. Confirm presence of medical order for shaving the patient, if required by facility policy.	Identifying limitations prevents patient discomfort and injury. In some settings, a medical order is required for shaving a patient with certain health problems or taking medications that affect coagulation.
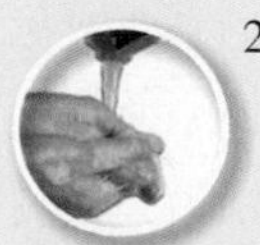 2. Perform hand hygiene. Put on PPE, as indicated.	Hand hygiene and PPE prevent the spread of microorganisms. PPE is required based on transmission precautions.
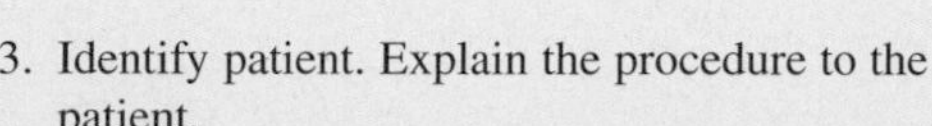 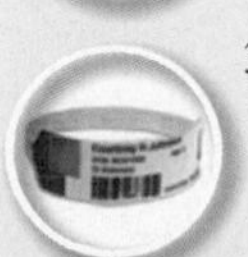 3. Identify patient. Explain the procedure to the patient.	Identifying the patient ensures the right patient receives the intervention and helps prevent errors. Explanation facilitates cooperation.

(continued)

SKILL 7-8 ASSISTING THE PATIENT TO SHAVE continued

ACTION	RATIONALE
4. Assemble equipment on overbed table within reach.	Organization facilitates performance of task.
5. Close the curtains around the bed and close the door to the room, if possible.	Provides for patient privacy.
6. Raise bed to a comfortable working position, usually elbow height of the caregiver (VISN 8 Patient Safety Center, 2009). Lower side rail. Cover patient's chest with a towel or waterproof pad. Fill bath basin with comfortably warm (100°F to less than 120°F to 125°F) water. Put on gloves. Press a warm washcloth on the area to be shaved.	Proper bed height helps reduce back strain while performing the procedure. Adjusting the water temperature to 100°F to less than 120°F to 125°F decreases risk of burns and drying of the skin. The lower temperature is recommended for children and adults over 65 years of age (Burn Foundation, 2012). Warm water is comfortable and relaxing for the patient. Moistens skin and softens hair. Gloves prevent the spread of microorganisms. Warm water softens the hair, making the process easier.
7. Dispense shaving cream into palm of hand. Apply cream to area to be shaved in a layer about 0.5 inch thick (Figure 1).	Using shaving cream helps to prevent skin irritation and prevents hair from pulling.
8. With one hand, pull the skin taut at the area to be shaved. Using a smooth stroke, begin shaving. *If shaving the face,* shave with the direction of hair growth in short strokes (Figure 2). *If shaving a leg,* shave against the hair in upward, short strokes. *If shaving an underarm,* pull skin taut and use short, upward strokes.	The skin on the face is more sensitive and needs to be shaved with the direction of hair growth to prevent discomfort.
9. Remove residual shaving cream with wet washcloth (Figure 3).	Shaving cream can lead to irritation if left on the skin.

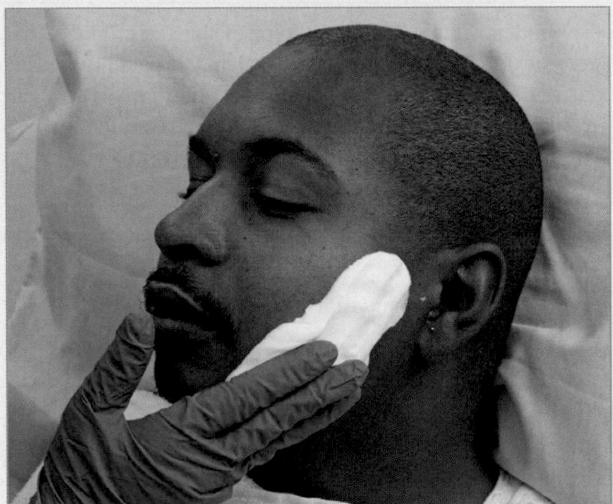

FIGURE 1 Applying shaving cream to face.

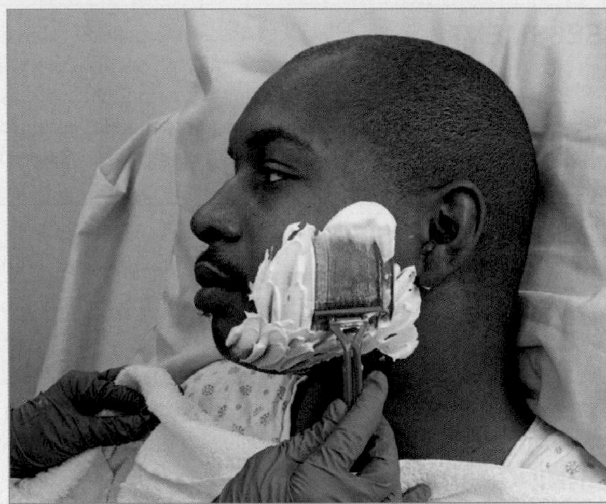

FIGURE 2 Shaving face.

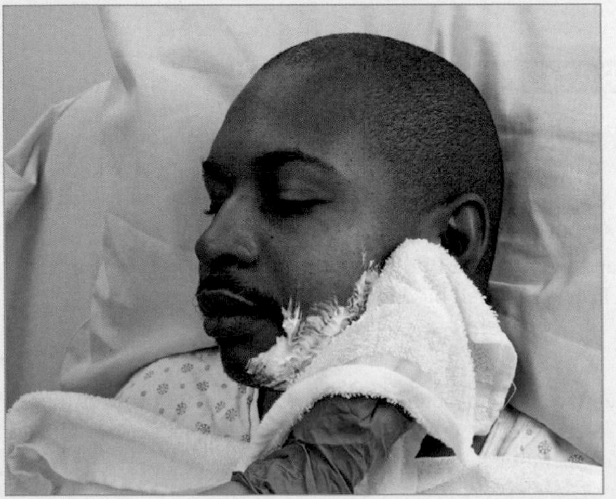

FIGURE 3 Using a wet washcloth to remove remaining shaving cream.

ACTION	RATIONALE
10. If patient requests, apply aftershave or lotion to area shaved.	Aftershave and lotion can reduce skin irritation.
11. Remove equipment and return patient to a position of comfort. Remove your gloves. Raise side rail and lower bed.	Promotes patient comfort and safety. Removing gloves properly reduces the risk for infection transmission and contamination of other items.
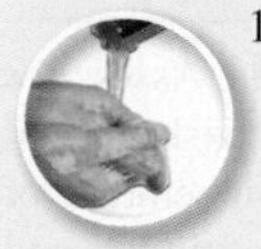 12. Remove additional PPE, if used. Perform hand hygiene.	Removing PPE properly reduces the risk for infection transmission and contamination of other items. Hand hygiene deters spread of microorganisms.

EVALUATION

The expected outcome is met when the patient is clean-shaven without evidence of trauma, irritation, or redness. In addition, the patient verbalizes feeling refreshed and demonstrates improved self-esteem.

DOCUMENTATION

Shaving a patient does not usually require documentation. However, if your skin assessment reveals any unusual findings, document your assessment and the procedure. If the patient or nurse breaks the skin while shaving, document the occurrence and your assessment of the patient.

UNEXPECTED SITUATIONS AND ASSOCIATED INTERVENTIONS

- *Patient is cut and bleeds during shave:* Apply pressure with gauze or towel to injured area. Do not release pressure for 2 to 3 minutes. After bleeding has stopped, resume shaving. The water basin may need to be rewarmed before washing off the shaving cream. Document the occurrence and assessment of area after the shave.
- *Patient has large amount of hair to be shaved:* If hair is longer, it may need to be trimmed with scissors before shaving to prevent pulling of hair when shaving.

SPECIAL CONSIDERATIONS

- *Patient is brought to hospital with full beard:* Do not shave patient's beard without consent unless it is an emergency situation, such as insertion of an endotracheal tube. For this procedure, shave only the area needed and leave the rest of the beard.

SKILL 7-9 PROVIDING NAIL CARE

Care of the nails is important to prevent pain and infection. Long, roughened nails that have not been trimmed or filed may increase the occurrence of traumatic nail injury, such as damage to the nail that may result in the nail plate being torn from the nail bed (Malkin & Berridge, 2009). Poor toenail care may lead to poor mobility. The nurse should document and report to the patient's primary care provider any changes to nail color, such as discoloration of the entire nail or a dark streak under the nail; changes in nail shape, such as curled nails; thinning or thickening of the nails; separation of the nail from the surrounding skin; bleeding around the nails; and redness, swelling, or pain around the nails (Mayo Foundation for Medical Education and Research, 2011c).

DELEGATION CONSIDERATIONS

Depending on the organization's policies and procedures, the care of a patient's nails may be delegated to nursing assistive personnel (NAP) or to unlicensed assistive personnel (UAP) after assessment by the registered nurse. The care of a patient's nails may be delegated to licensed practical/vocational nurses (LPN/LVNs). The decision to delegate must be based on careful analysis of the patient's needs and circumstances, as well as the qualifications of the person to whom the task is being delegated. Refer to the Delegation Guidelines in Appendix A.

(continued)

SKILL 7-9 PROVIDING NAIL CARE continued

EQUIPMENT

- Nail file
- Nail clipper
- Cuticle scissors
- Orangewood stick or cuticle stick
- Emollient
- Disposable waterproof pad
- Towel
- Wash basin and skin cleanser, or commercially prepared bathing system
- Disposable gloves
- Additional PPE, if indicated

ASSESSMENT

Assess the patient's nail care preferences: frequency, time of day, and type of products. Assess for any physical activity limitations. Assess for conditions that may put the patient at high risk for nail problems, such as diabetes and peripheral vascular disease. Assess the color and temperature of fingers and toes. Assess adequacy of pulses to area and capillary refill. Assess the skin of fingers and toes for dryness, cracking, or inflammation. Assess the nails and surrounding skin for changes in nail color, changes in nail shape, thinning or thickening of the nails, separation of the nail from the surrounding skin, bleeding around the nails, and redness, swelling, or pain around the nails. Nails should appear intact, smooth, firmly attached to nail bed, pink in color, with white crescent visible at the base. Dark streaks running lengthwise in nails are a normal variation for patients with darker skin tones. Assess the patient's ability for self-care of nails or assist with the procedure.

NURSING DIAGNOSIS

Determine related factors for the nursing diagnoses based on the patient's current status. Appropriate nursing diagnoses may include:

- Risk for Injury
- Bathing Self-Care Deficit
- Impaired Physical Mobility

OUTCOME IDENTIFICATION AND PLANNING

The expected outcome to achieve when assisting the patient with care of the nails is nails are trimmed and clean with smooth edges and intact cuticles, without evidence of trauma to nails or surrounding skin. Other outcomes that may be appropriate include the patient verbalizes feelings of improved self-esteem.

IMPLEMENTATION

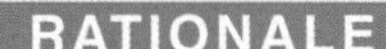

ACTION	RATIONALE
1. Review health record for any limitations in physical activity, or contraindications to the procedure. Confirm presence of medical order for nail care, if required by facility policy.	Identifying limitations prevents patient discomfort and injury. In some settings, a medical order is required for nail care, particularly for a patient with certain health problems.
2. Perform hand hygiene. Put on PPE, as indicated.	Hand hygiene and PPE prevent the spread of microorganisms. PPE is required based on transmission precautions.
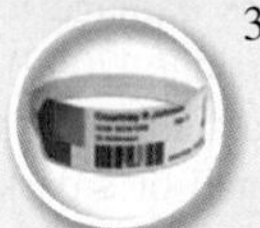 3. Identify patient. Explain procedure to the patient.	Identifying the patient ensures the right patient receives the intervention and helps prevent errors. Explanation facilitates cooperation.
4. Assemble equipment on overbed table within reach.	Organization facilitates performance of task.
5. Close the curtains around the bed and close the door to the room, if possible.	Provides for patient privacy.
6. Raise bed to a comfortable working position, usually elbow height of the caregiver (VISN 8 Patient Safety Center, 2009). Lower side rail. Place a towel or waterproof pad under the patient's hand or foot.	Proper bed height helps reduce back strain while performing the procedure. Waterproof pad protects bed linens and surrounding surfaces.
7. Put on gloves. Wash patient's hands or feet, depending on care to be given.	Gloves prevent the spread of microorganisms. Washing removes surface dirt and softens nails and skin, making it easier to trim and care for cuticles (Mayo Foundation for Medical Education and Research, 2011c).

ACTION	RATIONALE
8. Gently clean under the nails using the cuticle or orangewood stick (Figure 1). Wash hand or foot.	Washing removes debris and dirt dislodged from under nails.
9. Clip nail, if necessary. Avoid cutting the whole nail in one attempt. Use the tip of the nail clipper and take small cuts (Malkin & Berridge, 2009). Cut the nail straight across (Figure 2). Do not trim so far down on the sides that the skin and cuticle are injured. **Only file, do not cut, the nails of patients with diabetes or circulatory problems.**	Cutting entire nail in one attempt may lead to splitting the nail. Prevents injury to nail, cuticle, and finger or toe and reduces risk for in-growing nails (Mayo Foundation for Medical Education and Research, 2011a; Mayo Foundation for Medical Education and Research, 2011c; Malkin & Berridge, 2009).
10. File the nail straight across, then round the tips in a gentle curve, to shape the nail. Do not trim so far down on the sides that the skin and cuticle are injured. **Only file, do not cut, the nails of patients with diabetes or circulatory problems.**	Smoothes the nail. Prevents injury to nail, cuticle, and finger or toe and reduces risk for in-growing nails (Mayo Foundation for Medical Education and Research, 2011a; Mayo Foundation for Medical Education and Research, 2011c; Malkin & Berridge, 2009).
11. Remove hangnails, which are broken pieces of cuticle, by carefully trimming them off with cuticle scissors. Avoid injury to tissue with the cuticle scissors.	Removes dead cuticle. Reduces hangnail formation. Tearing of hangnail can cause injury to live tissue.
12. Gently push cuticles back off the nail using the orangewood stick or towel (Figure 3).	Keeps cuticles and nails neat and prevents cracking and drying of cuticles.
13. Dry hand or foot thoroughly, taking care to be sure to dry between fingers or toes (Figure 4). Apply an emollient to the hand or foot, rubbing it into the nails and cuticles. Do not moisturize between the toes of patients with peripheral artery disease.	Thorough drying reduces risk of maceration, damage from overly and consistently wet skin. Maceration increases risk for injury from rubbing or friction, and risk for fungal and bacterial infections. Moisturizing between the toes of patients with peripheral artery disease can encourage fungal growth (Mayo Foundation for Medical Education and Research, 2012).

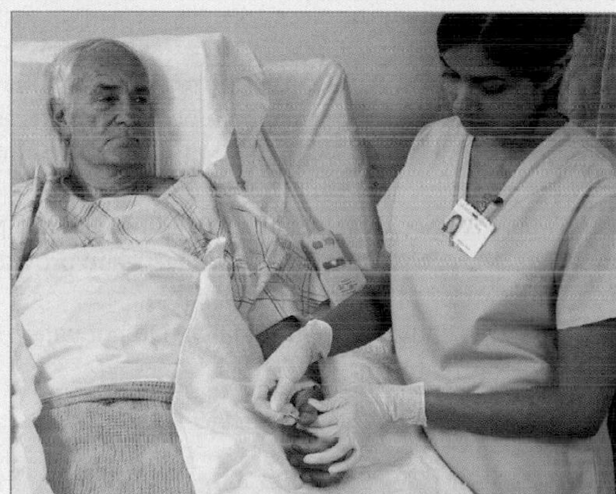

FIGURE 1 Gently cleaning under nails.

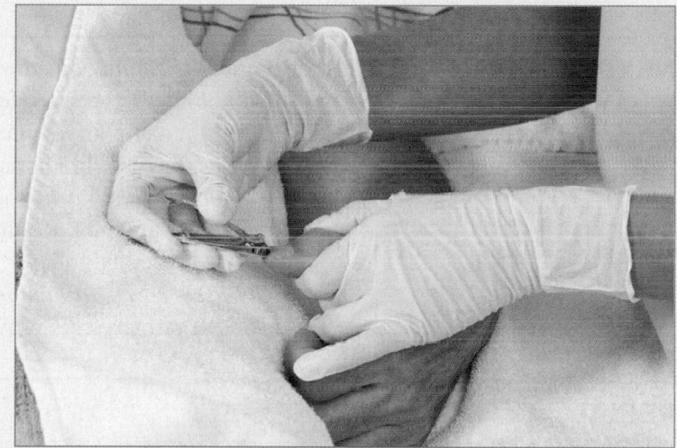

FIGURE 2 Trimming straight across nails with clipper.

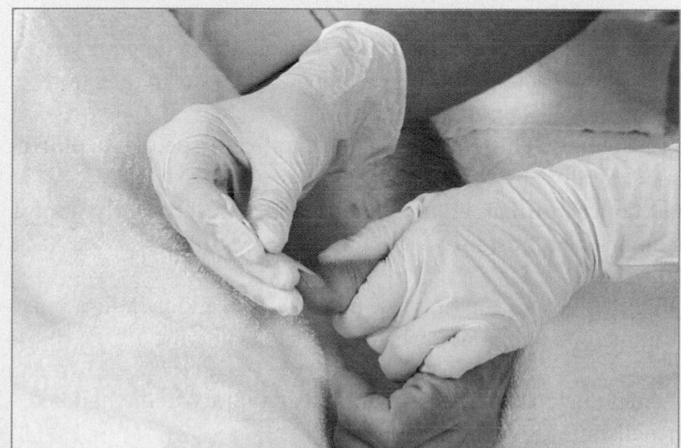

FIGURE 3 Gently pushing cuticles back off nail.

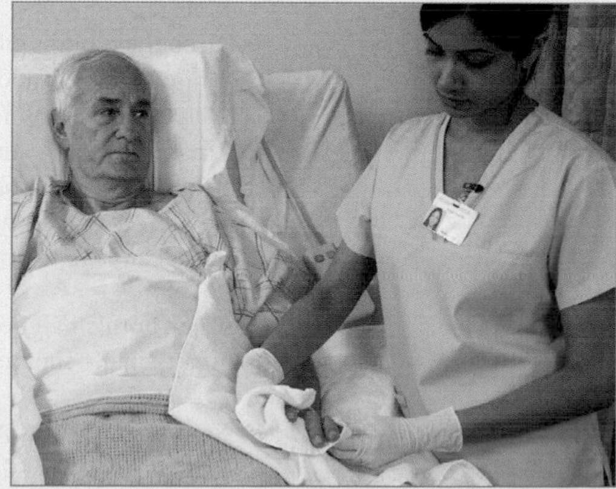

FIGURE 4 Drying hand thoroughly.

(continued)

SKILL 7-9 PROVIDING NAIL CARE continued

ACTION	RATIONALE
14. Repeat Steps 7-13 for other extremity or extremities.	
15. Remove equipment and return patient to a position of comfort. Remove your gloves. Raise side rail and lower bed.	Promotes patient comfort and safety. Removing gloves properly reduces the risk for infection transmission and contamination of other items.
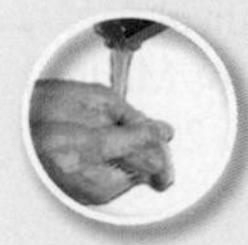 16. Remove additional PPE, if used. Perform hand hygiene.	Removing PPE properly reduces the risk for infection transmission and contamination of other items. Hand hygiene deters spread of microorganisms.

EVALUATION

The expected outcome is met when the patient's nails are trimmed and clean with smooth edges and intact cuticles, and are without evidence of trauma to nails or surrounding skin. In addition, the patient verbalizes feeling refreshed and demonstrates improved self-esteem.

DOCUMENTATION

Guidelines

Record your assessment, significant observations, and unusual findings, such as broken nails or inflammation. Document any teaching done. Document procedure and patient response. Nail care is often recorded on routine flow sheet.

Sample Documentation

7/17/15 2030 Nail care performed for fingernails. Nails intact, supple, pink in color, with white crescent visible at the base. Significant amount of old food removed from under nails. Skin on fingers and hands dry and cracked; emollient applied.

—J. Lyman, RN

UNEXPECTED SITUATIONS AND ASSOCIATED INTERVENTIONS

- *Patient is cut and bleeds during nail care:* Apply pressure with gauze or towel to injured area. Do not release pressure for 2 to 3 minutes. Assess the area. Document the occurrence and assessment of area; notify primary care provider according to facility policy. Continue to monitor area for bleeding and inflammation.
- *Cuticles, fingers, or toes are inflamed and tender:* Assess area. Document findings. Notify primary care provider. Resume care as appropriate after consultation with primary care provider and based on facility policy.
- *Calluses, corns, or bunions are present:* Assess area and document findings. Do not cut or file. Consult primary care provider and/or podiatrist for treatment.

SPECIAL CONSIDERATIONS

General Considerations

- Advise patient to avoid using fingernails as tools to pick, poke, or pry things to prevent nail damage.
- Discourage biting of nails or picking at cuticles. These habits can damage the nail bed. Even a minor cut alongside a fingernail can allow bacteria or fungi to enter and cause an infection (Mayo Foundation for Medical Education and Research, 2011c).
- Advise patients to avoid pulling off hangnails. This can cause injury to live tissue that is pulled off along with the hangnail. Instead, carefully clip off hangnails.
- Advise patients to wear appropriate footwear. Break in new shoes gradually. Improperly fitting shoes can lead to corns, calluses, bunions, and blisters.

Infant and Child Considerations

- A newborn's nail beds may be cyanotic (blue) for the first few hours of life, and then turn pink.
- Infants' nails should be carefully trimmed on a regular basis to prevent scratching.

Older Adult Considerations

- Nails may have lengthwise ridges, due to decreased nail growth rate and injury to the nail bed.
- Nails may be brittle or peeling. Toenails may be thickened.

Home Care Considerations

- Advise patients with diabetes or peripheral vascular disease to inspect feet daily for blisters, cuts, cracks, sores, redness, tenderness, or swelling. Encourage patients to report problems to primary care provider for early intervention.
- Encourage patients with diabetes or peripheral vascular disease to schedule regular foot checkups with their primary care provider or podiatrist. Schedule foot exams at least once a year or more often if recommended by primary care provider.
- Discourage patients with some conditions, such as diabetes and peripheral vascular diseases, from doing toenail care at home (Lyman & Vlahovic, 2010). Encourage patients with these diseases to see a podiatrist for treatment related to bunions, corns, or calluses (MFMER, 2011a).

SKILL 7-10 MAKING AN UNOCCUPIED BED

Usually bed linens are changed after the bath, but some agencies change linens only when soiled. If the patient can get out of bed, the nurse should make the bed while it is unoccupied to decrease stress on the patient and the nurse. The following procedure explains how to make the bed using a fitted bottom sheet. Some facilities do not provide fitted bottom sheets, or sometimes a fitted bottom sheet may not be available. If this is the case, refer to the accompanying Skill Variation for using a flat bottom sheet, instead of a fitted sheet.

DELEGATION CONSIDERATIONS

The making of an unoccupied bed may be delegated to nursing assistive personnel (NAP) or to unlicensed assistive personnel (UAP), as well as to licensed practical/vocational nurses (LPN/LVNs). The decision to delegate must be based on careful analysis of the patient's needs and circumstances, as well as the qualifications of the person to whom the task is being delegated. Refer to the Delegation Guidelines in Appendix A.

EQUIPMENT

- One large flat sheet
- One fitted sheet
- Drawsheet (optional)
- Blankets
- Bedspread
- Pillowcases
- Linen hamper or bag
- Bedside chair
- Waterproof protective pad (optional)
- Disposable gloves
- Additional PPE, as indicated

ASSESSMENT

Assess the patient's preferences regarding linen changes. Assess for any physical activity limitations. Check for any patient belongings that may have accidentally been placed in the bed linens, such as eyeglasses or prayer cloths.

NURSING DIAGNOSIS

Determine related factors for the nursing diagnoses based on the patient's current status. Appropriate nursing diagnoses may include:

- Risk for Impaired Skin Integrity
- Risk for Activity Intolerance
- Impaired Physical Mobility

OUTCOME IDENTIFICATION AND PLANNING

The expected outcome to achieve when making an unoccupied bed is that the bed linens will be changed without injury to the nurse or patient.

(continued)

SKILL 7-10 MAKING AN UNOCCUPIED BED continued

IMPLEMENTATION

ACTION	RATIONALE
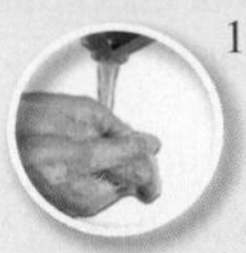 1. Perform hand hygiene. Put on PPE, as indicated.	Hand hygiene and PPE prevent the spread of microorganisms. PPE is required based on transmission precautions.
2. Explain to the patient what you are going to do and the reason for doing it, if the patient is present in room.	Explanation facilitates cooperation.
3. Assemble necessary equipment to the bedside stand or overbed table.	Arranging items nearby is convenient, saves time, and avoids unnecessary stretching and twisting of muscles on the part of the nurse.
4. Adjust the bed to a comfortable working height, usually elbow height of the caregiver (VISN 8 Patient Safety Center, 2009). Drop the side rails.	Having the bed at the proper height prevents back and muscle strain. Having the side rails down reduces strain on the nurse while working.
5. Disconnect call bell or any tubes from bed linens.	Disconnecting devices prevents damage to the devices.
6. Put on gloves. Loosen all linen as you move around the bed, from the head of the bed on the far side to the head of the bed on the near side.	Gloves prevent the spread of microorganisms. Loosening the linen helps prevent tugging and tearing on linen. Loosening the linen and moving around the bed systematically reduce strain caused by reaching across the bed.
7. Fold reusable linens, such as sheets, blankets, or spread, in place on the bed in fourths and hang them over a clean chair.	Folding saves time and energy when reusable linen is replaced on the bed. Folding linens while they are on the bed reduces strain on the nurse's arms. Some facilities change linens only when soiled.
8. Snugly roll all the soiled linen inside the bottom sheet and place directly into the laundry hamper (Figure 1). **Do not place on floor or furniture. Do not hold soiled linens against your uniform.**	Rolling soiled linens snugly and placing them directly into the hamper helps prevent the spread of microorganisms. The floor is heavily contaminated; soiled linen will further contaminate furniture. Soiled linen contaminates the nurse's uniform, and this may spread organisms to another patient.
9. If possible, shift mattress up to head of bed. If mattress is soiled, clean and dry according to facility policy before applying new sheets.	This allows more foot room for the patient.
10. Remove your gloves, unless indicated for transmission-based precautions. Place the bottom sheet with its centerfold in the center of the bed. Open the sheet and fan-fold to the center (Figure 2).	Gloves are not necessary to handle clean linen. Removing gloves properly reduces the risk for infection transmission and contamination of other items. Opening linens on the bed reduces strain on the nurse's arms and diminishes the spread of microorganisms. Centering the sheet ensures sufficient coverage for both sides of the mattress.
11. Pull the bottom sheet over the corners at the head and foot of the mattress. (See accompanying Skill Variation for using a flat bottom sheet, instead of a fitted sheet.)	Making the bed on one side and then completing the bedmaking on the other side saves time. Having bottom linens free of wrinkles reduces patient discomfort.

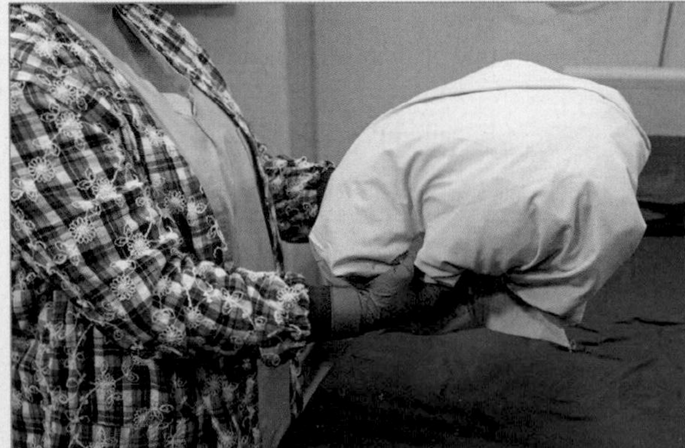

FIGURE 1 Bundling soiled linens in bottom sheet and holding them away from body.

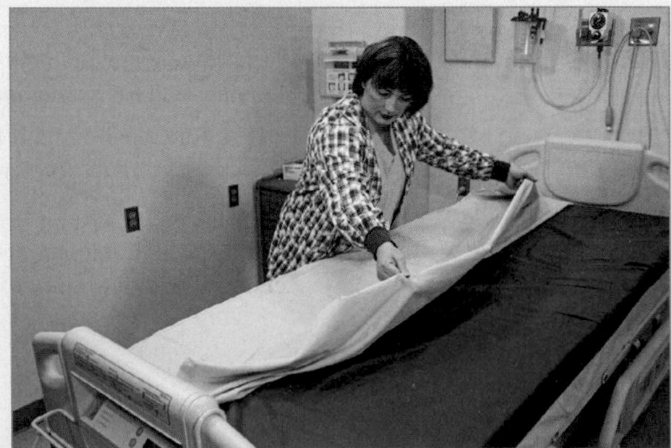

FIGURE 2 Opening bottom sheet and fan-folding to center of bed.

ACTION	RATIONALE
12. If using, place the drawsheet with its centerfold in the center of the bed and positioned so it will be located under the patient's midsection. Open the drawsheet and fan-fold to the center of the mattress (Figure 3). If a protective pad is used, place it over the drawsheet in the proper area and open to the centerfold. Not all facilities use drawsheets routinely. The nurse may decide to use one. In some institutions, the protective pad doubles as a drawsheet. Tuck the drawsheet securely under the mattress.	If the patient soils the bed, drawsheet and pad can be changed without the bottom and top linens on the bed. Having all bottom linens in place before tucking them under the mattress avoids unnecessary moving about the bed. A drawsheet can aid moving the patient in bed.
13. Move to the other side of the bed to secure bottom linens. Pull the bottom sheet tightly and secure over the corners at the head and foot of the mattress. Pull the drawsheet tightly and tuck it securely under the mattress.	This removes wrinkles from the bottom linens, which can cause patient discomfort and promote skin breakdown.
14. Place the top sheet on the bed with its centerfold in the center of the bed and with the hem even with the head of the mattress. Unfold the top sheet. Follow same procedure with top blanket or spread, placing the upper edge about 6 inches below the top of the sheet.	Opening linens by shaking them spreads organisms into the air. Holding linens overhead to open them causes strain on the nurse's arms.
15. Tuck the top sheet and blanket under the foot of the bed on the near side. Miter the corners (Figure 4). (Also, see accompanying Skill Variation.)	This saves time and energy and keeps the top linen in place.
16. Fold the upper 6 inches of the top sheet down over the spread and make a cuff.	This makes it easier for the patient to get into bed and pull up the covers.
17. Move to the other side of the bed and follow the same procedure for securing top sheets under the foot of the bed and making a cuff (Figure 5).	Working on one side of the bed at a time saves energy and is more efficient.

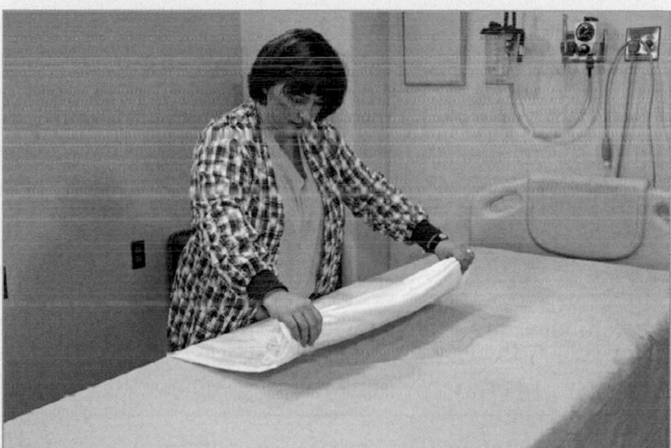

FIGURE 3 Placing drawsheet on bed.

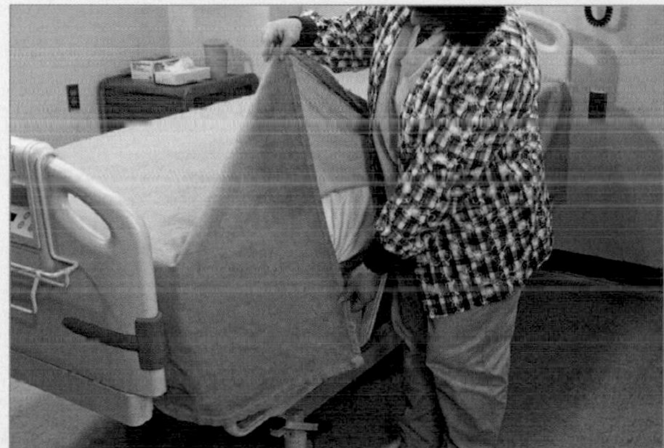

FIGURE 4 Mitering corner of top sheet and blanket.

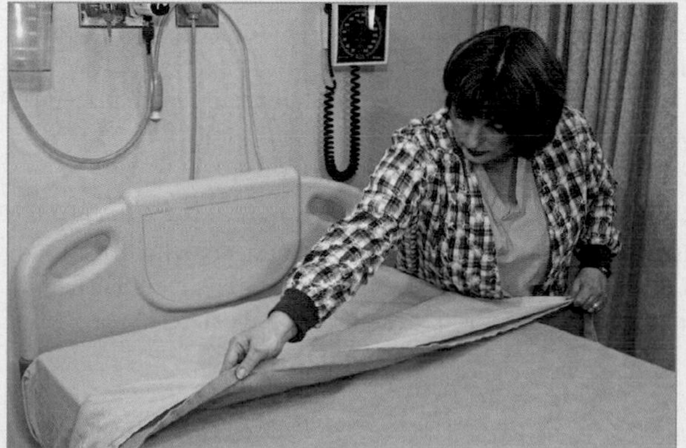

FIGURE 5 Cuffing top linens.

(continued)

SKILL 7-10 MAKING AN UNOCCUPIED BED continued

ACTION	RATIONALE
18. Place the pillows on the bed. Open each pillowcase in the same manner as you opened other linens. Gather the pillowcase over one hand toward the closed end. Grasp the pillow with the hand inside the pillowcase. Keep a firm hold on the top of the pillow and pull the cover onto the pillow. Place the pillow at the head of the bed (Figure 6).	Opening linens by shaking them causes organisms to be carried on air currents. Covering the pillow while it rests on the bed reduces strain on the nurse's arms and back.

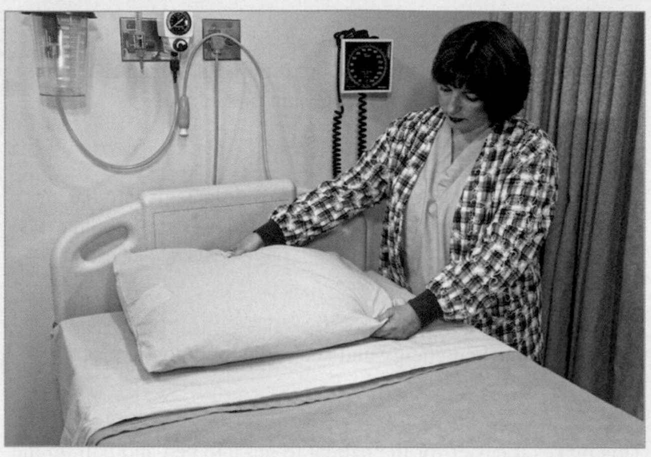

FIGURE 6 Placing pillow on bed.

ACTION	RATIONALE
19. Fan-fold or pie-fold the top linens.	Having linens opened makes it more convenient for the patient to get into bed.
20. Secure the signal device on the bed, according to facility policy.	The patient will be able to call for assistance as necessary. Promotes patient comfort and safety.
21. Raise side rail and lower bed.	Promotes patient comfort and safety.
22. Dispose of soiled linen according to facility policy.	Deters the spread of microorganisms.
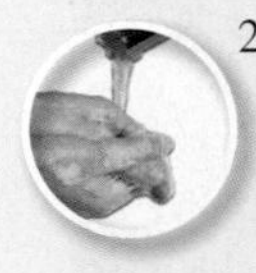 23. Remove any other PPE, if used. Perform hand hygiene.	Removing PPE properly reduces the risk for infection transmission and contamination of other items. Hand hygiene prevents the spread of microorganisms.

EVALUATION

The expected outcome is met when the bed linens are changed without any injury to the patient or nurse.

DOCUMENTATION

Changing of bed linens does not require documentation. The use of a specialty bed, or bed equipment, such as Balkan frame or foot cradle, should be documented.

UNEXPECTED SITUATIONS AND ASSOCIATED INTERVENTIONS

- *Drawsheet is not available:* A flat sheet can be folded in half to substitute for a drawsheet, but extra care must be taken to avoid wrinkles in the bed.
- *Patient is frequently incontinent of stool or urine:* More than one protective pad can be placed under the patient to protect the bed, but take care to ensure that the patient is not lying on wrinkles from linens.

SPECIAL CONSIDERATIONS

- Many different types of specialty beds are available for use as part of treatment and prevention of many health issues, such as treatment of pressure ulcers. Refer to manufacturer's recommendations and instructions on use of specialty lines and products with this equipment.

SKILL VARIATION Making a Bed With a Flat Bottom Sheet

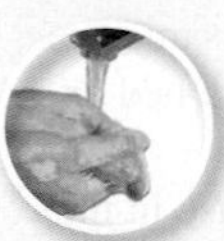

1. Perform hand hygiene and put on PPE, if indicated.
2. Explain what you are going to do and the reason for doing it to the patient, if the patient is present in room.
3. Assemble necessary equipment on the bedside stand or overbed table. Two large flat sheets are needed.
4. Raise bed to a comfortable working position, usually elbow height of the caregiver (VISN 8 Patient Safety Center, 2009). Disconnect call bell or any tubes from bed linens.
5. Put on gloves. Loosen all linen as you move around the bed, from the head of the bed on the far side to the head of the bed on the near side.
6. Fold reusable linens, such as sheets, blankets, or spread, in place on the bed in fourths and hang them over a clean chair.
7. Snugly roll all the soiled linen inside the bottom sheet and place directly into the laundry hamper. Do not place on floor or furniture. Do not hold soiled linens against your uniform.
8. If possible, shift mattress up to head of bed.
9. Remove your gloves. Place the bottom sheet with its centerfold in the center of the bed and high enough to be able to tuck it under the head of the mattress. Open the sheet and fan-fold to the center.
10. If using, place the drawsheet with its centerfold in the center of the bed and positioned so it will be located under the patient's midsection. Open the drawsheet and fan-fold it to the center of the mattress. If a protective pad is used, place it over the drawsheet in the proper area and open it to the centerfold.
11. Tuck the bottom sheet securely under the head of the mattress on one side of the bed, making a corner. Corners are usually mitered. Grasp the side edge of the sheet about 18 inches down from the mattress top (Figure A). Lay the sheet on top of the mattress to form a triangular, flat fold (Figure B). Tuck the portion of the sheet that is hanging loose below the mattress under the mattress without pulling on the triangular fold (Figure C). Pick the top of the triangle fold and place it over the side of the mattress (Figure D). Tuck this loose portion of the sheet under the mattress. Continue tucking the remaining bottom sheet and drawsheet

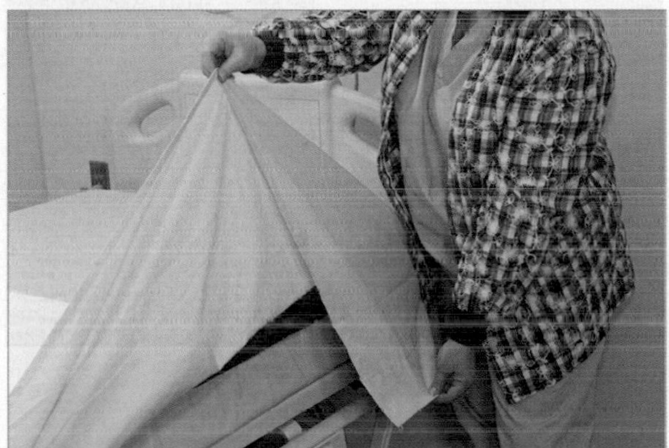

FIGURE A Grasping side edge of sheet and lifting up to form a triangle.

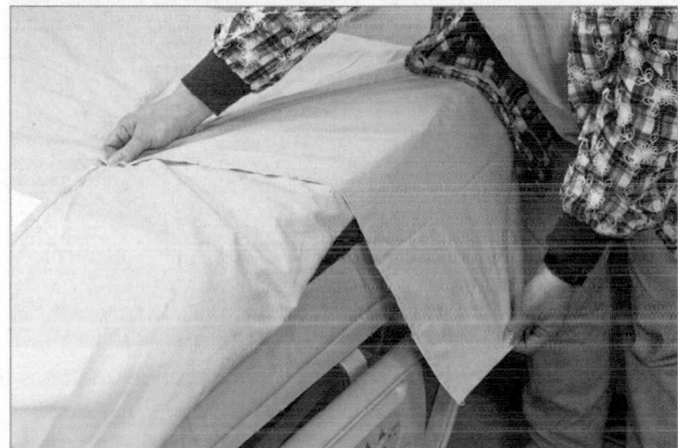

FIGURE B Laying sheet on top of bed to make triangular, flat fold.

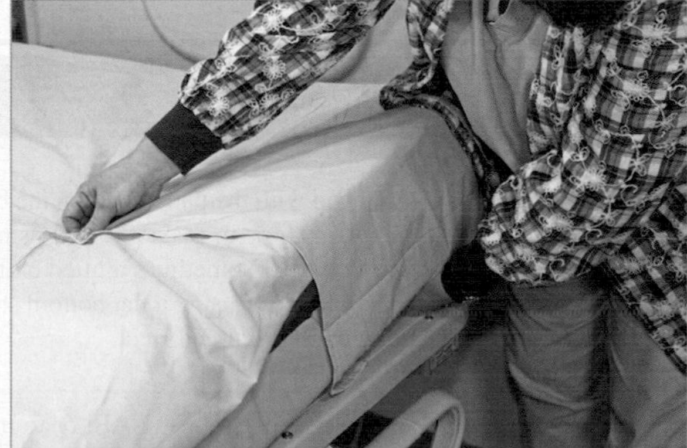

FIGURE C Tucking sheet under mattress.

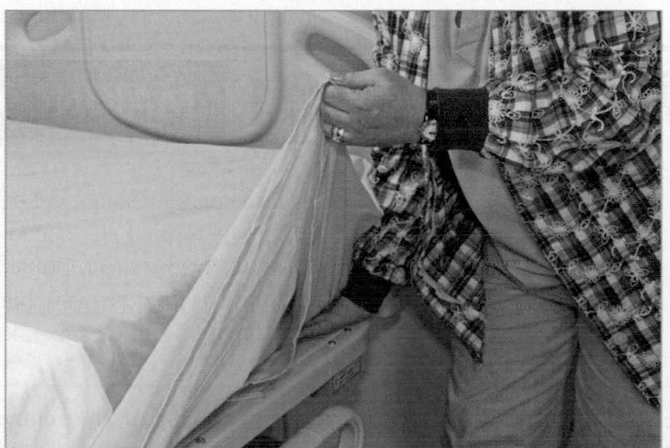

FIGURE D Placing top of triangular fold over mattress side.

(continued)

SKILL 7-10 MAKING AN UNOCCUPIED BED continued

SKILL VARIATION Making a Bed With a Flat Bottom Sheet continued

securely under the mattress (Figure E). Move to the other side of the bed to secure bottom linens. Pull the sheets across the mattress from the centerfold. Secure the bottom of the sheet under the head of the bed and miter the corner. Pull the remainder of the sheet and the drawsheet tightly and tuck under the mattress, starting at the head of the bed and moving toward the foot (Figure F).

12. Place the top sheet on the bed with its centerfold in the center of the bed and with the hem even with the head of the mattress. Unfold the top sheet. Follow same procedure with top blanket or spread, placing the upper edge about 6 inches below the top of the sheet.
13. Tuck the top sheet and blanket under the foot of the bed on the near side. Miter the corners.
14. Fold the upper 6 inches of the top sheet down over the spread and make a cuff.
15. Move to the other side of the bed and follow the same procedure for securing top sheet under the foot of the bed and making a cuff.
16. Place the pillows on the bed. Open each pillowcase in the same manner as you opened other linens. Gather the pillowcase over one hand toward the closed end. Grasp the pillow with the hand inside the pillowcase. Keep a firm hold on the top of the pillow and pull the cover onto the pillow. Place the pillow at the head of the bed.
17. Fan-fold or pie-fold the top linens. Remove gloves.
18. Secure the signal device on the bed according to facility policy.
19. Adjust bed to low position. Raise rail.

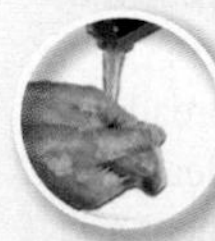

20. Dispose of soiled linen according to agency policy. Perform hand hygiene.

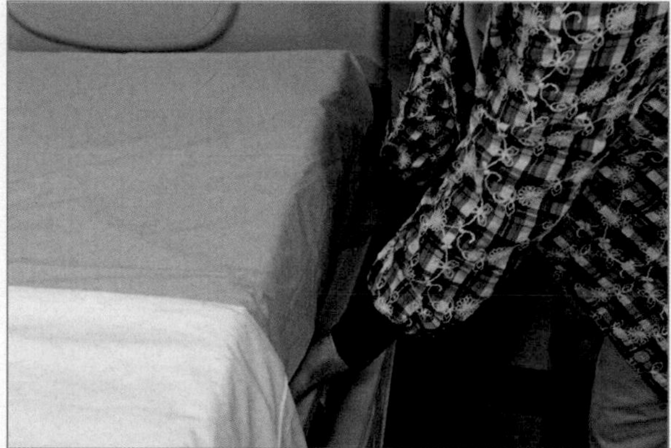

FIGURE E Tucking end of triangular linen fold under mattress to complete mitered corner.

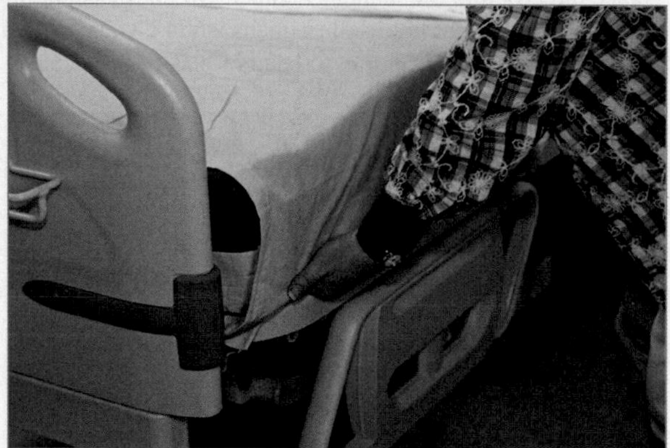

FIGURE F Tucking sheet snugly under mattress.

SKILL 7-11 MAKING AN OCCUPIED BED

If the patient cannot get out of bed, the linens may need to be changed with the patient still in the bed. This is termed an "occupied" bed. The following procedure explains how to make the bed using a fitted bottom sheet. Some facilities do not provide fitted bottom sheets, or sometimes a fitted bottom sheet may not be available. If this is the case, refer to the Skill Variation for using a flat bottom sheet instead of a fitted sheet, located at the end of Skill 7-10, Making an Unoccupied Bed.

DELEGATION CONSIDERATIONS

The making of an occupied bed may be delegated to nursing assistive personnel (NAP) or to unlicensed assistive personnel (UAP), as well as to licensed practical/vocational nurses (LPN/LVNs). The decision to delegate must be based on careful analysis of the patient's needs and circumstances, as well as the qualifications of the person to whom the task is being delegated. Refer to the Delegation Guidelines in Appendix A.

EQUIPMENT

- One large flat sheet
- One fitted sheet
- Drawsheet (optional)
- Blankets
- Bedspread
- Pillowcases
- Linen hamper or bag
- Bedside chair
- Protective pad (optional)
- Disposable gloves
- Additional PPE, as indicated

ASSESSMENT

Assess the patient's preferences regarding linen changes. Assess for any precautions or activity restrictions for the patient. Check the bed for any patient belongings that may have accidentally been placed or fallen there, such as eyeglasses or prayer cloths. Note the presence and position of any tubes or drains that the patient may have.

NURSING DIAGNOSIS

Determine related factors for the nursing diagnoses based on the patient's current status. Appropriate nursing diagnoses may include:

- Risk for Impaired Skin Integrity
- Impaired Physical Mobility
- Impaired Bed Mobility

OUTCOME IDENTIFICATION AND PLANNING

The expected outcome to achieve when making an occupied bed is that the bed linens are applied without injury to the patient or nurse. Other possible outcomes may include patient participates in moving from side to side, and patient verbalizes feelings of increased comfort.

IMPLEMENTATION

ACTION	RATIONALE
1. Check health care record for limitations on patient's physical activity.	This facilitates patient cooperation, determines level of activity, and promotes patient safety.
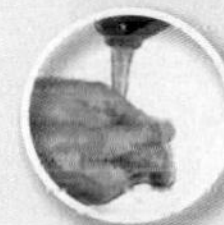 2. Perform hand hygiene. Put on PPE, as indicated.	Hand hygiene and PPE prevent the spread of microorganisms. PPE is required based on transmission precautions.
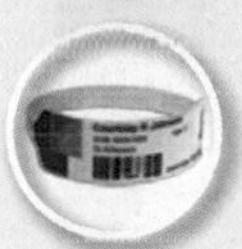 3. Identify the patient. Explain what you are going to do.	Patient identification validates the correct patient and correct procedure. Discussion and explanation allay anxiety and prepare the patient for what to expect.
4. Assemble equipment on overbed table within reach.	Organization facilitates performance of task.
5. Close the curtains around the bed and close the door to the room, if possible.	This ensures the patient's privacy.
6. Adjust the bed to a comfortable working height, usually elbow height of the caregiver (VISN 8 Patient Safety Center, 2009).	Having the bed at the proper height prevents back and muscle strain.
7. Lower side rail nearest you, leaving the opposite side rail up. Place bed in flat position unless contraindicated.	Having the mattress flat makes it easier to prepare a wrinkle-free bed.
8. Put on gloves. Check bed linens for patient's personal items. **Disconnect the call bell or any tubes/drains from bed linens.**	Gloves prevent the spread of microorganisms. It is costly and inconvenient when personal items are lost. Disconnecting tubes from linens prevents discomfort and accidental dislodging of the tubes.

(continued)

SKILL 7-11 MAKING AN OCCUPIED BED continued

ACTION	RATIONALE
9. Place a bath blanket over the patient. Have the patient hold on to bath blanket while you reach under it and remove top linens (Figure 1). Leave top sheet in place if a bath blanket is not used. Fold linen that is to be reused over the back of a chair. Discard soiled linen in laundry bag or hamper. **Do not place on floor or furniture. Do not hold soiled linens against your uniform.**	The blanket provides warmth and privacy. Placing linens directly into the hamper helps prevent the spread of microorganisms. The floor is heavily contaminated; soiled linen will further contaminate furniture. Soiled linen contaminates the nurse's uniform, and this may spread organisms to another patient.
10. If possible, and another person is available to assist, grasp mattress securely and shift it up to head of bed.	This allows more foot room for the patient.
11. Assist patient to turn toward opposite side of the bed, and reposition pillow under patient's head.	This allows the bed to be made on the vacant side.
12. Loosen all bottom linens from head, foot, and side of bed.	This facilitates removal of linens.
13. Fan-fold or roll soiled linens as close to the patient as possible (Figure 2).	This makes it easier to remove linens when the patient turns to the other side.
14. Use clean linen and make the near side of the bed. Place the bottom sheet with its centerfold in the center of the bed (Figure 3). Open the sheet and fan-fold to the center, positioning it under the old linens (Figure 4). Pull the bottom sheet over the corners at the head and foot of the mattress.	Opening linens on the bed reduces strain on the nurse's arms and diminishes the spread of microorganisms. Centering the sheet ensures sufficient coverage for both sides of the mattress. Positioning under the old linens makes it easier to remove linens.

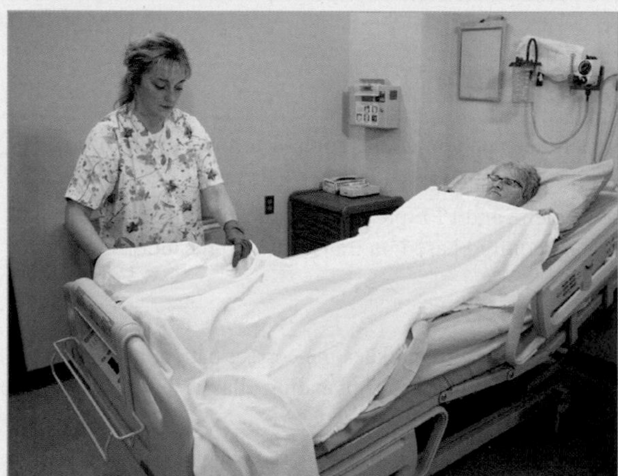

FIGURE 1 Removing top linens from under bath blanket.

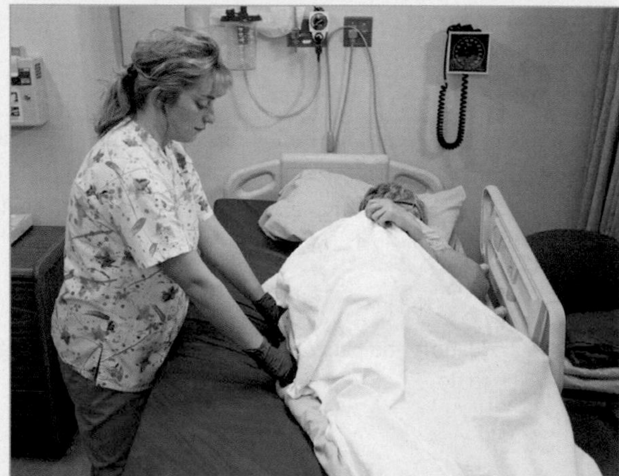

FIGURE 2 Moving soiled linen as close to patient as possible.

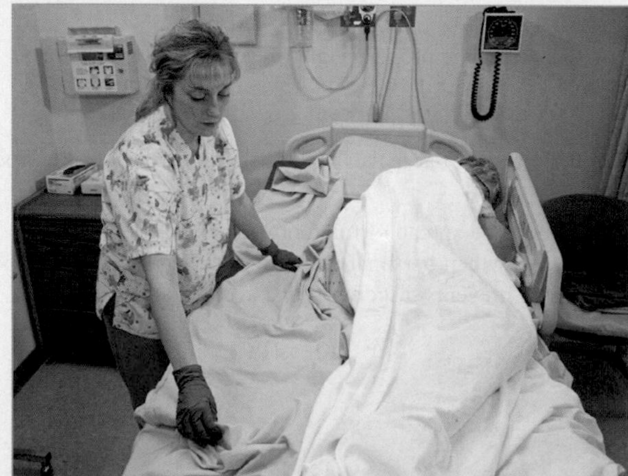

FIGURE 3 Placing bottom sheet with centerfold in center of bed.

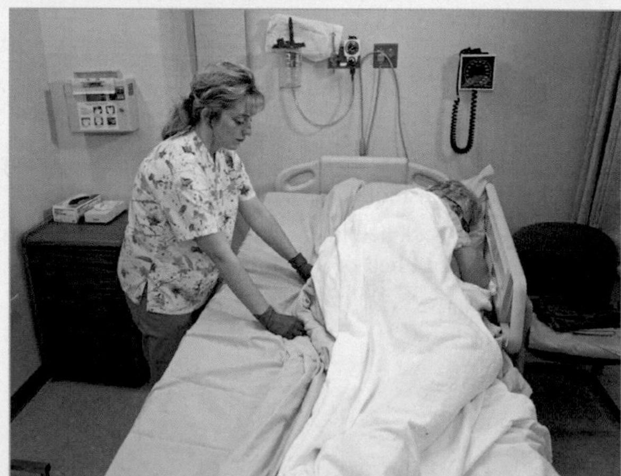

FIGURE 4 Fan-folding bottom sheet to center, positioning it under old linens.

ACTION	RATIONALE
15. If using, place the drawsheet with its centerfold in the center of the bed and positioned so it will be located under the patient's midsection. Open the drawsheet and fan-fold it to the center of the mattress. Tuck the drawsheet securely under the mattress (Figure 5). If a protective pad is used, place it over the drawsheet in the proper area and open to the centerfold. Not all facilities use drawsheets routinely. The nurse may decide to use one.	If the patient soils the bed, drawsheet and pad can be changed without the bottom and top linens on the bed. A drawsheet can aid in moving the patient in bed.
16. Raise side rail. Assist patient to roll over the folded linen in the middle of the bed toward you. Reposition pillow and bath blanket or top sheet. Move to other side of the bed and lower side rail.	This ensures patient safety. The movement allows the bed to be made on the other side. The bath blanket provides warmth and privacy.
17. Loosen and remove all bottom linen (Figure 6). Discard soiled linen in laundry bag or hamper. **Do not place on floor or furniture. Do not hold soiled linens against your uniform.**	Placing linens directly into the hamper helps prevent the spread of microorganisms. The floor is heavily contaminated; soiled linen will further contaminate furniture. Soiled linen contaminates the nurse's uniform, and this may spread organisms to another patient.

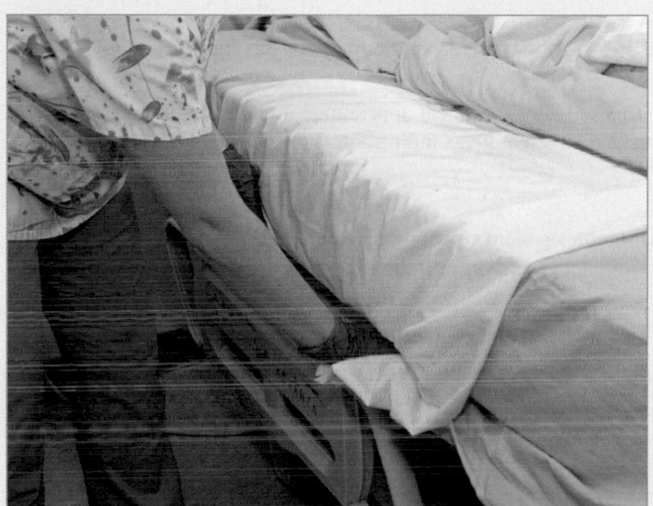

FIGURE 5 Tucking drawsheet tightly.

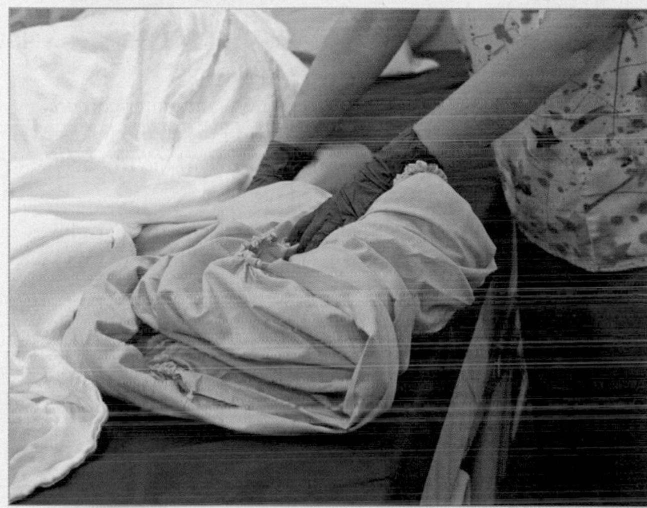

FIGURE 6 Removing soiled bottom linens from other side of bed.

ACTION	RATIONALE
18. Ease clean linen from under the patient. Pull the bottom sheet taut and secure at the corners at the head and foot of the mattress. Pull the drawsheet tight and smooth. Tuck the drawsheet securely under the mattress.	This removes wrinkles and creases in the linens, which are uncomfortable to lie on.
19. Assist patient to turn back to the center of bed. Remove pillow and change pillowcase. Open each pillowcase in the same manner as you opened other linens. Gather the pillowcase over one hand toward the closed end. Grasp the pillow with the hand inside the pillowcase. Keep a firm hold on the top of the pillow and pull the cover onto the pillow. Place the pillow under the patient's head.	Opening linens by shaking them causes organisms to be carried on air currents.

(continued)

SKILL 7-11 MAKING AN OCCUPIED BED continued

ACTION	RATIONALE
20. Apply top linen, sheet, and blanket, if desired, so that it is centered. Fold the top linens over at the patient's shoulders to make a cuff. Have patient hold on to top linen and remove the bath blanket from underneath (Figure 7).	This allows bottom hems to be tucked securely under the mattress and provides for privacy.

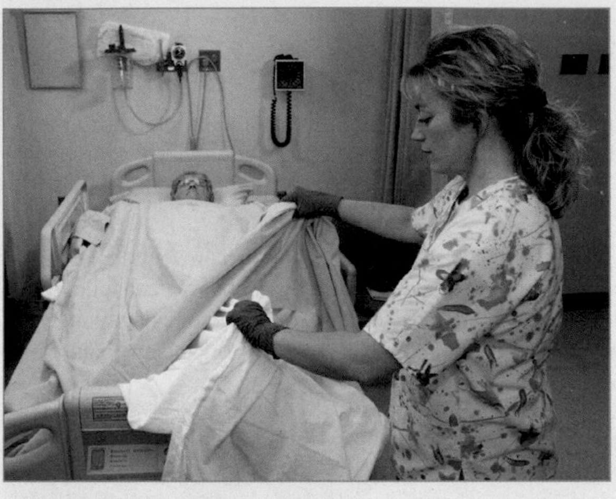

FIGURE 7 Removing bath blanket from under top linens.

ACTION	RATIONALE
21. Secure top linens under foot of mattress and miter corners. (Refer to Skill Variation in Skill 7-10.) Loosen top linens over patient's feet by grasping them in the area of the feet and pulling gently toward foot of bed.	This provides for a neat appearance. Loosening linens over the patient's feet gives more room for movement.
22. Return patient to a position of comfort. Remove your gloves. Raise side rail and lower bed. Reattach call bell.	Promotes patient comfort and safety. Removing gloves properly reduces the risk for infection transmission and contamination of other items.
23. Dispose of soiled linens according to agency policy.	Deters the spread of microorganisms.
24. Remove any other PPE, if used. Perform hand hygiene.	Removing PPE properly reduces the risk for infection transmission and contamination of other items. Hand hygiene prevents the spread of microorganisms.

EVALUATION

The expected outcome is met when the bed linens are changed, and the patient and nurse remain free of injury. In addition, the patient assists in moving from side to side and states feelings of increased comfort after the bed is changed.

DOCUMENTATION

Changing of bed linens does not require documentation. The use of a specialty bed, or bed equipment, such as Balkan frame or foot cradle, should be documented. Document any significant observations and communication.

UNEXPECTED SITUATIONS AND ASSOCIATED INTERVENTIONS

- *Dirty linens are grossly contaminated with urinary or fecal drainage:* Obtain an extra towel or protective pad. Place the pad under and over the soiled linens so that new linens will not be in contact with soiled linens. Clean and dry the mattress according to facility policy before applying new sheets.

SPECIAL CONSIDERATIONS

Older Adult Considerations

- Using a soft bath blanket or a flannelette blanket as a bottom sheet may solve the problem of "coldness" for older adult patients with vascular problems or arthritis.

ENHANCE YOUR UNDERSTANDING

FOCUSING ON PATIENT CARE: DEVELOPING CLINICAL REASONING

Consider the case scenarios at the beginning of the chapter as you answer the following questions to enhance your understanding and apply what you have learned.

QUESTIONS

1. Denasia Kerr, the 6-year-old on bed rest, needs her hair shampooed. It is now several days after surgery. How would you accomplish this task?
2. Cindy Vortex, the 34-year-old woman who is now in a coma after a car accident, is wearing contact lenses. What information would be important to gather before attempting to remove the contact lenses?
3. Carl Sheen, 76 years of age, asks you, "How can I clean my dentures with my right hand all tied up with this IV?" How best could you help Mr. Sheen with this hygiene activity while still fostering his independence?

You can find suggested answers after the Bibliography at the end of this chapter.

INTEGRATED CASE STUDY CONNECTION

The case studies in the back of the book are designed to focus on integrating concepts. Refer to the following case studies to enhance your understanding of the concepts related to the skills in this chapter.

- Basic Case Studies: Joe LeRoy, page 1072.
- Intermediate Case Studies: Victoria Holly, page 1079.

TAYLOR SUITE RESOURCES

Explore these additional resources to enhance learning for this chapter:

- NCLEX-Style Questions and other resources on thePoint, http://thePoint.lww.com/Lynn4e
- *Skill Checklists for Taylor's Clinical Nursing Skills,* 4e
- *Taylor's Video Guide to Clinical Nursing Skills:* Hygiene
- *Fundamentals of Nursing:* Chapter 30, Hygiene

Bibliography

Ackley, B.J., & Ladwig, G.B. (2011). *Nursing diagnosis handbook* (9th ed.). St. Louis: Mosby/Elsevier.

Agency for Healthcare Research and Quality. National Guideline Clearinghouse. (2011). *Prevention of pressure ulcers.* Available http://guideline.gov/syntheses/synthesis.aspx?id=25078&search=prevent+pressure+ulcers.

Ahluwalia, S.C., Gill, T.M., Baker, D.I., et al. (2010). Perspectives of older persons on bathing and bathing disability: A qualitative study. *Journal of the American Geriatrics Society, 58*(3), 450–456.

American Association of Critical-Care Nurses (AACN). (2010). *Practice Alert: Oral care in the critically ill.* Available http://aacn.org/WD/Practice/Content/practicealerts.content?menu=Practice. Accessed July 18, 2012.

American Dental Association (ADA). (2012). *Mouthrinses.* Available http://www.ada.org/1319.aspx. Accessed July 9, 2012.

Ames, N.J., Sulima, P., Yates, J.M., et al. (2011). Effects of systematic oral care in critically ill patients: A multicenter study. *American Journal of Critical Care, 20*(5), e103–e113. Available http://ajcc.aacnjournals.org/content/20/5/e103.full.pdf+html. Accessed July 10, 2012.

Bloomfield, J., & Pegram, A. (2012). Physical healthcare needs: Oral hygiene in the mental health setting. *Mental Health Practice, 15*(6), 32–38.

Bloomfield, J., Pegram, A., & Jones, A. (2008). Recommended procedure for bedmaking in hospital. *Nursing Standard, 22*(23), 41–44.

Brown, A., & Butcher, M. (2005). A guide to emollient therapy. *Nursing Standard, 19*(24), 68–75.

Burn Foundation. (2012). *Burn prevention. Safety facts on scald burns.* Available http://www.burnfoundation.org/programs/resource.cfm?c=1&a=3. Accessed July 14, 2012.

Boltz, M., Capezuti, E., Fulmer, T., et al. (Eds.) (2012). *Evidence-based geriatric nursing protocols for best practice* (4th ed.). New York: Springer Publishing Company.

Bulechek, G.M, Butcher, H.K., Dochterman, J.M., et al. (Eds.). (2013). *Nursing interventions classification (NIC)* (6th ed.). St. Louis: Mosby Elsevier.

Burn Foundation. (2012). *Burn prevention. Safety facts on scald burns.* Available http://www.burnfoundation.org/programs/resource.cfm?c=1&a=3. Accessed July 14, 2012.

Centers for Disease Control and Prevention (CDC). (2011a). *Chronic disease prevention and health promotion. Oral health.* Available http://www.cdc.gov/chronicdisease/resources/publications/AAG/doh.htm. Accessed July 7, 2012.

Chan, E.Y., Lee, Y.K., Poh, T.H., et al. (2011). Translating evidence into nursing practice: Oral hygiene for care dependent adults. *International Journal of Evidence-Based Healthcare, 9*(2), 172–183.

Ciancio, S. (2008). Mouth rinses and their impact on oral hygiene. *Access, 22*(5), 24–29.

Cleveland Clinic. (2009). *Contact lens care.* Available http://my.clevelandclinic.org/eye/patients/products/soft_contact_lenses.aspx. Accessed July 18, 2012.

Cleveland Clinic. (2009). *Patient information. Soft contact lenses.* Available http://my.clevelandclinic.org/devices/vision_correction/Contact_Lenses/hic_Contact_Lens_Care.aspx. Accessed July 16, 2012.

Coate, D. (2010). The ABCs of bathing. *Advance for Long-Term Care Management, 13*(3), 21. Available http://long-term-care.advanceweb.com/Archives/Article-Archives/The-ABCs-of-Bathing.aspx. Accessed July 10, 2012.

Cowdell, F. (2011). Older people, personal hygiene, and skin care. *MEDSURGNursing, 20*(5), 235–240.

Durgude, Y., & Cocks, N. (2011). Nurse's knowledge of the provision of oral care for patients with dysphagia. *British Journal of Community Nursing, 16*(12), 604–610.

Dyble, T., & Ashton, J. (2011). Use of emollients in the treatment of dry skin conditions. *British Journal of Community Nursing, 16*(5), 214–220.

Gaspard, G., & Cox, L. (2012). Bathing people with dementia: When education is not enough. *Journal of Gerontological Nursing, 38*(9), 43–51.

Geraghty, J. (2011). Introducing a new skin-care regimen for the incontinent patient. *British Journal of Nursing, 20*(7), 409–410, 412, 414–415.

Herter, R., & Wallace Kazer, M. (2010). Best practices in urinary catheter. *Home Healthcare Nurse, 28*(6), 342–349.

Hess, C.T. (2013). *Clinical guide to skin & wound care.* (7th ed.). Philadelphia: Wolters Kluwer Health/Lippincott Williams & Wilkins.

Hinkle, J.L., & Cheever, K.H. (2014). *Brunner & Suddarth's textbook of medical-surgical nursing* (13th ed.). Philadelphia: Wolters Kluwer Health/Lippincott Williams & Wilkins.

Hogan-Quigley, B., Palm, M.L., & Bickley, L. (2012). *Bates' nursing guide to physical examination and history taking.* Philadelphia: Wolters Kluwer Health/Lippincott Williams & Wilkins.

Holman, C., Roberts, S., & Nicol, M. (2005). Practice update: Clinical skills with older people. Promoting oral hygiene. *Nursing Older People, 16*(10), 37–38.

Jablonski, R.A., Therrien, B., & Kolanowski, A. (2011). No more fighting and biting during mouth care: Applying the theoretical constructs of threat perception to clinical practice. *Research and Theory for Nursing Practice: An International Journal, 25*(3), 163–175.

Jarvis, C. (2012). *Physical examination & health assessment.* (6th ed.). St. Louis: Saunders/Elsevier.

Jensen, S. (2011.) *Nursing health assessment. A best practice approach.* Philadelphia: Wolters Kluwer-Health/Lippincott Williams & Wilkins.

Johnson, R.H. (2011). Practical care: Creative strategies for bathing. *Nursing & Residential Care, 13*(8), 392–394.

Kanjirath, P.P., Kim, S.E., & Inglehart, M.R. (2011). Diabetes and oral health: The importance of oral health-related behavior. *The Journal of Dental Hygiene, 85*(4), 264–272.

Keefe, S. (2010). Bath safety and dementia. *Advance for long-term care management.* Available http://long-term-care.advanceweb.com/Features/Articles/Bath-Safety-and-Dementia.aspx. Accessed July 13, 2012.

Kelly, T., Timmis, S., & Twelvetree, T. (2010). Review of the evidence to support oral hygiene in stroke patients. *Nursing Standard, 24*(37), 35–38.

Kyle, T., & Carman, S. (2013). *Essentials of pediatric nursing* (2nd ed.). Philadelphia: Wolters Kluwer Health/Lippincott Williams & Wilkins.

Lyman, T.P., & Vlahovic, T.C. (2010). Foot care from A to Z. *Dermatology Nursing, 22*(5), 2–8.

Malkin, B., & Berridge, P. (2009). Guidance on maintaining personal hygiene in nail care. *Nursing Standard, 23*(41), 35–38.

Massa, J. (2010). Improving efficiency, reducing infection, and enhancing experience. *British Journal of Nursing, 19*(22), 1408–1414.

Mayo Foundation for Medical Education and Research (MFMER). (2012). *Peripheral artery disease (PAD). Lifestyle and home remedies.* Available http://www.mayoclinic.com/health/peripheral-arterial-disease/DS00537/DSECTION=lifestyle-and-home-remedies. Accessed July 9, 2012.

Mayo Foundation for Medical Education and Research (MFMER). (2011a). *Amputation and diabetes: How to protect your feet.* Available http://www.mayoclinic.com/health/amputation-and-diabetes/DA00140. Accessed July 9, 2012.

Mayo Foundation for Medical Education and Research (MFMER). (2011b). *Denture care: How do I clean dentures?* Available http://www.mayoclinic.com/health/denture-care/AN02028/. Accessed July 9, 2012.

Mayo Foundation for Medical Education and Research (MFMER). (2011c). *Fingernails: Do's and don'ts for healthy nails.* Available http://www.mayoclinic.com/health/nails/WO00020. Accessed July 31, 2012.

Mayo Foundation for Medical Education and Research (MFMER). (2011d). *Oral health: Brush up on dental care basics.* Available at www.mayoclinic.com/health/dental/DE00003. Accessed July 9, 2012.

Mayo Foundation for Medical Education and Research (MFMER). (2011e). *Skin care: 5 tips for healthy skin.* Available http://www.mayoclinic.com/health/skin-care/SN00003/NSECTIONGROUP=2. Accessed July 16, 2012.

MedlinePlus. (2012). *Penis care (uncircumcised).* Available at http://www.nlm.nih.gov/medlineplus/ency/article/001917.htm. Accessed July 31, 2012.

Moorhead, S., Johnson, M., Maas, M.L., et al. (Eds.). (2013). *Nursing outcomes classification (NOC).* (5th ed.). St. Louis: Mosby Elsevier.

National Institute on Aging (NIA). (2012). *Age page. Foot care.* Available http://www.nia.nih.gov/health/publication/foot-care. Accessed July 9, 2012.

NANDA International. (2012). *Nursing diagnoses: Definitions & classification 2012–2014.* West Sussex, UK: Wiley-Blackwell.

Papa, K.S. (2011). A dignified bathing experience. *Advance for Long-Term Care Management, 14*(6), 16.

Pegram, A., Bloomfield, J., & Jones, A. (2007). Clinical skills: Bed bathing and personal hygiene needs of patients. *British Journal of Nursing, 16*(6), 356–358.

Pellatt, G. (2007). Clinical skills: Bed making and patient positioning. *British Journal of Nursing, 16*(5), 302–305.

Polovich, M., White, J., & Kelleher, L. (Eds.). (2009). *Chemotherapy and biotherapy guidelines and recommendations for practice* (3rd ed.). Pittsburgh, PA: Oncology Nursing Society.

Ritter, L.A., & Hoffman, N.A. (2010). *Multicultural health.* Boston: Jones and Bartlett.

Ritz, J., Pashnik, B., Padula, C., et al. (2012). Effectiveness of 2 methods of chlorhexidine bathing. *Journal of Nursing Care Quality, 27*(2), 171–175.

Sievert, D., Armola, R., & Halm, M.A. (2011). Chlorhexidine gluconate bathing: Does it decrease hospital-acquired infections? *American Journal of Critical Care, 20*(2), 166–170.

Spector, R.E. (2009). *Cultural diversity in health and illness* (7th ed.). Upper Saddle River, NJ: Pearson/Prentice Hall.

Society of Urologic Nurses and Associates (SUNA). (2010). *Prevention & control of catheter-associated urinary tract infection (CAUTI). Clinical practice guideline.* Available https://www.suna.org/sites/default/files/download/cautiGuideline.pdf.

Tabloski, P.A. (2010). *Gerontological nursing* (2nd ed.). Upper Saddle River, NJ: Pearson.

Tada, A., & Miura, H. (2012). Prevention of aspiration pneumonia with oral care. *Archives of Gerontology & Geriatrics, 55*(1), 16–21.

Taylor, C.R, Lillis, C., & Lynn, P. (2015). *Fundamentals of nursing.* (8th ed.). Philadelphia: Wolters Kluwer Health/Lippincott Williams & Wilkins.

U.S. Food and Drug Administration (FDA). (2010). *A guide to bed safety. Bed rails in hospitals, nursing homes and home health care: The facts.* Available http://www.fda.gov/MedicalDevices/ProductsandMedicalProcedures/GeneralHospitalDevicesandSupplies/HospitalBeds/ucm123676.htm. Accessed July 9, 2012.

VISN 8 Patient Safety Center. (2009). *Safe patient handling and movement algorithms.* Tampa, FL: Author. Available at http://www.visn8.va.gov/patientsafetycenter/safePtHandling. Accessed April 23, 2010.

Voegeli, D. (2012). Moisture-associated skin damage: Aetiology, prevention and treatment. *British Journal of Nursing, 21*(9), 517–521.

Voegeli, D. (2010). Care or harm: Exploring essential components in skin care regimens. *British Journal of Nursing, 19*(13), 812,814,816,818–819.

SUGGESTED ANSWERS FOR FOCUSING ON PATIENT CARE: DEVELOPING CLINICAL REASONING

1. Before Denasia's hair is washed, assess the situation. Assess the patient's hygiene preferences: frequency, time of day, and type of shampoo products. Assess for any physical activity limitations. Assess the patient's ability to get out of bed to have her hair washed. If the medical orders allow it and the patient is physically able to wash her hair in the shower, the patient may prefer to do so. Otherwise, the shampoo could take place at the sink, if available. If the patient cannot tolerate being out of bed or is not allowed to do so, or a sink is not available, perform a bed shampoo. Assess for any activity or positioning limitations. Inspect the patient's scalp for any cuts, lesions, or bumps. Note any flaking, drying, or excessive oiliness. Find out if Denasia would prefer a family member to shampoo her hair. If shampooing in bed, a shampoo cap can be used. Otherwise, use a bed shampoo with water.

2. Before removing Ms. Vortex's contacts assess the following: Assess both eyes for contact lenses, because some people wear them in only one eye. Determine the type of contact lenses worn. Assess eyes for any redness or drainage, which may indicate an eye infection or an allergic response. Assess for any eye injury. If an injury is present, notify the primary care provider about the presence of the contact lens. Do not try to remove the contact lens in this situation due to the risk for additional eye injury.

3. Assess the patient's oral hygiene preferences: frequency, time of day, and type of hygiene products. Assess for any physical activity limitations. Assess the patient's ability to perform own care. Determine if the IV site can be covered with water-protecting material, such as a glove or plastic wrap, to allow Mr. Sheen the ability to care for his dentures. Explore the possibility of discontinuing the IV infusion for a short period of time to keep the IV tubing from interfering with oral hygiene. If this is a possibility, review facility policy and determine the need for medical clearance to implement this option. Encourage Mr. Sheen to do as much as he can; offer assistance, as needed. Patients are often afraid they will damage the IV or hurt themselves. Reinforce the fact that normal range of motion and activity are acceptable and should not interfere with the IV infusion.

8 Skin Integrity and Wound Care

FOCUSING ON PATIENT CARE

This chapter will help you develop some of the skills related to skin integrity and wound care necessary to care for the following patients:

LORI DOWNS, a patient with diabetes mellitus, is being treated in the outpatient wound center for a chronic ulcer on her left foot.

TRAN NGUYEN, diagnosed with breast cancer, has had a modified radical mastectomy and is three days post-op.

ARTHUR LOWES, has an appointment with his surgeon today for a follow-up examination and removal of surgical staples following a colon resection.

Refer to Focusing on Patient Care: Developing Clinical Reasoning at the end of the chapter to apply what you learn.

LEARNING OBJECTIVES

After studying this chapter, you will be able to:

1. Clean a wound and apply a dry, sterile dressing.
2. Apply a saline-moistened dressing.
3. Apply a hydrocolloid dressing.
4. Perform wound irrigation.
5. Collect a wound culture.
6. Apply Montgomery straps.
7. Provide care to a Penrose drain.
8. Provide care to a T-tube drain.
9. Provide care to a Jackson-Pratt drain.
10. Provide care to a Hemovac drain.
11. Apply negative pressure wound therapy.
12. Remove sutures.
13. Remove surgical staples.
14. Apply an external heating pad.
15. Apply a warm sterile compress to an open wound.
16. Assist with a sitz bath.
17. Apply cold therapy.

KEY TERMS

approximated wound edges: edges of a wound that are lightly pulled together; epithelialization of wound margins; edges touch, wound is closed

debridement: removal of devitalized tissue and foreign material from a wound

dehiscence: accidental separation of wound edges, especially a surgical wound

ecchymosis: discoloration of an area resulting from infiltration of blood into the subcutaneous tissue

edema: accumulation of fluid in the interstitial tissues

epithelialization: stage of wound healing in which epithelial cells move across the surface of a wound margin (approximation); tissue color ranges from the color of "ground glass" to pink

erythema: redness or inflammation of an area as a result of dilation and congestion of capillaries

eschar: a thick, leathery scab or dry crust composed of dead cells and dried plasma

exudate: fluid that accumulates in a wound; may contain serum, cellular debris, bacteria, and white blood cells

granulation tissue: new tissue that is deep pink/red composed of fibroblasts and small blood vessels that fill an open wound when it starts to heal; characterized by irregular surface-like raspberries

health care-associated infection: infections caused by a wide variety of common and unusual bacteria, fungi, and viruses during the course of receiving medical care (CDC, 2012)

ischemia: insufficient blood supply to a body part due to obstruction of circulation

jaundice: condition characterized by yellowness of the skin, whites of eyes, mucous membranes, and body fluids as a result of deposition of bile pigment resulting from excess bilirubin in the blood

maceration: softening of tissue due to excessive moisture

necrosis: localized tissue death

nonsterile (clean) technique: strategies used in patient care to reduce overall number of microorganisms or to prevent or reduce the risk of transmission of microorganisms from one person to another or from one place to another. Involves meticulous handwashing, maintaining a clean environment by preparing a clean field, using clean gloves and sterile instruments, and preventing direct contamination of materials and supplies (WOCN, 2012)

pathogens: microorganisms that can harm humans

pressure ulcer: a wound with a localized area of injury to the skin and/or underlying tissue; the underlying cause is pressure, caused when soft tissue is compressed between a bony prominence and an external surface for a prolonged period of time, or when soft tissue undergoes pressure in combination with shear and/or friction (Hess, 2013; NPUAP, 2012a).

sinus tract: cavity or channel underneath a wound that has the potential for infection

sterile technique: strategies used in patient care to reduce exposure to microorganisms and maintain objects and areas as free from microorganisms as possible. Involves meticulous handwashing, use of a sterile field, use of sterile gloves for application of a sterile dressing, and use of sterile instruments (WOCN, 2012).

surgical staples: stainless-steel wire (shaped like a staple) used to close a surgical wound

surgical sutures: thread or wire used to hold tissue and skin together

tunneling: passageway or opening that may be visible at skin level, but with most of the tunnel under the surface of the skin

undermining: areas of tissue destruction underneath intact skin along the margins of a wound; associated with stage 3 or 4 pressure ulcers

vasoconstriction: narrowing of the lumen of a blood vessel

vasodilation: an increase in the diameter of a blood vessel

A disruption in the normal integrity and function of the skin and underlying tissues is called a wound. This disruption creates a potentially dangerous and possibly life-threatening situation. The patient is at risk for wound complications such as infection, hemorrhage, **dehiscence**, and evisceration (Fundamentals Review 8-1). These complications increase the risk for generalized illness and death, lengthen the time that the patient needs health care interventions, and add to health care costs. **Pressure ulcers**, a type of wound caused by unrelieved pressure that results in damage to underlying tissue and one of the most common skin and tissue disruptions, are costly in terms of health care expenditures (see Fundamentals Review 8-2 for staging of pressure ulcers).

Nursing responsibilities related to skin integrity involve assessment of the patient and the wound (Fundamentals Review 8-3), followed by the development of the nursing plan of care, including the identification of appropriate outcomes, nursing interventions, and evaluation of the nursing care. Depending upon the patient's individualized plan of care, specific wound care skills may be needed.

Carelessness in practicing asepsis when providing wound care is a cause of **health care-associated infections**. It is extremely important to use appropriate aseptic technique. Follow *Standard Precautions* and, if needed, *Transmission-Based Precautions* in providing wound care. Chronic wounds and pressure ulcers may be treated using clean technique. Refer to Chapter 4 for a discussion of infection control precautions, **sterile technique**, and clean technique.

Additionally, ongoing assessment for possible skin or wound complications will be required. Many wound care products/dressings are available, each with distinctive actions, as well as indications, contraindications, advantages, and disadvantages. It is very important for the nurse to be aware of the products available in a particular facility and be familiar with the indications for, and correct use of, each type of dressing and wound care product. Fundamentals Review 8-4 outlines the purposes and uses for several wound dressing/product categories. In addition, it is often appropriate and necessary to consult with a wound care specialist, often a wound certified nurse specialist, to plan and coordinate the most effective care for the patient.

In addition to caring for wounds, nurses must also be skilled in assessing the patient for pain and employing strategies to minimize the patient's pain experience. Some patients may experience both physiologic and psychological pain related to dressing changes and wound care.

This chapter will cover skills to assist the nurse in providing care related to skin integrity and wounds. In addition to the Fundamentals Review boxes in this chapter, refer to those found in Chapter 1 for a quick review of critical knowledge to assist you in understanding the skills related to skin integrity and wound care.

FUNDAMENTALS REVIEW 8-1

WOUND HEALING AND COMPLICATIONS

- Wounds heal by primary, secondary, or tertiary intention.
- Wounds healing by primary intention form a clean, straight line with little loss of tissue. The wound edges are well approximated with sutures. These wounds usually heal rapidly with minimal scarring.
- Wounds healing by secondary intention are large wounds with considerable tissue loss. The edges are not approximated. Healing occurs by formation of **granulation tissue**. These wounds have a longer healing time, a greater chance of infection, and larger scars.
- Wounds healing by primary intention that become infected heal by secondary intention. These wounds generate a greater inflammatory reaction and more granulation tissue. They have large scars and are less likely to shrink to a flat line as they heal.
- Wounds healing by delayed primary intention or tertiary intention are left open for several days to allow **edema** or infection to resolve or **exudates** to drain. They are then closed.
- Wound complications include infection, hemorrhage, dehiscence, and evisceration. These problems increase the risk for generalized illness, lengthen the time during which the patient needs health care interventions, increase the cost of health care, and can result in death.
- Multiple psychological effects can occur as a result of trauma to the integumentary system. Actual and potential emotional stressors are common in patients with wounds. Pain is part of almost every wound. In addition, anxiety and fear play a large role in a patient's recovery from a wound. Many patients must deal with changes in body image, body structure, and function related to a wound.

FUNDAMENTALS REVIEW 8-2

COMPARISON OF STAGES OF PRESSURE ULCERS

SUSPECTED DEEP TISSUE INJURY

Purple or maroon localized area of discolored intact skin or blood-filled blister due to damage of underlying soft tissue from pressure and/or shear. Deep tissue injury may be difficult to detect in individuals with dark skin tones. The area may be preceded by tissue that is painful, firm, boggy, warmer, or cooler as compared to adjacent tissue. Evolution may include a thin blister over a dark wound bed. The wound may further evolve and become covered by a thin **eschar**. Evolution may be rapid, exposing additional layers of tissue even with optimal treatment.

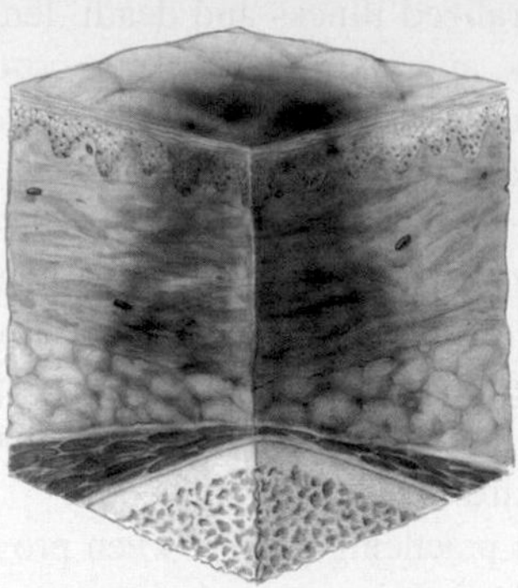

Suspected deep tissue injury.

STAGE I

Intact skin with non-blanchable redness of a localized area usually over a bony prominence. Darkly pigmented skin may not have visible blanching; its color may differ from the surrounding area. The area may be painful, firm, soft, warmer, or cooler as compared to adjacent tissue. Stage I may be difficult to detect in individuals with dark skin tones. Stage I may indicate "at risk" persons.

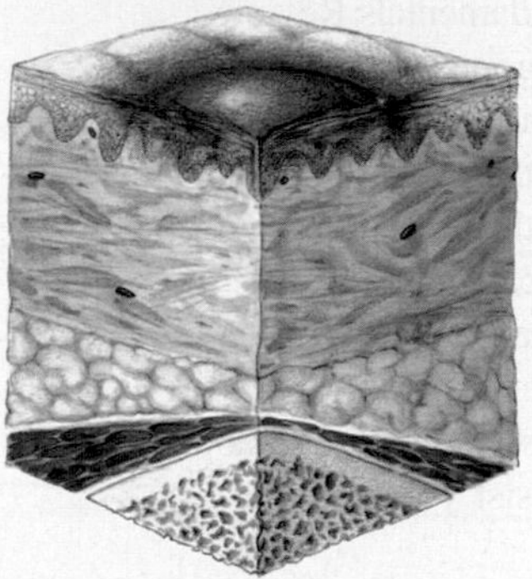

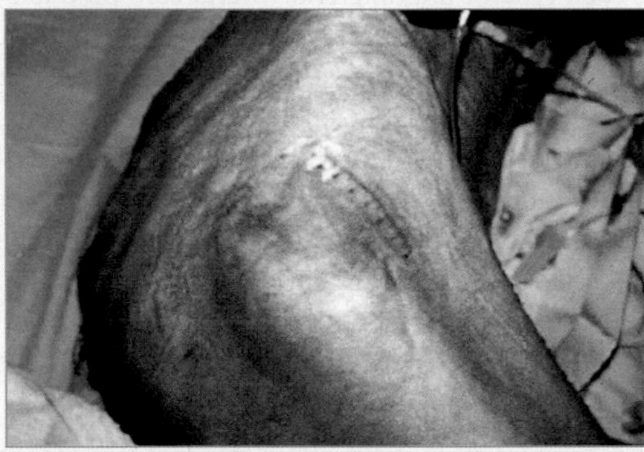

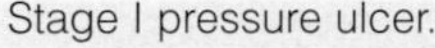

Stage I pressure ulcer.

STAGE II

Partial-thickness loss of dermis presenting as a shallow open ulcer with a red pink wound bed, without slough. Presents as a shiny or dry shallow ulcer without slough or bruising (which indicates suspected deep tissue injury). May also present as an intact or open/rupture serum-filled blister. This stage should not be used to describe skin tears, tape burns, perineal dermatitis, **maceration**, or excoriation.

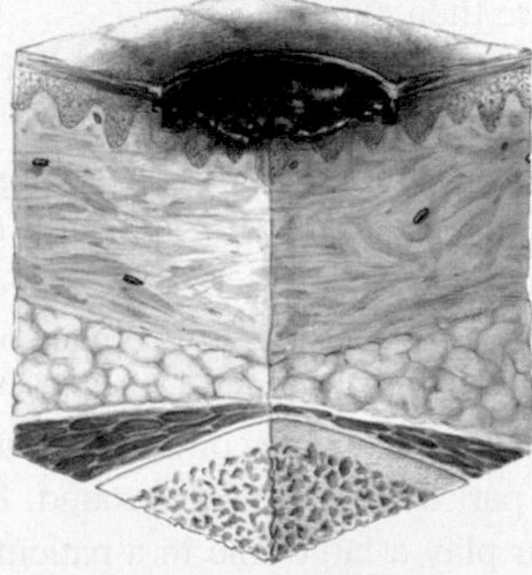

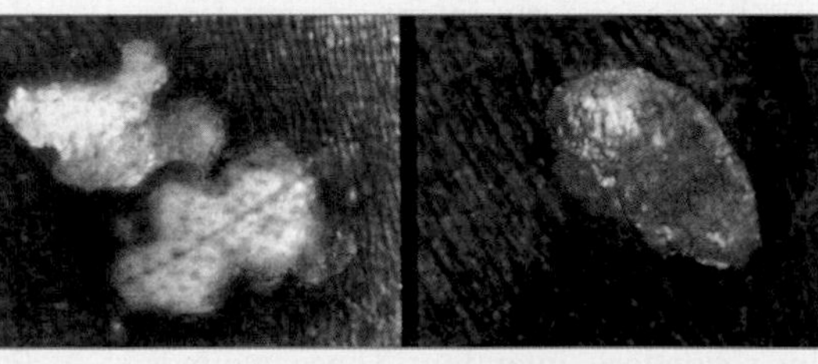

Stage II pressure ulcer.

(continued)

FUNDAMENTALS REVIEW 8-2 continued

COMPARISON OF STAGES OF PRESSURE ULCERS

STAGE III

Full-thickness tissue loss. Subcutaneous fat may be visible, but bone, tendon, or muscle is not exposed. Bone/tendon is not visible or directly palpable. Slough may be present, but does not obscure the depth of tissue loss. May include **undermining** and **tunneling**. The depth of a stage III pressure ulcer varies by anatomic location. The bridge of the nose, ear, occiput, and malleolus do not have subcutaneous tissue and stage II ulcers at these locations can be shallow. In contrast, areas with significant adipose tissue can develop extremely deep stage III pressure ulcers.

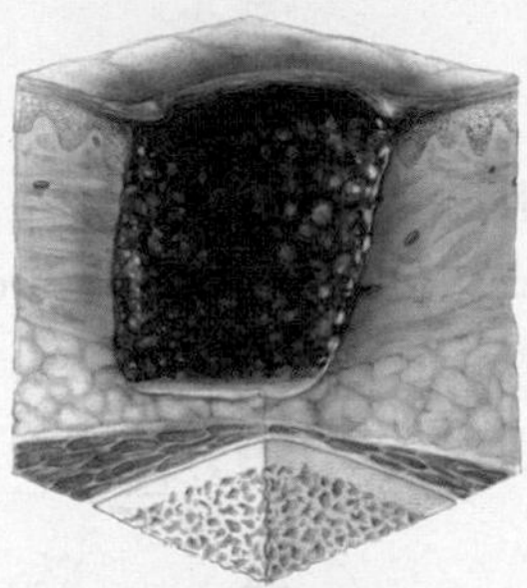

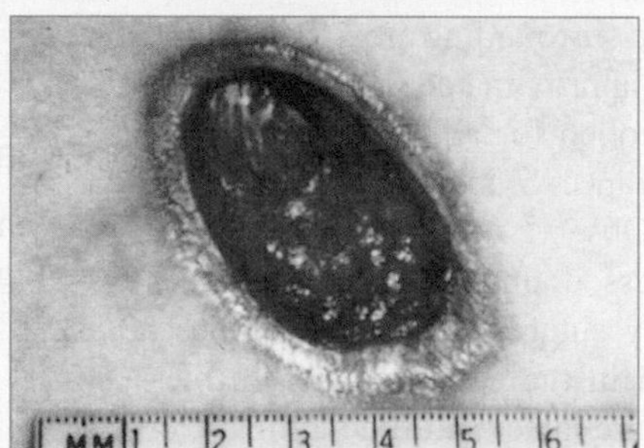

Stage III pressure ulcer.

STAGE IV

Full-thickness tissue loss with exposed bone, tendon, or muscle. Exposed bone/tendon is visible or directly palpable. Slough or eschar may be present on some parts of the wound bed. Often includes undermining and tunneling. The depth of a stage IV pressure ulcer varies by anatomic location. The bridge of the nose, ear, occiput, and malleolus do not have subcutaneous tissue and these ulcers can be shallow at these locations. Stage IV ulcers can extend into muscle and/or supporting structures (e.g., fascia, tendon, or joint capsule), making osteomyelitis possible.

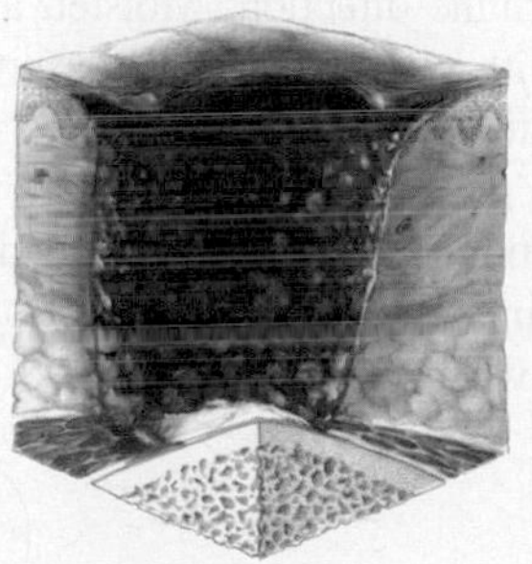

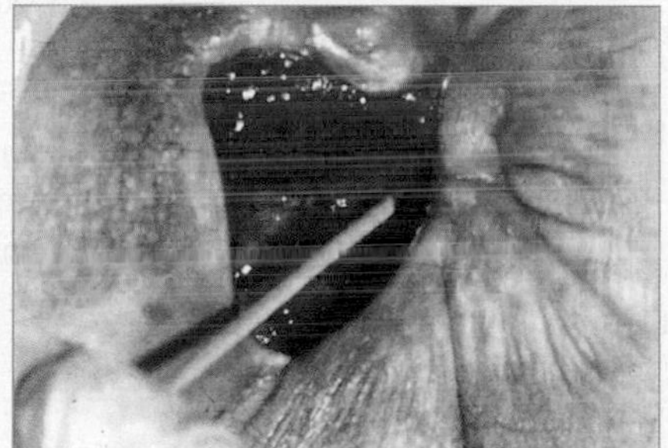

Stage IV pressure ulcer.

UNSTAGEABLE

Full-thickness tissue loss in which the base of the ulcer is covered by slough (yellow, tan, gray, green, or brown) and/or eschar (tan, brown, or black) in the wound bed. Until enough slough and/or eschar is removed to expose the base of the wound, the true depth, and therefore stage, cannot be determined. Stable (dry, adherent, intact, without **erythema** or movement) eschar on the heels serves as "the body's natural (biological) cover" and should not be removed.

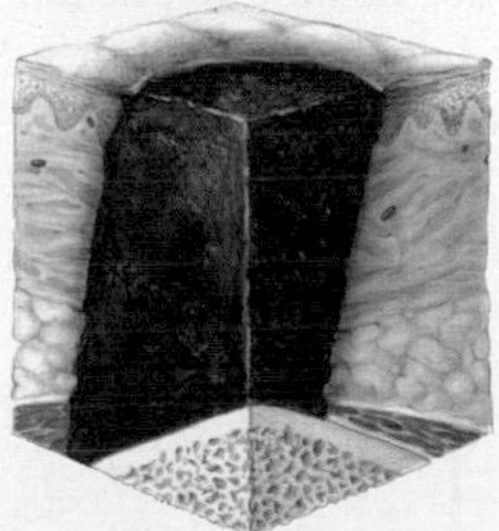

Unstageable pressure ulcer.

(From National Pressure Ulcer Advisory Panel (NPUAP). (2012a). *Educational and clinical resources Pressure ulcer stages/categories.* Available http://www.npuap.org/resources/educational-and-clinical-resources/npuap-pressure-ulcer-stagescategories/; and Porth, C., & Matfin, G. (2009). *Pathophysiology: Concepts of altered health states* (8th ed.). Philadelphia: Wolters Kluwer Health/Lippincott Williams & Wilkins.) (Illustrations from National Pressure Ulcer Advisory Panel (NPUAP). (2012b). *Educational and clinical resources. Pressure ulcer staging/illustrations.* Available http://www.npuap.org/resources/educational-and-clinical-resources/pressure-ulcer-categorystaging-illustrations/. Used with permission of the National Pressure Ulcer Advisory Panel 2012b.)

FUNDAMENTALS REVIEW 8-3

WOUND ASSESSMENT

Wounds are assessed for appearance, size, drainage, pain, presence of sutures, drains, and tubes, and the evidence of complications.

PERFORMING GENERAL WOUND ASSESSMENT

- Assess the wound's appearance by inspecting and palpating. Look for the approximation of the edges and the color of the wound and surrounding area. The edges should be clean and well approximated. Edges may be reddened and slightly swollen for about a week, then closer to normal in appearance. Skin around the wound may be bruised initially. Observe for signs of infection (increased swelling, redness, drainage, and/or warmth).
- Note the presence of any sutures, drains, and tubes. These areas are assessed in the same manner as the incision. Make sure they are intact and functioning.
- Assess the amount, color, odor, and consistency of any wound drainage.
- Assess the patient's pain, using an objective scale. Incisional pain is usually most severe for the first 2 to 3 days, after which it progressively diminishes. Increased or constant pain, especially an acute change in pain, requires further assessment. It can be a sign of delayed healing, infection, or other complication.
- Assess the patient's general condition for signs and symptoms of infection and hemorrhage.

MEASURING WOUNDS AND PRESSURE ULCERS

Size of the Wound

- Draw the shape and describe it.
- Measure the length, width, and diameter (if circular).

Depth of the Wound

- Perform hand hygiene. Put on gloves.
- Moisten a sterile, flexible applicator with saline and insert it gently into the wound at a 90-degree angle, with the tip down (Figure A).

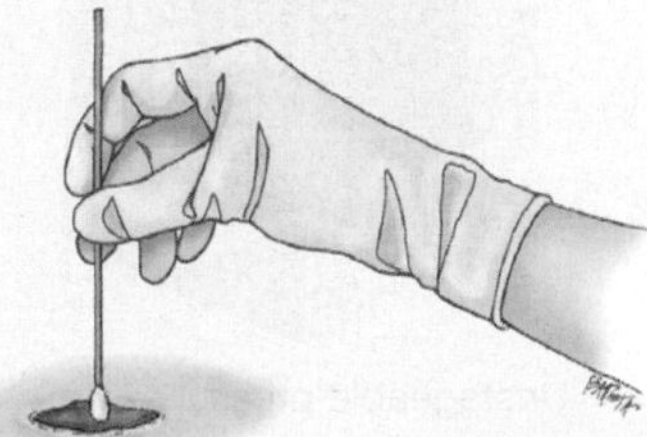

FIGURE A

- Mark the point on the swab that is even with the surrounding skin surface, or grasp the applicator with the thumb and forefinger at the point corresponding to the wound's margin (Figure B).

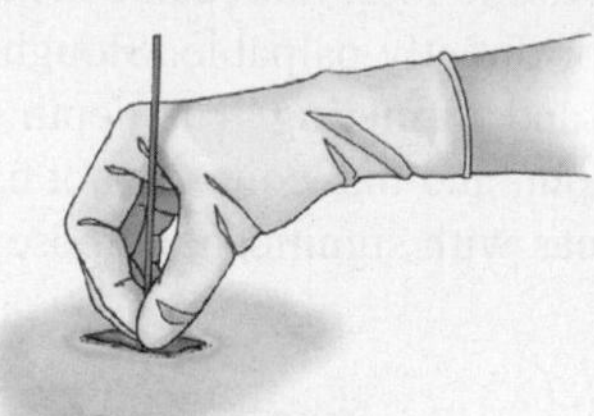

FIGURE B

- Remove the swab and measure the depth with a ruler (Figure C).

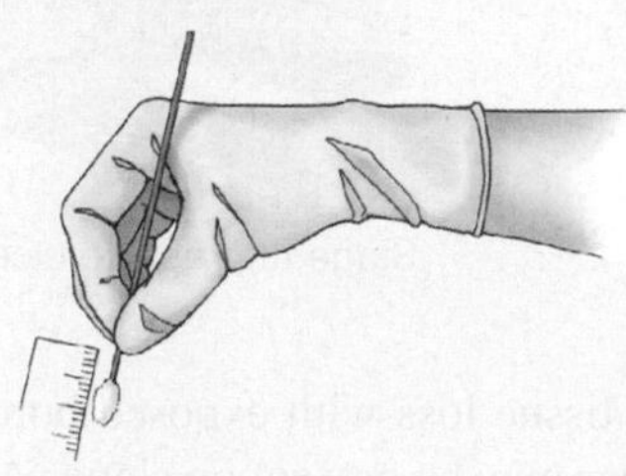

FIGURE C

Wound Tunneling

- Perform hand hygiene. Put on gloves.
- Determine direction: Moisten a sterile, flexible applicator with saline and gently insert a sterile applicator into the site where tunneling occurs. View the direction of the applicator as if it were the hand of a clock (Figure D). The direction of the patient's head represents 12 o'clock. Moving in a clockwise direction, document the deepest sites where the wound tunnels.

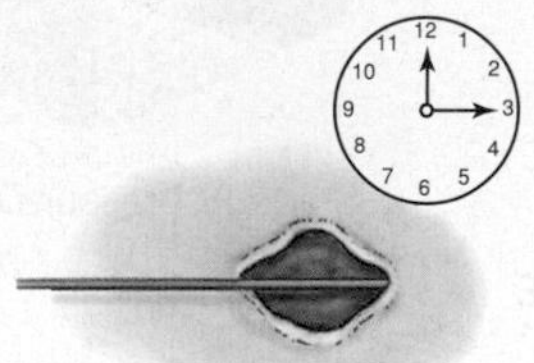

FIGURE D

- Determine the depth: While the applicator is inserted into the tunneling, mark the point on the swab that is even with the wound's edge, or grasp the applicator with the thumb and forefinger at the point corresponding to the wound's margin. Remove the swab and measure the depth with a ruler (see Figure C).
- Document both the direction and depth of tunneling.

(Adapted from Hess, C. [2013]. *Clinical guide to skin and wound care* (7th ed., pp. 17–21). Philadelphia: Wolters Kluwer Health/Lippincott Williams & Wilkins.)

FUNDAMENTALS REVIEW 8-4

EXAMPLES OF WOUND DRESSINGS/PRODUCTS

Type	Purposes	Use
Transparent films, such as: Bioclusive DermaView Mefilm Polyskin Uniflex OpSite Tegaderm	• Allow exchange of oxygen between wound and environment • Are self-adhesive • Protect against contamination; waterproof • Prevent loss of wound fluid • Maintain a moist wound environment • Facilitate autolytic **debridement** • No absorption of drainage • Allow visualization of wound • May remain in place for 24 to 72 hours, resulting in less interference with healing	• Wounds with minimal drainage • Wounds that are small; partial-thickness • Stage I pressure ulcers • Cover dressings for gels, foams, and gauze • Secure intravenous catheters, nasal cannulas, chest tube dressing, central venous access devices
Hydrocolloid dressings, such as: DuoDerm Comfeel PrimaCol Ultec Exuderm	• Are occlusive or semi-occlusive, limiting exchange of oxygen between wound and environment • Minimal to moderate absorption of drainage • Maintain a moist wound environment • Are self-adhesive • Provide cushioning • Facilitate autolytic debridement • Protect against contamination • May be left in place for 3 to 7 days, resulting in less interference with healing	• Partial- and full-thickness wounds • Wounds with light to moderate drainage • Wounds with necrosis or slough • Not for use with wounds that are infected
Hydrogels, such as: IntraSite Gel Aquasorb ClearSite Hypergel ActiformCool	• Maintain a moist wound environment • Minimal absorption of drainage • Facilitate autolytic debridement • Do not adhere to wound • Reduce pain • Most require a secondary dressing to secure	• Partial- and full-thickness wounds • Necrotic wounds • Burns • Dry wounds • Wounds with minimal exudate • Infected wounds
Alginates, such as: Sorbsan Algicell Curasorb AQUACEL KALGINATE Melgisorb	• Absorb exudate • Maintain a moist wound environment • Facilitate autolytic debridement • Require secondary dressing • Can be left in place for 1 to 3 days	• Infected and noninfected wounds • Wounds with moderate to heavy exudate • Partial- and full-thickness wounds • Tunneling wounds • Moist red and yellow wounds • Not for use with wounds with minimal drainage or dry eschar

(continued)

FUNDAMENTALS REVIEW 8-4 continued

EXAMPLES OF WOUND DRESSINGS/PRODUCTS

Type	Purposes	Use
Foams, such as: LYOfoam Allevyn Biatain Mepilex Optifoam	• Maintain a moist wound environment • Do not adhere to wound • Insulate wound • Highly absorbent • Can be left in place up to 7 days • Some products need a secondary dressing to secure	• Absorb light to heavy amounts of drainage • Use around tubes and drains • Not for use with wounds with dry eschar
Antimicrobials, such as: Silvasorb Acticoat Excilon Silverlon	• Antimicrobial or antibacterial action • Reduce infection • Prevent infection	• Draining, exuding, and nonhealing wounds to protect from bacterial contamination and reduce bacterial contamination • Acute and chronic wounds
Collagens, such as: BGC Matrix Stimulen PROMOGRAN Matrix	• Absorbent • Maintain a moist wound environment • Do not adhere to wound • Compatible with topical agents • Conform well to the wound surface • Require secondary dressing to secure	• Partial- or full-thickness wounds • Infected and noninfected wounds • Skin grafts • Donor sites • Tunneling wounds • Moist red and yellow wounds • Wounds with minimal to heavy exudate
Contact layers, such as: Adaptic Touch Profore WCL Telfa Clear	• Placed in contact with base of wound, protecting base from trauma during dressing change • Allow exudate to pass to a secondary dressing • Not intended to be changed with every dressing change • May be used with topical medication, wound filler, or gauze dressings • Requires secondary dressing	• Partial- and full-thickness wounds • Shallow, dehydrated wounds • Wounds with eschar • Wounds with viscous exudate
Composites, such as: Alldress Covaderm Stratasorb	• Combine two or more physically distinct products in a single dressing with several functions • Allow exchange of oxygen between wound and environment • May facilitate autolytic debridement • Provide physical bacterial barrier and absorptive layer • Semiadherent or nonadherent • Primary or secondary dressing	• Partial- and full-thickness wounds • Wounds with minimal to heavy exudate • Necrotic tissue • Mixed (granulation and necrotic tissue) wounds • Infected wounds

(Adapted from Anderson, I. (2010). Key principles involved in applying and removing wound dressings. *Nursing Standard, 25*(10), 51–57; White, R. (2011). Wound dressings and other topical treatment modalities in bioburden control. *Journal of Wound Care, 20*(9), 431–439; Baranoski, S., & Ayello, E.A. (2012). *Wound care essentials.* (3rd ed.). Wolters Kluwer Health/Lippincott Williams & Wilkins; and Hess, C. (2013). *Skin & wound care* (7th ed.). Philadelphia: Wolters Kluwer Health/Lippincott Williams & Wilkins.)

SKILL 8-1 CLEANING A WOUND AND APPLYING A DRY, STERILE DRESSING

The goal of wound care is to promote tissue repair and regeneration to restore skin integrity. Often, wound care includes cleaning of the wound and the use of a dressing as a protective covering over the wound. Wound cleansing is performed to remove debris, contaminants, and excess exudate. Sterile normal saline or a commercially prepared cleanser is the preferred cleansing solution.

There is no standard frequency for how often dressings should be changed. It depends on the amount of drainage, the primary practitioner's preference, the nature of the wound, and the particular wound care product being used. It is customary for the surgeon or other advanced practice professional to perform the first dressing change on a surgical wound, usually within 24 to 48 hours after surgery.

DELEGATION CONSIDERATIONS

Wound care and procedures requiring the use of a sterile field and other sterile items are not delegated to nursing assistive personnel (NAP) or unlicensed assistive personnel (UAP). Depending on the state's nurse practice act and the organization's policies and procedures, these procedures may be delegated to licensed practical/vocational nurses (LPN/LVNs). The decision to delegate must be based on careful analysis of the patient's needs and circumstances, as well as the qualifications of the person to whom the task is being delegated. Refer to the Delegation Guidelines in Appendix A.

EQUIPMENT

- Sterile gloves
- Clean, disposable gloves
- Additional PPE, as indicated
- Gauze dressings
- Surgical or abdominal pads
- Sterile dressing set or suture set (for the sterile scissors and forceps)
- Sterile cleaning solution as ordered (commonly 0.9% normal saline solution, or a commercially prepared wound cleanser)
- Sterile basin (may be optional)
- Sterile drape (may be optional)
- Plastic bag or other appropriate waste container for soiled dressings
- Waterproof pad and bath blanket
- Tape or ties
- Bath blanket or other linens for draping patient
- Additional dressings and supplies needed or required by the primary care provider's order

ASSESSMENT

Assess the situation to determine the need for wound cleaning and a dressing change. Confirm any medical orders relevant to wound care and any wound care included in the nursing plan of care. Assess the patient's level of comfort and the need for analgesics before wound care. Assess if the patient experienced any pain related to prior dressing changes and the effectiveness of interventions employed to minimize the patient's pain. Assess the current dressing to determine if it is intact. Assess for excess drainage, bleeding, or saturation of the dressing. Inspect the wound and the surrounding tissue. Assess the appearance of the wound for the approximation of wound edges, the color of the wound and surrounding area, and signs of dehiscence. Assess for the presence of sutures, staples, or adhesive closure strips. Note the stage of the healing process and characteristics of any drainage. Also assess the surrounding skin for color, temperature, and edema, **ecchymosis**, or maceration.

NURSING DIAGNOSIS

Determine the related factors for the nursing diagnoses based on the patient's current status. Appropriate nursing diagnoses may include:

- Risk for Infection
- Disturbed Body Image
- Acute Pain
- Impaired Skin Integrity
- Delayed Surgical Recovery

OUTCOME IDENTIFICATION AND PLANNING

The expected outcome to achieve when cleaning a wound and applying a dry, sterile dressing is that the wound is cleaned and protected with a dressing without contaminating the wound area, causing trauma to the wound, and/or causing the patient to experience pain or discomfort. Other outcomes that are appropriate include the following: the wound continues to show signs of progression of healing, and the patient demonstrates an understanding of the need for wound care and dressing change.

(continued)

SKILL 8-1 CLEANING A WOUND AND APPLYING A DRY, STERILE DRESSING continued

IMPLEMENTATION

ACTION	RATIONALE
1. Review the medical order for wound care or the nursing plan of care related to wound care. Gather necessary supplies.	Reviewing the order and plan of care validates the correct patient and correct procedure. Preparation promotes efficient time management and an organized approach to the task.
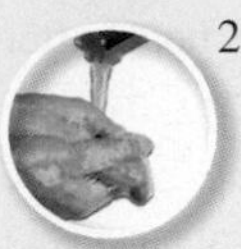 2. Perform hand hygiene and put on PPE, if indicated.	Hand hygiene and PPE prevent the spread of microorganisms. PPE is required based on transmission precautions.
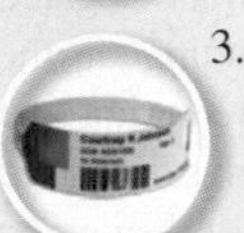 3. Identify the patient.	Identifying the patient ensures the right patient receives the intervention and helps prevent errors.
4. Assemble equipment on overbed table within reach.	Organization facilitates performance of the task.
5. Close the curtains around the bed and close the door to the room, if possible. Explain to the patient what you are going to do and why you are going to do it.	This ensures the patient's privacy. Explanation relieves anxiety and facilitates cooperation.
6. Assess the patient for the possible need for nonpharmacologic pain-reducing interventions or analgesic medication before wound care dressing change. Administer appropriate prescribed analgesic. Allow enough time for the analgesic to achieve its effectiveness.	Pain is a subjective experience influenced by past experience. Wound care and dressing changes may cause pain for some patients.
7. Place a waste receptacle or bag at a convenient location for use during the procedure.	Having a waste container handy means the soiled dressing may be discarded easily, without the spread of microorganisms.
8. Adjust the bed to a comfortable working height, usually elbow height of the caregiver (VISN 8, 2009).	Having the bed at the proper height prevents back and muscle strain.
9. Assist the patient to a comfortable position that provides easy access to the wound area. Use the bath blanket to cover any exposed area other than the wound. Place a waterproof pad under the wound site.	Patient positioning and use of a bath blanket provide for comfort and warmth. Waterproof pad protects underlying surfaces.
10. Check the position of drains, tubes, or other adjuncts before removing the dressing. Put on clean, disposable gloves and loosen tape on the old dressings (Figure 1). If necessary, use an adhesive remover to help get the tape off.	Checking ensures that a drain is not removed accidentally if one is present. Gloves protect the nurse from contaminated dressings and prevent the spread of microorganisms. Adhesive-tape remover helps reduce patient discomfort during dressing removal.

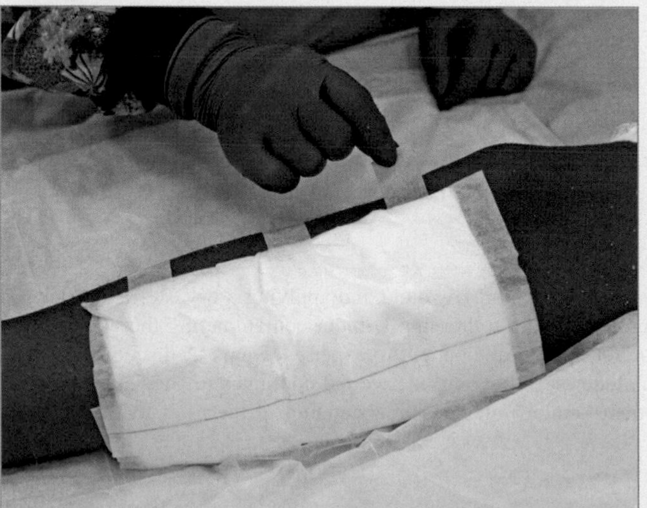

FIGURE 1 Loosening dressing tape.

ACTION	RATIONALE
11. Carefully remove the soiled dressings (Figure 2). If there is resistance, use a silicone-based adhesive remover to help remove the tape. If any part of the dressing sticks to the underlying skin, use small amounts of sterile saline to help loosen and remove it (Figure 3).	Cautious removal of the dressing is more comfortable for the patient and ensures that any drain present is not removed. A silicone-based adhesive remover allows for the easy, rapid, and painless removal without the associated problems of skin stripping (Denyer, 2011; Benbow, 2011). Sterile saline moistens the dressing for easier removal and minimizes damage and pain.

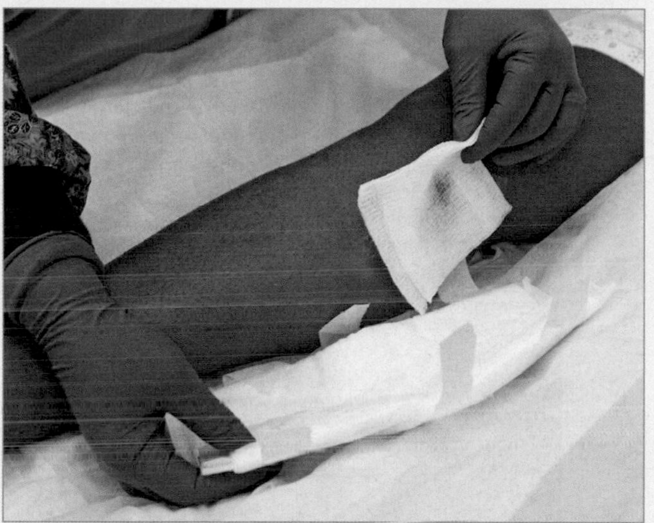

FIGURE 2 Removing soiled dressing.

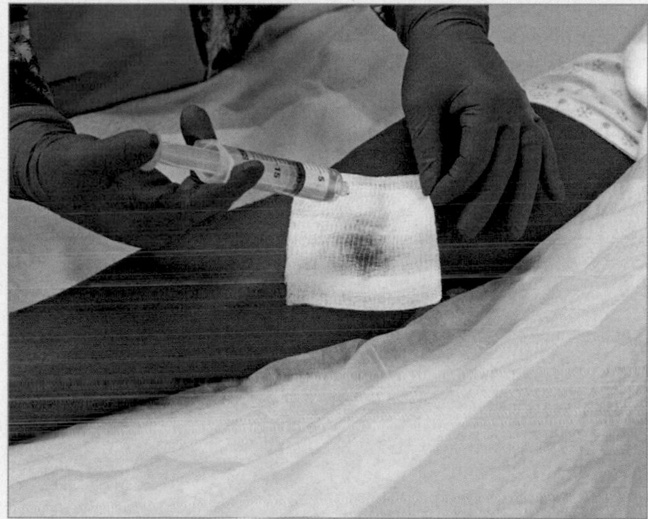

FIGURE 3 Using saline to aid in removing dressing.

ACTION	RATIONALE
12. After removing the dressing, note the presence, amount, type, color, and odor of any drainage on the dressings (Figure 4). Place soiled dressings in the appropriate waste receptacle. Remove your gloves and dispose of them in an appropriate waste receptacle (Figure 5).	The presence of drainage should be documented. Proper disposal of soiled dressings and used gloves prevents the spread of microorganisms.

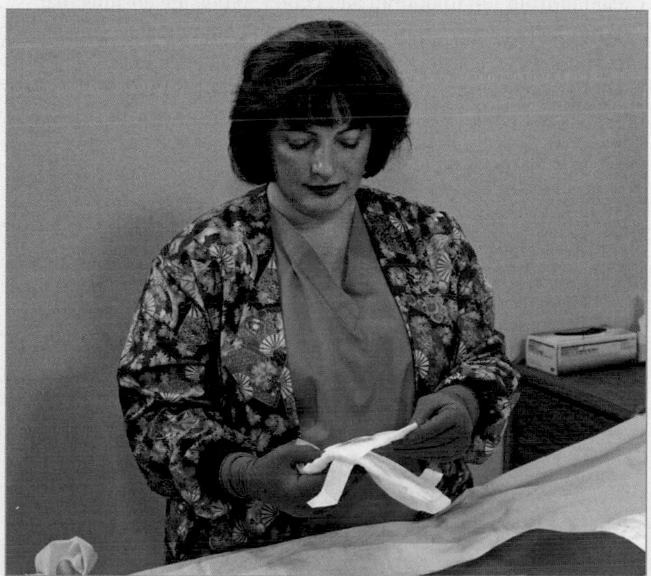

FIGURE 4 Assessing dressing that has been removed.

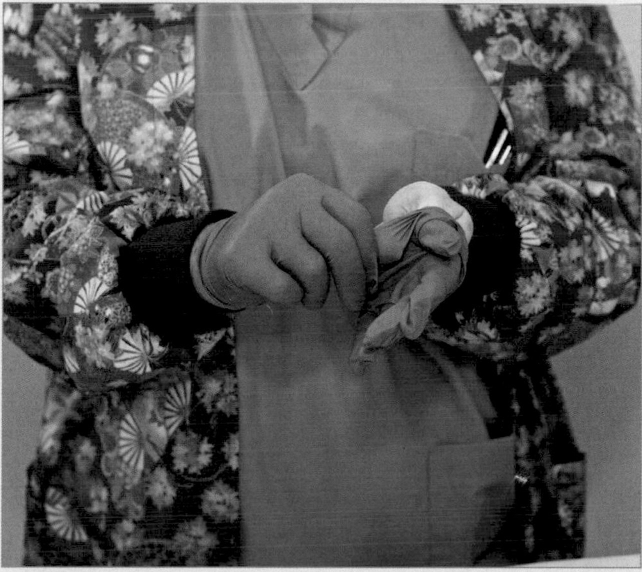

FIGURE 5 Removing gloves.

(continued)

SKILL 8-1 CLEANING A WOUND AND APPLYING A DRY, STERILE DRESSING continued

ACTION	RATIONALE
13. Inspect the wound site for size, appearance, and drainage. Assess if any pain is present. Check the status of sutures, adhesive closure strips, staples, and drains or tubes, if present. Note any problems to include in your documentation.	Wound healing or the presence of irritation or infection should be documented.
14. **Using sterile technique, prepare a sterile work area and open the needed supplies (Figure 6).**	Supplies are within easy reach and sterility is maintained.
15. Open the sterile cleaning solution. Depending on the amount of cleaning needed, the solution might be poured directly over gauze sponges over a container for small cleaning jobs, or into a basin for more complex or larger cleaning.	Sterility of dressings and solution is maintained.
16. Put on sterile gloves (Figure 7). Alternately, clean gloves (clean technique) may be used when cleaning a chronic wound or pressure ulcer.	Use of sterile gloves maintains surgical asepsis and sterile technique and reduces the risk for spreading microorganisms. Clean technique is appropriate for cleaning chronic wounds or pressure ulcers.

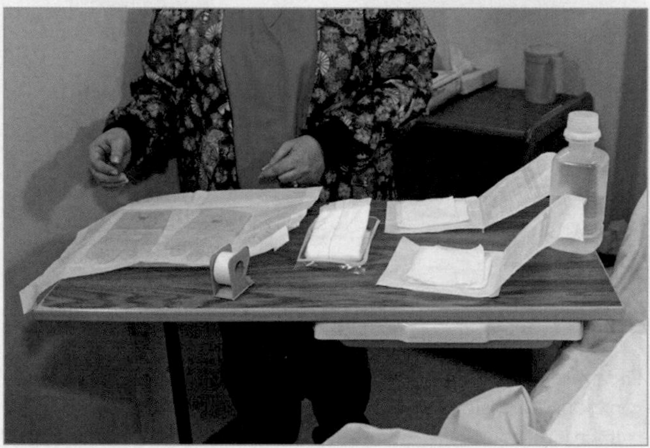

FIGURE 6 Setting up sterile field.

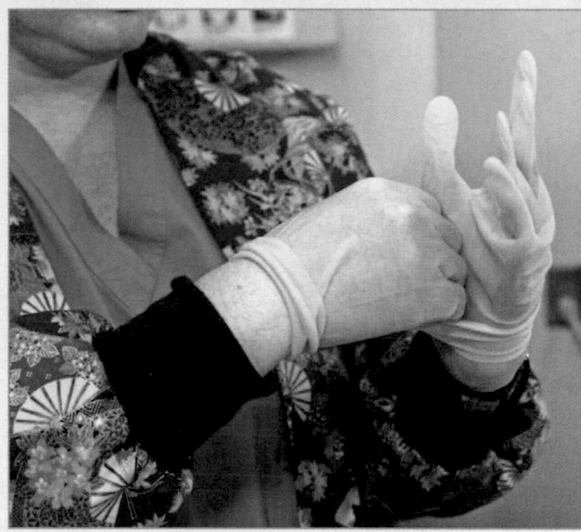

FIGURE 7 Putting on sterile gloves.

ACTION	RATIONALE
17. Clean the wound. **Clean the wound from top to bottom and from the center to the outside (Figure 8).** Following this pattern, use new gauze for each wipe, placing the used gauze in the waste receptacle. Alternately, spray the wound from top to bottom with a commercially prepared wound cleanser.	Cleaning from top to bottom and center to outside ensures that cleaning occurs from the least to most contaminated area and a previously cleaned area is not contaminated again. Using a single gauze for each wipe ensures that the previously cleaned area is not contaminated again.

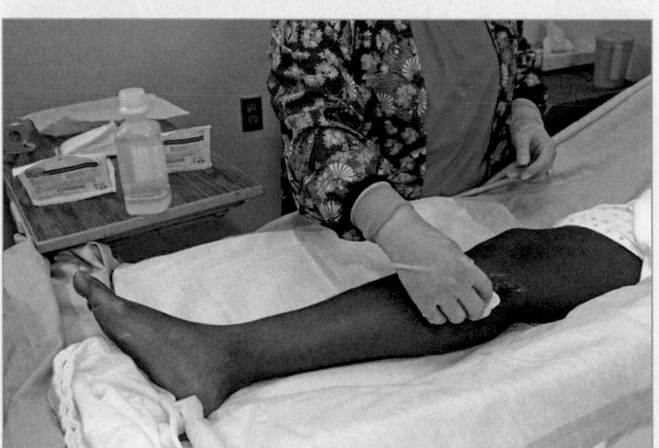

FIGURE 8 Cleaning wound with dampened gauze.

ACTION	RATIONALE
18. Once the wound is cleaned, dry the area using a gauze sponge in the same manner. Apply ointment or perform other treatments, as ordered (Figure 9).	Moisture provides a medium for growth of microorganisms. The growth of microorganisms may be inhibited and the healing process improved with the use of ordered ointments or other applications.
19. If a drain is in use at the wound location, clean around the drain. Refer to Skills 8-7, 8-8, 8-9, and 8-10.	Cleaning the insertion site helps prevent infection.
20. Apply a layer of dry, sterile dressing over the wound (Figure 10). Forceps may be used to apply the dressing.	Primary dressing serves as a wick for drainage. Use of forceps helps ensure that sterile technique is maintained.
21. Place a second layer of gauze over the wound site, as necessary.	A second layer provides for increased absorption of drainage.
22. Apply a surgical or abdominal pad (ABD) over the gauze at the site of the outermost layer of the dressing, as necessary (Figure 11).	The dressing acts as additional protection for the wound against microorganisms in the environment and increased absorption of drainage.

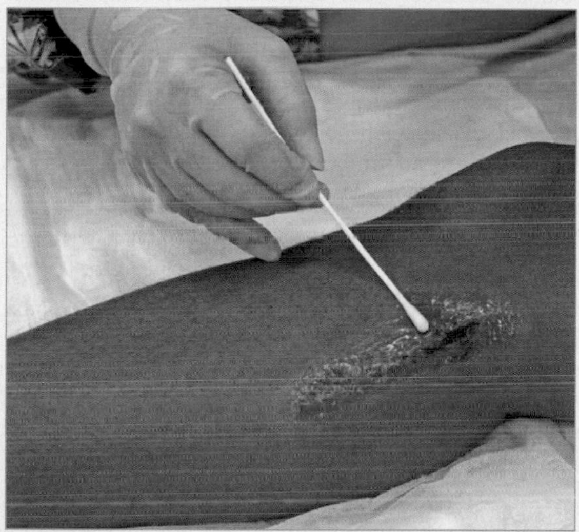

FIGURE 9 Applying antimicrobial ointment to wound with cotton applicator.

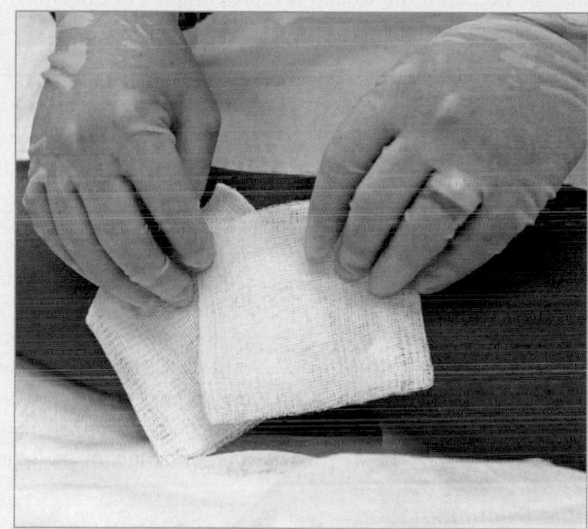

FIGURE 10 Applying dry dressing to site.

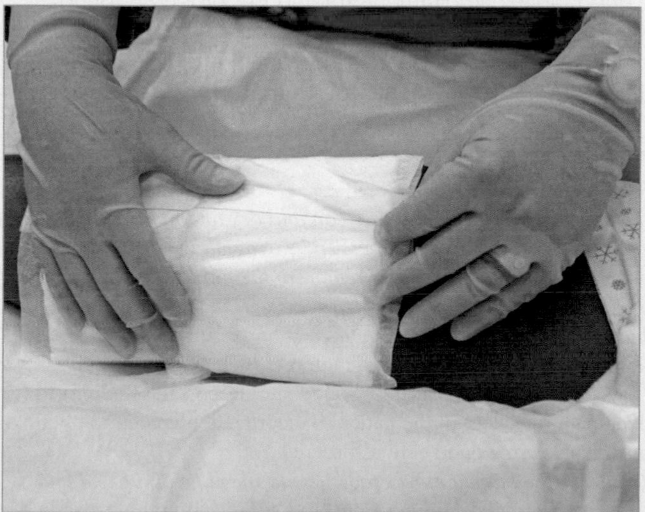

FIGURE 11 Applying a surgical pad over dressing and securing with tape.

(continued)

SKILL 8-1 CLEANING A WOUND AND APPLYING A DRY, STERILE DRESSING continued

ACTION	RATIONALE
23. Remove and discard gloves. Apply tape, Montgomery straps, or roller gauze to secure the dressings. Alternately, many commercial wound products are self-adhesive and do not require additional tape.	Proper disposal of gloves prevents the spread of microorganisms. Tape or other securing products are easier to apply after gloves have been removed.
24. After securing the dressing, label it with date and time. Remove all remaining equipment; place the patient in a comfortable position, with side rails up and bed in the lowest position.	Recording date and time provides communication and demonstrates adherence to plan of care. Proper patient and bed positioning promotes safety and comfort.
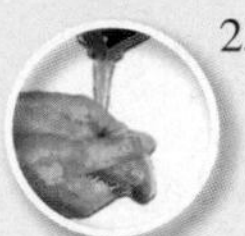 25. Remove PPE, if used. Perform hand hygiene.	Removing PPE properly reduces the risk for infection transmission and contamination of other items. Hand hygiene prevents the spread of microorganisms.
26. Check all wound dressings every shift. More frequent checks may be needed if the wound is more complex or dressings become saturated quickly.	Checking dressings ensures the assessment of changes in patient condition and timely intervention to prevent complications.

EVALUATION

The expected outcome is met when the patient exhibits a clean, intact wound with a clean dressing in place; the wound is free of contamination and trauma; the patient reports little to no pain or discomfort during care; and the patient demonstrates signs and symptoms of progressive wound healing.

DOCUMENTATION

Guidelines

Document the location of the wound and that the dressing was removed. Record your assessment of the wound, including approximation of wound edges; presence of sutures, staples, or adhesive closure strips; and the condition of the surrounding skin. Note if redness, edema, or drainage is observed. Document cleansing of the incision with normal saline and any application of antibiotic ointment as ordered. Record the type of dressing that was reapplied. Note pertinent patient and family education and any patient reaction to this procedure, including patient's pain level and effectiveness of nonpharmacologic interventions or analgesia if administered.

Sample Documentation

Lippincott DocuCare **Practice documenting wound care in *Lippincott DocuCare*.**

9/8/15 0600 Dressing removed from left lateral calf incision. Scant purulent secretions noted on dressing. Incision edges approximately 1 mm apart, red, with ecchymosis and edema present. Small amount of purulent drainage from wound noted. Area cleansed with normal saline, dried, antibiotic ointment applied per order. Surrounding tissue red and ecchymotic. Redressed with nonadhering dressing, gauze, and wrapped with stretch gauze. Patient reports adequate pain control after preprocedure analgesic; states pain is dull ache, 1/10 on pain scale.

—N. Joiner, RN

UNEXPECTED SITUATIONS AND ASSOCIATED INTERVENTIONS

- *The previous wound assessment states that the incision was clean and dry and the wound edges were approximated, with the staples and surgical drain intact. The surrounding tissue was without inflammation, edema, or erythema. After the dressing is removed, the nurse notes the incision edges are not approximated at the distal end, multiple staples are evident in the old dressing, the surrounding skin tissue is red and swollen, and purulent drainage is on the dressing and leaking from the wound:* Assess the patient for any other signs and symptoms, such as pain, malaise, fever, and paresthesias. Place a dry sterile dressing over the wound site. Report the findings to the primary care provider and document the event in the patient's record. Be prepared to obtain a wound culture and implement any changes in wound care as ordered.
- *After the nurse has put on sterile gloves, the patient moves too close to the edge of the bed and the nurse must support her with his hands to prevent the patient from falling:* If nothing else in the sterile field was touched, remove the contaminated gloves and put on new sterile gloves. If you did not bring a second pair, use the call bell to summon a coworker to provide a new pair of gloves.

• *The nurse has set up dressing supplies, removed the old dressing, and put on sterile gloves to clean the wound. The nurse then realizes that a necessary piece of dressing material has been forgotten:* Ask the patient to press the call bell to summon a coworker to provide the missing supplies.

SPECIAL CONSIDERATIONS

General Considerations

• Instruct the patient, if appropriate, and ancillary staff members to observe for excessive drainage that may overwhelm the dressing. They should also report when dressings become soiled or loosened from the skin.

Older Adult Considerations

• The skin of older adults is less elastic and more sensitive; use paper tape, Montgomery straps (Refer to Skill 8-6), or roller gauze (on extremities) to prevent tearing of the skin.

SKILL 8-2 APPLYING A SALINE-MOISTENED DRESSING

Gauze or other dressing materials can be moistened with saline to keep the surface of open wounds moist. A saline-moistened dressing promotes moist wound healing and protects the wound from contamination and trauma. A moist wound surface enhances the cellular migration necessary for tissue repair and healing. It is important that the dressing material be moist, not wet, when placed in open wounds. Dressing materials are soaked in normal saline solution and squeezed to remove excess saline so that the dressing is only slightly moist. The dressing can be loosely packed in the wound bed, if appropriate, and then covered with a secondary dressing to absorb drainage.

In addition, many commercially prepared wound care products are also available to maintain a moist wound environment. These dressing and wound care products are applied in a similar manner. It is very important for the nurse to be aware of the products available in a particular facility and to be familiar with the indications for, and correct use of, each type of dressing and wound care product (see Fundamentals Review 8-4).

DELEGATION CONSIDERATIONS

Wound care and procedures requiring the use of a sterile field and other sterile items are not delegated to nursing assistive personnel (NAP) or to unlicensed assistive personnel (UAP). Depending on the state's nurse practice act and the organization's policies and procedures, these procedures may be delegated to licensed practical/vocational nurses (LPN/LVNs). The decision to delegate must be based on careful analysis of the patient's needs and circumstances, as well as the qualifications of the person to whom the task is being delegated. Refer to the Delegation Guidelines in Appendix A.

EQUIPMENT

- Clean, disposable gloves
- Sterile gloves, if indicated
- Additional PPE, as indicated
- Sterile dressing set or suture set (for the sterile scissors and forceps)
- Sterile thin-mesh gauze dressing for packing, if ordered
- Sterile gauze dressings
- Surgical or abdominal pads
- Skin-protectant wipes
- Sterile basin
- Sterile cleaning solution as ordered (commonly 0.9% normal saline solution)
- Sterile saline
- Tape or ties
- Plastic bag or other appropriate waste container for soiled dressings
- Sterile cotton-tipped applicators
- Supplies for wound cleansing or irrigation, as necessary
- Waterproof pad and bath blanket

(continued)

SKILL 8-2 APPLYING A SALINE-MOISTENED DRESSING continued

ASSESSMENT

Assess the situation to determine the need for a dressing change. Confirm any medical orders relevant to wound care and any wound care included in the nursing plan of care. Assess the patient's level of comfort and the need for analgesics before wound care. Assess if the patient experienced any pain related to previous dressing changes and the effectiveness of interventions employed to minimize the patient's pain. Assess the current dressing to determine if it is intact. Assess for excess drainage or bleeding or saturation of the dressing. Inspect the wound and the surrounding tissue. Assess the location, appearance of the wound, wound stage (if appropriate), drainage, and types of tissue present in the wound. Measure the wound. Note the stage of the healing process and characteristics of any drainage. Also assess the surrounding skin for color, temperature, and edema, ecchymosis, or maceration.

NURSING DIAGNOSIS

Determine the related factors for the nursing diagnoses based on the patient's current health status. Appropriate nursing diagnoses may include:

- Disturbed Body Image
- Impaired Skin Integrity
- Acute Pain
- Impaired Tissue Integrity

OUTCOME IDENTIFICATION AND PLANNING

The expected outcome to achieve when applying a saline-moistened dressing (or similar dressing) is that the procedure is accomplished without contaminating the wound area, causing trauma to the wound, and/or causing the patient to experience pain or discomfort. Other outcomes that are appropriate include wound healing is promoted; the surrounding skin is without signs of irritation, infection, and maceration; and the wound continues to show signs of progression of healing.

IMPLEMENTATION

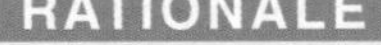

ACTION	RATIONALE
1. Review the medical orders for wound care or the nursing plan of care related to wound care. Gather necessary supplies.	Reviewing the order and plan of care validates the correct patient and correct procedure. Preparation promotes efficient time management and an organized approach to the task.
2. Perform hand hygiene and put on PPE, if indicated.	Hand hygiene and PPE prevent the spread of microorganisms. PPE is required based on transmission precautions.
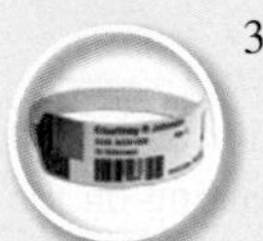 3. Identify the patient.	Identifying the patient ensures the right patient receives the intervention and helps prevent errors.
4. Assemble equipment on overbed table within reach.	Organization facilitates performance of the task.
5. Close the curtains around the bed and close the door to the room, if possible. Explain what you are going to do and why you are going to do it to the patient.	This ensures the patient's privacy. Explanation relieves anxiety and facilitates cooperation.
6. Assess the patient for possible need for nonpharmacologic pain-reducing interventions or analgesic medication before wound care dressing change. Administer appropriate prescribed analgesic. Allow enough time for the analgesic to achieve its effectiveness.	Pain is a subjective experience influenced by past experience. Wound care and dressing changes may cause pain for some patients.
7. Place a waste receptacle or bag at a convenient location for use during the procedure.	Having a waste container handy means the soiled dressing may be discarded easily, without the spread of microorganisms.
8. Adjust the bed to a comfortable working height, usually elbow height of the caregiver (VISN 8, 2009).	Having the bed at the proper height prevents back and muscle strain.

ACTION	RATIONALE
9. Assist the patient to a comfortable position that provides easy access to the wound area. Position the patient so the wound cleanser or irrigation solution will flow from the clean end of the wound toward the dirtier end, if being used (see Skill 8-1 for wound cleansing and Skill 8-4 for irrigation techniques). Use the bath blanket to cover any exposed area other than the wound. Place a waterproof pad under the wound site.	Patient positioning and use of a bath blanket provide for comfort and warmth. Gravity directs the flow of liquid from the least contaminated to the most contaminated area. Waterproof pad protects underlying surfaces.
10. Put on clean gloves. Carefully and gently remove the soiled dressings. If there is resistance, use a silicone-based adhesive remover to help remove the tape. If any part of the dressing sticks to the underlying skin, use small amounts of sterile saline to help loosen and remove it.	Gloves protect the nurse from handling contaminated dressings. Cautious removal of the dressing is more comfortable for the patient and ensures that any drain present is not removed. A silicone-based adhesive remover allows for the easy, rapid, and painless removal without the associated problems of skin stripping (Denyer, 2011; Benbow, 2011). Sterile saline moistens the dressing for easier removal and minimizes damage and pain.
11. After removing the dressing, note the presence, amount, type, color, and odor of any drainage on the dressings. Place soiled dressings in the appropriate waste receptacle.	The presence of drainage should be documented. Discarding dressings appropriately prevents the spread of microorganisms.
12. Assess the wound for appearance, stage, the presence of eschar, granulation tissue, **epithelialization**, undermining, tunneling, necrosis, **sinus tract**, and drainage. Assess the appearance of the surrounding tissue. Measure the wound. Refer to Fundamentals Review 8-3.	This information provides evidence about the wound healing process and/or the presence of infection.
13. Remove your gloves and put them in the receptacle.	Discarding gloves prevents the spread of microorganisms.
14. Using sterile technique, open the supplies and dressings. Place the fine-mesh gauze into the basin and pour the ordered solution over the mesh to saturate it.	Gauze touching the wound surface must be moistened to increase the absorptive ability and promote healing.
15. Put on sterile gloves. Alternately, clean gloves (clean technique) may be used to clean a chronic wound or pressure ulcer.	Sterile gloves maintain surgical asepsis. Clean technique is appropriate when cleaning chronic wounds and pressure ulcers.
16. Clean the wound. Refer to Skill 8-1. Alternately, irrigate the wound, as ordered or required (see Skill 8-4).	Cleaning the wound removes previous drainage and wound debris.
17. Dry the surrounding skin with sterile gauze dressings.	Moisture provides a medium for growth of microorganisms.
18. Apply a skin protectant to the surrounding skin, if needed.	A skin protectant prevents skin irritation and breakdown.
19. If not already on, put on sterile gloves. Squeeze excess fluid from the gauze dressing. Unfold and fluff the dressing.	Sterile gloves prevent contamination of the dressing material. The gauze provides a thin, moist layer to contact all the wound surfaces.
20. Gently press to loosely pack the moistened gauze into the wound (Figure 1). If necessary, use the forceps or cotton-tipped applicator to press the gauze into all wound surfaces (Figure 2).	The dressing provides a moist environment for all wound surfaces. Avoid overpacking the gauze; loosely pack to prevent too much pressure in the wound bed, which could impede wound healing.

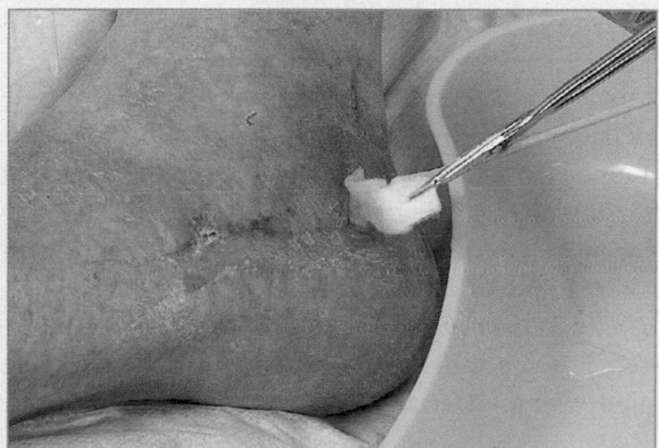

FIGURE 1 Gently pressing gauze into wound.

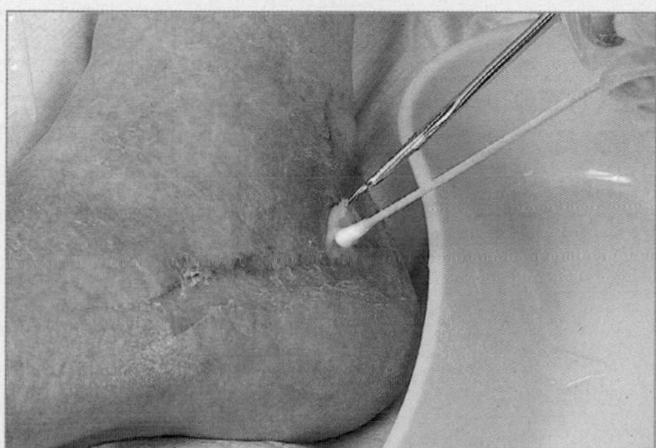

FIGURE 2 Using a cotton-tipped applicator to press gauze into all wound surfaces.

(continued)

SKILL 8-2 APPLYING A SALINE-MOISTENED DRESSING continued

ACTION	RATIONALE
21. Apply several dry, sterile gauze pads over the wet gauze.	Dry gauze absorbs excess moisture and drainage.
22. Place the ABD pad over the gauze.	The ABD pad prevents contamination.
23. Remove and discard gloves. Apply tape, Montgomery straps, or roller gauze to secure the dressings. Alternately, many commercial wound products are self-adhesive and do not require additional tape.	Proper disposal of gloves prevents the spread of microorganisms. Tape or other securing products are easier to apply after gloves have been removed.
24. After securing the dressing, label dressing with date and time. Remove all remaining equipment; place the patient in a comfortable position, with side rails up and bed in the lowest position.	Recording date and time provides communication and demonstrates adherence to plan of care. Proper patient and bed positioning promotes safety and comfort.
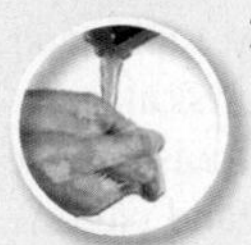 25. Remove PPE, if used. Perform hand hygiene.	Removing PPE properly reduces the risk for infection transmission and contamination of other items. Hand hygiene prevents the spread of microorganisms.
26. Check all wound dressings every shift. More frequent checks may be needed if the wound is more complex or dressings become saturated quickly.	Checking dressings ensures the assessment of changes in patient condition and timely intervention to prevent complications.

EVALUATION

The expected outcome when applying a saline-moistened dressing is met when the procedure is accomplished without contaminating the wound area, causing trauma to the wound, and/or causing the patient to experience pain or discomfort. Other outcomes are met when sterile technique is maintained (if appropriate); wound healing is promoted; the surrounding skin is without signs of irritation, infection, and maceration; and the wound continues to show signs of progression of healing.

DOCUMENTATION

Guidelines

Document the location of the wound and that the dressing was removed. Record your assessment of the wound, including evidence of granulation tissue, presence of necrotic tissue, stage (if appropriate), and characteristics of drainage. Include the appearance of the surrounding skin. Document the cleansing or irrigation of the wound and solution used. Record the type of dressing that was reapplied. Note pertinent patient and family education and any patient reaction to this procedure, including patient's pain level and effectiveness of nonpharmacologic interventions or analgesia if administered.

Sample Documentation

11/20/15 1645 Healing abdominal incision with granulating tissue noted. Open area 2 cm × 4 cm × 0.5 cm depth in center of incision. No evidence of necrosis or tunneling. Scant amount of serous drainage. Saline-moistened dressing applied to open wound; covered loosely with ABD dressing. Patient denies pain from incision. Instructed patient that moist saline gauze will facilitate the healing process and to notify nurse for any discomfort related to incision.

—R. Dobbins, RN

UNEXPECTED SITUATIONS AND RELATED INTERVENTIONS

- *When removing a patient's dressing, the assessment reveals eschar in the wound:* Notify the primary care provider or wound care specialist; a different treatment modality and/or debridement may be necessary. The presence of eschar in a wound precludes staging the wound. The eschar must be removed for adequate pressure ulcer staging to be done. However, note that stable (dry, adherent, intact, without erythema or movement) eschar on the heels serves as "the body's natural (biological) cover" and should not be removed (NPUAP, 2012a).
- *The wound assessment reveals several depressions or crater-like areas on inspection of a wound:* Notify the primary care provider or wound care specialist, who may order the wound to be packed. Pack wound cavities loosely with dressing material. Overpacking may increase pressure and interfere with tissue healing.
- *The nurse notes that the wound dressing is dry upon removal:* Reduce the time interval between changes to prevent drying of the materials, which may disrupt healing tissue.

SPECIAL CONSIDERATIONS

- Make sure ancillary staff understand the importance of reporting excessive drainage from the dressing, and any soiled or loose dressings.
- Guidelines from the Wound, Ostomy, Continence Nurses Society (WOCN) recommend that clean gloves may be used to treat chronic wounds and pressure ulcers as long as infection-control procedures are followed. The *no-touch technique* may be used within these guidelines. Clean gloves are used to handle dressing material. Irrigants and dressings are sterile. The wound is redressed by picking up dressing materials by the corner and placing the untouched side over the wound (WOCN, 2012).
- Many products are available to treat chronic wounds and pressure ulcers. Treatment varies based on facility policy, nursing protocol, clinical specialist referrals, primary care provider orders, and product in use.

EVIDENCE FOR PRACTICE ▶

CHRONIC WOUNDS AND DRESSING TECHNIQUES

Wound, Ostomy and Continence Nurses Society (WOCN). (2012). Clean vs. sterile dressing techniques for management of chronic wounds. A fact sheet. *Journal of Wound, Ostomy and Continence Nursing, 39*(2S) (Supplement), S30–S34.

These guidelines are a collaborative effort of the Association for Professionals in Infection Control and Epidemiology (APIC) and the Wound, Ostomy, Continence Nurses Society (WOCN). Approaches for chronic wound care management are presented, including the definitions of, and indications for, 'clean' and 'sterile' technique. Cleansing of chronic wounds requires the use of handwashing, clean (nonsterile) gloves, sterile cleansing solution, and irrigation with a sterile device. Routine dressing change without debridement requires the use of handwashing, clean (nonsterile) gloves, sterile solutions, sterile dressing supplies, and sterile instruments.

Refer to thePoint for additional research on related nursing topics.

SKILL 8-3 APPLYING A HYDROCOLLOID DRESSING

Hydrocolloid dressings are wafer-shaped dressings that come in many shapes, sizes, and thicknesses. An adhesive backing provides adherence to the wound and surrounding skin. They absorb drainage, maintain a moist wound surface, and decrease the risk for infection by covering the wound surface (refer to Fundamentals Review 8-4). Many commercially prepared dressing and wound care products are applied in a similar manner. It is very important for the nurse to be aware of the products available in a particular facility and be familiar with the indications for, and correct use of, each type of dressing and wound care product.

DELEGATION CONSIDERATIONS

Wound care and procedures requiring the use of a sterile field and other sterile items are not delegated to nursing assistive personnel (NAP) or to unlicensed assistive personnel (UAP). In some settings, such as long-term care, the application of a wound dressing using clean technique for a chronic wound may be delegated to NAP/UAPs. However, the assessment of the wound is performed by the RN. Depending on the state's nurse practice act and the organization's policies and procedures, these procedures may be delegated to licensed practical/vocational nurses (LPN/LVNs). The decision to delegate must be based on careful analysis of the patient's needs and circumstances, as well as the qualifications of the person to whom the task is being delegated. Refer to the Delegation Guidelines in Appendix A.

EQUIPMENT

- Hydrocolloid dressing
- Clean, disposable gloves
- Sterile gloves, if indicated
- Additional PPE, as indicated
- Sterile dressing instrument set or suture set (for the scissors and forceps)
- Sterile cleaning solution, as ordered (commonly 0.9% normal saline solution)

(continued)

SKILL 8-3 APPLYING A HYDROCOLLOID DRESSING continued

- Skin-protectant wipes
- Additional supplies needed for wound cleansing
- Sterile cotton-tipped applicators
- Waterproof pad
- Bath blanket
- Measuring tape or other supplies, such as sterile flexible applicator, for assessing wound measurements, as indicated

ASSESSMENT

Assess the situation to determine the need for a dressing change. Check the date when the current dressing (if present) was placed. Confirm any medical orders relevant to wound care and any wound care included in the nursing plan of care. Assess the current dressing to determine if it is intact. Assess the patient's level of comfort and the need for analgesics before wound care.

Assess if the patient experienced any pain related to prior dressing changes and the effectiveness of interventions employed to minimize the patient's pain. Assess for excess drainage or bleeding or saturation of the dressing. Inspect the wound and the surrounding tissue. Assess the location, appearance of the wound, stage (if appropriate), drainage, and types of tissue present in the wound. Measure the wound. Note the stage of the healing process and characteristics of any drainage. Also assess the surrounding skin for color, temperature, and edema, ecchymosis, or maceration.

NURSING DIAGNOSIS

Determine the related factors for the nursing diagnoses based on the patient's current status. Appropriate nursing diagnoses may include:

- Impaired Skin Integrity
- Chronic Pain
- Impaired Tissue Integrity

OUTCOME IDENTIFICATION AND PLANNING

The expected outcome to achieve when applying a hydrocolloid dressing is that the procedure is accomplished without contaminating the wound area, causing trauma to the wound, and/or causing the patient to experience pain or discomfort. Other outcomes that are appropriate include sterile technique is maintained (if appropriate); wound healing is promoted; the surrounding skin is without signs of irritation, infection, and maceration; and the wound continues to show signs of progression of healing.

IMPLEMENTATION

ACTION	RATIONALE
1. Review the medical orders for wound care or the nursing plan of care related to wound care. Gather necessary supplies.	Reviewing the order and plan of care validates the correct patient and correct procedure. Preparation promotes efficient time management and an organized approach to the task.
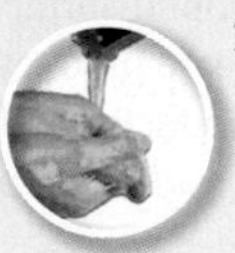 2. Perform hand hygiene and put on PPE, if indicated.	Hand hygiene and PPE prevent the spread of microorganisms. PPE is required based on transmission precautions.
 3. Identify the patient.	Identifying the patient ensures the right patient receives the intervention and helps prevent errors.
4. Assemble equipment on overbed table within reach.	Organization facilitates performance of the task.
5. Close the curtains around the bed and close the door to the room, if possible. Explain what you are going to do and why you are going to do it to the patient.	This ensures the patient's privacy. Explanation relieves anxiety and facilitates cooperation.
6. Assess the patient for possible need for nonpharmacologic pain-reducing interventions or analgesic medication before wound care dressing change. Administer appropriate prescribed analgesic. Allow enough time for the analgesic to achieve its effectiveness before beginning the procedure.	Pain is a subjective experience influenced by past experience. Wound care and dressing changes may cause pain for some patients.
7. Place a waste receptacle or bag at a convenient location for use during the procedure.	Having a waste container handy means the soiled dressing may be discarded easily, without the spread of microorganisms.

ACTION	RATIONALE
8. Adjust the bed to comfortable working height, usually elbow height of the caregiver (VISN 8, 2009).	Having the bed at the proper height prevents back and muscle strain.
9. Assist the patient to a comfortable position that provides easy access to the wound area. Position the patient so the wound cleanser or irrigation solution will flow from the clean end of the wound toward the dirtier end, if being used. (See Skill 8-1 for wound cleansing and Skill 8-4 for irrigation techniques.) Use the bath blanket to cover any exposed area other than the wound. Place a waterproof pad under the wound site.	Patient positioning and use of a bath blanket provide for comfort and warmth. Gravity directs the flow of liquid from the least contaminated to the most contaminated area. Waterproof pad protects underlying surfaces.
10. Put on clean gloves. Carefully and gently remove the soiled dressings. If there is resistance, use a silicone-based adhesive remover to help remove the tape. If any part of the dressing sticks to the underlying skin, use small amounts of sterile saline to help loosen and remove it.	Gloves protect the nurse from handling contaminated dressings. Cautious removal of the dressing is more comfortable for the patient and ensures that any drain present is not removed. A silicone-based adhesive remover allows for the easy, rapid, and painless removal without the associated problems of skin stripping (Denyer, 2011; Benbow, 2011). Sterile saline moistens the dressing for easier removal and minimizes damage and pain.
11. After removing the dressing, note the presence, amount, type, color, and odor of any drainage on the dressings. Place soiled dressings in the appropriate waste receptacle.	The presence of drainage should be documented. Discarding dressings appropriately prevents the spread of microorganisms.
12. Assess the wound for appearance, stage, presence of eschar, granulation tissue, epithelialization, undermining, tunneling, necrosis, sinus tract, and drainage. Assess the appearance of the surrounding tissue. Measure the wound. Refer to Fundamentals Review 8-3.	This information provides evidence about the wound healing process and/or the presence of infection.
13. Remove your gloves and put them in the receptacle.	Discarding gloves prevents the spread of microorganisms.
14. Set up a sterile field, if indicated, and wound cleaning supplies. Put on sterile gloves. Alternately, clean gloves (clean technique) may be used when cleaning a chronic wound or pressure ulcer.	Sterile gloves maintain surgical asepsis. Clean technique is appropriate for cleaning chronic wounds or pressure ulcers.
15. Clean the wound. Refer to Skill 8-1. Alternately, irrigate the wound, as ordered or required (see Skill 8-4).	Cleaning the wound removes previous drainage and wound debris.
16. Dry the surrounding skin with gauze dressings.	Moisture provides a medium for growth of microorganisms. Excess moisture can contribute to skin irritation and breakdown.
17. Apply a skin protectant to the surrounding skin.	A skin protectant prevents skin irritation and breakdown.
18. Cut the dressing to size, if indicated, using sterile scissors. Size the dressing generously, allowing at least a 1-inch margin of healthy skin around the wound to be covered with the dressing.	These actions ensure proper adherence, coverage of the wound, and wear of the dressing.
19. Remove the release paper from the adherent side of the dressing. Apply the dressing to the wound without stretching the dressing. Smooth wrinkles as the dressing is applied (Figure 1).	Proper application prevents shearing force on the wound and minimizes irritation.

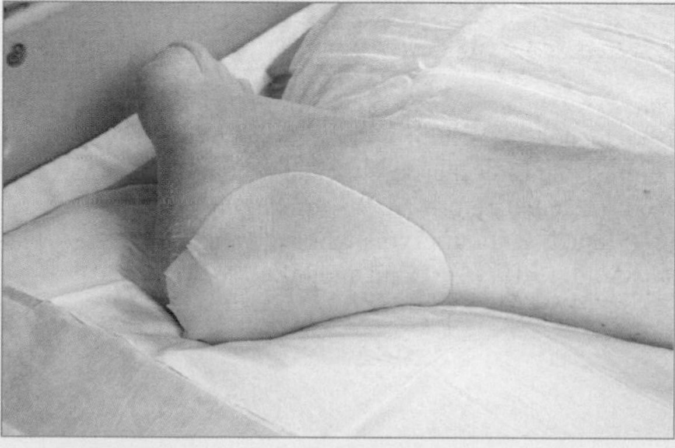

FIGURE 1 Hydrocolloid dressing in place.

(continued)

SKILL 8-3 APPLYING A HYDROCOLLOID DRESSING continued

ACTION	RATIONALE
20. If necessary, secure the dressing edges with tape. Apply additional skin barrier to the areas to be covered with tape, if necessary. Dressings that are near the anus need to have the edges taped. Apply additional skin barrier to the areas to be covered with tape, if necessary.	Taping helps keep the dressing intact. Skin protectant prevents surrounding skin irritation and breakdown. Taping the edges of dressings near the anus prevents wound contamination from fecal material.
21. After securing the dressing, label it with date and time. Remove all remaining equipment; place the patient in a comfortable position, with side rails up and bed in the lowest position.	Recording date and time provides communication and demonstrates adherence to plan of care. Proper patient and bed positioning promotes safety and comfort.
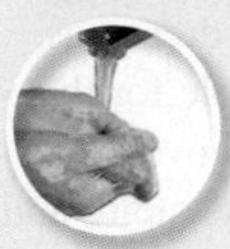 22. Remove PPE, if used. Perform hand hygiene.	Removing PPE properly reduces the risk for infection transmission and contamination of other items. Hand hygiene prevents the spread of microorganisms.
23. Check all wound dressings every shift. More frequent checks may be needed if the wound is more complex or dressings become saturated quickly.	Checking dressings ensures the assessment of changes in patient condition and timely intervention to prevent complications.

EVALUATION

The expected outcome when applying a hydrocolloid dressing is met when the procedure is accomplished without contaminating the wound area, causing trauma to the wound, and/or causing the patient to experience pain or discomfort. Other outcomes are met when sterile technique is maintained (if appropriate); wound healing is promoted; surrounding skin is without signs of irritation, infection, and maceration; and the wound continues to show signs of progression of healing.

DOCUMENTATION

Guidelines

Document the location of the wound and that the dressing was removed. Record your assessment of the wound, including evidence of granulation tissue, presence of necrotic tissue, stage (if appropriate), and characteristics of drainage. Include the appearance of the surrounding skin. Document the cleansing or irrigation of the wound and solution used. Record the type of hydrocolloid dressing that was applied. Note pertinent patient and family education and any patient reaction to this procedure, including the patient's pain level and effectiveness of nonpharmacologic interventions or analgesia if administered.

Sample Documentation

11/4/15 0930 Stage III wound on right hip area (3 × 2 × 2 cm) assessed. Granulation tissue about 50%, no necrosis, undermining, or tunneling present. Minimal serous drainage on old dressing. Wound cleansed with normal saline. Hydrocolloid dressing applied. Due to be changed in 5 days. Skin barrier applied to surrounding intact skin. Prior to dressing change, patient was medicated with Tylenol 650 mg PO for anticipated pain. Patient tolerated dressing change. Stated "pain not so bad," about a "3." Instructed patient to call for nurse for any discomfort related to dressing.

—M. Semet, RN

UNEXPECTED SITUATIONS AND RELATED INTERVENTION

- *When removing a patient's dressing, the assessment reveals eschar in the wound:* Notify the primary care provider or wound care specialist, as a different treatment modality and/or debridement may be necessary. The presence of eschar in a wound precludes staging the wound. The eschar must be removed for adequate pressure ulcer staging to be done. However, note that stable (dry, adherent, intact, without erythema or movement) eschar on the heels serves as "the body's natural (biological) cover" and should not be removed (NPUAP, 2012a).

SPECIAL CONSIDERATIONS

- Guidelines from the Wound, Ostomy, Continence Nurses Society (WOCN) recommend that clean gloves may be used to treat chronic wounds and pressure ulcers as long as the infection-control procedures are followed. The *no-touch technique* may be used within these guidelines. Clean gloves are used to handle dressing material. Irrigants and dressings are sterile. The wound is redressed by picking up dressing materials by the corner and placing the untouched side over the wound (WOCN, 2012).
- Many products are available to treat chronic wounds and pressure ulcers. Treatment varies based on facility policy, nursing protocol, clinical specialist referrals, and primary care provider orders.

EVIDENCE FOR PRACTICE ▶

CHRONIC WOUNDS AND DRESSING TECHNIQUES

Wound, Ostomy and Continence Nurses Society (WOCN). (2012). Clean vs. sterile dressing techniques for management of chronic wounds. A fact sheet. *Journal of Wound, Ostomy and Continence Nursing, 39*(2S) (Supplement), S30–S34.

See the Evidence for Practice in Skill 8-2 for detailed information regarding these guidelines, and refer to thePoint for additional research on related nursing topics.

SKILL 8-4 PERFORMING IRRIGATION OF A WOUND

Irrigation is a directed flow of solution over tissues. Wound irrigations are ordered to clean the area of **pathogens** and other debris and to promote wound healing. Irrigation procedures may also be ordered to apply heat or antiseptics locally. If the wound edges are approximated, clean technique may be used; if the wound edges are not approximated, sterile equipment and solutions are used for irrigation. Normal saline is often the solution of choice when irrigating wounds.

DELEGATION CONSIDERATIONS

Irrigation of a wound and procedures requiring the use of a sterile field and other sterile items are not delegated to nursing assistive personnel (NAP) or to unlicensed assistive personnel (UAP). Depending on the state's nurse practice act and the organization's policies and procedures, these procedures may be delegated to licensed practical/vocational nurses (LPN/LVNs). The decision to delegate must be based on careful analysis of the patient's needs and circumstances, as well as the qualifications of the person to whom the task is being delegated. Refer to the Delegation Guidelines in Appendix A.

EQUIPMENT

- A sterile irrigation set, including a basin, irrigant container, and irrigation syringe
- Sterile irrigation solution as ordered, warmed to body temperature, commonly 0.9% normal saline solution
- Plastic bag or other waste container to dispose of soiled dressings
- Sterile gloves
- Sterile drape (may be optional)
- Clean, disposable gloves
- Moisture-proof gown, mask, and eye protection
- Additional PPE, as indicated
- Sterile dressing set or suture set (for the sterile scissors and forceps)
- Waterproof pad and bath blanket, as needed
- Sterile gauze dressings
- Sterile packing gauze, as needed
- Tape or ties
- Skin-protectant wipes

ASSESSMENT

Assess the situation to determine the need for wound irrigation. Confirm any medical orders relevant to wound care and any wound care included in the nursing plan of care. Assess the current dressing to determine if it is intact. Assess the patient's level of comfort and the need for analgesics before wound care. Assess if the patient experienced any pain related to previous dressing changes and the effectiveness of interventions employed to minimize the patient's pain. Assess for excess drainage or bleeding or saturation of the dressing. Inspect the wound and the surrounding tissue. Assess the location, appearance of the wound, stage (if appropriate), drainage, and types of tissue present in the wound. Measure

(*continued*)

SKILL 8-4 PERFORMING IRRIGATION OF A WOUND continued

the wound. Note the stage of the healing process and characteristics of any drainage. Also assess the surrounding skin for color, temperature, and edema, ecchymosis, or maceration.

NURSING DIAGNOSIS

Determine the related factors for the nursing diagnoses based on the patient's current health status. Appropriate nursing diagnoses may include:

- Risk for Infection
- Acute Pain
- Impaired Skin Integrity
- Impaired Tissue Integrity

OUTCOME IDENTIFICATION AND PLANNING

The expected outcome to achieve when irrigating a wound is that the wound is cleaned without contamination or trauma and without causing the patient to experience pain or discomfort. Other outcomes that might be appropriate include the following: the wound continues to show signs of progression of healing, and the patient demonstrates an understanding of the need for wound irrigation.

IMPLEMENTATION

ACTION	RATIONALE
1. Review the medical orders for wound care or the nursing plan of care related to wound care. Gather necessary supplies.	Reviewing the order and plan of care validates the correct patient and correct procedure. Preparation promotes efficient time management and an organized approach to the task.
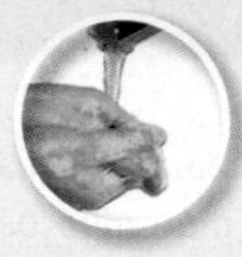 2. Perform hand hygiene and put on PPE, if indicated.	Hand hygiene and PPE prevent the spread of microorganisms. PPE is required based on transmission precautions.
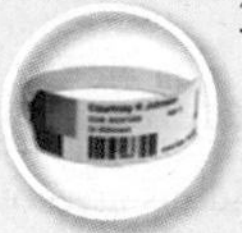 3. Identify the patient.	Identifying the patient ensures the right patient receives the intervention and helps prevent errors.
4. Assemble equipment on overbed table within reach.	Organization facilitates performance of the task.
5. Close the curtains around the bed and close the door to the room if possible. Explain what you are going to do and why you are going to do it to the patient.	This ensures the patient's privacy. Explanation relieves anxiety and facilitates cooperation.
6. Assess the patient for possible need for nonpharmacologic pain-reducing interventions or analgesic medication before wound care and/or dressing change. Administer appropriate prescribed analgesic. Allow enough time for the analgesic to achieve its effectiveness before beginning the procedure.	Pain is a subjective experience influenced by past experience. Wound care and dressing changes may cause pain for some patients.
7. Place a waste receptacle or bag at a convenient location for use during the procedure.	Having a waste container handy means the soiled dressing may be discarded easily, without the spread of microorganisms.
8. Adjust the bed to a comfortable working height, usually elbow height of the caregiver (VISN 8, 2009).	Having the bed at the proper height prevents back and muscle strain.
9. Assist the patient to a comfortable position that provides easy access to the wound area. Position the patient so the irrigation solution will flow from the clean end of the wound toward the dirtier end. Use the bath blanket to cover any exposed area other than the wound. Place a waterproof pad under the wound site.	Patient positioning and use of a bath blanket provide for comfort and warmth. Gravity directs the flow of liquid from the least contaminated to the most contaminated area. Waterproof pad protects underlying surfaces.
10. Put on a gown, mask, and eye protection.	Using PPE, such as gowns, masks, and eye protection, is part of *Standard Precautions.* A gown protects clothes from contamination should splashing occur. Goggles protect mucous membranes of eyes from contact with irrigant fluid or wound drainage.

ACTION	RATIONALE
11. Put on clean gloves. Carefully and gently remove the soiled dressings. If there is resistance, use a silicone-based adhesive remover to help remove the tape. If any part of the dressing sticks to the underlying skin, use small amounts of sterile saline to help loosen and remove it.	Gloves protect the nurse from handling contaminated dressings. Cautious removal of the dressing is more comfortable for the patient and ensures that any drain present is not removed. A silicone-based adhesive remover allows for the easy, rapid, and painless removal without the associated problems of skin stripping (Denyer, 2011; Benbow, 2011). Sterile saline moistens the dressing for easier removal and minimizes damage and pain.
12. After removing the dressing, note the presence, amount, type, color, and odor of any drainage on the dressings. Place soiled dressings in the appropriate waste receptacle.	The presence of drainage should be documented. Discarding dressings appropriately prevents the spread of microorganisms.
13. Assess the wound for appearance, stage, presence of eschar, granulation tissue, epithelialization, undermining, tunneling, necrosis, sinus tract, and drainage. Assess the appearance of the surrounding tissue. Measure the wound. Refer to Fundamentals Review 8-3.	This information provides evidence about the wound healing process and/or the presence of infection.
14. Remove your gloves and put them in the receptacle.	Discarding gloves prevents the spread of microorganisms.
15. Set up a sterile field, if indicated, and wound cleaning supplies. Pour warmed sterile irrigating solution into the sterile container. Put on the sterile gloves. Alternately, clean gloves (clean technique) may be used when irrigating a chronic wound or pressure ulcer.	Using warmed solution prevents chilling the patient and may minimize patient discomfort. Sterile technique and gloves maintain surgical asepsis. Clean technique is appropriate for irrigating chronic wounds or pressure ulcers.
16. Position the sterile basin below the wound to collect the irrigation fluid.	Patient and bed linens are protected from contaminated fluid.
17. Fill the irrigation syringe with solution (Figure 1). **Using your nondominant hand, gently apply pressure to the basin against the skin below the wound to form a seal with the skin (Figure 2).**	The solution will collect in the basin and prevent the irrigant from running down the skin. Patient and bed linens are protected from contaminated fluid.

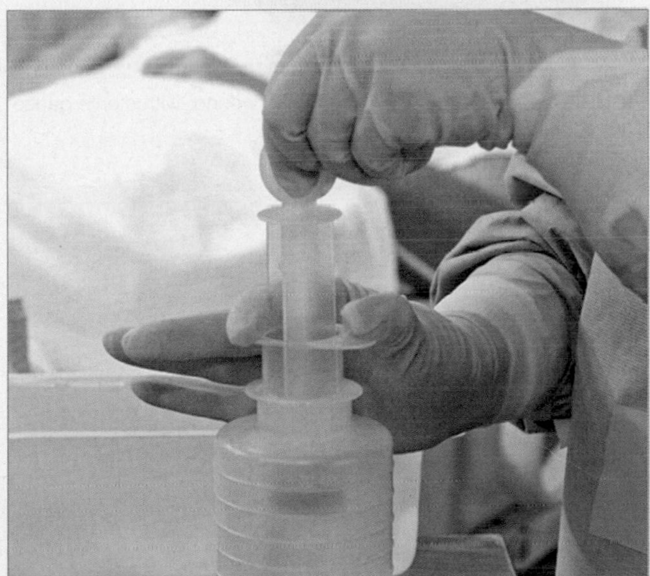

FIGURE 1 Drawing up sterile solution from sterile container into irrigation syringe.

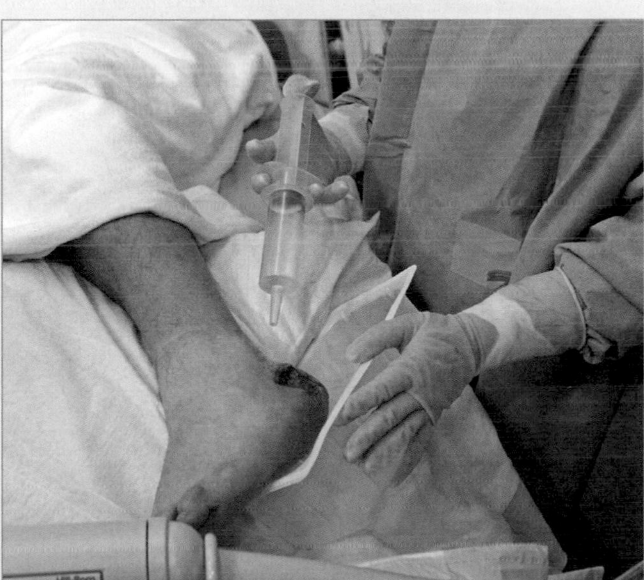

FIGURE 2 Patient lying on side with wound exposed, sterile collection container placed against skin, bed protected with waterproof pad.

(continued)

SKILL 8-4 PERFORMING IRRIGATION OF A WOUND continued

ACTION	RATIONALE
18. **Gently direct a stream of solution into the wound (Figure 3). Keep the tip of the syringe at least 1 inch above the upper tip of the wound. When using a catheter tip, insert it gently into the wound until it meets resistance. Gently flush all wound areas.**	Debris and contaminated solution flow from the least contaminated to most contaminated area. High-pressure irrigation flow may cause patient discomfort as well as damage granulation tissue. A catheter tip allows the introduction of irrigant into a wound with a small opening or one that is deep.
19. Watch for the solution to flow smoothly and evenly. When the solution from the wound flows out clear, discontinue irrigation.	Irrigation removes exudate and debris.
20. Dry the surrounding skin with gauze dressings (Figure 4).	Moisture provides a medium for growth of microorganisms. Excess moisture can contribute to skin irritation and breakdown.
21. Apply a skin protectant to the surrounding skin.	A skin protectant prevents skin irritation and breakdown.
22. Apply a new dressing to the wound (see Skills 8-1, 8-2, 8-3) (Figure 5).	Dressings absorb drainage, protect the wound, and promote healing.

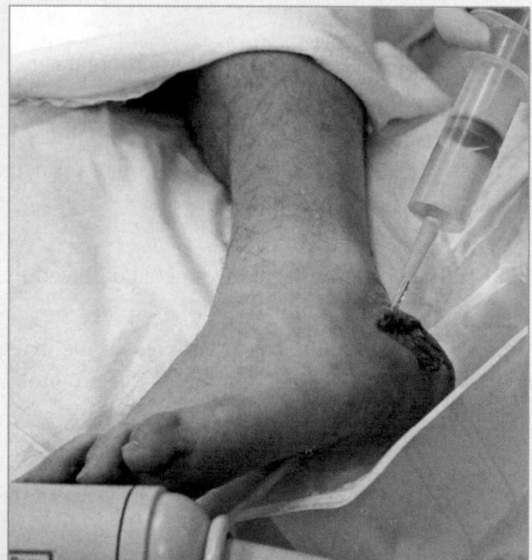

FIGURE 3 Irrigating wound with a gentle stream of solution. Solution drains into collection container.

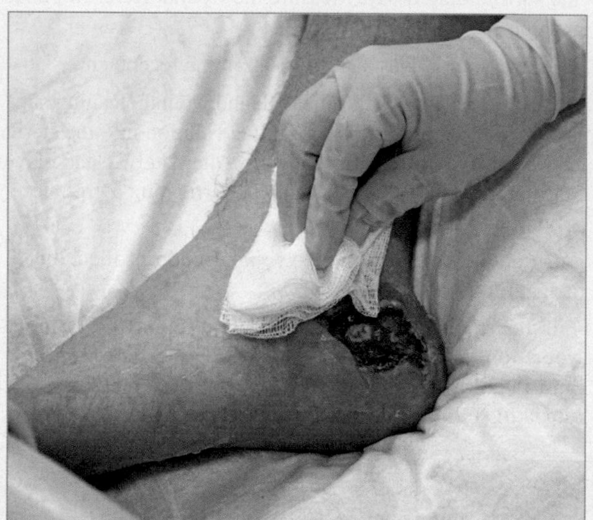

FIGURE 4 Drying around wound, not in wound, with sterile gauze pad.

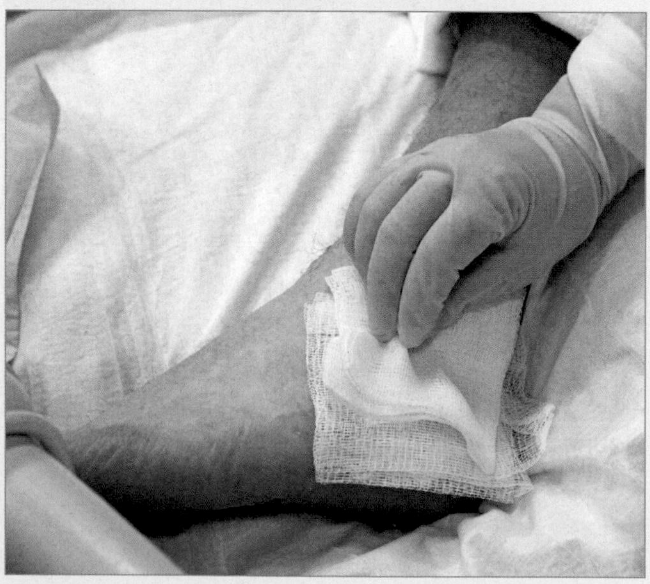

FIGURE 5 Applying a new dressing.

ACTION	RATIONALE
23. Remove and discard gloves. Apply tape, Montgomery straps, or roller gauze to secure the dressing. Alternately, many commercial wound products are self-adhesive and do not require additional tape.	Tape or other securing products are easier to apply after gloves have been removed. Proper disposal of gloves prevents the spread of microorganisms.
24. After securing the dressing, label it with date and time. Remove all remaining equipment; place the patient in a comfortable position, with side rails up and bed in the lowest position.	Recording date and time provides communication and demonstrates adherence to plan of care. Proper patient and bed positioning promotes safety and comfort.
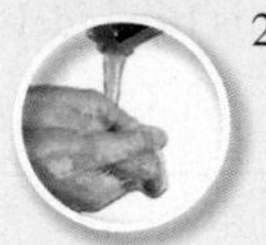 25. Remove remaining PPE. Perform hand hygiene.	Removing PPE properly reduces the risk for infection transmission and contamination of other items. Hand hygiene prevents the spread of microorganisms.
26. Check all wound dressings every shift. More frequent checks may be needed if the wound is more complex or dressings become saturated quickly.	Checking dressings ensures the assessment of changes in patient condition and timely intervention to prevent complications.

EVALUATION

The expected outcome is met when the wound irrigation is completed without contamination and trauma; the patient verbalizes little to no pain or discomfort; the patient verbalizes understanding of the need for irrigation; and the wound continues to show signs of progression of healing.

DOCUMENTATION

Guidelines

Document the location of the wound and that the dressing was removed. Record your assessment of the wound, including evidence of granulation tissue, presence of necrotic tissue, stage (if appropriate), and characteristics of drainage. Include the appearance of the surrounding skin. Document the irrigation of the wound and solution used. Record the type of dressing that was applied. Note pertinent patient and family education and any patient reaction to this procedure, including patient's pain level and effectiveness of nonpharmacologic interventions or analgesia if administered.

Sample Documentation

3/5/15 1700 Dressing removed from left outer heel area. Minimal serosanguineous drainage noted on dressings. Wound 4 × 5 × 2 cm, pink, with granulation tissue evident. Surrounding skin tone consistent with patient's skin, no edema or redness noted. Irrigated with normal saline and hydrogel dressing applied.

—J. Lark, RN

UNEXPECTED SITUATIONS AND ASSOCIATED INTERVENTIONS

- *The patient experiences pain when the wound irrigation is begun:* Stop the procedure and administer an analgesic, as ordered. Obtain new sterile supplies and begin the procedure after an appropriate amount of time has elapsed to allow the analgesic to begin working. Note the patient's pain on the nursing plan of care so that pain medication can be given before future wound treatments.
- *During the wound irrigation, the nurse notes bleeding from the wound. This has not been documented as happening with previous irrigations:* Stop the procedure. Assess the patient for other symptoms. Obtain vital signs. Report the findings to the primary care provider and document the event in the patient's record.

EVIDENCE FOR PRACTICE ▶

CHRONIC WOUNDS AND DRESSING TECHNIQUES

Wound, Ostomy and Continence Nurses Society (WOCN). (2012). Clean vs. sterile dressing techniques for management of chronic wounds. A fact sheet. *Journal of Wound, Ostomy and Continence Nursing, 39*(2S) (Supplement), S30–S34.

See Evidence for Practice in Skill 8-2 for detailed information regarding these guidelines, and refer to thePoint for additional research on related nursing topics.

SKILL 8-5 COLLECTING A WOUND CULTURE

A wound culture may be ordered to identify the causative organism of an infected wound. Identifying the invading microorganism will provide useful information for selecting the most appropriate therapy. A nurse or other primary care provider can perform a wound culture. Maintaining strict asepsis is crucial so that only the pathogen present in the wound is isolated. It is essential to use the correct swab, based on the tests ordered, for collection of a specimen to isolate aerobic and/or anaerobic organisms.

DELEGATION CONSIDERATIONS

Collection of a wound culture is not delegated to nursing assistive personnel (NAP) or to unlicensed assistive personnel (UAP). Depending on the state's nurse practice act and the organization's policies and procedures, collection of a wound culture may be delegated to licensed practical/vocational nurses (LPN/LVNs). The decision to delegate must be based on careful analysis of the patient's needs and circumstances, as well as the qualifications of the person to whom the task is being delegated. Refer to the Delegation Guidelines in Appendix A.

EQUIPMENT

- A sterile Culturette kit (aerobic or anaerobic) with swab, or a culture tube with individual sterile swabs
- Sterile gloves
- Clean, disposable gloves
- Additional PPE, as indicated
- Plastic bag or appropriate waste receptacle
- Patient label for the sample tube
- Biohazard specimen bag
- Bath blanket (if necessary to drape the patient)
- Supplies to clean the wound and reapply a sterile dressing after obtaining the culture. (Refer to Skills 8-1 through 8-4.)

ASSESSMENT

Assess the situation to determine the need for wound culture. Confirm any medical orders relevant to obtaining a wound culture, as well as wound care, and/or any wound care included in the nursing plan of care. Assess the patient's level of comfort and the need for analgesics before obtaining the wound culture. Inspect the wound and the surrounding tissue. Assess the location, appearance of the wound, stage (if appropriate), drainage, and types of tissue present in the wound. Measure the wound. Note the stage of the healing process and characteristics of any drainage. Also assess the surrounding skin for color, temperature, and edema, ecchymosis, or maceration.

NURSING DIAGNOSIS

Determine the related factors for the nursing diagnoses based on the patient's current health status. Appropriate nursing diagnoses may include:

- Impaired Skin Integrity
- Impaired Tissue Integrity
- Disturbed Body Image

OUTCOME IDENTIFICATION AND PLANNING

The expected outcome to achieve when collecting a wound culture is that the culture is obtained without evidence of contamination, exposing the patient to additional pathogens, or causing discomfort for the patient.

IMPLEMENTATION

ACTION	RATIONALE
1. Review the medical orders for obtaining a wound culture. Gather necessary supplies.	Reviewing the order and plan of care validates the correct patient and correct procedure. Preparation promotes efficient time management and an organized approach to the task.
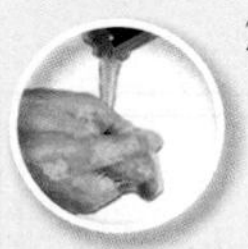 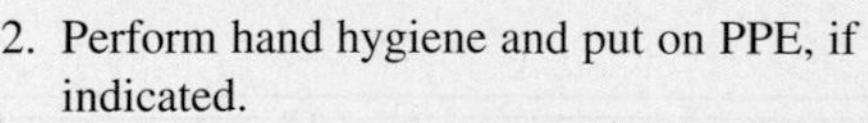 2. Perform hand hygiene and put on PPE, if indicated.	Hand hygiene and PPE prevent the spread of microorganisms. PPE is required based on transmission precautions.
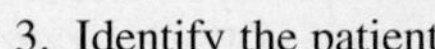 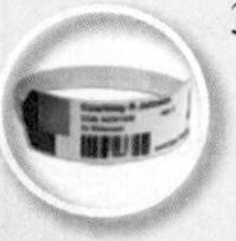 3. Identify the patient.	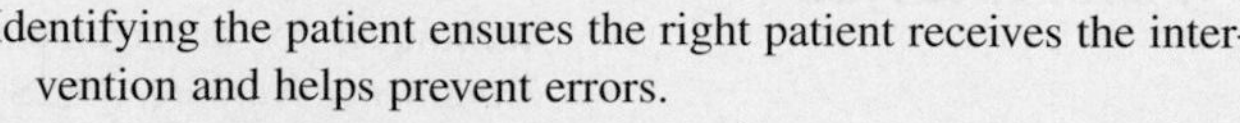 Identifying the patient ensures the right patient receives the intervention and helps prevent errors.

ACTION	RATIONALE
4. Assemble equipment on overbed table within reach.	Organization facilitates performance of the task.
5. Close the curtains around the bed and close the door to the room, if possible. Explain what you are going to do and why you are going to do it to the patient.	This ensures the patient's privacy. Explanation relieves anxiety and facilitates cooperation.
6. Assess the patient for possible need for nonpharmacologic pain-reducing interventions or analgesic medication before obtaining the wound culture. Administer appropriate prescribed analgesic. Allow enough time for the analgesic to achieve its effectiveness before beginning the procedure.	Pain is a subjective experience influenced by past experience. Wound care and dressing changes may cause pain for some patients.
7. Place an appropriate waste receptacle within easy reach for use during the procedure.	Having the waste container handy means that soiled materials may be discarded easily, without the spread of microorganisms.
8. Adjust bed to comfortable working height, usually elbow height of the caregiver (VISN 8, 2009).	Having the bed at the proper height prevents back and muscle strain.
9. Assist the patient to a comfortable position that provides easy access to the wound. If necessary, drape the patient with the bath blanket to expose only the wound area. Place a waterproof pad under the wound site. Check the culture label against the patient's identification bracelet (Figure 1).	Patient positioning and use of a bath blanket provide for comfort and warmth. Checking the culture label with the patient's identification ensures the correct patient and the correct procedure.

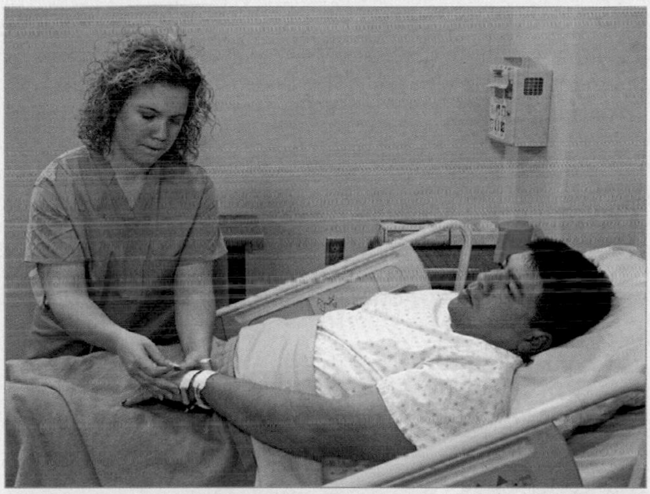

FIGURE 1 Checking culture label with the patient's identification band.

ACTION	RATIONALE
10. If there is a dressing in place on the wound, put on clean gloves. Carefully and gently remove the soiled dressings. If there is resistance, use a silicone-based adhesive remover to help remove the tape. If any part of the dressing sticks to the underlying skin, use small amounts of sterile saline to help loosen and remove it.	Gloves protect the nurse from handling contaminated dressings. Cautious removal of the dressing is more comfortable for the patient and ensures that any drain present is not removed. A silicone-based adhesive remover allows for the easy, rapid, and painless removal without the associated problems of skin stripping (Denyer, 2011; Benbow, 2011). Sterile saline moistens the dressing for easier removal and minimizes damage and pain.
11. After removing the dressing, note the presence, amount, type, color, and odor of any drainage on the dressings. Place soiled dressings in the appropriate waste receptacle.	The presence of drainage should be documented. Discarding dressings appropriately prevents the spread of microorganisms.

(continued)

SKILL 8-5 COLLECTING A WOUND CULTURE continued

ACTION	RATIONALE
12. Assess the wound for appearance, stage, presence of eschar, granulation tissue, epithelialization, undermining, tunneling, necrosis, sinus tract, and drainage. Assess the appearance of the surrounding tissue. Measure the wound. Refer to Fundamentals Review 8-3.	This information provides evidence about the wound healing process and/or the presence of infection.
13. Remove your gloves and put them in the receptacle.	Discarding gloves prevents the spread of microorganisms.
14. Set up a sterile field, if indicated, and wound cleaning supplies. Put on the sterile gloves. Alternately, clean gloves (clean technique) may be used when cleaning a chronic wound.	Sterile gloves maintain surgical asepsis. Clean technique is appropriate when cleaning chronic wounds.
15. Clean the wound. Refer to Skill 8-1. Alternately, irrigate the wound, as ordered or required (see Skill 8-4).	Cleaning the wound removes previous drainage and wound debris, which could introduce extraneous organisms into the collected specimen, resulting in inaccurate results.
16. Dry the surrounding skin with gauze dressings. Put on clean gloves.	Moisture provides a medium for growth of microorganisms. Excess moisture can contribute to skin irritation and breakdown. The use of a culture swab does not require immediate contact with the skin or wound, so clean gloves are appropriate to protect the nurse from contact with blood and/or body fluids.
17. Twist the cap to loosen the swab on the Culturette tube, or open the separate swab and remove the cap from the culture tube. **Keep the swab and inside of the culture tube sterile (Figure 2).**	Supplies are ready to use and within easy reach, and aseptic technique is maintained.
18. If contact with the wound is necessary to separate wound margins to permit insertion of the swab deep into the wound, put a sterile glove on one hand to manipulate the wound margins. Clean gloves may be appropriate for contact with pressure ulcers and chronic wounds.	If contact with the wound is necessary to collect the specimen, a sterile glove is necessary to prevent contamination of the wound.
19. **Carefully insert the swab into the wound. Press and rotate the swab several times over the wound surfaces. Avoid touching the swab to intact skin at the wound edges (Figure 3). Use another swab if collecting a specimen from another site.**	Cotton tip absorbs wound drainage. Contact with skin could introduce extraneous organisms into the collected specimen, resulting in inaccurate results. Using another swab at a different site prevents cross-contamination of the wound.

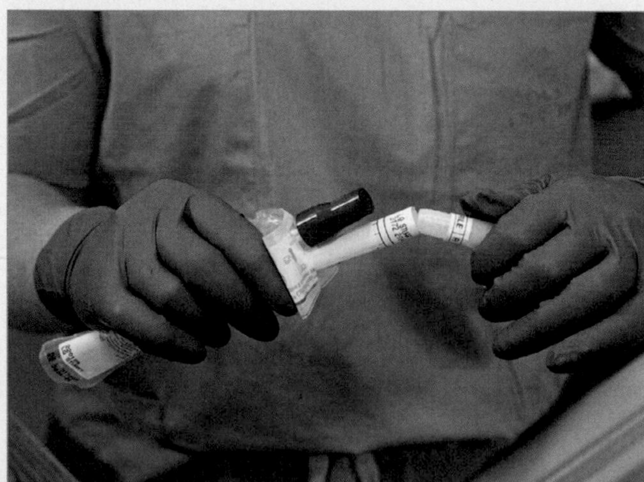

FIGURE 2 Removing cap from culture tube.

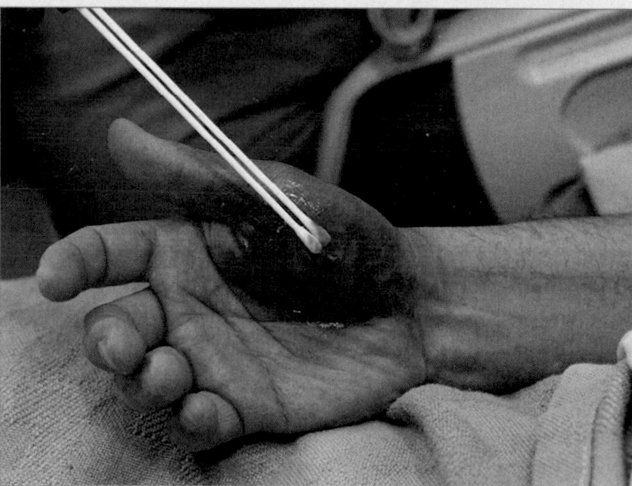

FIGURE 3 Rotating swab several times over wound surfaces.

ACTION	RATIONALE
20. Place the swab back in the culture tube (Figure 4). **Do not touch the outside of the tube with the swab.** Secure the cap. Some swab containers have an ampule of medium at the bottom of the tube. It might be necessary to crush this ampule to activate. Follow the manufacturer's instructions for use.	The outside of the container is protected from contamination with microorganisms, and the sample is not contaminated with organisms not in the wound. Surrounding the swab with culture medium is necessary for accurate culture results.
21. Remove gloves and discard them accordingly.	Removing gloves properly reduces the risk for infection transmission and contamination of other items.
22. Put on gloves. Place a dressing on the wound, as appropriate, based on medical orders and/or the nursing plan of care. Refer to Skills 8-1 through 8-3. Remove gloves.	Wound dressings protect, absorb drainage, provide a moist environment, and promote wound healing. Removing gloves properly reduces the risk for infection transmission and contamination of other items.
23. After securing the dressing, label dressing with date and time. Remove all remaining equipment; place the patient in a comfortable position, with side rails up and bed in the lowest position.	Recording date and time provides communication and demonstrates adherence to plan of care. Proper patient and bed positioning promotes safety and comfort.
24. Label the specimen according to your institution's guidelines and send it to the laboratory in a biohazard bag (Figure 5).	Proper labeling ensures proper identification of the specimen.

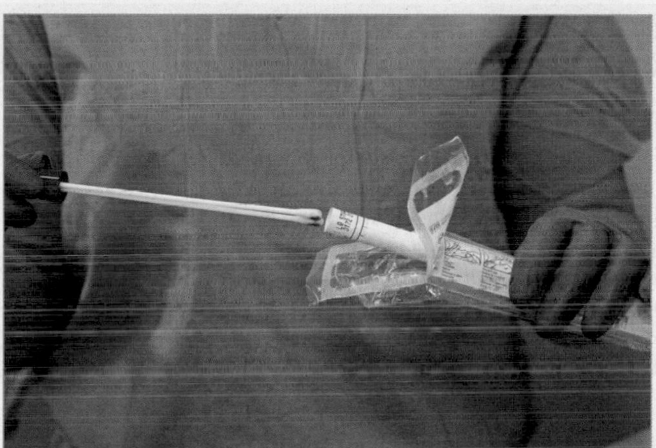

FIGURE 4 Placing swab in culture tube.

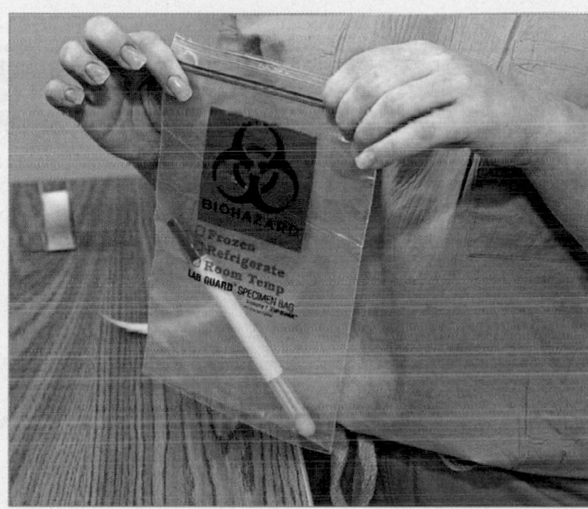

FIGURE 5 Labeled culture container in biohazard bag.

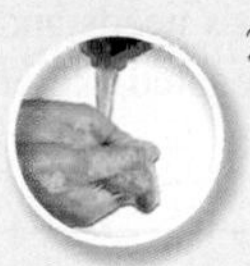

25. Remove PPE, if used. Perform hand hygiene.	Removing PPE properly reduces the risk for infection transmission and contamination of other items. Hand hygiene prevents the spread of microorganisms.

EVALUATION

The expected outcome is met when the patient's wound is cultured without evidence of contamination, and the patient remains free of exposure to additional pathogens.

DOCUMENTATION

Guidelines

Document the location of the wound, the assessment of the wound, including type of tissue present, presence of necrotic tissue, stage (if appropriate), and characteristics of drainage. Include the appearance of the surrounding skin. Document cleansing of the wound and obtaining the culture. Record any skin care and/or dressing applied. Note pertinent patient and family education and any patient reaction to this procedure, including patient's pain level and effectiveness of nonpharmacologic interventions or analgesia, if administered.

(continued)

SKILL 8-5 COLLECTING A WOUND CULTURE continued

Sample Documentation

6/22/15 2100 Wound noted on patient's hand; 2 cm × 3 cm × 1 cm, red, tender, with purulent drainage present. Edges macerated, without erythema and tenderness. Wound cleaned with normal saline, culture obtained. Skin barrier applied to surrounding area, wound packed with moist saline gauze, dressed with dry gauze and Kling. Hand elevated. Culture labeled and sent to lab.

—J. Wentz, RN

UNEXPECTED SITUATIONS AND ASSOCIATED INTERVENTIONS

- *The nurse has inserted the culture swab into the patient's wound to obtain the specimen and realizes that the wound was not cleaned:* Discard this swab. Obtain the additional supplies needed to clean the wound according to facility policy and a new culture swab. Cleaning the wound prior to obtaining a specimen for culture removes previous drainage, wound debris, and skin flora, which could introduce extraneous organisms into the specimen, resulting in inaccurate results. Clean the wound and then proceed to obtain the culture specimen.
- *As the nurse prepares to insert the culture swab into the wound, the nurse inadvertently touches the swab to the patient's bedclothes:* Discard this swab, obtain a new culture swab, and collect the specimen.

SKILL 8-6 APPLYING MONTGOMERY STRAPS

Montgomery straps are prepared strips of nonallergenic tape with ties inserted through holes at one end. One set of straps is placed on either side of a wound, and the straps are tied like shoelaces to secure the dressings. When it is time to change the dressing, the straps are untied, the wound is cared for, and then the straps are retied to hold the new dressing. Often a skin barrier is applied before the straps to protect the skin. The straps or ties need to be changed only if they become loose or soiled.

Montgomery straps are recommended to secure dressings on wounds that require frequent dressing changes, such as wounds with increased drainage. These straps allow the nurse to perform wound care without the need to remove adhesive strips, such as tape, with each dressing change, thus decreasing the risk of skin irritation and injury.

DELEGATION CONSIDERATIONS

Application of Montgomery Straps is not delegated to nursing assistive personnel (NAP) or to unlicensed assistive personnel (UAP). Depending on the state's nurse practice act and the organization's policies and procedures, this procedure may be delegated to licensed practical/vocational nurses (LPN/LVNs). The decision to delegate must be based on careful analysis of the patient's needs and circumstances, as well as the qualifications of the person to whom the task is being delegated. Refer to the Delegation Guidelines in Appendix A.

EQUIPMENT

- Clean, disposable gloves
- Additional PPE, as indicated
- Dressings for wound care, as ordered
- Commercially available Montgomery straps or 2- to 3-inch hypoallergenic tape and strings for ties
- Cleansing solution, usually normal saline
- Gauze pads
- Skin-protectant wipe
- Skin-barrier sheet (hydrocolloidal or nonhydrocolloidal)

ASSESSMENT

Assess the situation to determine the need for wound cleaning and a dressing change. Assess the integrity of any straps currently in use. Replace loose or soiled straps or ties. Confirm any medical orders relevant to wound care and any wound care included in the nursing plan of care. Assess the patient's level of comfort and the need for analgesics before wound care. Assess if the patient experienced any pain related to prior dressing changes and the effectiveness of interventions employed to minimize the patient's pain. Assess the current dressing to determine if it is intact. Assess for excess drainage or bleeding or saturation of the dressing. Inspect the wound and the surrounding tissue. Assess the appearance of the wound for the approximation of wound edges, the color of the wound and surrounding area, and signs of dehiscence. Assess for the presence of sutures, staples, or adhesive closure strips. Note the stage of the healing process and characteristics of any drainage. Also assess the surrounding skin for color, temperature, and edema, ecchymosis, or maceration.

NURSING DIAGNOSIS

Determine the related factors for the nursing diagnoses based on the patient's current health status. Appropriate nursing diagnoses may include:

- Impaired Skin Integrity
- Acute Pain
- Delayed Surgical Recovery
- Risk for Infection

OUTCOME IDENTIFICATION AND PLANNING

The expected outcome to achieve when applying Montgomery straps is that the patient's skin is free from irritation and injury. Other outcomes that may be appropriate include that the care is accomplished without contaminating the wound area, causing trauma to the wound, and/or causing the patient to experience pain or discomfort, and the wound continues to show signs of progression of healing.

IMPLEMENTATION

ACTION	RATIONALE
1. Review the medical orders for wound care or the nursing plan of care related to wound care. Gather necessary supplies.	Reviewing the order and plan of care validates the correct patient and correct procedure. Preparation promotes efficient time management and an organized approach to the task.
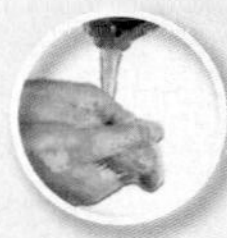 2. Perform hand hygiene and put on PPE, if indicated.	Hand hygiene and PPE prevent the spread of microorganisms. PPE is required based on transmission precautions.
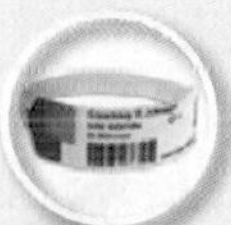 3. Identify the patient.	Identifying the patient ensures the right patient receives the intervention and helps prevent errors.
4. Assemble equipment on overbed table within reach.	Organization facilitates performance of the task.
5. Close the curtains around the bed and close the door to the room, if possible. Explain what you are going to do and why you are going to do it to the patient.	This ensures the patient's privacy. Explanation relieves anxiety and facilitates cooperation.
6. Assess the patient for possible need for nonpharmacologic pain-reducing interventions or analgesic medication before wound care dressing change. Administer appropriate prescribed analgesic. Allow enough time for the analgesic to achieve its effectiveness before beginning the procedure.	Pain is a subjective experience influenced by past experience. Wound care and dressing changes may cause pain for some patients.
7. Place a waste receptacle at a convenient location for use during the procedure.	Having a waste container handy means that the soiled dressing may be discarded easily, without the spread of microorganisms.
8. Adjust bed to comfortable working height, usually elbow height of the caregiver (VISN 8, 2009).	Having the bed at the proper height prevents back and muscle strain.
9. Assist the patient to a comfortable position that provides easy access to the wound area. Use a bath blanket to cover any exposed area other than the wound. Place a waterproof pad under the wound site.	Patient positioning and use of a bath blanket provide for comfort and warmth. Waterproof pad protects underlying surfaces.
10. Perform wound care and a dressing change as outlined in Skills 8-1 through 8-4, as ordered.	Wound care aids in healing and protects the wound.

(continued)

SKILL 8-6 APPLYING MONTGOMERY STRAPS continued

ACTION	RATIONALE
11. Put on clean gloves. Clean the skin on either side of the wound with the gauze, moistened with normal saline. Dry the skin.	Gloves prevent the spread of microorganisms. Cleaning and drying the skin prevents irritation and injury.
12. **Apply a skin protectant to the skin where the straps will be placed.**	Skin protectant minimizes the risk for skin breakdown and irritation.
13. Remove gloves.	Tape is easier to handle without gloves. Wound is covered with the dressing.
14. Cut the skin barrier to the size of the tape or strap. Apply the skin barrier to the patient's skin, near the dressing. Apply the sticky side of each tape or strap to the skin barrier sheet, so the openings for the strings are at the edge of the dressing (Figure 1). Repeat for the other side.	Skin barrier prevents skin irritation and breakdown.
15. Thread a separate string through each pair of holes in the straps, if not already in place. Tie one end of the string in the hole. Fasten the other end with the opposing tie, like a shoelace (Figure 2). **Do not secure too tightly.** Repeat according to the number of straps needed. If commercially prepared straps are used, tie strings like a shoelace. Note date and time of application on strap (Figure 3).	Ties hold the dressing in place. Tying too tightly puts additional stress on the surrounding skin. Recording date and time provides a baseline for changing straps.

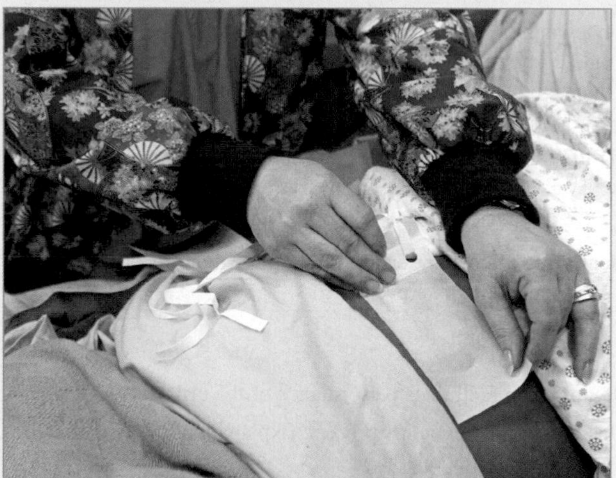

FIGURE 1 Applying Montgomery straps to skin barrier sheet on patient's abdomen.

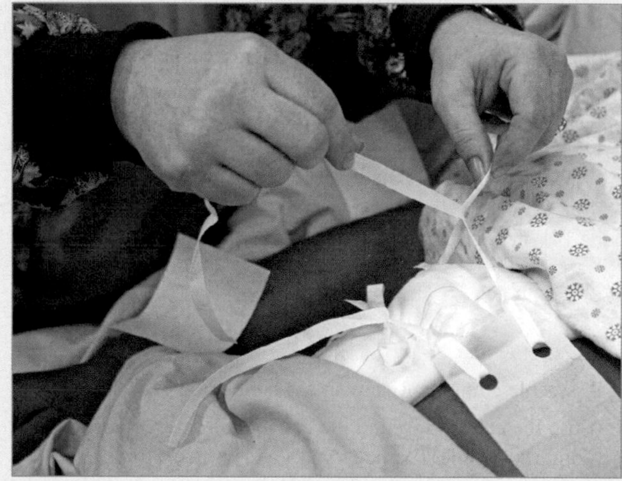

FIGURE 2 Tying Montgomery straps.

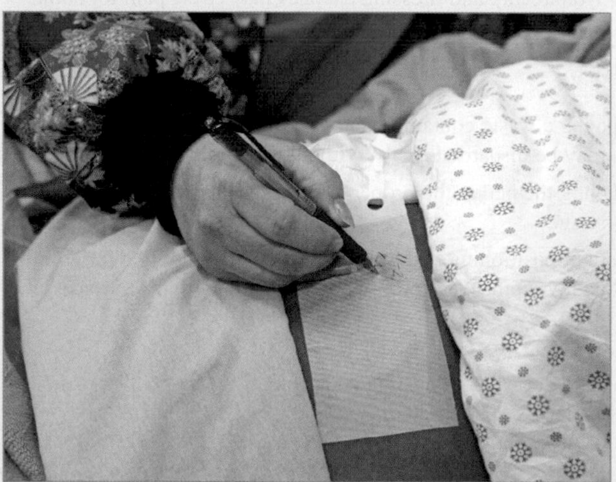

FIGURE 3 Labeling Montgomery straps.

ACTION	RATIONALE
16. After securing the dressing, label dressing with date and time. Remove all remaining equipment; place the patient in a comfortable position, with side rails up and bed in the lowest position.	Recording date and time provides communication and demonstrates adherence to plan of care. Proper patient and bed positioning promotes safety and comfort.
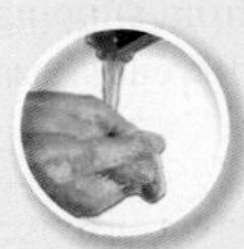 17. Remove additional PPE, if used. Perform hand hygiene.	Removing PPE properly reduces the risk for infection transmission and contamination of other items. Hand hygiene prevents the spread of microorganisms.
18. Check all wound dressings every shift. More frequent checks may be needed if the wound is more complex or dressings become saturated quickly.	Checking dressings ensures the assessment of changes in patient condition and timely intervention to prevent complications.
19. Replace the ties and straps whenever they are soiled, or every 2 to 3 days. Straps can be reapplied onto skin barrier. Skin barrier can remain in place up to 7 days. Use a silicone-based adhesive remover to help remove the skin barrier.	Replacing soiled ties and straps prevents growth of pathogens. Minimizing removal of skin barrier prevents skin irritation and breakdown. A silicone-based adhesive remover allows for the easy, rapid, and painless removal without the associated problems of skin stripping (Denyer, 2011; Benbow, 2011).

EVALUATION

The expected outcome when applying Montgomery straps is met when the patient's skin is clean, dry, intact, and free from irritation and injury. Other outcomes are met when the patient exhibits a clean wound area free of contamination and trauma. In addition, the patient verbalizes minimal to no pain or discomfort, and the patient exhibits signs and symptoms indicative of progressive wound healing.

DOCUMENTATION

Guidelines

Document the procedure, the patient's response, and your assessment of the area before and after application of Montgomery straps. Record a description of the wound, amount and character of the wound drainage, and an assessment of the surrounding skin. Note the type of dressing that was applied, including the application of skin protectant and a skin barrier. Document that Montgomery straps were applied to secure the dressings. Record the patient's response to the dressing care and associated pain assessment. Include any pertinent patient and family education.

Sample Documentation

10/20/15 1930 Patient's abdominal wound has large amounts of serosanguineous drainage, saturating multiple layers of gauze and ABDs, requiring dressing changes at least q3h. Surrounding skin cleansed, skin protectant applied, and Montgomery straps applied to secure wound dressings.

—D. Rightner, RN

UNEXPECTED SITUATION AND ASSOCIATED INTERVENTION

- *A patient has had an abdominal wound for several weeks. Despite careful wound and skin care, the nurse observes signs of redness and irritation where the tape for the dressings has been repeatedly placed:* Obtain the supplies listed in this skill. Apply Montgomery straps, being sure to move the skin barrier sheet at least 1 inch away from the area of irritation.

SKILL 8-7 CARING FOR A PENROSE DRAIN

Drains are inserted into or near a wound when it is anticipated that a collection of fluid in a closed area would delay healing. A Penrose drain is a hollow, open-ended rubber tube. It allows fluid to drain via capillary action into absorbent dressings. Penrose drains are commonly used after a surgical procedure or for drainage of an abscess. After a surgical procedure, the surgeon places one end of the drain in or near the area to be drained. The other end passes through the skin, directly through the incision or through a separate opening referred to as a stab wound. A Penrose drain is not sutured. A large safety pin is usually placed in the part outside the wound to prevent the drain from slipping back into the incised area. This type of drain can be advanced or shortened to drain different areas. The patency and placement of the drain are included in the wound assessment.

DELEGATION CONSIDERATIONS

Care for a Penrose drain insertion site and wound care is not delegated to nursing assistive personnel (NAP) or to unlicensed assistive personnel (UAP). Depending on the state's nurse practice act and the organization's policies and procedures, these procedures may be delegated to licensed practical/vocational nurses (LPN/LVNs). The decision to delegate must be based on careful analysis of the patient's needs and circumstances, as well as the qualifications of the person to whom the task is being delegated. Refer to the Delegation Guidelines in Appendix A.

EQUIPMENT

- Sterile gloves
- Gauze dressings
- Sterile cotton-tipped applicators, if appropriate
- Sterile drain sponges
- Surgical or abdominal pads
- Sterile dressing set or suture set (for the sterile scissors and forceps)
- Sterile cleaning solution as ordered (commonly 0.9% normal saline solution)
- Sterile container to hold cleaning solution
- Clean safety pin
- Clean, disposable gloves
- Plastic bag or other appropriate waste container for soiled dressings
- Waterproof pad and bath blanket
- Tape or ties
- Skin-protectant wipes, if needed
- Additional dressings and supplies needed or as required for ordered wound care

ASSESSMENT

Assess the situation to determine the necessity for wound cleaning and a dressing change. Confirm any medical orders relevant to drain care and any drain care included in the nursing plan of care. Assess the patient's level of comfort and the need for analgesics before wound care. Assess if the patient experienced any pain related to prior dressing changes and the effectiveness of interventions employed to minimize the patient's pain. Assess the current dressing to determine if it is intact, and assess for the presence of excess drainage, bleeding, or saturation of the dressing. Assess the patency of the Penrose drain.

Inspect the wound and the surrounding tissue. Assess the appearance of the wound for the approximation of wound edges, the color of the wound and surrounding area, and signs of dehiscence. Note the stage of the healing process and the characteristics of any drainage. Assess the surrounding skin for color, temperature, and the presence of edema, ecchymosis, or maceration.

NURSING DIAGNOSIS

Determine the related factors for the nursing diagnoses based on the patient's current health status. Appropriate nursing diagnoses may include:

- Risk for Infection
- Disturbed Body Image
- Deficient Knowledge

OUTCOME IDENTIFICATION AND PLANNING

The expected outcome to achieve when performing care for a Penrose drain is that the Penrose drain remains patent and intact; the care is accomplished without contaminating the wound area, or causing trauma to the wound, and without causing the patient to experience pain or discomfort. Other outcomes that are appropriate may include the following: the wound shows signs of progressive healing without evidence of complications, and the patient demonstrates an understanding of drain care.

IMPLEMENTATION

ACTION	RATIONALE
1. Review the medical orders for wound care or the nursing plan of care related to wound/drain care. Gather necessary supplies.	Reviewing the order and plan of care validates the correct patient and correct procedure. Preparation promotes efficient time management and an organized approach to the task.
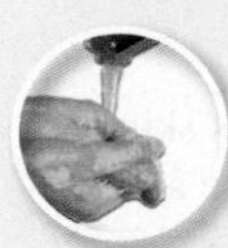 2. Perform hand hygiene and put on PPE, if indicated.	Hand hygiene and PPE prevent the spread of microorganisms. PPE is required based on transmission precautions.
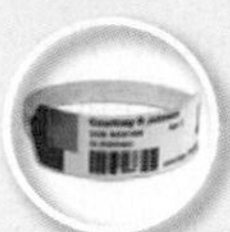 3. Identify the patient.	Identifying the patient ensures the right patient receives the intervention and helps prevent errors.
4. Assemble equipment on overbed table within reach.	Organization facilitates performance of the task.
5. Close the curtains around the bed and close the door to the room, if possible. Explain what you are going to do and why you are going to do it to the patient.	This ensures the patient's privacy. Explanation relieves anxiety and facilitates cooperation.
6. Assess the patient for possible need for nonpharmacologic pain-reducing interventions or analgesic medication before wound care dressing change. Administer appropriate prescribed analgesic. Allow enough time for the analgesic to achieve its effectiveness before beginning procedure.	Pain is a subjective experience influenced by past experience. Wound care and dressing changes may cause pain for some patients.
7. Place a waste receptacle at a convenient location for use during the procedure.	Having a waste container handy means that the soiled dressing may be discarded easily, without the spread of microorganisms.
8. Adjust bed to comfortable working height, usually elbow height of the caregiver (VISN 8, 2009).	Having the bed at the proper height prevents back and muscle strain.
9. Assist the patient to a comfortable position that provides easy access to the drain and/or wound area. Use a bath blanket to cover any exposed area other than the wound. Place a waterproof pad under the wound site.	Patient positioning and use of a bath blanket provide for comfort and warmth. Waterproof pad protects underlying surfaces.
10. Put on clean gloves. Check the position of the drain or drains before removing the dressing. Carefully and gently remove the soiled dressings. If there is resistance, use a silicone-based adhesive remover to help remove the tape. If any part of the dressing sticks to the underlying skin, use small amounts of sterile saline to help loosen and remove it.	Gloves protect the nurse from handling contaminated dressings. Checking the position ensures that a drain is not removed accidentally if one is present. Cautious removal of the dressing is more comfortable for the patient and ensures that any drain present is not removed. A silicone-based adhesive remover allows for the easy, rapid, and painless removal without the associated problems of skin stripping (Denyer, 2011; Benbow, 2011). Sterile saline moistens the dressing for easier removal and minimizes damage and pain.
11. After removing the dressing, note the presence, amount, type, color, and odor of any drainage on the dressings. Place soiled dressings in the appropriate waste receptacle.	The presence of drainage should be documented. Discarding dressings appropriately prevents the spread of microorganisms.
12. Inspect the drain site for appearance and drainage. Assess if any pain is present.	The wound healing process and/or the presence of irritation or infection must be documented.
13. Using sterile technique, prepare a sterile work area and open the needed supplies.	Supplies are within easy reach and sterility is maintained.
14. Open the sterile cleaning solution. Pour it into the basin. Add the gauze sponges.	Sterility of dressings and solution is maintained.
15. Put on sterile gloves.	Sterile gloves help to maintain surgical asepsis and sterile technique and prevent the spread of microorganisms.

(continued)

SKILL 8-7 CARING FOR A PENROSE DRAIN continued

ACTION	RATIONALE
16. Cleanse the drain site with the cleaning solution. Use the forceps and the moistened gauze or cotton-tipped applicators. **Start at the drain insertion site, moving in a circular motion toward the periphery (Figure 1). Use each gauze sponge or applicator only once.** Discard and use new gauze if additional cleansing is needed.	Using a circular motion ensures that cleaning occurs from the least to most contaminated area and a previously cleaned area is not contaminated again.
17. Dry the skin with a new gauze pad in the same manner. Apply skin protectant to the skin around the drain; extend out to include the area of skin that will be taped. Place a pre-split drain sponge under and around the drain (Figure 2). Closely observe the safety pin in the drain. If the pin or drain is crusted, replace the pin with a new sterile pin. **Take care not to dislodge the drain.**	Drying prevents skin irritation. Skin protectant prevents skin irritation and breakdown. The gauze absorbs drainage and prevents the drainage from accumulating on the patient's skin. Microorganisms grow more easily in a soiled environment. The safety pin ensures proper placement because the drain is not sutured in place.
18. Apply gauze pads over the drain (Figure 3). Apply ABD pads over the gauze.	The gauze absorbs drainage. Pads provide both extra absorption for excess drainage and a moisture barrier.

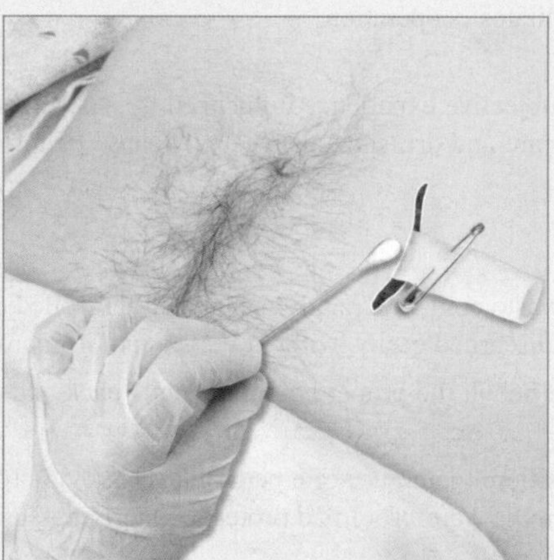

FIGURE 1 Cleaning drain site in circular motion toward periphery.

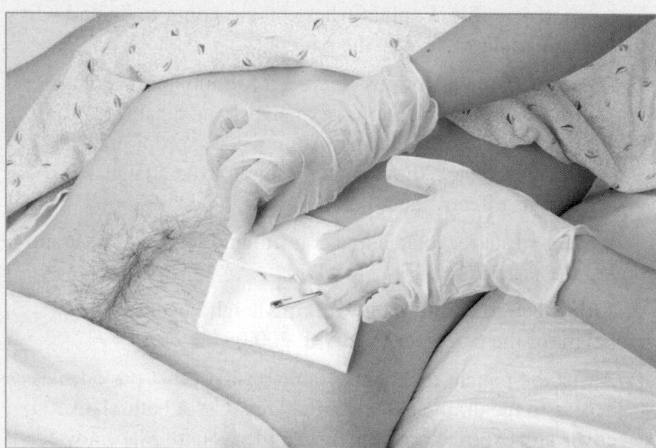

FIGURE 2 Placing pre-split dressing around Penrose drain.

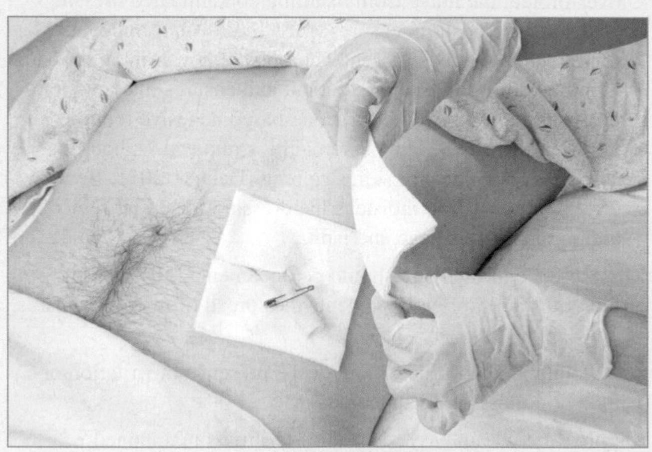

FIGURE 3 Applying gauze pads over drain.

ACTION	RATIONALE
19. Remove and discard gloves. Apply tape, Montgomery straps, or roller gauze to secure the dressings.	Proper disposal of gloves prevents the spread of microorganisms. Tape or other securing products are easier to apply after gloves have been removed.
20. After securing the dressing, label dressing with date and time. Remove all remaining equipment; place the patient in a comfortable position, with side rails up and bed in the lowest position.	Recording date and time provides communication and demonstrates adherence to plan of care. Proper patient and bed positioning promotes safety and comfort.

ACTION	RATIONALE
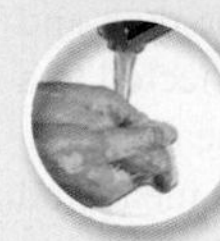 21. Remove additional PPE, if used. Perform hand hygiene.	Removing PPE properly reduces the risk for infection transmission and contamination of other items. Hand hygiene prevents the spread of microorganisms.
22. Check all wound dressings every shift. More frequent checks may be needed if the wound is more complex or dressings become saturated quickly.	Checking dressings ensures the assessment of changes in patient condition and timely intervention to prevent complications.

EVALUATION

The expected outcome is met when the patient exhibits a wound that is clean, dry, and intact, with a patent, intact Penrose drain. Other outcomes that are appropriate may include the following: the patient remains free of wound contamination and trauma; the patient reports minimal to no pain or discomfort; the patient exhibits signs and symptoms of progressive wound healing; and the patient verbalizes an understanding of the rationale for and/or the technique for drain care.

DOCUMENTATION

Guidelines

Document the location of the wound and drain, the assessment of the wound and drain site, and intactness of the Penrose drain. Document the presence of drainage and characteristics on the old dressing upon removal. Include the appearance of the surrounding skin. Document cleansing of the drain site. Record any skin care and the dressing applied. Note pertinent patient and family education and any patient reaction to this procedure, including patient's pain level and effectiveness of nonpharmacologic interventions or analgesia if administered.

Sample Documentation

3/13/15 1400 Patient medicated with morphine 3 mg IV, as ordered, prior to dressing change. Dressing to right forearm removed. Dressings noted with small amount of serosanguineous drainage. Forearm with gross edema and erythema. Penrose drain intact, with safety pin in place. Incision edges approximated, staples intact. Area irrigated with normal saline, dried, and redressed with gauze, ABD pads, and stretch gauze. Reinforced the importance of keeping arm elevated on pillows, with patient verbalizing understanding.

—*P. Towns, RN*

UNEXPECTED SITUATIONS AND ASSOCIATED INTERVENTIONS

- *Assessment of the drain site reveals significantly increased edema, erythema, and drainage from the site, in addition to drainage via the drain:* Cleanse the site, as ordered, or per the nursing plan of care. Obtain vital signs, including the patient's temperature. Document care and assessments. Notify the primary care provider of the findings.
- *Assessment of the drain site reveals that the drain has slipped back into the incision:* Follow facility policy and the medical orders related to advancing Penrose drains. Document assessments and interventions. Notify the primary care provider of the findings and interventions.
- *When preparing to change a dressing on a Penrose drain site, the nurse's assessment reveals that the drain is completely out, lying in the dressing material:* Assess the site and the patient for symptoms of pain, increased edema/erythema/drainage. Provide site care, as ordered. Notify the primary care provider. Often, depending on the patient's stage of recovery, the drain is left out. Document the findings and interventions.

SPECIAL CONSIDERATIONS

- Evaluate a sudden increase in the amount of drainage or bright red drainage and notify the primary care provider of these findings.
- Wound care is often uncomfortable, and patients may experience significant pain. Assess the patient's comfort level and past experiences with wound care. Offer analgesics, as ordered, to maintain the patient's level of comfort.

SKILL 8-8 CARING FOR A T-TUBE DRAIN

A biliary drain, or T-tube, (Figure 1) is sometimes placed in the common bile duct after removal of the gallbladder (cholecystectomy) or a portion of the bile duct (choledochostomy). The tube drains bile while the surgical site is healing. A portion of the tube is inserted into the common bile duct and the remaining portion is anchored to the abdominal wall, passed through the skin, and connected to a closed drainage system. Often, a three-way valve is inserted between the drain tube and the drainage system to allow for clamping and flushing of the tube, if necessary. The drainage amount is measured every shift, recorded, and included in output totals.

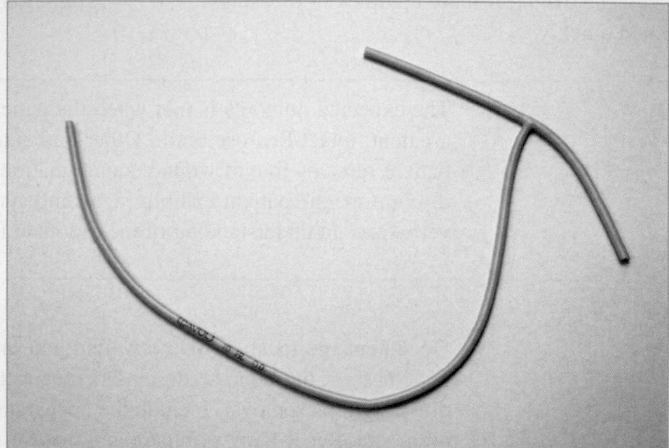

FIGURE 1 T-tube.

DELEGATION CONSIDERATIONS

Care for a T-tube drain insertion site is not delegated to nursing assistive personnel (NAP) or to unlicensed assistive personnel (UAP). Depending on the organization's policies and procedures, the drain may be emptied and reconstituted by nursing assistive personnel (NAP) or unlicensed assistive personnel (UAP). Depending on the state's nurse practice act and the organization's policies and procedures, these procedures may be delegated to licensed practical/vocational nurses (LPN/LVNs). The decision to delegate must be based on careful analysis of the patient's needs and circumstances, as well as the qualifications of the person to whom the task is being delegated. Refer to the Delegation Guidelines in Appendix A.

EQUIPMENT

- Sterile gloves
- Clean, disposable gloves
- Additional PPE, as indicated
- Sterile gauze pads
- Sterile drain sponges
- Cleansing solution, usually sterile normal saline
- Sterile cotton-tipped applicators (if appropriate)
- Transparent dressing
- Graduated collection container
- Waste receptacle
- Sterile basin
- Sterile forceps
- Tape
- Skin-protectant wipes
- Waterproof pad and bath blanket, if needed

ASSESSMENT

Assess the situation to determine the need for wound cleaning, a dressing change, or emptying of the drain. Confirm any medical orders relevant to drain care and any drain care included in the nursing plan of care. Assess the patient's level of comfort and the need for analgesics before wound care. Assess if the patient experienced any pain related to prior dressing changes and the effectiveness of interventions employed to minimize the patient's pain. Assess the current dressing to determine if it is intact, and assess for evidence of excessive drainage or bleeding or saturation of the dressing. Assess the patency of the T-tube and the drain site. Note the characteristics of the drainage in the collection bag.

Inspect the wound and the surrounding tissue. Assess the appearance of the incision for the approximation of wound edges, the color of the wound and surrounding area, and signs of dehiscence. Note the stage of the healing process and characteristics of any drainage. Assess the surrounding skin for color, temperature, and edema, ecchymosis, or maceration.

NURSING DIAGNOSIS

Determine the related factors for the nursing diagnoses based on the patient's current health status. Appropriate nursing diagnoses may include:

- Risk for Infection
- Deficient Knowledge
- Disturbed Body Image
- Impaired Skin Integrity

OUTCOME IDENTIFICATION AND PLANNING

The expected outcome to achieve when performing care for a T-tube drain is that the drain remains patent and intact; drain care is accomplished without contaminating the wound area and/or without causing trauma to the wound; and the patient does not experience pain or discomfort. Other outcomes that are appropriate may include the following: the wound continues to show signs of progression of healing; the drainage amounts are measured accurately at the frequency required by facility policy and recorded as part of the intake and output record; and the patient demonstrates an understanding of drain care.

IMPLEMENTATION

ACTION	RATIONALE
1. Review the medical orders for wound care or the nursing plan of care related to wound/drain care. Gather necessary supplies.	Reviewing the order and plan of care validates the correct patient and correct procedure. Preparation promotes efficient time management and an organized approach to the task.
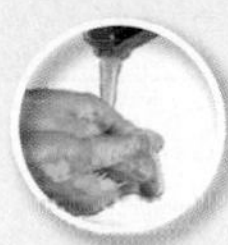 2. Perform hand hygiene and put on PPE, if indicated.	Hand hygiene and PPE prevent the spread of microorganisms. PPE is required based on transmission precautions.
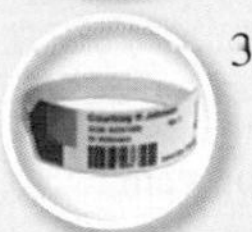 3. Identify the patient.	Identifying the patient ensures the right patient receives the intervention and helps prevent errors.
4. Assemble equipment on overbed table within reach.	Organization facilitates performance of the task.
5. Close the curtains around the bed and close the door to the room, if possible. Explain what you are going to do and why you are going to do it to the patient.	This ensures the patient's privacy. Explanation relieves anxiety and facilitates cooperation.
6. Assess the patient for possible need for nonpharmacologic pain-reducing interventions or analgesic medication before wound care dressing change. Administer appropriate prescribed analgesic. Allow enough time for the analgesic to achieve its effectiveness before beginning the procedure.	Pain is a subjective experience influenced by past experience. Wound care and dressing changes may cause pain for some patients.
7. Place a waste receptacle at a convenient location for use during the procedure.	Having a waste container handy means that the soiled dressing may be discarded easily, without the spread of microorganisms.
8. Adjust bed to comfortable working height, usually elbow height of the caregiver (VISN 8, 2009).	Having the bed at the proper height prevents back and muscle strain.
9. Assist the patient to a comfortable position that provides easy access to the drain and/or wound area. Use a bath blanket to cover any exposed area other than the wound. Place a waterproof pad under the wound site.	Patient positioning and use of a bath blanket provide for comfort and warmth. Waterproof pad protects underlying surfaces.
Emptying Drainage	
10. Put on clean gloves; put on mask or face shield, as indicated.	Gloves prevent the spread of microorganisms; mask reduces the risk of transmission should splashing occur.
11. Using sterile technique, open a gauze pad, making a sterile field with the outer wrapper.	Using sterile technique deters the spread of microorganisms.

(continued)

SKILL 8-8 CARING FOR A T-TUBE DRAIN continued

ACTION	RATIONALE
12. Place the graduated collection container under the outlet valve of the drainage bag. **Without touching the outlet, pull off the cap and empty the bag's contents completely into the container (Figure 2). Use the gauze to wipe the outlet, and replace the cap (Figure 3).**	Draining contents into a container allows for accurate measurement of the drainage. Touching the outlet with gloves or other surface contaminates the valve, potentially introducing pathogens. Wiping the outlet with gauze prevents contamination of the valve. Recapping prevents the spread of microorganisms.

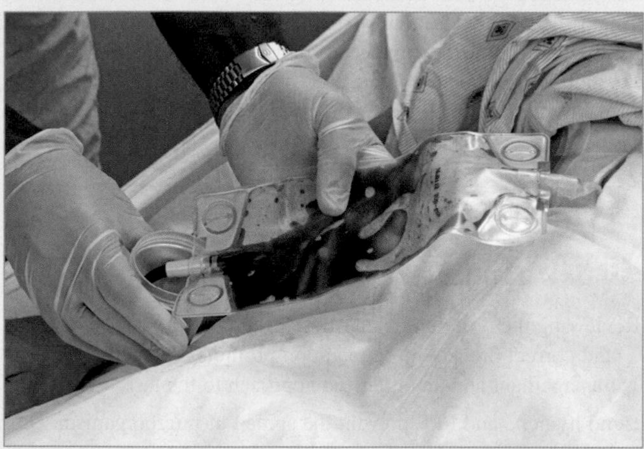

FIGURE 2 Emptying bag's contents into collection container.

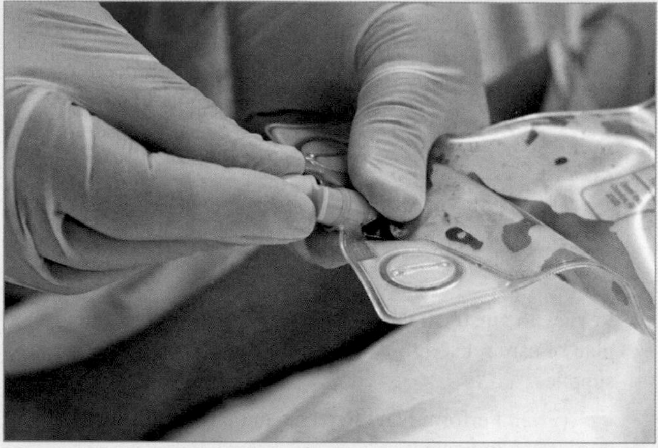

FIGURE 3 Replacing outlet cap.

ACTION	RATIONALE
14. Remove gloves and perform hand hygiene.	Proper glove removal and performing hand hygiene prevent spread of microorganisms.
ly measure and note the characteristics of the drainage. Discard the drainage according to facility policy.	Documentation promotes continuity of care and communication. Appropriate disposal of biohazard material reduces the risk for microorganism transmission.

Cleaning the Drain Site

ACTION	RATIONALE
15. Put on clean gloves. Check the position of the drain or drains before removing the dressing. Carefully and gently remove the soiled dressings. If there is resistance, use a silicone-based adhesive remover to help remove the tape. If any part of the dressing sticks to the underlying skin, use small amounts of sterile saline to help loosen and remove it. Do not reach over the drain site.	Gloves protect the nurse from handling contaminated dressings. Checking the position ensures that a drain is not removed accidentally if one is present. Cautious removal of the dressing is more comfortable for the patient and ensures that any drain present is not removed. A silicone-based adhesive remover allows for the easy, rapid, and painless removal without the associated problems of skin stripping (Denyer, 2011; Benbow, 2011). Sterile saline moistens the dressing for easier removal and minimizes damage and pain.
16. After removing the dressing, note the presence, amount, type, color, and odor of any drainage on the dressings. Place soiled dressings in the appropriate waste receptacle. Remove gloves and dispose of them in appropriate waste receptacle.	The presence of drainage should be documented. Proper disposal of gloves prevents spread of microorganisms.
17. Inspect the drain site for appearance and drainage. Assess if any pain is present.	Wound healing process and/or the presence of irritation or infection should be documented.
18. Using sterile technique, prepare a sterile work area and open the needed supplies.	Preparing a sterile work area ensures that supplies are within easy reach and sterility is maintained.
19. Open the sterile cleaning solution. Pour it into the basin. Add the gauze sponges.	Sterility of dressings and solution is maintained.
20. Put on sterile gloves.	Use of sterile gloves maintains surgical asepsis and sterile technique and reduces the risk of microorganism transmission.

ACTION	RATIONALE
21. Cleanse the drain site with the cleaning solution. Use the forceps and the moistened gauze or cotton-tipped applicators. **Start at the drain insertion site, moving in a circular motion toward the periphery. Use each gauze sponge only once.** Discard and use new gauze if additional cleansing is needed. (Refer to Figure 1 in Skill 8-7.)	Cleaning is done from the least to most contaminated area so that a previously cleaned area is not contaminated again.
22. Dry with new sterile gauze in the same manner. Apply skin protectant to the skin around the drain; extend out to include the area of skin that will be taped.	Drying prevents skin irritation. Skin protectant prevents skin irritation and breakdown.
23. Place a pre-split drain sponge under the drain. (Refer to Figure 2 in Skill 8-7.) Apply gauze pads over the drain. Remove and discard gloves.	The gauze absorbs drainage and prevents the drainage from accumulating on the patient's skin. Proper disposal of gloves prevents spread of microorganisms.
24. Secure the dressings with tape, as needed. Alternatively, before removing gloves, place a transparent dressing over the tube and insertion site. **Be careful not to kink the tubing.**	Kinked tubing could block drainage. Type of dressing used is often determined by facility policy.
25. After securing the dressing, label it with date and time. Remove all remaining equipment; place the patient in a comfortable position, with side rails up and bed in the lowest position.	Recording date and time provides communication and demonstrates adherence to plan of care. Proper patient and bed positioning promotes safety and comfort.
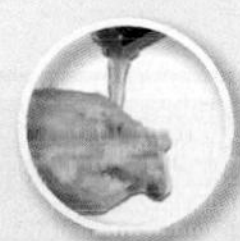 26. Remove additional PPE, if used. Perform hand hygiene.	Removing PPE properly reduces the risk for infection transmission and contamination of other items. Hand hygiene prevents the spread of microorganisms.
27. Check drain status at least every 4 hours. Check all wound dressings every shift. Perform more frequent checks if the wound is more complex or dressings become saturated quickly.	Checking drain ensures proper functioning and early detection of problems. Checking dressings ensures the assessment of changes in patient condition and timely intervention to prevent complications.

EVALUATION

The expected outcome is met when the patient exhibits a patent and intact T-tube drain with a wound area that is free of contamination and trauma. The patient verbalizes minimal to no pain or discomfort. Other outcomes that are appropriate may include the following: the patient exhibits signs and symptoms of progressive wound healing, with drainage being measured accurately at the frequency required by facility policy, and amounts recorded as part of the intake and output record; and the patient verbalizes an understanding of the rationale for and/or the technique for drain care.

DOCUMENTATION

Guidelines

Document the location of the wound and drain, the assessment of the wound and drain site, and patency of the drain. Note if sutures are intact. Document the presence and characteristics of drainage on the old dressing upon removal. Include the appearance of the surrounding skin. Document cleansing of the drain site. Record any skin care and the dressing applied. Note pertinent patient and family education and any patient reaction to this procedure, including patient's pain level and effectiveness of nonpharmacologic interventions or analgesia, if administered. Document the amount of bile drainage obtained from the drainage bag on the appropriate intake and output record.

Sample Documentation

<u>8/9/15</u> 1500 Dressing removed from T-tube site. No drainage noted on dressings. Drain site without redness, edema, drainage, or ecchymosis. Suture intact. Exit site cleaned with normal saline, dried, skin protectant applied, and redressed with dry dressing. Patient denies pain. Emptied collection bag of 20 mL bile-colored drainage.

—L. Saunders, RN

(continued)

SKILL 8-8 CARING FOR A T-TUBE DRAIN continued

UNEXPECTED SITUATIONS AND ASSOCIATED INTERVENTIONS

- *A patient's T-tube has been consistently draining 30 to 50 mL a shift, but now there is no output for the current shift. You check the tubing and site and do not observe kinks or other exterior obstructions:* Assess for signs of obstructed bile flow, including chills, fever, tachycardia, nausea, right upper quadrant fullness and pain, **jaundice**, dark foamy urine, and clay-colored stools. Obtain vital signs. Notify the primary care provider of the situation and findings and document the event in the patient's record. Flushing of the tube with sterile saline via the three-way valve may be ordered as part of the patient's care.
- *Patient had a T-tube placed after surgery. The surgeon has asked that the tube be clamped for 1 hour before and after meals:* This diverts bile into the duodenum to aid in digestion and is accomplished by turning the three-way access valve so the drain is closed to the drainage bag or occluding the tube with a clamp. Monitor the patient's response to clamping the tube. If the patient reports new symptoms, such as right upper quadrant pain, nausea, or vomiting, unclamp the tube. Assess for other symptoms and obtain vital signs. Report the findings to the surgeon and document the intervention in the patient's record.

SPECIAL CONSIDERATIONS

- When the patient with a drain is ready to ambulate, empty and compress the drain before activity. Secure the drain to the patient's gown below the wound, making sure there is no tension on the drainage tubing. This removes excess drainage, maintains maximum suction, and avoids strain on the drain's suture line.

SKILL 8-9 CARING FOR A JACKSON-PRATT DRAIN

A Jackson-Pratt (J-P) or grenade drain collects wound drainage in a bulblike device that is compressed to create gentle suction (Figure 1). It consists of perforated tubing connected to a portable vacuum unit. After a surgical procedure, the surgeon places one end of the drain in or near the area to be drained. The other end passes through the skin via a separate incision. These drains are usually sutured in place. The site may be treated as an additional surgical wound, but often these sites are left open to air 24 hours after surgery. They are typically used with breast and abdominal surgery.

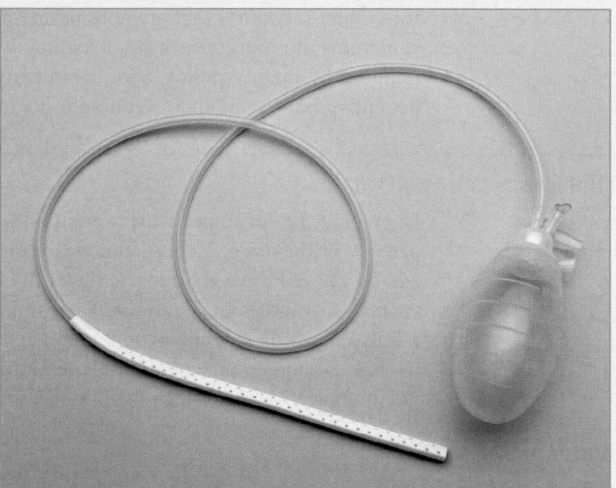

FIGURE 1 Jackson-Pratt drain.

As the drainage accumulates in the bulb, the bulb expands and suction is lost, requiring recompression. Typically, these drains are emptied every 4 to 8 hours, and when they are half full of drainage or air. However, based on nursing assessment and judgment, the drain could be emptied and recompressed more frequently.

DELEGATION GUIDELINES

Care for a Jackson-Pratt drain insertion site is not delegated to nursing assistive personnel (NAP) or to unlicensed assistive personnel (UAP). Depending on the organization's policies and procedures, the drain may be emptied and reconstituted by nursing assistive personnel (NAP) or unlicensed assistive personnel (UAP). Depending on the state's nurse practice act and the organization's policies and procedures, these procedures may be delegated to licensed practical/vocational nurses (LPN/LVNs). The decision to delegate must be based on careful analysis of the patient's needs and circumstances, as well as the qualifications of the person to whom the task is being delegated. Refer to the Delegation Guidelines in Appendix A.

EQUIPMENT

- Graduated container for measuring drainage
- Clean, disposable gloves
- Additional PPE, as indicated
- Cleansing solution, usually sterile normal saline
- Sterile gauze pads
- Skin-protectant wipes
- Dressing materials for site dressing, if used

ASSESSMENT

Assess the situation to determine the need for wound cleaning, a dressing change, or emptying of the drain. Assess the patient's level of comfort and the need for analgesics before wound care. Assess if the patient experienced any pain related to prior dressing changes and the effectiveness of interventions employed to minimize the patient's pain. Assess the current dressing. Assess for the presence of excess drainage or bleeding or saturation of the dressing. Assess the patency of the Jackson-Pratt drain and the drain site. Note the characteristics of the drainage in the collection bag.

Inspect the wound and the surrounding tissue. Assess the appearance of the incision for the approximation of wound edges, the color of the wound and surrounding area, and signs of dehiscence. Note the stage of the healing process and characteristics of any drainage. Also assess the surrounding skin for color, temperature, and edema, ecchymosis, or maceration.

NURSING DIAGNOSIS

Determine the related factors for the nursing diagnoses based on the patient's current health status. Appropriate nursing diagnoses may include:

- Risk for Infection
- Impaired Skin Integrity
- Disturbed Body Image
- Deficient Knowledge

OUTCOME IDENTIFICATION AND PLANNING

The expected outcome to achieve when performing care for a Jackson-Pratt drain is that the drain is patent and intact; drain care is accomplished without contaminating the wound area and/or without causing trauma to the wound; and the patient does not experience pain or discomfort. Other outcomes that are appropriate may include the following: the wound continues to show signs of progression of healing; the drainage amounts are measured accurately at the frequency required by facility policy and recorded as part of the intake and output record; and the patient demonstrates an understanding of drain care.

IMPLEMENTATION

ACTION	RATIONALE
1. Review the medical orders for wound care or the nursing plan of care related to wound/drain care. Gather necessary supplies.	Reviewing the order and plan of care validates the correct patient and correct procedure. Preparation promotes efficient time management and organized approach to the task.
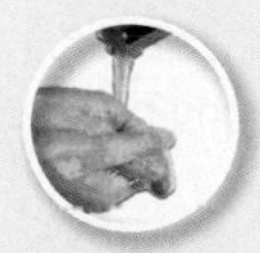 2. Perform hand hygiene and put on PPE, if indicated.	Hand hygiene and PPE prevent the spread of microorganisms. PPE is required based on transmission precautions.
 3. Identify the patient.	Identifying the patient ensures the right patient receives the intervention and helps prevent errors.

(continued)

SKILL 8-9 CARING FOR A JACKSON-PRATT DRAIN continued

ACTION	RATIONALE
4. Assemble equipment on overbed table within reach.	Organization facilitates performance of the task.
5. Close the curtains around the bed and close the door to the room, if possible. Explain what you are going to do and why you are going to do it to the patient.	This ensures the patient's privacy. Explanation relieves anxiety and facilitates cooperation.
6. Assess the patient for possible need for nonpharmacologic pain-reducing interventions or analgesic medication before wound care dressing change. Administer appropriate prescribed analgesic. Allow enough time for the analgesic to achieve its effectiveness before beginning the procedure.	Pain is a subjective experience influenced by past experience. Wound care and dressing changes may cause pain for some patients.
7. Place a waste receptacle at a convenient location for use during the procedure.	Having a waste container handy means that the soiled dressing may be discarded easily, without the spread of microorganisms.
8. Adjust bed to comfortable working height, usually elbow height of the caregiver (VISN 8, 2009).	Having the bed at the proper height prevents back and muscle strain.
9. Assist the patient to a comfortable position that provides easy access to the drain and/or wound area. Use a bath blanket to cover any exposed area other than the wound. Place a waterproof pad under the wound site.	Patient positioning and use of a bath blanket provide for comfort and warmth. Waterproof pad protects underlying surfaces.
10. Put on clean gloves; put on mask or face shield, as indicated.	Gloves prevent the spread of microorganisms; mask reduces the risk of transmission should splashing occur.
11. Place the graduated collection container under the drain outlet. Without contaminating the outlet valve, pull off the cap. The chamber will expand completely as it draws in air. **Empty the chamber's contents completely into the container (Figure 2). Use the gauze pad to clean the outlet. Fully compress the chamber with one hand and replace the cap with your other hand (Figure 3).**	Emptying the drainage allows for accurate measurement. Cleaning the outlet reduces the risk of contamination and helps prevent the spread of microorganisms. Compressing the chamber reestablishes the suction.

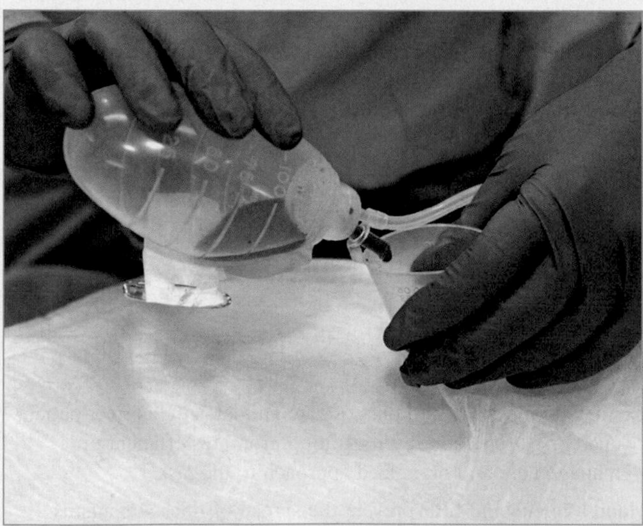

FIGURE 2 Emptying contents of Jackson-Pratt drain into collection container.

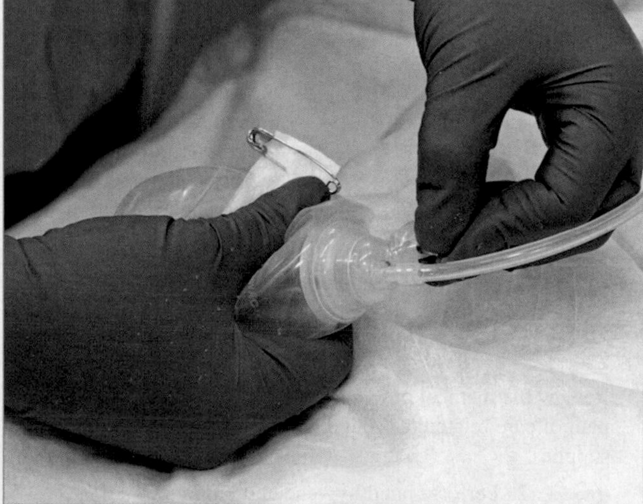

FIGURE 3 Compressing Jackson-Pratt drain and replacing cap.

ACTION	RATIONALE
12. Check the patency of the equipment. **Make sure the tubing is free from twists and kinks.**	Patent, untwisted, or unkinked tubing promotes appropriate wound drainage.
13. Secure the Jackson-Pratt drain to the patient's gown below the wound with a safety pin, **making sure that there is no tension on the tubing.**	Securing the drain prevents injury to the patient and accidental removal of the drain.

ACTION	RATIONALE
14. Carefully measure and record the character, color, and amount of the drainage. Discard the drainage according to facility policy. Remove gloves.	Documentation promotes continuity of care and communication. Appropriate disposal of biohazard material reduces the risk for microorganism transmission.
15. Put on clean gloves. If the drain site has a dressing, redress the site as outlined in Skill 8-1. Include cleaning of the sutures with the gauze pad moistened with normal saline. Dry sutures with gauze before applying new dressing.	Dressing protects the site. Cleaning and drying sutures deters growth of microorganisms.
16. If the drain site is open to air, observe the sutures that secure the drain to the skin. Look for signs of pulling, tearing, swelling, or infection of the surrounding skin. Gently clean the sutures with the gauze pad moistened with normal saline. Dry with a new gauze pad. Apply skin protectant to the surrounding skin, if needed.	Early detection of problems leads to prompt intervention and prevents complications. Gentle cleaning and drying prevent the growth of microorganisms. Skin protectant prevents skin irritation and breakdown.
17. Remove and discard gloves. Remove all remaining equipment; place the patient in a comfortable position, with side rails up and bed in the lowest position.	Proper removal of gloves prevents spread of microorganisms. Proper patient and bed positioning promotes safety and comfort.
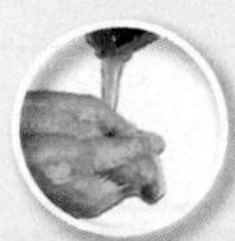 18. Remove additional PPE, if used. Perform hand hygiene.	Removing PPE properly reduces the risk for infection transmission and contamination of other items. Hand hygiene prevents the spread of microorganisms.
19. Check drain status at least every 4 hours. Check all wound dressings every shift. Perform more frequent checks if the wound is more complex or dressings become saturated quickly.	Checking drain ensures proper functioning and early detection of problems. Checking dressings ensures the assessment of changes in patient condition and timely intervention to prevent complications.

EVALUATION

The expected outcome is met when the patient exhibits a patent and intact Jackson-Pratt drain with a wound area that is free of contamination and trauma. The patient verbalizes minimal to no pain or discomfort. Other outcomes that are appropriate may include the following: the patient exhibits signs and symptoms of progressive wound healing, with drainage being measured accurately at the frequency required by facility policy, and amounts recorded as part of the intake and output record; and the patient verbalizes an understanding of the rationale for and/or the technique for drain care.

DOCUMENTATION

Guidelines

Document the location of the wound and drain, the assessment of the wound and drain site, and patency of the drain. Note if sutures are intact. Document the presence and characteristics of drainage on the old dressing upon removal. Include the appearance of the surrounding skin. Document cleansing the drain site. Record any skin care and the dressing applied. Note that the drain was emptied and recompressed. Note pertinent patient and family education and any patient reaction to this procedure, including patient's pain level and effectiveness of nonpharmacologic interventions or analgesia, if administered. Document the amount and characteristics of drainage obtained on the appropriate intake and output record.

Sample Documentation

2/7/15 2400 Right chest incision and drain open to air. Wound edges approximated, slight ecchymosis, no edema, redness, or drainage. Steri-Strips intact. J-P drain patent and secured with suture. Exit site without edema, drainage, or redness. Drain emptied and recompressed. 40 mL sanguineous drainage recorded.

—*Carol White, RN*

UNEXPECTED SITUATIONS AND ASSOCIATED INTERVENTIONS

- *A patient has a Jackson-Pratt drain in the right lower quadrant following abdominal surgery. The record indicates it has been draining serosanguineous fluid, 40 to 50 mL every shift. While performing your initial assessment, you note that the dressing around the drain site is saturated with serosanguineous secretions and there is minimal drainage in the collection chamber:*

(continued)

SKILL 8-9 CARING FOR A JACKSON-PRATT DRAIN continued

Inspect the tubing for kinks or obstruction. Assess the patient for changes in condition. Remove the dressing and assess the site. Often, if the tubing becomes blocked with a blood clot or drainage particles, the wound drainage will leak around the exit site of the drain. Cleanse the area and redress the site. Notify the primary care provider of the findings and document the event in the patient's record.

- *Your patient calls you to the room and says, "I found this in the bed when I went to get up." He has his Jackson-Pratt drain in his hand. It is completely removed from the patient:* Assess the patient for any new and abnormal signs or symptoms, and assess the surgical site and drain site. Apply a sterile dressing with gauze and tape to the drain site. Notify the primary care provider of the findings and document the event in the patient's record.

SPECIAL CONSIDERATIONS

- Often patients have more than one Jackson-Pratt drain. Number or letter the drains for easy identification. Record the drainage from each drain separately, identified by the number or letter, on the intake and output record.
- When the patient with a drain is ready to ambulate, empty and compress the drain before activity. Secure the drain to the patient's gown below the wound, making sure there is no tension on the drainage tubing. This removes excess drainage, maintains maximum suction, and avoids strain on the drain's suture line.

SKILL 8-10 CARING FOR A HEMOVAC DRAIN

A Hemovac drain is placed into a vascular cavity where blood drainage is expected after surgery, such as with abdominal and orthopedic surgery. The drain consists of perforated tubing connected to a portable vacuum unit (Figure 1). Suction is maintained by compressing a spring-like device in the collection unit. After a surgical procedure, the surgeon places one end of the drain in or near the area to be drained. The other end passes through the skin via a separate incision. These drains are usually sutured in place. The site may be treated as an additional surgical wound, but often these sites are left open to air 24 hours after surgery.

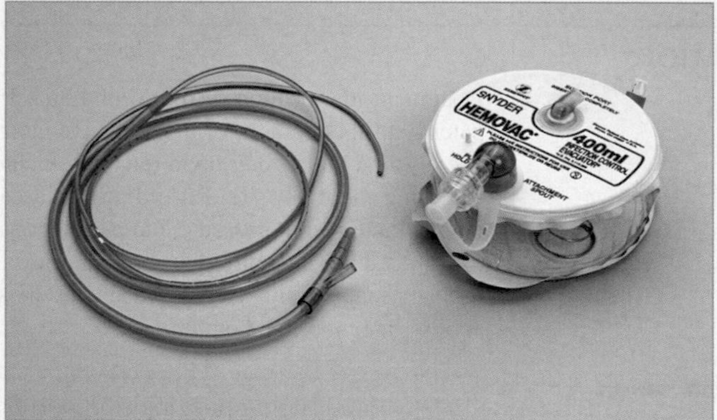

FIGURE 1 Hemovac drain.

As the drainage accumulates in the collection unit, it expands and suction is lost, requiring recompression. Typically, the drain is emptied every 4 or 8 hours and when it is half full of drainage or air. However, based on the medical orders and nursing assessment and judgment, it could be emptied and recompressed more frequently.

DELEGATION GUIDELINES

Care for a Hemovac drain insertion site is not delegated to nursing assistive personnel (NAP) or to unlicensed assistive personnel (UAP). Depending on the organization's policies and procedures, the drain may be emptied and reconstituted by nursing assistive personnel (NAP) or to unlicensed assistive personnel (UAP). Depending on the state's nurse practice act and the organization's policies and procedures, these procedures may be delegated to licensed practical/vocational nurses (LPN/LVNs). The decision to delegate must be based on careful analysis of the patient's needs and circumstances, as well as the qualifications of the person to whom the task is being delegated. Refer to the Delegation Guidelines in Appendix A.

EQUIPMENT

- Graduated container for measuring drainage
- Clean, disposable gloves
- Additional PPE, as indicated
- Cleansing solution, usually sterile normal saline
- Sterile gauze pads
- Skin-protectant wipes
- Dressing materials for site dressing, if used

ASSESSMENT

Assess the situation to determine the need for wound cleaning, a dressing change, or emptying of the drain. Assess the patient's level of comfort and the need for analgesics before wound care. Assess if the patient experienced any pain related to prior dressing changes and the effectiveness of interventions employed to minimize the patient's pain. Assess the current dressing. Assess for the presence of excess drainage or bleeding or saturation of the dressing. Assess the patency of the Hemovac drain and the drain site. Note the characteristics of the drainage in the collection bag.

Inspect the wound and the surrounding tissue. Assess the appearance of the incision for the approximation of wound edges, the color of the wound and surrounding area, and signs of dehiscence. Note the stage of the healing process and characteristics of any drainage. Also assess the surrounding skin for color, temperature, and edema, ecchymosis, or maceration.

NURSING DIAGNOSIS

Determine the related factors for the nursing diagnoses based on the patient's current health status. Appropriate nursing diagnoses may include:

- Risk for Infection
- Disturbed Body Image
- Impaired Skin Integrity
- Deficient Knowledge

OUTCOME IDENTIFICATION AND PLANNING

The expected outcome to achieve when performing care for a Hemovac drain is that the drain is patent and intact; drain care is accomplished without contaminating the wound area and/or without causing trauma to the wound; and the patient does not experience pain or discomfort. Other outcomes that are appropriate may include the following: the wound continues to show signs of progression of healing; the drainage amounts are measured accurately at the frequency required by facility policy and recorded as part of the intake and output record; and the patient demonstrates an understanding of drain care.

IMPLEMENTATION

ACTION	RATIONALE
1. Review the medical orders for wound care or the nursing plan of care related to wound/drain care. Gather necessary supplies.	Reviewing the order and plan of care validates the correct patient and correct procedure. Preparation promotes efficient time management and an organized approach to the task.
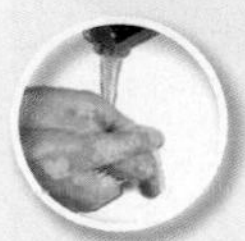 2. Perform hand hygiene and put on PPE, if indicated.	Hand hygiene and PPE prevent the spread of microorganisms. PPE is required based on transmission precautions.
3. Identify the patient.	Identifying the patient ensures the right patient receives the intervention and helps prevent errors.

(continued)

SKILL 8-10 CARING FOR A HEMOVAC DRAIN continued

ACTION	RATIONALE
4. Assemble equipment on overbed table within reach.	Organization facilitates performance of the task.
5. Close the curtains around the bed and close the door to the room, if possible. Explain what you are going to do and why you are going to do it to the patient.	This ensures the patient's privacy. Explanation relieves anxiety and facilitates cooperation.
6. Assess the patient for possible need for nonpharmacologic pain-reducing interventions or analgesic medication before wound care dressing change. Administer appropriate prescribed analgesic. Allow enough time for analgesic to achieve its effectiveness before beginning the procedure.	Pain is a subjective experience influenced by past experience. Wound care and dressing changes may cause pain for some patients.
7. Place a waste receptacle at a convenient location for use during the procedure.	Having a waste container handy means that the soiled dressing may be discarded easily, without the spread of microorganisms.
8. Adjust bed to comfortable working height, usually elbow height of the caregiver (VISN 8, 2009).	Having the bed at the proper height prevents back and muscle strain.
9. Assist the patient to a comfortable position that provides easy access to the drain and/or wound area. Use a bath blanket to cover any exposed area other than the wound. Place a waterproof pad under the wound site.	Patient positioning and use of a bath blanket provide for comfort and warmth. Waterproof pad protects underlying surfaces.
10. Put on clean gloves; put on mask or face shield, as indicated.	Gloves prevent the spread of microorganisms; mask reduces the risk of transmission should splashing occur.
11. Place the graduated collection container under the drain outlet. **Without contaminating the outlet, pull off the cap.** The chamber will expand completely as it draws in air. **Empty the chamber's contents completely into the container (Figure 2). Use the gauze pad to clean the outlet. Fully compress the chamber by pushing the top and bottom together with your hands. Keep the device tightly compressed while you apply the cap (Figure 3).**	Emptying the drainage allows for accurate measurement. Cleaning the outlet reduces the risk of contamination and helps prevent the spread of microorganisms. Compressing the chamber reestablishes the suction.

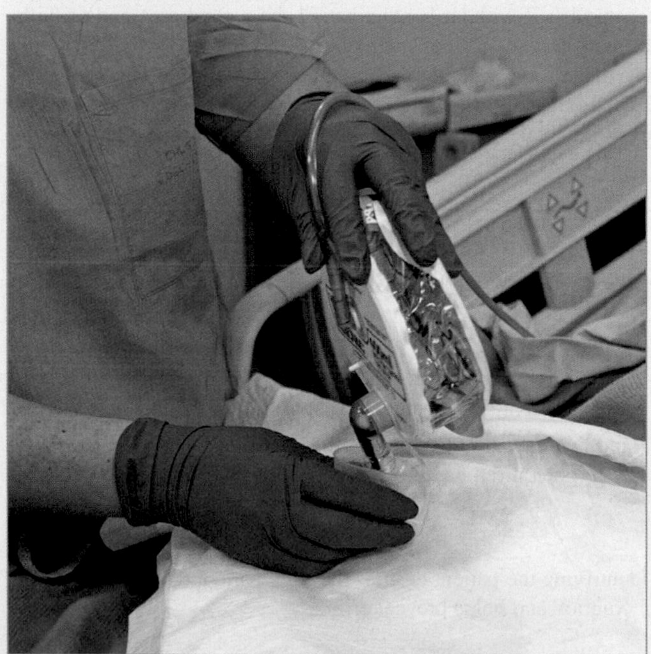
FIGURE 2 Emptying Hemovac drain into collection container.

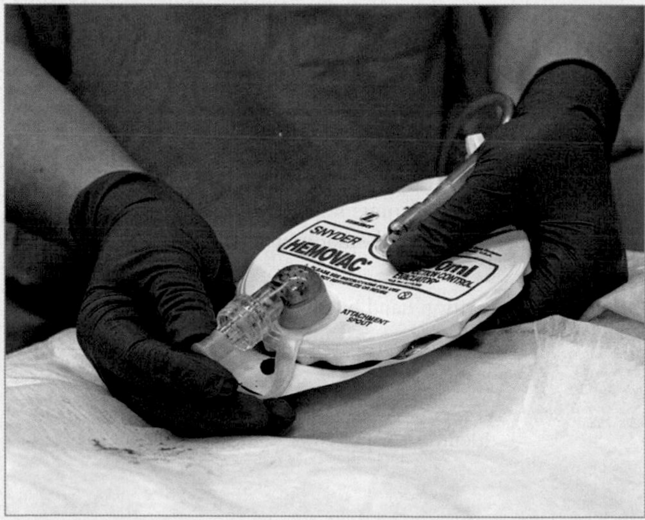

FIGURE 3 Compressing Hemovac and securing cap.

ACTION	RATIONALE
12. Check the patency of the equipment. **Make sure the tubing is free from twists and kinks.**	Patent, untwisted, or unkinked tubing promotes appropriate drainage from wound.
13. Secure the Hemovac drain to the patient's gown below the wound with a safety pin, **making sure that there is no tension on the tubing.**	Securing the drain prevents injury to the patient and accidental removal of the drain.
14. Carefully measure and record the character, color, and amount of the drainage. Discard the drainage according to facility policy.	Documentation promotes continuity of care and communication. Appropriate disposal of biohazard material reduces the risk for microorganism transmission. Proper disposal of gloves deters transmission of microorganisms.
15. Put on clean gloves. If the drain site has a dressing, redress the site as outlined in Skill 8-1. Include cleaning of the sutures with the gauze pad moistened with normal saline. Dry sutures with gauze before applying new dressing.	Dressing protects the site. Cleaning and drying sutures deters growth of microorganisms.
16. If the drain site is open to air, observe the sutures that secure the drain to the skin. Look for signs of pulling, tearing, swelling, or infection of the surrounding skin. Gently clean the sutures with the gauze pad moistened with normal saline. Dry with a new gauze pad. Apply skin protectant to the surrounding skin, if needed.	Early detection of problems leads to prompt intervention and prevents complications. Gentle cleaning and drying prevent the growth of microorganisms. Skin protectant prevents skin irritation and breakdown.
17. Remove and discard gloves. Remove all remaining equipment; place the patient in a comfortable position, with side rails up and bed in the lowest position.	Proper removal and disposal of gloves prevents spread of microorganisms. Proper patient and bed positioning promotes safety and comfort.
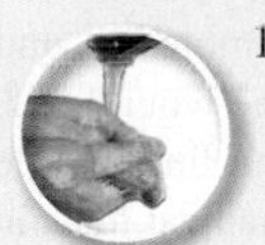 18. Remove additional PPE, if used. Perform hand hygiene.	Removing PPE properly reduces the risk for infection transmission and contamination of other items. Hand hygiene prevents the spread of microorganisms.
19. Check drain status at least every 4 hours. Check all wound dressings every shift. More frequent checks may be needed if the wound is more complex or dressings become saturated quickly.	Checking drain ensures proper functioning and early detection of problems. Checking dressings ensures the assessment of changes in patient condition and timely intervention to prevent complications.

EVALUATION

The expected outcome is met when the patient exhibits a patent and intact Hemovac drain with a wound area that is free of contamination and trauma. The patient verbalizes minimal to no pain or discomfort. Other outcomes that are appropriate may include the following: the patient exhibits signs and symptoms of progressive wound healing, with drainage being measured accurately at the frequency required by facility policy, and amounts recorded as part of the intake and output record; and the patient verbalizes an understanding of the rationale for and/or the technique for drain care.

DOCUMENTATION

Guidelines

Document the location of the wound and drain, the assessment of the wound and drain site, and patency of the drain. Note if sutures are intact. Document the presence and characteristics of drainage on the old dressing upon removal. Include the appearance of the surrounding skin. Document cleansing of the drain site. Record any skin care and any dressing applied. Note that the drain was emptied and recompressed. Note pertinent patient and family education and any patient reaction to this procedure, including patient's pain level and effectiveness of nonpharmacologic interventions or analgesia, if administered. Document the amount and characteristics of drainage obtained on the appropriate intake and output record.

Sample Documentation

1/18/15 1000 Hemovac drain in place in left lower extremity, site open to air. Suture intact; exit site slightly pink, without redness, edema, or drainage. Surrounding skin without edema, ecchymosis, or redness. Exit site and suture cleansed with normal saline. Hemovac emptied of 90 mL sanguineous secretions and recompressed.

—*A. Smith, RN*

(continued)

SKILL 8-10 CARING FOR A HEMOVAC DRAIN continued

UNEXPECTED SITUATIONS AND ASSOCIATED INTERVENTIONS

- *A patient has a Hemovac drain placed in the left knee following surgery. The record indicates it has been draining serosanguineous secretions, 40 to 50 mL, every shift. While performing your initial assessment, you note that the collection chamber is completely expanded. The nurse empties the device and compresses to resume suction. A short time later, the nurse observes that the chamber is completely expanded again:* Inspect the tubing for kinks or obstruction. Inspect the device, looking for breaks in the integrity of the chamber. Make sure the cap is in place and closed. Assess the patient for changes in condition. Remove the dressing and assess the site. Make sure the drainage tubing has not advanced out of the wound, exposing any of the perforations in the tubing. If you are not successful in maintaining the suction, notify the primary care provider of the findings and interventions and document the event in the patient's record.

SPECIAL CONSIDERATIONS

- When the patient with a drain is ready to ambulate, empty and compress the drain before activity. Secure the drain to the patient's gown below the wound, making sure there is no tension on the drainage tubing. This removes excess drainage, maintains maximum suction, and avoids strain on the drain's suture line.

SKILL 8-11 APPLYING NEGATIVE-PRESSURE WOUND THERAPY

Negative-pressure wound therapy (NPWT) (or topical negative pressure [TNP]) promotes wound healing and wound closure through the application of uniform negative pressure on the wound bed. NPWT results in reduction in bacteria in the wound and the removal of excess wound fluid, while providing a moist wound healing environment. The negative pressure results in mechanical tension on the wound tissues, stimulating cell proliferation, blood flow to wounds, and the growth of new blood vessels. An open-cell foam dressing or gauze is applied in the wound. A fenestrated tube is connected to the foam, allowing the application of the negative pressure. The dressing and distal tubing are covered by a transparent, occlusive, air-permeable dressing that provides a seal, allowing the application of the negative pressure. Excess wound fluid is removed through tubing into a collection container. NPWT also acts to pull the wound edges together. Refer to Figure 1 for an example of the components of a NPWT system.

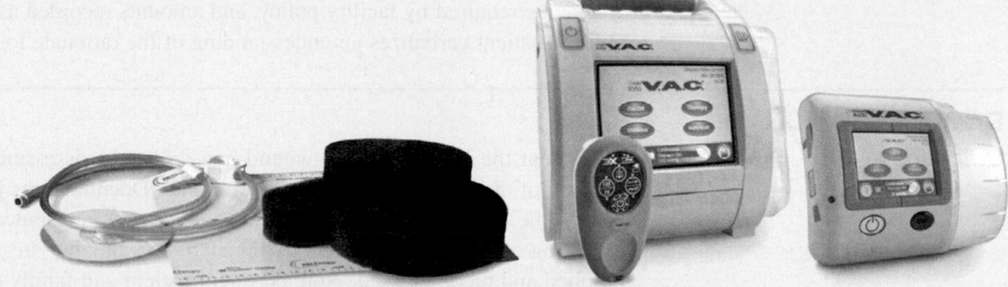

FIGURE 1 Example of components of a NPWT system. (From Hess, C. (2013). *Clinical guide to skin & wound care* (7th ed.). Philadelphia: Wolters Kluwer Health/Lippincott Williams & Wilkins, p. 482 and 484.)

NPWT is used to treat a variety of acute or chronic wounds, wounds with heavy drainage, wounds failing to heal, or wounds healing slowly. Examples of such wounds include pressure ulcers; arterial, venous, and diabetic ulcers; dehisced surgical wounds; infected wounds; skin graft sites; and burns. NPWT is not considered for use in the presence of active bleeding; wounds with exposed blood vessels, organs, or nerves; malignancy in wound tissue; presence of dry/necrotic tissue; or with fistulas of unknown origin (Hess, 2013; Martindell, 2012; Preston, 2008; Thompson, 2008).

Cautious use is indicated in the presence of unrelieved pressure, anticoagulant therapy, poor nutritional status, and immunosuppressant therapy (Martindell, 2012; Preston, 2008). Candidates must be assessed for preexisting bleeding disorders, use of anticoagulants and other medications, or use of supplements that prolong bleeding times, such as aspirin or ginkgo biloba (Malli, 2005; Preston, 2008). NPWT dressings are changed every 48 to 72 hours, depending on the manufacturer's specifications and medical orders. Infected wounds may require dressing changes every 12 to 24 hours. The following Skill outlines the procedure for vacuum-assisted closure (V.A.C.) therapy (KCl), as an example of NPWT. There are many manufacturers of negative pressure wound therapy systems. **The nurse should be familiar with the components of, and procedures related to, the particular system in use for an individual patient.**

DELEGATION CONSIDERATIONS

The application of negative-pressure wound therapy is not delegated to nursing assistive personnel (NAP) or to unlicensed assistive personnel (UAP). Depending on the state's nurse practice act and the organization's policies and procedures, the application of negative–pressure wound therapy may be delegated to licensed practical/vocational nurses (LPN/LVNs). The decision to delegate must be based on careful analysis of the patient's needs and circumstances, as well as the qualifications of the person to whom the task is being delegated. Refer to the Delegation Guidelines in Appendix A.

EQUIPMENT

- Negative pressure unit (V.A.C. ATS Unit)
- Evacuation/collection canister
- V.A.C. Foam dressing
- V.A.C. Drape
- T.R.A.C. Pad
- Skin-protectant wipes
- Sterile gauze sponge
- Sterile irrigation set, including a basin, irrigant container, and irrigation syringe
- Sterile irrigation solution as ordered, warmed to body temperature
- Waste receptacle to dispose of contaminated materials
- Sterile gloves (2 pairs)
- Sterile scissors
- Clean, disposable gloves
- Gown, mask, eye protection
- Additional PPE, as indicated
- Sterile scissors
- Waterproof pad and bath blanket

ASSESSMENT

Confirm the medical order for the application of NPWT. Check the patient's chart and question the patient about current treatments and medications that may make the application contraindicated. Assess the situation to determine the need for a dressing change. Confirm any medical orders relevant to wound care and any wound care included in the nursing plan of care. Assess the patient's level of comfort and the need for analgesics before wound care. Assess if the patient experienced any pain related to prior dressing changes and the effectiveness of interventions employed to minimize the patient's pain. Assess the current dressing to determine if it is intact. Assess for excess drainage or bleeding or saturation of the dressing. Inspect the wound and the surrounding tissue. Assess the location, appearance of the wound, stage (if appropriate), drainage, and types of tissue present in the wound. Measure the wound. Note the stage of the healing process and characteristics of any drainage. Also assess the surrounding skin for color, temperature, and edema, ecchymosis, or maceration.

NURSING DIAGNOSIS

Determine the related factors for the nursing diagnoses based on the patient's current status. An appropriate nursing diagnosis is Impaired Skin Integrity. Other nursing diagnoses that may be appropriate or require the use of this skill include:

- Anxiety
- Acute Pain
- Impaired Tissue Integrity
- Disturbed Body Image
- Deficient Knowledge

OUTCOME IDENTIFICATION AND PLANNING

The expected outcome to achieve when applying NPWT is that the therapy is accomplished without contaminating the wound area, causing trauma to the wound, and/or causing the patient to experience pain or discomfort. Other outcomes that may be appropriate include the following: the negative-pressure device functions correctly; the appropriate and ordered pressure is maintained throughout therapy; and the wound exhibits progression in healing.

(continued)

SKILL 8-11 APPLYING NEGATIVE-PRESSURE WOUND THERAPY continued

IMPLEMENTATION

ACTION	RATIONALE
1. Review the medical order for the application of NPWT therapy, including the ordered pressure setting for the device. Gather necessary supplies.	Reviewing the order validates the correct patient and correct procedure. Preparation promotes efficient time management and an organized approach to the task.
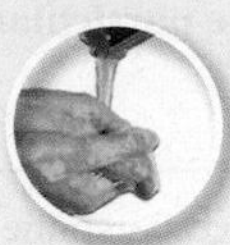 2. Perform hand hygiene and put on PPE, if indicated.	Hand hygiene and PPE prevent the spread of microorganisms. PPE is required based on transmission precautions.
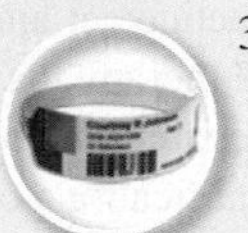 3. Identify the patient.	Identifying the patient ensures the right patient receives the intervention and helps prevent errors.
4. Assemble equipment on overbed table within reach.	Organization facilitates performance of task.
5. Close the curtains around the bed and close the door to the room, if possible. Explain what you are going to do and why you are going to do it to the patient.	This ensures the patient's privacy. Explanation relieves anxiety and facilitates cooperation.
6. Assess the patient for possible need for nonpharmacologic pain-reducing interventions or analgesic medication before wound care dressing change. Administer appropriate prescribed analgesic. Allow enough time for the analgesic to achieve its effectiveness before beginning the procedure.	Pain is a subjective experience influenced by past experience. Wound care and dressing changes may cause pain for some patients.
7. Adjust bed to comfortable working height, usually elbow height of the caregiver (VISN 8, 2009).	Having the bed at the proper height prevents back and muscle strain.
8. Assist the patient to a comfortable position that provides easy access to the wound area. Position the patient so the irrigation solution will flow from the clean end of the wound toward the dirty end. Expose the area and drape the patient with a bath blanket, if needed. Put a waterproof pad under the wound area.	Patient positioning and draping provide for comfort and warmth. Gravity directs the flow of liquid from the least contaminated to the most contaminated area. Waterproof pad protects the patient and the bed linens.
9. Have the disposal bag or waste receptacle within easy reach for use during the procedure.	Having a waste container handy allows for easy disposal of the soiled dressings and supplies, without the spread of microorganisms.
10. Using sterile technique, prepare a sterile field and add all the sterile supplies needed for the procedure to the field. Pour warmed, sterile irrigating solution into the sterile container.	Proper preparation ensures that supplies are within easy reach and sterility is maintained. Warmed solution may result in less discomfort.
11. Put on a gown, mask, and eye protection.	Use of PPE is part of *Standard Precautions.* A gown protects your clothes from contamination if splashing should occur. Goggles protect mucous membranes of your eyes from contact with irrigant fluid.
12. Put on clean gloves. Carefully and gently remove the dressing. If there is resistance, use a silicone-based adhesive remover to help remove the drape. **Note the number of pieces of foam removed from the wound. Compare with the documented number from the previous dressing change.**	Gloves protect the nurse from handling contaminated dressings. A silicone-based adhesive remover allows for the easy, rapid, and painless removal without the associated problems of skin stripping (Denyer, 2011; Benbow, 2011). Counting the number of pieces of foam assures the removal of all foam that was placed during the previous dressing change.
13. Discard the dressings in the receptacle. Remove your gloves and put them in the receptacle.	Proper disposal of dressings and used gloves prevents the spread of microorganisms.
14. Put on sterile gloves. Using sterile technique, irrigate the wound (see Skill 8-4).	Irrigation removes exudate and debris.

ACTION	RATIONALE
15. Clean the area around the wound with normal saline. Dry the surrounding skin with a sterile gauze sponge.	Moisture provides a medium for growth of microorganisms.
16. Assess the wound for appearance, stage, presence of eschar, granulation tissue, epithelialization, undermining, tunneling, necrosis, sinus tract, and drainage. Assess the appearance of the surrounding tissue. Measure the wound. Refer to Fundamentals Review 8-3.	This information provides evidence about the wound healing process and/or the presence of infection.
17. **Wipe intact skin around the wound with a skin-protectant wipe and allow it to dry well.**	Skin protectant provides a barrier against irritation and breakdown.
18. **Using sterile scissors, cut the foam to the shape and measurement of the wound. Do not cut foam over the wound.** More than one piece of foam may be necessary if the first piece is cut too small. Carefully place the foam in the wound. **Ensure foam-to-foam contact if more than one piece is required. Note the number of pieces of foam placed in the wound.**	Aseptic technique maintains sterility of items to come in contact with wound. Foam should fill the wound, but not cover intact surrounding skin. Foam fragments may fall into the wound if cutting is performed over the wound. Foam-to foam contact allows for even distribution of negative pressure. Recording the number of pieces of foam aids in assuring the removal of all foam with next dressing change.
19. Trim and place the V.A.C. Drape to cover the foam dressing and an additional 3 to 5 cm border of intact periwound tissue. V.A.C. Drape may be cut into multiple pieces for easier handling.	The occlusive air-permeable V.A.C. Drape provides a seal, allowing the application of the negative pressure.
20. Choose an appropriate site to apply the T.R.A.C. Pad.	T.R.A.C. Pad should be placed in the area where the greatest fluid flow and optimal drainage is anticipated. Avoid placing over bony prominences or within creases in the tissue.
21. Pinch the drape and cut a 2-cm hole through it. Apply the T.R.A.C. Pad (Figure 2). Remove V.A.C. Canister from package and insert into the V.A.C. Therapy Unit until it locks into place. Connect T.R.A.C. Pad tubing to canister tubing (Figure 3) and check that the clamps on each tube are open. Turn on the power to the V.A.C. Therapy Unit and select the prescribed therapy setting.	A hole in the drape allows for removal of fluid and/or exudate. The canister provides a collection chamber for drainage.

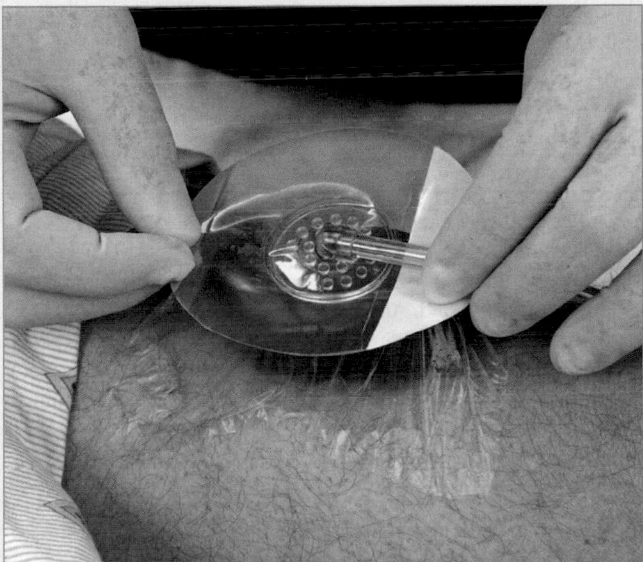

FIGURE 2 Applying T.R.A.C. Pad.

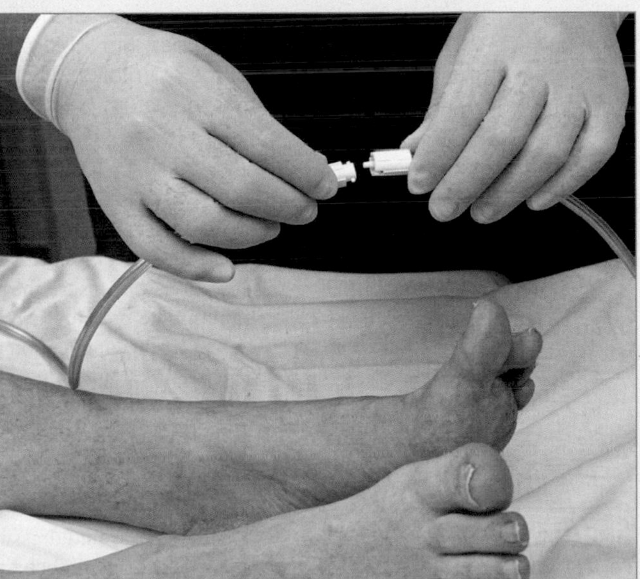

FIGURE 3 Connecting T.R.A.C. tubing to collection canister tubing.

(continued)

SKILL 8-11 APPLYING NEGATIVE-PRESSURE WOUND THERAPY continued

ACTION	RATIONALE
22. **Assess the dressing to ensure seal integrity. The dressing should be collapsed, shrinking to the foam and skin.**	Shrinkage confirms a good seal, allowing for accurate application of pressure and treatment.
23. Remove and discard gloves.	Proper disposal of gloves prevents the spread of microorganisms.
24. Label dressing with date and time. Remove all remaining equipment; place the patient in a comfortable position, with side rails up and bed in the lowest position.	Recording date and time provides communication and demonstrates adherence to plan of care. Proper patient and bed positioning promotes safety and comfort.
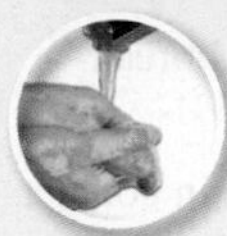 25. Remove PPE, if used. Perform hand hygiene.	Removing PPE properly reduces the risk for infection transmission and contamination of other items. Hand hygiene prevents the spread of microorganisms.
26. Check all wound dressings every shift. More frequent checks may be needed if the wound is more complex or dressings become saturated quickly.	Checking dressings ensures the assessment of changes in patient condition and timely intervention to prevent complications.

EVALUATION

The expected outcome is met when applying negative-pressure wound therapy is accomplished without contaminating the wound area, causing trauma to the wound, and/or causing the patient to experience pain or discomfort. In addition, the vacuum device functions correctly; the appropriate and ordered pressure is maintained throughout therapy; and the wound exhibits progression in healing.

DOCUMENTATION

Guidelines

Record your assessment of the wound, including evidence of granulation tissue, presence of necrotic tissue, stage (if appropriate), and characteristics of drainage. Include the appearance of the surrounding skin. Document the cleansing or irrigation of the wound and solution used. Document the application of the NPWT, noting the pressure setting, patency, and seal of the dressing. Describe the color and characteristics of the drainage in the collection chamber. Record pertinent patient and family education and any patient reaction to this procedure, including the presence of pain and effectiveness or ineffectiveness of pain interventions.

Sample Documentation

4/5/15 0800 NPWT dressing intact with good seal maintained, V.A.C. system patent, pressure setting 50 mm Hg. Purulent, sanguineous drainage noted in collection chamber and tubing. Surrounding tissue without edema, redness, ecchymosis, or signs of irritation. Patient verbalizes an understanding of movement limitations related to the system.

—*B. Clark, RN*

UNEXPECTED SITUATIONS AND ASSOCIATED INTERVENTIONS

- *While assessing the patient, the nurse notes that the seal between the transparent dressing and the foam and skin is not tight:* Check the dressing seals, tubing connections, and canister insertion, and ensure the clamps are open. If a leak in the transparent dressing is identified, the appropriate pressure is not being applied to the wound. Apply additional transparent dressing to reseal. If this application does not correct the break, change the dressing.
- *The patient complains of acute pain while NPWT is operating:* Assess the patient for other symptoms, obtain vital signs, assess the wound, and assess the vacuum device for proper functioning. Report your findings to the primary care provider and document the event in the patient's record. Administer analgesics, as ordered. Continue or change the wound therapy, as ordered.

SPECIAL CONSIDERATIONS

- Change the wound dressing initially 48 hours after beginning treatment, then two to three times per week for noninfected wounds, as indicated by the wound's response to the intervention (Baranoski & Ayello, 2012). Time dressing changes to allow for wound assessment by the other members of the health care team.
- Monitor infected wounds often; dressings may need to be changed more often than 48 to 72 hours (Hess, 2013).

- Measure and record the amount of drainage each shift as part of the intake and output record.
- Check the fluid level in the canister periodically. Depending on the particular device in use, replace canister whenever full or nearly full.
- Be alert for audible and visual alarms on the vacuum device to alert you to problems, such as tipping of the device greater than 45 degrees, a full collection canister, an air leak in the dressing, or dislodgment of the canister.
- NPWT should operate for 24 hours a day. It should not be shut off for more than 2 hours in a 24-hour period. When NPWT is restarted, irrigate the wound per medical order or facility policy, and apply a new NPWT dressing.
- When maceration of the surrounding skin beneath the occlusive dressing occurs, this may be treated by placing a barrier/wafer dressing beneath the transparent dressing to protect the skin. Verify with facility policy, as needed.

EVIDENCE FOR PRACTICE ▶

NEGATIVE-PRESSURE WOUND THERAPY AND PATIENT PERSPECTIVES

Because the skin is a sensory organ and plays a major role in communication with others and self-image, wounds and pressure ulcers require emotional as well as physical adaptation. Although stress and adaptation vary greatly among individuals, actual and potential emotional stressors are common in all patients with wounds. Therapies related to wound care are also a source of stress. These stressors impact the quality of life of the patient and caregivers and include pain, anxiety, fear, activities of daily living, and changes in body image.

Related Research

Bolas, N., & Holloway, S. (2012). Negative pressure wound therapy: A study on patient perspectives. *Wound Care, 17*(3 Suppl), S30–S35.

This observational study explored patients' lived experience of using NPWT. Participants used NPWT for a minimum of 4 weeks. Semistructured interviews were transcribed verbatim and investigated for common themes in the participants' experiences. The three most common themes were identified as altered sense of self, a new culture of technology, and leading a restricted life. The authors' stated that the themes associated with an altered sense of self and leading a restricted life were in keeping with other wound care studies. Barriers, such as managing technical difficulties, and the impact of the technology on the practicalities of daily living were identified.

Relevance for Nursing Practice

Using the best treatment for a wound or pressure ulcer is important. However, the best treatment may not produce the best patient experience, if the patient's emotional needs are not met. Nurses need to be holistic in their approach with patients receiving wound care and be aware of patient experiences related to any prescribed treatments for wounds and pressure ulcers. Interventions, including patient education, support, and encouragement, can foster hope and reduce anxiety for patients.

Refer to thePoint for additional research on related nursing topics.

SKILL 8-12 REMOVING SUTURES

Skin sutures are used to hold tissue and skin together. Sutures may be black silk, synthetic material, or fine wire. **Surgical sutures** are removed when enough tensile strength has developed to hold the wound edges together during healing. The time frame varies depending on the patient's age, nutritional status, and wound location. Frequently, after skin sutures are removed, adhesive wound closure strips are applied across the wound to give additional support as it continues to heal. The removal of sutures may be done by the primary care provider or by the nurse with a medical order.

(*continued*)

SKILL 8-12 REMOVING SUTURES continued

DELEGATION CONSIDERATIONS

The removal of surgical sutures is not delegated to nursing assistive personnel (NAP) or to unlicensed assistive personnel (UAP). Depending on the state's nurse practice act and the organization's policies and procedures, the removal of surgical sutures may be delegated to licensed practical/vocational nurses (LPN/LVNs). The decision to delegate must be based on careful analysis of the patient's needs and circumstances, as well as the qualifications of the person to whom the task is being delegated. Refer to the Delegation Guidelines in Appendix A.

EQUIPMENT

- Suture removal kit or forceps and scissors
- Gauze
- Wound cleansing agent, according to facility policy
- Clean, disposable gloves
- Additional PPE, as indicated
- Adhesive wound closure strips
- Skin protectant wipes

ASSESSMENT

Inspect the surgical incision and the surrounding tissue. Assess the appearance of the wound for the approximation of wound edges, the color of the wound and surrounding area, presence of wound drainage noting color, volume, and odor, and for signs of dehiscence. Note the stage of the healing process and characteristics of any drainage. Assess the surrounding skin for color, temperature, and the presence of edema, maceration, or ecchymosis.

NURSING DIAGNOSIS

Determine the related factors for the nursing diagnoses based on the patient's current health status. Appropriate nursing diagnoses may include:

- Deficient Knowledge
- Risk for Infection
- Impaired Skin Integrity

OUTCOME IDENTIFICATION AND PLANNING

The expected outcome to achieve when removing surgical sutures is that the sutures are removed without contaminating the incisional area, causing trauma to the wound, and/or causing the patient to experience pain or discomfort. In addition, other outcomes that are appropriate include the following: the patient remains free of complications that would delay recovery; and the patient verbalizes an understanding of the procedure.

IMPLEMENTATION

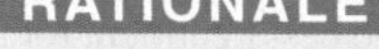

ACTION	RATIONALE
1. Review the medical orders for suture removal. Gather necessary supplies.	Reviewing the order and plan of care validates the correct patient and correct procedure. Preparation promotes efficient time management and an organized approach to the task.
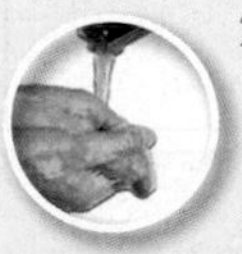 2. Perform hand hygiene and put on PPE, if indicated.	Hand hygiene and PPE prevent the spread of microorganisms. PPE is required based on transmission precautions.
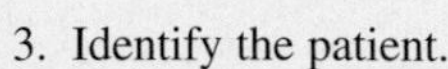 3. Identify the patient.	Identifying the patient ensures the right patient receives the intervention and helps prevent errors.
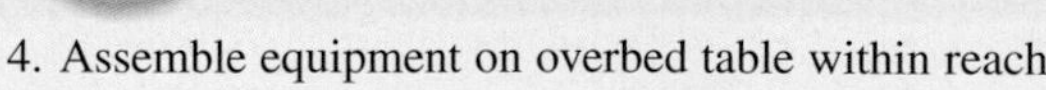 4. Assemble equipment on overbed table within reach.	Organization facilitates performance of task.
5. Close the curtains around the bed and close the door to the room, if possible. Explain what you are going to do and why you are going to do it to the patient. Describe the sensation of suture removal as a pulling or slightly uncomfortable experience.	This ensures the patient's privacy. Explanation relieves anxiety and facilitates cooperation.

ACTION	RATIONALE
6. Assess the patient for possible need for nonpharmacologic pain-reducing interventions or analgesic medication before beginning the procedure. Administer appropriate prescribed analgesic. Allow enough time for the analgesic to achieve its effectiveness before beginning the procedure.	Pain is a subjective experience influenced by past experience. Wound care and dressing changes may cause pain for some patients.
7. Place a waste receptacle at a convenient location for use during the procedure.	Having a waste container handy means that the soiled dressing may be discarded easily, without the spread of microorganisms.
8. Adjust bed to comfortable working height, usually elbow height of the caregiver (VISN 8, 2009).	Having the bed at the proper height prevents back and muscle strain.
9. Assist the patient to a comfortable position that provides easy access to the incision area. Use a bath blanket to cover any exposed area other than the incision. Place a waterproof pad under the incision site.	Patient positioning and use of a bath blanket provide for comfort and warmth. Waterproof pad protects underlying surfaces.
10. Put on clean gloves. Carefully and gently remove the soiled dressings. If there is resistance, use a silicone-based adhesive remover to help remove the tape. If any part of the dressing sticks to the underlying skin, use small amounts of sterile saline to help loosen and remove it. Inspect the incision area (Figure 1).	Gloves protect the nurse from handling contaminated dressings. Cautious removal of the dressing is more comfortable for the patient and ensures that any drain present is not removed. A silicone-based adhesive remover allows for the easy, rapid, and painless removal without the associated problems of skin stripping (Denyer, 2011; Benbow, 2011). Sterile saline moistens the dressing for easier removal and minimizes damage and pain.
11. Clean the incision using the wound cleanser and gauze, according to facility policies and procedures.	Incision cleaning prevents the spread of microorganisms and contamination of the wound.
12. Using the forceps, grasp the knot of the first suture and gently lift the knot up off the skin.	Raising the suture knot prevents accidental injury to the wound or skin when cutting.
13. Using the scissors, cut one side of the suture below the knot, close to the skin (Figure 2). Grasp the knot with the forceps and pull the cut suture through the skin. **Avoid pulling the visible portion of the suture through the underlying tissue.**	Pulling the cut suture through the skin helps reduce the risk for contamination of the incision area and resulting infection.
14. Remove every other suture to be sure the wound edges are healed. If they are, remove the remaining sutures, as ordered. Dispose of sutures according to facility policy.	Removing every other suture allows for inspection of the wound, while leaving adequate suture in place to promote continued healing if the edges are not totally approximated. Follow *Standard Precautions* in disposing of sutures.

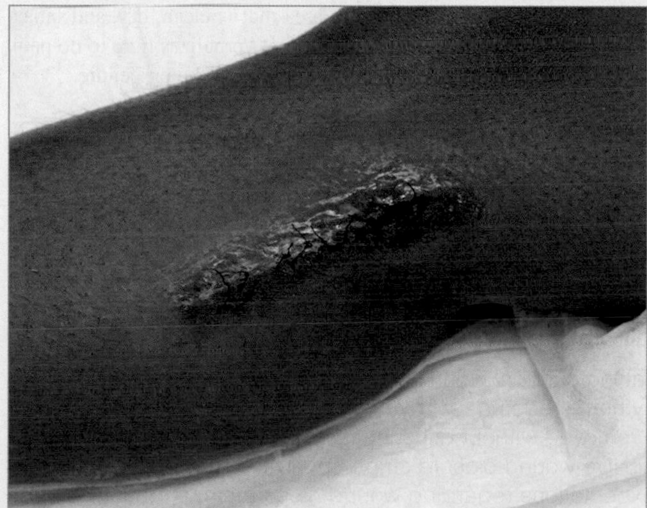

FIGURE 1 Incision with sutures.

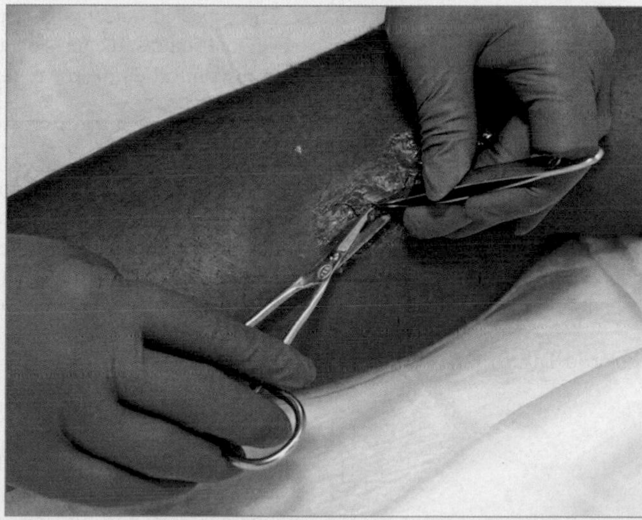

FIGURE 2 Using gloved hands to pull up on a suture with forceps and cutting suture with sterile scissors.

(continued)

SKILL 8-12 REMOVING SUTURES continued

ACTION	RATIONALE
15. If wound closure strips are to be used, apply skin protectant to skin around incision. **Do not apply to incision.** Apply adhesive closure strips (Figure 3). Take care to handle the strips by the paper backing.	Skin protectant helps adherence of closure strips and prevents skin irritation. Adhesive wound closure strips provide additional support to the wound as it continues to heal. Handling by the paper backing avoids contamination.

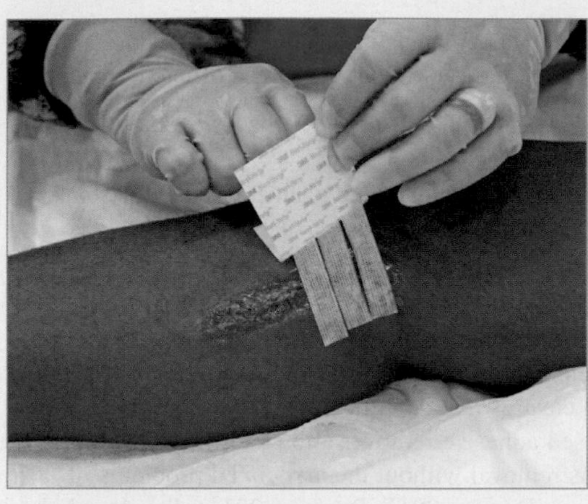

FIGURE 3 Applying adhesive closure strips on incision.

ACTION	RATIONALE
16. Reapply the dressing, depending on the medical orders and facility policy.	A new dressing protects the wound. Some policies advise leaving the area uncovered.
17. Remove gloves and discard. Remove all remaining equipment; place the patient in a comfortable position, with side rails up and bed in the lowest position.	Proper removal of gloves prevents spread of microorganisms. Proper patient and bed positioning promotes safety and comfort.
18. Remove additional PPE, if used. Perform hand hygiene.	Removing PPE properly reduces the risk for infection transmission and contamination of other items. Hand hygiene prevents the spread of microorganisms.
19. Assess all wounds every shift. More frequent checks may be needed if the wound is more complex.	Checking wound and dressings ensures the assessment of changes in patient condition and timely intervention to prevent complications.

EVALUATION

The expected outcome is met when the patient exhibits an incision area that is clean, dry, and intact without sutures; the incision area is free of trauma and infection; the patient verbalizes little to no pain or discomfort during the removal; and the patient verbalizes an understanding of the procedure.

DOCUMENTATION

Guidelines

Document the location of the incision and the assessment of the site. Include the appearance of the surrounding skin. Document cleansing of the site and suture removal. Record any skin care, application of wound closure strips, and the dressing applied, if appropriate. Note pertinent patient and family education and any patient reaction to this procedure, including patient's pain level and effectiveness of nonpharmacologic interventions or analgesia if administered.

Sample Documentation

3/4/13 1800 Right lower lateral leg surgical wound appears healed. Incision edges are approximated, without erythema, edema, ecchymosis, or drainage. Skin warm with consistent tone. Sutures removed without difficulty; skin protectant applied to skin surrounding incision and adhesive wound closure strips applied. Patient instructed in how to care for wound and expectations regarding wound closure strips; patient and wife verbalized an understanding of information and asked appropriate questions.

—L. Downs, RN

UNEXPECTED SITUATIONS AND ASSOCIATED INTERVENTIONS

- *Sutures are crusted with dried blood or secretions, making them difficult to remove:* Moisten sterile gauze with sterile saline and gently loosen crusts before removing sutures.
- *Resistance is met when attempting to pull suture through the tissue:* Use a gentle, continuous pulling motion to remove the suture. If the suture still does not come out, do not use excessive force. Report findings to the primary care provider and document the event in the patient's record.

SPECIAL CONSIDERATIONS

- After suture removal, continue to encourage the patient to splint chest and abdominal wounds during activity, such as changing position, ambulating, coughing, and sneezing. This provides increased support for the skin and underlying tissues and can decrease discomfort.

SKILL 8-13 REMOVING SURGICAL STAPLES

Skin staples made of stainless steel are used to hold tissue and skin together. Staples decrease the risk of infection and allow for faster wound closure. **Surgical staples** are removed when enough tensile strength has developed to hold the wound edges together during healing. The time frame for removal varies depending on the patient's age, nutritional status, and wound location. After skin staples are removed, adhesive wound closure strips are applied across the wound to keep the skin edges approximated as it continues to heal. The removal of surgical staples may be done by the primary care provider or by the nurse with a medical order.

DELEGATION CONSIDERATIONS

The removal of surgical staples is not delegated to nursing assistive personnel (NAP) or to unlicensed assistive personnel (UAP). Depending on the state's nurse practice act and the organization's policies and procedures, the removal of surgical staples may be delegated to licensed practical/vocational nurses (LPN/LVNs). The decision to delegate must be based on careful analysis of the patient's needs and circumstances, as well as the qualifications of the person to whom the task is being delegated. Refer to the Delegation Guidelines in Appendix A.

EQUIPMENT

- Staple remover
- Gauze
- Wound cleansing agent, according to facility policy
- Clean, disposable gloves
- Additional PPE, as indicated
- Adhesive wound closure strips
- Skin protectant wipes

ASSESSMENT

Inspect the surgical incision and the surrounding tissue. Assess the appearance of the wound for the approximation of wound edges, the color of the wound and surrounding area, and signs of dehiscence. Note the stage of the healing process and the characteristics of any drainage. Assess the surrounding skin for color, temperature, and the presence of edema or ecchymosis.

NURSING DIAGNOSIS

Determine the related factors for the nursing diagnoses based on the patient's current health status. Appropriate nursing diagnoses may include:

- Impaired Skin Integrity
- Acute Pain
- Delayed Surgical Recovery

OUTCOME IDENTIFICATION AND PLANNING

The expected outcome to achieve when removing surgical staples is that the staples are removed without contaminating the incisional area, causing trauma to the wound, and/or causing the patient to experience pain or discomfort. In addition, other outcomes that are appropriate include the following: the patient remains free of complications that would delay recovery; and the patient verbalizes an understanding of the procedure.

(continued)

SKILL 8-13 REMOVING SURGICAL STAPLES continued

IMPLEMENTATION

ACTION	RATIONALE
1. Review the medical order for staple removal. Gather necessary supplies.	Reviewing the order and plan of care validates the correct patient and correct procedure. Preparation promotes efficient time management and an organized approach to the task.
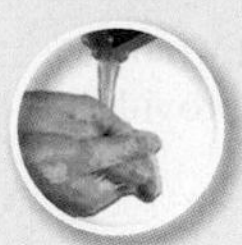 2. Perform hand hygiene and put on PPE, if indicated.	Hand hygiene and PPE prevent the spread of microorganisms. PPE is required based on transmission precautions.
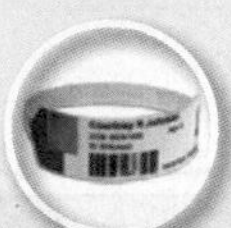 3. Identify the patient.	Identifying the patient ensures the right patient receives the intervention and helps prevent errors.
4. Assemble equipment on overbed table within reach.	Organization facilitates performance of task.
5. Close the curtains around the bed and close the door to the room, if possible. Explain what you are going to do and why you are going to do it to the patient. Describe the sensation of staple removal as a pulling experience.	This ensures the patient's privacy. Explanation relieves anxiety and facilitates cooperation.
6. Assess the patient for possible need for nonpharmacologic pain-reducing interventions or analgesic medication before beginning the procedure. Administer appropriate prescribed analgesic. Allow enough time for the analgesic to achieve its effectiveness before beginning procedure.	Pain is a subjective experience influenced by past experience. Wound care and dressing changes may cause pain for some patients.
7. Place a waste receptacle at a convenient location for use during the procedure.	Having a waste container handy means that the soiled dressing may be discarded easily, without the spread of microorganisms.
8. Adjust bed to comfortable working height, usually elbow height of the caregiver (VISN 8, 2009).	Having the bed at the proper height prevents back and muscle strain.
9. Assist the patient to a comfortable position that provides easy access to the incision area. Use a bath blanket to cover any exposed area other than the incision. Place a waterproof pad under the incision site.	Patient positioning and use of a bath blanket provide for comfort and warmth. Waterproof pad protects underlying surfaces.
10. Put on clean gloves. Carefully and gently remove the soiled dressings. If there is resistance, use a silicone-based adhesive remover to help remove the tape. If any part of the dressing sticks to the underlying skin, use small amounts of sterile saline to help loosen and remove it. Inspect the incision area (Figure 1).	Gloves protect the nurse from handling contaminated dressings. Cautious removal of the dressing is more comfortable for the patient and ensures that any drain present is not removed. A silicone-based adhesive remover allows for the easy, rapid, and painless removal without the associated problems of skin stripping (Denyer, 2011; Benbow, 2011). Sterile saline moistens the dressing for easier removal and minimizes damage and pain.

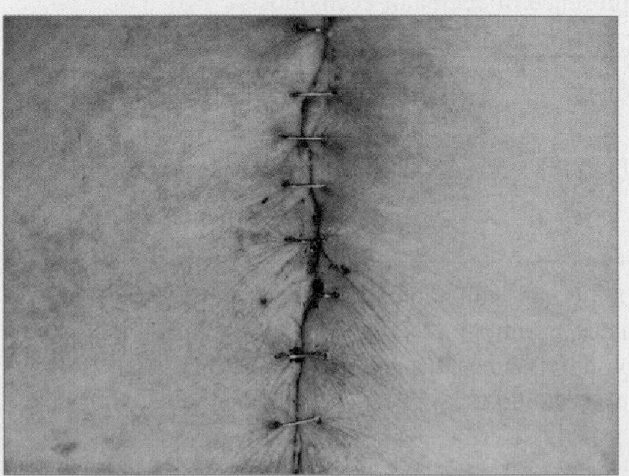

FIGURE 1 Incision with surgical staples.

ACTION	RATIONALE
11. Clean the incision using the wound cleanser and gauze, according to facility policies and procedures.	Incision cleaning prevents the spread of microorganisms and contamination of the wound.
12. Grasp the staple remover (Figure 2). **Position the staple remover under the staple to be removed. Firmly close the staple remover.** The staple will bend in the middle and the edges will pull up out of the skin.	Correct use of the staple remover prevents accidental injury to the wound and contamination of the incision area and resulting infection.

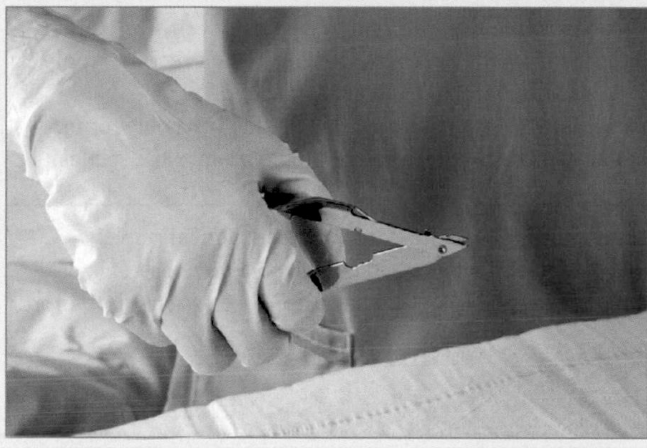

FIGURE 2 Grasping staple remover.

ACTION	RATIONALE
13. Remove every other staple to be sure the wound edges are healed. If they are, remove the remaining staples, as ordered. Dispose of staples in the sharps container.	Removing every other staple allows for inspection of the wound, while leaving an adequate number of staples in place to promote continued healing if the edges are not totally approximated.
14. If wound closure strips are to be used, apply skin protectant to skin around incision. **Do not apply to incision.** Apply adhesive closure strips. Take care to handle the strips by the paper backing.	Skin protectant helps adherence of closure strips and prevents skin irritation. Adhesive wound closure strips provide additional support to the wound as it continues to heal. Handling by the paper backing avoids contamination.
15. Reapply the dressing, depending on the medical orders and facility policy.	A new dressing protects the wound. Some policies advise leaving the area uncovered.
16. Remove gloves and discard. Remove all remaining equipment; place the patient in a comfortable position, with side rails up and bed in the lowest position.	Proper removal of gloves prevents spread of microorganisms. Proper patient and bed positioning promotes safety and comfort.
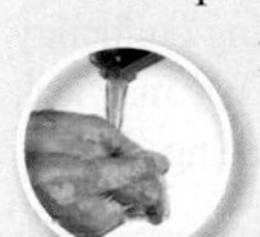 17. Remove additional PPE, if used. Perform hand hygiene.	Removing PPE properly reduces the risk for infection transmission and contamination of other items. Hand hygiene prevents the spread of microorganisms.
18. Assess all wounds every shift. More frequent checks may be needed if the wound is more complex.	Checking wound and dressings ensures the assessment of changes in patient condition and timely intervention to prevent complications.

EVALUATION

The expected outcome is met when the patient exhibits an incision area that is clean, dry, and intact without staples; the incision area is free of trauma and infection; the patient verbalizes little to no pain or discomfort during the removal; and the patient verbalizes an understanding of the procedure.

DOCUMENTATION

Guidelines

Document the location of the incision and the assessment of the site. Include the appearance of the surrounding skin. Document cleansing of the site and staple removal. Record any skin care and the dressing applied, if appropriate. Note pertinent patient and family education and any patient reaction to this procedure, including patient's pain level and effectiveness of nonpharmacologic interventions or analgesia if administered.

(*continued*)

SKILL 8-13 REMOVING SURGICAL STAPLES continued

Sample Documentation

3/4/15 1800 Left upper lateral leg surgical wound appears healed. Incision edges are approximated, without erythema, edema, ecchymosis, or drainage. Skin warm with consistent tone. Staples removed without difficulty; skin protectant applied to skin surrounding incision and adhesive wound closure strips applied. Patient instructed in how to care for wound and expectations regarding wound closure strips; patient and wife verbalized an understanding of information and asked appropriate questions.
—*S. Hoffman, RN*

UNEXPECTED SITUATIONS AND ASSOCIATED INTERVENTIONS

- *The wound edges appear approximated before staple removal but pull apart afterward:* Report the findings to the primary care provider and document the event in the patient's record. Apply adhesive wound closure strips according to facility policy or medical order.
- *The staples are stuck to the wound because of dried blood or secretions:* Per facility policy or medical order, apply moist saline compresses to loosen crusts before attempting to remove the staples.

SPECIAL CONSIDERATIONS

- Encourage the patient to splint chest and abdominal wounds (before and after surgical staple removal) during activity, such as changing position, ambulating, coughing, and sneezing. This provides increased support for the skin and underlying tissues and can help decrease patient discomfort.

SKILL 8-14 APPLYING AN EXTERNAL HEATING PAD

Heat applications accelerate the inflammatory response, promoting healing. Heat is also used to reduce muscle tension, and to relieve muscle spasm and joint stiffness. Heat also helps relieve pain. It is used to treat infections, surgical wounds, inflammation, arthritis, joint pain, muscle pain, and chronic pain.

Heat is applied by moist and dry methods. The medical order should include the type of application, the body area to be treated, the frequency of application, and the length of time for the applications. Water used for heat applications needs to be at the appropriate temperature to avoid skin damage: 115°F to 125°F for older children and adults and 105°F to 110°F for infants, young children, older adults, and patients with diabetes or those who are unconscious.

Common types of external heating devices include Aquathermia pads (one brand) and crushable, microwaveable hot packs. Aquathermia pads are used in health care agencies and are safer to use than heating pads. The temperature setting for an Aquathermia pad should not exceed 105°F to 109.4°F, depending on facility policy. Microwaveable packs are easy and inexpensive to use, but have several disadvantages. They may leak and pose a danger from burns related to improper use. They are used most often in the home setting.

DELEGATION CONSIDERATIONS

The application of an external heating pad may be delegated to nursing assistive personnel (NAP) or to unlicensed assistive personnel (UAP), as well as to licensed practical/vocational nurses (LPN/LVNs). The decision to delegate must be based on careful analysis of the patient's needs and circumstances, as well as the qualifications of the person to whom the task is being delegated. Refer to the Delegation Guidelines in Appendix A.

EQUIPMENT

- Aquathermia heating pad (or other brand) with electronic unit
- Distilled water
- Cover for the pad, if not part of pad
- Gauze bandage or tape to secure the pad
- Bath blanket
- PPE, as indicated

ASSESSMENT

Assess the situation to determine the appropriateness for the application of heat. Assess the patient's physical and mental status and the condition of the body area to be treated with heat. Confirm the medical order for heat therapy, including frequency, type of therapy, body area to be treated, and length of time for the application. Check the equipment to be used, including the condition of cords, plugs, and heating elements. Look for fluid leaks. Once the equipment is turned on, make sure there is a consistent distribution of heat and the temperature is within safe limits.

NURSING DIAGNOSIS

Determine the related factors for the nursing diagnoses based on the patient's current health status. Appropriate nursing diagnoses may include:

- Chronic Pain
- Acute Pain
- Risk for Impaired Skin Integrity

OUTCOME IDENTIFICATION AND PLANNING

The expected outcome to achieve when applying an external heat source depends on the patient's nursing diagnosis. Outcomes that may be appropriate include the following: the patient experiences increased comfort; the patient experiences decreased muscle spasms; the patient exhibits improved wound healing; the patient demonstrates a reduction in inflammation; and the patient remains free from injury.

IMPLEMENTATION

ACTION	RATIONALE
1. Review the medical order for the application of heat therapy, including frequency, type of therapy, body area to be treated, and length of time for the application. Gather necessary supplies.	Reviewing the order and plan of care validates the correct patient and correct procedure. Preparation promotes efficient time management and an organized approach to the task.
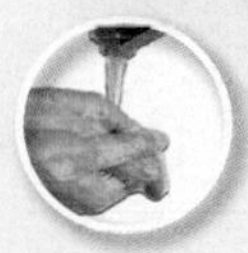 2. Perform hand hygiene and put on PPE, if indicated.	Hand hygiene and PPE prevent the spread of microorganisms. PPE is required based on transmission precautions.
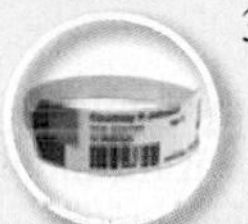 3. Identify the patient.	Identifying the patient ensures the right patient receives the intervention and helps prevent errors.
4. Assemble equipment on overbed table within reach.	Organization facilitates performance of task.
5. Close the curtains around the bed and close the door to the room, if possible. Explain what you are going to do and why you are going to do it to the patient.	This ensures the patient's privacy. Explanation relieves anxiety and facilitates cooperation.
6. Adjust bed to comfortable working height, usually elbow height of the caregiver (VISN 8, 2009).	Having the bed at the proper height prevents back and muscle strain.
7. Assist the patient to a comfortable position that provides easy access to the area where the heat will be applied; use a bath blanket to cover any other exposed area.	Patient positioning and use of a bath blanket provide for comfort and warmth.
8. Assess the condition of the skin where the heat is to be applied.	Assessment supplies baseline data for post-treatment comparison and identifies conditions that may contraindicate the application.
9. Check that the water in the electronic unit (Figure 1) is at the appropriate level. Fill the unit two-thirds full or to the fill mark, with distilled water, if necessary. Check the temperature setting on the unit to ensure it is within the safe range.	Sufficient water in the unit is necessary to ensure proper function of the unit. Tap water leaves mineral deposits in the unit. Checking the temperature setting helps to prevent skin or tissue damage.

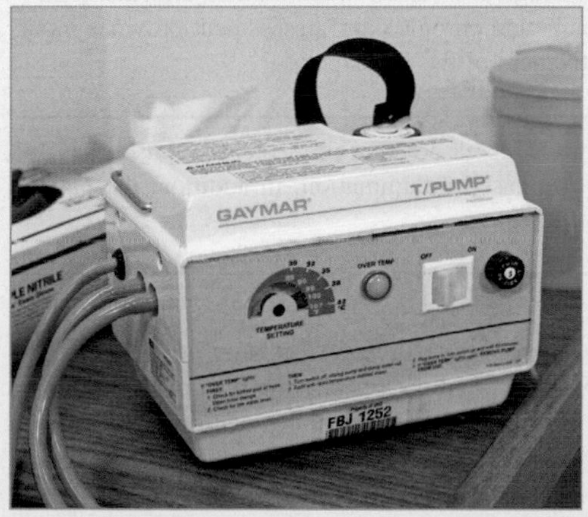

FIGURE 1 External heating pad electronic unit.

(continued)

SKILL 8-14 APPLYING AN EXTERNAL HEATING PAD continued

ACTION	RATIONALE
10. Attach pad tubing to the electronic unit tubing (Figure 2).	Allows flow of warmed water through the heating pad.
11. Plug in the unit and warm the pad before use. Apply the heating pad to the prescribed area (Figure 3). Secure with gauze bandage or tape.	Plugging in the pad readies it for use. Heat travels by conduction from one object to another. Gauze bandage or tape holds the pad in position; **do not use pins, as they may puncture and damage the pad.**

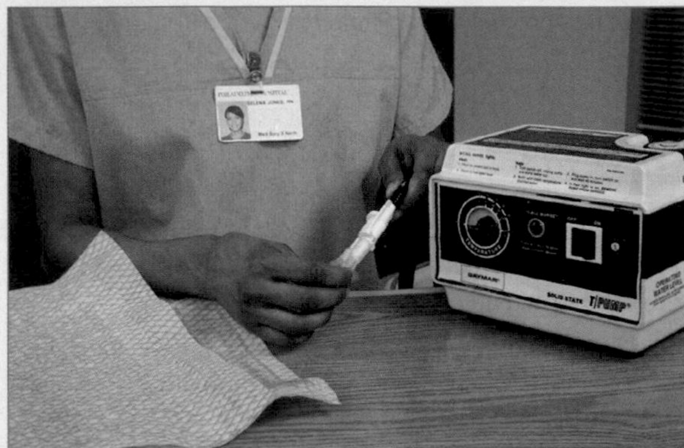

FIGURE 2 Attaching pad tubing to electronic unit tubing.

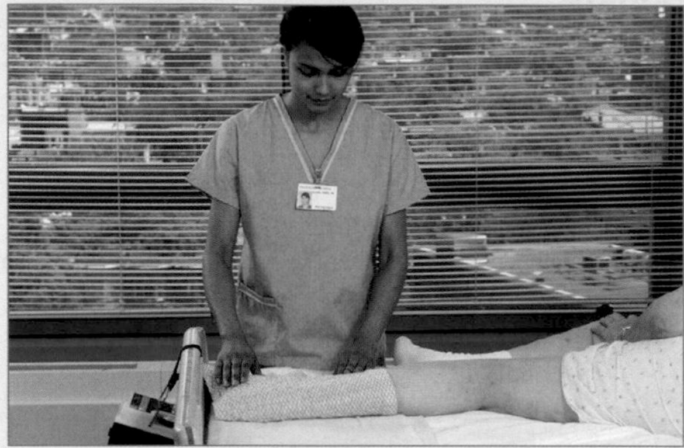

FIGURE 3 Applying heating pad.

ACTION	RATIONALE
12. **Assess the condition of the skin and the patient's response to the heat at frequent intervals, according to facility policy. Do not exceed the prescribed length of time for the application of heat.**	Maximum **vasodilation** and therapeutic effects from the application of heat occur within 20 to 30 minutes. Using heat for more than 45 minutes results in tissue congestion and **vasoconstriction**, known as the rebound phenomenon. Also, prolonged heat application may result in an increased risk of burns.
13. Remove gloves and discard. Remove all remaining equipment; place the patient in a comfortable position, with side rails up and bed in the lowest position.	Proper removal of gloves prevents spread of microorganisms. Proper patient and bed positioning promotes safety and comfort.
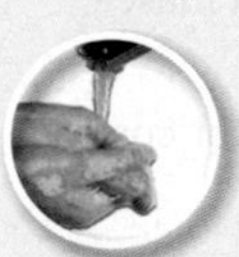 14. Remove additional PPE, if used. Perform hand hygiene.	Removing PPE properly reduces the risk for infection transmission and contamination of other items. Hand hygiene prevents the spread of microorganisms.
15. **Monitor the time the heating pad is in place to prevent burns and skin/tissue damage. Monitor the condition of the patient's skin and the patient's response at frequent intervals.**	Extended use of heat results in an increased risk for burns from the heat. Impaired circulation may affect the patient's sensitivity to heat.
16. Remove the pad after the prescribed amount of time (up to 30 minutes). Reassess the patient and area of application, noting the effect and presence of adverse effects.	Removal reduces risk of injury due to prolonged heat application. Heat applications are used to promote healing; reduce muscle tension; relieve muscle spasm, joint stiffness, and pain; and treat infections, surgical wounds, inflammation, arthritis, joint pain, muscle pain, and chronic pain. Assessment provides input as to the effectiveness of the treatment.

EVALUATION

The expected outcome is met when the patient exhibits increased comfort, decreased muscle spasm, decreased pain, improved wound healing, and/or decreased inflammation. In addition, the patient remains free of injury.

DOCUMENTATION

Guidelines

Document the rationale for application of heat therapy. If the patient is receiving heat therapy for pain, document the assessment of pain pre- and post-intervention. Specify the type of heat therapy and location where it is applied, as well as length of time applied. Record the condition of the skin, noting any redness or irritation before the heat application and after the application. Document the patient's reaction to the heat therapy. Record any appropriate patient or family education.

Sample Documentation

<u>9/13/15</u> 2300 Patient complaining of pain, rating it 5 of 10. Aquathermia pad applied to patient's lower back for 30 minutes; now rating pain as 2 of 10. Skin without signs of redness or irritation before and after application.

—M. Martinez, RN

UNEXPECTED SITUATIONS AND ASSOCIATED INTERVENTIONS

- *When performing a periodic assessment of the site during the application of heat, the nurse notes excessive swelling and redness at the site and the patient complains of pain that was not present prior to the application of heat:* Remove the heat source. Assess the patient for other symptoms and obtain vital signs. Report your findings to the primary care provider and document the interventions in the patient's record.

SPECIAL CONSIDERATIONS

General Considerations

- Direct heat treatment is contraindicated for patients at risk for bleeding, patients with a sprained limb in the acute stage, or patients with a condition associated with acute inflammation. Use cautiously with children and older adults. Patients with diabetes, stroke, spinal cord injury, and peripheral neuropathy are at risk for thermal injury, as are patients with very thin or damaged skin. Be extremely careful when applying to heat-sensitive areas, such as scar tissue and stomas.
- Instruct the patient not to lean or lie directly on the heating device, as this reduces air space and increases the risk of burns.
- Check the water level in the Aquathermia unit periodically. Evaporation may occur. If the unit runs dry, it could become damaged. Refill with distilled water periodically.

Older Adult Considerations

- Older adults are more at risk for skin and tissue damage because of their thin skin, loss of heat sensation, decreased subcutaneous tissue, and changes in the body's ability to regulate temperature. Check these patients more frequently during therapy.

Home Care Considerations

- A hot water bag or commercially prepared hot pack may be used in the home to apply heat. If using a hot water bag, fill with hot tap water to warm the bag, then empty it to detect any leaks. Check the temperature of the water with the bath thermometer or test on your inner wrist, adjusting the temperature as ordered (usually 115°F to 125°F for adults). Checking the temperature ensures that the heat applied is within the acceptable range of temperatures. Fill the bag one-half to two-thirds full. Partial filling keeps the bag lightweight and flexible so that it can be molded to the treatment area. Squeeze the bag until the water reaches the neck; this expels air, which would make the bag inflexible and would reduce heat conduction. Fasten the top and cover the bag with an absorbent cloth. The covering protects the skin from direct contact with the bag. If using a commercially prepared hot pack, follow manufacturer's directions and carefully assess skin before and after heat application.

SKILL 8-15 APPLYING A WARM COMPRESS

Warm, moist compresses are used to help promote circulation, encourage healing, decrease edema, promote consolidation of exudate, and decrease pain and discomfort. Moist heat softens crusted material and is less drying to the skin. Moist heat also penetrates tissues more deeply than dry heat.

The heat of a warm compress dissipates quickly, so the compresses must be changed frequently. If a constant warm temperature is required, a heating device such as an Aquathermia pad (refer to Skill 8-14) is applied over the compress. However, **because moisture conducts heat, a low temperature setting is needed on the heating device.** Many facilities have warming devices to heat the dressing package to an appropriate temperature for the compress. These devices help reduce the risk of burning or skin damage.

(continued)

SKILL 8-15 APPLYING A WARM COMPRESS continued

DELEGATION CONSIDERATIONS

The application of a warm compress may be delegated to nursing assistive personnel (NAP) or to unlicensed assistive personnel (UAP), as well as to licensed practical/vocational nurses (LPN/LVNs). The decision to delegate must be based on careful analysis of the patient's needs and circumstances, as well as the qualifications of the person to whom the task is being delegated. Refer to the Delegation Guidelines in Appendix A.

EQUIPMENT

- Prescribed solution to moisten the compress material, warmed to 105°F to 110°F
- Container for solution
- Gauze dressings or compresses
- Alternately, obtain the appropriate number of commercially packaged, prewarmed dressings from the warming device
- Clean, disposable gloves
- Additional PPE, as indicated
- Waterproof pad and bath blanket
- Dry bath towel
- Tape or ties
- Aquathermia or other external heating device, if ordered or required to maintain the temperature of the compress

ASSESSMENT

Assess for circulatory compromise in the area where the compress will be applied, including skin color, pulses distal to the site, evidence of edema, and the presence of sensation. Assess the situation to determine the appropriateness for the application of heat. Confirm the medical order for the compresses, including the solution to be used, frequency, body area to be treated, and length of time for the application. Assess the equipment to be used, if necessary, including the condition of cords, plugs, and heating elements. Look for fluid leaks. Once the equipment is turned on, make sure there is a consistent distribution of heat and the temperature is within safe limits. Assess the application site frequently during the treatment, as tissue damage can occur.

NURSING DIAGNOSIS

Determine the related factors for the nursing diagnoses based on the patient's current health status. Appropriate nursing diagnoses may include:

- Impaired Tissue Integrity
- Chronic Pain
- Risk for Impaired Skin Integrity

OUTCOME IDENTIFICATION AND PLANNING

The expected outcome to achieve when applying warm compresses is that the patient shows signs such as decreased inflammation, decreased muscle spasms, or decreased pain that indicate problems have been relieved. Other outcomes that may be appropriate include the following: the patient experiences improved healing, and the patient remains free from injury.

IMPLEMENTATION

ACTION	RATIONALE
1. Review the medical order for the application of a moist warm compress, including frequency and length of time for the application. Gather necessary supplies.	Reviewing the order and plan of care validates the correct patient and correct procedure. Preparation promotes efficient time management and an organized approach to the task.
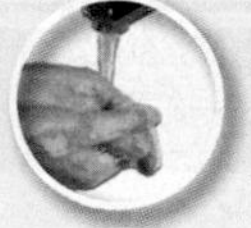 2. Perform hand hygiene and put on PPE, if indicated.	Hand hygiene and PPE prevent the spread of microorganisms. PPE is required based on transmission precautions.
 3. Identify the patient.	Identifying the patient ensures the right patient receives the intervention and helps prevent errors.
4. Assemble equipment on overbed table within reach.	Organization facilitates performance of task.
5. Assess the patient for possible need for nonpharmacologic pain-reducing interventions or analgesic medication before beginning the procedure. Administer appropriate analgesic, as ordered, and allow enough time for the analgesic to achieve its effectiveness before beginning the procedure.	Pain is a subjective experience influenced by past experience. Depending on the site of application, manipulation of the area may cause pain for some patients.

ACTION	RATIONALE
6. Close the curtains around the bed and close the door to the room, if possible. Explain what you are going to do and why you are going to do it to the patient.	This ensures the patient's privacy. Explanation relieves anxiety and facilitates cooperation.
7. If using an electronic heating device, check that the water in the unit is at the appropriate level. Fill the unit two-thirds full with distilled water, or to the fill mark, if necessary. Check the temperature setting on the unit to ensure it is within the safe range (refer to Skill 8-14).	Sufficient water in the unit is necessary to ensure proper function of the unit. Tap water leaves mineral deposits in the unit. Checking the temperature setting helps to prevent skin or tissue damage.
8. Assist the patient to a comfortable position that provides easy access to the area. Use a bath blanket to cover any exposed area other than the intended site. Place a waterproof pad under the site.	Patient positioning and use of a bath blanket provide for comfort and warmth. Waterproof pad protects underlying surfaces.
9. Place a waste receptacle at a convenient location for use during the procedure.	Having a waste container handy means that the used materials may be discarded easily, without the spread of microorganisms.
10. Pour the warmed solution into the container and drop the gauze for the compress into the solution. Alternately, if commercially packaged, prewarmed gauze is used, open packaging.	Prepares compress for application.
11. Put on clean gloves. Assess the application site for inflammation, skin color, and ecchymosis.	Gloves protect the nurse from potential contact with microorganisms. Assessment provides information about the area, the healing process, and the presence of infection, and allows for documentation of the condition of the area before the compress is applied.
12. Retrieve the compress from the warmed solution, squeezing out any excess moisture (Figure 1). Alternately, remove prewarmed gauze from open package. **Apply the compress by gently and carefully molding it to the intended area. Ask the patient if the application feels too hot.**	Excess moisture may contaminate the surrounding area and is uncomfortable for the patient. Molding the compress to the skin promotes retention of warmth around the site.

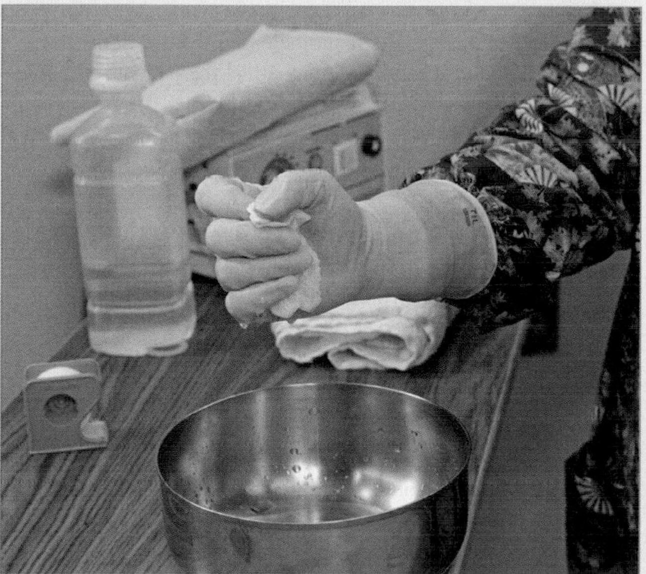

FIGURE 1 Squeezing excess solution out of compress material.

(continued)

SKILL 8-15 APPLYING A WARM COMPRESS continued

ACTION	RATIONALE
13. Cover the site with a single layer of gauze (Figure 2) and with a clean dry bath towel (Figure 3); secure in place with tape or roller gauze, if necessary.	Towel provides extra insulation.

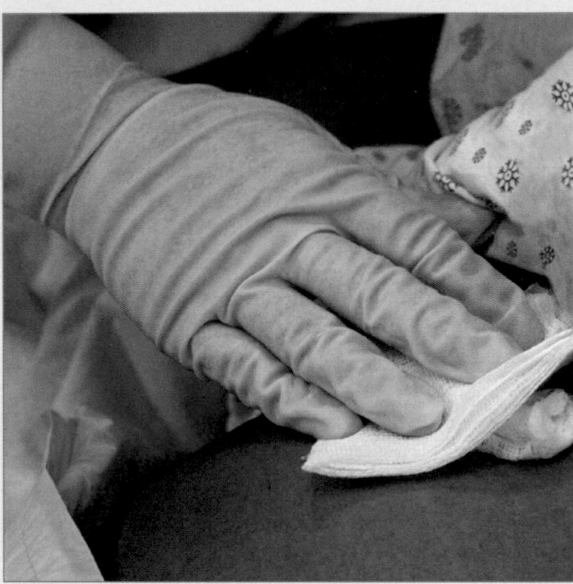

FIGURE 2 Applying single layer of gauze.

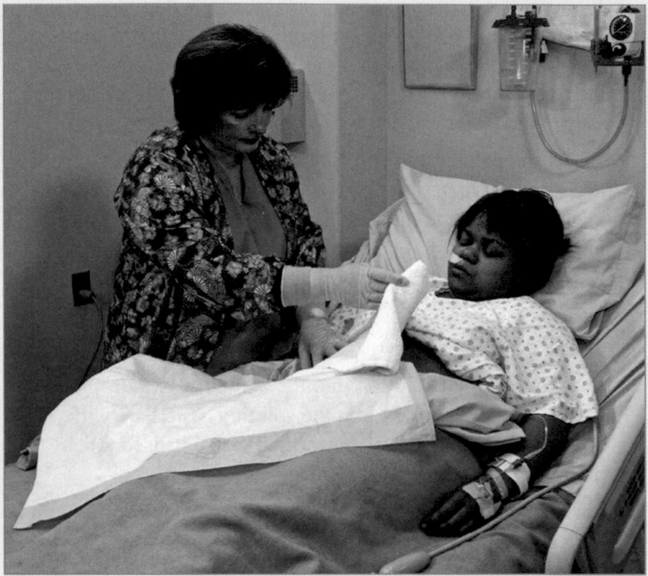

FIGURE 3 Applying clean bath towel.

ACTION	RATIONALE
14. Place the Aquathermia or heating device, if used, over the towel.	Use of heating device maintains the temperature of the compress and extends the therapeutic effect.
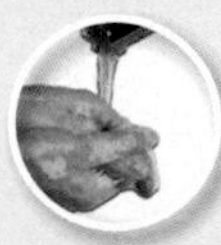 15. Remove gloves and discard them appropriately. Perform hand hygiene and remove additional PPE, if used.	Hand hygiene prevents the spread of microorganisms. Removing PPE properly reduces the risk for infection transmission and contamination of other items.
16. **Monitor the time the compress is in place to prevent burns and skin/tissue damage. Monitor the condition of the patient's skin and the patient's response at frequent intervals.**	Extended use of heat results in an increased risk for burns from the heat. Impaired circulation may affect the patient's sensitivity to heat.
17. After the prescribed time for the treatment (up to 30 minutes), remove the external heating device (if used). Put on gloves.	Gloves protect the nurse from potential contact with microorganisms.
18. Carefully remove the compress while assessing the skin condition around the site and observing the patient's response to the heat application. Note any changes in the application area.	Assessment provides information about the healing process; the presence of irritation or infection should be documented.
19. Remove gloves. Place the patient in a comfortable position. Lower the bed. Dispose of any other supplies appropriately.	Repositioning promotes patient comfort and safety.
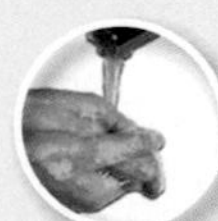 20. Remove additional PPE, if used. Perform hand hygiene.	Removing PPE properly reduces the risk for infection transmission and contamination of other items. Hand hygiene prevents the spread of microorganisms.

EVALUATION

The expected outcome is met when the patient reports relief of symptoms, such as decreased inflammation, pain, or muscle spasms. In addition, the patient remains free of signs and symptoms of injury.

DOCUMENTATION

Guidelines

Document the procedure, the length of time the compress was applied, including any use of an Aquathermia pad. Record the temperature of the Aquathermia pad and length of application time. Include a description of the application area, noting any edema, redness, or ecchymosis. Document the patient's reaction to the procedure including pain assessment. Record any patient and family education provided.

Sample Documentation

> 7/6/15 0900 Left forearm with positive radial pulse, sensation and movement within normal limits, skin pale with brisk capillary refill. Left medial forearm (IV access infiltration site) positive for redness, edema; no evidence of maceration or drainage. Moist saline compress applied with Aquathermia pad set at 100°F for 30 min. Site assessed every 10 min; no evidence of injury noted. Left arm elevated on pillows.
>
> —*S. Tran, RN*

UNEXPECTED SITUATIONS AND ASSOCIATED INTERVENTIONS

- *The nurse is monitoring a patient with a warm compress. Procedure requires that the nurse check the area of application every 5 minutes for tissue tolerance. The nurse notes excessive redness and slight maceration of the surrounding skin, and the patient verbalizes increased discomfort:* Stop the heat application. Remove the compress. Assess the patient for other symptoms. Obtain vital signs. Report the findings to the primary care provider and document the event in the patient's record.

SPECIAL CONSIDERATIONS

- Patients with diabetes, stroke, spinal cord injury, and peripheral neuropathy are at risk for thermal injury, as are patients with very thin or damaged skin.
- Be extremely careful when applying to heat-sensitive areas, such as scar tissue and stomas.

Older Adult Considerations

- Older adults are more at risk for skin and tissue damage because of their thin skin, loss of heat sensation, decreased subcutaneous tissue, and changes in the body's ability to regulate temperature. Check these patients more frequently during therapy.

SKILL 8-16 ASSISTING WITH A SITZ BATH

Sitz baths are a method of applying tepid or warm water to the perineal or rectal areas by sitting in a basin filled with this water. A sitz bath can help relieve pain and discomfort in the perineal area, such as after childbirth or surgery, and can increase circulation to the tissues, promoting healing.

DELEGATION CONSIDERATIONS

Assisting with a sitz bath may be delegated to nursing assistive personnel (NAP) or to unlicensed assistive personnel (UAP), as well as to licensed practical/vocational nurses (LPN/LVNs). The decision to delegate must be based on careful analysis of the patient's needs and circumstances, as well as the qualifications of the person to whom the task is being delegated. Refer to the Delegation Guidelines in Appendix A.

EQUIPMENT

- Clean gloves
- Additional PPE, as indicated
- Towel
- Adjustable IV pole
- Disposable sitz bath bowl with water bag

ASSESSMENT

Review any orders related to the sitz bath. Determine patient's ability to ambulate to the bathroom and maintain a sitting position for 15 to 20 minutes. Prior to the sitz bath, inspect perineal/rectal area for swelling, drainage, redness, warmth, and tenderness. Assess bladder fullness and encourage patient to void before sitz bath.

(continued)

SKILL 8-16 ASSISTING WITH A SITZ BATH continued

NURSING DIAGNOSIS

Determine related factors for the nursing diagnoses based on the patient's current status. Possible nursing diagnoses may include:

- Acute Pain
- Risk for Infection
- Impaired Tissue Integrity

OUTCOME IDENTIFICATION AND PLANNING

The expected outcome to achieve when administering a sitz bath is that the patient states an increase in comfort. Other outcomes that may be appropriate include the following: the patient experiences a decrease in healing time, maintains normal body temperature, remains free of any signs and symptoms of infection, and exhibits signs and symptoms of healing.

IMPLEMENTATION

ACTION	RATIONALE
1. Review the medical order for the application of a sitz bath, including frequency and length of time for the application. Gather necessary supplies.	Reviewing the order and plan of care validates the correct patient and correct procedure. Preparation promotes efficient time management and an organized approach to the task.
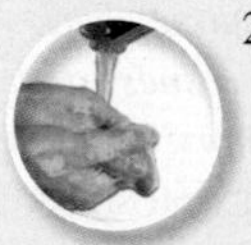 2. Perform hand hygiene and put on PPE, if indicated.	Hand hygiene and PPE prevent the spread of microorganisms. PPE is required based on transmission precautions.
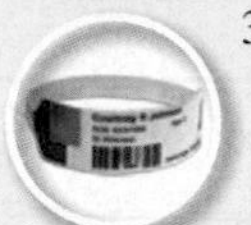 3. Identify the patient.	Identifying the patient ensures the right patient receives the intervention and helps prevent errors.
4. Close the curtains around the bed and close the door to the room, if possible.	This ensures the patient's privacy.
5. Put on gloves. Assemble equipment either at the bedside if using a bedside commode or in the bathroom.	Gloves prevent exposure to blood and body fluids. Organization facilitates performance of task.
6. Raise lid of toilet or commode. Place bowl of sitz bath, with drainage ports to rear and infusion port in front, in the toilet (Figure 1). Fill bowl of sitz bath about halfway full with tepid to warm water (98°F to 115°F [37°C to 46°C]).	Sitz bath will not drain appropriately if placed in toilet backwards. Tepid water can promote relaxation and help with edema; warm water can help with circulation.

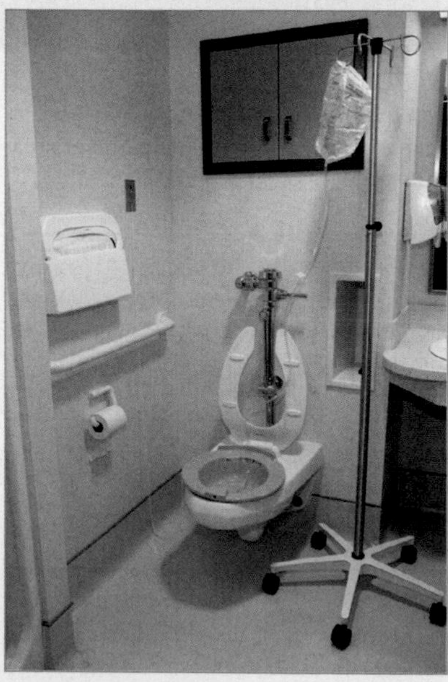

FIGURE 1 Disposable sitz bath.

ACTION	RATIONALE
7. Clamp tubing on bag. Fill bag with same temperature water as mentioned above. Hang bag above patient's shoulder height on the IV pole.	If bag is hung lower, the flow rate will not be sufficient and water may cool too quickly.
8. Assist patient to sit on toilet or commode. The patient should be able to sit in the basin or tub with the feet flat on the floor without any pressure on the sacrum or thighs. Wrap a blanket around the shoulders and provide extra draping, if needed. Insert tubing into the infusion port of the sitz bath. Slowly unclamp tubing and allow the sitz bath to fill.	Excessive pressure on sacrum or thighs could cause tissue injury. Blanket and draping protects from chilling and exposure. If tubing is placed into the sitz bath before the patient sits on the toilet, the patient may trip over tubing. Filling the sitz bath ensures that the tissue is submerged in water.
9. Clamp tubing once sitz bath is full. Instruct patient to open clamp when water in bowl becomes cool. **Ensure that call bell is within reach. Instruct patient to call if he or she feels light-headed or dizzy or has any problems. Instruct patient not to try standing without assistance.**	Cool water may produce hypothermia. Patient may become light-headed due to vasodilation, so call bell should be within reach.
10. Remove gloves and perform hand hygiene.	Hand hygiene deters the spread of microorganisms.
11. When patient is finished (in about 15 to 20 minutes, or prescribed time), put on clean gloves. Assist the patient to stand and gently pat perineal area dry. Remove gloves. Assist patient to bed or chair. Ensure that call bell is within reach.	Gloves prevent contact with blood and body fluids. Patient may be light-headed and dizzy due to vasodilation. Patient should not stand alone, and bending over to dry self may cause patient to fall.
12. Put on gloves. Empty and disinfect sitz bath bowl according to agency policy.	Proper equipment cleaning deters the spread of microorganisms.
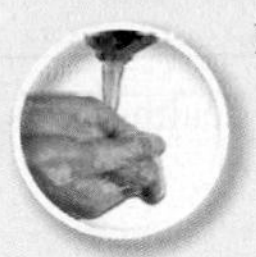 13. Remove gloves and any additional PPE, if used. Perform hand hygiene.	Removing PPE properly reduces the risk for infection transmission and contamination of other items. Hand hygiene prevents the spread of microorganisms.

EVALUATION

The expected outcomes are met when the patient verbalizes a decrease in pain or discomfort, patient tolerates sitz bath without incident, area remains clean and dry, and patient demonstrates signs of healing.

DOCUMENTATION

Guidelines

Document administration of the sitz bath, including water temperature and duration. Document patient response, and assessment of perineum before and after administration.

Sample Documentation

7/30/15 1620 Perineum assessed. Episiotomy mediolateral; edges well approximated, no drainage noted. Patient assisted to sitz bath. Patient took warm water sitz bath (temperature 99°F) for 20 minutes. Denies feeling light-headed or dizzy. Assisted back to bed after bath. Patient states pain level has dropped "from a 5 to a 2."

—*C. Stone, RN*

UNEXPECTED SITUATIONS AND ASSOCIATED INTERVENTIONS

- *Patient complains of feeling light-headed or dizzy during sitz bath:* Stop sitz bath. Do not attempt to ambulate patient alone. Use call bell to summon help. Let patient sit on toilet until feeling subsides or help has arrived to assist patient back to bed.
- *Temperature of water is uncomfortable:* The water may be too warm or cold, depending on the patient's preference. If this happens, clamp the tubing, disconnect the water bag, and refill it with water that is comfortable for the patient, but no warmer than 115°F (46°C).

SKILL 8-17 APPLYING COLD THERAPY

Cold constricts the peripheral blood vessels, reducing blood flow to the tissues and decreasing the local release of pain-producing substances. Cold reduces the formation of edema and inflammation, reduces muscle spasm, and promotes comfort by slowing the transmission of pain stimuli. The application of cold therapy (hypothermia therapy) reduces bleeding and hematoma formation. The application of cold, using ice, is appropriate after direct trauma, for dental pain, for muscle spasms, after muscle sprains, and for the treatment of chronic pain. Ice can be used to apply cold therapy, usually in the form of an ice bag or ice collar, or in a glove. Commercially prepared cold packs are also available. For electronically controlled cooling devices, see the accompanying Skill Variation.

DELEGATION CONSIDERATIONS

The application of cold therapy may be delegated to nursing assistive personnel (NAP) or to unlicensed assistive personnel (UAP), as well as to licensed practical/vocational nurses (LPN/LVNs). The decision to delegate must be based on careful analysis of the patient's needs and circumstances, as well as the qualifications of the person to whom the task is being delegated. Refer to the Delegation Guidelines in Appendix A.

EQUIPMENT

- Ice
- Ice bag, ice collar, glove
- Commercially prepared cold packs
- Small towel or washcloth
- PPE, as indicated
- Disposable waterproof pad
- Gauze wrap or tape
- Bath blanket

ASSESSMENT

Assess the situation to determine the appropriateness for the application of cold therapy. Assess the patient's physical and mental status and the condition of the body area to be treated with the cold therapy. Confirm the medical order, including frequency, type of therapy, body area to be treated, and length of time for the application. Assess the equipment to be used to make sure it will function properly.

NURSING DIAGNOSIS

Determine the related factors for the nursing diagnoses based on the patient's current health status. Appropriate nursing diagnoses may include:

- Acute Pain
- Delayed Surgical Recovery
- Chronic Pain

OUTCOME IDENTIFICATION AND PLANNING

The expected outcome to achieve when applying an external cold source depends on the patient's nursing diagnosis. Outcomes that may be appropriate include the following: the patient experiences increased comfort; the patient experiences decreased muscle spasms; the patient experiences decreased inflammation; and the patient does not show signs of bleeding or hematoma at the treatment site.

IMPLEMENTATION

ACTION	RATIONALE
1. Review the medical order or nursing plan of care for the application of cold therapy, including frequency, type of therapy, body area to be treated, and length of time for the application. Gather necessary supplies.	Reviewing the order validates the correct patient and correct procedure. Preparation promotes efficient time management and an organized approach to the task.
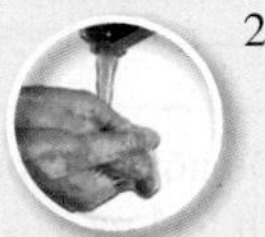 2. Perform hand hygiene and put on PPE, if indicated.	Hand hygiene and PPE prevent the spread of microorganisms. PPE is required based on transmission precautions.
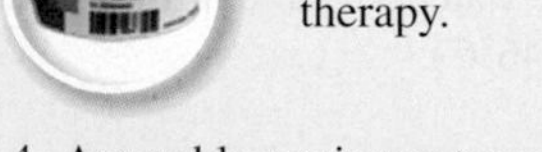 3. Identify the patient. Determine if the patient has had any previous adverse reaction to hypothermia therapy.	Identifying the patient ensures the right patient receives the intervention and helps prevent errors. Individual differences exist in tolerating specific therapies.
4. Assemble equipment on overbed table within reach.	Organization facilitates performance of task.
5. Close the curtains around the bed and close the door to the room, if possible. Explain what you are going to do and why you are going to do it to the patient.	This ensures the patient's privacy. Explanation relieves anxiety and facilitates cooperation.

ACTION	RATIONALE
6. Assess the condition of the skin where the cold is to be applied.	Assessment supplies baseline data for post-treatment comparison and identifies any conditions that may contraindicate the application.
7. Assist the patient to a comfortable position that provides easy access to the area to be treated. Expose the area and drape the patient with a bath blanket, if needed. Put the waterproof pad under the wound area, if necessary.	Patient positioning and use of a bath blanket provide for comfort and warmth. Waterproof pad protects the patient and the bed linens.
8. Prepare device: Fill the bag, collar, or glove about three-fourths full with ice (Figure 1). **Remove any excess air from the device.** Securely fasten the end of the bag or collar; tie the glove closed, checking for holes and leakage of water. Prepare commercially prepared ice pack, according to manufacturer's directions, if appropriate.	Ice provides a cold surface. Excess air interferes with cold conduction. Fastening the end prevents leaks.
9. **Cover the device with a towel or washcloth; commercially prepared devices may come with a cover (Figure 2).** (If the device has a cloth exterior, this is not necessary.)	The cover protects the skin and absorbs condensation.
10. Position cooling device on top of designated area and lightly secure in place, as needed (Figure 3).	Proper positioning ensures the cold therapy to the specified body area.

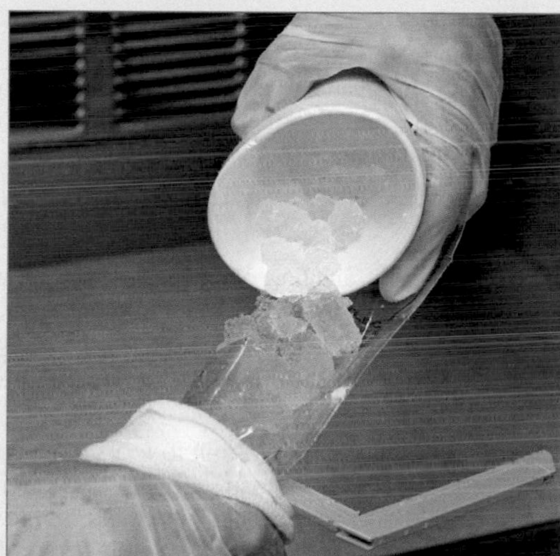
FIGURE 1 Filling ice bag with ice.

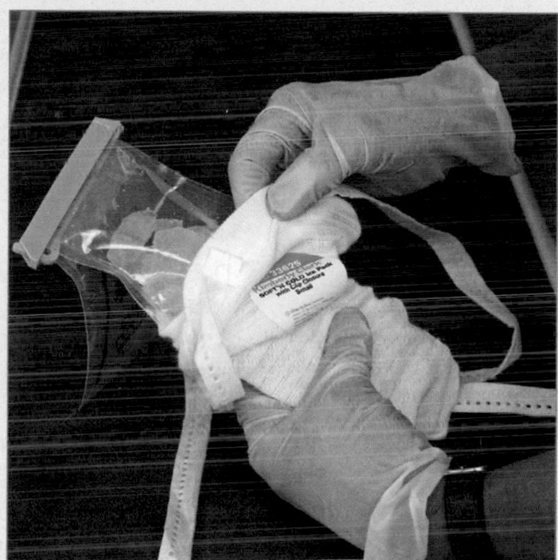
FIGURE 2 Wrapping ice bag with cover.

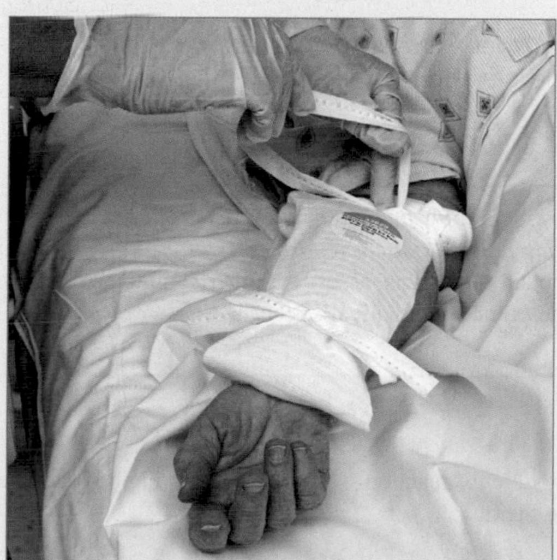
FIGURE 3 Applying cloth-wrapped bag and securing in place.

(continued)

SKILL 8-17 APPLYING COLD THERAPY continued

ACTION	RATIONALE
11. **Remove the ice and assess the site for redness after 30 seconds. Ask the patient about the presence of burning sensations.**	These actions prevent tissue injury.
12. Replace the device snugly against the site if no problems are evident. Secure it in place with gauze wrap, ties, or tape.	Wrapping or taping stabilizes the device in the proper location.
13. Reassess the treatment area every 5 minutes or according to facility policy.	Assessment of the patient's skin is necessary for early detection of adverse effects, thereby allowing prompt intervention to avoid complications.
14. **After 20 minutes or the prescribed amount of time, remove the ice and dry the skin.**	Limiting the time of application prevents injury due to overexposure to cold. Prolonged application of cold may result in decreased blood flow with resulting tissue **ischemia**. A compensatory vasodilation or rebound phenomenon may occur as a means to provide warmth to the area.
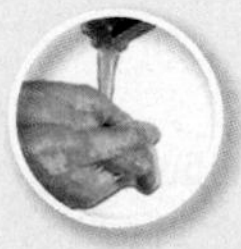 15. Remove PPE, if used. Perform hand hygiene.	Removing PPE properly reduces the risk for infection transmission and contamination of other items. Hand hygiene prevents the spread of microorganisms.

EVALUATION

The expected outcome is met when the patient reports relief of pain and increased comfort. Other outcomes that may be appropriate include the following: patient verbalizes a decrease in muscle spasms; the patient exhibits a reduction in inflammation; and the patient remains free of any injury, including signs of bleeding or hematoma at the treatment site.

DOCUMENTATION

Guidelines

Document the location of the application, time of placement, and time of removal. Record the assessment of the area where the cold therapy was applied, including the patient's mobility, sensation, color, temperature, and any presence of numbness, tingling, or pain. Document the patient's response, such as any decrease in pain or change in sensation. Include any pertinent patient and family education.

Sample Documentation

11/1/15 1430 Swelling noted on right lower extremity from mid-calf to foot. Toes warm, pink, positive sensation and movement, negative for numbness, tingling, and pain. Ice bags wrapped in cloth applied to right ankle and lower calf. Patient instructed to communicate any changes in sensation or pain; verbalizes an understanding of information.

—L. Semet, RN

11/1/15 1450 Ice removed from right lower extremity; neurovascular assessment unchanged. Right lower extremity elevated on two pillows.

—L. Semet, RN

UNEXPECTED SITUATIONS AND ASSOCIATED INTERVENTIONS

- *When performing a skin assessment during therapy, the nurse notes increased pallor at the treatment site and sluggish capillary refill, and the patient reports alterations in sensation at the application site:* Discontinue therapy, obtain vital signs, assess for other symptoms, notify the primary care provider, and document the event in the patient's record.

SPECIAL CONSIDERATIONS

General Considerations

- The patient may experience a secondary defense reaction, vasodilation, causing body temperature to rebound, defeating the purpose of the therapy.

Older Adult Considerations

- Older adults are more at risk for skin and tissue damage because of their thin skin, loss of cold sensation, decreased subcutaneous tissue, and changes in the body's ability to regulate temperature. Check these patients more frequently during therapy.

SKILL VARIATION Applying an Electronically Controlled Cooling Device

Electronically controlled cooling devices are used in situations to deliver a constant cooling effect. After orthopedic surgery, those patients as well as other patients with acute musculoskeletal injuries may benefit from this therapy. A medical order is required for use of this device. Initial assessment of the extremity is involved, as well as ongoing assessment throughout the period of use. As with application of any electronic device, ongoing monitoring for proper functioning and temperature regulation is necessary.

1. Gather equipment and verify the medical order.

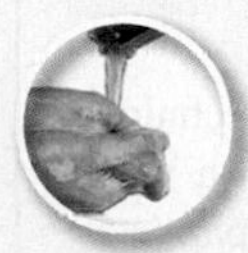

2. Perform hand hygiene. Put on PPE, as indicated.

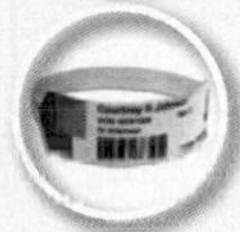

3. Identify the patient and explain the procedure.
4. Assess the involved extremity or body part.
5. Set the correct temperature on the device.
6. Wrap the cooling water-flow pad around the involved body part.
7. Wrap an Ace bandage or gauze pads around the water-flow pads.
8. Assess to ensure that the cooling pads are functioning properly.

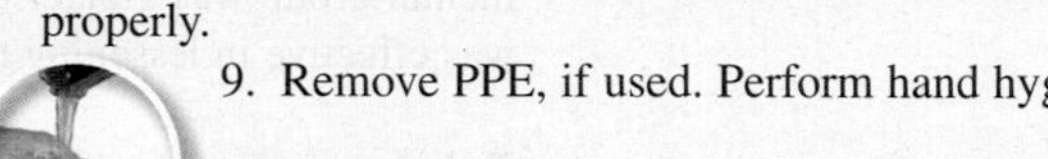

9. Remove PPE, if used. Perform hand hygiene.
10. Recheck frequently to ensure proper functioning of equipment.
11. Unwrap at intervals to assess skin integrity of the body part.

EVIDENCE FOR PRACTICE ▶

COLD APPLICATION AND PAIN RELIEF

Chest tube removal is a painful procedure for many, if not most, patients. Pharmacologic and nonpharmacologic interventions have been used to decrease patients' discomfort during this procedure.

Related Research

Ertuğ, N., & Ülker, S. (2011). The effect of cold application on pain due to chest tube removal. *Journal of Clinical Nursing, 21*(5/6), 784–790.

The objective of this study was to determine whether the application of cold to the chest wall had an effect on pain related to chest tube removal. The study was conducted with 140 patients, divided evenly between an experimental group and a control group. Data were collected regarding the patient's demographic and health history. Skin temperature and pain intensity, using a Visual Analogue Scale, was measured at various points before and after the tube removal process. There were significant differences related to pain between the two groups. Age, gender, the number of days the chest tube was inserted had no effect on the pain related to chest tube removal. This study concluded that the application of cold is effective in reducing the pain related to removal of a chest tube.

Relevance for Nursing Practice

Nursing interventions related to decreasing pain and increasing patient comfort are an important nursing responsibility. Interventions should include the use of nonpharmacologic interventions, in addition to the administration of analgesics. The application of cold to the chest wall could significantly decrease the pain and discomfort experienced by a patient during removal of a chest tube. Nurses could easily incorporate this simple intervention as part of nursing care for these patients.

Refer to thePoint for additional research on related nursing topics.

(continued)

SKILL 8-17 APPLYING COLD THERAPY continued

EVIDENCE FOR PRACTICE ▶

COLD APPLICATION AND PAIN RELIEF

Pain is commonly experienced by patients after invasive procedures, such as arthroscopy. Pain management is an important nursing intervention.

Related Research

Fang, L., Hung, C.H., Wu, S.L., et al. (2011). The effects of cryotherapy in relieving postarthroscopy pain. *Journal of Clinical Nursing, 21*(5/6), 636–643.

Commercial devices can be used to provide compression and cold therapy for the postoperative patient. The objective of this study was to determine if the simple application of ice in a plastic bag was effective in relieving postarthroscopy pain. Patients (N = 59) who received arthroscopy were assigned to receive cryotherapy (experimental group) or no cryotherapy (control group). The experimental group received three 10-minute sessions of ice packing over a 3-hour period, with 50-minute intervals between each session. The first session of ice packing was applied immediately after recovery from anesthesia. The decrease of pain level in the experimental group was greater than that in the control group. Cryotherapy using ice in a plastic bag was effective in lessening the degree of pain in patients after arthroscopy.

Relevance for Nursing Practice

Cryotherapy with ice in a plastic bag is a simple, readily attainable, and cost-effective technique for relieving postarthroscopy pain. Nurses should consider the use of cold application when planning interventions for patients experiencing postoperative pain and other types of pain.

Refer to thePoint for additional research on related nursing topics.

ENHANCE YOUR UNDERSTANDING

FOCUSING ON PATIENT CARE: DEVELOPING CLINICAL REASONING

Consider the case scenarios at the beginning of the chapter as you answer the following questions to enhance your understanding and apply what you have learned.

QUESTIONS

1. While providing wound care for Lori Downs' foot ulcer, you note that the drainage, which was scant and yellow 2 days ago, is now green and has saturated the old dressing. Should you continue with the prescribed wound care?
2. Three days ago Tran Nguyen underwent a modified radical mastectomy. She has three Jackson-Pratt drains at her surgical site. She has started asking questions about her surgery and has anticipated discharge home. Until this morning, she has avoided looking at her surgical site. You are helping her with her bathing and dressing. As you help her remove her gown, she becomes visibly upset and anxious and exclaims, "Oh no! What's wrong? I'm bleeding from the cuts!" You realize she is looking at her drains. How should you respond?
3. Arthur Lowes has come to his surgeon's office today for a follow-up examination after a colon resection. After he sees the physician, you, the treatment nurse, will remove the surgical staples from the incision and apply adhesive wound strips. As you prepare to remove the staples, Mr. Lowes comments, "I hope my stomach doesn't pop out now!" What should you tell him?

You can find suggested answers after the Bibliography at the end of this chapter

INTEGRATED CASE STUDY CONNECTION

The case studies in the back of the book are designed to focus on integrating concepts. Refer to the following case studies to enhance your understanding of the concepts related to the skills in this chapter.

- Basic Case Studies: Tula Stillwater, page 1075.
- Intermediate Case Studies: Tula Stillwater, page 1081.
- Advanced Case Studies: Robert Espinoza, page 1097.

TAYLOR SUITE RESOURCES

Explore these additional resources to enhance learning for this chapter:

- NCLEX-Style Questions and other resources on thePoint, http://thePoint.lww.com/Lynn4e
- *Skill Checklists for Taylor's Clinical Nursing Skills,* 4e
- *Taylor's Video Guide to Clinical Nursing Skills:* Skin Integrity and Wound Care
- *Fundamentals of Nursing:* Chapter 31, Skin Integrity and Wound Care
- *Lippincott DocuCare* Fundamentals cases

Bibliography

Ackley, B.J., & Ladwig, G.B. (2011). *Nursing diagnosis handbook* (9th ed.). St. Louis: Mosby/Elsevier.

Agency for Healthcare Research and Quality (AHRQ). National Guideline Clearinghouse. (2011). *Pressure ulcer treatment recommendations. In: Prevention and treatment of pressure ulcers: Clinical practice guideline.* Available http://www.guideline.gov/content.aspx?id=25139&search=pressure+ulcer+treatment#Section420.

Anderson, I. (2010). Key principles involved in applying and removing wound dressings. *Nursing Standard, 25*(10), 51–57.

Association of Operating Room Nurses (AORN). (2006). Recommended practices for maintaining a sterile field. *AORN Journal, 83*(2), 402–416.

Baranoski, S., & Ayello, E.A. (2012). *Wound care essentials. Practice principles.* (3rd ed.). Philadelphia: Wolters Kluwer Health/Lippincott Williams & Wilkins.

Benbow, M. (2011). Addressing pain in wound care and dressing removal. *Nursing & Residential Care, 13*(10), 474, 476, 478.

Benbow, M. (2008a). Exploring the concept of moist wound healing and its application in practice. *British Journal of Nursing, (Tissue Viability Supplement), 17*(15), S4–S16.

Benbow, M. (2008b). Pressure ulcer prevention and pressure-relieving surfaces. *British Journal of Nursing, 17*(13), 830–835.

Bergstrom, N., Braden, B., Laguzza, A., et al. (1987). The Braden scale for predicting pressure sore risk. *Nursing Research, 36*(4), 205–210.

Bolas, N., & Holloway, S. (2012). Negative pressure wound therapy: A study on patient perspectives. *Wound Care, 17*(3 Suppl), S30–S35.

Boltz, M., Capezuti, E., Fulmer, T., et al. (Eds.). (2012). *Evidence-based geriatric nursing protocols for best practice* (4th ed.). New York: Springer Publishing Company.

Borgquist, O., Ingemansson, R., & Malmsjö, M. (2011). Individualizing the use of negative pressure wound therapy for optimal wound healing: A focused review of the literature. *Ostomy Wound Management, 57*(4), 44–54.

Braden, B., & Maklebust, J. (2005). Preventing pressure ulcers with the Braden scale. *American Journal of Nursing, 105*(6), 70–72.

Bulechek, G.M, Butcher, H.K., Dochterman, J.M., et al. (Eds.). (2013). *Nursing interventions classification (NIC)* (6th ed.). St. Louis: Mosby Elsevier.

Centers for Disease Control and Prevention (CDC). (2012). *Healthcare-associated infections (HAIs).* Available http://www.cdc.gov/hai/.

Centers for Disease Control and Prevention (CDC). (2010). *Healthcare-associated infections (HAIs). Frequently asked questions about surgical site infections.* Available http://www.cdc.gov/HAI/ssi/faq_ssi.html.

Cowdell, F. (2010). Promoting skin health in older people. *Nursing Older People, 22*(10), 21–26.

Denyer, J. (2011). Reducing pain during the removal of adhesive and adherent products. *British Journal of Nursing, 20*(15) (*Tissue Viability Supplement*), S28–S35.

Downie, F., Egdell, S., Bielby, A., et al. (2010). Barrier dressings in surgical site infection prevention strategies. *British Journal of Nursing, 19*(20) (*Tissue Viability Supplement*), S42–S46.

Dudek, S. (2014). *Nutrition essentials for nursing practice* (7th ed.). Philadelphia: Wolters Kluwer Health/Lippincott Williams & Wilkins.

Durai, R., & Ng, P.C.H. (2010). Surgical vacuum drains: Types, uses and complications. *AORN Journal, 91*(2), 266–274.

Dyble, T., & Ashton, J. (2011). Use of emollients in the treatment of dry skin conditions. *British Journal of Community Nursing, 16*(5), 214–220.

Elliott, J. (2011). Applying pressure ulcer prevention theory to practice. *Nursing & Residential Care, 13*(6), 276–279.

Ertuğ, N., & Ülker, S. (2011). The effect of cold application on pain due to chest tube removal. *Journal of Clinical Nursing, 21*(5/6), 784–790.

Fang, L., Hung, C.H., Wu, S.L., et al. (2011). The effects of cryotherapy in relieving postarthroscopy pain. *Journal of Clinical Nursing, 21*(5/6), 636–643.

Flores, A. (2008). Sterile versus non-sterile glove use and aseptic technique. *Nursing Standard, 23*(6), 35–39.

Geraghty, J. (2011). Introducing a new skin-care regimen for the incontinent patient. *British Journal of Nursing, 20*(7), 409–415.

Gould, D. (2012). Causes, prevention and management of surgical site infection. *Nursing Standard, 26*(47), 47–56.

Gupta, S., & Ichioka, S. (2010). Optimal use of negative pressure wound therapy in treating pressure ulcers. *International Wound Journal, 9*(Suppl 1), 8–16.

Harvey, C. (2005). Wound healing. *Orthopaedic Nursing, 24*(2), 143–157.

Hess, C. (2013). *Clinical guide to skin & wound care* (7th ed.). Philadelphia: Wolters Kluwer Health/Lippincott Williams & Wilkins.

Hinkle, J.L., & Cheever, K.H. (2014). *Brunner & Suddarth's textbook of medical-surgical nursing* (13th ed.). Philadelphia: Wolters Kluwer Health/Lippincott Williams & Wilkins.

Hogan-Quigley, B., Palm, M.L., & Bickley, L. (2012). *Bates' nursing guide to physical examination and history taking.* Philadelphia: Wolters Kluwer Health/Lippincott Williams & Wilkins.

Huether, S.E., & McCance, K.L. (2012.) *Understanding pathophysiology* (5th ed.). St. Louis: Elsevier.

Jarvis, C. (2012). *Physical examination & health assessment.* (6th ed.). St. Louis: Saunders/Elsevier.

Jensen, S. (2011.) *Nursing health assessment. A best practice approach.* Philadelphia: Wolters Kluwer Health/Lippincott Williams & Wilkins.

Kelly, J. (2010). Methods of wound debridement: A case study. *Nursing Standard, 25*(25), 51–56, 58–59.

Krasner, D. (1995). Wound care: How to use the red-yellow-black system. *American Journal of Nursing, 5*(95), 44–47.

Kyle, T., & Carman, S. (2013). *Essentials of pediatric nursing* (2nd ed.). Philadelphia: Wolters Kluwer Health/Lippincott Williams & Wilkins.

Lloyd Jones, M. (2012a). Choosing the appropriate barrier product. *Nursing & Residential Care, 14*(4), 184–188.

Lloyd Jones, M. (2012b). Prevention and treatment of superficial pressure damage. *Nursing & Residential Care, 14*(1), 14, 16, 18, 20.

Lloyd Jones, M. (2008). Assessing and managing wound pain during dressing changes. *Nursing & Residential Care, 10*(7), 325–330.

Malarkey, L.M., & McMorrow, M.E. (2012). *Saunders nursing guide to laboratory and diagnostic tests* (2nd ed.). St. Louis: Elsevier Saunders.

Malli, S. (2005). Device safety. Keep a close eye on vacuum-assisted wound closure. *Nursing, 35*(7), 25.

Martindell, D. (2012). Safety monitor. The safe use of negative-pressure wound therapy. *American Journal of Nursing, 112*(6), 59–63.

Medlin, S. (2012). Nutrition for wound healing. *British Journal of Nursing, 21*(12) (*Tissue Viability Supplement*), 511–513.

Moorhead, S., Johnson, M., Maas, M.L., et al. (Eds.). (2013). *Nursing outcomes classification (NOC).* (5th ed.). St. Louis: Mosby Elsevier.

NANDA International. (2012). *Nursing diagnoses: Definitions & classification 2012–2014.* West Sussex, UK: Wiley-Blackwell.

National Pressure Ulcer Advisory Panel (NPUAP). (2012a). *Educational and clinical resources. Pressure ulcer stages/categories.* Available http://www.npuap.org/resources/educational-and-clinical-resources/npuap-pressure-ulcer-stagescategories/.

National Pressure Ulcer Advisory Panel (NPUAP). (2012b). *Educational and clinical resources. Pressure ulcer staging/illustrations.* Available http://www.npuap.org/resources/educational-and-clinical-resources/pressure-ulcer-categorystaging-illustrations/.

National Pressure Ulcer Advisory Panel (NPUAP). (2012c). *Educational and clinical resources. PUSH tool.* Available http://www.npuap.org/resources/educational-and-clinical-resources/push-tool/.

National Pressure Ulcer Advisory Panel (NPUAP). (2012d). *Educational and clinical resources. Pressure ulcer prevention points.* Available at http://www.npuap.org/resources/educational-and-clinical-resources/pressure-ulcer-prevention-points/.

Nilsson, S., & Renning, A-C. (2012). Pain management during wound dressing in children. *Nursing Standard, 26*(32), 50–55.

O'Tuathall, C., & Taqi, R. (2011). Evaluation of three commonly used pressure ulcer risk assessment scales. *British Journal of Nursing, 20*(6) (*Tissue Viability Supplement*), S27–S34.

Parnham, A. (2012). Pressure ulcer risk assessment and prevention in children. *Nursing Children and Young People, 24*(2), 24–29.

Pegram, A., & Bloomfield, J. (2010). Wound care: Principles of aseptic technique. *Mental Health Practice, 14*(2), 14–18.

Perry, S.E., Hockenberry, M.J., Lowdermilk, D.L., et al. (2010). *Maternal child nursing care* (4th ed.). Maryland Heights, MO: Mosby/Elsevier.

Porth, C., & Matfin, G. (2009). *Pathophysiology: Concepts of altered health states* (8th ed.). Philadelphia: Wolters Kluwer Health/Lippincott Williams & Wilkins.

Posthauer, M.E. (2012). Nutrition strategies for wound healing. *Journal of Legal Nurse Consulting, 23*(1), 15–23.

Preston, G. (2008). An overview of topical negative pressure therapy in wound care. *Nursing Standard, 23*(7), 62–68.

Ritter, L.A., & Hoffman, N.A. (2010). *Multicultural health.* Boston: Jones and Bartlett.

Rudoni, C. (2008). A service evaluation of the use of silicone-based adhesive remover. *British Journal of Nursing, (Stoma Care Supplement), 17*(2), S4, S6, S8–S9.

Spear, M. (2012). Wound exudate: The good, the bad, and the ugly. *Plastic Surgical Nursing, 32*(2), 77–79.

Spector, R.E. (2009). *Cultural diversity in health and illness* (7th ed.). Upper Saddle River, NJ: Pearson/Prentice Hall.

Sprigle, S., & Sonenblum, S. (2011). Assessing the evidence supporting redistribution of pressure for pressure ulcer prevention: A review. *Journal of Rehabilitation Research & Development, 48*(3), 203–214.

Stephen-Hayes, J. (2012). Skin tears: Achieving positive clinical and financial outcomes. *British Journal of Community Nursing,* (3 Suppl), S6–S16.

Stephen-Hayes, J. (2011). Managing exudate and the key requirements of absorbent dressings. *British Journal of Nursing, 16*(Suppl), S44–S49.

Stephen-Haynes, J. (2008). Skin integrity and silicone: APPEEL 'no-sting' medical adhesive remover. *British Journal of Nursing, 17*(12), 792–795.

Stotts, N. (1990). Seeing red, yellow and black: The three-color concept of wound care. *Nursing, 20*(2), 59–61.

Sullivan, J.M. (2011). Caring for older adults after surgery. *Nursing, 41*(4), 48–51.

Tabloski, P. (2010). *Gerontological nursing* (2nd ed.). Upper Saddle River, NJ: Pearson.

Taylor, C., Lillis, C., & Lynn, P. (2015). *Fundamentals of nursing.* (7th ed.). Philadelphia: Wolters Kluwer Health/Lippincott Williams & Wilkins.

Taylor, J.J., & Cohen, B.J. (2013). *Memmler's structure and function of the human body* (10th ed.). Philadelphia: Wolters Kluwer Health/Lippincott Williams & Wilkins.

Thompson, G. (2008). An overview of negative pressure wound therapy (NPWT). *Wound Care,* 13(6), S23–S24, S26, S28–S30.

VISN 8 Patient Safety Center. (2009). *Safe patient handling and movement algorithms.* Tampa, FL: Author. Available at http://www.visn8.va.gov/patientsafetycenter/safePtHandling. Accessed April 23, 2010.

Voegeli, D. (2012). Moisture-associated skin damage: Aetiology, prevention and treatment. *British Journal of Nursing, 21*(9), 517–518, 520–521.

Voegeli, D. (2010). Care or harm: Exploring essential components in skin care regimens. *British Journal of Nursing, 19*(13), 810, 812, 814, 816, 818–819.

Walker, J. (2007). Patient preparation for safe removal of surgical drains. *Nursing Standard, 21*(49), 39–41.

White, R. (2011). Wound dressings and other topical treatment modalities in bioburden control. *Journal of Wound Care, 20*(9), 431–439.

Woo, K.Y. (2012). Exploring the effects of pain and stress on wound healing. *Advances in Skin & Wound Care, 25*(1), 38–44.

The Wound Healing and Management Node Group. Joanna Briggs Institute. (2011). Wet-to-dry saline moistened gauze for wound dressing. *Wound Practice and Research, 19*(1), 48–49.

Wound, Ostomy and Continence Nurses Society (WOCN). (2012). Clean vs. sterile dressing techniques for management of chronic wounds. A fact sheet. *Journal of Wound, Ostomy and Continence Nursing, 39* (2S) (Suppl), S30–S34.

SUGGESTED ANSWERS FOR FOCUSING ON PATIENT CARE: DEVELOPING CLINICAL REASONING

1. This is a significant change in the patient's assessment. Perform a thorough wound assessment and obtain vital signs. Assess the patient for any new symptoms, such as increased pain, chills, or abnormal sensation (e.g., numbness, tingling). Report findings to the primary care provider; a change in wound care, additional assessments (e.g., diagnostic tests, laboratory tests), or change/addition of medication may be required.
2. Reassure the patient regarding her wound status. Explain what the drains are, how they work, and their intended purpose. Provide information regarding wound care, drain care, and recording of drainage amounts. Discuss anticipated care requirements at home and potential arrangements to ensure required care is performed, either by the patient or significant other.
3. Reassure the patient regarding his wound status. Explain the purpose of the staples, the process of wound healing, and the purpose of adhesive wound strips. Discuss the patient's responsibilities for wound care at this point in his healing.

9 Activity

FOCUSING ON PATIENT CARE

This chapter will help you develop some of the skills related to activity necessary to care for the following patients:

BOBBY ROWDEN, age 8, was knocked down during soccer practice and has come to the emergency room with pain, swelling, and deformity of his right forearm. He is diagnosed with a fracture.

ESTHER LEVITZ, age 58, has been admitted to the hospital with nausea, anorexia, debilitating fatigue, and weight loss. Her underlying diagnosis of lymphoma and inactivity put her at risk for thrombus formation.

MANUEL ESPOSITO, age 72, is scheduled for surgery tomorrow to repair a fractured hip. His physician has ordered skin traction to immobilize the injury before surgery.

Refer to Focusing on Patient Care: Developing Clinical Reasoning at the end of the chapter to apply what you learn.

LEARNING OBJECTIVES

After studying this chapter, you will be able to:

1. Assist a patient with turning in bed.
2. Move a patient up in bed with the assistance of another caregiver.
3. Transfer a patient from the bed to a stretcher.
4. Transfer a patient from the bed to a chair.
5. Transfer a patient using a full-powered body sling lift.
6. Provide range-of-motion exercises.
7. Assist a patient with ambulation.
8. Assist a patient with ambulation using a walker.
9. Assist a patient with ambulation using crutches.
10. Assist a patient with ambulation using a cane.
11. Apply and remove graduated compression stockings.
12. Apply pneumatic compression devices.
13. Apply a continuous passive motion device.
14. Apply a sling.
15. Apply a figure-eight bandage.
16. Assist with a cast application.
17. Care for a patient with a cast.
18. Apply and care for a patient in skin traction.
19. Care for a patient in skeletal traction.
20. Care for a patient with an external fixation device.

KEY TERMS

abduction: movement away from the center or median line of the body
adduction: movement toward the center or median line of the body
arthroplasty: surgical formation or reformation of a joint
compartment syndrome: occurs when there is increased tissue pressure within a limited space; leads to compromises in the circulation and the function of the involved tissue
contracture: permanent shortening or tightening of a muscle due to spasm or paralysis
contusion: an injury in which the skin is not broken; a bruise
deep-vein thrombosis: a blood clot in a blood vessel originating in the large veins of the legs
extension: the return movement from flexion; the joint angle is increased
flexion: bending of a joint so that the angle of the joint diminishes
fracture: a break in the continuity of a bone
goniometer: an apparatus to measure joint movement and angles
hyperextension: extreme or abnormal extension
orthostatic hypotension: an abnormal drop in blood pressure that occurs as a person changes from a supine to a standing position
patient care ergonomics: the practice of designing equipment and work tasks to conform to the capability of the worker in relation to patient care. It provides a means for adjusting the work environment and work practices to prevent injuries before they occur and is part of best practices for providing safe patient care (VISN 8 Patient Safety Center, 2009; Occupational Safety & Health Administration [OSHA], 2003).
peripheral vascular disease: pathologic conditions of the vascular system characterized by reduced blood flow through the peripheral blood vessels
pronation: the act of lying face downward; the act of turning the hand so the palm faces downward or backward
rotation: process of turning on an axis; twisting or revolving
shearing force: force created by the interplay of gravity and friction on the skin and underlying tissues; shear causes tissue layers to slide over one another and blood vessels to stretch and twist and disrupts the microcirculation of the skin and subcutaneous tissue
supination: turning of the palm or foot upward
thrombophlebitis: a blood clot that accompanies vein inflammation
thrombosis: the formation or development of a blood clot
venous stasis: decrease in blood flow in the venous system related to dysfunctional valves or inactivity of the muscles of the affected extremity

The ability to move is closely related to the fulfillment of other basic human needs. Regular exercise contributes to the healthy functioning of each body system. Conversely, lack of exercise and immobility affect each body system negatively. A summary of the effects of immobility on the body is outlined in Fundamentals Review 9-1. An important nursing role is to encourage activity and exercise to promote wellness, prevent illness, and restore health.

Nursing interventions are directed at preventing potential problems and treating actual problems related to a patient's activity and mobility status. Strategies designed to promote correct body alignment, mobility, and fitness are important parts of nursing care. Nurses use knowledge of body mechanics, mobility, and safe patient-handling techniques along with specific nursing interventions to promote fitness and to resolve mobility problems. See Fundamentals Review 9-2: Principles of Body Mechanics.

Nurses lift, carry, push, pull, and move objects and people routinely in the course of their work. Performing these actions correctly is necessary to avoid musculoskeletal strain and injury. Body mechanics include proper body movement in daily activities, the prevention and correction of problems associated with posture, and the enhancement of coordination and endurance. When promoting activity for a patient, the safety of the patient and the nurse is extremely important. Research has shown that body mechanics and lifting techniques alone are not enough to establish a safe environment of care for nurses and patients to prevent musculoskeletal disorders and injuries related to patient handling tasks (American Nurses Association [ANA], 2013; VISN 8 Patient Safety Center, 2009; Waters et al., 2009). **Patient care ergonomics** is the practice of designing equipment and work tasks to conform to the capability of the worker in relation to patient care. It provides a means for adjusting the work environment and work practices to prevent injuries before they occur and is part of best practices for providing safe patient care (VISN 8 Patient Safety Center, 2009). It is imperative to use principles of body mechanics and ergonomics in conjunction with safe patient handling and movement techniques and aids when handling and moving patients. An effective approach to safe patient transfers is thought to include patient assessment criteria; algorithms for patient handling and movement decisions; specialized patient handling equipment, used properly, and operated using good body mechanics; and the use of lift teams (Nelson, Motacki, & Menzel, 2009). The Occupational Safety and Health Administration (OSHA, 2012) recommends a no lift policy for all health care facilities. Instead, it recommends using patient handling aids and mechanical lifting equipment on patients who are unable to assist in their transfer. Always check institution practices and guidelines and available equipment related to safe patient handling and movement. Samples of algorithms to aid decision-making to prevent injury to staff and patients during patient movement and handling are provided in the appropriate skills. When using any equipment, check for proper functioning before using with the patient. Fundamentals Review 9-3 presents guidelines for safe patient handling and movement. Fundamentals Review 9-4 discusses examples of equipment and assistive devices that are available to aid with safe patient movement and handling. Fundamentals Review 9-5 provides an example of an assessment tool to aid in patient assessment and decision-making regarding safe patient handling and movement.

This chapter covers skills to assist the nurse in providing care related to activity, inactivity, and health care problems related to the musculoskeletal system.

FUNDAMENTALS REVIEW 9-1

EFFECTS OF IMMOBILITY ON THE BODY

- Decreased muscle strength and tone, decreased muscle size
- Decreased joint mobility and flexibility
- Limited endurance and activity intolerance
- Bone demineralization
- Lack of coordination and altered gait
- Decreased ventilatory effort and increased respiratory secretions, atelectasis, respiratory congestion
- Increased cardiac workload, **orthostatic hypotension**, venous **thrombosis**
- Impaired circulation and skin breakdown
- Decreased appetite, constipation
- Urinary stasis, infection
- Altered sleep patterns, pain, depression, anger, anxiety

FUNDAMENTALS REVIEW 9-2

PRINCIPLES OF BODY MECHANICS

- Correct body alignment is important to prevent undue strain on joints, muscles, tendons, and ligaments while maintaining balance.
- Face the direction of your movement. Avoid twisting your body.
- Maintaining balance involves keeping the spine in vertical alignment, body weight close to the center of gravity, and feet spread for a broad base of support.
- Using the body's major muscle groups and natural levers and fulcrums allows for coordinated movement to avoid musculoskeletal strain and injury.
- Assess the situation before acting so that you can plan to use good body mechanics.
- Use the large muscle groups in the legs to provide force for movement. Keep the back straight, with hips and knees bent. Slide, roll, push, or pull rather than lift an object.
- Perform work at the appropriate height for your body position, close to your center of gravity.
- Use mechanical lifts and/or assistance to ease the movement.

FUNDAMENTALS REVIEW 9-3

GUIDELINES FOR SAFE PATIENT HANDLING AND MOVEMENT

Keep the patient in good alignment and protect from injury while being moved. Follow these recommended guidelines when moving and lifting patients:

- Assess the patient. Know the patient's medical diagnosis, capabilities, and any movement not allowed. Put in place braces or any device the patient wears before helping the patient from the bed.
- Assess the patient's ability to assist with the planned movement. Encourage the patient to assist in own transfers. Encouraging the patient to perform tasks that are within his or her capabilities promotes independence. Eliminating or reducing unnecessary tasks by the nurse reduces the risk of injury.
- Assess the patient's ability to understand instructions and cooperate with the staff to achieve the movement. (See Box 9-1 in Skill 9-1 for general guidelines related to mobility and safe handling of people with dementia.)
- During any patient transferring task, if any caregiver is required to lift more than 35 pounds of a patient's weight, consider the patient to be fully dependent and use assistive devices for the transfer.
- Ensure sufficient staff is available and present to move the patient safely.
- Assess the area for clutter, accessibility to the patient and availability of devices. Remove any obstacles that may make moving and lifting inconvenient.
- Decide which equipment to use. Use handling aids whenever possible to help reduce risk of injury to the nurse and patient.
- Plan carefully what you will do before moving or lifting a patient. Assess the mobility of attached equipment. You may injure the patient or yourself if you have not planned well. If necessary, enlist the support of another nurse. This reduces the strain on everyone involved. Communicate the plan with staff and the patient, to ensure coordinated movement.
- Explain to the patient what you plan to do. Then, use what abilities the patient has to assist you. This technique often decreases the effort required and the possibility of injury to you.
- If the patient is in pain, administer the prescribed analgesic sufficiently in advance of the transfer to allow the patient to participate in the move comfortably.
- Elevate the bed, as necessary, so that you are working at a height that is comfortable and safe for you.
- Lock the wheels of the bed, wheelchair, or stretcher so that they do not slide while you are moving the patient.
- Observe the principles of body mechanics to prevent injuring yourself while you work.
- Be sure the patient is in good body alignment while being moved and lifted to protect the patient from strain and muscle injury.
- Support the patient's body properly. Avoid grabbing and holding an extremity by its muscles.
- Use friction-reducing devices, whenever possible, especially during lateral transfers.
- Move your body and the patient in a smooth, rhythmic motion. Jerky movements tend to put extra strain on muscles and joints and are uncomfortable for the patient.
- Use mechanical devices, such as lifts, slides, transfer chairs, or gait belts, for moving patients. Be sure that you understand how the device operates and that the patient is properly secured and informed of what will occur. If you are not comfortable with the operation of

FUNDAMENTALS REVIEW 9-3 continued

GUIDELINES FOR SAFE PATIENT HANDLING AND MOVEMENT

the equipment, obtain assistance from a caregiver who is. Patients who do not understand or are afraid may be unable to cooperate and may cause injury to the staff as well as suffer injury as a result.

- Assure equipment used meets weight requirements. Bariatric patients (body mass index [BMI] greater than 50) require bariatric transfer aids and equipment.

FUNDAMENTALS REVIEW 9-4

EQUIPMENT AND ASSISTIVE DEVICES

Many devices and equipment are available to aid in transferring, repositioning, and lifting patients. It is important to use the right equipment and appropriate device based on patient assessment and desired movement.

GAIT BELTS

A gait belt is a belt, often with handles. It is placed around the patient's waist and secured. The handles can be placed in a variety of configurations so the caregiver can have better access to, improved grasp, and control of the patient. Some belts are hand-held slings that go around the patient, providing a firm grasp for the caregiver and facilitating the transfer (VISN 8 Patient Safety Center, 2009). Do not use gait belts on patients with abdominal or thoracic incisions (Blocks, 2005). (See Figure A for a gait belt.)

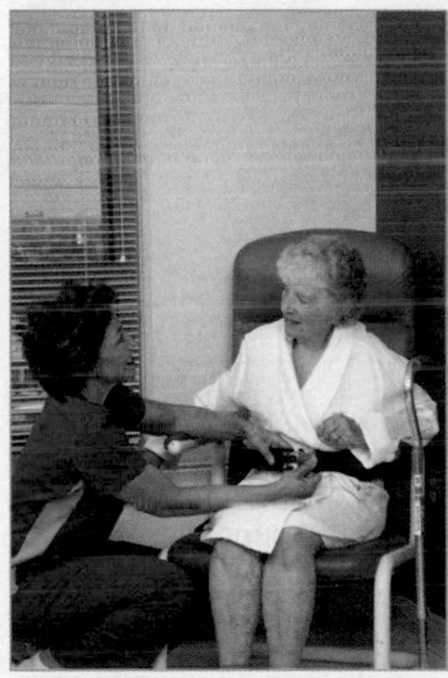

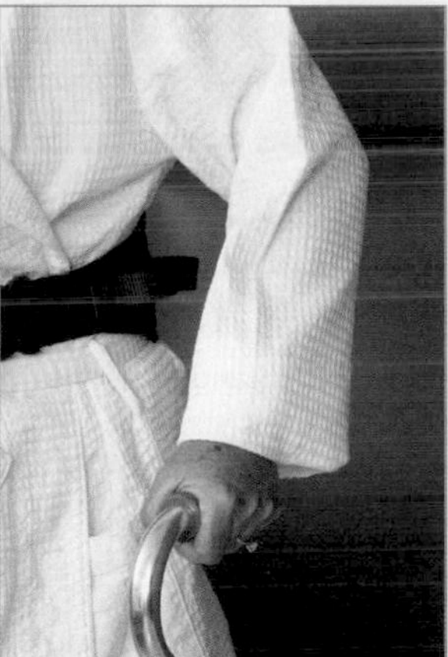

FIGURE A Using a gait belt.

STAND-ASSIST AND REPOSITIONING AIDS

Some patients need minimal assistance to stand up. With an appropriate support to grasp, they can lift themselves. Many types of secure devices can help a patient to stand. These devices are freestanding or attach to the bed or wheelchair. One type of stand-assist aid attaches to the bed. Other aids have a pull bar to assist the patient to stand, and then a seat unfolds under the patient. After sitting on the seat, the device can be wheeled to the toilet, chair, shower, or bed.

LATERAL-ASSIST DEVICES

Lateral-assist devices reduce patient-surface friction during lateral transfers. Roller boards, slide boards, transfer boards, inflatable mattresses, and friction-reducing, lateral-assist devices are examples of these devices that make transfers safer and more comfortable for the patient. An inflatable lateral-assist device is a flexible mattress that is placed under the patient. An attached, portable air supply inflates the mattress, which provides a layer of air under the patient. This air cushion allows nursing staff to perform the move with much less effort (Baptiste et al., 2006), but have been found to place the care providers at an increased risk of injury because of the horizontal reach required, posture adopted during transfer, and lack of handles (Nelson & Baptiste, 2004). Transfer boards are placed under the patient. They provide a slick surface for the patient during transfers, reducing friction and the force required to move the patient. Transfer boards are made of smooth, rigid, low-friction material, such as coated wood or plastic. Another lateral sliding aid is made of a special fabric that reduces friction. Some devices have long handles that reduce reaching by staff, to improve safety and make the transfer easier (Figure B).

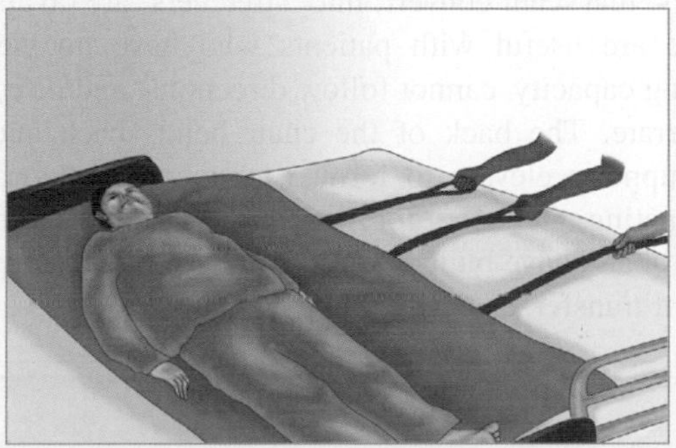

FIGURE B Lateral-assist device with long handles to reduce reaching by staff.

(continued)

FUNDAMENTALS REVIEW 9-4 continued

EQUIPMENT AND ASSISTIVE DEVICES

FRICTION-REDUCING SHEETS

Friction-reducing sheets can be used under patients to prevent skin shearing when moving a patient in the bed and to assist with lateral transfers. The use of these sheets when moving the patient up in bed, turning, and repositioning reduces friction and the force required to move the patient.

MECHANICAL LATERAL-ASSIST DEVICES

Mechanical lateral-assist devices eliminate the need to slide the patient manually. Some devices are motorized and some use a hand crank (Figure C). A portion of the device moves from the stretcher to the bed, sliding under the patient, bridging the bed and stretcher. The device is then returned to the stretcher, effectively moving the patient without pulling by staff members.

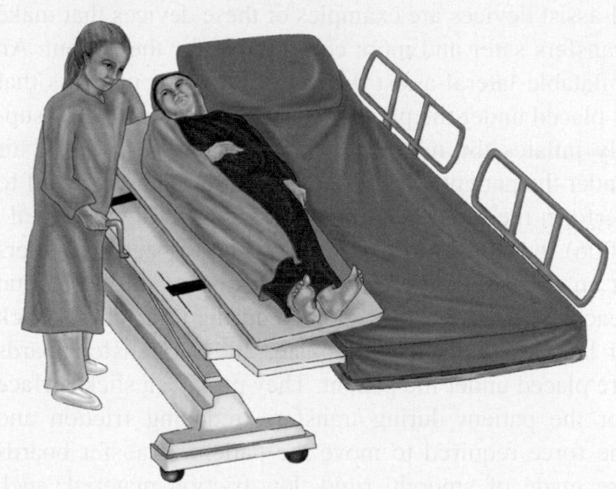

FIGURE C Mechanical lateral-assist device.

TRANSFER CHAIRS

Chairs that can convert into stretchers are available. These are useful with patients who have no weight-bearing capacity, cannot follow directions, and/or cannot cooperate. The back of the chair bends back and the leg supports elevate to form a stretcher configuration, eliminating the need for lifting the patient. Some of these chairs have built-in mechanical aids to perform the patient transfer, as detailed above.

POWERED STAND-ASSIST AND REPOSITIONING LIFTS

Powered stand-assist and repositioning devices can be used with patients who have weight-bearing ability in at least one leg, who can follow directions, and are cooperative. A simple sling is placed around the patient's back and under the arms (Figure D). The patient's feet rest on the device's footrest and then places his or her hands on the handle. The device mechanically assists the patient to stand, without any lifting by the nurse. Once the patient is standing, the device can be wheeled to a chair, the toilet, or bed. Some devices have removable footrests and can be used as a walker. Some have scales incorporated into the device that can be used to weigh the patient.

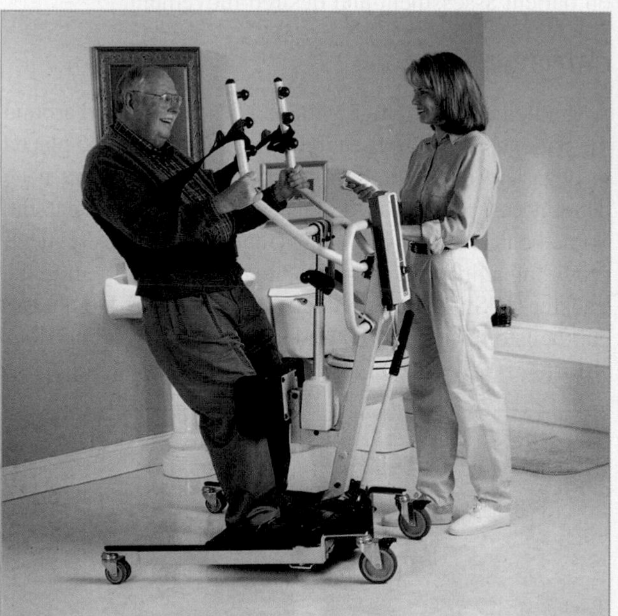

FIGURE D Stand-assist device.

POWERED FULL-BODY LIFTS

Powered full-body lifts are used with patients who cannot bear any weight to move them out of bed, into and out of a chair, and to a commode or stretcher. A full-body sling is placed under the patient's body, including head and torso, and then the sling is attached to the lift. The device slowly lifts the patient. Some devices can be lowered to the floor to pick up a patient who has fallen. These devices are available on portable bases and ceiling-mounted tracks.

FUNDAMENTALS REVIEW 9-5

ASSESSMENT CRITERIA AND CARE PLAN FOR SAFE PATIENT HANDLING AND MOVEMENT

I. Patient's Level of Assistance:

_____ Independent—Patient performs task safely, with or without staff assistance, with or without assistive devices.

_____ Partial Assist—Patient requires no more help than standby, cueing, or coaxing, or caregiver is required to lift no more than 35 lbs. of a patient's weight.

_____ Dependent—Patient requires nurse to lift more than 35 lbs. of the patient's weight, or patient is unpredictable in the amount of assistance offered. In this case, assistive devices should be used.

An assessment should be made prior to each task if the patient has varying levels of ability to assist due to medical reasons, fatigue, medications, etc. When in doubt, assume the patient cannot assist with the transfer/repositioning.

II. Weight-Bearing Capability

_____ Full

_____ Partial

_____ None

III. Bilateral Upper-Extremity Strength

_____ Yes

_____ No

IV. Patient's level of cooperation and comprehension:

_____ Cooperative—May need prompting; able to follow simple commands.

_____ Unpredictable or varies (patient whose behavior changes frequently should be considered as unpredictable), not cooperative, or unable to follow simple commands.

V. Weight: _________ **Height:** ___________

Body Mass Index (BMI) [needed if patient's weight is over 300 lbs.][1]: ___________

If BMI exceeds 50, institute Bariatric Algorithms

The presence of the following conditions are likely to affect the transfer/repositioning process and should be considered when identifying equipment and technique needed to move the patient.

VI. Check applicable conditions likely to affect transfer/repositioning techniques.

_____ Hip/Knee/Shoulder Replacements

_____ History of Falls

_____ Paralysis/Paresis

_____ Unstable Spine

_____ Severe Edema

_____ Very Fragile Skin

_____ Respiratory/Cardiac Compromise

_____ Wounds Affecting Transfer/Positioning

_____ Amputation

_____ Urinary/Fecal Stoma

_____ **Contractures**/Spasms

_____ Tubes (e.g., IV, Chest)

_____ Fractures

_____ Splints/Traction

_____ Severe Osteoporosis

_____ Severe Pain/Discomfort

_____ Postural Hypotension

Comments: ____

____

____

VII. Appropriate Lift/Transfer Devices Needed:

Vertical Lift: ____

____

Horizontal Lift: ____

____

Other Patient Handling Devices Needed: ____

____

Sling Type: Seated _____ Seated (Amputee) _____ Standing _____ Supine _____ Ambulation _____ Limb Support _____

Sling Size: ____________

Signature: ____ **Date:** ____________

[1]If patient's weight is over 300 lbs., the BMI is needed. For Online BMI table and calculator see: http://www.nhlbi.nih.gov/guidelines/obesity/bmi_tbl.htm

(VISN 8 Patient Safety Center. (2009). *Safe patient handling and movement algorithms.* Tampa, FL: Author. Available. http://www.visn8.va.gov/visn8/patientsafetycenter/safePtHandling/default.asp)

SKILL 9-1 ASSISTING A PATIENT WITH TURNING IN BED

People who are forced into inactivity by illness or injury are at high risk for serious health complications. One of the most common skills that you can use involves helping patients who cannot turn themselves in bed without assistance. You need to use your knowledge of correct body alignment and assistive devices to turn the patient in bed. Figure 1, Safe Patient Handling Algorithm 4, can help you make decisions about safe patient handling and movement. Mastering and using these techniques will help you maintain a turn schedule to prevent complications for a patient who is immobile. If a patient requires logrolling, please refer to Skill 17-1, Logrolling a Patient. During any patient-handling task, if any caregiver is required to lift more than 35 pounds of a patient's weight, consider the patient to be fully dependent and use assistive devices (Waters, 2007). Refer to Box 9-1 for general guidelines related to mobility and safe handling of people with dementia.

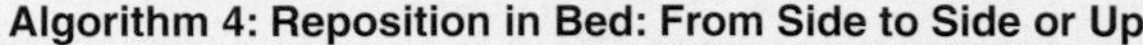

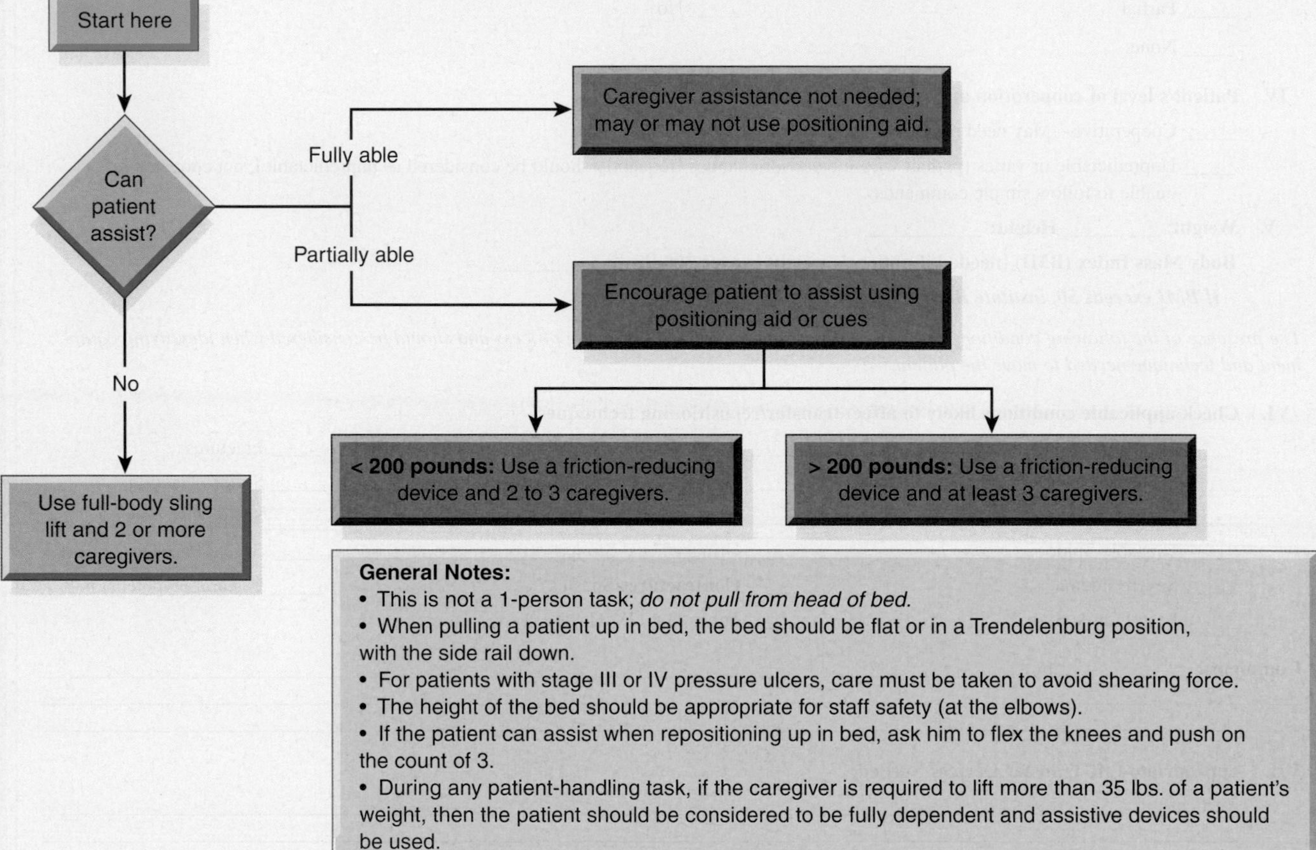

FIGURE 1 Step-by-step procedure or algorithm used to outline safe technique for repositioning a patient in bed. The first decision point is whether the patient can assist. If he or she is fully able, caregiver assistance is not needed, and the patient may or may not use a positioning aid. If the patient weighs less than 200 pounds, use a friction-reducing device and two to three caregivers. If the patient weighs more than 200 pounds, use a friction-reducing device and at least three caregivers. If the patient is not able to assist, use a full-body sling lift and two or more caregivers. (From VISN 8 Patient Safety Center. (2009). *Safe patient handling and movement algorithms*. Tampa, FL: Author. Available at http://www.visn8.va.gov/visn8/patientsafetycenter/safePtHandling/default.asp.)

DELEGATION CONSIDERATIONS

Assisting a patient to turn in bed may be delegated to nursing assistive personnel (NAP) or to unlicensed assistive personnel (UAP), as well as to licensed practical/vocational nurses (LPN/LVN). The decision to delegate must be based on careful analysis of the patient's needs and circumstances, as well as the qualifications of the person to whom the task is being delegated. Refer to the Delegation Guidelines in Appendix A.

BOX 9-1 SAFE HANDLING OF PATIENTS WITH DEMENTIA

- Be aware that communication problems and weakness can make the handling of patients with dementia challenging.
- Face the patient when speaking.
- Use clear, short sentences.
- Call patient by name.
- Use calm, reassuring tone of voice.
- Offer simple, step-by-step instructions.
- Use positive instructions ("stay standing") rather than negative ("don't sit down"). Positive instructions are more likely to result in successful maneuvers.
- Repeat verbal cues and prompts, as necessary. This assists when thought processes are delayed.
- Determine if the patient experiencing dementia has receptive aphasia. This inability to understand what is being said results in noncompliance with verbal instructions.
- Phrase instructions positively. For example, remind the patient to "Stand up" until the chair is correctly positioned, instead of saying "Don't sit down." The patient may not register the "Don't" and will try to sit too early. Positive instructions are more likely to result in successful maneuvers.
- Ask one question at a time, allow the patient to answer, and repeat the question, if necessary.
- Allow the patient to focus on the task; avoid correcting the process of the action unless it would be dangerous to the patient not to do so.
- Identify the patient's established patterns of behavior, customs, traits, and everyday habits and try to incorporate these habits into desired activities. For instance, a patient with dementia may resist or become frightened when a morning shower is attempted if the patient was accustomed to evening baths. Another individual may have difficulty getting out of bed in the morning for the simple reason that he is being asked to get out on what he considers the wrong side of the bed.

(Adapted from Varnam, W. (2011). How to mobilize patients with dementia to a standing position. *Nursing Older People, 23*(8), 31–36; Miller, C. (2008). Communication difficulties in hospitalized older adults with dementia: Try these techniques to make communicating with patients easier and more effective. *American Journal of Nursing, 108*(3), 58–66; and Wright, K. (2005). Mobility and safe handling of people with dementia. *Nursing Times, 101*(17), 38–40.)

EQUIPMENT

- Friction-reducing sheet or draw sheet
- Bed surface that inflates to aid in turning
- Pillows or other supports to help the patient maintain the desired position after turning and to maintain correct body alignment for the patient
- Additional caregivers and/or safe handling equipment to assist, based on assessment
- Nonsterile gloves, if indicated; other PPE as indicated

ASSESSMENT

Before moving a patient, check the medical record for any conditions or orders that will limit mobility. Perform a pain assessment before the time for the activity. If the patient reports pain, administer the prescribed medication in sufficient time to allow for the full effect of the analgesic. Assess the patient's ability to assist with moving, the need for assistive devices, and the need for a second or third person to assist with the activity. Determine the need for bariatric equipment. Assess the patient's skin for signs of irritation, redness, edema, or blanching.

NURSING DIAGNOSIS

Determine the related factors for the nursing diagnoses based on the patient's current status. Appropriate nursing diagnoses may include:

- Activity Intolerance
- Impaired Bed Mobility
- Acute Pain

OUTCOME IDENTIFICATION AND PLANNING

The expected outcome to achieve when assisting a patient with turning in bed is that the activity takes place without injury to patient or nurse. An additional outcome is that the patient is comfortable and in proper body alignment.

IMPLEMENTATION

ACTION	RATIONALE
1. Review the medical orders and nursing plan of care for patient activity. Identify any movement limitations and the ability of the patient to assist with turning. **Consult patient handling algorithm, if available, to plan appropriate approach to moving the patient.**	Checking the medical orders and plan of care validates the correct patient and correct procedure. Identification of limitations and ability along with use of an algorithm helps to prevent injury and aids in determining the best plan for patient movement.

(*continued*)

SKILL 9-1 ASSISTING A PATIENT WITH TURNING IN BED continued

ACTION	RATIONALE
2. Gather any positioning aids or supports, if necessary.	Having aids readily available promotes efficient time management.
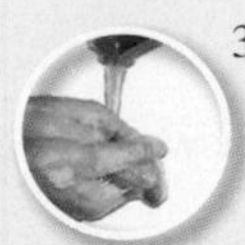 3. Perform hand hygiene. Put on PPE, as indicated.	Hand hygiene and PPE prevent the spread of microorganisms. PPE is required based on transmission precautions.
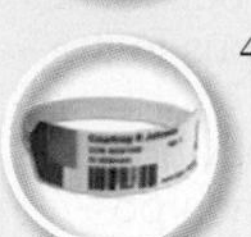 4. Identify the patient. Explain the procedure to the patient.	Patient identification validates the correct patient and correct procedure. Discussion and explanation help allay anxiety and prepare the patient for what to expect.
5. Close the curtains around the bed and close the door to the room, if possible. Position at least one nurse on either side of the bed. Place pillows, wedges, or any other support to be used for positioning within easy reach. Place the bed at an appropriate and comfortable working height, usually elbow height of the caregiver (VISN 8 Patient Safety Center, 2009). Lower both side rails.	Closing the door or curtain provides privacy. Proper bed height helps reduce back strain while performing the procedure. Proper positioning and lowering of the side rails facilitates moving the patient and minimizes strain on the nurses.
6. If not already in place, position a friction-reducing sheet under the patient.	Friction-reducing sheets aid in preventing shearing and in reducing friction and the force required to move the patient.
7. Using the friction-reducing sheet, move the patient to the edge of the bed, opposite the side to which he or she will be turned. Raise the side rails.	With this placement, the patient will be on the center of the bed after turning is accomplished. Raising side rails ensures patient safety.
8. If the patient is able, have the patient grasp the side rail on the side of the bed toward which he or she is turning (Figure 2). Alternately, place the patient's arms across his or her chest and cross his or her far leg over the leg toward which they are turning.	This encourages the patient to assist as much as possible with the movement. This facilitates the turning motion and protects the patient's arms during the turn.

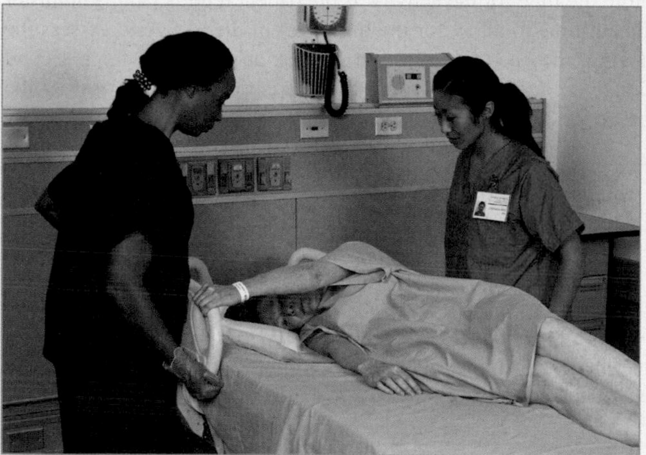

FIGURE 2 Having patient grasp side rail on side of bed toward which he or she is turning. *(Note: Patient's covers have been pulled back in this series of photos to show skill action. Covers should be folded back just enough to work, not to expose patients unnecessarily.) (Photo by B. Proud.)*

ACTION	RATIONALE
9. If available, activate the bed turn mechanism to inflate the side of the bed behind the patient's back.	Activating the turn mechanism inflates the side of the bed for approximately 10 seconds, aiding in propelling the patient to turn, and reducing the work required by the nurse. This helps avoid straining the nurse's lower back.

ACTION	RATIONALE
10. The nurse on the side of the bed toward which the patient is turning should stand opposite the patient's center with his or her feet spread about shoulder width and with one foot ahead of the other (Figure 3). Tighten your gluteal and abdominal muscles and flex your knees. Use your leg muscles to do the pulling. The other nurse should position his or her hands on the patient's shoulder and hip, assisting to roll the patient to the side. Instruct the patient to pull on the bed rail at the same time. Use the friction-reducing sheet to gently pull the patient over on his or her side (Figure 4).	Each nurse is in a stable position with good body alignment and prepared to use large muscle masses to turn the patient. These maneuvers support the patient's body and use the nurses' weight to assist with turning.
11. Use a pillow or other support behind the patient's back. Pull the shoulder blade forward and out from under the patient.	Pillow will provide support and help the patient maintain the desired position. Positioning the shoulder blade removes pressure from the bony prominence.

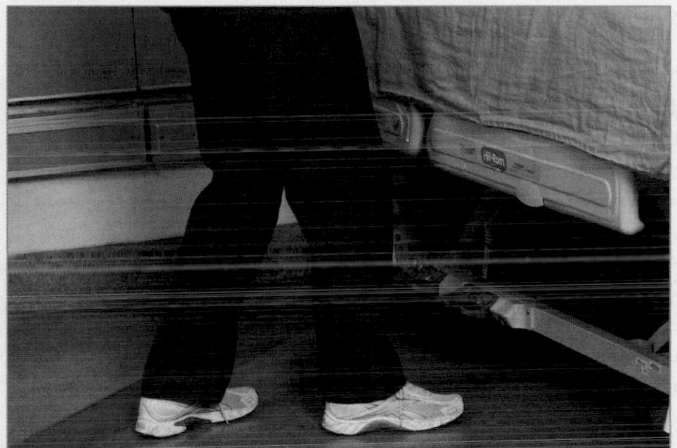

FIGURE 3 Standing opposite patient's center with feet spread about shoulder width and with one foot ahead of the other. *(Photo by B. Proud.)*

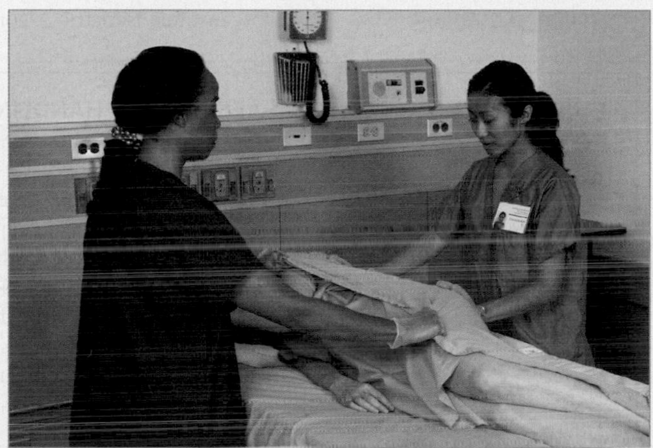

FIGURE 4 Using friction-reducing sheet to pull patient over on her side. *(Photo by B. Proud.)*

ACTION	RATIONALE
12. Make the patient comfortable and position in proper alignment, using pillows or other supports under the leg and arm, as needed. Readjust the pillow under the patient's head. Elevate the head of the bed as needed for comfort.	Positioning in proper alignment with supports ensures that the patient will be able to maintain the desired position and will be comfortable.
13. Place the bed in the lowest position, with the side rails up, as indicated. Make sure the call bell and other necessary items are within easy reach.	Adjusting the bed height ensures patient safety. Having the call bell and essential items readily available helps promote safety.
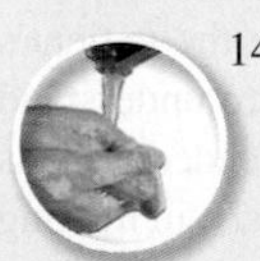 14. Clean transfer aids, per facility policy, if not indicated for single patient use. Remove gloves and other PPE, if used. Perform hand hygiene.	Proper cleaning of equipment between patient use prevents the spread of microorganisms. Removing PPE properly reduces the risk for infection transmission and contamination of other items. Hand hygiene prevents the spread of microorganisms.

EVALUATION

The expected outcome is met when the patient is turned and repositioned without injury to patient or nurse. The patient demonstrates proper body alignment and verbalizes comfort.

DOCUMENTATION

Guidelines

Many facilities provide areas on the bedside flow sheet to document repositioning. Be sure to document the time the patient's position was changed, use of supports, and any pertinent observations, including skin assessment. Document the patient's tolerance of the position change. Document aids used to facilitate movement.

(continued)

SKILL 9-1 ASSISTING A PATIENT WITH TURNING IN BED continued

Sample Documentation

11/10/15 1130 Patient repositioned from right side to left side; alignment maintained with wedge support behind back and pillow between legs. Skin on pressure points on right side without signs of irritation, edema, or redness. Patient reports no pain with movement. Friction-reducing sheet used to facilitate transfer and left in place under patient. Three caregivers required for repositioning.

—*B. Clapp, RN*

UNEXPECTED SITUATIONS AND ASSOCIATED INTERVENTIONS

- *You are turning a patient by yourself, but you realize that the patient cannot help as much as you thought and is heavier than you anticipated:* Use the call bell to summon assistance from a coworker. Alternatively, cover the patient, make sure all rails are up, lower the bed to the lowest position, and get someone to assist you. Consider using a friction-reducing sheet and two to three additional caregivers.

SPECIAL CONSIDERATIONS

- Calculate the Body Mass Index (BMI) for patients weighing over 300 pounds. If BMI exceeds 50, institute Bariatric Algorithms.

EVIDENCE FOR PRACTICE ▶

SAFE PATIENT HANDLING AND MOVEMENT

VISN 8 Patient Safety Center. (2009). *Safe patient handling and movement algorithms.* Tampa, FL: Author. Available http://www.visn8.va.gov/visn8/patientsafetycenter/safePtHandling/default.asp.

Derived from best practices within and outside health care, this guide outlines a comprehensive program to eradicate job-related musculoskeletal injuries in nursing. The program elements described in this guidebook have been tested within the Veterans Health Administration (VHA). Data from VHA and outside organizations suggest a decrease in the frequency and severity of injuries to caregivers through the use of this approach. In the long run, a decrease in the costs associated with such injuries, reductions in musculoskeletal pain, improved quality of life, and reductions in disability are anticipated.

Refer to thePoint for additional research on related nursing topics.

SKILL 9-2 MOVING A PATIENT UP IN BED WITH THE ASSISTANCE OF ANOTHER CAREGIVER

When a patient needs to be moved up in bed, it is important to avoid injuring yourself and the patient. The patient is at risk for injuries from **shearing forces** while being moved. Evaluate the patient's condition, any activity restrictions, the patient's ability to assist with positioning and to understand directions, and the patient's body weight to decide how much additional assistance is needed. This is not a one-person task. Safe Patient Handling Algorithm 4 (Figure 1 in Skill 9-1) can assist in making decisions about patient handling and movement. Using assistance, appropriate lifting and repositioning devices, good body mechanics, and correct technique are important to avoid injuries to yourself and the patient. During any patient-handling task, if any caregiver is required to lift more than 35 pounds of a patient's weight, consider the patient to be fully dependent and use assistive devices (Waters, 2007). Fundamentals Review 9-4 reviews examples of equipment and assistive devices that are available to aid in patient movement and handling. Box 9-1 in Skill 9-1 outlines general guidelines related to mobility and safe handling of people with dementia. The procedure below describes moving a patient using a friction-reducing sheet; the Skill Variation at the end of the skill discusses using a full-body sling to reposition the patient.

DELEGATION CONSIDERATIONS

Moving a patient up in bed may be delegated to nursing assistive personnel (NAP) or to unlicensed assistive personnel (UAP), as well as to licensed practical/vocational nurses (LPN/LVNs). The decision to delegate must be based on careful analysis of the patient's needs and circumstances, as well as the qualifications of the person to whom the task is being delegated. Refer to the Delegation Guidelines in Appendix A.

EQUIPMENT

- Friction-reducing sheet or other friction-reducing device
- Nonsterile gloves, if indicated; other PPE, as indicated
- Additional caregivers to assist, based on assessment
- Full-body sling lift and cover sheet, if necessary, based on assessment

ASSESSMENT

Assess the situation to determine the need to move the patient up in the bed. Review the medical record and nursing plan of care for conditions that may influence the patient's ability to move or to be positioned. Assess for tubes, IV lines, incisions, or equipment that may alter the positioning procedure. Assess the patient's level of consciousness, ability to understand and follow directions, and ability to assist with moving. Assess the patient's weight and your strength to determine the number of caregivers required to assist with the activity. Determine the need for bariatric equipment. Assess the patient's skin for signs of irritation, redness, edema, or blanching.

NURSING DIAGNOSIS

Determine the related factors for the nursing diagnoses based on the patient's current status. Appropriate nursing diagnoses may include:

- Activity Intolerance
- Risk for Injury
- Impaired Bed Mobility

OUTCOME IDENTIFICATION AND PLANNING

The expected outcome to achieve when moving a patient up in bed with the assistance of another caregiver is that the patient remains free from injury and maintains proper body alignment. Additional outcomes may include the following: the patient reports improved comfort; and the patient's skin is clean, dry, and intact, and without any redness, irritation, or breakdown.

IMPLEMENTATION

ACTION	RATIONALE
1. Review the medical record and nursing plan of care for conditions that may influence the patient's ability to move or to be positioned. Assess for tubes, IV lines, incisions, or equipment that may alter the positioning procedure. Identify any movement limitations. **Consult patient handling algorithm, if available, to plan appropriate approach to moving the patient.**	Reviewing the order and plan of care validates the correct patient and correct procedure. Identification of limitations and ability and use of an algorithm helps to prevent injury and aids in determining best plan for patient movement.
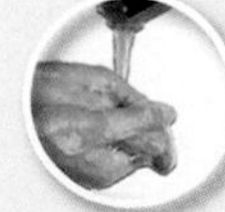 2. Perform hand hygiene and put on PPE, if indicated.	Hand hygiene and PPE prevent the spread of microorganisms. PPE is required based on transmission precautions.
 3. Identify the patient. Explain the procedure to the patient.	Patient identification validates the correct patient and correct procedure. Discussion and explanation help allay anxiety and prepare the patient for what to expect.
4. Close the curtains around the bed and close the door to the room, if possible. Place the bed at an appropriate and comfortable working height, usually elbow height of the caregiver (VISN 8 Patient Safety Center, 2009). Adjust the head of the bed to a flat position or as low as the patient can tolerate. Place the bed in slight Trendelenburg position, if the patient is able to tolerate it.	Closing the door or curtain provides for privacy. Proper bed height helps reduce back strain while you are performing the procedure. Flat positioning helps to decrease the gravitational pull of the upper body. Placing the bed in slight Trendelenburg position aids movement.
5. Remove all pillows from under the patient. Leave one at the head of the bed, leaning upright against the headboard.	Removing pillows from under the patient facilitates movement; placing a pillow at the head of the bed prevents accidental head injury against the top of the bed.

(*continued*)

SKILL 9-2 MOVING A PATIENT UP IN BED WITH THE ASSISTANCE OF ANOTHER CAREGIVER continued

ACTION	RATIONALE
6. Position at least one nurse on either side of the bed, and lower both side rails.	Proper positioning and lowering the side rails facilitate moving the patient and minimize strain on the nurses.
7. If a friction-reducing sheet (or device) is not in place under the patient, place one under the patient's midsection.	A friction-reducing device supports the patient's weight and reduces friction during the repositioning.
8. Ask the patient (if able) to bend his or her legs and put his or her feet flat on the bed to assist with the movement.	Patient can use major muscle groups to push. Even if the patient is too weak to push on the bed, placing the legs in this fashion will assist with movement and prevent skin shearing on the heels.
9. Have the patient fold the arms across the chest. Have the patient (if able) lift the head with chin on chest.	Positioning in this manner provides assistance, reduces friction, and prevents **hyperextension** of the neck.
10. One nurse should be positioned on each side of the bed, at the patient's midsection, with feet spread shoulder width apart and one foot slightly in front of the other.	Doing so positions each nurse opposite the center of the body mass, lowers the center of gravity, and reduces the risk for injury.
11. If available on bed, engage mechanism to make the bed surface firmer for repositioning.	Decreases friction and effort needed to move the patient.
12. Grasp the friction-reducing sheet securely, close to the patient's body.	Having the sheet close to the body brings the patient's center of gravity closer to each nurse and provides for a secure hold.
13. Flex your knees and hips. Tighten your abdominal and gluteal muscles and keep your back straight.	Using the legs' large muscle groups and tightening muscles during transfer prevent back injury.
14. If possible, the patient can assist with the move by pushing with the legs. Shift your weight back and forth from your back leg to your front leg and count to three (Figure 1). On the count of three, move the patient up in bed (Figure 2). Repeat the process, if necessary, to get the patient to the right position.	If the patient assists, the nurses exert less effort. The rocking motion uses the nurses' weight to counteract the patient's weight. Rocking develops momentum, which provides a smooth lift with minimal exertion by the nurses.

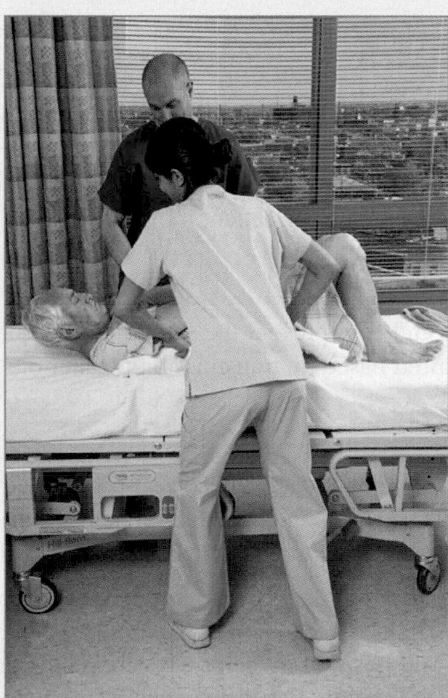

FIGURE 1 Nurses positioned at patient's midsection, shifting weight from back leg to front leg in preparation for move. *(Note: Patient's covers have been pulled back in this series of photos to show skill action. Covers should be folded back just enough to work, not expose patients unnecessarily.)*

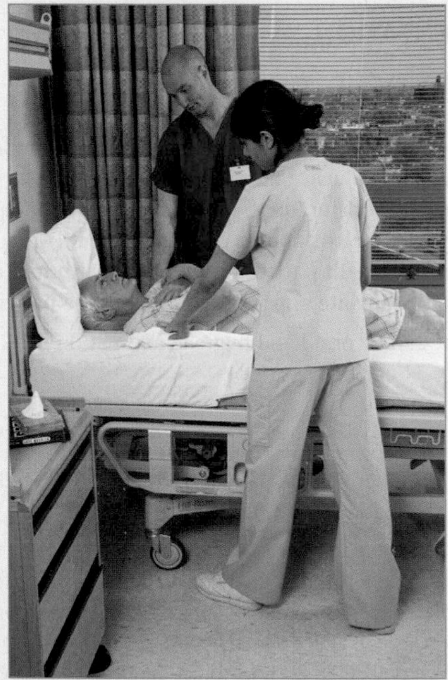

FIGURE 2 Patient moved up in bed.

ACTION	RATIONALE
15. Assist the patient to a comfortable position and readjust the pillows and supports, as needed. Take bed out of Trendelenburg position and return bed surface to normal setting, if necessary. Raise the side rails. Place the bed in the lowest position (Figure 3). Make sure the call bell and other necessary items are within easy reach.	Readjusting the bed and adjusting the bed height ensures patient safety and comfort. Having the call bell and essential items readily available helps promote safety.

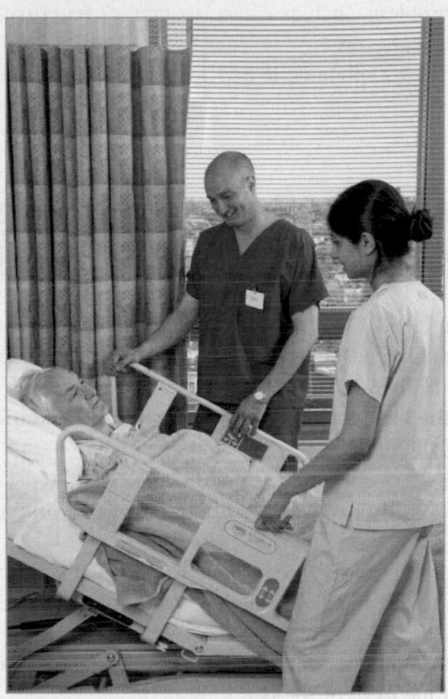

FIGURE 3 Adjusting bed to a safe and comfortable position.

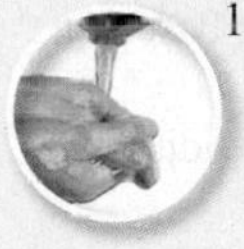

16. Clean transfer aids, per facility policy, if not indicated for single patient use. Remove gloves or other PPE, if used. Perform hand hygiene.	Proper cleaning of equipment between patient use prevents the spread of microorganisms. Removing PPE properly reduces the risk for infection transmission and contamination of other items. Hand hygiene prevents the spread of microorganisms.

EVALUATION

The expected outcome is met when the patient is moved up in bed without injury and maintains proper body alignment, is comfortable, and demonstrates intact skin without evidence of any breakdown.

DOCUMENTATION

Guidelines

Many facilities provide areas on the bedside flow sheet to document repositioning. Document the time the patient's position was changed, use of supports, and any pertinent observations, including skin assessment. Document the patient's tolerance of the position change. Document aids used to facilitate movement.

Sample Documentation

11/10/15 1130 Patient repositioned from right side to left side; alignment maintained with wedge support behind back and pillow between legs. Skin on pressure points on right side without signs of irritation, edema, or redness. Patient reports no pain with movement.

—B. Clapp, RN

(continued)

SKILL 9-2 MOVING A PATIENT UP IN BED WITH THE ASSISTANCE OF ANOTHER CAREGIVER continued

UNEXPECTED SITUATIONS AND ASSOCIATED INTERVENTIONS

- *You are attempting to move a patient up in the bed with another nurse. Your first attempt is unsuccessful, and you realize the patient is too heavy for only two people to move:* Obtain the assistance of at least two other coworkers. Make use of available friction-reducing devices. Use full-body lift, if available. Position opposing pairs at the patient's shoulders and buttocks to distribute the weight. If necessary, have a fifth person lift the patient's legs or heels. The movement of a very large patient is aided by putting the bed in a slight Trendelenburg position temporarily, provided the patient can tolerate it.

SPECIAL CONSIDERATIONS

- When moving a patient with a leg or foot problem, such as a cast, wound, or **fracture**, one assistant should be assigned to lift and move that extremity.
- Calculate the BMI for patients weighing over 300 pounds. If BMI exceeds 50, institute Bariatric Algorithms.

SKILL VARIATION Using Full-Body Sling to Reposition Patient

1. Review the medical record and nursing plan of care for conditions that may influence the patient's ability to move or to be positioned. Assess for tubes, IV lines, incisions, or equipment that may alter the positioning procedure. Identify any movement limitations. **Consult patient handling algorithm, if available, to plan appropriate approach to moving the patient (see Figure 1 in Skill 9-1).**
2. Check equipment for proper functioning.

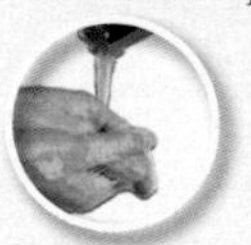

3. Perform hand hygiene and put on gloves and/or other PPE, as indicated.

4. Identify the patient. Explain the procedure to the patient.
5. Close the curtains around the bed and close the door to the room, if possible. Place the bed at an appropriate and comfortable working height. Adjust the head of the bed to a flat position or as low as the patient can tolerate.
6. Remove all pillows from under the patient. Leave one at the head of the bed, leaning upright against the headboard.
7. Position at least one nurse on either side of the bed, and lower both side rails.
8. Place cover sheet on sling surface. Place sling under patient.
9. Roll the base of the lift under the side of the bed nearest to the chair. **Center the frame over the patient. Lock the wheels of the lift.**
10. **Using the base-adjustment lever, widen the stance of the base of the device.**
11. Position yourself and the other caregiver at the patient's midsection. If necessary, additional staff can support the patient's legs.
12. Crank or engage the mechanism to raise the sling, with the patient, up off the bed. Raise the patient just high enough to clear the bed surface.
13. Guide the sling and relocate the patient to the appropriate place at the head of the bed.
14. Release the sling slowly or activate the lowering device on the lift and slowly lower the patient to the bed surface.
15. Remove the sling or leave in place for future use, based on facility policy.
16. Assist the patient to a comfortable position and readjust the pillows and supports, as needed.
17. Raise the side rails. Place the bed in the lowest position. Make sure the call bell and other necessary items are within easy reach.

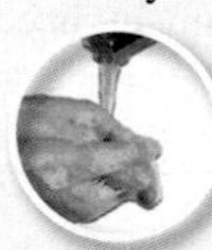

18. Clean transfer aids, per facility policy, if not indicated for single patient use. Remove gloves and any other PPE, if used, and perform hand hygiene.

EVIDENCE FOR PRACTICE ▶

SAFE PATIENT HANDLING AND MOVEMENT

VISN 8 Patient Safety Center. (2009). *Safe patient handling and movement algorithms.* Tampa, FL: Author. Available. http://www.visn8.va.gov/visn8/patientsafetycenter/safePtHandling/default.asp.

Refer to details in Skill 9-1, Evidence for Practice, and refer to thePoint for additional research on related nursing topics.

SKILL 9-3 TRANSFERRING A PATIENT FROM THE BED TO A STRETCHER

While in the hospital, patients are often transported by stretcher to other areas for tests or procedures. Considerable care must be taken when moving someone from a bed to a stretcher or from a stretcher to a bed to prevent injury to the patient or staff. Refer to Figure 1, Safe Patient Handling Algorithm 2, to help in making decisions about safe patient handling and movement. Using assistance, appropriate lifting and repositioning devices, good body mechanics, and correct technique are important to avoid injuries to self and to the patient. During any patient-handling task, if any caregiver is required to lift more than 35 pounds of a patient's weight, consider the patient to be fully dependent and use assistive devices (Waters, 2007). Be familiar with the proper way to use lateral-assist devices, based on the manufacturer's directions. Fundamentals Review 9-4 reviews examples of equipment and assistive devices that are available to aid in patient movement and handling. Box 9-1 in Skill 9-1 outlines general guidelines to consider related to mobility and safe handling of people with dementia.

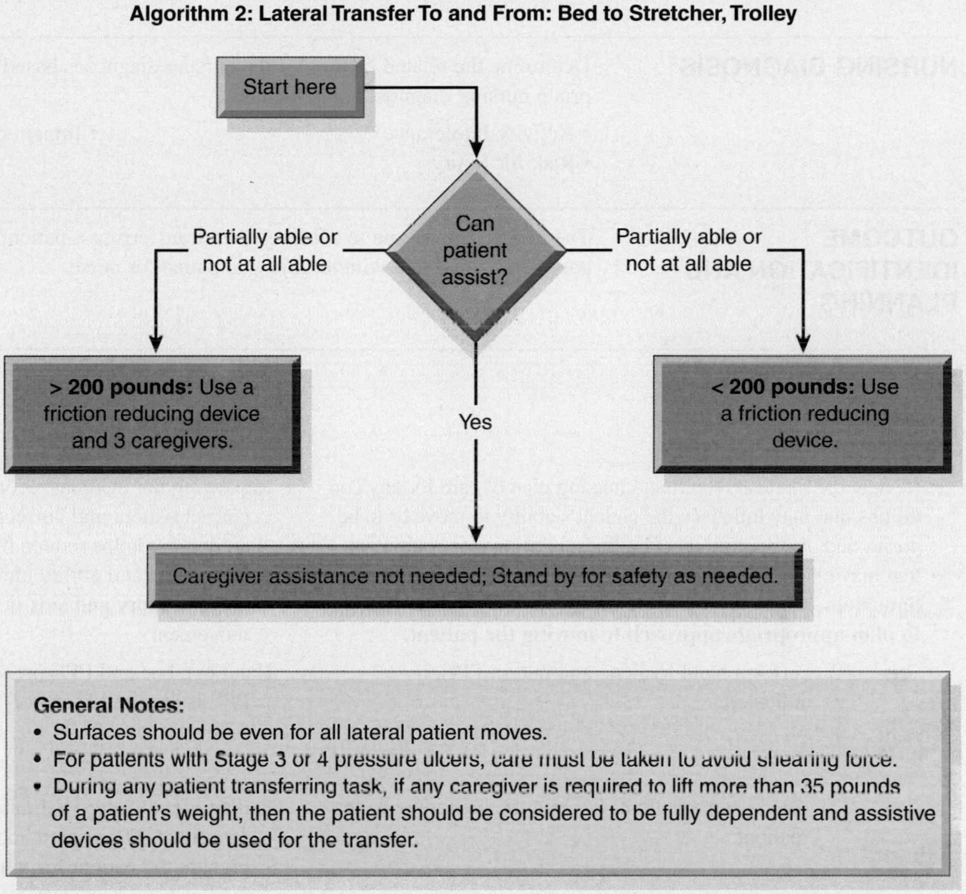

Algorithm 2: Lateral Transfer To and From: Bed to Stretcher, Trolley

Start here

Can patient assist?

Partially able or not at all able → **> 200 pounds:** Use a friction reducing device and 3 caregivers.

Partially able or not at all able → **< 200 pounds:** Use a friction reducing device.

Yes → Caregiver assistance not needed; Stand by for safety as needed.

General Notes:

- Surfaces should be even for all lateral patient moves.
- For patients with Stage 3 or 4 pressure ulcers, care must be taken to avoid shearing force.
- During any patient transferring task, if any caregiver is required to lift more than 35 pounds of a patient's weight, then the patient should be considered to be fully dependent and assistive devices should be used for the transfer.

FIGURE 1 Step-by-step procedure or algorithm used to outline safe technique for transferring a patient from bed to a stretcher. The first decision point in this algorithm is whether or not the patient can assist. If the patient is partially able or not at all able and weighs less than 200 pounds, use a friction-reducing device and three caregivers. If the patient can assist, caregiver assistance is not needed, but caregivers should stand by for safety. (From VISN 8 Patient Safety Center. (2009). *Safe patient handling and movement algorithms.* Tampa, FL: Author. Available. http://www.visn8.va.gov/visn8/patientsafetycenter/safePtHandling/default.asp).

DELEGATION CONSIDERATIONS

The transfer of a patient from bed to stretcher may be delegated to nursing assistive personnel (NAP) or to unlicensed assistive personnel (UAP), as well as to licensed practical/vocational nurses (LPN/LVNs). The decision to delegate must be based on careful analysis of the patient's needs and circumstances, as well as the qualifications of the person to whom the task is being delegated. Refer to the Delegation Guidelines in Appendix A.

(*continued*)

SKILL 9-3 TRANSFERRING A PATIENT FROM THE BED TO A STRETCHER continued

EQUIPMENT

- Transport stretcher
- Friction-reducing sheet
- Lateral-assist device, such as a transfer board, roller board, or mechanical lateral-assist device, if available
- Bath blanket
- Regular blanket
- At least two assistants, depending on the patient's condition
- Nonsterile gloves and/or other PPE, as indicated

ASSESSMENT

Review the medical record and nursing plan of care for conditions that may influence the patient's ability to move or to be transferred. Assess for tubes, IV lines, incisions, or equipment that may alter the transfer process. Assess the patient's level of consciousness, ability to understand and follow directions, and ability to assist with the transfer. Assess the patient's weight and your strength to determine if a fourth individual (or more) is required to assist with the activity. Determine a need for bariatric equipment. Assess the patient's comfort level; if needed, medicate, as ordered, with analgesics.

NURSING DIAGNOSIS

Determine the related factors for the nursing diagnoses based on the patient's current status. Appropriate nursing diagnoses may include:

- Activity Intolerance
- Risk for Injury
- Impaired Transfer Ability

OUTCOME IDENTIFICATION AND PLANNING

The expected outcome to achieve when transferring a patient from the bed to a stretcher is that the patient is transferred without injury to patient or nurse.

IMPLEMENTATION

ACTION	RATIONALE
1. Review the medical record and nursing plan of care for any conditions that may influence the patient's ability to move or to be positioned. Assess for tubes, IV lines, incisions, or equipment that may alter the positioning procedure. Identify any movement limitations. **Consult patient handling algorithm, if available, to plan appropriate approach to moving the patient.**	Reviewing the medical record and plan of care validates the correct patient and correct procedure. Checking for interfering equipment helps reduce the risk for injury. Identification of limitations and ability along with use of an algorithm helps to prevent injury and aids in determining the best plan for patient movement.
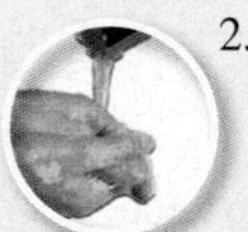 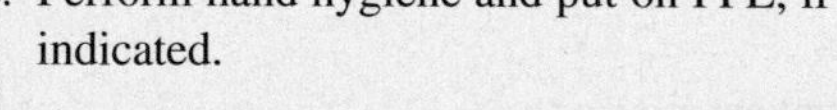 2. Perform hand hygiene and put on PPE, if indicated.	Hand hygiene and PPE prevent the spread of microorganisms. PPE is required based on transmission precautions.
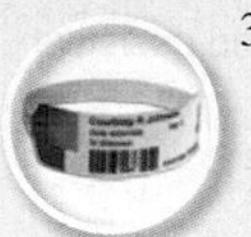 3. Identify the patient. Explain the procedure to the patient.	Patient identification validates the correct patient and correct procedure. Discussion and explanation help allay anxiety and prepare the patient for what to expect.
4. Close the curtains around the bed and close the door to the room, if possible. Adjust the head of the bed to a flat position or as low as the patient can tolerate. Raise the bed to a height that is even with the transport stretcher (VISN 8 Patient Safety Center, 2009). Lower the side rails, if in place.	Closing the door or curtain provides privacy. Proper bed height and lowering side rails make transfer easier and decrease the risk for injury.
5. Place the bath blanket over the patient and remove the top covers from underneath.	Bath blanket provides privacy and warmth.
6. If a friction-reducing transfer sheet is not in place under the patient, place one under the patient's midsection. Have patient fold arms against chest and move chin to chest. Use the friction-reducing sheet to move the patient to the side of the bed where the stretcher will be placed. Alternately, place a lateral-assist device under the patient. Follow manufacturer's directions for use.	A friction-reducing sheet supports the patient's weight, reduces friction during the lift, and provides for a secure hold. Positioning with chin to chest and arms folded provides assistance, reduces friction, and prevents hyperextension of the neck. A transfer board or other lateral-assist device makes it easier to move the patient and minimizes the risk for injury to the patient and nurses.

ACTION	RATIONALE
7. Position the stretcher next (and parallel) to the bed. **Lock the wheels on the stretcher and the bed.**	Positioning equipment makes the transfer easier and decreases the risk for injury. Locking the wheels keeps the bed and stretcher from moving.
8. Two nurses should stand on the stretcher side of the bed. A third nurse should stand on the side of the bed without the stretcher.	Team coordination provides for patient safety during transfer.
9. Use the friction-reducing sheet to roll the patient away from the stretcher (Figure 2). Place the transfer board across the space between the stretcher and the bed, partially under the patient (Figure 3). Roll the patient onto his or her back, so that the patient is partially on the transfer board.	The transfer board or other lateral-assist device reduces friction, easing the workload to move patient.

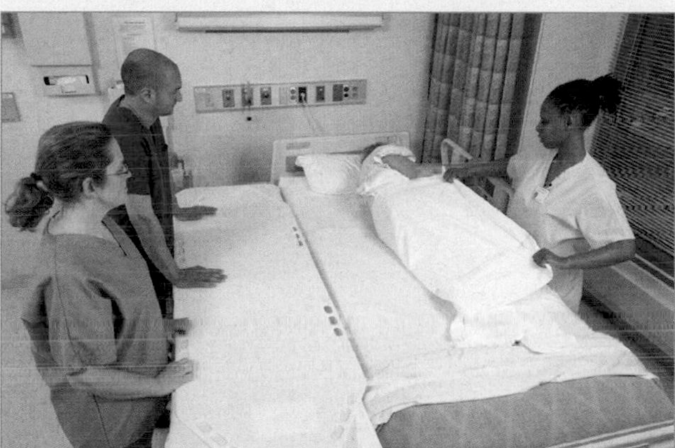

FIGURE 2 Using sheet to roll patient away from stretcher.

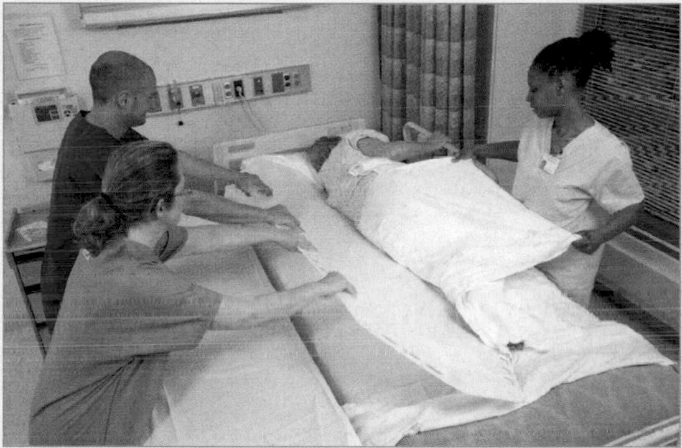

FIGURE 3 Positioning transfer board under patient.

ACTION	RATIONALE
10. The nurse on the side of the bed without the stretcher should grasp the friction-reducing sheet at the head and chest areas of the patient. The nurse on the stretcher side of the bed should grasp the friction-reducing sheet at the head and chest, and the other nurse on that side should grasp the friction-reducing sheet at the chest and leg areas of the patient.	Grasping the friction-reducing sheet at these locations evenly supports the patient.
11. **At a signal given by one of the nurses, have the nurses standing on the stretcher side of the bed pull the friction-reducing sheet. At the same time, the nurse (or nurses) on the other side push, transferring the patient's weight toward the transfer board, and pushing the patient from the bed to the stretcher (Figure 4).**	Working in unison distributes the work of moving the patient and facilitates the transfer.

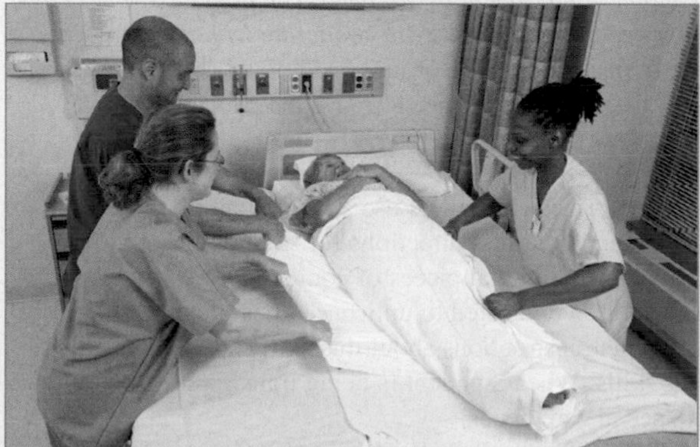

FIGURE 4 Transferring patient onto stretcher.

(continued)

SKILL 9-3 TRANSFERRING A PATIENT FROM THE BED TO A STRETCHER continued

ACTION	RATIONALE
12. Once the patient is transferred to the stretcher, remove the transfer board, and secure the patient until the side rails are raised (Figure 5). Raise the side rails. To ensure the patient's comfort, cover the patient with blanket and remove the bath blanket from underneath. Leave the friction-reducing sheet in place for the return transfer. Make sure the call bell and other necessary items are within easy reach.	Side rails promote safety. Blanket promotes comfort and warmth. Having the call bell and essential items readily available helps promote safety.
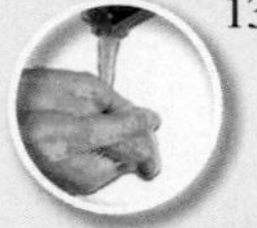 13. Clean transfer aids, per facility policy, if not indicated for single patient use. Remove gloves and any other PPE, if used. Perform hand hygiene.	Proper cleaning of equipment between patient use prevents the spread of microorganisms. Removing PPE properly reduces the risk for infection transmission and contamination of other items. Hand hygiene prevents the spread of microorganisms.

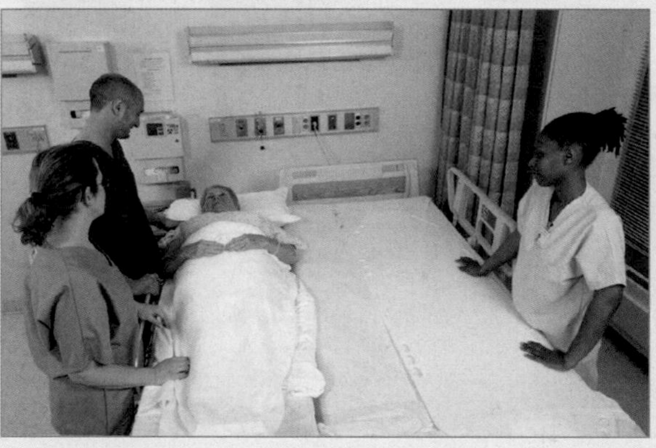

FIGURE 5 Securing patient on stretcher.

EVALUATION

The expected outcome is met when the patient is transferred to the stretcher without injury to patient or nurse.

DOCUMENTATION

Guidelines

Document the time and method of transport, and patient's destination, according to facility policy. Document the use of transfer aids and number of staff required for transfer.

Sample Documentation

5/12/15 1005 Patient transferred to stretcher via three-person assistance and lateral-assist transfer sheet. Transported to radiology for chest x-ray.

—M. Joliet, RN

UNEXPECTED SITUATIONS AND ASSOCIATED INTERVENTIONS

- *Your patient needs to be transported to another department by stretcher. The patient is very heavy and somewhat confused, so you are concerned about his ability to cooperate with the transfer:* Consult a Bariatric Algorithm. Obtain the assistance of three or more additional coworkers. Use a mechanical lateral-transfer device or air-assisted transfer device to move the patient.

SPECIAL CONSIDERATIONS

- Some mechanical lateral-transfer aids are motorized and others use a hand crank. If a mechanical lateral-assist device is used, follow the manufacturer's directions for safe movement of the patient. Be familiar with weight restrictions for individual pieces of equipment.
- Keep in mind that the transfer of patients is often delegated to unlicensed personnel. Before moving patients, all personnel need to complete instructions about this skill and must be able to provide return demonstrations of transfer skills. When a patient is being transferred, communicate clearly any mobility restrictions or special care needs.
- Calculate the BMI for patients weighing over 300 pounds. If BMI exceeds 50, institute Bariatric Algorithms.

EVIDENCE FOR PRACTICE ▶

SAFE PATIENT HANDLING AND MOVEMENT

VISN 8 Patient Safety Center. (2009). *Safe patient handling and movement algorithms.* Tampa, FL: Author. Available. http://www.visn8.va.gov/visn8/patientsafetycenter/safePtHandling/default.asp.

Refer to details in Skill 9-1, Evidence for Practice, and refer to thePoint for additional research on related nursing topics.

SKILL 9-4 TRANSFERRING A PATIENT FROM THE BED TO A CHAIR

Often, moving a patient from the bed to a chair helps him or her begin engaging in physical activity. Also, changing a patient's position will help prevent complications related to immobility. Safety and comfort are key concerns when assisting the patient out of bed. Assessing the patient's response to activity is a major nursing responsibility. Before performing the transfer, identify any restrictions related to the patient's condition and determine how activity levels may be affected. Figure 1, Safe Patient Handling Algorithm 1, can assist in making decisions about safe patient handling and movement. Using assistance, appropriate lifting and repositioning devices, good body mechanics, and correct technique are important to avoid injuries to yourself and the patient. During any patient-handling task, if any caregiver is required to lift more than 35 pounds of a patient's weight, consider the patient to be fully dependent and use assistive devices (Waters, 2007). Fundamentals Review 9-4 reviews examples of equipment and assistive devices that are available to aid in patient movement and handling. Box 9-1 in Skill 9-1 outlines general guidelines to consider related to mobility and safe handling of people with dementia.

DELEGATION CONSIDERATIONS

The transfer of a patient from bed to a chair may be delegated to nursing assistive personnel (NAP) or to unlicensed assistive personnel (UAP), as well as to licensed practical/vocational nurses (LPN/LVNs). The decision to delegate must be based on careful analysis of the patient's needs and circumstances, as well as the qualifications of the person to whom the task is being delegated. Refer to the Delegation Guidelines in Appendix A.

EQUIPMENT

- Chair or wheelchair
- Gait belt
- Stand-assist aid, if available
- Additional staff person to assist
- Blanket to cover the patient in the chair
- Nonsterile gloves and/or other PPE, as indicated

ASSESSMENT

Assess the situation to determine the need to get the patient out of bed. Review the medical record and nursing plan of care for conditions that may influence the patient's ability to move or to be transferred. Check for tubes, IV lines, incisions, or equipment that may require modifying the transfer procedure. Assess the patient's level of consciousness, ability to understand and follow directions, and ability to assist with the transfer. Assess the patient's weight and your strength to determine if additional assistance is needed. Determine the need for bariatric equipment. Assess the patient's comfort level; if needed, medicate as ordered with analgesics. If the patient is able to bear only partial weight, consider a second staff person to assist. If the patient is unable to bear even partial weight, or is uncooperative, use a full-body sling lift to move the patient.

NURSING DIAGNOSIS

Determine the related factors for the nursing diagnoses based on the patient's current status. Appropriate nursing diagnoses may include:

- Activity Intolerance
- Risk for Falls
- Impaired Physical Mobility

(continued)

SKILL 9-4 TRANSFERRING A PATIENT FROM THE BED TO A CHAIR continued

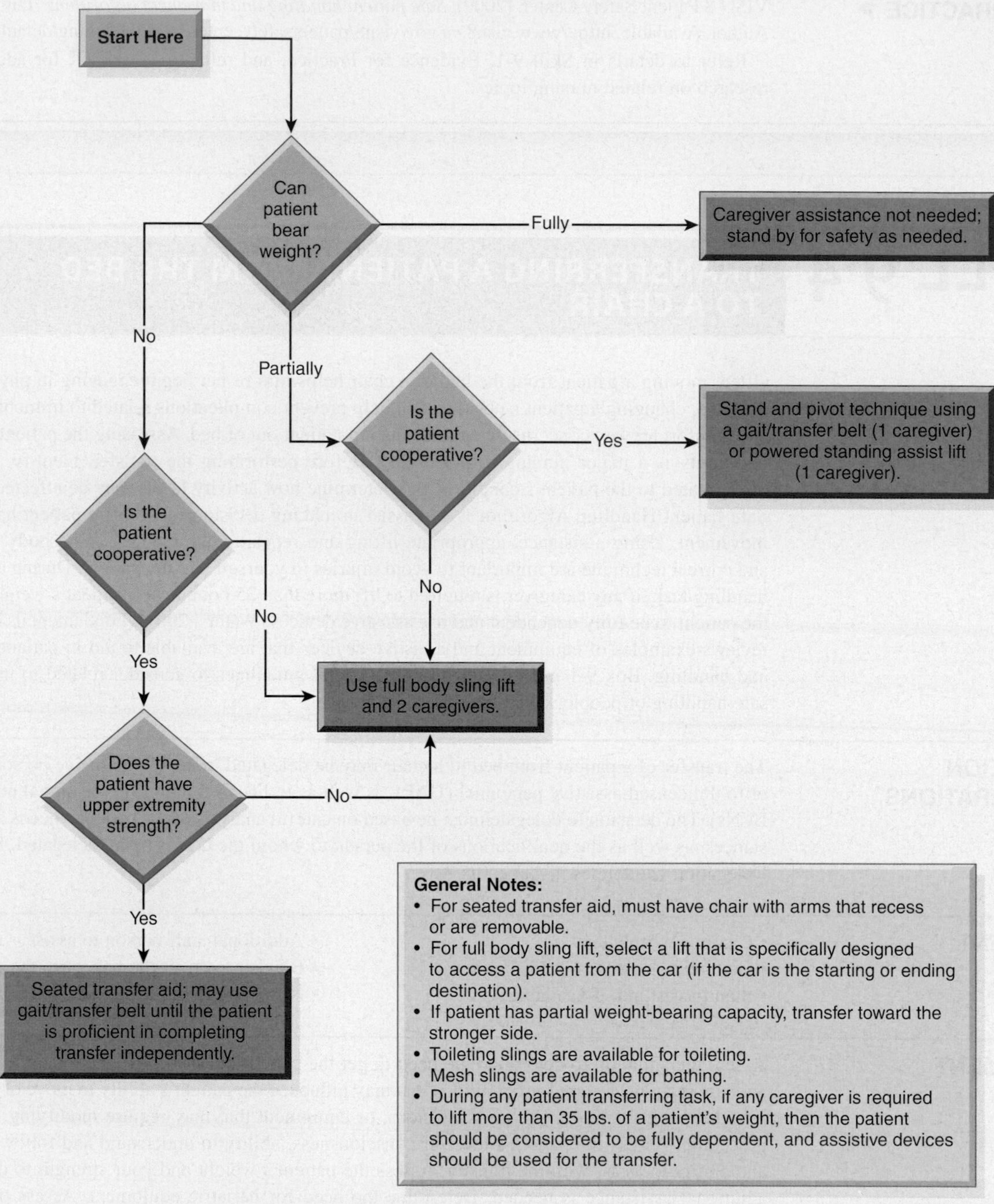

FIGURE 1 Step-by-step procedure or algorithm used to outline safe techniques for transferring a patient to and from bed to chair. The algorithm starts with a decision whether the patient can bear weight fully, partially, or not at all. If the patient can bear weight fully, caregiver assistance is not needed, but caregivers should stand by for safety. If the patient can bear weight partially, the next decision point is whether or not the patient is cooperative. If cooperative, then the stand and pivot technique should be used with a gait/transfer belt or a powered stand-assist lift (one caregiver needed). If not cooperative, a full-body sling lift and two caregivers should be used. If the patient cannot bear weight, the next decision point is whether or not the patient is cooperative. If the patient is not, a full-body sling lift and two to three caregivers should be used. If cooperative, the next decision point is whether or not the patient has upper extremity strength. If the patient does not, again a full-body sling lift and two to three caregivers should be used. If the patient has upper body strength, then a seated transfer aid should be used. A gait/transfer belt can also be used until the patient is proficient in completing the transfer independently. (From VISN 8 Patient Safety Center. (2009). *Safe patient handling and movement algorithms*. Tampa, FL: Author. Available. http://www.visn8.va.gov/visn8/patientsafetycenter/safePtHandling/default.asp.)

OUTCOME IDENTIFICATION AND PLANNING

The expected outcome to achieve when transferring a patient from the bed to a chair is that the transfer is accomplished without injury to patient or nurse and the patient remains free of any complications of immobility.

IMPLEMENTATION

ACTION	RATIONALE
1. Review the medical record and nursing plan of care for conditions that may influence the patient's ability to move or to be positioned. Assess for tubes, IV lines, incisions, or equipment that may alter the positioning procedure. Identify any movement limitations. **Consult patient-handling algorithm, if available, to plan appropriate approach to moving the patient.**	Reviewing the medical record and plan of care validates the correct patient and correct procedure. Identification of limitations and ability and use of an algorithm help to prevent injury and aid in determining best plan for patient movement.
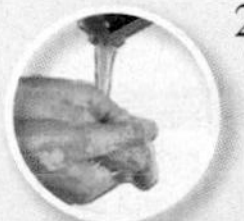 2. Perform hand hygiene and put on PPE, as indicated.	Hand hygiene and PPE prevent spread of microorganisms. PPE is required based on transmission precautions.
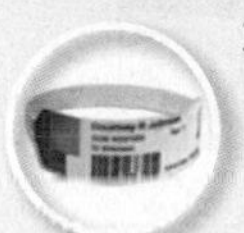 3. Identify the patient. Explain the procedure to the patient.	Patient identification validates the correct patient and correct procedure. Discussion and explanation help allay anxiety and prepare the patient for what to expect.
4. If needed, move equipment to make room for the chair. Close the curtains around the bed and close the door to the room, if possible.	A clear pathway from the bed to the chair facilitates the transfer. Closing the door or curtain provides for privacy.
5. Place the bed in the lowest position. Raise the head of the bed to a sitting position, or as high as the patient can tolerate.	Proper bed height and positioning facilitate the transfer. The amount of energy needed to move from a sitting position or elevated position to a sitting position is decreased.
6. **Make sure the bed brakes are locked. Put the chair next to the bed. If available, lock the brakes of the chair. If the chair does not have brakes, brace the chair against a secure object.**	Locking brakes or bracing the chair prevents movement during transfer and increases stability and patient safety.
7. Encourage the patient to make use of a stand-assist aid, either freestanding or attached to the side of the bed, if available, to move to the side of the bed and to a side-lying position, facing the side of the bed on which the patient will sit.	Encourages independence, reduces strain for staff, and decreases risk for patient injury.
8. Lower the side rail, if necessary, and stand near the patient's hips. Stand with your legs shoulder width apart with one foot near the head of the bed, slightly in front of the other foot.	The nurse's center of gravity is placed near the patient's greatest weight to assist the patient to a sitting position safely.
9. Encourage the patient to make use of the stand-assist device. Assist the patient to sit up on the side of the bed; ask the patient to swing his or her legs over the side of the bed. At the same time, pivot on your back leg to lift the patient's trunk and shoulders. Keep your back straight; avoid twisting.	Gravity lowers the patient's legs over the bed. The nurse transfers weight in the direction of motion and protects his or her back from injury.

(continued)

SKILL 9-4 TRANSFERRING A PATIENT FROM THE BED TO A CHAIR continued

ACTION	RATIONALE
10. **Stand in front of the patient, and assess for any balance problems or complaints of dizziness (Figure 2). Allow the patient's legs to dangle a few minutes before continuing.**	Standing in front of the patient prevents falls or injuries from orthostatic hypotension. The sitting position facilitates transfer to the chair and allows the circulatory system to adjust to a change in position.
11. Assist the patient to put on a robe, as necessary, and nonskid footwear.	Robe provides warmth and privacy. Nonskid soles reduce the risk for falling.
12. Wrap the gait belt around the patient's waist, based on assessed need and facility policy (Figure 3).	Gait belts improve the caregiver's grasp, reducing the risk of musculoskeletal injuries to staff and the patient. Provides firmer grasp for the caregiver if patient should lose his or her balance.

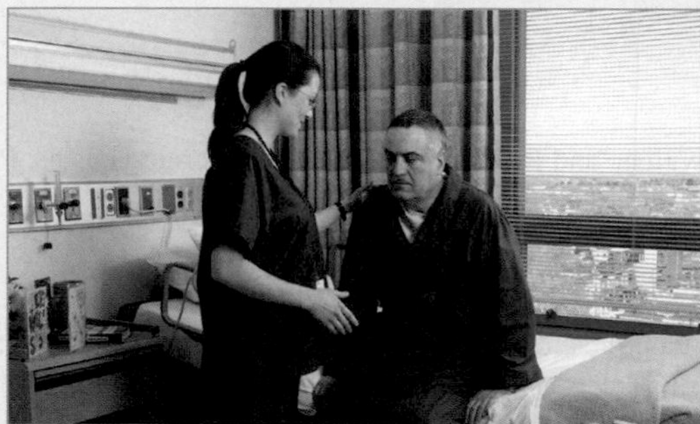

FIGURE 2 Standing in front of patient, and assessing for any balance problems or complaints of dizziness.

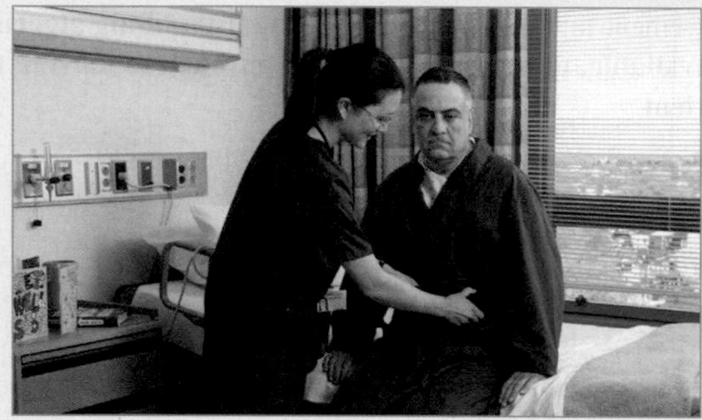

FIGURE 3 Wrapping gait belt around patient's waist.

ACTION	RATIONALE
13. Stand facing the patient. Spread your feet about shoulder width apart and flex your hips and knees.	This position provides stability and allows for smooth movement using the legs' large muscle groups.
14. Ask the patient to slide his or her buttocks to the edge of the bed until the feet touch the floor. Position yourself as close as possible to the patient, with your foot positioned on the outside of the patient's foot. If a second staff person is assisting, have him or her assume a similar position. Grasp the gait belt (Figure 4).	Doing so provides balance and support.
15. Encourage the patient to make use of the stand-assist device. If necessary, have second staff person grasp the gait belt on opposite side. Rock back and forth while counting to three. **On the count of three, using the gait belt and your legs (not your back), assist the patient to a standing position (Figure 5).** If indicated, brace your front knee against the patient's weak extremity as he or she stands. Assess the patient's balance and leg strength. If the patient is weak or unsteady, return the patient to bed.	Holding at the gait belt prevents injury to the patient. Bracing your knee against a weak extremity prevents a weak knee from buckling and the patient from falling. Assessing balance and strength helps to identify the need for additional assistance to prevent falling.

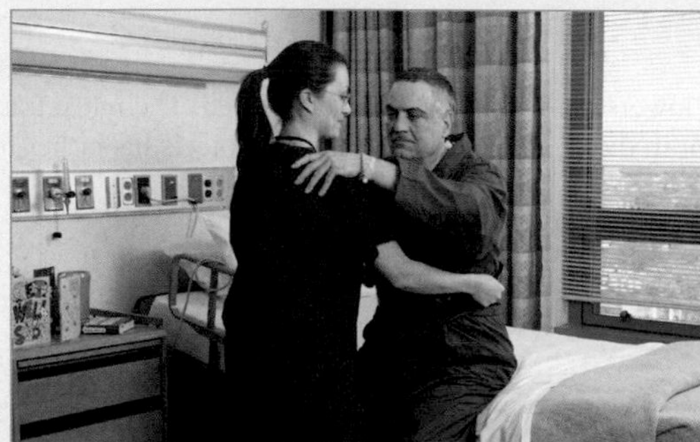

FIGURE 4 Standing close to patient and grasping gait belt.

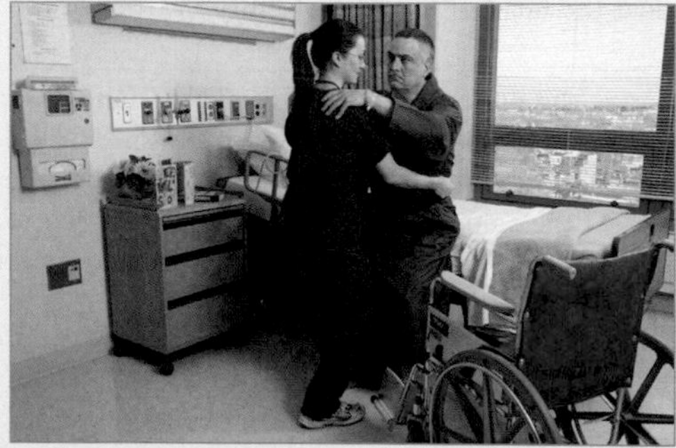

FIGURE 5 Nurse using gait belt and her legs to help raise the patient to a standing position.

ACTION	RATIONALE
16. Pivot on your back foot and assist the patient to turn until the patient feels the chair against his or her legs.	This action ensures proper positioning before sitting.
17. Ask the patient to use his arm to steady himself on the arm of the chair while slowly lowering to a sitting position. Continue to brace the patient's knees with your knees and hold the gait belt. Flex your hips and knees when helping the patient sit in the chair (Figure 6).	The patient uses his or her own arm for support and stability. Flexing hips and knees uses major muscle groups to aid in movement and to reduce strain on the nurse's back.

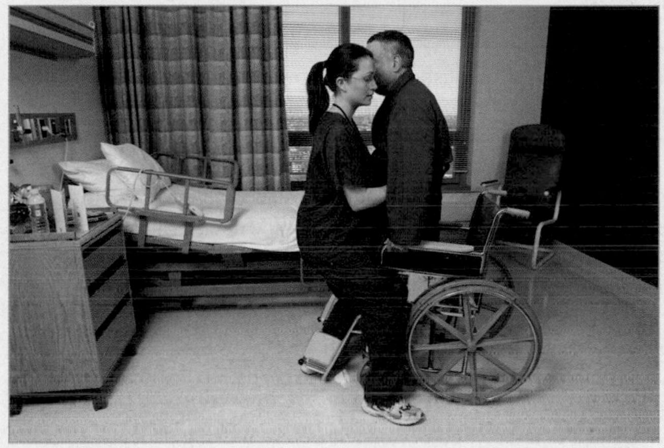

FIGURE 6 Assisting patient to sit.

ACTION	RATIONALE
18. Assess the patient's alignment in the chair. Remove gait belt, if desired. Depending on patient comfort, it could be left in place to use when returning to bed. Cover with a blanket, if needed. Make sure call bell and other essential items are within easy reach.	Assessment promotes comfort; blanket provides warmth and privacy; having the call bell and other essential items readily available helps promote safety.
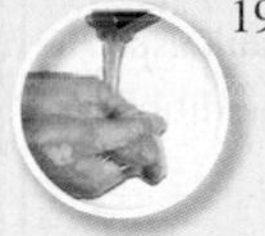 19. Clean transfer aids, per facility policy, if not indicated for single patient use. Remove gloves and any other PPE, if used. Perform hand hygiene.	Proper cleaning of equipment between patient use prevents the spread of microorganisms. Removing PPE properly reduces the risk for infection transmission and contamination of other items. Hand hygiene prevents the spread of microorganisms.

EVALUATION

The expected outcome is met when the patient transfers from the bed to the chair without injury and exhibits no signs and symptoms of problems or complications related to immobility. In addition, the nurse remains free of injury during the transfer.

DOCUMENTATION

Guidelines

Document the activity, including the length of time the patient sat in the chair, any other pertinent observations, and the patient's tolerance of and reaction to the activity. Document the use of transfer aids and number of staff required for transfer.

Sample Documentation

5/13/15 1135 Patient dangled at side of bed for 5 minutes without complaints of dizziness or light-headedness. Patient assisted out of bed to chair with minimal difficulty; gait belt in place. Tolerated sitting in chair for 30 minutes. Assisted back to bed, in semi-Fowler's position. Both upper side rails up.

—J. Minkins, RN

(continued)

SKILL 9-4 TRANSFERRING A PATIENT FROM THE BED TO A CHAIR continued

UNEXPECTED SITUATIONS AND ASSOCIATED INTERVENTIONS

- *You are assisting a patient out of bed. The previous times the patient has gotten up, you have not had any difficulty helping him by yourself, so you are working alone this time. The patient is positioned on the side of the bed. You flex your hips and knees to help him stand. As you move to pivot to the chair, the patient becomes very lightheaded and weak and his knees buckle. The patient is too heavy for you to lift to the chair:* Do not continue the move to the chair. Lower the patient back to the side of the bed. Pivot him back into bed, cover him, and raise the side rails. Check vital signs and assess for any other symptoms. After his symptoms have subsided and you are ready to get him up again, arrange for the assistance of another staff member. Have the patient dangle his legs for a longer period of time before standing. Assess for light-headedness or dizziness before helping him to stand. Notify the primary care provider if there are any significant findings or if his symptoms persist.

SPECIAL CONSIDERATIONS

- Transfer of a patient to a chair or toilet can be accomplished using a powered stand-assist and repositioning lift, if available. These devices can be used with patients who have weight-bearing ability on at least one leg and who can follow directions and are cooperative. A simple sling is placed around the patient's back and under the arms. The patient rests feet on the device's footrest and places his or her hands on the handle. The device mechanically assists the patient to stand, without any lifting by the nurse. (See Fundamentals Review 9-4.) Once the patient is standing, the device can be wheeled to a chair, the toilet, or bed. Some devices have removable footrests and can be used as a walker. Some have scales incorporated into the device that can be used to weigh the patient.
- Patients who are unable to bear partial weight or full weight or who are uncooperative, as well as bariatric patients, should be transferred using a full-body sling lift. (Refer to Skill 9-5.)
- Calculate the BMI for patients weighing over 300 pounds. If BMI exceeds 50, institute Bariatric Algorithms.
- The transfer of patients is often delegated to unlicensed personnel. Before moving patients, all personnel need to complete instructions and must be able to provide return demonstrations of transfer skills. Before the transfer, communicate clearly any mobility restrictions or special care needs.

EVIDENCE FOR PRACTICE ▶

SAFE PATIENT HANDLING AND MOVEMENT

VISN 8 Patient Safety Center. (2009). *Safe patient handling and movement algorithms.* Tampa, FL: Author. Available. http://www.visn8.va.gov/visn8/patientsafetycenter/safePtHandling/default.asp.

Refer to details in Skill 9-1, Evidence for Practice, and refer to thePoint for additional research on related nursing topics.

SKILL 9-5 TRANSFERRING A PATIENT USING A POWERED FULL-BODY SLING LIFT

When it has been determined through the use of a transfer assessment and/or the patient cannot bear any weight, use a powered full-body sling lift device to move him or her up in or out of bed, into and out of a chair, and to a commode or stretcher. (Refer to Fundamentals Review 9-5.) During any patient-handling task, if any caregiver is required to lift more than 35 pounds of a patient's weight, consider the patient to be fully dependent and use assistive devices (Waters, 2007). A full-body sling is placed under the patient's body, including head and torso, and then the sling is attached to the lift. The device slowly lifts the patient. Some devices can be lowered to the floor to pick up a patient who has fallen. These devices are available on portable bases and ceiling-mounted tracks. Each manufacturer's device is slightly different, so review the instructions for your particular device. (See Fundamentals Review 9-4.) Box 9-1 in Skill 9-1 outlines general guidelines related to mobility and safe handling of people with dementia.

DELEGATION CONSIDERATIONS

The transfer of a patient from bed to a chair may be delegated to nursing assistive personnel (NAP) or to unlicensed assistive personnel (UAP), as well as to licensed practical/vocational nurses (LPN/LVNs). The decision to delegate must be based on careful analysis of the patient's needs and circumstances, as well as the qualifications of the person to whom the task is being delegated. Refer to the Delegation Guidelines in Appendix A.

EQUIPMENT

- Powered full-body sling lift
- Sheet or pad to cover the sling, if sling is not dedicated to only one patient
- Chair or wheelchair
- One or more caregivers for assistance, based on assessment
- Nonsterile gloves and/or other PPE, as indicated

ASSESSMENT

Assess the situation to determine the need to use the lift. Review the medical record and nursing plan of care for conditions that may influence the patient's ability to move or to be transferred. Determine the need for bariatric equipment. Assess for tubes, IV lines, incisions, or equipment that may alter the transfer procedure. Assess the patient's level of consciousness and ability to understand and follow directions. Assess the patient's comfort level; if needed, medicate, as ordered, with analgesics. Assess the condition of the equipment to ensure proper functioning before using with the patient.

NURSING DIAGNOSIS

Determine the related factors for the nursing diagnoses based on the patient's current status. Nursing diagnoses that may be appropriate include:

- Risk for Injury
- Impaired Transfer Ability
- Risk for Falls

OUTCOME IDENTIFICATION AND PLANNING

The expected outcome to achieve when transferring a patient using a powered full-body sling lift is that the transfer is accomplished without injury to patient or nurse and the patient is free of any complications of immobility.

IMPLEMENTATION

ACTION	RATIONALE
1. Review the medical record and nursing plan of care for conditions that may influence the patient's ability to move or to be positioned. Assess for tubes, IV lines, incisions, or equipment that may alter the positioning procedure. Identify any movement limitations. **Consult patient-handling algorithm, if available, to plan appropriate approach to moving the patient.**	Reviewing the medical record and plan of care validates the correct patient and correct procedure. Checking for equipment and limitations reduces the risk for injury during the transfer.
2. Perform hand hygiene and put on PPE, if indicated.	Hand hygiene and PPE prevent the spread of microorganisms. PPE is required based on transmission precautions.
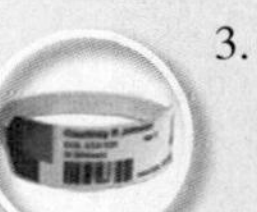 3. Identify the patient. Explain the procedure to the patient.	Patient identification validates the correct patient and correct procedure. Discussion and explanation allay anxiety and prepare the patient for what to expect.
4. If needed, move the equipment to make room for the chair. Close the curtains around the bed and close the door to the room, if possible.	Moving equipment out of the way provides a clear path and facilitates the transfer. Closing the door or curtain provides for privacy.
5. Adjust the bed to a comfortable working height, usually elbow height of the caregiver (VISN 8 Patient Safety Center, 2009). **Lock the bed brakes.**	Having the bed at the proper height prevents back and muscle strain. Locking the brakes prevents bed movement and ensures patient safety.

(continued)

SKILL 9-5 TRANSFERRING A PATIENT USING A POWERED FULL-BODY SLING LIFT continued

ACTION	RATIONALE
6. Lower the side rail, if in use, on the side of the bed you are working. If the sling is for use with more than one patient, place a cover or pad on the sling. Place the sling evenly under the patient. Roll the patient to one side and place half of the sling with the sheet or pad on it under the patient from shoulders to mid-thigh (Figure 1). Raise the rail and move to the other side. Lower the rail, if necessary. Roll the patient to the other side and pull the sling under the patient (Figure 2). Raise the side rail.	Lowering the side rail prevents strain on the nurse's back. Covering the sling prevents transmission of microorganisms. Some facilities, such as long-term care institutions, provide each patient with own transport sling. Rolling the patient positions the patient on the sling with minimal movement. Even distribution of the patient's weight in the sling provides for patient comfort and safety.
7. Bring the chair to the side of the bed. **Lock the wheels, if present.**	Bringing the chair close to the bed minimizes the distance needed for transfer. Locking the wheels prevents chair movement and ensures patient safety.
8. Lower the side rail on the chair side of the bed. Roll the base of the lift under the side of the bed nearest to the chair. **Center the frame over the patient. Lock the wheels of the lift.**	Lowering the rail allows for ease of transfer. Doing so reduces the distance necessary for transfer. Centering the frame helps maintain the balance of the lift. Locking the lift's wheels prevents the lift from rolling.
9. **Using the base-adjustment lever, widen the stance of the base (Figure 3).**	A wider stance provides greater stability and prevents tipping.
10. Lower the arms close enough to attach the sling to the frame (Figure 4).	Lowering the arms is necessary to allow for the attachment of the sling's hooks.

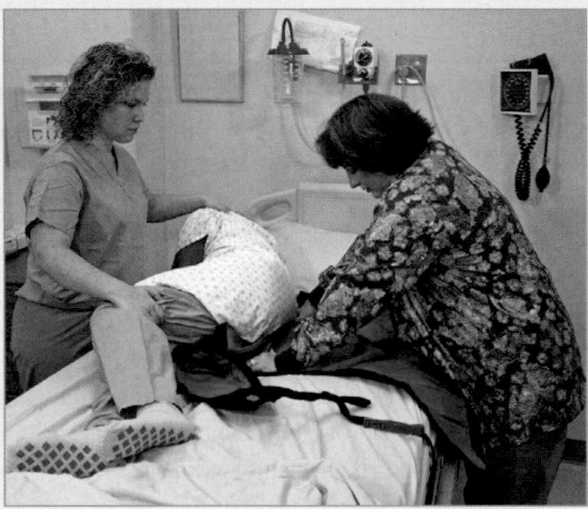

FIGURE 1 Rolling patient to one side and placing rolled sling underneath patient.

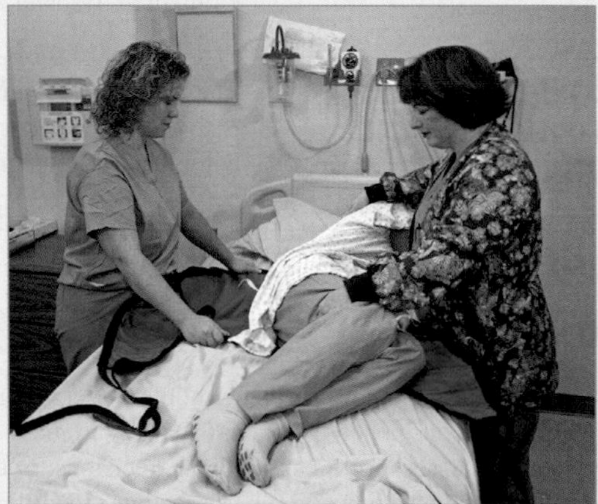

FIGURE 2 Rolling patient to opposite side and pulling sling under patient.

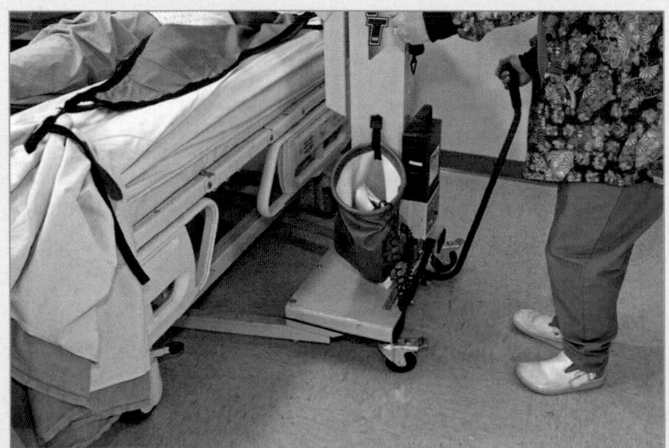

FIGURE 3 Widening stance of lift base.

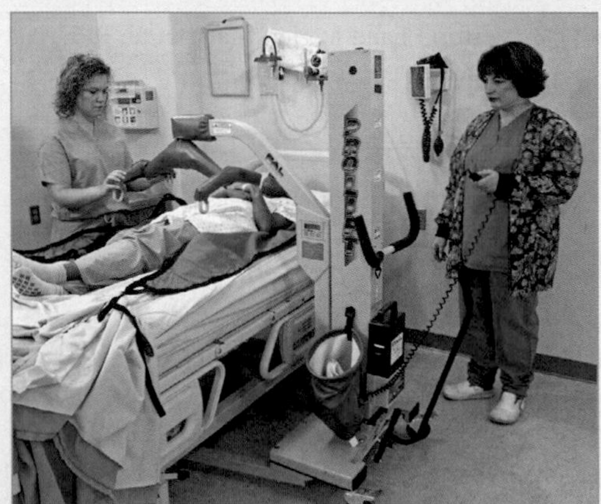

FIGURE 4 Lowering lift arms.

ACTION	RATIONALE
11. Attach the straps on the sling to the hooks on the frame (Figure 5). Short straps attach behind the patient's back and long straps attach at the other end of the sling. Check the patient to make sure the straps are not pressing into the skin. Some lifts have straps or chains with hooks that attach to holes in the sling. Check the manufacturer's instructions for each lift.	Connecting the straps or chains permits attachment of the sling to the lift. Checking the patient's skin for pressure from the hooks prevents injury.
12. Check all equipment, lines, and drains attached to the patient so that they are not interfering with the device. Have the patient fold his or her arms across the chest.	Ensuring that equipment and lines are free of the device prevents dislodgement and possible injury.
13. With a person standing on each side of the lift, tell the patient that he or she will be lifted from the bed. Support injured limbs as necessary. Engage the pump to raise the patient about 6 inches above the bed (Figure 6).	Having the necessary people available provides for safety. Supporting injured limbs helps maintain stability. Informing the patient about what will occur reassures the patient and reduces fear.
14. Unlock the wheels of the lift. **Carefully wheel the patient straight back and away from the bed. Support the patient's limbs, as needed.**	Moving in this manner promotes stability and safety.
15. Position the patient over the chair with the base of the lift straddling the chair (Figure 7). Lock the wheels of the lift.	Proper positioning of the patient and device promotes stability and safety.
16. Gently lower the patient to the chair until the hooks or straps are slightly loosened from the sling or frame (Figure 8). Guide the patient into the chair with your hands as the sling lowers.	Gently lowering the patient in this manner places the patient fully in the chair and reduces the risk for injury.

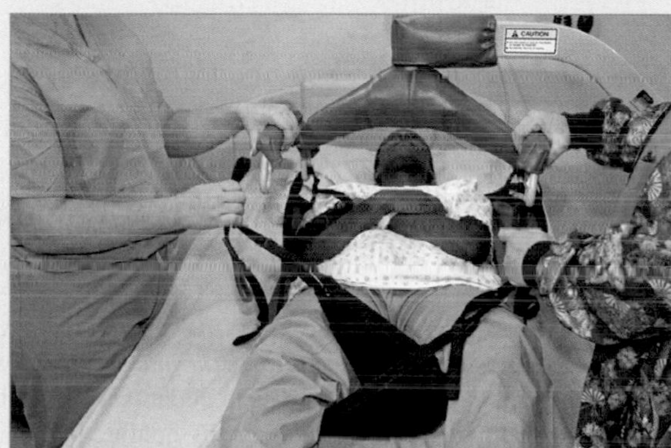

FIGURE 5 Connecting lift straps.

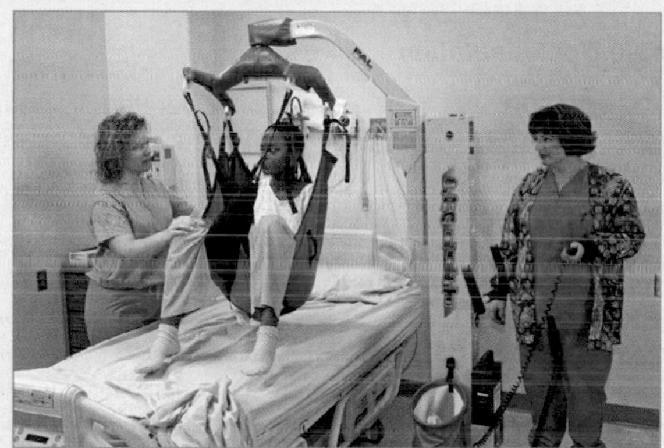

FIGURE 6 Raising patient 6 inches above bed.

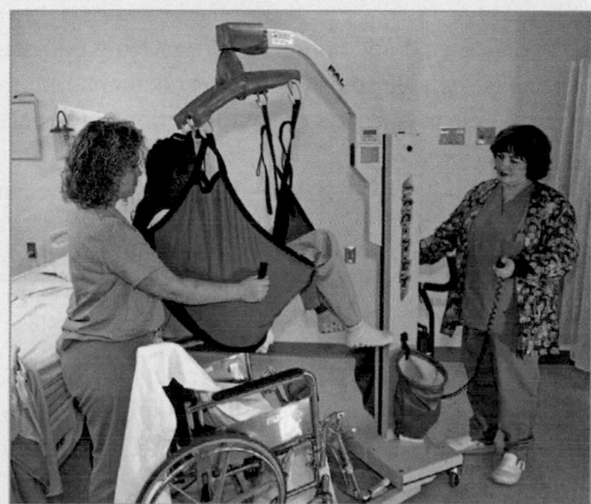

FIGURE 7 Positioning patient in sling over chair.

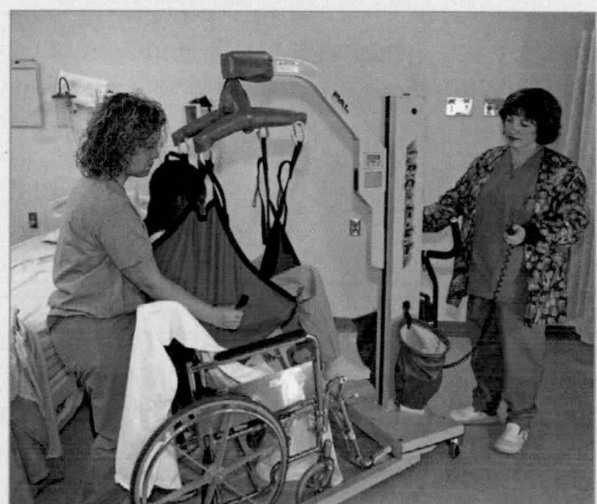

FIGURE 8 Lowering patient in sling into chair.

(continued)

SKILL 9-5 TRANSFERRING A PATIENT USING A POWERED FULL-BODY SLING LIFT continued

ACTION	RATIONALE
17. Disconnect the hooks or strap from the frame. Keep the sling in place under the patient.	Disconnecting the hooks or straps allows the patient to be supported by the chair and promotes comfort. The sling will need to be reattached to the lift to move the patient back to bed.
18. Adjust the patient's position, using pillows, if necessary. Check the patient's alignment in the chair. Cover the patient with a blanket, if necessary. Make sure call bell and other essential items are within easy reach. When it is time for the patient to return to bed, reattach the hooks or straps and reverse the steps.	Pillows and proper alignment provide for patient safety and comfort. Having the call bell and other essential items readily available helps promote safety. Reattaching the hooks or straps allows the lift to support the patient for transfer back to bed.
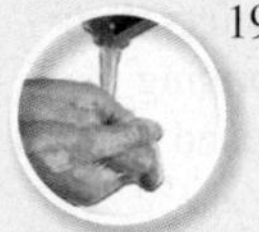 19. Clean transfer aids, per facility policy, if not indicated for single patient use. Remove gloves and any other PPE, if used. Perform hand hygiene.	Proper cleaning of equipment between patient use prevents the spread of microorganisms. Removing PPE properly reduces the risk for infection transmission and contamination of other items. Hand hygiene prevents the spread of microorganisms.

EVALUATION

The expected outcome is met when the transfer is accomplished without injury to patient or nurse, and the patient exhibits no evidence of complications of immobility.

DOCUMENTATION

Guidelines

Document the activity, transfer, any other pertinent observations, the patient's tolerance of the procedure, and the length of time in the chair. Document the use of transfer aids and number of staff required for transfer.

Sample Documentation

5/13/15 1430 Patient transferred out of bed to chair using powered full-body sling lift. Tolerated sitting in chair for 25 minutes without complaints of dizziness or pain. Assisted back to bed via lift. Left sitting in semi-Fowler's position with all four side rails up.

—*P. Jefferson, RN*

UNEXPECTED SITUATIONS AND ASSOCIATED INTERVENTIONS

- *You are preparing to move a patient using a powered full-body sling lift. After you apply the sling and attach it to the frame, the patient becomes anxious and tells you she is afraid:* Acknowledge the patient's feelings and explain the procedure again. Reassure the patient about the safety of the device. Obtain an additional person to support the patient during the move by holding her hand or supporting her head. If possible, plan the transfer when a family member or friend is present to offer support.

SPECIAL CONSIDERATIONS

- The transfer of patients is often delegated to unlicensed personnel. Before moving patients, all personnel need to complete instructions and must be able to provide return demonstrations of transfer skills. Before the transfer, communicate clearly any mobility restrictions or special care needs.
- Calculate the BMI for patients weighing over 300 pounds. If BMI exceeds 50, institute Bariatric Algorithms.

EVIDENCE FOR PRACTICE ▶

SAFE PATIENT HANDLING AND MOVEMENT

VISN 8 Patient Safety Center. (2009). *Safe patient handling and movement algorithms.* Tampa, FL: Author. Available. http://www.visn8.va.gov/visn8/patientsafetycenter/safePtHandling/default.asp.

Refer to details in Skill 9-1, Evidence for Practice, and refer to thePoint for additional research on related nursing topics.

SKILL 9-6 PROVIDING RANGE-OF-MOTION EXERCISES

Range of motion (ROM) is the complete extent of movement of which a joint is normally capable. When a person performs routine activities of daily living (ADLs), he or she is using muscle groups that help to keep many joints in an effective range of motion. When all or some of the normal ADLs are impossible due to illness or injury, it is important to give attention to the joints not being used or to those that have limited use. When the patient does the exercise for him- or herself, it is referred to as *active range of motion.* Exercises performed by the nurse without participation by the patient are referred to as *passive range of motion.* Exercises should be as active as the patient's physical condition permits. Allow the patient to do as much individual activity as his or her condition permits. Initiate ROM exercises as soon as possible because body changes can occur after only 3 days of impaired mobility.

DELEGATION CONSIDERATIONS

Patient teaching regarding range-of-motion exercises cannot be delegated to nursing assistive personnel (NAP) or to unlicensed assistive personnel (UAP). Reinforcement or implementation of ROM exercises may be delegated to NAP or UAP, as well as to licensed practical/vocational nurses (LPN/LVNs). The decision to delegate must be based on careful analysis of the patient's needs and circumstances, as well as the qualifications of the person to whom the task is being delegated. Refer to the Delegation Guidelines in Appendix A.

EQUIPMENT

No special equipment or supplies are necessary to perform ROM exercises. Wear nonsterile gloves and/or other PPE, as appropriate.

ASSESSMENT

Review the medical record and nursing plan of care for any conditions or orders that will limit mobility. Perform a pain assessment before the time for the exercises. If the patient reports pain, administer the prescribed medication in sufficient time to allow for the full effect of the analgesic. Assess the patient's ability to perform ROM exercises. Inspect and palpate joints for redness, tenderness, pain, swelling, or deformities.

NURSING DIAGNOSIS

Determine the related factors for the nursing diagnoses based on the patient's current status. Appropriate nursing diagnoses may include:

- Impaired Physical Mobility
- Fatigue
- Deficient Knowledge

OUTCOME IDENTIFICATION AND PLANNING

The expected outcome to achieve when performing ROM exercises is that the patient maintains joint mobility. Other outcomes include improving or maintaining muscle strength, and preventing muscle atrophy and contractures.

IMPLEMENTATION

ACTION	RATIONALE
1. Review the medical orders and nursing plan of care for patient activity. Identify any movement limitations.	Reviewing the order and plan of care validates the correct patient and correct procedure. Identification of limitations prevents injury.
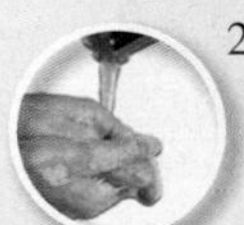 2. Perform hand hygiene and put on PPE, if indicated.	Hand hygiene and PPE prevent the spread of microorganisms. PPE is required based on transmission precautions.
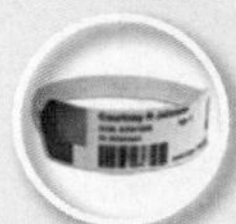 3. Identify the patient. Explain the procedure to the patient.	Patient identification validates the correct patient and correct procedure. Discussion and explanation help allay anxiety and prepare the patient for what to expect.

(continued)

SKILL 9-6 PROVIDING RANGE-OF-MOTION EXERCISES continued

ACTION	RATIONALE
4. Close the curtains around the bed and close the door to the room, if possible. Place the bed at an appropriate and comfortable working height, usually elbow height of the caregiver (VISN 8 Patient Safety Center, 2009). Adjust the head of the bed to a flat position or as low as the patient can tolerate.	Closing the door or curtains provides privacy. Proper bed height helps reduce back strain while performing the procedure.
5. Stand on the side of the bed where the joints are to be exercised. Lower side rail on that side, if in place. Uncover only the limb to be used during the exercise.	Standing on the side to be exercised and lowering the side rail prevent strain on the nurse's back. Proper draping provides for privacy and warmth.
6. Perform the exercises slowly and gently, providing support by holding the areas proximal and distal to the joint. Repeat each exercise two to five times, moving each joint in a smooth and rhythmic manner. **Stop movement if the patient complains of pain or if you meet resistance.**	Slow, gentle movements with support prevent discomfort and muscle spasms resulting from jerky movements. Repeated movement of muscles and joints improves flexibility and increases circulation to the body part. Pain may indicate the exercises are causing damage.
7. While performing the exercises, begin at the head and move down one side of the body at a time. **Encourage the patient to do as many of these exercises independently as possible.**	Proceeding from head to toe, one side at a time, promotes efficient time management and an organized approach to the task. Both active and passive exercises improve joint mobility and increase circulation to the affected part, but only active exercise increases muscle mass, tone, and strength and improves cardiac and respiratory functioning.
8. Move the chin down to rest on the chest (Figure 1). Return the head to a normal upright position (Figure 2). Tilt the head as far as possible toward each shoulder (Figure 3).	These movements provide for **flexion, extension**, and lateral flexion of the head and neck.
9. Move the head from side to side, bringing the chin toward each shoulder (Figure 4).	These movements provide for **rotation** of neck.

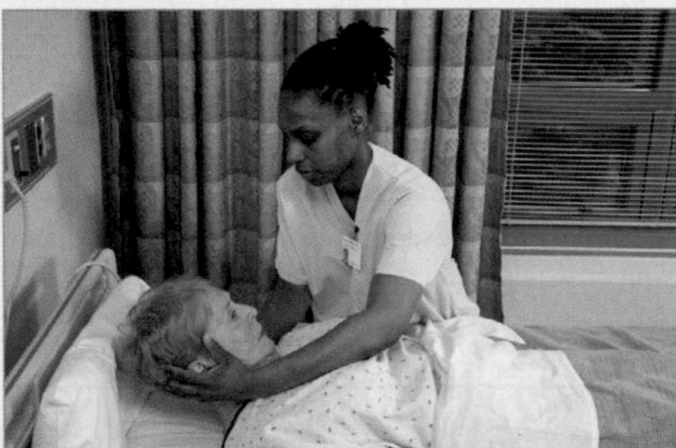

FIGURE 1 Moving patient's chin down to rest on chest.

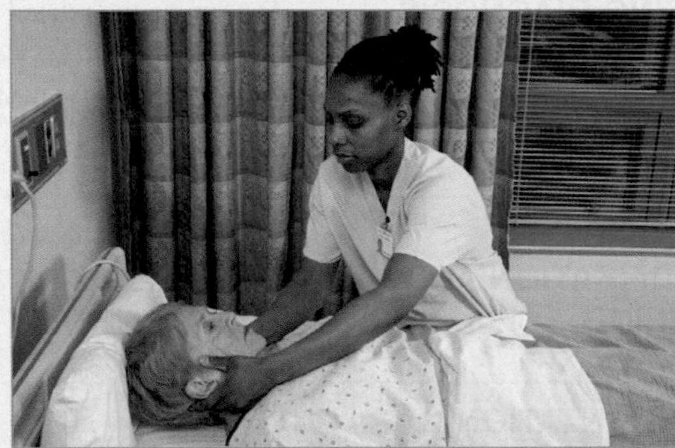

FIGURE 2 Holding patient's head upright and centered.

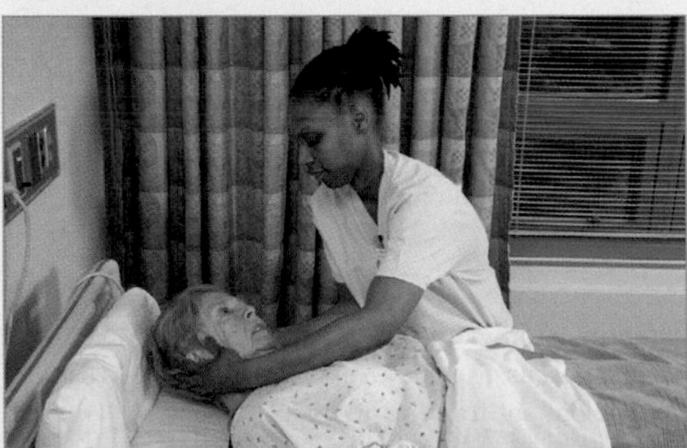

FIGURE 3 Moving patient's head to one shoulder.

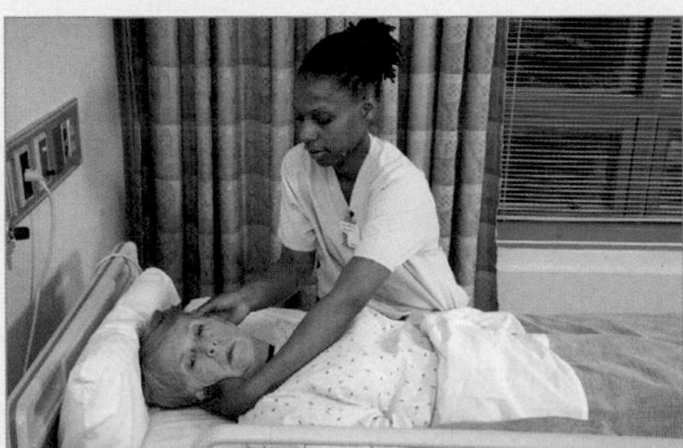

FIGURE 4 Moving patient's chin toward one shoulder.

ACTION	RATIONALE
10. Start with the arm at the patient's side (Figure 5) and lift the arm forward to above the head (Figure 6). Return the arm to the starting position at the side of the body.	These movements provide for flexion and extension of the shoulder.
11. With the arm back at the patient's side, move the arm laterally to an upright position above the head (Figure 7), and then return it to the original position. Move the arm across the body as far as possible (Figure 8).	These movements provide for **abduction** and **adduction** of the shoulder.
12. Raise the arm at the side until the upper arm is in line with the shoulder. Bend the elbow at a 90-degree angle (Figure 9) and move the forearm upward and downward, then return the arm to the side.	These movements provide for internal and external rotation of the shoulder.
13. Bend the elbow and move the lower arm and hand upward toward the shoulder (Figure 10). Return the lower arm and hand to the original position while straightening the elbow.	These movements provide for flexion and extension of the elbow.

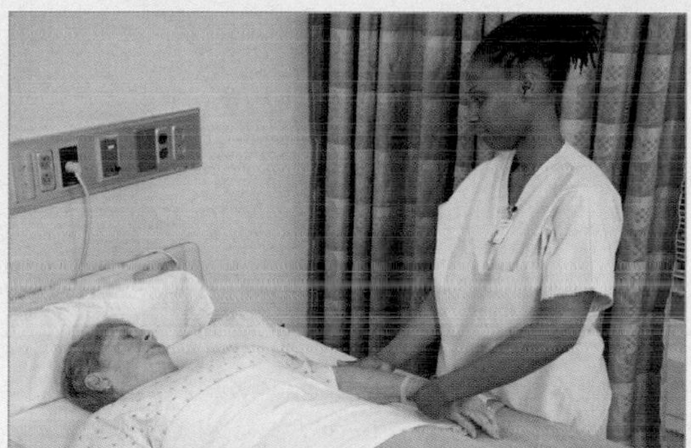

FIGURE 5 Holding patient's arm at side.

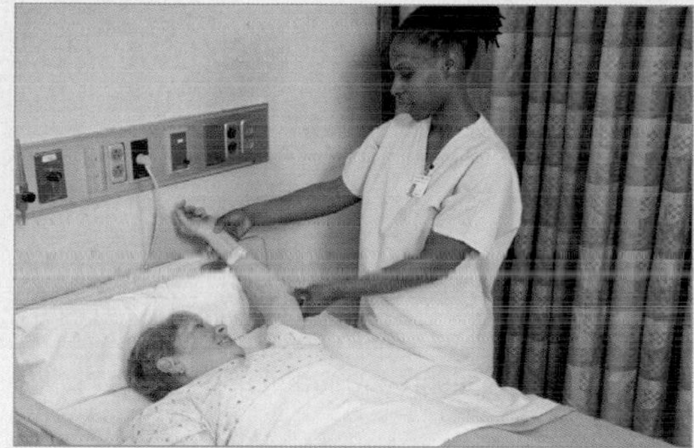

FIGURE 6 Lifting patient's arm above patient's head.

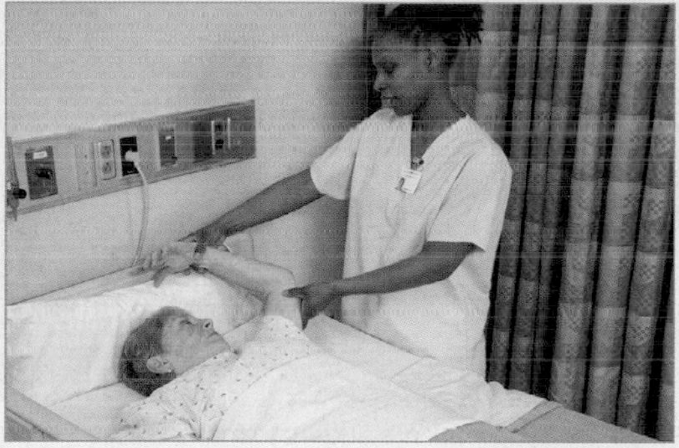

FIGURE 7 Moving patient's arm laterally to an upright position above patient's head.

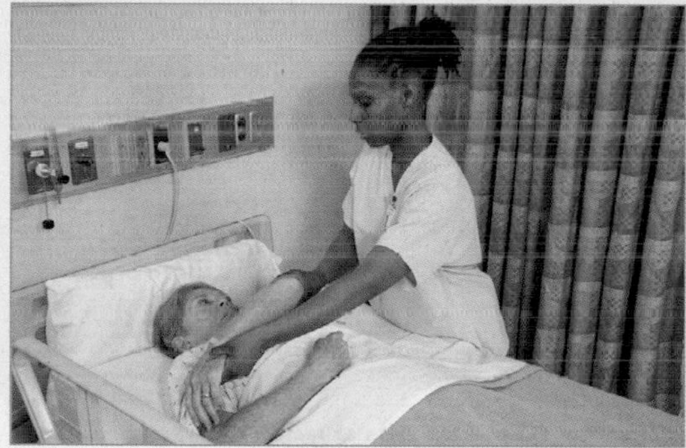

FIGURE 8 Moving arm across patient's body as far as possible.

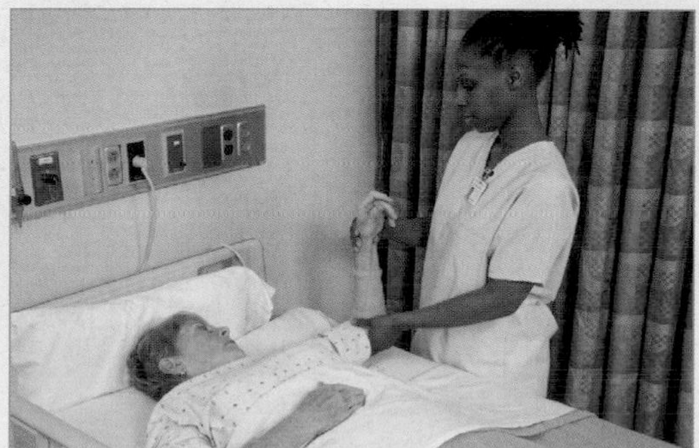

FIGURE 9 Raising patient's arm until upper arm is in line with patient's shoulder, with elbow bent.

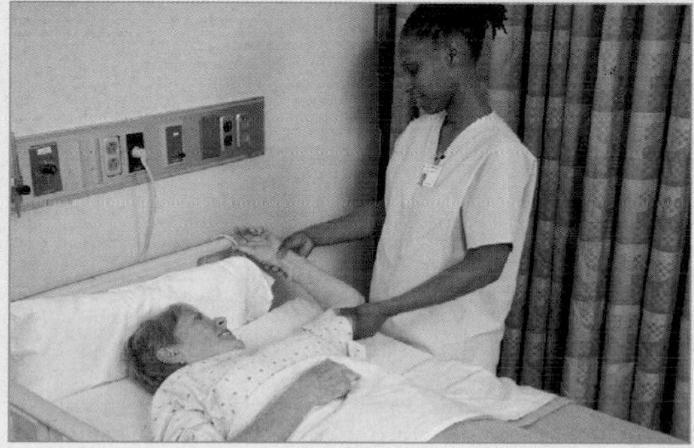

FIGURE 10 Bending patient's elbow, lower arm, and hand upward toward shoulder.

(continued)

SKILL 9-6 PROVIDING RANGE-OF-MOTION EXERCISES continued

ACTION	RATIONALE
14. Rotate the lower arm and hand so the palm is up (Figure 11). Rotate the lower arm and hand so the palm of the hand is down.	These movements provide for **supination** and **pronation** of the forearm.
15. Move the hand downward toward the inner aspect of the forearm (Figure 12). Return the hand to a neutral position even with the forearm (Figure 13). Then move the dorsal portion of the hand backward as far as possible.	These movements provide for flexion, extension, and hyperextension of the wrist.
16. Bend the fingers to make a fist (Figure 14), and then straighten them out (Figure 15). Spread the fingers apart (Figure 16) and return them back together. Touch the thumb to each finger on the hand (Figure 17).	These movements provide for flexion, extension, abduction, and adduction of the fingers.

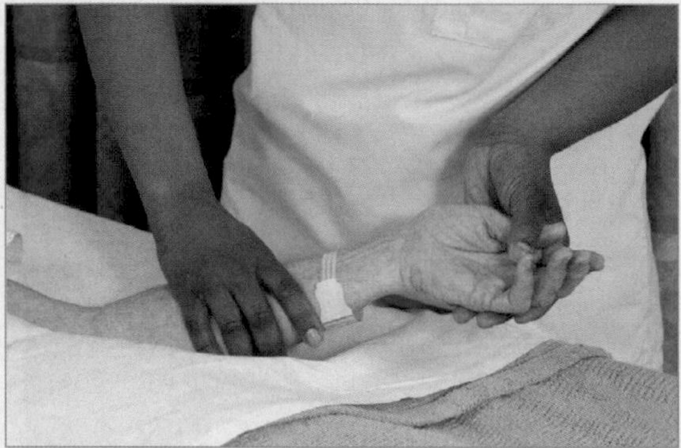

FIGURE 11 Rotating patient's lower arm and hand so palm is up.

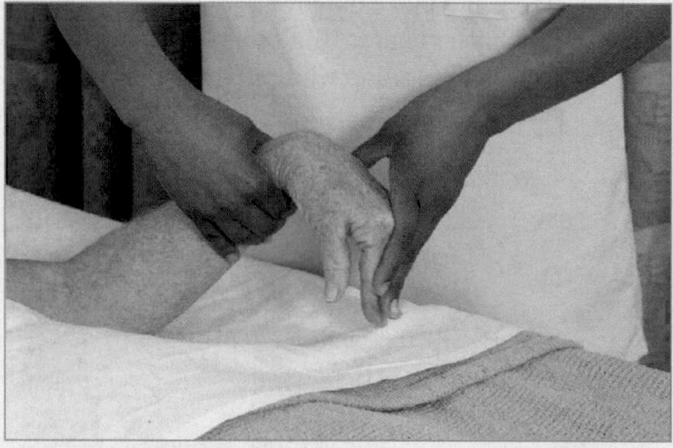

FIGURE 12 Moving patient's hand downward toward inner aspect of forearm.

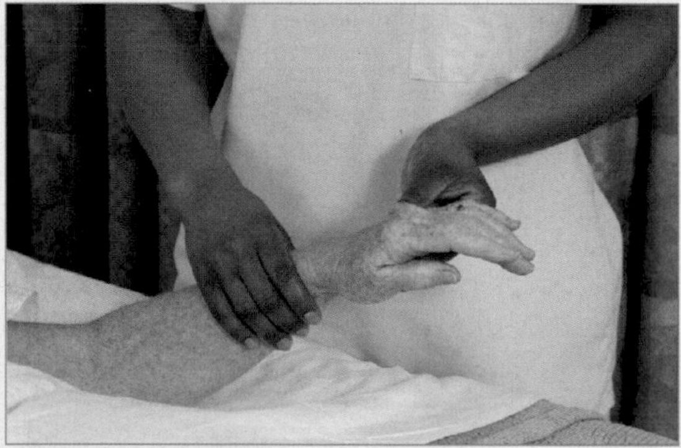

FIGURE 13 Returning hand to neutral position.

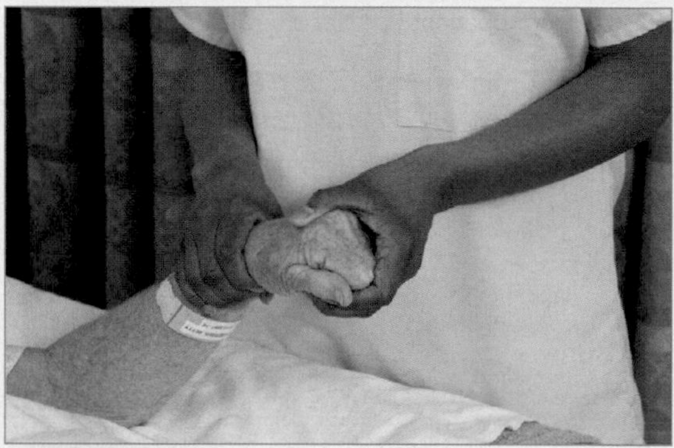

FIGURE 14 Bending patient's fingers to make a fist.

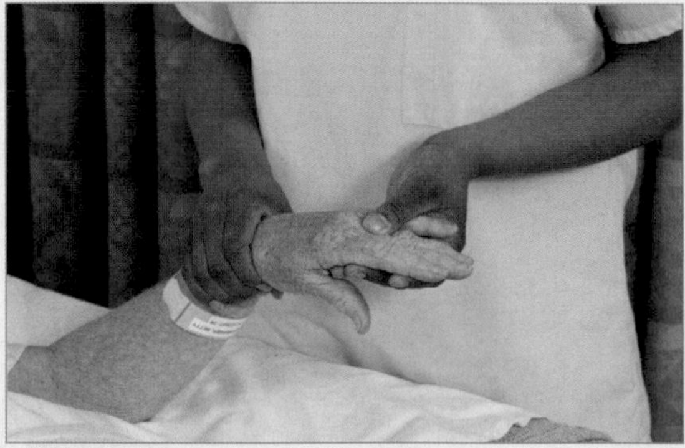

FIGURE 15 Straightening out patient's fingers.

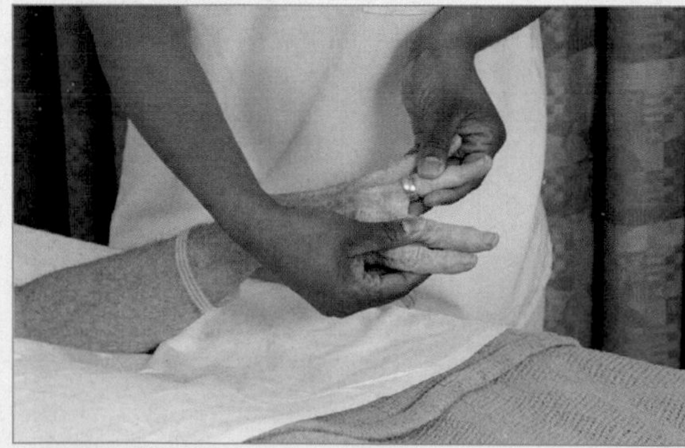

FIGURE 16 Spreading patient's fingers apart.

ACTION | RATIONALE

17. Extend the leg and lift it upward (Figure 18). Return the leg to the original position beside the other leg.

These movements provide for flexion and extension of the hip.

18. Lift the leg laterally away from the patient's body (Figure 19). Return the leg back toward the other leg and try to extend it beyond the midline (Figure 20).

These movements provide for abduction and adduction of the hip.

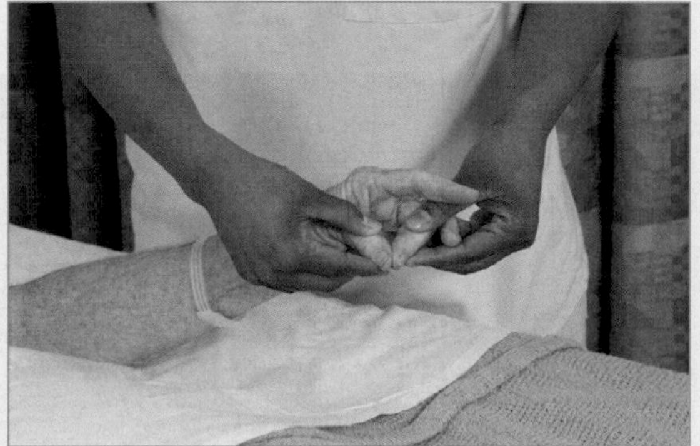

FIGURE 17 Assisting patient to touch thumb to each finger on hand.

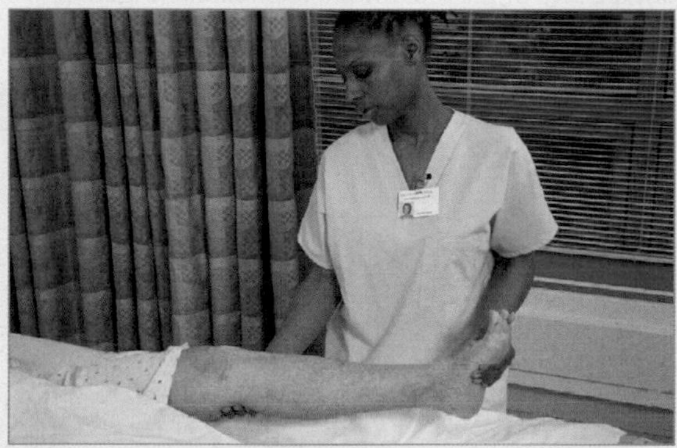

FIGURE 18 Extending and lifting patient's leg.

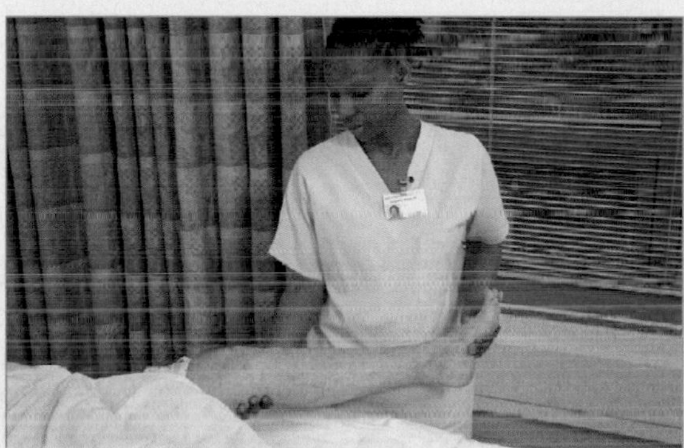

FIGURE 19 Lifting patient's leg laterally away from body (abduction).

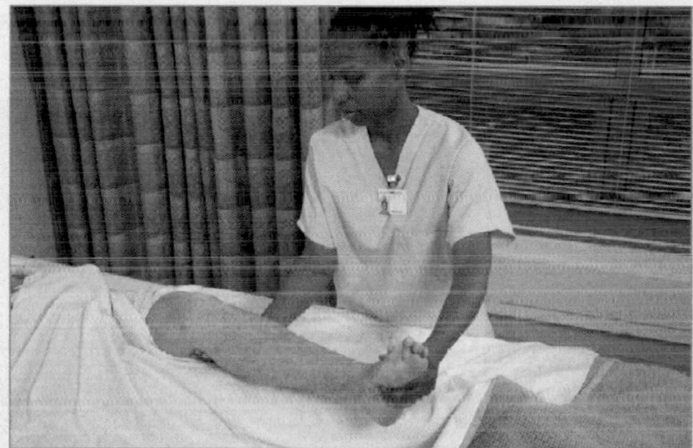

FIGURE 20 Returning leg back toward other leg and trying to extend it beyond midline, if possible.

19. Turn the foot and leg toward the opposite leg to rotate it internally (Figure 21). Turn the foot and leg outward away from the opposite leg to rotate it externally (Figure 22).

These movements provide for internal and external rotation of the hip.

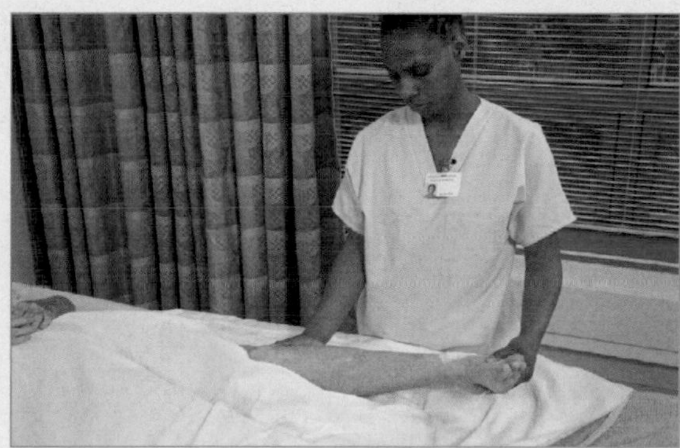

FIGURE 21 Turning patient's foot and leg toward opposite leg to rotate it internally.

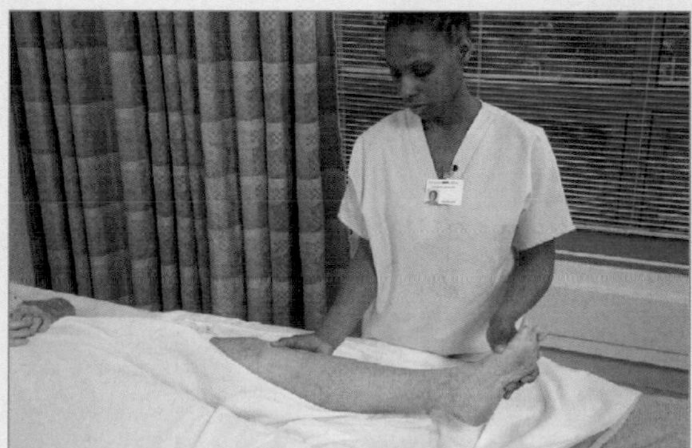

FIGURE 22 Turning patient's foot and leg outward, away from opposite leg, to rotate it externally.

(continued)

SKILL 9-6 PROVIDING RANGE-OF-MOTION EXERCISES continued

ACTION	RATIONALE
20. Bend the leg and bring the heel toward the back of the leg (Figure 23). Return the leg to a straight position (Figure 24).	These movements provide for flexion and extension of the knee.
21. At the ankle, move the foot up and back until the toes are upright (Figure 25). Move the foot with the toes pointing downward (Figure 26).	These movements provide for dorsiflexion and plantar flexion of the ankle.
22. Turn the sole of the foot toward the midline (Figure 27). Turn the sole of the foot outward (Figure 28).	These movements provide for inversion and eversion of the ankle.

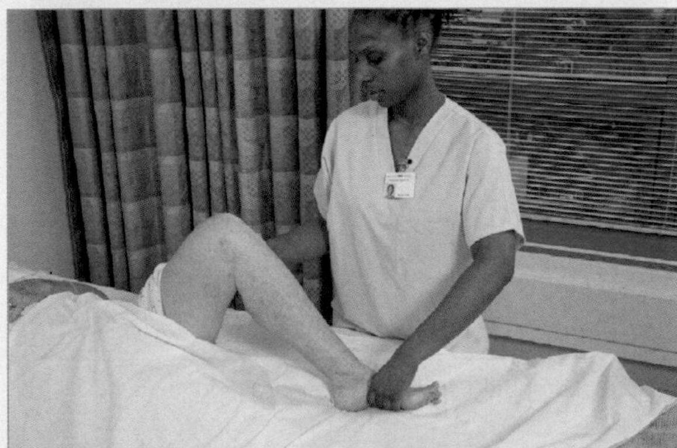

FIGURE 23 Bending patient's leg and bringing heel toward back of leg.

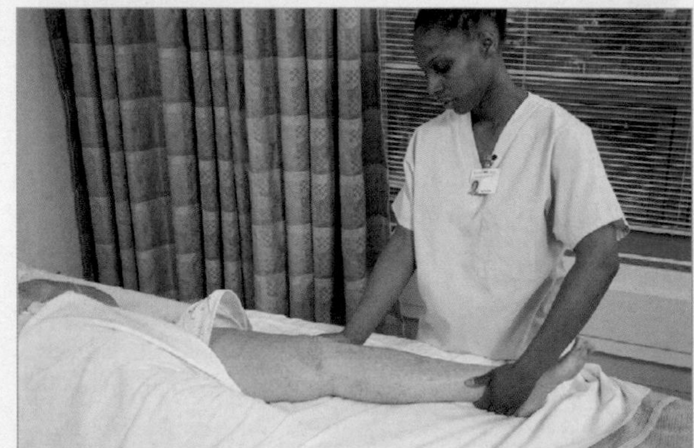

FIGURE 24 Returning leg to a straight position.

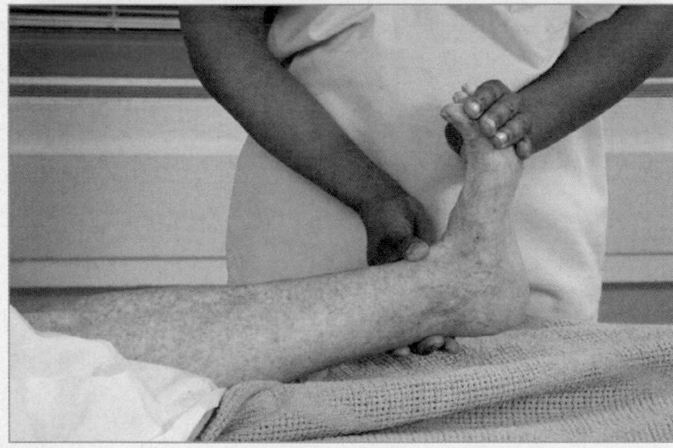

FIGURE 25 At the ankle, moving patient's foot up and back until toes are upright.

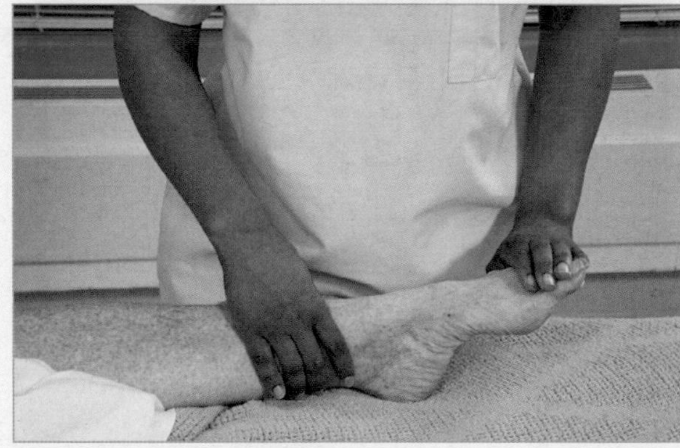

FIGURE 26 Moving patient's foot with toes pointing down.

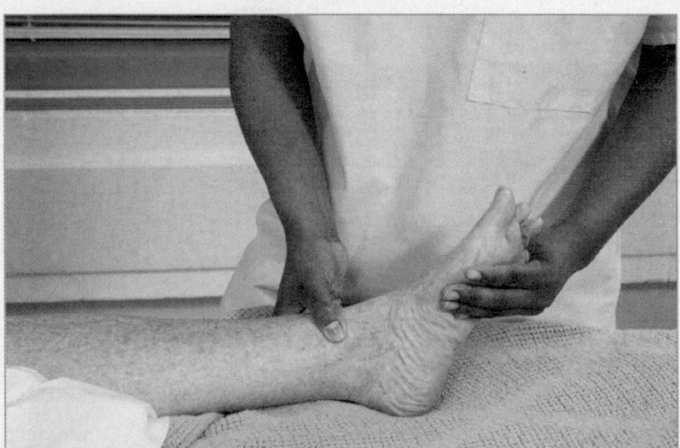

FIGURE 27 Turning sole toward midline.

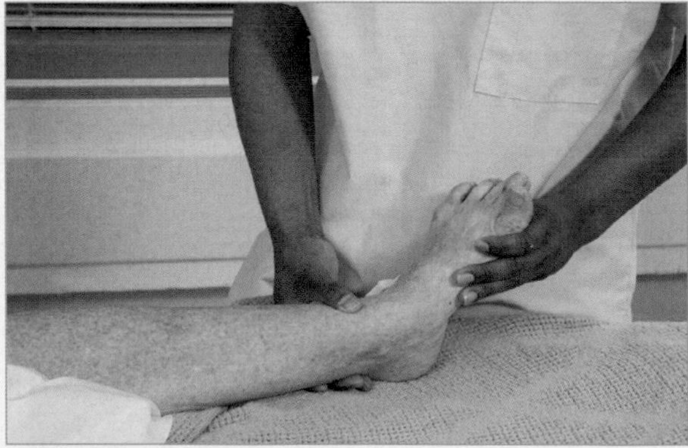

FIGURE 28 Turning sole outward.

ACTION | RATIONALE

23. Curl the toes downward (Figure 29), and then straighten them out (Figure 30). Spread the toes apart (Figure 31) and bring them together (Figure 32).

These movements provide for flexion, extension, abduction, and adduction of the toes.

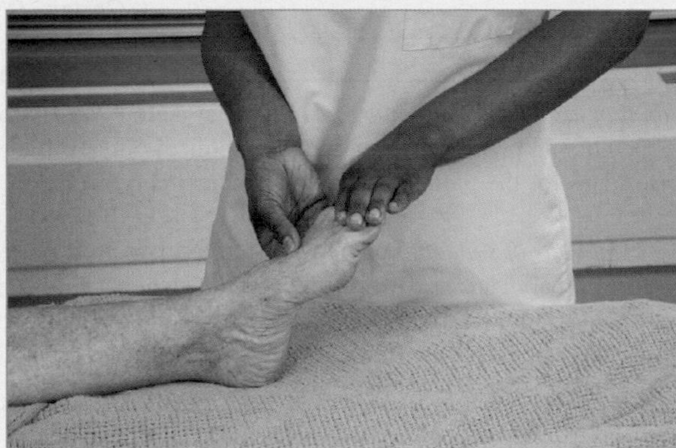

FIGURE 29 Curling patient's toes downward.

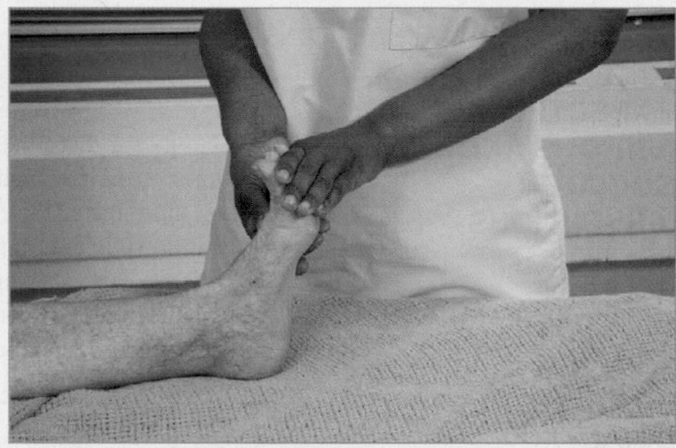

FIGURE 30 Straightening patient's toes.

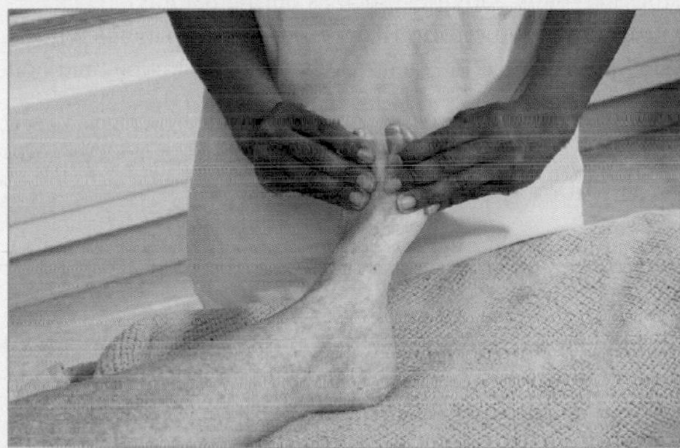

FIGURE 31 Spreading patient's toes apart.

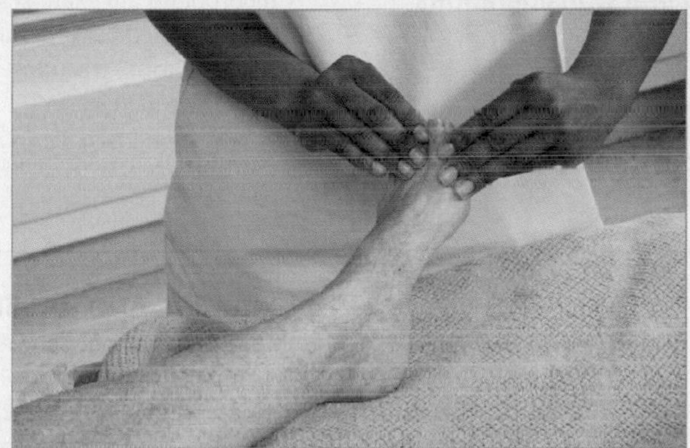

FIGURE 32 Bringing patient's toes together.

24. Repeat these exercises on the other side of the body. Encourage the patient to do as many of these exercises independently as possible.

Repeating motions on the other side provides exercise for the entire body. Self-esteem, self-care, and independence are encouraged through the patient performing the exercises on his or her own.

25. When finished, make sure the patient is comfortable, with the side rails up and the bed in the lowest position. Place call bell and other essential items within reach.

Proper positioning with raised side rails and proper bed height provide for patient comfort and safety. Having the call bell and other essential items within reach promotes safety.

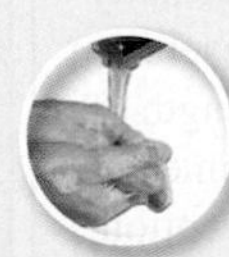

26. Remove gloves and any other PPE, if used. Perform hand hygiene.

Removing PPE properly reduces the risk for infection transmission and contamination of other items. Hand hygiene prevents the spread of microorganisms.

EVALUATION

The expected outcome is met when the patient maintains or improves joint mobility and muscle strength, and muscle atrophy and contractures are prevented.

DOCUMENTATION

Guidelines

Document the exercises performed, any significant observations, and the patient's reaction to the activities.

(continued)

SKILL 9-6 PROVIDING RANGE-OF-MOTION EXERCISES continued

Sample Documentation

5/1/15 0945 Range-of-motion exercises performed to all joints. Patient able to perform active ROM of head, neck, shoulders, and arms. Required moderate assistance with ROM to lower extremities. Denied any complaints of pain during exercises. Patient tolerated exercise session well. Sitting in semi-Fowler's position with side rails up, watching television.

—J. Chrisp, RN

UNEXPECTED SITUATIONS AND ASSOCIATED INTERVENTIONS

- *While you are performing range-of-motion exercises, the patient complains of feeling tired:* Stop the activity for that time. Reevaluate the nursing plan of care. Space the exercises out at different times of the day. Schedule exercise times for the parts of the day the patient is typically feeling more rested.
- *While exercising your patient's leg, he complains of sudden, sharp pain:* Stop the exercises. Assess the patient for other symptoms. Notify the primary care provider of the event, the patient's uncomfortable reaction, and your assessment findings. Joints should be moved until there is resistance, but not pain. Report uncomfortable reactions and halt exercises. Revise activity plan if necessary.

SPECIAL CONSIDERATIONS

General Considerations

- Incorporate the exercises when possible into daily activities, such as during bathing.
- Obtain a medical order and specific instructions to perform ROM exercises for patients with acute arthritis, fractures, torn ligaments, joint dislocation, acute myocardial infarction, and bone tumors or metastases.

Older Adult Considerations

- Avoid neck hyperextension and attempts to achieve full range of motion in all joints with older patients.

EVIDENCE FOR PRACTICE ▶

EXERCISE AND IMPAIRED MOBILITY

Stroke is major public health concern and many survivors experience moderate to severe levels of permanent physical disability as a result. Range-of-motion exercises improve joint mobility; increase circulation, muscle mass, muscle tone, and muscle strength; and improve cardiac and respiratory functioning. Exercises should be as active as the patient's physical condition permits. ROM exercises should be initiated as soon as possible as part of a patient's plan of care because body changes can occur after only a few days of impaired mobility. The benefits of physical rehabilitation for stroke survivors have been established. Nurses are in ideal positions to discuss the effects of exercise with patients and include exercise programs in the plan of care.

Related Research

Kim, G., Kwon, G., Hur, H.K., et al. (2012). Effects of muscle strengthening exercise program on muscle strength, activities of daily living, health perception, and depression in post-stroke elders. *Korean Journal of Adult Nursing, 24*(3), 1.

This trial evaluated the effects of an exercise program on muscle strength, activities of daily living (ADL), health perception, and depression among post-stroke older adults. The exercise program consisted of deep breathing, range of motion, and muscle exercises. Muscle strength of the shoulder ($P = 0.001$), leg ($P = 0.002$), and health perception ($P = 0.01$) in the experimental group was significantly higher compared to the control group, at 12 weeks of post-intervention. Self-rated symptoms of depression scores were significantly lower in the experimental group compared to the control group at 6 weeks ($P = 0.021$) and at 12 weeks ($P = 0.006$) of the exercise program. By applying this program, older adults showed increases in muscle strength and a decrease in depression as well as improvement of health perception after a stroke.

Relevance for Nursing Practice

An exercise program that includes ROM exercises can generate positive effects in enhancing physical and psychological function of older adult stroke survivors. Methods to assist patients in maintaining or increasing physical activity should be a part of routine nursing care.

Refer to thePoint for additional research on related nursing topics.

SKILL 9-7 ASSISTING A PATIENT WITH AMBULATION

Walking exercises most of the body's muscles and increases joint flexibility. It improves respiratory and gastrointestinal function. Ambulating also reduces the risk for complications of immobility. However, even a short period of immobility can decrease a person's tolerance for ambulating. If necessary, make use of appropriate equipment and assistive devices to aid in patient movement and handling. (Refer to Fundamentals Review 9-4 for examples of assistive equipment and devices.) Box 9-1 in Skill 9-1 outlines general guidelines related to mobility and safe handling of people with dementia.

DELEGATION CONSIDERATIONS

Assisting a patient with ambulation may be delegated to nursing assistive personnel (NAP) or to unlicensed assistive personnel (UAP), as well as to licensed practical/vocational nurses (LPN/LVNs). The decision to delegate must be based on careful analysis of the patient's needs and circumstances, as well as the qualifications of the person to whom the task is being delegated. Refer to the Delegation Guidelines in Appendix A.

EQUIPMENT

- Gait belt, as necessary
- Nonskid shoes or slippers
- Nonsterile gloves and/or other PPE, as indicated
- Stand-assist device, as necessary, if available
- Additional staff for assistance, as needed

ASSESSMENT

Assess the patient's ability to walk and the need for assistance. Review the patient's record for conditions that may affect ambulation. Perform a pain assessment before the time for the activity. If the patient reports pain, administer the prescribed medication in sufficient time to allow for the full effect of the analgesic. Take vital signs and assess the patient for dizziness or light-headedness with position changes.

NURSING DIAGNOSIS

Determine the related factors for the nursing diagnoses based on the patient's current status. Appropriate nursing diagnoses may include:

- Impaired Physical Mobility
- Activity Intolerance
- Risk for Falls
- Impaired Walking

OUTCOME IDENTIFICATION AND PLANNING

The expected outcome to achieve when assisting a patient with ambulation is that the patient ambulates safely, without falls or injury. Additional appropriate outcomes include the patient demonstrates improved muscle strength and joint mobility; the patient's level of independence increases; and the patient remains free of complications of immobility.

IMPLEMENTATION

ACTION	RATIONALE
1. Review the medical record and nursing plan of care for conditions that may influence the patient's ability to move and ambulate. Assess for tubes, IV lines, incisions, or equipment that may alter the procedure for ambulation. Identify any movement limitations.	Reviewing the medical record and plan of care validates the correct patient and correct procedure. Checking for equipment and limitations reduces the risk for patient injury.
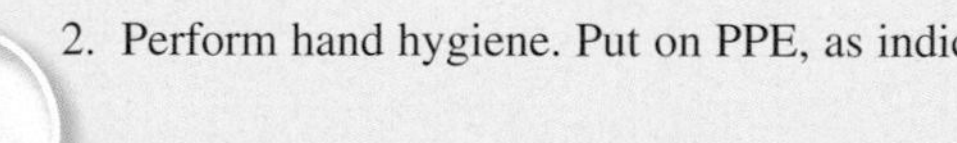 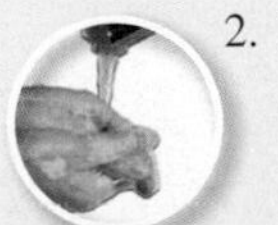 2. Perform hand hygiene. Put on PPE, as indicated.	Hand hygiene and PPE prevent the spread of microorganisms. PPE is required based on transmission precautions.
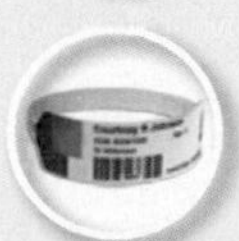 3. Identify the patient. Explain the procedure to the patient. Ask the patient to report any feelings of dizziness, weakness, or shortness of breath while walking. Decide how far to walk.	Patient identification validates the correct patient and correct procedure. Discussion and explanation help allay anxiety and prepare the patient for what to expect.

(continued)

SKILL 9-7 ASSISTING A PATIENT WITH AMBULATION continued

ACTION	RATIONALE
4. Place the bed in the lowest position.	Proper bed height ensures safety when getting the patient out of bed.
5. Encourage the patient to make use of a stand-assist aid, either freestanding or attached to the side of the bed, if available, to move to the side of the bed. Assist the patient to the side of the bed, if necessary.	Encourages independence, reduces strain for staff, and decreases risk for patient injury.
6. Have the patient sit on the side of the bed for several minutes and assess for dizziness or light-headedness. Have the patient stay sitting until he or she feels secure.	Having the patient sit at the side of the bed minimizes the risk for blood pressure changes (orthostatic hypotension) that can occur with position change. Allowing the patient to sit until he or she feels secure reduces anxiety and helps prevent injury.
7. Assist the patient to put on footwear and a robe, if desired.	Doing so ensures safety and patient warmth.
8. Wrap the gait belt around the patient's waist, based on assessed need and facility policy.	Gait belts improve the caregiver's grasp, reducing the risk of musculoskeletal injuries to staff and the patient. The belt also provides a firmer grasp for the caregiver if the patient should lose his or her balance.
9. Encourage the patient to make use of the stand-assist device. Assist the patient to stand, using the gait belt, if necessary. Assess the patient's balance and leg strength. If the patient is weak or unsteady, return the patient to the bed or assist to a chair.	Use of gait belt prevents injury to the nurse and to the patient. Assessing balance and strength helps to identify the need for additional assistance to prevent falling.
10. If you are the only person assisting, position yourself to the side and slightly behind the patient. Support the patient by the waist or transfer belt (Figure 1).	Positioning to the side and slightly behind the patient encourages the patient to stand and walk erect. It also places the nurse in a safe position if the patient should lose his or her balance or begin to fall.
• When two caregivers assist, position yourself to the side and slightly behind the patient, supporting the patient by the waist or gait belt. Have the other caregiver carry or manage equipment or provide additional support from the other side.	Gait belts improve the caregiver's grasp, reducing the risk of musculoskeletal injuries to staff and the patient, and allow for a firmer grasp for the caregiver if the patient should lose his or her balance.
• Alternately, when two caregivers assist, stand at the patient's sides (one nurse on each side) with near hands grasping the gait belt and far hands holding the patient's lower arm or hand.	Gait belts improve the caregiver's grasp, reducing the risk of musculoskeletal injuries to staff and the patient, and allow for a firmer grasp for the caregiver if the patient should lose his or her balance.

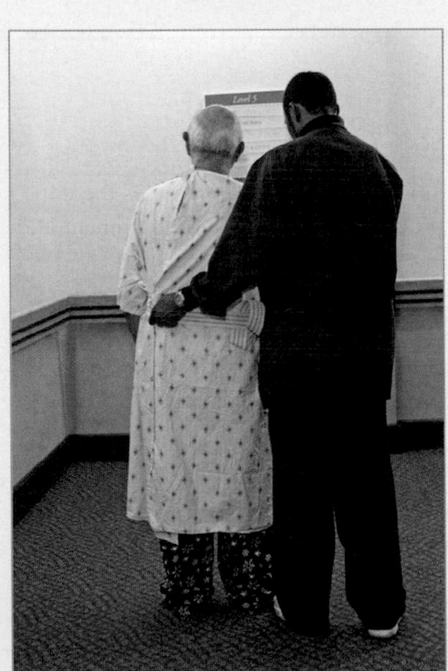

FIGURE 1 Nurse positioned to side and slightly behind patient while walking, supporting patient by gait belt or waist.

ACTION	RATIONALE
11. Take several steps forward with the patient. Continue to assess the patient's strength and balance. Remind the patient to stand erect.	Taking several steps with the patient and standing erect promote good balance and stability. Continued assessment helps maintain patient safety.
12. Continue with ambulation for the planned distance and time. Return the patient to the bed or chair based on the patient's tolerance and condition. Remove gait belt.	Ambulation as prescribed promotes activity and prevents fatigue.
13. Ensure the patient is comfortable, with the side rails up and the bed in the lowest position, as necessary. Place call bell and other essential items within reach.	Proper positioning with raised side rails and proper bed height provide for patient comfort and safety. Having the call bell and other essential items within reach promotes safety.
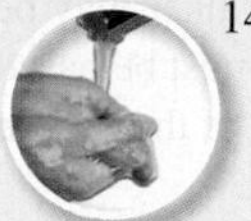 14. Clean transfer aids per facility policy, if not indicated for single patient use. Remove gloves and any other PPE, if used. Perform hand hygiene.	Proper cleaning of equipment between patient use prevents the spread of microorganisms. Removing PPE properly reduces the risk for infection transmission and contamination of other items. Hand hygiene prevents the spread of microorganisms.

EVALUATION

The expected outcome is met when the patient ambulates safely for the prescribed distance and time and remains free from falls or injury. Additional outcomes are met when the patient exhibits increasing muscle strength, joint mobility, and independence; and the patient remains free of any signs and symptoms of immobility.

DOCUMENTATION

Guidelines

Document the activity, any other pertinent observations, the patient's tolerance of the procedure, and the distance walked. Document the use of transfer aids and number of staff required for transfer.

Sample Documentation

5/14/15 1720 Patient ambulated with assistance in hallway for a distance of approximately 15 feet. Patient tolerated ambulation well; denied any complaints of dizziness, pain, or fatigue. Ambulated back to room and sitting in chair listening to music.

—J. Minkins, RN

UNEXPECTED SITUATIONS AND ASSOCIATED INTERVENTIONS

- *You are walking with a patient in the hallway. She tells you she feels faint and begins to lean over as if she is going to fall:* Place your feet wide apart, with one foot in front. Rock your pelvis out on the side nearest the patient. This widens and stabilizes the base of support. Grasp the gait belt. This ensures a safe hold on the patient. Support the patient by pulling her weight backward against your body. Gently slide her down your body to the floor, protecting her head. This enables you to support the patient's weight with large muscle groups and protects you from back strain. Stay with the patient. Call for help. If another staff member was assisting you with ambulation, each of you should use one hand to grasp the gait belt and grasp the patient's hand or wrist with your other hand. Slowly lower her to the floor.

SPECIAL CONSIDERATIONS

Secure all equipment, such as indwelling urinary catheters, drains, or IV infusions, to a pole for ambulation. Do not carry equipment while helping the patient. Your hands should be free to provide support.

SKILL 9-8 ASSISTING A PATIENT WITH AMBULATION USING A WALKER

A walker is a lightweight metal frame with four legs. Walkers provide stability and security for patients with insufficient strength and balance to use other ambulatory aids. There are several kinds of walkers; the choice of which to use is based on the patient's arm strength and balance. Regardless of the type used, the patient stands between the back legs of the walker with arms relaxed at the side; the top of the walker should line up with the crease on the inside of the patient's wrist. When the patient's hands are placed on the grips, elbows should be flexed about 30 degrees (Mayo Clinic, 2011c). Usually, the legs of the walker can be adjusted to the appropriate height. Box 9-1 in Skill 9-1 outlines general guidelines related to mobility and safe handling of people with dementia.

DELEGATION CONSIDERATIONS

Patient teaching regarding use of a walker cannot be delegated to nursing assistive personnel (NAP) or to unlicensed assistive personnel (UAP). Reinforcement or implementation of ambulation using a walker may be delegated to NAP or UAP. Assisting a patient with ambulation using a walker may be delegated to licensed practical/vocational nurses (LPN/LVNs). The decision to delegate must be based on careful analysis of the patient's needs and circumstances, as well as the qualifications of the person to whom the task is being delegated. Refer to the Delegation Guidelines in Appendix A.

EQUIPMENT

- Walker, adjusted to the appropriate height
- Nonskid shoes or slippers
- Nonsterile gloves and/or other PPE, as indicated
- Additional staff for assistance, as needed
- Stand-assist device, as necessary, if available
- Gait belt, based on assessment

ASSESSMENT

Assess the patient's ability to walk and the need for assistance. Review the patient's record for conditions that may affect ambulation. Perform a pain assessment before the time for the activity. If the patient reports pain, administer the prescribed medication in sufficient time to allow for the full effect of the analgesic. Take vital signs and assess the patient for dizziness or light-headedness with position changes. Assess the patient's knowledge regarding the use of a walker. Ensure that the walker is at the appropriate height for the patient.

NURSING DIAGNOSIS

Determine the related factors for the nursing diagnoses based on the patient's current status. Appropriate nursing diagnoses may include:

- Risk for Falls
- Impaired Walking
- Deficient Knowledge
- Activity Intolerance

OUTCOME IDENTIFICATION AND PLANNING

The expected outcome is met when the patient ambulates safely with the walker and is free from falls or injury. Additional appropriate outcomes include the following: the patient demonstrates proper use of the walker and states the need for the walker; the patient demonstrates increasing muscle strength, joint mobility, and independence; and the patient remains free of complications of immobility.

IMPLEMENTATION

ACTION	RATIONALE
1. Review the medical record and nursing plan of care for conditions that may influence the patient's ability to move and ambulate, and for specific instructions for ambulation, such as distance. Assess for tubes, IV lines, incisions, or equipment that may alter the procedure for ambulation. Assess the patient's knowledge and previous experience regarding the use of a walker. Identify any movement limitations.	Reviewing the medical record and plan of care validates the correct patient and correct procedure. Checking for equipment and limitations helps minimize the risk for injury.
2. Perform hand hygiene. Put on PPE, if indicated.	Hand hygiene and PPE prevent the spread of microorganisms. PPE is required based on transmission precautions.

ACTION	RATIONALE
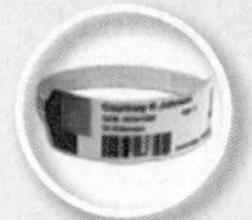 3. Identify the patient. Explain the procedure to the patient. Tell the patient to report any feelings of dizziness, weakness, or shortness of breath while walking. Decide how far to walk.	Patient identification validates the correct patient and correct procedure. Discussion and explanation help allay anxiety and prepare the patient for what to expect.
4. Place the bed in the lowest position, if the patient is in bed.	Proper bed height ensures safety when getting the patient out of bed.
5. Encourage the patient to make use of a stand-assist aid, either free-standing or attached to the side of the bed, if available, to move to the side of the bed.	Use of assistive devices encourages independence, reduces strain for staff, and decreases risk for patient injury.
6. Assist the patient to the side of the bed, if necessary. Have the patient sit on the side of the bed. Assess for dizziness or light-headedness. Have the patient stay seated until he or she feels secure.	Having the patient sit on the side of the bed minimizes the risk for blood pressure changes (orthostatic hypotension) that can occur with position change. Assessing patient complaints helps prevent injury.
7. Assist the patient to put on footwear and a robe, if desired.	Doing so ensures safety and warmth.
8. Wrap the gait belt around the patient's waist, based on assessed need and facility policy.	Gait belts improve the caregiver's grasp, reducing the risk of musculoskeletal injuries to staff and the patient and provide for a firmer grasp if patient should lose his or her balance.
9. Place the walker directly in front of the patient (Figure 1). Ask the patient to push him- or herself off the bed or chair; make use of the stand-assist device, or assist the patient to stand (Figure 2). Once the patient is standing, have him or her hold the walker's handgrips firmly and equally. Stand slightly behind the patient, on one side.	Proper positioning with the walker ensures balance. Standing within the walker and holding the handgrips firmly provide stability when moving the walker and helps ensure safety. Positioning to the side and slightly behind the patient encourages the patient to stand and walk erect. It also places the nurse in a safe position if the patient should lose his or her balance or begin to fall.

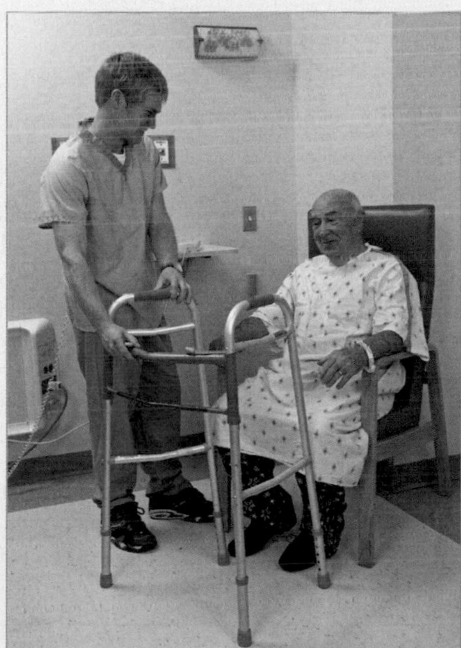

FIGURE 1 Setting walker in front of a seated patient.

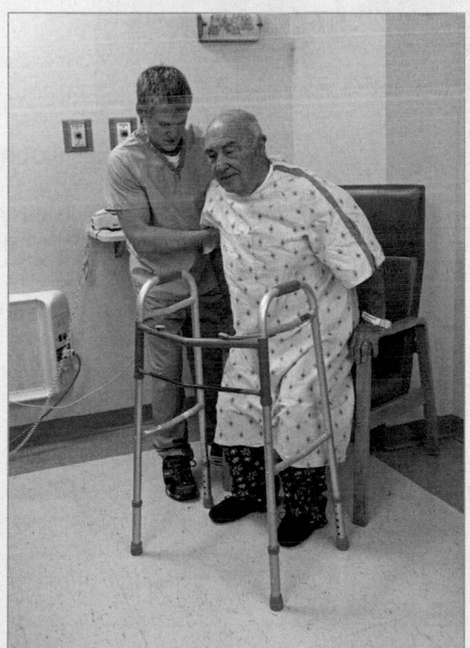

FIGURE 2 Assisting patient to stand.

(continued)

SKILL 9-8 ASSISTING A PATIENT WITH AMBULATION USING A WALKER continued

ACTION	RATIONALE
10. Have the patient move the walker forward 6 to 8 inches and set it down, making sure all four feet of the walker stay on the floor. Then, tell the patient to step forward with either foot into the walker, supporting him- or herself on his or her arms. Follow through with the other leg.	Having all four feet of the walker on the floor provides a broad base of support. Moving the walker and stepping forward moves the center of gravity toward the walker, ensuring balance and preventing tipping of the walker.
11. Move the walker forward again, and continue the same pattern. Continue with ambulation for the planned distance and time (Figure 3). Return the patient to the bed or chair based on the patient's tolerance and condition, ensuring that the patient is comfortable. Remove gait belt.	Moving the walker promotes activity. Continuing for the planned distance and time prevents the patient from becoming fatigued.

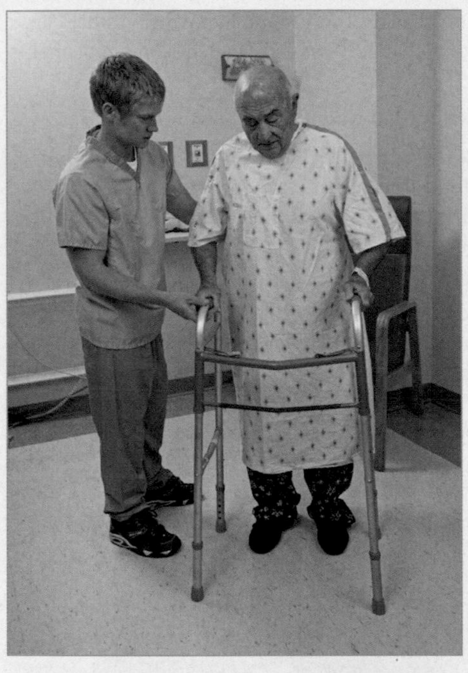

FIGURE 3 Assisting patient to walk with walker.

ACTION	RATIONALE
12. Ensure the patient is comfortable, with the side rails up and the bed in the lowest position, as necessary. Place call bell and other essential items within reach.	Proper positioning with raised side rails and proper bed height provides for patient comfort and safety. Having the call bell and other essential items within reach promotes safety.
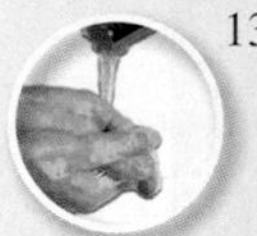 13. Clean transfer aids per facility policy, if not indicated for single patient use. Remove gloves and any other PPE, if used. Perform hand hygiene.	Proper cleaning of equipment between patient use prevents the spread of microorganisms. Removing PPE properly reduces the risk for infection transmission and contamination of other items. Hand hygiene prevents the spread of microorganisms.

EVALUATION

The expected outcome is met when the patient uses the walker to ambulate safely and remains free of injury. Other outcomes are met when the patient exhibits increased muscle strength, joint mobility, and independence; demonstrates independent walker use; and exhibits no evidence of complications of immobility.

DOCUMENTATION

Guidelines

Document the activity, any other pertinent observations, the patient's ability to use the walker, the patient's tolerance of the procedure, and the distance walked. Document the use of transfer aids and number of staff required for transfer.

Sample Documentation

5/15/15 0900 Patient ambulated with walker from bed to bathroom for morning care with minimal assistance; demonstrated proper steps in using walker. Able to ambulate back to bed using walker independently.

—P. Collins, RN

UNEXPECTED SITUATIONS AND ASSOCIATED INTERVENTIONS

- *You are assisting a patient ambulating in the hallway using a walker. She becomes extremely tired and says she cannot pick up the walker anymore ("it's too heavy"). However, she cannot walk without the walker:* Call for assistance. Have a coworker obtain a wheelchair to transport the patient back to her room. Assess the patient for other symptoms, if necessary. In the future, plan to ambulate for shorter distances to prevent the patient from becoming fatigued.

SPECIAL CONSIDERATIONS

- Never use a walker on the stairs.
- Wear nonskid shoes or slippers.
- Some walkers have wheels on the front legs. These walkers are best for patients with a gait that is too fast for a walker without wheels and for patients who have difficulty lifting a walker. This type of walker is rolled forward while the patient walks as normally as possible. Because lifting repeatedly is not required, energy expenditure and stress to the back and upper extremities is less than with a standard walker (Mayo, 2011c).
- Keep in mind, walkers often prove to be difficult to maneuver through doorways and congested areas.
- Advise the patient to check the walker before use for signs of damage, frame deformity, or loose or missing parts.
- Teach patients to use the arms of the chair or a stand-assist device for leverage when getting up from a chair. Explain to patients that they should not pull on the walker to get up; the walker could tip or become unbalanced.

SKILL 9-9 ASSISTING A PATIENT WITH AMBULATION USING CRUTCHES

Crutches enable a patient to walk and remove weight from one or both legs. The patient uses the arms to support the body weight. Crutches can be used for the short or the long term. This section will discuss short-term crutch use. Crutches must be fitted to each person. Have the patient stand up straight with the palm of the hand pressed against the body under the arm. The hand should fit between the top of the crutches and the armpit. When using crutches, the elbow should be slightly bent at about 30 degrees and the hands, not the armpits, should support the patient's weight. Weight on the armpits can cause nerve damage. If anything needs to be carried, it is best to use a backpack (University of Iowa Hospitals and Clinics, 2008). A physical therapist usually teaches the procedure for crutch walking, but it is important for the nurse to be knowledgeable about the patient's progress and the gait being taught. Be prepared to guide the patient at home or in the hospital after the initial teaching is completed. Remind the patient that the support of body weight should be primarily on the hands and arms while using the crutches. There are a number of different ways to walk using crutches, based on how much weight the patient is allowed to bear on one or both legs.

DELEGATION CONSIDERATIONS

Patient teaching regarding use of crutches cannot be delegated to nursing assistive personnel (NAP) or unlicensed assistive personnel (UAP). Reinforcement or implementation of the use of crutches may be delegated to NAP or UAP. Assisting a patient with ambulation using crutches may be delegated to licensed practical/vocational nurses (LPN/LVNs). The decision to delegate must be based on careful analysis of the patient's needs and circumstances, as well as the qualifications of the person to whom the task is being delegated. Refer to the Delegation Guidelines in Appendix A.

(*continued*)

SKILL 9-9 ASSISTING A PATIENT WITH AMBULATION USING CRUTCHES continued

EQUIPMENT

- Crutches with axillary pads, handgrips, and rubber suction tips
- Nonskid shoes or slippers
- PPE, as indicated
- Stand-assist device, as necessary, if available
- Gait belt, based on assessment

ASSESSMENT

Review the patient's record and nursing plan of care to determine the reason for using crutches and instructions for weight bearing. Check for specific instructions from physical therapy. Perform a pain assessment before the time for the activity. If the patient reports pain, administer the prescribed medication in sufficient time to allow for the full effect of the analgesic. Determine the patient's knowledge regarding the use of crutches and assess the patient's ability to balance on the crutches. Assess for muscle strength in the legs and arms. Determine the appropriate gait for the patient to use.

NURSING DIAGNOSIS

Determine the related factors for the nursing diagnosis based on the patient's current status. Appropriate nursing diagnoses may include:

- Impaired Walking
- Deficient Knowledge
- Risk for Falls

OUTCOME IDENTIFICATION AND PLANNING

The expected outcome to achieve when assisting a patient with ambulation using crutches is that the patient ambulates safely without experiencing falls or injury. Additional appropriate outcomes include the following: the patient demonstrates proper crutch-walking technique; the patient demonstrates increased muscle strength and joint mobility; and the patient exhibits no evidence of injury related to crutch use.

IMPLEMENTATION

ACTION	RATIONALE
1. Review the medical record and nursing plan of care for conditions that may influence the patient's ability to move and ambulate. Assess for tubes, IV lines, incisions, or equipment that may alter the procedure for ambulation. Assess the patient's knowledge and previous experience regarding the use of crutches. Determine that the appropriate size crutch has been obtained.	Reviewing the medical record and plan of care validates the correct patient and correct procedure. Assessment helps identify problem areas to minimize the risk for injury.
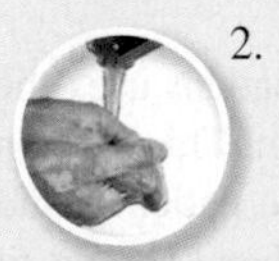 2. Perform hand hygiene. Put on PPE, if indicated.	Hand hygiene and PPE prevent the spread of microorganisms. PPE is required based on transmission precautions.
3. Identify the patient. Explain the procedure to the patient. Tell the patient to report any feelings of dizziness, weakness, or shortness of breath while walking. Decide how far to walk.	Patient identification validates the correct patient and correct procedure. Discussion and explanation help allay anxiety and prepare the patient for what to expect.
4. Place the bed in the lowest position, if the patient is in bed.	Proper bed height ensures safety when getting the patient out of bed.
5. Encourage the patient to make use of a stand-assist aid, either free-standing or attached to the side of the bed, if available, to move to the side of the bed.	Use of assistive devices encourages independence, reduces strain for staff, and decreases risk for patient injury.
6. Assist the patient to the side of the bed, if necessary. Have the patient sit on the side of the bed. Assess for dizziness or lightheadedness. Have the patient stay seated until he or she feels secure.	Having the patient sit on the side of the bed minimizes the risk for blood pressure changes (orthostatic hypotension) that can occur with position change. Assessing patient complaints helps prevent injury.
7. Assist the patient to put on footwear and a robe, if desired.	Doing so ensures safety and warmth.

ACTION	RATIONALE
8. Wrap the gait belt around the patient's waist, based on assessed need and facility policy.	Gait belts improve the caregiver's grasp, reducing the risk of musculoskeletal injuries to staff and the patient and provide for a firmer grasp if patient should lose his or her balance.
9. Assist the patient to stand erect, face forward in the tripod position (Figure 1). This means the patient holds the crutches 12 inches in front of, and 12 inches to the side of, each foot.	Positioning the crutches in this manner provides a wide base of support to increase stability and balance.

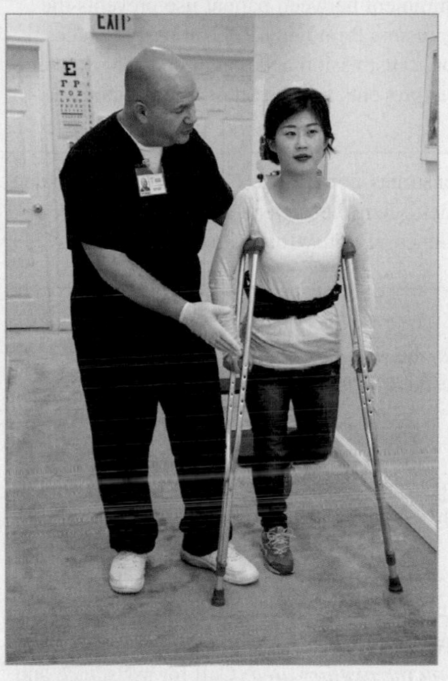

FIGURE 1 Assisting patient to stand erect facing forward in tripod position.

ACTION	RATIONALE
10. For the four-point gait: a. Have the patient move the right crutch forward 12 inches and then move the left foot forward to the level of the right crutch. b. Then have the patient move the left crutch forward 12 inches and then move the right foot forward to the level of the left crutch.	This movement ensures stability and safety.
11. For the three-point gait: a. Have the patient move the affected leg and both crutches forward about 12 inches. b. Have the patient move the stronger leg forward to the level of the crutches.	Patient bears weight on the stronger leg.
12. For the two-point gait: a. Have the patient move the left crutch and the right foot forward about 12 inches at the same time. b. Have the patient move the right crutch and left leg forward to the level of the left crutch at the same time.	Patient bears partial weight on both feet.
13. For the swing-to gait: a. Have the patient move both crutches forward about 12 inches. b. Have the patient lift the legs and swing them to the crutches, supporting his or her body weight on the crutches.	Swing-to gait provides mobility for patients with weakness or paralysis of the hips or legs.

(continued)

SKILL 9-9 ASSISTING A PATIENT WITH AMBULATION USING CRUTCHES continued

ACTION	RATIONALE
14. Continue with ambulation for the planned distance and time. Return the patient to the bed or chair based on the patient's tolerance and condition. Remove gait belt.	Continued ambulation promotes activity. Adhering to the planned distance and time prevents the patient from becoming fatigued.
15. Ensure the patient is comfortable, with the side rails up and the bed in the lowest position, as necessary. Place call bell and other essential items within reach.	Proper positioning with raised side rails and proper bed height provide for patient comfort and safety. Having the call bell and other essential items within reach promotes safety.
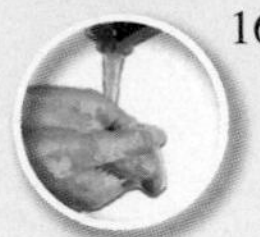 16. Clean transfer aids per facility policy, if not indicated for single patient use. Remove gloves and any other PPE, if used. Perform hand hygiene.	Proper cleaning of equipment between patient use prevents the spread of microorganisms. Removing PPE properly reduces the risk for infection transmission and contamination of other items. Hand hygiene prevents the spread of microorganisms.

EVALUATION

The expected outcome is met when the patient demonstrates correct use of crutches to ambulate safely and without injury. Additional outcomes are met when the patient demonstrates increased muscle strength and joint mobility and exhibits no evidence of injury related to crutch use.

DOCUMENTATION

Guidelines

Document the activity, any other pertinent observations, the patient's ability to use the crutches, the patient's tolerance of the procedure, and the distance walked. Document the use of transfer aids and number of staff required for transfer.

Sample Documentation

5/10/15 1830 Patient instructed in crutch walking using four-point gait. Patient return-demonstrated gait, ambulating for approximately 15 feet in hallway, without difficulty.
—*H. Pointer, RN*

UNEXPECTED SITUATIONS AND ASSOCIATED INTERVENTIONS

- *You are assisting a patient ambulating in the hallway using crutches when the patient reports fatigue. You notice that the patient is bearing weight on the axillary area:* Call for assistance and have a coworker obtain a wheelchair to transport the patient back to the room. Once the patient is back in bed, reinforce instructions about avoiding pressure on the axillary area. In the future, plan to ambulate for a shorter distance to prevent the patient from becoming fatigued. Talk with the multidisciplinary health care team about possible exercises for upper-extremity strengthening.

SPECIAL CONSIDERATIONS

- Crutches can be used when climbing stairs. The patient grasps both crutches as one on one side of the body and uses the stair railing. Have the patient stand in the tripod position facing the stairs. The patient transfers his or her weight to the crutches and holds the railing. The patient places the unaffected leg on the first stair tread. The patient then transfers his or her weight to the unaffected leg, moving up onto the stair tread. The patient moves the crutches and affected leg up to the stair tread and continues to the top of the stairs. Using this process, the crutches always support the affected leg.
- Long-term use of the swing-to gait can lead to atrophy of the hips and legs. Include appropriate exercises in the patient's plan of care to avoid this complication.
- Patients should not lean on the crutches. Prolonged pressure on the axillae can damage the brachial nerves, causing brachial nerve palsy, with resulting loss of sensation and inability to move the upper extremities.
- Patients using crutches should perform arm- and shoulder-strengthening exercises to aid with crutch walking.

SKILL 9-10 ASSISTING A PATIENT WITH AMBULATION USING A CANE

Canes are useful for patients who can bear weight, but need support for balance. They are also useful for patients who have decreased strength in one leg. Canes provide an additional point of support during ambulation. Canes are made of wood or metal and often have a rubberized cap on the tip to prevent slipping. Canes come in three variations: single-ended canes with half-circle handles (recommended for patients requiring minimal support and for those who will be using stairs frequently); single-ended canes with straight handles (recommended for patients with hand weakness because the handgrip is easier to hold, but not recommended for patients with poor balance); and canes with three (tripod) or four prongs (quad cane) or legs to provide a wide base of support (recommended for patients with poor balance). The cane should rise from the floor to the height of the person's waist, and the elbow should be flexed about 30 degrees when holding the cane. The patient holds the cane in the hand opposite the weak or injured leg. Box 9-1 in Skill 9-1 outlines general guidelines to consider related to mobility and safe handling of people with dementia.

DELEGATION CONSIDERATIONS

Patient teaching regarding use of a cane cannot be delegated to nursing assistive personnel (NAP) or unlicensed assistive personnel (UAP). Reinforcement or implementation of the use of a cane may be delegated to NAP or UAP. Assisting a patient with ambulation using a cane may be delegated to licensed practical/vocational nurses (LPN/LVNs). The decision to delegate must be based on careful analysis of the patient's needs and circumstances, as well as the qualifications of the person to whom the task is being delegated. Refer to the Delegation Guidelines in Appendix A.

EQUIPMENT

- Cane of appropriate size with rubber tip
- Nonskid shoes or slippers
- Nonsterile gloves and/or other PPE, as indicated
- Stand-assist aid, if necessary and available
- Gait belt, based on assessment

ASSESSMENT

Assess the patient's upper body strength, ability to bear weight and to walk, and the need for assistance. Review the patient's record for conditions that may affect ambulation. Perform a pain assessment before the time for the activity. If the patient reports pain, administer the prescribed medication in sufficient time to allow for the full effect of the analgesic. Take vital signs and assess the patient for dizziness or light-headedness with position changes. Assess the patient's knowledge regarding the use of a cane.

NURSING DIAGNOSIS

Determine the related factors for the nursing diagnoses based on the patient's current status. Appropriate nursing diagnoses may include:

- Risk for Falls
- Impaired Walking
- Deficient Knowledge
- Activity Intolerance

OUTCOME IDENTIFICATION AND PLANNING

The expected outcome to achieve when assisting a patient with ambulation using a cane is that the patient ambulates safely without falls or injury. Additional appropriate outcomes include the following: the patient demonstrates proper use of the cane; the patient demonstrates increased muscle strength, joint mobility, and independence; and the patient exhibits no evidence of injury from use of the cane.

IMPLEMENTATION

ACTION	RATIONALE
1. Review the medical record and nursing plan of care for conditions that may influence the patient's ability to move and ambulate. Assess for tubes, IV lines, incisions, or equipment that may alter the procedure for ambulation.	Review of the medical record and plan of care validates the correct patient and correct procedure. Identification of equipment and limitations helps reduce the risk for injury.
2. Perform hand hygiene. Put on PPE, as indicated.	Hand hygiene and PPE prevent the spread of microorganisms. PPE is required based on transmission precautions.

(continued)

SKILL 9-10 ASSISTING A PATIENT WITH AMBULATION USING A CANE continued

ACTION	RATIONALE
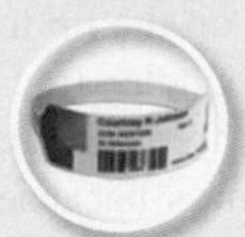 3. Identify the patient. Explain the procedure to the patient. Tell the patient to report any feelings of dizziness, weakness, or shortness of breath while walking. Decide how far to walk.	Patient identification validates the correct patient and correct procedure. Discussion and explanation help allay anxiety and prepare the patient for what to expect.
4. Place the bed in the lowest position, if the patient is in bed.	Proper bed height ensures safety when getting the patient out of bed.
5. Encourage the patient to make use of a stand-assist aid, either free-standing or attached to the side of the bed, if available, to move to the side of the bed.	Use of assistive devices encourages independence, reduces strain for staff, and decreases risk for patient injury.
6. Assist the patient to the side of the bed, if necessary. Have the patient sit on the side of the bed. Assess for dizziness or lightheadedness. Have the patient stay seated until he or she feels secure.	Having the patient sit on the side of the bed minimizes the risk for blood pressure changes (orthostatic hypotension) that can occur with position change. Assessing patient complaints helps prevent injury.
7. Assist the patient to put on footwear and a robe, if desired.	Doing so ensures safety and warmth.
8. Wrap the gait belt around the patient's waist, based on assessed need and facility policy.	Gait belts improve the caregiver's grasp, reducing the risk of musculoskeletal injuries to staff and the patient and provide firmer grasp for the caregiver if patient should lose his or her balance.
9. Encourage the patient to make use of the stand-assist device to stand with weight evenly distributed between the feet and the cane.	A stand-assist device reduces strain for caregiver and decreases risk for patient injury. Evenly distributed weight provides a broad base of support and balance.
10. Have the patient hold the cane on his or her stronger side, close to the body, while the nurse stands to the side and slightly behind the patient (Figure 1).	Holding the cane on the stronger side helps to distribute the patient's weight away from the involved side and prevents leaning. Positioning to the side and slightly behind the patient encourages the patient to stand and walk erect. It also places the nurse in a safe position if the patient should lose his or her balance or begin to fall.

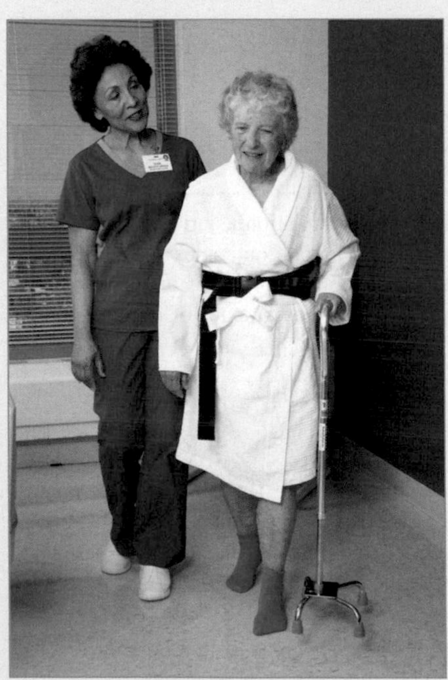

FIGURE 1 Nurse stands slightly behind patient. Cane is held on patient's stronger side, close to body.

ACTION	RATIONALE
11. Tell the patient to advance the cane 4 to 12 inches (10 to 30 cm) and then, while supporting his or her weight on the stronger leg and the cane, advance the weaker foot forward, parallel with the cane.	Moving in this manner provides support and balance.
12. While supporting his or her weight on the weaker leg and the cane, have the patient advance the stronger leg forward ahead of the cane (heel slightly beyond the tip of the cane).	Moving in this manner provides support and balance.
13. Tell the patient to move the weaker leg forward until it is even with the stronger leg, and then advance the cane again.	This motion provides support and balance.
14. Continue with ambulation for the planned distance and time. Return the patient to the bed or chair based on the patient's tolerance and condition. Remove gait belt.	Continued ambulation promotes activity. Adhering to the planned distance and time prevents the patient from becoming fatigued.
15. Ensure the patient is comfortable, with the side rails up and the bed in the lowest position, as necessary. Place call bell and other essential items within reach.	Proper positioning with raised side rails and proper bed height provides for patient comfort and safety. Having the call bell and other essential items within reach promotes safety.
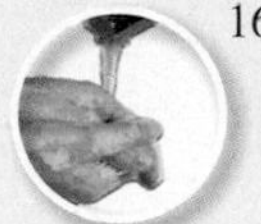 16. Clean transfer aids per facility policy, if not indicated for single patient use. Remove gloves and any other PPE, if used. Perform hand hygiene.	Proper cleaning of equipment between patient use prevents the spread of microorganisms. Removing PPE properly reduces the risk for infection transmission and contamination of other items. Hand hygiene prevents the spread of microorganisms.

EVALUATION

The expected outcome is met when the patient uses the cane to ambulate safely and is free from falls or injury. Additional outcomes are met when the patient demonstrates proper use of the cane; the patient exhibits increased muscle strength, joint mobility, and independence; and the patient experiences no injury related to cane use.

DOCUMENTATION

Guidelines

Document the activity, any other pertinent observations, the patient's ability to use the cane, the patient's tolerance of the procedure, and the distance walked. Document the use of transfer aids and the number of staff required for transfer.

Sample Documentation

5/14/15 1330 Patient instructed in cane use. Patient return demonstrated gait, ambulating approximately 10 feet in room. Patient needed continued reminders about leaning to one side. Requires continued instruction in cane use. Another teaching session planned for early evening.

—*J. Phelps, RN*

UNEXPECTED SITUATIONS AND ASSOCIATED INTERVENTIONS

- *You are assisting a patient ambulating in the hallway using a cane when the patient says she "can't walk any more"*: Call for assistance. Have a coworker obtain a wheelchair to transport the patient back to her room. Assess the patient for possible causes, such as anxiety, fatigue, or a change in her condition. In the future, plan shorter distances to prevent the patient from becoming fatigued. Anticipate the need for referral to physical therapy for muscle strengthening.

SPECIAL CONSIDERATIONS

- Patients with bilateral weakness should not use a cane. Crutches or a walker would be more appropriate.
- To climb stairs, the patient should advance the stronger leg up the stair first, followed by the cane and weaker leg. To descend, reverse the process.
- When less support is required from the cane, the patient can advance the cane and weaker leg forward simultaneously while the stronger leg supports the patient's weight.
- Teach patients to position their canes within easy reach when they sit down so that they can rise easily.

SKILL 9-11 APPLYING AND REMOVING GRADUATED COMPRESSION STOCKINGS

Graduated compression stockings are often used for patients at risk for **deep-vein thrombosis** (DVT) and pulmonary embolism, and to help prevent phlebitis. Manufactured by several companies, graduated compression stockings are made of elastic material and are available in either knee-high or thigh-high length. By applying pressure, graduated compression stockings increase the velocity of blood flow in the superficial and deep veins and improve venous valve function in the legs, promoting venous return to the heart. A physician's order is required for their use.

Be prepared to apply the stockings in the morning before the patient is out of bed and while the patient is supine. If the patient is sitting or has been up and about, have the patient lie down with legs and feet elevated for at least 15 minutes before applying the stockings. Otherwise, the leg vessels are congested with blood, reducing the effectiveness of the stockings.

DELEGATION CONSIDERATIONS

The application and removal of graduated compression stockings may be delegated to nursing assistive personnel (NAP) or to unlicensed assistive personnel (UAP), as well as to licensed practical/vocational nurses (LPN/LVNs). The decision to delegate must be based on careful analysis of the patient's needs and circumstances, as well as the qualifications of the person to whom the task is being delegated. Refer to the Delegation Guidelines in Appendix A.

EQUIPMENT

- Elastic graduated compression stockings in ordered length in correct size. See Assessment for appropriate measurement procedure.
- Measuring tape
- Talcum powder (optional)
- Skin cleanser, basin, towel
- PPE, as indicated

ASSESSMENT

Assess the skin condition and neurovascular status of the legs. Report any abnormalities before continuing with the application of the stockings. Assess patient's legs for any redness, swelling, warmth, tenderness, or pain that may indicate DVT. If any of these symptoms are noted, notify the physician before applying stockings. Measure the patient's legs to obtain the correct size stocking. For knee-high length: Measure around the widest part of the calf and the leg length from the bottom of the heel to the back of the knee, at the bend. For thigh-high length: Measure around the widest part of the calf and the thigh. Measure the length from the bottom of the heel to the gluteal fold. Follow the manufacturer's specifications to select the correct sized stockings. Each leg should have a correctly fitted stocking; if measurements differ, then two different sizes of stocking need to be ordered to ensure correct fitting on each leg (Walker & Lamont, 2008).

NURSING DIAGNOSIS

Determine related factors for the nursing diagnose based on the patient's current status. Appropriate nursing diagnoses may include:

- Ineffective Peripheral Tissue Perfusion
- Risk for Impaired Skin Integrity
- Deficient Knowledge

OUTCOME IDENTIFICATION AND PLANNING

The expected outcome to achieve when applying and removing graduated compression stockings is that the stockings will be applied and removed with minimal discomfort to the patient. Other outcomes that may be appropriate include the following: edema will decrease in the lower extremities; patient will understand the rationale for stocking application; and patient will remain free of DVT.

IMPLEMENTATION

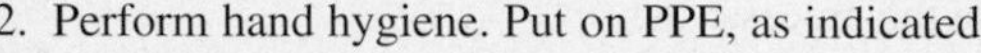

ACTION	RATIONALE
1. Review the medical record and medical orders to determine the need for graduated compression stockings.	Reviewing the medical record and order validates the correct patient and correct procedure.
2. Perform hand hygiene. Put on PPE, as indicated.	Hand hygiene and PPE prevent the spread of microorganisms. PPE is required based on transmission precautions.

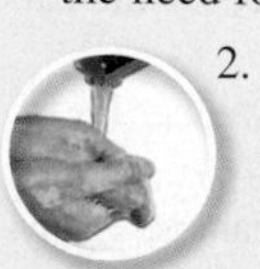

ACTION	RATIONALE
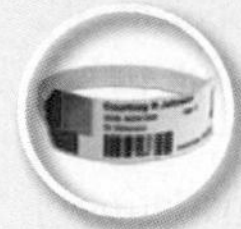 3. Identify the patient. Explain what you are going to do and the rationale for use of elastic stockings.	Patient identification validates the correct patient and correct procedure. Discussion and explanation allay anxiety and prepare the patient for what to expect.
4. Close the curtains around the bed and close the door to the room, if possible.	This ensures the patient's privacy.
5. Adjust the bed to a comfortable working height, usually elbow height of the caregiver (VISN 8 Patient Safety Center, 2009).	Having the bed at the proper height prevents back and muscle strain.
6. Assist patient to supine position. If patient has been sitting or walking, have him or her lie down with legs and feet well elevated for at least 15 minutes before applying stockings.	Dependent position of legs encourages blood to pool in the veins, reducing the effectiveness of the stockings if they are applied to congested blood vessels.
7. Expose legs one at a time. Wash and dry legs, if necessary. Powder the leg lightly unless patient has a respiratory problem, dry skin, or sensitivity to the powder. If the skin is dry, a lotion may be used. Powders and lotions are not recommended by some manufacturers; check the package material for manufacturer specifications.	Helps maintain patient's privacy. Powder and lotion reduce friction and make application of stockings easier.
8. Stand at the foot of the bed. Place hand inside stocking and grasp heel area securely. Turn stocking inside-out to the heel area, leaving the foot inside the stocking leg (Figure 1).	Inside-out technique provides for easier application; bunched elastic material can compromise extremity circulation.
9. With the heel pocket down, ease the stocking foot over the foot and heel (Figure 2). Check that patient's heel is centered in heel pocket of stocking (Figure 3).	Wrinkles and improper fit interfere with circulation.

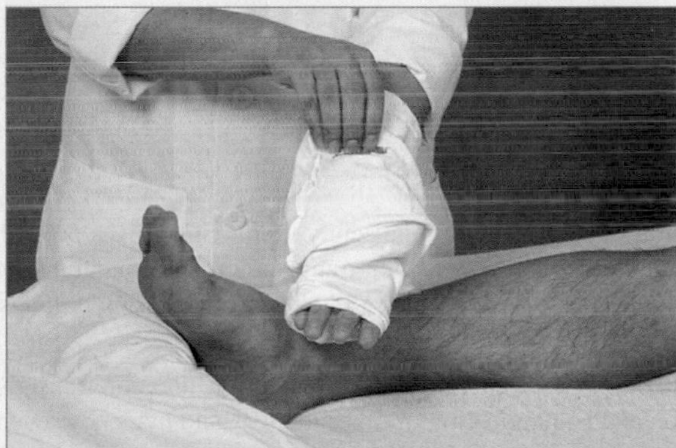

FIGURE 1 Pulling graduated compression stocking inside-out.

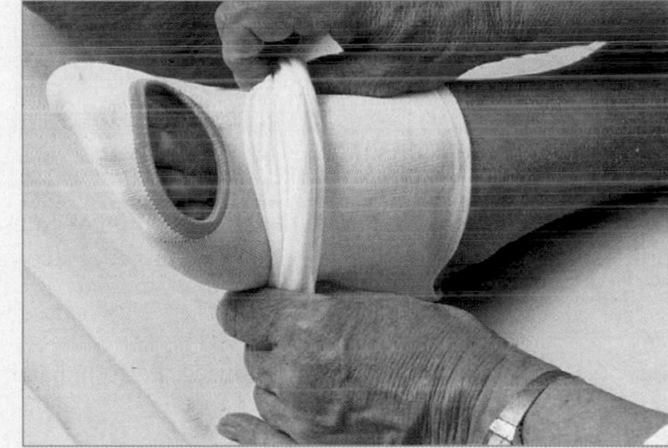

FIGURE 2 Putting foot of stocking onto patient.

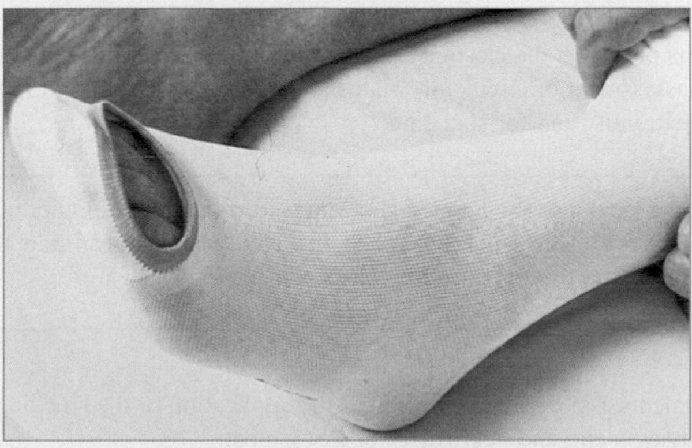

FIGURE 3 Ensuring heel is centered after stocking is on foot.

(*continued*)

SKILL 9-11 APPLYING AND REMOVING GRADUATED COMPRESSION STOCKINGS continued

ACTION	RATIONALE
10. Using your fingers and thumbs, carefully grasp edge of stocking and pull it up smoothly over ankle and calf, toward the knee (Figure 4). Make sure it is distributed evenly.	Easing the stocking carefully into position ensures proper fit of the stocking to the contour of the leg. Even distribution prevents interference with circulation.
11. Pull forward slightly on toe section. If the stocking has a toe window, make sure it is properly positioned. Adjust if necessary to ensure material is smooth.	Ensures toe comfort and prevents interference with circulation.
12. If the stockings are knee-length, make sure each stocking top is 1 to 2 inches below the patella. Make sure the stocking does not roll down.	Prevents pressure and interference with circulation. Rolling stockings may have a constricting effect on veins.
13. If applying thigh-length stocking, continue the application. Flex the patient's leg. Stretch the stocking over the knee.	This ensures even distribution.
14. Pull the stocking over the thigh until the top is 1 to 3 inches below the gluteal fold (Figure 5). Adjust the stocking, as necessary, to distribute the fabric evenly. Make sure the stocking does not roll down.	Prevents excessive pressure and interference with circulation. Rolling stockings may have a constricting effect on veins.

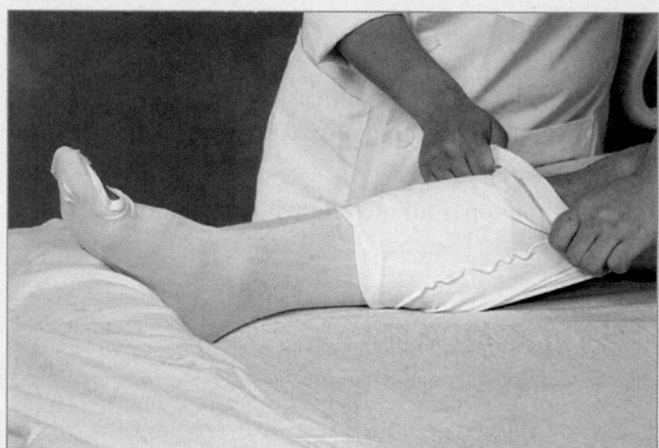

FIGURE 4 Pulling stocking up leg.

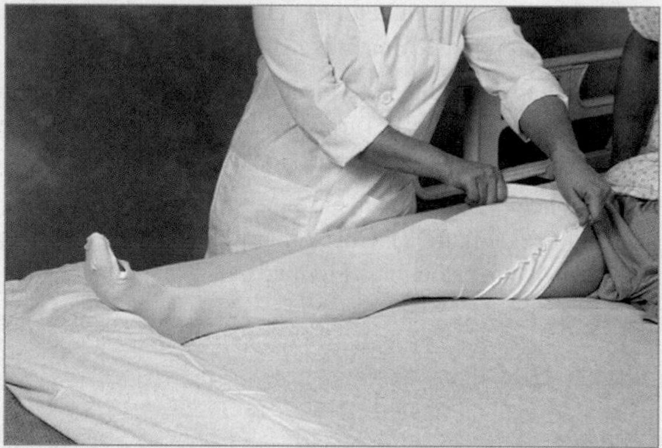

FIGURE 5 Pulling stocking up over thigh.

ACTION	RATIONALE
15. Remove equipment and return patient to a position of comfort. Remove gloves. Raise side rail and lower bed. Place call bell and other essential items within reach.	Promotes patient comfort and safety. Removing gloves properly reduces the risk for infection transmission and contamination of other items. Having the call bell and other essential items within reach promotes safety.
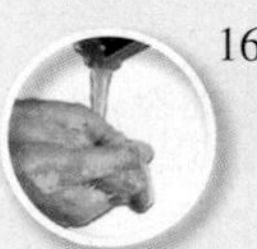 16. Remove any other PPE, if used. Perform hand hygiene.	Removing PPE properly reduces the risk for infection transmission and contamination of other items. Hand hygiene prevents the spread of microorganisms.
Removing Stockings	
17. To remove stocking, grasp top of stocking with your thumb and fingers and smoothly pull stocking off inside-out to heel. Support foot and ease stocking over it.	This preserves the elasticity and contour of the stocking. It allows assessment of circulatory status and condition of skin on lower extremity and for skin care.

EVALUATION

The expected outcome is met when the stockings are applied and removed, as indicated. Other outcomes are met when the patient exhibits a decrease in peripheral edema, and the patient can state the reason for using the stockings, and give an accurate return demonstration, as indicated.

DOCUMENTATION

Guidelines

Document the patient's leg measurements as a baseline. Document the application of the stockings, size stocking applied, skin and leg assessment, and neurovascular assessment.

Sample Documentation

7/22/15 0945 Leg measurements: calf 14½ inches, length heel to knee 16 inches. Measurements equal bilaterally. Knee-high graduated compression stockings (medium/regular) applied bilaterally. Posterior tibial and dorsalis pedal pulses +2 bilaterally; capillary refill less than 2 seconds and skin on toes consistent with rest of skin and warm. Skin on lower extremities is intact bilaterally.

—*C. Stone, RN*

UNEXPECTED SITUATIONS AND ASSOCIATED INTERVENTIONS

- *Patient's leg measurements are outside the guidelines for the available sizes:* Notify prescriber. Patient may require custom-fitted stockings.
- *Patient has a lot of pain with application of stockings:* If pain is expected (e.g., if the patient has a leg incision), it may be necessary to premedicate the patient and apply the stockings once the medication has had time to take effect. If the pain is unexpected, notify the primary care provider because the patient may be developing a DVT.
- *Patient has an incision on the leg:* When applying and removing stockings, be careful not to hit the incision. If the incision is draining, apply a small bandage to the incision so that it does not drain onto the stockings. If the stockings become soiled by drainage, wash and dry according to instructions.
- *Patient is to ambulate with stockings:* Place skid-resistant socks or slippers on before patient attempts to ambulate.

SPECIAL CONSIDERATIONS

General Considerations

- Remove stockings once every shift for 20 to 30 minutes. Wash and air-dry, as necessary, according to manufacturer's directions.
- Assess patient at least every shift for skin color, temperature, sensation, swelling, and the ability to move. If complications are evident, remove the stockings and notify the primary care provider.
- Evaluate stockings to ensure the top or toe opening does not roll with movement. Rolled stocking edges can cause excessive pressure and interfere with circulation.
- Despite the use of elastic stockings, a patient may develop DVT or phlebitis. Unilateral swelling, redness, tenderness, pain, and warmth are possible indicators of these complications. Notify the primary care provider of the presence of any symptoms.

Home Care Considerations

- Make sure that the patient has an extra pair of stockings ordered during hospitalization before discharge (for payment and convenience purposes).
- Stockings may be laundered with other "white" clothing. Avoid excessive bleach. Remove from dryer as soon as "low heat" cycle is complete to avoid shrinkage. Stockings may also be air-dried. Check manufacturer's directions.

EVIDENCE FOR PRACTICE ▶

VENOUS THROMBOEMBOLISM PREVENTION

American Association of Critical Care Nurses. (2010). *Venous Thromboembolism prevention.* Available at http://www.aacn.org/WD/Practice/Docs/PracticeAlerts/VTE%20Prevention%2004-2010%20final.pdf

The American Association of Critical Care Nurses provides Practice Alerts. Practice Alerts, are succinct, dynamic directives that are supported by authoritative evidence to ensure excellence in practice and a safe and humane work environment. Almost all hospitalized patients have at least one risk factor for VTE. VTE, a common complication, contributes to excess length of stay, excess charges, and mortality. Their Venous Thromboembolism Prevention Practice Alert supports the use of mechanical methods of prophylaxis, including graduated compression stockings, to reduce the risk of venous thromboembolism. Nurses must select the correct size of stockings, properly apply them, and ensure that they are removed for only a short time each day.

Refer to thePoint for additional research on related nursing topics.

(continued)

SKILL 9-11 APPLYING AND REMOVING GRADUATED COMPRESSION STOCKINGS continued

EVIDENCE FOR PRACTICE ▶

VENOUS THROMBOEMBOLISM PREVENTION

Geerts, W.H., Bergqvist, D., Pineo, G.F., et al.(2008). Prevention of venous embolism: American College of Chest Physicians Evidence-based clinical practice guidelines (8th ed.). *Chest, 133*(6) (Suppl), 381S–453S.

This evidence-based guideline outlines best practices for the prevention of venous thromboembolism (VTE). The use of mechanical methods of prophylaxis is included in the discussion.

Refer to thePoint for additional research on related nursing topics.

SKILL 9-12 APPLYING PNEUMATIC COMPRESSION DEVICES

Pneumatic compression devices (PCD) consist of fabric sleeves containing air bladders that apply brief pressure to the legs. Intermittent compression pushes blood from the smaller blood vessels into the deeper vessels and into the femoral veins. This action enhances blood flow and venous return and promotes fibrinolysis, deterring venous thrombosis. The sleeves are attached by tubing to an air pump. The sleeve may cover the entire leg or may extend from the foot to the knee.

Pneumatic compression devices may be used in combination with graduated compression stockings (antiembolism stockings) and anticoagulant therapy to prevent thrombosis formation. They can be used preoperatively and postoperatively with patients at risk for blood clot formation. They are also prescribed for patients with other risk factors for clot formation, including inactivity or immobilization, chronic venous disease, and malignancies.

DELEGATION CONSIDERATIONS

The application and removal of pneumatic compression devices may be delegated to nursing assistive personnel (NAP) or unlicensed assistive personnel (UAP), as well as to licensed practical/vocational nurses (LPN/LVNs). The decision to delegate must be based on careful analysis of the patient's needs and circumstances, as well as the qualifications of the person to whom the task is being delegated. Refer to the Delegation Guidelines in Appendix A.

EQUIPMENT

- Compression sleeves of appropriate size based on the manufacturer's guidelines
- Inflation pump with connection tubing
- PPE, as indicated

ASSESSMENT

Assess the patient's history, medical record, and current condition and status to identify risk for development of DVT. Assess lower extremity skin integrity. Identify any leg conditions that would be exacerbated by the use of the compression device or would contraindicate its use.

NURSING DIAGNOSIS

Determine the related factors for the nursing diagnoses based on the patient's current status. Appropriate nursing diagnoses may include:

- Impaired Physical Mobility
- Risk for Peripheral Neurovascular Dysfunction
- Delayed Surgical Recovery

OUTCOME IDENTIFICATION AND PLANNING

The expected outcome to achieve when applying PCD is that the patient maintains adequate circulation in extremities and is free from symptoms of neurovascular compromise.

IMPLEMENTATION

ACTION	RATIONALE
1. Review the medical record and nursing plan of care to determine the need for a pneumatic compression device (PCD) and for conditions that may contraindicate its use.	Reviewing the medical record and plan of care validates the correct patient and correct procedure and minimizes the risk for injury.
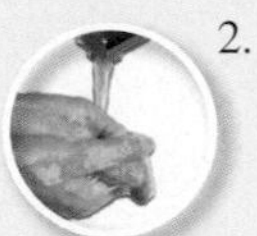 2. Perform hand hygiene. Put on PPE, as indicated.	Hand hygiene and PPE prevent the spread of microorganisms. PPE is required based on transmission precautions.
 3. Identify the patient. Explain the procedure to the patient.	Patient identification validates the correct patient and correct procedure. Discussion and explanation help allay anxiety and prepare the patient for what to expect.
4. Close the curtains around the bed and close the door to the room, if possible. Place the bed at an appropriate and comfortable working height, usually elbow height of the caregiver (VISN 8 Patient Safety Center, 2009).	Closing the door or curtains provides privacy. Proper bed height helps reduce back strain.
5. Hang the compression pump on the foot of the bed and plug it into an electrical outlet (Figure 1). Attach the connecting tubing to the pump.	Equipment preparation promotes efficient time management and provides an organized approach to the task.
6. Remove the compression sleeves from the package and unfold them. Lay the unfolded sleeves on the bed with the cotton lining facing up. **Note the markings indicating the correct placement for the ankle and popliteal areas.**	Proper placement of the sleeves prevents injury.
7. Apply graduated compression stockings, if ordered. Place a sleeve under the patient's leg with the tubing toward the heel (Figure 2). Each one fits either leg. **For total leg sleeves, place the behind-the-knee opening at the popliteal space to prevent pressure there. For knee-high sleeves, make sure the back of the ankle is over the ankle marking.**	Proper placement prevents injury.

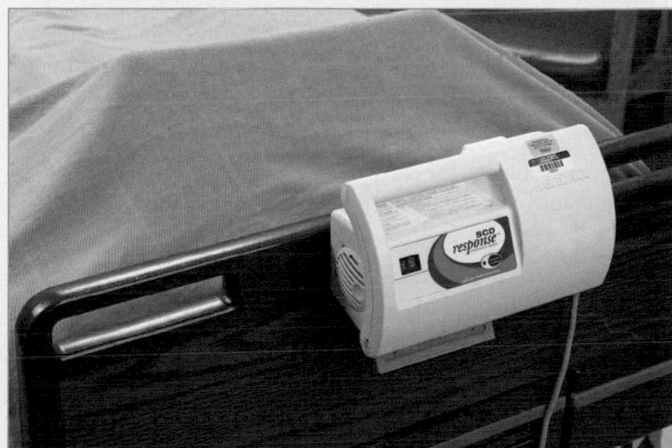

FIGURE 1 PCD machine at foot of bed.

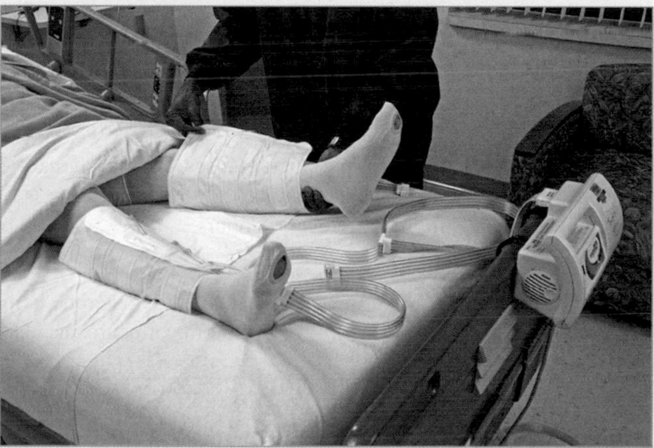

FIGURE 2 Placing PCD sleeves under patient's legs with tubing toward heel.

(continued)

SKILL 9-12 APPLYING PNEUMATIC COMPRESSION DEVICES continued

ACTION	RATIONALE
8. Wrap the sleeve snugly around the patient's leg so that two fingers fit between the leg and the sleeve. Secure the sleeve with the Velcro fasteners. Repeat for the second leg, if bilateral therapy is ordered. Connect each sleeve to the tubing, following manufacturer's recommendations (Figure 3).	Correct placement ensures appropriate, but not excessive, compression of the extremity.

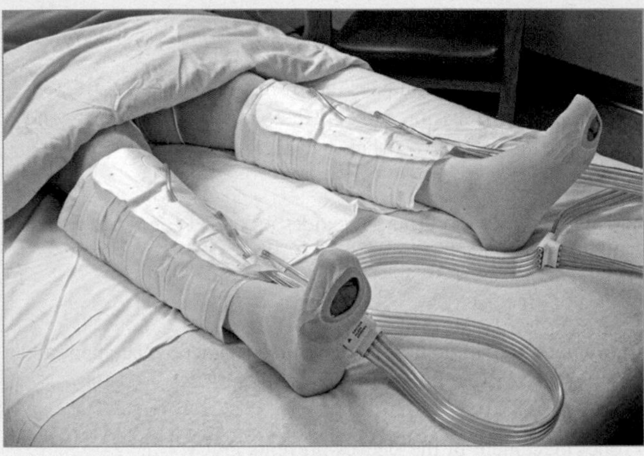

FIGURE 3 PCD sleeves snugly around patient's legs with sleeve tubing connected to device.

ACTION	RATIONALE
9. Set the pump to the prescribed maximal pressure (usually 35 to 55 mm Hg). Make sure the tubing is free from kinks. Check that the patient can move about without interrupting the airflow. Turn on the pump. Initiate cooling setting, if available.	Proper pressure setting ensures patient safety and prevents injury. Some devices have a cooling setting available to increase patient comfort.
10. **Observe the patient and the device during the first cycle. Check the audible alarms. Check the sleeves and pump at least once per shift or per facility policy.**	Observation and frequent checking ensure proper fit and inflation and reduce the risk for injury from the device.
11. Place the bed in the lowest position. Make sure the call bell and other essential items are within easy reach.	Returning the bed to the lowest position and having the call bell and other essential items readily available promote patient safety.
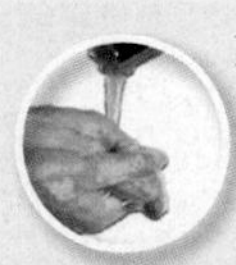 12. Remove PPE, if used. Perform hand hygiene.	Removing PPE properly reduces the risk for infection transmission and contamination of other items. Hand hygiene prevents the spread of microorganisms.
13. Assess the extremities for peripheral pulses, edema, changes in sensation, and movement. Remove the sleeves and assess and document skin integrity every 8 hours.	Assessment provides for early detection and prompt intervention for possible complications, including skin irritation.

EVALUATION

The expected outcome is met when the patient exhibits adequate circulation in extremities without symptoms of neurovascular compromise.

DOCUMENTATION

Guidelines

Document the time and date of application of the PCD, the patient's response to the therapy, and the patient's understanding of the therapy. Document the status of the alarms and pressure settings. Note the use of the cooling setting, if appropriate.

Sample Documentation

4/27/15 1615 Patient instructed regarding reason for PCD therapy; verbalizes understanding of therapy. Knee-high PCD applied to both lower extremities; pressure set at 45 mm Hg, as ordered. Patient denies any complaints of numbness or tingling. Feet and toes warm and pink; quick capillary refill; bilateral pedal pulses present and equal. Alarms and cooling settings as ordered.

—J. Trotter, RN

UNEXPECTED SITUATIONS AND ASSOCIATED INTERVENTIONS

- *Your postoperative patient is wearing PCD on both legs. While you are performing a routine assessment, he tells you that he has started to have pain in his left leg, along with tingling and numbness:* Remove the PCD and assess both lower extremities. Perform skin and neurovascular assessments. Assess the extremities for peripheral pulses, edema, changes in sensation, and movement. Report the patient's symptoms and assessment to the physician.

SPECIAL CONSIDERATIONS

- PCD are contraindicated in patients with suspected or existing DVT. They should not be used for patients with arterial occlusive disease, severe edema, cellulitis, phlebitis, a skin graft, or an infection of the extremity.
- Use the cooling setting, if the unit has one. The skin under the sleeve can become wet with diaphoresis, which can increase the risk for impaired skin integrity.
- Generally, the PCD should be worn continuously. It may be removed for bathing, walking, and physical therapy. Use is usually discontinued when the patient is ambulating consistently.
- The risk for DVT formation and injury is greater if the sleeves are not applied correctly.

EVIDENCE FOR PRACTICE ▶

VENOUS THROMBOEMBOLISM PREVENTION

American Association of Critical Care Nurses. (2010). *Venous Thromboembolism prevention.* Available http://www.aacn.org/WD/Practice/Docs/PracticeAlerts/VTE%20Prevention%2004-2010%20final.pdf

Refer to details in Skill 9-11, Evidence for Practice, and refer to thePoint for additional research on related nursing topics.

EVIDENCE FOR PRACTICE ▶

VENOUS THROMBOEMBOLISM PREVENTION

Geerts, W.H., Bergqvist, D., Pineo, G.F., et al. (2008). Prevention of venous embolism: American College of Chest Physicians Evidence-based clinical practice guidelines (8th ed.). *Chest, 133*(6) (Suppl), 381S–453S.

Refer to details in Skill 9-11, Evidence for Practice, and refer to thePoint for additional research on related nursing topics.

SKILL 9-13 APPLYING A CONTINUOUS PASSIVE MOTION DEVICE

A continuous passive motion (CPM) device passively moves a joint within a certain ROM (Viswanathan & Kidd, 2010). It is frequently prescribed after total knee **arthroplasty** as well as after surgery on other joints, such as shoulders. The degree of flexion and extension of the joint and the cycle rate (the number of revolutions per minute) are determined by the prescriber, but nurses place the patient in and out of the device and monitor the patient's response to the therapy.

(continued)

SKILL 9-13 APPLYING A CONTINUOUS PASSIVE MOTION DEVICE continued

DELEGATION CONSIDERATIONS

The application and removal of a continuous passive motion (CPM) device is not delegated to nursing assistive personnel (NAP) or to unlicensed assistive personnel (UAP). The application and removal of a continuous passive motion (CPM) device may be delegated to licensed practical/vocational nurses (LPN/LVNs). The decision to delegate must be based on careful analysis of the patient's needs and circumstances, as well as the qualifications of the person to whom the task is being delegated. Refer to the Delegation Guidelines in Appendix A.

EQUIPMENT

- CPM device
- Single-patient use soft-goods kit
- Tape measure
- Goniometer
- Nonsterile gloves and/or other PPE, if indicated

ASSESSMENT

Review the medical record and nursing plan of care for orders for degrees of flexion and extension. Assess the neurovascular status of the involved extremity. Perform a pain assessment. Administer the prescribed medication in sufficient time to allow for the full effect of the analgesic before starting the device. Assess for proper alignment of the joint in the CPM device. Assess the patient's ability to tolerate the prescribed treatment.

NURSING DIAGNOSIS

Determine the related factors for the nursing diagnoses based on the patient's current status. Appropriate nursing diagnoses may include:

- Impaired Physical Mobility
- Risk for Peripheral Neurovascular Dysfunction
- Risk for Impaired Skin Integrity
- Risk for Injury

OUTCOME IDENTIFICATION AND PLANNING

The expected outcome to achieve when applying a CPM device is that the patient experiences increased joint mobility. Other outcomes include the following: the patient displays improved or maintained muscle strength; muscle atrophy and contractures are prevented; circulation is promoted in the affected extremity; effects of immobility are decreased; and healing is stimulated.

IMPLEMENTATION

ACTION	RATIONALE
1. Review the medical record and nursing plan of care for the appropriate degrees of flexion and extension, the cycle rate, and the length of time the CPM is to be used.	Reviewing the medical record and plan of care validates the correct patient and correct procedure and reduces the risk for injury.
2. Obtain equipment. Apply the soft goods to the CPM device.	Equipment preparation promotes efficient time management and provides an organized approach to the task. The soft goods help to prevent friction to the extremity during motion.
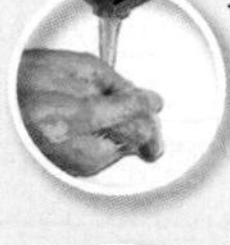 3. Perform hand hygiene. Put on PPE, as indicated.	Hand hygiene and PPE prevent the spread of microorganisms. PPE is required based on transmission precautions.
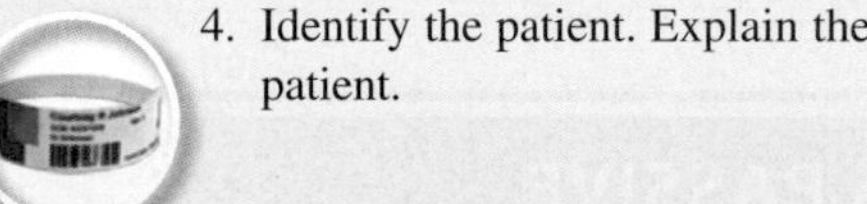 4. Identify the patient. Explain the procedure to the patient.	Patient identification validates the correct patient and correct procedure. Discussion and explanation help allay anxiety and prepare the patient for what to expect.
5. Close the curtains around the bed and close the door to the room, if possible. Place the bed at an appropriate and comfortable working height, usually elbow height of the caregiver (VISN 8 Patient Safety Center, 2009).	Closing the door or curtains provides privacy. Proper bed height helps reduce back strain.
6. Using the tape measure, determine the distance between the gluteal crease and the popliteal space.	The thigh length on the CPM device is adjusted based on this measurement.
7. Measure the leg from the knee to 14 inches beyond the bottom of the foot.	The position of the footplate is adjusted based on this measurement.

ACTION	RATIONALE
8. Position the patient in the middle of the bed. Make sure the affected extremity is in a slightly abducted position.	Proper positioning promotes correct body alignment and prevents pressure on the unaffected extremity.
9. Support the affected extremity and elevate it, placing it in the padded CPM device (Figure 1).	Support and elevation assist in movement of the affected extremity without injury.
10. **Make sure the knee is at the hinged joint of the CPM device.**	Proper positioning in the device prevents injury.
11. **Adjust the footplate to maintain the patient's foot in a neutral position (Figure 2). Assess the patient's position to make sure the leg is not internally or externally rotated.**	Adjustment helps ensure proper positioning and prevents injury.
12. Apply the restraining straps under the CPM device and around the leg. **Check that two fingers fit between the strap and the leg (Figure 3).**	Restraining straps maintain the leg in position. Leaving a space between the strap and leg prevents injury from excessive pressure from the strap.
13. Explain the use of the STOP/GO button to the patient. Set the controls to the prescribed levels of flexion and extension and cycles per minute. Turn on the power to the CPM.	Explanation decreases anxiety by allowing the patient to participate in care.
14. Set the device to ON and start the therapy by pressing the GO button. Observe the patient and the device during the first cycle. Determine the angle of flexion when the device reaches its greatest height using the goniometer (Figure 4). Compare with prescribed degree.	Observation ensures that the device is working properly, thereby ensuring patient safety. Measuring with a **goniometer** ensures the device is set to the prescribed parameters.
15. Check the patient's level of comfort and perform skin and neurovascular assessments at least every 8 hours or per facility policy.	Frequent assessments provide for early detection and prompt intervention should problems arise.
16. Place the bed in the lowest position, with the side rails up. Make sure the call bell and other essential items are within easy reach.	Having the bed at the proper height and having the call bell and other items handy ensure patient safety.

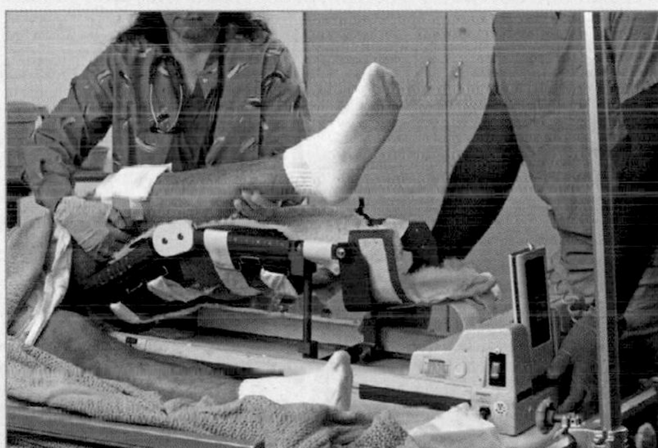

FIGURE 1 Placing patient's leg into CPM machine.

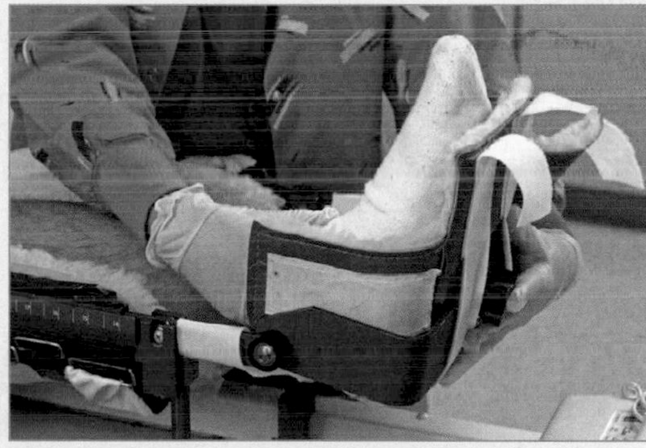

FIGURE 2 Adjusting footplate to maintain patient's foot in a neutral position.

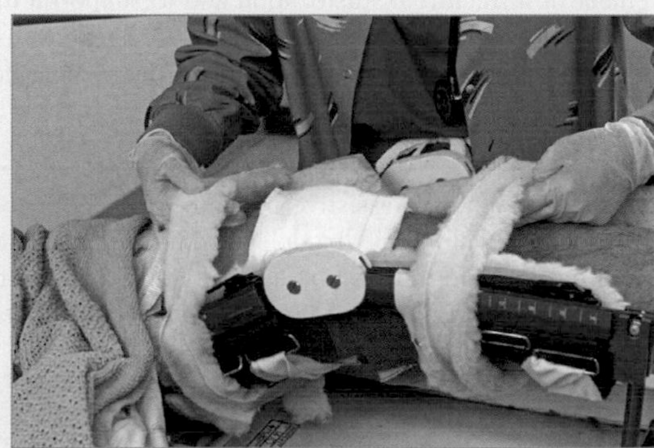

FIGURE 3 Using two fingers to check fit between straps and leg.

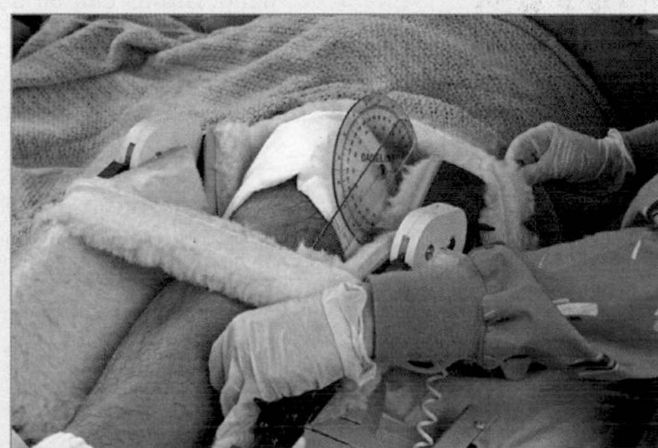

FIGURE 4 Determining angle of joint flexion, using goniometer.

(continued)

SKILL 9-13 APPLYING A CONTINUOUS PASSIVE MOTION DEVICE continued

ACTION	RATIONALE
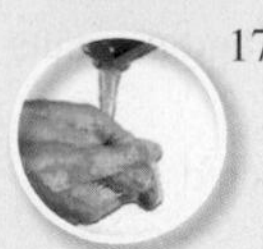 17. Remove PPE, if used. Perform hand hygiene.	Removing PPE properly reduces the risk for infection transmission and contamination of other items. Hand hygiene prevents the spread of microorganisms.

EVALUATION

The expected outcome is met when the patient demonstrates increased joint mobility. In addition, the patient exhibits improved muscle strength without evidence of atrophy or contractures.

DOCUMENTATION

Guidelines

Document the time and date of application of the CPM, the extension and flexion settings, the speed of the device, the patient's response to the therapy, and your assessment of the extremity.

Sample Documentation

5/03/15 1430 Right knee incision clean and dry; dressing intact. Right toes pink and warm, with brisk capillary refill; equal to left. Pedal pulses present and equal bilaterally. CPM device applied with range of motion at 30 degrees of knee flexion, for five cycles per minute for 30 minutes. Patient complains of slight increase in pain from a rating of 4/10 to 5/10, but states, "I don't want anything for the pain right now." Plan to reassess in 15 minutes and offer analgesic as ordered.

—K. Dugas, RN

UNEXPECTED SITUATIONS AND ASSOCIATED INTERVENTIONS

- *A patient is prescribed therapy with a CPM device. After you initiate the prescribed flexion and extension of the joint, the patient complains of sudden pain in the joint:* Stop the CPM device. Check the settings to make sure the device is set correctly for the prescribed therapy. Assess the patient for other signs and symptoms and obtain vital signs. Perform a neurovascular assessment of the affected extremity. Notify the primary care provider of the patient's pain and any other findings. When therapy is resumed, evaluate the need for premedication with analgesics. Continue pain intervention with analgesics, as prescribed.

SKILL 9-14 APPLYING A SLING

A sling is a bandage that can provide support for an arm or immobilize an injured arm, wrist, or hand. Slings can be used to restrict movement of a fracture or dislocation and to support a muscle sprain. They may also be used to support a splint or secure dressings. Health care agencies usually use commercial slings. The sling should distribute the supported weight over a large area, not the back of the neck, to prevent pressure on the cervical spinal nerves.

DELEGATION CONSIDERATIONS

The application of a sling may not be delegated to nursing assistive personnel (NAP) or to unlicensed assistive personnel (UAP). The application of a sling may be delegated to licensed practical/vocational nurses (LPN/LVNs). The decision to delegate must be based on careful analysis of the patient's needs and circumstances, as well as the qualifications of the person to whom the task is being delegated. Refer to the Delegation Guidelines in Appendix A.

EQUIPMENT

- Commercial arm sling
- ABD gauze pad
- Nonsterile gloves and/or other PPE, as indicated

ASSESSMENT

Assess the situation to determine the need for a sling. Assess the affected limb for pain and edema. Perform a neurovascular assessment of the affected extremity. Assess body parts distal to the site for cyanosis, pallor, coolness, numbness, tingling, swelling, and absent or diminished pulses.

NURSING DIAGNOSIS

Determine the related factors for the nursing diagnoses based on the patient's current status. Appropriate nursing diagnoses may include:

- Impaired Physical Mobility
- Risk for Impaired Skin Integrity
- Risk for Peripheral Neurovascular Dysfunction

OUTCOME IDENTIFICATION AND PLANNING

The expected outcome to achieve when applying a sling is that the arm is immobilized, and the patient maintains muscle strength and joint range of motion. In addition, the patient shows no evidence of contractures, **venous stasis**, thrombus formation, or skin breakdown.

IMPLEMENTATION

ACTION	RATIONALE
1. Review the medical record and nursing plan of care to determine the need for the use of a sling.	Reviewing the medical record and plan of care validates the correct patient and correct procedure and prevents injury.
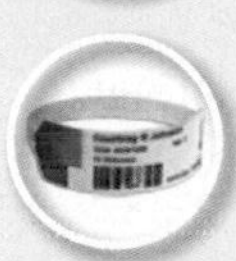 2. Perform hand hygiene. Put on PPE, as indicated.	Hand hygiene and PPE prevent the spread of microorganisms. PPE is required based on transmission precautions.
3. Identify the patient. Explain the procedure to the patient.	Patient identification validates the correct patient and correct procedure. Discussion and explanation help allay anxiety and prepare the patient for what to expect.
4. Close the curtains around the bed and close the door to the room, if possible. Place the bed at an appropriate and comfortable working height, usually elbow height of the caregiver (VISN 8 Patient Safety Center, 2009).	Closing the door or curtain provides privacy. Proper bed height helps reduce back strain.
5. Assist the patient to a sitting position. Place the patient's forearm across the chest with the elbow flexed and the palm against the chest. Measure the sleeve length, if indicated.	Proper positioning facilitates sling application. Measurement ensures proper sizing of the sling and proper placement of the arm.
6. Enclose the arm in the sling, making sure the elbow fits into the corner of the fabric (Figure 1). Run the strap up the patient's back and across the shoulder opposite the injury, then down the chest to the fastener on the end of the sling (Figure 2).	This position ensures adequate support and keeps the arm out of a dependent position, preventing edema.

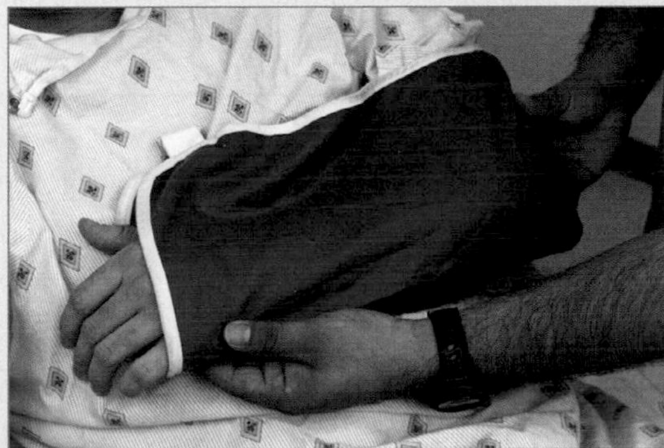

FIGURE 1 Placing patient's arm into canvas sling with elbow flush in corner of sling.

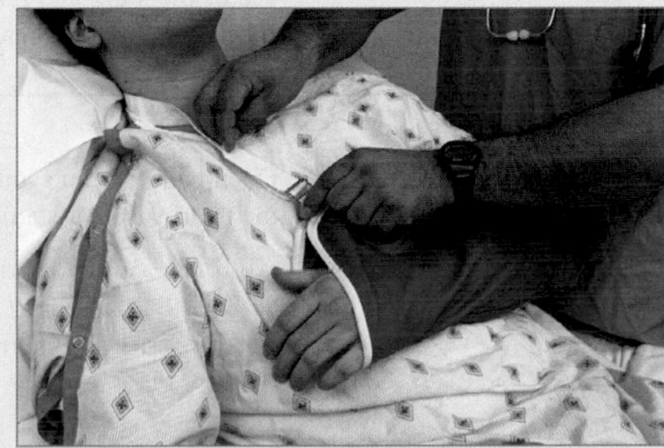

FIGURE 2 Placing strap around patient's neck.

(continued)

SKILL 9-14 APPLYING A SLING continued

ACTION	RATIONALE
7. Place the ABD pad under the strap, between the strap and the patient's neck (Figure 3). **Ensure that the sling and forearm are slightly elevated and at a right angle to the body (Figure 4).**	Padding prevents skin irritation and reduces pressure on the neck. Proper positioning ensures alignment, provides support, and prevents edema.

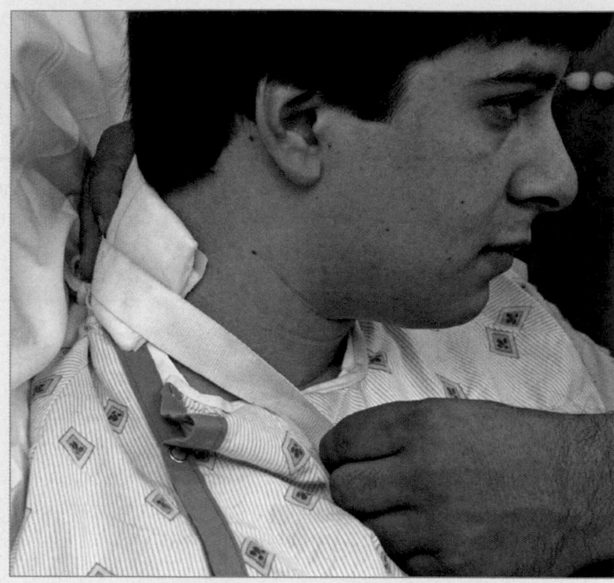

FIGURE 3 Placing padding between strap and patient's neck.

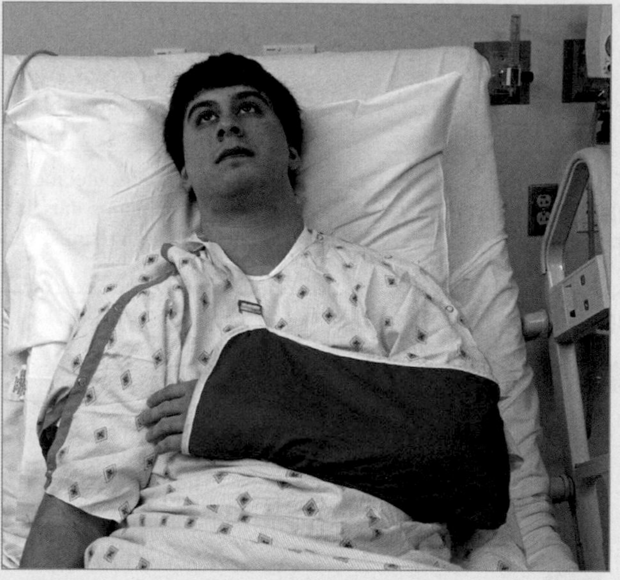

FIGURE 4 Patient with sling in place.

ACTION	RATIONALE
8. Place the bed in the lowest position, with the side rails up. Make sure the call bell and other essential items are within easy reach.	Having the bed at proper height and leaving the call bell and other items within reach ensure patient safety.
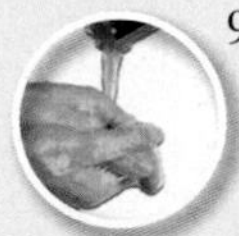 9. Remove PPE, if used. Perform hand hygiene.	Removing PPE properly reduces the risk for infection transmission and contamination of other items. Hand hygiene prevents the spread of microorganisms.
10. Check the patient's level of comfort, arm positioning, and neurovascular status of the affected limb every 4 hours or according to facility policy. Assess the axillary and cervical skin frequently for irritation or breakdown.	Frequent assessment ensures patient safety, prevents injury, and provides early intervention for skin irritation and other complications.

EVALUATION

The expected outcome is met when the patient demonstrates the extremity in proper alignment with adequate muscle strength and joint range of motion. In addition, the patient demonstrates proper use of the sling and remains free of complications, including contractures, venous stasis, thrombus formation, or skin breakdown.

DOCUMENTATION

Guidelines

Document the time and date the sling was applied. Document the patient's response to the sling and the neurovascular status of the extremity.

Sample Documentation

5/22/15 2015 Sling applied to left arm, as ordered. Left hand and fingers warm to touch and pink. Brisk capillary refill. Left radial pulse present and equal to right. Patient denies any complaints of numbness, pain, or tingling of left upper extremity.

—*P. Peterson, RN*

UNEXPECTED SITUATIONS AND ASSOCIATED INTERVENTIONS

- *Your patient needs a sling to support a wrist fracture, but you cannot obtain a commercially prepared sling:* Make a sling using a triangular bandage or cloth. Place the cloth or bandage on the chest with a corner of the cloth at the elbow. Place the affected arm across the chest with the elbow flexed and the palm on the chest. Wrap the end closest to the head around the neck, on the opposite side from the injured arm. Bring the end of the cloth that is farthest from the head up over the injured arm and tie it at the side of the neck. Make sure that the sling and forearm are slightly elevated and at a right angle to the body.

SPECIAL CONSIDERATIONS

- Be sure that the patient's wrist is enclosed in the sling. Do not allow it to hang out and down over the edge. This prevents pressure on nerves and blood vessels and prevents muscle contractures, deformity, and discomfort.
- Assess circulation and comfort at regular intervals.

SKILL 9-15 APPLYING A FIGURE-EIGHT BANDAGE

Bandages are used to apply pressure over an area, immobilize a body part, prevent or reduce edema, and secure splints and dressings. Bandages can be elasticized or made of gauze, flannel, or muslin. In general, narrow bandages are used to wrap feet, the lower legs, hands, and arms, and wider bandages are used for the thighs and trunk. A roller bandage is a continuous strip of material wound on itself to form a roll. The free end is anchored and the roll is passed or rolled around the body part, maintaining equal tension with all turns. The bandage is unwound gradually and only as needed. The bandage should overlap itself evenly and by one-half to two-thirds the width the bandage. The figure-eight turn consists of oblique overlapping turns that ascend and descend alternately. It is used around the knee, elbow, ankle, and wrist.

DELEGATION CONSIDERATIONS

The application of a figure eight bandage may not be delegated to nursing assistive personnel (NAP) or to unlicensed assistive personnel (UAP). The application of a figure-eight bandage may be delegated to licensed practical/vocational nurses (LPN/LVNs). The decision to delegate must be based on careful analysis of the patient's needs and circumstances, as well as the qualifications of the person to whom the task is being delegated. Refer to the Delegation Guidelines in Appendix A.

EQUIPMENT

- Elastic or other bandage of the appropriate width
- Tape, pins, or self-closures
- Gauze pads
- Nonsterile gloves and/or other PPE, as indicated

ASSESSMENT

Review the medical record and nursing plan of care and assess the situation to determine the need for a bandage. Assess the affected limb for pain and edema. Perform a neurovascular assessment of the affected extremity. Assess body parts distal to the site for evidence of cyanosis, pallor, coolness, numbness, tingling, and swelling and absent or diminished pulses. Assess the distal circulation of the extremity after the bandage is in place and at least every 4 hours thereafter.

NURSING DIAGNOSIS

Determine the related factors for the nursing diagnoses based on the patient's current status. Appropriate nursing diagnoses may include:

- Impaired Physical Mobility
- Risk for Peripheral Neurovascular Dysfunction
- Risk for Impaired Skin Integrity

OUTCOME IDENTIFICATION AND PLANNING

The expected outcome to achieve when applying a figure-eight bandage is that the bandage is applied correctly without injury or complications. Other outcomes that may be appropriate include the following: patient maintains circulation to the affected part and remains free of neurovascular complications.

(continued)

SKILL 9-15 APPLYING A FIGURE-EIGHT BANDAGE continued

IMPLEMENTATION

ACTION	RATIONALE
1. Review the medical record and nursing plan of care to determine the need for a figure-eight bandage.	Reviewing the medical record and plan of care validates the correct patient and correct procedure and reduces risk for injury.
2. Perform hand hygiene. Put on PPE, as indicated.	Hand hygiene and PPE prevent the spread of microorganisms. PPE is required based on transmission precautions.
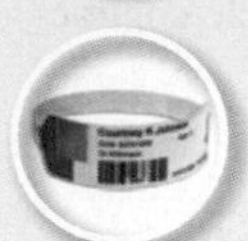 3. Identify the patient. Explain the procedure to the patient.	Patient identification validates the correct patient and correct procedure. Discussion and explanation help allay anxiety and prepare the patient for what to expect.
4. Close the curtains around the bed and close the door to the room, if possible. Place the bed at an appropriate and comfortable working height, usually elbow height of the caregiver (VISN 8 Patient Safety Center, 2009).	Closing the door or curtains provides privacy. Proper bed height helps reduce back strain.
5. Assist the patient to a comfortable position, with the affected body part in a normal functioning position.	Keeping the body part in a normal functioning position promotes circulation and prevents deformity and discomfort.
6. Hold the bandage roll with the roll facing upward in one hand while holding the free end of the roll in the other hand. Make sure to hold the bandage roll so it is close to the affected body part.	Proper handling of the bandage allows application of even tension and pressure.
7. Wrap the bandage around the limb twice, below the joint, to anchor it (Figure 1).	Anchoring the bandage ensures that it will stay in place.
8. Use alternating ascending and descending turns to form a figure eight (Figure 2). Overlap each turn of the bandage by one-half to two-thirds the width of the strip (Figure 3).	Making alternating ascending and descending turns helps to ensure the bandage will stay in place on a moving body part.

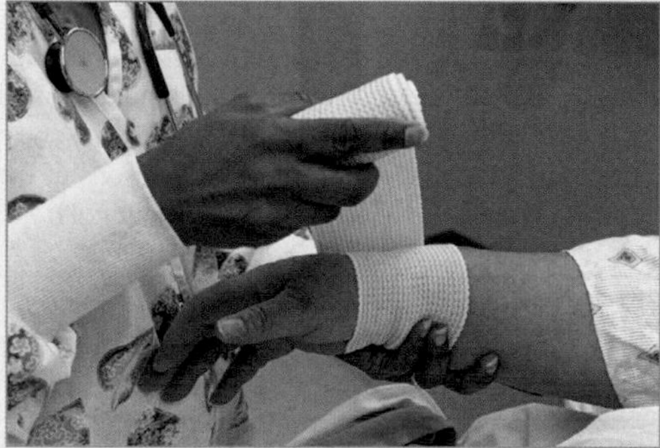

FIGURE 1 Wrapping bandage around patient's limb twice, below joint, to anchor it.

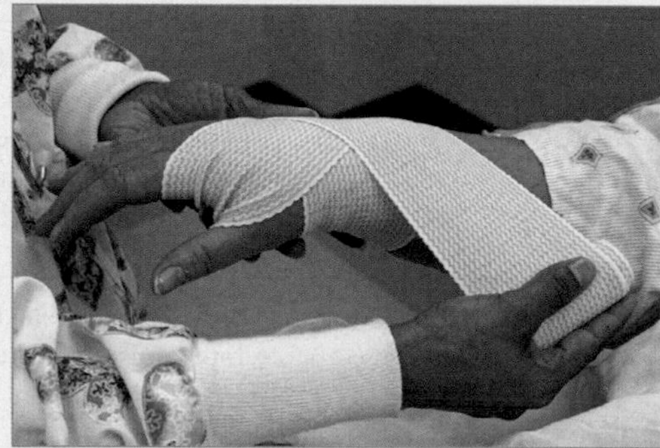

FIGURE 2 Using alternating ascending and descending turns to form a figure eight.

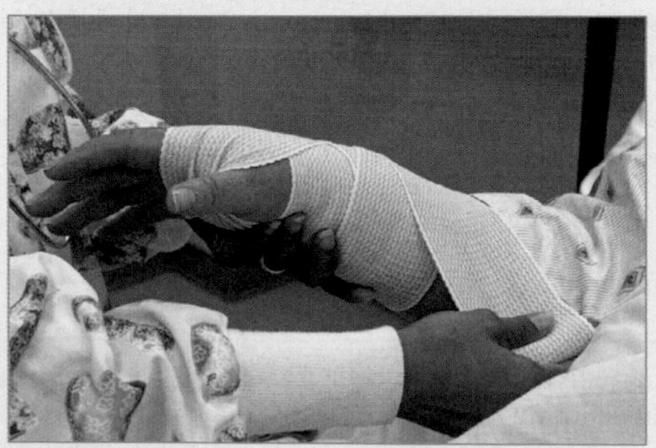

FIGURE 3 Overlapping each turn of bandage by one-half to two-thirds strip width.

ACTION | **RATIONALE**

9. Unroll the bandage as you wrap, not before wrapping.

Unrolling the bandage with wrapping prevents uneven pressure, which could interfere with blood circulation.

10. **Wrap firmly, but not tightly. Assess the patient's comfort as you wrap. If the patient reports tingling, itching, numbness, or pain, loosen the bandage.**

Firm wrapping is necessary to provide support and prevent injury, but wrapping too tightly interferes with circulation. Patient complaints are helpful indicators of possible circulatory compromise.

11. After the area is covered, wrap the bandage around the limb twice, above the joint, to anchor it (Figure 4). Secure the end of the bandage with tape, pins, or self-closures. Avoid metal clips.

Anchoring at the end ensures the bandage will stay in place. Metal clips can cause injury.

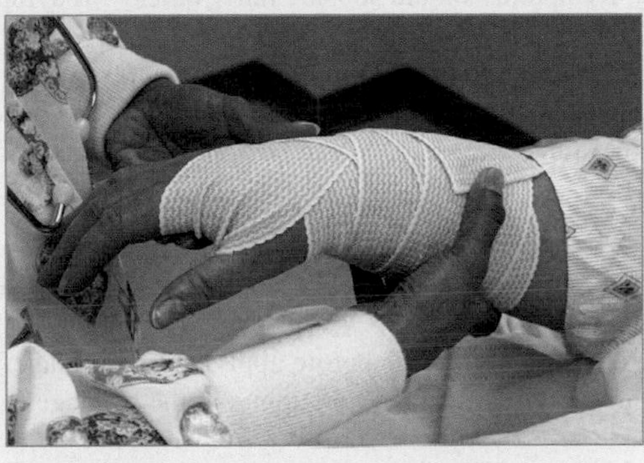

FIGURE 4 Wrapping bandage around patient's limb twice, above joint, to anchor it.

12. Place the bed in the lowest position, with the side rails up. Make sure the call bell and other necessary items are within easy reach.

Repositioning the bed and having items nearby ensure patient safety.

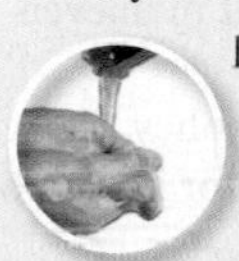

13. Remove PPE, if used. Perform hand hygiene.

Removing PPE properly reduces the risk for infection transmission and contamination of other items. Hand hygiene prevents the spread of microorganisms.

14. Elevate the wrapped extremity for 15 to 30 minutes after application of the bandage.

Elevation promotes venous return and reduces edema.

15. Assess the distal circulation after the bandage is in place.

Elastic may tighten as it is wrapped. Frequent assessment of distal circulation ensures patient safety and prevents injury.

16. Lift the distal end of the bandage and assess the skin for color, temperature, and integrity. Assess for pain and perform a neurovascular assessment of the affected extremity after applying the bandage and at least every 4 hours thereafter, or per facility policy.

Assessment aids in prompt detection of compromised circulation and allows for early intervention for skin irritation and other complications.

EVALUATION

The expected outcome is achieved when the patient exhibits a bandage that is applied correctly, without causing injury or neurovascular compromise. In addition, the patient demonstrates proper alignment of the bandaged body part; the patient remains free of evidence of complications; and the patient demonstrates an understanding of signs and symptoms to report immediately.

DOCUMENTATION

Guidelines

Document the time, date, and site that the bandage was applied and the size of the bandage used. Include the skin assessment and care provided before application. Document the patient's response to the bandage and the neurovascular status of the extremity.

(continued)

SKILL 9-15 APPLYING A FIGURE-EIGHT BANDAGE continued

Sample Documentation

> 5/27/15 1615 3-inch bandage applied to right knee using figure-eight technique. Skin pink, warm, and dry, with quick capillary refill; pedal and dorsalis pedis pulses present and equal bilaterally. Patient denies any complaints of pain, numbness, or tingling. Patient instructed to report any complaints immediately. Right lower extremity resting on two pillows at present.
>
> —J. Wilkins, RN

UNEXPECTED SITUATIONS AND ASSOCIATED INTERVENTIONS

- *After you have applied a figure-eight bandage to a patient's elbow to hold dressings in place, the patient reports tingling, numbness, and pain in his hand during a routine assessment:* Remove the bandage, wait 30 minutes, and reapply the bandage with less tension. Continue to monitor the neurovascular status of the extremity. Symptoms should subside fairly quickly. If symptoms persist, notify the physician.
- *You remove the bandage on a patient's ankle and note the bandage is limp and less elastic than when it was applied:* Obtain a new bandage and apply it to the ankle. Launder the old bandage to restore its elasticity. Keep two bandages at the bedside: One can be applied while the other is being laundered.

SPECIAL CONSIDERATIONS

- Keep in mind that a figure-eight bandage may be contraindicated if skin breakdown or lesions are present on the area to be wrapped.
- When wrapping an extremity, elevate it for 15 to 30 minutes before applying the bandage, if possible. This promotes venous return and prevents edema. Avoid applying the bandage to a dependent extremity.
- Place gauze pads or cotton between skin surfaces, such as toes and fingers, to prevent skin irritation. Skin surfaces should not touch after the bandage is applied.
- Include the heel when wrapping the foot, but do not wrap the toes or fingers unless necessary. Assess distal body parts to detect impaired circulation.
- Avoid leaving gaps in bandage layers or leaving skin exposed, because this may result in uneven pressure on the body part.
- Remove and change the bandage at least once a day, or per medical order or facility policy. Cleanse the skin and dry thoroughly before applying a new bandage. Assess the skin for irritation and breakdown.

SKILL 9-16 ASSISTING WITH CAST APPLICATION

A cast is a rigid external immobilizing device that encases a body part. Casts are used to immobilize a body part in a specific position and to apply uniform pressure on the encased soft tissue. They may be used to treat injuries, correct a deformity, stabilize weakened joints, or promote healing after surgery. Casts generally allow the patient mobility while restricting movement of the affected body part. Casts may be made of plaster or synthetic materials, such as fiberglass. Each material has advantages and disadvantages. Nonplaster casts set in 15 minutes and can sustain weight bearing or pressure in 15 to 30 minutes. Plaster casts can take 24 to 72 hours to dry, and weight bearing or pressure is contraindicated during this period. Patient safety is of utmost importance during the application of a cast. Typically, a physician or other advanced practice professional applies the cast. Nursing responsibilities include preparing the patient and equipment and assisting during the application. The nurse provides skin care to the affected area before, during, and after the cast is applied. In some settings, nurses with special preparation may apply or change casts.

DELEGATION CONSIDERATIONS

Assisting with the application of a cast may not be delegated to nursing assistive personnel (NAP) or to unlicensed assistive personnel (UAP). Depending on the state's nurse practice act and the organization's policies and procedures, assisting with the application of a cast may be delegated to licensed practical/vocational nurses (LPN/LVNs). The decision to delegate must be based on careful analysis of the patient's needs and circumstances, as well as the qualifications of the person to whom the task is being delegated. Refer to the Delegation Guidelines in Appendix A.

EQUIPMENT

- Casting materials, such as plaster rolls or fiberglass, depending on the type of cast being applied
- Padding material, such as stockinette, sheet wadding, or Webril, depending on the type of cast being applied
- Plastic bucket or basin filled with warm water
- Disposable, nonsterile gloves and aprons
- Scissors
- Waterproof, disposable pads
- PPE, as indicated

ASSESSMENT

Assess the skin condition in the affected area, noting redness, **contusions**, or open wounds. Assess the neurovascular status of the affected extremity, including distal pulses, color, temperature, presence of edema, capillary refill to fingers or toes, weakness, sensation, and motion. Perform a pain assessment. If the patient reports pain, administer the prescribed analgesic in sufficient time to allow for the full effect of the medication. Assess for muscle spasms and administer the prescribed muscle relaxant in sufficient time to allow for the full effect of the medication. Assess for the presence of disease processes that may contraindicate the use of a cast or interfere with wound healing, including skin diseases, **peripheral vascular disease**, diabetes mellitus, and open or draining wounds.

NURSING DIAGNOSIS

Determine the related factors for the nursing diagnoses based on the patient's current status. Appropriate nursing diagnoses may include:

- Risk for Impaired Skin Integrity
- Impaired Physical Mobility
- Risk for Peripheral Neurovascular Dysfunction
- Ineffective Peripheral Tissue Perfusion

OUTCOME IDENTIFICATION AND PLANNING

The expected outcome to achieve when assisting with a cast application is that the cast is applied without interfering with neurovascular function and that healing occurs. Other outcomes that may be appropriate include that the patient is free from complications; the patient has knowledge of the treatment regimen; and the patient experiences increased comfort.

IMPLEMENTATION

ACTION	RATIONALE
1. Review the medical record and medical orders to determine the need for the cast.	Reviewing the medical record and order validates the correct patient and correct procedure.
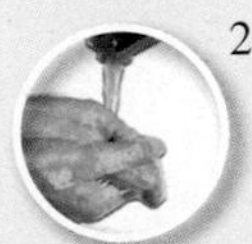 2. Perform hand hygiene. Put on gloves and/or other PPE, as indicated.	Hand hygiene and PPE prevent the spread of microorganisms. PPE is required based on transmission precautions.
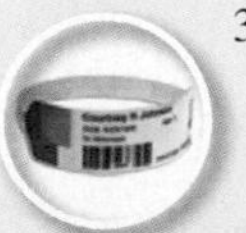 3. Identify the patient. Explain the procedure to the patient and verify area to be casted.	Patient identification validates the correct patient and correct procedure. Discussion and explanation help allay anxiety and prepare the patient for what to expect.
4. Perform a pain assessment and assess for muscle spasm. Administer prescribed medications in sufficient time to allow for the full effect of the analgesic and/or muscle relaxant.	Assessment of pain and analgesic administration ensures patient comfort and enhances cooperation.
5. Close the curtains around the bed and close the door to the room, if possible. Place the bed at an appropriate and comfortable working height, usually elbow height of the caregiver (VISN 8 Patient Safety Center, 2009).	Closing the door or curtains provides privacy. Proper bed height helps reduce back strain while you are performing the procedure.

(continued)

SKILL 9-16 ASSISTING WITH CAST APPLICATION continued

ACTION	RATIONALE
6. Position the patient, as needed, depending on the type of cast being applied and the location of the injury. Support the extremity or body part to be casted.	Proper positioning minimizes movement, maintains alignment, and increases patient comfort.
7. Drape the patient with the waterproof pads.	Draping provides warmth and privacy and helps protect other body parts from contact with casting materials.
8. Cleanse and dry the affected body part.	Skin care before cast application helps prevent skin breakdown.
9. Position and maintain the affected body part in the position indicated by the physician or advanced practice professional as the stockinette, sheet wadding, and padding are applied (Figure 1). The stockinette should extend beyond the ends of the cast. As the wadding is applied, check for wrinkles.	Stockinette and other materials protect the skin from casting materials and create a smooth, padded edge, protecting the skin from abrasion. Padding protects the skin, tissues, and nerves from the pressure of the cast.
10. Continue to position and maintain the affected body part in the position indicated by the physician or advanced practice professional as the casting material is applied (Figure 2). Assist with finishing by folding the stockinette or other padding down over the outer edge of the cast.	Smooth edges lessen the risk for skin irritation and abrasion.
11. **Support the cast during hardening**. Handle hardening plaster casts with the palms of hands, not fingers (Figure 3). Support the cast on a firm, smooth surface. Do not rest it on a hard surface or sharp edges. Avoid placing pressure on the cast.	Proper handling avoids denting of the cast and development of pressure areas.

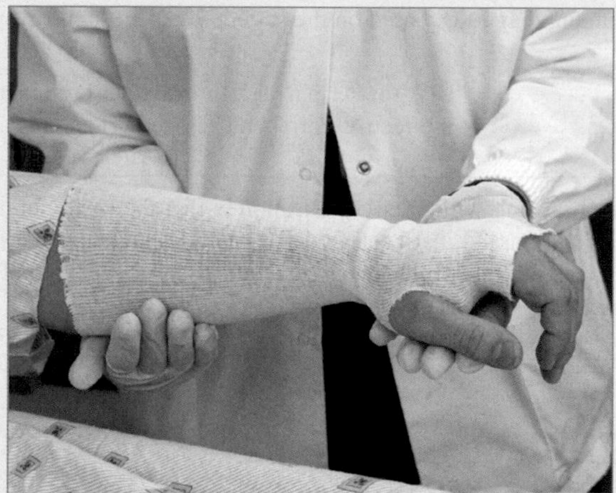

FIGURE 1 Stockinette in place.

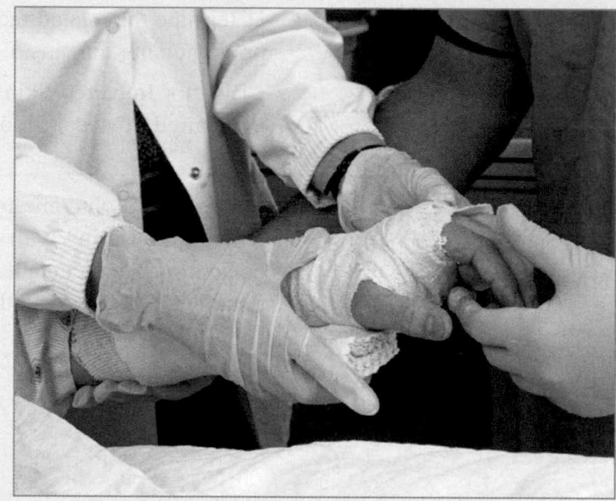

FIGURE 2 Casting material being applied.

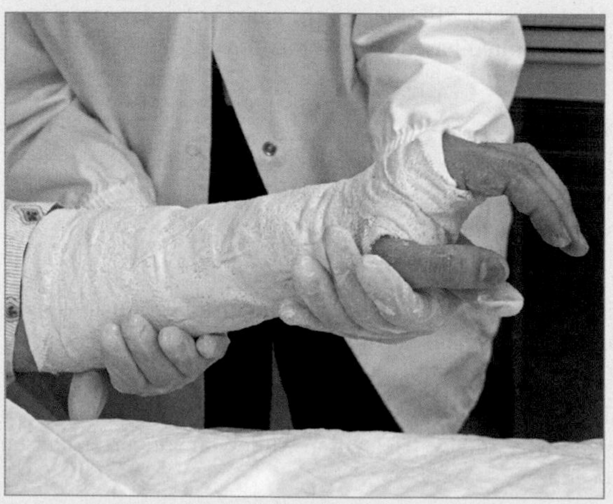

FIGURE 3 Using palms to handle casted limb.

ACTION	RATIONALE
12. **Elevate the injured limb at heart level with pillow or bath blankets, as ordered, making sure pressure is evenly distributed under the cast.**	Elevation promotes venous return. Evenly distributed pressure prevents molding and denting of the cast and development of pressure areas.
13. Place the bed in the lowest position, with the side rails up. Make sure the call bell and other essential items are within easy reach.	Having the bed at proper height and leaving the call bell and other items within reach ensure patient safety.
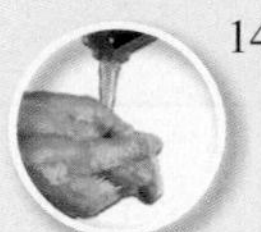 14. Remove gloves and any other PPE, if used. Perform hand hygiene.	Removing PPE properly reduces the risk for infection transmission and contamination of other items. Hand hygiene prevents the spread of microorganisms.
15. Obtain x-rays, as ordered.	X-rays identify that the affected area is positioned properly.
16. Instruct the patient to report pain, odor, drainage, changes in sensation, abnormal sensation, or the inability to move fingers or toes of the affected extremity.	Pressure within a cast may increase with edema and lead to compartment syndrome. Patient complaints allow for early detection of, and prompt intervention for, complications such as skin irritation or impaired tissue perfusion.
17. Leave the cast uncovered and exposed to the air. Reposition the patient every 2 hours. Depending on facility policy, a fan may be used to dry the cast.	Keeping the cast uncovered promotes drying. Repositioning prevents development of pressure areas. Using a fan helps increase airflow and speeds drying.

EVALUATION

The expected outcome is achieved when neurovascular function is maintained and healing occurs. In addition, the patient is free from complications, has knowledge of the treatment regimen, and experiences increased comfort

DOCUMENTATION

Guidelines

Document the time, date, and site that the cast was applied. Include the skin assessment and care provided before application. Document the patient's response to the cast and the neurovascular status of the extremity.

Sample Documentation

6/1/15 1245 Fiberglass cast applied to right forearm from mid-upper arm to middle of hand. Cast clean and dry; edges padded. No signs of irritation noted. Patient able to move fingers freely. Fingers pale pink, warm, and dry. Capillary refill less than 2 seconds. Patient denies any numbness, tingling, or pain. Right forearm resting on two pillows. Patient instructed to report any complaints of pain, pressure, numbness, tingling, or decreased ability to move fingers.

—P. Collins, RN

Unexpected Situations and Associated Interventions

- *Your patient, who has a cast on his hand and forearm, has been experiencing pain relief in the extremity with ice application and oral analgesics. He now reports pain unrelieved by the analgesic and a feeling of tightness in his arm. In addition, his fingers are cool, with sluggish capillary refill:* **Compartment syndrome** may be developing. Adjust the position of the arm so that it is no higher than heart level. This enhances arterial perfusion and controls edema. Notify the primary care provider of the situation immediately. Prepare for bivalving of the cast (cutting of the cast in half longitudinally) to relieve pressure.

SPECIAL CONSIDERATIONS

General Considerations

- Perform frequent, regular assessment of neurovascular status. Early recognition of diminished circulation and nerve function is essential to prevent loss of function. Be alert for the presence of compartment syndrome.
- Fiberglass casts dry quickly, usually within 5 to 15 minutes.

(continued)

SKILL 9-16 ASSISTING WITH CAST APPLICATION continued

- If a fiberglass cast was applied, remove any fiberglass resin residue on the skin with alcohol or acetone.
- Synthetic casts are lightweight, easy to clean, and somewhat water-resistant. If a Gore-Tex liner is used when the cast is applied, the cast may be immersed in water without affecting the cast integrity.

Infant and Child Considerations

- Synthetic casts come in different colors and with designs, such as cartoons and stripes. These features may make the experience more pleasant for a child.

SKILL 9-17 CARING FOR A CAST

A cast is a rigid external immobilizing device that encases a body part. Casts, made of plaster or synthetic materials, such as fiberglass, are used to immobilize a body part in a specific position and to apply uniform pressure on the encased soft tissue. They may be used to treat injuries, correct a deformity, stabilize weakened joints, or promote healing after surgery. Casts generally allow the patient mobility while restricting movement of the affected body part. Nursing responsibilities after the cast is in place include maintaining the cast, preventing complications, and providing patient teaching related to cast care.

DELEGATION CONSIDERATIONS

Care of a cast may not be delegated to nursing assistive personnel (NAP) or to unlicensed assistive personnel (UAP). Depending on the state's nurse practice act and the organization's policies and procedures, care of a cast may be delegated to licensed practical/vocational nurses (LPN/LVNs). The decision to delegate must be based on careful analysis of the patient's needs and circumstances, as well as the qualifications of the person to whom the task is being delegated. Refer to the Delegation Guidelines in Appendix A.

EQUIPMENT

- Washcloth
- Towel
- Skin cleanser
- Basin of warm water
- Waterproof pads
- Tape
- Pillows
- PPE, as indicated

ASSESSMENT

Review the patient's medical record and nursing plan of care to determine the need for cast care and care of the affected area. Perform a pain assessment and administer the prescribed medication in sufficient time to allow for the full effect of the analgesic before starting care. Assess the neurovascular status of the affected extremity, including distal pulses, color, temperature, presence of edema, capillary refill to fingers or toes, and sensation and motion. Assess the skin distal to the cast. Note any indications of infection, including any foul odor from the cast, pain, fever, edema, and extreme warmth over an area of the cast. Assess for complications of immobility, including alterations in skin integrity, reduced joint movement, decreased peristalsis, constipation, alterations in respiratory function, and signs of **thrombophlebitis**. Inspect the condition of the cast. Be alert for cracks, dents, or the presence of drainage from the cast. Assess the patient's knowledge of cast care.

NURSING DIAGNOSIS

Determine the related factors for the nursing diagnoses based on the patient's current status. Appropriate nursing diagnoses may include:

- Risk for Peripheral Neurovascular Dysfunction
- Self-Care Deficit (bathing, feeding, dressing, or toileting)
- Risk for Impaired Skin Integrity

OUTCOME IDENTIFICATION AND PLANNING

The expected outcome to achieve when caring for a patient with a cast is that the cast remains intact, and the patient does not experience neurovascular compromise. Other outcomes include that the patient is free from infection; the patient experiences only mild pain and slight edema or soreness; the patient experiences only slight limitations of range of joint motion; the skin around the cast edges remains intact; the patient participates in ADLs; and the patient demonstrates appropriate cast-care techniques.

IMPLEMENTATION

ACTION	RATIONALE
1. Review the medical record and the nursing plan of care to determine the need for cast care and care for the affected body part.	Reviewing the medical record and plan of care validates the correct patient and correct procedure.
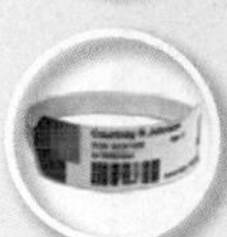 2. Perform hand hygiene. Put on PPE, as indicated.	Hand hygiene and PPE prevent the spread of microorganisms. PPE is required based on transmission precautions.
3. Identify the patient. Explain the procedure to the patient.	Patient identification validates the correct patient and correct procedure. Discussion and explanation help allay anxiety and prepare the patient for what to expect.
4. Close the curtains around the bed and close the door to the room, if possible. Place the bed at an appropriate and comfortable working height, usually elbow height of the caregiver (VISN 8 Patient Safety Center, 2009).	Closing the door or curtains provides privacy. Proper bed height helps reduce back strain while you are performing the procedure.
5. If a plaster cast was applied, handle the casted extremity or body area with the palms of your hands for the first 24 to 36 hours, until the cast is fully dry.	Proper handling of a plaster cast prevents dents in the cast, which may create pressure areas on the inside of the cast.
6. If the cast is on an extremity, elevate the affected area on pillows covered with waterproof pads. **Maintain the normal curvatures and angles of the cast (Figure 1).**	Elevation helps reduce edema and enhances venous return. Use of a waterproof pad prevents soiling of linen. Maintaining curvatures and angles maintains proper joint alignment, helps prevent flattened areas on the cast as it dries, and prevents pressure areas.

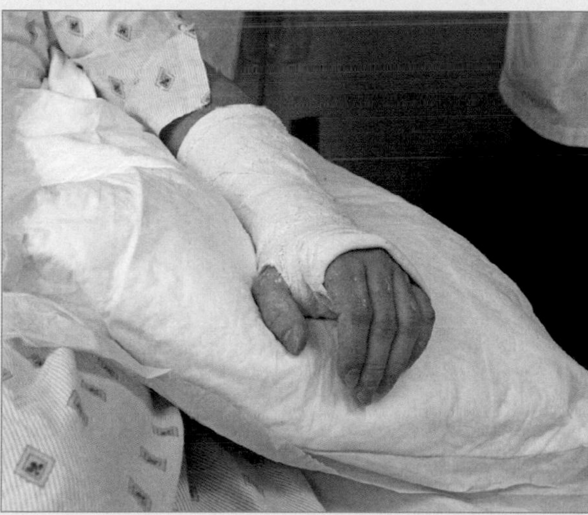

FIGURE 1 Elevating casted limb, maintaining normal curvatures and angles of the cast.

(*continued*)

SKILL 9-17 CARING FOR A CAST continued

ACTION	RATIONALE
7. Keep cast (plaster) uncovered until fully dry.	Keeping the cast uncovered allows heat and moisture to dissipate and air to circulate to speed drying.
8. Assess the condition of the cast (Figure 2). Be alert for cracks, dents, or the presence of drainage from the cast. Perform skin and neurovascular assessments according to facility policy, as often as every 1 to 2 hours. **Check for pain, edema, inability to move body parts distal to the cast, pallor, pulses, and abnormal sensations. If the cast is on an extremity, compare it with the noncasted extremity (Figure 3).**	Assessment helps detect abnormal neurovascular function or infection and allows for prompt intervention. Assessing the neurovascular status determines the circulation and oxygenation of tissues. Pressure within a cast may increase with edema and lead to compartment syndrome.
9. If breakthrough bleeding or drainage is noted on the cast, mark the area on the cast, according to facility policy (Figure 4). Indicate the date and time next to the area. Follow medical orders or facility policy regarding the amount of drainage that needs to be reported to the primary care provider.	Marking the area provides a baseline for monitoring the amount of bleeding or drainage.

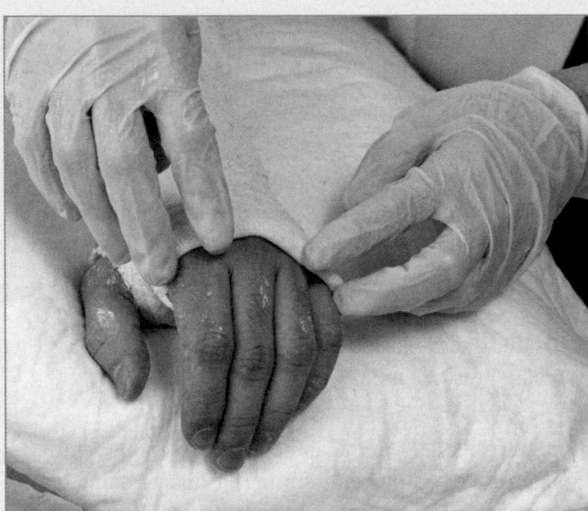

FIGURE 2 Assessing condition of cast.

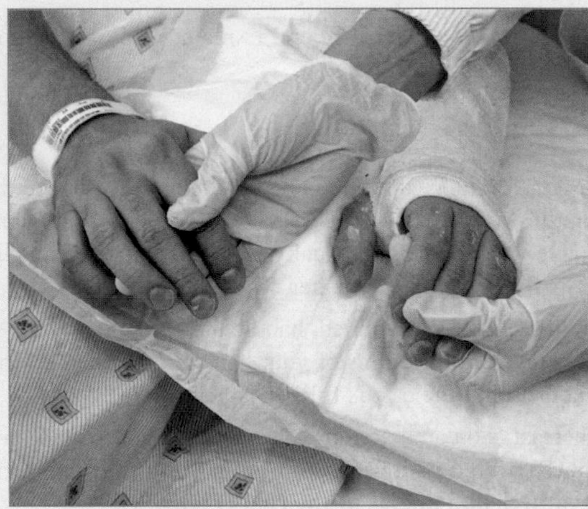

FIGURE 3 Assessing skin and neurovascular function, comparing with noncasted extremity.

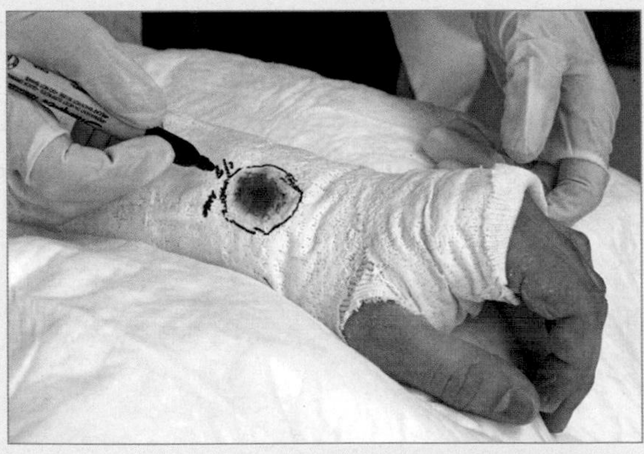

FIGURE 4 Marking any breakthrough bleeding on cast, indicating date and time.

ACTION	RATIONALE
10. Assess for signs of infection. Monitor the patient's temperature. Assess for a foul odor from the cast, increased pain, or extreme warmth over an area of the cast.	Infection deters healing. Assessment allows for early detection and prompt intervention.

ACTION	RATIONALE
11. Reposition the patient every 2 hours. Provide back and skin care frequently. Encourage ROM exercises for unaffected joints. Encourage the patient to cough and breathe deeply.	Repositioning promotes even drying of the cast and reduces the risk for the development of pressure areas under the cast. Frequent skin and back care prevents patient discomfort and skin breakdown. ROM exercises maintain joint function of unaffected areas. Coughing and deep breathing reduce the risk for respiratory complications associated with immobility.
12. Instruct the patient to report pain, odor, drainage, changes in sensation, abnormal sensation, or the inability to move fingers or toes of the affected extremity.	Pressure within a cast may increase with edema and lead to compartment syndrome. The patient's understanding of signs and symptoms allows for early detection and prompt intervention.
13. Place the bed in the lowest position, with the side rails up. Make sure the call bell and other essential items are within easy reach.	Having the bed at proper height and leaving the call bell and other items within reach ensures patient safety.
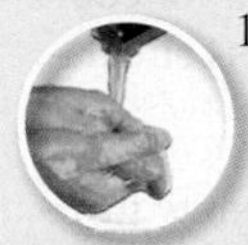 14. Remove PPE, if used. Perform hand hygiene.	Removing PPE properly reduces the risk for infection transmission and contamination of other items. Hand hygiene prevents the spread of microorganisms.

EVALUATION

The expected outcome is achieved when the patient exhibits a cast that is intact without evidence of neurovascular compromise to the affected body part. Other expected outcomes include the following: the patient remains free from infection; the patient verbalizes only mild pain and slight edema or soreness; the patient maintains range of joint motion; the patient demonstrates intact skin at cast edges; the patient is able to perform ADLs; and the patient demonstrates appropriate cast-care techniques.

DOCUMENTATION

Guidelines

Document all assessments and care provided. Document the patient's response to the cast, repositioning, and any teaching.

Sample Documentation

9/1/15 0845 Fiberglass cast in place on right lower extremity from just below knee to toes. Patient repositioned from right side to back. Cast clean and dry; edges padded. No signs of irritation noted. Patient able to move toes freely. Skin tone on right toes somewhat paler tone compared with left toes; toes warm and dry. Capillary refill less than 2 seconds. Patient denies any numbness, tingling, or pain. Right lower extremity elevated on two pillows. Patient instructed to report any complaints of pain, pressure, numbness, tingling, or decreased ability to move toes

—P. Collins, RN

UNEXPECTED SITUATIONS AND ASSOCIATED INTERVENTIONS

- *Your patient, who has a cast on his hand and forearm, has been experiencing pain relief in the extremity with ice application and oral analgesics. He now reports pain unrelieved by the analgesic and a feeling of tightness in his arm. In addition, his fingers are cool, with sluggish capillary refill:* Compartment syndrome may be developing. Adjust the arm so that it is no higher than heart level. This enhances arterial perfusion and controls edema. Notify the primary care provider of the situation immediately. Prepare for bivalving of the cast (cutting of the cast in half longitudinally) to relieve pressure.

SPECIAL CONSIDERATIONS

General Considerations

- Explain that itching under the cast is normal, but the patient should not stick objects down or in the cast to scratch.
- Begin patient teaching immediately after the cast is applied and continue until the patient or a significant other can provide care.

(continued)

SKILL 9-17 CARING FOR A CAST continued

- If a cast is applied after surgery or trauma, monitor vital signs (the most accurate way to assess for bleeding).
- Synthetic casts are lightweight, easy to clean, and somewhat water-resistant. If a Gore-Tex liner is used when the cast is applied, the cast may be immersed in water without affecting the cast integrity.

Infant and Child Considerations

- Do not allow the child to put anything inside the cast.
- Remove toys, hazardous floor rugs, pets, or other items that might cause the child to stumble.
- Keep in mind that synthetic casts come in different colors and with designs, such as cartoons and stripes. These features may make the experience more pleasant for a child.
- Cover a synthetic cast with a plastic bag for bathing.
- Instruct the parents/guardians of a child with a cast not to alter standard car seats to accommodate a cast. Specially designed car seats and restraints are available for travel in a car.

Older Adult Considerations

- Older adults may experience changes in circulation related to their age. They may have slow or poor capillary refill related to peripheral vascular disease. Obtain baseline information for comparison after the cast is applied. Use more than one neurovascular assessment to assess circulation. Compare extremities or sides of the body for symmetry.

Home Care Considerations

- Instruct patients to rest the extremity, apply ice to the extremity, and elevate the extremity to prevent pain and swelling after the application of the cast (Satryb et al., 2011).
- To control itching after the cast is dry, teach patients to tap on the outside of the cast with a pen or use a hair dryer on cool setting to blow cool air into the cast. Instruct patients to never insert an object into the cast and immediately to report a wet cast to their health care provider (Satryb, et al., 2011).

SKILL 9-18 APPLYING SKIN TRACTION AND CARING FOR A PATIENT IN SKIN TRACTION

Traction is the application of a pulling force to a part of the body. It is used to reduce fractures, treat dislocations, correct or prevent deformities, improve or correct contractures, or decrease muscle spasms. It must be applied in the correct direction and magnitude to obtain the therapeutic effects desired.

With traction, the affected body part is immobilized by pulling with equal force on each end of the injured area, mixing traction and counter traction. Weights provide the pulling force or traction. The use of additional weights or positioning the patient's body weight against the traction pull provides the counter traction. Skin traction is applied directly to the skin, exerting indirect pull on the bone. The force may be applied using adhesive or nonadhesive traction tape or a boot, belt, or halter. Skin traction immobilizes a body part intermittently. See Box 9-2 Principles of Effective Traction.

Types of skin traction for adults include Buck's extension traction (lower leg), a cervical head halter, and the pelvic belt. Nursing care for skin traction includes setting the traction up, applying the traction, monitoring the application and patient response, and preventing complications from the therapy and immobility.

BOX 9-2 PRINCIPLES OF EFFECTIVE TRACTION

- Countertraction must be applied for effective traction.
- Traction must be continuous to be effective.
- Skeletal traction is never interrupted unless a life-threatening emergency occurs.
- Weights are not removed unless intermittent traction is prescribed.
- Patient must maintain good body alignment in the center of the bed.
- Ropes must be unobstructed.
- Weights must hang free.

(Adapted from Hinkle, J.L., & Cheever, K.H. (2014). *Brunner & Suddarth's textbook of medical-surgical nursing* (13th ed.). Philadelphia: Wolters Kluwer Health/Lippincott Williams & Wilkins.)

DELEGATION CONSIDERATIONS

The application of, and care for a patient with, skin traction may not be delegated to nursing assistive personnel (NAP) or unlicensed assistive personnel (UAP). Depending on the state's nurse practice act and the organization's policies and procedures, this care may be delegated to licensed practical/vocational nurses (LPN/LVNs). The decision to delegate must be based on careful analysis of the patient's needs and circumstances, as well as the qualifications of the person to whom the task is being delegated. Refer to the Delegation Guidelines in Appendix A.

EQUIPMENT

- Bed with traction frame and trapeze
- Weights
- Velcro straps or other straps
- Rope and pulleys
- Boot with footplate
- Graduated compression stocking, as appropriate
- Nonsterile gloves and/or other PPE, as indicated
- Skin cleansing supplies

ASSESSMENT

Assess the patient's medical record and the nursing plan of care to determine the type of traction, traction weight, and line of pull. Assess the traction equipment to ensure proper function, including inspecting the ropes for fraying and proper positioning. Assess the patient's body alignment. Perform skin and neurovascular assessments. Assess for complications of immobility, including alterations in respiratory function, skin integrity, urinary and bowel elimination, and muscle weakness, contractures, thrombophlebitis, pulmonary embolism, and fatigue.

NURSING DIAGNOSIS

Determine the related factors for the nursing diagnoses based on the patient's current status. Appropriate nursing diagnoses may include:

- Risk for Injury
- Impaired Physical Mobility
- Self-Care Deficit (bathing, feeding, dressing, or toileting)
- Risk for Impaired Skin Integrity

OUTCOME IDENTIFICATION AND PLANNING

The expected outcome to achieve when applying and caring for a patient in skin traction is that the traction is maintained with the appropriate counterbalance and the patient is free from complications of immobility. Other outcomes that may be appropriate include that the patient maintains proper body alignment; the patient reports an increased level of comfort; and the patient is free from injury.

IMPLEMENTATION

ACTION	RATIONALE
1. Review the medical record and the nursing plan of care to determine the type of traction being used and care for the affected body part.	Reviewing the medical record and plan of care validates the correct patient and correct procedure.
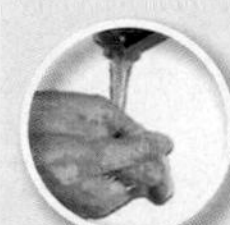 2. Perform hand hygiene. Put on PPE, as indicated.	Hand hygiene and PPE prevent the spread of microorganisms. PPE is required based on transmission precautions.
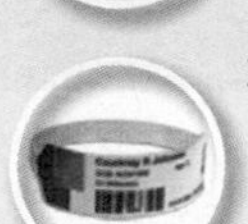 3. Identify the patient. Explain the procedure to the patient, emphasizing the importance of maintaining counterbalance, alignment, and position.	Patient identification validates the correct patient and correct procedure. Discussion and explanation help allay anxiety and prepare the patient for what to expect.
4. Perform a pain assessment and assess for muscle spasm. Administer prescribed medications in sufficient time to allow for the full effect of the analgesic and/or muscle relaxant.	Assessing pain and administering analgesics promote patient comfort.
5. Close the curtains around the bed and close the door to the room, if possible. Place the bed at an appropriate and comfortable working height, usually elbow height of the caregiver (VISN 8 Patient Safety Center, 2009).	Closing the door or curtains provides for privacy. Proper bed height prevents back and muscle strain.

(continued)

SKILL 9-18 APPLYING SKIN TRACTION AND CARING FOR A PATIENT IN SKIN TRACTION continued

ACTION	RATIONALE
Applying Skin Traction	
6. Ensure the traction apparatus is attached securely to the bed. Assess the traction setup.	Assessment of traction setup and weights promotes safety.
7. Check that the ropes move freely through the pulleys. Check that all knots are tight and are positioned away from the pulleys. Pulleys should be free from the linens.	Checking ropes and pulleys ensures that weight is being applied correctly, promoting accurate counterbalance and traction function.
8. Place the patient in a supine position with the foot of the bed elevated slightly. The patient's head should be near the head of the bed and in alignment.	Proper patient positioning maintains proper counterbalance and promotes safety.
9. Cleanse the affected area. Place the elastic stocking on the affected limb, as appropriate.	Skin care aids in preventing skin breakdown. Use of graduated compression stockings prevents edema and neurovascular complications.
10. Place the traction boot over the patient's leg (Figure 1). Be sure the patient's heel is in the heel of the boot. Secure the boot with the straps.	The boot provides a means for attaching traction; proper application ensures proper pull.
11. Attach the traction cord to the boot footplate. Pass the rope over the pulley fastened at the end of the bed. Attach the weight to the hook on the rope, usually 5 to 10 pounds for an adult (Figure 2). Gently let go of the weight. **The weight should hang freely, not touching the bed or the floor.**	Weight attachment applies the pull for the traction. Gently releasing the weight prevents a quick pull on the extremity and possible injury and pain. Properly hanging weights and correct patient positioning ensure accurate counterbalance and traction function.
12. **Check the patient's alignment with the traction.**	Proper alignment is necessary for proper counterbalance and ensures patient safety.
13. **Check the boot for placement and alignment. Make sure the line of pull is parallel to the bed and not angled downward.**	Misalignment causes ineffective traction and may interfere with healing. A properly positioned boot prevents pressure on the heel.

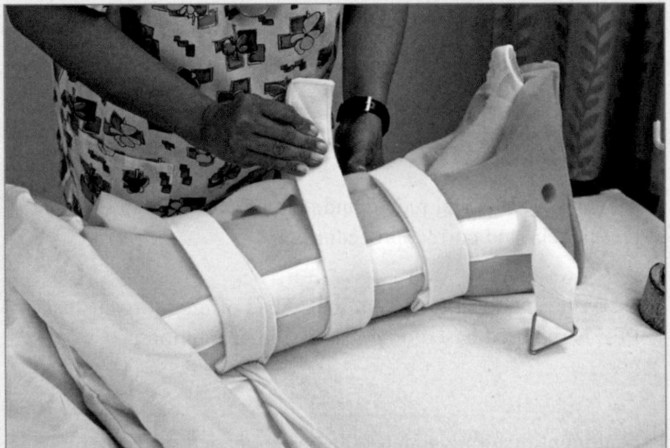

FIGURE 1 Applying traction boot with an elastic stocking in place on leg.

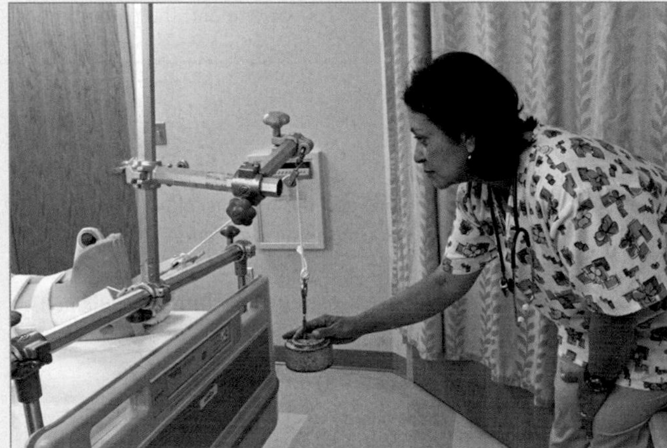

FIGURE 2 Applying weight for skin traction.

ACTION	RATIONALE
14. Place the bed in the lowest position that still allows the weight to hang freely. Make sure the call bell and other essential items are within easy reach.	Proper bed positioning ensures effective application of traction without patient injury. Having call bell and other items in easy reach contributes to patient safety.
15. Remove PPE, if used. Perform hand hygiene.	Removing PPE properly decreases the risk for infection transmission and contamination of other items. Hand hygiene prevents the spread of microorganisms.

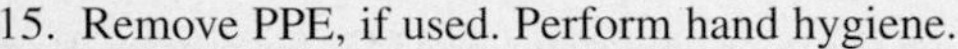

ACTION | RATIONALE

Caring for a Patient with Skin Traction

16. Perform a skin-traction assessment per facility policy. This assessment includes checking the traction equipment, examining the affected body part, maintaining proper body alignment, and performing skin and neurovascular assessments.

Assessment provides information to determine proper application and alignment, thereby reducing the risk for injury. Misalignment causes ineffective traction and may interfere with healing.

17. Remove the straps every 4 hours per the physician's order or facility policy. Check bony prominences for skin breakdown, abrasions, and pressure areas. Remove the boot, per medical order or facility policy, every 8 hours. Put on gloves and wash, rinse, and thoroughly dry the skin.

Removing the straps provides assessment information for early detection and prompt intervention of potential complications should they arise. Washing the area enhances circulation to skin; thorough drying prevents skin breakdown. Using gloves prevents transfer of microorganisms.

18. Assess the extremity distal to the traction for edema, and assess peripheral pulses (Figure 3). Assess the temperature, color, and capillary refill (Figure 4), and compare with the unaffected limb. Check for pain, inability to move body parts distal to the traction, pallor, and abnormal sensations. Assess for indicators of DVT, including calf tenderness, and swelling.

Doing so helps detect signs of abnormal neurovascular function and allows for prompt intervention. Assessing neurovascular status determines the circulation and oxygenation of tissues. Pressure within the traction boot may increase with edema.

19. Replace the traction; remove gloves and dispose of them appropriately.

Replacing traction is necessary to provide immobilization and facilitate healing. Proper disposal of gloves prevents the transmission of microorganisms.

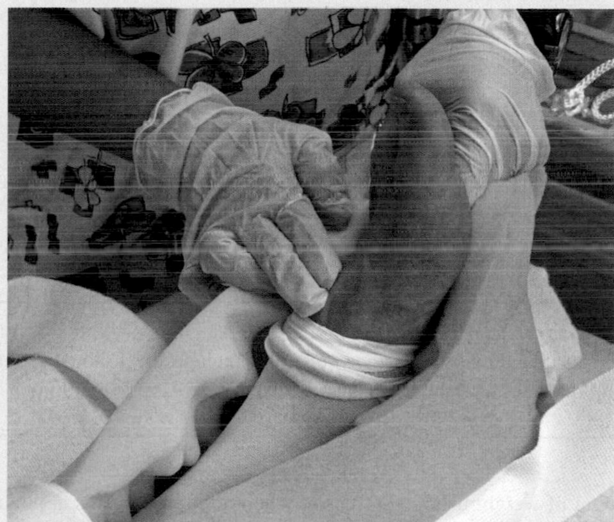

FIGURE 3 Assessing distal pulses.

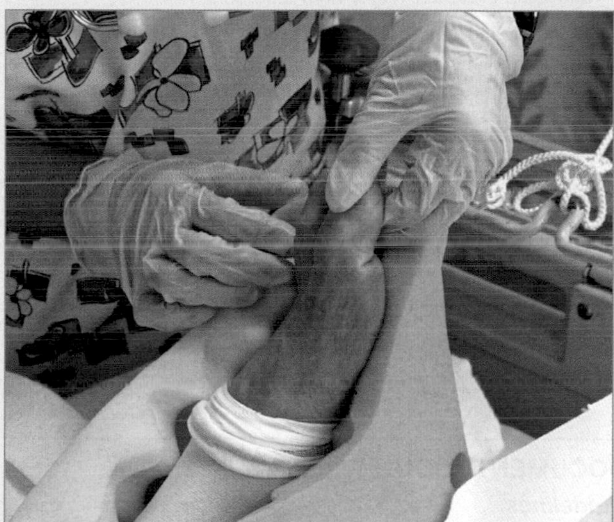

FIGURE 4 Assessing capillary refill.

20. Check the boot for placement and alignment. **Make sure the line of pull is parallel to the bed and not angled downward.**

Misalignment causes ineffective traction and may interfere with healing. A properly positioned boot prevents pressure on the heel.

21. **Ensure the patient is positioned in the center of the bed, with the affected leg aligned with the trunk of the patient's body. Check overall alignment of the patient's body.**

Misalignment interferes with the effectiveness of traction and may lead to complications.

(*continued*)

SKILL 9-18 APPLYING SKIN TRACTION AND CARING FOR A PATIENT IN SKIN TRACTION continued

ACTION	RATIONALE
22. Examine the weights and pulley system. **Weights should hang freely, off the floor and bed. Knots should be secure. Ropes should move freely through the pulleys. The pulleys should not be constrained by knots (Figure 5).**	Checking the weights and pulley system ensures proper application and reduces the risk for patient injury from traction application.

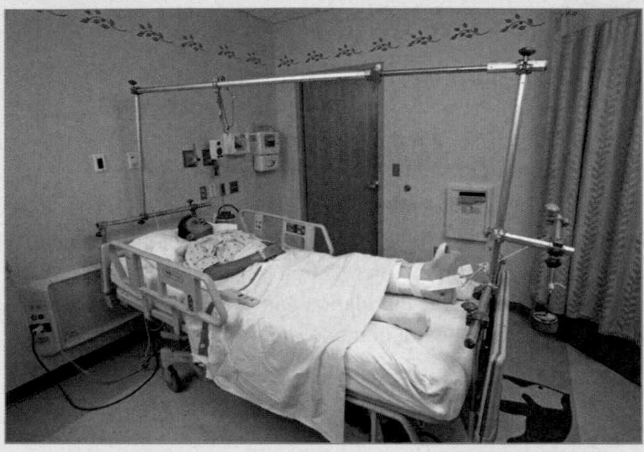

FIGURE 5 Skin traction in place.

ACTION	RATIONALE
23. Perform range-of-motion exercises on all unaffected joint areas, unless contraindicated. Encourage the patient to cough and deep breathe every 2 hours.	ROM exercises maintain joint function. Coughing and deep breathing help to reduce the risk for respiratory complications related to immobility.
24. Raise the side rails. Place the bed in the lowest position that still allows the weight to hang freely. Make sure the call bell and other essential items are within easy reach.	Raising the side rails promotes patient safety. Proper bed positioning ensures effective application of traction without patient injury. Having call bell and other items in easy reach contributes to patient safety.
25. Remove PPE, if used. Perform hand hygiene.	Removing PPE properly decreases the risk for infection transmission and contamination of other items. Hand hygiene prevents the spread of microorganisms.

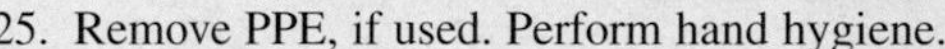
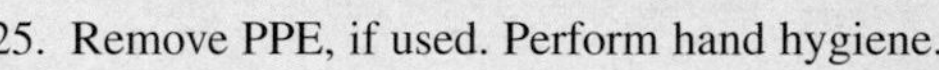

EVALUATION

The expected outcome is met when the patient demonstrates proper body alignment with traction applied and maintained with appropriate counterbalance. Other outcomes include the following: the patient verbalizes pain relief, with pain rated at lower numbers, and the patient remains free of injury.

DOCUMENTATION

Guidelines

Document the time, date, type, amount of weight used, and the site where the traction was applied. Include the skin assessment and care provided before application. Document the patient's response to the traction and the neurovascular status of the extremity.

Sample Documentation

6/3/15 1500 Patient complaining of pain in left hip due to fracture, rating it 7/10. Administered oxycodone (2 tablets), as ordered. Pain rated 3/10, 30 minutes later. Buck's extension traction with 5 pounds of weight applied to left extremity. Skin intact. Pedal pulses present and equal, feet pale pink, warm, and dry, with brisk capillary refill bilaterally. Patient able to wiggle toes freely. Denies numbness or tingling. Patient lying flat in bed with head of bed elevated approximately 15 degrees. Surgery planned for tomorrow.

—L. James, RN

UNEXPECTED SITUATIONS AND ASSOCIATED INTERVENTIONS

- *Your patient in Buck's traction reports pain in the heel of the affected leg:* Remove traction and perform skin and neurovascular assessments. Reapply the traction and reassess the neurovascular status in 15 to 20 minutes. Notify the primary care provider.

SPECIAL CONSIDERATIONS

General Considerations

- Unless contraindicated, encourage the patient to do active flexion–extension ankle exercise and calf-pumping exercises at regular intervals to decrease venous stasis.
- Be alert for pressure on peripheral nerves with skin traction. Take care with Buck's traction to avoid pressure on the peroneal nerve at the point where it passes around the neck of the fibula just below the knee.
- Assess patients who are in traction for extended periods for the development of helplessness, isolation, confinement, and loss of control. Diversional activities, therapeutic communication, and frequent visits by staff and significant others are an important part of care.

Older Adult Considerations

- Be extra vigilant with older adults in skin traction. Older patients are susceptible to alterations in skin integrity due to a decreased amount of subcutaneous fat and thinner, drier, more fragile skin.

EVIDENCE FOR PRACTICE ▶

PREOPERATIVE SKIN TRACTION FOR A FRACTURED HIP

Following a hip fracture, traction may be applied to the injured limb before surgery. What is the effectiveness of this intervention?

Related Research

Handoll, H.H., Queally, J.M., & Parker, M.J. (2011). Pre-operative traction for hip fractures in adults. *The Cochrane Database of Systematic Reviews.* Issue 12. Art. No.: CD000168. DOI: 10.1002/14651858.CD000168.pub3.

The objective of this literature review was to evaluate the effects of traction applied to an injured limb prior to surgery for a fractured hip. All randomized or quasi-randomized trials comparing either skin or skeletal traction with no traction, or skin traction with skeletal traction for patients with an acute hip fracture prior to surgery were considered. At least two authors independently assessed trial quality and extracted data. In all, 11 trials (six were randomized and five were quasi-randomized), involving a total of 1,654 predominantly elderly patients with hip fractures, were included in the review. Most trials were at risk of bias, particularly bias resulting from inadequate allocation concealment, lack of assessor blinding, and incomplete outcome assessment. Only very limited data pooling was possible. Ten trials compared predominantly skin traction with no traction. The available data provided no evidence of benefit from traction either in the relief of pain, ease of fracture reduction, or quality of fracture reduction at time of surgery. There were inconclusive data for pressure sores and other complications, including fracture fixation failure. Three minor adverse effects (sensory disturbance and skin blisters) related to skin traction were reported. One of the above trials included both skin and skeletal traction groups. This trial and one other compared skeletal traction with skin traction and found no important differences between these two methods, although the initial application of skeletal traction was noted as being more painful and more costly. The authors concluded that the routine use of traction (either skin or skeletal) prior to surgery for a hip fracture does not appear to have any benefit. However, the evidence is also insufficient to rule out the potential advantages for traction, in particular for specific fracture types, or to confirm additional complications due to traction use. Given the increasing lack of evidence for the use of preoperative traction, the authors also concluded that the use of preoperative skin traction should not be implemented on a routine basis or it should only be used in the context of a well-designed randomized controlled trial.

Relevance for Nursing Practice

This research review suggests that routine use of traction prior to surgery following hip fracture may not decrease a patient's pain, nor improve patient outcomes. Nurses have a responsibility to consider current evidence related to patient care and take a proactive role in examining policies and procedures, as necessary.

Refer to thePoint for additional research on related nursing topics.

SKILL 9-19 CARING FOR A PATIENT IN SKELETAL TRACTION

Skeletal traction provides pull to a body part by attaching weight directly to the bone, using pins, screws, wires, or tongs. It is used to immobilize a body part for prolonged periods. This method of traction is used to treat fractures of the femur, tibia, and cervical spine. Box 9-2 in Skill 9-18 outlines principles of effective traction. Nursing responsibilities related to skeletal traction include maintaining the traction, maintaining body alignment, monitoring neurovascular status, promoting exercise, preventing complications from the therapy and immobility, and preventing infection by providing pin-site care. A growing evidence base supports effective management of pin sites, but no clear consensus (Walker, 2012; Lagerquist et al., 2012). Pin-site care often varies based on primary care provider and facility policy. Dressings are often applied for the first 48 to 72 hours, and then sites may be left open to air. Pin site care may be performed frequently in the first 48 to 72 hours after application, when drainage may be heavy; other evidence suggests pin care should begin after the first 48 to 72 hours. Pin-site care may be done daily or weekly (Timms & Pugh, 2012; Lagerquist et al., 2012). Refer to specific patient medical orders and facility guidelines.

DELEGATION CONSIDERATIONS

The care of a patient with skeletal traction may not be delegated to nursing assistive personnel (NAP) or to unlicensed assistive personnel (UAP). Depending on the state's nurse practice act and the organization's policies and procedures, care for these patients may be delegated to licensed practical/vocational nurses (LPN/LVNs). The decision to delegate must be based on careful analysis of the patient's needs and circumstances, as well as the qualifications of the person to whom the task is being delegated. Refer to the Delegation Guidelines in Appendix A.

EQUIPMENT

- Sterile gloves
- Sterile applicators
- Cleansing agent for pin care, usually sterile normal saline or chlorhexidine, per primary care provider order or facility policy
- Sterile container
- Antimicrobial ointment, per primary care provider order or facility policy
- Sterile gauze or dressing, per primary care provider order or facility policy
- Analgesic, as ordered
- Sterile gloves for performing pin care, depending on facility policy
- Additional PPE, as indicated

ASSESSMENT

Review the patient's medical record and nursing plan of care to determine the type of traction, traction weight, and line of pull. Assess the traction equipment to ensure proper function, including inspecting the ropes for fraying and proper positioning. Assess the patient's body alignment. Assess the patient's pain and need for analgesia before providing care. Perform skin and neurovascular assessments. Inspect the pin insertion sites for inflammation and infection, including swelling, cloudy or offensive drainage, pain, or redness. Assess for complications of immobility, including alterations in respiratory function, constipation, alterations in skin integrity, alterations in urinary elimination, and muscle weakness, contractures, thrombophlebitis, pulmonary embolism, and fatigue.

NURSING DIAGNOSIS

Determine the related factors for the nursing diagnoses based on the patient's current status. Appropriate nursing diagnoses may include:

- Self-Care Deficit (toileting, bathing, or dressing)
- Anxiety
- Deficient Knowledge
- Risk for Infection

OUTCOME IDENTIFICATION AND PLANNING

The expected outcome to achieve when caring for a patient in skeletal traction is that the traction is maintained appropriately and that the patient is free from complications of immobility and infection. Other outcomes that may be appropriate include the following: the patient maintains proper body alignment; the patient reports an increased level of comfort; and the patient is free from injury.

IMPLEMENTATION

ACTION	RATIONALE
1. Review the medical record and the nursing plan of care to determine the type of traction being used and the prescribed care.	Reviewing the medical record and plan of care validates the correct patient and correct procedure.
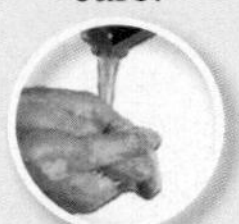 2. Perform hand hygiene. Put on PPE, as indicated.	Hand hygiene and PPE prevent the spread of microorganisms. PPE is required based on transmission precautions.
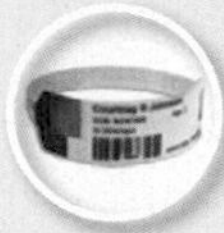 3. Identify the patient. Explain the procedure to the patient, emphasizing the importance of maintaining counterbalance, alignment, and position.	Patient identification validates the correct patient and correct procedure. Discussion and explanation help allay anxiety and prepare the patient for what to expect.
4. Perform a pain assessment and assess for muscle spasm. Administer prescribed medications in sufficient time to allow for the full effect of the analgesic and/or muscle relaxant.	Assessing for pain and administering analgesics promote patient comfort.
5. Close the curtains around the bed and close the door to the room, if possible. Place the bed at an appropriate and comfortable working height, usually elbow height of the caregiver (VISN 8 Patient Safety Center, 2009).	Closing the door or curtains provides for privacy. Proper bed height prevents back and muscle strain.
6. Ensure the traction apparatus is attached securely to the bed. Assess the traction setup, including application of the ordered amount of weight. **Be sure that the weights hang freely, not touching the bed or the floor.**	Proper traction application reduces the risk of injury by promoting accurate counterbalance and traction function.
7. **Check that the ropes move freely through the pulleys. Check that all knots are tight and are positioned away from the pulleys. Pulleys should be free from the linens.**	Free ropes and pulleys ensure accurate counterbalance and traction function.
8. Check the alignment of the patient's body, as prescribed.	Proper alignment maintains an effective line of pull and prevents injury.
9. Perform a skin assessment. Pay attention to pressure points, including the ischial tuberosity, popliteal space, Achilles' tendon, sacrum, and heel.	Skin assessment provides early intervention for skin irritation, impaired tissue perfusion, and other complications.
10. Perform a neurovascular assessment. Assess the extremity distal to the traction for edema and peripheral pulses. Assess the temperature and color and compare with the unaffected limb. Check for pain, inability to move body parts distal to the traction, pallor, and abnormal sensations. Assess for indicators of DVT, including calf tenderness, and swelling.	Neurovascular assessment aids in early identification and allows for prompt intervention should compromised circulation and oxygenation of tissues develop.
11. Assess the site at and around the pins for redness, edema, and odor. Assess for skin tenting, prolonged or purulent drainage, elevated body temperature, elevated pin site temperature, and bowing or bending of the pins.	Pin sites provide a possible entry for microorganisms. Skin inspection allows for early detection and prompt intervention should complications develop.
12. Provide pin-site care.	Performing pin-site care prevents crusting at the site that could lead to fluid buildup, infection, and osteomyelitis.
a. Using sterile technique, open the applicator package and pour the cleansing agent into the sterile container.	Using sterile technique reduces the risk for transmission of microorganisms.
b. Put on the sterile gloves.	Gloves prevent contact with blood and/or body fluids.
c. Place the applicators into the solution.	

(continued)

SKILL 9-19 CARING FOR A PATIENT IN SKELETAL TRACTION continued

ACTION	RATIONALE
d. **Clean the pin site, starting at the insertion area and working outward, away from the pin site (Figure 1).**	Cleaning from the center outward ensures movement from the least to most contaminated area.
e. **Use each applicator once. Use a new applicator for each pin site.**	Using an applicator once reduces the risk of transmission of microorganisms.

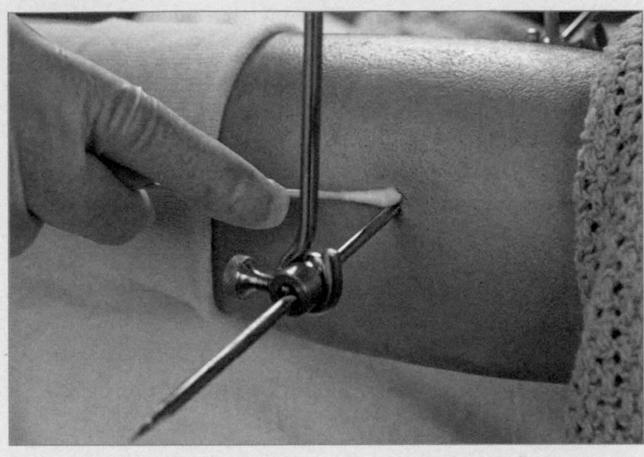

FIGURE 1 Cleaning around pin sites with normal saline on an applicator.

ACTION	RATIONALE
13. Depending on medical order and facility policy, apply the antimicrobial ointment to pin sites and apply a dressing. Remove gloves and dispose of them appropriately.	Antimicrobial ointment helps reduce the risk of infection. A dressing aids in protecting the pin sites from contamination and in containing any drainage. Disposing of gloves reduces the risk of microorganism transmission.
14. Perform ROM exercises on all joint areas, unless contraindicated. Encourage the patient to cough and deep breathe every 2 hours.	Range-of-motion exercises promote joint mobility. Coughing and deep breathing reduce the risk of respiratory complications related to immobility.
15. Place the bed in the lowest position that still allows the weight to hang freely. Make sure the call bell and other essential items are within easy reach.	Proper bed positioning ensures effective application of traction without patient injury. Having call bell and other items in easy reach contributes to patient safety.
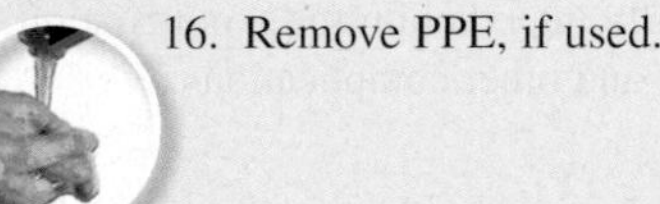 16. Remove PPE, if used. Perform hand hygiene.	Removing PPE properly reduces the risk for infection transmission and contamination of other items. Hand hygiene prevents the spread of microorganisms.

EVALUATION

The expected outcome is met when the patient demonstrates maintenance of skeletal traction with pin sites free of infection. In addition, the patient maintains proper body alignment and joint function; patient verbalizes pain relief; patient states signs and symptoms to report; and patient remains free of injury.

DOCUMENTATION

Guidelines

Document the time, date, type of traction, and the amount of weight used. Include skin and pin site assessments, and pin-site care. Document the patient's response to the traction and the neurovascular status of the extremity.

Sample Documentation

6/5/12 1020 Pin-site care performed. Pin sites cleaned with normal saline and open to the air. Sites slightly red with serosanguineous crusting noted. Neurovascular status intact. Balanced suspension skeletal traction maintained as ordered.

—M. Leroux, RN

UNEXPECTED SITUATIONS AND ASSOCIATED INTERVENTIONS

- *While performing a pin site assessment for your patient with skeletal traction, you note that several of the pins move and slide in the pin tract:* Assess the patient for other symptoms, including signs of infection at the pin sites, pain, and fever. Assess for neurovascular changes. Notify the primary care provider of the findings.

SPECIAL CONSIDERATIONS

- If a pin site becomes unusually painful or tender, or if you notice any fluid discharge, it may be a signal that the pin has loosened or become infected. In the event of unusual pain or irritation, notify the primary care provider (AANN, 2012). Pin loosening may also be indicated by a "tight" feeling or a "clicking" sound (Lagerquist et al., 2012).
- If mechanical looseness or early signs of infection (swelling, cloudy or offensive drainage, pain or redness) are present, increase the frequency of pin-site care (Baird Holmes & Brown, 2005).
- Assess the patient for chronic conditions, such as diabetes mellitus, peripheral vascular disease, and chronic obstructive pulmonary disease, which can significantly increase a patient's risk for complications when skeletal traction is in use.
- Never remove the weights from skeletal traction unless a life-threatening situation occurs. Removal of the weights interferes with therapy and can result in injury to the patient.
- Inspect the pin sites for inflammation and evidence of infection at least every 8 hours. Prevention of osteomyelitis is of utmost importance.

EVIDENCE FOR PRACTICE ▶

EXTERNAL FIXATOR PIN SITES-CLINICAL EVIDENCE REVIEW

Lagerquist, D., Dabrowski, M., Dock, C., et al. (2012). Clinical evidence review. Care of external fixator pin sites. *American Journal of Critical Care, 21*(4), 288–292.

This clinical evidence review was conducted in CINAHL and MEDLINE, using the search terms *external fixator pin sites, pin sites, and pin site infections,* and included articles from 2003 to 2011. Ten studies were retrieved, including two prospective observational studies, seven randomized controlled trials, and one systematic review. Studies demonstrated mixed approaches to pin-site care. Recommendations for practice based on the evidence review and considerations for practice in the absence of stronger conclusive evidence are provided. The studies addressed solutions for pin-site care, frequency of pin-site management, site dressings, and showering by patients.

Refer to thePoint for additional research on related nursing topics.

SKILL 9-20 CARING FOR A PATIENT WITH AN EXTERNAL FIXATION DEVICE

External fixation devices are used to manage open fractures with soft-tissue damage. They consist of one of a variety of frames to hold pins that are drilled into or through bones. External fixators provide stable support for severely crushed or splintered fractures and access to, and treatment for, soft-tissue injuries. The use of these devices allows treatment of the fracture and damaged soft tissues while promoting patient comfort, early mobility, and active exercise of adjacent uninvolved joints. Complications related to disuse and immobility are minimized. Nursing responsibilities include reassuring the patient, maintaining the device, monitoring neurovascular status, promoting exercise, preventing complications from the therapy, preventing infection by providing pin-site care, and providing teaching to ensure compliance and self-care. A growing evidence base supports effective management of pin sites, but no clear consensus (Walker, 2012; Lagerquist et al., 2012). Pin-site care often varies based on primary care provider and facility policy. Dressings are often applied for the first 48 to 72 hours, and then sites may be left open to air. Pin-site care may be performed frequently in the first 48 to 72 hours after application, when drainage may be heavy; other evidence suggests pin care should begin after the first 48 to 72 hours. Pin-site care may be done daily or weekly (Timms & Pugh, 2012; Lagerquist et al., 2012). Refer to specific patient medical orders and facility guidelines.

(continued)

SKILL 9-20 CARING FOR A PATIENT WITH AN EXTERNAL FIXATION DEVICE continued

Nurses play a major role in preparing the patient psychologically for the application of an external fixator. The devices appear clumsy and large. In addition, the nurse needs to clarify misconceptions regarding pain and discomfort associated with the device.

DELEGATION CONSIDERATIONS

The care of a patient with an external fixator device may not be delegated to nursing assistive personnel (NAP) or to unlicensed assistive personnel (UAP). Depending on the state's nurse practice act and the organization's policies and procedures, care for these patients may be delegated to licensed practical/vocational nurses (LPN/LVNs). The decision to delegate must be based on careful analysis of the patient's needs and circumstances, as well as the qualifications of the person to whom the task is being delegated. Refer to the Delegation Guidelines in Appendix A.

EQUIPMENT

Equipment varies with the type of fixator and the type and location of the fracture, but may include:

- Sterile applicators
- Cleansing solution, usually sterile normal saline or chlorhexidine, per primary care provider order or facility policy
- Ice bag
- Antimicrobial ointment, per primary care provider order or facility policy
- Sterile gauze or dressing, per primary care provider order or facility policy
- Analgesic, as ordered
- Sterile gloves for performing pin care, depending on facility policy
- Additional PPE, as indicated

ASSESSMENT

Review the patient's medical record and the nursing plan of care to determine the type of device being used and prescribed care. Assess the patient's pain and need for analgesia before providing care. Assess the external fixator to ensure proper function and position. Perform skin and neurovascular assessments. Inspect the pin insertion sites for signs of inflammation and infection, including swelling, cloudy or offensive drainage, pain, or redness. Assess the patient's knowledge regarding the device and self-care activities and responsibilities.

NURSING DIAGNOSIS

Determine the related factors for the nursing diagnoses based on the patient's current status. Appropriate nursing diagnoses may include:

- Risk for Infection
- Anxiety
- Acute Pain
- Self-Care Deficit (toileting, bathing, or dressing)

OUTCOME IDENTIFICATION AND PLANNING

The expected outcome to achieve when caring for a patient with an external fixator device is that the patient shows no evidence of complication, such as infection, contractures, venous stasis, thrombus formation, or skin breakdown. Additional outcomes that may be appropriate include that the patient shows signs of healing; the patient experiences relief from pain; and the patient is free from injury.

IMPLEMENTATION

ACTION	RATIONALE
1. Review the medical record and the nursing plan of care to determine the type of device being used and prescribed care.	Reviewing the medical record and plan of care validates the correct patient and correct procedure.
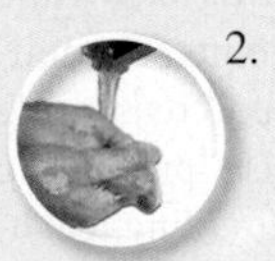 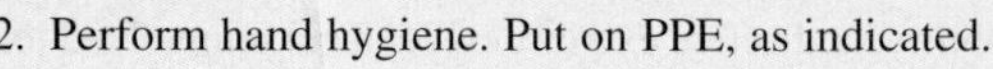 2. Perform hand hygiene. Put on PPE, as indicated.	Hand hygiene and PPE prevent the spread of microorganisms. PPE is required based on transmission precautions.
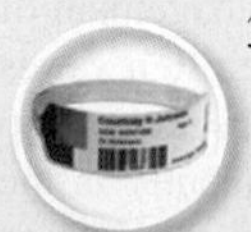 3. Identify the patient. Explain the procedure to the patient. Assure the patient that there will be little pain after the fixation device is in place. Reinforce that the patient will be able to adjust to the device and will be able to move about with the device, allowing him or her to resume normal activities more quickly.	Patient identification validates the correct patient and correct procedure. Discussion and explanation allay anxiety and prepare the patient psychologically for the application of the device.

ACTION	RATIONALE
4. **After the fixation device is in place, apply ice to the surgical site, as ordered or per facility policy (Figure 1). Elevate the affected body part, if appropriate.**	Ice and elevation help reduce swelling, relieve pain, and reduce bleeding.
5. Perform a pain assessment and assess for muscle spasm. Administer prescribed medications in sufficient time to allow for the full effect of the analgesic and/or muscle relaxant.	Pain assessment and analgesic administration help promote patient comfort.
6. Administer analgesics, as ordered, before exercising or mobilizing the affected body part.	Administration of analgesics promotes patient comfort and facilitates movement.
7. Perform neurovascular assessments, per facility policy or medical order, usually every 2 to 4 hours for 24 hours, then every 4 to 8 hours. Assess the affected body part for color, motion, sensation, edema, capillary refill, and pulses. If appropriate, compare with the unaffected side. Assess for pain not relieved by analgesics, and for burning, tingling, and numbness.	Assessment promotes early detection and prompt intervention for abnormal neurovascular function, nerve damage, or circulatory impairment. Assessment of neurovascular status determines the circulation and oxygenation of tissues.
8. Close the curtains around the bed and close the door to the room, if possible. Place the bed at an appropriate and comfortable working height, usually elbow height of the caregiver (VISN 8 Patient Safety Center, 2009).	Closing the door or curtains provides for privacy. Proper bed height prevents back and muscle strain.
9. Assess the pin site for redness, tenting of the skin, prolonged or purulent drainage, swelling, and bowing, bending, or loosening of the pins. Monitor body temperature.	Assessing pin sites aids in early detection of infection and stress on the skin and allows for appropriate intervention.
10. Perform pin-site care.	Performing pin-site care prevents crusting at the site that could lead to fluid buildup, infection, and osteomyelitis.
a. Using sterile technique, open the applicator package and pour the cleansing agent into the sterile container.	Using sterile technique reduces the risk for transmission of microorganisms.
b. Put on the sterile gloves.	Gloves prevent contact with blood and/or body fluids.
c. Place the applicators into the solution.	
d. **Clean the pin site starting at the insertion area and working outward, away from the pin site (Figure 2).**	Cleaning from the center outward promotes movement from the least to most contaminated area.
e. **Use each applicator once. Use a new applicator for each pin site.**	Using each applicator only once prevents transfer of microorganisms.

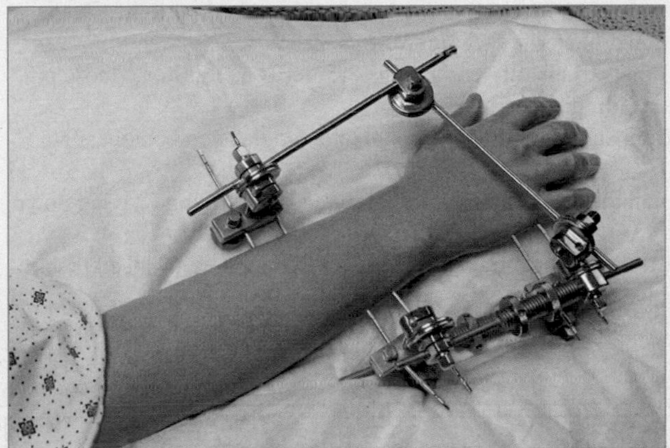

FIGURE 1 External fixation device in place.

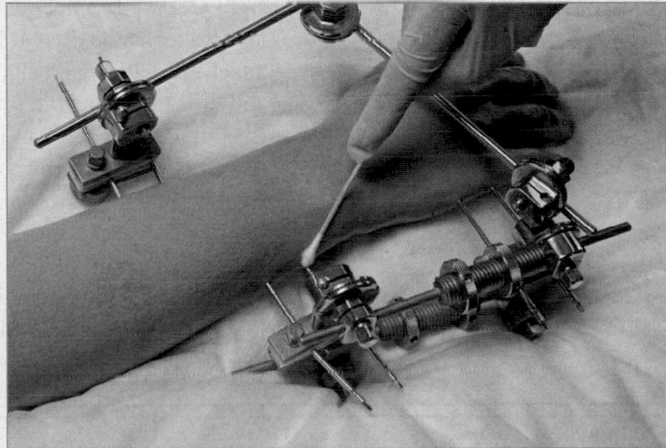

FIGURE 2 Cleaning around pin sites with normal saline on an applicator.

(continued)

SKILL 9-20 CARING FOR A PATIENT WITH AN EXTERNAL FIXATION DEVICE continued

ACTION	RATIONALE
11. Depending on medical order and facility policy, apply the antimicrobial ointment to pin sites and apply a dressing. Remove gloves and dispose of them appropriately.	Antimicrobial ointment helps reduce the risk of infection. A dressing aids in protecting the pin sites from contamination and containing any drainage. Disposing of gloves reduces the risk of microorganism transmission.
12. Perform ROM exercises on all joint areas, unless contraindicated. Encourage the patient to cough and deep breathe every 2 hours.	Range-of-motion exercises promote joint mobility. Coughing and deep breathing reduce the risk of respiratory complications related to immobility.
13. Place the bed in the lowest position that still allows the weight to hang freely, with the side rails up. Make sure the call bell and other essential items are within easy reach.	Proper bed positioning ensures effective application of traction without patient injury. Leaving the call bell and other items within reach ensures patient safety.
14. Remove PPE, if used. Perform hand hygiene.	Removing PPE properly reduces the risk for infection transmission and contamination of other items. Hand hygiene prevents the spread of microorganisms.

EVALUATION

The expected outcome is met when the patient exhibits an external fixation device in place with pin sites that are clean, dry, and intact, without evidence of infection. The patient remains free of complications, such as contractures, venous stasis, thrombus formation, or skin breakdown; the patient verbalizes pain relief; the patient remains free of injury, and the patient demonstrates knowledge of pin-site care.

DOCUMENTATION

Guidelines

Document the time, date, and type of device in place. Include the skin assessment, pin site assessment, and pin-site care. Document the patient's response to the device and the neurovascular status of the affected area.

Sample Documentation

7/6/15 1020 External fixator in place on left forearm. Pin-site care performed. Pin sites cleaned with normal saline and open to the air. Sites slightly red with serosanguineous crusting noted. Neurovascular status intact. Instruction given regarding ROM exercises to left fingers and elbow; patient verbalizes an understanding and is able to demonstrate.

—*B. Clapp, RN*

SPECIAL CONSIDERATIONS

- Teach the patient and significant others how to provide pin-site care and how to recognize the signs of pin-site infection. External fixator devices are in place for prolonged periods. Clean technique can be used at home instead of sterile technique.
- Teach the patient and significant others to identify early signs of infection, signs of a loose pin, and how to contact the orthopedic team, if necessary.
- Encourage the patient to refrain from smoking, if appropriate, to avoid delayed bone healing (Baird Holmes & Brown, 2005).
- Reinforce the importance of keeping the affected body part elevated when sitting or lying down to prevent edema.
- Do not adjust the clamps on the external fixator frame. It is the physician's or advanced practice professional's responsibility to adjust the clamps.
- Fractures often require additional treatment and stabilization with a cast or molded splint after the fixator device is removed.

EVIDENCE FOR PRACTICE ▶

EXTERNAL FIXATOR PIN SITES—CLINICAL EVIDENCE REVIEW

Lagerquist, D., Dabrowski, M., Dock, C., et al. (2012). Clinical evidence review. Care of external fixator pin sites. *American Journal of Critical Care, 21*(4), 288–292.

Refer to details in Skill 9-19, Evidence for Practice, and refer to thePoint for additional research on related nursing topics.

ENHANCE YOUR UNDERSTANDING

FOCUSING ON PATIENT CARE: DEVELOPING CLINICAL REASONING

Consider the case scenarios at the beginning of the chapter as you answer the following questions to enhance your understanding and apply what you have learned.

QUESTIONS

1. You are preparing to discharge Bobby Rowden from the emergency room. Discuss the teaching you should include for Bobby and his parents related to his injury and his plaster cast.
2. A pneumatic compression device has been ordered as part of the admission orders for Esther Levitz. You bring the pump and sleeves into the room, and she asks, "What is that? It looks like a torture machine!" How will you respond?
3. You are caring for Manuel Esposito the evening before his surgery. Your assessment of his affected extremity reveals skin that is warm to the touch, rapid capillary refill, and positive sensation and movement. What other assessments should you perform as part of your care for Mr. Esposito?

You can find suggested answers after the Bibliography at the end of this chapter.

INTEGRATED CASE STUDY CONNECTION

The case studies in the back of the book are designed to focus on integrating concepts. Refer to the following case studies to enhance your understanding of the concepts related to the skills in this chapter.

- Basic Case Studies: Abigail Cantonelli, page 1063.
- Intermediate Case Studies: Jason Brown, page 1083; Kent Clark, page 1085.

TAYLOR SUITE RESOURCES

Explore these additional resources to enhance learning for this chapter:

- NCLEX-Style Questions and other resources on thePoint, http://thePoint.lww.com/Lynn4e
- *Skill Checklists for Taylor's Clinical Nursing Skills*, 4e
- *Taylor's Video Guide to Clinical Nursing Skills:* Activity
- *Fundamentals of Nursing:* Chapter 32, Activity

Bibliography

Ackley, B.J., & Ladwig, G.B. (2011). *Nursing diagnosis handbook* (9th ed.). St. Louis: Mosby/Elsevier.

American Academy of Orthopaedic Surgeons. (2011). *Care of casts and splints.* Available http://orthoinfo.aaos.org/topic.cfm?topic=A00095

American Association of Critical Care Nurses. (2010). *Venous Thromboembolism prevention.* Available http://www.aacn.org/WD/Practice/Docs/PracticeAlerts/VTE%20Prevention%2004-2010%20final.pdf.

American Association of Neuroscience Nurses (AANN). (2012). Cervical spine surgery. A guide to preoperative and postoperative patient care. *AANN Reference Series for Clinical Practice.* Glenview, IL: Author.

American Geriatric Society. (2012). *Choosing the right cane or walker.* Available http://www.healthinaging.org/files/documents/tipsheets/canes_walkers.pdf.

American Nurses Association (ANA). (2013). *Safe patient handling.* Available http://www.nursingworld.org/MainMenuCategories/OccupationalandEnvironmental/occupationalhealth/handlewithcare.aspx.

American Nurses Association. (2004). *Handle with care®.* Available http://www.nursingworld.org/MainMenuCategories/WorkplaceSafety/SafePatient/hwc.pdf.

Baird Holmes, S., & Brown, S. (2005). National Association of Orthopaedic Nurses. Guidelines for orthopaedic nursing: Skeletal pin site care. *Orthopaedic Nursing, 24*(2), 99–107.

Baptiste, A. (2011). An evaluation of nursing tasks. *Work, 40*(2), 115–124.

Baptiste, A., Boda, S., Nelson, A., et al. (2006). Friction-reducing devices for lateral patient transfers: A clinical evaluation. *AAOHN Journal, 54*(4), 173–180.

Black, T.R., Shah, S.M., Busch, A.J., et al. (2011). Effect of transfer, lifting, and repositioning (TLR) injury prevention program on musculoskeletal injury among direct care workers. (2011). *Journal of Occupational and Environmental Hygiene, 8*(4), 226–235.

Blocks, M. (2005). Practical solutions for safe patient handling. *Nursing, 35*(10), 44–45.

Boltz, M., Capezuti, E., Fulmer, T., et al. (Eds.) (2012). *Evidence-based geriatric nursing protocols for best practice* (4th ed.). New York: Springer Publishing Company.

Bolz, M., Resnick, B., Capezuti, E., et al. (2012). Functional decline in hospitalized older adults: Can nursing make a difference? *Geriatric Nursing, 33*(4), 272–279.

Bulechek, G.M, Butcher, H.K., Dochterman, J.M., et al. (Eds.). (2013). *Nursing interventions classification (NIC)* (6th ed.). St. Louis: Mosby Elsevier.

Conway, D., Quatrara, B., & Rodriguez, L. (2012). A better fit. Industry collaboration with nurse-clinicians in the development and redesign of a pneumatic compression device. *Orthopaedic Nursing, 31*(6), 348–354.

Fernandes, T. (2006). Moving and handling: Hoists and slings. *Nursing and Residential Care, 8*(12), 548–551.

Fernandes, T. (2006). Suitable moving and handling equipment: A guide. *International Journal of Therapy and Rehabilitation, 13*(10), 477–481.

Gait belt handle helps during transfers. (2010). *Journal of Gerontological Nursing, 36*(12), 8.

Geerts, W.H., Bergqvist, D., Pineo, G.F., et al. (2008). Prevention of venous embolism: American College of Chest Physicians Evidence-based clinical practice guidelines (8th ed.). *Chest, 133* (6) (Suppl), 381S–453S.

Green, D. (2012). Moving and positioning individuals. *Nursing & Residential Care, 14*(10), 506–509.

Haglund, K., Kyle, J., & Finkelstein, M. (2010). Pediatric safe patient handling. *Journal of Pediatric Nursing, 25*(2), 98–107.

Handoll, H.H., Queally, J.M., & Parker, M.J. (2011). Pre-operative traction for hip fractures in adults. *The Cochrane Database of Systematic Reviews.* Issue 12. Art. No.: CD000168. DOI: 10.1002/14651858.CD000168.pub3.

Hinkle, J.L., & Cheever, K.H. (2014). *Brunner & Suddarth's textbook of medical-surgical nursing* (13th ed.). Philadelphia: Wolters Kluwer Health/Lippincott Williams & Wilkins.

Hogan-Quigley, B., Palm, M.L., & Bickley, L. (2012). *Bates' nursing guide to physical examination and history taking.* Philadelphia: Wolters Kluwer Health/Lippincott Williams & Wilkins.

Jarvis, C. (2012). *Physical examination & health assessment* (6th ed.). St. Louis: Saunders/Elsevier.

Jensen, S. (2011.) *Nursing health assessment. A best practice approach.* Philadelphia: Wolters Kluwer Health/Lippincott Williams & Wilkins.

Jitramontree, N. (2010). Evidence-based practice guideline. Exercise promotion: Walking in elders. *Journal of Gerontological Nursing, 36*(11), 10–18.

Kim, G., Kwon, G., Hur, H.K., et al. (2012). Effects of muscle strengthening exercise program on muscle strength, activities of daily living, health perception, and depression in post-stroke elders. *Korean Journal of Adult Nursing, 24*(3), 1.

Kyle, T., & Carman, S. (2013). *Essentials of pediatric nursing* (2nd ed.). Philadelphia: Wolters Kluwer Health/Lippincott Williams & Wilkins.

Lagerquist, D., Dabrowski, M., Dock, C., et al. (2012). Clinical evidence review. Care of external fixator pin sites. *American Journal of Critical Care, 21*(4), 288–292.

Mayo Clinic. (2011a). *Adult health. Back pain at work: Preventing pain and injury.* Available www.mayoclinic.com/health/back-pain/HQ00955.

Mayo Clinic. (2011b). *Fitness. Exercise: 7 benefits of regular physical activity.* Available www.mayoclinic.com/health/exercise/HQ01676.

Mayo Clinic. (2011c). *How to choose and use a walker.* Available www.mayoclinic.com/health/walker/HA00060.

Menzel, N.N., & Nelson, A.L. (2010). Strengthening your evidence base: Focus on safe patient handling. *American Nurse Today, 5*(7), 38–40.

Miller, C. (2008). Communication difficulties in hospitalized older adults with dementia: Try these techniques to make communicating with patients easier and more effective. *American Journal of Nursing, 108*(3), 58–66.

Mincer, A. (2007). Assistive devices for the adult patient with orthopaedic dysfunction: Why physical therapists choose what they do. *Orthopaedic Nursing, 26*(4), 226–233.

Moorhead, S., Johnson, M., Maas, M.L., et al. (Eds.). (2013). *Nursing outcomes classification (NOC).* (5th ed.). St. Louis: Mosby Elsevier.

Murphy Dawson, J., & Harrington, S. (2012). Embracing safe patient handling. *Nursing Management, 43*(10), 15–17.

NANDA-I International. (2012). *Nursing diagnoses: Definitions & classification 2012–2014.* West Sussex, UK: Wiley-Blackwell.

Nelson, A., & Baptiste, A. (2004). Evidence-based practices for safe patient handling and movement. *Online Journal of Issues in Nursing, 9*(3), Manuscript 3. Available at www.nursingworld.org/ojin/topic25/tpc25_3.htm.

Nelson, A., Motacki, K., & Menzel, N. (2009). *The illustrated guide to safe patient handling and movement.* New York: Springer Publishing Company.

NIOSH sets 35-lb limit as the max for safe lifts. (2007). *Hospital Employee Health, 26*(12), 136–137.

Nolen, J., Liu, H., Liu, H., et al. (2010). Comparison of gait characteristics with a single-tip cane, tripod cane, and quad cane. *Physical & Occupational Therapy in Geriatrics, 28*(4), 387–395.

Occupational Safety & Health Administration (OSHA), U.S. Department of Labor. (2009). *Guidelines for Nursing Homes. Ergonomics for the prevention of musculoskeletal disorders.* Washington, DC: Author. Available www.osha.gov/ergonomics/guidelines/nursinghome/final_nh_guidelines.pdf.

Occupational Safety & Health Administration (OSHA), U.S. Department of Labor. (2012). *Safe patient handling.* Washington, DC: Author. Available www.osha.gov/SLTC/healthcarefacilities/safepatienthandling.html.

Pellatt, G. (2005). Safe handling. The safety and dignity of patients and nurses during patient handling. *British Journal of Nursing, 14*(21), 1150–1156.

Perry, S.E., Hockenberry, M.J., Lowdermilk, D.L., et al. (2010). *Maternal child nursing care* (4th ed.). Maryland Heights, MO: Mosby/Elsevier.

Pullen, R. (2004). Logrolling a patient. *Nursing, 34*(2), 22.

Qaseem, A., Chou, R., Humphrey, L.L., et al. (2011). American College of Physicians Clinical Guidelines Committee. Venous thromboembolism prophylaxis in hospitalized patients: A clinical practice guideline from the American College of Physicians. *Annals of Internal Medicine, 155*(9), 625–632.

Santy-Tomlinson, J., Vincent, M., Glossop, N., et al. (2011). Calm, irritated or infected? The experience of the inflammatory states and symptoms of pin site infection and irritation during external fixation: A grounded theory study. *Journal of Clinical Nursing, 20*(21/22), 3163–3173.

Satryb, S.A., Wilson, T.J., & Patterson, J.M. (2011). Casting: all wrapped up. *Orthopaedic Nursing, 30*(1), 37–43.

Spotted Horse, J. (2010). Improving clinical outcomes with continuous passive motion: An interactive education approach. *Orthopaedic Nursing, 29*(1), 27–35.

Tabloski, P. (2010). *Gerontological nursing* (2nd ed.). Upper Saddle River, NJ: Pearson.

Taylor, C., Lillis, C., & Lynn, P. (2015). *Fundamentals of nursing. The art & science of nursing care.* (8th ed.). Philadelphia: Wolters Kluwer Health/Lippincott Williams & Wilkins.

Taylor, J.J., & Cohen, B.J. (2013). *Memmler's structure and function of the human body* (10th ed.). Philadelphia: Wolters Kluwer Health/Lippincott Williams & Wilkins.

Timms, A., & Pugh, H. (2012). Pin site care: Guidance and key recommendations. *Nursing Standard, 27*(1), 50–55.

University of Iowa Hospitals and Clinics. (2008). *Using crutches safely.* Iowa City, Iowa: Author. Available at www.uihealthcare.com/topics/bonesjointsmuscles/bone3458.html.

U.S. Department of Labor. Occupational Safety & Health Administration (OSHA). (2013). *Healthcare wide hazards module—Ergonomics.* Washington, DC: Author. Available at www.osha.gov/SLTC/etools/hospital/hazards/ergo/ergo.html.

U.S. National Library of Medicine. National Institutes of Health. (2012). MedlinePlus. *How to make a sling.* Available http://www.nlm.nih.gov/medlineplus/ency/article/000017.htm.

Varnam, W. (2011). How to mobilize patients with dementia to a standing position. *Nursing Older People, 23*(8), 31–36.

VISN 8 Patient Safety Center. (2009). *Safe patient handling and movement algorithms.* Tampa, FL: Author. Available. http://www.visn8.va.gov/visn8/patientsafetycenter/safePtHandling/default.asp.

Viswanathan, P., & Kidd, M. (2010). Effect of continuous passive motion following total knee arthroplasty on knee range of motion and function: a systematic review. *New Zealand Journal of Physiotherapy, 38* (1), 14–22.

Walker, J. (2012). Pin site infection in orthopaedic external fixation devices. *British Journal of Nursing, 21*(3), 148–151.

Walker, L., & Lamont, S. (2008). Graduated compression stockings to prevent deep vein thrombosis. *Nursing Standard, 22*(40), 35–38.

Wanless, S., & Wanless, S. (2012). Hoisting a patient: principles and advice for safer practice. *Nursing & Residential Care, 14*(6), 306–310.

Waters, T.R. (2007). When is it safe to manually lift a patient. *American Journal of Nursing, 107*(8), 53–58.

Waters, T.R., Nelson, A., Hughes, N., et al. (2009). Department of Health and Human Services (DHHS). Centers for Disease Control and Prevention (CDC). National Institute for Occupational Safety and Health (NIOSH). *Safe patient handling training for schools of nursing. Curricular materials.* Available http://www.cdc.gov/niosh/docs/2009-127/pdfs/2009-127.pdf.

Winslow, E.H., & Brosz, D.L. (2010). Unraveling the mystery of graduated compression stockings. *OR Nurse, 4*(3), 56.

Wright, K. (2005). Mobility and safe handling of people with dementia. *Nursing Times, 101*(17), 38–40.

Zisberg, A., Shadmi, E., Sinoff, G., et al. (2011). Low mobility during hospitalization and functional decline in older adults. *Journal of the American Geriatrics Society, 59*(2), 266–273.

SUGGESTED ANSWERS FOR FOCUSING ON PATIENT CARE: DEVELOPING CLINICAL REASONING

1. Teaching that should be included for Bobby and his parents related to his injury and his plaster cast includes the following: keeping the extremity elevated on pillows to reduce edema; handling the cast with the palm of the hands for the first 24 to 36 hours; keeping the cast uncovered until fully dry; reporting pain, odor, drainage, changes in sensation, abnormal sensation, or the inability to move his fingers; and avoiding putting anything in the cast.

2. Reassure the patient, Esther Levitz, that the device will not hurt. Explain how the pneumatic compression device works and the rationale for its use. In addition, describe potential adverse symptoms, such as pain or discomfort in the legs and changes in sensation, that the patient should report while the pneumatic compression device is in use.

3. Additional assessments that should be performed as part of Mr. Esposito's care include the following: assessing the traction equipment to ensure proper function, including inspecting the ropes for fraying and proper positioning; assessing the patient's body alignment; performing skin and neurovascular assessments; assessing for complications of immobility, including alterations in respiratory function, skin integrity, urinary and bowel elimination, and muscle weakness, contractures, thrombophlebitis, pulmonary embolism, and fatigue.

10 Comfort and Pain Management

FOCUSING ON PATIENT CARE

This chapter will help you develop the skills needed to meet the comfort needs of the following patients:

MILDRED SIMPSON, is a 75-year-old woman recovering from a total hip replacement.

JOSEPH WATKINS, comes to the emergency department because of acute pain in his lower back that started when he was moving furniture.

JEROME BATISTE, age 60, has been diagnosed with bone cancer and is being discharged with an order for patient-controlled analgesia (PCA) at home.

Refer to Focusing on Patient Care: Developing Clinical Reasoning at the end of the chapter to apply what you learn.

LEARNING OBJECTIVES

After studying this chapter, you will be able to:

1. Promote patient comfort.
2. Give a back massage.
3. Apply and care for a patient using a transcutaneous electrical nerve stimulation (TENS) unit.
4. Care for a patient receiving PCA.
5. Care for a patient receiving epidural analgesia.
6. Care for a patient receiving continuous wound perfusion pain management.

KEY TERMS

acute pain: pain that is generally rapid in onset and varies in intensity from mild to severe

adjuvant: substances or treatments that enhance the effect of another treatment, especially substances that enhance the effect of drugs

analgesic: agent used to relieve pain

breakthrough pain: a temporary flare-up of moderate to severe pain that occurs even when the patient is taking around-the-clock medication for persistent pain

caregiver-controlled analgesia (CCA): a method of pain control in which a consistently available and competent person is authorized by a prescriber and properly educated to activate the dosing button of an analgesic infusion pump in response to a patient's pain when that patient is unable to do so; the authorized agent is a nonprofessional person (e.g., parent, significant other) (Wuhrman et al., 2007).

chronic pain: pain that may be limited, intermittent, or persistent, but lasts beyond the normal healing period

continuous wound perfusion pain management system: device that delivers a continuous infusion of local analgesia to a surgical wound bed

epidural route: administration of analgesia via an infusion catheter placed in the epidural space

intractable pain: pain that is resistant to therapy and persists despite a variety of interventions

neuropathic pain: pain that results from an injury to, or abnormal functioning of, peripheral nerves or the central nervous system

nonpharmacologic interventions: interventions without the use of medicine or drugs; interventions in addition to the use of medicines or drugs

nurse-controlled analgesia (NCA): a method of pain control in which a consistently available and competent person is authorized by a prescriber and properly educated to activate the dosing button of an analgesic infusion pump in response to a patient's pain when that patient is unable to do so; the authorized agent is the nurse responsible for the patient (Wuhrman et al., 2007)

pain threshold: the lowest intensity of a stimulus that causes the subject to recognize pain

pain tolerance: point beyond which a person is no longer willing to endure pain

perineural route: administration of local anesthetic for pain management via an infusion catheter placed along most or all of the length of a wound

Comfort is an important need, and ensuring a patient's comfort is a major nursing responsibility. Providing comfort can be as simple as straightening the patient's bed linens, offering to hold the patient's hand, or assisting with hygiene needs. Often, providing comfort includes providing pain relief. The classic definition of pain that is probably of greatest benefit to nurses and patients is that offered by McCaffery (1979, p. 11): "Pain is whatever the experiencing person says it is, existing whenever he (or she) says it does." This definition rests on the belief that the only one who can be a real authority on whether, and how, a person is experiencing pain is that person. The International Association for the Study of Pain (IASP) further defines pain as an unpleasant sensory and emotional experience associated with actual or potential tissue damage (IASP, 1994).

Differences in individual pain perception and response to pain, as well as the multiple and diverse causes of pain, require the use of highly specialized abilities to promote comfort and relieve pain. The most important of these are the nurse's belief that the patient's pain is real, a willingness to become involved in the patient's pain experience, and competence in developing effective pain management regimens.

Any indication of pain requires a thorough pain assessment. Fundamentals Review 10-1 outlines factors to include in a pain assessment. Because pain is subjective, self-report is generally considered the most reliable way to assess pain and the nurse should use this method whenever possible. According to Pasero and McCaffery (2011), additional methods to assess a person's pain include the following: report of a family member, other person close to the patient, or caregiver who is familiar with the patient; nonverbal behaviors (restlessness, grimacing, crying, clenching fists, protecting the painful area); and physiologic measures (increased blood pressure and pulse), although most research verifies that reliance on vital signs to indicate the presence of pain should be minimized. **The absence of an increase in vital signs does not mean that pain is not present.** Infants, young children, patients who are nonverbal or have difficulty communicating verbally, and cognitively impaired adults, such as those with dementia, are at high risk for inadequate pain management as they are unable to describe their pain and may be poorly assessed (Baldridge & Andrasik, 2010; Horgas et al., 2012).

A pain measurement scale should be part of the initial assessment and the continued assessment of pain and evaluation of pain control measures. Choosing an appropriate tool for patient assessment is necessary to obtain an accurate assessment and valid pain ratings. Fundamentals Review 10-2 is an example of a pain assessment tool. Fundamentals Review 10-3 provides a listing of pain assessment scales that can be used in adults and children who can self-report, as well as scales that can be used to assess pain in adults and children who cannot self-report discomfort and pain. Fundamentals Review 10-4 is an example of a scale that can be used to assess discomfort and pain in patients who are unable to self-report.

This chapter covers skills to assist the nurse in providing for patient comfort, including pain relief. Fundamentals Review 10-5 and 10-6 provide a summary of additional information to assist in understanding the skills related to comfort and pain relief. Refer to a fundamentals of nursing textbook for further, in-depth discussions of the physiology, assessment, and treatment of pain.

FUNDAMENTALS REVIEW 10-1

GENERAL GUIDELINES FOR PAIN ASSESSMENT

Factors to Assess	Questions and Approaches
Characteristics of the pain Location	"Where is your pain? Is it external or internal?" (Asking the patient with **acute pain** to point to the painful area with one finger may help to localize the pain. Patients with **chronic pain** may have difficulty trying to localize their pain, however.)
Duration	"How long have you been experiencing pain? How long does a pain episode last? How often does a pain episode occur?"
Intensity/Quantity	Ask the patient to indicate the degree (amount) of pain currently experienced on the scale below: 0 1 2 3 4 5 6 7 8 9 10 0 = No Pain; 2 = Mild; 4–5 = Moderate; 7 = Severe; 10 = Pain as bad as it can be It is also helpful to ask how much pain the patient has (on the same scale) when the pain is at its least and at its worst: Least_______ Worst_______
Quality	"What words would you use to describe your pain?"
Chronology	"How does the pain develop and progress?" (If a pattern can be identified, interventions early in a pain sequence will often be far more effective than those used after the pain is well established.) "Has the pain changed since it first began? If so, how?"
Aggravating factors	"What makes the pain occur or increase in intensity?"
Alleviating factors	"What makes the pain go away or lessen? What methods of relief have you tried in the past? How long were they used? How effective were they?" (Methods of relief currently in effect for hospitalized patients should be apparent from the chart. It is important to verify the use of current orders and their effectiveness with the patient. Outpatients may need to be asked to record a medication profile, a thorough and accurate account of all medications they are taking.)
Associated phenomena	"Are there any other factors that seem to relate consistently to your pain? Any other symptoms that occur just before the pain begins?"
Physiologic responses Vital signs (blood pressure, pulse, respirations) Skin color Perspiration Pupil size Nausea	Signs of sympathetic stimulation can occur with acute pain, but need not be present to verify the presence of pain. Signs of parasympathetic stimulation (decreased blood pressure and pulse, rapid and regular respirations, pupil constriction, nausea and vomiting, and warm, dry skin) may occur, especially with prolonged, severe pain, visceral, or deep pain.

(continued)

FUNDAMENTALS REVIEW 10-1

GENERAL GUIDELINES FOR PAIN ASSESSMENT continued

Factors to Assess	Questions and Approaches
Muscle tension	Observe. Ask the patient whether he or she is aware of any tight, tense muscles.
Anxiety	Are signs of anxiety evident? (May include decreased attention span or ability to follow directions, frequent asking questions, shifting topics of conversation, avoiding discussion of feelings, acting out, somatizing.)
Behavioral responses	
Posture, gross motor activities	Does patient rub or support a particular area? Make frequent position changes? Walk, pace, kneel, or assume a rolled-up position? Does patient rest a particular body part? Protect an area from stimulation? Lie quietly? (In acute pain, postural and gross motor activities are often altered; in chronic pain, the only signs of change may be postures characteristic of withdrawal.)
Facial features	Does the patient have a pinched look? Are there facial grimaces? Knotted brow? Overall taut, anxious appearance? (A look of fatigue is more characteristic of chronic pain.)
Verbal expressions	Does the patient sigh, moan, scream, cry, or repetitively use the same words?
Affective responses	
Anxiety	"Do you feel anxious? Are you afraid? If so, how bad are these feelings?"
Depression	"Do you feel depressed, down, or low? If so, how bad are these feelings? Are your feelings about yourself mostly good or bad? Do you have feelings of failure? Do you see yourself or your illness as a burden to those you care about?"
Interactions with others	How does the patient act when he or she is in pain in the presence of others? How does the patient respond to others when he or she is not in pain? How do significant others and caregivers respond to the patient when the patient is in pain? When the patient is not in pain?
Degree to which pain interferes with patient's life (use past performance as baseline)	"Does the pain interfere with sleep? If so, to what extent? Is fatigue a major factor in the pain experience? Is the conduct of intimate or peer relationships affected by the pain? Is work function affected? Participation in recreational–diversional activities?" (An activity diary is often helpful—sometimes crucial. One to several weeks of hourly activity recorded by the patient may be necessary. Pain level, food intake, and sleep–rest periods are noted along with activities performed. Separate diaries for inpatient and outpatient episodes may be necessary because hospitalization markedly affects the nature and type of activities performed.)
Perception of pain and meaning to patient	"Are you worried about your illness? Do you see any connection between your pain and the nature or course of illness? If so, how do you see them as related? Do you find any meaning in your pain? If so, is this beneficial or detrimental to you? Are you struggling to find some meaning for your pain?"
Adaptive mechanisms used to cope with pain	"What do you usually do to relieve stress? How well do these things work? What techniques do you use at home to help cope with the pain? How well have they worked? Do you use these in the hospital? If not, why not?"
Outcomes	"What would you like to be doing right now, this week, this month, if the pain were better controlled? How much would the pain have to decrease (on the 0-to-10 scale) for you to begin to accomplish these goals?"
Factors that affect expression of pain	Patterned attitudes related to cultural and social group; gender; spirituality; religious heritage; age

FUNDAMENTALS REVIEW 10-2

PAIN ASSESSMENT TOOL

Date ______

Patient's name ______ Age ______ Room ______

Diagnosis ______ Physician ______

Nurse ______

1. LOCATION: Patient or nurse marks drawing.

Right Left Right Left Left Right Right Left R L L R

Left Right Left

Right Right Left

2. INTENSITY: Patient rates the pain. Scale used ______

Present: ______

Worst pain gets: ______

Best pain gets: ______

Acceptable level of pain: ______

3. QUALITY: (Use patient's own words, e.g., prick, ache, burn, throb, pull, sharp) ______

4. ONSET, DURATION, VARIATION, RHYTHMS: ______

5. MANNER OF EXPRESSING PAIN: ______

6. WHAT RELIEVES THE PAIN? ______

7. WHAT CAUSES OR INCREASES THE PAIN? ______

8. EFFECTS OF PAIN: (Note decreased function, decreased quality of life.)

- Accompanying symptoms (e.g., nausea) ______
- Sleep ______
- Appetite ______
- Physical activity ______
- Relationship with others (e.g., irritability) ______
- Emotions (e.g., anger, suicidal, crying) ______
- Concentration ______
- Other ______

9. OTHER COMMENTS: ______

10. PLAN: ______

FUNDAMENTALS REVIEW 10-3

PAIN ASSESSMENT SCALES

Resource	Web Site	Indications
COMFORT Scale	http://painconsortium.nih.gov/pain_scales/COMFORT_scale.pdf	Infants, children, adults who are unable to use Numeric Rating Scale or Wong-Baker Faces Pain Rating Scale
CRIES Pain Scale	http://painconsortium.nih.gov/pain_scales/CRIESPainScale.pdf	Neonates (0–6 months)
FLACC Scale	http://painconsortium.nih.gov/pain_scales/FLACCScale.pdf	Infants and children (2 months–7 years) who are unable to validate the presence of or quantify the severity of pain
Wong-Baker Faces Pain Rating Scale	http://painconsortium.nih.gov/pain_scales/wong-Baker_Faces.pdf	Adults and children (>3 years) in all patient care settings
0–10 Numeric Rating Scale	http://painconsortium.nih.gov/pain_scales/NumericRatingScale.pdf	Adults and children (>9 years) in all patient care settings who are able to use numbers to rate the intensity of their pain
Checklist of Nonverbal Indicators	http://painconsortium.nih.gov/pain_scales/checklistofNonverbal.pdf	Adults who are unable to validate the presence of or quantify the severity of pain using either the Numeric Rating Scale or Wong-Baker Faces Pain Rating Scale
Oucher Pain Scale	http://www.oucher.org/history.html	Young children who can point to a face to indicate their level of pain
PAINAD Scale	web.missouri.edu/~proste/tool/cog/painad.pdf	Patients whose dementia is so advanced that they cannot verbally communicate
FPS-R (Faces Pain Scale, Revised)	http://www.iasp-pain.org/Content/NavigationMenu/GeneralResourceLinks/FacesPainScaleRevised/default.htm	Young children in parallel with numerical self-rating scales (0–10). Patients choose the depiction of a facial expression that best corresponds with their pain.
Payen Behavioral Pain Scale	www.consensus-conference.org/data/Upload/Consensus/1/pdf/1670.pdf	Can be used with intubated, critically ill patients; measures bodily indicators of pain and tolerance of intubation.

FUNDAMENTALS REVIEW 10-4

FLACC BEHAVIORAL SCALE

This display presents two ways of demonstrating the FLACC Behavioral Scale.

Categories	Scoring 0	1	2
Face	No particular expression or smile	Occasional grimace or frown, withdrawn, disinterested	Frequent to constant frown, clenched jaw, quivering chin
Legs	Normal position or relaxed	Uneasy, restless, tense	Kicking, or legs drawn up
Activity	Lying quietly, normal position, moves easily	Squirming, shifting back and forth, tense	Arched, rigid, or jerking
Cry	No cry (awake or asleep)	Moans or whimpers, occasional complaint	Crying steadily, screams or sobs, frequent complaints
Consolability	Content, relaxed	Reassured by occasional touching, hugging, or being talked to, distractible	Difficult to console or comfort

Each of the five categories **(F)** Face; **(L)** Legs; **(A)** Activity; **(C)** Cry; **(C)** Consolability is scored from 0–2, which results in a total score between 0 and 10.

Patients who are awake: Observe for at least 1 to 2 minutes. Observe legs and body uncovered. Reposition the patient or observe activity; assess body for tenseness and tone. Initiate consoling interventions, if needed.

Patients who are asleep: Observe for at least 2 minutes or longer. Observe body and legs uncovered. If possible, reposition the patient. Touch the body and assess for tenseness and tone.

Face

Score 0 points if patient has a relaxed face, eye contact, and interest in surroundings.

Score 1 point if patient has a worried look to face, with eyebrows lowered, eyes partially closed, cheeks raised, mouth pursed.

Score 2 points if patient has deep furrows in forehead, with closed eyes, open mouth, and deep lines around the nose/lips.

Legs

Score 0 points if patient has usual tone and motion to limbs (legs and arms).

Score 1 point if patient has increased tone; rigidity; tense, intermittent flexion/extension of limbs.

Score 2 points if patient has hypertonicity, legs pulled tight, exaggerated flexion/extension of limbs, tremors.

Activity

Score 0 points if patient moves easily and freely, with normal activity/restrictions.

Score 1 point if patient shifts positions, is hesitant to move or is guarding, has tense torso, pressure on body part.

Score 2 points if patient is in fixed position, rocking, has side-to-side head movements, is rubbing body part.

Cry

Score 0 points if patient has no cry/moan (awake or asleep).

Score 1 point if patient has occasional moans, cries, whimpers, sighs.

Score 2 points if patient has frequent/continuous moans, cries, grunts.

Consolability

Score 0 points if patient is calm and does not require consoling.

Score 1 point if patient responds to comfort by touch or talk in 30 seconds to a minute.

Score 2 points if patient requires constant consoling or is unable to be consoled after an extended time.

Whenever feasible, behavioral measurement of pain should be used in conjunction with self-report. When self-report is not possible, interpretation of pain behaviors and decision making regarding treatment of pain requires careful consideration of the context in which pain behaviors were observed.

Each category is scored on the 0–2 scale, which results in a total score of 0–10.

Assessment of Behavioral Scale

0 = Relaxed and comfortable

1–3 = Mild discomfort

4–6 = Moderate pain

7–10 = Severe discomfort/pain

FUNDAMENTALS REVIEW 10-5

ADDITIONAL TERMS USED BY PATIENTS TO DESCRIBE PAIN

QUALITY

Term	Description
Sharp	Pain that is sticking in nature and is intense.
Dull	Pain that is not as intense or acute as sharp pain, possibly more annoying than painful. It is usually more diffuse than sharp pain.
Diffuse	Pain that covers a large area. Usually, the patient is unable to point to a specific area without moving the hand over a large surface, such as the entire abdomen.
Shifting	Pain that moves from one area to another, such as from the lower abdomen to the area over the stomach.

Other terms used to describe the quality of pain include sore, stinging, pinching, cramping, gnawing, cutting, throbbing, shooting, and viselike pressure.

SEVERITY

Term	Description
Severe or excruciating Moderate Slight or mild	These terms depend on the patient's interpretation of pain. Behavioral and physiologic signs help assess the severity of pain. On a scale of 1 to 10, slight pain could be described as being between about 1 and 3; moderate pain, between about 4 and 7; and severe pain, between about 8 and 10.

PERIODICITY

Term	Description
Continuous	Pain that does not stop.
Intermittent	Pain that stops and starts again.
Brief or transient	Pain that passes quickly.

FUNDAMENTALS REVIEW 10-6

COMMON RESPONSES TO PAIN

BEHAVIORAL (VOLUNTARY) RESPONSES

Moving away from painful stimuli

Grimacing, moaning, and crying

Restlessness

Protecting the painful area and refusing to move

PHYSIOLOGIC (INVOLUNTARY) RESPONSES

Typical Sympathetic Responses When Pain Is Moderate and Superficial

Increased blood pressure*

Increased pulse and respiratory rates*

Pupil dilation

Muscle tension and rigidity

Pallor (peripheral vasoconstriction)

Increased adrenaline output

Increased blood glucose

Typical Parasympathetic Responses When Pain Is Severe and Deep

Nausea and vomiting

Fainting or unconsciousness

Decreased blood pressure

Decreased pulse rate

Prostration

Rapid and irregular breathing

AFFECTIVE (PSYCHOLOGICAL) RESPONSES

Exaggerated weeping and restlessness	Fear
	Anger
Withdrawal	Anorexia
Stoicism	Fatigue
Anxiety	Hopelessness
Depression	Powerlessness

---

*Research has indicated that increases in vital signs may occur briefly in acute pain and may be absent in chronic pain (D'Arcy, 2008b). Reliance on vital signs to indicate the presence of pain should be minimized. **Absence of an increase in vital signs does not mean that pain is not present** (Pasero & McCaffery, 2011).

SKILL 10-1 PROMOTING PATIENT COMFORT

The nurse can promote increased comfort and relieve patient discomfort and pain through various pain management therapies. Interventions can include the administration of **analgesics**, emotional support, comfort measures, and **nonpharmacologic interventions**. Nonpharmacologic methods of pain management can diminish the emotional components of pain, strengthen coping abilities, give patients a sense of control, contribute to pain relief, decrease fatigue, and promote sleep (see Evidence for Practice). The following skill identifies potential interventions related to discomfort and pain. The interventions are listed sequentially for teaching purposes; the order is not sequential and should be adjusted based on patient assessment and nursing judgment. Not every intervention discussed will be appropriate for every patient. Additional interventions for discomfort and pain are discussed in other chapters. Refer to Chapter 5, Medications, for nursing skills related to administering topical medications for pain relief. The application of heat or cold therapy is discussed in Chapter 8, Skin Integrity and Wound Care.

DELEGATION CONSIDERATIONS

The assessment of a patient's pain is not delegated to nursing assistive personnel (NAP) or to unlicensed assistive personnel (UAP). The assessment of a patient's pain may be delegated to licensed practical/vocational nurses (LPN/LVNs). The use of nonpharmacologic interventions related to patient comfort may be delegated to nursing assistive personnel (NAP) or to unlicensed assistive personnel (UAP), as well as to licensed practical/vocational nurses (LPN/LVNs). The decision to delegate must be based on careful analysis of the patient's needs and circumstances, as well as the qualifications of the person to whom the task is being delegated. Refer to the Delegation Guidelines in Appendix A.

EQUIPMENT

- Pain assessment tool and pain scale
- Oral hygiene supplies
- Nonsterile gloves, if necessary
- Additional PPE, as indicated

ASSESSMENT

Review the patient's medical record and plan of care for information about the patient's status and contraindications to any of the potential interventions. Inquire about any allergies. Assess the patient's level of discomfort. Assess the patient's pain using an appropriate assessment tool and pain scale. Assess the characteristics of any pain and for other symptoms that often occur with the pain, such as headache or restlessness. Ask the patient what interventions have and have not been successful in the past to promote comfort and relieve pain. Assess the patient's vital signs. Check the patient's medication administration record for the time an analgesic was last administered. Assess cultural beliefs related to pain. Assess the patient's response to a particular intervention to evaluate effectiveness and presence of adverse effects.

NURSING DIAGNOSIS

Determine the related factors for the nursing diagnoses based on the patient's current status. Nursing diagnoses that may be appropriate include:

- Acute Pain
- Chronic Pain
- Disturbed Sleep Pattern

OUTCOME IDENTIFICATION AND PLANNING

The expected outcome to achieve is that the patient experiences relief from discomfort and/or pain without adverse effect. Other outcomes that may be appropriate include the patient experiences decreased anxiety and improved relaxation; is able to participate in activities of daily living (ADLs); verbalizes an understanding of, and satisfaction with, the pain management plan.

IMPLEMENTATION

ACTION	RATIONALE
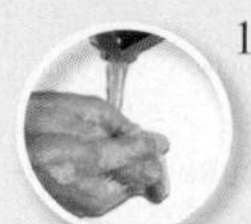 1. Perform hand hygiene and put on PPE, if indicated.	Hand hygiene and PPE prevent the spread of microorganisms. PPE is required based on transmission precautions.
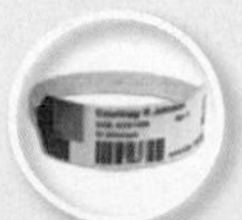 2. Identify the patient.	Identifying the patient ensures the right patient receives the intervention and helps prevent errors.

(continued)

SKILL 10-1 PROMOTING PATIENT COMFORT continued

ACTION	RATIONALE
3. Discuss pain with the patient, acknowledging that the patient's pain exists. Explain how pain medications and other pain management therapies work together to provide pain relief. Allow the patient to help choose interventions for pain relief.	Pain discussion and patient involvement strengthen the nurse–patient relationship and promote pain relief (Taylor et al., 2015). Explanation encourages patient understanding and cooperation and reduces apprehension.
4. Assess the patient's pain, using an appropriate assessment tool and measurement scale (see Fundamentals Review 10-1 through 10-5).	Accurate assessment is necessary to guide treatment/relief interventions and evaluate the effectiveness of pain control measures.
5. Provide pharmacologic interventions, if indicated and ordered.	Analgesics and **adjuvant** drugs reduce perception of pain and alter responses to discomfort.
6. Adjust the patient's environment to promote comfort.	The environment can improve or detract from the patient's sense of well-being and can be a source of stimulation that aggravates pain and reduces comfort.
a. Adjust and maintain the room temperature per the patient's preference.	A too warm or too cool environment can be a source of stimulation that aggravates pain and reduces comfort.
b. Reduce harsh lighting, but provide adequate lighting per the patient's preference.	Harsh lighting can be a source of stimulation that aggravates pain and reduces comfort.
c. Reduce harsh and unnecessary noise. Avoid having conversations immediately outside the patient's room.	Noise, including talking, can be a source of stimuli that aggravates pain and reduces comfort.
d. Close the room door and/or curtain whenever possible.	Closing the door or curtain provides privacy and reduces noise and other extraneous stimuli that may aggravate pain and reduce comfort.
e. Provide good ventilation in the patient's room. Reduce unpleasant odors by promptly emptying bedpans, urinals, and emesis basins after use. Remove trash and laundry promptly.	Odors can be a source of stimuli that aggravate pain and reduce comfort.
7. Prevent unnecessary interruptions and coordinate patient activities to group activities together. Allow for and plan rest periods without disturbance.	Frequent interruptions and disturbances for assessment or treatment can be a source of stimuli that aggravate pain and reduce comfort. Fatigue reduces tolerance for pain and can increase the pain experience.
8. Assist the patient to change position frequently. Assist the patient to a comfortable position, maintaining good alignment and supporting extremities, as needed. Raise the head of the bed as appropriate. (See Chapter 9 for more information on positioning.)	Positioning in proper alignment with supports ensures that the patient will be able to maintain the desired position and reduces pressure.
9. Provide oral hygiene as often as necessary (e.g., every 1 to 2 hours) to keep the mouth and mucous membranes clean and moist. This is especially important for patients who cannot drink or are not permitted fluids by mouth. (See Chapter 7 for additional information about mouth care.)	Moisture helps maintain the integrity of mucous membranes. Dry mucous membranes can be a source of stimuli that aggravate pain and reduce comfort.
10. Ensure the availability of appropriate fluids for drinking, unless contraindicated. Make sure the patient's water pitcher is filled and within reach. Have other fluids of the patient's choice available.	Thirst and dry mucous membranes can be sources of stimuli that reduce comfort and aggravate pain.
11. Remove physical situations that might cause discomfort.	
a. Change soiled and/or wet dressings; replace soiled and/or wet bed linens.	Moisture can cause discomfort and irritation to skin.
b. Smooth wrinkles in bed linens.	Wrinkled bed linens apply pressure to skin and can cause discomfort and irritation to skin.
c. Ensure patient is not lying or sitting on tubes, tubing, wires, or other equipment.	Tubing and equipment apply pressure to skin and can cause discomfort and irritation to skin.

ACTION	RATIONALE
12. Assist the patient, as necessary, with ambulation, and active or passive range-of-motion exercises (ROM), as appropriate. (See Chapter 9 for more information about activity.)	Activity prevents stiffness and loss of mobility, which can reduce comfort and aggravate pain.
13. Assess the patient's spiritual needs related to the pain experience. Ask the patient if her or she would like a spiritual counselor to visit.	Some people's spiritual beliefs facilitate positive coping with the effects of illness, including pain.
14. Consider the use of distraction. Distraction requires the patient to focus on something other than the pain.	Conscious attention often appears to be necessary to experience pain. Preoccupation with other things has been observed to distract the patient from pain. Distraction is thought to raise the threshold of pain and/or increase **pain tolerance** (Taylor et al., 2015).
a. Have the patient recall a pleasant experience or focus attention on an enjoyable experience.	
b. Offer age or developmentally appropriate games, toys, books, audiobooks, access to television, and/or videos, or other items of interest to the patient.	
c. Encourage the patient to hold or stroke a loved person, pet, or toy.	
d. Offer access to music the patient prefers. Turn on the music when pain begins, or before anticipated painful stimuli. The patient can close his or her eyes and concentrate on listening. Raising or lowering the volume as pain increases or decreases can be helpful.	
15. Consider the use of guided imagery.	Guided imagery helps the patient gradually become less aware of the discomfort or pain. Positive emotions evoked by the image help reduce the pain experience.
a. Help the patient to identify a scene or experience that the patient describes as happy, pleasant, or peaceful.	
b. Encourage the patient to begin with several minutes of focused breathing, relaxation, or meditation. (Refer to specific information in steps 16 and 17.)	
c. Help the patient concentrate on the peaceful, pleasant image.	
d. If indicated, read a description of the identified scene or experience, using a soothing, soft voice.	
e. Encourage the patient to concentrate on the details of the image, such as its sight, sounds, smells, tastes, and touch.	
16. Consider the use of relaxation activities, such as deep breathing.	Relaxation techniques reduce skeletal muscle tension and lessen anxiety, both of which can reduce comfort and aggravate pain. Relaxation can also be a distraction, providing help in reducing the pain experience (Kwekkeboom et al., 2008; Taylor et al., 2015).
a. Have the patient sit or recline comfortably and place hands on stomach. Close the eyes.	
b. Ask the patient to mentally count to maintain a comfortable rate and rhythm. Have the patient inhale slowly and deeply while letting the abdomen expand as much as possible. Have the patient hold his or her breath for a few seconds.	
c. Tell the patient to exhale slowly through the mouth, blowing through puckered lips. Have the patient continue to count to maintain comfortable rate and rhythm, concentrating on the rise and fall of the abdomen.	

(continued)

SKILL 10-1 PROMOTING PATIENT COMFORT continued

ACTION	RATIONALE
d. When the patient's abdomen feels empty, have the patient begin again with a deep inhalation.	
e. Encourage patient to practice at least twice a day, for 10 minutes, and then use the technique, as needed, to assist with pain management.	
17. Consider the use of relaxation activities, such as progressive muscle relaxation.	Relaxation techniques reduce skeletal muscle tension and lessen anxiety, both of which can reduce comfort and aggravate pain. Relaxation can also be a distraction, providing help in reducing the pain experience (Kwekkeboom et al., 2008; Taylor et al., 2015).
a. Assist the patient to a comfortable position.	
b. Direct the patient to focus on a particular muscle group. Start with the muscles of the jaw, then repeat with the muscles of the neck, shoulder, upper and lower arm, hand, abdomen, buttocks, thigh, lower leg, and foot.	
c. Ask the patient to tighten the muscle group and note the sensation that the tightened muscles produce. After 5 to 7 seconds, tell the patient to relax the muscles all at once and concentrate on the sensation of the relaxed state, noting the difference in feeling in the muscles when contracted and relaxed.	
d. Have the patient continue to tighten–hold–relax each muscle group until the entire body has been covered.	
e. Encourage the patient to practice at least twice a day, for 10 minutes, and then use the technique, as needed, to assist with pain management.	
18. Consider the use of cutaneous stimulation, such as the intermittent application of heat or cold, or both. (See Chapter 8 for additional information on heat and cold therapy.)	Heat helps relieve pain by stimulating specific nerve fibers, closing the gate that allows the transmission of pain stimuli to centers in the brain. Heat accelerates the inflammatory response to promote healing, and reduces muscle tension to promote relaxation and help to relieve muscle spasms and joint stiffness. Cold reduces blood flow to tissues and decreases the local release of pain-producing substances, such as histamine, serotonin, and bradykinin, and reduces the formation of edema and inflammation. Cold reduces muscle spasm, alters tissue sensitivity (producing numbness), and promotes comfort by slowing the transmission of pain stimuli (Taylor et al., 2015).
19. Consider the use of cutaneous stimulation, such as massage (see Skill 10-2).	Cutaneous stimulation techniques stimulate the skin's surface, closing the gating mechanism in the spinal cord, decreasing the number of pain impulses that reach the brain for perception.
20. Discuss the potential for use of cutaneous stimulation, such as TENS, with the patient and primary care provider. (See Skill 10-3.)	Cutaneous stimulation techniques stimulate the skin's surface, closing the gating mechanism in the spinal cord, decreasing the number of pain impulses that reach the brain for perception.
21. Remove equipment and return patient to a position of comfort. Remove gloves, if used. Raise side rail and lower bed.	Equipment removal and repositioning promote patient comfort. Removing gloves properly reduces the risk for infection transmission and contamination of other items. Lowering bed promotes patient safety.
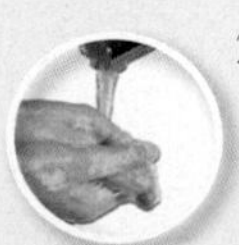 22. Remove additional PPE, if used. Perform hand hygiene.	Removing PPE properly reduces the risk for infection transmission and contamination of other items. Hand hygiene prevents transmission of microorganisms.
23. Evaluate the patient's response to interventions. Reassess level of discomfort or pain using original assessment tools. Reassess and alter plan of care, as appropriate.	Evaluation allows for individualization of plan of care and promotes optimal patient comfort.

EVALUATION

The expected outcome is met when the patient experiences relief from discomfort and/or pain without adverse effect; the patient experiences decreased anxiety and improved relaxation; the patient is able to participate in ADLs; and the patient verbalizes an understanding of, and satisfaction with, the pain management plan.

DOCUMENTATION

Guidelines

Document pain assessment and other significant assessments. Document pain relief therapies used and patient responses. Record alternative treatments to consider, if appropriate. Document reassessment of pain and comfort after interventions, at an appropriate interval, based on specific interventions used.

Sample Documentation

5/12/15 2030 Patient reports increased pain in lower extremities, rating the pain at 5/10, and described it as burning and constant, consistent with previous pain. Medicated with oxycodone 5 mg P.O. as ordered for **breakthrough pain**. Patient using relaxation and deep-breathing techniques, as well as listening to music. Reviewed instructions for use of relaxation and deep breathing; patient verbalized understanding.

—R. Curry, RN

5/12/15 2145 Patient reports pain reduced to 2/10. OOB to solarium with family.

—R. Curry, RN

UNEXPECTED SITUATIONS AND ASSOCIATED INTERVENTIONS

- *Patient reports or assessment reveals ineffective/or lack of pain relief:* Reassess pain and evaluate response to implemented therapies. Implement additional or alternate interventions until desired level of comfort is achieved.
- *Intervention increases patient discomfort or pain:* Immediately stop intervention. Document intervention used and the effect. Communicate changes in the patient's condition to the primary care provider, as appropriate. Revise plan of care, noting adverse effect of intervention, so other caregivers avoid using same intervention.

SPECIAL CONSIDERATIONS

General Considerations

- The use of alternate and adjunct therapies is often a 'try and see' process. Many interventions can be tried to achieve the best combination for a particular patient. People respond to pain differently; what works for one person may not help another.

Infant and Child Considerations

- Assessment, measurement, and treatment of discomfort and pain in infants and children frequently involve the use of more than one technique. Communication with parents, guardians, or significant others is vital for accurate pediatric pain assessment and management.
- Nonpharmacologic therapies can be very beneficial in decreasing acute and chronic pain, as well as pain related to procedures, in infants and children (Kyle & Carman, 2013; Perry et al., 2010; Taylor et al., 2015).

Older Adult Considerations

- Older patients may report that their pain level is tolerable and that it only hurts when they move. These patients are at risk for developing conditions related to immobility. Provide effective pain relief to allow movement and participation in ADLs. The nursing plan of care should also include interventions related to 'risk for impaired skin integrity' (Tabloski, 2010).
- Older adults often view pain as a natural component of the aging process. They may not complain of pain due to fear of potential treatment or because they have accepted the pain as a part of their life; again, a part of the aging process (Taylor et al., 2015). Be vigilant in performing pain assessment and in forming a plan of care for these patients. Effective pain management will allow the patient to maintain dignity, functional capacity, and quality of life (American Geriatrics Society, 2002).

(*continued*)

SKILL 10-1 PROMOTING PATIENT COMFORT continued

EVIDENCE FOR PRACTICE ▶

HEALING TOUCH AND PAIN IN OLDER ADULTS

Pain is often under-assessed and under-treated, particularly in older adults residing in long-term care facilities. Most of this population suffers from chronic pain, with estimates varying from 20% to 80%. Analgesics used to treat chronic pain can have adverse effects on older adults. In addition, their medication regimens are more complicated, leading to the potential for drug interactions. Many factors affect a person's reaction to pain, including previous pain experience and its effect on quality of life. The addition of a complementary nonpharmacologic approach to pain management, such as Healing Touch, addresses the subjective component of pain and provides an additional method to use to ease pain for people in this setting.

Related Research

Wardell, D., Decker, S. & Engebretson, J. (2012). Healing touch for older adults with persistent pain. *Holistic Nursing Practice*, *26*(4), 194–202.

The goal of this research was to explore the effect that Healing Touch (HT) had on older adults with chronic pain living in a long-term care facility. Healing Touch is an alternative energy therapy that is thought to rebalance the system and promote healing. This was a secondary study meant as a follow-up to previous research. Twelve residents of five long-term care facilities participated in this study and had an HT intervention three times per week for 30 minutes over 2 weeks, followed by a closing session with one of the three certified Healing Touch practitioners (CHTPs) who each had at least 5 years of experience and conducted the research sessions. The residents were at least 60 years of age, able to complete self-report data instruments, and had multiple painful chronic conditions and multiple medication regimens. Pain assessments, including quality of life, were completed pre- and post-intervention. A participant's level of pain was measured using the Verbal Descriptor Scale, and a tool for observational behavioral assessment of pain was also utilized. Only one of the participants did not have a positive response to the HT and none of the older adults had an adverse or negative response. There were varying degrees of response to HT in regard to pain relief. Initially, all the participants believed that HT would not help their "long-standing problems," but usually by the third session, they verified that HT did provide some level of a positive effect on their pain. The researchers concluded that since pain has a subjective component and is an individualized experience, it is difficult to measure objectively the effects of HT on pain. They suggest, though, that HT may offer a benefit to this population and provide positive outcomes.

Relevance to Nursing Practice

Healing Touch is just one of the nonpharmacologic, nontraditional nursing measures that might individualize care and take into account the varying complexities of aging and pain. Many patients, as well as health care practitioners, are unaware of the potential benefits of alternative approaches to pain management. Although it is difficult to measure and quantify, HT may offer a benefit to older adults with chronic pain issues. Coupled with nursing assessments, observations, and traditional treatments for pain, this complementary therapy provides an additional treatment modality as nurses strive to provide holistic care to their patients.

Refer to thePoint for additional research on related nursing topics.

EVIDENCE FOR PRACTICE ▶

MUSIC AND PATIENT COMFORT

Conscious attention often appears to be necessary to experience pain. Preoccupation with other things has been observed to distract the patient from pain. Distraction is thought to raise the threshold of pain and/or increase pain tolerance. Listening to music has been offered as a type of distraction. Does listening to music help decrease pain and increase patient comfort?

Related Research

Vaajoki, A., Pietilä, A-M., Kankkunen, P., et al. (2011). Effects of listening to music on pain intensity and pain distress after surgery: An intervention. *Journal of Clinical Nursing, 21*(5/6), 708–717.

This study evaluated the effects of listening to music on pain intensity and pain distress on the first and second postoperative days, as well as the long-term effects of music on the third postoperative day in patients having had abdominal surgery. Patients undergoing elective abdominal surgery were divided into either a music group or a control group. Patients in the music group listened to music seven times between the operation day and the second postoperative day. The participants were given the music they liked to listen to. Patients assessed their pain intensity and pain distress in bed rest, during deep breathing, and in shifting position once in the evening of the operation day. These assessments were repeated on the first and second postoperative days in the morning, at noon, and in the evening. Patients assessed their pain intensity and pain distress once on the third postoperative day. In the music group, the patients' pain intensity and pain distress in bed rest, during deep breathing, and in shifting position were significantly lower on the second postoperative day compared with the control group of patients. On the third postoperative day, when long-term effects of music on pain intensity and pain distress were assessed, no significant differences were found between music and control groups. The authors concluded the study demonstrated that the use of music alleviates pain intensity and pain distress in bed rest, during deep breathing, and in shifting position after abdominal surgery. Music intervention is safe, inexpensive, and easily used to improve the healing environment for patients after abdominal surgery.

Relevance to Nursing Practice

Nurses should consider music as an additional intervention in pain management. Nurses should consider individual patient preferences when offering music as an addition to analgesics for postoperative pain.

Refer to thePoint for additional research on related nursing topics.

EVIDENCE FOR PRACTICE ▶

COLD APPLICATION AND PAIN RELIEF

Stimulation of the skin's surface (cutaneous stimulation) has been identified as a way to decrease pain. The application of cold to the skin is one form of cutaneous stimulation. Does the application of cold to the skin decrease pain?

Related Research

Chailler, M., Ellis, J., Stolarik, A., et al. (2010). Cold therapy for the management of pain associated with deep breathing and coughing post-cardiac surgery. *Canadian Journal of Cardiovascular Nursing, 20*(2), 18–24.

Coughing after cardiac surgery is an important intervention for preventing postoperative respiratory complications. Postoperative chest wall pain may prevent patients from performing deep breathing and coughing. This study examined the effect of the application of cold (a frozen gel pack) to the sternal incision dressing of patients after coronary bypass graft surgery before performing deep breathing and coughing exercises. Pain scores were rated using a numeric scale from 0 to 10 at rest and compared with pain scores after deep breathing and coughing, with and without the gel pack. Participants also described their sensations with the frozen gel pack, as well as their preferences for gel pack application. The results revealed a significant reduction in pain scores between pre- and post-application of the gel pack. Of participants, 69% preferred the application of the gel pack compared with no gel pack. All (100%) participants stated they would reapply the gel pack in the future. The authors concluded cold therapy can be used to manage sternal incisional pain when performing deep breathing and coughing exercises in the postoperative period.

Relevance to Nursing Practice

Nursing interventions related to decreasing pain and increasing patient comfort are an important nursing responsibility. Interventions should include the use of nonpharmacologic interventions, in addition to the administration of analgesics. The application of cold to the chest wall could significantly decrease the pain and discomfort experienced by a patient during deep breathing and coughing after cardiac surgery. Nurses could easily incorporate this simple intervention as part of nursing care for these patients.

Refer to thePoint for additional research on related nursing topics.

SKILL 10-2 GIVING A BACK MASSAGE

Massage has many benefits, including general relaxation and increased circulation. Massage can help alleviate pain (The Joint Commission, 2008) (see Evidence for Practice). A back massage can be incorporated into the patient's bath, as part of care before bedtime, or at any time to promote increased patient comfort. Some nurses do not always give back massages to patients because they do not think they have sufficient time. However, giving a back massage provides an opportunity for the nurse to observe the skin for signs of breakdown. It also improves circulation; decreases pain, symptom distress, and anxiety; improves sleep quality; and provides a means of communicating with the patient through the use of touch. A back massage also provides cutaneous stimulation as a method of pain relief.

Because some patients consider the back massage a luxury and may be reluctant to accept it, communicate its importance and value to the patient. An effective back massage should take 4 to 6 minutes to complete. A lotion is usually applied; warm it before applying to the back. Be aware of the patient's medical diagnosis when considering giving a back massage. A back massage is contraindicated, for example, when the patient has had back surgery or has fractured ribs. Position the patient on the abdomen or, if this is contraindicated, on the side for a back massage.

DELEGATION CONSIDERATIONS

Providing a back massage may be delegated to nursing assistive personnel (NAP) or to unlicensed assistive personnel (UAP), as well as to licensed practical/vocational nurses (LPN/LVNs). The decision to delegate must be based on careful analysis of the patient's needs and circumstances, as well as the qualifications of the person to whom the task is being delegated. Refer to the Delegation Guidelines in Appendix A.

EQUIPMENT

- Pain assessment tool and pain scale
- Powder, if not contraindicated
- Bath blanket
- Towel
- Nonsterile gloves, if indicated
- Additional PPE, as indicated

ASSESSMENT

Review the patient's medical record and plan of care for information about the patient's status and contraindications to back massage. Question the patient about any conditions that might require modifications or that might contraindicate a massage. Inquire about any allergies, such as to lotions or scents. Ask if the patient has any preferences for lotion or has his or her own lotion. Assess the patient's level of pain. Check the patient's medication administration record for the time an analgesic was last administered. If appropriate, administer an analgesic early enough so that it has time to take effect.

NURSING DIAGNOSIS

Determine the related factors for the nursing diagnoses based on the patient's current status. Appropriate nursing diagnoses may include:

- Acute Pain
- Chronic Pain
- Disturbed Sleep Pattern

OUTCOME IDENTIFICATION AND PLANNING

The expected outcomes to achieve are that the patient reports increased comfort and/or decreased pain, and that the patient is relaxed. Other outcomes that may be appropriate include the patient displays decreased anxiety and improved relaxation; patient is free of skin breakdown; and patient verbalizes an understanding of the reasons for back massage.

IMPLEMENTATION

ACTION	RATIONALE
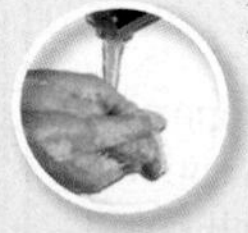 1. Perform hand hygiene and put on PPE, if indicated.	Hand hygiene and PPE prevent the spread of microorganisms. PPE is required based on transmission precautions.
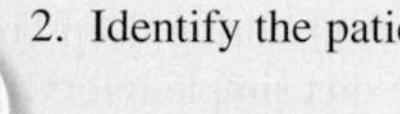 2. Identify the patient.	Identifying the patient ensures the right patient receives the intervention and helps prevent errors.

ACTION	RATIONALE
3. Offer a back massage to the patient and explain the procedure.	Explanation encourages patient understanding and cooperation and reduces apprehension.
4. Put on gloves, if indicated.	Gloves are not usually necessary. Gloves prevent contact with blood and body fluid.
5. Close the room door and/or the curtain around the bed.	Closing the door or curtain provides privacy, promotes relaxation, and reduces noise and stimuli that may aggravate pain and reduce comfort.
6. Assess the patient's pain, using an appropriate assessment tool and measurement scale. (See Fundamentals Review 10-1 through 10-6.)	Accurate assessment is necessary to guide treatment and pain relief interventions and to evaluate the effectiveness of pain control measures.
7. Raise the bed to a comfortable working position, usually elbow height of the caregiver (VISN 8 Patient Safety Center, 2009), and lower the side rail.	Having the bed at the proper height prevents back and muscle strain.
8. Assist the patient to a comfortable position, preferably the prone or side-lying position. Remove the covers and move the patient's gown just enough to expose the patient's back from the shoulders to sacral area. Drape the patient, as needed, with the bath blanket.	This position exposes an adequate area for massage. Draping the patient provides privacy and warmth.
9. Warm the lubricant or lotion in the palm of your hand, or place the container in small basin of warm water. **During massage, observe the patient's skin for reddened or open areas. Pay particular attention to the skin over bony prominences.** (See Chapter 8 for detailed information regarding skin assessment.)	Cold lotion causes chilling and discomfort. Pressure may interfere with circulation and lead to pressure ulcers.
10. Using light, gliding strokes (*effleurage*), apply lotion to patient's shoulders, back, and sacral area (Figure 1).	Effleurage relaxes the patient and lessens tension.
11. Place your hands beside each other at the base of the patient's spine and stroke upward to the shoulders and back downward to the buttocks in slow, continuous strokes (Figure 2). Continue for several minutes.	Continuous contact is soothing and stimulates circulation and muscle relaxation.

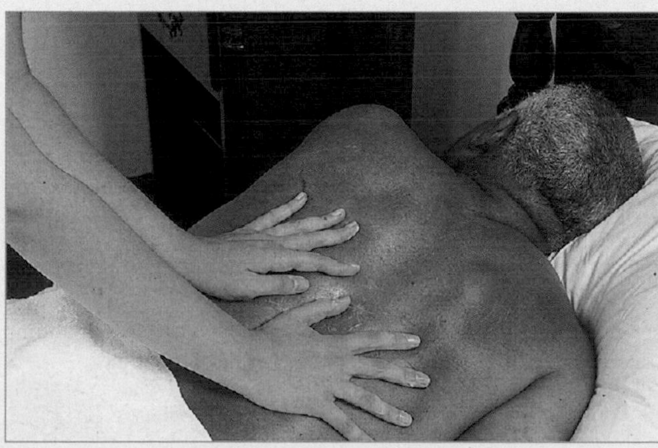

FIGURE 1 Using effleurage on a patient's back.

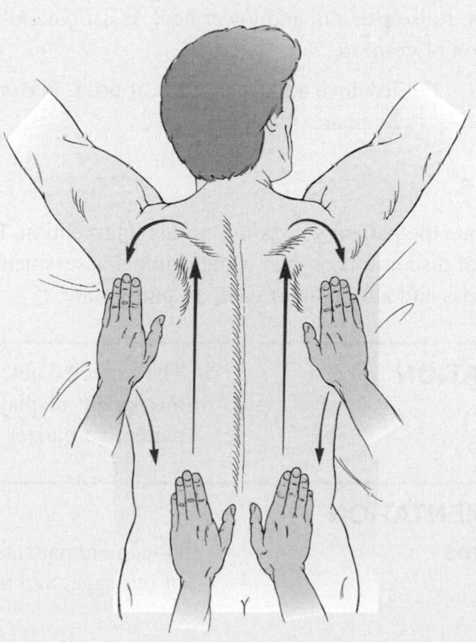

FIGURE 2 Stroking upward to shoulders.

(*continued*)

SKILL 10-2 GIVING A BACK MASSAGE continued

ACTION	RATIONALE
12. Massage the patient's shoulders, entire back, areas over iliac crests, and sacrum with circular stroking motions. **Keep your hands in contact with the patient's skin.** Continue for several minutes, applying additional lotion, as necessary.	A firm stroke with continuous contact promotes relaxation.
13. Knead the patient's skin by gently alternating grasping and compression motions (*pétrissage*) (Figure 3).	Kneading increases blood circulation.
14. Complete the massage with additional long, stroking movements that eventually become lighter in pressure (Figure 4).	Long, stroking motions are soothing and promote relaxation; continued stroking with gradual lightening of pressure helps extend the feeling of relaxation.

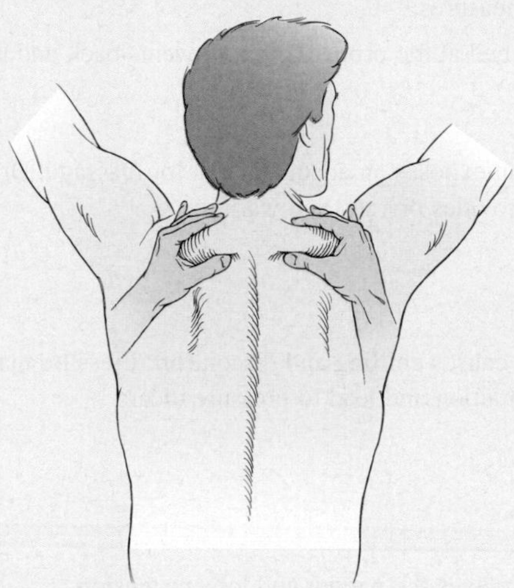

FIGURE 3 Using pétrissage.

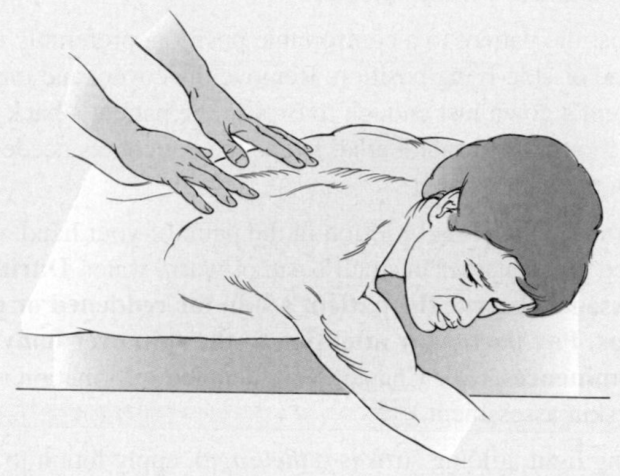

FIGURE 4 Using light strokes with lessening pressure.

ACTION	RATIONALE
15. Use the towel to pat the patient dry and to remove excess lotion.	Drying provides comfort and reduces the feeling of moisture on the back.
16. Remove gloves, if worn. Reposition patient's gown and covers. Raise side rail and lower bed. Assist patient to a position of comfort.	Repositioning bedclothes, linens, and the patient helps to promote patient comfort and safety.
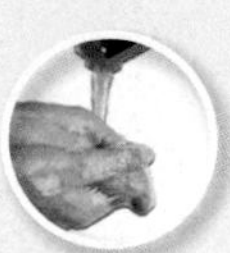 17. Remove additional PPE, if used. Perform hand hygiene.	Removing PPE properly reduces the risk for infection transmission and contamination of other items. Hand hygiene prevents transmission of microorganisms.
18. Evaluate the patient's response to this intervention. Reassess level of discomfort or pain using original assessment tools. Reassess and alter plan of care, as appropriate.	Reassessment allows for individualization of the patient's plan of care and promotes optimal patient comfort.

EVALUATION

The expected outcome is achieved when the patient reports increased comfort and/or decreased pain; the patient displays decreased anxiety and improved relaxation; skin breakdown is absent; and the patient verbalizes an understanding of the reasons for back massage.

DOCUMENTATION

Guidelines

Document pain assessment and other significant assessments. Document massage use, length of time of massage, and patient response. Record alternative treatments to consider, if appropriate.

Sample Documentation

12/6/15 2330 Patient reports inability to sleep and increased pain at surgical site, rated 3/10. Medicated with propoxyphene 100 mg and acetaminophen 650 mg, as ordered. Back massage administered ×10 minutes. Skin intact without redness. Patient reports increased comfort and relaxation; "I feel like I could sleep now."

—*B. Black, RN*

12/6/15 2400 Patient reports pain level 0/10.

—*B. Black, RN*

UNEXPECTED SITUATIONS AND ASSOCIATED INTERVENTIONS

- *The patient cannot lie prone, so you are giving him a back massage while he is lying on his side. However, as you begin to massage the back, the patient cannot maintain the side-lying position:* If possible, have the patient hold on to the side rail on the side to which he is facing. If this is not possible or the patient cannot assist, use pillows and bath blankets to prevent the patient from rolling. If necessary, enlist the help of another person to maintain the patient's position. If possible, experiment with other positions based on the patient's condition and comfort, such as leaning forward against a pillow on the bedside table while sitting in a chair.
- *While massaging the patient's back, you notice a 2-inch reddened area on the patient's sacrum:* Note this observation in the patient's medical record and report it to the physician. Do not massage the area. When the back massage is completed, position the patient off the sacral area, using pillows to maintain the patient's position, and institute a turning schedule.

SPECIAL CONSIDERATIONS

General Considerations

- Before giving a back massage, assess the patient's body structure and skin condition, and tailor the duration and intensity of the massage accordingly. If you are giving a back massage at bedtime, have the patient ready for bed beforehand so the massage can help him or her fall asleep.
- If the patient has oily skin, substitute a talcum powder or lotion of the patient's choice. However, to avoid aspiration, do not use powder if the patient has an endotracheal or tracheal tube in place. Avoid using powder and lotion together because this can lead to skin maceration.
- When massaging the patient's back, stand with one foot slightly forward and your knees slightly bent to allow effective use of your arm and shoulder muscles.

Infant and Child Considerations

- Hold infants and small children in a comfortable, well-supported position, such as against the chest or across the lap.

Older Adult Considerations

- Be gentle with massage. The skin on older adults is often fragile and dry.

EVIDENCE FOR PRACTICE ▶

MASSAGE AND PAIN RELIEF

Patient comfort is attained through management of many factors. Achieving pain relief and/or pain control is a large contributor to achieving patient comfort. Pharmacologic interventions alone may not address all of the factors involved in the pain experience. Do alternative approaches to managing pain that supplement medication administration help achieve effective pain management?

Related Research

Abbaspoor, Z., Akbari, M., & Najar, S. (2013). Effect of foot and hand massage in post-cesarean section pain control: A randomized control trial. *Pain Management Nursing*. Available PubMed. DOI: 10.1016/j.pmn.2012.07.008.

One of the problems for mothers in the post-cesarean section period is pain, which disturbs the early relationship between mothers and newborns. Timely pain management prevents the side effects of pain, facilitates the patient's recovery, reduces the costs of treatment by minimizing or eliminating the mother's distress, and increases mother–infant interactions. The aim of this study was to determine the effect of hand and foot massage on post-cesarean section pain. This

(*continued*)

SKILL 10-2 GIVING A BACK MASSAGE continued

study was carried out on 80 women who had an elective cesarean section. A visual analog scale was used to determine the pain intensity before, immediately, and 90 minutes after conducting 5 minutes of foot and hand massage. Vital signs were measured and recorded. Pain intensity was found to be significantly reduced after intervention compared with the intensity before the intervention, in women who received the massage interventions when compared with women who did not receive massage interventions. There was also a significant difference between groups in terms of the pain intensity and requesting for analgesic. The authors concluded foot and hand massage can be considered as a complementary method to reduce the pain of cesarean section effectively and to decrease the amount of medications required, and their side effects.

Relevance to Nursing Practice

Massage is an economical intervention that is easily incorporated into nursing practice. As nursing activities and responsibilities have grown, however, the inclusion of patient massage has diminished in daily nursing care. Evidence indicates that massage can be an important part of decreasing pain and increasing comfort. Nurses should consider making time to incorporate this intervention into their practice.

Refer to thePoint for additional research on related nursing topics.

SKILL 10-3 APPLYING AND CARING FOR A PATIENT USING A TENS UNIT

Transcutaneous electrical nerve stimulation (TENS) is a noninvasive technique for providing pain relief that involves the electrical stimulation of large-diameter fibers to inhibit the transmission of painful impulses carried over small-diameter fibers. The TENS unit consists of a battery-powered portable unit, lead wires, and cutaneous electrode pads that are applied to or around the painful area (Figure 1). It is most beneficial when used to treat pain that is localized, and it requires an order from the primary care provider. The TENS unit can be applied intermittently throughout the day or worn for extended periods.

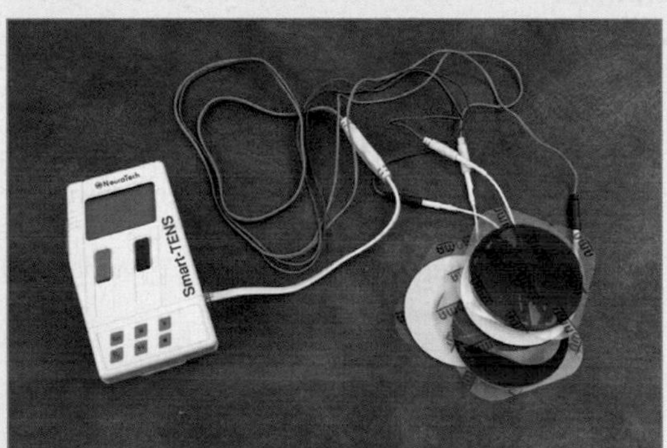

FIGURE 1 TENS unit.

DELEGATION CONSIDERATIONS

The application of and care for a TENS unit is not delegated to nursing assistive personnel (NAP) or unlicensed assistive personnel (UAP). Depending on the state's nurse practice act and the organization's policies and procedures, the application of, and care for, a TENS unit may be delegated to licensed practical/vocational nurses (LPN/LVNs). The decision to delegate must be based on careful analysis of the patient's needs and circumstances, as well as the qualifications of the person to whom the task is being delegated. Refer to the Delegation Guidelines in Appendix A.

EQUIPMENT

- TENS unit
- Electrodes
- Electrode gel (if electrodes are not pre-gelled)
- Tape (if electrodes are not self-adhesive)
- Pain assessment tool and pain scale
- Skin cleanser and water
- Towel and washcloth
- PPE, as indicated

ASSESSMENT

Review the patient's medical record and plan of care for specific instructions related to TENS therapy, including the order and conditions indicating the need for therapy. Review the patient's history for conditions that might contraindicate therapy, such as pacemaker insertion, cardiac monitoring, or electrocardiography. Determine the location of electrode placement in consultation with the ordering practitioner and on the patient's report of pain. Assess the patient's understanding of TENS therapy and the rationale for its use.

Inspect the skin of the area designated for electrode placement for irritation, redness, or breakdown. Assess the patient's pain and level of discomfort using an appropriate assessment tool. Assess the characteristics of any pain. Assess for other symptoms that often occur with the pain, such as headache or restlessness. Ask the patient what interventions have and have not been successful in the past to promote comfort and relieve pain. Assess the patient's vital signs. Check the patient's medication administration record for the time an analgesic was last administered. Assess the patient's response to a particular intervention to evaluate effectiveness and presence of any adverse effect.

Check the unit to ensure proper functioning and review the manufacturer's instructions for use.

NURSING DIAGNOSIS

Determine the related factors for the nursing diagnoses based on the patient's current status. Appropriate nursing diagnoses may include:

- Acute Pain
- Chronic Pain
- Deficient Knowledge

OUTCOME IDENTIFICATION AND PLANNING

The expected outcome to achieve is that the patient verbalizes decreased discomfort and pain, without experiencing any injury or skin irritation or breakdown. Other appropriate outcomes may include patient displays decreased anxiety, improved coping skills, and an understanding of the therapy and the reason for its use.

IMPLEMENTATION

ACTION	RATIONALE
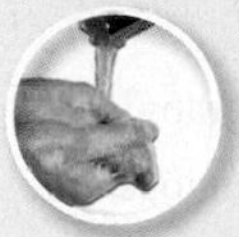 1. Perform hand hygiene and put on PPE, if indicated.	Hand hygiene and PPE prevent the spread of microorganisms. PPE is required based on transmission precautions.
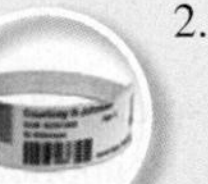 2. Identify the patient.	Identifying the patient ensures that the right patient receives the intervention and helps prevent errors.
3. Show the patient the device, and explain its function and the reason for its use.	Explanation encourages patient understanding and cooperation and reduces apprehension.
4. Assess the patient's pain, using an appropriate assessment tool and measurement scale. (See Fundamentals Review 10-1 through 10-6.)	Accurate assessment is necessary to guide treatment and relief interventions and evaluate the effectiveness of pain control measures.
5. Inspect the area where the electrodes are to be placed. Clean the patient's skin, using skin cleanser and water. Dry the area thoroughly.	Inspection ensures that the electrodes will be applied to intact skin. Cleaning and drying help ensure that the electrodes will adhere.

(*continued*)

SKILL 10-3 APPLYING AND CARING FOR A PATIENT USING A TENS UNIT continued

ACTION	RATIONALE
6. Remove the adhesive backing from the electrodes and apply them to the specified location (Figure 2). If the electrodes are not pre-gelled, apply a small amount of electrode gel to the bottom of each electrode. If the electrodes are not self-adhering, tape them in place.	Application to the proper location enhances the success of the therapy. Gel is necessary to promote conduction of the electrical current.
7. **Check the placement of the electrodes; leave at least a 2-inch (5-cm) space (about the width of one electrode) between them.**	Proper spacing is necessary to reduce the risk of burns due to the proximity of the electrodes.
8. **Check the controls on the TENS unit to make sure that they are off.** Connect the wires to the electrodes (if not already attached) and plug them into the unit.	Having controls off prevents flow of electricity. This connection completes the electrical circuit necessary to stimulate the nerve fibers.
9. Turn on the unit and adjust the intensity setting to the lowest intensity and determine if the patient can feel a tingling, burning, or buzzing sensation (Figure 3). Then adjust the intensity to the prescribed amount or the setting most comfortable for the patient. Secure the unit to the patient.	Using the lowest setting at first introduces the patient to the sensations. Adjusting the intensity is necessary to provide the proper amount of stimulation.

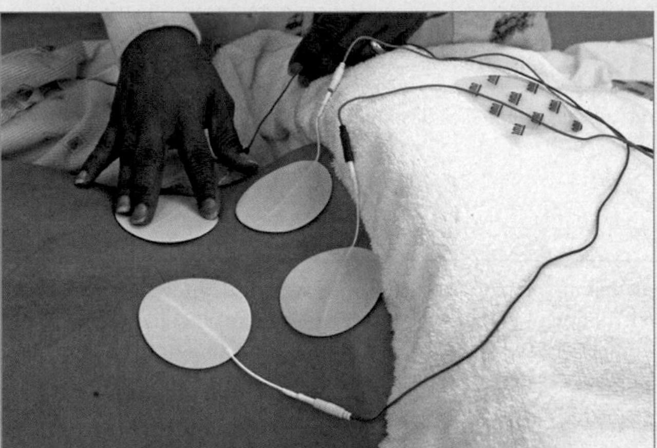

FIGURE 2 Applying TENS electrodes.

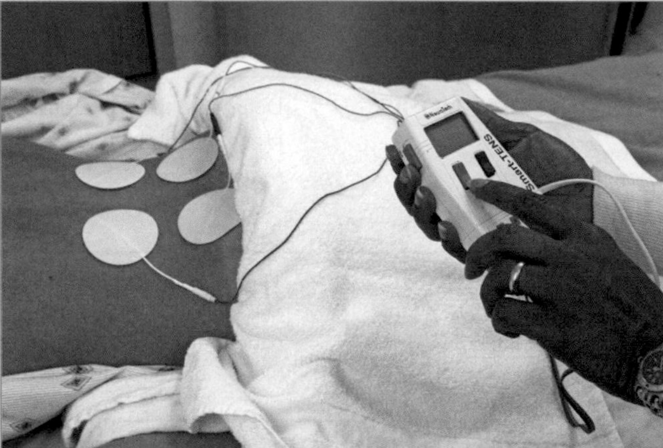

FIGURE 3 Turning on TENS unit.

ACTION	RATIONALE
10. Set the pulse width (duration of the each pulsation) as indicated or recommended.	The pulse width determines the depth and width of the stimulation.
11. Assess the patient's pain level during therapy.	Pain assessment helps evaluate the effectiveness of therapy.
a. If intermittent use is ordered, turn the unit off after the specified duration of treatment and remove the electrodes. Provide skin care to the area.	TENS therapy can be ordered for intermittent or continuous use. Skin care reduces the risk for irritation and breakdown.
b. If continuous therapy is ordered, periodically remove the electrodes from the skin (after turning off the unit) to inspect the area and clean the skin, according to facility policy. Reapply the electrodes and continue therapy. Change the electrodes according to manufacturer's directions.	Periodic removal of electrodes allows for skin assessment. Skin care reduces the risk for irritation and breakdown. Reapplication ensures continued therapy.
12. When therapy is discontinued, turn off the unit and remove the electrodes. Clean the patient's skin. Clean the unit and replace the batteries.	Turning off the unit and removing electrodes when therapy is discontinued reduces the risk of injury to the patient. Cleaning the unit and replacing the batteries ensures that the unit is ready for future use.
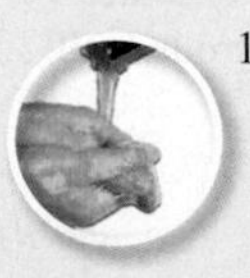 13. Remove PPE, if used. Perform hand hygiene.	Removing PPE properly reduces the risk for infection transmission and contamination of other items. Hand hygiene prevents transmission of microorganisms.

EVALUATION

The expected outcome is achieved when the patient verbalizes pain relief. In addition, the patient remains free of signs and symptoms of skin irritation and breakdown, and injury. The patient reports decreased anxiety and increased ability to cope with pain. The patient verbalizes information related to the functioning of the unit and the reasons for its use.

DOCUMENTATION

Guidelines

Document the date and time of application; patient's initial pain assessment; skin assessment; electrode placement location; intensity and pulse width; duration of therapy; pain assessments during therapy and patient's response; and time of removal or discontinuation of therapy.

Sample Documentation

5/28/15 1105 Patient complaining of severe lower back pain, rating it as 9/10 on pain scale. Identified lower sacral area as site of pain. TENS therapy ordered for 30 to 45 minutes. Electrodes applied to right and left sides of sacral area. Intensity initially set at 80 pulses per second with pulse width of 80 microseconds. Pain rating at 7/10 after 15 minutes of therapy. Intensity increased to 100 pulses per second, with a pulse width increased to 100 microseconds. Pain rating at 5/10 after 15 minutes at increased settings. Therapy continued for an additional 15 minutes and discontinued. Patient rated pain at 3/10 at end of session. Skin on lower sacral area clean, dry, and intact without evidence of irritation or breakdown. Patient instructed to report increasing pain.

—*K. Lewin, RN*

UNEXPECTED SITUATIONS AND ASSOCIATED INTERVENTIONS

- *While receiving TENS therapy, the patient reports pain and intolerable paresthesia:* Check the settings, connections, and placement of the electrodes. Adjust the settings and reposition the electrodes, as necessary.
- *During a TENS therapy session, the patient reports muscle twitching:* Assess the patient and check the intensity setting. Readjust the intensity to a lower setting, because the patient is most likely experiencing overstimulation.
- *While assessing the skin where the electrodes are placed for a patient receiving continuous TENS therapy, you notice some irritation and redness:* Clean and dry the area thoroughly. Reposition the electrodes in the same area, but avoid the irritated and reddened area.

SPECIAL CONSIDERATIONS

- Because TENS is noninvasive, it is easy to discontinue if the patient does not feel it is helping manage pain (D'Arcy, 2011, p.34)
- Never place electrodes over the carotid sinus nerves, laryngeal or pharyngeal muscles, the eyes, or the uterus of a pregnant woman.
- Do not use TENS when the etiology of the pain is unknown because it may mask a new pathology.
- Whenever electrodes are being repositioned or removed, first turn off the unit.

SKILL 10-4 CARING FOR A PATIENT RECEIVING PATIENT-CONTROLLED ANALGESIA

Patient-controlled analgesia (PCA) allows patients to control the administration of their own medication within predetermined safety limits. This approach can be used with oral analgesic agents as well as with infusions of opioid analgesic agents by intravenous, subcutaneous, **epidural**, and **perineural routes** (Hinkle & Cheever, 2014; Cranwell-Bruce, 2009; D'Arcy, 2008a; Hicks et al., 2012). PCA provides effective individualized analgesia and comfort. This drug delivery system can be used to manage acute and chronic pain in a health care facility or the home.

The PCA pump permits the patient to self-administer medication (bolus doses) with episodes of increased pain or painful activities. A timing device electronically controls the PCA pump. The PCA

(*continued*)

SKILL 10-4 CARING FOR A PATIENT RECEIVING PATIENT-CONTROLLED ANALGESIA continued

system consists of a portable infusion pump containing a reservoir or chamber for a syringe or other reservoir that is prefilled with the prescribed medication, usually an opioid, or dilute anesthetic solutions in the case of epidural administration (Hinkle & Cheever, 2014; Cranwell-Bruce, 2009; D'Arcy, 2008a; Hicks et al., 2012). When pain occurs, the patient pushes a button that activates the PCA device to deliver a small, preset bolus dose of the analgesic. A lockout interval that is programmed into the PCA unit prevents reactivation of the pump and administration of another dose during that period of time. The pump mechanism can also be programmed to deliver only a specified amount of analgesic within a given time interval (basal rate; most commonly every hour or, occasionally, every 4 hours). These safeguards limit the risk for overmedication and allow the patient to evaluate the effect of the previous dose. PCA pumps also have a locked safety system that prohibits tampering with the device.

Nursing responsibilities for patients receiving medications via a PCA pump include patient/family teaching, initial device setup, monitoring the device to ensure proper functioning, and frequent assessment of the patient's response, including pain and discomfort control and presence of adverse effects (see Evidence for Practice). Box 10-1 outlines guidelines for safe and effective use of PCA. Additional information related to epidural infusions is discussed in Skill 10-5.

BOX 10-1 GUIDELINES FOR SAFE AND EFFECTIVE USE OF PATIENT-CONTROLLED ANALGESIA

Safe patient-controlled analgesia (PCA) use requires proper patient selection, education, assessment, and monitoring (D'Arcy, 2008a). Use the following tips as guidelines to ensure optimal patient comfort and safety when caring for patients receiving PCA.

- Be aware of patient groups who generally are not good candidates for PCA, including infants and young children, confused older adults; patients who are obese or have asthma or sleep apnea when their condition is a significant risk factor for oversedation; patients taking other drugs that potentiate opioids, such as muscle relaxants, antiemetics, and sleeping medications.
- Use standard medical order sets and prefilled syringes with standard drug concentrations.
- Check PCA orders ensuring that they include the medication, the dose, demand (bolus), and dose and lockout intervals.
- Be familiar with the particular PCA pumps in use at a facility. Use smart infusion pump technology, when possible.
- Ensure that PCA pumps are programmed correctly. Check pump settings at least once every 4 hours. Two nurses should verify PCA programming when initiating infusion or making a change in infusion settings.
- Place warning signs on all PCA pumps that say "For patient use only."
- Assess pain level, alertness, pulse oximetry, capnography, and vital signs, including respiratory rate and quality, at least every 4 hours or more often as needed, such as during the first 24 hours of treatment and at night, when nocturnal hypoxia may develop.
- Assess for sedation using minimal spoken and tactile stimulation.
- Teach patients and family members about the danger of PCA use by anyone other than the patient (PCA by proxy).
- Keep in mind that when the number of patient attempts to activate the PCA is twice the number of actual delivered doses, pain control may be inadequate. Consider increasing the dose according to standing orders or request an order for a dose increase or shorter dose interval.

(Adapted from Capnography: New standard of care for sedation? (2012). *OR Manager, 28*(3), 17–20; D'Arcy, Y. (2007). Eyeing capnography to improve PCA safety. *Nursing, 37*(9), 18–19; D'Arcy, Y. (2008a). Keep your patient safe during PCA. *Nursing, 38*(1), 50–55; The Joint Commission. (2012). *Sentinel event alert issue 49: Safe use of opioids in hospitals.* Available http://www.jointcommission.org/sea_issue_49/; and Institute for Safe Medication Practices (ISMP). (2006). *Patient-controlled analgesia: Making it safer for patients.* Available http://www.ismp.org/profdevelopment/PCAMonograph.pdf)

DELEGATION CONSIDERATIONS

The care related to patient-controlled analgesia is not delegated to nursing assistive personnel (NAP) or to unlicensed assistive personnel (UAP). Depending on the state's nurse practice act and the organization's policies and procedures, specific aspects of the care related to PCA, such as monitoring the infusion and assessment of patient response, may be delegated to licensed practical/vocational nurses (LPN/LVNs). The decision to delegate must be based on careful analysis of the patient's needs and circumstances, as well as the qualifications of the person to whom the task is being delegated. Refer to the Delegation Guidelines in Appendix A.

EQUIPMENT

- PCA system
- Syringe (or appropriate reservoir for device) filled with medication
- PCA system tubing
- Antimicrobial swabs

- Appropriate label for syringe and tubing, based on facility policy and procedure
- Second nurse to verify medication and programmed pump information, if necessary, according to facility policy
- Pain assessment tool and pain scale
- Computerized medication administration record (CMAR) or medication administration record (MAR)
- Gloves
- Additional PPE, as indicated

ASSESSMENT

Review the patient's medical record and plan of care for specific instructions related to PCA therapy, including the primary care provider's orders and conditions indicating the need for therapy. Check the medical order for the prescribed drug, initial loading dose, dose for self-administration, and lockout interval. Check to ensure proper functioning of the unit. Assess the patient's level of consciousness and understanding of PCA therapy and the rationale for its use.

Review the patient's history for conditions that might contraindicate therapy, such as respiratory limitations, history of substance abuse, or psychiatric disorder. Review the patient's medical record and assess for factors contributing to an increased risk for respiratory depression, such as the use of a basal infusion, the patient's age, obesity, upper abdominal or thoracic surgery, sleep apnea, history of smoking, concurrent CNS depressants, and impaired major organ functioning (The Joint Commission, 2012; Jarzyna et al., 2011). Determine the prescribed route for administration. Inspect the site to be used for the infusion for signs of infiltration or infection. If the route is via an IV infusion, ensure that the line is patent and the current solution is compatible with the drug ordered.

Assess the patient's pain and level of discomfort using an appropriate assessment tool and pain scale. (Refer to Fundamentals Review 10-1 through 10-6.) Assess the characteristics of any pain, and for other symptoms that often occur with the pain, such as headache or restlessness. Ask the patient what interventions have and have not been successful in the past to promote comfort and relieve pain. Assess the patient's vital signs. Assess the patient's respiratory status, including rate, depth, and rhythm; oxygen saturation level using pulse oximetry; and level of carbon dioxide concentration using capnography. Assess the patient's sedation score (Table 10-1). Determine the patient's response to the intervention to evaluate effectiveness and for the presence of adverse effects.

Table 10-1 PASERO OPIOID-INDUCED SEDATION SCALE (POSS)

PATIENT ASSESSMENT CHARACTERISTICS	SEDATION SCORE	ACTION
Sleeping, easy to arouse	S	
Awake and alert	1	No action needed
Slightly drowsy, easily aroused	2	No action needed
Frequently drowsy, arousable, drifts off during conversation	3	Requires action; decrease dose
Somnolent, minimal or no response to physical stimulation	4	Unacceptable, stop opioid, consider administering naloxone

(Used with permission. Copyright 1994, Chris Pasero. Pasero, C., & McCaffery, M. (2011). *Pain Assessment and Pharmacologic Management*, p. 510. St. Louis, Mosby/Elsevier.)

NURSING DIAGNOSIS

Determine the related factors for the nursing diagnoses based on the patient's current status. Appropriate nursing diagnoses may include:

- Acute Pain
- Chronic Pain
- Deficient Knowledge

OUTCOME IDENTIFICATION AND PLANNING

The expected outcome to achieve is that the patient reports increased comfort and/or decreased pain, without adverse effects, oversedation, and respiratory depression. Other appropriate outcomes may include the patient displays decreased anxiety, improved coping skills, and an understanding of the therapy and the reason for its use.

(*continued*)

SKILL 10-4 CARING FOR A PATIENT RECEIVING PATIENT-CONTROLLED ANALGESIA continued

IMPLEMENTATION

ACTION	RATIONALE
1. Gather equipment. Check the medication order against the original order in the medical record, according to facility policy. Clarify any inconsistencies. Check the patient's medical record for allergies.	This comparison helps to identify errors that may have occurred when orders were transcribed. The physician's order is the legal record-of-medication order for each agency.
2. Know the actions, special nursing considerations, safe dose ranges, purpose of administration, and adverse effects of the medications to be administered. Consider the appropriateness of the medication for this patient.	This knowledge aids the nurse in evaluating the therapeutic effect of the medication in relation to the patient's disorder and can also be used to educate the patient about the medication.
3. Prepare the medication syringe or other container for administration, based on facility policy. (See Chapter 5 for additional information.)	Proper preparation and administration procedures prevent errors.
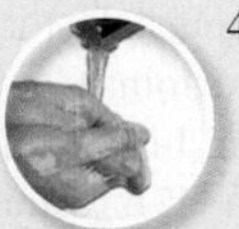 4. Perform hand hygiene and put on PPE, if indicated.	Hand hygiene and PPE prevent the spread of microorganisms. PPE is required based on transmission precautions.
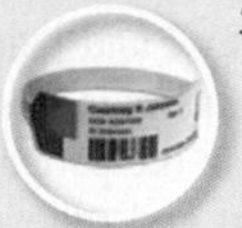 5. Identify the patient.	Identifying the patient ensures that the right patient receives the intervention and helps prevent errors.
6. Show the patient the device, and explain its function and the reason for use. Explain the purpose and action of the medication to the patient.	Explanation encourages patient understanding and cooperation and reduces apprehension.
7. Plug the PCA device into the electrical outlet, if necessary. Check status of battery power, if appropriate.	The PCA device requires a power source (electricity or battery) to run. Most units will alarm to acknowledge a low battery state.
8. Close the door to the room or pull the bedside curtain.	Closing the door or pulling the curtain provides patient privacy.
9. Complete necessary assessments before administering medication. Check allergy bracelet or ask patient about allergies. Assess the patient's pain, using an appropriate assessment tool and measurement scale. (See Fundamentals Review 10-1 through 10-6.)	Assessment is a prerequisite to medication administration. Accurate assessment is necessary to guide treatment and relief interventions and to evaluate the effectiveness of pain control measures.
10. **Check the label on the prefilled drug syringe or reservoir with the medication record and patient identification (Figure 1).** Obtain verification of information from a second nurse, according to facility policy.	This action verifies that the correct drug and dosage will be administered to the correct patient. Confirmation of information by a second nurse helps prevent errors (D'Arcy, 2008a).

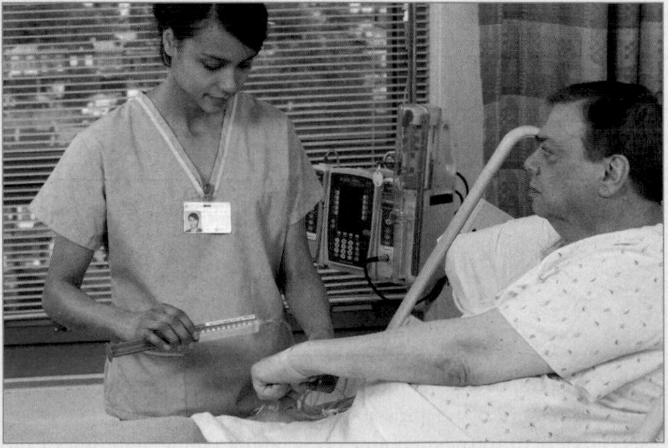

FIGURE 1 Checking label on prefilled drug syringe with patient identification.

ACTION	RATIONALE
11. Scan the patient's barcode on the identification band, if required.	This provides an additional check to ensure that the medication is given to the right patient.
12. Connect tubing to prefilled syringe and place the syringe into the PCA device (Figure 2). **Prime the tubing.**	Doing so prepares the device to deliver the drug. Priming the tubing purges air from the tubing and reduces the risk for air embolism.
13. Set the PCA device to administer the loading dose, if ordered, and then program the device based on the medical order for medication dosage, dose interval, and lockout interval (Figure 3). Obtain verification of information from a second nurse, according to facility policy.	These actions ensure that the appropriate drug dosage will be administered. Confirmation of information by a second nurse helps prevent errors.
14. Put on gloves. Using an antimicrobial swab, clean connection port on IV infusion line or other site access, based on route of administration. Connect the PCA tubing to the patient's IV infusion line or appropriate access site, based on the specific site used. Secure the site per facility policy and procedure. Remove gloves. Initiate the therapy by activating the appropriate button on the pump. Lock the PCA device, per facility policy.	Gloves prevent contact with blood and body fluids. Cleaning the connection port reduces the risk of infection. Connection and initiation are necessary to allow drug delivery to the patient. Locking the device prevents tampering with the settings.
15. Remind the patient to press the button each time he or she needs relief from pain (Figure 4).	Instruction promotes correct use of the device.

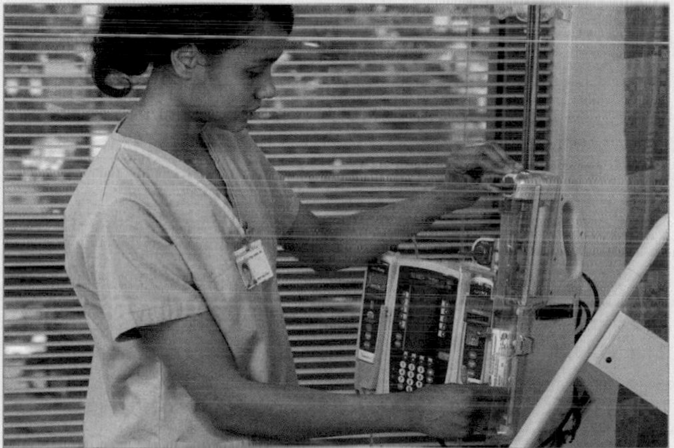

FIGURE 2 Placing syringe into PCA device.

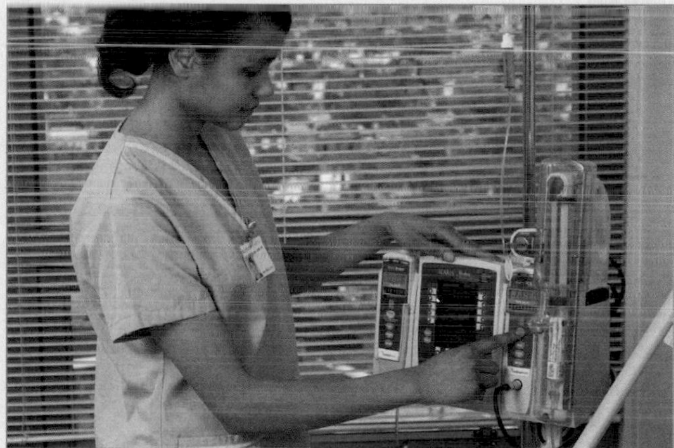

FIGURE 3 Programming PCA device.

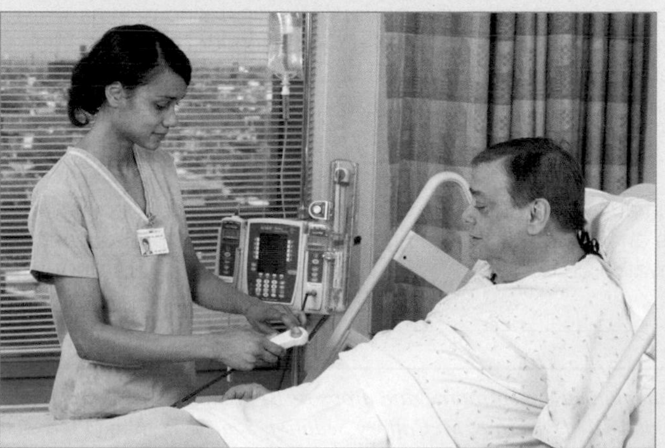

FIGURE 4 Reminding patient to press button to administer pain medication.

(*continued*)

SKILL 10-4 CARING FOR A PATIENT RECEIVING PATIENT-CONTROLLED ANALGESIA continued

ACTION	RATIONALE
16. Assess the patient's pain at least every 4 hours or more often, as needed, based on patient's individual risk factors. Monitor vital signs, especially respiratory status, including oxygen saturation at least every 4 hours or more often, as needed, based on patient's individual risk factors.	Continued assessment at frequent intervals helps evaluate the effectiveness of the drug and reduce the risk for complications (Jarzyna et al., 2011; D'Arcy, 2008a; D'Arcy, 2007a).
17. Assess the patient's sedation score (Table 10-1) and end-tidal carbon dioxide level (capnography) at least every 4 hours or more often, as needed, based on patient's individual risk factors.	Sedation occurs before clinically significant respiratory depression (D'Arcy, 2008a). Respiratory depression can occur with the use of narcotic analgesics. Capnography is a more reliable indicator of respiratory depression (Capnography, 2012; Hicks et al., 2012; Jarzyna et al., 2011; Johnson et al., 2011).
18. Assess the infusion site periodically, according to facility policy and nursing judgment. Assess the patient's use of the medication, noting number of attempts and number of doses delivered. Replace the drug syringe when it is empty.	Continued assessment of the infusion site is necessary for early detection of problems. Continued assessment of the patient's use of medication and effect is necessary to ensure adequate pain control without adverse effect. Replacing the syringe ensures continued drug delivery.
19. Make sure the patient control (dosing button) is within the patient's reach.	Easy access to the control is essential for the patients to use the device.
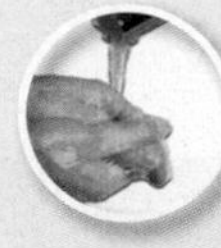 20. Remove gloves and additional PPE, if used. Perform hand hygiene.	Removing PPE properly reduces the risk for infection transmission and contamination of other items. Hand hygiene prevents transmission of microorganisms.

EVALUATION

The expected outcome is achieved when the patient reports increased comfort and/or decreased pain, without adverse effects, oversedation, and respiratory depression; the patient displays decreased anxiety and improved coping skills; and the patient verbalizes an understanding of the therapy and the reason for its use.

DOCUMENTATION

Guidelines

Document the date and time PCA therapy was initiated, initial pain assessment, drug and loading dose administered, if appropriate, and individual dosing and time interval. Document continued pain, sedation level, vital signs and assessments, and patient's response to therapy.

Sample Documentation

6/1/15 0645 Patient returned from surgery with PCA therapy with morphine sulfate 1 mg/mL in place via IV infusion. Device programmed to deliver 0.1 mg at 10-minute lockout intervals. Patient complaining of moderate to severe abdominal pain, rating pain as 6–8/10 on a pain rating scale. Patient instructed to press PCA button for pain relief. Vital signs within acceptable parameters. Respiratory rate 16 breaths per minute. Oxygen saturation 96%; partial pressure end-tidal CO_2 ($PetCO_2$) 36%. IV of 1,000 mL D5LR infusing at 100 mL/min; IV site clean and dry without evidence of infiltration or infection.

—*P. Joyner, RN*

6/1/15 0700 Patient rates pain at 4/10. Respirations 16 breaths per minute. Encouraged patient to take deep breaths and cough. Lying on right side with the support of two pillows and head of bed elevated 30 degrees.

—*P. Joyner, RN*

UNEXPECTED SITUATIONS AND ASSOCIATED INTERVENTIONS

- *While receiving PCA therapy, the patient's respiratory rate drops to 10 breaths per minute, with a sedation score of 3 via sedation scale (Pasero & McCaffery Sedation Scale):* Stop the PCA infusion if basal infusion is present. Notify the primary care provider. Discontinue the basal infusion; if no basal infusion is being used, then reduce the medication dosage. Increase the frequency of sedation and respiratory rate monitoring to every 15 minutes. Arouse the patient every 15 minutes and encourage deep breathing (D'Arcy, 2008a; Chumbley & Mountford, 2010; Jarzyna et al., 2011; Pasero & McCaffery, 2005a).

- *While receiving PCA therapy, the patient is somnolent, with a sedation score of 4 via sedation scale (Pasero & McCaffery Sedation Scale):* Stop the medication infusion immediately. Notify the primary care provider. Prepare to administer oxygen and a narcotic antagonist, such as naloxone (Narcan). Because naloxone reverses all analgesia, as well as the respiratory depression, patients will experience extremely severe pain once awake and alert (D'Arcy, 2008a; Pasero & McCaffery, 2005a).
- *The patient's IV infusion line becomes infiltrated:* Stop the PCA infusion and IV infusion. Remove the IV catheter and restart the IV line in another site. Once the site is established, resume the IV and PCA infusion.
- *The patient's subcutaneous infusion site becomes infiltrated:* Stop the PCA infusion. Remove the administration device. Obtain new administration equipment and restart the infusion at another site. Once the site is established, resume the PCA infusion.

SPECIAL CONSIDERATIONS

General Considerations

- A wide variety of PCA devices are available on the market. Check the manufacturer's instructions before using the device.
- Adults and children who are cognitively and physically able to use the PCA equipment and are able to understand that pressing a button can result in pain relief are appropriate candidates for PCA therapy (D'Arcy, 2008a; Pasero & McCaffery, 2011).
- The analgesic administered most often administered PCA is an opioid, which causes sedation before respiratory depression. A sedated patient cannot self-administer a dose, reducing the risk of an overdose (D'Arcy, 2008a; Pasero & McCaffery, 2005a).
- Family members and nurses may need to remind the patient to push the button. If someone other than the patient delivers a dose, the risk for oversedation is increased (D'Arcy, 2008a; Pasero & McCaffery, 2005a; Wuhrman et al., 2007).
- Some facilities have developed clinical practice guidelines for **authorized agent-controlled analgesia (AACA).** In these cases, one family member (**caregiver-controlled analgesia [CCA]**) or primary nurse (**nurse-controlled analgesia [NCA]**) is designated as the primary pain manager and only that person can press the PCA button for the patient. In the case of family members, the primary pain manager must be chosen carefully and taught to asses for pain and the adverse effect of the medication. Additionally, nursing staff must be vigilant in assessing the patient's need for and response to the medication, following the same assessment guidelines previously discussed. It is very important to follow facility guidelines to ensure safe administration (D'Arcy, 2007a; Pasero & McCaffery, 2005a; Wuhrman et al., 2007). Box 10-2 outlines guidelines for safe implementation of AACA.

BOX 10-2 GUIDELINES FOR SAFE IMPLEMENTATION OF AUTHORIZED AGENT-CONTROLLED ANALGESIA

Authorized agent-controlled analgesia (AACA) can be implemented to provide prompt, safe, and effective pain relief for the patient who, because of cognitive or physical limitations, is unable to self-administer analgesics using an analgesic pump (Wuhrman et al., 2007). Use the following tips as guidelines to ensure optimal patient comfort and safety when caring for patients receiving AACA.

- Limit the number of authorized agents to one at a given time; alternative authorized agents may be designated to provide respite and/or coverage.
- Use standard AACA medical order sets.
- Provide patient and family education regarding the principles of AACA, requirements of an authorized agent, specific policies and procedures related to AACA, and the negative consequences of unauthorized activation of the analgesic infusion pump dosing button.
- Document the identity of the authorized agent(s) and caregiver authorized agent, as well as education provided and feedback.
- Ensure that authorized agents only activate the dosing button if the patient is awake and/or the patient's words or behavior indicate that the patient is in pain or pain is anticipated. Authorized agents should verbalize an understanding of how to recognize pain, sedation, and respiratory depression.

(Adapted with permission from Wuhrman, E., Cooney, M., Dunwoody, C., et al. (2007). Authorized and unauthorized ("PCA by proxy") dosing of analgesic infusion pumps: Position statement with clinical practice recommendations. *Pain Management Nursing, 8*(1), 4–11.)

(*continued*)

SKILL 10-4 CARING FOR A PATIENT RECEIVING PATIENT-CONTROLLED ANALGESIA continued

- If using a device that provides continuous and bolus doses, the cumulative doses per hour should not exceed the total hourly dose ordered by the physician.
- Vital-sign monitoring is crucial, especially when initiating therapy. Encourage the patient to practice coughing and deep breathing to promote ventilation and prevent pooling of secretions.
- A narcotic antagonist, such as naloxone (Narcan), must be readily available in case the patient develops respiratory complications related to drug therapy.
- A fentanyl patient-controlled transdermal system (PCTS) is another patient-controlled delivery technique for pain medication. The small device contains the medication in a reservoir in a patch that attaches to the patient's upper arm or chest with adhesive. When the patient pushes the button on the device, the medication is delivered by iontophoresis, an electrical current that introduces the medication into the tissues. The device is preprogrammed to deliver fixed 40-µg doses of fentanyl. Each patch holds 80 doses, with a minimum time between doses of 10 minutes. The device will deliver the maximum 80 doses or will operate for 24 hours from the first dose, whichever occurs first. The patch then shuts off. If continued use is required, it is replaced with a new device, in another location. It is not for use in patients with burns or patients with implanted devices, such as cardioverter defibrillators or demand (Gevirtz, 2010a).

Infant and Child Considerations

- PCA can be an effective method of pain control for a child. When determining the appropriateness of this therapy for a child, consider the child's chronologic age and developmental level, ability to understand (cognitive level), and motor skills (Pasero & McCaffery, 2011).
- PCA has been shown to be very effective for adolescents because it gives them an increased feeling of control over the situation.

Home Care Considerations

- Be sure that the patient understands how to use the PCA device properly. Teach the patient how the device works, when to contact the physician, and signs and symptoms of adverse reactions and of drug tolerance.
- Advise the patient to change positions gradually to prevent orthostatic hypotension, which can result from use of a narcotic analgesic.
- Ensure that a reliable adult is available who can provide backup assistance should the patient have difficulty.
- Consider a referral to a home health care agency to continue teaching and provide assessment of the therapy.

EVIDENCE FOR PRACTICE ▶

PATIENT KNOWLEDGE AND PCA

Explanation encourages patient understanding and cooperation and reduces apprehension. It is important that patients and their caregivers have accurate and appropriate information to achieve optimal pain relief and prevent adverse effects. PCA therapy is not always universally effective in providing high-quality analgesia for postoperative patients. Inadequate preoperative patient education regarding the optimal use of the PCA approach to postoperative analgesia is thought to contribute to the lack of adequate pain management. What effect does preoperative patient education regarding PCA use have on postoperative pain control?

Related Research

Hong, S.J., & Lee, E. (2012). Effects of a structured educational programme on patient-controlled analgesia (PCA) for gynaecological patients in South Korea. *Journal of Clinical Nursing, 21*(23/24), 3546–3555.

This study evaluated the effects of a structured educational program on the PCA device related to postoperative pain, doses of analgesics used, adverse reactions, patient knowledge and attitudes of PCA, and patient satisfaction with postoperative pain management among gynecologic patients in South Korea. Participants were patients receiving gynecologic surgery under general anesthesia. Patients were assigned to the experimental group and to the control group. A day before surgery, 40 minutes of structured education on the PCA device was provided individually to the patients in the experimental group using computer-based information and a brochure. Pain level and adverse reactions were significantly lower in the experimental group than in the control group. In addition, the analgesic dose administered and the level of patient satisfaction with postoperative pain management increased significantly in the experimental group compared with the control group. The authors concluded a structured educational program related to PCA can be an effective nursing intervention for pain management for gynecologic patients.

Relevance to Nursing Practice

Patient education is an important nursing responsibility and preoperative education seems to improve the patient's knowledge regarding PCA and pain management. Nursing interventions to decrease the number of problems related to PCA should be adopted into clinical practice. Nurses should provide patient education related to PCA to increase knowledge of pain management, improved postoperative pain management, and patient satisfaction with pain management, as well as more effective management of adverse reactions caused by PCA.

Refer to thePoint for additional research on related nursing topics.

SKILL 10-5 CARING FOR A PATIENT RECEIVING EPIDURAL ANALGESIA

Epidural analgesia is being used more commonly to provide pain relief during the immediate postoperative phase (particularly after thoracic, abdominal, orthopedic, and vascular surgery), procedural pain, trauma pain, and for chronic pain situations (Sawhney, 2012). Epidural pain management is also being used with infants and children (Kyle & Carman, 2013). The anesthesiologist or radiologist usually inserts the catheter in the mid-lumbar region into the epidural space that exists between the walls of the vertebral canal and the dura mater or outermost connective tissue membrane surrounding the spinal cord. For temporary therapy, the catheter exits directly over the spine, and the tubing is positioned over the patient's shoulder with the end of the catheter taped to the chest. For long-term therapy, the catheter is usually tunneled subcutaneously and exits on the side of the body or on the abdomen (Figure 1).

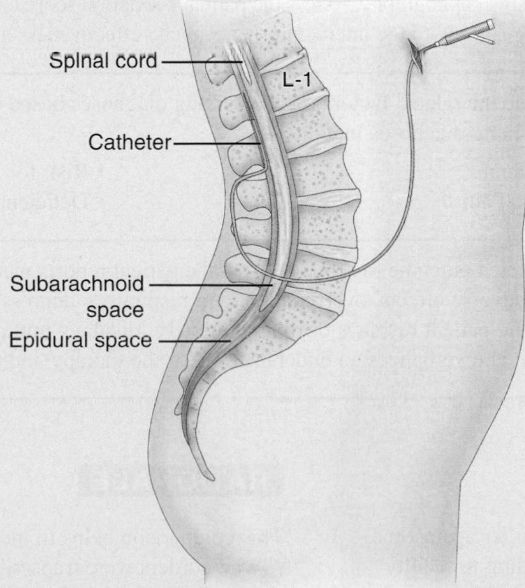

FIGURE 1 Placement of an epidural catheter for long-term use.

(continued)

SKILL 10-5 CARING FOR A PATIENT RECEIVING EPIDURAL ANALGESIA continued

The epidural analgesia can be administered as a bolus dose (either one time or intermittently), via a continuous infusion pump, or by a patient-controlled epidural analgesia (PCEA) pump (Taylor et al., 2015) (see Evidence for Practice). Additional information specific to PCA administration was discussed in Skill 10-4. Epidural catheters used for the management of acute pain are typically removed 36 to 72 hours after surgery, when oral medication can be substituted for pain relief.

DELEGATION CONSIDERATIONS

The care related to epidural analgesia is not delegated to nursing assistive personnel (NAP) or to unlicensed assistive personnel (UAP). Depending on the state's nurse practice act and the organization's policies and procedures, specific aspects of the care related to epidural analgesia, such as monitoring the infusion and assessment of patient response, may be delegated to licensed practical/vocational nurses (LPN/LVNs). The decision to delegate must be based on careful analysis of the patient's needs and circumstances, as well as the qualifications of the person to whom the task is being delegated. Refer to the Delegation Guidelines in Appendix A.

EQUIPMENT

- Volume infusion device
- Epidural infusion tubing
- Prescribed epidural analgesic solutions
- Computerized medication administration record (CMAR) or medication administration record (MAR)
- Pain assessment tool and/or measurement scale
- Transparent dressing or gauze pads
- Labels for epidural infusion line
- Tape
- Emergency drugs and equipment, such as naloxone, oxygen, endotracheal intubation set, handheld resuscitation bag, per facility policy
- Gloves
- Additional PPE, as indicated

ASSESSMENT

Review the patient's medical record and plan of care for specific instructions related to epidural analgesia therapy, including the medical order for the drug and conditions indicating the need for therapy. Review the patient's history for conditions that might contraindicate therapy, such as local or systemic infections, increased intracranial pressure, neurologic disease, coagulopathy or use of anticoagulant therapy, spinal arthritis or spinal deformity, hypotension, marked hypertension, allergy to the prescribed medication, or psychiatric disorder. Check to ensure proper functioning of the unit. Assess the patient's level of consciousness and understanding of epidural analgesia therapy and the rationale for its use.

Assess the patient's level of discomfort and pain using an appropriate assessment tool. Assess the characteristics of any pain. Assess for other symptoms that often occur with the pain, such as headache or restlessness. Ask the patient what interventions have and have not been successful in the past to promote comfort and relieve pain. Assess the patient's vital signs and respiratory status, including rate, depth, and rhythm, oxygen saturation level using pulse oximetry, and level of carbon dioxide concentration using capnography. Assess the patient's sedation score (see Table 10-1 in Skill 10-4). Assess the patient's response to the intervention to evaluate effectiveness and for the presence of adverse effects.

NURSING DIAGNOSIS

Determine the related factors for the nursing diagnoses based on the patient's current status. Appropriate nursing diagnoses may include:

- Acute Pain
- Chronic Pain
- Risk for Infection
- Deficient Knowledge

OUTCOME IDENTIFICATION AND PLANNING

The expected outcome to achieve is that the patient reports increased comfort and/or decreased pain, without adverse effects, oversedation, and respiratory depression. Other appropriate outcomes may include the patient displays decreased anxiety; displays improved coping skills; remains free from infection; and verbalizes an understanding of the therapy and the reason for its use.

IMPLEMENTATION

ACTION	RATIONALE
1. Gather equipment. Check the medication order against the original order in the medical record, according to facility policy. Clarify any inconsistencies. Check the patient's medical record for allergies.	This comparison helps to identify errors that may have occurred when orders were transcribed. The medical order is the legal record-of-medication order for each agency.

ACTION	RATIONALE
2. Know the actions, special nursing considerations, safe dose ranges, purpose of administration, and adverse effects of the medications to be administered. Consider the appropriateness of the medication for this patient.	This knowledge aids the nurse in evaluating the therapeutic effect of the medication in relation to the patient's disorder and can also be used to educate the patient about the medication.
3. Prepare the medication syringe or other container for administration, based on facility policy. (See Chapter 5 for additional information.)	Proper preparation and administration prevents errors.
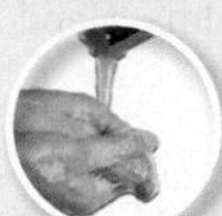 4. Perform hand hygiene and put on PPE, if indicated.	Hand hygiene and PPE prevent the spread of microorganisms. PPE is required based on transmission precautions.
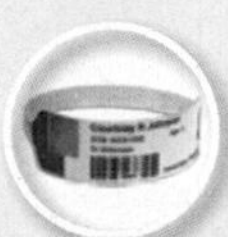 5. Identify the patient.	Identifying the patient ensures that the right patient receives the intervention and helps prevent errors.
6. Show the patient the device, and explain the function of the device and the reason for its use. Explain the purpose and action of the medication to the patient.	Explanation encourages patient understanding and cooperation and reduces apprehension.
7. Close the door to the room or pull the bedside curtain.	Closing the door or curtain provides patient privacy.
8. Complete necessary assessments before administering the medication. Check allergy bracelet or ask the patient about allergies. Assess the patient's pain, using an appropriate assessment tool and measurement scale. (See Fundamentals Review 10-1 through 10-6.) Put on gloves.	Assessment is a prerequisite to administration of medications. Accurate assessment is necessary to guide treatment and relief interventions and to evaluate the effectiveness of pain control measures. Gloves are indicated for potential contact with blood or body fluids.
9. **Have an ampule of 0.4 mg naloxone (Narcan) and a syringe at the bedside.**	Naloxone reverses the respiratory depressant effect of opioids.
10. After the catheter has been inserted and the infusion initiated by the anesthesiologist or radiologist, **check the label on the medication container and rate of infusion with the medication record and patient identification (Figure 2).** Obtain verification of information from a second nurse, according to facility policy. If using a barcode administration system, scan the barcode on the medication label, if required.	This action verifies that the correct drug and dosage will be administered to the correct patient. Confirmation of information by a second nurse helps prevent errors. Scanning the barcode provides an additional check to ensure that the medication is given to the right patient.

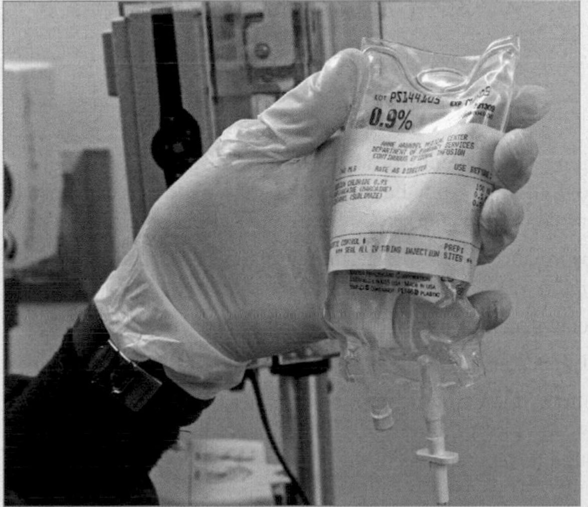

FIGURE 2 Checking label on medication container.

(*continued*)

SKILL 10-5 CARING FOR A PATIENT RECEIVING EPIDURAL ANALGESIA continued

ACTION	RATIONALE
11. Tape all connection sites. Label the bag, tubing, and pump apparatus "For Epidural Infusion Only." **Do not administer any other narcotics or adjuvant drugs without the approval of the clinician responsible for the epidural injection.**	Taping prevents accidental dislodgement. Labeling prevents inadvertent administration of other IV medications through this setup. Additional medication may potentiate the action of the opioid, increasing the risk for respiratory depression.
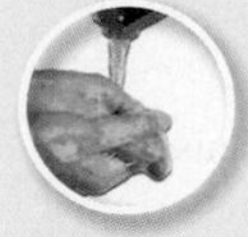 12. Assess the catheter exit site and apply a transparent dressing over the catheter insertion site, if not already in place (Figure 3). Remove gloves and additional PPE, if used. Perform hand hygiene.	The transparent dressing protects the site while still allowing assessment. Removing PPE properly reduces the risk for infection transmission and contamination of other items. Hand hygiene reduces transmission of microorganisms.

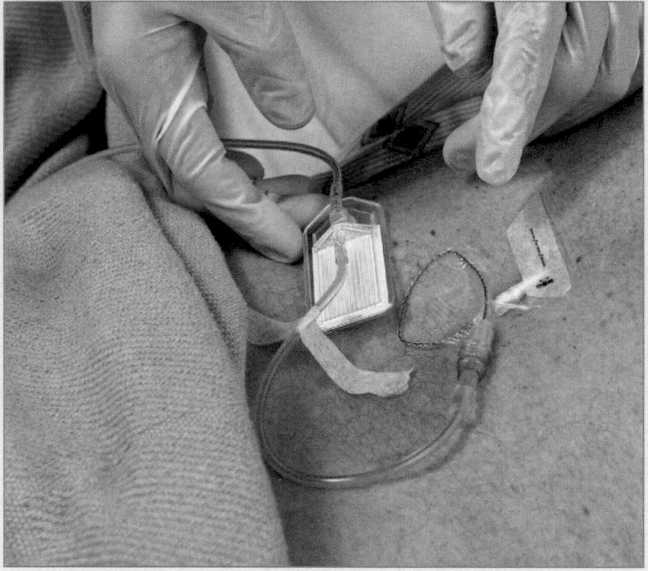

FIGURE 3 Assessing exit site.

ACTION	RATIONALE
13. Monitor the infusion rate according to facility policy. Assess and record sedation level (see Table 10-1 in Skill 10-4) and respiratory status, including the patient's oxygen saturation, continuously for the first 20 minutes after initiation, then at least every hour for the first 12 hours, every 2 hours up to 24 hours, then at 4-hour intervals (or according to facility policy) (Sawhney, 2012). **Notify the physician if the sedation rating is 3 or 4, the respiratory depth decreases, or the respiratory rate falls below 10 breaths per minute.** Also monitor end-tidal carbon dioxide level (capnography) for patients at high risk of respiratory depression (Sawhney, 2012).	Monitoring the infusion rate prevents incorrect administration of the medication. Opioids can depress the respiratory center in the medulla. A change in the level of consciousness is usually the first sign of altered respiratory function.
14. Keep the head of bed elevated 30 degrees unless contraindicated.	Elevation of the patient's head minimizes upward migration of the opioid in the spinal cord, thus decreasing the risk for respiratory depression.
15. Assess the patient's level of pain and the effectiveness of pain relief.	This information helps in determining the need for subsequent *breakthrough* pain medication.
16. Monitor the patient's blood pressure and pulse.	Hypotension can result from the use of epidural analgesia.
17. Monitor urinary output and assess for bladder distention.	Opioids can cause urinary retention.
18. Assess motor strength and sensation every 4 hours.	The catheter may migrate into the intrathecal space and allow opioids to block the transmission of nerve impulses completely through the spinal cord to the brain.

ACTION	RATIONALE
19. Monitor for adverse effects (pruritus, nausea, and vomiting).	Opioids may spread into the trigeminal nerve, causing itching, or resulting in nausea and vomiting owing to slowed gastrointestinal function or stimulation of a chemoreceptor trigger zone in the brain. Medications are available to treat these adverse effects.
20. Assess for signs of infection at the insertion site.	Inflammation or local infection can develop at the catheter insertion site.
21. Assess the catheter-site dressing for drainage, based on facility policy. Notify the anesthesia provider or pain management team immediately of any abnormalities. Change the dressing over the catheter exit site per facility policy using aseptic technique. Change the infusion tubing every 48 hours or as specified by facility policy.	Catheter-site dressing should remain clean, dry, and intact. Abnormalities in the dressing may indicate leakage of cerebrospinal fluid or catheter dislodgement. Dressing and tubing changes using aseptic technique reduce the risk for infection.

EVALUATION

The expected outcome is achieved when the patient verbalizes pain relief. In addition, the patient exhibits a dry, intact dressing, and the catheter exit site is free of signs and symptoms of complications, injury, or infection. The patient reports a decrease in anxiety and increased ability to cope with pain. The patient verbalizes information related to the functioning of the epidural catheter and the reasons for its use.

DOCUMENTATION

Guidelines

Document catheter patency; the condition of the insertion site and dressing; sedation score, oxygen saturation, vital signs, and assessment information; any change in infusion rate, solution, or tubing; analgesics administered; and the patient's response.

Sample Documentation

6/3/15 0935 Continuous morphine infusion via epidural catheter in place; see medication administration record. Exit site clean and slightly moist. Transparent dressing in place. Patient rates pain 2/10. Temperature 98.2°F; pulse, 76 beats per minute; respirations 16 breaths per minute and effortless; blood pressure, 110/70 mm Hg. Pulse oximetry 96% on oxygen via nasal cannula at 2 L/min. Patient alert and quickly responds to verbal stimuli. Sedation score of 1. Bladder nonpalpable; urine output of 100 mL over the last 2 hours. Denies nausea, vomiting, or itching. Able to detect sensation of cold in lower extremities bilaterally. Able to wiggle toes and flex and dorsiflex feet bilaterally. Lower extremity muscle strength equal and moderately strong bilaterally.

—T. James, RN

UNEXPECTED SITUATIONS AND ASSOCIATED INTERVENTIONS

- *While receiving epidural analgesia, the patient's sedation score drops below 3 and/or has a respiratory rate of ≤8 breaths, or has shallow respirations:* Immediately notify the anesthesiologist. Stop the epidural infusion, if indicated, according to facility procedure. Encourage the patient to take deep, slow breaths, if possible. Prepare to administer oxygen and a narcotic antagonist, such as naloxone (Narcan), via a peripheral IV site.
- *The patient demonstrates weakness and loss of sensation in the lower extremities while receiving epidural analgesia:* Reassess the patient's lower extremities for motor and sensory function. If positive for sensorimotor loss, notify the physician and expect to decrease the epidural infusion.
- *While receiving epidural analgesia, the patient suddenly develops a severe headache. Inspection of the catheter site reveals clear drainage on the dressing:* Stop the epidural infusion and notify the physician immediately. The catheter may have migrated and entered the dura.

SPECIAL CONSIDERATIONS

- Notify the anesthesiologist or pain management team immediately if the patient exhibits any of the following: respiratory rate below 10 breaths per minute, continued complaints of unmanaged pain, leakage at the insertion site, fever, inability to void, paresthesia, itching, or headache (Roman & Cabaj, 2005).

(continued)

SKILL 10-5 CARING FOR A PATIENT RECEIVING EPIDURAL ANALGESIA continued

- Do not administer other sedatives or analgesics unless ordered by the anesthesiologist or pain management team to avoid oversedation (Roman & Cabaj, 2005).
- Always ensure that the patient receiving epidural analgesia has a peripheral IV line in place, either as a continuous IV infusion or as an intermittent infusion device, to allow immediate administration of emergency drugs, if warranted.
- Keep in mind that drugs given via the epidural route diffuse slowly and can cause adverse reactions, including excessive sedation, for up to 12 hours after the infusion has been discontinued.
- Typically, an anesthesiologist orders analgesics and removes the catheter. However, facility policy may allow a specially trained nurse to remove the catheter.
- Be aware that no resistance should be felt during the removal of an epidural catheter.

EVIDENCE FOR PRACTICE ▶

PATIENT KNOWLEDGE AND PCA

Postoperative pain after cesarean birth, a major postpartum problem, contributes to decreased mobility (increasing risk of thromboembolic disease) and interferes with effective breastfeeding and infant caring activities and interactions. For women who plan to breastfeed, early initiation and experiences during the days after birth influence the continuation and success of breastfeeding. Many options exist to provide analgesia after a cesarean birth. Is there a better way to provide effective pain management and support effective, successful breastfeeding?

Related Research

Woods, A.B., Crist, B., Kowalewski, S., et al. (2012). A cross-sectional analysis of the effect of patient-controlled epidural analgesia versus patient controlled analgesia on postcesarean pain and breastfeeding. *Journal of Obstetric, Gynecologic & Neonatal Nursing, 41*(3), 339–346.

This retrospective study assesses the effectiveness of pain management (patient controlled epidural analgesia [PCEA] versus patient controlled analgesia [PCA] postcesarean birth and to determine the impact of these postoperative analgesic interventions on breastfeeding behavior in the first 24 hours postpartum. Medical records for all women with cesarean births of at least 34 weeks gestational age during one year (621 patients) were examined and analyzed. Women with PCEA reported significantly less average pain and required significantly less analgesic adjuvant medication doses than women with PCA. Statistically significant negative correlations were found for average total pain score with number of breastfeeding sessions. Women with PCEA experienced milder pain compared with PCA. Women with mild pain, a term neonate, breastfeeding within 2 hours, and no supplemental feedings had significantly greater odds of breastfeeding six or more times in the first 24 hours. The authors concluded PCEA provides greater pain control compared with PCA and women with less pain breastfeed sooner and more frequently than women with greater pain levels in the first 24 hours postcesarean. Women with greater pain are less likely to breastfeed six or more times within the first 24 hours and this could potentially affect success and duration of breastfeeding.

Relevance to Nursing Practice

The importance of adequate maternal pain management postcesarean birth is crucial for mothers and neonates and an important nursing responsibility. Adequate pain management results in greater odds of more frequent breastfeeding in the first 24 hours postpartum. Nurses should work to provide a comprehensive, interdisciplinary approach toward improving maternal and neonatal outcomes postcesarean birth.

Refer to thePoint for additional research on related nursing topics.

SKILL 10-6 CARING FOR A PATIENT RECEIVING CONTINUOUS WOUND PERFUSION PAIN MANAGEMENT

Continuous wound perfusion pain management systems deliver a continuous infusion of local analgesia to surgical wound beds. These systems are used as an adjuvant in the management of postoperative pain in a wide range of surgical procedures, such as cardiothoracic and orthopedic procedures. The system consists of a balloon type pump filled with local anesthetic and a catheter placed near an incision, in a nerve close to a surgical site, or in a wound bed (Figure 1). The catheter delivers a consistent flow rate and uniform distribution to the surgical site. Continuous wound perfusion catheters decrease postoperative pain and opioid use and side effects, and have been associated with decreased postoperative nausea and vomiting (D'Arcy, 2012; Charous, 2008). The catheter is placed during surgery and is not sutured into place; the site dressing holds it in place.

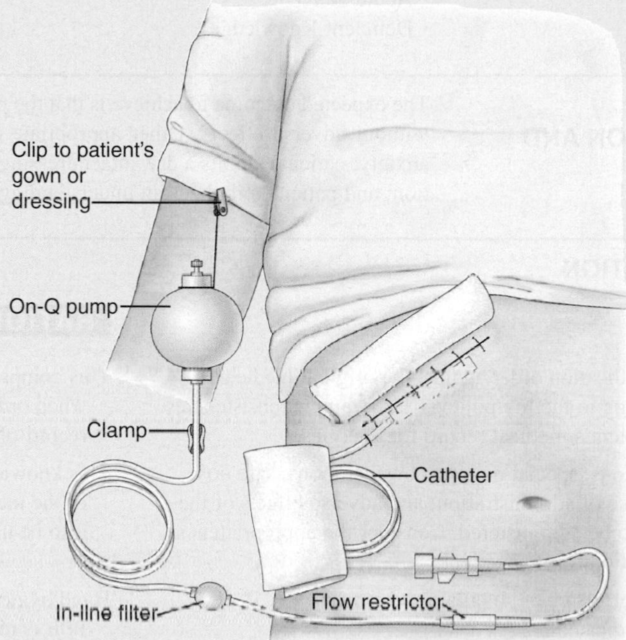

FIGURE 1 Wound perfusion pain management system consists of a balloon (pump), filter, and catheter that delivers a specific amount of prescribed local anesthetic at the rate determined by the prescriber. (Redrawn from I-Flow LLC, a Kimberly-Clark Health Care Company, with permission.)

DELEGATION CONSIDERATIONS

Care related to continuous wound perfusion pain management systems is not delegated to nursing assistive personnel (NAP) or to unlicensed assistive personnel (UAP). Depending on the state's nurse practice act and the organization's policies and procedures, specific aspects of the care related to continuous wound perfusion pain management systems, such as monitoring the infusion and assessment of patient response, may be delegated to licensed practical/vocational nurses (LPN/LVNs). The decision to delegate must be based on careful analysis of the patient's needs and circumstances, as well as the qualifications of the person to whom the task is being delegated. Refer to the Delegation Guidelines in Appendix A.

EQUIPMENT

- Computerized medication administration record (CMAR) or medication administration record (MAR)
- Pain assessment tool and pain scale
- Gauze and tape, or other dressing, based on facility policy
- Gloves
- Additional PPE, as indicated

ASSESSMENT

Review the patient's medical record and plan of care for specific instructions related to continuous perfusion analgesia therapy, including the medical order for the drug and conditions indicating the need for therapy. Review the patient's history for allergy to the prescribed medication. Assess the patient's understanding of a continuous wound perfusion pain management system and the rationale

(continued)

SKILL 10-6 CARING FOR A PATIENT RECEIVING CONTINUOUS WOUND PERFUSION PAIN MANAGEMENT continued

for its use. Assess the patient's level of discomfort and pain using an appropriate assessment tool. Assess the characteristics of any pain. Assess for other symptoms that often occur with the pain, such as headache or restlessness. Assess the surgical site (see Chapter 8). Assess the catheter insertion site dressing. Assess the patient's vital signs and respiratory status, including rate, depth, and rhythm, and oxygen saturation level using pulse oximetry. Assess the patient's response to the intervention to evaluate its effectiveness and for the presence of adverse effects.

NURSING DIAGNOSIS

Determine the related factors for the nursing diagnoses based on the patient's current status. Appropriate nursing diagnoses may include:

- Acute Pain
- Deficient Knowledge
- Risk for Infection

OUTCOME IDENTIFICATION AND PLANNING

The expected outcome to achieve is that the patient reports increased comfort and/or decreased pain, without adverse effects. Other appropriate outcomes may include the patient displays decreased anxiety; patient exhibits a dry, intact dressing with catheter in place; patient remains free from infection; and patient verbalizes an understanding of the therapy and the reason for its use.

IMPLEMENTATION

ACTION	RATIONALE
1. Check the medication order against the original medical order, according to facility policy. Clarify any inconsistencies. Check the patient's medical record for allergies.	This comparison helps to identify errors that may have occurred when orders were transcribed. The medical order is the legal record-of-medication order for each agency.
2. Know the actions, special nursing considerations, safe dose ranges, purpose of administration, and adverse effects of the medications to be administered. Consider the appropriateness of the medication for this patient.	This knowledge aids the nurse in evaluating the therapeutic effect of the medication in relation to the patient's disorder and can also be used to educate the patient about the medication.
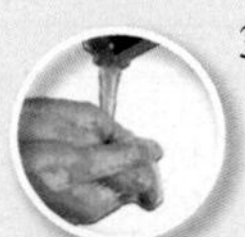 3. Perform hand hygiene and put on PPE, if indicated.	Hand hygiene and PPE prevent the spread of microorganisms. PPE is required based on transmission precautions.
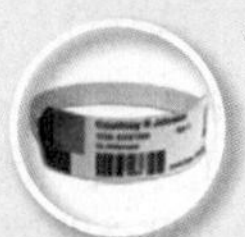 4. Identify the patient.	Identifying the patient ensures that the right patient receives the intervention and helps prevent errors.
5. Close the door to the room or pull the bedside curtain.	Closing the door or curtain provides patient privacy.
6. Assess the patient's pain. Administer postoperative analgesic, as ordered.	Continuous wound perfusion pain management is an adjuvant therapy; patients will likely require postoperative pain medication, with reduced frequency.
7. Check the medication label attached to the pain management system balloon. Compare it with the medical order and MAR, per facility policy. Assess the patient for perioral numbness or tingling, numbness or tingling of fingers or toes, blurred vision, ringing in the ears, metallic taste in the mouth, confusion, seizures, drowsiness, nausea and/or vomiting. Assess the patient's vital signs.	Checking the medication label with the order and MAR ensures correct therapy for the patient. These symptoms may indicate local anesthetic toxicity (I-Flow, 2012; D'Arcy, 2007b). Changes in vital signs may indicate adverse effect. Cardiac dysrhythmias and hypertension are possible adverse effects (Layzell, 2008).
8. Put on gloves. Assess the wound perfusion system. Inspect tubing for kinks; check that the white tubing clamps are open. If tubing appears crimped, massage area on tubing to facilitate flow. Check filter in tubing, which should be unrestricted and free from tape.	Gloves prevent contact with blood and body fluids. Tubing must be unclamped and free of kinks and/or crimping to maintain consistent flow of analgesic. Tape over filter interferes with properly functioning system.

ACTION	RATIONALE
9. Check the flow restrictor to ensure it is in contact with the patient's skin. Tape in place, as necessary (see Figure 1).	Checking the flow restrictor for adequate contact ensures accurate flow rate.
10. Check the insertion site dressing. Ensure that it is intact. Assess for leakage and dislodgement. Assess for redness, warmth, swelling, pain at site, and drainage.	Transparent dressing holds the catheter in place. Dressing must stay in place to prevent accidental dislodgement or removal. These symptoms may indicate infection.
11. Review the device with the patient. Review the function of the device and reason for its use. Reinforce the purpose and action of the medication to the patient.	Explanation encourages patient understanding and cooperation and reduces apprehension.
To Remove the Catheter	
12. Check to ensure that infusion is complete. Infusion is complete when the delivery time has passed and the balloon is no longer inflated.	Depending on the size and volume of the balloon, the infusion typically lasts 2 to 5 days. Infusion time should be recorded in the operative note or postoperative instructions. The balloon will no longer appear full, the outside bag will be flat, and a hard tube can be felt in the middle of the balloon (I-Flow, 2010).
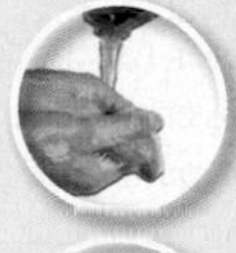 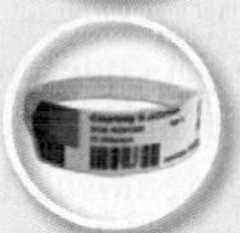 13. Perform hand hygiene. Identify the patient. Put on gloves. Remove the catheter site dressing. Loosen adhesive skin closure strips at the catheter site.	Hand hygiene and use of gloves reduce the risk of infection transmission. Identifying the patient ensures that the right patient receives the intervention and helps prevent errors. Loosening of materials allows the catheter to be free of constraints.
14. Grasp the catheter close to the patient's skin at the insertion site. Gently pull catheter to remove. Catheter should be easy to remove and not painful. Do not tug or quickly pull on the catheter during removal. Check the distal end of the catheter for the black marking.	Gentle removal prevents patient discomfort and accidental breakage of the catheter. Checking for the black mark at the distal end ensures the entire catheter was removed.
15. Cover puncture site with a dry dressing, according to facility policy.	Covering the wound prevents contamination.
16. Dispose of the balloon, tubing, and catheter, according to facility policy.	Proper disposal reduces the risk for infection transmission and contamination of other items.
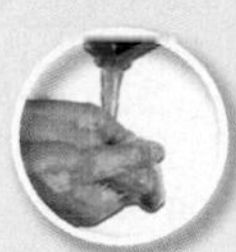 17. Remove gloves and additional PPE, if used. Perform hand hygiene.	Removing PPE properly reduces the risk for infection transmission and contamination of other items. Hand hygiene prevents transmission of microorganisms.

EVALUATION

The expected outcome is achieved when the patient verbalizes pain relief. In addition, the patient exhibits a dry, intact dressing, and the catheter exit site is free of signs and symptoms of complications, injury, or infection. The patient reports a decrease in anxiety and an increased ability to cope with pain. The patient verbalizes information related to the functioning of the system and the reasons for its use.

DOCUMENTATION

Guidelines

Document system patency, the condition of the insertion site and dressing, vital signs and assessment information, analgesics administered, and the patient's response.

(continued)

SKILL 10-6 CARING FOR A PATIENT RECEIVING CONTINUOUS WOUND PERFUSION PAIN MANAGEMENT continued

Sample Documentation

6/3/15 0935 Continuous wound perfusion pain management system in place. Exit site clean and dry. Transparent dressing in place. Temperature 98.7°F; pulse, 82 beats per minute; respirations, 14 breaths per minute and effortless; blood pressure, 112/74 mm Hg. Pulse oximetry 96% on room air. Patient alert and quickly responds to verbal stimuli. Denies nausea, vomiting, vision changes, paraesthesias, dizziness, or ringing in ears. Patient rates pain in RLE 3/10. Ibuprofen 800 mg po given as ordered.

—T. James, RN

6/3/15 1035 Patient reports pain in RLE 1/10. OOB to ambulate length of hall with wife.

—T. James, RN

UNEXPECTED SITUATIONS AND ASSOCIATED INTERVENTIONS

- *Patient reports and/or your assessment identifies the following symptoms: increase in pain; redness, swelling, pain, and/or discharge at the catheter site; dizziness, light-headedness; blurred vision; ringing, buzzing in ears; metal taste in mouth; numbness and/or tingling around the mouth, fingers, or toes; drowsiness; and/or confusion:* Close the clamp on the system tubing to stop the infusion. Report the symptoms to the patient's physician immediately. The presence of any of these symptoms may indicate local anesthetic toxicity (I-Flow, 2012; D'Arcy, 2007b; Layzell, 2008).
- *The catheter and tubing are accidentally pulled out:* Check the distal end of the catheter for the black marking to ensure the entire catheter was removed. Assess the insertion site. Cover the site with a dry, sterile dressing. Notify the patient's physician. Assess the patient's level of pain and administer analgesic, as ordered.
- *Resistance is encountered and/or the catheter stretches during its removal:* Stop. Do not continue to try to remove the catheter. Wait 30 to 60 minutes and attempt to remove the catheter again. The patient's body movements may relieve constriction on the catheter to allow easier removal. If catheter is still difficult to remove, contact the patient's physician. Do not forcefully remove the catheter. Do not continue to apply tension if the catheter begins to stretch (I-Flow, 2011).

SPECIAL CONSIDERATIONS

- Be aware that a change in the appearance and size of the pump may not be evident for more than 24 hours after surgery owing to the slow flow rate of the device.
- Do not expect to observe a fluid level line in the balloon and fluid moving through the system tubing.
- Over time, expect to see the outside bag on the balloon becoming looser, with creases beginning to form in the bag.
- Know that as the medication is delivered, the balloon will gradually become smaller.
- Do not forcefully remove the catheter.
- Do not reuse or refill balloon. System is intended for one-time use.
- Protect the balloon and catheter site from water.
- Clip the balloon to the patient's clothing or dressing to prevent the application of tension on the system and site.
- Avoid placing cold therapy in the area of the flow restrictor. Contact with cold therapy will decrease flow rate.

ENHANCE YOUR UNDERSTANDING

FOCUSING ON PATIENT CARE: DEVELOPING CLINICAL REASONING

Consider the case scenarios at the beginning of the chapter as you answer the following questions to enhance your understanding and apply what you have learned.

QUESTIONS

1. Since her surgery, Mildred Simpson has been spending most of her time in bed. A special pillow is placed between her legs to keep her hips in abduction. The nurse offers to give Mrs. Simpson a back massage. What areas would be most important for the nurse to address when performing this skill?
2. The physician decides to admit Joseph Watkins to the hospital for evaluation of his back pain. Intermittent TENS therapy is ordered and is to be started in the emergency department. How would the nurse initiate this therapy?
3. Jerome Batiste and his wife are concerned about using the PCA device at home. What information would the nurse provide to help alleviate their concerns?

You can find suggested answers after the Bibliography at the end of this chapter.

INTEGRATED CASE STUDY CONNECTION

The case studies in the back of the book are designed to focus on integrating concepts. Refer to the following case studies to enhance your understanding of the concepts related to the skills in this chapter.

- Basic Case Studies: Claudia Tran, page 1070; Kate Townsend, 1073
- Advanced Case Studies: Cole McKean, page 1093; Robert Espinoza, 1097

TAYLOR SUITE RESOURCES

Explore these additional resources to enhance learning for this chapter:

- NCLEX-Style Questions and other resources on thePoint, http://thePoint.lww.com/Lynn4e
- *Skill Checklists for Taylor's Clinical Nursing Skills*, 4e
- *Fundamentals of Nursing:* Chapter 34, Comfort and Pain Management

Bibliography

Abbaspour, Z., Akbari, M., & Najar, S. (2013). Effect of foot and hand massage in post cesarean section pain control: A randomized control trial. Pain Management Nursing. Available PubMed. DOI: 10.1016/j.pmn.2012.07.008.

Ackley, B.J., & Ladwig, G.B. (2011). *Nursing diagnosis handbook* (9th ed.). St. Louis: Mosby/Elsevier.

American Geriatrics Society (AGS). Panel on the pharmacological management of persistent pain in older persons. (2009). Pharmacological management of persistent pain in older persons. *Journal of the American Geriatrics Society, 57*(8), 1331–1346.

American Geriatrics Society (AGS). Panel on chronic pain in older persons. (2002). The management of persistent pain in older persons. *Journal of the American Geriatrics Society, 50*, (Suppl 6), S205–S224.

Arnstein, P. (2011). Multimodal approaches to pain management. *Nursing, 41*(3), 60–61.

Aschenbrenner, D., & Venable, S. (2012). *Drug therapy in nursing* (4th ed.). Philadelphia: Wolters Kluwer Health/Lippincott Williams & Wilkins.

Baldridge, K., & Andrasik, F. (2010). Pain assessment in people with intellectual or developmental disabilities. *American Journal of Nursing, 110*(12), 29–37.

Baulch, I. (2010). Assessment and management of pain in the paediatric patient. *Nursing Standard, 25*(10), 35–40.

Beyer, J., Denyes, M.J., & Villarruel, A.M. (1992). The creation, validation, and continuing development of the Oucher: A measure of pain intensity in children. *Journal of Pediatric Nursing, 7*(5), 335.

Birrer, K.L., Anderson, R.L., Liu-DeRyke, X., et al. (2011). Measures to improve safety of an elastomeric infusion system for pain management. *American Journal of Health-System Pharmacy, 68*(13), 1251–1255.

Bulechek, G.M, Butcher, H.K., Dochterman, J.M., et al. (Eds.). (2013). *Nursing interventions classification (NIC)* (6th ed.). St. Louis: Mosby Elsevier.

Capnography: New standard of care for sedation? (2012). *OR Manager, 28*(3), 17–20.

Chailler, M., Ellis, J., Stolarik, A., et al. (2010). Cold therapy for the management of pain associated with deep breathing and coughing post-cardiac surgery. *Canadian Journal of Cardiovascular Nursing, 20*(2), 18–24.

Chapman, S. (2010). Managing pain in the older person. *Nursing Standard, 25*(11), 35–39.

Charous, S. (2008). Use of the ON-Q pain pump management system in the head and neck Preliminary report. *Otolaryngology-Head and Neck Surgery, 138*(1), 110–112.

Chatterjee, J. (2012). Improving pain assessment for patients with cognitive impairment: Development of a pain assessment toolkit. *International Journal of Palliative Nursing, 18*(12), 581–590.

Chumbley, G., & Mountford, L. (2010). Patient-controlled analgesia infusion pumps for adults. *Nursing Standard, 25*(8), 35–40.

Cranwell-Bruce, L.A. (2009). PCA delivery systems. *MEDSURGNursing, 18*(2), 127–129, 133.

D'Arcy, Y. (2012). Treating acute pain in the hospitalized patient. *The Nurse Practitioner, 37*(8), 22–30.

D'Arcy, Y. (2011a). New criteria for assessing and treating neuropathic pain. *Nursing, 41*(12), 61–62.

D'Arcy, Y. (2011b). New thinking about postoperative pain management. *OR Nurse, 5*(6), 28-36.

D'Arcy, Y. (2010a). Is continuous subcutaneous infusion a good route for pain medication? *Nursing, 40*(10), 59–60.

D'Arcy, Y. (2010b). Managing chronic pain in acute care: Getting it right. *Nursing, 40*(4), 49–51.

D'Arcy, Y. (2008a). Keep your patient safe during PCA. *Nursing, 38*(1), 50–55.

D'Arcy, Y. (2008b). Pain management survey report. *Nursing, 38*(6), 42–50.

D'Arcy, Y. (2007a). Eyeing capnography to improve PCA safety. *Nursing, 37*(9), 18–19.

D'Arcy, Y. (2007b). New pain management options: Delivery systems and techniques. *Nursing, 37*(2), 26–27.

Fouladbakhsh, J.M., Szczesny, S., Jenuwine, E.S., et al. (2011). Nondrug therapies for pain management among rural older adults. *Pain Management Nursing, 12*(2), 70–81.

Flaherty, E. (2012). *Try this: Best practices in nursing care to older adults. Pain assessment for older adults.* Available http://consultgerirn.org/uploads/File/trythis/try_this_7.pdf.

Galloway, K, Buckenmaier, C., & Polomano, R. (2011). Understanding pain and pain responses. *American Nurse Today*, September, 3–7.

Gevirtz, C. (2010a). Getting current with iontophoretic fentanyl. *Nursing, 40*(2), 65.

Gevirtz, C. (2010b). Controlling pain. Infection control for patients with implanted pain management devices. *Nursing, 40*(6), 62–63.

Herr, K., Coyne, P.J., McCaffery, M., et al. (2011). American Society for Pain Management Nursing. *Pain assessment in the patient unable to self-report.* Available http://www.aspmn.org/organization/documents/UPDATED_NonverbalRevisionFinalWEB.pdf.

Hicks, R.W., Hernandez, J., & Wanzer, L.J. (2012). Perioperative pharmacology: Patient-controlled analgesia. *AORN Journal, 95*(2), 255–262.

Hinkle, J.L., & Cheever, K.H. (2014). *Brunner & Suddarth's textbook of medical-surgical nursing* (13th ed.). Philadelphia: Wolters Kluwer Health/Lippincott Williams & Wilkins.

Hong, S.J., & Lee, E. (2012). Effects of a structured educational programme on patient-controlled analgesia

(PCA) for gynaecological patients in South Korea. *Journal of Clinical Nursing, 21*(23/24), 3546–3555.

Horgas, A.L. (2012). *Try this: Best practices in nursing care to older adults with dementia. Assessing pain in older adults with dementia.* Available http://consultgerirn.org/uploads/File/trythis/try_this_d2.pdf.

Horgas, A.L., Yoon, S.L., & Grall, M. (2012). *Pain. Nursing standard of practice protocol: Pain management in older adults.* Available http://consultgerirn.org/topics/pain/want_to_know_more.

I-Flow Corporation. (2012). *On-Q pain relief system. Patient guidelines.* Available http://www.iflo.com/pdf/products/1307136A.pdf.

I-Flow Corporation. (2010). *On-Q PainBuster postoperative pain relief system. Floor nurse guide.* Available http://www.iflo.com/prod_onq_classic.php.

I-Flow Corporation. (2011). *On-Q pain catheter. Patient guideline insert.* Available http://www.iflo.com/pdf/products/1307133a.pdf.

Institute for Safe Medication Practices (ISMP). (2006). *Patient-controlled analgesia: Making it safer for patients.* Available http://www.ismp.org/profdevelopment/PCAMonograph.pdf.

Institute for Safe Medication Practices (ISMP). (2003). *Medication safety alert. Part II: How to prevent errors. Safety issues with patient-controlled analgesia.* Available http://www.ismp.org/newsletters/acutecare/articles/20030724.asp.

Institute of Medicine (IOM). (2011). *Relieving pain in America.* Washington, D.C.: The National Academies Press.

International Association for the Study of Pain (IASP). (1994). Part III: Pain terms, a current list with definitions and notes on usage. In: Merskey, H., & Bogduk. (Eds.). *Classification of chronic pain* (2nd ed.). Seattle, WA: IASP Press, 209–214.

Jablonski, A., DuPen, A., & Ersek, M. (2011). The use of algorithms in assessing and managing persistent pain in older adults. *American Journal of Nursing, 111*(3), 34–45.

Jarvis, C. (2012). *Physical examination & health assessment* (6th ed.). St. Louis: Saunders/Elsevier.

Jarzyna, D., Jungquist, C.R., Pasero, C., et al. (2011). American Society for Pain Management nursing guidelines on monitoring for opioid-induced sedation and respiratory depression. *Pain Management Nursing, 12*(3), 118–145.

Johnson, A., Schweitzer, D., & Ahrens, T. (2011). Time to throw away your stethoscope? Capnography: Evidence-based patient monitoring technology. *Journal of Radiological Nursing, 30*(1), 25–34.

The Joint Commission. (2013). *Facts about pain management.* Available http://www.jointcommission.org/pain_management/.

The Joint Commission. (2012). Sentinel event alert issue 49: Safe use of opioids in hospitals. Available http://www.jointcommission.org/sea_issue_49/.

The Joint Commission. (2008). Speak Up. What you should know about pain management. Available http://ωωω.jointcommission.org/topics/speakup_brochures.aspx. www.jointcommission.org/PatientSafety/SpeakUp. Accessed December 17, 2008.

Kwekkeboom, K., Hau, H., Wanta, B., et al. (2008). Patients' perceptions of the effectiveness of guided imagery and progressive muscle relaxation interventions used for cancer pain. *Complementary Therapies in Clinical Practice, 14*(3), 185–194.

Kyle, T., & Carman, S. (2013). *Essentials of pediatric nursing* (2nd ed.). Philadelphia: Wolters Kluwer Health/Lippincott Williams & Wilkins.

Layzell, M. (2008). Current interventions and approaches to postoperative pain management. *British Journal of Nursing, 17*(7), 414–419.

McCaffery, M. (1979). *Nursing management of the patient with pain.* (2nd ed.). Philadelphia: JB Lippincott.

McCaffery, M., & Beebe, A. (1989). *Pain: Clinical manual for nursing practice.* St. Louis: CV Mosby.

McCaffery, M., & Pasero, C. (1999). *Pain clinical manual.* (2nd ed.). St. Louis: Mosby.

McHugh, M.E., Miller-Saultz, D., Wuhrman, E., et al. Interventional pain management in the palliative care patient. *International Journal of Palliative Nursing, 18*(9), 426–428, 430–433.

Merkel, S., Voepel-Lewis, T., & Malviya, S. (2002). Pain assessment in infants and young children: The FLACC Scale: A behavioral tool to measure pain in young children. *American Journal of Nursing, 102*(10), 55–58.

Moorhead, S., Johnson, M., Maas, M.L., et al. (Eds.). (2013). *Nursing outcomes classification (NOC).* (5th ed.). St. Louis: Mosby Elsevier.

NANDA International. (2012). *Nursing diagnoses: Definitions & classification 2012–2014.* West Sussex, UK: Wiley-Blackwell.

Nurse Advise-ERR. (2005). Safety issues with patient-controlled analgesia (PCA). Part II. Practical error-reduction strategies. *Institute for Safe Medication Practices Safety Alert, 3*(2), 1–3.

Pasero, C., & McCaffery, M. (2005a). Authorized and unauthorized use of PCA pumps: Clarifying the use of patient-controlled analgesia, in light of recent alerts. *American Journal of Nursing, 105*(7), 30–32.

Pasero, C. & McCaffery, M. (2011). *Pain assessment and pharmacological management.* St. Louis: Mosby Elsevier.

Pasero, C., & McCaffery, M. (2005b). No self-report means no pain-intensity rating: Assessing pain in patients who cannot provide a report. *American Journal of Nursing, 105*(10), 50–53.

Perry, S.E., Hockenberry, M.J., Lowdermilk, D.L., et al. (2010). *Maternal child nursing care* (4th ed.). Maryland Heights, MO: Mosby/Elsevier.

Pfeifer, G. (2011). Transforming pain care: An IOM report. *American Journal of Nursing, 111*(9), 18.

Porth, C., & Matfin, G. (2014). *Pathophysiology: Concepts of altered health states* (9th ed.). Philadelphia: Wolters Kluwer Health/Lippincott Williams & Wilkins.

Roman, M., & Cabaj, T. (2005). Epidural analgesia. *MEDSURG Nursing, 14*(4), 257–259.

Running, A., & Turnbeaugh, E. (2011). Oncology pain and complementary therapy. *Clinical Journal of Oncology Nursing, 15*(4), 374–379.

Sawhney, M. (2012). Epidural analgesia: What nurses need to know. *Nursing, 42*(8), 36–42.

Tabloski, P. (2010). *Gerontological nursing* (2nd ed.). Upper Saddle River, NJ: Pearson.

Taylor, C., Lillis, C., & Lynn, P. (2015). *Fundamentals of nursing* (8th ed.). Philadelphia: Wolters Kluwer Health/Lippincott Williams & Wilkins.

Taylor, S.A. (2010). Safety and satisfaction provided by patient-controlled analgesia. *Dimensions of Critical Care Nursing, 29*(4), 163–166.

Vaajoki, A., Pietilä, A-M., Kankkunen, P., et al. (2011). Effects of listening to music on pain intensity and pain distress after surgery: An intervention. *Journal of Clinical Nursing, 21*(5/6), 708–717.

VISN 8 Patient Safety Center. (2009). *Safe patient handling and movement algorithms.* Tampa, FL. Available at www.visn8.va.gov/patientsafetycenter/safePtHandling/default.asp. Accessed April 23, 2010.

Wardell, D., Decker, S., & Engebretson, J. (2012). Healing touch for older adults with persistent pain. *Holistic Nursing Practice, 26*(4), 194–202.

Westbrook, G., & D'Arcy, Y. (2012). Pain management basics. *Nurse.com, 21*(3), 28–33.

Woods, A.B., Crist, B., Kowalewski, S., et al. (2012). A cross-sectional analysis of the effect of patient-controlled epidural analgesia versus patient controlled analgesia on postcesarean pain and breastfeeding. *Journal of Obstetric, Gynecologic & Neonatal Nursing, 41*(3), 339–346.

Wuhrman, E., Cooney, M., Dunwoody, C., et al. (2007). Authorized and unauthorized ("PCA by proxy") dosing of analgesic infusion pumps: Position statement with clinical practice recommendations. *Pain Management Nursing, 8*(1), 4–11.

SUGGESTED ANSWERS FOR FOCUSING ON PATIENT CARE: DEVELOPING CLINICAL REASONING

1. Review the patient's medical record and plan of care for information about the patient's status and contraindications to back massage, and review the medical orders for the patient's activity level. Because of her surgery, it will probably be difficult for Mrs. Simpson to lie in a prone position; assess her ability to turn to her side for the massage. It will be necessary to maintain the position of the abductor pillow, to prevent adduction of her hip. Assess the patient's level of pain. Check the patient's medication administration record for the time an analgesic was last administered. If appropriate, administer an analgesic sufficiently early so it has time to take effect before beginning the massage. Assess for the need to obtain assistance of another caregiver to assist the patient to her side and maintain that position for the massage. Include an assessment of the patient's skin integrity, because of the increased risk for impaired skin integrity.

2. Review the patient's medical record and plan of care for specific instructions related to TENS therapy, including the order and conditions indicating the need for therapy, and ordered settings. Review the patient's history for conditions that might contraindicate therapy, such as pacemaker insertion, cardiac monitoring, or electrocardiography. Determine the location of electrode placement in consultation with the ordering practitioner and on the patient's report of pain. Assess the patient's understanding of TENS therapy and the rationale for its use. Explain the rationale for the use of TENS therapy and patient instructions.

   Before initiating therapy, inspect the skin of the area designated for electrode placement for irritation, redness, or breakdown. Assess the patient's pain and level of discomfort using an appropriate assessment tool. Check the unit to ensure proper functioning and review the manufacturer's instructions for use.

3. Provide teaching for Mr. Batiste and his wife concerning the rationale for the use of a PCA and how a PCA works. Show the patient and his wife the equipment as part of the explanation and provide a written copy of the information. Include information regarding safety mechanisms built into the device, as well as guidelines for adverse effects. Instruct the patient and his wife regarding symptoms that should be reported to the physician. They should be aware that a home care nurse will be consulted to continue support at home. The patient and/or his wife should be able to verbalize an understanding of information.

11 Nutrition

FOCUSING ON PATIENT CARE

This chapter will help you develop some of the skills related to nutrition needed to care for the following patients:

PAULA WILLIAMS, age 78, who is recovering from a cerebrovascular accident (CVA), or stroke. The nurse needs to help her with breakfast.

JACK MASON, a 62-year-old man who has severe dysphagia related to progressive muscle weakness. He is NPO and receiving enteral nutrition through a nasogastric tube. He and his wife are considering the placement of a gastrostomy tube for long-term nutrition.

COLE BRENAU, age 12, has cystic fibrosis and needs to increase his caloric intake through gastrostomy tube feedings at nighttime.

Refer to Focusing on Patient Care: Developing Clinical Reasoning at the end of the chapter to apply what you learn.

LEARNING OBJECTIVES

After studying this chapter, you will be able to:

1. Assist a patient with eating.
2. Insert a nasogastric tube.
3. Administer a tube feeding.
4. Remove a nasogastric tube.
5. Care for a gastrostomy tube.

KEY TERMS

aspiration: the misdirection of oropharyngeal secretions or gastric contents into the larynx and lower respiratory tract

body mass index (BMI): ratio of height to weight that more accurately reflects total body fat stores in the general population (weight in kg/height^2 in meters)

calorie: measure of heat, or energy; kilocalorie, commonly referred to as a calorie, is defined as the amount of heat required to raise 1 kg of water by 1°C

carbohydrate: organic compounds (commonly known as sugars and starches) that are composed of carbon, hydrogen, and oxygen; the most abundant and least expensive source of calories in the diet worldwide

cholesterol: fatlike substance, found only in animal tissues, that is important for cell membrane structure, a precursor of steroid hormones, and a constituent of bile

dysphagia: difficulty swallowing or the inability to swallow

enteral nutrition: alternate form of feeding that involves passing a tube into the gastrointestinal tract to allow instillation of the appropriate formula

ketosis: catabolism of fatty acids that occurs when a person's carbohydrate intake is not adequate; without adequate glucose, the catabolism is incomplete and ketones are formed, resulting in increased ketones

lipids: group name for fatty substances, including fats, oils, waxes, and related compounds

nasogastric (NG) tube: a tube inserted through the nose and into the stomach

nasointestinal (NI) tube: a tube inserted through the nose and into the upper portion of the small intestine

NPO (nothing by mouth): nothing can be consumed by mouth, including medications, unless ordered otherwise

nutrient: specific biochemical substance used by the body for growth, development, activity, reproduction, lactation, health maintenance, and recovery from illness or injury

nutrition: study of the nutrients and how they are handled by the body, as well as the impact of human behavior and environment on the process of nourishment

obesity: weight greater than 20% above ideal body weight

percutaneous endoscopic gastrostomy tube (PEG): a surgically or laparoscopically placed gastrostomy tube

percutaneous endoscopic jejunostomy tube (PEJ): a surgically or laparoscopically placed jejunostomy tube

protein: vital component of every living cell; composed of carbon, hydrogen, oxygen, and nitrogen

residual: as applied to tube feeding, the amount of gastric contents in the stomach after the administration of a tube feeding

vitamins: organic substances needed by the body in small amounts to help regulate body processes; they are susceptible to oxidation and destruction

Good nutrition is vital for life and health. Important **nutrients**, found in food, are needed for the body to function. A varied diet is necessary to provide all of the essential nutrients that a person needs. Poor nutrition can seriously decrease a person's level of wellness. Refer to Fundamentals Review 11-1 for sources and functions of **carbohydrates, protein**, and fats.

This chapter discusses the skills necessary to care for patients with nutritional needs. Because of the significant influence that adequate **nutrition** plays in maintaining health and disease prevention, the nurse integrates nutritional assessment into the care of the patient (Fundamentals Review 11-2). Ongoing data collection through various methods, such as history taking, the physical examination, and laboratory data analysis (Fundamentals Review 11-3), can provide pertinent information for directing the nursing plan of care. Factors that may affect nutritional status are discussed in Fundamentals Review 11-4.

FUNDAMENTALS REVIEW 11-1

SOURCES, FUNCTIONS, AND SIGNIFICANCE OF CARBOHYDRATES, PROTEIN, AND FAT

Nutrient	Sources	Functions	Significance
Carbohydrates Simple sugars and starch	Fruits Vegetables Grains: rice, pasta, breads, cereals Dried peas and beans Milk (lactose) Sugars: white and brown sugar, honey, molasses, syrup	Provide energy Spare protein so it can be used for other functions Prevent **ketosis** from inefficient fat metabolism	An adequate intake for total fiber is 25 g/day (women) and 38 g/day (men); maximum level of 25% of total **calories** or less from added sugars. Low carbohydrate intake can cause ketosis; high simple sugar intake increases the risk for dental caries
Cellulose and other water-insoluble fibers	Whole wheat flour and wheat bran Vegetables: cabbage, peas, green beans, wax beans, broccoli, brussels sprouts, cucumber skins, peppers, carrots Apples	Absorb water to increase fecal bulk Decrease intestinal transit time	Is nondigestible; therefore, it is excreted Helps relieve constipation North Americans are urged to eat more of all types of fiber Excess intake can cause gas, distention, and diarrhea
Water-soluble fibers	Oat bran and oatmeal Dried peas and beans Vegetables Prunes, pears, apples, bananas, oranges	Slow gastric emptying Lower serum **cholesterol** level Delay glucose absorption	Help improve glucose tolerance in diabetics
Protein	Milk and milk products Meat, poultry, fish Eggs Dried peas and beans Nuts	Tissue growth and repair Component of body framework: bones, muscles, tendons, blood vessels, skin, hair, nails Component of body fluids: hormones, enzymes, plasma proteins, neurotransmitters, mucus Helps regulate fluid balance through oncotic pressure Helps regulate acid–base balance Detoxifies harmful substances Forms antibodies Transports fat and other substances through the blood Provides energy when carbohydrate intake is inadequate	Experts recommend that we eat less animal protein and more vegetable protein. Protein deficiency is characterized by edema, retarded growth and maturation, muscle wasting, changes in the hair and skin, permanent damage to physical and mental development (in children), diarrhea, malabsorption, numerous secondary nutrient deficiencies, fatty infiltration of the liver, increased risk for infections, and high mortality Protein malnutrition occurs secondary to chronic diseases, such as cancer, AIDS, and COPD; it may also result from acute critical illnesses such as trauma and sepsis. It may also be seen in the homeless, older adults, fad dieters, adults addicted to drugs or alcohol, and people with eating disorders.

(continued)

FUNDAMENTALS REVIEW 11-1 continued

SOURCES, FUNCTIONS, AND SIGNIFICANCE OF CARBOHYDRATES, PROTEIN, AND FAT

Nutrient	Sources	Functions	Significance
Fat	Butter, oils, margarine, lard, salt pork, salad dressings, mayonnaise, bacon Whole milk and whole milk products High-fat meats Nuts	Provides energy Provides structure Insulates the body Cushions internal organs Necessary for the absorption of fat-soluble **vitamins**	High-fat diets increase the risk for heart disease and **obesity** and are correlated with an increased risk for colon and breast cancers

(Dudek, S. G. [2014]. *Nutrition essentials for nursing practice* [7th ed.]. Philadelphia: Lippincott Williams & Wilkins|Wolters Kluwer Heath.)

FUNDAMENTALS REVIEW 11-2

CLINICAL OBSERVATIONS FOR NUTRITIONAL ASSESSMENT

Body Area	Signs of Good Nutritional Status	Signs of Poor Nutritional Status
General appearance	Alert, responsive	Listless, apathetic, and cachexic
General vitality	Endurance, energetic, sleeps well, vigorous	Easily fatigued, no energy, falls asleep easily, looks tired, apathetic
Weight	Normal for height, age, body build	Overweight or underweight
Hair	Shiny, lustrous, firm, not easily plucked, healthy scalp	Dull and dry, brittle, loss of color, easily plucked, thin and sparse
Face	Uniform skin color; healthy appearance, not swollen	Dark skin over cheeks and under eyes, flaky skin, facial edema (moon face), pale skin color
Eyes	Bright, clear, moist; no sores at corners of eyelids; membranes moist and healthy pink color; no prominent blood vessels	Pale eye membranes, dry eyes (xerophthalmia), Bitot's spots, increased vascularity, cornea soft (keratomalacia), small yellowish lumps around eyes (xanthelasma), dull or scarred cornea
Lips	Good pink color, smooth, moist, not chapped or swollen	Swollen and puffy (cheilosis); angular lesion at corners of mouth or fissures or scars (stomatitis)
Tongue	Deep red, surface papillae present	Smooth appearance, beefy red or magenta colored, swollen, hypertrophy or atrophy

FUNDAMENTALS REVIEW 11-2 continued

CLINICAL OBSERVATIONS FOR NUTRITIONAL ASSESSMENT

Body Area	Signs of Good Nutritional Status	Signs of Poor Nutritional Status
Teeth	Straight, no crowding, no cavities, no pain, bright, no discoloration, well-shaped jaw	Cavities, mottled appearance (fluorosis), malpositioned, missing teeth
Gums	Firm, good pink color, no swelling or bleeding	Spongy, bleed easily, marginal redness, recessed, swollen and inflamed
Glands	No enlargement of the thyroid, face not swollen	Enlargement of the thyroid (goiter), enlargement of the parotid (swollen cheeks)
Skin	Smooth, good color, slightly moist; no signs of rashes, swelling, or color irregularities	Rough, dry, flaky, swollen, pale, pigmented, lack of fat under the skin, fat deposits around the joints (xanthomas), bruises, petechiae
Nails	Firm, pink	Spoon shaped (koilonychia), brittle, pale, ridged
Skeleton	Good posture, no malformations	Poor posture, beading of the ribs, bowed legs or knock-knees, prominent scapulas, chest deformity at diaphragm
Muscles	Well developed, firm, good tone, some fat under the skin	Flaccid, poor tone, wasted, underdeveloped, difficulty walking
Extremities	No tenderness	Weak and tender, presence of edema
Abdomen	Flat	Swollen
Nervous system	Normal reflexes, psychological stability	Decrease in or loss of ankle and knee reflexes, psychomotor changes, mental confusion, depression, sensory loss, motor weakness, loss of sense of position, loss of vibration, burning and tingling of the hands and feet (paresthesia)
Cardiovascular system	Normal heart rate and rhythm, no murmurs, normal blood pressure for age	Cardiac enlargement, tachycardia, elevated blood pressure
GI system	No palpable organs or masses (liver edge may be palpable in children)	Hepatosplenomegaly, enlarged liver or spleen

(Adapted from Dudek, S. G. [2014]. *Nutrition essentials for nursing practice* [7th ed.]. Philadelphia: Lippincott Williams & Wilkins; and Jarvis, C. [2012]. *Physical examination & health assessment* [6th ed.]. St. Louis: Saunders Elsevier.)

FUNDAMENTALS REVIEW 11-3

BIOCHEMICAL DATA WITH NUTRITIONAL IMPLICATIONS

- Hemoglobin (normal = 12–18 g/dL) decreased → anemia
- Hematocrit (normal = 40%–50%) decreased → anemia increased → dehydration
- Serum albumin (normal = 3.3–5 g/dL) decreased → high risk for morbidity, mortality, and malnutrition (prolonged protein depletion), malabsorption
- Transferrin (normal = 240–480 mg/dL) decreased → anemia, protein deficiency
- Total lymphocyte count (normal = greater than 1,800) decreased → impaired nutritional intake, severe debilitating disease
- Blood urea nitrogen (normal = 17–18 mg/dL) increased → starvation, high protein intake, severe dehydration decreased → malnutrition, overhydration
- Creatinine (normal = 0.4–1.5 mg/dL) increased → dehydration decreased → reduction in total muscle mass, severe malnutrition

(From Dudek, S. (2014). *Nutrition essentials for nursing practice* [7th ed.]. Philadelphia: Lippincott Williams & Wilkins/ Wolters Kluwer Health; and Van Leeuwen, A.M., Poelhuis-Leth, D., & Bladh, M.L. (2011). *Davis's comprehensive handbook of laboratory & diagnostic tests with nursing implications* (4th ed.). Philadelphia: F.A. Davis.)

FUNDAMENTALS REVIEW 11-4

FACTORS THAT MAY AFFECT NUTRITIONAL STATUS

- Socioeconomic status
- Psychosocial factors (meaning of food)
- Medical conditions that involve malabsorption, such as Crohn's disease or cystic fibrosis
- Age
- Medical conditions that may affect desire to eat, such as chemotherapy treatment or pregnancy accompanied by morning sickness
- Conditions that involve physical limitations, weakness, and/or fatigue
- Dysphagia
- Culture
- Medications
- Alcohol abuse
- Religion
- Megadoses of nutrient substances
- Alterations in mental status
- Illiteracy
- Language barriers
- Lack of caregiver or social support
- Knowledge of nutrition

SKILL 11-1 ASSISTING A PATIENT WITH EATING

The primary care provider will order a diet for the patient, based on the patient's condition. Many patients can independently meet their nutritional needs by feeding themselves. Other patients, especially the very young and some older adult patients, such as people with arthritis of the hands, may have some difficulty opening juice containers, and so on. Patients with paralysis of the hands or advanced dementia may be unable to feed themselves. For these patients, the nurse should provide assistance, as needed. This skill is frequently delegated to nursing assistants. However, the nurse is responsible for the initial and ongoing assessment of the patient for potential complications related to feeding. Before this skill can be delegated, it is paramount for the nurse to make sure that the nursing assistant has been educated to observe for any swallowing difficulties and has knowledge of aspiration precautions. Box 11-1 outlines special considerations and interventions for feeding patients with dementia or other alterations in cognition. Box 11-2 discusses special considerations and interventions for feeding patients with **dysphagia**.

BOX 11-1 SPECIAL CONSIDERATIONS AND INTERVENTIONS FOR FEEDING PATIENTS WITH DEMENTIA OR OTHER ALTERATIONS IN COGNITION

- Change the environment in which meals are eaten.
- Assess the area where meals are served. Create a home-like environment by preparing food close to the place where it will be served to stimulate senses.
- Observe as many former rituals as possible, such as handwashing and saying a blessing.
- Avoid clutter and distractions.
- Maintain a pleasant, well-lighted room. Play calming music.
- Keep food as close to its original form as possible.
- Serve meals in the same place at the same time.
- Closely supervise mealtime.
- Check food temperatures to prevent accidental mouth burns.
- Assist, as needed. Be alert for cues from the patient. Turning away may signal the patient has had enough to eat or that he or she needs to slow down. Leaning forward with an open mouth usually means the patient is ready for more food.
- Stroking the underside of the chin may help promote swallowing.
- Provide one food at a time. Offer small, frequent eating opportunities. A whole tray of food may be overwhelming.
- Ensure that the patient has glasses and that hearing aid is working properly.
- Demonstrate what you want the patient to do. State the goal clearly, and then mimic the action with exaggerated motions.
- Provide between-meal snacks that are easy to consume using the hands.
- Use adaptive feeding equipment, as needed, such as weighted utensils, large-handled cups, and larger or smaller silverware than standard.
- Promote family involvement to encourage eating.

Adapted from Cole, D. (2012). Optimising nutrition for older people with dementia. *Nursing Standard, 26*(20), 41–48; Dudek, S. (2014). *Nutrition essentials for nursing practice* (7th ed.). Philadelphia: Lippincott Williams & Wilkins/Wolters Kluwer Health; Lin, L., Watson, R., & Wu, S. (2010). What is associated with low food intake in older people with dementia? *Journal of Clinical Nursing, 19*(1–2), 53–59; Tabloski, P. (2010). *Gerontological nursing* (2nd ed.). Upper Saddle River, NJ: Pearson; and Dunne, A. (2010). Nutrition and dementia. *Nursing & Residential Care, 12*(3), 112, 114, 116.

BOX 11-2 SPECIAL CONSIDERATIONS AND INTERVENTIONS FOR FEEDING PATIENTS WITH DYSPHAGIA

- Provide at least a 30-minute rest period prior to mealtime. A rested person will likely have less difficulty swallowing.
- Sit the patient upright, preferably in a chair. If bed rest is mandatory, elevate the head of the bed to a 90-degree angle.
- Provide mouth care immediately before meals to enhance the sense of taste.
- Avoid rushed or forced feeding. Adjust the rate of feeding and size of bites to the patient's tolerance.
- Collaborate to obtain a speech therapy consult for swallowing evaluation.
- Initiate a nutrition consult for appropriate diet modification such as chopping, mincing, or pureeing of foods and liquid consistency (thin, nectar thick, honey-like, spoon-thick).
- Keep in mind that some patients may find thickened liquids unpalatable and thus drink insufficient fluids.
- Reduce or eliminate distractions at mealtime so patient can focus attention on swallowing.
- Alternate solids and liquids.
- Assess for signs of aspiration during eating: sudden appearance of severe coughing; choking; cyanosis; voice change, hoarseness, and/or gurgling after swallowing; frequent throat clearing after meals; or regurgitation through the nose or mouth.
- Inspect oral cavity for retained food.
- Avoid or minimize the use of sedatives and hypnotics because these agents may impair the cough reflex and swallowing.

Adapted from Metheny, N. (2012). Try this: Best practices in nursing care to older adults. The Hartford Institute for Geriatric Nursing. Preventing aspiration in older adults with dysphagia. Issue Number 20. Available http://consultgerirn.org/uploads/File/trythis/try_this_20.pdf; Eisenstadt, E.S. (2010). Dysphagia and aspiration pneumonia in older adults. *Journal of the American Academy of Nurse Practitioners, 22*(1), 17–22; and Dudek, S. (2014). *Nutrition essentials for nursing practice* (7th ed.). Philadelphia: Lippincott Williams & Wilkins/Wolters Kluwer Health.

DELEGATION CONSIDERATIONS

Assisting patients to eat may be delegated to nursing assistive personnel (NAP) or to unlicensed assistive personnel (UAP), as well as to licensed practical/vocational nurses (LPN/LVNs). See previous discussion. The decision to delegate must be based on careful analysis of the patient's needs and circumstances, as well as the qualifications of the person to whom the task is being delegated. Refer to the Delegation Guidelines in Appendix A.

EQUIPMENT

- Patient tray of food, based on prescribed diet
- Wet wipes for hand hygiene
- Mouth care materials
- Patient's dentures, eyeglasses, hearing aid, if needed
- Special adaptive utensils, as needed
- Napkins, protective covering, or towel
- PPE, as indicated

(continued)

SKILL 11-1 ASSISTING A PATIENT WITH EATING continued

ASSESSMENT

Before assisting the patient, confirm the type of diet that has been ordered for the patient. Also, it is important to assess for any food allergies and religious or cultural preferences, as appropriate. Check to make sure the patient does not have any scheduled laboratory or diagnostic studies that may impact whether he or she is able to eat a meal. Before beginning the feeding, assess for any swallowing difficulties. Assess the patient's abdomen.

NURSING DIAGNOSIS

Determine the related factors for the nursing diagnoses based on the patient's current status. Possible nursing diagnoses may include:

- Feeding Self-Care Deficit
- Risk for Aspiration
- Impaired Swallowing

OUTCOME IDENTIFICATION AND PLANNING

The expected outcome to achieve when assisting a patient with feeding is that the patient consumes 50% to 60% of the contents of the meal tray. Other outcomes include that the patient does not aspirate during or after the meal and the patient expresses contentment related to eating, as appropriate.

IMPLEMENTATION

ACTION	RATIONALE
1. Check the medical order for the type of diet prescribed for the patient.	Ensures the correct diet for the patient.
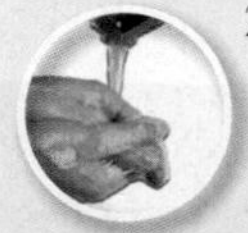 2. Perform hand hygiene and put on PPE, if indicated.	Hand hygiene and PPE prevent the spread of microorganisms. PPE is required based on transmission precautions.
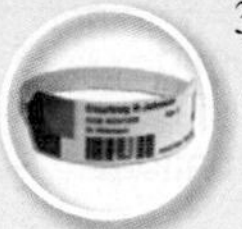 3. Identify the patient.	Identifying the patient ensures the right patient receives the intervention and helps prevent errors.
4. Explain the procedure to the patient.	Explanations provide reassurance and facilitate cooperation of the patient.
5. **Assess level of consciousness, for any physical limitations, decreased hearing or visual acuity. If patient uses a hearing aid or wears glasses or dentures, provide, as needed. Ask if the patient has any cultural or religious preferences and food likes and dislikes, if possible.**	Alertness is necessary for the patient to swallow and consume food. Using a hearing aid, glasses, and dentures for chewing facilitates the intake of food. Patient preferences should be considered in food selection as much as possible to increase the intake of food and maximize the benefit of the meal.
6. Pull the patient's bedside curtain. Assess the abdomen. Ask the patient if he or she has any nausea. Ask the patient if he or she has any difficulty swallowing. Assess the patient for nausea or pain and administer an antiemetic or analgesic, as needed.	Provides for privacy. A functioning GI tract is essential for digestion. The presence of pain or nausea will diminish appetite. If the patient is medicated, wait for the appropriate time for absorption of the medication before beginning the feeding.
7. Offer to assist the patient with any elimination needs.	Promotes comfort and may avoid interruptions for toileting during meals.
8. Provide hand hygiene and mouth care, as needed.	May improve appetite and promote comfort.
9. Remove any bedpans or undesirable equipment and odors, if possible, from the vicinity where the meal will be eaten. Perform hand hygiene.	Unpleasant odors and equipment may decrease the patient's appetite. Hand hygiene prevents the spread of microorganisms.
10. Open the patient's bedside curtain. Assist to, or position the patient in, a high Fowler's or sitting position in the bed or chair. Position the bed in the low position if the patient remains in bed.	Proper positioning improves swallowing ability and reduces the risk of aspiration.
11. Place protective covering or towel over the patient if desired.	Prevents soiling of the patient's gown.

ACTION	RATIONALE
12. Check tray to make sure that it is the correct tray before serving. Place tray on the overbed table so the patient can see the food, if able. Ensure that hot foods are hot and cold foods are cold. Use caution with hot beverages, allowing sufficient time for cooling, if needed. Ask the patient for his/her preference related to what foods are desired first. Cut food into small pieces, as needed. Observe swallowing ability throughout the meal.	Ensures that the correct tray is given to the patient. Encouraging the patient choice promotes patient dignity and respect. Close observation is necessary to assess for signs of aspiration or difficulty with meal.
13. If possible, sit facing the patient while feeding is taking place (Figure 1). If the patient is able, encourage him or her to hold finger foods and feed self as much as possible. Converse with patient during the meal, as appropriate. If, however, the patient has **dysphagia**, limit questioning or conversation that would require patient response during eating. Play relaxation music if patient desires.	In general, optimal mealtime involves social interaction and conversation. Talking during eating is contraindicated for patients with dysphagia, because of increased risk for aspiration.

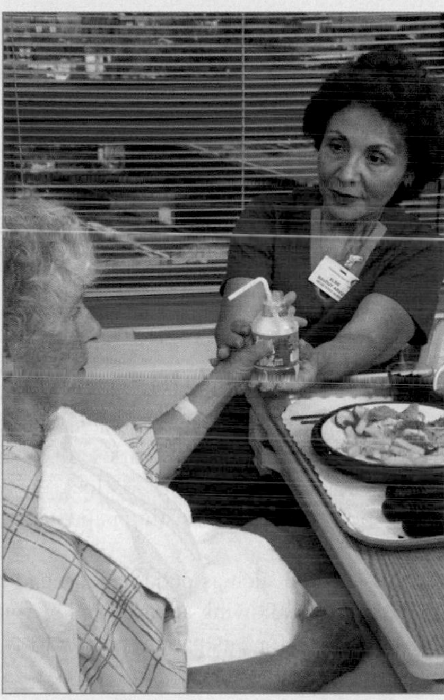

FIGURE 1 Assisting patient with eating.

ACTION	RATIONALE
14. Allow enough time for the patient to chew and swallow the food adequately. The patient may need to rest for short periods during eating.	Eating requires energy and many medical conditions can weaken patients. Rest can restore energy for eating.
15. When the meal is completed or the patient is unable to eat any more, remove the tray from the room. **Note the amount and types of food consumed. Note the volume of liquid consumed.**	Nutrition plays an important role in healing and overall health. If the patient is not eating enough to meet nutritional requirements, alternative methods need to be considered.
16. Reposition the overbed table, remove the protective covering, offer hand hygiene, as needed, and offer the bedpan. Assist the patient to a position of comfort and relaxation.	Promotes the comfort of the patient, meets possible elimination needs, and facilitates digestion.
17. Remove PPE, if used. Perform hand hygiene.	Removing PPE properly reduces the risk for infection transmission and contamination of other items. Hand hygiene prevents the spread of microorganisms.

(continued)

SKILL 11-1 ASSISTING A PATIENT WITH EATING continued

EVALUATION

The expected outcomes are met when the patient consumes an adequate amount of nutrients. In addition, the patient expresses an appetite for the food, relating likes and dislikes. Additionally, the patient experiences no nausea, vomiting, or aspiration episodes.

DOCUMENTATION

Guidelines

Document the condition of the abdomen. Record that the head of bed was elevated to at least 30 to 45 degrees. Note any swallowing difficulties and the patient's response to the meal. Document the percentage of the intake from the meal. If the patient had a poor intake, document the need for further consultation with the primary care provider and dietitian, as needed. Record any pertinent teaching that was conducted. Record liquids consumed on intake and output record, as appropriate.

Sample Documentation

12/23/15 0730 Patient's abdomen soft, nondistended, positive bowel sounds. HOB elevated to 45 degrees. Gag reflex intact. Awake. Fed full liquid tray; consumed about 50%; ate most of the oatmeal, 4 oz. of cranberry juice. Some conversation during the meal. Patient remains with HOB elevated, watching TV. Call bell in reach.

—*S. Essner, RN*

UNEXPECTED SITUATIONS AND ASSOCIATED INTERVENTIONS

- *The patient states that he does not want to eat anything on the tray:* Explore with the patient the reason why he does not want to eat anything on the tray. Assess for psychological factors that impact nutrition. Malnutrition is sometimes found with depression in the older adult population. Mutually develop a plan to address the lack of nutritional intake and consult the dietitian, as needed.
- *The patient states that she feels nauseated and cannot eat:* Remove the tray from the patient's room. Explore with the patient the desirability of eating small amounts of foods or liquids, such as crackers or ginger ale, if the patient's diet permits. Administer antiemetic as prescribed, and encourage patient to retry small amounts of food after medication has had time to take effect.

SPECIAL CONSIDERATIONS

- For patients with arthritis of the hands, special utensils with modified handles that facilitate an easier grip are available. Contact an occupational therapist for guidance on adaptive equipment.
- A visually impaired patient may be guided to feed him- or herself through use of a "clock" pattern. For example, the chicken is placed at 6 o'clock; the vegetables at 3 o'clock.
- Refer to Box 11-1 for interventions and considerations related to assisting patients with alterations in cognition.
- For the patient with dysphagia, suggest small bites of food such as puddings, ground meat, or cooked vegetables. Advise the patient not to talk while swallowing and to swallow twice after each bite. Refer to Box 11-2 for additional considerations for this patient population.

WATCH & LEARN SKILL 11-2 INSERTING A NASOGASTRIC (NG) TUBE

The **nasogastric (NG) tube** is passed through the nose and into the stomach. This type of tube permits the patient to receive nutrition through a tube feeding using the stomach as a natural reservoir for food. Another purpose of an NG tube may be to decompress or to drain unwanted fluid and air from the stomach. This application would be used, for example, to allow the intestinal tract to rest and promote healing after bowel surgery. The NG tube can also be used to monitor bleeding in the gastrointestinal (GI) tract, to remove undesirable substances (lavage) such as poisons, or to help treat an intestinal obstruction. Refer to Chapter 13, Bowel Elimination.

DELEGATION CONSIDERATIONS

The insertion of an NG tube is not delegated to nursing assistive personnel (NAP) or to unlicensed assistive personnel (UAP). Depending on the state's nurse practice act and the organization's policies and procedures, insertion of an NG tube may be delegated to licensed practical/vocational nurses (LPN/LVNs). The decision to delegate must be based on careful analysis of the patient's needs and circumstances, as well as the qualifications of the person to whom the task is being delegated. Refer to the Delegation Guidelines in Appendix A.

EQUIPMENT

- Nasogastric tube of appropriate size (8–18 French)
- Stethoscope
- Water-soluble lubricant
- Normal saline solution or sterile water, for irrigation, depending on facility policy
- Tongue blade
- Irrigations set, including a Toomey (20–50 mL)
- Flashlight
- Nonallergenic tape (1 inch wide)
- Tissues
- Glass of water with straw
- Topical anesthetic—lidocaine spray or gel (optional)
- Clamp
- Suction apparatus (if ordered)
- Bath towel or disposable pad
- Emesis basin
- Safety pin and rubber band
- Nonsterile, disposable gloves
- Additional PPE, as indicated
- Tape measure, or other measuring device
- Skin barrier
- pH paper

ASSESSMENT

Assess the patency of the patient's nares by asking the patient to occlude one nostril and breathe normally through the other. Select the nostril through which air passes more easily. Also, assess the patient's history for any recent facial trauma, polyps, blockages, or surgeries. Patients with facial fractures or facial surgeries present a higher risk for misplacement of the tube into the brain. Many facilities require a physician to place NG tubes in these patients. Inspect the abdomen for distention and firmness; auscultate for bowel sounds or peristalsis and palpate the abdomen for distention and tenderness. If the abdomen is distended, consider measuring the abdominal girth at the umbilicus to establish a baseline.

NURSING DIAGNOSIS

Determine the related factors for the nursing diagnoses based on the patient's current status. Nursing diagnoses may vary depending on the reason for the NG tube insertion. Possible nursing diagnoses may include:

- Imbalanced Nutrition, Less than Body Requirements
- Impaired Swallowing
- Risk for Aspiration

OUTCOME IDENTIFICATION AND PLANNING

The expected outcome to achieve when inserting an NG tube is that the tube is passed into the patient's stomach without any complications. Other outcomes may include the following: the patient demonstrates weight gain, indicating improved nutrition; the patient exhibits no signs and symptoms of aspiration; the patient rates pain as decreased from prior to insertion; and the patient verbalizes an understanding of the reason for NG tube insertion.

IMPLEMENTATION

ACTION	RATIONALE
1. Verify the medical order for insertion of an NG tube. Gather equipment, including selection of the appropriate NG tube.	Ensures the patient receives the correct treatment. Assembling equipment provides for an organized approach to the task. NG tubes should be radiopaque, contain clearly visible markings for measurement, and may have multiple ports for aspiration.
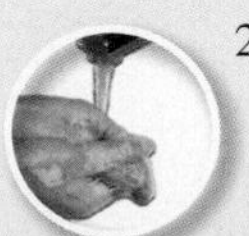 2. Perform hand hygiene and put on PPE, if indicated.	Hand hygiene and PPE prevent the spread of microorganisms. PPE is required based on transmission precautions.

(continued)

SKILL 11-2 INSERTING A NASOGASTRIC (NG) TUBE continued

ACTION	RATIONALE
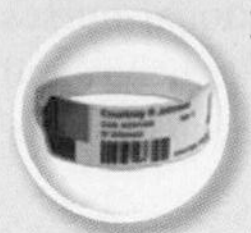 3. Identify the patient.	Identifying the patient ensures the right patient receives the intervention and helps prevent errors.
4. Explain the procedure to the patient, including the rationale for why the tube is needed. Discuss the associated discomforts that may be experienced and possible interventions that may allay this discomfort. Answer any questions, as needed.	Explanation facilitates patient cooperation. Some patient surveys report that of all routine procedures, the insertion of an NG tube is considered the most painful. Lidocaine gel or sprays are possible options to decrease discomfort during NG tube insertion.
5. Assemble equipment on overbed table within reach.	Arranging items nearby is convenient, saves time, and avoids unnecessary stretching and twisting of muscles on the part of the nurse.
6. Close the patient's bedside curtain or door. Raise the bed to a comfortable working position, usually elbow height of the caregiver (VISN 8, 2009). Assist the patient to high Fowler's position or elevate the head of the bed 45 degrees if the patient is unable to maintain an upright position (Figure 1). Drape chest with bath towel or disposable pad. Have emesis basin and tissues handy.	Closing curtains or door provides for patient privacy. Having the bed at the proper height prevents back and muscle strain. Upright position is more natural for swallowing and protects against bronchial intubation aspiration, if the patient should vomit. Passage of tube may stimulate gagging and tearing of eyes.
7. **Measure the distance to insert the tube by placing tube tip at the patient's nostril and extending it to tip of earlobe (Figure 2) and then to tip of xiphoid process (Figure 3).** Mark tube with an indelible marker.	Measurement ensures that tube will be long enough to enter patient's stomach.

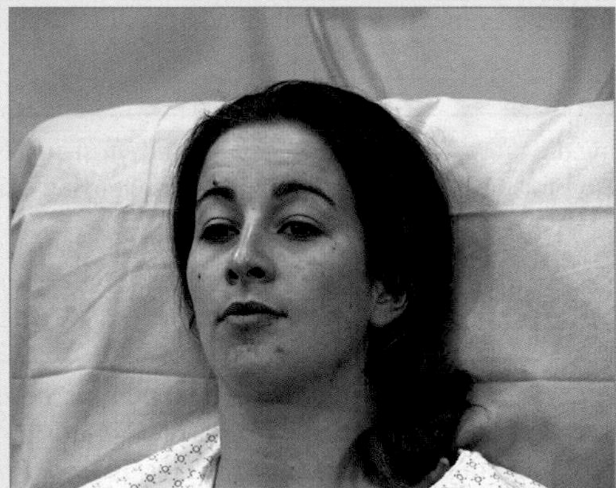

FIGURE 1 Placing patient in semi- to high Fowler's position in preparation for tube insertion.

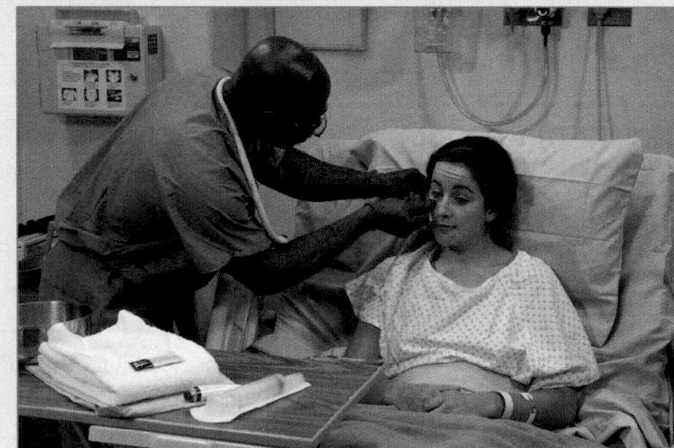

FIGURE 2 Measuring NG tube from nostril to tip of earlobe.

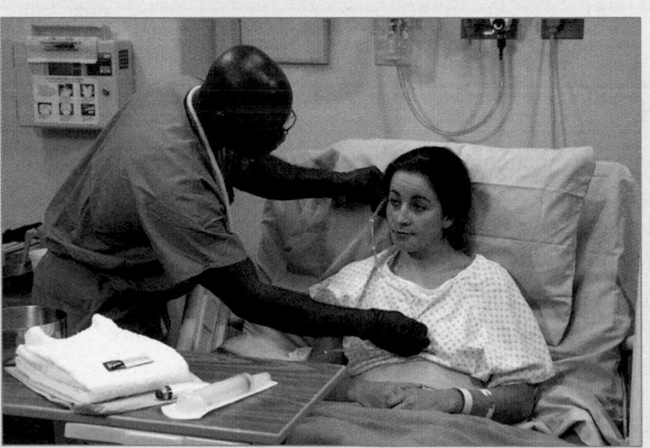

FIGURE 3 Measuring NG tube from tip of earlobe to xiphoid process.

ACTION	RATIONALE
8. Put on gloves. Lubricate tip of tube (at least 2 to 4 inches) with water-soluble lubricant. Apply topical anesthetic to nostril and oropharynx, as appropriate.	Lubrication reduces friction and facilitates passage of the tube into the stomach. Water-soluble lubricant will not cause pneumonia if the tube accidentally enters the lungs. Topical anesthetics act as local anesthetics, reducing discomfort. Consult the physician for an order for a topical anesthetic, such as lidocaine gel or spray, if needed.
9. After selecting the appropriate nostril, ask the patient to flex the head slightly back against the pillow. Gently insert the tube into the nostril while directing the tube upward and backward along the floor of the nose (Figure 4). Patient may gag when tube reaches pharynx. Provide tissues for tearing or watering of eyes. Offer comfort and reassurance to the patient.	Following the normal contour of the nasal passage while inserting the tube reduces irritation and the likelihood of mucosal injury. The tube stimulates the gag reflex readily. Tears are a natural response as the tube passes into the nasopharynx. Many patients report that gagging and throat discomfort can be more painful than the tube passing through the nostrils.
10. When pharynx is reached, instruct the patient to touch chin to chest. Encourage the patient to sip water through a straw or swallow even if no fluids are permitted. Advance tube in downward and backward direction when patient swallows (Figure 5). Stop when the patient breathes. **If gagging and coughing persist, stop advancing the tube and check placement of tube with tongue blade and flashlight.** If tube is curled, straighten the tube and attempt to advance again. Keep advancing the tube until pen marking is reached. **Do not use force.** Rotate the tube if it meets resistance.	Bringing the head forward helps close the trachea and open the esophagus. Swallowing helps advance the tube, causes the epiglottis to cover the opening of the trachea, and helps to eliminate gagging and coughing. Excessive coughing and gagging may occur if the tube has curled in the back of throat. Forcing the tube may injure mucous membranes.
11. **Discontinue the procedure and remove the tube if there are signs of distress, such as gasping, coughing, cyanosis, and inability to speak or hum.**	The tube is in the airway if the patient shows signs of distress and cannot speak or hum. If after three attempts, NG insertion is unsuccessful, another nurse may try or the patient should be referred to another health care professional.

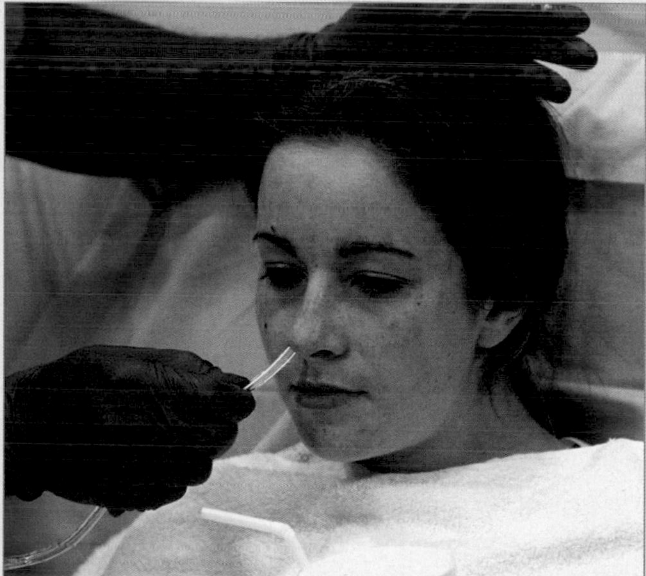

FIGURE 4 Beginning insertion with patient positioned with head slightly flexed back.

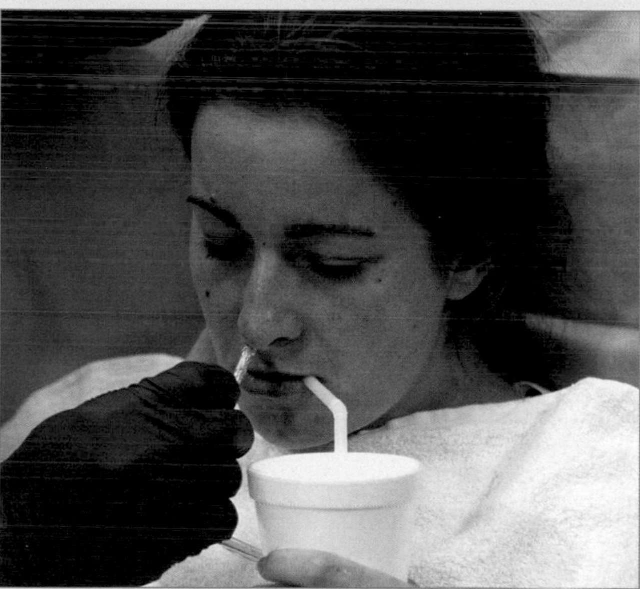

FIGURE 5 Advancing tube after patient drops chin to chest and while swallowing.

(continued)

SKILL 11-2 INSERTING A NASOGASTRIC (NG) TUBE continued

ACTION	RATIONALE
12. Secure the tube loosely to the nose or cheek until it is determined that the tube is in the patient's stomach:	Securing with tape stabilizes the tube while position is being determined.
a. Attach syringe to end of tube and aspirate a small amount of stomach contents.	The tube is in the stomach if its contents can be aspirated: pH of aspirate can then be tested to determine gastric placement. If unable to obtain a specimen, reposition the patient and flush the tube with 30 mL of air. This action may be necessary several times. Current literature recommends that the nurse ensures proper placement of the NG tube by relying on multiple methods and not on one method alone.
b. Measure the pH of aspirated fluid using pH paper or a meter. Place a drop of gastric secretions onto pH paper or place small amount in a plastic cup and dip the pH paper into it. Within 30 seconds, compare the color on the paper with the chart supplied by the manufacturer (Figure 6).	Current research demonstrates that the use of pH is predictive of correct placement. The pH of gastric contents is acidic (less than 5.5). If the patient is taking an acid-inhibiting agent, the range may be 4.0 to 6.0. The pH of intestinal fluid is 7.0 or higher. The pH of respiratory fluid is 6.0 or higher. This method will not effectively differentiate between intestinal fluid and pleural fluid.
c. Visualize aspirated contents, checking for color and consistency.	Gastric fluid can be green with particles, off-white, or brown if old blood is present. Intestinal aspirate tends to look clear or straw-colored to a deep golden-yellow color. Also, intestinal aspirate may be greenish-brown if stained with bile. Respiratory or tracheobronchial fluid is usually off-white to tan and may be tinged with mucus. A small amount of blood-tinged fluid may be seen immediately after NG insertion.
d. Obtain radiograph (x-ray) of placement of tube, based on facility policy (and ordered by physician).	The x-ray is considered the most reliable method for identifying the position of the NG tube.
13. Apply skin barrier to tip and end of nose and allow to dry. Remove gloves and secure tube with a commercially prepared device (follow manufacturer's directions) or tape to patient's nose. To secure with tape:	Skin barrier improves adhesion and protects skin. Constant pressure of the tube against the skin and mucous membranes may cause tissue injury. Securing tube prevents migration of the tube inward and outward.
a. Cut a 4-inch piece of tape and split bottom 2 inches (Figure 7) or use packaged nose tape for NG tubes.	
b. Place unsplit end over bridge of patient's nose (Figure 8).	
c. Wrap split ends under and around NG tube (Figure 9). **Be careful not to pull tube too tightly against nose.**	

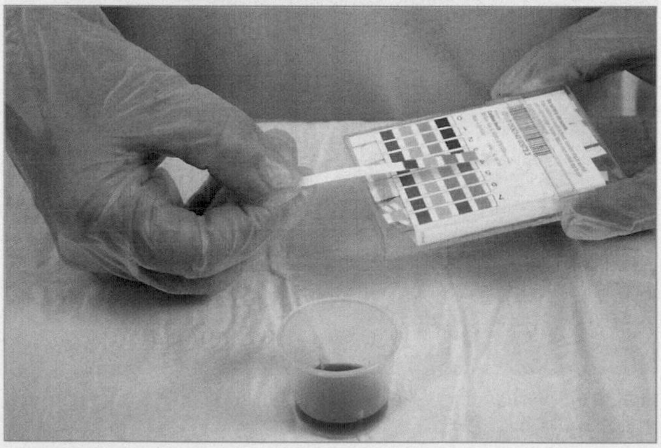

FIGURE 6 Checking pH of gastric fluid.

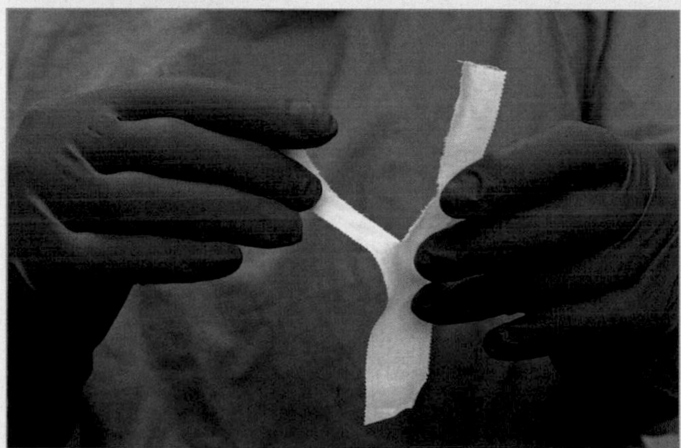

FIGURE 7 Making a 2-inch cut into a 4-inch strip of tape.

ACTION | RATIONALE

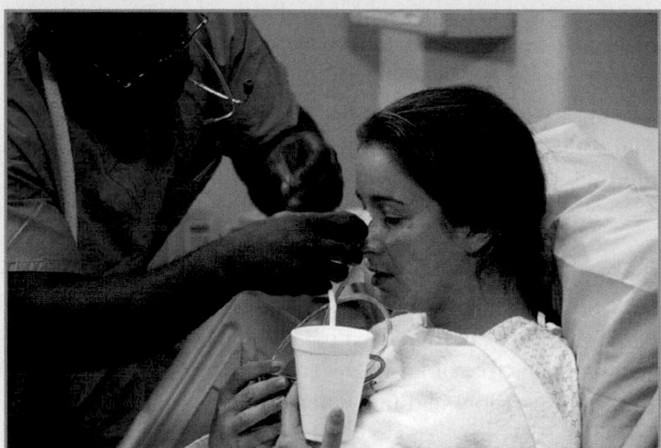
FIGURE 8 Applying tape to patient's nose.

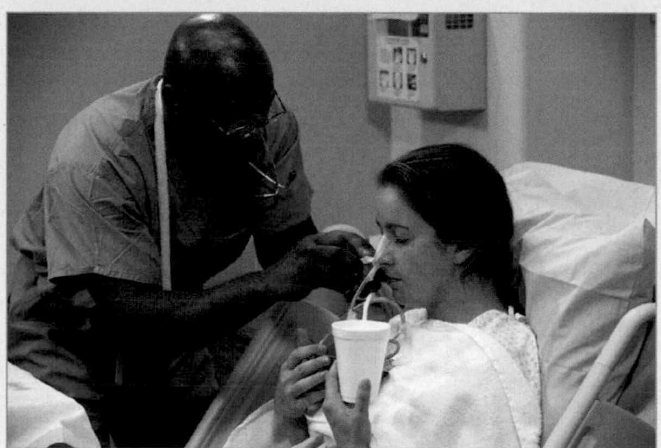
FIGURE 9 Wrapping split ends around NG tube.

14. Put on gloves. Clamp tube and remove the syringe. Cap the tube or attach tube to suction (Figure 10) according to the medical orders (see Chapter 13).

Suction provides for decompression of stomach and drainage of gastric contents.

15. Measure length of exposed tube. Reinforce marking on tube at nostril with indelible ink. Ask the patient to turn his/her head to the side opposite the nostril in which the tube is inserted. Secure tube to patient's gown by using rubber band or tape and safety pin. For additional support, tape the tube onto patient's cheek using a piece of tape. **If a double-lumen tube (e.g., Salem sump) is used, secure the vent above stomach level.** Attach the vent at shoulder level (Figure 11).

Tube length should be checked and compared with this initial measurement, in conjunction with pH measurement and visual assessment of aspirate. An increase in the length of the exposed tube may indicate dislodgement (AACN, 2010; Bourgault et al., 2007; Hinkle & Cheever, 2014). The tube should be marked with an indelible marker at the nostril. This marking should be assessed each time the tube is used to ensure the tube has not become displaced. Securing prevents tension and tugging on the tube. Turning the head ensures adequate slack in the tubing to prevent tension when the patient turns the head. Securing the double-lumen tube above stomach level prevents seepage of gastric contents and keeps the lumen clear for venting air.

16. Assist with or provide oral hygiene at 2- to 4-hour intervals. Lubricate the lips generously and clean nares and lubricate, as needed. Offer analgesic throat lozenges or anesthetic spray for throat irritation, if needed.

Oral hygiene keeps mouth clean and moist, promotes comfort, and reduces thirst.

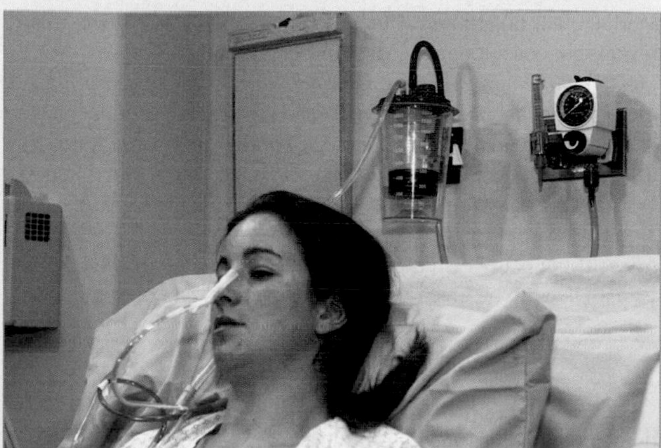
FIGURE 10 NG tube attached to wall suction.

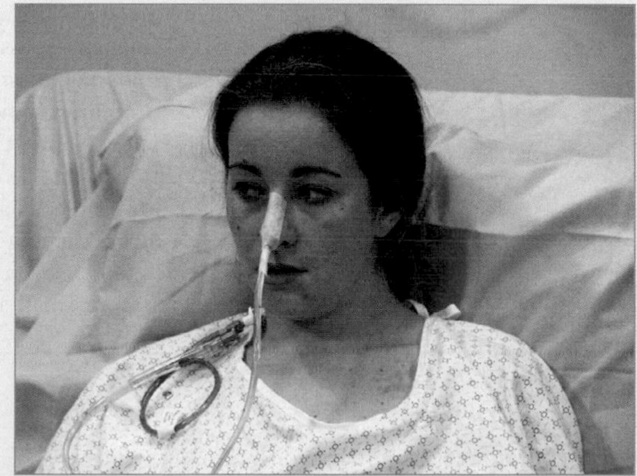
FIGURE 11 Patient with Salem sump tube (NG) secured. Note blue vent at patient's shoulder.

(continued)

SKILL 11-2 INSERTING A NASOGASTRIC (NG) TUBE continued

ACTION	RATIONALE
17. Remove equipment and return patient to a position of comfort. Remove gloves. Raise side rail and lower bed.	Promotes patient comfort and safety. Removing gloves properly reduces the risk for infection transmission and contamination of other items.
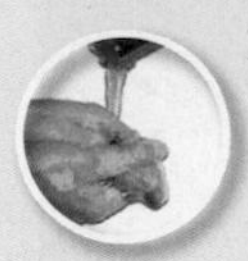 18. Remove additional PPE, if used. Perform hand hygiene.	Removing PPE properly reduces the risk for infection transmission and contamination of other items. Hand hygiene prevents transmission of microorganisms.

EVALUATION

The expected outcome is met when patient exhibits a nasogastric tube placed into the stomach without any complications. In addition, other outcomes are met when patient demonstrates weight gain, indicating improved nutrition; the patient remains free of any signs and symptoms of aspiration; the patient rates pain as decreased from prior to insertion; and the patient verbalizes an understanding of the reason for NG tube insertion.

DOCUMENTATION

Guidelines

Document the size and type of NG tube that was inserted and the measurement from tip of the nose to the end of the exposed tube. Also, document the results of the x-ray that was taken to confirm the tube position, if applicable. Record a description of the gastric contents, including the pH of the contents. Document the naris where the tube is placed and the patient's response to the procedure. Include assessment data, both subjective and objective, related to the abdomen. Record the patient teaching that was discussed.

Sample Documentation

Lippincott DocuCare Practice documenting NG tube insertion in *Lippincott DocuCare.*

10/4/15 0945 Abdomen slightly distended and taut; hypoactive bowel sounds. Patient reports transient nausea. 14-Fr Levin tube inserted via R naris, 20 cm of tube from naris to end of tube; gastric contents aspirated, pH 4, contents light green; patient tolerated without incident.

—*S. Essner, RN*

UNEXPECTED SITUATIONS AND ASSOCIATED INTERVENTIONS

- *As a tube is passing through the pharynx, patient begins to retch and gag:* This is common during placement of an NG tube. Ask the patient if he or she wants the nurse to stop the procedure, which will allow the patient to gain composure from the gagging episode. Continue to advance the tube when the patient relates that he or she is ready. Have the emesis basin nearby in case patient begins to vomit.
- *The nurse is unable to pass the tube after trying a second time down the one nostril:* If the patient's condition permits, inspect the other nostril and attempt to pass the NG tube down this nostril. If unable to pass down this nostril, consult another health professional.
- *As tube is passing through pharynx, the patient begins to cough and shows signs of respiratory distress:* **Stop advancing the tube.** The tube is most likely entering the trachea. Pull tube back into nasal area. Support patient as he or she regains normal breathing ability and composure. If the patient feels that he or she can tolerate another attempt, ask the patient to keep chin on chest and swallow as tube is advanced to help prevent the tube from entering the trachea. Begin to advance tube, watching for any signs of respiratory distress.
- *No gastric contents can be aspirated:* If the patient is comatose, check oral cavity. If the tube is in a gastric area, small air boluses may need to be given until gastric contents can be aspirated.

SPECIAL CONSIDERATIONS

General Considerations

To promote patient safety when administering a tube feeding, be sure to do the following:

- Check tube placement before administering any fluids, medications, or feedings. Use multiple techniques: x-ray, external length marking/measurement, pH testing, and aspirate characteristics.

- Some patients require a **nasointestinal tube**. To insert a nasointestinal tube:
  - Measure tube from tip of nose to earlobe and from earlobe to xiphoid process. Add 8 to 10 inches for intestinal placement. Mark tubing at desired point.
  - Place patient on his/her right side. Nasointestinal tube is usually placed in the stomach and allowed to advance through peristalsis through the pyloric sphincter (may take up to 24 hours).
  - Administer medications to enhance GI motility, such as metoclopramide (Reglan), if ordered.
  - Test pH of aspirate when tube has advanced to marked point to confirm placement in intestine. Confirm position by radiograph. Secure with tape once placement is confirmed.
- Monitoring for carbon dioxide to determine NG tube position and/or dislodgement has been investigated (Gilbert & Burns, 2012; Munera-Seeley et al., 2008). This involves the use of a capnograph or a colorimetric end-tidal CO_2 detector to detect the presence of carbon dioxide, which would indicate tube positioning in the patient's airway instead of the stomach.

Infant and Child Considerations

- Infants are obligate nose breathers; insertion of the tube via the mouth may be appropriate (orogastric tube) (Perry et al., 2010).
- Age-specific equations are available to predict insertion distance and are the best method to determine insertion distance based on age and height for infants and children, 2 weeks to 19 years of age. Other methods to determine insertion distance include the nose or mouth to ear-mid-xiphoid-umbilicus span. The accuracy of these methods has been challenged (Freeman et al., 2012).

EVIDENCE FOR PRACTICE ▶

ACCURATE PLACEMENT OF NASOGASTRIC FEEDING TUBES AND CARBON DIOXIDE DETECTION

Inadvertent placement of nasogastric feeding tubes into the tracheopulmonary system during insertion and displacement at a time following initial insertion are potential life-threatening problems. The only absolutely reliable method to determine accurate placement is radiography. However, repeated radiographic testing is not practical or safe. Several methods of bedside testing, including evaluation of tube aspirate, measurement of aspirate pH, and measurement of exposed tube length, are in use; there is a continued need to strive for more conclusive methods to determine tube placement. Can a device to detect the presence of carbon dioxide be used to detect inadvertent placement into the airway instead of the stomach?

Related Research

Gilbert, R.T., & Burns, S.M. (2012). Increasing the safety of blind gastric tube placement in pediatric patients: The design and testing of a procedure using a carbon dioxide detection device. *Journal of Pediatric Nursing, 27*(5), 528–532.

This study evaluated the use of a new commercial CO_2 sensor that was developed to assist in evaluating the placement of NG feeding tubes. Prior to each feeding tube placement, the nurse took two measurements of tube length. One was from the point of entry (nose or mouth) to the ear to the level of the carina. The other was from the point of entry to the ear to the xiphoid process. The data collector then placed a CO_2nfirm Now™ device on the distal end of the feeding tube prior to placement. As the tube was placed, both the bedside nurse and the study investigator monitored for signs of respiratory distress; if any signs of distress were observed, then the tube was immediately removed. If there were no signs of distress, then the tube was placed to the premeasured depth of the carina. The CO_2nfirm Now™ was assessed for color change from purple to yellow, which indicated the presence of carbon dioxide. If there was color change from purple to yellow but the patient was clinically stable, the investigator disconnected the CO_2nfirm Now™ from the feeding tube and flushed the device with room air using a 5-mL syringe until the purple color returned. This step was necessary due to the potential for carbon dioxide being in the mouth or back of the throat during feeding tube placement. CO_2nfirm Now™ was then reattached to the gastric tube. The data collector flushed the feeding tube through the CO_2nfirm Now™ with 3 mL room air, and a small volume of air was aspirated from the gastric tube through the CO_2nfirm Now™ device. This process was necessary because the pediatric gastric tubes used in this population have smaller internal diameters than those used in the adult population. Total reliance on the passive flow of gases entering or exiting the tubes was not possible. Thus, our procedure required both the active flushing and then aspiration of gases past the CO_2nfirm Now™

(*continued*)

SKILL 11-2 INSERTING A NASOGASTRIC (NG) TUBE continued

device, as described. If having done this flushing step, there continued to be a yellow color change on the device, it was determined that the gastric tube had been inadvertently placed into the airway and the tube was withdrawn. If there was no color change, the bedside nurse continued to advance the tube to the premeasured gastric level. The tube was secured, and an abdominal x-ray was obtained to determine if tube placement was in the esophagus, stomach, or postpyloric. This step was done to verify tube placement per a standing PICU guideline. Sixty devices were tested on 42 patients over a period of 15 months. Three of the feeding tubes were removed as a result of a color change, indicating the detection of carbon dioxide during tube placement, and three were removed for other reasons. The ability of the colorimetric device to detect the presence of carbon dioxide was 100% accurate in all cases where the tube was in contact with carbon dioxide. The authors concluded the use of a carbon dioxide sensing device during the blind placement of gastric tubes in pediatric patients may be a beneficial innovation to pediatric practices. The procedure presents little to no additional risk and it increased the safety of the procedure.

Relevance for Nursing Practice

The CO_2 sensor is a helpful bedside tool to use in conjunction with clinical methods during NG feeding tube insertions. Nurses should consider investigating the use of these devices in their individual clinical facilities.

Refer to thePoint for additional research on related nursing topics.

EVIDENCE FOR PRACTICE ▶

ESTIMATING GASTRIC TUBE INSERTION LENGTH IN CHILDREN

An accurate external method for predicting the internal distance to the esophagogastric junction or to locations within the stomach in children is a necessary condition for correctly placed orogastric and nasogastric tubes, particularly in circumstances where radiographic visualization is not available. Studies have indicated that commonly used distances to determine insertion length are frequently inaccurate. Is there a more effective way to estimate insertion length for infants?

Related Research

Freeman, D., Saxton, V., & Holberton, J. (2012). A weight-based formula for the estimation of gastric tube insertion length in newborns. *Advances in Neonatal Care, 12*(3), 179–182.

Safe and effective functioning of nasogastric and orogastric tubes in the neonatal intensive care unit (NICU) is achieved by ensuring their correct placement within the stomach. Studies have indicated that commonly used distances to determine insertion length are frequently inaccurate. This study aimed to evaluate the frequency of correct tube placement and to determine a weight-based formula for estimation of insertion length. A prospective study was performed over a 6-month period in a tertiary NICU. Infants with gastric tubes who required radiography for clinical reasons were included. The infant's weight and the type and length of tube were documented. A radiologist assessed the tube position to be high, borderline, correct, or long. A total of 218 radiographs of infants weighing 397 to 4,131 g were included. Correct tube position was achieved on 74% of occasions. By analyzing data for correct tube positions, formulas were derived to predict tube insertion length in centimeters: orogastric = [3 × weight (kg) + 12] and nasogastric = [3 × weight (kg) + 13]. The formulas correctly predicted 60% of misplaced orogastric tubes and 100% of misplaced nasogastric tubes. The authors proposed a novel weight-based formula for estimation of gastric tube insertion length in infants that could be used in association with current methods to improve the accuracy of this routine procedure.

Relevance for Nursing Practice

This study confirms that traditional methods of estimating NG and orogastric tube insertion length in newborn infants produce a reasonably high rate of error that is consistent with published studies. Nurses have a responsibility to continually strive to improve professional practice through evidence as it becomes available and to initiate investigation of possible improvements in nursing care. Nurses should consider proposals to examine these findings and for possible inclusion in facility policy and procedure, to ensure safe care for patients with these devices.

Refer to thePoint for additional research on related nursing topics.

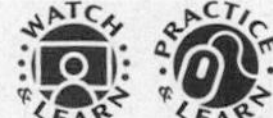

SKILL 11-3 ADMINISTERING A TUBE FEEDING

Depending on the patient's physical and psychosocial condition and nutritional requirements, a feeding through the NG tube or other GI tube might be ordered. The steps for administering feedings are similar regardless of the tube used. Feeding can be provided on an intermittent or continuous basis. Intermittent feedings are delivered at regular intervals, using gravity for instillation or a feeding pump to administer the formula over a set period of time. Intermittent feedings might also be given as a bolus, using a syringe to instill the formula quickly in one large amount. Intermittent feedings are the preferred method, introducing the formula over a set period of time via gravity or pump. If the order calls for continuous feeding, an external feeding pump is needed to regulate the flow of formula. Continuous feedings permit gradual introduction of the formula into the GI tract, promoting maximal absorption. However, there is a risk of both reflux and aspiration with this method. Feeding intolerance is less likely to occur with smaller volumes. Hanging smaller amounts of feeding also reduces the risk for bacteria growth and contamination of feeding at room temperature (when using open systems).

The procedure below describes using open systems and a feeding pump; the skill variation at the end of the skill describes using a closed system.

DELEGATION CONSIDERATIONS

The administration of a tube feeding is not usually delegated to nursing assistive personnel (NAP) or to unlicensed assistive personnel (UAP) in the acute care setting. The administration of a tube feeding in some settings may be delegated to NAP or UAP who have received appropriate training, after assessment of tube placement and patency by the registered nurse. Depending on the state's nurse practice act and the organization's policies and procedures, the administration of a tube feeding may be delegated to licensed practical/vocational nurses (LPN/LVNs). The decision to delegate must be based on careful analysis of the patient's needs and circumstances, as well as the qualifications of the person to whom the task is being delegated. Refer to the Delegation Guidelines in Appendix A.

EQUIPMENT

- Prescribed tube feeding formula at room temperature
- Feeding bag or prefilled tube feeding set
- Stethoscope
- Nonsterile gloves
- Additional PPE, as indicated
- Alcohol preps
- Disposable pad or towel
- Asepto or Toomey syringe
- Enteral feeding pump (if ordered)
- Rubber band
- Clamp (Hoffman or butterfly)
- IV pole
- Water for irrigation and hydration, as needed
- pH paper
- Tape measure, or other measuring device

ASSESSMENT

Assess the abdomen by inspecting for presence of distention, auscultate for bowel sounds, and palpate the abdomen for firmness or tenderness. If the abdomen is distended, consider measuring the abdominal girth at the umbilicus. If the patient reports any tenderness or nausea, exhibits any rigidity or firmness of the abdomen, and if bowel sounds are absent, confer with physician before administering the tube feeding. Assess for patient and/or family understanding, if appropriate, for the rationale for the tube feeding and address any questions or concerns expressed by the patient and family members. Consult physician, if needed, for further explanation.

NURSING DIAGNOSIS

Determine the related factors for the nursing diagnoses based on the patient's current status. Possible nursing diagnoses may include:

- Risk for Aspiration
- Deficient Knowledge
- Imbalanced Nutrition, Less than Body Requirements

OUTCOME IDENTIFICATION AND PLANNING

The expected outcome to achieve when administering a tube feeding is that the patient will receive the tube feeding without complaints of nausea, episodes of vomiting, gastric distention, or diarrhea. Additional expected outcomes may include the following: the patient demonstrates an increase in weight; the patient exhibits no signs and symptoms of aspiration; and the patient verbalizes knowledge related to tube feeding.

(continued)

SKILL 11-3 ADMINISTERING A TUBE FEEDING continued

IMPLEMENTATION

ACTION	RATIONALE
1. Gather equipment. Check amount, concentration, type, and frequency of tube feeding in the patient's medical record. Check formula expiration date.	This provides for an organized approach to the task. Checking ensures that correct feeding will be administered. Outdated formula may be contaminated.
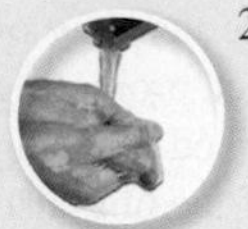 2. Perform hand hygiene and put on PPE, if indicated.	Hand hygiene and PPE prevent the spread of microorganisms. PPE is required based on transmission precautions.
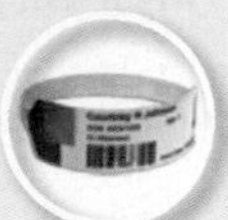 3. Identify the patient.	Identifying the patient ensures the right patient receives the intervention and helps prevent errors.
4. Explain the procedure to the patient and why this intervention is needed. Answer any questions, as needed.	Explanation facilitates patient cooperation.
5. Assemble equipment on overbed table within reach.	Organization facilitates performance of the task.
6. Close the patient's bedside curtain or door. Raise the bed to a comfortable working position, usually elbow height of the caregiver (VISN 8, 2009). Perform key abdominal assessments as described above.	Closing curtains or door provides for patient privacy. Having the bed at the proper height prevents back and muscle strain. Due to changes in the patient's condition, assessment is vital before initiating the intervention.
7. **Position the patient with HOB elevated at least 30 to 45 degrees or as near normal position for eating as possible.**	This position minimizes possibility of aspiration into the trachea. Patients who are considered at high risk for aspiration should be assisted to at least a 45-degree position.
8. Put on gloves. Unpin the tube from the patient's gown. Verify the position of the marking on the tube at the nostril. Measure length of exposed tube and compare with the documented length.	Gloves prevent contact with blood and body fluids. The tube should be marked with an indelible marker at the nostril. This marking should be assessed each time the tube is used to ensure the tube has not become displaced. Tube length should be checked and compared with this initial measurement, in conjunction with pH measurement and visual assessment of aspirate. An increase in the length of the exposed tube may indicate dislodgement (AACN, 2010; Bourgault et al., 2007; Hinkle & Cheever, 2014).
9. Attach syringe to end of tube and aspirate a small amount of stomach contents, as described in Skill 11-2 (Figure 1).	The tube is in the stomach if its contents can be aspirated: pH of aspirate can then be tested to determine gastric placement. If unable to obtain a specimen, reposition the patient and flush the tube with 30 mL of air. This action may be necessary several times. Current literature recommends that the nurse ensures proper placement of the NG tube by relying on multiple methods and not on one method alone.

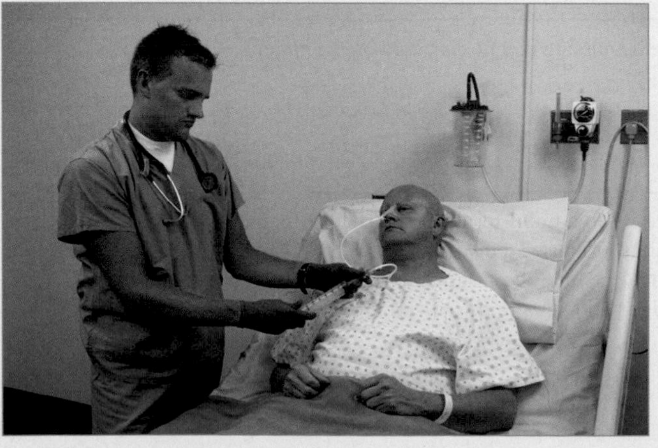

FIGURE 1 Aspirating gastric contents.

ACTION	RATIONALE
10. Check the pH as described in Skill 11-2 (Figure 2).	Current research demonstrates that the use of pH is predictive of correct placement. The pH of gastric contents is acidic (less than 5.5). If the patient is taking an acid-inhibiting agent, the range may be 4.0 to 6.0. The pH of intestinal fluid is 7.0 or higher. The pH of respiratory fluid is 6.0 or higher. This method will not effectively differentiate between intestinal fluid and pleural fluid. Testing for pH before the next feeding in intermittent feedings is conducted since the stomach has been emptied of the feeding formula. However, if the patient is receiving continuous feedings, the pH measurement is not as useful, since the formula raises the pH.

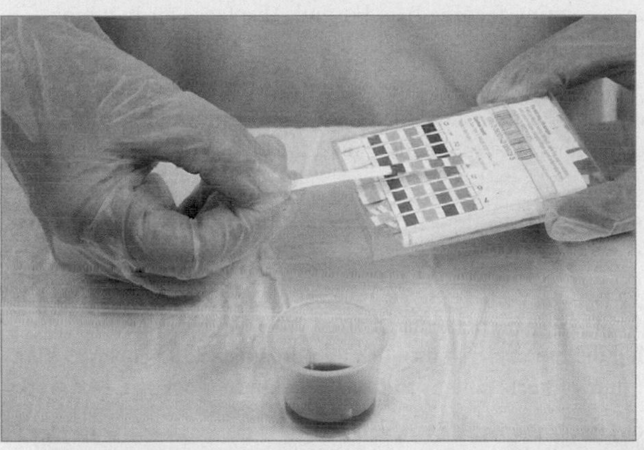

FIGURE 2 Checking pH of gastric fluid.

ACTION	RATIONALE
11. Visualize aspirated contents, checking for color and consistency.	Gastric fluid can be green, with particles, off white, or brown if old blood is present. Intestinal aspirate tends to look clear or straw colored to a deep golden-yellow color. Also, intestinal aspirate may be greenish-brown if stained with bile. Respiratory or tracheobronchial fluid is usually off-white to tan and may be tinged with mucus. A small amount of blood-tinged fluid may be seen immediately after NG insertion.
12. If it is not possible to aspirate contents; assessments to check placement are inconclusive, the exposed tube length has changed; or there are any other indications that the tube is not in place, check placement by x-ray.	The x-ray is considered the most reliable method for identifying the position of the NG tube.
13. After multiple steps have been taken to ensure that the feeding tube is located in the stomach or small intestine, **aspirate all gastric contents with the syringe and measure to check for gastric residual—the amount of feeding remaining in the stomach.** Return the residual based on facility policy. Proceed with feeding if amount of residual does not exceed agency policy or the limit indicated in the medical record.	Checking for residual before each feeding or every 4 to 6 hours during a continuous feeding according to institutional policy is implemented to identify delayed gastric emptying. High gastric residual volumes (200 to 250 mL or greater) can be associated with high risk for aspiration and aspiration-related pneumonia (Bourgault et al., 2007; Metheny, 2008). Some experts now recommend that the patient's pattern of residual is more important than the amount (ASPEN, 2011; Bourgault et al., 2007; Metheny, 2008). Feedings should be held if residual volumes exceed 200 mL on two successive assessments (ASPEN, 2011). Research findings are inconclusive on the benefit of returning gastric volumes to the stomach or intestine to avoid fluid or electrolyte imbalance, which has been accepted practice. Consult facility policy concerning this practice.

(continued)

SKILL 11-3 ADMINISTERING A TUBE FEEDING continued

ACTION	RATIONALE
14. Flush tube with 30 mL of water for irrigation. Disconnect syringe from tubing and cap end of tubing while preparing the formula feeding equipment. Remove gloves.	Flushing tube prevents occlusion (ASPEN, 2011; Bourgault et al., 2007; Metheny, 2008). Capping the tube deters the entry of microorganisms and prevents leakage onto the bed linens.
15. Put on gloves before preparing, assembling, and handling any part of the feeding system.	Gloves prevent contact with blood and body fluids and deter transmission of contaminants to feeding equipment and/or formula.
16. Administer feeding.	
When Using a Feeding Bag (Open System)	
a. Label bag and/or tubing with date and time. Hang bag on IV pole and adjust to about 12 iches above the stomach. Clamp tubing.	Labeling date and time of first use allows for disposal within 24 hours, to deter growth of microorganisms. Proper feeding bag height reduces risk of formula being introduced too quickly.
b. Check the expiration date of the formula. Cleanse top of feeding container with a disinfectant before opening it (Figure 3). Pour formula into feeding bag and allow solution to run through tubing. Close clamp.	Cleansing container top with alcohol minimizes risk for contaminants entering feeding bag. Formula displaces air in tubing.
c. Attach feeding setup to feeding tube (Figure 4), open clamp, and regulate drip according to the medical order, or allow feeding to run in over 30 minutes.	Introducing formula at a slow, regular rate allows the stomach to accommodate to the feeding and decreases GI distress.
d. **Add 30 to 60 mL (1 to 2 oz.) of water for irrigation to feeding bag when feeding is almost completed (Figure 5) and allow it to run through the tube.**	Water rinses the feeding from the tube and helps to keep it patent.
e. Clamp tubing immediately after water has been instilled. Disconnect feeding setup from feeding tube. Clamp tube and cover end with cap (Figure 6).	Clamping the tube prevents air from entering the stomach. Capping the tube deters entry of microorganisms and covering end of tube protects patient and linens from fluid leakage from tube.

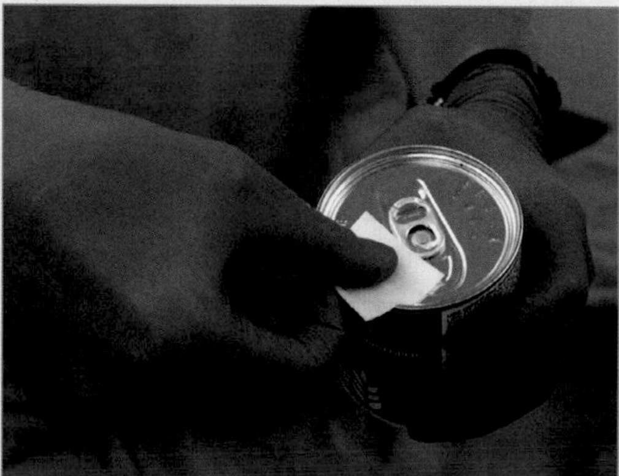

FIGURE 3 Cleaning top of feeding container with alcohol before opening it.

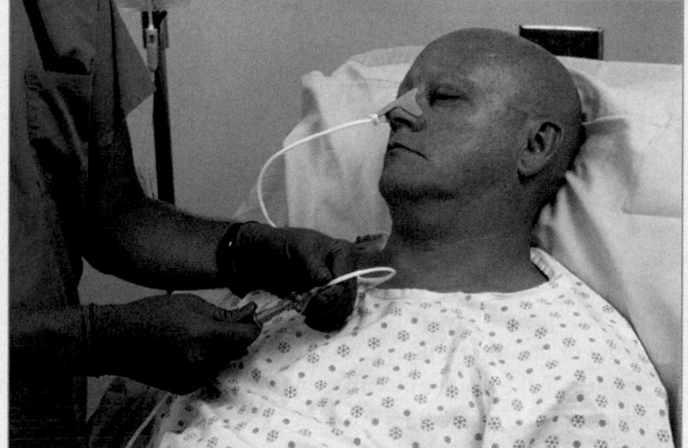

FIGURE 4 Attaching feeding bag tubing to NG tube.

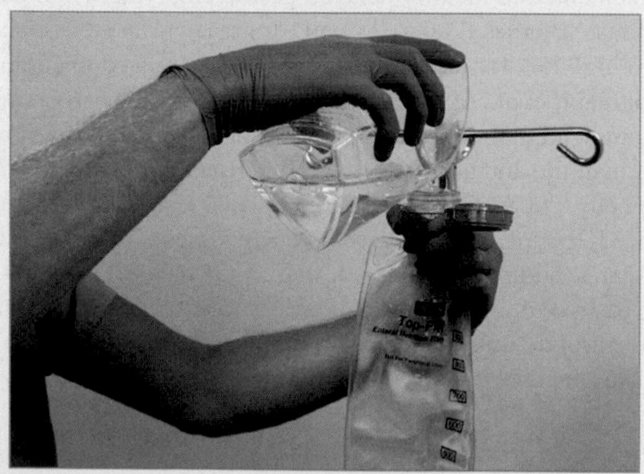

FIGURE 5 Pouring water into feeding bag.

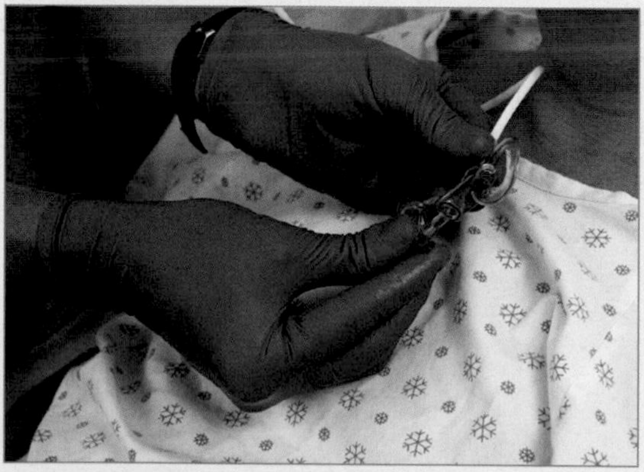

FIGURE 6 Capping NG tube after it is clamped.

ACTION	RATIONALE
When Using a Large Syringe (Open System)	
a. Remove plunger from 30- or 60-mL syringe (Figure 7).	Introducing the formula at a slow, regular rate allows the stomach to accommodate to the feeding and decreases GI distress. The higher the syringe is held, the faster the formula flows.
b. Attach syringe to feeding tube, pour premeasured amount of tube feeding formula into syringe (Figure 8), open clamp, and allow food to enter tube. Regulate rate, fast or slow, by height of the syringe. **Do not push formula with syringe plunger.**	
c. **Add 30 to 60 mL (1 to 2 oz.) of water for irrigation to syringe (Figure 9) when feeding is almost completed, and allow it to run through the tube.**	Water rinses the feeding from the tube and helps to keep it patent.
d. When syringe has emptied, hold syringe high and disconnect from tube. Clamp tube and cover end with cap.	By holding syringe high, the formula will not backflow out of tube and onto patient. Clamping the tube prevents air from entering the stomach. Capping end of tube deters entry of microorganisms. Covering the end protects patient and linens from fluid leakage from tube.

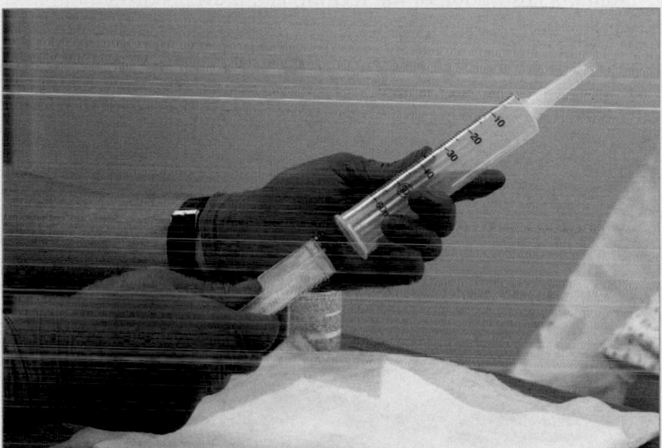

FIGURE 7 Removing plunger from a 60-mL syringe.

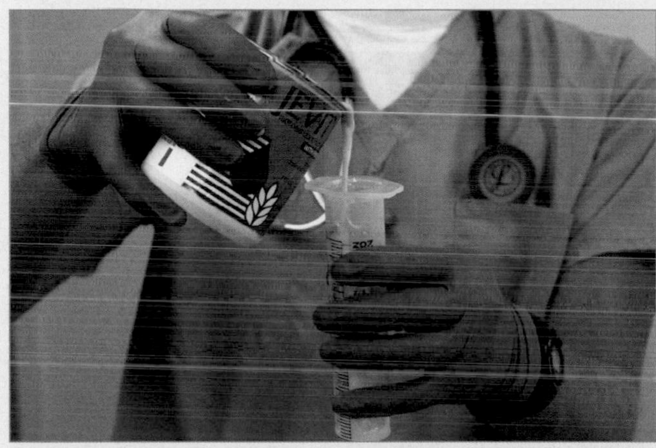

FIGURE 8 Pouring formula into syringe.

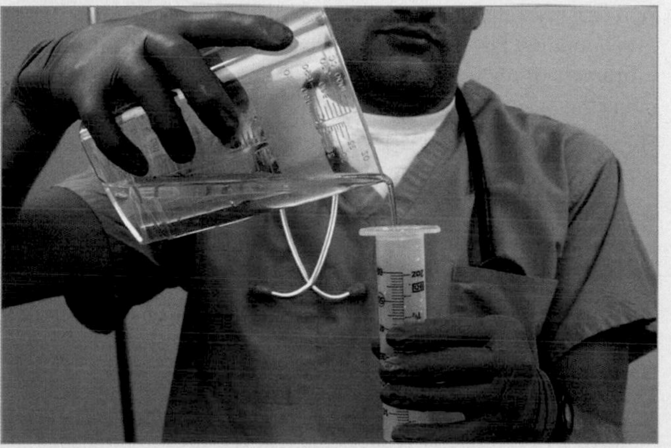

FIGURE 9 Pouring water into almost-empty syringe.

(*continued*)

SKILL 11-3 ADMINISTERING A TUBE FEEDING continued

ACTION	RATIONALE
When Using an Enteral Feeding Pump	
a. Close flow-regulator clamp on tubing and fill feeding bag with prescribed formula. Amount used depends on agency policy. Place label on container with patient's name, date, and time the feeding was hung.	Closing clamp prevents formula from moving through tubing until nurse is ready. Labeling date and time of first use allows for disposal within 24 hours, to deter growth of microorganisms.
b. Hang feeding container on IV pole. Allow solution to flow through tubing.	This prevents air from being forced into the stomach or intestines.
c. Connect to feeding pump, following manufacturer's directions. Set rate (Figure 10). Maintain the patient in the upright position throughout the feeding. If the patient needs to lie flat temporarily, pause the feeding. Resume the feeding after the patient's position has been changed back to at least 30 to 45 degrees.	Feeding pumps vary. Some of the newer pumps have built-in safeguards that protect the patient from complications. Safety features include cassettes that prevent free-flow of formula, automatic tube flush, safety tips that prevent accidental attachment to an IV setup, and various audible and visible alarms. Feedings are started at full strength rather than diluted, which was recommended previously. A smaller volume, 10 to 40 mL, of feeding infused per hour and gradually increased has been shown to be more easily tolerated by patients.
d. **Check placement of tube and gastric residual every 4 to 6 hours.**	Checking placement (Steps 9–12) verifies that the tube has not moved out of the stomach. Checking gastric residual (Step 13) monitors absorption of the feeding and prevents distention, which could lead to aspiration.

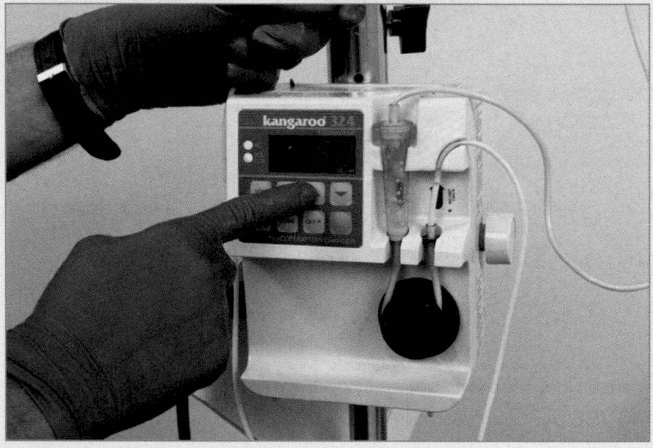

FIGURE 10 Setting up feeding pump with feeding bag and primed tubing.

ACTION	RATIONALE
17. Observe the patient's response during and after tube feeding and assess the abdomen at least once a shift.	Pain or nausea may indicate stomach distention, which may lead to vomiting. Physical signs, such as abdominal distention and firmness or regurgitation of tube feeding, may indicate intolerance.
18. **Have patient remain in upright position for at least 1 hour after feeding.**	This position minimizes risk for backflow and discourages aspiration, if any reflux or vomiting should occur.
19. Remove equipment and return patient to a position of comfort. Remove gloves. Raise side rail and lower bed.	Promotes patient comfort and safety. Removing gloves properly reduces the risk for infection transmission and contamination of other items.
20. Put on gloves. Wash and clean equipment or replace according to agency policy. Remove gloves.	This prevents contamination and deters spread of microorganisms. Reusable systems are cleansed with soap and water with each use and replaced every 24 hours. Refer to agency's policy and manufacturer's guidelines for specifics on equipment care.
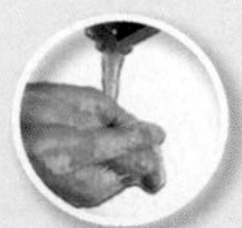 21. Remove additional PPE, if used. Perform hand hygiene.	Removing PPE properly reduces the risk for infection transmission and contamination of other items. Hand hygiene prevents transmission of microorganisms.

EVALUATION

The expected outcome is achieved when the patient receives the ordered tube feeding without complaints of nausea, episodes of vomiting, gastric distension, or diarrhea; the patient demonstrates an increase in weight; the patient remains free of any signs and symptoms of aspiration; and the patient voices knowledge related to tube feeding.

DOCUMENTATION

Guidelines

Document the type of NG tube or gastrostomy/jejunostomy tube that is present. Record the criteria that were used to confirm proper placement before feeding was initiated, such as the tube length in inches or centimeters compared to the length on initial insertion. Document the aspiration of gastric contents and pH of the gastric contents when intermittent feeding is used. Note the components of the abdominal assessment, such as observation of the abdomen, presence of distention or firmness, and presence of bowel sounds. Include subjective data, such as any reports from the patient of abdominal pain or nausea or any other patient response. Record the amount of gastric residual volume that was obtained. Document the position of the patient, the type of feeding, and the method and the amount of feeding. Include any relevant patient teaching.

Sample Documentation

10/29/15 1015 Position of NG tube was compared with initial measurement on insertion. Abdomen nondistended and soft; patient denies pain or nausea. HOB raised to 45 degrees. Thirty (30) mL residual aspirated prior to feeding; pH 3.9. Aspirate returned to stomach; aspirate yellow with dark flecks. 150 mL of Jevity 1.2 Cal. administered via bolus feeding. Tube flushed with 60 mL water with ease. Patient instructed to call for nurse for pain or nausea or other concerns related to feeding.

—*S. Essner, RN*

UNEXPECTED SITUATIONS AND ASSOCIATED INTERVENTIONS

- *Tube is found not to be in stomach or intestine:* Tube must be in the stomach before feeding. If the tube is in the esophagus, the patient is at increased risk for aspiration. See Skill 11-2 for steps to replace tube.
- *When checking for residual, the nurse aspirates a large amount:* Before discarding or replacing residual, check with the primary care provider and facility policy. Replacing a large amount may increase the patient's risk for vomiting and aspiration, whereas discarding a large amount may increase the patient's risk for metabolic alkalosis. At times, the primary care provider may instruct the nurse to replace half of the residual and recheck in a set amount of time.
- *Patient complains of nausea after tube feeding:* Ensure that the HOB remains elevated and that suction equipment is at the bedside. Check medication record to see if any antiemetics have been ordered for the patient. Consider notifying the primary care provider for an order for an antiemetic.
- *When attempting to aspirate contents, the nurse notes that tube is clogged:* Most obstructions are caused by coagulation of formula. Try using warm water and gentle pressure to remove the clog. Carbonated sodas, such as colas, and meat tenderizers have not been shown effective in removing clogs in feeding tubes. Never use a stylet to unclog tubes. Tube may have to be replaced. To prevent clogs, ensure that adequate flushing is completed after each feeding.

SPECIAL CONSIDERATIONS

- Checking for the residual amount of feeding in the stomach is explained in Step 13. High gastric residual volumes (200 to 250 mL or greater) can be associated with high risk for aspiration and aspiration-related pneumonia (Bourgault et al., 2007; Metheny, 2008). For patients who are experiencing gastric dysfunction or decreased level of consciousness, feedings may be held for smaller residual amounts (less than 400 mL) (Bourgault et al., 2007; Keithley & Swanson, 2004; Metheny). Also, research findings are inconclusive on the benefit of returning gastric volumes to the stomach or intestine to avoid fluid or electrolyte imbalance, which has been accepted practice. Consult agency policy concerning this practice. Some researchers point out that high residual volumes are not indicative of intolerance to the tube feeding. In contrast, low residual volumes do not guarantee that patients are tolerating enteral tube feedings and are not at risk for aspiration (McClave et al., 2005). Monitoring for trends in gradually increasing amounts of residual volumes and assessing for other signs of intolerance, such as gastric pain or distention, should be implemented (ASPEN, 2011; Bourgault et al.; Metheny). Feedings should be held if residual volumes exceed 200 mL on two successive assessments (ASPEN).

(*continued*)

SKILL 11-3 ADMINISTERING A TUBE FEEDING continued

- When the patient with dementia and/or family is deciding on whether to agree to tube feeding nutrition, inform them that research is recommending that tube feedings not be used for this population of patients because they do not increase survival or prevent malnutrition or aspiration. It is suggested to use such methods as increasing feeding assistance and changing food consistency, as well as respecting patient preferences, as needed (American Dietetic Association [ADA], 2008).
- Some feeding equipment allows for the addition of water for flushes to a second feeding container, which enters the system through a second set of tubing. The feeding pump will automatically administer the pre-set volume of flush at the pre-set frequency.

SKILL VARIATION Using a Prefilled Tube-Feeding Set (Closed System)

Prefilled tube-feeding sets, which are considered closed systems, are frequently used to provide patient nourishment (Figure A). Closed systems contain sterile feeding solutions in ready-to-hang containers. This method reduces the opportunity for bacterial contamination of the feeding formula. In general, these prefilled feedings are administered via an enteral pump.

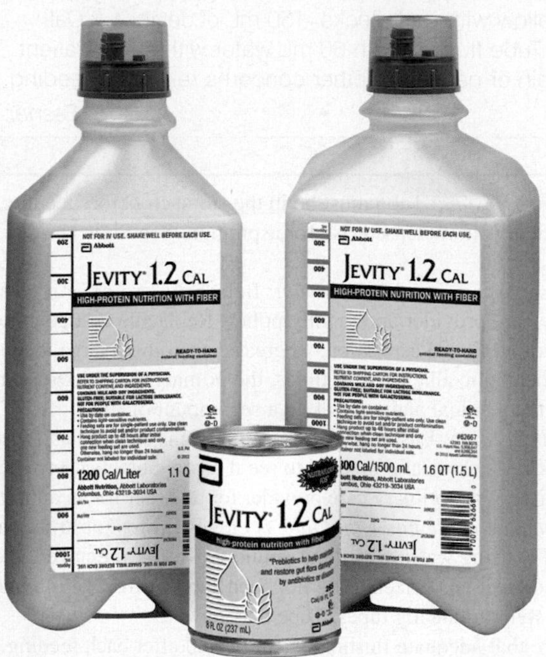

FIGURE A Prefilled tube feedings in plastic containers and ready-to-use feeding in a can. (Reprinted with permission from Abbott Nutrition, a division of Abbott Laboratories.)

1. Check amount, concentration, type, and frequency of tube feeding in the patient's medical record.
2. Gather all equipment, checking the feeding solution and container for correct solution and expiration date. Label with patient's name, type of solution, and prescribed rate.
3. Perform hand hygiene. Put on PPE, as indicated.

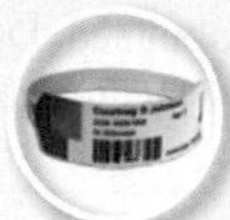

4. Identify the patient and explain the procedure.
5. Put on gloves.
6. Ensure the correct placement of the feeding tube by checking marking on tube at nose (if NG tube), length of exposed tube, aspiration of stomach contents, and gastric or intestinal pH.
7. Check for residual amount of feeding in the stomach and return residual, as ordered.
8. Flush tube with 30 mL of water.
9. Put on nonsterile gloves; remove screw on cap and attach administration setup with drip chamber and tubing.
10. Hang feeding container on IV pole and connect to feeding pump, allowing solution to flow through tubing, following manufacturer's directions.
11. Attach the feeding setup to the patient's feeding tube.
12. Open the clamp of the patient's feeding tube.
13. Turn on the pump.
14. Set the pump at the prescribed rate of flow and remove the nonsterile gloves.
15. Observe the patient's response during the tube feeding.
16. Continue to assess the patient for signs and symptoms of gastrointestinal distress, such as nausea, abdominal distention, or absence of bowel sounds.
17. Have the patient remain in the upright position throughout the feeding and for at least 1 hour after feeding. If patient's position needs to be changed to a supine position or turned in bed, pause the feeding pump during this time.
18. After the prescribed amount of feeding has been administrated or according to agency policy, turn off the pump, put on nonsterile gloves, clamp the feeding tube, and disconnect it from the feeding set tube, capping the end of the feeding set.
19. Draw up 30 to 60 mL of water using a syringe.
20. Attach the syringe to the feeding tube; unclamp the feeding tube and instill the 30 to 60 mL of water into it.
21. Clamp the feeding tube.
22. Remove equipment, according to facility policy.
23. Provide for any patient needs.
24. Remove gloves and additional PPE, if used. Perform hand hygiene.

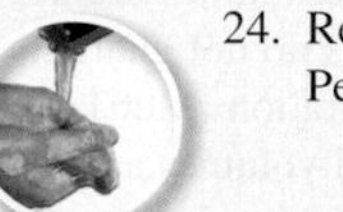

EVIDENCE FOR PRACTICE ▶

VERIFICATION OF FEEDING TUBE PLACEMENT

American Association of Critical-Care Nurses (AACN). (2010). *Practice alert: Verification of feeding tube placement.* Available http://www.aacn.org/wd/practice/content/feeding-tube-practice-alert.pcms?menu=practice

Practice alerts are directives from AACN that are supported by authoritative evidence to ensure excellence in practice and a safe and humane work environment. These directives provide guidance and standardize practice, as well as identify/inform about new advances and trends. The AACN has provided a directive regarding best practice for verification of feeding tube placement. Expected practice includes radiographic confirmation of correct tube placement on all critically ill patients who are to receive feedings or medications via blindly inserted gastric or small bowel tubes prior to initial use. The tube's exit site from the nose or mouth should be marked and length documented immediately after radiographic confirmation of correct tube placement. The mark should be observed routinely to assess for a change in length of the external portion of the tube. Bedside techniques to assess tube location should be used at regular intervals to determine if the tube has remained in its intended position. These bedside techniques include measuring the pH and observing the appearance of fluid withdrawn from the tube.

Refer to thePoint for additional research on related nursing topics.

SKILL 11-4 REMOVING A NASOGASTRIC TUBE

When the NG tube is no longer necessary for treatment, the primary care provider will order the tube to be removed. The NG tube is removed as carefully as it was inserted, to provide as much comfort as possible for the patient and to prevent complications. When the tube is removed, the patient must hold his/her breath to prevent aspiration of any secretions or fluid left in the tube as it is removed.

DELEGATION CONSIDERATIONS

The removal of a nasogastric (NG) tube is not delegated to nursing assistive personnel (NAP) or to unlicensed assistive personnel (UAP). Depending on the state's nurse practice act and the organization's policies and procedures, removal of an NG tube may be delegated to licensed practical/vocational nurses (LPN/LVNs). The decision to delegate must be based on careful analysis of the patient's needs and circumstances, as well as the qualifications of the person to whom the task is being delegated. Refer to the Delegation Guidelines in Appendix A.

EQUIPMENT

- Tissues
- 50-mL syringe
- Nonsterile gloves
- Additional PPE, as indicated
- Stethoscope
- Disposable plastic bag
- Bath towel or disposable pad
- Normal saline solution for irrigation (optional)
- Emesis basin

ASSESSMENT

Perform an abdominal assessment by inspecting for presence of distention, auscultating for bowel sounds, and palpating the abdomen for firmness or tenderness. If the abdomen is distended, consider measuring the abdominal girth at the umbilicus. If the patient reports any tenderness or nausea, exhibits any rigidity or firmness with distention, and if bowel sounds are absent, confer with the physician before discontinuing the NG tube.

Also assess any output from the NG tube, noting amount, color, and consistency.

NURSING DIAGNOSIS

Determine the related factors for the nursing diagnoses based on the patient's current status. Possible nursing diagnoses may include:

- Readiness for Enhanced Nutrition
- Risk for Aspiration

(continued)

SKILL 11-4 REMOVING A NASOGASTRIC TUBE continued

OUTCOME IDENTIFICATION AND PLANNING

The expected outcome to achieve when removing an NG tube is that the tube is removed with minimal discomfort to the patient, and the patient maintains an adequate nutritional intake. In addition, the abdomen remains free from distention and tenderness.

IMPLEMENTATION

ACTION	RATIONALE
1. Check medical record for the order for removal of NG tube.	This ensures correct implementation of primary care provider's order.
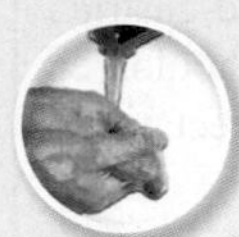 2. Perform hand hygiene and put on PPE, if indicated.	Hand hygiene and PPE prevent the spread of microorganisms. PPE is required based on transmission precautions.
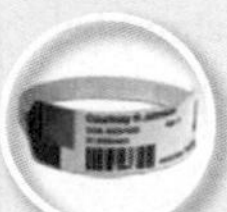 3. Identify the patient.	Identifying the patient ensures the right patient receives the intervention and helps prevent errors.
4. Explain the procedure to the patient and why this intervention is warranted. Describe that it will entail a quick few moments of discomfort. Perform key abdominal assessments as described above.	Patient cooperation is facilitated when explanations are provided. Due to changes in a patient's condition, assessment is vital before initiating intervention.
5. Pull the patient's bedside curtain. Raise the bed to a comfortable working position; usually elbow height of the caregiver (VISN 8, 2009). Assist the patient into a 30- to 45-degree position. Place towel or disposable pad across the patient's chest (Figure 1). Give tissues and emesis basin to patient.	Provides for privacy. Appropriate working height facilitates comfort and proper body mechanics for the nurse. Towel or pad protects the patient from contact with gastric secretions. Emesis basin is helpful if patient vomits or gags. Tissues are necessary if patient wants to blow his/her nose when tube is removed.
6. Put on gloves. Discontinue suction and separate tube from suction. Unpin tube from patient's gown and carefully remove adhesive tape from patient's nose.	Gloves prevent contact with blood and body fluids. Disconnecting tube from suction and the patient allows for its unrestricted removal.
7. Check placement (as outlined in Skill 11-2) and attach syringe and **flush with 10 mL of water or normal saline solution (optional) or clear with 30 to 50 mL of air (Figure 2).**	Air or saline solution clears the tube of secretions, feeding, or debris.

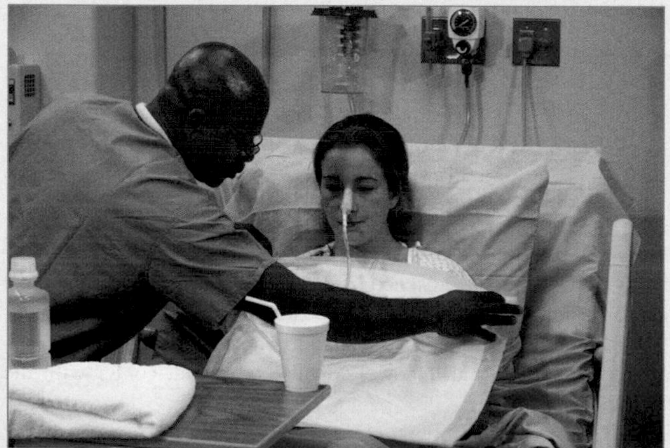

FIGURE 1 Placing towel or disposable pad across patient's chest.

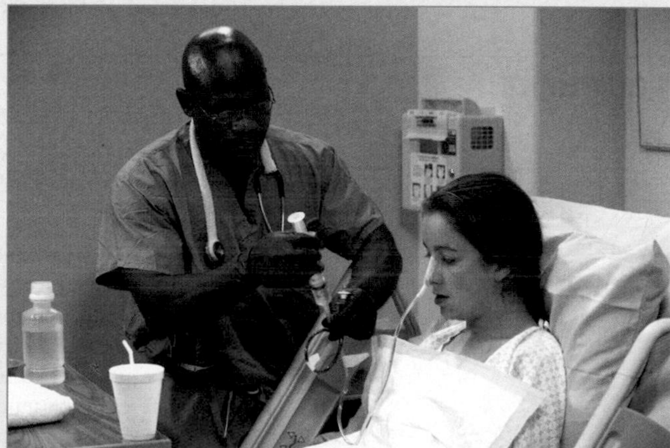

FIGURE 2 Flushing NG tube with 10 mL saline.

ACTION | RATIONALE

8. Clamp tube with fingers by doubling tube on itself (Figure 3). **Instruct patient to take a deep breath and hold it. Quickly and carefully remove tube while patient holds breath.** Coil the tube in the disposable pad as you remove it from the patient.

Clamping prevents drainage of gastric contents into the pharynx and esophagus. The patient holds breath to prevent accidental aspiration of gastric secretions in tube. Careful removal minimizes trauma and discomfort for the patient. Containing the tube in a towel while removing it prevents leakage onto the patient.

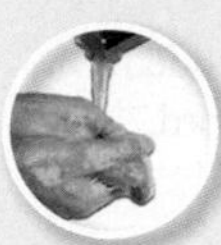

9. Dispose of tube per facility policy. Remove gloves. Perform hand hygiene.

This prevents contamination with microorganisms.

10. Offer mouth care to the patient and facial tissue to blow nose. Lower the bed and assist the patient to a position of comfort, as needed.

These interventions promote patient comfort.

11. Remove equipment and raise side rail and lower bed.

Promotes patient comfort and safety.

12. Put on gloves and measure the amount of nasogastric drainage in the collection device. Record the measurement on the output flow record, subtracting irrigant fluids if necessary (Figure 4). Add solidifying agent to nasogastric drainage and dispose of drainage according to facility policy.

Irrigation fluids are considered intake. To obtain the true nasogastric drainage, irrigant fluid amounts are subtracted from the total nasogastric drainage. Nasogastric drainage is recorded as part of the output of fluids from the patient. Solidifying agents added to liquid nasogastric drainage facilitate safe biohazard disposal.

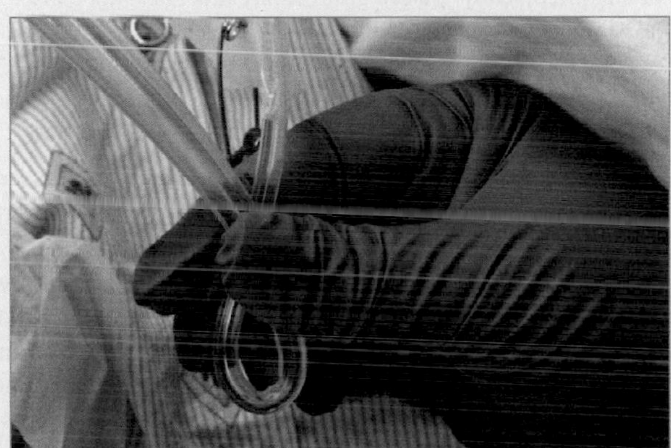

FIGURE 3 Doubling tube on itself.

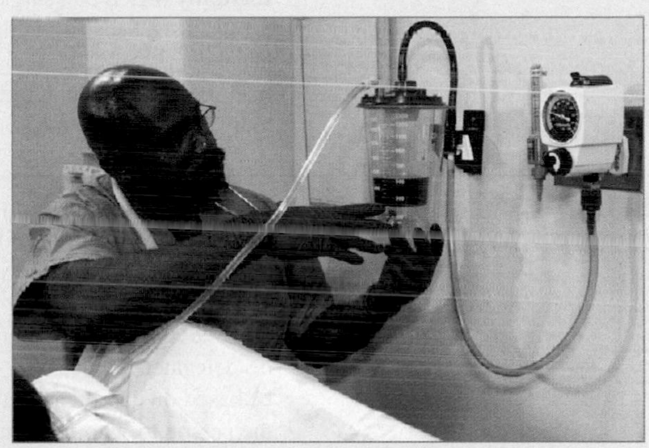

FIGURE 4 Measuring the amount of nasogastric drainage in collection device.

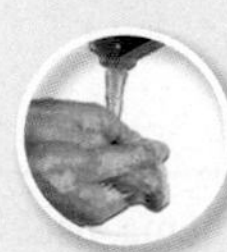

13. Remove additional PPE, if used. Perform hand hygiene.

Removing PPE properly reduces the risk for infection transmission and contamination of other items. Hand hygiene prevents transmission of microorganisms.

EVALUATION

The expected outcome is met when the patient experiences minimal discomfort and pain on NG tube removal. In addition, the patient's abdomen remains free from distention and tenderness, and the patient verbalizes measures to maintain an adequate nutritional intake.

DOCUMENTATION

Guidelines

Document assessment of the abdomen. If an abdominal girth reading was obtained, record this measurement. Document the removal of the NG tube from the naris where it had been placed. Note if there is any irritation to the skin of the naris. Record the amount of NG drainage in the suction container on the patient's intake-and-output record as well as the color of the drainage. Record any pertinent teaching, such as instruction to the patient to notify the nurse if he or she experiences any nausea, abdominal pain, or bloating.

(continued)

SKILL 11-4 REMOVING A NASOGASTRIC TUBE continued

Sample Documentation

10/29/15 1320 NG tube removed from L naris without incident. 600 mL of dark brown liquid emptied from NG tube. Patient's abdomen is 66 cm; abdomen is soft, nontender with hypoactive bowel sounds in all 4 quadrants.

—S. Essner, RN

UNEXPECTED SITUATIONS AND ASSOCIATED INTERVENTIONS

- *Within 2 hours after NG tube removal, the patient's abdomen is showing signs of distention:* Notify primary care provider. Anticipate order to reinsert NG tube.
- *Epistaxis occurs with removal of NG tube:* Occlude both nares until bleeding has subsided. Ensure that patient is in upright position. Document epistaxis in patient's medical record.

SKILL 11-5 CARING FOR A GASTROSTOMY TUBE

When long-term enteral feeding is required, an enterostomal tube may be placed through an opening created into the stomach (gastrostomy) or into the jejunum (jejunostomy). Placement of a tube into the stomach can be accomplished by a surgeon or gastroenterologist via a **percutaneous endoscopic gastrostomy** (PEG) or a surgically (open or laparoscopically) placed gastrostomy tube. PEG tube insertion is often used because, unlike a traditional, surgically placed gastrostomy tube, it usually does not require general anesthesia. Use of a PEG tube or other type of gastrostomy tube requires an intact, functional GI tract. Providing care at the insertion site is a nursing responsibility. Site care is the same for a jejunostomy (enterostomal tube placed through an opening created into the jejunum).

DELEGATION CONSIDERATIONS

The care of a gastrostomy tube, in the postoperative period, is not delegated to nursing assistive personnel (NAP) or to unlicensed assistive personnel (UAP) in the acute care setting. The care of a healed gastrostomy tube site in some settings may be delegated to NAP or UAP who have received appropriate training, after assessment of tube by the registered nurse. Depending on the state's nurse practice act and the organization's policies and procedures, the care of a gastrostomy tube may be delegated to licensed practical/vocational nurses (LPN/LVNs). The decision to delegate must be based on careful analysis of the patient's needs and circumstances, as well as the qualifications of the person to whom the task is being delegated. Refer to the Delegation Guidelines in Appendix A.

EQUIPMENT

- Nonsterile gloves
- Additional PPE, as indicated
- Washcloth, towel, and soap
- Cotton-tipped applicators
- Sterile saline solution
- Gauze (if needed)

ASSESSMENT

Assess gastrostomy or jejunostomy tube site, noting any drainage, skin breakdown, or erythema. Measure the length of exposed tube, comparing it with the initial measurement after insertion. Alternately, mark the tube at the skin with indelible marker; mark should be at skin level at the insertion site. Check to ensure that the tube is securely stabilized and has not become dislodged. Also, assess the tension of the tube. If there is not enough tension, the tube may leak gastric or intestinal drainage around exit site. If the tension is too great, the internal anchoring device may erode through the skin.

NURSING DIAGNOSIS

Determine the related factors for the nursing diagnoses based on the patient's current status. Possible nursing diagnoses may include:

- Imbalanced Nutrition, Less than Body Requirements
- Impaired Skin Integrity
- Risk for Infection

OUTCOME IDENTIFICATION AND PLANNING

The expected outcome to achieve when caring for a gastrostomy tube is that the patient ingests an adequate diet and exhibits no signs and symptoms of irritation, excoriation, or infection at the tube insertion site. Also, that the patient verbalizes little discomfort related to tube placement. In addition, the patient will be able to verbalize the care needed for the gastrostomy tube.

IMPLEMENTATION

ACTION	RATIONALE
1. Gather equipment. Verify the medical order or facility policy and procedure regarding site care.	Assembling equipment provides for an organized approach to the task. Verification ensures the patient receives the correct intervention.
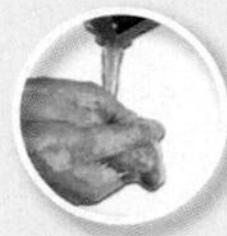 2. Perform hand hygiene and put on PPE, if indicated.	Hand hygiene and PPE prevent the spread of microorganisms. PPE is required based on transmission precautions.
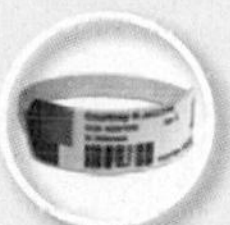 3. Identify the patient.	Identifying the patient ensures the right patient receives the intervention and helps prevent errors.
4. Explain the procedure to the patient and why this intervention is needed. Answer any questions, as needed.	Explanation facilitates patient cooperation.
5. Assess the patient for presence of pain at the tube insertion site. If pain is present, offer the patient analgesic medication per the medical order and wait for medication absorption before beginning insertion site care.	Feeding tubes can be uncomfortable, especially in the first few days after insertion. Analgesic medication may permit the patient to tolerate the insertion site care more easily. After the first few days, it has been reported that the need for pain medication decreases.
6. Pull the patient's bedside curtain. Assemble equipment on the bedside table, within reach. Raise bed to a comfortable working position, usually elbow height of the caregiver (VISN 8, 2009).	Provide for privacy. Assembling equipment provides for organized approach to the task. Appropriate working height facilitates comfort and proper body mechanics for the nurse.
7. Put on gloves. If gastrostomy tube is new and still has sutures holding it in place, dip a cotton-tipped applicator into sterile saline solution and gently clean around the insertion site, removing any crust or drainage (Figure 1). **Avoid adjusting or lifting the external disk for the first few days after placement, except to clean the area.** If the gastric tube insertion site has healed and the sutures are removed, wet a washcloth and apply a small amount of soap onto washcloth. Gently cleanse around the insertion, removing any crust or drainage (Figure 2). Rinse site, removing all soap.	Cleaning new site with sterile saline solution prevents the introduction of microorganisms into the wound. Crust and drainage can harbor bacteria and lead to skin breakdown. Removing soap helps to prevent skin irritation. If able, the patient may shower and cleanse the site with soap and water.

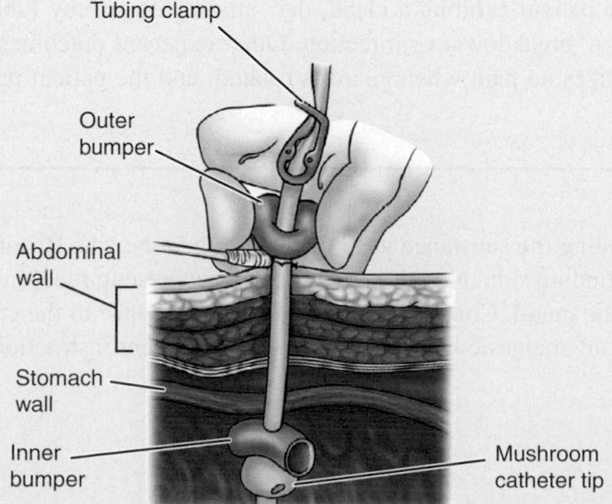

FIGURE 1 Wiping gastric tube site with cotton-tipped applicators.

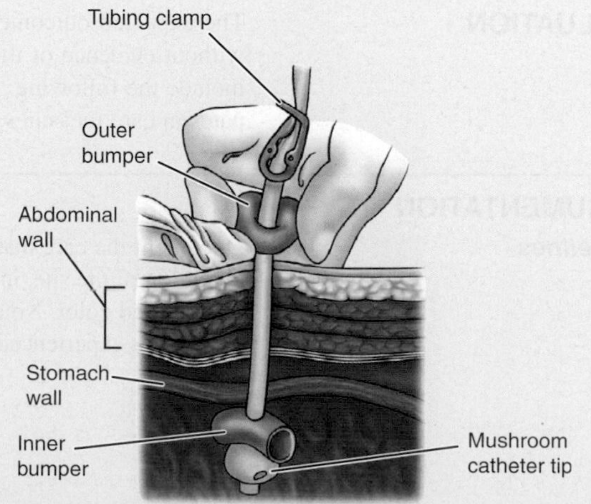

FIGURE 2 Cleaning site with soap, water, and washcloth.

(continued)

SKILL 11-5 CARING FOR A GASTROSTOMY TUBE continued

ACTION	RATIONALE
8. Pat skin around insertion site dry.	Drying the skin thoroughly prevents skin breakdown.
9. If the sutures have been removed, **gently rotate the guard or external bumper 90 degrees at least once a day (Figure 3). Assess that the guard or external bumper is not digging into the surrounding skin. Avoid placing any tension on the tube.**	Rotation of the guard or external bumper prevents skin breakdown and pressure ulcers. The risk of dislodgement is decreased when the tube has an external anchoring or bumper device.

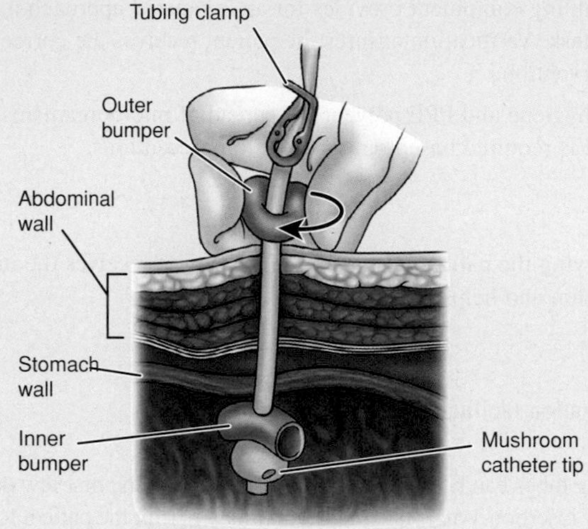

FIGURE 3 Gently turning or rotating guard or bumper 90 degrees.

ACTION	RATIONALE
10. Leave the site open to air unless there is drainage. If drainage is present, place one thickness of a precut gauze pad or drain sponge under the external bumper and change, as needed, to keep the area dry. Use a skin protectant or barrier cream to prevent skin breakdown.	The digestive enzymes from the gastric secretions may cause skin breakdown. Under normal conditions, expect only a minimal amount of drainage on a feeding tube dressing. Increased amounts of drainage should be explored for causes such as a possible gastric fluid leak.
11. Remove gloves. Lower the bed and assist the patient to a position of comfort, as needed.	Removing gloves reduces the risk for infection transmission and contamination of other items. Lowering bed and assisting patient ensure patient safety and comfort.
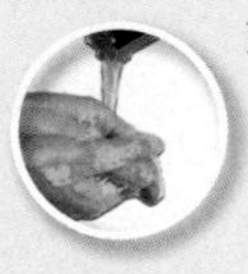 12. Remove additional PPE, if used. Perform hand hygiene.	Removing PPE properly reduces the risk for infection transmission and contamination of other items. Hand hygiene prevents transmission of microorganisms.

EVALUATION

The expected outcome is met when the patient exhibits a clean, dry, intact gastrostomy tube site without evidence of irritation, excoriation, breakdown, or infection. Other expected outcomes may include the following: the patient verbalizes no pain when guard is rotated; and the patient participates in care measures.

DOCUMENTATION

Guidelines

Document the care that was given, including the substance used to cleanse the tube site. Record the condition of the site, including the surrounding skin. Note if any drainage was present, recording the amount and color. Note the rotation of the guard. Comment on the patient's response to the care, if the patient experienced any pain, and if an analgesic was given. Record any patient instruction that was given.

Sample Documentation

> 10/10/15 1145 Gastrostomy tube site cleansed with soap and water. Guard rotated. Site is of consistent tone with surrounding skin, without any signs of skin breakdown. Small amount of clear crust noted on tube. Patient tolerated without incident. Wife at bedside, actively participating in tube care.
>
> —S. Essner, RN

UNEXPECTED SITUATIONS AND ASSOCIATED INTERVENTIONS

- *Gastrostomy tube is leaking large amount of drainage:* Check tension of tube. If there is a large amount of slack between the internal guard and the external bumper, drainage can leak out of site. Apply gentle pressure to tube while pressing the external bumper closer to the skin. If the tube has an internal balloon holding it in place (similar to a urinary catheter balloon), check to make sure that the balloon is inflated properly.
- *Skin irritation is noted around insertion site:* If the skin is erythematosus and appears to be broken down, gastric fluids may be leaking from the site. Gastric fluids have a low pH and are very acidic. Stop the leakage, as described above, and apply a skin barrier. If the skin has a patchy, red rash, the cause could be candidiasis (yeast). Notify the primary care provider for an order to apply an antifungal powder. Ensure that the site is kept dry.
- *Site appears erythematosus and patient complains of pain at site:* Notify primary care provider; patient could be developing cellulitis at the site.

SPECIAL CONSIDERATIONS

General Considerations

- Do not place a dressing between the skin and external fixation device unless drainage is present. Change the dressing immediately when soiled, to prevent skin complications.
- If length of exposed tube has changed or marking on tube is not visible, do not use the tube. Notify the patient's primary care provider of the finding.

Home Care Considerations

- Instruct patients on appropriate actions if the tube comes out. In the event the gastrostomy tube is pulled out, teach the patient to clean the area with water, cover the opening with a clean dressing, tape in place, and call the primary care provider immediately (Tracey & Patterson, 2006).

ENHANCE YOUR UNDERSTANDING

FOCUSING ON PATIENT CARE: DEVELOPING CLINICAL REASONING

Consider the case scenarios at the beginning of the chapter as you answer the following questions to enhance your understanding and apply what you have learned.

QUESTIONS

1. Ms. Williams tells the nurse that she hates hospital food and is too tired to eat. How can the nurse help Ms. Williams maintain her nutritional intake while recovering from her stroke?
2. Mr. Mason confides he is having "a lot of pain" in his throat and his nose feels "really sore." What assessments and nursing interventions should be a part of Mr. Mason's nursing care while he has the nasogastric tube?
3. The nurse is responsible for providing information to Cole and his family regarding home management of his gastrostomy tube and tube feedings. What information will the nurse include in the patient teaching?

You can find suggested answers after the Bibliography at the end of this chapter.

ENHANCE YOUR UNDERSTANDING (continued)

INTEGRATED CASE STUDY CONNECTION

The case studies in the back of the book are designed to focus on integrating concepts. Refer to the following case studies to enhance your understanding of the concepts related to the skills in this chapter.

- Basic Case Studies: Claudia Tran, 1070; Kate Townsend, 1073.
- Advanced Case Studies: Cole McKean, 1093; Robert Espinoza, 1097.

TAYLOR SUITE RESOURCES

Explore these additional resources to enhance learning for this chapter:

- NCLEX-Style Questions and other resources on thePoint, http://thePoint.lww.com/Lynn4e
- *Skill Checklists for Taylor's Clinical Nursing Skills,* 4e
- *Taylor's Video Guide to Clinical Nursing Skills:* Nutrition
- *Fundamentals of Nursing:* Chapter 35, Nutrition
- *Lippincott DocuCare* Fundamentals cases

Bibliography

Ackley, B.J., & Ladwig, G.B. (2011). *Nursing diagnosis handbook* (9th ed.). St. Louis: Mosby/Elsevier.

Amella, E.J., & Lawrence, J.F. (2007). *Try this: Best practices in nursing care to older adults. The Hartford Institute for Geriatric Nursing. Eating and feeding issues in older adults with dementia. Part II: Interventions.* Issue Number D11.2. Available http://consultgerirn.org/uploads/File/trythis/try_this_d11_2.pdf.

American Association of Critical-Care Nurses (AACN). (2010). *Practice alert: Verification of feeding tube placement.* Available http://aacn.org/WD/Practice/Docs/PracticeAlerts/Verification_of_Feeding_Tube_Placement_05-2005.pdf.

American Association of Critical-Care Nurses (AACN). (2012). Practice alert. Prevention of aspiration. *CriticalCareNurse, 32*(3), 71–73.

American Dietetic Association (ADA). (2008). Position of the American Dietetic Association: Ethical and legal issues in nutrition, hydration, and feeding. *Journal of the American Dietetic Association, 108*(5), 873–882.

American Society for Parenteral and Enteral Nutrition (ASPEN.) (2011). *Guidelines: Access for administration of nutrition support.* Available http://www.nutritioncare.org/Professional_Resources/Guidelines_and_Standards/Guidelines/Access_for_Administration_of_Nutrition_Support/.

American Society for Parenteral and Enteral Nutrition (ASPEN) (2009a). *Enteral nutrition practice recommendations. Enteral access devices: Selection, insertion, and maintenance considerations.* Available http://www.nutritioncare.org/Professional_Resources/Guidelines_and_Standards/Guidelines/2009_ENPR_-_Section_V_Enteral_Access_Devices/#Section_C.

American Society for Parenteral and Enteral Nutrition (ASPEN.) (2009b). *Enteral nutrition practice recommendations. Enteral nutrition administration.* Available http://www.nutritioncare.org/Professional_Resources/Guidelines_and_Standards/Guidelines/2009_ENPR_-_Section_VI_Enteral_Nutrition_Administration/.

American Society for Parenteral and Enteral Nutrition (ASPEN.) (2009c). *Enteral nutrition practice recommendations. Medication administration.* Available http://www.nutritioncare.org/Professional_Resources/Guidelines_and_Standards/Guidelines/2009_ENPR_-_Section_VII_Medication_Administration/.

Aselage, M.B. (2012). Measuring mealtime difficulties: Eating, feeding and meal behaviours in older adults with dementia. *Journal of Clinical Nursing, 19*(5–6), 621–631.

Beckstrand, J., Cirgin Ellet, M., & McDaniel, A. (2007). Predicting internal distance to the stomach for positioning nasogastric and orogastric feeding tubes in children. *Journal of Advanced Nursing, 59*(3), 274–289.

Best, C. (2005). Caring for the patient with a nasogastric tube. *Nursing Standard, 20*(3), 59–65.

Best, C., & Summers, J. (2010). Strategies for nutritional care in acute settings. *Nursing Older People, 22*(6), 27–31.

Best, C., & Wilson, N. (2011). Advice on safe administration of medications via enteral feeding tubes. *British Journal of Community Nursing, Nutrition Supplement* (Nov), S6–S10.

Bloomfield, J., & Pegram, A. (2012). Improving nutrition and hydration in the hospital: The nurse's responsibility. *Nursing Standard, 26*(34), 52–56.

Boltz, M., Capezuti, E., Fulmer, T., et al. (Eds.) (2012). *Evidence-based geriatric nursing protocols for best practice* (4th ed.). New York: Springer Publishing Company.

Bourgault, A., Ipe, L., Weaver, J., et al. (2007). Development of evidence-based guidelines and critical care nurses' knowledge of enteral feeding. *Critical Care Nurse, 27*(4), 17–29.

Bulechek, G.M, Butcher, H.K., Dochterman, J.M., et al. (Eds.). (2013). *Nursing interventions classification (NIC)* (6th ed.). St. Louis: Mosby Elsevier.

Dudek, S. (2014). *Nutrition essentials for nursing practice* (7th ed.). Philadelphia: Wolters Kluwer Health/Lippincott Williams & Wilkins.

Dunne, A. (2010). Nutrition and dementia. *Nursing & Residential Care, 12*(3), 112, 114, 116.

Eisenstadt, E.S. (2010). Dysphagia and aspiration pneumonia in older adults. *Journal of the American Academy of Nurse Practitioners, 22*(1), 17–22.

Ellet, M. (2004). What is known about methods of correctly placing gastric tubes in adults and children. *Gastroenterology Nursing, 27*(6), 253–261.

Forest-Lalande, L. (2012). The management of feeding gastrostomies. *Gastrointestinal Nursing, 10*(3), 28–35.

Fluids & electrolytes made incredibly easy. (2011). (5th ed.). Philadelphia: Wolters Kluwer Health/Lippincott Williams & Wilkins.

Freeman, D., Saxton, V., & Holberton, J. (2012). A weight-based formula for the estimation of gastric tube insertion length in newborns. *Advances in Neonatal Care, 12* (3), 179–182.

Gilbert, R.T., & Burns, S.M. (2012). Increasing the safety of blind gastric tube placement in pediatric patients: The design and testing of a procedure using a carbon dioxide detection device. *Journal of Pediatric Nursing, 27*(5), 528–532.

Grossman, S., & Porth, C.M. (2014). Porth's pathophysiology: concepts of altered health states. (9th ed.). Philadelphia: Wolters Kluwer Health/Lippincott Williams & Wilkins.

Hinkle, J.L., & Cheever, K.H. (2014). *Brunner & Suddarth's textbook of medical-surgical nursing* (13th ed.). Philadelphia: Wolters Kluwer Health/Lippincott Williams & Wilkins.

Hogan-Quigley, B., Palm, M.L., & Bickley, L. (2012). *Bates' nursing guide to physical examination and history taking.* Philadelphia: Wolters Kluwer Health/Lippincott Williams & Wilkins.

Jarvis, C. (2012). *Physical examination & health assessment.* (6th ed.). St. Louis: Saunders/Elsevier.

Kenny, D.J., & Goodman, P. (2010). Care of the patient with enteral tube feeding. An evidence-based practice protocol. *Nursing Research, 59*(1S), S22–S31.

Khair, J. (2005). Guidelines for testing the placing of nasogastric tubes. *Nursing Times, 101*(20), 26–27.

Kyle G. (2011). Managing dysphagia in older people with dementia. *British Journal of Community Nursing, 16*(1), 6–10.

Kyle, T., & Carman, S. (2013). *Essentials of pediatric nursing* (2nd ed.). Philadelphia: Wolters Kluwer Health/Lippincott Williams & Wilkins.

Lin, L., Watson, R., & Wu, S. (2010). What is associated with low food intake in older people with dementia? *Journal of Clinical Nursing, 19*(1–2), 53–59.

Malarkey, L.M., & McMorrow, M.E. (2012). *Saunders nursing guide to laboratory and diagnostic tests* (2nd ed.). St. Louis: Elsevier Saunders.

McClave, S., Lukan, J., Stefater, J., et al. (2005). Poor validity of residual volumes as a marker for risk of aspiration in critically ill patients. *Critical Care Medicine, 33*(2), 324–330.

Medlin, S. (2012). Recent developments in enteral feeding for adults: An update. *British Journal of Nursing, 21*(18), 1061–1067.

Metheny, N.M. (2012). *Fluid and electrolyte balance. Nursing considerations* (5th ed.). Sudbury, MA: Jones & Bartlett Learning.

Metheny, N. (2012). *Try this: Best practices in nursing care to older adults. The Hartford Institute for Geriatric Nursing. Preventing aspiration in older adults with dysphagia.* Issue Number 20. Available http://consultgerirn.org/uploads/File/trythis/try_this_20.pdf.

Metheny, N. (2008). Residual volume measurement should be retained in enteral feeding protocols. *American Journal of Critical Care, 17*(1), 62–64.

Metheny, N.A., Mills, A.C., & Stewart, B.J. (2012). Monitoring for intolerance to gastric tube feedings: A national survey. *American Journal of Critical Care, 21*(2), e33–e40.

Metheny, N., & Meert, K. (2004). Monitoring feeding tube placement. *Nutrition in Clinical Practice, 19*(5), 487–542.

Metheny, N., Schnelker, R., McGinnis, J., et al. (2005). Indicators of tubesite during feedings. *Journal of Neuroscience Nursing, 37*(6), 320–325.

Metheny, N., & Stewart, B. (2002). Testing feeding tube placement during continuous tube feedings. *Applied Nursing Research, 15*(4), 254–258.

Metheny, N., & Titler, M. (2001). Assessing placement of feeding tubes. *American Journal of Nursing, 101*(5), 36–45.

Miller, C. (2008). Communication difficulties in hospitalized older adults with dementia: Try these techniques to make communicating with patients easier and more effective. *American Journal of Nursing, 108*(3), 58–66.

Miller, S. (2011). Capnometry vs. pH testing in nasogastric tube placement. *Gastrointestinal Nursing, 9*(2), 30–33.

Moorhead, S., Johnson, M., Maas, M.L., et al. (Eds.). (2013). *Nursing outcomes classification (NOC)* (5th ed.). St. Louis: Mosby Elsevier.

Munera-Seeley, V., Ochoa, J., Brown, N., et al. (2008). Use of a colorimetric carbon dioxide sensor for nasoenteric feeding tube placement in critical care patients compared with clinical methods and radiography. *Nutrition in Clinical Practice, 23*(3), 318–321.

NANDA-I International. (2012). *Nursing diagnoses: Definitions & classification 2012–2014.* West Sussex, UK: Wiley-Blackwell.

Ojo, O., & Bowden, J. (2012). Infection control in enteral feed and feeding systems in the community. *British Journal of Nursing, 21*(18), 1070–1075.

Palmer, J., & Metheny, N. (2008). Preventing aspiration during nasogastric, nasointestinal, or gastrostomy tube feedings. *American Journal of Nursing, 108*(2).

Perry, S.E., Hockenberry, M.J., Lowdermilk, D.L., et al. (2010). *Maternal child nursing care* (4th ed.). Maryland Heights, MO: Mosby/Elsevier.

Ritter, L.A., & Hoffman, N.A. (2010). *Multicultural health.* Boston: Jones and Bartlett.

Spector, R.E. (2009). *Cultural diversity in health and illness* (7th ed.). Upper Saddle River, NJ: Pearson/Prentice Hall.

Stayner, J.L., Bhatnagar, A., McGinn, A.N., et al. (2012). Feeding tube placement: Errors and complications. *Nutrition in Clinical Practice, 27*(6), 738–748.

Stepter, C.R. (2012). Maintaining placement of temporary enteral feeding tubes in adults: A critical appraisal of the evidence. *MEDSURGNursing, 21*(2), 61–69.

Tabloski, P. (2010). *Gerontological nursing* (2nd ed.). Upper Saddle River, NJ: Pearson.

Taylor, C., Lillis, C., & Lynn, P. (2015). *Fundamentals of nursing* (8th ed.). Philadelphia: Wolters Kluwer Health/Lippincott Williams & Wilkins.

Tracey, D., & Patterson, G. (2006). Care of the gastrostomy tube in the home. *Home Healthcare Nurse, 24*(6), 381–386.

Turgay, A.S., & Khorshid, L. (2010). Effectiveness of the auscultatory and pH methods in predicting feeding tube placement. *Journal of Clinical Nursing, 19*(11–12), 1553–1559.

Van Leeuwen, A.M., Poelhuis-Leth, D., & Bladh, M.L. (2011). *Davis's comprehensive handbook of laboratory & diagnostic tests with nursing implications* (4th ed.). Philadelphia: F.A. Davis.

VISN 8 Patient Safety Center. (2009). *Safe patient handling and movement algorithms.* Tampa, FL: Author. Available http://www.visn8.va.gov/visn8/patientsafetycenter/safePtHandling/default.asp.

SUGGESTED ANSWERS FOR FOCUSING ON PATIENT CARE: DEVELOPING CLINICAL REASONING

1. Explore the patient's usual food preferences and habits. Choose foods that the patient prefers from facility menus. In addition, encourage Ms. Williams' family to bring favorite foods from home. Food choices should focus on foods that are easy to eat and nutrient dense. Provide rest periods before mealtimes, so she is not overly tired. Assist the patient to a comfortable position for meals, help her with hand hygiene, and ensure she has clean dentures in place, and her glasses, as appropriate. Encourage her family to visit during mealtimes, to provide as normal a social environment as possible. Cut food and open packages as necessary, to limit the amount of exertion by the patient. Suggest she eat small portions, keeping some food items to snack on as the day progresses. Frequent small servings are not as tiring. Allow enough time for the patient to chew and swallow the food adequately. The patient may need to rest for short periods during eating. If Ms. Williams is agreeable, feed her a portion of the meal, to avoid overtiring.

2. Assess the patient's level of comfort every 4 hours and prn. Offer analgesic as prescribed. Offer oral hygiene at least every 4 hours or more often. Discuss the potential for topical analgesic, such as analgesic throat spray, with the patient's physician. Reassess pain after interventions. Assess the patient's oral and nasal mucous membranes, as well as nasal skin, at least every shift. Ensure the tape anchoring the tube is not pulled taut, creating pressure on the nose. Retape/secure the NG tube with new commercially prepared device or tape every 24 hours; clean skin thoroughly and apply skin barrier. Retape in a slightly different position to prevent excessive pressure in one area of nostril.

3. Patients who are caring for a gastrostomy tube at home should understand the care of the tube, tube site, nutritional feeding routine, and potential adverse effects, with the accompanying actions. Provide Cole and his family with the date his tube was placed, the procedure used to place the tube, the tube size, how the tube is anchored, and the calibration measurement at skin level or the length of the external tube. Discuss, provide written information, and obtain a return demonstration for the care of the tube and tube site, as well as the feeding procedure. Teaching should include the formula type, frequency, rate of infusion, checking tube placement, and checking gastric residual, based on physician direction. Review infection control measures, such as handwashing before starting, refrigerating formula between use, disposing of unused formula after 24 hours, and measuring out only 4 hours of formula at a time. The length of the tube or calibration mark at the skin should be checked prior to each feeding or use of the tube. Cole should be in a sitting position for the feeding and for 1 hour afterward. Skin care for tube site includes washing the area with the cleansing agent identified by the physician or facility policy, rinsing and patting dry. Cole should assess the site daily for swelling, redness, or yellow/green drainage. Cole and his family should verbalize an understanding of these instructions, as well as a knowledge of signs and symptoms that should be reported to their physician. These include the presence of nausea or vomiting, pain, fever, and residual in excess of identified limits. Cole and his family should also understand proper procedure if the gastrostomy tube should come out or become dislodged.

12 Urinary Elimination

FOCUSING ON PATIENT CARE

This chapter will help you develop some of the skills related to urinary elimination necessary to care for the following patients:

RALPH BELLOWS, age 73 years, has been admitted with a stroke. Due to incontinence and skin breakdown, Ralph's nurse has decided to include the application of a condom catheter in his plan of care.

GRACE HALLIGAN, age 24, is pregnant and has been placed on bed rest. She needs to void, but cannot get out of bed.

MIKE WIMMER, age 36, receives peritoneal dialysis. Mike has noticed that the insertion site around his catheter is becoming tender and reddened.

Refer to Focusing on Patient Care: Developing Clinical Reasoning at the end of the chapter to apply what you learn.

LEARNING OBJECTIVES

After studying this chapter, you will be able to:

1. Assist with the use of a bedpan.
2. Assist with use of a urinal.
3. Assist with use of a bedside commode.
4. Assess bladder volume using an ultrasound bladder scanner.
5. Apply an external condom catheter.
6. Catheterize a female patient's urinary bladder.
7. Catheterize a male patient's urinary bladder.
8. Remove an indwelling urinary catheter.
9. Administer intermittent closed-catheter irrigation.
10. Administer continuous closed-bladder irrigation.
11. Empty and change a stoma appliance on an ileal conduit.
12. Care for a suprapubic urinary catheter.
13. Care for a peritoneal dialysis catheter.
14. Care for hemodialysis access.

KEY TERMS

arteriovenous fistula: a surgically created passage connecting an artery and a vein; used in hemodialysis

arteriovenous graft: a surgically created connection between an artery and vein using synthetic material; used in hemodialysis

bruit: a sound caused by turbulent blood flow

external condom catheter: soft, pliable sheath made of silicone material, applied externally to the penis, connected to drainage tubing and a collection bag

fenestrated: having a window-like opening

hemodialysis: removal from the body, by means of blood filtration, of toxins and fluid that are normally removed by the kidneys

ileal conduit: a surgical diversion formed by bringing the ureters to the ileum; urine is excreted through a stoma

indwelling urethral catheter (retention or Foley catheter): a catheter (tube) through the urethra into the bladder for the purpose of continuous drainage of urine; a balloon is inflated to ensure that the catheter remains in the bladder once it is inserted

intermittent urethral catheter (straight catheter): a catheter through the urethra into the bladder to drain urine for a short period of time (5 to 10 minutes)

peritoneal dialysis: removal of toxins and fluid from the body by the principles of diffusion and osmosis; accomplished by introducing a solution (dialysate) into the peritoneal cavity

peritonitis: inflammation of the peritoneal membrane

sediment: precipitate found at the bottom of a container of urine

stoma: artificial opening on the body surface

suprapubic urinary catheter: a urinary catheter surgically inserted through a small incision above the pubic area into the bladder

symphysis pubis: the anterior midline junction of the pubic bones; the bony projection under the pubic hair

thrill: palpable feeling caused by turbulent blood flow

This chapter covers skills that the nurse may use to promote urinary elimination. An assessment of the urinary system is required as part of the assessment related to many of the skills. See Fundamentals Review 12-1 for a review of the male and female genitourinary tract. Fundamentals Review 12-2 summarizes factors that may affect urinary elimination.

FUNDAMENTALS REVIEW 12-1

ANATOMY OF THE GENITOURINARY TRACT

- The main components of the urinary tract are the kidneys, ureters, bladder, and urethra.
- The average female urethra is 1.5 to 2.5 inches (3.7 to 6.2 cm) long; the average male urethra is 7 to 8 inches (18 to 20 cm) long.
- The average age at which men begin to have prostatic enlargement is 50.

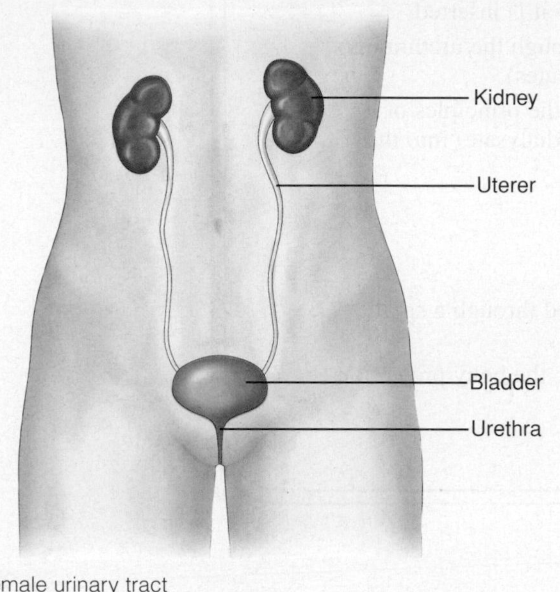

Female urinary tract

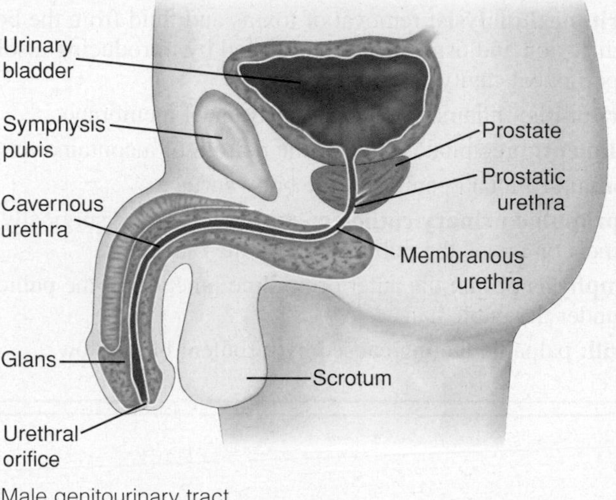

Male genitourinary tract.

FUNDAMENTALS REVIEW 12-2

FACTORS AFFECTING URINARY ELIMINATION

Numerous factors affect the amount and quality of urine produced by the body and the manner in which it is excreted.

EFFECTS OF AGING

- Diminished ability of kidneys to concentrate urine may result in nocturia.
- Decreased bladder muscle tone may reduce the capacity of the bladder to hold urine, resulting in increased frequency of urination.
- Decreased bladder contractility leading to urine retention and stasis with an increased risk of urinary tract infection (UTI).
- Neuromuscular problems, degenerative joint problems, alterations in thought processes, and weakness may interfere with voluntary control of urination and the ability to reach a toilet in time.

FOOD AND FLUID INTAKE

- Dehydration leads to increased fluid reabsorption by the kidneys, leading to decreased and concentrated urine production.
- Fluid overload leads to excretion of a large quantity of dilute urine.
- Consumption of alcoholic beverages leads to increased urine production due to their inhibition of antidiuretic hormone release.
- Ingestion of foods high in water content may increase urine production.
- Ingestion of foods and beverages high in sodium content leads to decreased urine formation due to sodium and water reabsorption and retention.
- Ingestion of certain foods (e.g., asparagus, onions, beets) may lead to alterations in the odor or color of urine.

FUNDAMENTALS REVIEW 12-2 continued

FACTORS AFFECTING URINARY ELIMINATION

PSYCHOLOGICAL VARIABLES

- Individual, family, and sociocultural variables may influence voiding habits.
- Patients may view voiding as a personal and private act. The need to ask for assistance may lead to embarrassment and/or anxiety.
- Stress may lead to voiding of smaller amounts of urine at more frequent intervals.
- Stress may lead to difficulty emptying the bladder due to its effects on relaxation of perineal muscles and the external urethral sphincter.

ACTIVITY AND MUSCLE TONE

- Regular exercise increases metabolism and optimal urine production and elimination.
- Prolonged periods of immobility may lead to poor urinary control and urinary stasis due to decreased bladder and sphincter tone.
- Use of indwelling urinary catheters leads to loss of bladder tone because the bladder muscle is not being stretched by filling with urine.
- Childbearing, muscle atrophy related to menopausal hormonal changes, and trauma-related muscle damage lead to decreased muscle tone.

PATHOLOGIC CONDITIONS

- Congenital urinary tract abnormalities, polycystic kidney disease, urinary tract infection, urinary calculi (kidney stones), hypertension, diabetes mellitus, gout, and certain connective tissue disorders lead to altered quantity and quality of urine.
- Diseases that reduce physical activity or lead to generalized weakness (e.g., arthritis, Parkinson's disease, degenerative joint disease) interfere with toileting.
- Cognitive deficits and psychiatric conditions may interfere with ability or desire to control urination voluntarily.
- Fever and diaphoresis (profuse perspiration) lead to conservation of body fluids.
- Other pathologic conditions, such as congestive heart failure, may lead to fluid retention and decreased urine output.
- High blood–glucose levels, such as with diabetes mellitus, may lead to increased urine output due to osmotic diuresis.

MEDICATIONS

- Abuse of analgesics, such as aspirin or ibuprofen (Advil), can cause kidney damage (nephrotoxic).
- Use of some antibiotics, such as gentamicin, can cause kidney damage.
- Use of diuretics can lead to moderate to severe increases in production and excretion of dilute urine, related to their prevention of water and certain electrolyte reabsorption in the renal tubules.
- Use of cholinergic medications may lead to increased urination due to stimulation of detrusor muscle contraction.
- Use of some analgesics, sedatives, and tranquilizers interferes with urination due to the diminished effectiveness of the neural reflex for voiding because of suppression of the central nervous system.
- Use of certain drugs causes changes to the color of urine. Anticoagulants may cause hematuria (blood in the urine) or a pink or red color. Diuretics can lighten the color of urine to pale yellow. Phenazopyridine (Pyridium) can cause orange or orange-red urine. Amitriptyline (Elavil) and B-complex vitamins can cause green or blue-green urine. Levodopa (L-dopa) and injectable iron compounds can cause brown or black urine.

SKILL 12-1 ASSISTING WITH THE USE OF A BEDPAN

Patients who cannot get out of bed because of physical limitations or medical orders need to use a bedpan or urinal for voiding. Male patients confined to bed usually prefer to use the urinal for voiding (see Skill 12-2) and the bedpan for defecation; female patients usually prefer to use the bedpan for both. Many patients find it difficult and embarrassing to use the bedpan. When a patient uses a bedpan, promote comfort and normalcy and respect the patient's privacy as much as possible. Be sure to maintain a professional manner. In addition, provide skin care, perineal hygiene, and hand hygiene after bedpan use.

Regular bedpans have a rounded, smooth upper end and a tapered, open lower end. The upper end fits under the patient's buttocks toward the sacrum, with the open end toward the foot of the bed (Figure 1). A special bedpan called a *fracture bedpan* is frequently used for patients with fractures of the femur or lower spine. Smaller and flatter than the ordinary bedpan, this type of bedpan is helpful for patients who cannot easily raise themselves onto the regular bedpan (see Figure 1). The fracture pan has a shallow, narrow upper end with a flat wide rim, and a deeper, open lower end. The upper end fits under the patient's buttocks toward the sacrum, with the deeper, open lower end toward the foot of the bed.

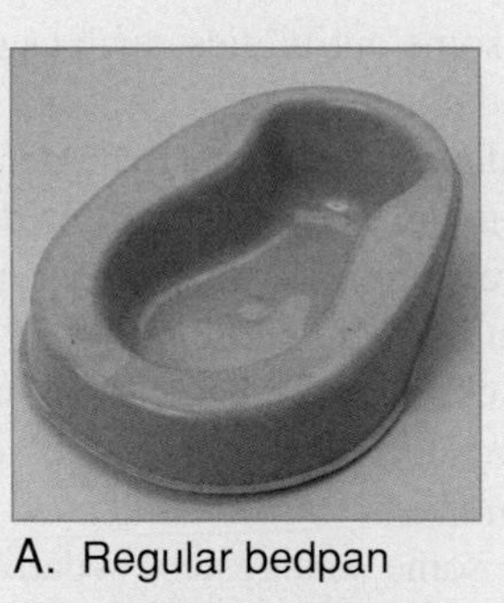

A. Regular bedpan

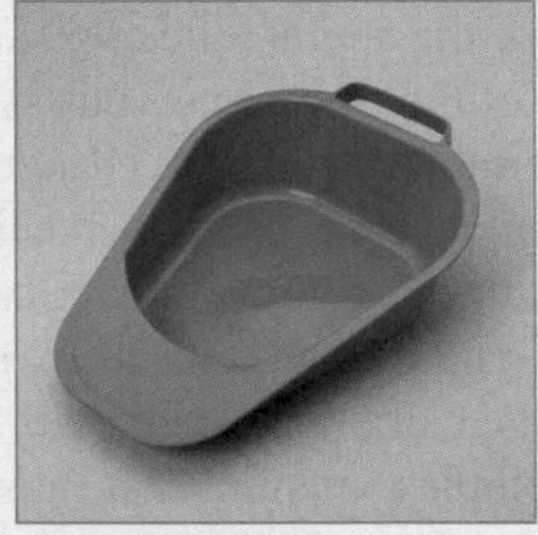

B. Fracture pan

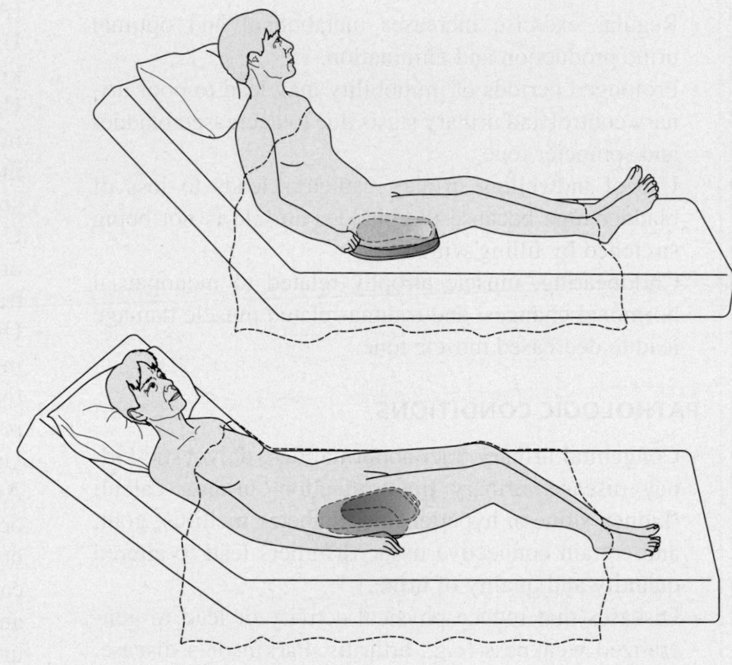

FIGURE 1 (**A**) Standard bedpan. Position a standard bedpan like a regular toilet seat—the buttocks are placed on the wide, rounded shelf, with the open end pointed toward the foot of the bed. (**B**) Fracture pan. Position a fracture pan with the thin edge toward the head of the bed.

DELEGATION CONSIDERATIONS

Assisting a patient with the use of a bedpan may be delegated to nursing assistive personnel (NAP) or to unlicensed assistive personnel (UAP), as well as to licensed practical/vocational nurses (LPN/LVNs). The decision to delegate must be based on careful analysis of the patient's needs and circumstances, as well as the qualifications of the person to whom the task is being delegated. Refer to the Delegation Guidelines in Appendix A.

EQUIPMENT

- Bedpan (regular or fracture)
- Toilet tissue
- Disposable clean gloves
- Additional PPE, as indicated
- Cover for bedpan or urinal (disposable waterproof pad or cover)
- Disposable washcloths and skin cleanser
- Moist towelettes, skin cleanser and water, or hand sanitizer

ASSESSMENT

Assess the patient's normal elimination habits. Determine why the patient needs to use a bedpan (e.g., a medical order for strict bed rest or immobilization). Also assess the patient's degree of limitation and ability to help with activity. Assess for activity limitations, such as hip surgery or spinal injury, which would contraindicate certain actions by the patient. Check for the presence of drains, dressings, intravenous fluid infusion sites/equipment, traction, or any other devices that could interfere with the patient's ability to help with the procedure or that could become dislodged. Assess the characteristics of the urine and the patient's skin.

NURSING DIAGNOSIS

Determine the related factors for the nursing diagnoses based on the patient's current status. Appropriate nursing diagnoses may include:

- Impaired Physical Mobility
- Impaired Urinary Elimination
- Toileting Self-Care Deficit

OUTCOME IDENTIFICATION AND PLANNING

The expected outcome to achieve when offering a bedpan is that the patient is able to void with assistance. Other appropriate outcomes may include the following: the patient maintains continence; the patient demonstrates how to use the bedpan with assistance; and the patient maintains skin integrity.

IMPLEMENTATION

ACTION	RATIONALE
1. Review the patient's medical record for any limitations in physical activity. (See Skill Variation: Assisting With Use of a Bedpan When the Patient Has Limited Movement.) Gather equipment.	Activity limitations may contraindicate certain actions by the patient. Assembling equipment provides for an organized approach to the task.
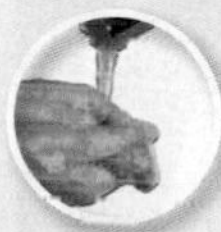 2. Perform hand hygiene and put on PPE, if indicated.	Hand hygiene and PPE prevent the spread of microorganisms. PPE is required based on transmission precautions.
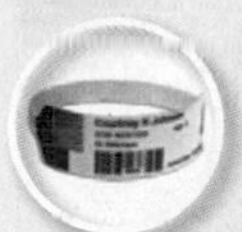 3. Identify the patient.	Identifying the patient ensures the right patient receives the intervention and helps prevent errors.
4. Assemble equipment on chair next to bed within reach.	Arranging items nearby is convenient, saves time, and avoids unnecessary stretching and twisting of muscles on the part of the nurse.
5. Close curtains around the bed and close the door to the room, if possible. Discuss the procedure with the patient and assess the patient's ability to assist with the procedure, as well as personal hygiene preferences.	This ensures the patient's privacy. Discussion promotes reassurance and provides knowledge about the procedure. Dialogue encourages patient participation and allows for individualized nursing care.
6. Unless contraindicated, apply powder to the rim of the bedpan. Place bedpan and cover on chair next to bed. Put on gloves.	Powder helps keep the bedpan from sticking to the patient's skin and makes it easier to remove. Powder is not applied if the patient has respiratory problems, is allergic to powder, or if a urine specimen is needed (could contaminate the specimen). The bedpan on the chair allows for easy access. Gloves prevent contact with blood and body fluids.
7. Adjust the bed to a comfortable working height, usually elbow height of the caregiver (VISN 8 Patient Safety Center, 2009). Place the patient in a supine position, with the head of the bed elevated about 30 degrees, unless contraindicated.	Having the bed at the proper height prevents back and muscle strain. Supine position is necessary for correct placement of patient on bedpan.

(continued)

SKILL 12-1 ASSISTING WITH THE USE OF A BEDPAN continued

ACTION	RATIONALE
8. Fold top linen back just enough to allow placement of bedpan. If there is no waterproof pad on the bed and time allows, consider placing a waterproof pad under patient's buttocks before placing the bedpan (Figure 2).	Folding back the linen in this manner minimizes unnecessary exposure while still allowing the nurse to place the bedpan. The waterproof pad will protect the bed should there be a spill.
9. Ask the patient to bend the knees. Have the patient lift his/her hips upward. Assist the patient, if necessary, by placing your hand that is closest to the patient palm up, under the lower back, and assist with lifting. Slip the bedpan into place with other hand (Figure 3).	The nurse uses less energy when the patient can assist by placing some of his/her weight on the heels.
10. **Ensure that the bedpan is in proper position and the patient's buttocks are resting on the rounded shelf of the regular bedpan or the shallow rim of the fracture bedpan.**	Having the bedpan in the proper position prevents spills onto the bed, ensures patient comfort, and prevents injury to the skin from a misplaced bedpan.
11. Raise head of bed as near to sitting position as tolerated, unless contraindicated. Cover the patient with bed linens.	This position makes it easier for the patient to void or defecate, avoids strain on the patient's back, and allows gravity to aid in elimination. Covering promotes warmth and privacy.
12. **Place call bell and toilet tissue within easy reach. Place the bed in the lowest position.** Leave patient if it is safe to do so. Use side rails appropriately (Figure 4).	Falls can be prevented if the patient does not have to reach for items he or she needs. Placing the bed in the lowest position promotes patient safety. Leaving the patient alone, if possible, promotes self-esteem and shows respect for privacy. Side rails assist the patient in repositioning.

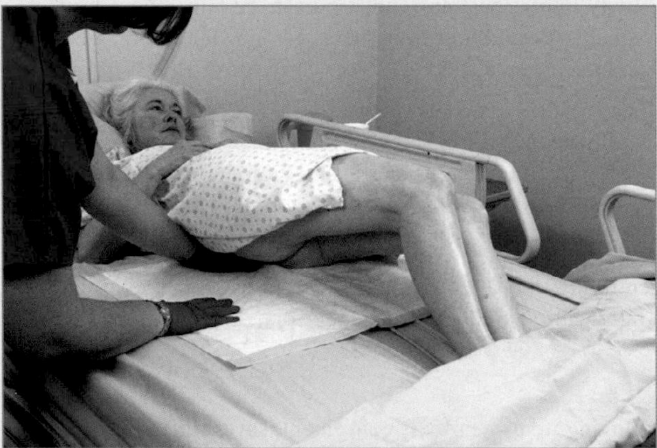

FIGURE 2 Placing waterproof pad under patient's buttocks. *(Note: Covers should be folded back just enough to work, not expose patient unnecessarily. Covers in this series of photos have been pulled back to show action.)*

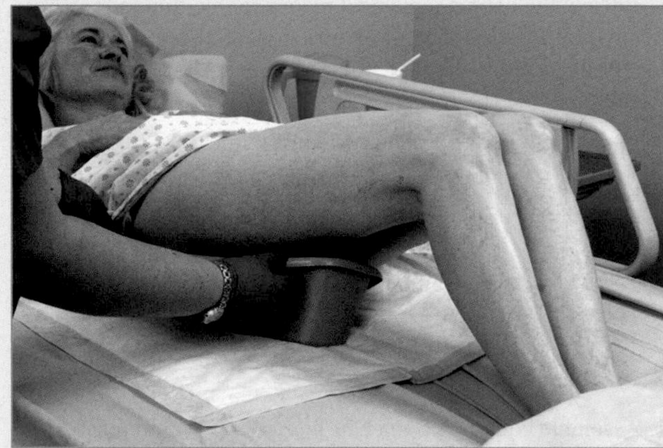

FIGURE 3 Assisting patient to raise self in bed to position bedpan. *(Note: Covers should be folded back just enough to work, not expose patient unnecessarily. Covers in this series of photos have been pulled back to show action.)*

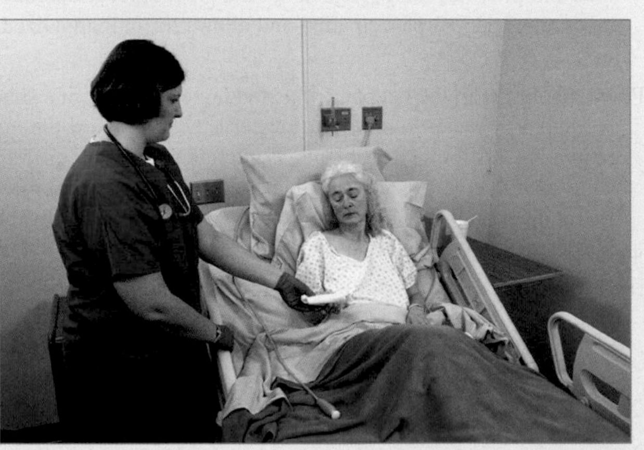

FIGURE 4 Placing call bell within patient's reach and handing patient toilet tissue.

ACTION	RATIONALE
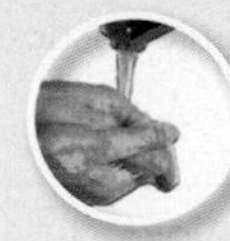 13. Remove gloves and additional PPE, if used. Perform hand hygiene.	Proper removal of PPE prevents transmission of microorganisms. Hand hygiene deters the spread of microorganisms.

Removing the Bedpan

ACTION	RATIONALE
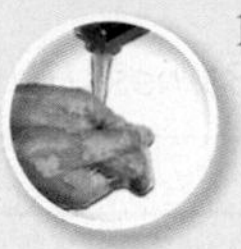 14. Perform hand hygiene and put on gloves and additional PPE, as indicated. Adjust the bed to a comfortable working height, usually elbow height of the caregiver (VISN 8 Patient Safety Center, 2009). Have a receptacle, such as plastic trash bag, handy for discarding tissue.	Hand hygiene deters the spread of microorganisms. Gloves prevent exposure to blood and body fluids. Having the bed at the proper height prevents back and muscle strain. Proper disposal of soiled tissue prevents transmission of microorganisms.
15. Lower the head of the bed, if necessary, to about 30 degrees. Remove bedpan in the same manner in which it was offered, being careful to hold it steady. Ask the patient to bend the knees and lift the buttocks up from the bedpan. Assist the patient, if necessary, by placing your hand that is closest to the patient palm up, under the lower back, and assist with lifting. Place the bedpan on the bedside chair and cover it.	Holding the bedpan steady prevents spills. The nurse uses less energy when the patient can assist by placing some of his/her weight on the heels. Covering the bedpan helps to prevent the spread of microorganisms.
16. If patient needs assistance with hygiene, wrap tissue around the hand several times, and wipe patient clean, using one stroke from the pubic area toward the anal area. Discard tissue. Use warm, moist disposable washcloth and skin cleanser to clean perineal area. Place patient on his or her side and spread buttocks to clean anal area.	Cleaning area from front to back minimizes fecal contamination of the vagina and urinary meatus. Cleaning the patient after he or she has used the bedpan prevents offensive odors and skin irritation.
17. Do not place toilet tissue in the bedpan if a specimen is required or if output is being recorded. Place toilet tissue in appropriate receptacle.	Mixing toilet tissue with a specimen makes laboratory examination more difficult and interferes with accurate output measurement.
18. Return the patient to a comfortable position. Make sure the linens under the patient are dry. Replace or remove pad under the patient, as necessary. Remove your gloves and ensure that the patient is covered.	Positioning helps to promote patient comfort. Removing contaminated gloves prevents spread of microorganisms.
19. Raise side rail. Lower bed height and adjust head of bed to a comfortable position. Reattach call bell.	These actions promote patient safety.
20. Offer patient supplies to wash and dry his/her hands, assisting as necessary.	Washing hands after using the urinal helps prevent the spread of microorganisms.
21. Put on clean gloves. Empty and clean the bedpan, measuring urine in graduated container, as necessary. Discard trash receptacle with used toilet paper per facility policy.	Gloves prevent exposure to blood and body fluids. Cleaning reusable equipment helps prevent the spread of microorganisms.
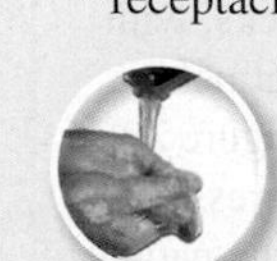 22. Remove additional PPE, if used. Perform hand hygiene.	Removing PPE properly reduces the risk for infection transmission and contamination of other items. Hand hygiene prevents the spread of microorganisms.

EVALUATION

The expected outcome is met when the patient voids using the bedpan. Other outcomes are met when the patient remains dry; the patient does not experience episodes of incontinence, the patient demonstrates measures to assist with using the bedpan; and the patient does not experience impaired skin integrity.

(continued)

SKILL 12-1 ASSISTING WITH THE USE OF A BEDPAN continued

DOCUMENTATION

Guidelines

Document the patient's tolerance of the activity. Record the amount of urine voided on the intake and output record, if appropriate. Document any other assessments, such as unusual urine characteristics or alterations in the patient's skin.

Sample Documentation

12/06/15 0730 Patient placed on fracture bedpan with a two-person assist. Voided 400 mL dark yellow urine; strong odor noted. Perineal skin intact, without redness or irritation. Specimen sent for urinalysis as ordered.

—S. Barnes, RN

SPECIAL CONSIDERATIONS

- A fracture bedpan is usually more comfortable for the patient, but it does not hold as large a volume as the regular bedpan (see Figure 1).
- Very thin or elderly patients often find it easier and more comfortable to use the fracture bedpan.
- Bedpan should not be left in place for extended periods because this can result in excessive pressure and irritation to the patient's skin.

SKILL VARIATION Assisting With Use of a Bedpan When the Patient Has Limited Movement

Patients who are unable to lift themselves onto the bedpan or who have activity limitations that prohibit the required actions can be assisted onto the bedpan in an alternate manner using these actions:

1. Review patient's chart for any limitations in physical activity. Gather equipment.
2. Put on PPE, as indicated, and perform hand hygiene. Check the patient's identification band.

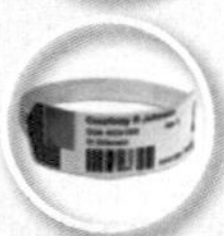

3. Place bedpan and cover on chair next to bed. Close curtains around the bed and close the door to the room, if possible.
4. Discuss procedure with the patient and assess the patient's ability to assist with the procedure, as well as personal hygiene preferences.
5. Unless contraindicated, apply powder to the rim of the bedpan.
6. Adjust the bed to a comfortable working height, usually elbow height of the caregiver (VISN 8 Patient Safety Center, 2009). Place the patient in a supine position, with the head of the bed elevated about 30 degrees, unless contraindicated. Put on disposable gloves.
7. Fold top linen just enough to turn the patient, while minimizing exposure. If no waterproof pad is on the bed and time allows, consider placing a waterproof pad under patient's buttocks before placing bedpan.
8. Assist the patient to roll to the opposite side or turn the patient into a side-lying position.

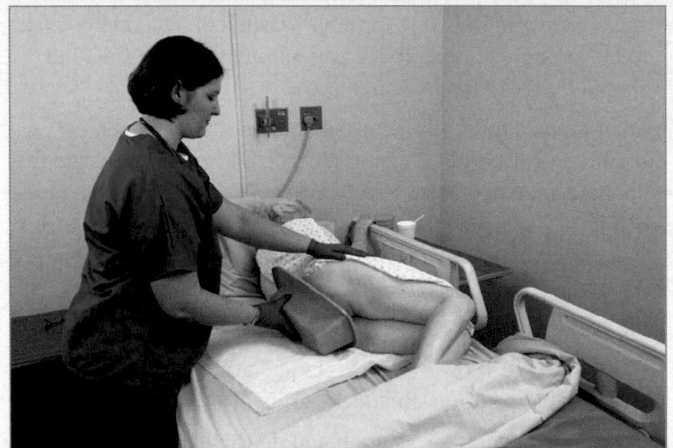

FIGURE A Rolling patient on side to place bedpan. *(Note: Covers should be folded back just enough to work, not expose patient unnecessarily. Covers in photo pulled back to show action for photo.)*

9. Hold the bedpan firmly against the patient's buttocks, with the upper end of the bedpan under the patient's buttocks toward the sacrum, and down into the mattress (Figure A).
10. Keep one hand against the bedpan. Apply gentle pressure to ensure the bedpan remains in place as you assist the patient to roll back onto the bedpan.
11. Ensure that the bedpan is in the proper position and the patient's buttocks are resting on rounded shelf of the regular bedpan or the shallow rim of the fracture bedpan.
12. Raise the head of bed as near to sitting position as tolerated, unless contraindicated. Cover the patient with bed linens.
13. Place call bell and toilet tissue within easy reach. Place the bed in the lowest position. Leave the patient if it is safe to do so. Use side rails appropriately.

SKILL VARIATION Assisting With Use of a Bedpan When the Patient Has Limited Movement continued

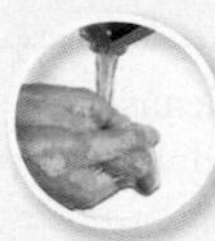

14. Remove gloves, and PPE, if used. Perform hand hygiene.
15. To remove the bedpan, perform hand hygiene and put on disposable gloves, and additional PPE, as indicated. Raise the bed to a comfortable working height. Have a receptacle handy for discarding tissue.
16. Lower the head of the bed. Grasp the closest side of the bedpan. Apply gentle pressure to hold the bedpan flat and steady. Assist the patient to roll to the opposite side or turn the patient into a side-lying position with the assistance of a second caregiver. Remove the bedpan and set on chair. Cover the bedpan.
17. If patient needs assistance with hygiene, wrap tissue around the hand several times, and wipe patient clean, using one stroke from the pubic area toward the anal area. Discard tissue. Use warm, moist disposable washcloth and skin cleanser to clean perineal area. Place patient on his/her side and spread buttocks to clean anal area.
18. Return the patient to a comfortable position. Make sure the linens under the patient are dry and that the patient is covered.
19. Remove your gloves. Offer the patient supplies to wash and dry his/her hands, assisting as necessary.
20. Raise side rail. Lower bed height and adjust head of bed to a comfortable position. Reattach call bell.

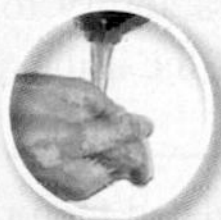

21. Put on clean gloves. Empty and clean the bedpan, measuring urine in graduated container, as necessary. Remove gloves and additional PPE, if used. Perform hand hygiene.

SKILL 12-2 ASSISTING WITH THE USE OF A URINAL

Male patients confined to bed usually prefer to use the urinal (Figure 1) for voiding as a matter of convenience. Use of a urinal in the standing position facilitates emptying of the bladder. Patients who are unable to stand alone may benefit from assistance when voiding into a urinal. If the patient is unable to stand, the urinal may be used in bed. Patients may also use a urinal in the bathroom to facilitate measurement of urinary output. Many patients find it embarrassing to use the urinal. Promote comfort and normalcy as much as possible, while respecting the patient's privacy. Provide skin care, perineal hygiene, and hand hygiene after urinal use and maintain a professional manner.

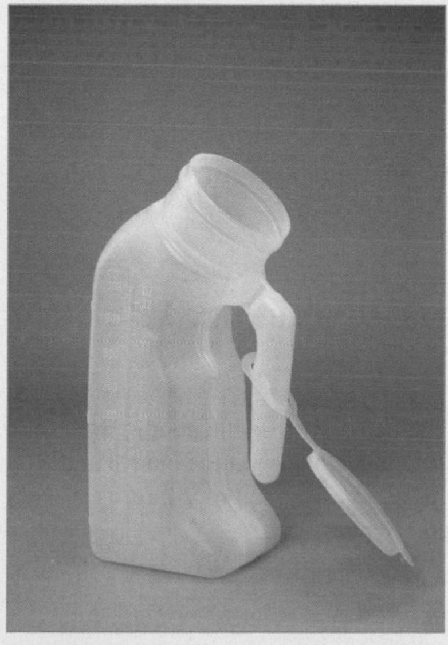

FIGURE 1 Urinal.

(continued)

SKILL 12-2 ASSISTING WITH THE USE OF A URINAL continued

DELEGATION CONSIDERATIONS

Assisting a patient with the use of a urinal may be delegated to nursing assistive personnel (NAP) or to unlicensed assistive personnel (UAP), as well as to licensed practical/vocational nurses (LPN/LVNs). The decision to delegate must be based on careful analysis of the patient's needs and circumstances, as well as the qualifications of the person to whom the task is being delegated. Refer to the Delegation Guidelines in Appendix A.

EQUIPMENT

- Urinal with end cover (usually attached)
- Toilet tissue
- Clean gloves
- Additional PPE, as indicated
- Disposable washcloths and skin cleanser
- Moist towelettes, skin cleanser and water, or hand sanitizer

ASSESSMENT

Assess the patient's normal elimination habits. Determine why the patient needs to use a urinal (e.g., a medical order for strict bed rest or immobilization). Also assess the patient's degree of limitation and ability to help with activity. Assess for activity limitations, such as hip surgery or spinal injury, which would contraindicate certain actions by the patient. Check for the presence of drains, dressings, intravenous fluid infusion sites/equipment, traction, or any other devices that could interfere with the patient's ability to help with the procedure or that could become dislodged. Assess the characteristics of the urine and the patient's skin.

NURSING DIAGNOSIS

Determine the related factors for the nursing diagnoses based on the patient's current status. Appropriate nursing diagnoses may include:

- Impaired Physical Mobility
- Impaired Urinary Elimination
- Toileting Self-Care Deficit

OUTCOME IDENTIFICATION AND PLANNING

The expected outcome to achieve when offering a urinal is that the patient is able to void with assistance. Other appropriate outcomes may include the following: the patient maintains continence; the patient demonstrates how to use the urinal; and the patient maintains skin integrity.

IMPLEMENTATION

ACTION	RATIONALE
1. Review the patient's medical record for any limitations in physical activity. Gather equipment.	Activity limitations may contraindicate certain actions by the patient. Assembling equipment provides for an organized approach to the task.
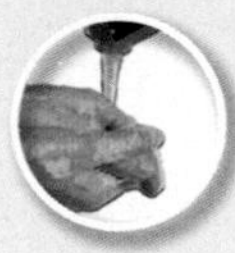 2. Perform hand hygiene and put on PPE, if indicated.	Hand hygiene and PPE prevent the spread of microorganisms. PPE is required based on transmission precautions.
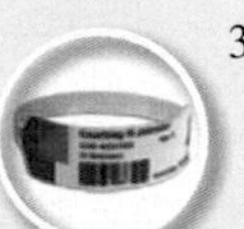 3. Identify the patient.	Identifying the patient ensures the right patient receives the intervention and helps prevent errors.
4. Assemble equipment on chair next to bed within reach.	Arranging items nearby is convenient, saves time, and avoids unnecessary stretching and twisting of muscles on the part of the nurse.
5. Close the curtains around the bed and close the door to the room, if possible. Discuss the procedure with the patient and assess the patient's ability to assist with the procedure, as well as personal hygiene preferences.	This ensures the patient's privacy. Discussion promotes reassurance and provides knowledge about the procedure. Dialogue encourages patient participation and allows for individualized nursing care.

ACTION	RATIONALE
6. Put on gloves.	Gloves prevent exposure to blood and body fluids.
7. Assist the patient to an appropriate position, as necessary: standing at the bedside, lying on one side or back, sitting in bed with the head elevated, or sitting on the side of the bed.	These positions facilitate voiding and emptying of the bladder.
8. If the patient remains in the bed, fold the linens just enough to allow for proper placement of the urinal.	Folding back the linen in this manner minimizes unnecessary exposure while still allowing the nurse to place the urinal.
9. If the patient is not standing, have him spread his legs slightly. **Hold the urinal close to the penis and position the penis completely within the urinal (Figure 2). Keep the bottom of the urinal lower than the penis. If necessary, assist the patient to hold the urinal in place.**	Slight spreading of the legs allows for proper positioning of the urinal. Placing penis completely within the urinal and keeping the bottom lower than the penis avoids urine spills.

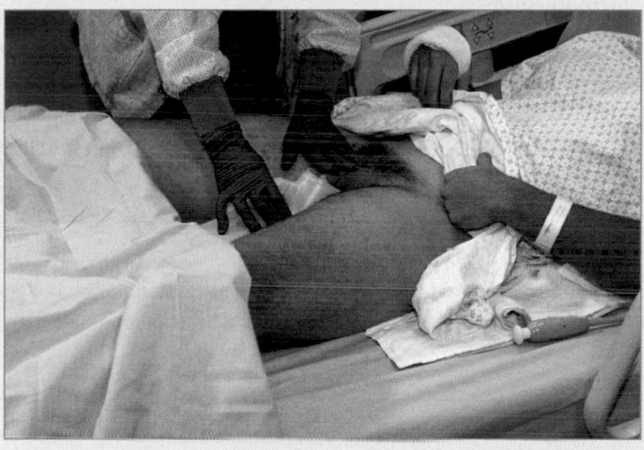

FIGURE 2 Positioning urinal in place for a male patient. (*Note: Covers should be folded back just enough to work, not expose patient unnecessarily. Covers have been pulled back to show action.*)

ACTION	RATIONALE
10. Cover the patient with the bed linens.	Covering promotes warmth and privacy.
11. Place call bell and toilet tissue within easy reach. Have a receptacle, such as plastic trash bag, handy for discarding tissue. Ensure the bed is in the lowest position. Leave patient if it is safe to do so. Use side rails appropriately.	Falls can be prevented if the patient does not have to reach for items he needs. Placing the bed in the lowest position promotes patient safety. Leaving the patient alone, if possible, promotes self-esteem and shows respect for privacy. Side rails assist the patient in repositioning.
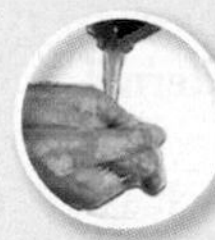 12. Remove gloves and additional PPE, if used. Perform hand hygiene.	Proper removal of PPE reduces transmission of microorganisms. Hand hygiene deters the spread of microorganisms.

Removing the Urinal

ACTION	RATIONALE
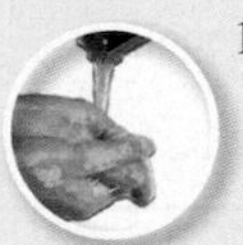 13. Perform hand hygiene. Put on gloves and additional PPE, as indicated.	Hand hygiene and PPE prevent the spread of microorganisms. Gloves prevent exposure to blood and body fluids. PPE is required based on transmission precautions.
14. Pull back the patient's bed linens just enough to remove the urinal. Remove the urinal. Cover the open end of the urinal. Place on the bedside chair. If the patient needs assistance with hygiene, wrap tissue around the hand several times, and wipe patient dry. Place tissue in receptacle. Use warm, moist disposable washcloth and skin cleanser to clean perineal area, as necessary, and as per patient request.	Covering the end of the urinal helps to prevent the spread of microorganisms. Cleaning the patient after he has used the urinal prevents offensive odors and skin irritation.

(*continued*)

SKILL 12-2 ASSISTING WITH THE USE OF A URINAL continued

ACTION	RATIONALE
15. Return the patient to a comfortable position. Make sure the linens under the patient are dry. Remove your gloves and ensure that the patient is covered.	Proper positioning promotes patient comfort. Removing contaminated gloves prevents spread of microorganisms.
16. Ensure patient call bell is in reach.	Promotes patient safety.
17. Offer patient supplies to wash and dry his hands, assisting as necessary.	Washing hands after using the urinal helps prevent the spread of microorganisms.
18. Put on clean gloves. Empty and clean the urinal, measuring urine in graduated container, as necessary. Discard trash receptacle with used toilet paper per facility policy.	Measurement of urine volume is required for accurate intake and output records.
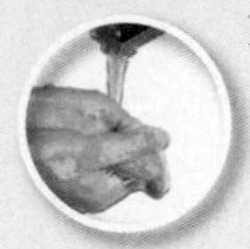 19. Remove gloves and additional PPE, if used, and perform hand hygiene.	Gloves prevent exposure to blood and body fluids. Removing PPE properly reduces the risk for infection transmission and contamination of other items. Hand hygiene prevents the spread of microorganisms.

EVALUATION

The expected outcome is met when the patient voids using the urinal. Other outcomes are met when the patient remains dry; the patient does not experience episodes of incontinence; the patient demonstrates measures to assist with using the urinal; and the patient does not experience impaired skin integrity.

DOCUMENTATION

Guidelines

Document the patient's tolerance of the activity. Record the amount of urine voided on the intake and output record, if appropriate. Document any other assessments, such as unusual urine characteristics or alterations in the patient's skin.

Sample Documentation

12/06/15 0730 Patient using urinal at bedside to void. Voided 600 mL yellow urine. Perineal skin intact, without redness or irritation. Reinforced need for continued use of urinal for recording accurate output. Patient verbalized an understanding of instructions.

—*S. Barnes, RN*

SPECIAL CONSIDERATIONS

- Urinal should not be left in place for extended periods because pressure and irritation to the patient's skin can result. If patient is unable to use alone or with assistance, consider other interventions, such as assisting the patient to use a bedside commode or applying an **external condom catheter** (see Skill 12-3 and Skill 12-5).
- It may be necessary to assist patients who have difficulty holding the urinal in place, such as those with limited upper extremity movement or alteration in mentation, to prevent spillage of urine.
- The urinal may also be used standing or sitting at the bedside or in the patient's bathroom, if patient is able to do so.

SKILL 12-3 ASSISTING WITH THE USE OF A BEDSIDE COMMODE

Patients who experience difficulty getting to the bathroom may benefit from the use of a bedside commode. Bedside commodes are portable toilet substitutes that can be used for voiding and defecation (Figure 1). A bedside commode can be placed close to the bed for easy use. Many have armrests attached to the legs that may interfere with ease of transfer. The legs usually have some type of end cap on the bottom to reduce movement, but care must be taken to prevent the commode from moving during transfer, resulting in patient injury or falls.

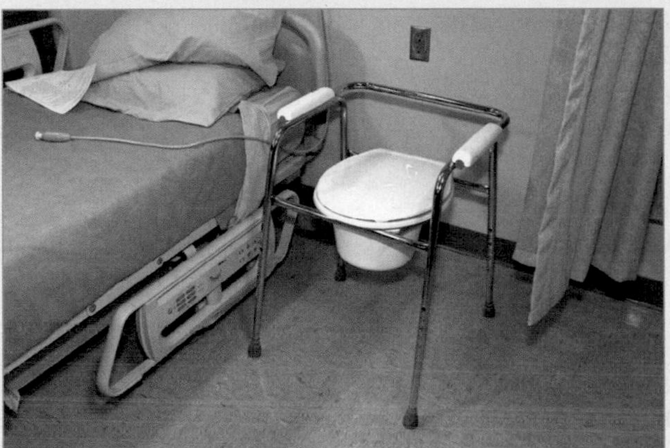

FIGURE 1 Bedside commode.

DELEGATION CONSIDERATIONS

Assisting a patient with the use of a commode may be delegated to nursing assistive personnel (NAP) or to unlicensed assistive personnel (UAP), as well as to licensed practical/vocational nurses (LPN/LVNs). The decision to delegate must be based on careful analysis of the patient's needs and circumstances, as well as the qualifications of the person to whom the task is being delegated. Refer to the Delegation Guidelines in Appendix A.

EQUIPMENT

- Commode with cover (usually attached)
- Toilet tissue
- Nonsterile gloves
- Additional PPE, as indicated
- Disposable washcloths and skin cleanser
- Moist towelettes, skin cleanser and water, or hand sanitizer

ASSESSMENT

Assess the patient's normal elimination habits. Determine why the patient needs to use a commode, such as weakness or unsteady gait. Assess the patient's degree of limitation and ability to help with the activity. Check for the presence of drains, dressings, intravenous fluid infusion sites/equipment, or other devices that could interfere with the patient's ability to help with the procedure or that could become dislodged. Assess the characteristics of the urine and the patient's skin.

NURSING DIAGNOSIS

Determine the related factors for the nursing diagnosis based on the patient's current status. Appropriate nursing diagnoses may include:

- Risk for Falls
- Impaired Urinary Elimination
- Toileting Self-Care Deficit

OUTCOME IDENTIFICATION AND PLANNING

The expected outcome to achieve when assisting with the use of a commode is that the patient is able to void with assistance. Other appropriate outcomes may include the following: the patient maintains continence; the patient demonstrates how to use the commode; the patient maintains skin integrity; and the patient remains free from injury.

(continued)

SKILL 12-3 ASSISTING WITH THE USE OF A BEDSIDE COMMODE continued

IMPLEMENTATION

ACTION	RATIONALE
1. Review the patient's chart for any limitations in physical activity. Gather equipment.	Physical limitations may require adaptations in performing the skill. Assembling equipment provides for an organized approach to the task.
2. Obtain assistance for patient transfer from another staff member, if necessary.	Assistance from another person may be required to transfer the patient safely to the commode.
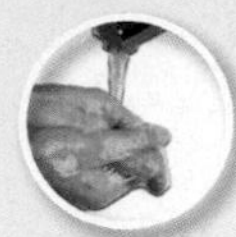 3. Perform hand hygiene and put on PPE, if indicated.	Hand hygiene and PPE prevent the spread of microorganisms. PPE is required based on transmission precautions.
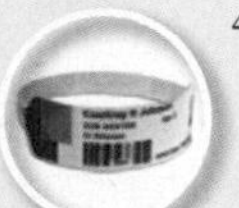 4. Identify the patient.	Identifying the patient ensures the right patient receives the intervention and helps prevent errors.
5. Close the curtains around the bed and close the door to the room, if possible. Discuss the procedure with the patient and assess the patient's ability to assist with the procedure, as well as personal hygiene preferences.	This ensures the patient's privacy. Discussion promotes reassurance and provides knowledge about the procedure. Dialogue encourages patient participation and allows for individualized nursing care.
6. Place the commode close to, and parallel with, the bed. Raise or remove the seat cover. (Refer to Figure 1, above.)	Allows for easy access.
7. Assist the patient to a standing position and then help the patient pivot to the commode. **While bracing one commode leg with your foot, ask the patient to place his/her hands one at a time on the armrests. Assist the patient to lower himself/herself slowly onto the commode seat.**	Standing and then pivoting ensures safe patient transfer. Bracing the commode leg with a foot prevents the commode from shifting while the patient is sitting down.
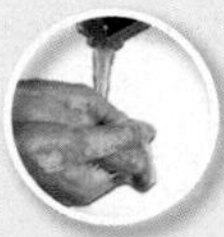 8. Cover the patient with a blanket. Place call bell and toilet tissue within easy reach. Leave patient if it is safe to do so. Remove PPE, if used, and perform hand hygiene.	Covering the patient promotes warmth. Falls can be prevented if the patient does not have to reach for items he or she needs. Leaving patient alone, if possible, promotes self-esteem and shows respect for privacy. Removing PPE properly reduces the risk for infection transmission and contamination of other items. Hand hygiene prevents the spread of microorganisms.
Assisting Patient Off Commode	
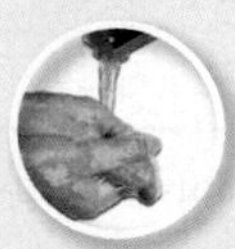 9. Perform hand hygiene. Put on gloves and additional PPE, as indicated.	Hand hygiene deters the spread of microorganisms. Gloves prevent exposure to blood and body fluids.
10. Assist the patient to a standing position. If the patient needs assistance with hygiene, wrap toilet tissue around your hand several times, and wipe the patient clean, using one stroke from the pubic area toward the anal area. Discard tissue in an appropriate receptacle, according to facility policy, and continue with additional tissue until patient is dry. Place tissue in receptacle. Use warm, moist disposable washcloth and skin cleanser to clean perineal area, as necessary, and as per patient request.	Cleaning area from front to back minimizes fecal contamination of the vagina and urinary meatus. Cleaning the patient after he or she has used the commode prevents offensive odors and irritation to the skin.

ACTION	RATIONALE
11. Do not place toilet tissue in the commode if a specimen is required or if output is being recorded. Replace or lower the seat cover.	Mixing toilet tissue with a specimen makes laboratory examination more difficult and interferes with accurate output measurement. Covering the commode helps to prevent the spread of microorganisms.
12. Remove your gloves. Return the patient to the bed or chair. If the patient returns to the bed, raise side rails, as appropriate. Ensure that the patient is covered and call bell is readily within reach.	Removing contaminated gloves prevents spread of microorganisms. Returning the patient to the bed or chair promotes patient comfort. Side rails assist with patient movement in the bed. Having the call bell readily available promotes patient safety.
13. Offer patient supplies to wash and dry his or her hands, assisting as necessary.	Washing hands after using the commode helps prevent the spread of microorganisms.
14. Put on clean gloves. Empty and clean the commode, measuring urine in graduated container, as necessary.	Gloves prevent exposure to blood and body fluids. Accurate measurement of urine is necessary for accurate intake and output records.
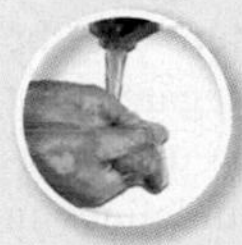 15. Remove gloves and additional PPE, if used. Perform hand hygiene.	Removing PPE properly reduces the risk for infection transmission and contamination of other items. Hand hygiene prevents the spread of microorganisms.

EVALUATION

The expected outcome is met when the patient successfully uses the bedside commode. Other outcomes are met when the patient remains dry, does not experience episodes of incontinence, demonstrates measures to assist with using the commode, and does not experience impaired skin integrity or falls.

DOCUMENTATION

Guidelines

Document the patient's tolerance of the activity, including his/her ability to use the commode. Record the amount of urine voided and/or stool passed on the intake and output record, if appropriate. Document any other assessments, such as unusual urine or stool characteristics or alterations in the patient's skin.

Sample Documentation

07/06/12 0730 Patient using commode at bedside to void with assistance of one for transfer. Voided 325 mL yellow urine. Perineal skin intact and slightly red. Perineal hygiene provided and skin protectant applied. Reinforced need for continued use of commode related to patient's unsteady gait. Patient verbalized an understanding of instructions and states she will call for assistance when getting up to use commode.

—*S. Barnes, RN*

SPECIAL CONSIDERATIONS

- Commode can be left within patient's reach, to be used without assistance, if appropriate and safe to do so, based on patient's activity limitations and mobility. Adjust room door or curtain to provide privacy for the patient in the event the commode is used.

SKILL 12-4 ASSESSING BLADDER VOLUME USING AN ULTRASOUND BLADDER SCANNER

A portable bladder ultrasound scanner is an accurate, reliable, and noninvasive device used to assess bladder volume. Bladder scanners do not pose a risk for the development of a urinary tract infection, unlike intermittent catheterization, which is also used to determine bladder volume. They are used when there is urinary frequency, absent or decreased urine output, bladder distention, or inability to void, and when establishing intermittent catheterization schedules. Protocols can be established to guide the decision to catheterize a patient. Some scanners offer the ability to print the scan results for documentation purposes.

Results are most accurate when the patient is in the supine position during the scanning. The device must be programmed for the gender of the patient by pushing the correct button on it. If a female patient has had a hysterectomy, the male button is pushed (Altschuler & Diaz, 2006). A postvoid residual (PVR) volume less than 50 mL indicates adequate bladder emptying. A PVR of greater than 150 mL is often recommended as the guideline for catheterization, because residual urine volumes of greater than 100 mL have been associated with the development of urinary tract infections (NKUDIC, 2012).

DELEGATION CONSIDERATIONS

The assessment of bladder volume using an ultrasound bladder scanner is not delegated to nursing assistive personnel (NAP) or to unlicensed assistive personnel (UAP). Depending on the state's nurse practice act and the organization's policies and procedures, this procedure may be delegated to licensed practical/vocational nurses (LPN/LVNs). The decision to delegate must be based on careful analysis of the patient's needs and circumstances, as well as the qualifications of the person to whom the task is being delegated. Refer to the Delegation Guidelines in Appendix A.

EQUIPMENT

- Bladder scanner
- Ultrasound gel or bladder scan gel pad
- Alcohol wipe or other sanitizer recommended by the scanner manufacturer and/or facility policy
- Clean gloves
- Additional PPE, as indicated
- Paper towel or washcloth

ASSESSMENT

Assess the patient for the need to check bladder volume, including signs of urinary retention, measurement of PVR volume, verification that the bladder is empty, identification of obstruction in an indwelling catheter, and evaluation of bladder distension to determine if catheterization is necessary. Verify medical order, if required by facility. Many facilities allow the use of a bladder scanner as a nursing judgment.

NURSING DIAGNOSIS

Determine the related factors for the nursing diagnoses based on the patient's current status. Appropriate nursing diagnoses may include:

- Impaired Urinary Elimination
- Urinary Retention

OUTCOME IDENTIFICATION AND PLANNING

The expected outcome to achieve when using a bladder scanner is that the volume of urine in the bladder will be accurately measured. Other appropriate outcomes may include the following: the patient's urinary elimination will be maintained, with a urine output of at least 30 mL/hour; and the patient's bladder will not be distended.

IMPLEMENTATION

ACTION	RATIONALE
1. Review the patient's medical record for any limitations in physical activity. Gather equipment.	Physical limitations may require adaptations in performing the skill. Assembling equipment provides for an organized approach to the task.
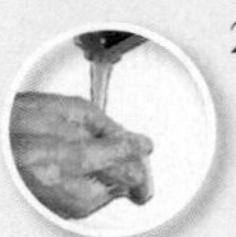 2. Perform hand hygiene and put on PPE, if indicated.	Hand hygiene and PPE prevent the spread of microorganisms. PPE is required based on transmission precautions.
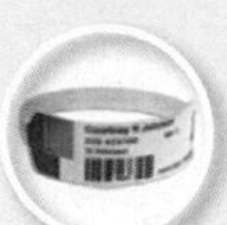 3. Identify the patient.	Identifying the patient ensures the right patient receives the intervention and helps prevent errors.
4. Close the curtains around the bed and close the door to the room, if possible. Discuss the procedure with the patient and assess the patient's ability to assist with the procedure, as well as personal hygiene preferences.	This ensures the patient's privacy. Discussion promotes reassurance and provides knowledge about the procedure. Dialogue encourages patient participation and allows for individualized nursing care.
5. Adjust the bed to a comfortable working height, usually elbow height of the caregiver (VISN 8 Patient Safety Center, 2009). Place the patient in a supine position. Drape patient. Stand on the patient's right side if you are right-handed, patient's left side if you are left-handed.	Having the bed at the proper height prevents back and muscle strain. Proper positioning allows accurate assessment of bladder volume. Keeping the patient covered as much as possible promotes patient comfort and privacy. Positioning allows for ease of use of dominant hand for the procedure.
6. Put on clean gloves.	Gloves prevent contact with blood and body fluids.
7. Press the ON button. Wait until the device warms up. Press the SCAN button to turn on the scanning screen.	Many devices require a few minutes to prepare the internal programs.
8. Press the appropriate gender button. The appropriate icon for male or female will appear on the screen (Figure 1).	The device must be programmed for the gender of the patient by pushing the correct button on it. If a female patient has had a hysterectomy, the male button is pushed (Altschuler & Diaz, 2006).
9. Clean the scanner head with the appropriate cleaner (Figure 2).	Cleaning the scanner head deters transmission of microorganisms.

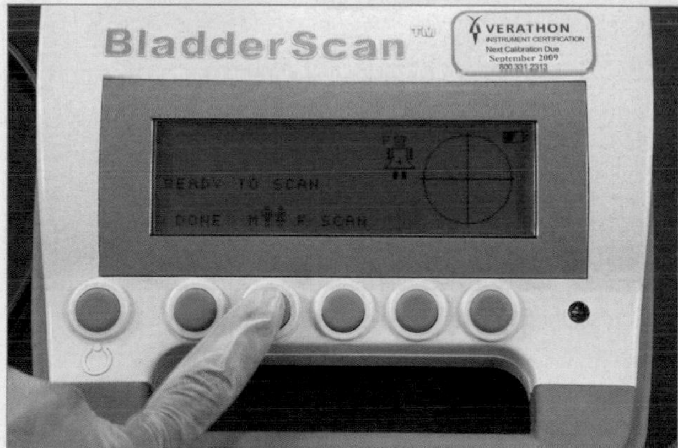

FIGURE 1 Identifying icon for patient's gender. (*Photo by B. Proud.*)

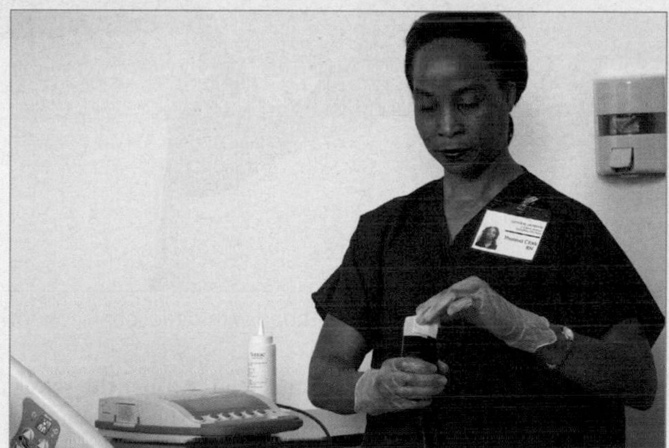
FIGURE 2 Cleaning scanner head. (*Photo by B. Proud.*)

(*continued*)

SKILL 12-4 ASSESSING BLADDER VOLUME USING AN ULTRASOUND BLADDER SCANNER continued

ACTION	RATIONALE
10. Gently palpate the patient's **symphysis pubis** (anterior midline junction of pubic bones). Place a generous amount of ultrasound gel or gel pad midline on the patient's abdomen, about 1 to 1.5 inches above the symphysis pubis (Figure 3).	Palpation identifies the proper location and allows for correct placement of the scanner head over the patient's bladder.
11. Place the scanner head on the gel or gel pad, **with the directional icon on the scanner head toward the patient's head. Aim the scanner head toward the bladder (point the scanner head slightly downward toward the coccyx) (Patraca, 2005).** Press and release the scan button (Figure 4).	Proper placement allows for accurate reading of urine in the bladder.

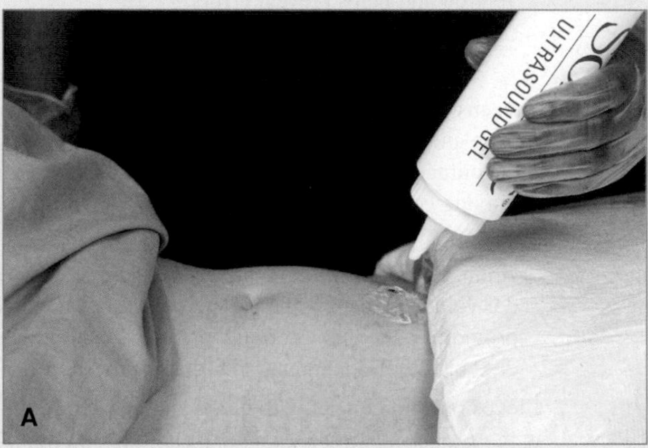

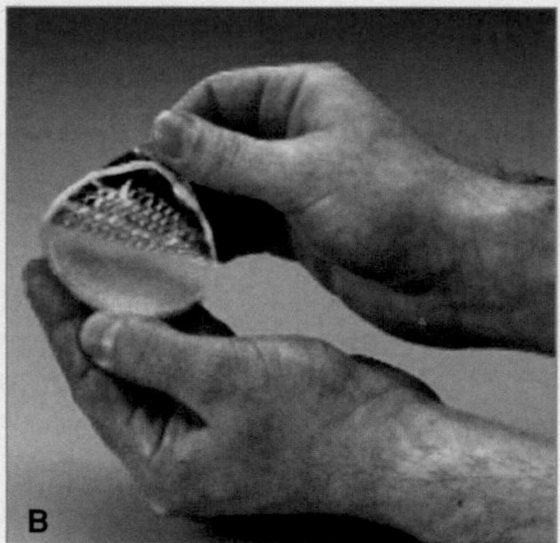

FIGURE 3 (**A**) Placing ultrasound gel about 1 to 1.5 inches above symphysis pubis. (*Photo by B. Proud.*) (**B**) Gel pad.

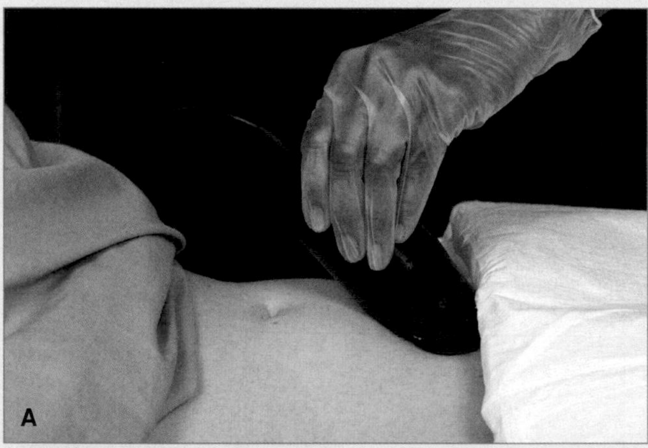

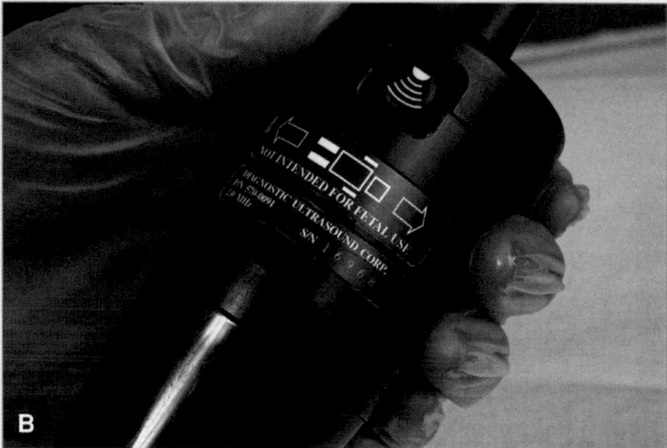

FIGURE 4 (**A**) Positioning scanner head with directional icon toward patient's bladder. (**B**) Scan button. (*Photos by B. Proud.*)

ACTION	RATIONALE
12. Observe the image on the scanner screen. **Adjust the scanner head to center the bladder image on the crossbars (Figure 5).**	This action allows for accurate reading of urine in the bladder.
13. Press and hold the DONE button until it beeps. Read the volume measurement on the screen. Print the results, if required, by pressing PRINT.	This action provides for accurate documentation of reading.

ACTION | RATIONALE

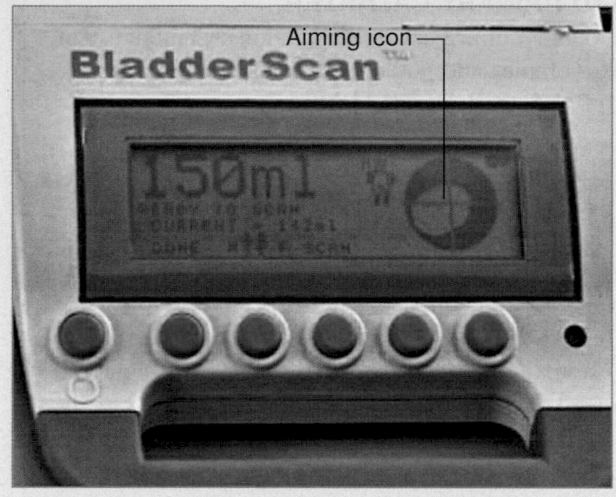

FIGURE 5 Centering image on crossbars. (From Patraca, K. (2005). Measure bladder volume without catheterization. *Nursing, 35*(4), 4.)

14. Use a washcloth or paper towel to remove remaining gel from the patient's skin. Alternately, gently remove gel pad from patient's skin. Return the patient to a comfortable position. Remove your gloves and ensure that the patient is covered.

    Removal of the gel promotes patient comfort. Removing contaminated gloves prevents spread of microorganisms.

15. Lower bed height and adjust head of bed to a comfortable position. Reattach call bell, if necessary.

    These actions promote patient safety.

16. Remove additional PPE, if used. Perform hand hygiene.

    Removing PPE properly reduces the risk for infection transmission and contamination of other items. Hand hygiene prevents the spread of microorganisms.

EVALUATION

The expected outcome is met when the volume of urine in the bladder is accurately measured; the patient's urinary elimination is maintained, with a urine output of at least 30 mL/hour; and the patient's bladder is not distended.

DOCUMENTATION

Guidelines

Document the assessment data that led to the use of the bladder scanner, relevant symptoms, the urine volume measured, and the patient's response.

Sample Documentation

7/06/15 1130 Patient has not voided 8 hours after catheter removal. Patient denies feelings of discomfort, pressure, and pain. Bladder not palpable. Bladder scanned for 120 mL of urine. Patient encouraged to increase oral fluid intake to eight 6-oz. glasses today. Dr. Liu notified of assessment. Orders received to rescan in 4 hours if patient does not void.

—*B. Clapp, RN*

UNEXPECTED SITUATIONS AND ASSOCIATED INTERVENTIONS

- *You press wrong icon for the patient's gender when initiating the scanner:* Turn scanner off and back on. Re-enter information using correct gender button.
- *You have reason to believe the bladder is full, based on assessment data, but scanner reveals little to no urine in bladder:* Ensure proper positioning of scanner head. Place a generous amount of ultrasound gel or gel pad midline on the patient's abdomen, about 1 to 1.5 inches above the symphysis pubis. Place the scanner head on the gel or gel pad, with the directional icon on the scanner head toward the patient's head. Aim the scanner head toward the bladder (point the scanner head slightly downward toward the coccyx). Ensure that the bladder image is centered on the crossbars.

(*continued*)

SKILL 12-4 ASSESSING BLADDER VOLUME USING AN ULTRASOUND BLADDER SCANNER continued

EVIDENCE FOR PRACTICE ▶

ULTRASONIC BLADDER SCANNING AND URINARY CATHETER

Urinary catheters are associated with the development of urinary tract infections. Can the use of ultrasonic bladder scanning to monitor bladder volumes and postvoid residuals help reduce the use of catheters, potentially reducing the risk of catheter-associated infections?

Related Research

Cutright, J. (2011). The effect of the bladder scanner policy on the number of urinary catheters inserted. *Journal of Wound Ostomy Continence Nursing, 38*(1), 71–76.

The aim of this study was to determine if use of an ultrasonic bladder-scanning device reduced the number of urinary catheters inserted in an acute care facility. This retrospective chart review evaluated 4 weeks of data from the medical records of adult patients who were scanned based on the facility's policy. The reasons for the use of the bladder scan, the results, and outcome were recorded. A total of 79 scans were performed on 47 patients (33 surgical patients, 14 medical patients). Of scans, 47% were performed on patients who were able to urinate on their own after removal of an indwelling catheter; the remaining patients were "unable to void," based on clinical observation. Of these patients, three (4%) required intermittent catheterization and eight (10%) required indwelling catheterization. Use of the bladder scanner resulted in an 87% reduction in catheterization, and an 80% reduction in re-catheterization (after removal of an indwelling catheter) among patients deemed "unable to void" based on clinical observation alone. The authors concluded the use of an ultrasonic bladder-scanning device reduced the number of urinary catheters inserted and was valuable when monitoring postoperative urinary retention.

Relevance for Nursing Practice

Current best-practice guidelines encourage a reduction in the use of urinary catheters to reduce catheter-associated urinary tract infections. Nurses should encourage the use of interventions to reduce the need for urinary catheters. The decrease in use of urethral catheters will result in less urethral trauma, less introduction of bacteria into the bladder, and ultimately fewer UTIs. The use of bladder scanning can reduce the need for catheterization and promote safe, early removal of urinary catheters.

Refer to thePoint for additional research on related nursing topics.

WATCH & LEARN SKILL 12-5 APPLYING AN EXTERNAL CONDOM CATHETER

When voluntary control of urination is not possible for male patients, an alternative to an indwelling catheter is the **external condom catheter**. This soft, pliable sheath made of silicone material is applied externally to the penis. Most devices are self-adhesive. The condom catheter is connected to drainage tubing and a collection bag. The collection bag may be a leg bag. The risk for UTI with a condom catheter is lower than the risk associated with an indwelling urinary catheter. Nursing care of a patient with a condom catheter includes vigilant skin care to prevent excoriation. This includes removing the condom catheter daily, washing the penis with skin cleanser and water and drying carefully, and inspecting the skin for irritation. In hot, humid weather, more frequent changing may be required. Always follow the manufacturer's instructions for applying the condom catheter because there are several variations. In all cases, take care to fasten the condom securely enough to prevent leakage, yet not so tightly as to constrict the blood vessels in the area. In addition, the tip of the tubing should be kept 1 to 2 inches (2.5 to 5 cm) beyond the tip of the penis to prevent irritation to the sensitive glans area.

Maintaining free urinary drainage is another nursing priority. Institute measures to prevent the tubing from becoming kinked and urine from backing up in the tubing. Urine can lead to excoriation of the glans, so position the tubing that collects the urine from the condom so that it draws urine away from the penis.

Always use a measuring or sizing guide supplied by the manufacturer to ensure the correct size of sheath is applied. Apply skin barriers, such as Cavilon™ or Skin Prep™, to the penis to protect penile skin from irritation and changes in integrity.

DELEGATION CONSIDERATIONS

The application of an external condom catheter may be delegated to nursing assistive personnel (NAP) or to unlicensed assistive personnel (UAP), as well as to licensed practical/vocational nurses (LPN/LVNs). The decision to delegate must be based on careful analysis of the patient's needs and circumstances, as well as the qualifications of the person to whom the task is being delegated. Refer to the Delegation Guidelines in Appendix A.

EQUIPMENT

- Condom sheath in appropriate size
- Skin protectant, such as Cavilon™ or Skin Prep™
- Velcro leg strap, catheter securing device, or tape
- Bath blanket
- Reusable leg bag with tubing or urinary drainage setup
- Basin of warm water and skin cleanser
- Disposable gloves
- Additional PPE, as indicated
- Washcloth and towel
- Scissors

ASSESSMENT

Assess the patient's knowledge of the need for catheterization. Ask the patient about any allergies, especially to latex or tape. Assess the size of the patient's penis to ensure that the appropriate-sized condom catheter is used. Inspect the skin in the groin and scrotal area, noting any areas of redness, irritation, or breakdown.

NURSING DIAGNOSIS

Determine the related factors for the nursing diagnoses based on the patient's current status. Possible nursing diagnoses may include:

- Impaired Urinary Elimination
- Functional Urinary Incontinence
- Risk for Impaired Skin Integrity

OUTCOME IDENTIFICATION AND PLANNING

The expected outcome to achieve when applying a condom catheter is that the patient's urinary elimination will be maintained, with a urine output of at least 30 mL/hour, and the bladder is not distended. Other outcomes may include the following: the patient's skin remains clean, dry, and intact, without evidence of irritation or breakdown.

IMPLEMENTATION

ACTION	RATIONALE
1. Gather equipment.	Assembling equipment provides for an organized approach to the task.
2. Perform hand hygiene and put on PPE, if indicated.	Hand hygiene and PPE prevent the spread of microorganisms. PPE is required based on transmission precautions.
3. Identify the patient.	Identifying the patient ensures the right patient receives the intervention and helps prevent errors.
4. Close the curtains around the bed and close the door to the room, if possible. Discuss the procedure with the patient. Ask the patient if he has any allergies, especially to latex.	This ensures the patient's privacy. Discussion promotes reassurance and provides knowledge about the procedure. Dialogue encourages patient participation and allows for individualized nursing care. Some condom catheters are made of latex.
5. Assemble equipment on overbed table within reach.	Arranging items nearby is convenient, saves time, and avoids unnecessary stretching and twisting of muscles on the part of the nurse.

(continued)

SKILL 12-5 APPLYING AN EXTERNAL CONDOM CATHETER continued

ACTION	RATIONALE
6. Adjust the bed to a comfortable working height, usually elbow height of the caregiver (VISN 8 Patient Safety Center, 2009). Stand on the patient's right side if you are right-handed, or on patient's left side if you are left-handed.	Having the bed at the proper height prevents back and muscle strain. Positioning on one side allows for ease of use of dominant hand for catheter application.
7. Prepare urinary drainage setup or reusable leg bag for attachment to the condom sheath.	Provides for an organized approach to the task.
8. Position the patient on his back with thighs slightly apart. Drape patient so that only the area around the penis is exposed. Slide waterproof pad under the patient.	Positioning allows access to the site. Draping prevents unnecessary exposure and promotes warmth. The waterproof pad will protect bed linens from moisture.
9. Put on disposable gloves. Trim any long pubic hair that is in contact with the penis.	Gloves prevent contact with blood and body fluids. Trimming pubic hair prevents pulling of hair by adhesive without the risk of infection associated with shaving.
10. Clean the genital area with washcloth, skin cleanser, and warm water. If patient is uncircumcised, retract foreskin and clean glans of penis. Replace foreskin. Clean the tip of the penis first, moving the washcloth in a circular motion from the meatus outward. Wash the shaft of the penis using downward strokes toward the pubic area. Rinse and dry. Remove gloves. Perform hand hygiene again.	Washing removes urine, secretions, and microorganisms. The penis must be clean and dry to minimize skin irritation. If the foreskin is left retracted, it may cause venous congestion in the glans of the penis, leading to edema.
11. Apply skin protectant to penis and allow to dry.	Skin protectant minimizes the risk of skin irritation from adhesive and moisture and increases the adhesive's ability to adhere to skin.
12. Roll condom sheath outward onto itself. Grasp penis firmly with nondominant hand. **Apply condom sheath by rolling it onto the penis with dominant hand (Figure 1). Leave 1 to 2 inches (2.5 to 5 cm) of space between the tip of the penis and the end of the condom sheath.**	Rolling the condom sheath outward allows for easier application. The space prevents irritation to tip of penis and allows free drainage of urine.
13. **Apply pressure to the sheath at the base of the penis for 10 to 15 seconds.**	Application of pressure ensures good adherence of adhesive with skin.
14. Connect condom sheath to drainage setup (Figure 2). Avoid kinking or twisting drainage tubing.	The collection device keeps the patient dry. Kinked tubing encourages backflow of urine.

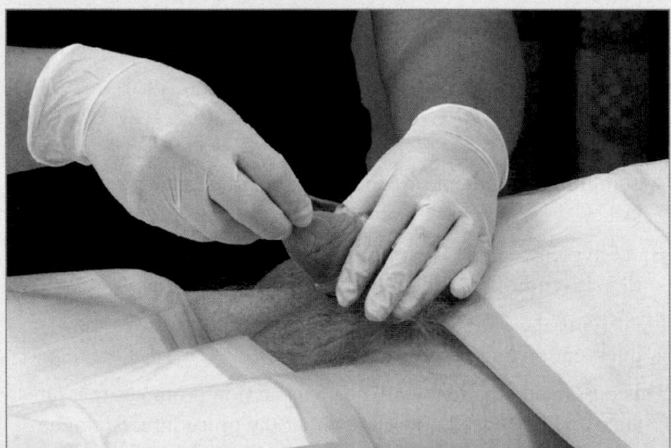

FIGURE 1 Unrolling sheath onto penis.

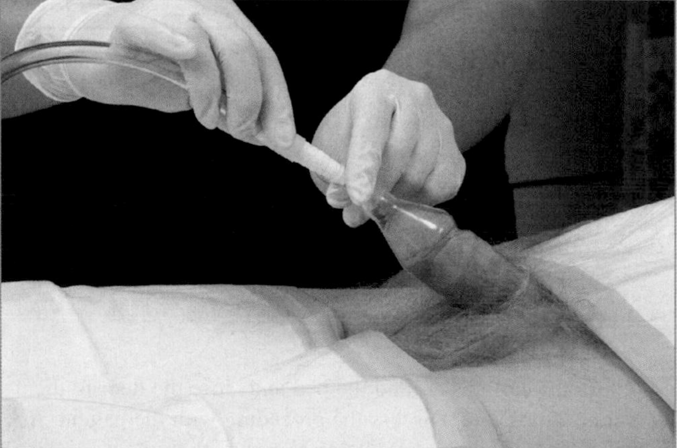

FIGURE 2 Connecting condom sheath to drainage setup.

ACTION	RATIONALE
15. Remove gloves. Secure drainage tubing to the patient's inner thigh with Velcro leg strap or tape. Leave some slack in tubing for leg movement.	Proper attachment prevents tension on the sheath and potential inadvertent removal.

ACTION	RATIONALE
16. Assist the patient to a comfortable position. Cover the patient with bed linens. Place the bed in the lowest position.	Positioning and covering provide warmth and promote comfort. Bed in the lowest position promotes patient safety.
17. Secure drainage bag below the level of the bladder. Check that drainage tubing is not kinked and that movement of side rails does not interfere with the drainage bag.	Facilitates drainage of urine and prevents the backflow of urine.
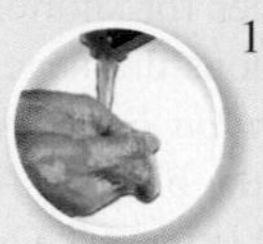 18. Remove equipment. Remove gloves and additional PPE, if used. Perform hand hygiene.	Proper disposal of equipment prevents transmission of microorganisms. Removing PPE properly reduces the risk for infection transmission and contamination of other items. Hand hygiene prevents the spread of microorganisms.

EVALUATION

The expected outcome is met when the condom catheter is applied without adverse effect; the patient's urinary elimination is maintained, with a urine output of at least 30 mL/hour; and the patient's skin remains clean, dry, and intact, without evidence of irritation or breakdown.

DOCUMENTATION

Guidelines

Document the assessment data supporting the decision to use a condom catheter, the application of the condom catheter, and the condition of the patient's skin. Record urine output on the intake and output record.

Sample Documentation

7/12/15 1910 Patient incontinent of urine; states: "It just comes too fast. I can't get to the bathroom in time." Perineal skin slightly reddened. Discussed rationale for use of condom catheter. Patient and wife agreeable to trying condom catheter. Medium-sized condom catheter applied; 200 mL of clear urine returned. Leg bag in place for daytime use. Patient verbalized understanding of need to call for assistance to empty drainage bag.

—B. Clapp, RN

UNEXPECTED SITUATIONS AND ASSOCIATED INTERVENTIONS

- *Condom catheter leaks with every voiding:* Check size of condom catheter. If it is too big or too small, it may leak. Check space between tip of penis and end of condom sheath. If this space is too small, the urine has no place to go and will leak out.
- *Condom catheter will not stay on patient:* Ensure that the condom catheter is correct size and that the penis is thoroughly dried before applying the condom catheter. Remind the patient that the condom catheter is in place, so that he does not tug at the tubing. If the patient has a retracted penis, a condom catheter may not be the best choice; there are pouches made for patients with a retracted penis.
- *When assessing the patient's penis, you find a break in skin integrity:* Do not reapply condom catheter. Allow skin to be open to air as much as possible. If your facility has a wound, ostomy, and continence nurse, arrange for a consult.

EVIDENCE FOR PRACTICE ▶

PREVENTION OF CATHETER-ASSOCIATED INFECTIONS

Centers for Disease Control and Prevention (CDC). (2012). *Healthcare-associated infections (HAIs). Catheter-associated urinary tract infections (CAUTI).* Available http://www.cdc.gov/HAI/ca_uti/uti.html.

This site provides resources for health care providers and patients, including the CDC guidelines for prevention of catheter-associated infections. These guidelines recommend considering use of alternatives to indwelling urethral catheterization in selected patients, when appropriate, such as the use of external catheters in cooperative male patients without urinary retention or bladder outlet obstruction.

Refer to thePoint for additional research on related nursing topics.

SKILL 12-6 CATHETERIZING THE FEMALE URINARY BLADDER

Urinary catheterization is the introduction of a catheter (tube) through the urethra into the bladder for the purpose of withdrawing urine. Catheter-associated UTIs are the most common hospital-acquired infection in the United States and is one reason catheterization should be avoided whenever possible. When it is deemed necessary, it should be performed using strict aseptic technique and left in place for the shortest length of time possible (Hooton et al., 2010). The duration of catheterization is the most important risk factor for the development of a urinary tract infection (Bernard et al., 2012).

Intermittent urethral catheters, or straight catheters, are used to drain the bladder for shorter periods (5 to 10 minutes) (Figure 1B). If a catheter is to remain in place for continuous drainage, an **indwelling urethral catheter** is used. Indwelling catheters are also called *retention* or *Foley catheters.* The indwelling urethral catheter is designed so that it does not slip out of the bladder. A balloon is inflated to ensure that the catheter remains in the bladder once it is inserted (Figure 1A).

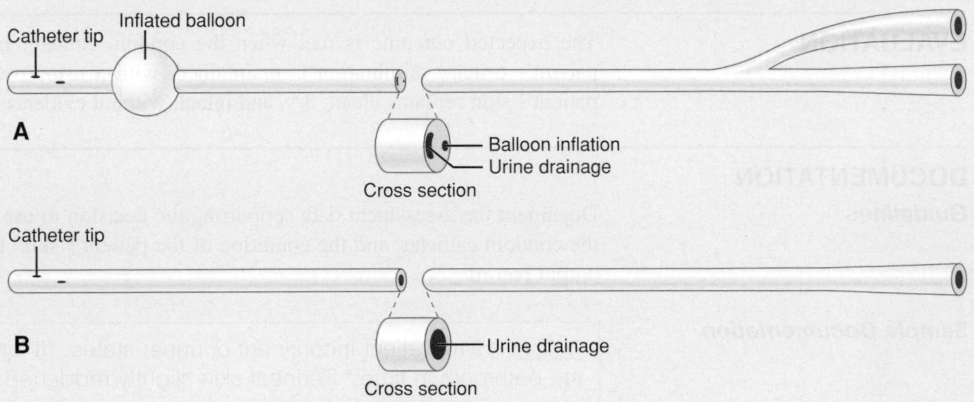

FIGURE 1 (**A**) Indwelling urethral catheter. (**B**) Intermittent urethral catheter.

Intermittent catheterization should be considered as an alternative to short-term or long-term indwelling urethral catheterization to reduce catheter-associated UTIs (Hooton et al., 2010). Intermittent catheterization is becoming the gold standard for the management of bladder-emptying dysfunctions and following surgical interventions. Certain advantages to intermittent catheterization, including the lower risks of catheter-associated UTI and complications, may make it a more desirable and safer option than indwelling catheterization (Herter & Wallace Kazer, 2010, p. 343–344).

The following procedure reviews insertion of an indwelling catheter. The procedure for an intermittent catheter follows as a Skill Variation. Guidelines for caring for a patient with an indwelling catheter are summarized in Box 12-1.

BOX 12-1 GUIDELINES FOR CARE OF THE PATIENT WITH AN INDWELLING CATHETER

- Use an indwelling catheter only when necessary. In addition, consider evidence-based practice guidelines and facility policy to ensure the catheter is removed at the earliest time possible, to limit use to the shortest duration possible (Adams et al., 2012; Bernard et al., 2012; Gokula et al., 2012; Hooton et al., 2010).
- Use strict hand hygiene principles.
- Use the smallest appropriate-size catheter.
- Use sterile technique when inserting a catheter.
- Secure the catheter properly to the patient's thigh or abdomen after insertion.
- Keep the drainage bag below the level of the patient's bladder to maintain drainage of urine and prevent the backflow of urine into the patient's bladder.
- Keep the drainage bag and tubing off the ground.
- Maintain a closed system whenever possible.
- If necessary, obtain urine samples using aseptic technique via a closed system.
- Keep the catheter free from obstruction to maintain free flow to the urine.
- Avoid irrigation unless needed to relieve or prevent obstruction (Herter & Wallace Kazer, 2010).
- Ensure that the patient maintains adequate fluid intake.
- Empty the drainage bag when one-half to two-thirds full or every 3 to 6 hours. (When emptying the drainage bag, do not touch drainage bag spout to the collection device.)
- Clean drainage bags daily using a commercial cleaning product or vinegar solution (1 part vinegar to 3 parts water).
- Provide daily routine personal hygiene as outlined in Chapter 7, Hygiene. Do not use powders and lotions after cleaning. Do not use antibiotic or other antimicrobial cleaners or betadine at the urethral meatus (Herter & Wallace Kazer, 2010; Society of Urologic Nurses and Associates [SUNA], 2010).

DELEGATION CONSIDERATIONS

The catheterization of the female urinary bladder is not delegated to nursing assistive personnel (NAP) or to unlicensed assistive personnel (UAP). Depending on the state's nurse practice act and the organization's policies and procedures, catheterization of the female urinary bladder may be delegated to licensed practical/vocational nurses (LPN/LVNs).The decision to delegate must be based on careful analysis of the patient's needs and circumstances, as well as the qualifications of the person to whom the task is being delegated. Refer to the Delegation Guidelines in Appendix A.

EQUIPMENT

- Sterile catheter kit that contains:
  - Sterile gloves
  - Sterile drapes (one of which is **fenestrated**)
  - Sterile catheter (Use the smallest appropriate-size catheter, usually a 14F to 16F catheter with a 5- to 10-mL balloon [Newman, 2008].)
  - Antiseptic cleansing solution and cotton balls or gauze squares; antiseptic swabs
  - Lubricant
  - Forceps
  - Prefilled syringe with sterile water (sufficient to inflate indwelling catheter balloon)
  - Sterile specimen container (if specimen is required)
- Flashlight or lamp
- Waterproof, disposable pad
- Sterile, disposable urine collection bag and drainage tubing (may be connected to catheter in catheter kit)
- Velcro leg strap, catheter securing device, or tape
- Disposable gloves
- Additional PPE, as indicated
- Washcloth, skin cleanser, and warm water to perform perineal hygiene before and after catheterization

ASSESSMENT

Assess the patient's normal elimination habits. Assess the patient's degree of limitations and ability to help with activity. Assess for activity limitations, such as hip surgery or spinal injury, which would contraindicate certain actions by the patient. Assess for the presence of any other conditions that may interfere with passage of the catheter or contraindicate insertion of the catheter, such as urethral strictures or bladder cancer. Check for the presence of drains, dressings, intravenous fluid infusion sites/equipment, traction, or any other devices that could interfere with the patient's ability to help with the procedure or that could become dislodged. Assess bladder fullness before performing the procedure, either by palpation or with a handheld bladder ultrasound device. Question patient about any allergies, especially to latex or iodine. Ask the patient if she has ever been catheterized. If she had an indwelling catheter previously, ask why and for how long it was used. The patient may have urethral strictures, which may make catheter insertion more difficult. Assess the characteristics of the urine and the patient's skin.

NURSING DIAGNOSIS

Determine the related factors for the nursing diagnoses based on the patient's current status. Appropriate nursing diagnoses may include:

- Impaired Urinary Elimination
- Urinary Retention
- Risk for Infection

OUTCOME IDENTIFICATION AND PLANNING

The expected outcome to achieve when inserting a female urinary catheter is that the patient's urinary elimination will be maintained, with a urine output of at least 30 mL/hour, and the patient's bladder will not be distended. Other appropriate outcomes may include the following: the patient's skin remains clean, dry, and intact, without evidence of irritation or breakdown; and the patient verbalizes an understanding of the purpose for, and care of, the catheter, as appropriate.

IMPLEMENTATION

ACTION	RATIONALE
1. Review the patient's chart for any limitations in physical activity. Confirm the medical order for indwelling catheter insertion.	Physical limitations may require adaptations in performing the skill. Verifying the medical order ensures that the correct intervention is administered to the right patient.
2. Gather equipment. Obtain assistance from another staff member, if necessary.	Assembling equipment provides for an organized approach to the task. Assistance from another person may be required to perform the intervention safely.

(continued)

SKILL 12-6 CATHETERIZING THE FEMALE URINARY BLADDER continued

ACTION	RATIONALE
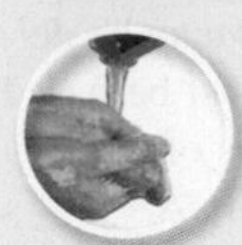 3. Perform hand hygiene and put on PPE, if indicated.	Hand hygiene and PPE prevent the spread of microorganisms. PPE is required based on transmission precautions.
 4. Identify the patient.	Identifying the patient ensures the right patient receives the intervention and helps prevent errors.
5. Close the curtains around the bed and close the door to the room, if possible. Discuss the procedure with the patient and assess the patient's ability to assist with the procedure. Ask the patient if she has any allergies, especially to latex or iodine.	This ensures the patient's privacy. Discussion promotes reassurance and provides knowledge about the procedure. Dialogue encourages patient participation and allows for individualized nursing care. Some catheters and gloves in kits are made of latex. Some antiseptic solutions contain iodine.
6. Provide good lighting. Artificial light is recommended (use of a flashlight requires an assistant to hold and position it). Place a trash receptacle within easy reach.	Good lighting is necessary to see the meatus clearly. A readily available trash receptacle allows for prompt disposal of used supplies and reduces the risk of contaminating the sterile field.
7. Assemble equipment on overbed table within reach.	Arranging items nearby is convenient, saves time, and avoids unnecessary stretching and twisting of muscles on the part of the nurse.
8. Adjust the bed to a comfortable working height, usually elbow height of the caregiver (VISN 8 Patient Safety Center, 2009). Stand on the patient's right side if you are right-handed, patient's left side if you are left-handed.	Having the bed at the proper height prevents back and muscle strain. Positioning allows for ease of use of dominant hand for catheter insertion.
9. Assist the patient to a dorsal recumbent position with knees flexed, feet about 2 feet apart, with her legs abducted. Drape patient (Figure 2). Alternately, the Sims', or lateral, position can be used. Place the patient's buttocks near the edge of the bed with her shoulders at the opposite edge and her knees drawn toward her chest (Figure 3). Allow the patient to lie on either side, depending on which position is easiest for the nurse and best for the patient's comfort. Slide waterproof pad under patient.	Proper positioning allows adequate visualization of the urinary meatus. Embarrassment, chilliness, and tension can interfere with catheter insertion; draping the patient will promote comfort and relaxation. The Sims' position may allow better visualization and be more comfortable for the patient, especially if hip and knee movements are difficult. The smaller area of exposure is also less stressful for the patient. The waterproof pad will protect bed linens from moisture.

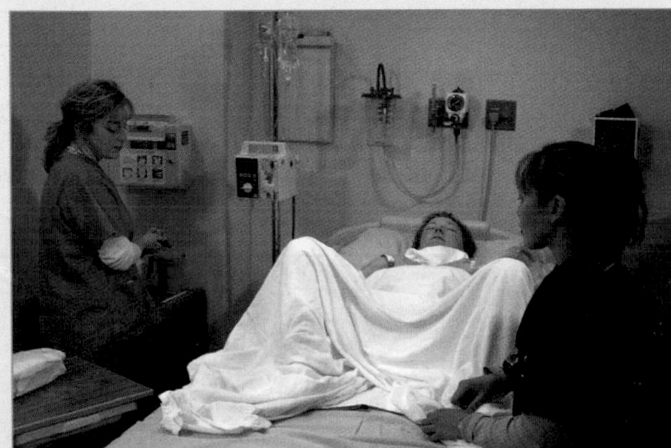

FIGURE 2 Patient in dorsal recumbent position and draped properly.

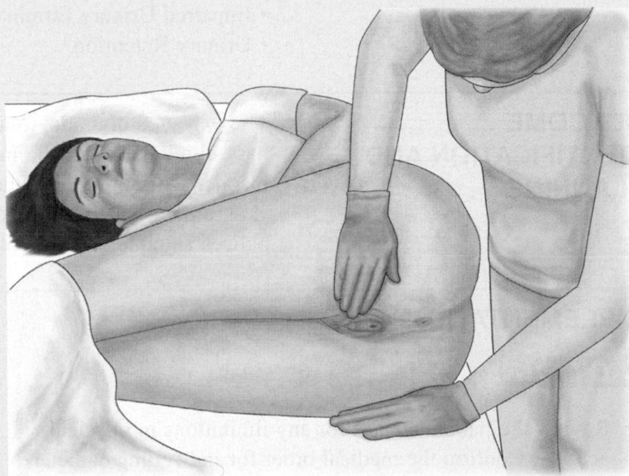

FIGURE 3 Demonstration of side-lying position.

ACTION	RATIONALE
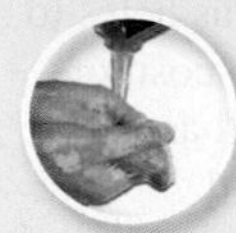 10. Put on clean gloves. Clean the perineal area with washcloth, skin cleanser, and warm water, using a different corner of the washcloth with each stroke. Wipe from above orifice downward toward sacrum (front to back). Rinse and dry. Remove gloves. Perform hand hygiene again.	Gloves reduce the risk of exposure to blood and body fluids. Cleaning reduces microorganisms near the urethral meatus and provides an opportunity to visualize the perineum and landmarks before the procedure. Hand hygiene reduces the spread of microorganisms.
11. Prepare urine drainage setup if a separate urine collection system is to be used. Secure to bed frame, according to manufacturer's directions.	This facilitates connection of the catheter to the drainage system and provides for easy access.
12. Open sterile catheterization tray on a clean overbed table using sterile technique.	Placement of equipment near the worksite increases efficiency. Sterile technique protects the patient and prevents transmission of microorganisms.
13. Put on sterile gloves. Grasp upper corners of drape and unfold drape without touching nonsterile areas. Fold back a corner on each side to make a cuff over gloved hands. Ask the patient to lift her buttocks and slide sterile drape under her with gloves protected by cuff.	The drape provides a sterile field close to the meatus. Covering the gloved hands will help keep the gloves sterile while placing the drape.
14. Based on facility policy, position the fenestrated sterile drape. Place a fenestrated sterile drape over the perineal area, exposing the labia (Figure 4). (*Note:* The fenestrated drape is not shown in the remaining illustrations in order to provide a clear view of the procedure.)	The drape expands the sterile field and protects against contamination. Use of a fenestrated drape may limit visualization and is considered optional by some practitioners and/or facility policies.

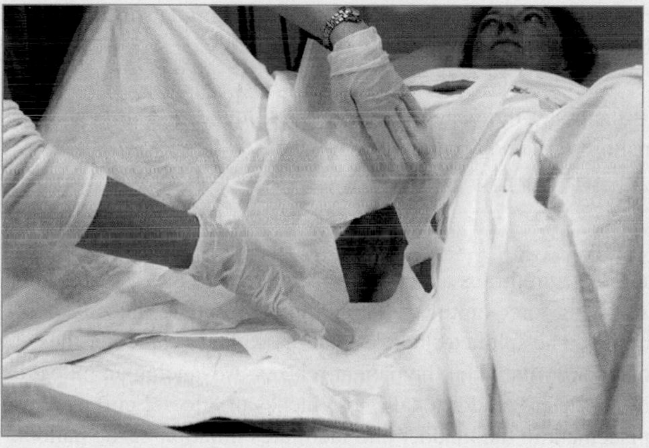

FIGURE 4 Patient with fenestrated drape in place over perineum.

ACTION	RATIONALE
15. Place sterile tray on drape between the patient's thighs.	Provides easy access to supplies.
16. Open all the supplies. Open package of antiseptic swabs. Alternately, fluff cotton balls in tray before pouring antiseptic solution over them. Open specimen container if specimen is to be obtained.	It is necessary to open all supplies and prepare for the procedure while both hands are sterile.
17. Lubricate 1 to 2 inches of catheter tip.	Lubrication facilitates catheter insertion and reduces tissue trauma.

(continued)

SKILL 12-6 CATHETERIZING THE FEMALE URINARY BLADDER continued

ACTION	RATIONALE
18. With thumb and one finger of nondominant hand, spread labia and identify meatus. **Be prepared to maintain separation of labia with one hand until catheter is inserted and urine is flowing well and continuously (Figure 5).** If the patient is in the side-lying position, lift the upper buttock and labia to expose the urinary meatus (Figure 6).	Smoothing the area immediately surrounding the meatus helps to make it visible. Allowing the labia to drop back into position may contaminate the area around the meatus, as well as the catheter. The nondominant hand is now contaminated.

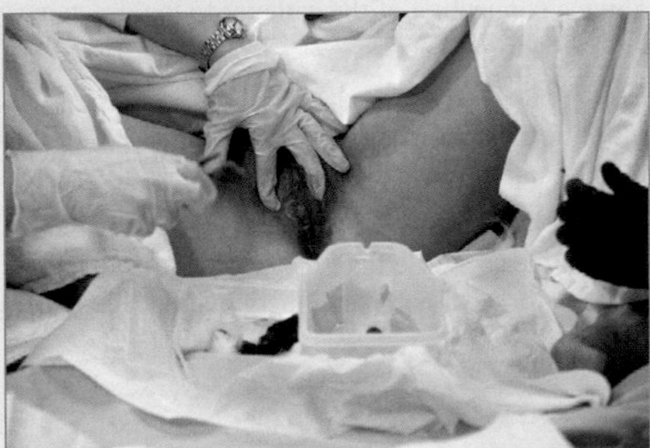

FIGURE 5 Using dominant hand to separate and hold labia open.

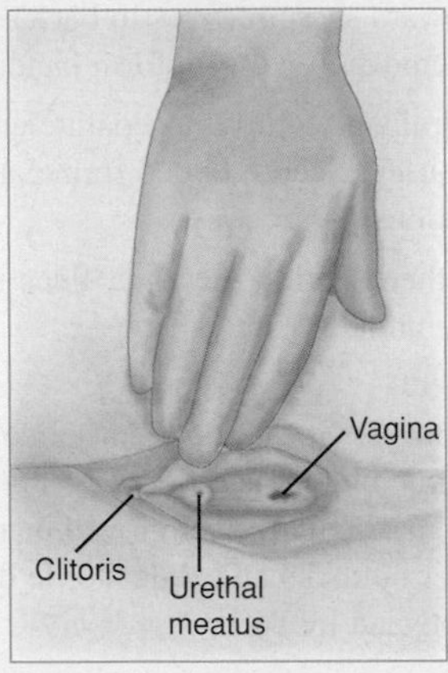

FIGURE 6 Exposing urinary meatus with patient in side-lying position.

ACTION	RATIONALE
19. Use the dominant hand to pick up an antiseptic swab or use forceps to pick up a cotton ball. **Clean one labial fold, top to bottom (from above the meatus down toward the rectum), then discard the cotton ball. Using a new cotton ball/swab for each stroke, continue to clean the other labial fold, then directly over the meatus (Figure 7).**	Moving from an area where there is likely to be less contamination to an area where there is more contamination helps prevent the spread of microorganisms. Cleaning the meatus last helps reduce the possibility of introducing microorganisms into the bladder.
20. With your noncontaminated, dominant hand, place the drainage end of the catheter in receptacle. If the catheter is pre-attached to sterile tubing and drainage container (closed drainage system), position catheter and setup within easy reach on sterile field. Ensure that the clamp on the drainage bag is closed.	This facilitates drainage of urine and minimizes risk of contaminating sterile equipment.
21. **Using your dominant hand, hold the catheter 2 to 3 inches from the tip and insert slowly into the urethra (Figure 8). Advance the catheter until there is a return of urine (approximately 2 to 3 inches [4.8 to 7.2 cm]). Once urine drains, advance catheter another 2 to 3 inches (4.8 to 7.2 cm). Do not force catheter through urethra into bladder.** Ask patient to breathe deeply, and rotate catheter gently if slight resistance is met as catheter reaches external sphincter.	The female urethra is about 1.5 to 2.5 inches (3.6 to 6.0 cm) long. Applying force on the catheter is likely to injure mucous membranes. The sphincter relaxes and the catheter can enter the bladder easily when the patient relaxes. Advancing an indwelling catheter an additional 2 to 3 inches (4.8 to 7.2 cm) ensures placement in the bladder and facilitates inflation of the balloon without damaging the urethra.

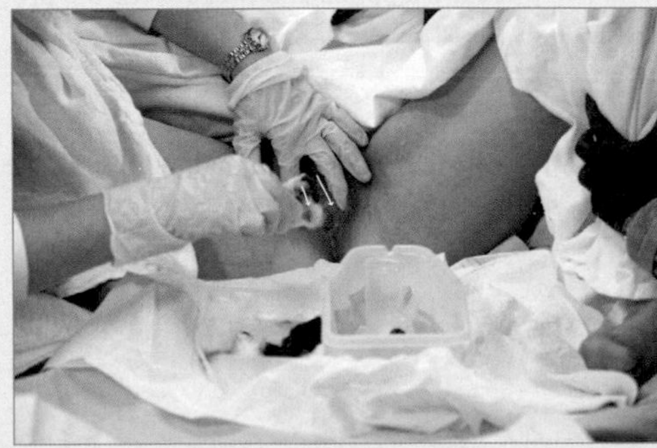

FIGURE 7 Wiping perineum with cotton ball held by forceps. Wipe in one direction—from top to bottom.

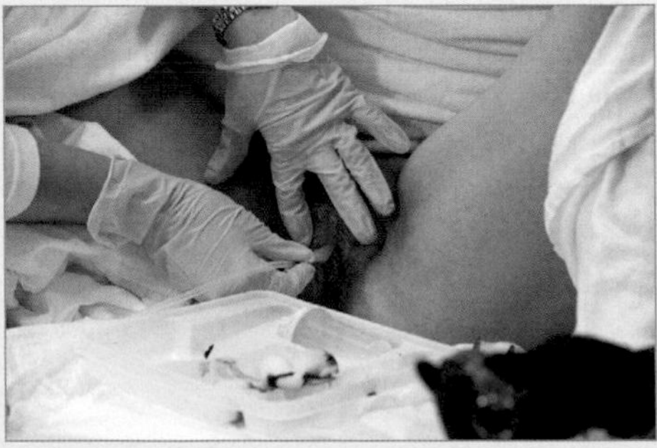

FIGURE 8 Inserting catheter with dominant hand while nondominant hand holds labia apart.

ACTION	RATIONALE
22. Hold the catheter securely at the meatus with your nondominant hand. Use your dominant hand to inflate the catheter balloon (Figure 9). Inject entire volume of sterile water supplied in prefilled syringe.	Bladder or sphincter contraction could push the catheter out. The balloon anchors the catheter in place in the bladder. Manufacturer provides appropriate amount of sterile water for the size of catheter in the kit; as a result, use entire syringe provided in the kit.
23. Pull gently on catheter after balloon is inflated to feel resistance.	Improper inflation can cause patient discomfort and malpositioning of catheter.
24. Attach catheter to drainage system if not already pre-attached (Figure 10).	Closed drainage system minimizes the risk for microorganisms being introduced into the bladder.
25. Remove equipment and dispose of it according to facility policy. Discard syringe in sharps container. Wash and dry the perineal area, as needed.	Proper disposal prevents the spread of microorganisms. Placing syringe in sharps container prevents reuse. Cleaning promotes comfort and appropriate personal hygiene.
26. Remove gloves. **Secure catheter tubing to the patient's inner thigh with Velcro leg strap, catheter securing device, or tape (Figure 11).** Leave some slack in catheter for leg movement.	Proper attachment prevents trauma to the urethra and meatus from tension on the tubing. Whether to tape the drainage tubing over or under the leg depends on gravity flow, patient's mobility, and patient's comfort.

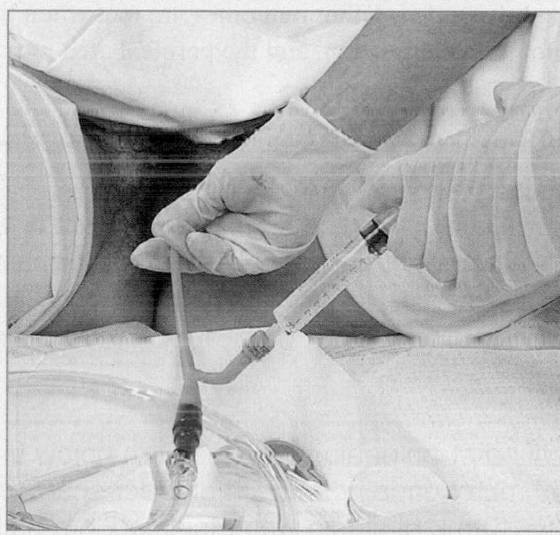

FIGURE 9 Inflating balloon of indwelling catheter.

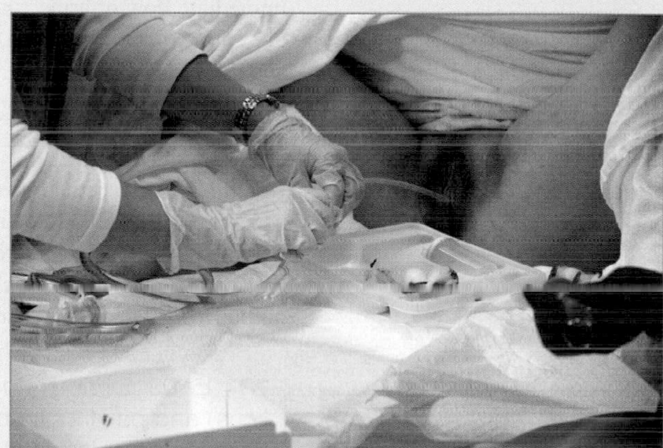

FIGURE 10 Attaching catheter to drainage bag.

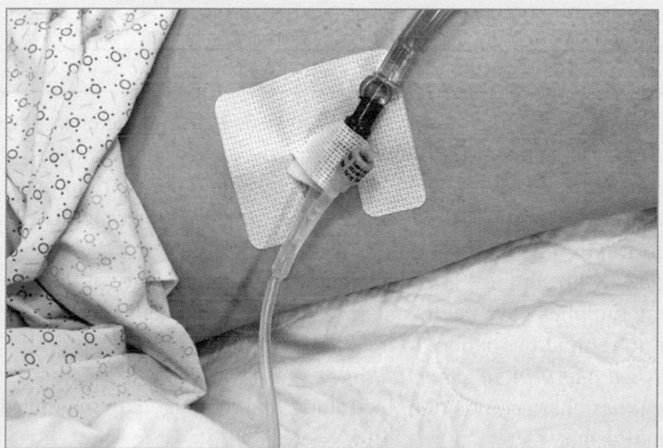

FIGURE 11 Catheter secured to leg.

(*continued*)

SKILL 12-6 CATHETERIZING THE FEMALE URINARY BLADDER continued

ACTION	RATIONALE
27. Assist the patient to a comfortable position. Cover the patient with bed linens. Place the bed in the lowest position.	Positioning and covering provides warmth and promotes comfort.
28. Secure drainage bag below the level of the bladder. Check that drainage tubing is not kinked and that movement of side rails does not interfere with catheter or drainage bag.	This facilitates drainage of urine and prevents the backflow of urine.
29. Put on clean gloves. Obtain urine specimen immediately, if needed, from drainage bag. Label specimen. Send urine specimen to the laboratory promptly or refrigerate it.	Catheter system is sterile. Obtaining a specimen immediately allows access to sterile system. Keeping urine at room temperature may cause microorganisms, if present, to grow and distort laboratory findings.
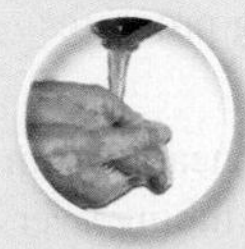 30. Remove gloves and additional PPE, if used. Perform hand hygiene.	Removing PPE properly reduces the risk for infection transmission and contamination of other items. Hand hygiene prevents the spread of microorganisms.

EVALUATION

The expected outcome is met when the catheter is inserted using sterile technique, results in the immediate flow of urine, and the bladder is not distended. Other outcomes are met when the patient does not experience trauma, reports little to no pain on insertion, and the perineal area remains clean and dry.

DOCUMENTATION

Guidelines

Document the type and size of catheter and balloon inserted, as well as the amount of fluid used to inflate the balloon. Document the patient's tolerance of the activity. Record the amount of urine obtained through the catheter and any specimen obtained. Document any other assessments, such as unusual urine characteristics or alterations in the patient's skin. Record urine amount on intake and output record, if appropriate.

Sample Documentation

Lippincott DocuCare Practice documenting catheterization of the female urinary bladder in *Lippincott DocuCare.*

7/14/15 0915 Primary care provider notified of palpable bladder (3 cm below umbilicus) and patient's inability to void; 750 mL of urine noted with bladder scan. A 16F Foley catheter inserted without difficulty; 10 mL of sterile water injected into balloon port; 700 mL clear yellow urine returned. Patient states, "Oh, I feel much better now." Bladder is no longer palpable. Patient tolerated procedure without adverse event.

—*B. Clapp, RN*

UNEXPECTED SITUATIONS AND ASSOCIATED INTERVENTIONS

- *No urine flow is obtained, and you note that catheter is in vaginal orifice:* Leave catheter in place as a marker. Obtain new sterile gloves and catheter kit. Start the procedure over and attempt to place new catheter directly above misplaced catheter. Once the new catheter is correctly in place, remove the catheter in the vaginal orifice. Because of the risk of cross-infection, never remove a catheter from the vagina and insert it into the urethra.
- *Patient moves legs during procedure:* If no supplies have been contaminated, ask patient to hold still and continue with procedure. If supplies have been contaminated, stop procedure and start over. If necessary, get an assistant to remind the patient to hold still.
- *Urine flow is initially well established and urine is clear, but after several hours flow dwindles:* Check tubing for kinking. If patient has changed position, the tubing and drainage bag may need to be moved to facilitate drainage of urine.
- *Patient complains of extreme pain when you are inflating the balloon:* Stop inflation of balloon. Balloon is most likely still in urethra. Withdraw the solution from the balloon. Insert catheter an additional 0.5 to 1 inch (1.2 to 2.4 cm) and slowly attempt to inflate balloon again.

- *Urine leaks out of meatus around the catheter:* Do not increase the size of the indwelling catheter. Make sure the smallest sized catheter with a 10-mL balloon is used. Large catheters cause bladder and urethral irritation and trauma. Large balloon-fill volumes occupy more space inside the bladder and put added weight on the base of the bladder. Irritation of the bladder wall and detrusor muscle can cause leakage. If leakage persists, consider an evaluation for urinary tract infection. Ensure that the correct amount of solution was used to inflate the balloon. Underfilling the balloon can cause the catheter to dislodge into the urethra, causing urethral spasm, pain, and discomfort. If you suspect underfill, do not attempt to push the catheter farther into the bladder. Remove the catheter and replace. Assess the patient for constipation. Bowel full of stool can cause pressure on the catheter lumen and prevent the drainage of urine. Implement interventions to prevent/treat constipation.

SPECIAL CONSIDERATIONS

General Considerations

- Be familiar with facility policy and/or primary practitioner guidelines for the maximum amount of urine to remove from the bladder at the time of insertion.
- If the patient is unable to lift buttocks or maintain required position for the procedure, the assistance of another staff member may be necessary to place the drape under the patient and to help the patient maintain the required position.
- Supplies can be opened and prepared on the overbed table, moving the tray onto the bed just before cleansing the patient.
- If there is not an immediate flow of urine after the catheter has been inserted, several measures may prove helpful:
  - Have the patient take a deep breath, which helps to relax the perineal and abdominal muscles.
  - Rotate the catheter slightly, because a drainage hole may be resting against the bladder wall.
  - Raise the head of the patient's bed to increase pressure in the bladder area.
  - Assess the patient's intake to ensure adequate fluid intake for urine production.
  - Assess the catheter and drainage tubing for kinks and occlusion.
- If the catheter cannot be advanced, have the patient take several deep breaths. Rotate the catheter half a turn and try to advance it. If you are still unable to advance, remove the catheter. Notify the primary care provider.
- Some catheter kits do not contain the catheter. This allows you to select a catheter and balloon size separately.

Infant and Child Considerations

- Size 5F to 8F is used for infants and young children. Size 8F to 12F catheters are commonly used for older children (Perry et al., 2010).
- Distraction, such as blowing bubbles, deep breathing, or singing a song, can help the child relax.
- Lidocaine jelly is often used to anesthetize and lubricate the area before insertion of the catheter, decreasing the child's discomfort and anxiety.

Home Care Considerations

- Intermittent catheterization, performed by the patient or a caregiver in the home, may be necessary for patients with spinal cord injuries or other neurologic conditions. Although the risk for UTI is always present, most research supports the use of clean, rather than sterile, technique in this environment. The procedure for self-catheterization is essentially the same as that used by the nurse to catheterize a patient. Self-catheterization is recommended at regular intervals to prevent over distention of the bladder and decreased blood flow through the wall of the bladder (Hinkle & Cheever, 2014; SUNA, 2010). Box 12-2 outlines important information related to patient intermittent self-catheterization.

(continued)

SKILL 12-6 CATHETERIZING THE FEMALE URINARY BLADDER continued

BOX 12-2 PATIENT INTERMITTENT SELF-CATHETERIZATION

- Explain the reason for self-catheterization and corresponding health issues related to the need for catheterization.
- Explain the consequences of not doing intermittent self-catheterization, such as upper urinary tract problems, urinary tract infections, and incontinence.
- Explain potential complications, such as bleeding and the risk of urinary tract infections, and what to do if they occur.
- Ensure privacy and dignity.
- Include discussion regarding the frequency of intermittent catheterization and how to incorporate it into usual daily routine.
- Explain the anatomy of the urinary tract, hygiene, and preparation of the catheter.
- Demonstrate how to open, hold, and use the catheter.
- Explain catheterization process; demonstrate process; observe return demonstration by patient.
- Explore process to obtain supplies, cleaning of reusable catheters, and storage.
- Provide information in an appropriate format (such as written materials or video, in appropriate language) to reinforce instruction.
- Allow the patient adequate time to ask questions.
- Provide information about how to recognize a urinary tract infection and other signs/symptoms to report to the primary health care provider.
- Explain that aids are available to help meet the challenges of intermittent self-catheterization for patients with poor eyesight, reduced mobility, and/or reduced manual dexterity.

Adapted from Logan, K. (2012). An overview of male intermittent self-catheterisation. *British Journal of Nursing, 21(*18), S18–S22; Mangnall, J. (2012). Key considerations of intermittent catheterisation. *British Journal of Nursing, 21*(7), 392, 394, 396–398; Newman, D.K., & Willson, M.M. (2011). Review of intermittent catheterization and current best practices. *Urologic Nursing, 31*(1), 12–28; Rantell, A. (2012). Intermittent self-catheterisation in women. *Nursing Standard, 26*(42), 61–68; and Stewart, E. (2011). Intermittent self-catheterization and infection reduction. *British Journal of Neuroscience Nursing, 7*(5), S4–S7.

SKILL VARIATION Intermittent Female Urethral Catheterization

1. Check the medical record for the order for intermittent urethral catheterization. Review the patient's chart for any limitations in physical activity. Gather equipment. Obtain assistance from another staff member, if necessary.
2. Perform hand hygiene. Put on PPE, as indicated, based on transmission precautions.

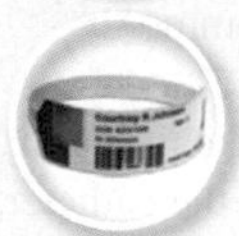

3. Identify the patient. Discuss the procedure with the patient and assess the patient's ability to assist with the procedure. Ask the patient if she has any allergies, especially to latex or iodine.
4. Close the curtains around the bed and close the door to the room, if possible.
5. Provide good lighting. Artificial light is recommended (use of a flashlight requires an assistant to hold and position it). Place a trash receptacle within easy reach.
6. Assemble equipment on overbed table within reach.
7. Raise the bed to a comfortable working height. Stand on the patient's right side if you are right-handed, patient's left side if you are left-handed.
8. Put on disposable gloves. Assist the patient to dorsal recumbent position with knees flexed, feet about 2 feet apart, with her legs abducted. Drape patient. Alternately, use the Sims', or lateral, position. Place the patient's buttocks near the edge of the bed with her shoulders at the opposite edge and her knees drawn toward her chest. Slide waterproof drape under patient.

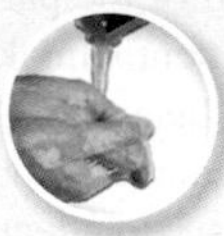

9. Put on clean gloves. Clean the perineal area with washcloth, skin cleanser, and warm water, using a different corner of the washcloth with each stroke. Wipe from above the orifice downward toward the sacrum (front to back). Rinse and dry. Remove gloves. Perform hand hygiene again.
10. Open sterile catheterization tray on a clean overbed table using sterile technique.
11. Put on sterile gloves. Grasp upper corners of drape and unfold drape without touching nonsterile areas. Fold back a corner on each side to make a cuff over gloved hands. Ask patient to lift her buttocks and slide sterile drape under her with gloves protected by cuff.
12. Place a fenestrated sterile drape over the perineal area, exposing the labia, if appropriate.
13. Place sterile tray on drape between patient's thighs.
14. Open all the supplies. Open package of antiseptic swabs. Alternately, fluff cotton balls in tray before pouring antiseptic solution over them. Open specimen container if specimen is to be obtained.
15. Lubricate 1 to 2 inches of catheter tip.
16. With thumb and one finger of nondominant hand, spread labia and identify meatus. If the patient is in the side-lying position, lift the upper buttock and labia to expose the urinary meatus. **Be prepared to maintain separation of labia with one hand until catheter is inserted and urine is flowing well and continuously.**

SKILL VARIATION Intermittent Female Urethral Catheterization continued

17. Use the dominant hand to pick up a cotton ball. **Clean one labial fold, top to bottom (from above the meatus down toward the rectum), then discard the cotton ball. Using a new cotton ball for each stroke, continue to clean the other labial fold, then directly over the meatus.**
18. With the noncontaminated, dominant hand, place drainage end of catheter in receptacle. If a specimen is required, place the end into the specimen container in the receptacle.
19. **Using the dominant hand, hold the catheter 2 to 3 inches from the tip and insert slowly into the urethra. Advance the catheter until there is a return of urine (approximately 2 to 3 inches [4.8 to 7.2 cm]). Do not force the catheter through the urethra into the bladder.** Ask the patient to breathe deeply, and rotate the catheter gently if slight resistance is met as the catheter reaches the external sphincter.
20. Hold the catheter securely at the meatus with the nondominant hand while the bladder empties. If a specimen is being collected, remove the drainage end of the tubing from the specimen container after required amount is obtained and allow urine to flow into the receptacle. Set specimen container aside and place lid on container.
21. Allow the bladder to empty. Withdraw catheter slowly and smoothly after urine has stopped flowing. Remove equipment and dispose of it according to facility policy. Discard syringe in sharps container to prevent reuse. Wash and dry the perineal area, as needed.
22. Remove gloves. Assist the patient to a comfortable position. Cover the patient with bed linens. Place the bed in the lowest position.
23. Put on clean gloves. Secure the container lid and label specimen. Send urine specimen to the laboratory promptly or refrigerate it.

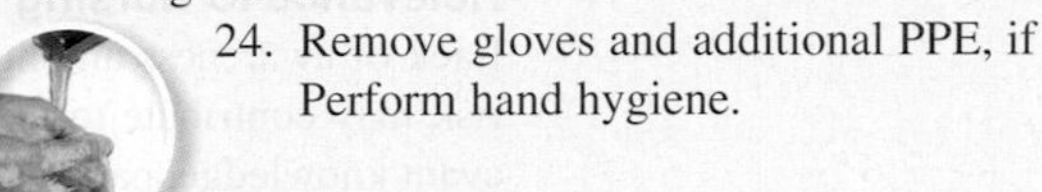

24. Remove gloves and additional PPE, if used. Perform hand hygiene.

Note: Intermittent catheterization in the home is performed using clean technique. The bladder's natural resistance to the microorganisms normally found in the home makes sterile technique unnecessary. Catheters are washed, dried, and stored for repeated use. Clean technique involves the use of cleansed reusable catheters, washing hands with soap and water, and daily cleansing of the perineum or more often only when fecal or other wastes are present (Newman, 2008, as cited in Herter & Wallace, 2010). Cleansing the perineal area to decrease bacteria in the surrounding area is highly recommended (Herter & Wallace, 2010).

EVIDENCE FOR PRACTICE ▶

PREVENTION AND CONTROL OF CATHETER-ASSOCIATED URINARY TRACT INFECTION

Society of Urologic Nurses and Associates (SUNA). (2010). *Prevention & control of catheter-associated urinary tract infection (CAUTI). Clinical practice guideline.* Available https://www.suna.org/sites/default/files/download/cautiGuideline.pdf.

These guidelines provide evidence-based recommendations to guide care for patients requiring catheterization of the urinary bladder to prevent CAUTI.

Refer to thePoint for additional research on related nursing topics.

EVIDENCE FOR PRACTICE ▶

POSTOPERATIVE URINARY CATHETERS

Preventing CAUTI is a health care priority. Routine placement of a urinary catheter for longer than 2 days postoperative had been found to increase the risk of infection. What factors may be contributing to increased duration of use?

Related Research

Bhardwaj, R., Pickard, R., Carrick-Sen, D., & Britain, K. (2012). Patients' perspectives on timing of urinary catheter removal after surgery. *British Journal of Nursing, 21*(18), S4, S6–S9.

The aims of this study were to explore patients' perceptions of the care process relating to perioperative catheterization and to identify patient factors that encourage early removal, reducing the number of postoperative CAUTIs. In this qualitative study, patients were asked about

(continued)

SKILL 12-6 CATHETERIZING THE FEMALE URINARY BLADDER continued

attitudes toward, and beliefs surrounding, perioperative catheterization and timing of catheter removal in terms of their past and current experience and future perception. Interviews were audio recorded and transcribed for analysis. Catheter duration ranged from 1 to 10 days. Major themes elicited included the following: lack of understanding of the purpose and catheterization process; loss of patient autonomy and dignity; and impact of environmental factors. The authors concluded that a lack of knowledge of the catheterization process among participants led to fears and concerns that may have contributed to delayed catheter removal. The authors suggest changes to patient care to reduce catheter duration, including ensuring the provision of preoperative information, greater patient involvement in catheter removal decisions, and provision of easily accessible toilet facilities.

Relevance to Nursing Practice

Lack of awareness among patients concerning the link between catheter duration and CAUTI risk may contribute to increased duration of postoperative catheter use. Once armed with relevant knowledge, patients could be more involved in decisions related to catheter use and could be motivated to contribute to planning the removal of their catheter. Nurses have a responsibility to provide accurate and appropriate patient education, and should consider this an important part of the plan of care whenever possible, resulting in improved patient care and decreased CAUTIs.

See additional Evidence for Practice related to urinary catheters at the end of Skill 12-5 and Skill 12-7, and refer to thePoint for additional research on related nursing topics.

SKILL 12-7 CATHETERIZING THE MALE URINARY BLADDER

Urinary catheterization is the introduction of a catheter (tube) through the urethra into the bladder for the purpose of withdrawing urine. Catheter-associated urinary tract infections are the most common hospital-acquired infection in the United States and is one reason catheterization should be avoided whenever possible. When it is deemed necessary, it should be performed using strict aseptic technique and left in place for the shortest length of time possible (Hooton et al., 2010). The duration of catheterization is the most important risk factor for the development of a UTI (Bernard et al., 2012).

Intermittent urethral catheters, or straight catheters, are used to drain the bladder for shorter periods. If a catheter is to remain in place for continuous drainage, an indwelling urethral catheter is used. Indwelling catheters are also called *retention* or *Foley* catheters. The indwelling urethral catheter is designed so that it does not slip out of the bladder. A balloon is inflated to ensure that the catheter remains in the bladder once it is inserted (Figure 1; Skill 12-6).

Intermittent catheterization should be considered as an alternative to short-term or long-term indwelling urethral catheterization to reduce catheter-associated urinary tract infections (Hooton et al., 2012). Intermittent catheterization is becoming the gold standard for the management of bladder-emptying dysfunctions and following surgical interventions. Certain advantages to intermittent catheterization, including the lower risks of CAUTI and complications, may make it a more desirable and safer option than indwelling catheterization (Herter & Wallace Kazer, 2010, p. 343–344).

The following procedure reviews insertion of an indwelling catheter into the male urinary bladder. The procedure for an intermittent catheter of a male bladder follows as a Skill Variation. Guidelines for caring for a patient with an indwelling catheter are summarized in Box 12-1, located within Skill 12-6.

DELEGATION CONSIDERATIONS

The catheterization of the male urinary bladder is not delegated to nursing assistive personnel (NAP) or to unlicensed assistive personnel (UAP). Depending on the state's nurse practice act and the organization's policies and procedures, catheterization of the male urinary bladder may be delegated to licensed practical/vocational nurses (LPN/LVNs). The decision to delegate must be based on careful analysis of the patient's needs and circumstances, as well as the qualifications of the person to whom the task is being delegated. Refer to the Delegation Guidelines in Appendix A.

EQUIPMENT

- Sterile catheter kit that contains:
  - Sterile gloves
  - Sterile drapes (one of which is **fenestrated**)
  - Sterile catheter (Use the smallest appropriate-size catheter, usually a 14F to 16F catheter with a 5- to 10-mL balloon [Newman, 2008].)
  - Antiseptic cleansing solution and cotton balls or gauze squares; antiseptic swabs
  - Lubricant
  - Forceps
  - Prefilled syringe with sterile water (sufficient to inflate indwelling catheter balloon)
  - Sterile basin (usually base of kit serves as this)
- Sterile specimen container (if specimen is required)
- Flashlight or lamp
- Waterproof, disposable pad
- Sterile, disposable urine collection bag and drainage tubing (may be connected to catheter in catheter kit)
- Velcro leg strap, catheter securing device, or tape
- Disposable gloves
- Additional PPE, as indicated
- Washcloth, skin cleanser, and warm water to perform perineal hygiene before and after catheterization

ASSESSMENT

Assess the patient's normal elimination habits. Assess the patient's degree of limitations and ability to help with activity. Assess for activity limitations, such as hip surgery or spinal injury, which would contraindicate certain actions by the patient. Assess for the presence of any other conditions that may interfere with passage of the catheter or contraindicate insertion of the catheter, such as urethral strictures or bladder cancer. Check for the presence of drains, dressings, intravenous fluid infusion sites/equipment, traction, or any other devices that could interfere with the patient's ability to help with the procedure or that could become dislodged. Assess bladder fullness before performing the procedure, either by palpation or with a handheld bladder ultrasound device, and question the patient about any allergies, especially to latex or iodine. Ask the patient if he has ever been catheterized. If he had an indwelling catheter previously, ask why and for how long it was used. The patient may have urethral strictures, which may make catheter insertion more difficult. If the patient is 50 years of age or older, ask if he has had any prostate problems. Prostate enlargement typically is noted around the age of 50 years. Assess the characteristics of the urine and the patient's skin.

NURSING DIAGNOSIS

Determine the related factors for the nursing diagnoses based on the patient's current status. Appropriate nursing diagnoses may include:

- Impaired Urinary Elimination
- Risk for Infection
- Urinary Retention

OUTCOME IDENTIFICATION AND PLANNING

The expected outcome to achieve when inserting a male urinary catheter is that the patient's urinary elimination will be maintained, with a urine output of at least 30 mL/hour, and the patient's bladder will not be distended. Other appropriate outcomes may include the following: the patient's skin remains clean, dry, and intact, without evidence of irritation or breakdown; and the patient verbalizes an understanding of the purpose for, and care of, the catheter, as appropriate.

(continued)

SKILL 12-7 CATHETERIZING THE MALE URINARY BLADDER continued

IMPLEMENTATION

ACTION	RATIONALE
1. Review chart for any limitations in physical activity. Confirm the medical order for indwelling catheter insertion.	Physical limitations may require adaptations in performing the skill. Verifying the medical order ensures that the correct intervention is administered to the right patient.
2. Gather equipment. Obtain assistance from another staff member, if necessary.	Assembling equipment provides for an organized approach to the task. Assistance from another person may be required to perform the intervention safely.
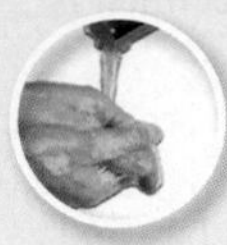 3. Perform hand hygiene and put on PPE, if indicated.	Hand hygiene and PPE prevent the spread of microorganisms. PPE is required based on transmission precautions.
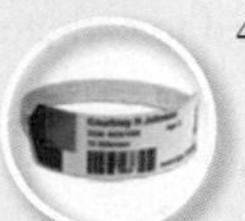 4. Identify the patient.	Identifying the patient ensures the right patient receives the intervention and helps prevent errors.
5. Close the curtains around the bed and close the door to the room, if possible. Discuss the procedure with the patient and assess the patient's ability to assist with the procedure. Ask the patient if he has any allergies, especially to latex or iodine.	This ensures the patient's privacy. Discussion promotes reassurance and provides knowledge about the procedure. Dialogue encourages patient participation and allows for individualized nursing care. Some catheters and gloves in kits are made of latex. Some antiseptic solutions contain iodine.
6. Provide good lighting. Artificial light is recommended (use of a flashlight requires an assistant to hold and position it). Place a trash receptacle within easy reach.	Good lighting is necessary to see the meatus clearly. A readily available trash receptacle allows for prompt disposal of used supplies and reduces the risk of contaminating the sterile field.
7. Assemble equipment on overbed table within reach.	Arranging items nearby is convenient, saves time, and avoids unnecessary stretching and twisting of muscles on the part of the nurse.
8. Adjust the bed to a comfortable working height, usually elbow height of the caregiver (VISN 8 Patient Safety Center, 2009). Stand on the patient's right side if you are right-handed, patient's left side if you are left-handed.	Having the bed at the proper height prevents back and muscle strain. Positioning allows for ease of use of dominant hand for catheter insertion.
9. Position the patient on his back with thighs slightly apart. Drape the patient so that only the area around the penis is exposed. Slide waterproof pad under the patient.	This prevents unnecessary exposure and promotes warmth. The waterproof pad will protect bed linens from moisture.
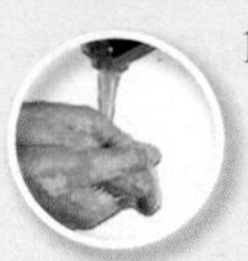 10. Put on clean gloves. Clean the genital area with washcloth, skin cleanser, and warm water. Clean the tip of the penis first, moving the washcloth in a circular motion from the meatus outward. Wash the shaft of the penis using downward strokes toward the pubic area. Rinse and dry. Remove gloves. Perform hand hygiene again.	Gloves reduce the risk of exposure to blood and body fluids. Cleaning the penis reduces microorganisms near the urethral meatus. Hand hygiene reduces the spread of microorganisms.
11. Prepare urine drainage setup if a separate urine collection system is to be used. Secure to bed frame according to manufacturer's directions.	This facilitates connection of the catheter to the drainage system and provides for easy access.
12. Open sterile catheterization tray on a clean overbed table, using sterile technique.	Placement of equipment near worksite increases efficiency. Sterile technique protects patient and prevents spread of microorganisms.

ACTION	RATIONALE
13. Put on sterile gloves. Open sterile drape and place on patient's thighs. Place fenestrated drape with opening over penis (Figure 1).	This maintains a sterile working area.

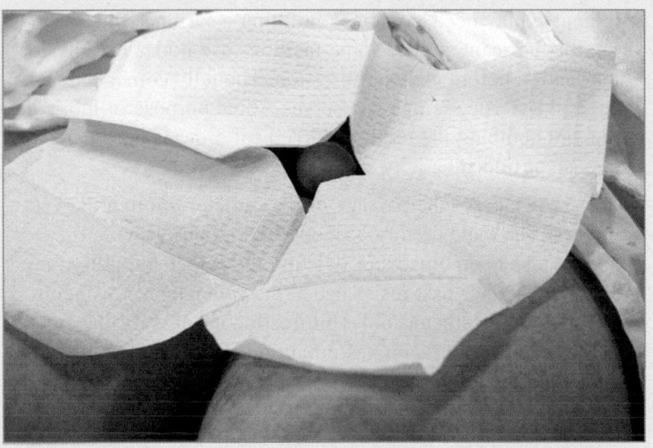

FIGURE 1 Patient lying supine with fenestrated drape over penis.

ACTION	RATIONALE
14. Place catheter setup on or next to patient's legs on sterile drape.	Sterile setup should be arranged so that the nurse's back is not turned to it, nor should it be out of the nurse's range of vision.
15. Open all the supplies. Open package of antiseptic swabs. Alternately, fluff cotton balls in tray before pouring antiseptic solution over them. Open specimen container if specimen is to be obtained. Remove cap from syringe prefilled with lubricant.	It is necessary to open all supplies and prepare for the procedure while both hands are sterile.
16. Place drainage end of catheter in receptacle. If the catheter is pre-attached to sterile tubing and drainage container (closed drainage system), position catheter and setup within easy reach on sterile field. Ensure that clamp on drainage bag is closed.	This facilitates drainage of urine and minimizes risk of contaminating sterile equipment.
17. Lift penis with nondominant hand. Retract foreskin in uncircumcised patient. **Be prepared to keep this hand in this position until the catheter is inserted and urine is flowing well and continuously. Use the dominant hand to pick up an antiseptic swab or use forceps to pick up a cotton ball. Using a circular motion, clean the penis, moving from the meatus down the glans of the penis (Figure 2). Repeat this cleansing motion two more times, using a new cotton ball/swab each time. Discard each cotton ball/swab after one use.**	The hand touching the penis becomes contaminated. Cleansing the area around the meatus and under the foreskin in the uncircumcised patient helps prevent infection. Moving from the meatus toward the base of the penis prevents bringing microorganisms to the meatus.

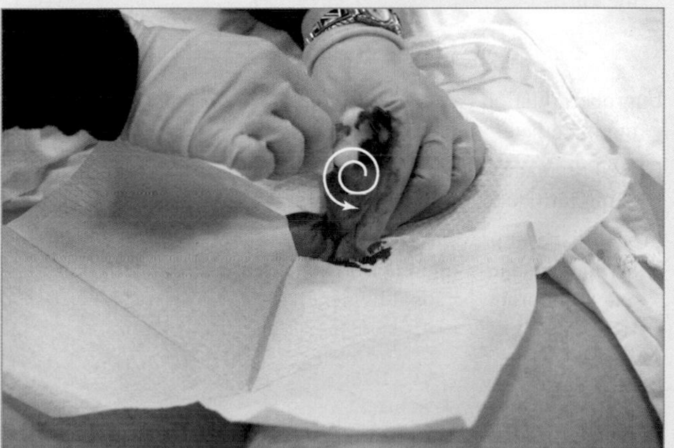

FIGURE 2 Lifting penis with gloved nondominant hand and cleaning meatus with cotton ball held with forceps in gloved dominant hand.

(continued)

SKILL 12-7 CATHETERIZING THE MALE URINARY BLADDER continued

ACTION	RATIONALE
18. Hold penis with slight upward tension and perpendicular to patient's body. Use the dominant hand to pick up the lubricant syringe. **Gently insert tip of syringe with lubricant into urethra and instill the 10 mL of lubricant** (Figure 3).	The lubricant causes the urethra to distend slightly and facilitates passage of the catheter without traumatizing the lining of the urethra (Society of Urologic Nurses and Associates, 2005c). If the prepackaged kit does not contain a syringe with lubricant, the nurse may need assistance in filling a syringe while keeping the lubricant sterile. Some facilities use lidocaine jelly for lubrication before catheter insertion. The jelly comes prepackaged in a sterile syringe and serves a dual purpose of lubricating and numbing the urethra. A medical order is necessary for the use of lidocaine jelly.
19. Use the dominant hand to pick up the catheter and hold it an inch or two from the tip. Ask the patient to bear down as if voiding. **Insert catheter tip into meatus (Figure 4). Ask the patient to take deep breaths. Advance the catheter to the bifurcation or "Y" level of the ports. Do not use force to introduce the catheter.** If the catheter resists entry, ask the patient to breathe deeply and rotate the catheter slightly.	Bearing down eases the passage of the catheter through the urethra. The male urethra is about 20 cm long. Having the patient take deep breaths or twisting the catheter slightly may ease the catheter past resistance at the sphincters. Advancing an indwelling catheter to the bifurcation ensures its placement in the bladder and facilitates inflation of the balloon without damaging the urethra.

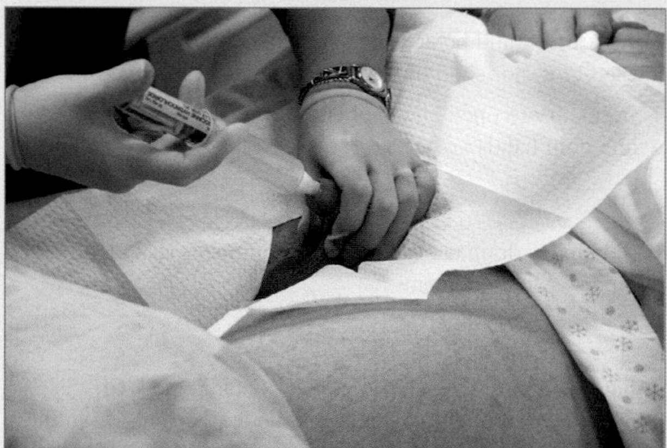

FIGURE 3 Inserting syringe into urethra and instilling lubricant.

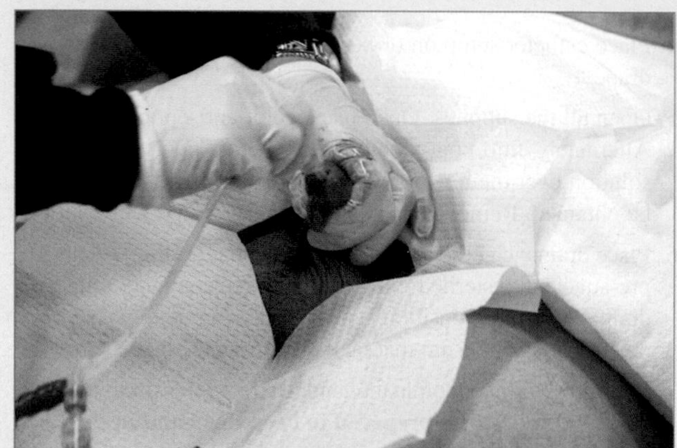

FIGURE 4 Inserting catheter using dominant hand.

ACTION	RATIONALE
20. Hold the catheter securely at the meatus with your nondominant hand. Use your dominant hand to inflate the catheter balloon. **Inject the entire volume of sterile water supplied in the prefilled syringe. Once the balloon is inflated, the catheter may be gently pulled back into place. Replace foreskin over the catheter.** Lower penis.	Bladder or sphincter contraction could push the catheter out. The balloon anchors the catheter in place in the bladder. Manufacturer provides appropriate amount of solution for the size of catheter in the kit; as a result, use entire syringe provided in the kit.
21. Pull gently on the catheter after the balloon is inflated to feel resistance.	Improper inflation can cause patient discomfort and malpositioning of catheter.
22. Attach catheter to drainage system, if necessary.	Closed drainage system minimizes the risk for microorganisms being introduced into the bladder.
23. Remove equipment and dispose of it according to facility policy. Discard syringe in sharps container. Wash and dry the perineal area, as needed.	Proper disposal prevents the spread of microorganisms. Placing syringe in sharps container prevents reuse. Promotes comfort and appropriate personal hygiene.

ACTION | **RATIONALE**

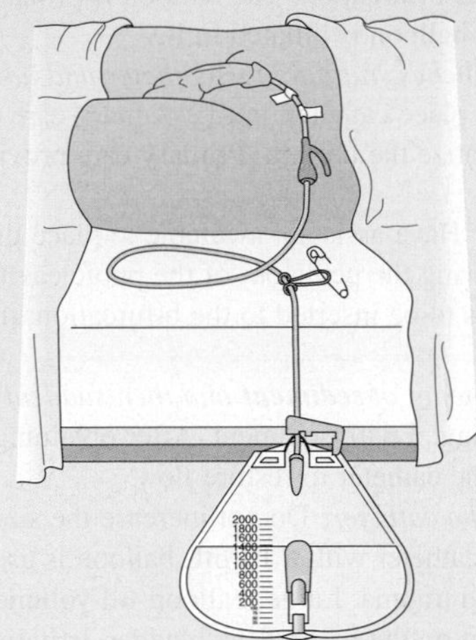

FIGURE 5 Securing tubing to patient's abdomen.

24. Remove gloves. Secure catheter tubing to the patient's inner thigh or lower abdomen (with the penis directed toward the patient's chest) with Velcro leg strap, catheter securing device, or tape (Figure 5). Leave some slack in catheter for leg movement.

    Proper attachment prevents trauma to the urethra and meatus from tension on the tubing. Whether to take the drainage tubing over or under the leg depends on gravity flow, patient's mobility, and comfort of the patient.

25. Assist the patient to a comfortable position. Cover the patient with bed linens. Place the bed in the lowest position.

    Positioning and covering provides warmth and promotes comfort.

26. Secure drainage bag below the level of the bladder. Check that drainage tubing is not kinked and that movement of side rails does not interfere with catheter or drainage bag.

    This facilitates drainage of urine and prevents the backflow of urine.

27. Put on clean gloves. Obtain urine specimen immediately, if needed, from drainage bag. Label specimen. Send urine specimen to the laboratory promptly or refrigerate it.

    Catheter system is sterile. Obtaining specimen immediately allows access to sterile system. Keeping urine at room temperature may cause microorganisms, if present, to grow and distort laboratory findings.

28. Remove gloves and additional PPE, if used. Perform hand hygiene.

    Removing PPE properly reduces the risk for infection transmission and contamination of other items. Hand hygiene prevents the spread of microorganisms.

EVALUATION

The expected outcome is met when the catheter is inserted using sterile technique, results in the immediate flow of urine, and the bladder is not distended. Other outcomes are met when the patient does not experience trauma, reports little to no pain on insertion, and the perineal area remains clean and dry.

DOCUMENTATION

Guidelines

Document the type and size of catheter and balloon inserted, as well as the amount of fluid used to inflate the balloon. Document the patient's tolerance of the activity. Record the amount of urine obtained through the catheter and any specimen obtained. Document any other assessments, such as unusual urine characteristics or alterations in the patient's skin. Record urine amount on intake and output record, if appropriate.

Sample Documentation

DocuCare Practice documenting catheterization of the male urinary bladder in *Lippincott DocuCare*.

7/14/15 1830 Patient unable to void for 8 hours and reports, "I feel like I have to go to the bathroom." Bladder scanned for 540 mL urine. Primary care provider notified; 10 mL 2% lidocaine jelly instilled before catheterization per order; 14F Foley catheter inserted without difficulty; 10 mL of sterile water injected into 5-mL balloon port; 525 mL clear yellow urine returned. Patient reports decreased bladder pressure. Patient tolerated procedure without adverse event.

—B. Clapp, RN

(continued)

SKILL 12-7 CATHETERIZING THE MALE URINARY BLADDER continued

UNEXPECTED SITUATIONS AND ASSOCIATED INTERVENTIONS

- *Patient complains of intense pain when you begin to inflate the balloon:* Stop inflation. Be sure to insert the catheter all the way into the bifurcation. The balloon is probably still in the urethra. Damage to the urethra can result if the balloon is inflated in it.
- *You cannot insert catheter past 3 to 4 inches; rotating the catheter and having patient breathe deeply are of no help:* If still unable to place catheter, notify primary care provider. Repeated catheter placement attempts can traumatize the urethra. Primary care provider may order and insert a Coude catheter.
- *Patient is obese or has retracted penis:* Have assistant available to place fingers on either side of the pubic area and press backward to bring the penis out of the pubic cavity. Hold patient's penis up and forward. The catheter still needs to be inserted to the bifurcation; the length of the urethra has not changed.
- *Urine flow initially contains a large amount of* ***sediment*** *and then suddenly stops; bladder remains palpable:* Catheter may be plugged with sediment. After obtaining an order from the primary care provider, gently irrigate the catheter to restore flow.
- *Urine leaks out of the meatus around the catheter:* Do not increase the size of the indwelling catheter. Make sure the smallest sized catheter with a 10-mL balloon is used. Large catheters cause bladder and urethral irritation and trauma. Large, balloon-fill volumes occupy more space inside the bladder and put added weight on the base of the bladder. Irritation of the bladder wall and detrusor muscle can cause leakage. If leakage persists, consider an evaluation for urinary tract infection. Ensure that the correct amount of solution was used to inflate the balloon. Underfilling the balloon can cause the catheter to dislodge into the urethra, causing urethral spasm, pain, and discomfort. If underfill is suspected, do not attempt to push the catheter farther into the bladder. Remove the catheter and replace it. Assess the patient for constipation. Bowel full of stool can cause pressure on the catheter lumen and prevent the drainage of urine. Implement interventions to prevent/treat constipation.
- *Urine flow is initially well established and urine is clear, but after several hours urine flow dwindles:* Check tubing for kinking. If patient has changed position, the tubing and drainage bag may need to be moved to facilitate drainage of urine.

SPECIAL CONSIDERATIONS

General Considerations

- Be familiar with facility policy and/or primary practitioner guidelines for the maximum amount of urine to remove from the bladder at the time of insertion.
- Supplies can be opened and prepared on the overbed table, moving the tray onto the bed just before cleansing the patient.
- If there is not an immediate flow of urine after the catheter has been inserted, several measures may prove helpful:
  - Have the patient take a deep breath, which helps to relax the perineal and abdominal muscles.
  - Rotate the catheter slightly, because a drainage hole may be resting against the bladder wall.
  - Raise the head of the patient's bed to increase pressure in the bladder area.
  - Assess the patient's intake to ensure adequate fluid intake for urine production.
  - Assess the catheter and drainage tubing for kinks and occlusion.
  - Urethral strictures, false passages, prostatic enlargement, and postsurgical bladder-neck contractures can make urethral catheterization difficult and may require the services of a urologist. With any question to the location of the catheter, such as no return of urine, do not inflate the balloon. Remove the catheter and notify the physician (Society of Urologic Nurses and Associates, 2005c).
- If the catheter cannot be advanced, having the patient take several deep breaths may be helpful. Rotate the catheter half a turn, and try to advance it. If you are still unable to advance it, remove the catheter. Notify the primary care provider.
- Some catheter kits do not contain the catheter. This allows you to select a catheter and balloon size separately.

Infant and Child Considerations

- Size 5F to 8F is used for infants and young children. Size 8F to 12F catheters are commonly used for older children (Perry et al., 2010).
- Distraction, such as blowing bubbles, deep breathing, or singing a song, can help the child relax.
- Lidocaine jelly is often used to anesthetize and lubricate the area before insertion of the catheter, decreasing the child's discomfort and anxiety.

Older Adult Considerations

- If resistance is met while inserting a catheter and rotating does not help, it is important to never force the catheter. The resistance may be caused by enlargement of the prostate gland, which is commonly seen in men over age 50 years. A special crook-tipped catheter called a Coude catheter, inserted by the physician or advanced practice nurse, may be required to maneuver past the prostate gland.

Home Care Considerations

- Intermittent catheterization, performed by the patient or a caregiver in the home, may be necessary for patients with spinal cord injuries or other neurologic conditions. Although the risk for UTI is always present, most research supports the use of clean, rather than sterile, technique in this environment. The procedure for self-catheterization is essentially the same as that used by the nurse to catheterize a patient. Self-catheterization is recommended at regular intervals to prevent over distention of the bladder and decreased blood flow through the wall of the bladder (Hinkle & Cheever, 2014; SUNA, 2010). Box 12-2 in Skill 12-6 outlines important information related to patient self-catheterization.

SKILL VARIATION Intermittent Male Urethral Catheterization

1. Check the medical record for the order for intermittent urethral catheterization. Review the patient's chart for any limitations in physical activity. Gather supplies. Obtain assistance from another staff member, if necessary.

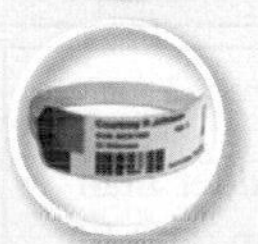

2. Perform hand hygiene. Put on PPE, as indicated, based on transmission precautions.
3. Identify the patient. Discuss the procedure with the patient and assess the patient's ability to assist with the procedure. Ask the patient if he has any allergies, especially to latex or iodine.
4. Close the curtains around the bed and close the door to the room, if possible.
5. Provide good lighting. Artificial light is recommended (use of a flashlight requires an assistant to hold and position it). Place a trash receptacle within easy reach.
6. Assemble equipment on overbed table within reach.
7. Raise the bed to a comfortable working height. Stand on the patient's right side if you are right-handed, patient's left side if you are left-handed.
8. Position patient on his back with thighs slightly apart. Drape patient so that only the area around the penis is exposed. Slide waterproof pad under patient.

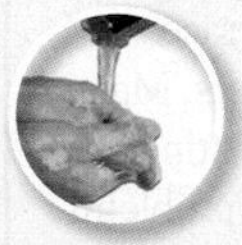

9. Put on clean gloves. Clean the genital area with washcloth, skin cleanser, and warm water. Clean the tip of the penis first, moving the washcloth in a circular motion from the meatus outward. Wash the shaft of the penis using downward strokes toward the pubic area. Rinse and dry. Remove gloves. Perform hand hygiene again.
10. Open sterile catheterization tray on a clean overbed table using sterile technique.
11. Put on sterile gloves. Open sterile drape and place on patient's thighs. Place fenestrated drape with opening over penis.
12. Place catheter setup on or next to patient's legs on sterile drape.
13. Open all the supplies. Open package of antiseptic swabs. Alternately, fluff cotton balls in tray before pouring antiseptic solution over them. Open specimen container if specimen is to be obtained.
14. Remove cap from syringe prefilled with lubricant.
15. Lift penis with nondominant hand. Retract foreskin in uncircumcised patient. **Be prepared to keep this hand in this position until catheter is inserted and urine is flowing well and continuously.**
16. **Use the dominant hand to pick up an antiseptic swab or use forceps to pick up a cotton ball. Using a circular motion, clean the penis, moving from the meatus down the glans of the penis. Repeat this cleansing motion two more times, using a new cotton ball/swab each time. Discard each cotton ball/swab after one use.**
17. Hold penis with slight upward tension and perpendicular to patient's body. Use the dominant hand to pick up the lubricant syringe. **Gently insert tip of syringe with lubricant into urethra and instill the 10 mL of lubricant.**
18. With the noncontaminated, dominant hand, place drainage end of catheter in receptacle. If a specimen is required, place the end into the specimen container in the receptacle.
19. Use the dominant hand to pick up the catheter and hold it an inch or two from the tip. Ask the patient to bear down as if voiding. Insert catheter tip into meatus. Ask the patient to take deep breaths as you advance the catheter 6 to 8 inches (14.4 to 19.2 cm) or until urine flows.
20. Hold the catheter securely at the meatus with the nondominant hand while the bladder empties. If a specimen is being collected, remove the drainage end of the tubing from the specimen container after the required amount is obtained and allow urine to flow into the receptacle. Set specimen container aside.
21. Allow the bladder to empty. Withdraw the catheter slowly and smoothly after urine has stopped flowing. Remove equipment and dispose of it according to facility policy. Discard syringe in sharps container to prevent reuse. Wash and

(*continued*)

SKILL 12-7 CATHETERIZING THE MALE URINARY BLADDER continued

SKILL VARIATION Intermittent Male Urethral Catheterization continued

dry the genital area, as needed. Replace foreskin in forward position, if necessary.

22. Remove gloves. Assist the patient to a comfortable position. Cover the patient with bed linens. Place the bed in the lowest position.
23. Put on clean gloves. Cover and label the specimen. Send the urine specimen to the laboratory promptly or refrigerate it.
24. Remove gloves and additional PPE, if used. Perform hand hygiene.

Note: Intermittent catheterization in the home is performed using clean technique. The bladder's natural resistance to the microorganisms normally found in the home makes sterile technique unnecessary. Catheters are washed, dried, and stored for repeated use. Clean technique involves the use of cleansed reusable catheters, washing hands with soap and water, and daily cleansing of the perineum or more often only when fecal or other wastes are present (Newman, 2008 as cited in Herter & Wallace Kazer, 2010). Cleansing the perineal area to decrease bacteria in the surrounding area is highly recommended (Herter & Wallace Kazer, 2010).

EVIDENCE FOR PRACTICE ▶

CATHETER-ASSOCIATED URINARY TRACT INFECTIONS

Centers for Disease Control and Prevention. (2012). *Healthcare-associated infections (HAIs). Catheter-associated urinary tract infections (CAUTI).* Available http://www.cdc.gov/HAI/ca_uti/uti.html.

Refer to details in Skill 12-5, Evidence for Practice, and refer to thePoint for additional research on related nursing topics.

EVIDENCE FOR PRACTICE ▶

LONG-TERM URINARY CATHETERS

Long-term urinary catheters may be appropriate for patients unable to use other bladder management methods, patients with a disability the makes it difficult to use the bathroom, and for patients with neurogenic bladder dysfunction. Living with an indwelling urinary catheter presents challenges that must be addressed on a daily basis. What issues do patients using a long-term indwelling catheter encounter?

Related Research

Wilde, M.H., McDonald, M.V., Brasch, J., McMahon, J.M., Fairbanks, E., et al. (2013). Long-term urinary catheter users self-care practices and problems. *Journal of Clinical Nursing, 22*(3/4), 356–367.

The aims of this study were to describe self-care practices and catheter problems in adult community-living long-term indwelling urinary catheter users and to explore relationships among catheter practices and problems. This descriptive and exploratory analysis utilized home interviews conducted with catheter users who provided information by self-reported recall over the previous 2 months. Data were analyzed by descriptive statistics and tests of association between demographics, catheter practices, and catheter problems. The sample was widely diverse in age, race, and medical diagnosis. Urethral catheters were used slightly more often than suprapubic catheters. Many participants were highly disabled, having difficulty in bathing, dressing, toileting, and getting out of bed. Participants also required assistance with eating. A high percentage of catheter problems were reported, including bypass leakage of urine, urinary tract infections, blockage of the catheter, catheter-associated pain, and accidental dislodgement of the catheter. Treatment of catheter-related problems contributed to additional health care utilization, including extra nurse or clinic visits, visits to the emergency department, or hospitalization. Symptoms of CAUTI most often included changes in the color or character of urine or generalized symptoms. The authors concluded catheter-related problems contribute to excess health problems and health care utilization and costs.

Relevance to Nursing Practice

Many of the catheter-related problems reported in this study could be prevented or minimized with more attention to catheter management, early identification of problems, and more evidence-based catheter practices. Nurses are often in the position of being the primary care provider and advocate for patients with long-term indwelling catheters. Nurses are in strategic positions to plan interventions to address the persistent catheter-related problems that affect large proportions of long-term indwelling urinary catheter users. Nurses have a responsibility to provide accurate and appropriate patient education, and should consider this an important part of the plan of care whenever possible, resulting in improved patient care.

See additional Evidence for Practice related to urinary catheters at the end of Skills 12-5 and 12-6, and refer to thePoint for additional research on related nursing topics.

SKILL 12-8 REMOVING AN INDWELLING CATHETER

Removal of an indwelling catheter is performed using clean technique. Take care to prevent trauma to the urethra during the procedure. Completely deflate the catheter balloon before catheter removal to avoid irritation and damage to the urethra and meatus. The patient may experience burning or irritation the first few times he or she voids after removal, due to urethral irritation. If the catheter was in place for more than a few days, decreased bladder muscle tone and swelling of the urethra may cause the patient to experience difficulty voiding or an inability to void. Monitor the patient for urinary retention. It is important to encourage adequate oral fluid intake to promote adequate urinary output. Check facility policy regarding the length of time the patient is allowed to accomplish successful voiding after catheter removal.

DELEGATION CONSIDERATIONS

Removal of an indwelling catheter is not delegated to nursing assistive personnel (NAP) or to unlicensed assistive personnel (UAP). Depending on the state's nurse practice act and the organization's policies and procedures, removal of an indwelling catheter may be delegated to licensed practical/vocational nurses (LPN/LVNs). The decision to delegate must be based on careful analysis of the patient's needs and circumstances, as well as the qualifications of the person to whom the task is being delegated. Refer to the Delegation Guidelines in Appendix A.

EQUIPMENT

- Syringe sufficiently large to accommodate the volume of solution used to inflate the balloon (balloon size/inflation volume is printed on the balloon inflation valve on the catheter at the bifurcation)
- Waterproof, disposable pad
- Disposable gloves
- Additional PPE, as indicated
- Washcloth, skin cleanser, and warm water to perform perineal hygiene after catheter removal

ASSESSMENT

Check the medical record for an order to remove the catheter. Assess for discharge or encrustation around the urethral meatus. Assess urine output, including color and current amount in drainage bag.

NURSING DIAGNOSIS

Determine the related factors for the nursing diagnoses based on the patient's current status. Appropriate nursing diagnoses may include:

- Impaired Urinary Elimination
- Risk for Injury
- Urinary Retention

OUTCOME IDENTIFICATION AND PLANNING

The expected outcome to achieve when removing an indwelling catheter is that the catheter will be removed without difficulty and with minimal patient discomfort. Other appropriate outcomes include the following: the patient voids without discomfort after catheter removal; the patient voids a minimum of 250 mL of urine within 6 to 8 hours of catheter removal; the patient's skin remains clean, dry, and intact, without evidence of irritation or breakdown; and the patient verbalizes an understanding of the need to maintain adequate fluid intake, as appropriate.

(continued)

SKILL 12-8 REMOVING AN INDWELLING CATHETER continued

IMPLEMENTATION

ACTION	RATIONALE
1. Confirm the order for catheter removal in the medical record. Gather equipment.	Verifying the medical order ensures that the correct intervention is administered to the right patient. Assembling equipment provides for an organized approach to the task.
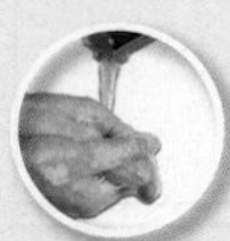 2. Perform hand hygiene and put on PPE, if indicated.	Hand hygiene and PPE prevent the spread of microorganisms. PPE is required based on transmission precautions.
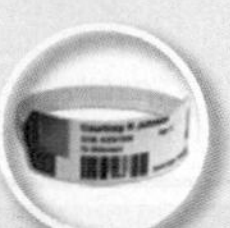 3. Identify the patient.	Identifying the patient ensures the right patient receives the intervention and helps prevent errors.
4. Close the curtains around the bed and close the door to the room, if possible. Discuss the procedure with the patient and assess the patient's ability to assist with the procedure.	This ensures the patient's privacy. Discussion promotes reassurance and provides knowledge about the procedure. Dialogue encourages patient participation and allows for individualized nursing care.
5. Adjust the bed to a comfortable working height, usually elbow height of the caregiver (VISN 8 Patient Safety Center, 2009). Stand on the patient's right side if you are right-handed, patient's left side if you are left-handed.	Having the bed at the proper height prevents back and muscle strain. Positioning allows for ease of use of dominant hand for catheter removal.
6. Position the patient as for catheter insertion. Drape the patient so that only the area around the catheter is exposed. Slide waterproof pad between the female patient's legs or over the male patient's thighs.	Positioning allows access to site. Draping prevents unnecessary exposure and promotes warmth. The waterproof pad will protect bed linens from moisture and serve as a receptacle for the used catheter after removal.
7. Remove the leg strap, tape, or other device used to secure the catheter to the patient's thigh or abdomen.	This action permits removal of catheter.
8. Insert the syringe into the balloon inflation port. Allow water to come back by gravity. Alternately, aspirate the entire amount of sterile water used to inflate the balloon (Figure 1). Refer to manufacturer's instructions for deflation. **Do not cut the inflation port.**	Removal of sterile water deflates the balloon to allow for catheter removal. All of the sterile water must be removed to prevent injury to the patient. Aspiration by pulling on the syringe plunger may result in collapse of the inflation lumen; contribute to the formation of creases, ridges, or cuffing at the balloon area; and increase the catheter balloon diameter size on deflation, resulting in difficult removal and urethral trauma.

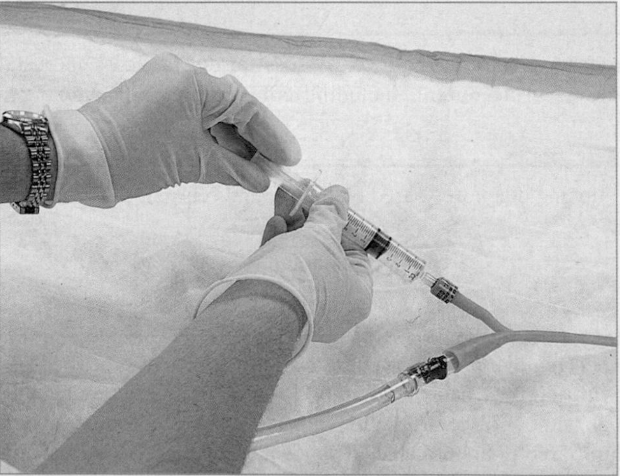

FIGURE 1 Removing fluid from balloon.

ACTION	RATIONALE
9. Ask the patient to take several slow deep breaths. **Slowly and gently remove the catheter.** Place it on the waterproof pad and wrap it in the pad.	Slow deep breathing helps to relax the sphincter muscles. Slow gentle removal prevents trauma to the urethra. Using a waterproof pad prevents contact with the catheter.
10. Wash and dry the perineal area, as needed.	Cleaning promotes comfort and appropriate personal hygiene.
11. Remove gloves. Assist the patient to a comfortable position. Cover the patient with bed linens. Place the bed in the lowest position.	These actions provide warmth and promote comfort and safety.
12. Put on clean gloves. Remove equipment and dispose of it according to facility policy. Note characteristics and amount of urine in drainage bag.	Proper disposal prevents the spread of microorganisms. Observing the characteristics ensures accurate documentation.
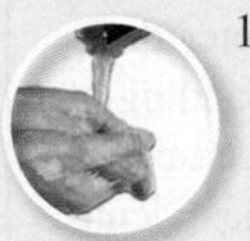 13. Remove gloves and additional PPE, if used. Perform hand hygiene.	Removing PPE properly reduces the risk for infection transmission and contamination of other items. Hand hygiene prevents the spread of microorganisms.

EVALUATION

The expected outcomes are met when the catheter is removed without difficulty and with minimal patient discomfort; the patient voids without discomfort after catheter removal; the patient voids a minimum of 250 mL of urine within 6 to 8 hours of catheter removal; the patient's skin remains clean, dry, and intact, without evidence of irritation or breakdown; and the patient verbalizes an understanding of the need to maintain adequate fluid intake, as appropriate.

DOCUMENTATION

Guidelines

Document the type and size of catheter removed and the amount of fluid removed from the balloon. Also document the patient's tolerance of the procedure. Record the amount of urine in the drainage bag. Note the time the patient is due to void. Document any other assessments, such as unusual urine characteristics or alterations in the patient's skin. Also record urine amount on intake and output record, if appropriate.

Sample Documentation

7/14/15 0800 Removed 15 mL fluid from catheter balloon; 14F Foley removed without difficulty; 500 mL of clear yellow urine noted in drainage bag at time of removal. Patient due to void by 1600. Patient instructed to drink 6 to 8 6-oz. glasses of fluid in the course of the day, and that it may take some time for the passage of urine on his own; patient verbalized understanding of instructions. Urinal placed at bedside, with patient demonstrating appropriate use.

—B. Clapp, RN

UNEXPECTED SITUATIONS AND ASSOCIATED INTERVENTIONS

- *Resistance is felt while attempting to pull out catheter:* Stop pulling the catheter. Reattach syringe to balloon inflation port and re-aspirate to make sure all the sterile water has been removed. Reattempt catheter removal. If resistance is still present, stop removal and notify the primary care provider.

SPECIAL CONSIDERATIONS

- Have alternate toileting measures available, as necessary, based on patient assessment. A bedside commode, urinal, or bedpan may be necessary if the patient is unable to get to the bathroom.
- Refer to facility policy and manufacturer's recommendation regarding balloon deflation. Aspiration by pulling on the syringe plunger may result in collapse of the inflation lumen; contribute to the formation of creases, ridges, or cuffing at the balloon area; and increase the catheter balloon diameter size on deflation, resulting in difficult removal and urethral trauma.

(continued)

SKILL 12-8 REMOVING AN INDWELLING CATHETER continued

EVIDENCE FOR PRACTICE ▶

EARLY REMOVAL OF INDWELLING URINARY CATHETERS

Indwelling urinary catheters should be left in place for the shortest length of time possible to reduce the risk for catheter-associated urinary tract infections. Are there patient factors that can be taken into consideration to facilitate early removal?

Related Research

Bhardwaj, R., Pickard, R., Carrick-Sen, D., & Brittain, K. (2012). Patients' perspectives on timing of urinary catheter removal after surgery. *British Journal of Nursing (Urology Supplement), 21*(18), S4–S9.

The aim of this qualitative study was to explore patients' perceptions of the care process relating to perioperative catheterization to identify patient factors that encourage early removal of urinary catheters. Semi-structured interviews were conducted, exploring patients' attitudes toward, and belief surrounding, perioperative catheterization and timing of catheter removal. Catheter duration ranged from 1 to 10 days. The main themes identified included the lack of understanding of the purpose of the catheter and the catheterization process, in particular related to uncertainties regarding the removal process, resulting in patient concerns and anxieties. Other themes identified included a lack of patient autonomy and dignity, and symptoms experienced after catheter removal, and patients' lack of awareness of infection risk related to catheterization. A lack of easily accessible toilet facilities was also cited by some participants. The authors concluded that a lack of knowledge of the catheterization process among participants led to fears and concerns that may have contributed to delayed catheter removal. The authors suggest changes to patient care to reduce catheter duration, including ensuring the provision of preoperative information, greater patient involvement in catheter removal decisions, and provision of easily accessible toilet facilities.

Relevance to Nursing Practice

Nurses should incorporate interventions to ensure compliance with best-practice guidelines to provide quality patient care. Nurses should provide appropriate patient teaching related to the use of urinary catheters, discuss/encourage alternative methods for urinary elimination, and advocate to include the patient in care decisions. These interventions can possibly lead to timely removal of urinary catheters and prevent associated infections.

See additional Evidence for Practice related to urinary catheters at the end of Skills 12-5, 12-6, and 12-7, and refer to thePoint for additional research on related nursing topics.

SKILL 12-9 PERFORMING INTERMITTENT CLOSED CATHETER IRRIGATION

Bladder irrigation is not recommended unless obstruction is anticipated, as might occur with bleeding after prostate or bladder surgery (SUNA, 2010, p. 9). Catheter irrigation should be avoided unless necessary to relieve or prevent obstruction (Herter & Wallace Kazer, 2010). If obstruction is anticipated, continuous irrigation is suggested to prevent obstruction (SUNA) (see Skill 12-10). However, intermittent irrigation is sometimes prescribed to restore or maintain the patency of the drainage system. Sediment or debris, as well as blood clots, might block the catheter, preventing the flow of urine out of the catheter. Irrigations might also be used to instill medications that will act directly on the bladder wall. Irrigating a catheter through a closed system is preferred to opening the catheter because opening the catheter could lead to contamination and infection.

DELEGATION CONSIDERATIONS

Intermittent closed catheter irrigation is not delegated to nursing assistive personnel (NAP) or to unlicensed assistive personnel (UAP). Depending on the state's nurse practice act and the organization's policies and procedures, intermittent closed catheter irrigation may be delegated to licensed practical/vocational nurses (LPN/LVNs). The decision to delegate must be based on careful analysis of the patient's needs and circumstances, as well as the qualifications of the person to whom the task is being delegated. Refer to the Delegation Guidelines in Appendix A.

EQUIPMENT

- Sterile basin or container
- Sterile irrigating solution (at room temperature or warmed to body temperature)
- 30- to 60-mL syringe (with 18- or 19-gauge blunt-end needle, if catheter access port is not a needleless system)
- Clamp for drainage tubing
- Bath blanket
- Disposable gloves
- Additional PPE, as indicated
- Waterproof pad
- Alcohol or other disinfectant swab

ASSESSMENT

Check the medical record for an order to irrigate the catheter, including the type and amount of solution to use for the irrigation. Before performing the procedure, assess catheter drainage and amount of urine in drainage bag. Also assess for bladder fullness, either by palpation or with a handheld bladder ultrasound device. Assess for signs of adverse effects, which may include pain, bladder spasm, bladder distension/fullness, or lack of drainage from the catheter.

NURSING DIAGNOSIS

Determine related factors for the nursing diagnoses based on the patient's current status. Appropriate nursing diagnoses may include:

- Impaired Urinary Elimination
- Risk for Infection

OUTCOME IDENTIFICATION AND PLANNING

The expected outcome to achieve when performing closed catheter irrigation is that the patient exhibits the free flow of urine through the catheter. Other outcomes may include the following: the patient's bladder is not distended; the patient remains free from pain; and the patient remains free of any signs and symptoms of infection.

IMPLEMENTATION

ACTION	RATIONALE
1. Confirm the order for catheter irrigation in the medical record.	Verifying the medical order ensures that the correct intervention is administered to the right patient.
2. Gather equipment.	Assembling equipment provides for an organized approach to the task.
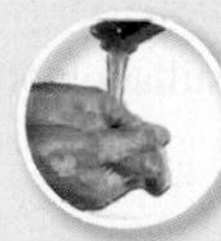 3. Perform hand hygiene and put on PPE, if indicated.	Hand hygiene and PPE prevent the spread of microorganisms. PPE is required based on transmission precautions.
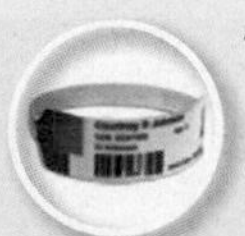 4. Identify the patient.	Identifying the patient ensures the right patient receives the intervention and helps prevent errors.
5. Close the curtains around the bed and close the door to the room, if possible. Discuss the procedure with the patient.	This ensures the patient's privacy. Discussion promotes reassurance and provides knowledge about the procedure. Dialogue encourages patient participation and allows for individualized nursing care.
6. Assemble equipment on overbed table within reach.	Arranging items nearby is convenient, saves time, and avoids unnecessary stretching and twisting of muscles on the part of the nurse.
7. Adjust the bed to a comfortable working height, usually elbow height of the caregiver (VISN 8 Patient Safety Center, 2009).	Having the bed at the proper height prevents back and muscle strain.

(continued)

SKILL 12-9 PERFORMING INTERMITTENT CLOSED CATHETER IRRIGATION continued

ACTION	RATIONALE
8. Put on gloves. Empty the catheter drainage bag and measure the amount of urine, noting the amount and characteristics of the urine. Remove gloves.	Gloves prevent contact with blood and body fluids. Emptying the drainage bag allows for accurate assessment of drainage after the irrigation solution is instilled. Assessment of urine provides a baseline for future comparison. Proper removal of PPE prevents transmission of microorganisms.
9. Assist the patient to a comfortable position and expose access port on catheter setup. Place waterproof pad under catheter and aspiration port. Remove catheter from device or tape anchoring catheter to the patient.	This provides adequate visualization. Waterproof pad protects patient and bed from leakage. Removing the catheter from the anchoring device or tape allows for manipulation of the catheter.
10. Open supplies, using aseptic technique. Pour sterile solution into sterile basin. Aspirate the prescribed amount of irrigant (usually 30 to 60 mL) into sterile syringe. Put on gloves.	Use of aseptic technique ensures sterility of irrigating fluid and prevents spread of microorganisms. Gloves prevent contact with blood and body fluids.
11. **Cleanse the access port on the catheter with antimicrobial swab (Figure 1).**	Cleaning the port reduces the risk of introducing organisms into the closed urinary system.
12. Clamp or fold catheter tubing below the access port (Figure 2).	This directs the irrigating solution into the bladder, preventing flow into the drainage bag.

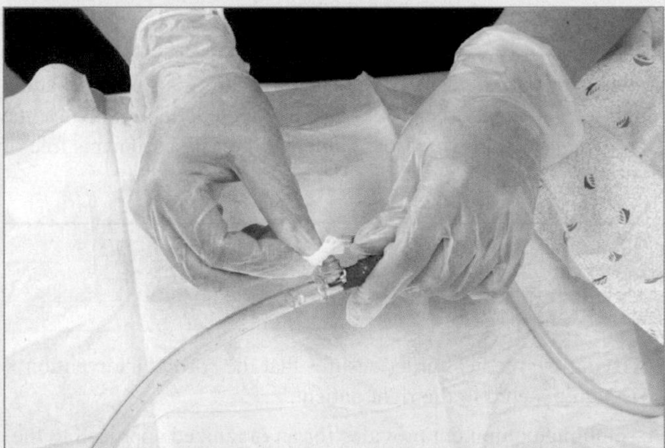

FIGURE 1 Cleansing access port on catheter.

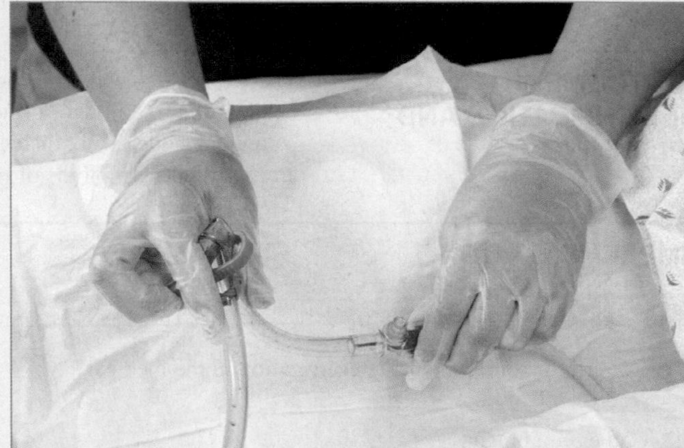

FIGURE 2 Clamping catheter below access port.

ACTION	RATIONALE
13. Attach the syringe to the access port on the catheter using a twisting motion (Figure 3). **Gently instill solution into catheter (Figure 4).**	Gentle irrigation prevents damage to bladder lining. Instillation of fluid dislodges material blocking the catheter.

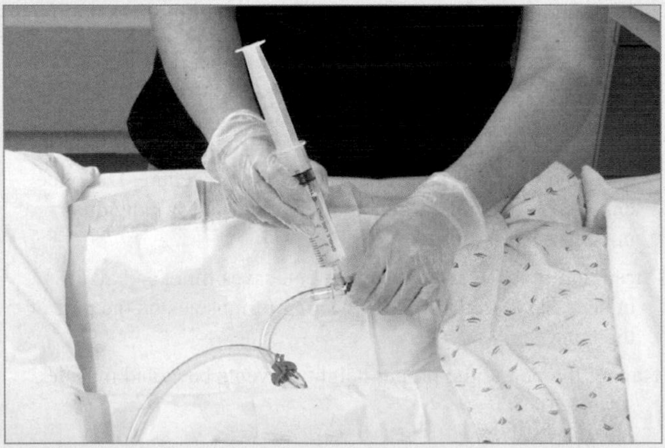

FIGURE 3 Attaching syringe to access port with twisting motion.

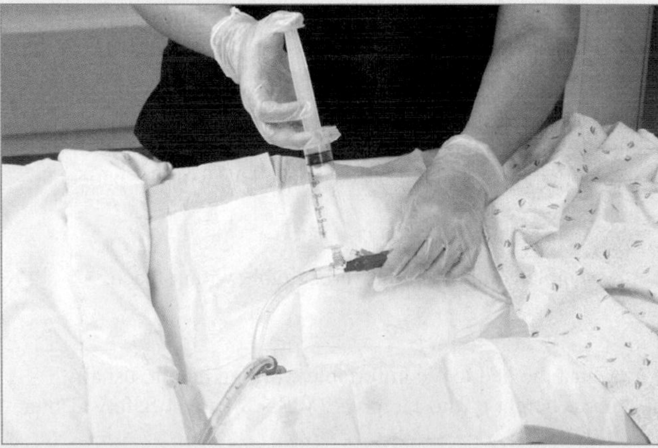

FIGURE 4 Gently instilling irrigation solution.

ACTION	RATIONALE
14. Remove syringe from access port (Figure 5). **Unclamp or unfold tubing and allow irrigant and urine to flow into the drainage bag.** Repeat procedure, as necessary.	Gravity aids drainage of urine and irrigant from the bladder.

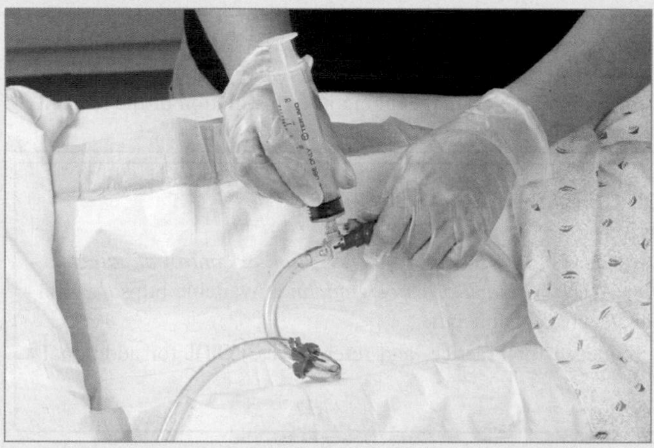

FIGURE 5 Removing syringe from access port.

15. Remove gloves. Secure catheter tubing to the patient's inner thigh or lower abdomen (if a male patient) with anchoring device or tape. Leave some slack in the catheter for leg movement.	Proper attachment prevents trauma to the urethra and meatus from tension on the tubing. Whether to take the drainage tubing over or under the leg depends on gravity flow and patient's mobility and comfort.
16. Assist the patient to a comfortable position. Cover the patient with bed linens. Place the bed in the lowest position.	Positioning and covering provide warmth and promote comfort. Lowering bed contributes to patient safety.
17. Secure drainage bag below the level of the bladder. Check that drainage tubing is not kinked and that movement of side rails does not interfere with catheter or drainage bag.	This facilitates drainage of urine and prevents the backflow of urine.
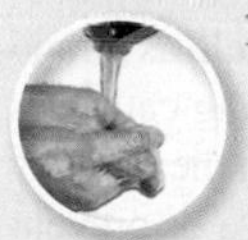 18. Remove equipment and discard syringe in appropriate receptacle. Remove gloves and additional PPE, if used. Perform hand hygiene.	Proper disposal of equipment prevents transmission of microorganisms. Removing PPE properly reduces the risk for infection transmission and contamination of other items. Hand hygiene prevents the spread of microorganisms.
19. Assess the patient's response to the procedure and the quality and amount of drainage after the irrigation.	This provides accurate assessment of the patient's response to the procedure.

EVALUATION

The expected outcome is met when the patient exhibits the free flow of urine through the catheter; the irrigant and urine are returned into the drainage bag; the patient's bladder is not distended; the patient remains free from pain; and the patient remains free of any signs and symptoms of infection.

DOCUMENTATION

Guidelines

Document baseline assessment of the patient. Document the amount and type of irrigation solution used and the amount and characteristics of drainage returned after the procedure. Document the ease of irrigation and the patient's tolerance of the procedure. Record urine amount emptied from the drainage bag before the procedure and the amount of irrigant used on intake and output record. Subtract irrigant amount from the urine output when totaling output to provide accurate recording of urine output.

Sample Documentation

7/22/15 1630 Urinary catheter irrigated with 60 mL of normal saline without difficulty. All of irrigation returned plus 200 mL of cloudy yellow urine. Patient tolerated procedure without adverse effect. Order received to notify physician if urine output is less than 30 mL/hour.

—*B. Clapp, RN*

(*continued*)

SKILL 12-9 PERFORMING INTERMITTENT CLOSED CATHETER IRRIGATION continued

UNEXPECTED SITUATIONS AND ASSOCIATED INTERVENTIONS

- *Irrigation solution will not enter the catheter:* Do not force the solution into the catheter. Notify primary care provider. Prepare to change catheter.
- *Tubing was not clamped before introducing irrigation solution:* Repeat irrigation, making sure to clamp the tube before introducing irrigation solution. If the tubing is not clamped, the irrigation solution will drain into the urinary drainage bag and not enter the catheter.

SPECIAL CONSIDERATIONS

- If irrigant is a medication intended for action in the bladder, be aware of specific dwell time included in the order or determined by the action of the medication. Allow the appropriate amount of time to lapse before unclamping the drainage tubing after instillation of the irrigant.

EVIDENCE FOR PRACTICE ▶

PREVENTION AND CONTROL OF CATHETER-ASSOCIATED URINARY TRACT INFECTIONS

Society of Urologic Nurses and Associates (SUNA). (2010). *Prevention & control of catheter-associated urinary tract infection (CAUTI). Clinical practice guideline.* Available https://www.suna.org/sites/default/files/download/cautiGuideline.pdf.

Refer to details in Skill 12-6, Evidence for Practice, and refer to thePoint for additional research on related nursing topics.

SKILL 12-10 ADMINISTERING A CONTINUOUS CLOSED BLADDER OR CATHETER IRRIGATION

Bladder irrigation is not recommended unless obstruction is anticipated, as might occur with bleeding after prostate or bladder surgery (SUNA, 2010, p. 9). Sediment or debris, as well as blood clots, might block the catheter, preventing the flow of urine out of the catheter. Indwelling catheters sometimes require continuous irrigation, or flushing, with solution to restore or maintain the patency of the drainage system. Catheter irrigation should be avoided unless necessary to relieve or prevent obstruction (Herter & Wallace Kazer, 2010). If obstruction is anticipated, continuous irrigation is suggested to prevent obstruction (SUNA, 2010).

Irrigations might also be used to instill medications that will act directly on the bladder wall. Irrigating a catheter through a closed system is preferred to opening the catheter because opening the catheter could lead to contamination and infection. A triple-lumen or three-way catheter (Figure 1) is used for a continuous irrigation in order to maintain a closed system (Figure 2).

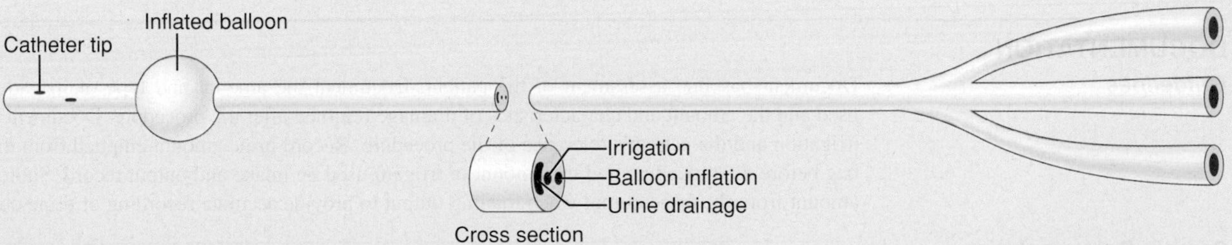

FIGURE 1 A triple-lumen catheter.

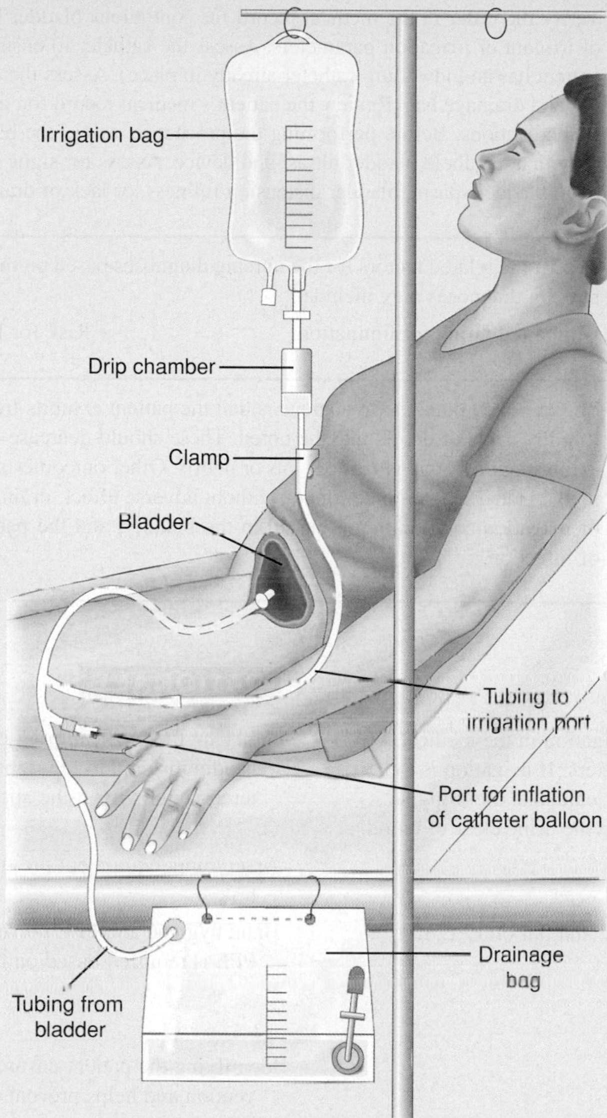

FIGURE 2 A continuous bladder irrigation (CBI) setup.

DELEGATION CONSIDERATIONS

The administration of continuous closed bladder irrigation is not delegated to nursing assistive personnel (NAP) or to unlicensed assistive personnel (UAP). Depending on the state's nurse practice act and the organization's policies and procedures, administration of continuous closed bladder irrigation may be delegated to licensed practical/vocational nurses (LPN/LVNs). The decision to delegate must be based on careful analysis of the patient's needs and circumstances, as well as the qualifications of the person to whom the task is being delegated. Refer to the Delegation Guidelines in Appendix A.

EQUIPMENT

- Sterile irrigating solution (at room temperature or warmed to body temperature)
- Sterile tubing with drip chamber and clamp for connection to irrigating solution
- IV pole
- IV pump (if bladder is being irrigated with a solution containing medication)
- Three-way indwelling catheter in place in patient's bladder
- Indwelling catheter drainage setup (tubing and collection bag)
- Alcohol or other disinfectant swab
- Bath blanket
- Disposable gloves
- Additional PPE, as indicated

(continued)

SKILL 12-10 ADMINISTERING A CONTINUOUS CLOSED BLADDER OR CATHETER IRRIGATION continued

ASSESSMENT

Verify the order in the medical record for continuous bladder irrigation, including type and amount of irrigant or irrigation parameters. Assess the catheter to ensure that it has an irrigation port (if the patient has an indwelling catheter already in place). Assess the characteristics of urine present in tubing and drainage bag. Review the patient's medical record for, and ask the patient about, any allergies to medications. Before performing the procedure, assess the bladder for fullness either by palpation or with a handheld bladder ultrasound device. Assess for signs of adverse effects, which may include pain, bladder spasm, bladder distension/fullness, or lack of drainage from the catheter.

NURSING DIAGNOSIS

Determine related factors for the nursing diagnoses based on the patient's current status. Appropriate nursing diagnoses may include:

- Impaired Urinary Elimination
- Risk for Infection

OUTCOME IDENTIFICATION AND PLANNING

The expected outcome to achieve is that the patient exhibits free-flowing urine through the catheter. Initially, clots or debris may be noted. These should decrease over time, with the patient ultimately exhibiting urine that is free of clots or debris. Other outcomes may include the following: the continuous bladder irrigation continues without adverse effect; drainage is greater than the hourly amount of irrigation solution being placed in the bladder; and the patient exhibits no signs and symptoms of infection.

IMPLEMENTATION

ACTION	RATIONALE
1. Confirm the order for catheter irrigation in the medical record, including infusion parameters. If irrigation is to be implemented via gravity infusion, calculate the drip rate. Often, orders are to infuse to keep the urine clear of blood.	Verifying the medical order ensures that the correct intervention is administered to the right patient. Solution must be administered via gravity at the appropriate rate as prescribed.
2. Gather equipment.	Assembling equipment provides for an organized approach to the task.
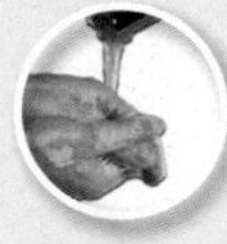 3. Perform hand hygiene and put on PPE, if indicated.	Hand hygiene and PPE prevent the spread of microorganisms. PPE is required based on transmission precautions.
4. Identify the patient.	Identifying the patient ensures the right patient receives the intervention and helps prevent errors.
5. Close the curtains around the bed and close the door to the room, if possible. Discuss the procedure with the patient.	This ensures the patient's privacy. Discussion promotes reassurance and provides knowledge about the procedure. Dialogue encourages patient participation and allows for individualized nursing care.
6. Assemble equipment on overbed table within reach.	Arranging items nearby is convenient, saves time, and avoids unnecessary stretching and twisting of muscles on the part of the nurse.
7. Adjust the bed to a comfortable working height, usually elbow height of the caregiver (VISN 8 Patient Safety Center, 2009).	Having the bed at the proper height prevents back and muscle strain.
8. Empty the catheter drainage bag and measure the amount of urine, noting the amount and characteristics of the urine.	Emptying the drainage bag allows for accurate assessment of drainage after the irrigation solution is instilled. Assessment of urine provides baseline for future comparison.
9. Assist the patient to a comfortable position and expose the irrigation port on the catheter setup. Place waterproof pad under the catheter and aspiration port.	This provides adequate visualization. Waterproof pad protects the patient and bed from leakage.

ACTION	RATIONALE
10. Prepare sterile irrigation bag for use as directed by manufacturer. Clearly label the solution as 'Bladder Irrigant.' Include the date and time on the label. Hang bag on IV pole 2.5 to 3 feet above the level of the patient's bladder. Secure tubing clamp and insert sterile tubing with drip chamber to container using aseptic technique (Figure 3). Release clamp and remove protective cover on end of tubing without contaminating it. Allow solution to flush tubing and remove air (Figure 4). Clamp tubing and replace end cover.	Proper labeling provides accurate information for caregivers. Sterile solution not used within 24 hours of opening should be discarded. Aseptic technique prevents contamination of solution irrigation system. Priming the tubing before attaching irrigation clears air from the tubing that might cause bladder distention.
11. Put on gloves. **Cleanse the irrigation port on the catheter with an alcohol swab. Using aseptic technique, attach irrigation tubing to irrigation port of three-way indwelling catheter (Figure 5).**	Aseptic technique prevents the spread of microorganisms into the bladder.
12. Check the drainage tubing to make sure clamp, if present, is open.	An open clamp prevents accumulation of solution in the bladder.
13. **Release clamp on irrigation tubing and regulate flow at determined drip rate, according to the ordered rate (Figure 6).** If the bladder irrigation is to be done with a medicated solution, use an electronic infusion device to regulate the flow.	This allows for continual gentle irrigation without causing discomfort to the patient. An electronic infusion device regulates the flow of the medication.

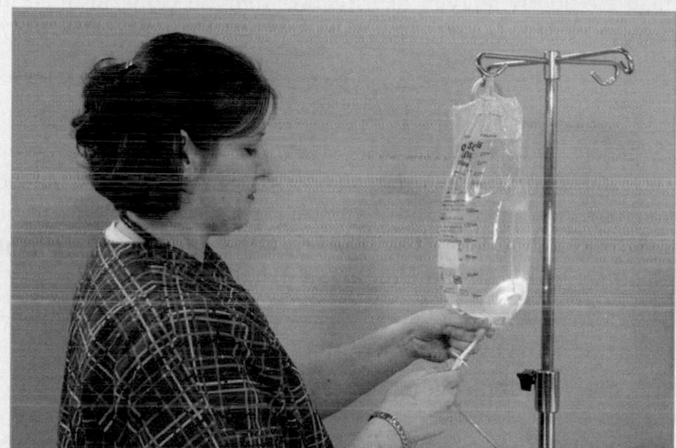
FIGURE 3 Inserting tubing into solution bag.

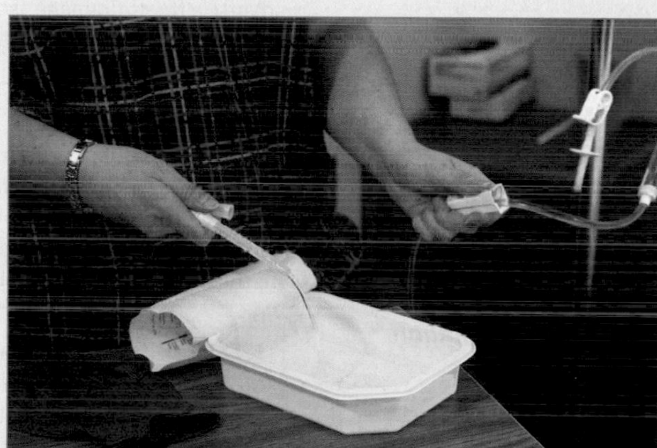
FIGURE 4 Removing air from irrigation tubing.

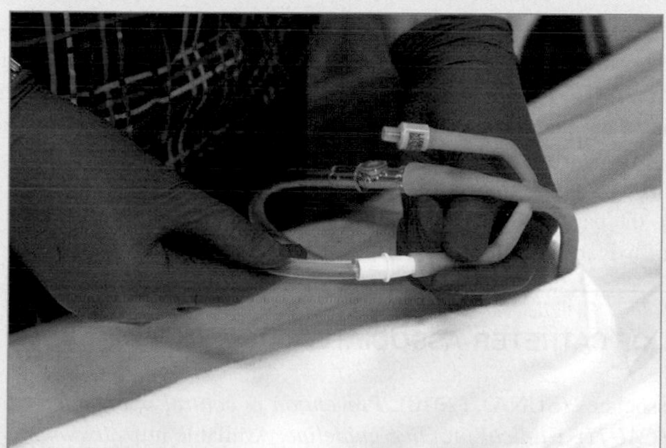
FIGURE 5 Attaching irrigation tubing to irrigation port on catheter.

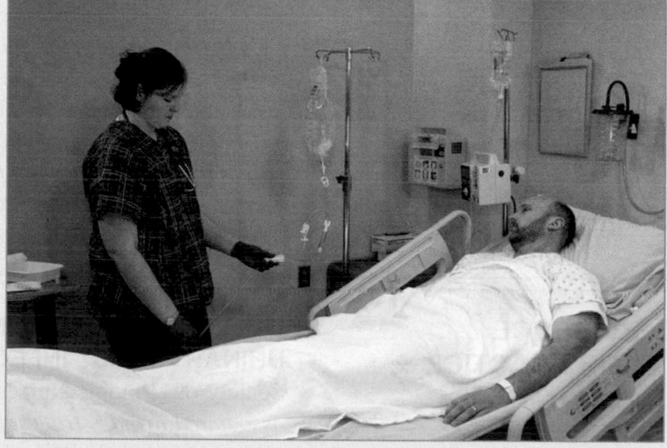
FIGURE 6 Regulating irrigation flow rate using flow clamp.

(*continued*)

SKILL 12-10 ADMINISTERING A CONTINUOUS CLOSED BLADDER OR CATHETER IRRIGATION continued

ACTION	RATIONALE
14. Remove gloves. Assist the patient to a comfortable position. Cover the patient with bed linens. Place the bed in the lowest position.	Positioning and covering provide warmth and promote comfort and safety.
15. Assess the patient's response to the procedure, and the quality and amount of drainage.	Assessment is necessary to determine the effectiveness of the intervention and to detect adverse effects.
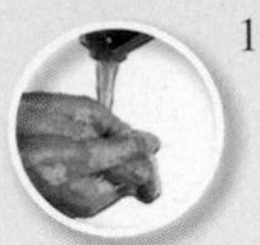 16. Remove equipment. Remove gloves and additional PPE, if used. Perform hand hygiene.	Proper disposal of equipment prevents transmission of microorganisms. Removing PPE properly reduces the risk for infection transmission and contamination of other items. Hand hygiene prevents the spread of microorganisms.
17. As irrigation fluid container nears empty, clamp the administration tubing. Do not allow drip chamber to empty. Disconnect empty bag and attach a new full irrigation solution bag.	This eliminates the need to separate tubing from the catheter and clear air from the tubing. Opening the drainage system provides access for microorganisms.
18. Put on gloves and empty drainage collection bag as each new container is hung and recorded.	Gloves protect against exposure to blood, body fluids, and microorganisms.

EVALUATION

The expected outcome is met when urine flows freely through the catheter. Effectiveness of therapy is determined by the urine characteristics. On completion of the therapy with continuous bladder irrigation, the patient should exhibit urine that is clear, without evidence of clots or debris. Other outcomes would include the following: the continuous bladder irrigation is administered without adverse effect; drainage is greater than the hourly amount of irrigation solution being instilled in bladder; and the patient exhibits no signs and symptoms of infection.

DOCUMENTATION

Guidelines

Document baseline assessment of the patient. Document the amount and type of irrigation solution used and the patient's tolerance of the procedure. Record urine amount emptied from the drainage bag before the procedure and the amount of irrigant used on intake and output record. Record the amount of urine and irrigant emptied from the drainage bag. **Subtract the amount of irrigant instilled from the total volume of drainage to obtain the volume of urine output.**

Sample Documentation

12/14/15 1330 Foley catheter replaced with 3-way Foley catheter. Bladder nonpalpable. Continuous bladder irrigation with normal saline initiated at 100 mL/hour. Patient tolerated procedure without adverse effect. Drainage from bladder slightly cloudy, light cherry colored. No evidence of clots.

—B. Clapp, RN

UNEXPECTED SITUATIONS AND ASSOCIATED INTERVENTIONS

- *Continuous bladder irrigation begins and hourly drainage is less than amount of irrigation being given:* Palpate for bladder distention. If the patient is lying supine, rolling the patient onto his/her side may help increase the amount of drainage. Check to make sure that the tubing is not kinked. If return flow remains decreased, notify primary care provider.
- *Bladder irrigation is not flowing at ordered rate, even with clamp wide open:* Check the tubing for kinks or pressure points. Raise the bag 3 to 6 inches and then check flow of irrigation solution. Frequently check flow rate of irrigation solution.

EVIDENCE FOR PRACTICE ▶

PREVENTION AND CONTROL OF CATHETER-ASSOCIATED URINARY TRACT INFECTION

Society of Urologic Nurses and Associates (SUNA). (2010). *Prevention & control of catheter-associated urinary tract infection (CAUTI). Clinical practice guideline.* Available https://www.suna.org/sites/default/files/download/cautiGuideline.pdf.

Refer to details in Skill 12-6, Evidence for Practice, and refer to thePoint for additional research on related nursing topics.

SKILL 12-11 EMPTYING AND CHANGING A STOMA APPLIANCE ON AN ILEAL CONDUIT

An **ileal conduit** is a cutaneous urinary diversion. An ileal conduit involves a surgical resection of the small intestine, with transplantation of the ureters to the isolated segment of small bowel. This separated section of the small intestine is then brought to the abdominal wall, where urine is excreted through a **stoma,** a surgically created opening on the body surface. Such diversions are usually permanent, and the patient wears an external appliance to collect the urine because urine elimination from the stoma cannot be controlled voluntarily. Appliances are available in a one-piece (barrier backing already attached to the pouch) or two-piece (separate pouch that fastens to the barrier backing) system; they are usually changed every 3 to 7 days, although they could be changed more often. Proper application minimizes the risk for skin breakdown around the stoma. This skill addresses changing a one-piece appliance. A one-piece appliance consists of a pouch with an integral adhesive section that adheres to the patient's skin. The adhesive flange is generally made from hydrocolloid. The accompanying Skill Variation addresses changing a two-piece appliance.

The appliance usually is changed after a time of low fluid intake, such as in the early morning. Urine production is less at this time, making changing the appliance easier. Proper application minimizes the risk for skin breakdown around the stoma. Box 12-3 summarizes guidelines for care of the patient with a urinary diversion.

Box 12-3 GUIDELINES FOR CARE OF THE PATIENT WITH A URINARY DIVERSION

- Keep the patient as free of odors as possible. If the patient has an external appliance, empty the appliance frequently.
- Inspect the patient's stoma regularly. It should be dark pink to red and moist. A pale stoma may indicate anemia, and a dark or purple-blue stoma may reflect compromised circulation or ischemia. Bleeding around the stoma and its stem should be minimal. Notify the primary care provider promptly if bleeding persists, is excessive, or if color changes occur in the stoma.
- Note the size of the stoma, which usually stabilizes within 6 to 8 weeks. Most stomas protrude 0.5 to 1 inch from the abdominal surface and may initially appear swollen and edematous. After 6 weeks, the edema usually subsides. If an abdominal dressing is in place at the incision site after surgery, check it frequently for drainage and bleeding.
- Keep the skin around the stoma site (peristomal area) clean and dry. If care is not taken to protect the skin around the stoma, irritation or infection may occur. A leaking appliance frequently causes skin erosion. Candida or yeast infections can also occur around the stoma if the area is not kept dry.
- Measure the patient's fluid intake and output. Careful monitoring of the patient's urinary output is necessary to monitor fluid balance.
- Monitor the return of intestinal function and peristalsis. Initially after surgery, peristalsis is inhibited. Remember, the patient had a bowel resection as part of the urinary diversion procedure.
- Watch for mucus in the urine from an ileal conduit, which is a normal finding. The isolated segment of small intestine continues to produce mucus as part of its normal functioning.
- Explain each aspect of care to the patient and explain what his/her role will be when he or she begins self-care. Patient teaching is one of the most important aspects of ostomy care and should include family members, when appropriate. Teaching can begin before surgery so that the patient has adequate time to absorb the information.
- Encourage the patient to participate in care and to look at the stoma. Patients normally experience emotional depression during the early postoperative period. Help the patient to cope by listening, explaining, and being available and supportive. A visit from a representative of the local ostomy support group may be helpful. Patients usually begin to accept their altered body image when they are willing to look at the stoma, make neutral or positive statements concerning the ostomy, and express interest in learning self-care.

DELEGATION CONSIDERATIONS

The empting of a stoma appliance on an ileal conduit may be delegated to nursing assistive personnel (NAP) or to unlicensed assistive personnel (UAP), as well as to licensed practical/vocational nurses (LPN/LVNs). The changing of a stoma appliance on an ileal conduit may be delegated to LPN/LVNs. The decision to delegate must be based on careful analysis of the patient's needs and circumstances, as well as the qualifications of the person to whom the task is being delegated. Refer to the Delegation Guidelines in Appendix A.

(continued)

SKILL 12-11 EMPTYING AND CHANGING A STOMA APPLIANCE ON AN ILEAL CONDUIT continued

EQUIPMENT

- Basin with warm water
- Skin cleanser, towel, washcloth
- Silicone-based adhesive remover
- Gauze squares
- Skin protectant, such as SkinPrep™
- Ostomy appliance
- Stoma measuring guide
- Graduated container
- Ostomy belt (optional)
- Disposable gloves
- Additional PPE, as indicated
- Waterproof, disposable pad
- Small plastic trash bag

ASSESSMENT

Assess current ileal conduit appliance, observing product style, condition of appliance, and stoma (if bag is clear). Note length of time the appliance has been in place. Determine the patient's knowledge of ileal conduit care, including level of self-care and ability to manipulate the equipment. After the appliance is removed, assess the skin surrounding the ileal conduit. Assess the condition of any abdominal scars or incisional areas, if surgery to create the urinary diversion was recent.

NURSING DIAGNOSIS

Determine the related factors for the nursing diagnoses based on the patient's current status. Possible nursing diagnoses may include:

- Disturbed Body Image
- Risk for Impaired Skin Integrity
- Deficient Knowledge

OUTCOME IDENTIFICATION AND PLANNING

The expected outcome to achieve when changing a patient's urinary stoma appliance is that the stoma appliance is applied correctly to the skin to allow urine to drain freely. Other outcomes may include the following: the patient exhibits a moist red stoma with intact skin surrounding the stoma; the patient demonstrates knowledge of how to apply the appliance; and the patient verbalizes positive self-image.

IMPLEMENTATION

ACTION	RATIONALE
1. Gather equipment.	Assembling equipment provides for an organized approach to the task.
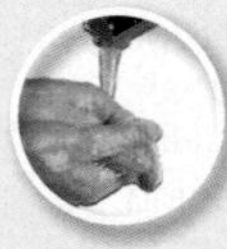 2. Perform hand hygiene and put on PPE, if indicated.	Hand hygiene and PPE prevent the spread of microorganisms. PPE is required based on transmission precautions.
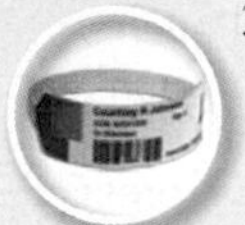 3. Identify the patient.	Identifying the patient ensures the right patient receives the intervention and helps prevent errors.
4. Close the curtains around the bed and close the door to the room, if possible. Explain what you are going to do and why you are going to do it to the patient. Encourage the patient to observe or participate, if possible.	This ensures the patient's privacy. Explanation relieves anxiety and facilitates cooperation. Discussion promotes cooperation and helps to minimize anxiety. Having the patient observe or assist encourages self-acceptance.
5. Assemble equipment on overbed table within reach.	Arranging items nearby is convenient, saves time, and avoids unnecessary stretching and twisting of muscles on the part of the nurse.
6. Assist the patient to a comfortable sitting or lying position in bed or a standing or sitting position in the bathroom. If the patient is in bed, adjust the bed to a comfortable working height, usually elbow height of the caregiver (VISN 8 Patient Safety Center, 2009). Place waterproof pad under the patient at the stoma site.	Either position should allow the patient to view the procedure in preparation for learning to perform it independently. Lying flat or sitting upright facilitates smooth application of the appliance. Having the bed at the proper height prevents back and muscle strain. A waterproof pad protects linens and the patient from moisture.

ACTION	RATIONALE
Emptying the Appliance	
7. Put on gloves. Hold end of appliance over a bedpan, toilet, or measuring device. Remove the end cap from the spout. Open the spout and empty the contents into the bedpan, toilet, or measuring device (Figure 1).	Gloves protect the nurse from exposure to blood and body fluids. Emptying the pouch before handling it reduces the likelihood of spilling the excretions.

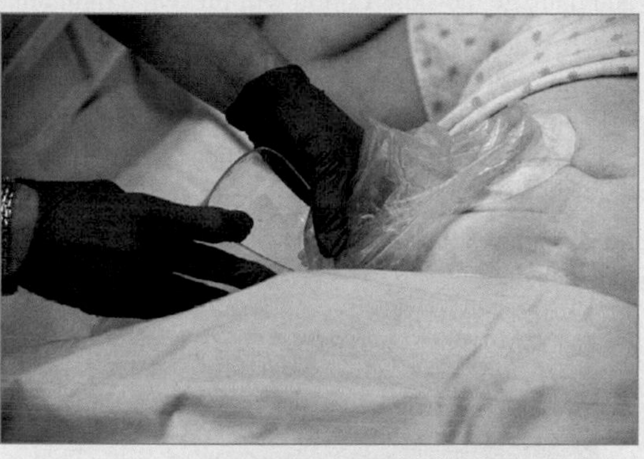

FIGURE 1 Emptying urine into graduated container.

ACTION	RATIONALE
8. Close the spout. Wipe the spout with toilet tissue. Replace the cap.	Drying the spout removes any urine.
9. Remove equipment. Remove gloves. Assist the patient to a comfortable position.	Proper removal of PPE prevents the transmission of microorganisms. Ensures patient comfort.
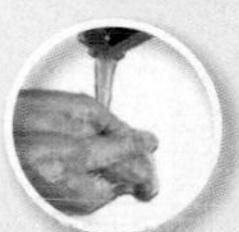 10. If appliance is not to be changed, place bed in lowest position. Remove additional PPE, if used. Perform hand hygiene.	Lowering the bed promotes patient safety. Removing PPE properly reduces the risk for infection transmission and contamination of other items. Hand hygiene prevents the spread of microorganisms.
Changing the Appliance	
11. Place a disposable waterproof pad on the overbed table or other work area. Set up the washbasin with warm water and the rest of the supplies. Place a trash bag within reach.	The pad protects the surface. Organization facilitates performance of the procedure.
12. Put on clean gloves. Place waterproof pad under the patient at the stoma site. Empty the appliance, if necessary, as described in steps 6–8.	Waterproof pad protects linens and patient from moisture. Emptying the contents before removal prevents accidental spillage of fecal material.
13. Gently remove the appliance faceplate, starting at the top and keeping the abdominal skin taut (Figure 2). Remove appliance faceplate from skin by pushing skin from appliance rather than pulling appliance from skin (Figure 3). Apply a silicone-based adhesive remover by spraying or wiping with the remover wipe, as needed.	The seal between the surface of the faceplate and the skin must be broken before the faceplate can be removed. Harsh handling of the appliance can damage the skin and impair the development of a secure seal in the future. Silicone-based adhesive remover allows for the rapid and painless removal of adhesives and prevents skin stripping (Rudoni, 2008; Stephen-Haynes, 2008).

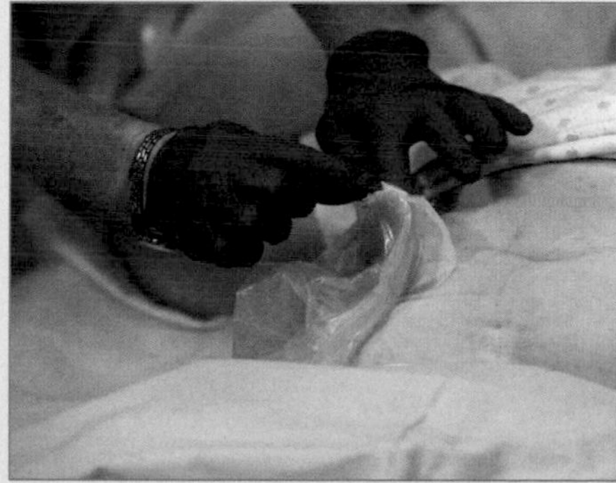

FIGURE 2 Gently removing appliance faceplate from skin.

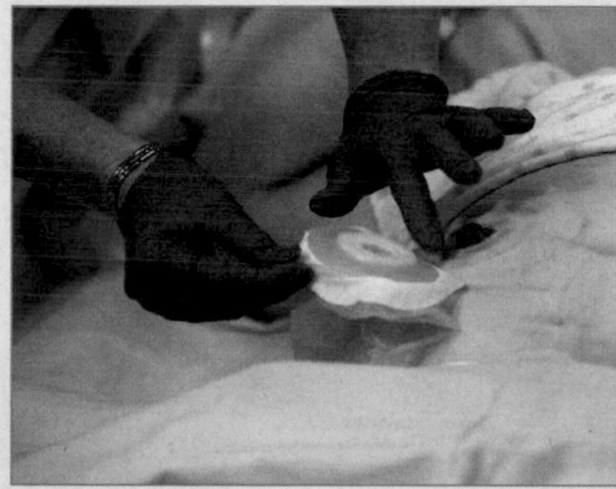

FIGURE 3 Pushing skin from appliance rather than pulling appliance from skin.

(*continued*)

SKILL 12-11 EMPTYING AND CHANGING A STOMA APPLIANCE ON AN ILEAL CONDUIT continued

ACTION	RATIONALE
14. Place the appliance in the trash bag, if disposable. If reusable, set aside to wash in lukewarm soap and water and allow to air dry after the new appliance is in place.	Thorough cleaning and airing of the appliance reduce odor and deterioration of appliance. For aesthetic and infection-control purposes, used appliances should be discarded appropriately.
15. Clean skin around stoma with mild skin cleanser and water or a cleansing agent and a washcloth (Figure 4). Remove all old adhesive from the skin; additional adhesive remover may be used. Do not apply lotion to the peristomal area.	Cleaning the skin removes excretions and old adhesive and skin protectant. Excretions or a buildup of other substances can irritate and damage the skin. Lotion will prevent a tight adhesive seal.
16. Gently pat area dry. **Make sure skin around stoma is thoroughly dry.** Assess stoma and condition of surrounding skin.	Careful drying prevents trauma to skin and stoma. An intact, properly applied urinary collection device protects skin integrity. Any change in color and size of the stoma may indicate circulatory problems.
17. Place one or two gauze squares over the stoma opening (Figure 5).	Continuous drainage must be absorbed to keep skin dry during appliance change.

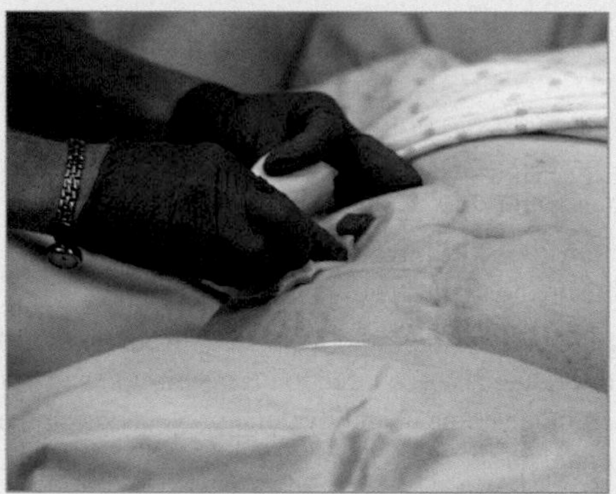

FIGURE 4 Cleaning stoma with cleansing agent and washcloth.

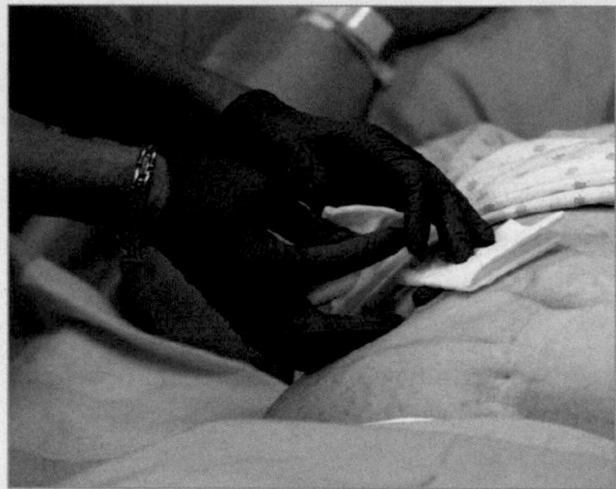

FIGURE 5 Placing one or two gauze squares over stoma opening.

ACTION	RATIONALE
18. Apply skin protectant to a 2-inch (5-cm) radius around the stoma, and allow it to dry completely, which takes about 30 seconds.	The skin needs protection from the potentially excoriating effect of the appliance adhesive. The skin must be perfectly dry before the appliance is placed to get good adherence and to prevent leaks.
19. Lift the gauze squares for a moment and measure the stoma opening, using the measurement guide. Replace the gauze. Trace the same size opening on the back center of the appliance. Cut the opening 1/8 inch larger than the stoma size (Figure 6). Use a finger to gently smooth the wafer edges after cutting. Check that the spout is closed and the end cap is in place.	The appliance should fit snugly around the stoma, with only 1/8 inch of skin visible around the opening. A faceplate opening that is too small can cause trauma to the stoma. If the opening is too large, exposed skin will be irritated by urine. Wafer edges may be uneven after cutting and could cause irritation to and/or pressure on the stoma. A closed spout and secured end cap prevent urine from leaking from the appliance.

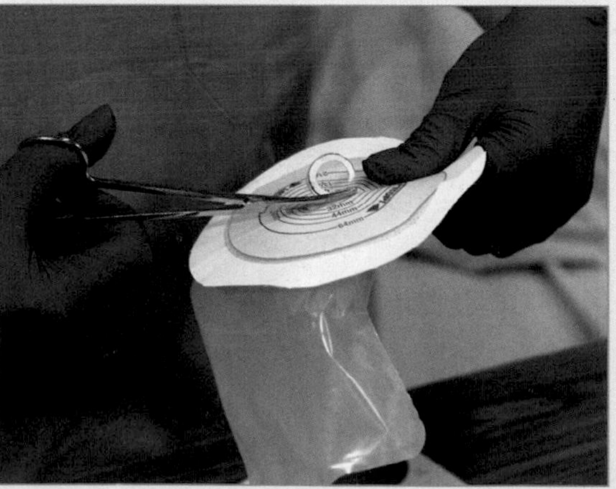

FIGURE 6 Cutting the faceplate opening 1/8 inch larger than stoma size.

ACTION	RATIONALE
20. Remove the paper backing from the appliance faceplate. Quickly remove the gauze squares and discard appropriately; ease the appliance over the stoma. Gently press onto the skin while smoothing over the surface (Figure 7). Apply gentle, even pressure to the appliance for approximately 30 seconds.	The appliance is effective only if it is properly positioned and adhered securely. Pressure on faceplate allows the faceplate to mold to the patient's skin and improves the seal.

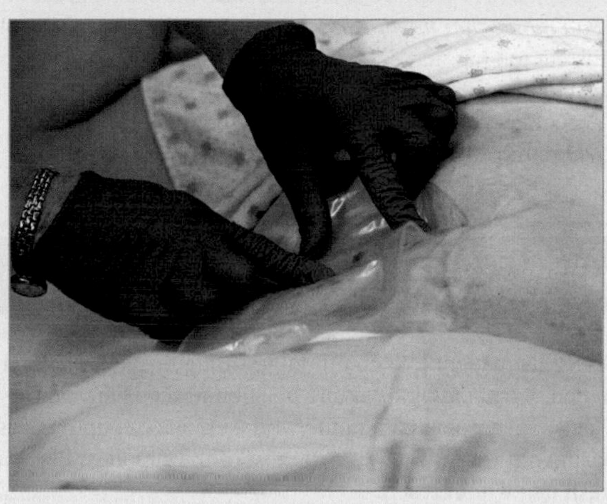

FIGURE 7 Applying faceplate over stoma.

ACTION	RATIONALE
21. Secure optional belt to appliance and around patient.	An elasticized belt helps support the appliance for some people.
22. Remove gloves. Assist the patient to a comfortable position. Cover the patient with bed linens. Place the bed in the lowest position.	Removing gloves reduces risk of transmission of microorganisms. Positioning and covering provide warmth and promote comfort. Bed in lowest position promotes patient safety.
23. Put on clean gloves. Remove or discard any remaining equipment and assess the patient's response to the procedure.	The patient's response may indicate acceptance of the ostomy as well as the need for health teaching.
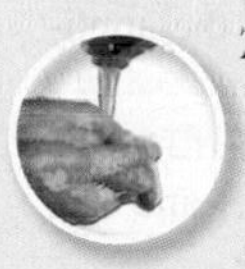 24. Remove gloves and additional PPE, if used. Perform hand hygiene.	Removing PPE properly reduces the risk for infection transmission and contamination of other items. Hand hygiene prevents the spread of microorganisms.

EVALUATION

The expected outcome is met when the ileal conduit appliance is changed without trauma to the stoma or peristomal skin, or leaking; urine is draining freely into the appliance; the skin surrounding the stoma is clean, dry, and intact; and the patient shows an interest in learning to perform the pouch change and verbalizes positive self-image.

DOCUMENTATION

Guidelines

Document the procedure, including the appearance of the stoma, condition of the peristomal skin, characteristics of the urine, the patient's response to the procedure, and pertinent patient teaching.

Sample Documentation

7/23/15 1245 Ileal conduit appliance changed. Mr. Jones present. Mrs. Jones asking questions about care for ileal conduit, states, "I don't know if I'll ever be able to care for this thing at home." Tearful at times. Patient encouraged to express feelings. Patient agreed to talk with wound, ostomy, and continence nurse about concerns. Mr. Jones very supportive, also asking appropriate questions. Patient states she would like to watch change one more time before she attempts to do it. Stoma is moist and red, peristomal skin intact, draining yellow urine with small amount of mucus.

—*B. Clapp, RN*

(*continued*)

SKILL 12-11 EMPTYING AND CHANGING A STOMA APPLIANCE ON AN ILEAL CONDUIT continued

UNEXPECTED SITUATIONS AND ASSOCIATED INTERVENTIONS

- *You remove appliance and find an area of skin excoriated:* Make sure that the appliance is not cut too large. Skin that is exposed inside of the ostomy appliance will become excoriated. Assess for the presence of a fungal skin infection. If present, consult with primary care provider to obtain appropriate treatment. Cleanse the skin thoroughly and pat dry. Apply products made for excoriated skin before placing appliance over stoma. Frequently check faceplate to ensure that a seal has formed and that there is no leakage. Confer with primary care provider for a wound, ostomy, and continence nurse consult to manage these issues. Document the excoriation in the patient's chart.
- *Faceplate is leaking after applying a new appliance:* Remove appliance, clean the skin, and start over.
- *You are ready to place the faceplate and notice that the opening is cut too large:* Discard appliance and begin over. A faceplate that is cut too big may lead to excoriation of the skin.
- *Stoma is dark brown or black:* Stoma should appear pink to red, shiny, and moist. Alterations indicate compromised circulation. If the stoma is dark brown or black, suspect ischemia and necrosis. Notify the primary care provider immediately.

SKILL VARIATION Applying a Two-Piece Appliance

A two-piece colostomy appliance is composed of a pouch and a separate adhesive faceplate that 'click' together (Figure A). The faceplate is left in place for a period of time, usually 3 to 7 days. During this period, when the appliance requires changing, only the bag needs to be replaced.

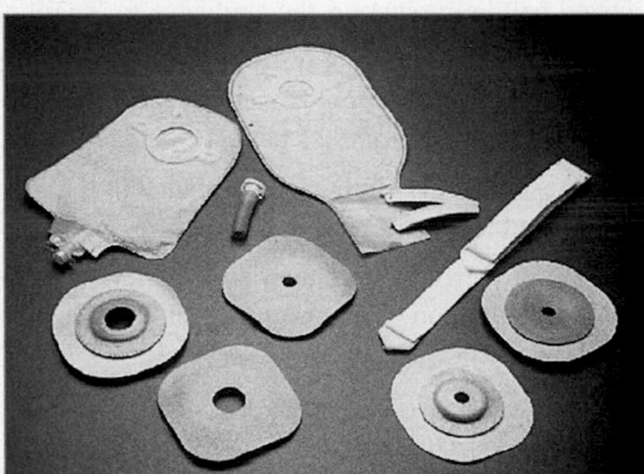

FIGURE A Two-piece appliances.

1. Gather necessary equipment.

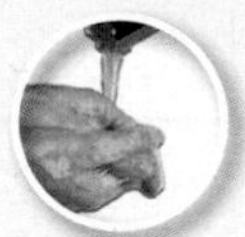

2. Perform hand hygiene and put on PPE, if indicated.

3. Identify the patient.

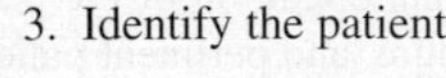

4. Close the curtains around the bed and close the door to room, if possible. Explain what you are going to do and why you are going to do it to the patient. Encourage the patient to observe or participate, if possible.
5. Assemble equipment on overbed table within reach.
6. Assist the patient to a comfortable sitting or lying position in bed or a standing or sitting position in the bathroom.
7. Place a disposable pad on the work surface. Set up the wash basin with warm water and the rest of the supplies. Place a trash bag within reach.
8. Put on gloves. Place waterproof pad under the patient at the stoma site. Empty the appliance as described previously in Skill 12-11.
9. Gently remove pouch faceplate from skin by pushing skin from appliance rather than pulling appliance from skin. Start at the top of the appliance, while keeping the abdominal skin taut. Apply a silicone-based adhesive remover by spraying or wiping with the remover wipe. Push the skin from the appliance rather than pulling the appliance from the skin.
10. Place the appliance in the trash bag, if disposable. If reusable, set aside to wash in lukewarm soap and water and allow to air dry after the new appliance is in place.
11. Clean skin around the stoma with a mild skin cleanser and water or a cleansing agent and a washcloth. Remove all old adhesive from skin; additional adhesive remover may be used. Do not apply lotion to peristomal area.
12. Gently pat area dry. Make sure skin around the stoma is thoroughly dry. Assess stoma and condition of surrounding skin. Place one or two gauze squares over stoma opening.
13. Apply skin protectant to a 2-inch (5 cm) radius around the stoma, and allow it to dry completely, which takes about 30 seconds
14. Lift the gauze squares for a moment and measure the stoma opening, using the measurement guide. Replace the gauze. Trace the same-size opening on the back center of the appliance faceplate. Cut the opening 1/8 inch larger than the stoma size. Use a finger to gently smooth the wafer edges after cutting.
15. Remove the backing from the faceplate. Quickly remove the gauze squares and ease the faceplate over the stoma. Gently press onto the skin while smoothing over the surface.

SKILL VARIATION Applying a Two-Piece Appliance continued

Apply gentle pressure to the faceplate for approximately 30 seconds (Figure B).

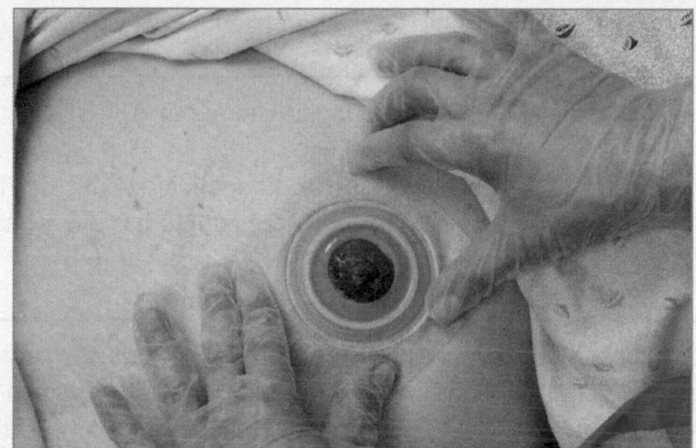

FIGURE B Gently pressing faceplate to skin.

16. Apply the appliance pouch to the faceplate following manufacturer's directions. Check that the spout is closed and the end cap is in place. If using a 'click' system, lay the ring on the pouch over the ring on the faceplate. Ask the patient to tighten stomach muscles, if possible. Beginning at one edge of the ring, push the pouch ring onto the faceplate ring. A 'click' should be heard when the pouch is secured onto the faceplate.
17. Remove gloves. Assist the patient to a comfortable position. Cover the patient with bed linens. Place the bed in the lowest position.
18. Put on clean gloves. Remove or discard equipment and assess the patient's response to the procedure.
19. Remove gloves and additional PPE, if used. Perform hand hygiene.

SKILL 12-12 CARING FOR A SUPRAPUBIC URINARY CATHETER

A **suprapubic urinary catheter** may be used for long-term continuous urinary drainage. This type of catheter is surgically inserted through a small incision above the pubic area (Figure 1). Suprapubic bladder drainage diverts urine from the urethra when injury, stricture, prostatic obstruction, or gynecologic or abdominal surgery has compromised the flow of urine through the urethra. A suprapubic catheter is often preferred over indwelling urethral catheters for long-term urinary drainage. Suprapubic catheters are associated with decreased risk of contamination with organisms from fecal material, elimination of damage to the urethra, a higher rate of patient satisfaction, and lower risk of catheter-associated urinary tract infections. The drainage tube is secured with sutures or tape. Care of the patient with a suprapubic catheter includes skin care around the insertion site; care of the drainage tubing and drainage bag is the same as for an indwelling catheter. (Refer to Box 12-1, in Skill 12-6.)

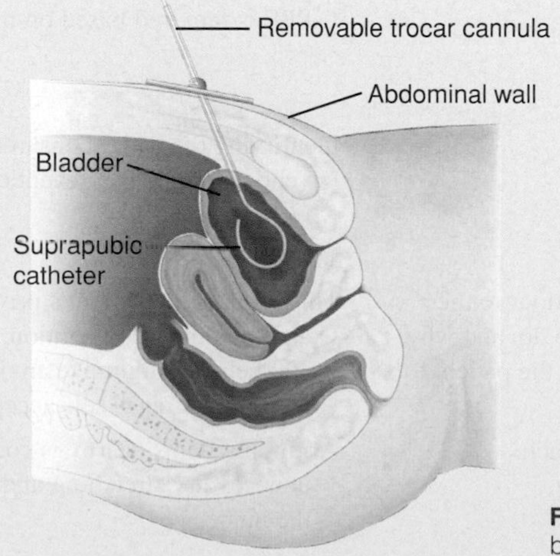

FIGURE 1 A suprapubic catheter positioned in bladder.

(continued)

SKILL 12-12 CARING FOR A SUPRAPUBIC URINARY CATHETER continued

DELEGATION CONSIDERATIONS

The care of a suprapubic urinary catheter, in the postoperative period, is not delegated to nursing assistive personnel (NAP) or to unlicensed assistive personnel (UAP) in the acute care setting. The care of a healed suprapubic catheter site in some settings may be delegated to NAP or UAP who have received appropriate training, after assessment of the catheter by the registered nurse. Depending on the state's nurse practice act and the organization's policies and procedures, the care of a suprapubic urinary catheter may be delegated to licensed practical/vocational nurses (LPN/LVNs). The decision to delegate must be based on careful analysis of the patient's needs and circumstances, as well as the qualifications of the person to whom the task is being delegated. Refer to the Delegation Guidelines in Appendix A.

EQUIPMENT

- Washcloth
- Skin cleanser and water
- Disposable gloves
- Additional PPE, as indicated
- Velcro tube holder or tape to secure tube
- Drainage sponge (if necessary)
- Plastic trash bag
- Sterile cotton-tipped applicators and sterile saline solution (if the patient has a new suprapubic catheter)

ASSESSMENT

Assess the suprapubic catheter and bag, observing the condition of the catheter and the drainage bag connected to the catheter, and the product style. If a dressing is in place at the insertion site, assess the dressing for drainage. Inspect the site around the suprapubic catheter, looking for drainage, erythema, or excoriation. Assess the method used to secure the catheter in place. If sutures are present, assess for intactness. Also, assess the characteristics of the urine in the drainage bag. Assess the patient's knowledge of caring for a suprapubic catheter.

NURSING DIAGNOSIS

Determine the related factors for the nursing diagnoses based on the patient's current status. Possible nursing diagnoses may include:

- Impaired Urinary Elimination
- Risk for Infection
- Deficient Knowledge

OUTCOME IDENTIFICATION AND PLANNING

The expected outcomes to be achieved when caring for a suprapubic catheter are that the patient's skin remains clean, dry, and intact, without evidence of irritation or breakdown; and the patient verbalizes an understanding of the purpose for, and care of, the catheter, as appropriate. Other appropriate outcomes include the following: the patient's urinary elimination is maintained, with a urine output of at least 30 mL/hour, and the patient's bladder is not distended.

IMPLEMENTATION

ACTION	RATIONALE
1. Gather equipment.	Assembling equipment provides for an organized approach to task.
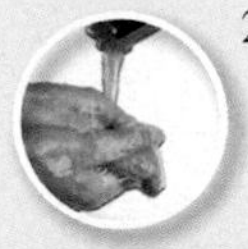 2. Perform hand hygiene and put on PPE, if indicated.	Hand hygiene and PPE prevent the spread of microorganisms. PPE is required based on transmission precautions.
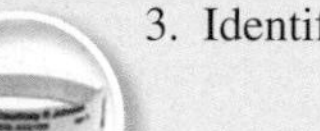 3. Identify the patient.	Identifying the patient ensures the right patient receives the intervention and helps prevent errors.
4. Close the curtains around the bed and close the door to the room, if possible. Explain what you are going to do, and why you are going to do it, to the patient. Encourage the patient to observe or participate, if possible.	This ensures the patient's privacy. Explanation relieves anxiety and facilitates cooperation. Discussion promotes cooperation and helps to minimize anxiety. Having the patient observe or assist encourages self-acceptance.
5. Assemble equipment on overbed table within reach.	Arranging items nearby is convenient, saves time, and avoids unnecessary stretching and twisting of muscles on the part of the nurse.

ACTION	RATIONALE
6. Adjust the bed to a comfortable working height, usually elbow height of the caregiver (VISN 8 Patient Safety Center, 2009). Assist the patient to a supine position. Place waterproof pad under the patient at the stoma site.	Having the bed at the proper height prevents back and muscle strain. The supine position is usually the best way to gain access to the suprapubic urinary catheter. A waterproof pad protects linens and patient from moisture.
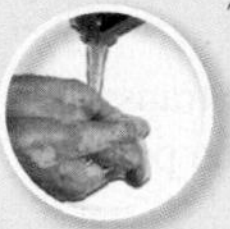 7. Put on clean gloves. Gently remove old dressing, if one is in place. Place dressing in trash bag. Remove gloves. Perform hand hygiene.	Gloves protect the nurse from blood, body fluids, and microorganisms. Proper disposal of contaminated dressing and hand hygiene deter the spread of microorganisms.
8. Assess the insertion site and surrounding skin.	Any changes in assessment could indicate potential infection.
9. Wet washcloth with warm water and apply skin cleanser. **Gently cleanse around suprapubic exit site (Figure 2).** Remove any encrustations. If this is a new suprapubic catheter, use sterile cotton-tipped applicators and sterile saline to clean the site until the incision has healed. Moisten the applicators with the saline. **Clean in circular motion from the insertion site outward (Figure 3).**	Using a gentle skin cleanser helps to protect the skin. The exit site is the most common area of skin irritation with a suprapubic catheter. If encrustations are left on the skin, they provide a medium for bacteria and an area of skin irritation.
10. Rinse area of all cleanser. Pat dry.	The skin needs to be kept dry to prevent any irritation.
11. If the exit site has been draining, place a small drain sponge around the catheter to absorb any drainage (Figure 4). Be prepared to change this sponge throughout the day, depending on the amount of drainage. Do not cut a 4 × 4 gauze to make a drain sponge.	A small amount of drainage from the exit site is normal. The sponge needs to be changed when it becomes soiled to prevent skin irritation and breakdown. The fibers from a cut 4 × 4 gauze may enter the exit site and cause irritation or infection.
12. Remove gloves. Form a loop in the tubing and anchor it on the patient's abdomen (Figure 5).	Anchoring the catheter and tubing absorbs any tugging, preventing tension on, and irritation to, the skin or bladder.

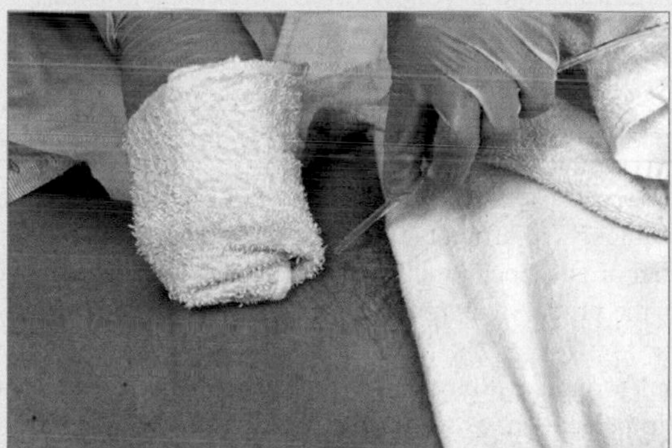

FIGURE 2 Cleaning area around catheter site with skin cleanser and water.

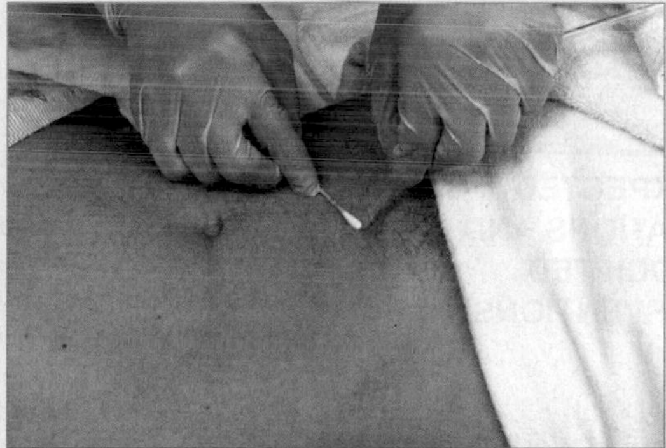

FIGURE 3 Using sterile cotton-tipped applicators for cleaning.

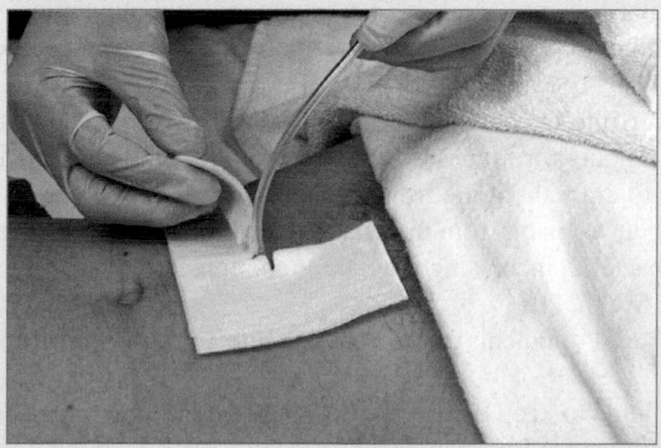

FIGURE 4 Applying small drain sponge around catheter.

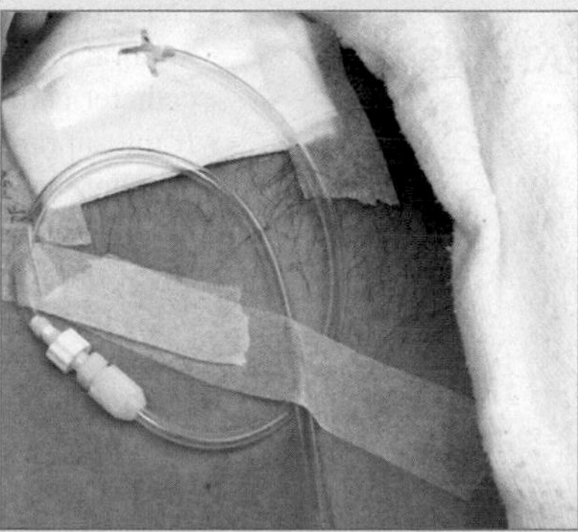

FIGURE 5 Forming a loop in tubing and taping to abdomen.

(continued)

SKILL 12-12 CARING FOR A SUPRAPUBIC URINARY CATHETER continued

ACTION	RATIONALE
13. Assist the patient to a comfortable position. Cover the patient with bed linens. Place the bed in the lowest position.	Positioning and covering provide warmth and promote comfort. Bed in lowest position promotes patient safety.
14. Put on clean gloves. Remove or discard equipment and assess the patient's response to the procedure.	Gloves prevent contact with blood and body fluids. The patient's response may indicate acceptance of the catheter or the need for health teaching.
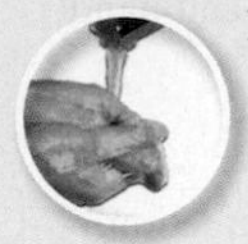 15. Remove gloves and additional PPE, if used. Perform hand hygiene.	Removing PPE properly reduces the risk for infection transmission and contamination of other items. Hand hygiene prevents the spread of microorganisms.

EVALUATION

The expected outcomes are met when the patient's skin remains clean, dry, and intact, without evidence of irritation or breakdown; the patient verbalizes an understanding of the purpose for, and care of, the catheter, as appropriate; the patient's urinary elimination is maintained, with a urine output of at least 30 mL/hour; and the patient's bladder is not distended.

DOCUMENTATION

Guidelines

Document the appearance of catheter exit site and surrounding skin, urine amount and characteristics, as well as patient's reaction to the procedure.

Sample Documentation

7/12/15 1845 Suprapubic catheter care performed. Patient assisted in care. Skin is slightly erythematous on R side where catheter was taped. Catheter taped to L side. Small amount of yellow, clear drainage noted on drain sponge. Patient would like to try to go without drain sponge at this time. Instructions given to call nurse if amount of drainage increases. Moderate amount of clear yellow urine continues to drain from catheter into collection bag.

—*B. Clapp, RN*

UNEXPECTED SITUATIONS AND ASSOCIATED INTERVENTIONS

- *When cleaning the site, the catheter becomes dislodged and pulls out:* Notify primary care provider. Site of insertion can close fairly quickly, so prompt attention is needed (Bullman, 2011). If this is a well-healed site, the physician or advanced practice nurse can replace a new catheter easily. If this is a new suprapubic tube, the primary care provider may want to assess for any trauma to the bladder wall.
- *Exit site is extremely excoriated:* Consult wound, ostomy, and incontinence nurse for evaluation. A skin protectant or barrier may need to be applied, as well as more frequent cleansing of the area and changing of the drain sponge (if applied).

SPECIAL CONSIDERATIONS

- Depending on the patient's situation, he or she may have both a suprapubic and indwelling urethral catheter. Urine will drain from both catheters; usually, drainage from the suprapubic catheter is the larger volume.
- If the suprapubic catheter is not draining into the bag but, instead, has a valve at the end of the catheter, open the valve at least every 6 hours (or more frequently depending on the order in the medical record or institutional policy) to drain the urine from the bladder.
- Remove dressings at the exit site when any oozing from the wound has diminished. Prolonged dressings around the site may harbor bacteria, increasing the risk of site infection, and contribute to over-granulation at the site (Rew & Smith, 2011).
- The use of antiseptics and petroleum-based ointments at the insertion site are not recommended (Bullman, 2011; Rew & Smith, 2011).
- Encourage patients to drink adequate fluids to keep the urine clear and free flowing; residual urine can lead to stone formation and infection (Bullman, 2011).

SKILL 12-13 CARING FOR A PERITONEAL DIALYSIS CATHETER

Peritoneal dialysis is a method of removing fluid and wastes from the body of a patient with kidney failure. A catheter inserted through the abdominal wall into the peritoneal cavity allows a special fluid (dialysate) to be infused and then drained from the body, removing waste products and excess fluid (Figure 1). The exit site should be protected and kept clean and dry to allow for healing, which will take approximately 2 to 3 weeks (Lee & Park, 2012). Exit site dressings are initially changed weekly, until the site is healed. Frequent dressing changes in the immediate postoperative period are not necessary unless there is excessive oozing, bleeding, or signs of infection, to decrease the risk of contamination and unnecessary movement of the catheter (Lee & Park, 2012). Once the exit site has healed, exit site care is an important part of patient care. The catheter insertion site is a site for potential infection, possibly leading to catheter tunnel infection and **peritonitis,** therefore, meticulous care is needed. The incidence of exit site infections can be reduced through a cleansing regimen by the patient or caregiver. Chronic exit site care is performed daily or every other day (Hain & Chan, 2013). In the postoperative period, catheter care is performed using aseptic technique, to reduce the risk for a health care-acquired infection. At home, clean technique can be used by the patient and caregivers.

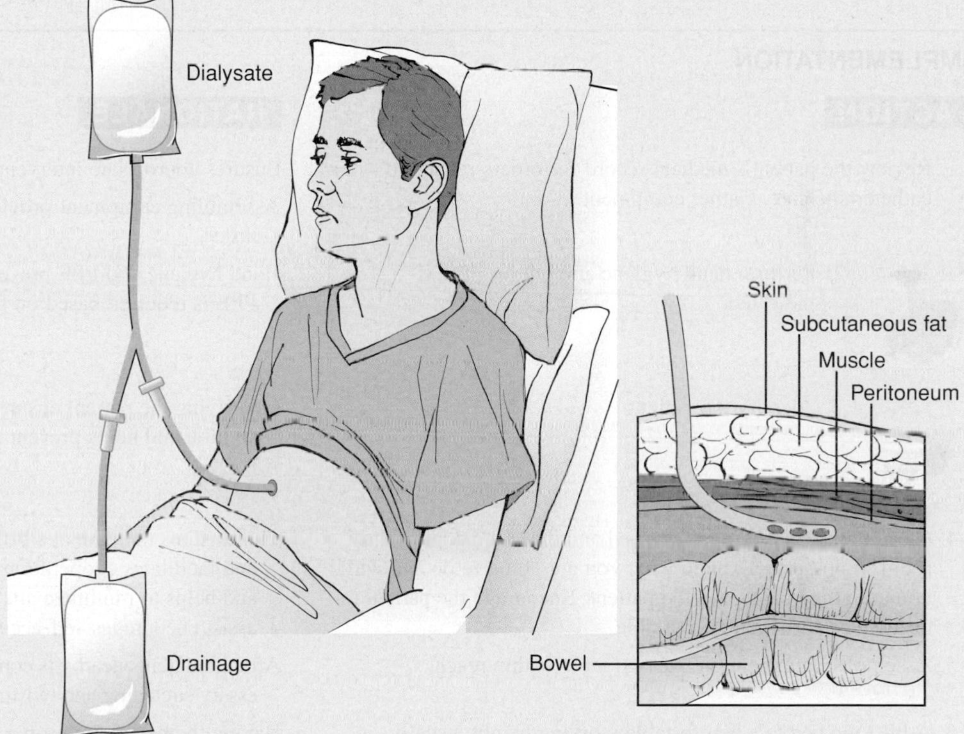

FIGURE 1 Position of catheter in peritoneal space. Patient is set up for peritoneal dialysis.

DELEGATION CONSIDERATIONS

The care of a peritoneal dialysis catheter is not delegated to nursing assistive personnel (NAP) or to unlicensed assistive personnel (UAP). Depending on the state's nurse practice act and the organization's policies and procedures, care of a peritoneal dialysis catheter may be delegated to licensed practical/vocational nurses (LPN/LVNs). The decision to delegate must be based on careful analysis of the patient's needs and circumstances, as well as the qualifications of the person to whom the task is being delegated. Refer to the Delegation Guidelines in Appendix A.

EQUIPMENT

- Face masks (2)
- Sterile gloves
- Nonsterile gloves
- Additional PPE, as indicated
- Antimicrobial cleansing agent, per facility policy
- Sterile gauze squares (4)
- Sterile basin
- Sterile drain sponge
- Transparent, occlusive site dressing
- Topical antibiotic, such as mupirocin or gentamicin, depending on order and policy
- Sterile applicator
- Plastic trash bag
- Bath blanket

(*continued*)

SKILL 12-13 CARING FOR A PERITONEAL DIALYSIS CATHETER continued

ASSESSMENT

Inspect the peritoneal dialysis catheter exit site for any erythema, drainage, bleeding, tenderness, swelling, skin irritation or breakdown, or leakage. These signs could indicate exit site or tunnel infection. Assess abdomen for tenderness, pain, and guarding. Assess the patient for nausea, vomiting, and fever, which could indicate peritonitis. Assess the patient's knowledge about measures used to care for the exit site.

NURSING DIAGNOSIS

Determine the related factors for the nursing diagnoses based on the patient's current status. Possible nursing diagnoses include:

- Risk for Impaired Skin Integrity
- Risk for Infection
- Deficient Knowledge

OUTCOME IDENTIFICATION AND PLANNING

The expected outcomes to achieve when performing care for a peritoneal dialysis catheter are as follows: the peritoneal dialysis catheter dressing change is completed using aseptic technique without trauma to the site or patient; the site is clean, dry, and intact, without evidence of inflammation or infection; and the patient exhibits fluid balance and participates in care, as appropriate.

IMPLEMENTATION

ACTION	RATIONALE
1. Review the patient's medical record for orders related to catheter site care. Gather equipment.	Ensures appropriate interventions for the patient. Assembling equipment provides for an organized approach to the task.
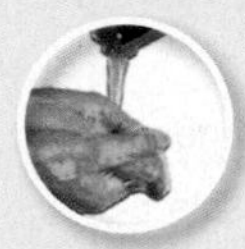 2. Perform hand hygiene and put on PPE, if indicated.	Hand hygiene and PPE prevent the spread of microorganisms. PPE is required based on transmission precautions.
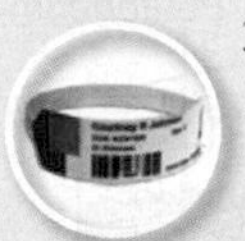 3. Identify the patient.	Identifying the patient ensures the right patient receives the intervention and helps prevent errors.
4. Close the curtains around the bed and close the door to the room, if possible. Explain what you are going to do and why you are going to do it to the patient. Encourage the patient to observe or participate if possible.	This ensures the patient's privacy. Explanation relieves anxiety and facilitates cooperation. Discussion promotes cooperation and helps to minimize anxiety. Having the patient observe or assist encourages self-acceptance.
5. Assemble equipment on overbed table within reach.	Arranging items nearby is convenient, saves time, and avoids unnecessary stretching and twisting of muscles on the part of the nurse.
6. Adjust the bed to a comfortable working height, usually elbow height of the caregiver (VISN 8 Patient Safety Center, 2009). Assist the patient to a supine position. Expose the abdomen, draping the patient's chest with the bath blanket, exposing only the catheter site.	Having the bed at the proper height prevents back and muscle strain. The supine position is usually the best way to gain access to the peritoneal dialysis catheter. Use of bath blanket provides patient warmth and avoids unnecessary exposure.
7. Put on nonsterile gloves. Put on one of the facemasks; have patient put on the other mask.	Gloves protect the nurse from contact with blood and bodily fluids. Use of facemasks deters the spread of microorganisms.
8. Gently remove old dressing, noting odor, amount, and color of drainage; leakage and condition of skin around the catheter. Discard dressing in appropriate container.	Drainage, leakage, and skin condition can indicate problems with the catheter, such as infection.
9. Remove gloves and discard. Set up sterile field. Open packages. Using aseptic technique, place two sterile gauze squares in basin with antimicrobial agent. Leave two sterile gauze squares opened on sterile field. Alternately (based on facility's policy), place sterile antimicrobial swabs on the sterile field. Place sterile applicator on field. Squeeze a small amount of the topical antibiotic on one of the gauze squares on the sterile field.	Until catheter site has healed, aseptic technique is necessary for site care to prevent infection.

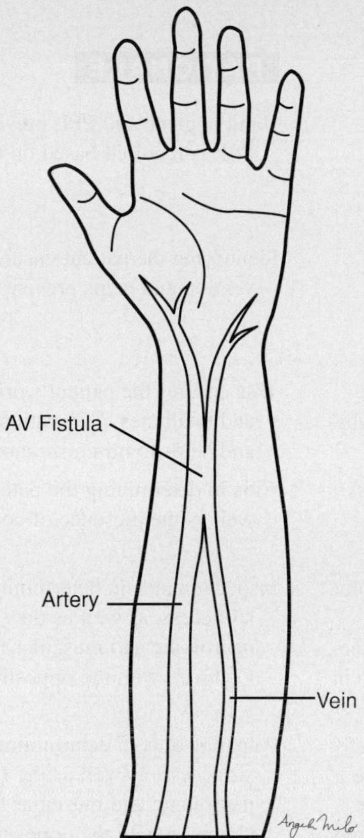

FIGURE 2 Arteriovenous fistula for hemodialysis

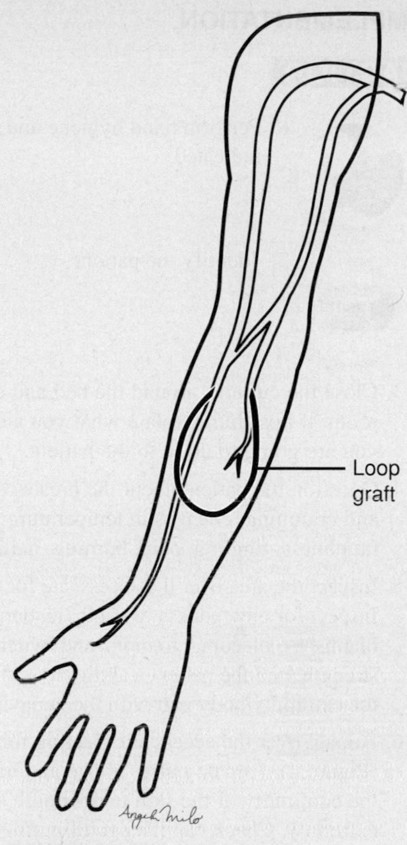

FIGURE 3 Arteriovenous graft for hemodialysis.

DELEGATION CONSIDERATIONS

The assessment of, and care for, a hemodialysis access is not delegated to nursing assistive personnel (NAP) or to unlicensed assistive personnel (UAP). Depending on the state's nurse practice act and the organization's policies and procedures, these procedures may be delegated to licensed practical/vocational nurses (LPN/LVNs). The decision to delegate must be based on careful analysis of the patient's needs and circumstances, as well as the qualifications of the person to whom the task is being delegated. Refer to the Delegation Guidelines in Appendix A.

EQUIPMENT

- Stethoscope
- PPE, as indicated

ASSESSMENT

Ask the patient how much he or she knows about caring for the site. Ask the patient to describe important observations to be made. Note the location of the access site. Assess the site for signs of infection, including inflammation, edema, and drainage; and for healing of the incision. Assess for patency by assessing for presence of **bruit** and **thrill** (refer to explanation in Step 4, below).

NURSING DIAGNOSIS

Determine the related factors for the nursing diagnoses based on the patient's current status. Possible nursing diagnoses include:

- Deficient Knowledge
- Risk for Injury

OUTCOME IDENTIFICATION AND PLANNING

The expected outcomes to achieve when caring for a hemodialysis catheter are that the graft or fistula remains patent, the patient verbalizes appropriate care measures and observations to be made, and the patient demonstrates appropriate care measures.

(continued)

SKILL 12-14 CARING FOR A HEMODIALYSIS ACCESS (ARTERIOVENOUS FISTULA OR GRAFT) continued

IMPLEMENTATION

ACTION	RATIONALE
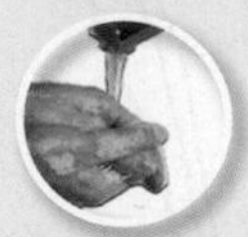 1. Perform hand hygiene and put on PPE, if indicated.	Hand hygiene and PPE prevent the spread of microorganisms. PPE is required based on transmission precautions.
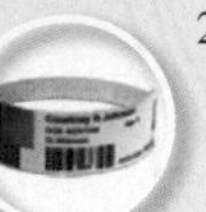 2. Identify the patient.	Identifying the patient ensures the right patient receives the intervention and helps prevent errors.
3. Close the curtains around the bed and close the door to the room, if possible. Explain what you are going to do, and why you are going to do it, to the patient.	This ensures the patient's privacy. Explanation relieves anxiety and facilitates cooperation. Discussion promotes cooperation and helps to minimize anxiety.
4. Question the patient about the presence of muscle weakness and cramping; changes in temperature; sensations, such as numbness, tingling, pain, burning, itchiness; and pain.	Aids in determining the patency of the hemodialysis access, as well as the presence of complications.
5. Inspect the area over the access site for continuity of skin color. Inspect for any redness, warmth, tenderness, edema, rash, blemishes, bleeding, tremors, and twitches. Inspect the muscle strength, and the patient's ability to perform range of motion in the extremity/body part with the hemodialysis access.	Inspection aids in determining the patency of the hemodialysis access, as well as the status of the patient's circulatory, neurologic and muscular function; and presence of infection. Compare with the opposite body area/part.
6. Palpate over the access site, feeling for a thrill or vibration (Figure 4). Palpate pulses above and below the site. Palpate the continuity of the skin temperature along and around the extremity. Check capillary refill in fingers or toes of extremity with the fistula or graft.	Palpation aids in determining the patency of the hemodialysis access, as well as the status of the patient's circulatory, neurologic and muscular function; and presence of infection. Compare with the opposite body area/part.

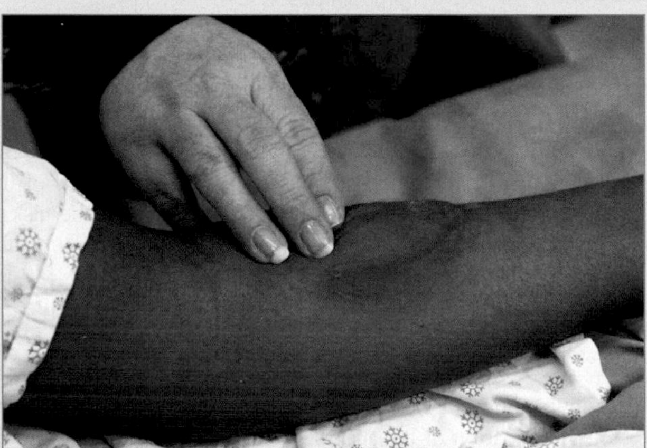

FIGURE 4 Palpating access site for thrill.

ACTION	RATIONALE
7. Auscultate over the access site with bell of stethoscope, listening for a bruit or vibration.	Palpation aids in determining the patency of the hemodialysis access.
8. Ensure that a sign is placed over the head of the bed informing the health care team which arm is affected. **Do not measure blood pressure, perform a venipuncture, or start an IV on the access arm.**	The affected arm should not be used for any other procedures, such as obtaining blood pressure, which could lead to clotting of the graft or fistula. Venipuncture or IV access could lead to an infection of the affected arm and could cause the loss of the graft or fistula.
9. Instruct the patient not to sleep with the arm with the access site under the head or body.	This could lead to clotting of the fistula or graft.
10. Instruct the patient not to lift heavy objects with, or put pressure on, the arm with the access site. Advise the patient not to carry heavy bags (including purses) on the shoulder of that arm.	This could lead to clotting of the fistula or graft.

ACTION

11. Remove PPE, if used. Perform hand hygiene.

RATIONALE

Removing PPE properly reduces the risk for infection transmission and contamination of other items. Hand hygiene prevents the spread of microorganisms.

EVALUATION

The expected outcome is met when the access site has an audible bruit and a palpable thrill; the site is intact without signs of adverse complications, or pain; and the patient verbalizes appropriate information about caring for the access site and observations to report.

DOCUMENTATION

Guidelines

Document assessment findings, including the presence or absence of a bruit and thrill. Document any patient education and patient response.

Sample Documentation

5/10/15 0830 Arteriovenous fistula patent in left upper arm. Area without redness, pain, or edema; skin at site similar to surrounding skin tone. Patient denies pain and tenderness. Positive bruit and thrill noted. Patient verbalized understanding the importance of avoiding venipuncture in left arm.

—B. Clapp, RN

Unexpected Situations and Associated Interventions

- *Thrill is diminished or not palpable and/or bruit is diminished or not audible:* Notify the primary care provider immediately. The thrill and bruit are caused by arterial blood flowing into the vein. If these signs are not present, the access may be clotting off.
- *Site is warm to touch, erythematous, or painful or has a skin blemish:* Notify the primary care provider. These signs can indicate a site infection.

EVIDENCE FOR PRACTICE ▶

HEMODIALYSIS AND PATIENT FATIGUE

Patients receiving chronic hemodialysis experience troubling symptoms that cause distress and adversely affect their quality of life. Fatigue is common and can be debilitating. What is the experience of patients receiving hemodialysis and how can nurses assist them in dealing with this issue?

Related Research

Horigan, A.E., Schneider, S.M., Docherty, S., & Barroso, J. (2013). The experience and self-management of fatigue in patients on hemodialysis. *Nephrology Nursing Journal, 40*(2), 113–122.

The aim of this qualitative descriptive study was to describe the experience and self-management of fatigue in patients on hemodialysis. Several themes were identified, including the nature of fatigue, management of fatigue, consequences of fatigue, and factors associated with fatigue. Patients described fatigue as having a lack of physical strength and energy, as well as mental fatigue, being not as mentally sharp as usual, unable to remember conversations, names of familiar individuals, and other short-term memory difficulties. Patients also described fatigue as difficult to manage, and expressed dissatisfaction with the degree of relief experienced with activities employed to alleviate fatigue. Fatigue also contributed to negative consequences affecting everyday life and activities, including having a negative effect on socialization, a decrease in the amount and quality of time spent with family members, and decreased participation in activities of daily living. Participants also reported poor sleep quality associated with fatigue, having trouble falling asleep, staying asleep, and difficulty staying awake in the daytime.

Relevance to Nursing Practice

This information can be valuable to nurses caring for these patients. The themes identified can be used to plan appropriate nursing interventions, and in planning areas in which nurses could be of support for patients with fatigue. The information can also be used to plan and implement appropriate patient education related to the fatigue associated with hemodialysis. Devising ways to manage symptoms is important to improve quality of life.

Refer to thePoint for additional research on related nursing topics.

ENHANCE YOUR UNDERSTANDING

FOCUSING ON PATIENT CARE: DEVELOPING CLINICAL REASONING

Consider the case scenarios at the beginning of the chapter as you answer the following questions to enhance your understanding and apply what you have learned.

QUESTIONS

1. When checking Ralph Bellow's condom catheter, you notice that, although the catheter is still in place, Mr. Bellow's bed is soaked with urine and there is very little urine in the catheter tubing. What should you do?
2. Grace Halligan is asking to go to the bathroom; she says, "I don't think I can go on a bedpan." You recheck the physician's orders and notice that Ms. Halligan is on strict bed rest. How can you help alleviate her concerns about using a bedpan?
3. Mike Wimmer notices that his peritoneal dialysis catheter insertion site is reddened and tender. He phones to ask what should be done. What should you tell Mike?

You can find suggested answers after the Bibliography at the end of this chapter.

INTEGRATED CASE STUDY CONNECTION

The case studies in Unit 3 are designed to focus on integrating concepts. Refer to the following case studies to enhance your understanding of the concepts related to the skills in this chapter.

- Basic Case Studies: Tiffany Jones, page 1064.
- Intermediate Case Studies: Lucille Howard, page 1086.
- Advanced Case Studies: Robert Espinoza, page 1097.

TAYLOR SUITE RESOURCES

Explore these additional resources to enhance learning for this chapter:

- NCLEX-Style Questions and other resources on thePoint, http://thePoint.lww.com/Lynn4e
- *Skill Checklists for Taylor's Clinical Nursing Skills,* 4e
- *Taylor's Video Guide to Clinical Nursing Skills:* Urinary Elimination and Indwelling and Intermittent Catheters
- *Fundamentals of Nursing:* Chapter 36, Urinary Elimination
- *Lippincott DocuCare* Fundamentals cases

Bibliography

Ackley, B.J., & Ladwig, G.B. (2011). *Nursing diagnosis handbook* (9th ed.). St. Louis: Mosby/Elsevier.

Adams, D., Bucior, H., Day, G., & Rimmer, J.A. (2012). HOUDINI: make that urinary catheter disappear - nurse-led protocol. *Journal of Infection Prevention, 13*(2), 44–46.

Altschuler, V., & Diaz, L. (2006). Bladder ultrasound. *MEDSURG Nursing, 15*(5), 317–318.

American Association of Critical Care Nurses (AACN). (2011). *AACN practice alert. Catheter-associated urinary tract infections.* Available http://www.aacn.org/WD/practice/docs/practicealerts/catheter-associated-uti-practice-alert.pdf.

American Cancer Society. (2011). *Urostomy.* Available http://www.cancer.org/treatment/treatmentsandsideeffects/physicalsideeffects/ostomies/urostomyguide/index.

Avent, Y. (2012). Wound wise: Understanding urinary diversions. *Nursing Made Incredibly Easy!, 10*(4), 47–52.

Bentley, A. (2012). Recommended practice. Stoma care: Older adults. *PACEsetterS, 9*(1), 23–25.

Bernard, M.S., Hunter, K.F., & Moore, K.N. (2012). Decrease the duration of indwelling urethral catheters and potentially reduce the incidence of catheter-associated urinary tract infections. *Urologic Nursing, 32*(1), 29–37.

Bernardini, J., Bender, F., Florio, T., et al. (2005). Randomized, double-blind trial of antibiotic exit site cream for prevention of exit site infection in peritoneal dialysis patients. *Journal of the American Society of Nephrology, 16*(2), 539–545.

Bhardwaj, R., Pickard, R., Carrick-Sen, D., & Brittain, K. (2012). Patients' perspectives on timing of urinary catheter removal after surgery. *British Journal of Nursing (Urology Supplement), 21*(18), S4–S9.

Boltz, M., Capezuti, E., Fulmer, T., & Zwicker, D. (Eds.). (2012). *Evidence-based geriatric nursing protocols for best practice* (4th ed.). New York: Springer Publishing Company.

Bourbonnais, F.F., & Tousignant, K.F. (2012). The pain experience of patients on maintenance hemodialysis. *Nephrology Nursing Journal, 39*(1), 13–19.

Bulechek, G.M, Butcher, H.K., Dochterman, J.M., & Wagner, C.M. (Eds.). (2013). *Nursing interventions classification (NIC)* (6th ed.). St. Louis, MO: Mosby Elsevier.

Bullman, S. (2011). Ins and outs of suprapubic catheters—a clinician's experience. *Urologic Nursing, 31*(5), 259–264.

Burch, J. (2011). Peristomal skin care and the use of accessories to promote skin health. *British Journal of Nursing, 20*(7), S4–S10.

Burch, J. (2010). Caring for peristomal skin: What every nurse should know. *British Journal of Nursing, 19*(3), 166–172.

Carrion, J. (2012). Vascular access devices for hemodialysis. *OR Nurse, 6*(1), 28–33.

Centers for Disease Control and Prevention (CDC). (2012). *Healthcare-associated infections (HAIs). Catheter-associated urinary tract infections (CAUTI).* Available http://www.cdc.gov/HAI/ca_uti/uti.html.

Cipa-Tatum, J., Kelly-Signs, M., & Afsart, K. (2011). Urethral erosion: A case for prevention. *Journal of Wound Ostomy & Continence Nursing, 38*(5), 581–583.

Cutright, J. (2011). The effect of the bladder scanner policy on the number of urinary catheters inserted. *Journal of Wound Ostomy Continence Nursing, 38*(1), 71–76.

Denyer, J. (2011). Reducing pain during the removal of adhesive and adherent products. *British Journal of Nursing, 20*(15) (Tissue Viability Supplement), S28–S35.

Gokula, M., Smolen, D., Gaspar, P.M., Hensley, S.J., Benninghoff, M.C., & Smith, M. (2012). Designing a protocol to reduce catheter-associated urinary tract infections among hospitalized patients. *American Journal of Infection Control, 40*(10), 1002–1004.

Gray, M.L. (2008). Securing the indwelling catheter. *American Journal of Nursing, 108*(12), 44–50.

Grossman, S., & Porth, C.M. (2014). Porth's pathophysiology: concepts of altered health states. (9th ed.). Philadelphia: Wolters Kluwer Health/Lippincott Williams & Wilkins.

Hain, D.J., & Chan, J. (2013). Best available evidence for peritoneal dialysis catheter exit-site care. *Nephrology Nursing Journal, 40*(1), 63–69.

Herter, R., & Wallace Kazer, M. (2010). Best practices in urinary catheter. *Home Healthcare Nurse, 28*(6), 342–349.

Hinkle, J.L., & Cheever, K.H. (2014). *Brunner & Suddarth's textbook of medical-surgical nursing* (13th ed.). Philadelphia: Wolters Kluwer Health/Lippincott Williams & Wilkins.

Hogan-Quigley, B., Palm, M.L., & Bickley, L. (2012). *Bates' nursing guide to physical examination and history taking.* Philadelphia: Wolters Kluwer Health/Lippincott Williams & Wilkins.

Hooton, T.M., Bradley, S.F., Cardenas, D.D., Colgan, R., Geerlings, S.E., Rice, J.C., et al. (2010). Diagnosis, prevention, and treatment of catheter-associated urinary tract infection in adults: 2009 international clinical practice guidelines from the Infectious Diseases Society of America. *Clinical Infectious Diseases, 50*(5), 625–663. Available http://www.idsociety.org/uploadedFiles/IDSA/Guidelines-Patient_Care/PDF_Library/Comp%20UTI.pdf.

Horigan, A.E., Schneider, S.M., Docherty, S., & Barroso, J. (2013). The experience and self-management of fatigue in patients on hemodialysis. *Nephrology Nursing Journal, 40*(2), 113–122.

Infusion Nurses Society (INS). (2011). Infusion nursing standards of practice. *Journal of Infusion Nursing, 34*(Suppl: 1S).

Jarvis, C. (2012). *Physical examination & health assessment* (6th ed.). St. Louis: Saunders/Elsevier.

The Joanna Briggs Institute. (2004). Clinical effectiveness of different approaches to peritoneal dialysis catheter exit-site care. *BestPractice, 8*(1), 1–7.

Kannankeril, A.J., Lam, H.T., Reyes, E.B., & McCartney, J. (2011). Urinary tract infection rates associated with re-use of catheters in clean intermittent catheterization of male veterans. *Urologic Nursing, 31*(1), 41–48.

Kyle, G. (2011). Reducing urethral catheterization trauma with urethral gels. *British Journal of Neuroscience Nursing, 7*(5), S8–S12.

Kyle, T., & Carman, S. (2013). *Essentials of pediatric nursing* (2nd ed.). Philadelphia: Wolters Kluwer Health/Lippincott Williams & Wilkins.

Lee, A., & Park, Y. (2012). Reducing peritoneal dialysis catheter exit site infections by implementing a standardized postoperative dressing protocol. *Renal Society of Australasia Journal, 8*(1), 18–22.

Logan, K. (2012). An overview of male intermittent self-catheterisation. *British Journal of Nursing, 21*(18), S18–S22.

Malarkey, L.M., & McMorrow, M.E. (2012). *Saunders nursing guide to laboratory and diagnostic tests* (2nd ed.). St. Louis: Elsevier Saunders.

Mangnall, J. (2012). Key considerations of intermittent catheterisation. *British Journal of Nursing, 21*(7), 392, 394, 396–398.

Mangnall, J. (2012). Promoting patient safety in continence care. *Nursing Standard, 26*(23), 49–56.

The Mayo Clinic. (2011a). *Hemodialysis.* Available http://www.mayoclinic.com/health/hemodialysis/MY00281.

The Mayo Clinic. (2011b). *Peritoneal dialysis.* Available http://www.mayoclinic.com/health/peritoneal-dialysis/MY00282.

Moorhead, S., Johnson, M., Maas, M.L., & Swanson, E. (Eds.). (2013). *Nursing outcomes classification (NOC)* (5th ed.). St. Louis: Mosby Elsevier.

NANDA-I International. (2012). *Nursing diagnoses: Definitions & classification 2012–2014.* West Sussex, UK: Wiley-Blackwell.

National Kidney and Urologic Diseases Information Clearinghouse (NKUDIC). (2012). *Urodynamic testing.* NIH publication No. 12-5106. Available http://kidney.niddk.nih.gov/KUDiseases/pubs/urodynamic/index.aspx.

National Kidney Foundation. (2006). *Peritoneal dialysis: What you need to know.* Publication No. 11-50-0215. Available http://www.kidney.org/atoz/pdf/peritonealdialysis.pdf.

Nazarko, L. (2012). Evaluating clinical indications for continued catheterisation. *Nursing & Residential Care, 14*(9), 450, 452, 454–455.

Newman, D.K., & Willson, M.M. (2011). Review of intermittent catheterization and current best practices. *Urologic Nursing, 31*(1), 12–28.

Newman, D. (2008). Internal and external urinary catheters: A primer for clinical practice. *Ostomy Wound Management, 54*(12), 18–20, 22–26, 28–38.

Patraca, K. (2005). Measure bladder volume without catheterization. *Nursing, 35*(4), 46–47.

Palese, A., Buchini, S., Deroma, L., & Barbone, F. (2010). The effectiveness of the ultrasound bladder scanner in reducing urinary tract infections: A meta-analysis. *Journal of Clinical Nursing, 19*(21/22), 2970–2979.

Perry, S.E., Hockenberry, M.J., Lowdermilk, D.L., & Wilson, D. (2010). *Maternal child nursing care* (4th ed.). Maryland Heights, MO: Mosby/Elsevier.

Rantell, A. (2012). Intermittent self-catheterisation in women. *Nursing Standard, 26*(42), 61–68.

Rew, M., & Smith, R. (2011). Reducing infection through the use of suprapubic catheters. *British Journal of Neuroscience Nursing, 7*(5), S13–S16.

Richard, C.J. (2011). Preservation of vascular access for hemodialysis in acute care settings. *Critical Care Nursing Quarterly, 34*(1), 76–83.

Rudoni, C. (2008). A service evaluation of the use of silicone-based adhesive remover. *British Journal of Nursing, Stoma Care Supplement, 17*(2), S4, S6, S8–S9.

Society of Urologic Nurses and Associates (SUNA). (2010). *Prevention & control of catheter-associated urinary tract infection (CAUTI). Clinical practice guideline.* Available https://www.suna.org/sites/default/files/download/cautiGuideline.pdf.

Society of Urologic Nurses and Associates. (2005a). *Care of the patient with an indwelling catheter: Clinical practice guideline.* Available at suna.org/resources/indwellingCatheter.pdf. Accessed November 15, 2005.

Society of Urologic Nurses and Associates. (2005b). *Female urethral catheterization: Clinical practice guideline.* Available at suna.org/resources/female Catheterization.pdf. Accessed November 15, 2005.

Society of Urologic Nurses and Associates. (2005c). *Male urethral catheterization: Clinical practice guideline.* Available at suna.org/resources/maleCatheterization.pdf. Accessed November 15, 2005.

Stephen-Haynes, J. (2008). Skin integrity and silicone: APPEEL 'no-sting' medical adhesive remover. *British Journal of Nursing, 17*(12), 792–795.

Stewart, E. (2011). Intermittent self-catheterization and infection reduction. *British Journal of Neuroscience Nursing, 7*(5), S4–S7.

Tabloski, P. (2010). *Gerontological nursing* (2nd ed.). Upper Saddle River, NJ: Pearson.

Taylor, C., Lillis, C., & Lynn P. (2015). *Fundamentals of nursing.* (8th ed.). Philadelphia: Wolters Kluwer Health/Lippincott Williams & Wilkins.

Taylor, J.J., & Cohen, B.J. (2013). *Memmler's structure and function of the human body* (10th ed.). Philadelphia: Wolters Kluwer Health/Lippincott Williams & Wilkins.

Turner, B., & Dickens, N. (2010). Long-term urethral catheterisation. *Primary Health Care, 21*(4), 32–38.

United Ostomy Association. (2004). *Urostomy guide.* Available www.uoaa.org/ostomy_info/pubs/uoa_urostomy_en.pdf. Accessed April 17, 2009.

VISN 8 Patient Safety Center. (2009). *Safe patient handling and movement algorithms.* Tampa, FL: Author. Available http://www.visn8.va.gov/visn8/patientsafetycenter/safePtHandling/default.asp.

Wilde, M.H., McDonald, M.V., Brasch, J., McMahon, J.M., Fairbanks, E., Shah, S., et al. (2013). Long-term urinary catheter users self-care practices and problems. *Journal of Clinical Nursing, 22*(3/4), 356–367.

Williams, J. (2011). Choosing devices for stoma patients. *Practice Nursing, 22*(12), 646, 648–649.

Williams, J. (2012). Considerations for managing stoma complications in the community. *British Journal of Community Nursing, 17*(6), 266–269.

Wilson, M. (2011). Addressing the problems of long term urethral catheterization: Part 1. *British Journal of Nursing, 20*(22), 1418, 1420–1424.

Winder, A. (2012). Good practice in catheter care. *Journal of Community Nursing, 26*(6), 15–16, 19–20.

Yates, A. (2012). Management of long-term urinary catheters. *Nursing & Residential Care, 14*(4), 172, 174, 176–178.

SUGGESTED ANSWERS FOR FOCUSING ON PATIENT CARE: DEVELOPING CLINICAL REASONING

1. Assess the patency of the condom sheath. Lack of adhesion of the sheath on the penis or resistance to gravity flow of urine would allow urine to leak around the sheath. You should assess for the presence of these conditions, as well as the condition of the patient's skin. Take care to fasten the condom securely enough to prevent leakage, yet not so tightly as to constrict the blood vessels in the area. In addition, the tip of the tubing should be kept 1 to 2 inches (2.5 to 5 cm) beyond the tip of the penis to prevent irritation to the sensitive glans area. Maintaining free urinary drainage is another nursing priority. Institute measures to prevent the tubing from becoming kinked and urine from backing up in the tubing. Urine can lead to excoriation of the glans, as well as separation of the sheath from the skin, so position the tubing that collects the urine from the condom so that it draws urine away from the penis.

   Always use a measuring or sizing guide supplied by the manufacturer to ensure the correct size of sheath is applied. Skin barriers, such as 3M™ or SkinPrep™, can be applied to the penis to protect penile skin from irritation and changes in integrity. In addition, nursing care of a patient with a condom catheter includes vigilant skin care to prevent excoriation. This includes removing the condom catheter daily, washing the penis with skin cleanser and water and drying carefully, and inspecting the skin for irritation. In hot and humid weather, more frequent changing may be required. Always follow the manufacturer's instructions for applying the condom catheter because there are several variations.

2. Begin by assessing what the patient understands about the reason she is required to use the bedpan for elimination. Based on this information, reinforce the rationale for the use of the bedpan. Promote comfort and normalcy as much as possible, while respecting the patient's privacy. Determine if a regular bedpan or a fracture pan would be most appropriate for Ms. Halligan. Also be sure to provide skin care and perineal hygiene after bedpan use and maintain a professional manner.

3. Obtain additional assessment data regarding the catheter site. Assessment data should include the presence of erythema, drainage, bleeding, tenderness, swelling, skin irritation or breakdown, or leakage. These signs could indicate exit site or tunnel infection. In addition, inquire about any tenderness, pain, and guarding of the abdomen, as well as nausea, vomiting, and fever, which could indicate peritonitis. Assess the patient's knowledge about measures to care for the exit site. Remind Mr. Wimmer that exit site and catheter care includes avoiding baths and public pools; the importance of good handwashing before self-care; and that he should be maintaining an occlusive dressing over the site.

   Because he is experiencing site redness and tenderness, which could indicate an infection, instruct Mr. Wimmer to contact his primary care provider for an appointment to have his catheter and exit site evaluated.

13 Bowel Elimination

FOCUSING ON PATIENT CARE

This chapter will help you develop some of the skills related to bowel elimination necessary to care for the following patients:

HUGH LEVENS, a 64-year-old man, has been placed on a bowel program after a fall left him paralyzed from the waist down.

ISAAC GREENBERG, age 9 years, has been having blood in his stools. He is scheduled for a colonoscopy as an outpatient. He and his mother need teaching about the preparation for the procedure, which includes a small-volume cleansing enema.

MARIA BLAKELY, age 26, has recently received an ileostomy. She is having problems with her appliances and is concerned about excoriation.

Refer to Focusing on Patient Care: Developing Clinical Reasoning at the end of the chapter to apply what you learn.

LEARNING OBJECTIVES

After studying this chapter, you will be able to:

1. Administer a large-volume cleansing enema.
2. Administer a small-volume cleansing enema.
3. Administer a retention enema.
4. Remove stool digitally.
5. Apply a fecal incontinence device.
6. Change and empty an ostomy appliance.
7. Irrigate a colostomy.
8. Irrigate a nasogastric tube connected to suction.

KEY TERMS

colostomy: artificial opening that permits feces from the colon to be eliminated through the stoma

constipation: dry, hard stool; persistently difficult passage of stool; and/or the incomplete passage of stool

defecation: emptying of the large intestine; also called a bowel movement

diarrhea: passage of more than three loose stools a day

enema: introduction of a solution into the large intestine

fecal impaction: prolonged retention or an accumulation of fecal material that forms a hardened mass in the rectum

fissure: linear break on the margin of the anus

flatus: intestinal gas; intestinal gas exiting anus
hemorrhoids: abnormally distended veins in the anal area
ileostomy: artificial opening created to allow liquid fecal content from the ileum to be eliminated through a stoma
ostomy: a surgically formed opening from the inside of an organ to the outside
stoma: the part of the ostomy that is attached to the skin; formed by suturing the mucosa to the skin
vagal stimulus or response: stimulation of the vagus nerve that causes an increase in parasympathetic stimulation, triggering a decrease in heart rate
Valsalva maneuver: voluntary contraction of the abdominal wall muscles, fixing of the diaphragm, and closing of the glottis that increases intra-abdominal pressure and aids in expelling feces

Elimination of the waste products of digestion is a natural process critical for human functioning. Patients differ widely in their expectations about bowel elimination, their usual pattern of **defecation**, and the ease with which they speak about bowel elimination or bowel problems. Although most people have experienced minor acute bouts of **diarrhea** or **constipation**, some patients experience severe or chronic bowel elimination problems affecting their fluid and electrolyte balance, hydration, nutritional status, skin integrity, comfort, and self-concept. Moreover, many illnesses, diagnostic tests, medications, and surgical treatments can affect bowel elimination. Nurses play an integral role in preventing and managing bowel elimination problems.

This chapter covers skills to assist the nurse in promoting and assisting with bowel elimination. Understanding the anatomy of the gastrointestinal (GI) system is integral to performing the skills in this chapter (Fundamentals Review 13-1). An abdominal assessment is required as part of the assessment related to many of the skills (Fundamentals Review 13-2). Fundamentals Review 13-3 summarizes factors that affect elimination. Fundamentals Review 18-1 in Chapter 18 reviews the characteristics of stool.

FUNDAMENTALS REVIEW 13-1

ANATOMY OF THE GASTROINTESTINAL TRACT

- The GI tract begins with the mouth and continues to the esophagus, the stomach, the small intestine, and the large intestine. It ends at the anus.
- From the mouth to the anus, the GI tract is approximately 9 m (30 feet) long.
- The small intestine consists of the duodenum, jejunum, and ileum.
- The large intestine consists of the cecum, colon (ascending, transverse, descending, and sigmoid), and rectum.
- Accessory organs of the GI tract include the teeth, salivary glands, gallbladder, liver, and pancreas.

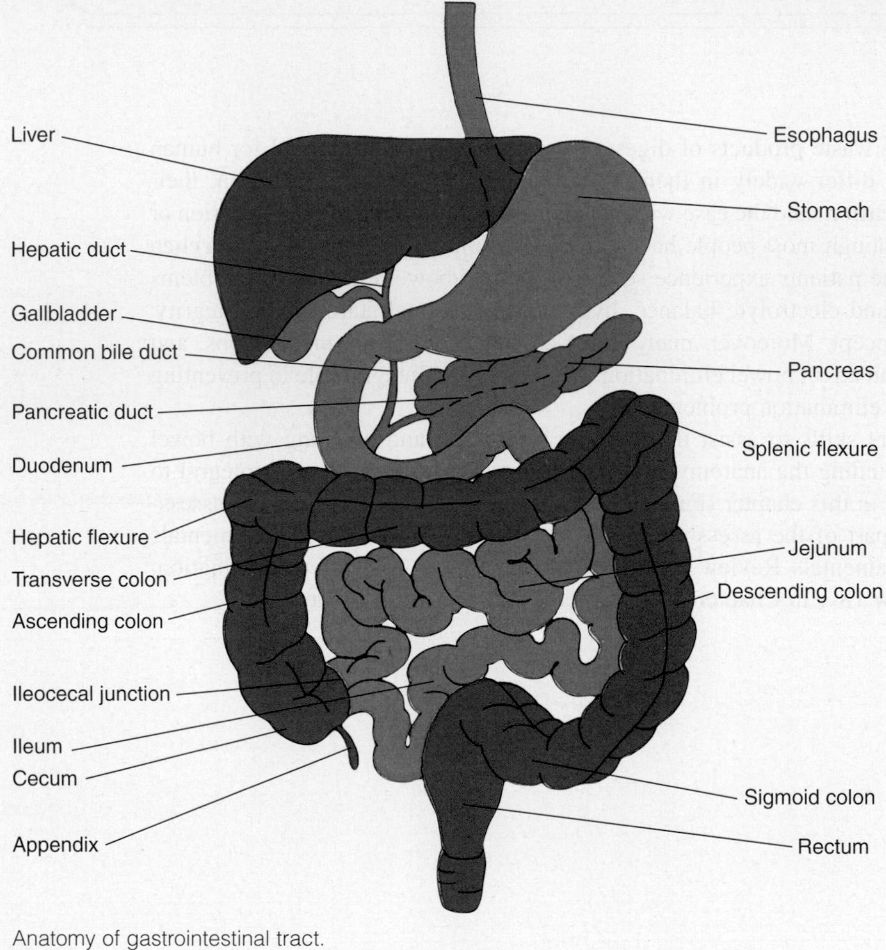

Anatomy of gastrointestinal tract.

FUNDAMENTALS REVIEW 13-2

ASSESSMENT TECHNIQUES FOR THE ABDOMEN

- Place patient in a supine position with knees slightly flexed.
- When assessing an infant or toddler, you may want to place the child on the parent's lap to prevent the child from becoming upset and crying.
- Perform the abdominal assessment in the following sequence: inspection, auscultation, percussion, palpation. Inspection and auscultation are performed before palpation because palpation may disturb normal peristalsis and bowel motility. Advanced practice professionals perform percussion and deep palpation of the abdomen. Refer to a health assessment text for details.
  - Inspection: Observe contour of abdomen; note any changes in skin or evidence of scars; inspect for any masses, bulges, or areas of distention. Observe the contour of the abdomen. Significant findings may include the presence of distention (inflation) or protrusion (projection).
  - Auscultation: Listen, using an orderly clockwise approach, in all abdominal quadrants with the diaphragm of the stethoscope; listen for bowel sounds (intermittent, soft click, and gurgles); note the frequency of bowel sounds (should be 5 to 30 sounds per minute) (Jensen, 2011).
  - Palpation: Lightly palpate over abdominal quadrants, first checking for any areas of pain or discomfort. Palpate each quadrant in a systematic manner, noting muscular resistance, tenderness, organ enlargement, or masses. If the patient complains of abdominal pain, palpate the area of pain last. If the patient's abdomen is distended, note the presence of firmness or tautness.

FUNDAMENTALS REVIEW 13-3

FACTORS THAT AFFECT BOWEL ELIMINATION

- Mobility: Regular exercise improves GI motility and muscle tone, whereas inactivity decreases both. Adequate tone in the abdominal muscles, the diaphragm, and the perineal muscles is essential for ease of defecation.
- Diet: Foods high in fiber help keep stool moving through the intestines. High fluid intake keeps stools from becoming dry and hard. Adequate fluid also helps fiber to keep stool soft and bulky and prevents dehydration from being a contributing factor to constipation.
- Medications: Antibiotics and laxatives may cause stool to become loose and more frequent. Diuretics may lead to dry, hard, and less frequent stools. Opioids decrease GI motility, leading to constipation.
- Intestinal diversions: Ileostomies normally have liquid, foul-smelling stool. Sigmoid colostomies normally have pasty, formed stool.

PRACTICE & LEARN SKILL 13-1 ADMINISTERING A LARGE-VOLUME CLEANSING ENEMA

Cleansing enemas are given to remove feces from the colon. Some of the reasons for administering a cleansing **enema** include relieving constipation or **fecal impaction**, preventing involuntary escape of fecal material during surgical procedures, promoting visualization of the intestinal tract by radiographic or instrument examination, and helping to establish regular bowel function during a bowel training program. Cleansing enemas are classified as either large-volume or small-volume. This skill addresses administering a large-volume enema. (Small-volume enemas are addressed in Skill 13-2.) Large-volume enemas are known as hypotonic or isotonic, depending on the solution used. Hypotonic (tap water) and isotonic (normal saline solution) enemas are large-volume enemas that result in rapid colonic emptying. However, using large volumes of solution (adults: 500 to 1,000 mL; infants: 150 to 250 mL) may be dangerous for patients with weakened intestinal walls, such as those with bowel inflammation or bowel infection. Large-volume enema solutions often require special preparation and equipment. See Table 13-1 for a list of commonly used enema solutions.

(continued)

SKILL 13-1 ADMINISTERING A LARGE-VOLUME CLEANSING ENEMA continued

Table 13-1 COMMONLY USED ENEMA SOLUTIONS

SOLUTION	AMOUNT	ACTION	TIME TO TAKE EFFECT	ADVERSE EFFECTS
Tap water (hypotonic)	500–1,000 mL	Distends intestine, increases peristalsis, softens stool	15 min	Fluid and electrolyte imbalance, water intoxication
Normal saline (isotonic)	500–1,000 mL	Distends intestine, increases peristalsis, softens stool	15 min	Fluid and electrolyte imbalance, sodium retention
Soap	500–1,000 mL (concentrate at 3–5 mL/1,000 mL)	Distends intestine, irritates intestinal mucosa, softens stool	10–15 min	Rectal mucosa irritation or damage
Hypertonic	70–130 mL	Distends intestine, irritates intestinal mucosa	5–10 min	Sodium retention
Oil (mineral, olive, or cottonseed oil)	150–200 mL	Lubricates stool and intestinal mucosa	30 min	

DELEGATION CONSIDERATIONS

The administration of some types of enemas may be delegated to nursing assistive personnel (NAP) or to unlicensed assistive personnel (UAP) who have received appropriate training. The administration of a large-volume cleansing enema may be delegated to licensed practical/vocational nurses (LPN/LVNs). The decision to delegate must be based on careful analysis of the patient's needs and circumstances, as well as the qualifications of the person to whom the task is being delegated. Refer to the Delegation Guidelines in Appendix A.

EQUIPMENT

- Enema solution as ordered at a temperature of 105°F to 110°F (40°C to 43°C) for adults in the prescribed amount. (Amount will vary depending on type of solution, patient's age, and patient's ability to retain the solution. Average cleansing enema for an adult may range from 750 to 1,000 mL)
- Disposable enema set, which includes a solution container and tubing
- Water-soluble lubricant
- IV pole
- Necessary additives, as ordered
- Waterproof pad
- Bath thermometer (if available)
- Bath blanket
- Bedpan and toilet tissue
- Disposable gloves
- Additional PPE, as indicated
- Paper towel
- Washcloth, skin cleanser, and towel

ASSESSMENT

Ask the patient when he or she had the last bowel movement. Assess the patient's abdomen, including auscultating for bowel sounds, and palpating for tenderness and/or firmness. Because the goal of a cleansing enema is to increase peristalsis, which should increase bowel sounds, assess the abdomen before and after the enema. Assess the rectal area for any **fissures**, **hemorrhoids**, sores, or rectal tears. If any of these are present, take added care while inserting the tube. Assess the results of the patient's laboratory work, specifically the platelet count and white blood cell (WBC) count. An enema is contraindicated for patients with a low platelet count or low WBC count. An enema may irritate or traumatize the GI mucosa, causing bleeding, bowel perforation, or infection in these patients. Any unnecessary procedures that would place the patient with a low platelet count or low WBC count at risk for bleeding or infection should not be performed. Assess for dizziness, light-headedness, diaphoresis, and clammy skin. The enema may stimulate a vagal response, which increases parasympathetic stimulation, causing a decrease in heart rate. Do not administer enemas to patients who have severe abdominal pain, bowel obstruction, bowel inflammation or bowel infection, or after rectal, prostate, or colon surgery.

NURSING DIAGNOSIS

Determine the related factors for the nursing diagnoses based on the patient's current status. Appropriate nursing diagnoses may include:

- Acute Pain
- Constipation
- Risk for Constipation

OUTCOME IDENTIFICATION AND PLANNING

The expected outcome to be met when administering a cleansing enema is that the patient expels feces. Other appropriate outcomes may include the following: the patient verbalizes decreased discomfort; abdominal distention is absent; and the patient remains free of any evidence of trauma to the rectal mucosa or other adverse effects.

IMPLEMENTATION

ACTION	RATIONALE
1. Verify the order for the enema. Gather equipment.	Verifying the medical order is crucial to ensuring that the proper enema is administered to the right patient. Assembling equipment provides for an organized approach to the task.
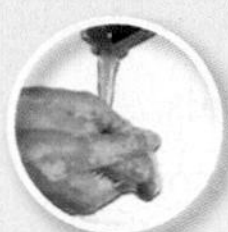 2. Perform hand hygiene and put on PPE, if indicated.	Hand hygiene and PPE prevent the spread of microorganisms. PPE is required based on transmission precautions.
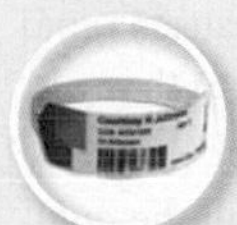 3. Identify the patient.	Identifying the patient ensures the right patient receives the intervention and helps prevent errors.
4. Explain the procedure to the patient and provide the rationale as to why the tube is needed. Discuss the associated discomforts that may be experienced and possible interventions that may allay this discomfort. Answer any questions, as needed.	Explanation facilitates patient cooperation and reduces anxiety.
5. Assemble equipment on overbed table within reach.	Arranging items nearby is convenient, saves time, and avoids unnecessary stretching and twisting of muscles on the part of the nurse.
6. Close the curtains around the bed and close the door to the room, if possible. Discuss where the patient will defecate. Have a bedpan, commode, or nearby bathroom ready for use.	This ensures the patient's privacy. Explanation relieves anxiety and facilitates cooperation. The patient is better able to relax and cooperate if he or she is familiar with the procedure and knows everything is in readiness when the urge to defecate is felt. Defecation usually occurs within 5 to 15 minutes.
7. Warm the enema solution in amount ordered, and check temperature with a bath thermometer, if available. If bath thermometer is not available, warm to room temperature or slightly higher, and test on inner wrist. If tap water is used, adjust temperature as it flows from the faucet (Figure 1).	Warming the solution prevents chilling the patient, adding to the discomfort of the procedure. Cold solution could cause cramping; a too-warm solution could cause trauma to intestinal mucosa.

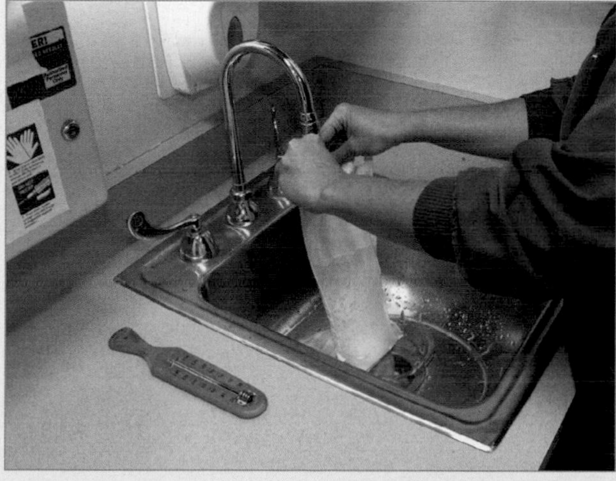

FIGURE 1 Preparing enema bag.

(continued)

SKILL 13-1 ADMINISTERING A LARGE-VOLUME CLEANSING ENEMA continued

ACTION	RATIONALE
8. Add enema solution to container. Release clamp and allow fluid to progress through tube before reclamping.	This causes any air to be expelled from the tubing. Although allowing air to enter the intestine is not harmful, it may further distend the intestine.
9. Adjust the bed to a comfortable working height, usually elbow height of the caregiver (VISN 8 Patient Safety Center, 2009). Position the patient on the left side (Sims' position), as dictated by patient comfort and condition. Fold top linen back just enough to allow access to the patient's rectal area. Drape the patient with the bath blanket, as necessary, to maintain privacy and warmth. Place a waterproof pad under the patient's hip.	Having the bed at the proper height prevents back and muscle strain. Sims' position facilitates flow of solution via gravity into the rectum and colon, optimizing solution retention. Folding back the linen in this manner minimizes unnecessary exposure and promotes the patient's comfort and warmth. The waterproof pad will protect the bed.
10. Put on gloves.	Gloves prevent contact with contaminants and body fluids.
11. Elevate solution so that it is no higher than 18 inches (45 cm) above level of anus (Figure 2). Plan to give the solution slowly over a period of 5 to 10 minutes. Hang the container on an IV pole or hold it at the proper height.	Gravity forces the solution to enter the intestine. The amount of pressure determines the rate of flow and pressure exerted on the intestinal wall. Giving the solution too quickly causes rapid distention and pressure, poor defecation, or damage to the mucous membrane.
12. Generously lubricate end of rectal tube 2 to 3 inches (5 to 7 cm). A disposable enema set may have a prelubricated rectal tube.	Lubrication facilitates passage of the rectal tube through the anal sphincter and prevents injury to the mucosa.
13. Lift buttock to expose anus. Ask patient to take several deep breaths. Slowly and gently insert the enema tube 3 to 4 inches (7 to 10 cm) for an adult. Direct it at an angle pointing toward the umbilicus, not the bladder (Figure 3).	Good visualization of the anus helps prevent injury to tissues. Deep breathing helps relax the anal sphincters. The anal canal is about 1 to 2 inches (2.5 to 5 cm) long. Insertion 3 to 4 inches ensures the tube is inserted past the external and internal anal sphincters; further insertion may damage intestinal mucous membrane. The suggested angle follows the normal intestinal contour and thus will help to prevent perforation of the bowel. Slow insertion of the tube minimizes spasms of the intestinal wall and sphincters.

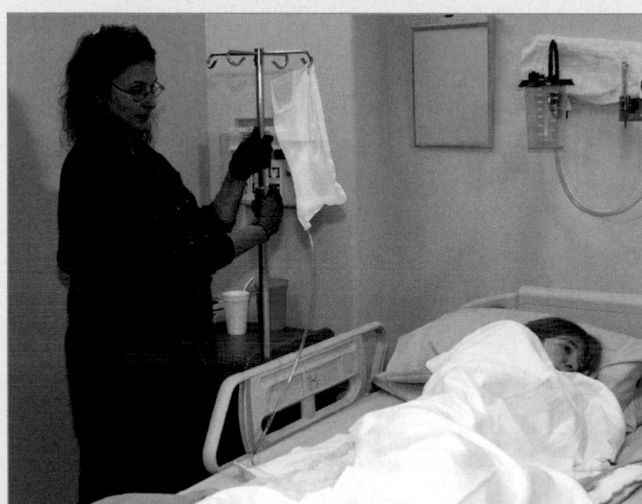

FIGURE 2 Adjusting height of solution container until it is no more than 18 inches above patient.

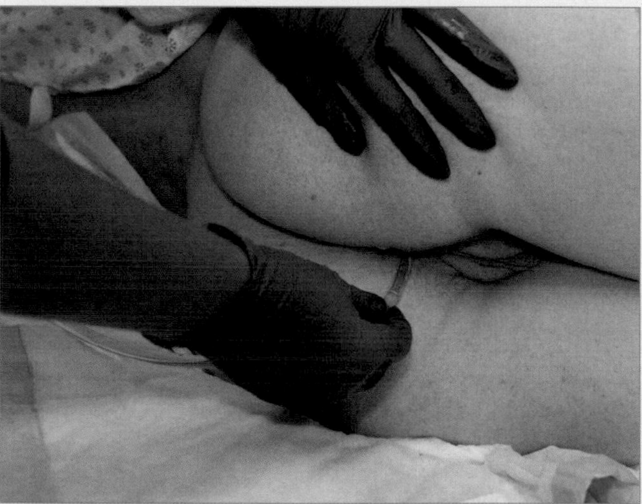

FIGURE 3 Inserting enema tip into anus, directing tip toward umbilicus.

ACTION	RATIONALE
14. If resistance is met while inserting the tube, permit a small amount of solution to enter, withdraw tube slightly, and then continue to insert it. **Do not force entry of the tube.** Ask the patient to take several deep breaths.	Resistance may be due to spasms of the intestine or failure of the internal sphincter to open. The solution may help to reduce spasms and relax the sphincter, thus making continued insertion of the tube safe. Forcing a tube may injure the intestinal mucosa wall. Taking deep breaths helps relax the anal sphincter.
15. Introduce solution slowly over a period of 5 to 10 minutes. Hold tubing all the time that solution is being instilled. Assess for dizziness, light-headedness, nausea, diaphoresis, and clammy skin during administration. **If the patient experiences any of these symptoms, stop the procedure immediately, monitor the patient's heart rate and blood pressure, and notify the primary care provider.**	Introducing the solution slowly helps prevent rapid distention of the intestine and a desire to defecate. Assessment allows for detection of a vagal response. The enema may stimulate a vagal response, which increases parasympathetic stimulation, causing a decrease in heart rate.
16. Clamp tubing or lower container if the patient has the urge to defecate or cramping occurs (Figure 4). Instruct the patient to take small, fast breaths or to pant.	These techniques help relax muscles and prevent premature expulsion of the solution.
17. After the solution has been given, clamp tubing (Figure 5) and remove tube. Have paper towel ready to receive tube as it is withdrawn.	Wrapping tube in paper towel prevents dripping of solution.

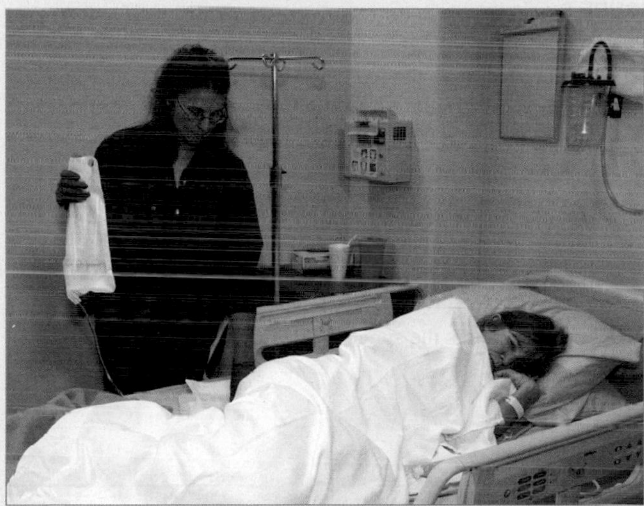

FIGURE 4 Holding bag lower to slow flow of enema solution.

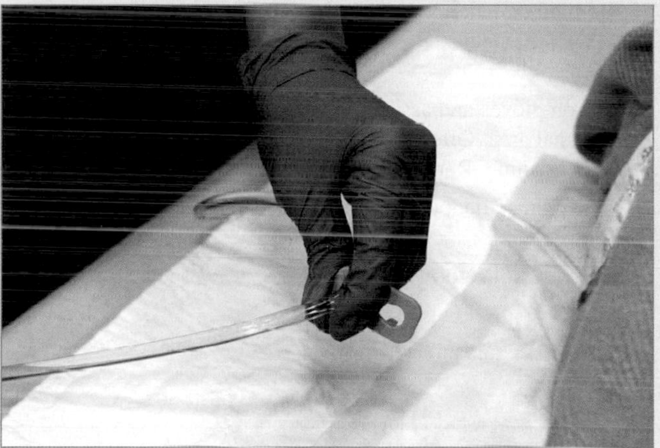

FIGURE 5 Clamping tubing before removing.

ACTION	RATIONALE
18. Return the patient to a comfortable position. Encourage the patient to hold the solution until the urge to defecate is strong, usually in about 5 to 15 minutes. Make sure the linens under the patient are dry. Remove your gloves and ensure that the patient is covered.	This amount of time usually allows muscle contractions to become sufficient to produce good results. Promotes patient comfort. Removing contaminated gloves prevents spread of microorganisms.
19. Raise side rail. Lower bed height and adjust head of bed to a comfortable position.	Promotes patient safety.
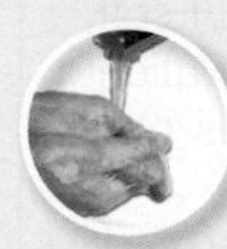 20. Remove additional PPE, if used. Perform hand hygiene.	Removing PPE properly reduces the risk for infection transmission and contamination of other items. Hand hygiene prevents the spread of microorganisms.

(continued)

SKILL 13-1 ADMINISTERING A LARGE-VOLUME CLEANSING ENEMA continued

ACTION	RATIONALE
21. When patient has a strong urge to defecate, place him or her in a sitting position on a bedpan or assist to commode or bathroom. Offer toilet tissues, if not in the patient's reach (Figure 6). Stay with the patient or have call bell readily accessible.	The sitting position is most natural and facilitates defecation. Fall prevention is a high priority due to the urgency of reaching the commode.

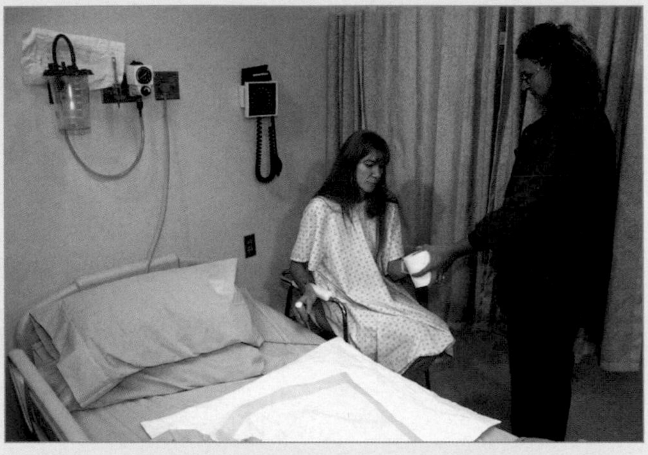

FIGURE 6 Offering toilet tissue to patient on bedside commode.

ACTION	RATIONALE
22. Remind patient not to flush the commode before you inspect results of enema.	The results need to be observed and recorded. Additional enemas may be necessary if the physician has ordered enemas "until clear." Refer to 'Special Considerations' below.
23. Put on gloves and assist patient, if necessary, with cleaning anal area. Offer washcloths, skin cleanser, and water for handwashing. Remove gloves.	Cleaning the anal area and proper hygiene deter the spread of microorganisms. Gloves prevent contact with contaminants and body fluids.
24. Leave the patient clean and comfortable. Care for equipment properly.	Bacteria that grow in the intestine can be spread to others if equipment is not properly cleaned.
25. Perform hand hygiene.	Hand hygiene deters the spread of microorganisms.

EVALUATION

The expected outcome is met when the patient expels feces; the patient verbalizes decreased discomfort; abdominal distention is absent; and the patient remains free of any evidence of trauma to the rectal mucosa or other adverse effect.

DOCUMENTATION

Guidelines

Document the amount and type of enema solution used; amount, consistency, and color of stool; pain assessment rating; assessment of perineal area for any irritation, tears, or bleeding; and the patient's reaction to the procedure.

Sample Documentation

7/22/15 1310 800 mL warm tap water enema given via rectum. Large amount of soft, brown stool returned. No irritation, tears, or bleeding noted in perineal area. Patient complained of "stomach cramping" relieved when enema was released. Rates pain as 0 after evacuation of enema.

—K. Sanders, RN

UNEXPECTED SITUATIONS AND ASSOCIATED INTERVENTIONS

- *Solution does not flow into rectum:* Reposition rectal tube. If solution will still not flow, remove tube and check for any fecal contents.
- *Patient cannot retain enema solution for adequate amount of time:* Patient may need to be placed on bedpan in the supine position while receiving the enema. The head of the bed may be elevated 30 degrees for the patient's comfort.
- *Patient cannot tolerate large amount of enema solution:* Amount and length of administration may have to be modified if patient begins to complain of pain.
- *Patient complains of severe cramping with introduction of enema solution:* Lower solution container and check temperature and flow rate. If the solution is too cold or flow rate too fast, severe cramping may occur.

SPECIAL CONSIDERATIONS

General Considerations

- Do not use rectal agents and rectal manipulation, including enemas, with patients who are myelosuppressed and/or patients at risk for myelosuppression and mucositis. These interventions can lead to development of bleeding, anal fissures, or abscesses, which are portals for infection (NCI, 2012).
- If the patient experiences fullness or pain or if fluid escapes around the tube, stop administration. Wait 30 seconds to a minute and then restart the flow at a slower rate. If symptoms persist, stop administration and contact the patient's physician.
- If the order states the enema is to be given "until clear," check with the primary care provider before administering more than three enemas. Severe fluid and electrolyte imbalances may occur if the patient receives more than three cleansing enemas. Results are considered clear whenever there are no more pieces of stool in enema return. The solution may be colored but still considered a clear return.

Infant and Child Considerations

- When administering an enema to a child, use isotonic solutions. Plain water is not used because it is hypotonic and can cause rapid fluid shift and fluid overload (Perry et al., 2010).
- Appropriate fluid volume for an enema (Perry et al., 2010):
  - Infant: 120 to 240 mL
  - 2 to 4 yr: 240 to 360 mL
  - 4 to 10 yr: 360 to 480 mL
  - 11 yr: 480 to 720 mL
- Insert tubing into the rectum 2 to 3 inches for children, 1 inch for infants.

Older Adult Considerations

- If the older adult patient cannot retain the enema solution, administer the enema with the patient on the bedpan in the supine position For comfort, elevate the head of the bed 30 degrees, if necessary, and use pillows appropriately.

SKILL 13-2 ADMINISTERING A SMALL-VOLUME CLEANSING ENEMA

Cleansing enemas are given to remove feces from the colon. Some of the reasons for administering a cleansing enema include relieving constipation or fecal impaction, preventing involuntary escape of fecal material during surgical procedures, promoting visualization of the intestinal tract by radiographic or instrument examination, and helping to establish regular bowel function during a bowel training program. Cleansing enemas are classified as either large-volume or small-volume. This skill addresses administering a small-volume enema. (Large-volume enemas are addressed in Skill 13-1.) Small-volume enemas (adult: 70 to 130 mL) are also known as hypertonic enemas. These hypertonic solutions work by drawing water into the colon, which stimulates the defecation reflex. They may be

(continued)

SKILL 13-2 ADMINISTERING A SMALL-VOLUME CLEANSING ENEMA continued

contraindicated in patients for whom sodium retention is a problem. They are also contraindicated for patients with renal impairment or reduced renal clearance, because these patients have compromised ability to excrete phosphate adequately, with resulting hyperphosphatemia (Jacobson et al., 2010; Bowers 2006).

DELEGATION CONSIDERATIONS

The administration of some types of enemas may be delegated to nursing assistive personnel (NAP) or to unlicensed assistive personnel (UAP) who have received appropriate training. The administration of a small-volume cleansing enema may be delegated to licensed practical/vocational nurses (LPN/LVNs). The decision to delegate must be based on careful analysis of the patient's needs and circumstances, as well as the qualifications of the person to whom the task is being delegated. Refer to the Delegation Guidelines in Appendix A.

EQUIPMENT

- Commercially prepared enema with rectal tip
- Water-soluble lubricant
- Waterproof pad
- Bath blanket
- Bedpan and toilet tissue
- Disposable gloves
- Additional PPE, as indicated
- Paper towel
- Washcloth, skin cleanser, and towel

ASSESSMENT

Assess the patient's abdomen, including auscultating for bowel sounds, and palpating the abdomen. Because the goal of a cleansing enema is to increase peristalsis, which should increase bowel sounds, assess the abdomen before and after the enema. Inspect the rectal area for any fissures, hemorrhoids, sores, or rectal tears. If any of these are noted, take added care while administering the enema. Check the results of the patient's laboratory work, specifically the platelet count and WBC count. A normal platelet count ranges from 150,000 to 400,000/mm^3. A platelet count of less than 20,000 may seriously compromise the patient's ability to clot blood. Therefore, do not perform any unnecessary procedures that would place the patient at risk for bleeding or infection. A low WBC count places the patient at risk for infection. Assess for dizziness, light-headedness, diaphoresis, nausea, and clammy skin. The enema may stimulate a vagal response, which increases parasympathetic stimulation, causing a decrease in heart rate. Do not administer enemas to patients who have severe abdominal pain, bowel obstruction, bowel inflammation or bowel infection, or after rectal, prostate, and colon surgery.

NURSING DIAGNOSIS

Determine the related factors for the nursing diagnoses based on the patient's current status. Appropriate nursing diagnoses may include:

- Acute Pain
- Constipation
- Risk for Constipation

OUTCOME IDENTIFICATION AND PLANNING

The expected outcome to be met when administering a cleansing enema is that the patient expels feces and reports a decrease in pain and discomfort. In addition, the patient remains free of any evidence of trauma to the rectal mucosa.

IMPLEMENTATION

ACTION	RATIONALE
1. Verify the order for the enema. Gather equipment.	Verifying the medical order is crucial to ensuring that the proper enema is administered to the right patient. Assembling equipment provides for an organized approach to the task.
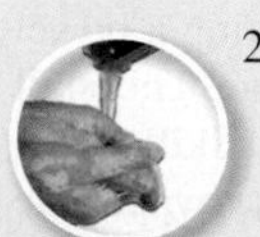 2. Perform hand hygiene and put on PPE, if indicated.	Hand hygiene and PPE prevent the spread of microorganisms. PPE is required based on transmission precautions.

ACTION	RATIONALE
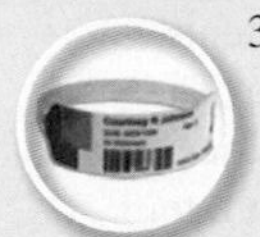 3. Identify the patient.	Identifying the patient ensures the right patient receives the intervention and helps prevent errors.
4. Explain the procedure to the patient and provide the rationale why the tube is needed. Discuss the associated discomforts that may be experienced and possible interventions that may allay this discomfort. Answer any questions, as needed.	Explanation facilitates patient cooperation and reduces anxiety.
5. Assemble equipment on overbed table within reach. Warm the enema solution to body temperature by placing the container in a bowl of warm water.	Arranging items nearby is convenient, saves time, and avoids unnecessary stretching and twisting of muscles on the part of the nurse. A cold solution can cause intestinal cramping.
6. Close the curtains around the bed and close the door to the room, if possible. Discuss where the patient will defecate. Have a bedpan, commode, or nearby bathroom ready for use.	This ensures the patient's privacy. Explanation relieves anxiety and facilitates cooperation. The patient is better able to relax and cooperate if he or she is familiar with the procedure and knows everything is in readiness when the urge to defecate is felt. Defecation usually occurs within 5 to 15 minutes.
7. Adjust the bed to a comfortable working height, usually elbow height of the caregiver (VISN 8 Patient Safety Center, 2009). Position the patient on the left side (Sims' position), as dictated by patient comfort and condition. Fold top linen back just enough to allow access to the patient's rectal area. Drape the patient with the bath blanket, as necessary, to maintain privacy and provide warmth. Place a waterproof pad under the patient's hip.	Having the bed at the proper height prevents back and muscle strain. Sims' position facilitates flow of solution via gravity into the rectum and colon, optimizing retention of solution. Folding back the linen in this manner minimizes unnecessary exposure and promotes the patient's comfort and warmth. The waterproof pad will protect the bed.
8. Put on gloves.	Gloves prevent contact with contaminants and body fluids.
9. Remove the cap (Figure 1) and generously lubricate end of rectal tube 2 to 3 inches (5 to 7 cm).	Lubrication facilitates passage of the rectal tube through the anal sphincter and prevents injury to the mucosa.
10. Lift buttock to expose anus. Ask the patient to take several deep breaths. Slowly and gently insert the rectal tube 3 to 4 inches (7 to 10 cm) for an adult. Direct it at an angle pointing toward the umbilicus, not bladder (Figure 2). **Do not force entry of the tube.**	Good visualization of the anus helps prevent injury to tissues. Deep breathing helps relax the anal sphincters. The anal canal is about 1 to 2 inches (2.5 to 5 cm) long. Insertion 3 to 4 inches ensures the tube is inserted past the external and internal anal sphincters; further insertion may damage intestinal mucous membrane. The suggested angle follows the normal intestinal contour, helping prevent perforation of the bowel. Forcing a tube may injure the intestinal mucosa wall.

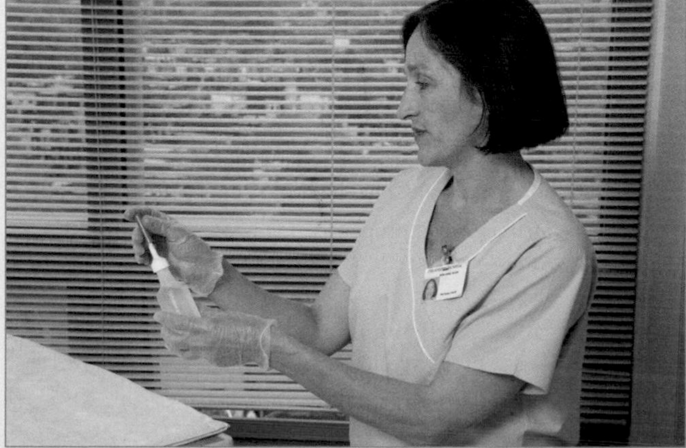

FIGURE 1 Removing cap from prepackaged enema solution container.

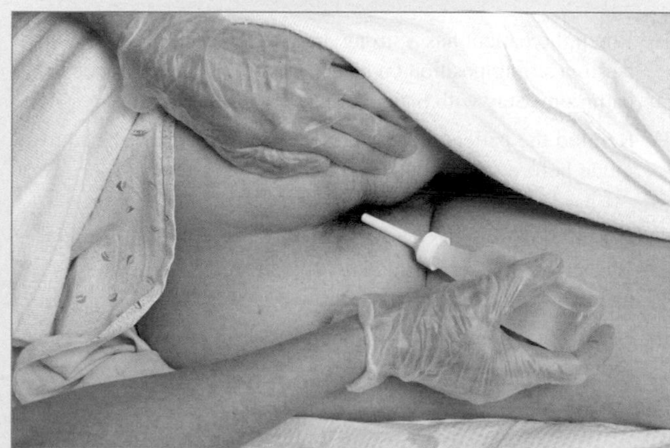

FIGURE 2 Inserting tube into rectum, directing toward umbilicus.

(continued)

SKILL 13-2 ADMINISTERING A SMALL-VOLUME CLEANSING ENEMA continued

ACTION	RATIONALE
11. Compress the container with your hands (Figure 3). Roll the end up on itself, toward the rectal tip. Administer all the solution in the container. Assess for dizziness, light-headedness, nausea, diaphoresis, and clammy skin during administration. **If the patient experiences any of these symptoms, stop the procedure immediately, monitor the patient's heart rate and blood pressure, and notify the primary care provider.**	Rolling the container aids administration of all its contents. Assessment allows for detection of a vagal response. The enema may stimulate a vagal response, which increases parasympathetic stimulation, causing a decrease in heart rate.

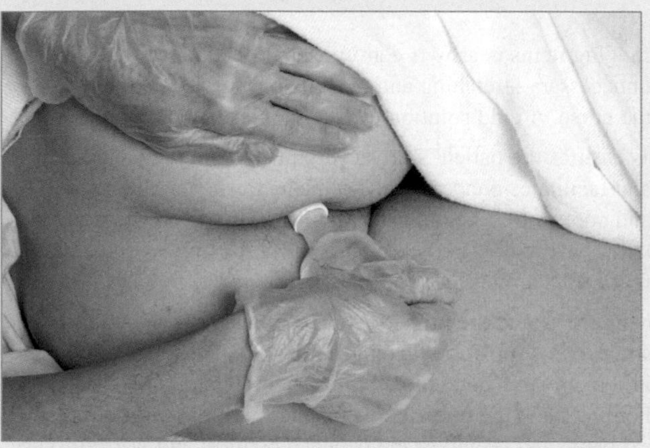

FIGURE 3 Compressing container.

ACTION	RATIONALE
12. After the solution has been given, remove the tube, **keeping the container compressed.** Have paper towel ready to receive tube as it is withdrawn. Encourage the patient to hold the solution until the urge to defecate is strong, usually in about 5 to 15 minutes.	If the container is released, a vacuum will form, allowing some of the enema solution to re-enter the container. This amount of time usually allows muscle contractions to become sufficient to produce good results.
13. Remove gloves. Return the patient to a comfortable position. Make sure the linens under the patient are dry. Ensure that the patient is covered.	Promotes patient comfort. Removing contaminated gloves prevents spread of microorganisms.
14. Raise side rail. Lower bed height and adjust head of bed to a comfortable position.	Promotes patient safety.
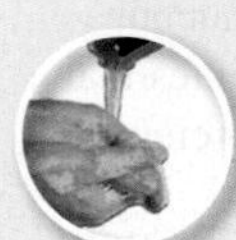 15. Remove additional PPE, if used. Perform hand hygiene.	Removing PPE properly reduces the risk for infection transmission and contamination of other items. Hand hygiene prevents the spread of microorganisms.
16. When the patient has a strong urge to defecate, place him or her in a sitting position on a bedpan or assist to commode or bathroom. Stay with patient or have call bell readily accessible.	The sitting position is most natural and facilitates defecation. Fall prevention is a high priority due to the urgency of reaching the commode.
17. Remind the patient not to flush the toilet or empty the commode before you inspect the results of the enema.	The results need to be observed and recorded. Additional enemas may be necessary if the physician has ordered enemas "until clear." Refer to 'Special Considerations' on the following page.
18. Put on gloves and assist patient, if necessary, with cleaning of anal area. Offer washcloths, skin cleanser, and water for handwashing. Remove gloves.	Cleaning the anal area and proper hygiene deter the spread of microorganisms.
19. Leave the patient clean and comfortable. Care for equipment properly.	Bacteria that grow in the intestine can be spread to others if equipment is not properly cleaned.
20. Perform hand hygiene.	Hand hygiene deters the spread of microorganisms.

EVALUATION

The expected outcome is met when the patient expels feces; the patient verbalizes decreased discomfort; abdominal distention is absent; and the patient remains free of any evidence of trauma to the rectal mucosa or other adverse effect.

DOCUMENTATION

Guidelines

Document the amount and type of enema solution used; amount, consistency, and color of stool; pain assessment rating; assessment of perineal area for any irritation, tears, or bleeding; and patient's reaction to the procedure.

Sample Documentation

7/22/15 1310 210-mL Fleet enema given via rectum. Large amount of soft, brown stool returned. No irritation, tears, or bleeding noted in perineal area. Patient states "stomach fullness" relieved when enema was released. Rates pain as 0 after evacuation of enema.

—K. Sanders, RN

UNEXPECTED SITUATIONS AND ASSOCIATED INTERVENTIONS

- *Patient cannot retain enema solution for adequate amount of time:* Patient may need to be placed on bedpan in the supine position while receiving the enema. The head of the bed may be elevated 30 degrees for the patient's comfort.

SPECIAL CONSIDERATIONS

General Considerations

- In patients who are myelosuppressed and/or patients at risk for myelosuppression and mucositis, rectal agents and manipulation, including enemas, are discouraged because they can lead to development of bleeding, anal fissures, or abscesses, which are portals for infection (NCI, 2012).
- If the enema has been ordered to be given "until clear," check with the primary care provider before administering more than three enemas. Severe fluid and electrolyte imbalances may occur if the patient receives more than three cleansing enemas. Results are considered clear whenever there are no more pieces of stool in enema return. The solution may be colored but still considered a clear return.

Infant and Child Considerations

- Position the infant or toddler on the abdomen with knees bent. Position the child or adolescent on the left side with the right leg flexed toward chest (Kyle & Carman, 2013).
- Insert tubing into the rectum 1 to 1.5 inches for infants and 2 to 3 inches for children (Kyle & Carman, 2013).
- Hold the child's buttocks together for 5 to 10 minutes if needed to encourage retention of the enema (Kyle & Carman, 2013).

Older Adult Considerations

- Use caution when giving enemas containing phosphates to frail older patients due to the potential for dehydration, electrolyte imbalances, and sodium phosphate toxicity (Bowers, 2006).

SKILL 13-3 ADMINISTERING A RETENTION ENEMA

Retention enemas are ordered for various reasons. *Oil-retention* enemas help to lubricate the stool and intestinal mucosa, making defecation easier. *Carminative* enemas help to expel **flatus** from the rectum and relieve distention secondary to flatus. *Medicated* enemas are used to administer a medication rectally. *Anthelmintic* enemas are administered to destroy intestinal parasites.

(*continued*)

SKILL 13-3 ADMINISTERING A RETENTION ENEMA continued

DELEGATION CONSIDERATIONS

The administration of some types of enemas may be delegated to nursing assistive personnel (NAP) or to unlicensed assistive personnel (UAP) who have received appropriate training. The administration of a retention enema may be delegated to licensed practical/vocational nurses (LPN/LVNs). The decision to delegate must be based on careful analysis of the patient's needs and circumstances, as well as the qualifications of the person to whom the task is being delegated. Refer to the Delegation Guidelines in Appendix A.

EQUIPMENT

- Enema solution (varies depending on reason for enema), often prepackaged, commercially prepared solutions
- Nonsterile gloves
- Additional PPE, as indicated
- Waterproof pad
- Bath blanket
- Washcloth, skin cleanser, and towel
- Bedpan or commode
- Toilet tissue
- Water-soluble lubricant

ASSESSMENT

Ask the patient when he or she had the last bowel movement. Assess the patient's abdomen, including auscultating for bowel sounds, and palpating. Because the goal of a cleansing enema is to increase peristalsis, which should increase bowel sounds, assess the abdomen before and after the enema. Assess the rectal area for any fissures, hemorrhoids, sores, or rectal tears. If present, added care should be taken while inserting the tube. Assess the results of the patient's laboratory work, specifically the platelet count and WBC count. An enema is contraindicated for patients with a low platelet count or low WBC count. An enema may irritate or traumatize the GI mucosa, causing bleeding, bowel perforation, or infection in these patients. Any unnecessary procedures that would place the patient with a low platelet count or low WBC count at risk for bleeding or infection should not be performed. Assess for dizziness, light-headedness, diaphoresis, nausea, and clammy skin. The enema may stimulate a vagal response, which increases parasympathetic stimulation, causing a decrease in heart rate. Do not administer enemas to patients who have severe abdominal pain, bowel obstruction, bowel inflammation or bowel infection, or after rectal, prostate, and colon surgery.

NURSING DIAGNOSIS

Determine the related factors for the nursing diagnoses based on the patient's current status. Appropriate nursing diagnoses may include:

- Constipation
- Acute Pain
- Risk for Injury

OUTCOME IDENTIFICATION AND PLANNING

The expected outcome to be met when administering a retention enema is that the patient retains the solution for the prescribed, appropriate length of time and experiences the expected therapeutic effect of the solution. Other appropriate outcomes may include the following: the patient verbalizes decreased discomfort; abdominal distention is absent; the patient demonstrates signs and symptoms indicative of a resolving infection; and the patient remains free of any evidence of trauma to the rectal mucosa or other adverse effect.

IMPLEMENTATION

ACTION	RATIONALE
1. Verify the order for the enema. Gather equipment.	Verifying the medical order is crucial to ensuring that the proper enema is administered to the right patient. Assembling equipment provides for an organized approach to the task.
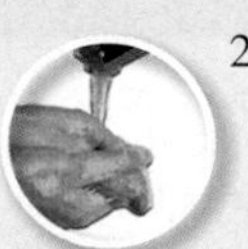 2. Perform hand hygiene and put on PPE, if indicated.	Hand hygiene and PPE prevent the spread of microorganisms. PPE is required based on transmission precautions.

ACTION	RATIONALE
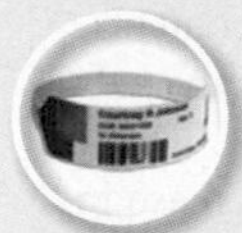 3. Identify the patient.	Identifying the patient ensures the right patient receives the intervention and helps prevent errors.
4. Explain the procedure to the patient and provide the rationale as to why the tube is needed. Discuss the associated discomforts that may be experienced and possible interventions that may allay this discomfort. Answer any questions, as needed.	Explanation facilitates patient cooperation and reduces anxiety.
5. Assemble equipment on overbed table within reach. Warm the enema solution to body temperature by placing the container in a bowl of warm water.	Arranging items nearby is convenient, saves time, and avoids unnecessary stretching and twisting of muscles on the part of the nurse. A cold solution can cause intestinal cramping.
6. Close the curtains around the bed and close the door to the room, if possible. Discuss where the patient will defecate. Have a bedpan, commode, or nearby bathroom ready for use.	This ensures the patient's privacy. Explanation relieves anxiety and facilitates cooperation. The patient is better able to relax and cooperate if he or she is familiar with the procedure and knows everything is in readiness if the urge to dispel the enema is felt.
7. Adjust the bed to a comfortable working height, usually elbow height of the caregiver (VISN 8 Patient Safety Center, 2009). Position the patient on the left side (Sims' position), as dictated by patient comfort and condition. Fold top linen back just enough to allow access to the patient's rectal area. Drape the patient with the bath blanket, as necessary, to maintain privacy and provide warmth. Place a waterproof pad under the patient's hip.	Having the bed at the proper height prevents back and muscle strain. Sims' position facilitates flow of solution via gravity into the rectum and colon, optimizing retention of the solution. Folding back the linen in this manner minimizes unnecessary exposure and promotes the patient's comfort and warmth. The waterproof pad will protect the bed.
8. Put on gloves.	Gloves prevent contact with blood and body fluids.
9. Remove cap of prepackaged enema solution. Apply a generous amount of lubricant to the tube.	Lubrication is necessary to minimize trauma on insertion.
10. Lift buttock to expose anus. Ask the patient to take several deep breaths. Slowly and gently insert the rectal tube 3 to 4 inches (7 to 10 cm) for an adult. Direct it at an angle pointing toward the umbilicus (Figure 1).	Good visualization of the anus helps prevent injury to tissues. Deep breathing helps relax the anal sphincters. The anal canal is about 1 to 2 inches (2.5 to 5 cm) long. Inserting 3 to 4 inches ensures the tube is inserted past the external and internal anal sphincters; further insertion may damage intestinal mucous membrane. The suggested angle follows the normal intestinal contour and thus will help to prevent perforation of the bowel. Slow insertion of the tube minimizes spasms of the intestinal wall and sphincters. Deep breathing helps relax the anal sphincters.

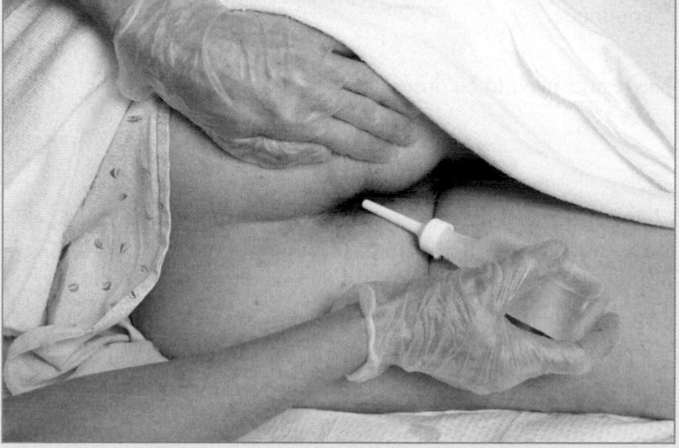

FIGURE 1 Inserting tube into rectum, directing toward umbilicus.

(continued)

SKILL 13-3 ADMINISTERING A RETENTION ENEMA continued

ACTION	RATIONALE
11. Compress the container with your hands (Figure 2). Roll the end up on itself, toward the rectal tip. Administer all the solution in the container. Assess for dizziness, light-headedness, nausea, diaphoresis, and clammy skin during administration. **If the patient experiences any of these symptoms, stop the procedure immediately, monitor the patient's heart rate and blood pressure, and notify the primary care provider.**	Rolling the container aids administration of all of the contents of the container. Assessment allows for detection of a vagal response. The enema may stimulate a vagal response, which increases parasympathetic stimulation, causing a decrease in heart rate.

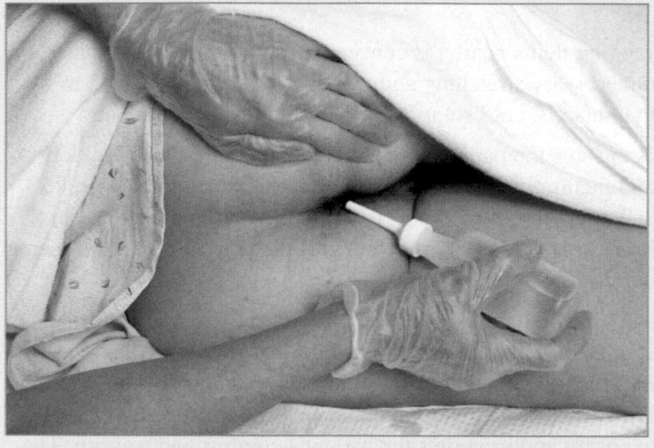

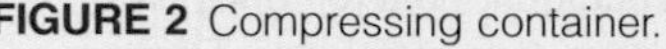

FIGURE 2 Compressing container.

ACTION	RATIONALE
12. **Remove the container while keeping it compressed.** Have paper towel ready to receive tube as it is withdrawn.	If container is released, a vacuum will form, allowing some of the enema solution to re-enter the container.
13. **Instruct the patient to retain the enema solution for at least 30 minutes or as indicated, per manufacturer's direction.**	Solution needs to dwell for at least 30 minutes, or per manufacturer's direction, to allow for its optimal action.
14. Remove gloves. Return the patient to a comfortable position. Make sure the linens under the patient are dry and ensure that the patient is covered.	Removing contaminated gloves prevents spread of microorganisms. Promotes patient comfort.
15. Raise side rail. Lower bed height and adjust head of bed to a comfortable position.	Promotes patient safety.
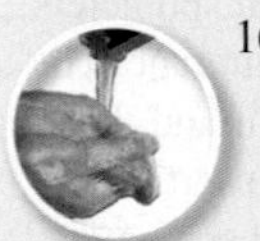 16. Remove additional PPE, if used. Perform hand hygiene.	Removing PPE properly reduces the risk for infection transmission and contamination of other items. Hand hygiene prevents the spread of microorganisms.
17. When the patient has a strong urge to dispel the solution, place him or her in a sitting position on bedpan or assist to commode or bathroom. Stay with the patient or have call bell readily accessible.	The sitting position is most natural and facilitates defecation. Fall prevention is a high priority due to the urgency of reaching the commode.
18. Remind the patient not to flush the commode before you inspect the results of the enema, if used for bowel evacuation. Record character of stool, as appropriate, and patient's reaction to the enema.	The results need to be observed and recorded.
19. Put on gloves and assist patient, if necessary, with cleaning of anal area. Offer washcloths, skin cleanser, and water for handwashing. Remove gloves.	Cleaning the anal area and proper hygiene deter the spread of microorganisms. Removing PPE properly reduces the risk for infection transmission and contamination of other items.
20. Leave patient clean and comfortable. Care for equipment properly.	Bacteria that grow in the intestine can be spread to others if equipment is not properly cleaned.
21. Perform hand hygiene.	Hand hygiene deters the spread of microorganisms.

EVALUATION

The expected outcome is met when the patient expels feces without evidence of trauma to the rectal mucosa. Depending on the reason for the retention enema, other outcomes met may include the patient verbalizes a decrease in pain after the enema; and the patient demonstrates signs and symptoms indicative of a resolving infection.

DOCUMENTATION

Guidelines

Document the amount and type of enema solution used; length of time retained by the patient; amount, consistency, and color of stool, as appropriate; pain assessment rating; assessment of perineal area for any irritation, tears, or bleeding; and the patient's reaction to the procedure.

Sample Documentation

6/26/15 2030 100 mL of mineral oil administered as enema via rectum. Small amount of firm, black stool returned. Small (approx. 1 cm) tear noted at 2 o'clock position on anus. No erythema or bleeding noted. Physician notified of tear and stool color. Reports pain as 2 on a 0-to10 rating scale after enema evacuated.

—*K. Sanders, RN*

UNEXPECTED SITUATIONS AND ASSOCIATED INTERVENTIONS

- *Solution does not flow into rectum:* Reposition rectal tube; if solution still will not flow, remove and check for any fecal contents.
- *Patient cannot retain enema solution for adequate amount of time:* Place patient on bedpan in supine position while receiving enema. Elevate the head of the bed 30 degrees for the patient's comfort. If still unable to retain, notify primary care provider.

SPECIAL CONSIDERATIONS

General Considerations

- In patients who are myelosuppressed and/or patients at risk for myelosuppression and mucositis, rectal agents and manipulation, including enemas, are discouraged because they can lead to development of bleeding, anal fissures, or abscesses, which are portals for infection (NCI, 2012).

Infant and Child Considerations

- Position the infant or toddler on the abdomen with knees bent. Position the child or adolescent on the left side with the right leg flexed toward chest (Kyle & Carman, 2013).
- Insert tubing into the rectum 1 to 1.5 inches for infants and 2 to 3 inches for children (Kyle & Carman, 2013).
- Hold the child's buttocks together for 5 to 10 minutes if needed to encourage retention of the enema (Kyle & Carman, 2013).

SKILL 13-4 DIGITAL REMOVAL OF STOOL

When a patient develops a fecal impaction (prolonged retention or an accumulation of fecal material that forms a hardened mass in the rectum), the stool must sometimes be broken up manually. However, before digital removal of feces is considered, dietary interventions, adequate fluids, and medication adjustment should be included in the patient's plan of care (Ness et al., 2012; Kyle et al., 2004). Digital removal of stool is very uncomfortable and may cause great discomfort to the patient as well as irritation of the rectal mucosa and bleeding. The primary care provider may order an oil-retention enema to be given before the procedure to soften stool. In addition, many patients find that a sitz bath or tub bath after this procedure soothes the irritated perineal area.

(*continued*)

SKILL 13-4 DIGITAL REMOVAL OF STOOL continued

DELEGATION CONSIDERATIONS

Digital removal of stool is not delegated to nursing assistive personnel (NAP) or to unlicensed assistive personnel (UAP). Depending on the state's nurse practice act and the organization's policies and procedures, the administration of a small-volume cleansing enema may be delegated to licensed practical/vocational nurses (LPN/LVNs). The decision to delegate must be based on careful analysis of the patient's needs and circumstances, as well as the qualifications of the person to whom the task is being delegated. Refer to the Delegation Guidelines in Appendix A.

EQUIPMENT

- Disposable gloves
- Additional PPE, as indicated
- Water-soluble lubricant
- Waterproof pad
- Bath blanket
- Bedpan
- Toilet paper, washcloth, skin cleanser, and towel
- Sitz bath (optional)

ASSESSMENT

Verify the time of the patient's last bowel movement by asking the patient and checking the patient's medical record. Assess the abdomen, including auscultating for bowel sounds, and palpating for tenderness and/or firmness. Inspect the rectal area for any fissures, hemorrhoids, sores, or rectal tears. If any of these are noted, consult the prescriber for the appropriateness of the intervention. Assess the results of the patient's laboratory work, specifically the platelet count and WBC count. Digital removal of stool is contraindicated for patients with a low platelet count or low WBC count. Digital removal of stool may irritate or traumatize the GI mucosa, causing bleeding, bowel perforation, or infection. Do not perform any unnecessary procedures that would place the patient at risk for bleeding or infection. Assess for dizziness, light-headedness, diaphoresis, and clammy skin. Assess pulse rate and blood pressure before and after the procedure. The procedure may stimulate a vagal response, which increases parasympathetic stimulation, causing a decrease in heart rate and blood pressure. Do not perform digital removal of stool on patients who have bowel inflammation or bowel infection, or after rectal, prostate, and colon surgery.

NURSING DIAGNOSIS

Determine the related factors for the nursing diagnoses based on the patient's current status. Appropriate nursing diagnoses may include:

- Constipation
- Acute Pain
- Risk for Injury

OUTCOME IDENTIFICATION AND PLANNING

The expected outcome to achieve when digitally removing stool is that the patient will expel feces with assistance. Other appropriate outcomes may include the patient verbalizes decreased discomfort; abdominal distention is absent; and the patient remains free of any evidence of trauma to the rectal mucosa or other adverse effect.

IMPLEMENTATION

ACTION	RATIONALE
1. Verify the order for digital removal of stool. Gather equipment.	Digital removal of stool is considered an invasive procedure and requires a medical order. Verifying the medical order is crucial to ensuring that the proper procedure is administered to the right patient. Assembling equipment provides for an organized approach to the task.
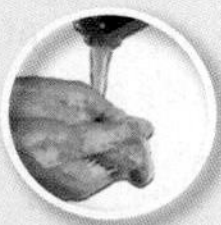 2. Perform hand hygiene and put on PPE, if indicated.	Hand hygiene and PPE prevent the spread of microorganisms. PPE is required based on transmission precautions.
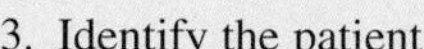 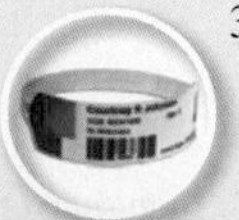 3. Identify the patient.	Identifying the patient ensures the right patient receives the intervention and helps prevent errors.

ACTION	RATIONALE
4. Explain the procedure to the patient and provide the rationale why the procedure is needed. Discuss the associated discomforts that may be experienced. Discuss signs and symptoms of a slow heart rate. Instruct the patient to alert you if any of these symptoms are felt during the procedure. Have a bedpan ready for use.	Explanation relieves anxiety and facilitates cooperation. The patient is better able to relax and cooperate if he or she is familiar with the procedure.
5. Assemble equipment on overbed table within reach.	Arranging items nearby is convenient, saves time, and avoids unnecessary stretching and twisting of muscles on the part of the nurse.
6. Close the curtains around the bed and close the door to the room, if possible. Discuss where the patient will defecate, if necessary. Have a bedpan, commode, or nearby bathroom ready for use.	This ensures the patient's privacy. Explanation relieves anxiety and facilitates cooperation. The patient is better able to relax and cooperate if he or she is familiar with the procedure and knows everything is in readiness if the urge to defecate is felt.
7. Adjust the bed to a comfortable working height, usually elbow height of the caregiver (VISN 8 Patient Safety Center, 2009). Position the patient on the left side (Sims' position), as dictated by patient comfort and condition. Fold top linen back just enough to allow access to the patient's rectal area. Drape the patient with the bath blanket, as necessary, to maintain privacy and provide warmth. Place a waterproof pad under the patient's hip.	Having the bed at the proper height prevents back and muscle strain. Sims' position facilitates access into the rectum and colon. Folding back the linen in this manner minimizes unnecessary exposure and promotes the patient's comfort and warmth. The waterproof pad will protect the bed.
8. Put on nonsterile gloves.	Gloves prevent contact with blood and body fluids, as well as feces.
9. Generously lubricate index finger of dominant hand with water-soluble lubricant and insert finger gently into anal canal, pointing toward the umbilicus (Figure 1).	Lubrication reduces irritation of the rectum. The presence of the finger added to the mass tends to cause discomfort for the patient if the work is not done slowly and gently.
10. Gently work the finger around and into the hardened mass to break it up (Figure 2) and then remove pieces of it. Instruct patient to bear down, if possible, while extracting feces to ease in removal. Place extracted stool in bedpan.	Fecal mass may be large and may need to be removed in smaller pieces.

FIGURE 1 Inserting lubricated forefinger of dominant hand into anal canal, pointing toward umbilicus.

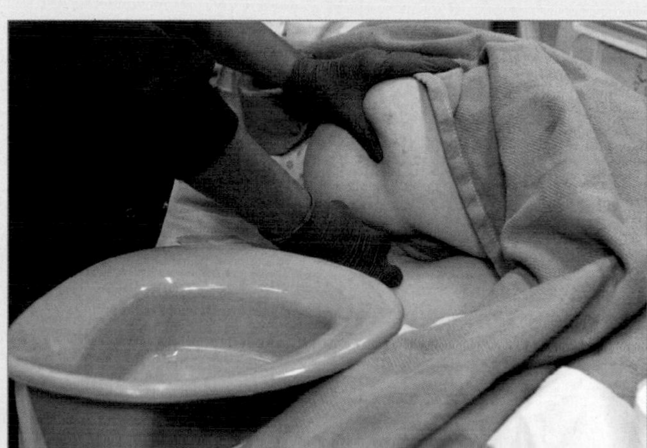

FIGURE 2 Gently working finger around to break up stool mass.

(continued)

SKILL 13-4 DIGITAL REMOVAL OF STOOL continued

ACTION	RATIONALE
11. Remove impaction at intervals if it is severe. **Instruct the patient to alert you if he or she begins to feel light-headed or nauseated. If patient reports either symptom, stop removal and assess the patient.**	Removal of stool in intervals helps to prevent discomfort and irritation, and vagal nerve stimulation. Assessment allows for detection of a vagal response. The enema may stimulate a vagal response, which increases parasympathetic stimulation, causing a decrease in heart rate.
12. When the procedure is completed, put on clean gloves. Assist the patient, if necessary, with cleaning of anal area (Figure 3). Offer washcloth, skin cleanser, and water for handwashing. If the patient is able, offer sitz bath.	Cleaning deters the transmission of microorganisms and promotes hygiene. Sitz bath may relieve the irritated perianal area.

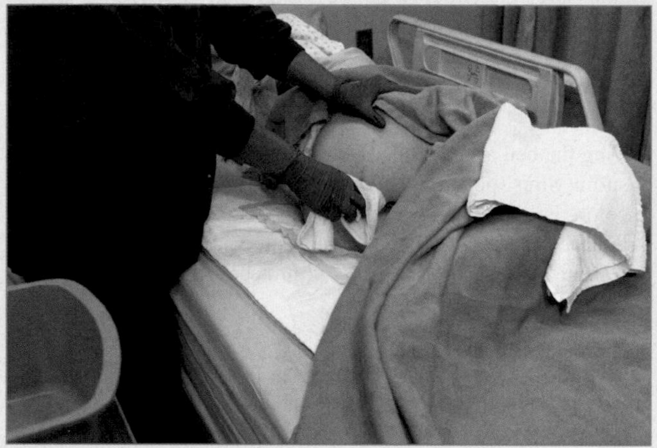

FIGURE 3 Cleaning anal area with washcloth and skin cleanser.

ACTION	RATIONALE
13. Remove gloves. Return the patient to a comfortable position. Make sure the linens under the patient are dry. Ensure that the patient is covered.	Removing contaminated gloves prevents spread of microorganisms. The other actions promote patient comfort.
14. Raise side rail. Lower bed height and adjust head of bed to a comfortable position.	These promote patient safety.
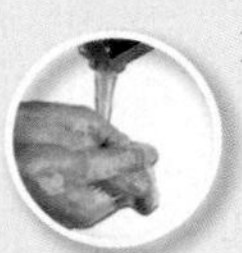 15. Remove additional PPE, if used. Perform hand hygiene.	Removing PPE properly reduces the risk for infection transmission and contamination of other items. Hand hygiene prevents the spread of microorganisms.

EVALUATION

The expected outcome is met when the fecal impaction is removed and the patient expels feces with assistance; the patient verbalizes decreased discomfort; abdominal distention is absent; and the patient remains free of any evidence of trauma to the rectal mucosa or other adverse effect.

DOCUMENTATION

Guidelines

Document the following: abdominal assessment; color, consistency, and amount of stool removed; condition of perianal area after the procedure; pain assessment rating; and the patient's reaction to the procedure.

Sample Documentation

6/29/15 1030 Digital removal of large amount of hard, brown stool. Abdomen soft, non-distended. Perineal area remains free from tears, erythema, or bleeding. Patient denied any light-headedness or nausea during procedure. Rates pain at 1 on a 0-to-10 scale.

—K. Sanders, RN

UNEXPECTED SITUATIONS AND ASSOCIATED INTERVENTIONS

- *Patient complains of being dizzy, light-headed, or nauseated or begins to vomit:* Stop digital stimulation immediately. Vagal nerve might have been stimulated. Assess heart rate and blood pressure. Notify primary care provider.
- *Patient experiences a large amount of pain during procedure:* Stop procedure and notify primary care provider.

SPECIAL CONSIDERATIONS

- In patients who are myelosuppressed and/or patients at risk for myelosuppression and mucositis, rectal agents and manipulation, including enemas, are discouraged because they can lead to development of bleeding, anal fissures, or abscesses, which are portals for infection (NCI, 2012).
- Recurrence of fecal impaction is common. It is important to help prevent and manage this condition by increasing dietary fiber content to 30 g/day, increasing water intake, and discontinuation of medications that can contribute to colonic hypomotility (Obokhare, 2012).

SKILL 13-5 APPLYING A FECAL INCONTINENCE DEVICE

A fecal incontinence device is used to protect the perianal skin from excoriation due to repeated exposure to liquid stool. This device reduces perineal skin damage by diverting liquid stool into a collection bag (Zimmaro Bliss & Norton, 2010). A skin barrier may be applied before the device to protect the patient's skin and improve adhesion. If excoriation is already present, the skin barrier should be applied before applying a device.

DELEGATION CONSIDERATIONS

Application of a fecal incontinence device may be delegated to nursing assistive personnel (NAP) or to unlicensed assistive personnel (UAP) who have received appropriate training. Application of a fecal incontinence device may be delegated to licensed practical/vocational nurses (LPN/LVNs). The decision to delegate must be based on careful analysis of the patient's needs and circumstances, as well as the qualifications of the person to whom the task is being delegated. Refer to the Delegation Guidelines in Appendix A.

EQUIPMENT

- Fecal incontinence device
- Disposable gloves
- Additional PPE, as indicated
- Washcloth, skin cleanser, and towel
- Drainage (Foley) bag
- Scissors (optional)
- Skin protectant or barrier
- Bath blanket

ASSESSMENT

Assess the amount and consistency of stool being passed. Also assess the frequency of bowel movements. Inspect the perianal area for any excoriation, wounds, or hemorrhoids.

NURSING DIAGNOSIS

Determine the related factors for the nursing diagnoses based on the patient's current status. Appropriate nursing diagnoses may include:

- Bowel Incontinence
- Risk for Impaired Skin Integrity
- Impaired Skin Integrity

OUTCOME IDENTIFICATION AND PLANNING

The expected outcome to achieve when applying a fecal incontinence device is that the patient expels feces into the device and maintains intact perianal skin. Other outcomes may include the following: the patient demonstrates a decrease in the amount and severity of excoriation; the patient verbalizes decreased discomfort; and the patient remains free of any signs and symptoms of infection.

(*continued*)

SKILL 13-5 APPLYING A FECAL INCONTINENCE DEVICE continued

IMPLEMENTATION

ACTION	RATIONALE
1. Gather equipment.	Assembling equipment provides for an organized approach to the task.
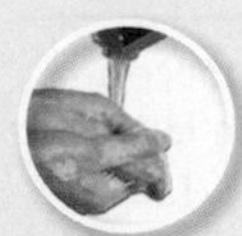 2. Perform hand hygiene and put on PPE, if indicated.	Hand hygiene and PPE prevent the spread of microorganisms. PPE is required based on transmission precautions.
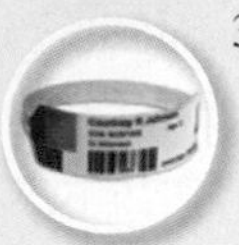 3. Identify the patient.	Identifying the patient ensures the right patient receives the intervention and helps prevent errors.
4. Close the curtains around the bed and close the door to the room, if possible. Explain what you are going to do and why you are going to do it to the patient.	This ensures the patient's privacy. Explanation relieves anxiety and facilitates cooperation. Discussion promotes cooperation and helps to minimize anxiety.
5. Assemble equipment on overbed table within reach.	Arranging items nearby is convenient, saves time, and avoids unnecessary stretching and twisting of muscles on the part of the nurse.
6. Adjust the bed to a comfortable working height, usually elbow height of the caregiver (VISN 8 Patient Safety Center, 2009). Position the patient on the left side (Sims' position), as dictated by patient comfort and condition. Fold top linen back just enough to allow access to the patient's rectal area. Drape the patient with the bath blanket, as necessary, to maintain privacy and provide warmth. Place a waterproof pad under the patient's hip.	Having the bed at the proper height prevents back and muscle strain. Sims' position facilitates access into the rectum. Folding back the linen in this manner minimizes unnecessary exposure and promotes the patient's comfort and warmth. The waterproof pad will protect the bed.
7. Put on gloves. Cleanse perianal area. Pat dry thoroughly.	Gloves protect the nurse from microorganisms in feces. Skin must be dry for device to adhere securely.
8. Trim perianal hair with scissors, if needed.	It may be uncomfortable if the perianal hair is pulled by adhesive from the fecal device. Trimming with scissors minimizes the risk for infection compared with shaving.
9. Apply the skin protectant or barrier and allow it to dry. Skin protectant may be contraindicated for use with some devices. Check manufacturer's recommendations before use.	Skin protectant aids in device adhesion and protects skin from irritation and injury from the adhesive. Skin must be dry for device to adhere securely.
10. If necessary, enlarge the opening in the adhesive skin barrier to fit the patient's anatomy. Do not cut beyond the printed line on the barrier. Remove paper backing from adhesive of device (Figure 1).	Cutting away too much of the adhesive backing will result in poor adhesion to the patient's skin. Removing the paper backing is necessary so that the device can adhere to the skin.

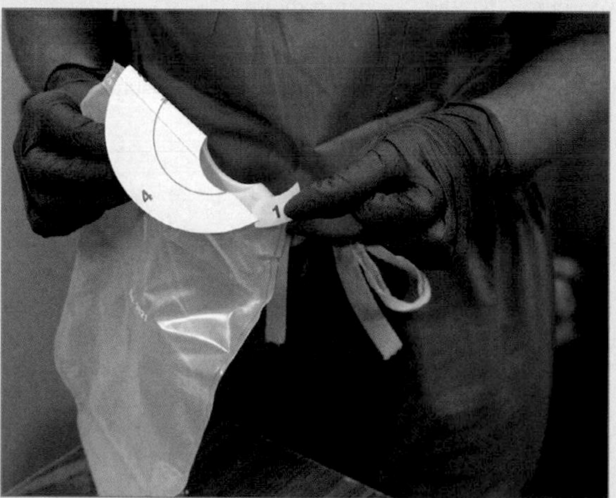

FIGURE 1 Removing paper backing from adhesive of rectal device.

ACTION

11. With nondominant hand, separate buttocks. Apply fecal device to anal area with dominant hand, ensuring that the bag opening is over anus (Figure 2). Hold the device in place for 30 seconds to achieve good adhesion.

RATIONALE

Opening should be over anus so that stool empties into bag and does not stay on patient's skin, which could lead to skin breakdown. The device is effective only if it is properly positioned and adhered securely.

12. Release buttocks. Attach connector of fecal incontinence device to drainage bag (Figure 3). Hang drainage bag below level of the patient (Figure 4).

Bag must be dependent for stool to drain into bag.

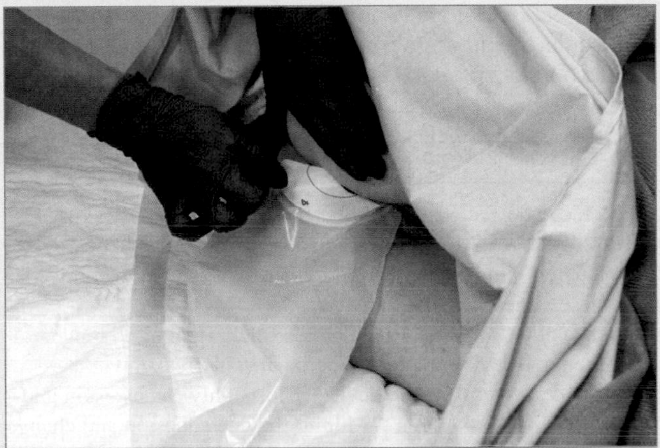

FIGURE 2 Applying device over anal opening.

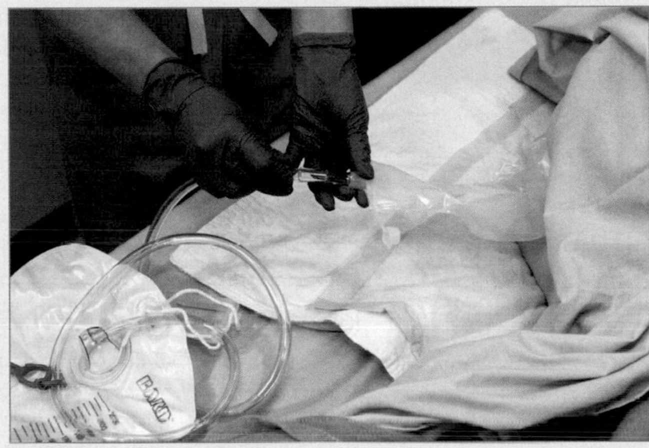

FIGURE 3 Attaching connector of fecal device to tubing of drainage bag.

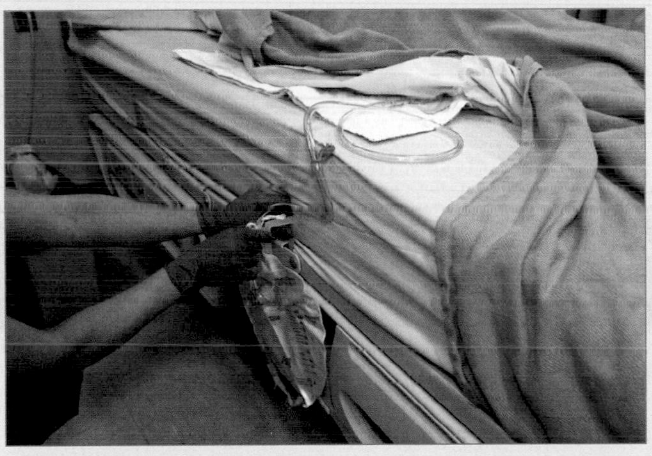

FIGURE 4 Checking that drainage bag is below level of patient.

13. Remove gloves. Return the patient to a comfortable position. Make sure the linens under the patient are dry. Ensure that the patient is covered.

Removing contaminated gloves prevents spread of microorganisms. Promotes patient comfort.

14. Raise side rail. Lower bed height and adjust head of bed to a comfortable position.

Promotes patient safety.

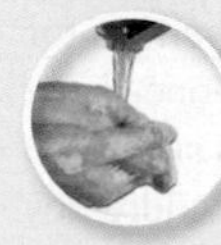

15. Remove additional PPE, if used. Perform hand hygiene.

Removing PPE properly reduces the risk for infection transmission and contamination of other items. Hand hygiene prevents the spread of microorganisms.

(*continued*)

SKILL 13-5 APPLYING A FECAL INCONTINENCE DEVICE continued

EVALUATION

The expected outcome is met when the patient expels feces into the device and maintains intact perianal skin; the patient demonstrates a decrease in the amount and severity of excoriation; the patient verbalizes decreased discomfort; and the patient remains free of any signs and symptoms of infection.

DOCUMENTATION

Guidelines

Document the date and time the fecal device was applied; appearance of perianal area; color of stool; intake and output (amount of stool out); and the patient's reaction to the procedure.

Sample Documentation

8/13/15 1210 Perianal area slightly erythematous. Fecal incontinence bag applied due to incontinence of large amounts of liquid stool and potential skin breakdown. Approximately 90 mL of liquid brown stool noted in drainage bag.

—K. Sanders, RN

UNEXPECTED SITUATIONS AND ASSOCIATED INTERVENTIONS

- *Perianal area becomes excoriated:* Remove device. Thoroughly cleanse skin and apply skin barrier. Allow to dry completely. Reapply device. Monitor device adhesion and change device as soon as there is a break in adhesion. Confer with primary care provider for a wound, ostomy, and continence nurse consult to manage these issues.
- *Stool does not drain from device into drainage bag:* Stool may be too thick. If stool no longer drains from device into drainage bag, remove device to prevent perianal skin breakdown.
- *Stool is leaking from around sides of fecal* device: Remove device. Thoroughly cleanse skin and apply skin barrier. Allow to dry completely. Reapply device. Monitor device adhesion and change device as soon as there is a break in adhesion.

SPECIAL CONSIDERATIONS

- Fecal collector may be left in place for up to 7 days as long as skin barrier is intact and adherent (Hollister, 2005). Remove fecal device based on manufacturer's recommendations; remove every 3 to 7 days to check for signs of skin breakdown.

SKILL 13-6 CHANGING AND EMPTYING AN OSTOMY APPLIANCE

The word *ostomy* is a term for a surgically formed opening from the inside of an organ to the outside. The intestinal mucosa is brought out to the abdominal wall, and a *stoma*, the part of the ostomy that is attached to the skin, is formed by suturing the mucosa to the skin. An *ileostomy* allows liquid fecal content from the ileum of the small intestine to be eliminated through the stoma. A *colostomy* permits formed feces in the colon to exit through the stoma. Colostomies are further classified by the part of the colon from which they originate. Ostomy appliances or pouches are applied to the opening to collect stool. They should be emptied promptly, usually when they are one-third to one-half full. If they are allowed to fill up, they may leak or become detached from the skin. Ostomy appliances are available in a one-piece (barrier backing already attached to the pouch) or two-piece (separate pouch that fastens to the barrier backing) system. Appliances are usually changed every 3 to 7 days, although they could be changed more often. Proper application minimizes the risk for skin breakdown around the stoma. This skill addresses changing a one-piece appliance. A one-piece appliance consists of a pouch with an integral adhesive section that adheres to the patient's skin. The adhesive flange is generally made from hydrocolloid. The accompanying Skill Variation addresses changing a two-piece appliance. Box 13-1 summarizes guidelines for care of the patient with a fecal diversion.

BOX 13-1 GUIDELINES FOR OSTOMY CARE

An ostomy requires specific physical care for which the nurse is initially responsible. Use the following guidelines to help promote the physical and psychological comfort of the patient with an ostomy:

- Keep the patient as free of odors as possible. Empty the ostomy appliance frequently.
- Inspect the patient's stoma regularly. It should be dark pink to red and moist. A pale stoma may indicate anemia, and a dark or purple-blue stoma may reflect compromised circulation or ischemia. Bleeding around the stoma and its stem should be minimal. Notify the primary care provider promptly if bleeding persists or is excessive, or if color changes occur in the stoma.
- Note the size of the stoma, which usually stabilizes within 6 to 8 weeks. Most stomas protrude 0.5 to 1 inch from the abdominal surface and may initially appear swollen and edematous. After 6 weeks, the edema has usually subsided. Depending on the surgical technique, the final stoma may be flush with the skin. Erosion of skin around the stoma area can also lead to a flush stoma. If an abdominal dressing is in place at the surgical incision, check it frequently for drainage and bleeding. The dressing is usually removed after 24 hours.
- Keep the skin around the stoma site (peristomal area) clean and dry. If care is not taken to protect the skin around the stoma, irritation or infection may occur. A leaking appliance frequently causes skin erosion. Candida or yeast infections can also occur around the stoma if the area is not kept dry.
- Measure the patient's fluid intake and output. Check the ostomy appliance for the quality and quantity of discharge. Initially after surgery, peristalsis may be inhibited. As peristalsis returns, stool will be eliminated from the stoma. Record intake and output every 4 hours for the first 3 days after surgery. If the patient's output decreases while intake remains stable, report the condition promptly.
- Explain each aspect of care to the patient and explain what his or her role will be when beginning self-care. Patient teaching is one of the most important aspects of colostomy care and should include family members and/or people identified by the patient to include in care, when appropriate. Teaching can begin before surgery, if possible, so that the patient has adequate time to absorb the information.
- Appliances can be either drainable or closed. A pouch that can be drained is emptied when it is one-third full and replaced every 3 to 7 days, or whenever the seal comes away from the skin. Nondrainable pouches require removal and changing when they are half full.
- Encourage the patient to participate in care and to look at the ostomy. Patients normally experience emotional depression during the early postoperative period. Help the patient cope by listening, explaining, and being available and supportive. A visit from a representative of the local ostomy support group may be helpful. Patients usually begin to accept their altered body image when they are willing to look at the stoma, make neutral or positive statements concerning the ostomy, and express interest in learning self-care.

DELEGATION CONSIDERATIONS

Emptying a stoma appliance on an ostomy may be delegated to nursing assistive personnel (NAP) or to unlicensed assistive personnel (UAP), as well as to licensed practical/vocational nurses (LPN/LVNs). Changing a stoma appliance on an ostomy may be delegated to an LPN/LVN. The decision to delegate must be based on careful analysis of the patient's needs and circumstances, as well as the qualifications of the person to whom the task is being delegated. Refer to the Delegation Guidelines in Appendix A.

EQUIPMENT

- Basin with warm water
- Skin cleanser, towel, washcloth
- Toilet tissue or paper towel
- Silicone-based adhesive remover
- Gauze squares
- Washcloth
- Skin protectant, such as SkinPrep
- One-piece ostomy appliance
- Closure clamp, if required, for appliance
- Stoma measuring guide
- Graduated container, toilet or bedpan
- Ostomy belt (optional)
- Disposable gloves
- Additional PPE, as indicated
- Small plastic trash bag
- Waterproof disposable pad

ASSESSMENT

Assess current ostomy appliance, looking at product style, condition of appliance, and stoma (if bag is clear). Note length of time the appliance has been in place. Determine the patient's knowledge of ostomy care. After removing the appliance, assess the stoma and the skin surrounding the stoma. Assess any abdominal scars, if surgery was recent. Assess the amount, color, consistency, and odor of stool from the ostomy.

(continued)

SKILL 13-6 CHANGING AND EMPTYING AN OSTOMY APPLIANCE continued

NURSING DIAGNOSIS

Determine the related factors for the nursing diagnoses based on the patient's current status. Appropriate nursing diagnoses may include:

- Risk for Impaired Skin Integrity
- Deficient Knowledge
- Disturbed Body Image

OUTCOME IDENTIFICATION AND PLANNING

The expected outcome to be met when changing and emptying an ostomy appliance is that the stoma appliance is applied correctly to the skin to allow stool to drain freely. Other outcomes may include the following: the patient exhibits a moist red stoma with intact skin surrounding the stoma; the patient demonstrates knowledge of how to apply the appliance; the patient demonstrates positive coping skills; the patient expels stool that is appropriate in consistency and amount for the ostomy location; and the patient verbalizes positive self-image.

IMPLEMENTATION

ACTION	RATIONALE
1. Gather equipment.	Assembling equipment provides for an organized approach to the task.
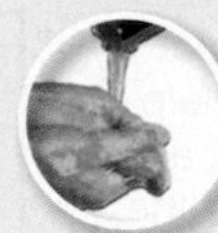 2. Perform hand hygiene and put on PPE, if indicated.	Hand hygiene and PPE prevent the spread of microorganisms. PPE is required based on transmission precautions.
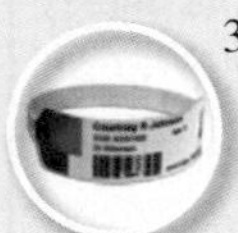 3. Identify the patient.	Identifying the patient ensures the right patient receives the intervention and helps prevent errors.
4. Close the curtains around the bed and close the door to the room, if possible. Explain what you are going to do and why you are going to do it to the patient. Encourage the patient to observe or participate, if possible.	This ensures the patient's privacy. Explanation relieves anxiety and facilitates cooperation. Discussion promotes cooperation and helps to minimize anxiety. Having the patient observe or assist encourages self-acceptance.
5. Assemble equipment on overbed table within reach.	Arranging items nearby is convenient, saves time, and avoids unnecessary stretching and twisting of muscles on the part of the nurse.
6. Assist the patient to a comfortable sitting or lying position in bed or a standing or sitting position in the bathroom. If the patient is in bed, adjust the bed to a comfortable working height, usually elbow height of the caregiver (VISN 8 Patient Safety Center, 2009). Place waterproof pad under the patient at the stoma site.	Either position should allow the patient to view the procedure in preparation to learn to perform it independently. Lying flat or sitting upright facilitates smooth application of the appliance. Having the bed at the proper height prevents back and muscle strain. A waterproof pad protects linens and patient from moisture.

Emptying an Appliance

ACTION	RATIONALE
7. Put on disposable gloves. Remove clamp and fold end of appliance or pouch upward like a cuff (Figure 1).	Gloves prevent contact with blood, body fluids, and microorganisms. Creating a cuff before emptying prevents additional soiling and odor.
8. Empty contents into bedpan, toilet, or measuring device (Figure 2).	Appliances do not need rinsing because rinsing may reduce appliance's odor barrier.
9. Wipe the lower 2 inches of the appliance or pouch with toilet tissue or paper towel (Figure 3).	Drying the lower section removes any additional fecal material, thus decreasing odor problems.

ACTION | RATIONALE

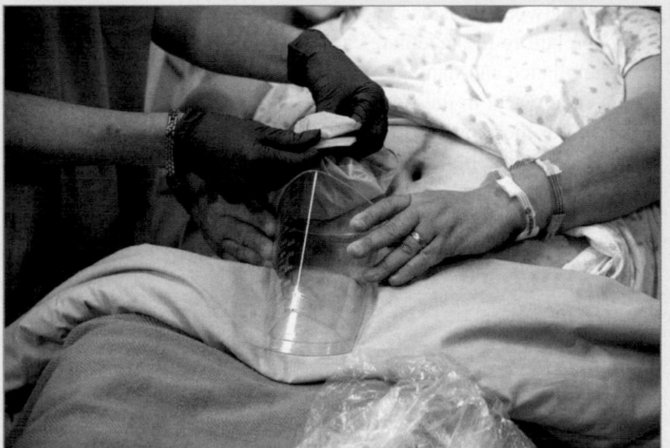
FIGURE 1 Removing clamp, getting ready to empty pouch.

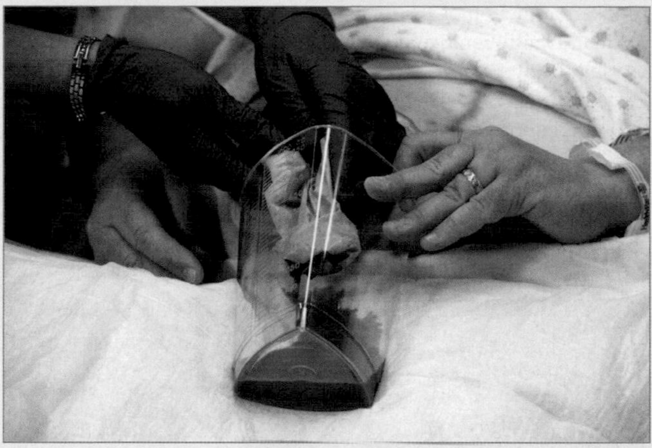
FIGURE 2 Emptying contents of appliance into a measuring device.

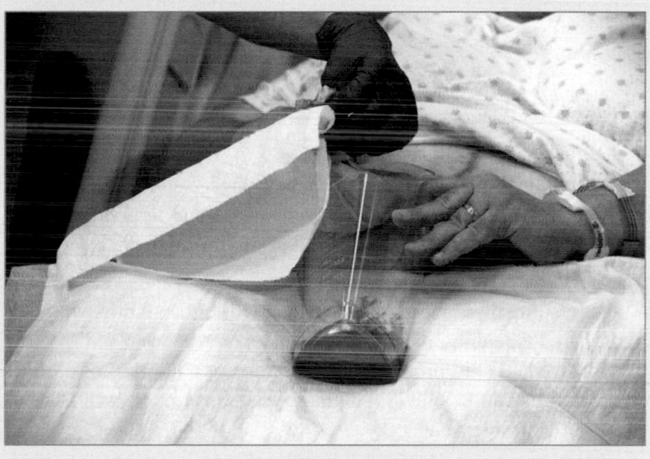
FIGURE 3 Wiping lower 2 inches of pouch with paper towel.

10. Uncuff edge of appliance or pouch and apply clip or clamp, or secure Velcro closure. Ensure the curve of the clamp follows the curve of the patient's body. Remove gloves. Assist the patient to a comfortable position.

The edge of the appliance or pouch should remain clean. The clamp secures closure. Hand hygiene deters spread of microorganisms. Ensures patient comfort.

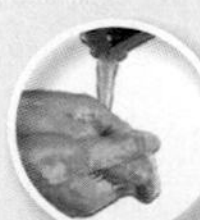
11. If appliance is not to be changed, remove additional PPE, if used. Perform hand hygiene.

Removing PPE properly reduces the risk for infection transmission and contamination of other items. Hand hygiene prevents the spread of microorganisms.

Changing an Appliance

12. Place a disposable pad on the work surface. Set up the washbasin with warm water and the rest of the supplies. Place a trash bag within reach.

Protects surface. Organization facilitates performance of procedure.

13. Put on clean gloves. Place waterproof pad under the patient at the stoma site. Empty the appliance as described previously.

Protects linens and patient from moisture. Emptying the contents before removal prevents accidental spillage of fecal material.

(*continued*)

SKILL 13-6 CHANGING AND EMPTYING AN OSTOMY APPLIANCE continued

ACTION	RATIONALE
14. Start at the top of the appliance and keep the abdominal skin taut. Gently remove pouch faceplate from skin by pushing skin from the appliance rather than pulling the appliance from skin (Figure 4). Apply a silicone-based adhesive remover by spraying or wiping with the remover wipe.	The seal between the surface of the faceplate and the skin must be broken before the faceplate can be removed. Harsh handling of the appliance can damage the skin and impair the development of a secure seal in the future. Silicone-based adhesive remover allows for the rapid and painless removal of adhesives and prevents skin stripping (Rudoni, 2008; Stephen-Haynes, 2008).

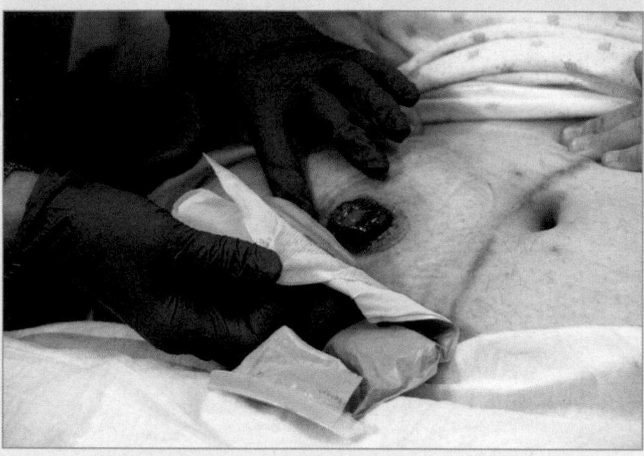

FIGURE 4 Removing appliance.

ACTION	RATIONALE
15. Place the appliance in the trash bag, if disposable. If reusable, set aside to wash in lukewarm soap and water and allow to air dry after the new appliance is in place.	Thorough cleaning and airing of the appliance reduce odor and deterioration of the appliance. For esthetic and infection-control purposes, discard used appliances appropriately.
16. Use toilet tissue to remove any excess stool from the stoma (Figure 5). Cover stoma with gauze pad. Clean skin around stoma with skin cleanser and water or a cleansing agent and a washcloth. Remove all old adhesive from skin; use an adhesive remover, as necessary. Do not apply lotion to the peristomal area.	Toilet tissue, used gently, will not damage the stoma. The gauze absorbs any drainage from the stoma while the skin is being prepared. Cleaning the skin removes excretions and old adhesive and skin protectant. Excretions or a buildup of other substances can irritate and damage the skin. Lotion will prevent a tight adhesive seal.
17. Gently pat area dry. **Make sure skin around stoma is thoroughly dry.** Assess stoma and condition of surrounding skin (Figure 6).	Careful drying prevents trauma to skin and stoma. An intact, properly applied fecal collection device protects skin integrity. Any change in color and size of the stoma may indicate circulatory problems. Refer to Box 13-1.

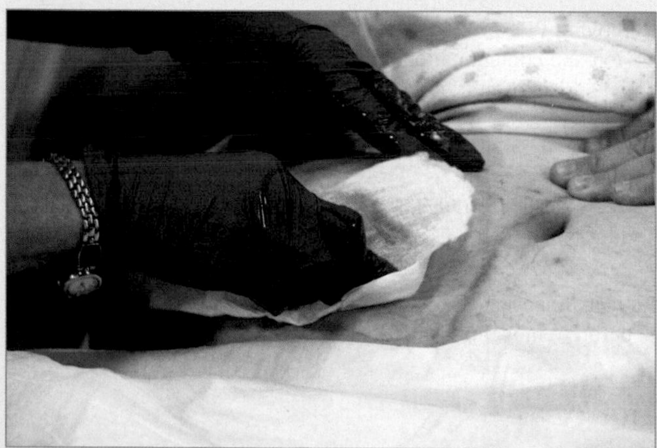

FIGURE 5 Using toilet tissue to wipe around stoma.

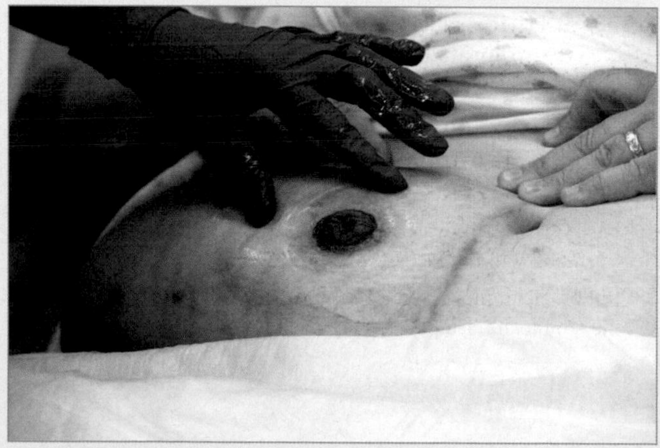

FIGURE 6 Assessing stoma and peristomal skin.

ACTION	RATIONALE
18. Apply skin protectant to a 2-inch (5 cm) radius around the stoma, and allow it to dry completely, which takes about 30 seconds.	The skin needs protection from the excoriating effect of the excretion and appliance adhesive. The skin must be perfectly dry before the appliance is placed to get good adherence and to prevent leaks.
19. Lift the gauze squares for a moment and measure the stoma opening, using the measurement guide (Figure 7). Replace the gauze. Trace the same-size opening on the back center of the appliance (Figure 8). Cut the opening 1/8 inch larger than the stoma size (Figure 9). Using a finger, gently smooth the wafer edges after cutting.	The appliance should fit snugly around the stoma, with only 1/8 inch of skin visible around the opening. A faceplate opening that is too small can cause trauma to the stoma. If the opening is too large, exposed skin will be irritated by stool. Wafer edges may be uneven after cutting and could cause irritation to, and/or pressure on, the stoma.

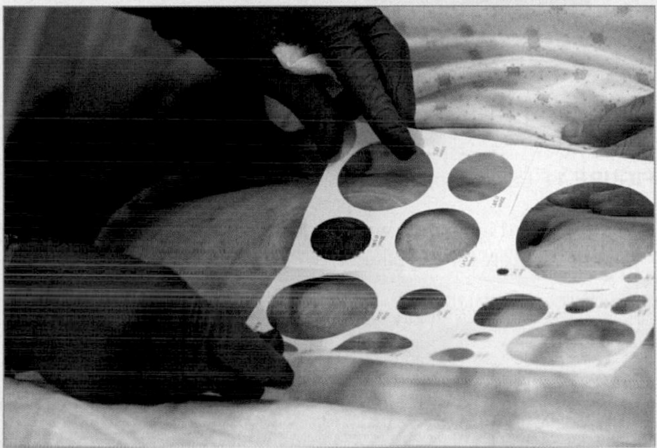

FIGURE 7 Using measurement guide to measure size of stoma.

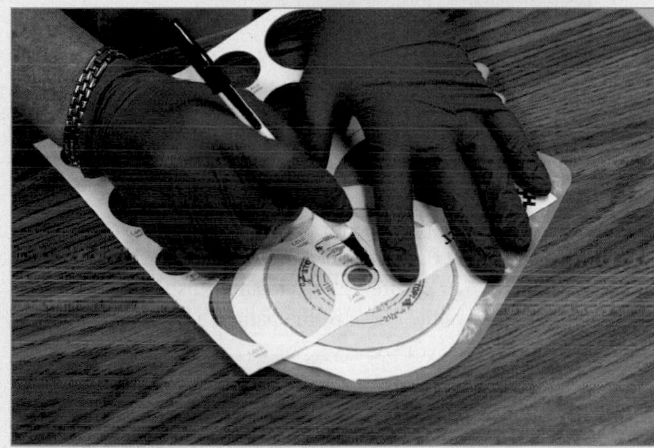

FIGURE 8 Tracing the same-sized circle on back and center of skin barrier.

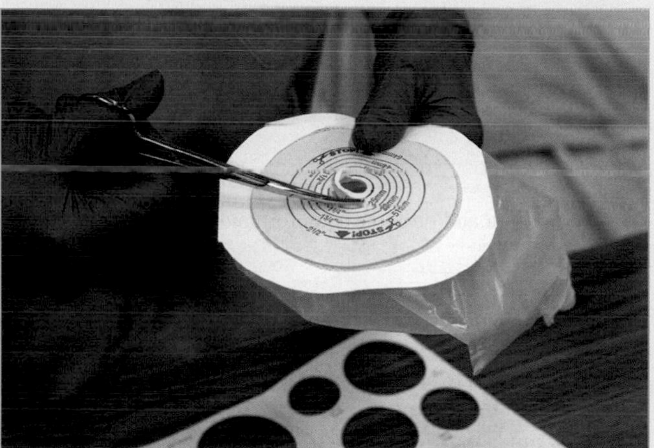

FIGURE 9 Cutting the opening 1/8 inch larger than stoma size.

(continued)

SKILL 13-6 CHANGING AND EMPTYING AN OSTOMY APPLIANCE continued

ACTION	RATIONALE
20. Remove the paper backing from the appliance faceplate (Figure 10). Quickly remove the gauze squares and ease the appliance over the stoma (Figure 11). Gently press onto the skin while smoothing over the surface. Apply gentle, even pressure to the appliance for approximately 30 seconds.	The appliance is effective only if it is properly positioned and adhered securely. Pressure on the appliance faceplate allows it to mold to the patient's skin and improve seal (Jones et al., 2011).

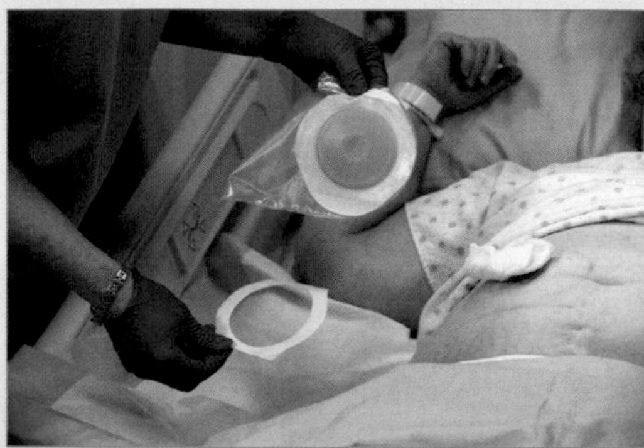

FIGURE 10 Removing paper backing on faceplate.

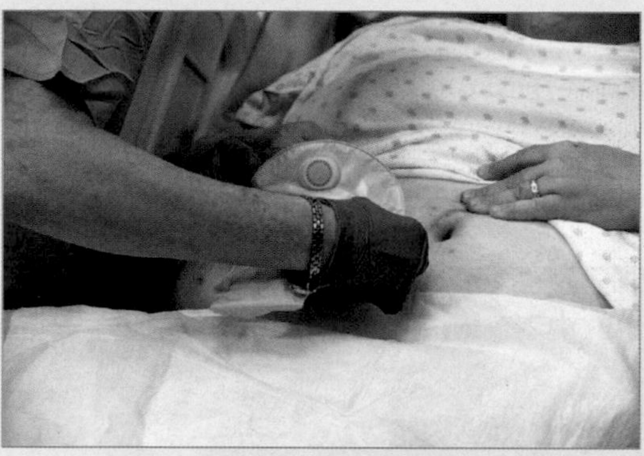

FIGURE 11 Easing appliance over stoma.

ACTION	RATIONALE
21. Close bottom of appliance or pouch by folding the end upward and using the clamp or clip that comes with the product (Figure 12), or secure Velcro closure. Ensure the curve of the clamp follows the curve of the patient's body.	A tightly sealed appliance will not leak and cause embarrassment and discomfort for the patient.

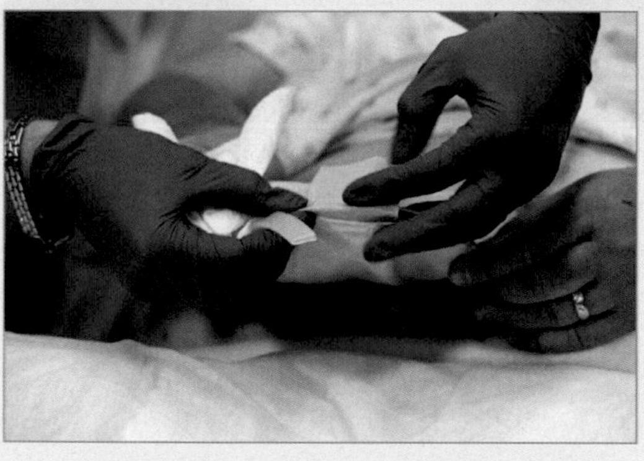

FIGURE 12 Using clip to close bottom of appliance.

ACTION	RATIONALE
22. Remove gloves. Assist the patient to a comfortable position. Cover the patient with bed linens. Place the bed in the lowest position.	Provides warmth and promotes comfort and safety.
23. Put on clean gloves. Remove or discard equipment and assess the patient's response to the procedure.	Gloves prevent contact with blood, body fluids, and microorganisms that contaminate the used equipment. The patient's response may indicate acceptance of the ostomy as well as the need for health teaching.
24. Remove gloves and additional PPE, if used. Perform hand hygiene.	Removing PPE properly reduces the risk for infection transmission and contamination of other items. Hand hygiene prevents the spread of microorganisms.

EVALUATION

The expected outcomes are met when the patient tolerates the procedure without pain and the peristomal skin remains intact without excoriation; odor is contained within the closed system; and the patient participates in ostomy appliance care, demonstrates positive coping skills, and expels stool that is appropriate in consistency and amount for the location of the ostomy.

DOCUMENTATION

Guidelines

Document appearance of stoma, condition of peristomal skin, characteristics of drainage (amount, color, consistency, unusual odor), the patient's reaction to procedure, and pertinent patient teaching.

Sample Documentation

Lippincott DocuCare Practice documenting changing and emptying an ostomy appliance in *Lippincott DocuCare.*

7/22/15 1630 Colostomy appliance changed due to leakage. Stoma is pink, moist, and flat against abdomen. No erythema or excoriation of surrounding skin. Moderate amount of pasty, brown stool noted in bag. Patient asking appropriate questions during appliance application. States, "I'm ready to try changing the next one."

—B. Clapp, RN

UNEXPECTED SITUATIONS AND ASSOCIATED INTERVENTIONS

- *Peristomal skin is excoriated or irritated:* Make sure that the appliance is not cut too large. Skin that is exposed inside of the ostomy appliance will become excoriated. Assess for the presence of a fungal skin infection. If present, consult with primary care provider to obtain appropriate treatment. Thoroughly cleanse skin and apply skin barrier. Allow to dry completely. Reapply pouch. Monitor pouch adhesion and change pouch as soon as there is a break in adhesion. Confer with primary care provider for a wound, ostomy, and continence nurse consult to manage these issues.
- *Patient continues to notice odor:* Check system for any leaks or poor adhesion. Clean outside of bag thoroughly when emptying.
- *Bag continues to come loose or fall off:* Thoroughly cleanse skin and apply skin barrier. Allow to dry completely. Reapply pouch. Monitor pouch adhesion and change pouch as soon as there is a break in adhesion.
- *Stoma is protruding into bag:* This is called a prolapse. Have patient rest for 30 minutes. If stoma is not back to normal size within that time, notify primary care provider. If stoma stays prolapsed, it may twist, resulting in impaired circulation to the stoma.
- *Stoma is dark brown or black:* Stoma should appear pink to red, shiny and moist. Alterations indicate compromised circulation. If the stoma is dark brown or black, suspect ischemia and necrosis. Notify the primary care provider immediately (Avent, 2012).

SKILL VARIATION Applying a Two-Piece Appliance

A two-piece colostomy appliance is composed of a pouch and a separate adhesive faceplate (Figure A). The faceplate is left in place for a period of time, usually 3 to 7 days. During this period, when the colostomy appliance requires changing, only the bag needs to be replaced. The two main types of two-piece appliance are (1) those that 'click' together and (2) those that 'adhere' together. The clicking Tupperware-type joining action provides extra security because there is a sensation when the appliance is secured, which the patient can feel. One problem with this type of system is that those with reduced manual dexterity may find it difficult to secure. Another disadvantage is that it is less discreet because the parts of the appliance that click together are more bulky than the one-piece system. Two-piece appliances with an adhesive system have the advantage that they are more discreet than conventional two-piece systems. They may also be simpler to use for those with poor manual dexterity. A potential disadvantage is that if the adhesive is not joined correctly and forms a crease, then feces or flatus may leak out, causing odor and embarrassment. Regardless of the type of two-piece appliance in use, the procedure to change is basically the same.

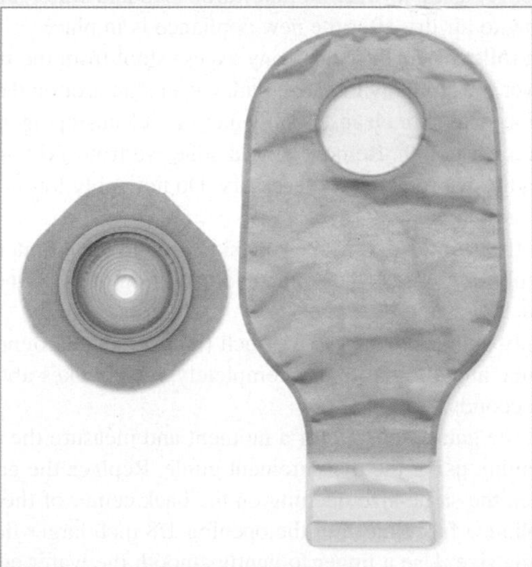

FIGURE A Two-piece appliances. (Courtesy of Hollister, Incorporated, Libertyville, Illinois.)

(continued)

SKILL 13-6 CHANGING AND EMPTYING AN OSTOMY APPLIANCE continued

SKILL VARIATION Applying a Two-Piece Appliance continued

1. Gather necessary equipment.

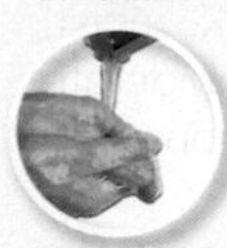

2. Perform hand hygiene and put on PPE, if indicated.

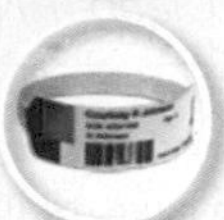

3. Identify the patient.
4. Close the curtains around the bed and close the door to the room, if possible. Explain what you are going to do and why you are going to do it to the patient. Encourage the patient to observe or participate, if possible.
5. Assemble equipment on overbed table within reach.
6. Assist the patient to a comfortable sitting or lying position in bed or a standing or sitting position in the bathroom.
7. Place a disposable pad on the work surface. Set up the washbasin with warm water and the rest of the supplies. Place a trash bag within reach.
8. Put on gloves. Place waterproof pad under the patient at the stoma site. Empty the appliance as described previously in Skill 13-6.
9. Starting at the top of the appliance, gently remove the pouch faceplate while keeping the abdominal skin taut. Apply a silicone-based adhesive remover by spraying or wiping with the remover wipe. Push the skin from the appliance rather than pulling the appliance from the skin.
10. Place the appliance in the trash bag, if disposable. If reusable, set aside to wash in lukewarm soap and water and allow to air dry after the new appliance is in place.
11. Use toilet tissue to remove any excess stool from the stoma. Cover the stoma with gauze pad. Clean skin around the stoma with skin cleanser and water or a cleansing agent and a washcloth. Remove all old adhesive from skin; use an adhesive remover as necessary. Do not apply lotion to peristomal area.
12. Gently pat area dry. Make sure skin around the stoma is thoroughly dry. Assess the stoma and condition of surrounding skin.
13. Apply skin protectant to a 2-inch (5 cm) radius around the stoma, and allow it to dry completely, which takes about 30 seconds.
14. Lift the gauze squares for a moment and measure the stoma opening, using the measurement guide. Replace the gauze. Trace the same-size opening on the back center of the appliance faceplate. Cut the opening 1/8 inch larger than the stoma size. Use a finger to gently smooth the wafer edges after cutting.
15. Remove the backing from the faceplate. Quickly remove the gauze squares and ease the faceplate over the stoma. Gently press onto the skin while smoothing over the surface. Apply gentle pressure to the faceplate for approximately 30 seconds (Figure B).

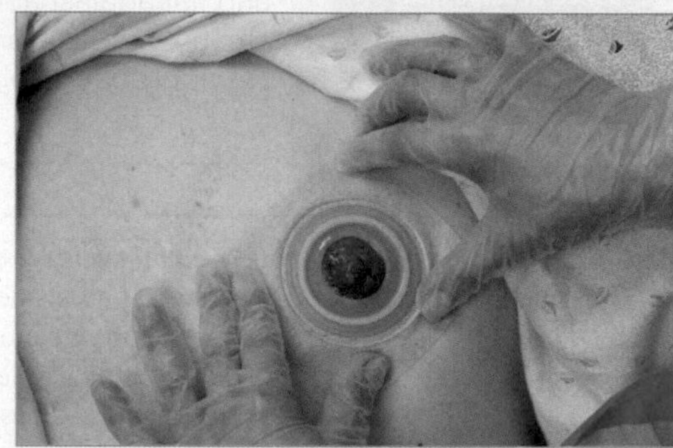

FIGURE B Gently press faceplate to skin.

16. Apply the appliance pouch to the faceplate following manufacturer's directions. If using a 'click' system, lay the ring on the pouch over the ring on the faceplate. Ask the patient to tighten stomach muscles, if possible. Beginning at one edge of the ring, push the pouch ring onto the faceplate ring (Figure C). A 'click' should be heard when the pouch is secured onto the faceplate.

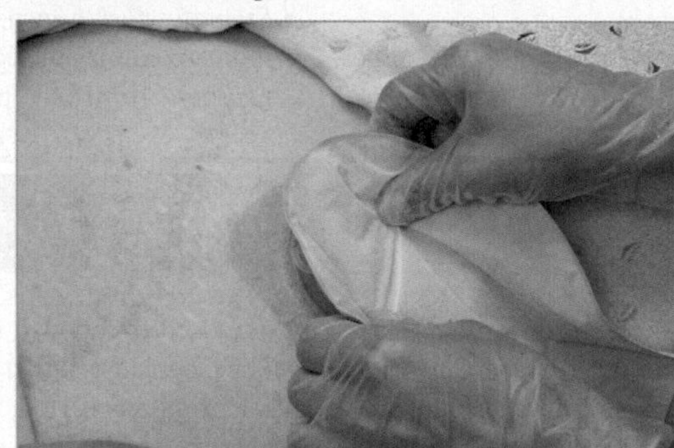

FIGURE C Applying appliance pouch to faceplate.

17. If using an 'adhere' system, remove the paper backing from the faceplate and pouch. Starting at one edge, carefully match the pouch adhesive with the faceplate adhesive. Press firmly and smooth the pouch onto the faceplate, taking care to avoid creases.
18. Close bottom of pouch by folding the end upward and using the clamp or clip that comes with the product, or secure Velcro closure. Ensure the curve of the clamp follows the curve of the patient's body.
19. Remove gloves. Assist the patient to a comfortable position. Cover the patient with bed linens. Place the bed in the lowest position.
20. Put on clean gloves. Remove or discard equipment and assess the patient's response to the procedure.

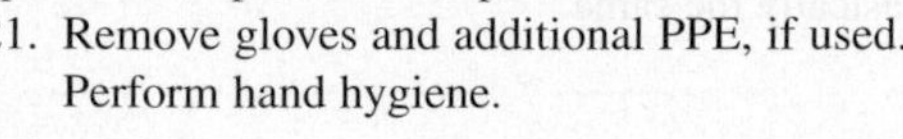

21. Remove gloves and additional PPE, if used. Perform hand hygiene.

EVIDENCE FOR PRACTICE ▶

LIVING WITH A COLOSTOMY

A stoma operation causes major changes in a patient's life because of the resulting physical damage, disfigurement, loss of bodily function, and change in personal hygiene. Such changes are a cause of major concern for patients and raise important issues for the provision of quality care.

Related Research

Notter, J., & Chalmers, F. (2012). Living with a colostomy: A pilot study. *Gastrointestinal Nursing, 10*(6), 16, 18, 20, 22–24.

This survey explored issues impacting on coping and quality of life for those living with a colostomy. Questionnaires were sent to 1,000 patients with ostomies who volunteered to participate in research studies. The response rate was 47%; of the 469 questionnaires returned, 369 were used for descriptive data analysis. The remaining 100 responses could not be analyzed, as they were incomplete. Over 97% of the respondents were over 50 years of age; almost 30% reported complications necessitating further admissions and/or more surgery. Restrictions on activities of daily living, including social activities with family and friends, were present for 40% of respondents. Problems with leakage were reported by 50% of the participants and 33% found emptying and/or disposal of used appliances to be a problem. Of men, 35%, and, of women, 37% reported emotional problems, such as body image and self-confidence, adjustment to the impact of major surgery, and depression. In addition, participants (30% of men and 27% of women) reported that intimacy with their partner had been adversely affected.

Relevance for Nursing Practice

Patients experiencing life-altering surgeries, such as colostomies and ileostomies, require much information and support to adapt and achieve an adequate standard of living. Nurses are the members of the health care team who typically spend the most time in direct contact with these patients. Nurses have a unique opportunity to provide the education and support these patients need, and improve the care provided to these patients. In addition to assisting patients to learn the physical care needs related to a stoma, nurses must address the psychosocial concerns of patients with ostomies as part of their nursing interventions. Assisting patients to adjust and encouraging social interactions should be part of the care routinely given to a patient with a stoma.

Refer to thePoint for additional research on related nursing topics.

SKILL 13-7 IRRIGATING A COLOSTOMY

Colostomy irrigation is a way of achieving fecal continence and control (Perston, 2010). Irrigations are used to promote regular evacuation of some colostomies. Colostomy irrigation may be indicated in patients who have a left-sided end colostomy in the descending or sigmoid colon, are mentally alert, have adequate vision, and have adequate manual dexterity needed to perform the procedure. Contraindications to colostomy irrigation include irritable bowel syndrome, peristomal hernia, post-radiation damage to the bowel, diverticulitis, and Crohn's disease (Carlsson et al., 2010). Ileostomies are not irrigated because the fecal content of the ileum is liquid and cannot be controlled.

Once the patient has established a routine and bowel continence has been established, a small appliance can be worn over the stoma. These 'stoma caps' are small capacity appliances with a pad to soak up discharge and a flatus filter (Perston, 2010). If a colostomy irrigation is to be implemented, the nurse should consult facility policy regarding the accepted procedure and, ideally, consult with a wound, ostomy, and continence nurse for patient education and support.

(*continued*)

SKILL 13-7 IRRIGATING A COLOSTOMY continued

DELEGATION CONSIDERATIONS

Colostomy irrigation is not delegated to nursing assistive personnel (NAP) or to unlicensed assistive personnel (UAP). Depending on the state's nurse practice act and the organization's policies and procedures, the administration of a small-volume cleansing enema may be delegated to licensed practical/vocational nurses (LPN/LVNs). The decision to delegate must be based on careful analysis of the patient's needs and circumstances, as well as the qualifications of the person to whom the task is being delegated. Refer to the Delegation Guidelines in Appendix A.

EQUIPMENT

- Disposable irrigation system and irrigation sleeve
- Waterproof pad
- Bedpan or toilet
- Water-soluble lubricant
- IV pole
- Disposable gloves
- Additional PPE, as indicated
- Solution at a temperature of 98.6°F (37°C) (normally tap water)
- Washcloth, skin cleanser, and towels
- Paper towel
- New ostomy appliance, if needed, or stoma cover

ASSESSMENT

Ask patient if he or she has been experiencing any abdominal discomfort. Ask the patient about the date of the last irrigation and whether there have been any changes in stool pattern or consistency. If the patient irrigates his or her colostomy at home, ask if he or she has any special routines during irrigation, such as reading the newspaper or listening to music. Also determine how much solution the patient typically uses for irrigation. The normal amount of irrigation fluid varies, but is usually around 500 mL to 1,000 mL for an adult. If this is a first irrigation, the normal irrigation volume is around 500 mL. Assess the ostomy, ensuring that the diversion is a colostomy. Note placement of colostomy on abdomen, color and size of ostomy, color and condition of stoma, and amount and consistency of stool.

NURSING DIAGNOSIS

Determine the related factors for the nursing diagnoses based on the patient's current status. Possible nursing diagnoses may include:

- Deficient Knowledge
- Anxiety
- Disturbed Body Image

OUTCOME IDENTIFICATION AND PLANNING

The expected outcome to be met when irrigating a colostomy is that the patient expels soft, formed stool. Other appropriate outcomes include the patient remains free of any evidence of trauma to the stoma and intestinal mucosa; the patient demonstrates the ability to participate in care; the patient voices increased confidence with ostomy care; and the patient demonstrates positive coping mechanisms.

IMPLEMENTATION

ACTION	RATIONALE
1. Verify the order for the irrigation. Gather equipment (Figure 1).	Verifying the medical order is crucial to ensuring that the proper treatment is administered to the right patient. Assembling equipment provides for an organized approach to the task.

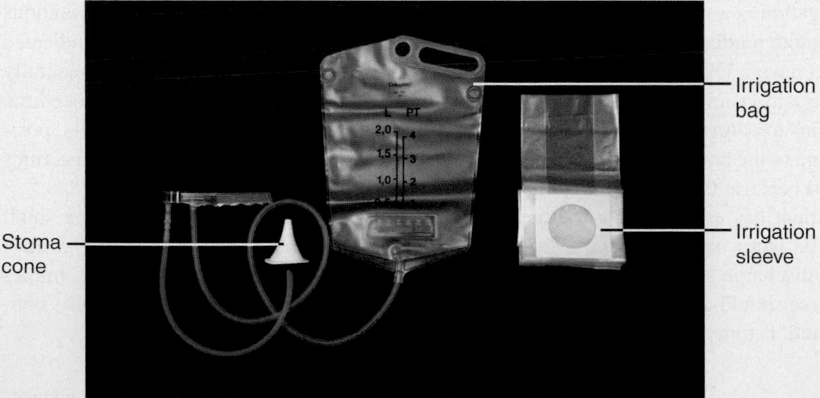

FIGURE 1 Irrigation sleeve and bag.

ACTION	RATIONALE
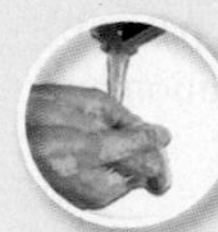 2. Perform hand hygiene and put on PPE, if indicated.	Hand hygiene and PPE prevent the spread of microorganisms. PPE is required based on transmission precautions.
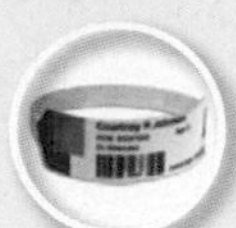 3. Identify the patient.	Identifying the patient ensures the right patient receives the intervention and helps prevent errors.
4. Close the curtains around the bed and close the door to the room, if possible. Explain what you are going to do and why you are going to do it to the patient. Plan where the patient will receive irrigation. Assist the patient onto bedside commode or into nearby bathroom.	This ensures the patient's privacy. Explanation relieves anxiety and facilitates cooperation. Discussion promotes cooperation and helps to minimize anxiety. The patient cannot hold the irrigation solution. A large immediate return of irrigation solution and stool usually occurs.
5. Assemble equipment on overbed table within reach.	Arranging items nearby is convenient, saves time, and avoids unnecessary stretching and twisting of muscles on the part of the nurse.
6. Warm solution in amount ordered and check temperature with a bath thermometer, if available. If bath thermometer is not available, warm to room temperature or slightly higher, and test on inner wrist. If tap water is used, adjust temperature as it flows from faucet.	If the solution is too cool, the patient may experience cramps or nausea. Solution that is too warm or too hot can cause irritation and trauma to intestinal mucosa.
7. Add irrigation solution to container. Release clamp and allow fluid to progress through tube before reclamping.	This causes any air to be expelled from the tubing. Although allowing air to enter the intestine is not harmful, it may further distend the intestine.
8. Hang container on IV pole so that bottom of bag will be at the patient's shoulder level when seated.	Gravity forces the solution to enter the intestine. The amount of pressure determines the rate of flow and pressure exerted on the intestinal wall.
9. Put on gloves.	Gloves prevent contact with blood, body fluids, and microorganisms.
10. Remove ostomy appliance and attach irrigation sleeve (Figure 2). Place drainage end into toilet bowl or commode.	The irrigation sleeve directs all irrigation fluid and stool into the toilet or bedpan for easy disposal.
11. Lubricate end of cone with water-soluble lubricant.	This facilitates passage of the cone into the stoma opening.

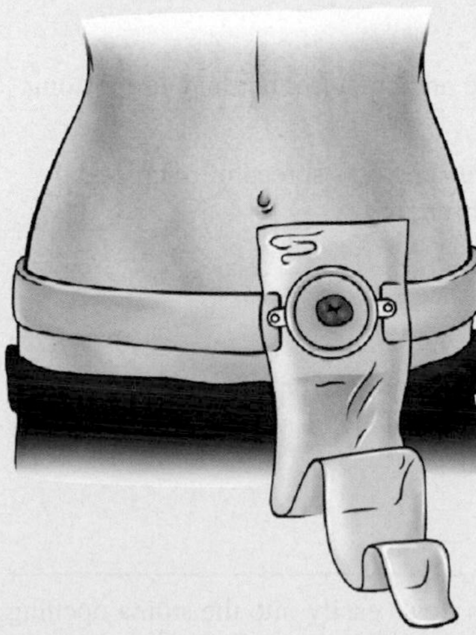

FIGURE 2 Positioning of irrigation sleeve on abdomen.

(*continued*)

SKILL 13-7 IRRIGATING A COLOSTOMY continued

ACTION	RATIONALE
12. Insert the cone through the top of the irrigation sleeve and into the stoma (Figure 3A). Introduce solution slowly over a period of 5 to 10 minutes. Hold cone and tubing (or if patient is able, allow patient to hold) all the time that solution is being instilled (Figure 3B). Control rate of flow by closing or opening the clamp.	If the irrigation solution is administered too quickly, the patient may experience nausea and cramps due to rapid distention and increased pressure in the intestine.

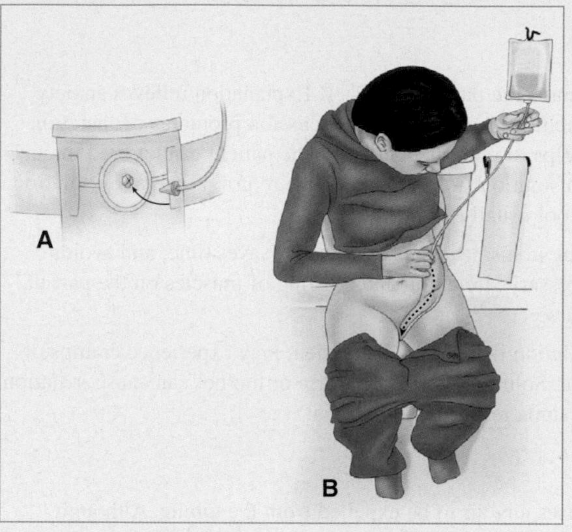

FIGURE 3 Colostomy irrigation. (**A**) Inserting irrigation cone. (**B**) Instilling irrigating fluid with sleeve in place.

ACTION	RATIONALE
13. Hold cone in place for an additional 10 seconds after the fluid is infused.	This will allow a small amount of dwell time for the irrigation solution.
14. Remove cone. Patient should remain seated on toilet or bedside commode.	An immediate return of solution and stool will usually occur, followed by a return in spurts for up to 45 more minutes.
15. After majority of solution has returned, allow the patient to clip (close) the bottom of irrigating sleeve and continue with daily activities.	An immediate return of solution and stool will usually occur, followed by a return in spurts for up to 45 more minutes. Leaving the sleeve in place allows the patient to continue with daily activities until return of solution is complete.
16. After solution has stopped flowing from stoma, put on clean gloves. Remove irrigating sleeve and cleanse skin around stoma opening with skin cleanser and water. Gently pat peristomal skin dry.	Gloves prevent contact with blood and body fluids. Peristomal skin must be clean and free of any liquid or stool before application of a new appliance.
17. Attach new appliance to stoma or stoma cover (see Skill 13-6), as needed.	Some patients will not require an appliance, but may use a stoma cover. Protects stoma.
18. Remove gloves. Return the patient to a comfortable position. Make sure the linens under the patient are dry, if appropriate. Ensure that the patient is covered.	Removing contaminated gloves prevents spread of microorganisms. Promotes patient comfort.
19. Raise side rail. Lower bed height and adjust head of bed to a comfortable position, as necessary.	Promotes patient safety.
20. Remove gloves and additional PPE, if used. Perform hand hygiene.	Removing PPE properly reduces the risk for infection transmission and contamination of other items. Hand hygiene prevents the spread of microorganisms.

EVALUATION

The expected outcome is achieved when the irrigation solution flows easily into the stoma opening and the patient expels soft, formed stool; the patient remains free of any evidence of trauma to the stoma and intestinal mucosa; the patient participates in irrigation with increasing confidence; and the patient demonstrates positive coping mechanisms.

DOCUMENTATION

Guidelines

Document the procedure, including the amount of irrigating solution used; color, amount, and consistency of stool returned; condition of stoma; degree of patient participation; and patient's reaction to irrigation.

Sample Documentation

> 8/1/15 0945 1,000 mL of warmed tap water used to irrigate colostomy. Large amount of soft, dark brown stool returned. Patient performed procedure with small amount of assistance from nurse. Stoma is pink and moist with no signs of bleeding. Patient tolerated procedure without incident. New ostomy appliance applied.
>
> *—B. Clapp, RN*

UNEXPECTED SITUATIONS AND ASSOCIATED INTERVENTIONS

- *Irrigation solution is not flowing or is flowing at a slow rate:* Check clamp on tubing to make sure that the tubing is open. Gently manipulate cone in stoma; if stool or tissue is blocking cone opening, this may block flow of fluid. Remove cone from stoma, clean the area, and gently reinsert. Alternately, assist the patient to a side-lying or sitting position in bed. Place a waterproof pad under the irrigation sleeve. Place the drainage end of the sleeve in a bedpan.
- *Patient experiences abdominal cramping:* Check the temperature of the irrigation fluid; decrease rate of irrigation fluid.
- *Patient experienced breakthrough evacuation of stool:* Increase frequency of colostomy irrigation if less than daily; ensure irrigation is performed at regular time intervals (Perston, 2010).

SPECIAL CONSIDERATIONS

- Irrigation is contraindicated for patients who are myelosuppressed and/or patients at risk for myelosuppression and mucositis. The stoma of a patient who is neutropenic should not be manipulated (NCI, 2012).

SKILL 13-8 IRRIGATING A NASOGASTRIC TUBE CONNECTED TO SUCTION

Nasogastric tubes (NGTs) may be inserted to decompress or drain the stomach of fluid or unwanted stomach contents, such as poison, medication, or air, and when conditions are present in which peristalsis is absent. Examples of such conditions include paralytic ileus and intestinal obstruction by tumor or hernia. Nasogastric tubes are also used to allow the GI tract to rest before or after abdominal surgery to promote healing; they are inserted to monitor GI bleeding. Historically, an NGT has often been used postoperatively as a routine part of care after major abdominal surgery, to rest the intestinal tract and promote healing. However, some research has suggested that the routine use of an NGT after abdominal surgery may serve no beneficial purpose and may actually delay the patient's progress, increasing the time required for flatus to occur and increasing pulmonary complications (Lafon & Lawson, 2012). It is suggested that selective decompression should be reserved for patients with nausea, vomiting, and abdominal distention after surgery (Brennan, 2008; Gannon, 2007; Nelson et al., 2007). The tube is usually attached to suction (intermittent or continuous) when used for these reasons or the tube may be clamped. The tube must be kept free from obstruction or clogging and is usually irrigated every 4 to 6 hours.

To promote patient safety when instilling solutions into a nasogastric tube, tube placement must be verified before administration of any fluids or medications. Radiographic examination, measurement of aspirate pH, visual assessment of aspirate, measurement of tube length and measurement of tube marking, and monitoring of carbon dioxide are used to confirm NGT placement. With the exception of radiographic examination, the use of several of these techniques in conjunction with each other increases the likelihood of correct tube placement. An old technique of auscultation of air injected into an NGT has proved unreliable and may result in tragic consequences if used as an indicator of tube placement (AACN, 2010; Best, 2005; Khair, 2005). Therefore, do not use it to confirm nasogastric tube placement.

(continued)

SKILL 13-8 IRRIGATING A NASOGASTRIC TUBE CONNECTED TO SUCTION continued

DELEGATION CONSIDERATIONS

The irrigation of a nasogastric tube (NGT) is not delegated to nursing assistive personnel (NAP) or to unlicensed assistive personnel (UAP). Depending on the state's nurse practice act and the organization's policies and procedures, irrigation of an NGT may be delegated to licensed practical/vocational nurses (LPN/LVNs). The decision to delegate must be based on careful analysis of the patient's needs and circumstances, as well as the qualifications of the person to whom the task is being delegated. Refer to the Delegation Guidelines in Appendix A.

EQUIPMENT

- NGT connected to continuous or intermittent suction
- Water or normal saline solution for irrigation (based on facility policy)
- Nonsterile gloves
- Additional PPE, as indicated
- Irrigation set (or a 60-mL catheter-tip syringe and cup for irrigating solution)
- Clamp
- Disposable waterproof pad or bath towel
- Emesis basin
- Tape measure, or other measuring device
- pH paper and measurement scale

ASSESSMENT

Assess abdomen by inspecting for presence of distention, auscultating for bowel sounds, and palpating the abdomen for firmness or tenderness. If the abdomen is distended, consider measuring the abdominal girth at the umbilicus. If the patient reports any tenderness or nausea, or exhibits any rigidity or firmness of the abdomen, confer with the primary care provider. If the NGT is attached to suction, assess suction to ensure that it is running at the prescribed pressure. Also, inspect drainage from NGT, including color, consistency, and amount.

NURSING DIAGNOSIS

Determine the related factors for the nursing diagnoses based on the patient's current status. Possible nursing diagnoses may include:

- Imbalanced Nutrition: Less than Body Requirements
- Risk for Injury
- Risk for Deficient Fluid Volume

OUTCOME IDENTIFICATION AND PLANNING

The expected outcome to achieve when irrigating a patient's NGT is that the tube will maintain patency with irrigation. In addition, the patient will not experience any trauma or injury.

IMPLEMENTATION

ACTION	RATIONALE
1. Gather equipment. Verify the medical order or facility policy and procedure regarding frequency of irrigation, solution type, and amount of irrigant. Check expiration dates on irrigating solution and irrigation set.	Assembling equipment provides for an organized approach to the task. Verification ensures the patient receives the correct intervention. Facility policy dictates safe interval for reuse of equipment.
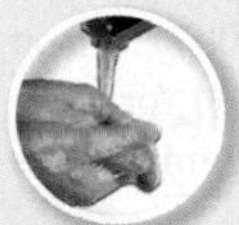 2. Perform hand hygiene and put on PPE, if indicated.	Hand hygiene and PPE prevent the spread of microorganisms. PPE is required based on transmission precautions.
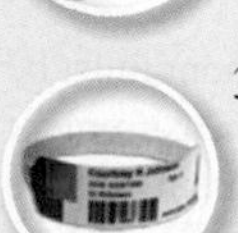 3. Identify the patient.	Identifying the patient ensures the right patient receives the intervention and helps prevent errors.
4. Explain the procedure to the patient and why this intervention is needed. Answer any questions, as needed. Perform key abdominal assessments as described above.	Explanation facilitates patient cooperation. Due to potential changes in a patient's condition, assessment is vital before initiating intervention.

ACTION	RATIONALE
5. Assemble equipment on overbed table within reach.	Organization facilitates performance of the task.
6. Pull the patient's bedside curtain. Raise bed to a comfortable working position, usually elbow height of the caregiver (VISN 8 Patient Safety Center, 2009). Assist patient to 30- to 45-degree position, unless this is contraindicated. Pour the irrigating solution into container.	Provides for privacy. Appropriate working height facilitates comfort and proper body mechanics for the nurse. This position minimizes risk for aspiration. Preparing the irrigation provides for an organized approach to the task.
7. Put on gloves. Place waterproof pad on the patient's chest, under connection of the nasogastric tube and suction tubing. **Check placement of NG tube.** (Refer to Skill 11-2.)	Gloves prevent contact with body fluids. Waterproof pad protects patient's clothing and bed linens from accidental leakage of gastric fluid. Checking placement before the instillation of fluid is necessary to prevent accidental instillation into the respiratory tract if the tube has become dislodged.
8. Draw up 30 mL of irrigation solution (or amount indicated in the order or policy) into syringe (Figure 1).	This delivers measured amount of irrigant through the tube. Saline solution (isotonic) may be used to compensate for electrolytes lost through nasogastric drainage.
9. Clamp nasogastric tube near connection site. Disconnect tube from suction apparatus (Figure 2) and lay on disposable pad or towel, or hold both tubes upright in nondominant hand (Figure 3).	Clamping prevents leakage of gastric fluid.

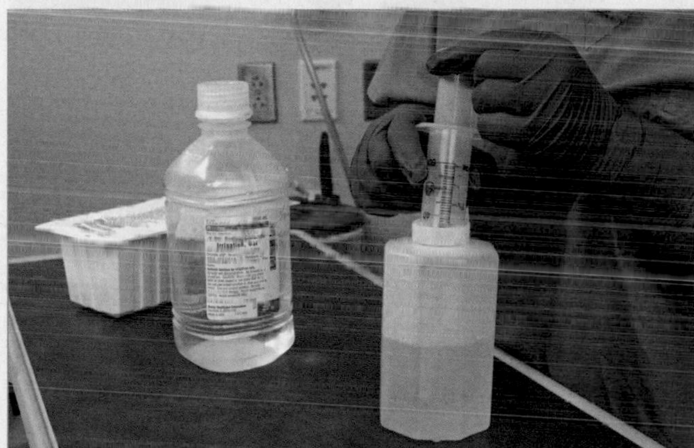
FIGURE 1 Preparing syringe with 30 mL of irrigation solution.

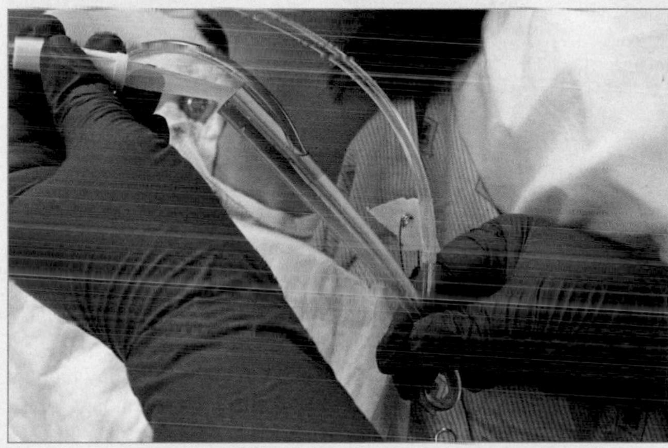
FIGURE 2 Clamping nasogastric tube while disconnecting.

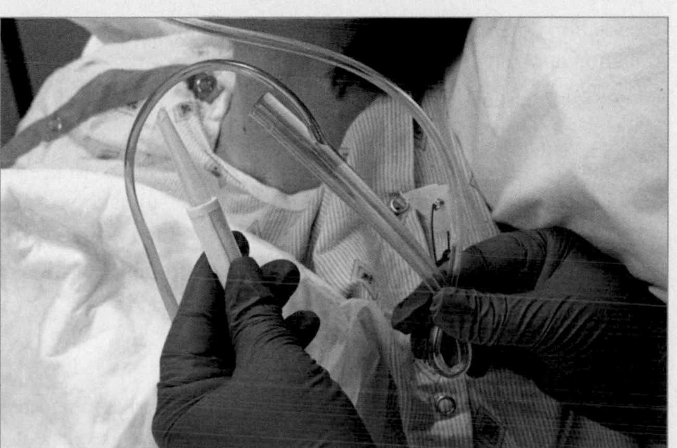
FIGURE 3 Holding both tubes upright to prevent leakage of gastric fluid.

(continued)

SKILL 13-8 IRRIGATING A NASOGASTRIC TUBE CONNECTED TO SUCTION continued

ACTION	RATIONALE
10. Place tip of syringe in tube. **If Salem sump or double-lumen tube is used, make sure that syringe tip is placed in the drainage port and not in blue air vent.** Hold syringe upright and gently insert the irrigant (Figure 4) (or allow solution to flow in by gravity if facility policy or medical order indicates). **Do not force solution into tube.**	Gentle insertion of saline solution (or gravity insertion) is less traumatic to gastric mucosa. The blue air vent acts to decrease pressure built up in the stomach when the Salem sump is attached to suction. It is not to be used for irrigation.
11. **If unable to irrigate tube, reposition patient and attempt irrigation again. Inject 10 to 20 mL of air and aspirate again (Figure 5). If repeated attempts to irrigate tube fail, consult with primary care provider or follow facility policy.**	Tube may be positioned against gastric mucosa, making it difficult to irrigate. Injection of air may reposition end of tube.

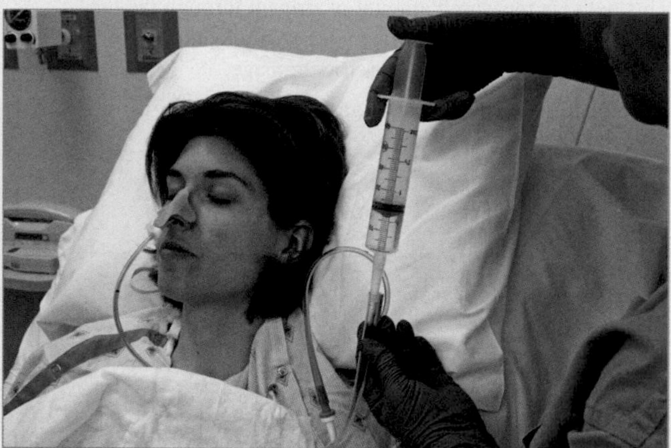

FIGURE 4 Gently instilling irrigation.

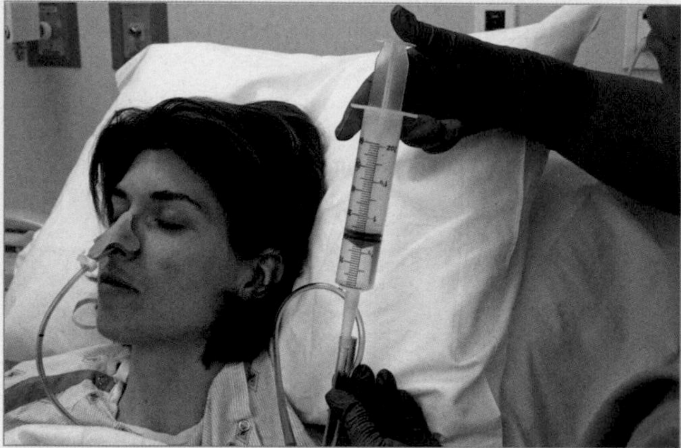

FIGURE 5 Injecting 10 to 20 mL of air into tube.

ACTION	RATIONALE
12. After irrigant has been instilled, hold end of NGT over irrigation tray or emesis basin. Observe for return flow of NG drainage into available container. Alternately, you may reconnect the NGT to suction and observe the return drainage as it drains into the suction container.	Return flow may be collected in an irrigating tray or other available container and measured. This amount will need to be subtracted from the irrigant to record the true NG drainage. A second method involves subtracting the total irrigant from the shift from the total NG drainage emptied over the entire shift, to find the true NG drainage. Check agency policy for guidelines. Observation determines tube patency and correct operation of suction apparatus.
13. If not already done, reconnect drainage port to suction, if ordered.	Allows for continued removal of gastric contents, as ordered.
14. Inject air into blue air vent after irrigation is complete. Position the blue air vent above the patient's stomach.	Following irrigation, the blue air vent is injected with air to keep it clear. Positioning the blue air vent above the stomach prevents the stomach contents from leaking from the NGT.
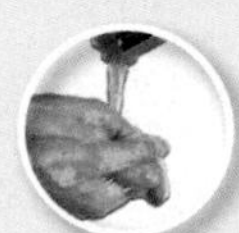 15. Remove gloves. Lower the bed and raise side rails, as necessary. Assist the patient to a position of comfort. Perform hand hygiene.	Lowering bed and assisting the patient to a comfortable position promote safety and comfort.
16. Put on gloves. Measure returned solution, if collected outside of suction apparatus. Rinse equipment if it will be reused. Label with the date, patient's name, room number, and purpose (for NGT/irrigation).	Gloves prevent contact with blood and body fluids. Irrigant placed in tube is considered intake; solution returned is recorded as output. Record on the intake and output record. Rinsing promotes cleanliness, infection control, and prepares equipment for next irrigation.

ACTION	RATIONALE
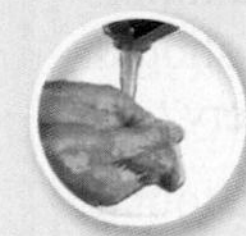 17. Remove gloves and additional PPE, if used. Perform hand hygiene.	Removing PPE properly reduces the risk for infection transmission and contamination of other items. Hand hygiene prevents transmission of microorganisms.

EVALUATION

The expected outcome is met when the patient demonstrates a patent and functioning NGT. In addition, the patient reports no distress with the irrigation. The patient remains free of any signs and symptoms of injury or trauma.

DOCUMENTATION

Guidelines

Document assessment of the patient's abdomen. Record if the patient's NGT is clamped or connected to suction, including the type of suction. Document the color and consistency of the NG drainage. Record the solution type and amount used to irrigate the NGT, as well as ease of irrigation or any difficulty related to the procedure. Record the amount of returned irrigant, if collected outside of the suction apparatus. Alternately, record irrigant amount so it can be subtracted from total NG drainage amount at the end of the shift. Record the patient's response to the procedure and any pertinent teaching points that were reviewed, such as instructions for the patient to contact the nurse for any feelings of nausea, bloating, or abdominal pain.

Sample Documentation

10/15/15 1100 Abdomen slightly distended but soft; absent bowel sounds, denies nausea. NG tube placement confirmed; gastric contents clear with brown flecks, pH 4; exposed NG tube 20 cm, consistent with documented length. NG tube irrigated with 30 mL of normal saline. NG tube reconnected to low intermittent suction. Clear drainage with brown flecks noted from tube. Patient tolerated irrigation without incident.

—S. Essner, RN

UNEXPECTED SITUATIONS AND ASSOCIATED INTERVENTIONS

- *Flush solution is meeting a lot of force when plunger is pushed:* Inject 20 to 30 mL of free air into the abdomen in attempt to reposition the tube and enable flushing of the tube.
- *Tube is connected to suction as ordered, but nothing is draining from tube:* First check the suction canister to ensure that the suction is working appropriately. Disconnect the NGT from suction and place your gloved thumb over the end of the suction tubing. If there is suction present, the problem lies in the tube itself. Next, attempt to flush the tube to ensure its patency.
- *After flushing the tube, the tube is not reconnected to suction as ordered:* Reconnect the tube to suction as soon as error is noticed. Assess the abdomen for distention and ask the patient if he or she is experiencing any nausea or any abdominal discomfort. Complete any paperwork per institutional policy, such as an incident report.

SPECIAL CONSIDERATIONS

- A one-way, anti-reflux valve may be used in the airflow lumen to prevent reflux of gastric contents through the airflow lumen (see Figure 5). When pressure from gastric contents enters the airflow tubing, the valve closes to prevent secretions from exiting the tube. This valve is removed before flushing the lumen with air, and then replaced.
- Monitoring for carbon dioxide to determine NG tube position and/or dislodgement has been investigated (Gilbert & Burns, 2012; Munera-Seeley et al., 2008). This involves the use of a capnograph or a colorimetric end-tidal CO_2 detector to detect the presence of carbon dioxide, which would indicate tube positioning in the patient's airway instead of the stomach.

ENHANCE YOUR UNDERSTANDING

FOCUSING ON PATIENT CARE: DEVELOPING CLINICAL REASONING

Consider the case scenarios at the beginning of the chapter as you answer the following questions to enhance your understanding and apply what you have learned.

QUESTIONS

1. While you are digitally removing feces from Hugh Levens, he suddenly complains of feeling light-headed. You note that he is now diaphoretic. What should you do?
2. Isaac Greenberg is afraid that the enema is going to hurt. His mother worries about being able to prepare properly for his sigmoidoscopy. What information should you include when teaching the steps to administer a small-volume enema? What interventions should you include to promote Isaac's comfort and safety?
3. Maria Blakely has noted that an area of peristomal skin is becoming erythematous and excoriated. She asks you whether she should cut her ostomy bag bigger so that the adhesive does not irritate this skin. How should you reply?

You can find suggested answers after the Bibliography at the end of this chapter.

INTEGRATED CASE STUDY CONNECTION

The case studies in Unit 3 are designed to focus on integrating concepts. Refer to the following case studies to enhance your understanding of the concepts related to the skills in this chapter.

- Intermediate Case Studies: Victoria Holly, page 1079.

TAYLOR SUITE RESOURCES

Explore these additional resources to enhance learning for this chapter:

- NCLEX-Style Questions and other resources on thePoint, http://thePoint.lww.com/Lynn4e
- *Skill Checklists for Taylor's Clinical Nursing Skills,* 4e
- *Taylor's Video Guide to Clinical Nursing Skills:* Bowel Elimination
- *Fundamentals of Nursing:* Chapter 37, Bowel Elimination
- *Lippincott DocuCare* Fundamentals cases

Bibliography

Ackley, B.J., & Ladwig, G.B. (2011). *Nursing diagnosis handbook* (9th ed.). St. Louis: Mosby/Elsevier.

American Association of Critical-Care Nurses (AACN). (2010). *Practice alert: Verification of feeding tube placement.* Available http://aacn.org/WD/Practice/Docs/PracticeAlerts/Verification_of_Feeding_Tube_Placement_05-2005.pdf.

Avent, Y. (2012). Understanding fecal diversions. *Nursing made incredibly easy! 10*(5), 11–16.

Best, C. (2005). Caring for the patient with a nasogastric tube. *Nursing Standard, 20*(3), 59–65.

Bisanz, A., Tucker, A.M., Amin, D.M., Patel, D., Calderon, B.B., Joseph, M.M., et al. (2010). Summary of the causative and treatment factors of diarrhea and the use of a diarrhea assessment and treatment tool to improve patient outcomes. *Gastroenterology Nursing, 33*(4), 269–281.

Bowers, B. (2006). Evaluating the evidence for administering phosphate enemas. *British Journal of Nursing, 15*(7), 378–381.

Brennan, M. (2008). Review: Routine NG decompression after abdominal surgery delays return of bowel function and increases pulmonary complications. *Evidence-Based Nursing, 11*(2), 55.

Bulechek, G.M, Butcher, H.K., Dochterman, J.M., & Wagner, C.M. (Eds.). (2013). *Nursing interventions classification (NIC)* (6th ed.). St. Louis: Mosby Elsevier.

Burch, J. (2011). Stoma management: Enhancing patient knowledge. *British Journal of Community Nursing, 16*(4), 162, 164, 166.

Burton, J., Allison, J., Smart, N, & Francis, N. (2011). Impact of stoma care on enhanced recovery after colorectal surgery. *Gastrointestinal Nursing, 9*(8), 15–16, 18–19.

Carlsson, E., Gylin, M., Nilsson, L., Svensson, K, Alverslid, I, & Persson, E. (2010). Positive and negative aspects of colostomy irrigation. *Journal of Wound, Ostomy, and Continence Nursing, 37*(5), 511–518.

Centers for Disease Control and Prevention (CDC). (2010). *Healthcare-associated infections (HAIs). Frequently asked questions about Clostridium difficile for healthcare providers.* Available http://www.cdc.gov/HAI/organisms/cdiff/Cdiff_faqs_HCP.html.

Chau, J.P.C., Lo, S.H.S., Thompson, D.R., Fernandez, R., & Griffiths, R. (2011). Use of end-tidal carbon dioxide detection to determine correct placement of nasogastric tube: A meta-analysis. *International Journal of Nursing Studies, 48*(4), 513–521.

Denyer, J. (2011). Reducing pain during the removal of adhesive and adherent products. *British Journal of Nursing, 20*(15) (Tissue Viability Supplement), S28–S35.

Dudek, S. (2014). *Nutrition essentials for nursing practice* (7th ed.). Philadelphia: Wolters Kluwer Health/Lippincott Williams & Wilkins.

Ellett, M. (2004). What is known about methods of correctly placing gastric tubes in adults and children. *Gastroenterology Nursing, 27*(6), 253–261.

Flynn Makic, M.B., VonRueden, K.T., Rauen, C.A., & Chadwick, J. (2011). Evidence-based practice habits: Putting more sacred cows out to pasture. *Critical Care Nurse, 31*(2), 38–44, 47–61.

Gannon, R. (2007). Current strategies for preventing or ameliorating postoperative ileus: A multimodal approach. *American Journal of Health-System Pharmacy, 64*(20), S8–S12.

Gilbert, R.T., & Burns, S.M. (2012). Increasing the safety of blind gastric tube placement in pediatric patients: The design and testing of a procedure using a carbon dioxide detection device. *Journal of Pediatric Nursing, 27*(5), 528–532.

Goldberg, M., Aukett, L.K., Carmel, J., Fellows, J., Folkedahl, B., & Pittman, J. (2010). Management of the patient with a fecal ostomy. Best practice guideline for clinicians. *Journal of Wound, Ostomy, and Continence Nursing, 37*(6), 596–598.

Grossman, S., & Porth, C.M. (2014). Porth's pathophysiology: concepts of altered health states. (9th ed.). Philadelphia: Wolters Kluwer Health/Lippincott Williams & Wilkins.

Higgins, D. (2008a). Patient assessment. Part 3: Measurement of gastric fluid pH. *Nursing Times, 104*(9), 26–27.

Higgins, D. (2008b). Specimen collection. Part 3: Collecting a stool specimen. *Nursing Times, 104*(19), 22–23.

Hinkle, J.L., & Cheever, K.H. (2014). *Brunner & Suddarth's textbook of medical-surgical nursing* (13th ed.). Philadelphia: Wolters Kluwer Health/Lippincott Williams & Wilkins.

Hockenberry, M., & Wilson, D. (2009). *Wong's essentials of pediatric nursing.* (8th ed.). St. Louis: Elsevier Mosby.

Hogan-Quigley, B., Palm, M.L., & Bickley, L. (2012). *Bates' nursing guide to physical examination and history taking.* Philadelphia: Wolters Kluwer Health/Lippincott Williams & Wilkins.

Hollister. (2005). *Drainable fecal incontinence collector. Protocol.* Libertyville, IL: Author. Available http://www.hollister.com/us/files/pdfs/907278-405.pdf.

Jacobson, R.M., Peery, J., Thompson, W.O., Kanapka, J.A., & Caswell, M. (2010). Serum electrolyte shifts following administration of sodium phosphates enema. *Gastroenterology Nursing, 33*(3), 191–201.

Jarvis, C. (2012). *Physical examination & health assessment* (6th ed.). St. Louis: Saunders/Elsevier.

Jensen, S. (2011.) *Nursing health assessment. A best practice approach.* Philadelphia: Wolters Kluwer Health/Lippincott Williams & Wilkins.

Jessee, M.A. (2010). Stool studies: Tried, true, and new. *Critical Care Nursing Clinics of North America, 22*(1), 129–145.

Jones, T., Springfield, T., Brudwich, M., & Ladd, A. (2011). Fecal ostomies. Practical management for the home health clinician. *Home Healthcare Nurse, 29*(5), 306–317.

Khair, J. (2005). Guidelines for testing the placing of nasogastric tubes. *Nursing Times, 101*(20), 26–27.

Kyle, G., Prynn, P., & Oliver, H. (2004). An evidence-based procedure for the digital removal of feces. *Nursing Times, 100*(48), 71.

Kyle, T., & Carman, S. (2013). *Essentials of pediatric nursing* (2nd ed.). Philadelphia: Wolters Kluwer Health/Lippincott Williams & Wilkins.

Lafon, C., & Lawson, L. (2012). Postoperative ileus in GI surgical patients: pathogenesis and interventions. *Gastrointestinal Nursing, 10*(2), 45–49.

Levin, B., Lieberman, D., McFarland, B., et al. (2008). Screening and surveillance for the early detection of colorectal cancer and adenomatous polyps, 2008: A joint guideline from the American Cancer Society, the US Multi-Society Task Force on Colorectal Cancer, and the American College of Radiology. *CA–A Cancer Journal for Clinicians, 58*(3), 130–160.

Massey, R.L. (2012). Return of bowel sounds indicating an end of postoperative ileus: Is it time to cease this long-standing nursing tradition? *MEDSURG Nursing, 21*(3), 146–150.

Mayo Foundation for Medical Education and Research (MFMER). (2011). *Constipation. Treatments and drugs.* Available http://www.mayoclinic.com/health/constipation/DS00063/DSECTION=symptoms.

Miller, S. (2011). Capnometry vs pH testing in nasogastric tube placement. *Gastrointestinal Nursing,* 9(2), 30–33.

Moorhead, S., Johnson, M., Maas, M.L., & Swanson, E. (Eds.). (2013). *Nursing outcomes classification (NOC)* (5th ed.). St. Louis: Mosby Elsevier.

Munera-Seeley, V., Ochoa, J., Brown, N., et al. (2008). Use of a colorimetric carbon dioxide sensor for nasoenteric feeding tube placement in critical care patients compared with clinical methods and radiography. *Nutrition in Clinical Practice, 23*(3), 318–321.

NANDA-I International. (2012). *Nursing diagnoses: Definitions & classification 2012–2014.* West Sussex, UK: Wiley-Blackwell.

National Cancer Institute (NCI). (2012). *Gastrointestinal complications (PDQ®). Constipation.* Available http://www.cancer.gov/cancertopics/pdq/supportivecare/gastrointestinalcomplications/HealthProfessional/page2#top.

National Institute of Diabetes and Digestive and Kidney Diseases (NIDDK). National Institutes of Health (NIH). (2012). National Digestive Diseases Information Clearinghouse (NDDIC). *Bowel diversion surgeries: Ileostomy, colostomy, ileoanal reservoir, and continent ileostomy.* Available http://digestive.niddk.nih.gov/ddiseases/pubs/ileostomy/.

National Institutes of Health. Clinical Center. (2007). *Patient education. Managing bowel dysfunction.* Available http://www.cc.nih.gov/ccc/patient_education/pepubs/bowel.pdf.

Nelson, R., Edwards, S., & Tse, B. (2007). Prophylactic nasogastric decompression after abdominal surgery. *Cochrane Database Systematic Review,* Issue 3. Art. No.: DOI: 10.1002/14651858.CD004929.pub3.

Ness, W., Hibberts, F., & Miles, S. (2012). Royal College of Nursing. *Management of lower bowel dysfunction, including DRE and DRF.* RCN guidance for nurses. London, U.K.: Royal College of Nursing.

Notter, J., & Chalmers, F. (2012). Living with a colostomy: A pilot study. *Gastrointestinal Nursing, 10*(6), 16, 18, 20, 22–24.

Obokhare, I. (2012). Fecal impaction: A cause for concern? *Clinics in Colon and Rectal Surgery, 25*(1), 53–57.

Perry, S.E., Hockenberry, M.J., Lowdermilk, D.L., & Wilson, D. (2010). *Maternal child nursing care* (4th ed.). Maryland Heights, MO: Mosby/Elsevier.

Perston, Y. (2010). Ensuring effective technique in colostomy irrigation to improve quality of life. *Gastrointestinal Nursing, 8*(4), 18–22.

Pontieri-Lewis, V. (2006). Basics of ostomy care. *MEDSURG Nursing, 15*(4), 199–202.

Rudoni, C. (2008). A service evaluation of the use of silicone-based adhesive remover. *British Journal of Nursing, Stoma Care Supplement, 17*(2), S4, S6, S8–S9.

Simons, S.R., & Abdallah, L.M. (2012). Bedside assessment of enteral tube placement: Aligning practice with evidence. *American Journal of Nursing, 112*(2), 40–46.

Stephen-Haynes, J. (2008). Skin integrity and silicone: APPEEL 'no-sting' medical adhesive remover. *British Journal of Nursing, 17*(12), 792–795.

Tabloski, P. (2010). *Gerontological nursing* (2nd ed.). Upper Saddle River, NJ: Pearson.

Taylor, C., Lillis, C., & Lynn, P. (2015). *Fundamentals of nursing.* (8th ed.). Philadelphia: Wolters Kluwer Health/Lippincott Williams & Wilkins.

Taylor, J.J., & Cohen, B.J. (2013). *Memmler's structure and function of the human body.* (10th ed.). Philadelphia: Wolters Kluwer Health/Lippincott Williams & Wilkins.

Toner, F., & Claros, E. (2012). Preventing, assessing, and managing constipation in older adults. *Nursing, 42*(12), 32–40.

U.S. National Library of Medicine. National Institutes of Health. (2013). MedlinePlus. *Bowel retraining.* Available http://www.nlm.nih.gov/medlineplus/ency/article/003971.htm.

VISN 8 Patient Safety Center. (2009). *Safe patient handling and movement algorithms.* Tampa, FL: Author. Available http://www.visn8.va.gov/visn8/patientsafetycenter/safePtHandling/default.asp.

Voegeli, D. (2012). Moisture-associated skin damage: Aetiology, prevention and treatment. *British Journal of Nursing, 21*(9), 517–518, 520–521.

Williams, J. (2011). Choosing devices for stoma patients. *Practice Nursing, 22*(12), 646, 648–649.

Williams, J., Gwillam, B., Sutherland, N., Matten, J., Hemmingway, J., Ilsey, H., et al. (2010). Evaluating skin care problems in people with stomas. *British Journal of Nursing, 19*(17), S6, S8, S10, S12 S15.

Woodward, S. (2012). Assessment and management of constipation in older people. *Nursing Older People, 24*(5), 21–26.

Zimmaro Bliss, D., & Norton, C. (2010). Conservative management of fecal incontinence. An evidence-based approach to controlling this life-altering condition. *American Journal of Nursing, 110*(9), 30–38.

SUGGESTED ANSWERS FOR FOCUSING ON PATIENT CARE: DEVELOPING CLINICAL REASONING

1. This procedure is very uncomfortable and may cause great discomfort to the patient as well as irritation of the rectal mucosa and bleeding. Digital removal of a fecal mass can stimulate the vagus nerve, resulting in a slowed heart rate, as well as nausea, diaphoresis, light-headedness, and/or dizziness. If the patient experiences any of these symptoms, stop the procedure immediately; monitor the patient's heart rate, blood pressure, and symptoms. Maintain the patient in a supine position, provide reassurance, and notify the primary care provider.

2. Hypertonic solution preparations are available commercially and are administered in smaller volumes (adult, 70 to 130 mL). These solutions draw water into the colon, which stimulates the defecation reflex. This enema is packaged in a flexible bottle containing hypertonic solution with an attached prelubricated firm tip about 2 to 3 inches (5 to 7.5 cm) long, and is easy to use. Explain the purpose and what they can expect. Use developmentally appropriate terms for a 9-year-old. Isaac and his mother should plan to administer the enema in or near the bathroom, so Isaac is not worried about being incontinent or getting to the toilet in time. Reinforce that the procedure will not hurt. Isaac will feel some pressure from the tube in his rectum, and in his belly. Explain that a child or adolescent should be positioned on the left side with the right leg flexed toward chest (Kyle & Carman, 2013). Explain to Isaac's mother that she should generously lubricate the end of the rectal tube 2 to 3 inches before administering. She should direct it at an angle pointing toward the umbilicus, not the bladder. She should ask Isaac to take several deep breaths when inserting it to help relax the anal sphincter. She should encourage Isaac to hold the solution until the urge to defecate is strong. Finally, the mother should hold the child's buttocks together if needed to encourage retention of the enema.

3. Explain that she should cut the opening only 1/8-inch larger than the stoma size. Creating a larger opening will expose the already irritated peristomal skin to further irritation from stool. Advise Maria to contact her ostomy nurse specialist or her physician to rule out a superimposed fungal infection, which would require treatment with an antifungal medication. Reinforce basic teaching with Maria. Ensure she understands the routine care of her ostomy. Explain that she should empty the ostomy

appliance frequently. This prevents excess pressure on the adhesive that could pull the adhesive plate off her skin and allow fecal material to come in contact with peristomal skin. Instruct Maria to keep the skin around the stoma site (peristomal area) clean and dry. If care is not taken to protect the skin around the stoma, irritation or infection may occur. A leaking appliance frequently causes skin erosion. Candida or yeast infections can also occur around the stoma if the area is not kept dry. If an appliance is leaking from underneath the skin barrier, ring, or wafer, the bag will have to be removed, the skin cleaned, and a new bag applied. The act of removing an appliance from the skin can result in skin stripping, removal of the outer, loosely bound, epidermal cell layers. This can be uncomfortable for the patient or, at worst, very painful. The cumulative effects of skin stripping over time can result in peristomal skin breakdown. The use of a silicone-based adhesive remover allows for the easy, rapid, and painless removal of a stoma pouch without the associated problems of skin stripping (Rudoni, 2008; Stephen-Haynes, 2008). Instruct Maria to use adhesive remover when removing her appliance, to prevent further skin damage. Explain that she should thoroughly cleanse the peristomal skin with a gentle cleanser, and then thoroughly dry it. The use of a skin barrier is important, as well as ensuring good adhesion when the appliance is replaced.

14 Oxygenation

FOCUSING ON PATIENT CARE

This chapter will help you develop some of the skills related to oxygenation necessary to care for the following patients:

SCOTT MINGUS, age 35, who has a chest drain after thoracic surgery.

SARANAM SRIVASTAVA, age 58, with a history of smoking, who is scheduled for a bowel resection and needs preoperative teaching regarding an incentive spirometer.

PAULA CUNNINGHAM, age 72, who is intubated and requires suctioning through her endotracheal tube.

Refer to Focusing on Patient Care: Developing Clinical Reasoning at the end of the chapter to apply what you learn.

LEARNING OBJECTIVES

After studying this chapter, you will be able to:

1. Use a pulse oximeter.
2. Teach a patient to use an incentive spirometer.
3. Administer oxygen by nasal cannula.
4. Administer oxygen by mask.
5. Use an oxygen hood.
6. Use an oxygen tent.
7. Suction the oropharynx and nasopharynx.
8. Insert an oropharyngeal airway.
9. Insert a nasopharyngeal airway.
10. Suction an endotracheal tube using an open system.
11. Suction an endotracheal tube using a closed system.
12. Secure an endotracheal tube.
13. Suction a tracheostomy.
14. Provide care of a tracheostomy tube.
15. Provide care of a chest drainage system.
16. Assist with chest tube removal.
17. Use a manual resuscitation bag and mask to deliver oxygen.

KEY TERMS

alveoli: small air sacs at the end of the terminal bronchioles that are the site of gas exchange

atelectasis: incomplete expansion or collapse of a part of the lungs

cilia: microscopic, hairlike projections that propel mucus toward the upper airway so it can be expectorated

dyspnea: difficult or labored breathing

endotracheal tube: polyvinylchloride airway that is inserted through the nose or mouth into the trachea, using a laryngoscope

expiration: act of breathing out

extubation: removal of a tube (in this case, an endotracheal tube)

hyperventilation: condition in which more than the normal amount of air is entering and leaving the lungs as a result of an increase in rate or depth of **respiration** or both

hypoventilation: decreased rate or depth of air movement into the lungs

hypoxia: inadequate amount of oxygen available to the cells

inspiration: act of breathing in

nasal cannula: disposable plastic device with two protruding prongs for insertion into the nostrils; used to administer oxygen

nasopharyngeal airway: a curved, soft rubber or plastic tube inserted into the back of the pharynx through the mouth

oropharyngeal airway: a semicircular tube of plastic or rubber inserted into the back of the pharynx through the mouth

pneumothorax: air in the pleural space

pulse oximetry: noninvasive technique that measures the oxygen saturation (SpO_2) of arterial blood

respiration: gas exchange between the atmospheric air in the alveoli and the blood in the capillaries

spirometer: instrument used to measure lung capacity and volume; one type is used to encourage deep breathing (incentive spirometry)

subcutaneous emphysema: small pockets of air trapped in the subcutaneous tissue; usually found around chest tube insertion sites

tachypnea: rapid breathing

tracheostomy tube: curved tube inserted into an artificial opening made into the trachea (tracheostomy); comes in varied angles and multiple sizes

ventilation (breathing): the movement of air into and out of the lungs

Life depends on a constant supply of oxygen. This demand for oxygen is met by the function of the respiratory and cardiovascular systems, also known as the **cardiopulmonary system**. Gas exchange, the intake of oxygen and the release of carbon dioxide, is made possible by the respiratory system (Figure 1). The cardiovascular system (Figure 2) delivers oxygen to the cells. Oxygenation of body tissues depends on essentially three factors:

- Integrity of the airway system to transport air to and from the lungs
- A properly functioning alveolar system in the lungs to oxygenate venous blood and to remove carbon dioxide from the blood
- A properly functioning cardiovascular system and blood supply to carry nutrients and wastes to and from body cells.

The air passages must remain patent (open) for oxygen to enter the system. Any condition that interferes with normal functioning must be minimized or eliminated to prevent pulmonary distress, which could lead to death. This chapter covers the skills necessary for the nurse to promote oxygenation. While performing skills related to oxygenation, keep in mind factors that affect cardiopulmonary (respiratory and cardiovascular systems) function, leading to impaired oxygenation, and how these factors might affect a particular patient (Fundamentals Review 14-1).

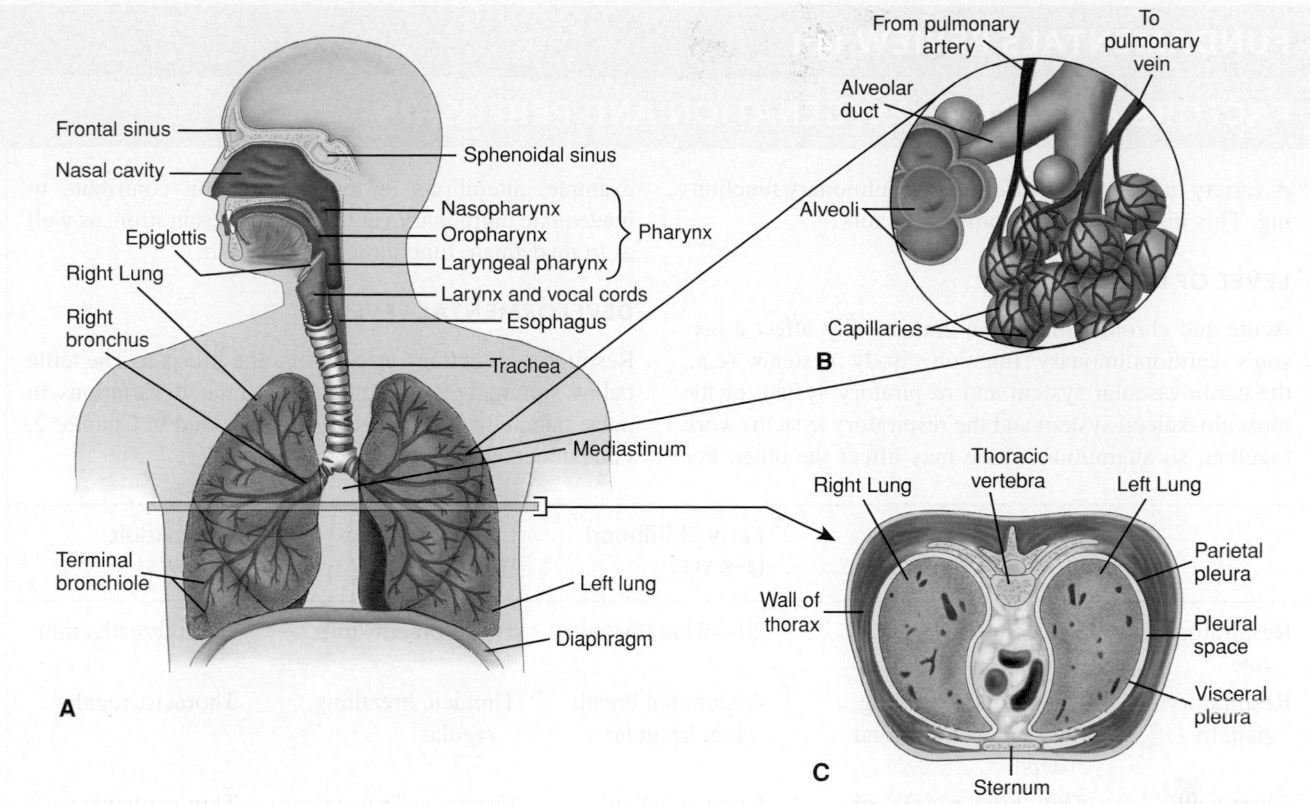

FIGURE 14-1 Organs of respiratory tract. (**A**) Overview. (**B**) Alveoli (air sacs) of lungs and blood capillaries. (**C**) Transverse section through lungs.

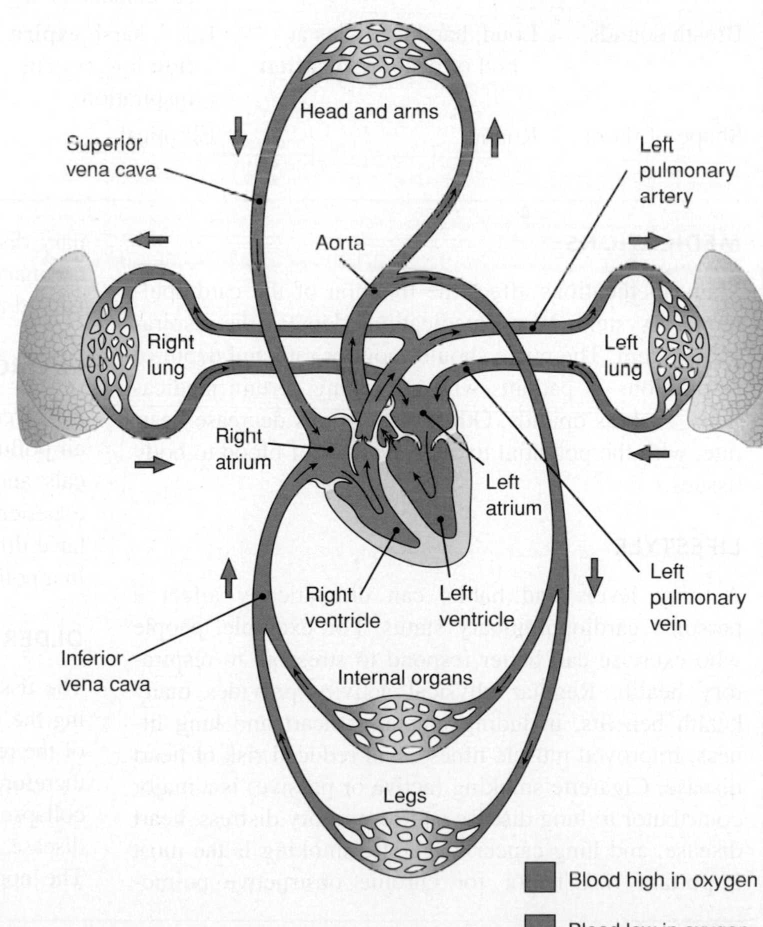

FIGURE 14-2 The right side of the heart pumps deoxygenated blood to the lungs, where oxygen is picked up and carbon dioxide released. The left side of the heart pumps oxygenated blood out to all other parts of the body. (From Taylor, J.J., & Cohen, B.J. (2013). *Memmler's structure and function of the human body.* (10th ed.). Philadelphia: Wolters Kluwer Health/Lippincott Williams & Wilkins.)

FUNDAMENTALS REVIEW 14-1

FACTORS AFFECTING OXYGENATION AND PERFUSION

A variety of factors can affect cardiopulmonary functioning. This display reviews common factors.

LEVEL OF HEALTH

Acute and chronic illness can dramatically affect a person's cardiopulmonary function. Body systems (e.g., the cardiovascular system and respiratory system or the musculoskeletal system and the respiratory system) work together, so alterations in one may affect the other. For example, alterations in muscle function contribute to inadequate pulmonary ventilation and respiration, as well as to inadequate functioning of the heart.

DEVELOPMENTAL LEVEL

Respiratory function varies across the lifespan. The table below summarizes variations. Age-related variations in pulse rate and blood pressure can be found in Chapter 2, Fundamentals Review 2-1.

	Infant (Birth–1 yr)	Early Childhood (1–5 yrs)	Late Childhood (6–12 yrs)	Aged Adult (65+ yrs)
Respiratory rate	30–55 breaths/min	20–40 breaths/min	18–26 breaths/min	16–20 breaths/min
Respiratory pattern	Abdominal breathing, irregular in rate and depth	Abdominal breathing, irregular	Thoracic breathing, regular	Thoracic, regular
Chest wall	Thin, little muscle, ribs and sternum easily seen	Same as infant's, but with more subcutaneous fat	Further subcutaneous fat deposited, structures less prominent	Thin, structures prominent
Breath sounds	Loud, harsh crackles at end of deep **inspiration**	Loud, harsh **expiration** longer than inspiration	Clear inspiration is longer than expiration	Clear
Shape of thorax	Round	Elliptical	Elliptical	Barrel-shaped or elliptical

MEDICATIONS

Many medications affect the function of the cardiopulmonary system. Many medications depress the respiratory system. The nurse should monitor rate and depth of respirations in patients who are taking certain medications, such as opioids. Other medications decrease heart rate, with the potential to alter the flow of blood to body tissues.

LIFESTYLE

Activity levels and habits can dramatically affect a person's cardiopulmonary status. For example, people who exercise can better respond to stressors to respiratory health. Regular physical activity provides many health benefits, including increased heart and lung fitness, improved muscle fitness, and reduced risk of heart disease. Cigarette smoking (active or passive) is a major contributor to lung disease and respiratory distress, heart disease, and lung cancer. Cigarette smoking is the most important risk factor for chronic obstructive pulmonary disease (COPD) (Macnee, 2007). Smoking causes coronary artery disease, the leading cause of death in the United States (CDC, 2010).

ENVIRONMENT

Research indicates that there is a high correlation between air pollution and occupational exposure to certain chemicals and lung disease. Additionally, people who have experienced an alteration in respiratory functioning often have difficulty continuing to perform self-care activities in a polluted environment.

OLDER ADULTS

The tissues and airways of the respiratory tract (including the alveoli) become less elastic with age. The power of the respiratory and abdominal muscles is reduced, and therefore the diaphragm moves less efficiently. Airways collapse more easily. These alterations increase the risk for disease, especially pneumonia and other chest infections. The normal aging heart can maintain adequate cardiac

FUNDAMENTALS REVIEW 14-1 continued

FACTORS AFFECTING OXYGENATION AND PERFUSION

output under ordinary circumstances, but may have a limited ability to respond to situations that cause physical or emotional stress (Hinkle & Cheever, 2014). Decreased physical activity, physical deconditioning, decreased elasticity of the blood vessels, and stiffening of the heart valves can lead to a decrease in the overall function of the heart, leading to decreased oxygenation of body tissues.

PSYCHOLOGICAL HEALTH

Many psychological factors can have an impact on the respiratory system. People responding to stress or anxiety may experience **hyperventilation**. In addition, patients with respiratory problems often develop some anxiety as a result of the **hypoxia** caused by the respiratory problem.

SKILL 14-1 USING A PULSE OXIMETER

Pulse oximetry is a noninvasive technique that measures the arterial oxyhemoglobin saturation (SaO_2 or SpO_2) of arterial blood. The reported result is a ratio, expressed as a percentage, between the actual oxygen content of the hemoglobin and the potential maximum oxygen-carrying capacity of the hemoglobin (Van Leeuwen et al., 2011). A sensor, or probe, uses a beam of red and infrared light that travels through tissue and blood vessels. One part of the sensor emits the light and another part receives the light. The oximeter then calculates the amount of light that has been absorbed by arterial blood. Oxygen saturation is determined by the amount of each light absorbed; nonoxygenated hemoglobin absorbs more red light and oxygenated hemoglobin absorbs more infrared light.

Sensors are available for use on a finger, a toe, a foot (infants), an earlobe, forehead, and the bridge of the nose. It is important to use the appropriate sensor for the intended site; use of a sensor on a site other than what it is intended can result in inaccurate or unreliable readings (Johnson et al., 2012). Circulation to the sensor site must be adequate to ensure accurate readings. Pulse oximeters also display a measured pulse rate.

It is important to know the patient's hemoglobin level before evaluating oxygen saturation because the test measures only the percentage of oxygen carried by the available hemoglobin. Thus, even a patient with a low hemoglobin level could appear to have a normal SpO_2 because most of that hemoglobin is saturated. However, the patient may not have enough oxygen to meet body needs. Also, take into consideration the presence of preexisting health conditions, such as COPD. Parameters for acceptable oxygen saturation readings may be different for these patients. Be aware of any medical orders regarding acceptable ranges and/or check with the patient's physician. A range of 95% to 100% is considered normal SpO_2. Values $\leq$ 90% are abnormal, indicating that oxygenation to the tissues is inadequate. It is important to investigate these low values for potential hypoxia or technical error.

Pulse oximetry is useful for monitoring patients receiving oxygen therapy, titrating oxygen therapy, monitoring those at risk for hypoxia, monitoring those at risk of hypoventilation (opioids use, neurologic compromise), and postoperative patients. Pulse oximetry does not replace arterial blood gas analysis. Desaturation (decreased level of SpO_2) indicates gas exchange abnormalities. Oxygen desaturation is considered a late sign of respiratory compromise in patients with reduced rate and depth of breathing (Johnson et al., 2011).

DELEGATION CONSIDERATIONS

The measurement of oxygen saturation using a pulse oximeter may be delegated to nursing assistive personnel (NAP) or to unlicensed assistive personnel (UAP), as well as to licensed practical/vocational nurses (LPN/LVNs). The decision to delegate must be based on careful analysis of the patient's needs and circumstances, as well as the qualifications of the person to whom the task is being delegated. Refer to the Delegation Guidelines in Appendix A.

(continued)

SKILL 14-1 USING A PULSE OXIMETER continued

EQUIPMENT

- Pulse oximeter with an appropriate sensor or probe
- Alcohol wipe(s) or disposable cleansing cloth
- Nail polish remover (if necessary)
- PPE, as indicated

ASSESSMENT

Assess the patient's skin temperature and color, including the color of the nail beds. Temperature is a good indicator of blood flow. Warm skin indicates adequate circulation. In a well-oxygenated patient, the skin and nail beds are usually pink. Skin that is bluish or dusky indicates hypoxia (inadequate amount of oxygen available to the cells). Also check capillary refill; prolonged capillary refill indicates a reduction in blood flow. Assess the quality of the pulse proximal to the sensor application site. Assess for edema of the sensor site. Avoid placing a sensor on edematous tissue; the presence of edema can interfere with readings. Auscultate the lungs (see Skill 3-5). Note the amount of oxygen and delivery method if the patient is receiving supplemental oxygen.

NURSING DIAGNOSIS

Determine the related factors for the nursing diagnoses based on the patient's current status. Appropriate nursing diagnoses may include:

- Impaired Gas Exchange
- Ineffective Airway Clearance
- Activity Intolerance

OUTCOME IDENTIFICATION AND PLANNING

The expected outcome to achieve when caring for a patient with a pulse oximeter is that the patient will exhibit oxygen saturation within acceptable parameters, or greater than 95%.

IMPLEMENTATION

ACTION	RATIONALE
1. Review health record for any health problems that would affect the patient's oxygenation status.	Identifying influencing factors aids in interpretation of results.
2. Bring necessary equipment to the bedside stand or overbed table.	Bringing everything to the bedside conserves time and energy. Arranging items nearby is convenient, saves time, and avoids unnecessary stretching and twisting of muscles on the part of the nurse.
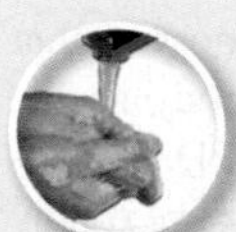 3. Perform hand hygiene and put on PPE, if indicated.	Hand hygiene and PPE prevent the spread of microorganisms. PPE is required based on transmission precautions.
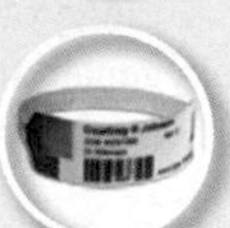 4. Identify the patient.	Identifying the patient ensures the right patient receives the intervention and helps prevent errors.
5. Close the curtains around the bed and close the door to the room, if possible. Explain what you are going to do and why you are going to do it to the patient.	This ensures the patient's privacy. Explanation relieves anxiety and facilitates cooperation.
6. Select an adequate site for application of the sensor.	Inadequate circulation can interfere with the oxygen saturation (SpO_2) reading.
a. Use the patient's index, middle, or ring finger (Figure 1).	Fingers are easily accessible.
b. Check the proximal pulse (Figure 2) and capillary refill (Figure 3) at the pulse closest to the site.	Brisk capillary refill and a strong pulse indicate adequate circulation to the site.

ACTION	RATIONALE

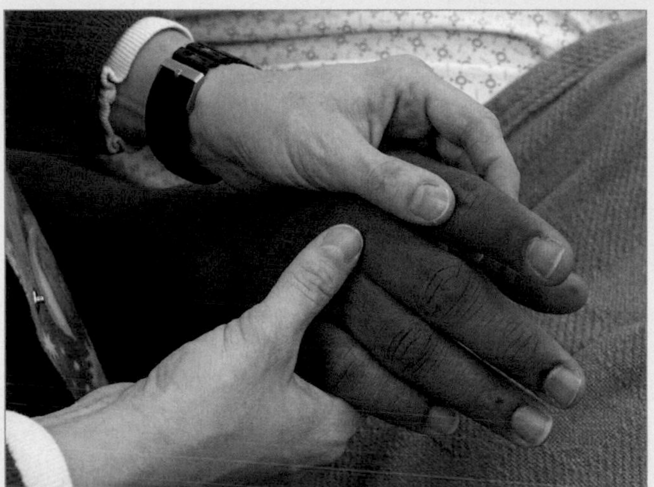

FIGURE 1 Selecting an appropriate finger.

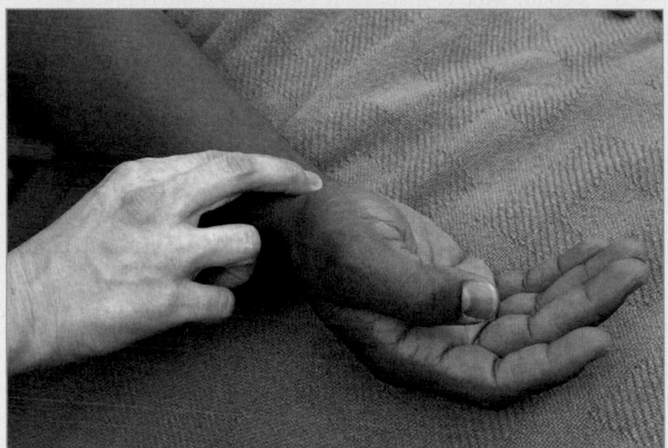

FIGURE 2 Assessing pulse.

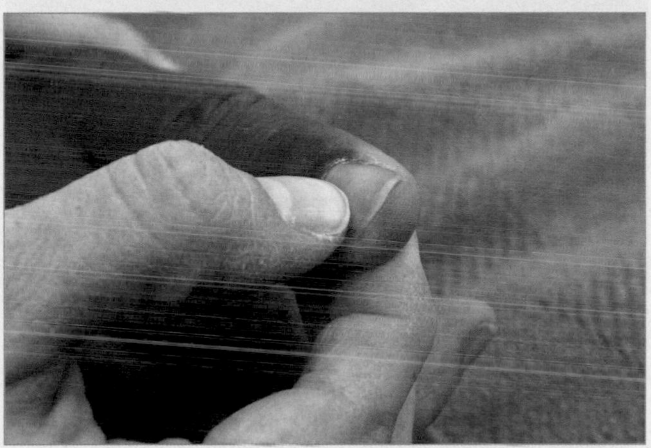

FIGURE 3 Assessing capillary refill.

ACTION	RATIONALE
c. If circulation to the site is inadequate, consider using the earlobe, forehead, or bridge of nose. Use the appropriate oximetry sensor for the chosen site.	These alternate sites are highly vascular alternatives. Correct use of appropriate equipment is vital for accurate results. The appropriate ear oximetry sensor should be used to obtain measurements from a patient's ear. The use of a finger sensor should be limited to use on the finger (Johnson et al., 2012).
d. Use a toe only if lower extremity circulation is not compromised.	Peripheral vascular disease is common in lower extremities.
7. Select proper equipment:	
a. If one finger is too large for the probe, use a smaller finger.	Inaccurate readings can result if probe or sensor is not attached correctly.
b. Use probes appropriate for patient's age and size. Use a pediatric probe for a small adult, if necessary.	Probes come in adult, pediatric, and infant sizes.
c. Check if patient is allergic to adhesive. A nonadhesive finger clip or reflectance sensor is available.	A reaction may occur if the patient is allergic to an adhesive substance.

(continued)

SKILL 14-1 USING A PULSE OXIMETER continued

ACTION	RATIONALE
8. Prepare the monitoring site. Cleanse the selected area with the alcohol wipe or disposable cleansing cloth (Figure 4). Allow the area to dry. If necessary, remove nail polish and artificial nails after checking pulse oximeter's manufacturer's instructions.	Skin oils, dirt, or grime on the site can interfere with the passage of light waves. Research is conflicting regarding the effect of dark color nail polish and artificial nails. It is prudent to remove nail polish (Hess et al., 2012). Refer to facility policy and pulse oximeter's manufacturer's instructions regarding nail polish and artificial nails for additional information (Collins & Andersen, 2007; DeMeulenaere, 2007).
9. **Attach probe securely to skin (Figure 5). Make sure that the light-emitting sensor and the light-receiving sensor are aligned opposite each other (not necessary to check if placed on forehead or bridge of nose).**	Secure attachment and proper alignment promote satisfactory operation of the equipment and an accurate recording of the SpO_2.

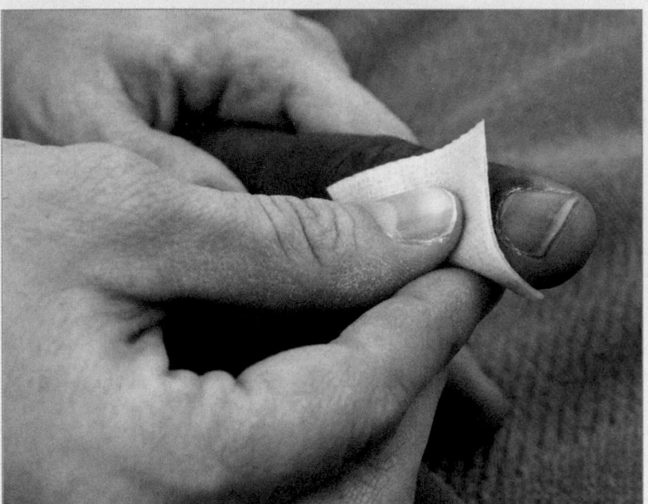

FIGURE 4 Cleaning area.

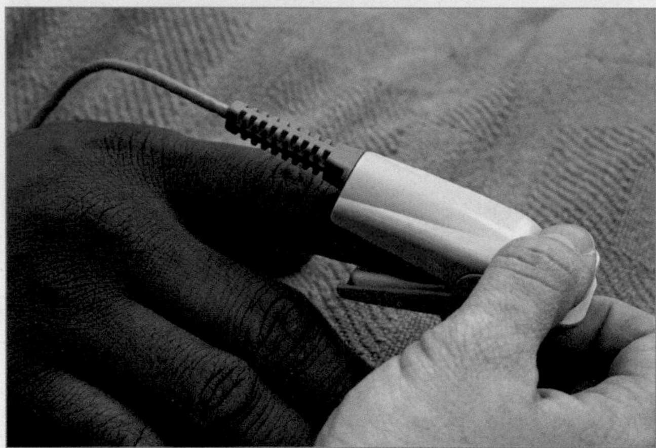

FIGURE 5 Attaching probe to patient's finger.

ACTION	RATIONALE
10. Connect the sensor probe to the pulse oximeter (Figure 6), turn the oximeter on, and check operation of the equipment (audible beep, fluctuation of bar of light or waveform on face of oximeter).	Audible beep represents the arterial pulse, and fluctuating waveform or light bar indicates the strength of the pulse. A weak signal will produce an inaccurate recording of the SpO_2. Tone of beep reflects SpO_2 reading. If SpO_2 drops, tone becomes lower in pitch.
11. Set alarms on pulse oximeter. Check manufacturer's alarm limits for high and low pulse rate settings (Figure 7).	Alarm provides additional safeguard and signals when high or low limits have been surpassed.

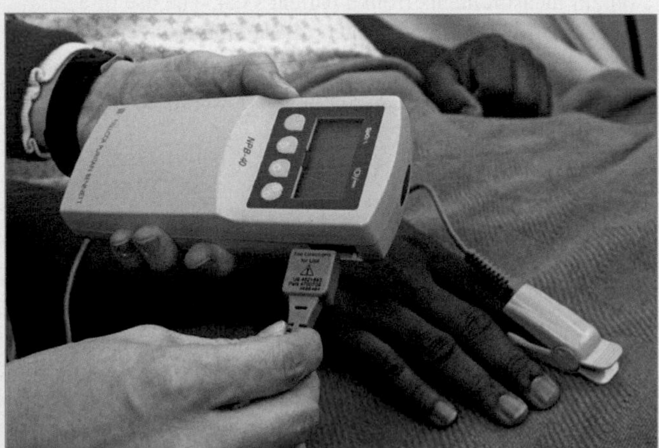

FIGURE 6 Connecting sensor probe to unit.

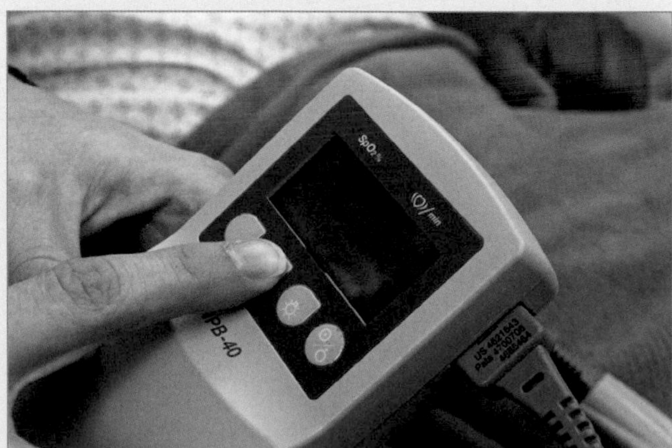

FIGURE 7 Checking alarms.

ACTION	RATIONALE
12. Check oxygen saturation at regular intervals, as ordered by primary care provider, nursing assessment, and signaled by alarms. Monitor hemoglobin level.	Monitoring SpO_2 provides ongoing assessment of patient's condition. A low hemoglobin level may be satisfactorily saturated yet inadequate to meet a patient's oxygen needs.
13. Remove sensor on a regular basis and check for skin irritation or signs of pressure (every 2 hours for spring-tension sensor or every 4 hours for adhesive finger or toe sensor).	Prolonged pressure may lead to tissue necrosis. Adhesive sensor may cause skin irritation.
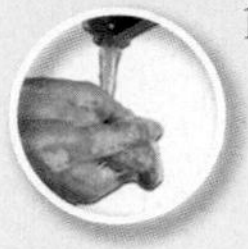 14. Clean nondisposable sensors according to the manufacturer's directions. Remove PPE, if used. Perform hand hygiene.	Cleaning equipment between patient use reduces the spread of microorganisms. Removing PPE properly reduces the risk for infection transmission and contamination of other items. Hand hygiene prevents the spread of microorganisms.

EVALUATION

The expected outcome is met when the patient exhibits an oxygen saturation level within acceptable parameters, or greater than 95%, and a heart rate that correlates with the pulse measurement.

DOCUMENTATION

Guidelines

Documentation should include the type of sensor and location used; assessment of the proximal pulse and capillary refill; pulse oximeter reading; the amount of oxygen and delivery method if the patient is receiving supplemental oxygen; lung assessment, if relevant; and any other relevant interventions required as a result of the reading.

Sample Documentation

9/03/15 Pulse oximeter placed on patient's index finger on right hand. Radial pulse present with brisk capillary refill. Pulse oximeter reading 98% on oxygen at 2 L via **nasal cannula**. Heart rate measured by oximeter correlates with the radial pulse measurement.

—C. Bausler, RN

UNEXPECTED SITUATIONS AND ASSOCIATED INTERVENTIONS

- *Absent or weak signal:* Check vital signs and patient condition. If satisfactory, check connections and circulation to site. Hypotension makes an accurate recording difficult. Equipment (restraint, blood pressure cuff) may compromise circulation to site and cause venous blood to pulsate, giving an inaccurate reading. If extremity is cold, cover with a warm blanket.
- *Inaccurate reading:* Check prescribed medications and history of circulatory disorders. Try device on a healthy person to see if problem is equipment-related or patient-related. Drugs that cause vasoconstriction interfere with accurate recording of oxygen saturation.
- *A bright light (sunlight or fluorescent light) is suspected of causing equipment malfunction:* Turn off light or cover probe with a dry washcloth. Bright light can interfere with operation of light sensors and cause an unreliable report.

SPECIAL CONSIDERATIONS

General Considerations

- Accuracy of readings can be influenced by conditions that decrease arterial blood flow, such as peripheral edema, hypotension, and peripheral vascular disease.
- Correlate the pulse reading on the pulse oximeter with the patient's heart rate. Variation between pulse and heart rate may indicate that not all pulsations are being detected and another sensor site may be required (Pullen, 2010).
- Excessive motion of sensor probe site, such as with extremity tremors or shivering, can also interfere with obtaining an accurate reading.
- Bradycardia and irregular cardiac rhythms may also cause inaccurate readings.
- In patients with low cardiac index (cardiac output in liters per minute divided by body surface area in square meters), the forehead sensor may be better than the digit sensor for pulse oximetry (Fernandez et al., 2007).

(continued)

SKILL 14-1 USING A PULSE OXIMETER continued

Infant and Child Considerations

- For infants, the oximeter probe may be placed on the toe or foot (Figure 8).

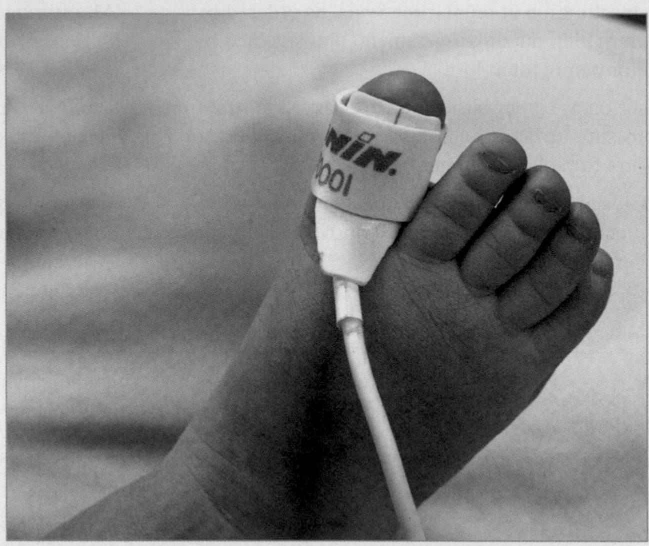

FIGURE 8 Oximetry probe on infant's toe.

Older Adult Considerations

- Careful attention to the patient's skin integrity and condition is necessary to prevent injury. Pressure or tension from the probe, as well as any adhesive used, can damage older, dry, thin skin.

Home Care Considerations

- Portable units are available for use in the home or in an outpatient setting.

EVIDENCE FOR PRACTICE ▶

PULSE OXIMETRY

Monitoring oxygen saturation by using pulse oximetry is a common method for assessing respiratory status in various clinical and home care situations. The patient's finger is used routinely as a site for this assessment. If the finger is unsuitable for measurement, the nurse might use the finger probe on the earlobe as an alternate measurement site. It is imperative that the nurse use the correct equipment for the site chosen to ensure accurate results.

Related Research

Johnson, C.L., Anderson, M.A., & Hill, P.D. (2012). Comparison of pulse oximetry measures in a healthy population. *MEDSURGNursing, 21*(2), 70–76.

In this study, finger and ear oximetry readings of 89 healthy people were compared. The findings do not support the common nursing practice of using a finger sensor to obtain a pulse oximetry reading from a person's ear if the finger is not usable.

Relevance for Nursing Practice

Nurses in the clinical setting should review procedures for obtaining pulse oximetry readings if the patient's fingers are not suitable. Correct use of appropriate equipment is vital for accurate results. The appropriate ear oximetry sensor should be used to obtain measurements from a patient's ear. A finger sensor should be limited to use on the finger. The oximetry measurement obtained during clinical assessment should include a record of the type of sensor used.

Refer to thePoint for additional research on related nursing topics.

SKILL 14-2 TEACHING A PATIENT TO USE AN INCENTIVE SPIROMETER

Incentive spirometry provides visual reinforcement for deep breathing by the patient. It assists the patient to breathe slowly and deeply, and to sustain maximal inspiration, while providing immediate positive reinforcement. Incentive spirometry encourages the patient to maximize lung inflation and prevent or reduce **atelectasis**. Optimal gas exchange is supported and secretions can be cleared and expectorated.

DELEGATION CONSIDERATIONS

Patient teaching related to the use of an incentive spirometer is not delegated to nursing assistive personnel (NAP), to unlicensed assistive personnel (UAP), or to licensed practical/vocational nurses (LPN/LVNs). Depending on the state's nurse practice act and the organization's policies and procedures, the LPN/LVN may reinforce and encourage the use of the incentive spirometer by the patient. The decision to delegate must be based on careful analysis of the patient's needs and circumstances, as well as the qualifications of the person to whom the task is being delegated. Refer to the Delegation Guidelines in Appendix A.

EQUIPMENT

- Incentive **spirometer**
- Stethoscope
- Folded blanket or pillow for splinting of chest or abdominal incision, if appropriate
- PPE, as indicated

ASSESSMENT

Assess the patient for pain and administer pain medication, as prescribed, if deep breathing may cause pain. Presence of pain may interfere with learning and performing required activities. Assess lung sounds before and after use to establish a baseline and to determine the effectiveness of incentive spirometry. Incentive spirometry encourages patients to take deep breaths, and lung sounds may be diminished before using the incentive spirometer. Assess vital signs and oxygen saturation to provide baseline data to evaluate patient response. Oxygen saturation may increase due to reinflation of **alveoli**.

NURSING DIAGNOSIS

Determine the related factors for the nursing diagnoses based on the patient's current status. Appropriate nursing diagnoses may include:

- Ineffective Breathing Pattern
- Risk for Infection
- Acute Pain
- Deficient Knowledge

OUTCOME IDENTIFICATION AND PLANNING

The expected outcome is that the patient accurately demonstrates the procedure for using the spirometer. Other outcomes that may be appropriate include the following: the patient demonstrates increased oxygen saturation level; the patient reports adequate control of pain during use; and the patient demonstrates increased lung expansion with clear breath sounds.

IMPLEMENTATION

ACTION	RATIONALE
1. Review the patient's health record for any health problems that would affect the patient's oxygenation status.	Identifying influencing factors aids in interpretation of results.
2. Bring necessary equipment to the bedside stand or overbed table.	Bringing everything to the bedside conserves time and energy. Arranging items nearby is convenient, saves time, and avoids unnecessary stretching and twisting of muscles on the part of the nurse.
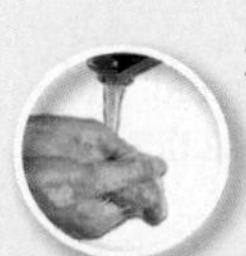 3. Perform hand hygiene and put on PPE, if indicated.	Hand hygiene and PPE prevent the spread of microorganisms. PPE is required based on transmission precautions.

(continued)

SKILL 14-2 TEACHING A PATIENT TO USE AN INCENTIVE SPIROMETER continued

ACTION	RATIONALE
4. Identify the patient. 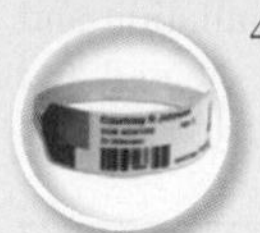	Identifying the patient ensures the right patient receives the intervention and helps prevent errors.
5. Close the curtains around the bed and close the door to the room, if possible. Explain what you are going to do and why you are going to do it to the patient. Using the chart provided with the device by the manufacturer, note the patient's inspiration target, based on the patient's height and age.	This ensures the patient's privacy. Explanation relieves anxiety and facilitates cooperation. Target for inspiration is based on the patient's height and age and provides an individualized target for each patient.
6. Assist the patient to an upright or semi-Fowler's position, if possible. Remove dentures if they fit poorly. Assess the patient's level of pain. Administer pain medication, as prescribed, if needed. Wait the appropriate amount of time for the medication to take effect. **If the patient has recently undergone abdominal or chest surgery, place a pillow or folded blanket over a chest or abdominal incision for splinting.**	Upright position facilitates lung expansion. Dentures may inhibit the patient from taking deep breaths if the patient is concerned that dentures may fall out. Pain may decrease the patient's ability to take deep breaths. Deep breaths may cause the patient to cough. Splinting the incision supports the area and helps reduce pain from the incision. (Refer to Skill 6-1.)
7. Demonstrate how to steady the device with one hand and hold the mouthpiece with the other hand (Figure 1). If the patient cannot use hands, assist the patient with the incentive spirometer.	This allows the patient to remain upright, visualize the volume of each breath, and stabilize the device.

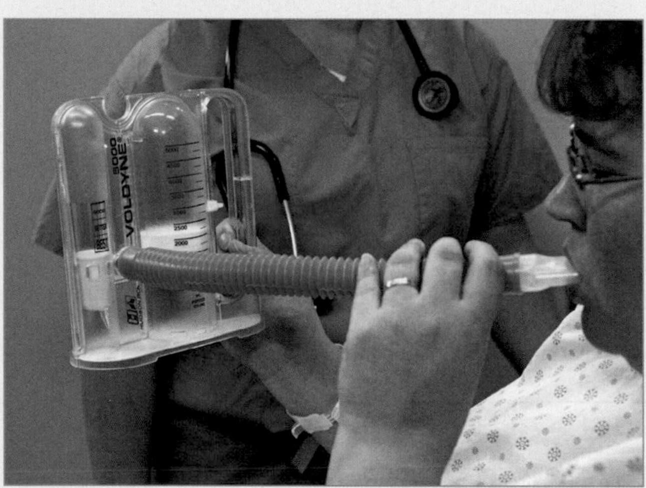

FIGURE 1 Patient using incentive spirometer.

ACTION	RATIONALE
8. Instruct the patient to exhale normally and then place lips securely around the mouthpiece.	Patient should fully empty lungs so that maximum volume may be inhaled. A tight seal allows for maximum use of the device.
9. **Instruct the patient to inhale slowly and as deeply as possible through the mouthpiece without using nose (if desired, a nose clip may be used).**	Inhaling through the nose would provide an inaccurate measurement of inhalation volume.
10. When the patient cannot inhale anymore, **the patient should hold his or her breath and count to three.** Check position of gauge to determine progress and level attained. If patient begins to cough, splint an abdominal or chest incision.	Holding breath for 3 seconds helps the alveoli to re-expand. Volume on incentive spirometry should increase with practice.

ACTION	RATIONALE
11. Instruct the patient to remove lips from mouthpiece and exhale normally. **If patient becomes light-headed during the process, tell him or her to stop and take a few normal breaths before resuming incentive spirometry.**	Deep breaths may change the CO_2 level, leading to light-headedness.
12. Encourage the patient to perform incentive spirometry 5 to 10 times every 1 to 2 hours, if possible.	This helps to reinflate the alveoli and prevent atelectasis due to **hypoventilation.**
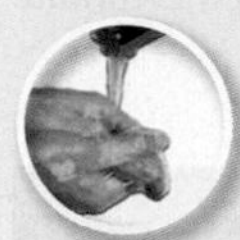 13. Clean the mouthpiece with water and shake to dry. Remove PPE, if used. Perform hand hygiene.	Cleaning equipment deters the spread of microorganisms and contaminants. Removing PPE properly reduces the risk for infection transmission and contamination of other items. Hand hygiene prevents the spread of microorganisms.

EVALUATION

The expected outcome is met when the patient demonstrates the steps for use of the incentive spirometer correctly and exhibits lung sounds that are clear and equal in all lobes. In addition, the patient demonstrates an increase in oxygen saturation levels, and verbalizes adequate pain control and the importance of, and need for, incentive spirometry.

DOCUMENTATION

Guidelines

Document that the incentive spirometer was used by the patient, the number of repetitions, and the average volume reached. Document patient teaching and patient response, if appropriate. If the patient coughs, document whether the cough is productive or nonproductive. If productive cough is present, include the characteristics of the sputum, including consistency, amount, and color.

Sample Documentation

9/8/15 Incentive spirometry performed × 10, volume 1,500 mL obtained. Patient with nonproductive cough during incentive spirometry.

—C. Bausler, RN

UNEXPECTED SITUATIONS AND ASSOCIATED INTERVENTIONS

- *Volume inhaled is decreasing:* Assess the patient's pain and anxiety level. Patient may have pain and not be inhaling fully, or patient may have experienced pain previously during incentive spirometry and have an increased anxiety level. If ordered, medicate patient when pain is present. Discuss fears with patient and encourage him or her to inhale fully or to increase the volume by 100 each time incentive spirometry is performed.
- *Patient attempts to blow into incentive spirometer:* Compare the incentive spirometer to a straw. Remind patient to exhale before beginning each time.

SPECIAL CONSIDERATIONS

General Considerations

- Reinforce importance of continued use by postoperative patients upon discharge.

Older Adult Considerations

- Older adults have decreased muscle function and fatigue more easily. Encourage rest periods between repetitions.

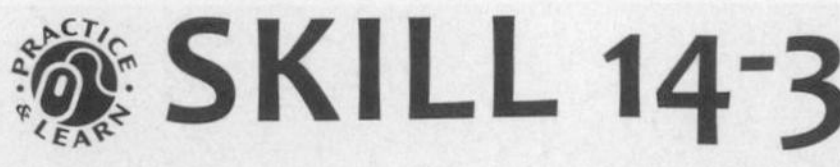

SKILL 14-3 ADMINISTERING OXYGEN BY NASAL CANNULA

A variety of devices are available for delivering oxygen to the patient. Each has a specific function and oxygen concentration. Device selection is based on the patient's condition and oxygen needs. A nasal cannula, also called nasal prongs, is the most commonly used oxygen delivery device. The cannula is a disposable plastic device with two protruding prongs for insertion into the nostrils. The cannula connects to an oxygen source with a flow meter and, many times, a humidifier. It is commonly used because the cannula does not impede eating or speaking and is used easily in the home. Disadvantages of this system are that it can be dislodged easily and can cause dryness of the nasal mucosa. In addition, if a patient breathes through the mouth, it is difficult to determine the amount of oxygen actually being received. A nasal cannula is used to deliver from 1 L/minute to 6 L/minute of oxygen. Table 14-1 compares amounts of delivered oxygen for these flow rates.

Table 14-1 OXYGEN DELIVERY SYSTEMS

METHOD	AMOUNT DELIVERED FiO_2 (FRACTION INSPIRED OXYGEN)	PRIORITY NURSING INTERVENTIONS
Nasal cannula	*Low Flow* 1–2 L/min = 23% to 30% 3–5 L/min = 30% to 40% 6 L/min = 42%	Check frequently that both prongs are in patient's nares. May be limited to no more than 2–3 L/min to patient with chronic lung disease.
Simple mask	*Low Flow* 6–8 L/min = 40% to 60% (5 L/min is minimum setting)	Monitor patient frequently to check mask placement. Support patient if claustrophobia is a concern. Secure physician's order to replace mask with nasal cannula during mealtime.
Partial rebreather mask	*Low Flow* 8–11 L/min = 50% to 75%	Set flow rate so that mask remains two-thirds full during inspiration. Keep reservoir bag free of twists or kinks.
Nonrebreather mask	*Low Flow* 12 L/min = 80% to 100%	Maintain flow rate so reservoir bag collapses only slightly during inspiration. Check that valves and rubber flaps are functioning properly (open during expiration and closed during inhalation). Monitor SaO_2 with pulse oximeter.
Venturi mask	*High Flow* 4–10 L/min = 24% to 40%	Requires careful monitoring to verify FiO_2 at flow rate ordered. Check that air intake valves are not blocked.

DELEGATION CONSIDERATIONS

The administration of oxygen by nasal cannula is not delegated to nursing assistive personnel (NAP) or to unlicensed assistive personnel (UAP). Reapplication of the nasal cannula during nursing care activities, such as during bathing, may be performed by NAP or UAP. Depending on the state's nurse practice act and the organization's policies and procedures, administration of oxygen by nasal cannula may be delegated to licensed practical/vocational nurses (LPN/LVNs). The decision to delegate must be based on careful analysis of the patient's needs and circumstances, as well as the qualifications of the person to whom the task is being delegated. Refer to the Delegation Guidelines in Appendix A.

EQUIPMENT

- Flow meter connected to oxygen supply
- Humidifier with sterile, distilled water (optional for low-flow system)
- Nasal cannula and tubing
- Gauze to pad tubing over ears (optional)
- PPE, as indicated

ASSESSMENT

Assess the patient's oxygen saturation level before starting oxygen therapy to provide a baseline for evaluating the effectiveness of oxygen therapy. Assess the patient's respiratory status, including respiratory rate, rhythm, effort, and lung sounds. Note any signs of respiratory distress, such as **tachypnea**, nasal flaring, use of accessory muscles, or **dyspnea**.

NURSING DIAGNOSIS	Determine the related factors for the nursing diagnoses based on the patient's current status. Appropriate nursing diagnoses may include: • Impaired Gas Exchange • Ineffective Breathing Pattern • Risk for Activity Intolerance
OUTCOME IDENTIFICATION AND PLANNING	The expected outcome is that the patient will exhibit an oxygen saturation level within acceptable parameters. Other outcomes that may be appropriate include the following: the patient will not experience dyspnea; and the patient will demonstrate effortless respirations in the normal range for age group, without evidence of nasal flaring or use of accessory muscles.

IMPLEMENTATION

ACTION	RATIONALE
1. Bring necessary equipment to the bedside stand or overbed table.	Bringing everything to the bedside conserves time and energy. Arranging items nearby is convenient, saves time, and avoids unnecessary stretching and twisting of muscles on the part of the nurse.
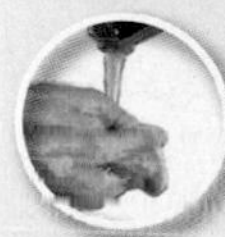 2. Perform hand hygiene and put on PPE, if indicated.	Hand hygiene and PPE prevent the spread of microorganisms. PPE is required based on transmission precautions.
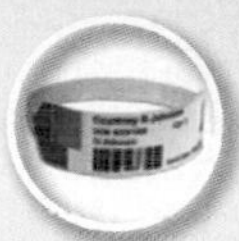 3. Identify the patient.	Identifying the patient ensures the right patient receives the intervention and helps prevent errors.
4. Close the curtains around the bed and close the door to the room, if possible.	This ensures the patient's privacy.
5. Explain what you are going to do and the reason for doing it to the patient. Review safety precautions necessary when oxygen is in use.	Explanation relieves anxiety and facilitates cooperation. Oxygen supports combustion; a small spark could cause a fire.
6. Connect nasal cannula to oxygen setup with humidification, if humidification is in use (Figure 1). Adjust flow rate as ordered (Figure 2). Check that oxygen is flowing out of prongs.	Oxygen forced through a water reservoir is humidified before it is delivered to the patient, thus preventing dehydration of the mucous membranes. Low-flow oxygen does not require humidification.

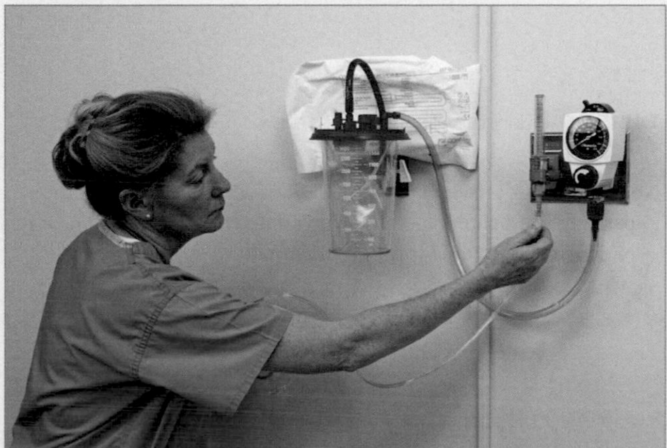

FIGURE 1 Connecting cannula to oxygen source.

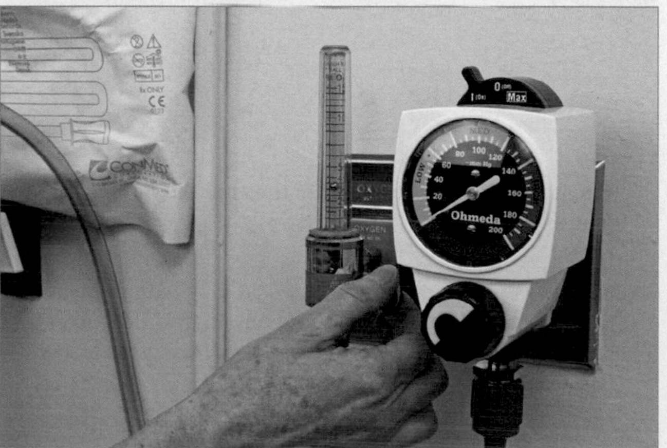

FIGURE 2 Adjusting flow rate.

(continued)

SKILL 14-3 ADMINISTERING OXYGEN BY NASAL CANNULA continued

ACTION	RATIONALE
7. Place prongs in patient's nostrils (Figure 3). Place tubing over and behind each ear with adjuster comfortably under chin. Alternately, the tubing may be placed around the patient's head, with the adjuster at the back or base of the head. Place gauze pads at ear beneath the tubing, as necessary (Figure 4).	Correct placement of the prongs and fastener facilitates oxygen administration and patient comfort. Pads reduce irritation and pressure and protect the skin.
8. Adjust the fit of the cannula, as necessary (Figure 5). Tubing should be snug but not tight against the skin.	Proper adjustment maintains the prongs in the patient's nose. Excessive pressure from tubing could cause irritation and pressure to the skin.

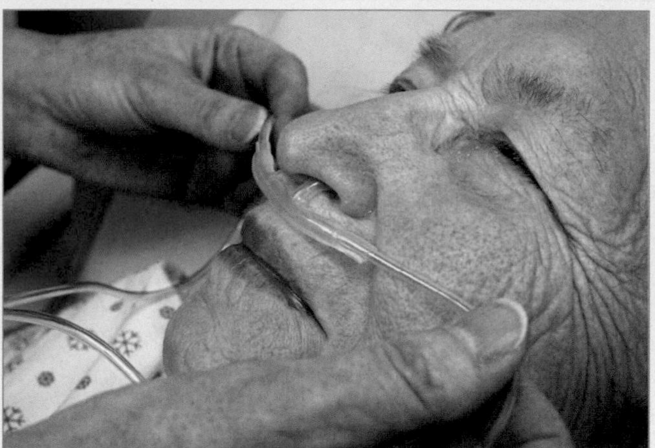

FIGURE 3 Applying cannula to nares.

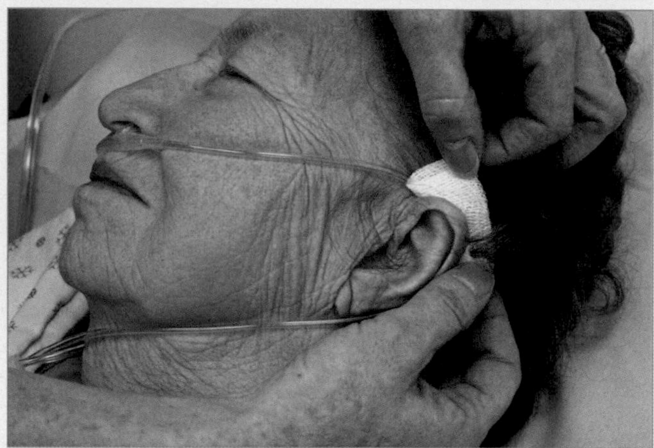

FIGURE 4 Placing gauze pad at ears.

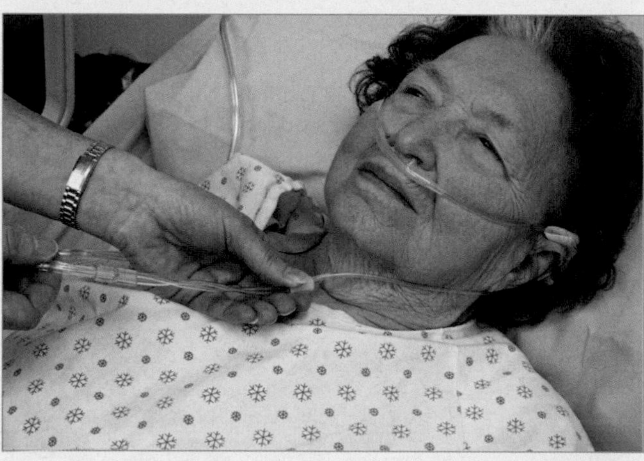

FIGURE 5 Adjusting cannula, if needed.

ACTION	RATIONALE
9. **Encourage patients to breathe through the nose, with the mouth closed.**	Nose breathing provides for optimal delivery of oxygen to the patient. The percentage of oxygen delivered can be reduced in patients who breathe through the mouth.
10. Reassess the patient's respiratory status, including respiratory rate, effort, and lung sounds. Note any signs of respiratory distress, such as tachypnea, nasal flaring, use of accessory muscles, or dyspnea.	Assesses the effectiveness of oxygen therapy.
11. Remove PPE, if used. Perform hand hygiene.	Removing PPE properly reduces the risk for infection transmission and contamination of other items. Hand hygiene prevents the spread of microorganisms.

ACTION	RATIONALE
12. Put on clean gloves. Remove and clean the cannula and assess nares at least every 8 hours, or according to agency recommendations (Figure 6). Check nares for evidence of irritation or bleeding.	The continued presence of the cannula causes irritation and dryness of the mucous membranes.

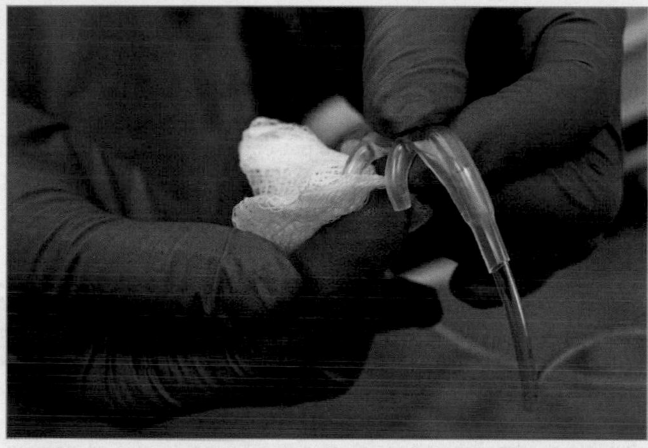

FIGURE 6 Cleaning cannula, when indicated.

EVALUATION

The expected outcome is met when the patient demonstrates an oxygen saturation level within acceptable parameters. In addition, the patient remains free of dyspnea, nasal flaring, or accessory muscle use and demonstrates respiratory rate and depth within normal ranges.

DOCUMENTATION

Guidelines

Document your assessment before and after intervention. Document the amount of oxygen applied, and the patient's respiratory rate, oxygen saturation, and lung sounds.

Sample Documentation

Lippincott DocuCare Practice documenting the administration of oxygen by nasal cannula in *Lippincott DocuCare*.

9/17/15 1300 Oxygen via nasal cannula applied at 2 L/min. Humidification in place. Pulse oximeter before placing oxygen 92%; after oxygen at 2 L/min 98%. Respirations even and unlabored. Chest rises symmetrically. No nasal flaring or retractions noted. Lung sounds clear and equal in all lobes.

—C. Bausler, RN

UNEXPECTED SITUATIONS AND ASSOCIATED INTERVENTIONS

- *Patient was fine on oxygen delivered by nasal cannula but now is cyanotic, and the pulse oximeter reading is less than 93%:* Check to see that the oxygen tubing is still connected to the flow meter and the flow meter is still on the previous setting. Someone may have stepped on the tubing, pulling it from the flow meter, or the oxygen may have accidentally been turned off. Assess lung sounds to note any changes. Report changes and assessment findings to primary care provider.
- *Areas over ear or back of head are reddened:* Ensure that areas are adequately padded and that tubing is not pulled too tight. If available, a skin care team may be able to offer some suggestions.
- *When dozing, the patient begins to breathe through the mouth:* Temporarily place the nasal cannula near the mouth. If this does not raise the pulse oximeter reading, you may need to obtain an order to switch the patient to a mask while sleeping.

(continued)

SKILL 14-3 ADMINISTERING OXYGEN BY NASAL CANNULA continued

SPECIAL CONSIDERATIONS

Home Care Considerations

- Oxygen administration may need to be continued in the home setting. Portable oxygen concentrators are used most frequently. Instruct caregivers about safety precautions with oxygen use and make sure they understand the rationale for the specific liter flow of oxygen.
- To prevent fires and injuries, take the following precautions:
  - Avoid open flames.
  - **Place "No Smoking" signs in conspicuous places in the patient's home.** Instruct the patient and visitors about the hazard of smoking when oxygen is in use.
  - Check to see that electrical equipment used in the room is in good working order and emits no sparks.
  - Avoid using oils in the area. Oil can ignite spontaneously in the presence of oxygen.

SKILL 14-4 ADMINISTERING OXYGEN BY MASK

When a patient requires a higher concentration of oxygen than a nasal cannula can deliver (6 L or 44% oxygen concentration), or is unable or unwilling to maintain a nasal cannula, use an oxygen mask. (See Table 14-1 in Skill 14-3 for a comparison of different types of oxygen delivery systems.) Fit the mask carefully to the patient's face to avoid oxygen leakage. The mask should be comfortably snug, but not tight against the face. Disposable and reusable face masks are available. The most commonly used types of masks are the simple face mask, the partial rebreather mask, the nonrebreather mask, and the Venturi mask. Figure 1 illustrates different types of oxygen masks.

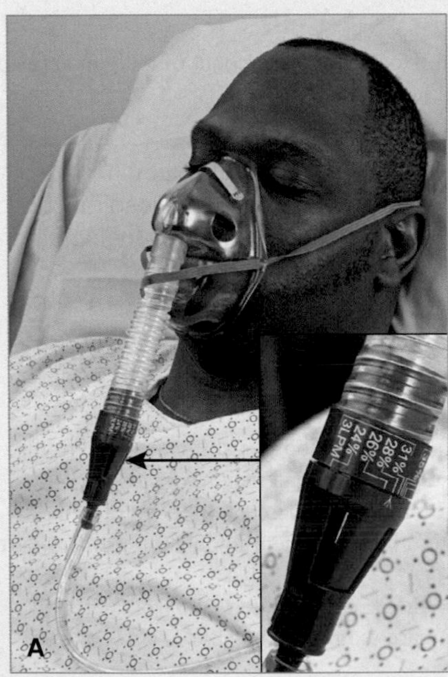

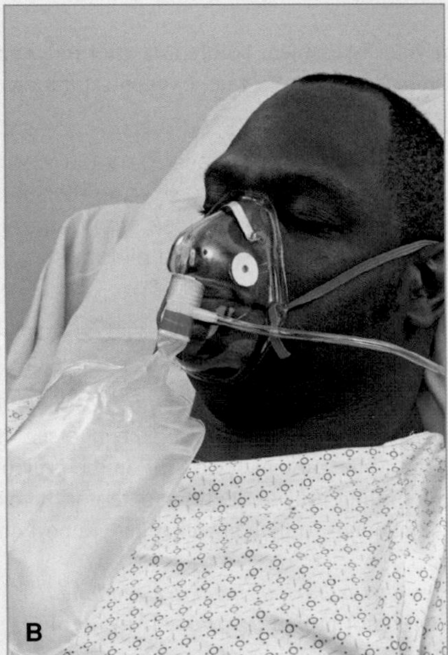

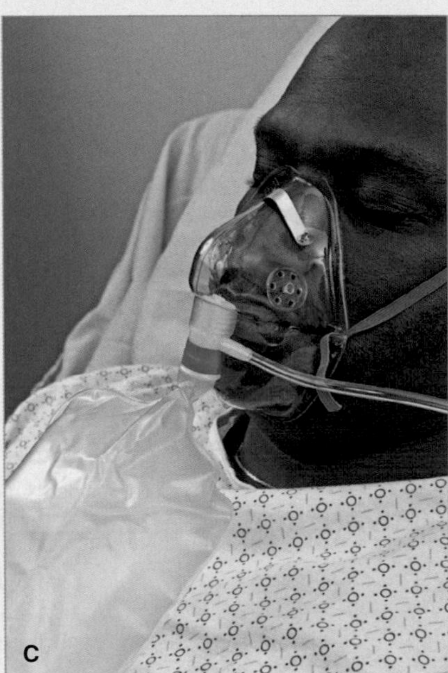

FIGURE 1 Types of oxygen masks. (**A**) Venturi mask. (**B**) Nonrebreather mask. (**C**) Partial rebreather mask. (*continued*)

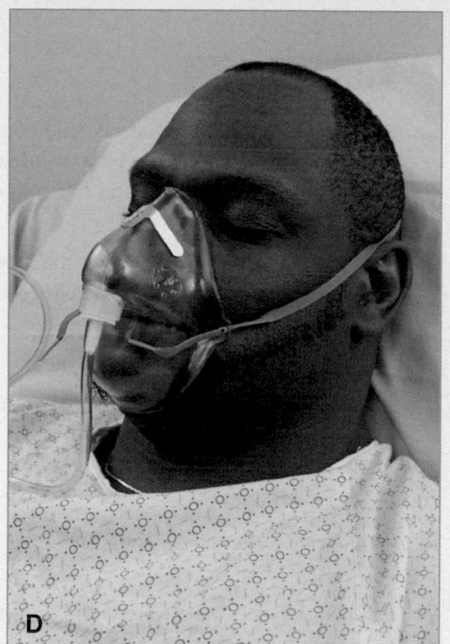
D

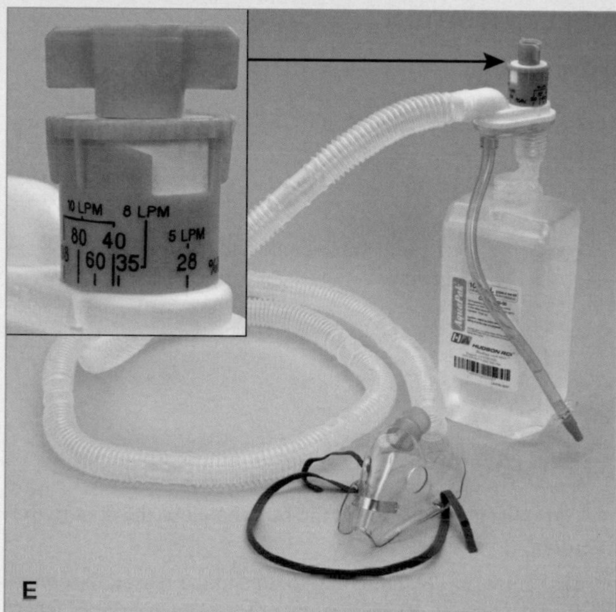

E

FIGURE 1 (*Continued*) (**D**) Simple face mask. (**E**) High-flow oxygen face mask and bottle.

DELEGATION CONSIDERATIONS

The administration of oxygen by a mask is not delegated to nursing assistive personnel (NAP) or to unlicensed assistive personnel (UAP). Reapplication of the mask during nursing care activities, such as during bathing, may be performed by NAP or UAP. Depending on the state's nurse practice act and the organization's policies and procedures, administration of oxygen by a mask may be delegated to licensed practical/vocational nurses (LPN/LVNs). The decision to delegate must be based on careful analysis of the patient's needs and circumstances, as well as the qualifications of the person to whom the task is being delegated. Refer to the Delegation Guidelines in Appendix A.

EQUIPMENT

- Flow meter connected to oxygen supply
- Humidifier with sterile distilled water, if necessary, for the type of mask prescribed
- Face mask, specified by medical order
- Gauze to pad elastic band (optional)
- PPE, as indicated

ASSESSMENT

Assess the patient's oxygen saturation level before starting oxygen therapy to provide a baseline for determining the effectiveness of therapy. Assess the patient's respiratory status, including respiratory rate, rhythm, effort, and lung sounds. Note any signs of respiratory distress, such as tachypnea, nasal flaring, use of accessory muscles, or dyspnea.

NURSING DIAGNOSIS

Determine the related factors for the nursing diagnoses based on the patient's current status. Appropriate nursing diagnoses may include:

- Impaired Gas Exchange
- Ineffective Breathing Pattern
- Ineffective Airway Clearance

OUTCOME IDENTIFICATION AND PLANNING

The expected outcome is that the patient exhibits an oxygen saturation level within acceptable parameters. Other outcomes that may be appropriate include the following: the patient will remain free of signs and symptoms of respiratory distress; and respiratory status, including respiratory rate and depth, will be in the normal range for the patient's age.

(*continued*)

SKILL 14-4 ADMINISTERING OXYGEN BY MASK continued

IMPLEMENTATION

ACTION	RATIONALE
1. Bring necessary equipment to the bedside stand or overbed table.	Bringing everything to the bedside conserves time and energy. Arranging items nearby is convenient, saves time, and avoids unnecessary stretching and twisting of muscles on the part of the nurse.
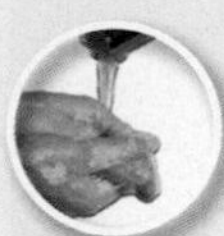 2. Perform hand hygiene and put on PPE, if indicated.	Hand hygiene and PPE prevent the spread of microorganisms. PPE is required based on transmission precautions.
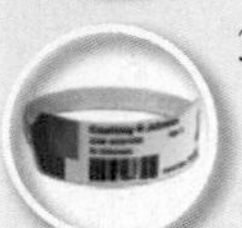 3. Identify the patient.	Identifying the patient ensures the right patient receives the intervention and helps prevent errors.
4. Close the curtains around the bed and close the door to the room, if possible.	This ensures the patient's privacy.
5. Explain what you are going to do and the reason for doing it to the patient. Review safety precautions necessary when oxygen is in use.	Explanation relieves anxiety and facilitates cooperation. Oxygen supports combustion; a small spark could cause a fire.
6. Attach face mask to oxygen source (with humidification, if appropriate, for the specific mask) (Figure 2). Start the flow of oxygen at the specified rate. For a mask with a reservoir, be sure to allow oxygen to fill the bag (Figure 3) before proceeding to the next step.	Oxygen forced through a water reservoir is humidified before it is delivered to the patient, thus preventing dehydration of the mucous membranes. A reservoir bag must be inflated with oxygen because the bag is the oxygen supply source for the patient.

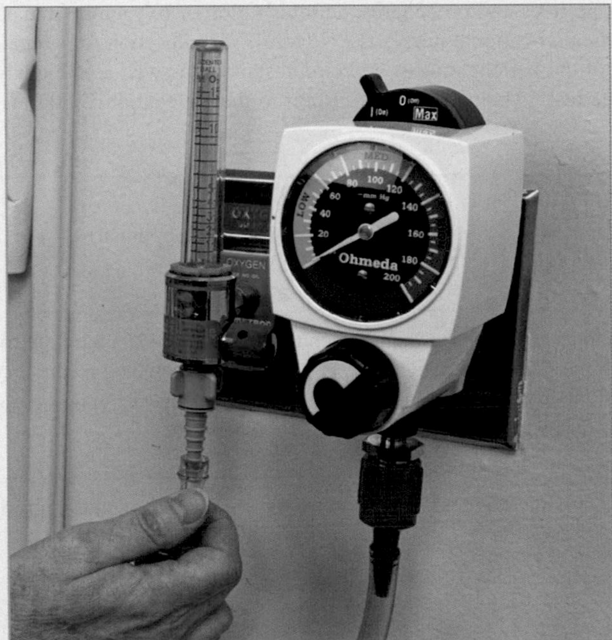

FIGURE 2 Connecting face mask to oxygen source.

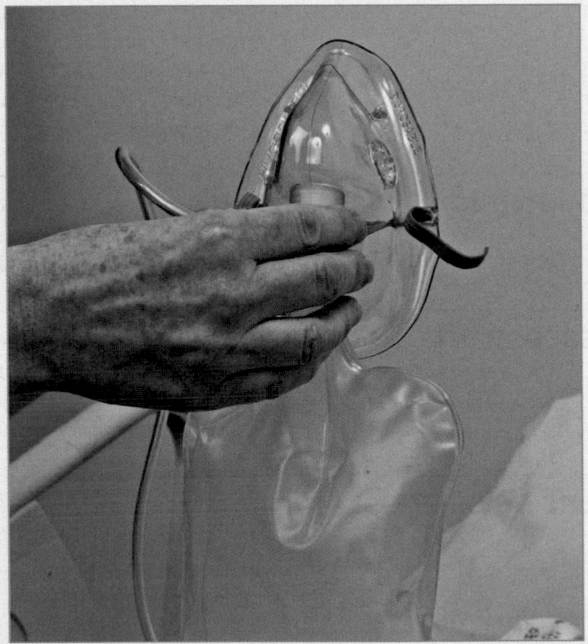

FIGURE 3 Allowing oxygen to fill bag.

ACTION

7. Position face mask over the patient's nose and mouth (Figure 4). Adjust the elastic strap so that the mask fits snugly but comfortably on the face (Figure 5). Adjust to the prescribed flow rate (Figure 6).

RATIONALE

A loose or poorly fitting mask will result in oxygen loss and decreased therapeutic value. Masks may cause a feeling of suffocation, and the patient needs frequent attention and reassurance.

ACTION

8. If the patient reports irritation or you note redness, use gauze pads under the elastic strap at pressure points to reduce irritation to ears and scalp.

RATIONALE

Pads reduce irritation and pressure and protect the skin.

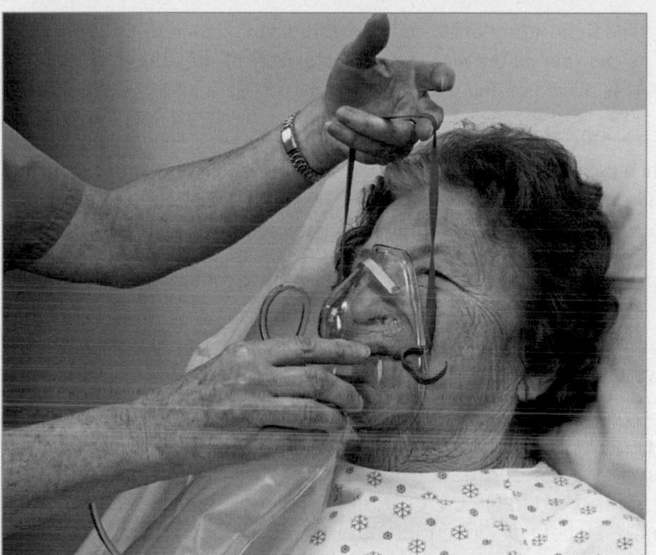

FIGURE 4 Applying face mask over nose and mouth.

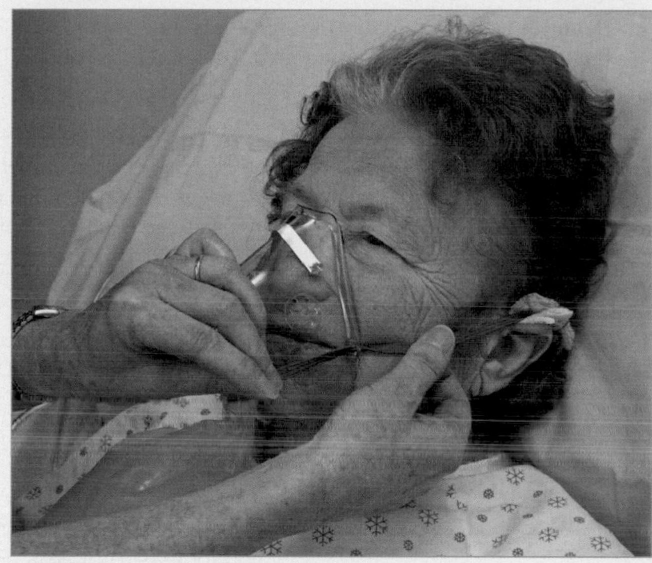

FIGURE 5 Adjusting elastic straps.

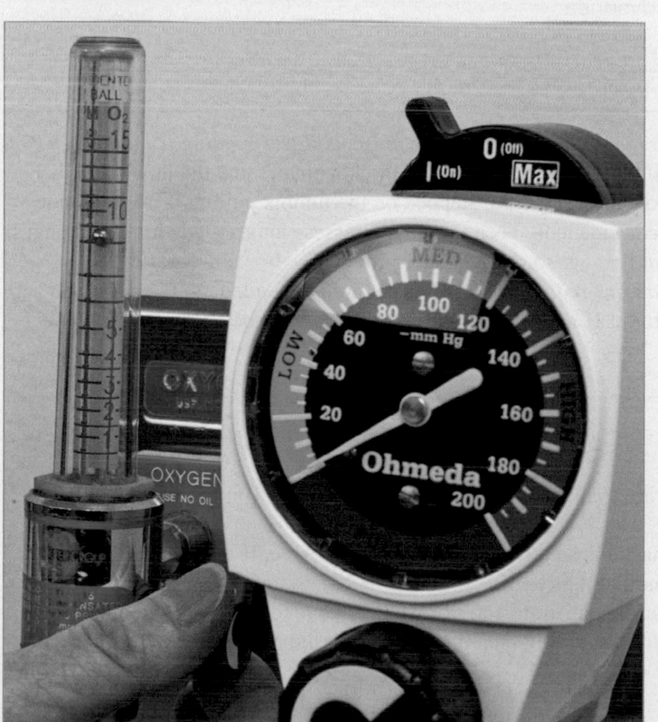

FIGURE 6 Adjusting flow rate.

(continued)

SKILL 14-4 ADMINISTERING OXYGEN BY MASK continued

ACTION	RATIONALE
9. Reassess the patient's respiratory status, including respiratory rate, effort, and lung sounds. Note any signs of respiratory distress, such as tachypnea, nasal flaring, use of accessory muscles, or dyspnea.	This helps assess the effectiveness of oxygen therapy.
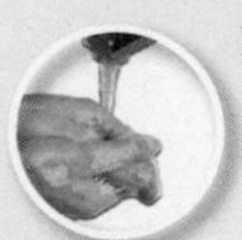 10. Remove PPE, if used. Perform hand hygiene.	Removing PPE properly reduces the risk for infection transmission and contamination of other items. Hand hygiene prevents the spread of microorganisms.
11. Remove the mask and dry the skin every 2 to 3 hours if the oxygen is running continuously. Do not use powder around the mask.	The tight-fitting mask and moisture from condensation can irritate the skin on the face. There is a danger of inhaling powder if it is placed on the mask.

EVALUATION

The expected outcome is met when the patient exhibits an oxygen saturation level within acceptable parameters. In addition, the patient demonstrates an absence of respiratory distress and accessory muscle use and exhibits respiratory rate and depth within normal parameters.

DOCUMENTATION

Guidelines

Document type of mask used, amount of oxygen used, oxygen saturation level, lung sounds, and rate/pattern of respirations. Document your assessment before and after intervention.

Sample Documentation

Lippincott DocuCare Practice documenting the administration of oxygen by mask in *Lippincott DocuCare.*

9/22/15 Patient reports feeling short of breath. Skin pale, respirations 30 breaths per minute and labored. Lung sounds decreased throughout. Oxygen saturation via pulse oximeter 88%. Findings reported to Dr. Lu. Oxygen via nonrebreather face mask applied at 12 L/min as ordered. Patient's skin is pink after O_2 applied. Oxygen saturation increased to 98%. Respirations even and unlabored. Chest rises symmetrically. Respiratory rate 18 breaths per minute. Lungs remain with decreased breath sounds throughout. Patient denies dyspnea.

—C. Bausler, RN

UNEXPECTED SITUATIONS AND ASSOCIATED INTERVENTIONS

- *Patient was previously fine but now is cyanotic, and the pulse oximeter reading is less than 93%:* Check to see that the oxygen tubing is still connected to the flow meter and the flow meter is still on the previous setting. Someone may have stepped on the tubing, pulling it from the flow meter, or the oxygen may have accidentally been turned off. Assess lung sounds for any changes. Report changes and assessment findings to primary care provider.
- *Areas over ear or back of head are reddened:* Ensure that areas are adequately padded and that tubing is not pulled too tight. If available, a skin-care team may be able to offer some suggestions.

SPECIAL CONSIDERATIONS

General Considerations

- Different types of face masks are available for use. (Refer to Table 14-1 in Skill 14-3 for more information.)
- It is important to ensure the mask fits snugly around the patient's face. If it is loose, it will not effectively deliver the right amount of oxygen.
- The mask must be removed for the patient to eat, drink, and take medications. Obtain an order for oxygen via nasal cannula for use during mealtimes and limit the amount of times the mask is removed to maintain adequate oxygenation.

SKILL VARIATION Using an Oxygen Hood

Oxygen hoods are generally used to deliver oxygen to infants. They can supply an oxygen concentration up to 80% to 90% (Kyle & Carman, 2013). The oxygen hood, a clear plastic cover, is placed over the infant's head and neck; it allows easy access to the chest and lower body. Continuous pulse oximetry allows for monitoring oxygenation and making adjustments according to the infant's condition (Perry et al., 2010). The infant must be removed from the hood for feeding; obtain an order for oxygen delivery for use during feeding times. Assessment of an infant should include assessment of skin color. A pale or cyanotic patient may not be receiving sufficient oxygen. Assess the patient's respiratory status, including respiratory rate, rhythm, effort, and lung sounds. Assessment should also include assessing the patient for any signs of respiratory distress, such as nasal flaring, grunting, or retractions; oxygen-depleted patients often exhibit these signs. Additional equipment required includes the oxygen hood, oxygen analyzer, and a humidification device.

1. Bring necessary equipment to the bedside stand or overbed table.

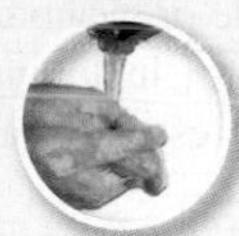

2. Perform hand hygiene and put on PPE, if indicated.

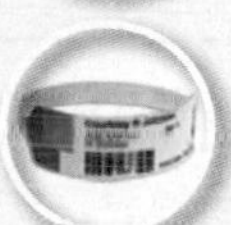

3. Identify the patient.
4. Close the curtains around the bed and close the door to the room, if possible.
5. Explain what you are going to do and the reason for doing it to the patient and parents/guardians. Review safety precautions necessary when oxygen is in use.
6. Calibrate the oxygen analyzer according to manufacturer's directions.
7. Place hood on crib. Connect humidifier to oxygen source in the wall. Connect the oxygen tubing to the hood. Adjust flow rate as ordered by physician. Check that oxygen is flowing into the hood.
8. Turn on analyzer. **Place oxygen analyzer probe in hood.**
9. Adjust oxygen flow, as necessary, based on sensor readings. Once oxygen levels reach the prescribed amount, place hood over patient's head (Figure A). The hood should not rub against the infant's neck, chin, or shoulder.

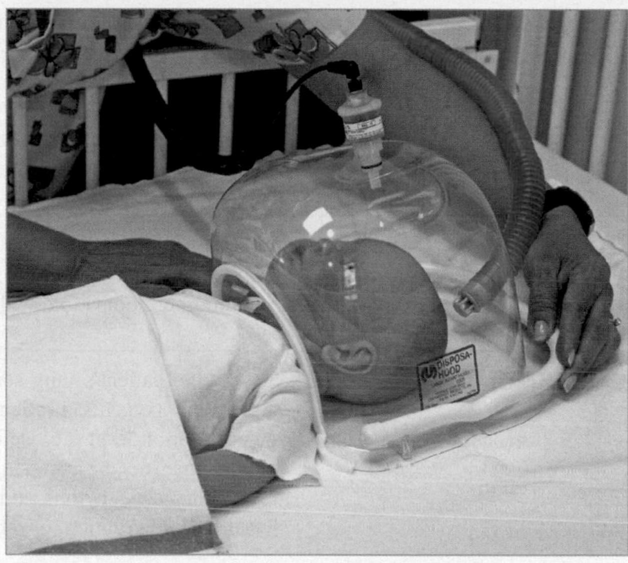

FIGURE A Placing oxygen hood over infant's head.

10. **Do not block hole in top of hood if present.**
11. Instruct family members not to raise edges of the hood.
12. Reassess the patient's respiratory status, including respiratory rate, effort, oxygen saturation, and lung sounds. Note any signs of respiratory distress, such as tachypnea, nasal flaring, grunting, retractions, or dyspnea.

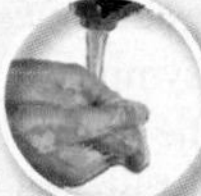

13. Remove PPE, if used. Perform hand hygiene.
14. **Frequently check bedding and patient's head for moisture. Change linen and dry the patient's skin, as needed, to keep the patient dry.**
15. **Monitor the patient's body temperature at regular intervals.**

SKILL 14-5 USING AN OXYGEN TENT

Oxygen tents are often used for children who will not leave a face mask or nasal cannula in place. The oxygen tent gives the patient freedom to move in the bed or crib while cool, highly humidified oxygen is being delivered. However, it is difficult to keep the tent closed because the child may want contact with his or her parents. It is also difficult to maintain a consistent level of oxygen and to deliver oxygen at a rate higher than 30% to 50% (Kyle & Carman, 2013). Frequent assessment of the child's temperature, pajamas, and bedding is necessary because the humidification quickly creates moisture, leading to damp clothing and linens, and, possibly, hypothermia.

DELEGATION CONSIDERATIONS

The application of an oxygen tent is not delegated to nursing assistive personnel (NAP) or to unlicensed assistive personnel (UAP). Depending on the state's nurse practice act and the organization's policies and procedures, the application of an oxygen tent may be delegated to licensed practical/vocational nurses (LPN/LVNs). The decision to delegate must be based on careful analysis of the patient's needs and circumstances, as well as the qualifications of the person to whom the task is being delegated. Refer to the Delegation Guidelines in Appendix A.

EQUIPMENT

- Oxygen source
- Oxygen tent
- Humidifier compatible with tent
- Oxygen analyzer
- Small blankets for blanket rolls
- PPE, as indicated

ASSESSMENT

Assess the patient's lung sounds. Secretions may cause the patient's oxygen demand to increase. Assess the oxygen saturation level. There will usually be an order for a baseline or goal for the oxygen saturation level (i.e., deliver oxygen to keep $SpO_2 \geq 95\%$). Assess skin color. A pale or cyanotic patient may not be receiving sufficient oxygen. Assess the patient's respiratory status, including respiratory rate, rhythm, and effort. Assess the patient for any signs of respiratory distress, such as nasal flaring, grunting, or retractions; oxygen-depleted patients often exhibit these signs.

NURSING DIAGNOSIS

Determine the related factors for the nursing diagnoses based on the patient's current status. Appropriate nursing diagnoses may include:

- Impaired Gas Exchange
- Ineffective Breathing Pattern
- Ineffective Airway Clearance
- Risk for Impaired Skin Integrity

OUTCOME IDENTIFICATION AND PLANNING

The expected outcome is that the patient exhibits an oxygen saturation level within acceptable parameters. Other outcomes that may be appropriate include the following: the patient will remain free of signs and symptoms of respiratory distress; respiratory status, including respiratory rate and depth, will be in the normal range for the patient's age; and the patient's skin will be warm, dry, and without evidence of breakdown.

IMPLEMENTATION

ACTION	RATIONALE
1. Bring necessary equipment to the bedside stand or overbed table.	Bringing everything to the bedside conserves time and energy. Arranging items nearby is convenient, saves time, and avoids unnecessary stretching and twisting of muscles on the part of the nurse.
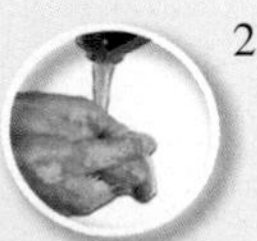 2. Perform hand hygiene and put on PPE, if indicated.	Hand hygiene and PPE prevent the spread of microorganisms. PPE is required based on transmission precautions.
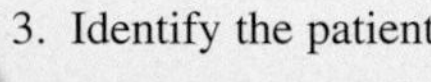 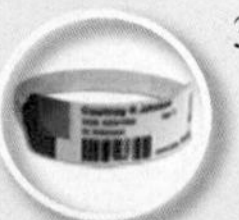 3. Identify the patient.	Identifying the patient ensures the right patient receives the intervention and helps prevent errors.

ACTION	RATIONALE
4. Close the curtains around the bed and close the door to the room, if possible.	This ensures the patient's privacy.
5. Explain what you are going to do and the reason for doing it to the patient and parents/guardians. Review safety precautions necessary when oxygen is in use.	Explanation relieves anxiety and facilitates cooperation. Oxygen supports combustion; a small spark could cause a fire.
6. Calibrate the oxygen analyzer according to manufacturer's directions.	Ensures accurate readings and appropriate adjustments to therapy.
7. Place tent over crib or bed. Connect the humidifier to the oxygen source in the wall and connect the tent tubing to the humidifier. Adjust flow rate as ordered by physician. Check that oxygen is flowing into the tent.	Oxygen forced through a water reservoir is humidified before it is delivered to the patient, thus preventing dehydration of the mucous membranes.
8. Turn on analyzer. Place oxygen analyzer probe in tent, out of patient's reach.	The analyzer will give an accurate reading of the concentration of oxygen in the crib or bed.
9. Adjust oxygen, as necessary, based on sensor readings (Figure 1). Once oxygen levels reach the prescribed amount, place the patient in the tent (Figure 2).	Patient will receive oxygen once placed in the tent.
10. Roll small blankets like a jelly roll and tuck tent edges under blanket rolls, as necessary (Figure 3).	The blanket helps keep the edges of the tent flap from coming up and letting oxygen out.

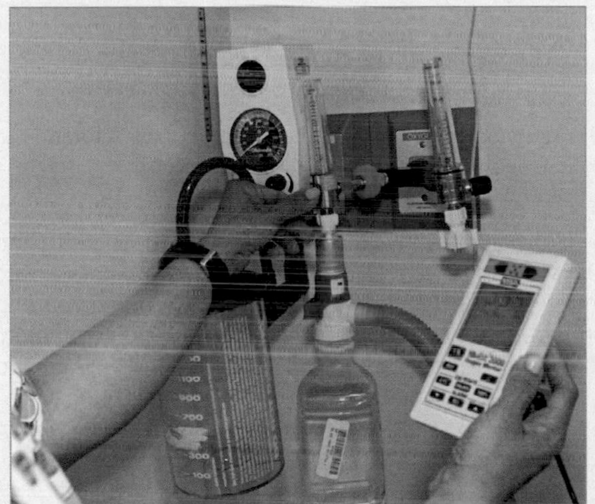

FIGURE 1 Adjusting oxygen flow.

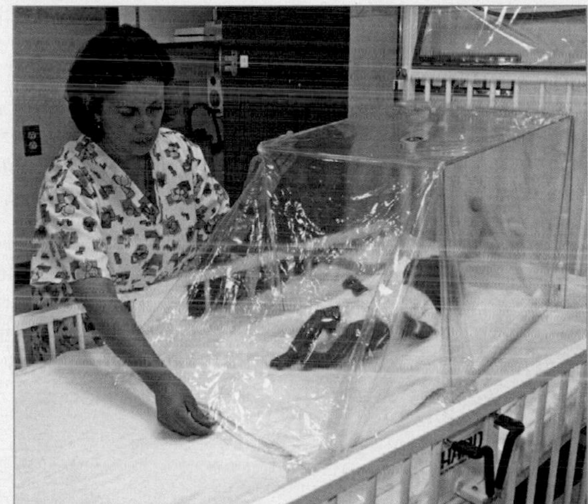

FIGURE 2 Placing patient in tent.

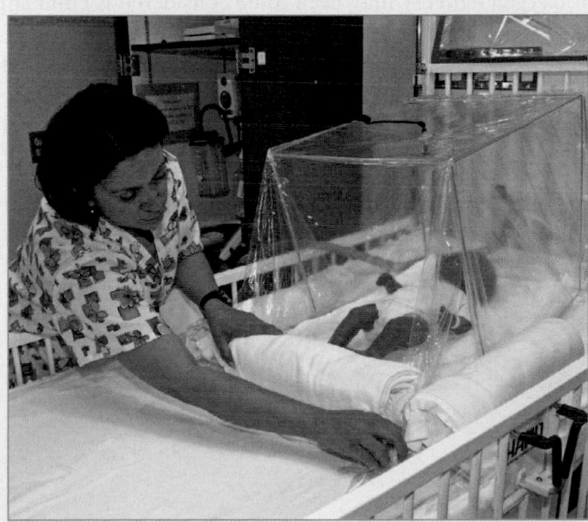

FIGURE 3 Tucking edges under blanket rolls.

(continued)

SKILL 14-5 USING AN OXYGEN TENT continued

ACTION	RATIONALE
11. **Encourage patient and family members to keep tent flap closed.**	Every time the tent flap is opened, oxygen is released.
12. Reassess the patient's respiratory status, including respiratory rate, effort, and lung sounds. Note any signs of respiratory distress, such as tachypnea, nasal flaring, use of accessory muscles, grunting, retractions, or dyspnea.	This assesses the effectiveness of oxygen therapy.
13. Remove PPE, if used. Perform hand hygiene.	Removing PPE properly reduces the risk for infection transmission and contamination of other items. Hand hygiene prevents the spread of microorganisms.
14. **Frequently check bedding and patient's pajamas for moisture. Change as needed to keep the patient dry. Monitor the patient's body temperature at regular intervals.**	The large amount of humidification delivered in an oxygen tent quickly makes cloth moist, which would be uncomfortable for the patient and may affect temperature regulation. The cool environment can cause hypothermia and cold stress (Perry et al., 2010).

EVALUATION

The expected outcome is met when the patient exhibits an oxygen saturation level within acceptable parameters. In addition, the patient remains free of dyspnea, nasal flaring, grunting, or use of accessory muscles when breathing; respirations remain in normal range for age; and body temperature remains within normal limits.

DOCUMENTATION

Guidelines

Document amount of oxygen applied; respiratory rate, rhythm, and effort; oxygen saturation level; and your assessment before and after intervention.

Sample Documentation

9/17/15 Patient noted to have nasal flaring and grunting. Lung sounds clear and equal. Pulse oximeter reading 92%. Respirations regular and deep, respiratory rate 52. Patient placed in oxygen tent at 45% per standing order. Pulse oximeter reading increased to 98% after placing in tent. Respirations even, unlabored, and symmetric. Respiratory rate 35. No nasal flaring or retractions noted. Lung sounds clear and equal in all lobes.

—C. Bausler, RN

UNEXPECTED SITUATIONS AND ASSOCIATED INTERVENTIONS

- *Child refuses to stay in tent:* Parent may play games in tent with child if this will help child to stay in tent. Alternative methods of oxygen delivery may need to be considered if child still refuses to stay in tent.
- *It is difficult to maintain an oxygen level above 40% in the tent:* Ensure that the flap is closed and edges of the tent are tucked under the blanket. Check oxygen delivery unit to ensure that the rate has not been changed. Encourage patient and family members to leave flaps closed. If still a problem, analyzer may need to be replaced or recalibrated.

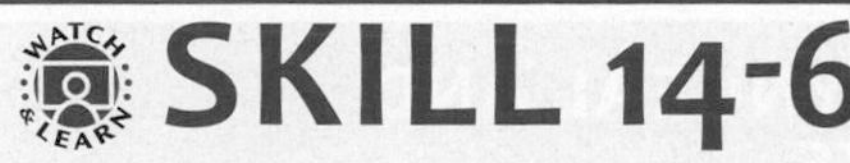

SKILL 14-6 SUCTIONING THE OROPHARYNGEAL AND NASOPHARYNGEAL AIRWAYS

Suctioning of the pharynx is indicated to maintain a patent airway and to remove saliva, pulmonary secretions, blood, vomitus, or foreign material from the pharynx. Suctioning helps a patient who cannot successfully clear his or her airway by coughing and expectorating (Sole et al., 2011). When performing suctioning, position yourself on the appropriate side of the patient. If you are right-handed, stand on the patient's right side; if left-handed, stand on the patient's left side. This allows for comfortable use of the dominant hand to manipulate the suction catheter. The following skill describes suctioning of the oropharyngeal airway. See the accompanying Skill Variation for a description of suctioning of the nasopharyngeal airway.

DELEGATION CONSIDERATIONS

The suctioning of the oropharyngeal airway may be delegated to nursing assistive personnel (NAP) or to unlicensed assistive personnel (UAP) who have received appropriate training. Depending on the state's nurse practice act and the organization's policies and procedures, the suctioning of the oropharyngeal and nasopharyngeal airways may be delegated to licensed practical/vocational nurses (LPN/LVNs). The decision to delegate must be based on careful analysis of the patient's needs and circumstances, as well as the qualifications of the person to whom the task is being delegated. Refer to the Delegation Guidelines in Appendix A.

EQUIPMENT

- Portable or wall suction unit with tubing
- A commercially prepared suction kit with an appropriate size catheter or
- Sterile suction catheter with Y-port in the appropriate size (Adult: 10F to 16F)
- Sterile disposable container
- Sterile gloves
- Sterile water or saline
- Towel or waterproof pad
- Goggles and mask or face shield
- Disposable, clean gloves
- Water-soluble lubricant
- Additional PPE, as indicated

ASSESSMENT

Assess lung sounds. Patients who need to be suctioned may have wheezes, crackles, or gurgling present. Assess oxygen saturation level. Oxygen saturation usually decreases when a patient needs to be suctioned. Assess respiratory status, including respiratory rate, rhythm, and depth. Patients may become tachypneic when they need to be suctioned. Assess the patient for signs of respiratory distress, such as nasal flaring, retractions, or grunting. Assess effectiveness of coughing and expectoration. Suctioning of the airway may be necessary for patients with an ineffective cough who are unable to expectorate secretions. Assess for history of deviated septum, nasal polyps, nasal obstruction, nasal injury, epistaxis (nasal bleeding), or nasal swelling. Assess for pain. Assess the characteristics and amount of secretions while suctioning.

NURSING DIAGNOSIS

Determine the related factors for the nursing diagnoses based on the patient's current status. Appropriate nursing diagnoses may include:

- Ineffective Airway Clearance
- Impaired Gas Exchange
- Ineffective Breathing Pattern
- Risk for Aspiration

OUTCOME IDENTIFICATION AND PLANNING

The expected outcome to achieve is that the patient will exhibit improved breath sounds and a clear, patent airway. Other outcomes that may be appropriate include the following: the patient will exhibit an oxygen saturation level within acceptable parameters; the patient will demonstrate a respiratory rate and depth within age-acceptable range; and the patient will remain free of any signs of respiratory distress, including retractions, nasal flaring, or grunting.

IMPLEMENTATION

ACTION	RATIONALE
1. Bring necessary equipment to the bedside stand or overbed table.	Bringing everything to the bedside conserves time and energy. Arranging items nearby is convenient, saves time, and avoids unnecessary stretching and twisting of muscles on the part of the nurse.

(continued)

SKILL 14-6 SUCTIONING THE OROPHARYNGEAL AND NASOPHARYNGEAL AIRWAYS continued

ACTION	RATIONALE
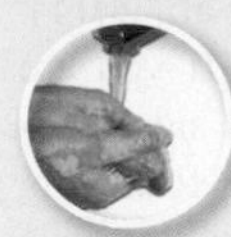 2. Perform hand hygiene and put on PPE, if indicated.	Hand hygiene and PPE prevent the spread of microorganisms. PPE is required based on transmission precautions.
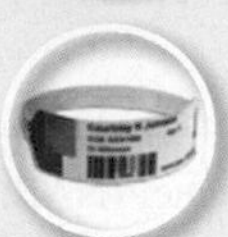 3. Identify the patient.	Identifying the patient ensures the right patient receives the intervention and helps prevent errors.
4. Close the curtains around the bed and close the door to the room, if possible.	This ensures the patient's privacy.
5. Determine the need for suctioning. Verify the suction order in the patient's medical record, if necessary. **Assess for pain or the potential to cause pain. Administer pain medication, as prescribed, before suctioning.**	To minimize trauma to airway mucosa, suctioning should be done only when secretions have accumulated or adventitious breath sounds are audible. Some facilities require an order for naso- and oropharyngeal suctioning. Suctioning stimulates coughing, which is painful for patients with surgical incisions and other conditions.
6. Explain what you are going to do and the reason for suctioning to the patient, even if the patient does not appear to be alert. Reassure the patient you will interrupt the procedure if he or she indicates respiratory difficulty.	Explanation alleviates fears. Even if the patient appears unconscious, explain what is happening. Any procedure that compromises respiration is frightening for the patient.
7. Adjust the bed to a comfortable working height, usually elbow height of the caregiver (VISN 8 Patient Safety Center, 2009). Lower side rail closest to you. **If conscious, place the patient in a semi-Fowler's position. If unconscious, place the patient in the lateral position, facing you.** Move the bedside table close to your work area and raise it to waist height.	Having the bed at the proper height prevents back and muscle strain. A sitting position helps the patient to cough and makes breathing easier. Gravity also facilitates catheter insertion. The lateral position prevents the airway from becoming obstructed and promotes drainage of secretions. The bedside table provides a work surface and helps maintain sterility of objects on the work surface.
8. Place towel or waterproof pad across the patient's chest.	This protects bed linens.
9. **Adjust suction to appropriate pressure (Figure 1).** For a wall unit for an adult: 100–150 mm Hg; neonates: 60–80 mm Hg; infants: 80–125 mm Hg; children: 80–125 mm Hg; adolescents: 80–150 mm Hg (Hess et al. 2012).	Higher pressures can cause excessive trauma, hypoxemia, and atelectasis.

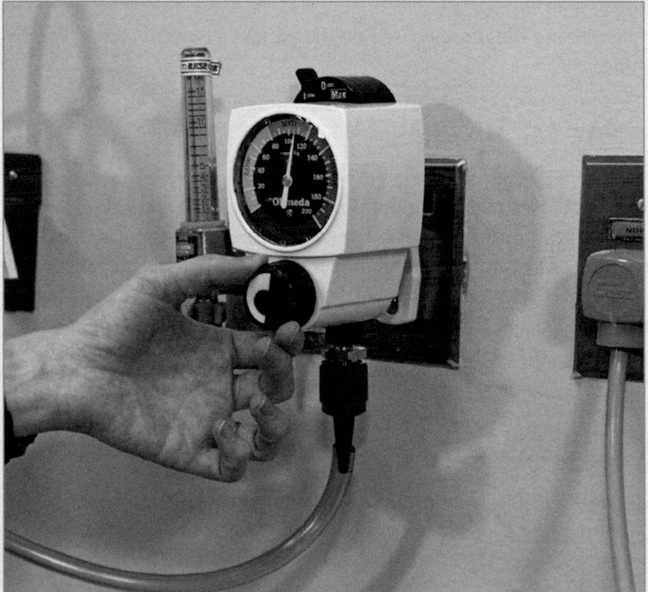

FIGURE 1 Adjusting wall suction.

ACTION	RATIONALE
For a portable unit for an adult: 10–15 cm Hg; neonates: 6–8 cm Hg; infants: 8–10 cm Hg; children: 8–10 cm Hg; adolescents: 8–15 cm Hg. **Put on a disposable, clean glove and occlude the end of the connecting tubing to check suction pressure.** Place the connecting tubing in a convenient location.	
10. Open sterile suction package using aseptic technique. The open wrapper or container becomes a sterile field to hold other supplies. Carefully remove the sterile container, touching only the outside surface. Set it up on the work surface and pour sterile saline into it.	Sterile normal saline or water is used to lubricate the outside of the catheter, minimizing irritation of mucosa during introduction. It is also used to clear the catheter between suction attempts.
11. Place a small amount of water-soluble lubricant on the sterile field, taking care to avoid touching the sterile field with the lubricant package.	Lubricant facilitates passage of the catheter and reduces trauma to mucous membranes.
12. Increase the patient's supplemental oxygen level or apply supplemental oxygen per facility policy or primary care provider order.	Suctioning removes air from the patient's airway and can cause hypoxemia. Hyperoxygenation can help prevent suction-induced hypoxemia.
13. Put on face shield or goggles and mask. Put on sterile gloves. **The dominant hand will manipulate the catheter and must remain sterile. The nondominant hand is considered clean rather than sterile and will control the suction valve (Y-port) on the catheter.** In the home setting and other community-based settings, maintenance of sterility is not necessary.	Gloves and other PPE protect the nurse from microorganisms. Handling the sterile catheter using a sterile glove helps prevent introducing organisms into the respiratory tract. In the home setting and other community-based settings, clean (instead of sterile) technique is used because the patient is not exposed to disease-causing organisms that may be found in health care settings, such as hospitals.
14. With dominant gloved hand, pick up sterile catheter. Pick up the connecting tubing with the nondominant hand and connect the tubing and suction catheter (Figure 2).	Sterility of the suction catheter is maintained.
15. Moisten the catheter by dipping it into the container of sterile saline (Figure 3). Occlude Y tube to check suction.	Lubricating the inside of the catheter with saline helps move secretions in the catheter. Checking suction ensures equipment is working properly.

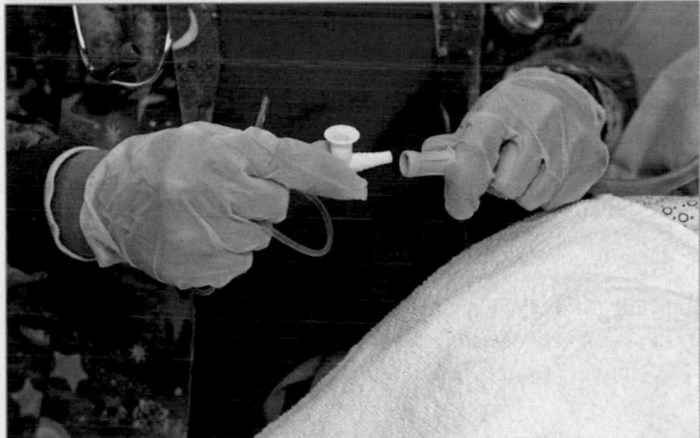

FIGURE 2 Connecting catheter to tubing.

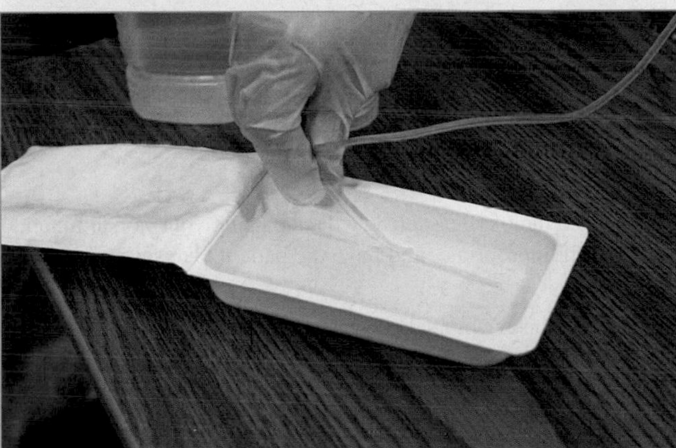

FIGURE 3 Dipping catheter into sterile saline.

ACTION	RATIONALE
16. Encourage the patient to take several deep breaths.	Hyperventilation can help prevent suction-induced hypoxemia.
17. Apply lubricant to the first 2 to 3 inches of the catheter, using the lubricant that was placed on the sterile field.	Lubricant facilitates passage of the catheter and reduces trauma to mucous membranes.

(continued)

SKILL 14-6 SUCTIONING THE OROPHARYNGEAL AND NASOPHARYNGEAL AIRWAYS continued

ACTION	RATIONALE
18. Remove the oxygen delivery device, if appropriate. Do not apply suction as the catheter is inserted. Hold the catheter between your thumb and forefinger.	Suctioning removes air from the patient's airway and can cause hypoxemia. Using suction while inserting the catheter can cause trauma to the mucosa and remove excessive oxygen from the respiratory tract.
19. Insert the catheter: a. **For nasopharyngeal suctioning,** gently insert catheter through the naris and along the floor of the nostril toward the trachea (Figure 4). Roll the catheter between your fingers to help advance it. Advance the catheter approximately 5 to 6 inches to reach the pharynx. b. **For oropharyngeal suctioning**, insert catheter through the mouth, along the side of the mouth toward the trachea. Advance the catheter 3 to 4 inches to reach the pharynx. (For nasotracheal suctioning, see the accompanying Skill Variation display.)	Correct distance for insertion ensures proper placement of the catheter. The general guideline for determining insertion distance for nasopharyngeal suctioning for an individual patient is to estimate the distance from the patient's earlobe to the nose.
20. **Apply suction by intermittently occluding the Y-port on the catheter with the thumb of your nondominant hand and gently rotating the catheter as it is being withdrawn (Figure 5). Do not suction for more than 10 to 15 seconds at a time.**	Turning the catheter as it is withdrawn minimizes trauma to the mucosa. Suctioning for longer than 10 to 15 seconds robs the respiratory tract of oxygen, which may result in hypoxemia. Suctioning too quickly may be ineffective at clearing all secretions.

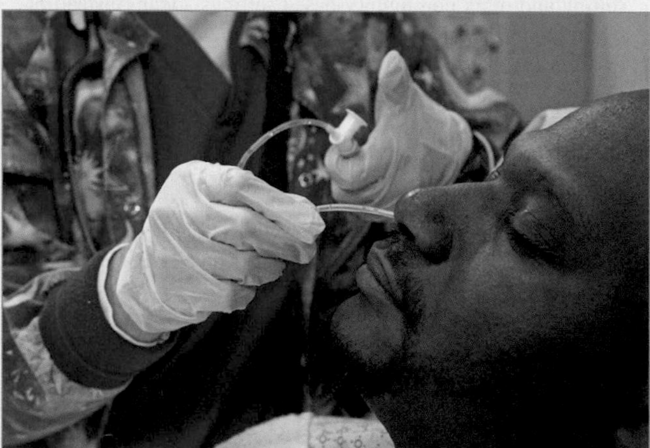

FIGURE 4 Inserting catheter into naris.

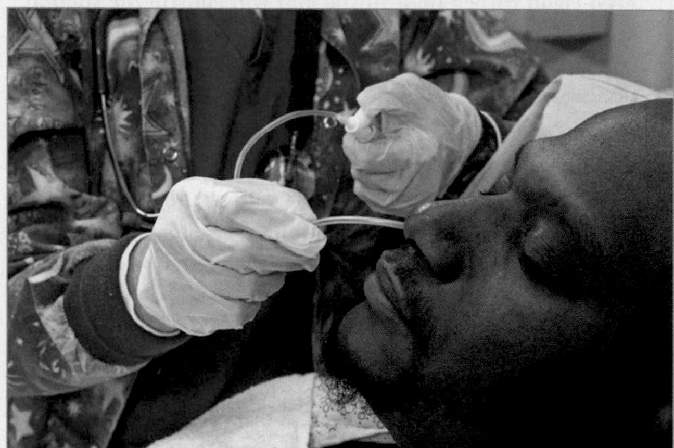

FIGURE 5 Suctioning nasopharynx.

ACTION	RATIONALE
21. Replace the oxygen delivery device using your nondominant hand, if appropriate, and have the patient take several deep breaths.	Suctioning removes air from the patient's airway and can cause hypoxemia. Hyperventilation can help prevent suction-induced hypoxemia.
22. Flush catheter with saline (Figure 6). Assess effectiveness of suctioning and repeat, as needed, and according to patient's tolerance. Wrap the suction catheter around your dominant hand between attempts.	Flushing clears the catheter and lubricates it for next insertion. Reassessment determines the need for additional suctioning. Wrapping prevents inadvertent contamination of the catheter.
23. **Allow at least a 30-second to 1-minute interval if additional suctioning is needed. No more than three suction passes should be made per suctioning episode. Alternate the nares, unless contraindicated, if repeated suctioning is required.** Do not force the catheter through the nares. Encourage the patient to cough and deep breathe between suctioning. **Suction the oropharynx after suctioning the nasopharynx.**	The interval allows for reventilation and reoxygenation of airways. Excessive suction passes contribute to complications. Alternating nares reduces trauma. Suctioning the oropharynx after the nasopharynx clears the mouth of secretions. More microorganisms are usually present in the mouth, so it is suctioned last to prevent transmission of contaminants.

ACTION	RATIONALE

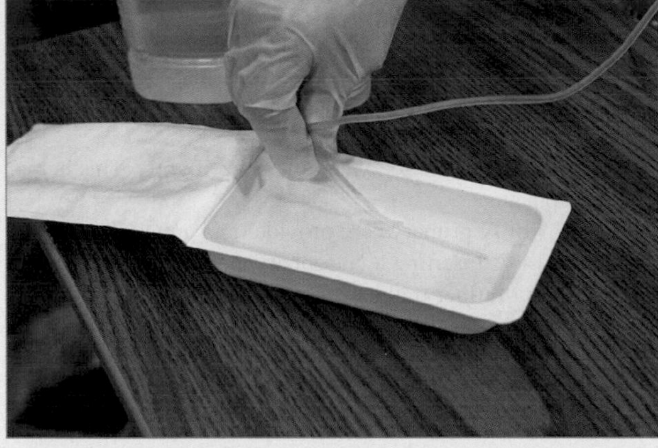

FIGURE 6 Rinsing catheter.

ACTION	RATIONALE
24. When suctioning is completed, remove gloves from dominant hand over the coiled catheter, pulling them off inside out. Remove glove from nondominant hand and dispose of gloves, catheter, and container with solution in the appropriate receptacle. Assist the patient to a comfortable position. Raise bed rail and place bed in the lowest position.	This technique reduces transmission of microorganisms. Proper positioning with raised side rails and proper bed height provide for patient comfort and safety.
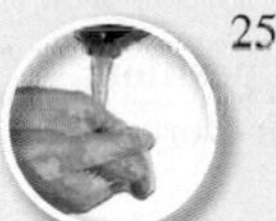 25. Turn off suction. Remove supplemental oxygen placed for suctioning, if appropriate. Remove face shield or goggles and mask. Perform hand hygiene.	Proper removal of PPE and hand hygiene reduces risk of transmission of microorganisms.
26. Offer oral hygiene after suctioning.	Respiratory secretions that are allowed to accumulate in the mouth are irritating to mucous membranes and unpleasant for the patient.
27. Reassess the patient's respiratory status, including respiratory rate, effort, oxygen saturation, and lung sounds.	This assesses effectiveness of suctioning and the presence of complications.
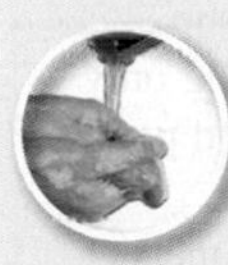 28. Remove additional PPE, if used. Perform hand hygiene.	Removing PPE properly reduces the risk for infection transmission and contamination of other items. Hand hygiene prevents the spread of microorganisms.

EVALUATION

The expected outcome is met when the patient exhibits improved breath sounds and a clear and patent airway. In addition, the oxygen saturation level is within acceptable parameters, and the patient does not exhibit signs or symptoms of respiratory distress or complications.

DOCUMENTATION

Guidelines

Document the time of suctioning, your assessments before and after intervention, reason for suctioning, route used, and the characteristics and amount of secretions.

Sample Documentation

9/17/15 1440 Patient with gurgling on inspiration and weak cough; unable to clear secretions. Lungs with rhonchi (sonorous wheezes) in upper airways. Nasopharyngeal suction completed with 12F catheter. Large amount of thick, yellow secretions obtained. After suctioning, lung sounds clear in all lobes, respirations 18 breaths per minute, no gurgling noted.

—C. Bausler, RN

SKILL 14-6 SUCTIONING THE OROPHARYNGEAL AND NASOPHARYNGEAL AIRWAYS continued

UNEXPECTED SITUATIONS AND ASSOCIATED INTERVENTIONS

- *The catheter or sterile glove touches an unsterile surface:* Stop the procedure. If the gloved hand is still sterile, call for assistance and have someone open another catheter or remove the gloves and restart the procedure.
- *Patient vomits during suctioning:* If the patient gags or becomes nauseated, remove the catheter; it has probably entered the esophagus inadvertently. If the patient needs to be suctioned again, change catheters, because it is probably contaminated. Turn patient to the side and elevate the head of the bed to prevent aspiration.
- *Secretions appear to be stomach contents:* Ask the patient to extend the neck slightly. This helps to prevent the tube from passing into the esophagus.
- *Epistaxis is noted with continued suctioning:* Notify primary care provider and anticipate the need for a nasal trumpet. (See Skill Variation 14-7: Inserting a Nasopharyngeal Airway.) The nasal trumpet will protect the nasal mucosa from further trauma related to suctioning.

SPECIAL CONSIDERATIONS

Infant and Child Considerations

- For infants, use a 5F to 6F catheter.
- For children, use a 6F to 10F catheter.

SKILL VARIATION Nasotracheal Suctioning

Nasotracheal suctioning is indicated to maintain a patent airway and remove saliva, pulmonary secretions, blood, vomitus, or foreign material from the trachea. Tracheal suctioning can lead to hypoxemia, cardiac dysrhythmias, trauma, atelectasis, infection, bleeding, and pain. It is imperative to be diligent in maintaining aseptic technique and following facility guidelines and procedures to prevent potential hazards. In the home setting and other community-based settings, clean technique is used because the patient is not exposed to disease-causing organisms that may be found in health care settings, such as hospitals. When performing suctioning, position yourself on the appropriate side of the patient. If you are right-handed, stand on the patient's right side; if left-handed, stand on the patient's left side. This allows for comfortable use of the dominant hand to manipulate the suction catheter. To perform nasotracheal suctioning:

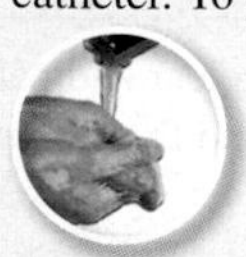

1. Perform hand hygiene. Put on PPE, as indicated.

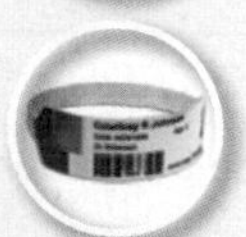

2. Identify the patient.
3. Determine the need for suctioning. **Assess for pain or the potential to cause pain. Administer pain medication, as prescribed, before suctioning.**
4. Explain to the patient what you are going to do and the reason for doing it, even if the patient does not appear to be alert.
5. Adjust bed to a comfortable working position. Lower the side rail closest to you. **If the patient is conscious, place him or her in a semi-Fowler's position. If the patient is unconscious, place him or her in the lateral position, facing you.** Move the overbed table close to your work area and raise to waist height.
6. Place a towel or waterproof pad across the patient's chest.
7. **Turn suction to appropriate pressure. Put on a disposable, clean glove and occlude the end of the connecting tubing to check suction pressure.** Place the connecting tubing in a convenient location.
8. Open sterile suction package using aseptic technique. The open wrapper becomes a sterile field to hold other supplies. Carefully remove the sterile container, touching only the outside surface. Set it up on the work surface and pour sterile saline into it.
9. Place a small amount of water-soluble lubricant on the sterile field, taking care to avoid touching the sterile field with the lubricant package.
10. Increase the patient's supplemental oxygen level or apply supplemental oxygen per facility policy or medical order.
11. Put on face shield or goggles and mask. Put on sterile gloves. **The dominant hand will manipulate the catheter and must remain sterile.** The nondominant hand is considered clean rather than sterile and will control the suction valve.
12. With dominant gloved hand, pick up the sterile catheter. Pick up the connecting tubing with the nondominant hand and connect the tubing and suction catheter.
13. Moisten the catheter by dipping it into the container of sterile saline. Occlude the Y-tube to check suction.
14. Encourage the patient to take several deep breaths.
15. Apply lubricant to the first 2 to 3 inches of the catheter, using the lubricant that was placed on the sterile field.

SKILL VARIATION Nasotracheal Suctioning continued

16. Remove the oxygen-delivery device, if appropriate. Do not apply suction as the catheter is inserted. Hold the catheter in your thumb and forefinger. Gently insert the catheter through the naris and along the floor of the nostril toward the trachea. Roll the catheter between your fingers to help advance it. Advance the catheter approximately 8 to 9 inches to reach the trachea. Resistance should not be met. If resistance is met, the carina or tracheal mucosa has been hit. Withdraw the catheter at least 12 inches before applying suction.
17. Apply suction by intermittently occluding the Y-port on the catheter with the thumb of your nondominant hand, and gently rotating the catheter as it is being withdrawn. **Do not suction for more than 10 to 15 seconds at a time.**
18. Replace the oxygen-delivery device using your nondominant hand and have the patient take several deep breaths.
19. Flush the catheter with saline. Assess effectiveness of suctioning and repeat, as needed, and according to patient's tolerance. Wrap the suction catheter around your dominant hand between attempts.
20. **Allow at least a 30-second to 1-minute interval if additional suctioning is needed. No more than three suction passes should be made per suctioning episode.** Alternate the nares, unless contraindicated, if repeated suctioning is required. Do not force catheter through the nares. Encourage the patient to cough and deep breathe between suctioning. Suction the oropharynx after suctioning the trachea.
21. When suctioning is completed, remove glove from dominant hand over the coiled catheter, pulling it off inside-out. Remove glove from nondominant hand and dispose of gloves, catheter, and container with solution in the appropriate receptacle. Remove face shield or goggles and mask. Perform hand hygiene.
22. Turn off suction. Remove supplemental oxygen placed for suctioning, if appropriate. Assist the patient to a comfortable position.
23. Offer oral hygiene after suctioning.
24. Reassess the patient's respiratory status, including respiratory rate, effort, oxygen saturation, and lung sounds.
25. Remove additional PPE, if used. Perform hand hygiene.
26. Document the time of suctioning, your assessments before and after intervention, the reason for suctioning, route used, and the characteristics and amount of secretions.

SKILL 14-7 INSERTING AN OROPHARYNGEAL AIRWAY

An **oropharyngeal airway** is a semicircular tube of plastic inserted into the back of the pharynx through the mouth in a patient who is breathing spontaneously. The oropharyngeal airway can help protect the airway of an unconscious patient by preventing the tongue from falling back against the posterior pharynx and blocking it. Once the patient regains consciousness, the oropharyngeal airway is removed. Tape is not used to hold the airway in place because the patient should be able to expel the airway once her or she becomes alert. The nurse can insert this device at the bedside with little to no trauma to the unconscious patient. Oropharyngeal airways may also be used to aid in ventilation during a code situation and to facilitate suctioning an unconscious or semiconscious patient. Alternately, airway support may be provided with a nasopharyngeal airway (Refer to the accompanying Skill Variation.)

DELEGATION CONSIDERATIONS

The insertion of an oropharyngeal airway is not delegated to nursing assistive personnel (NAP) or to unlicensed assistive personnel (UAP). Depending on the state's nurse practice act and the organization's policies and procedures, the insertion of an oropharyngeal airway may be delegated to licensed practical/vocational nurses (LPN/LVNs). The decision to delegate must be based on careful analysis of the patient's needs and circumstances, as well as the qualifications of the person to whom the task is being delegated. Refer to the Delegation Guidelines in Appendix A.

(continued)

SKILL 14-7 INSERTING AN OROPHARYNGEAL AIRWAY continued

EQUIPMENT

- Oropharyngeal airway of appropriate size
- Disposable gloves
- Suction equipment
- Goggles and mask or face shield (optional)
- Flashlight (optional)
- Additional PPE, as indicated

ASSESSMENT

Assess patient's level of consciousness and ability to protect the airway. Assess amount and consistency of oral secretions. Auscultate lung sounds. If the tongue is occluding the airway, lung sounds may be diminished. Assess for loose teeth or recent oral surgery, which may contraindicate the use of an oropharyngeal airway.

NURSING DIAGNOSIS

Determine related factors for the nursing diagnoses based on the patient's current status. Appropriate nursing diagnoses may include:

- Risk for Aspiration
- Ineffective Airway Clearance
- Risk for Injury

OUTCOME IDENTIFICATION AND PLANNING

The expected outcome is that the patient will maintain a patent airway and exhibit oxygen saturation within acceptable parameters, or greater than 95%. Another outcome that may be appropriate is that the patient remains free of aspiration and injury.

IMPLEMENTATION

ACTION	RATIONALE
1. Bring necessary equipment to the bedside stand or overbed table.	Bringing everything to the bedside conserves time and energy. Arranging items nearby is convenient, saves time, and avoids unnecessary stretching and twisting of muscles on the part of the nurse.
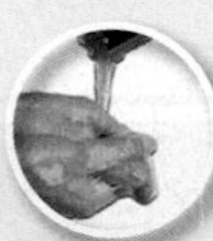 2. Perform hand hygiene and put on PPE, if indicated.	Hand hygiene and PPE prevent the spread of microorganisms. PPE is required based on transmission precautions.
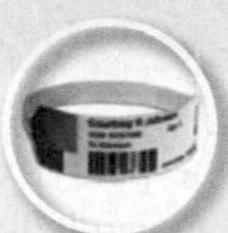 3. Identify the patient.	Identifying the patient ensures the right patient receives the intervention and helps prevent errors.
4. Close the curtains around the bed and close the door to the room, if possible.	This ensures the patient's privacy.
5. Explain to the patient what you are going to do and the reason for doing it, even if the patient does not appear to be alert.	Explanation alleviates fears. Even if a patient appears unconscious, the nurse should explain what is happening.
6. Put on disposable gloves; put on goggles and mask or face shield, as indicated.	Gloves and other PPE prevent contact with contaminants and body fluids.
7. Measure the oropharyngeal airway for correct size (Figure 1). Measure the oropharyngeal airway by holding the airway on the side of the patient's face. The airway should reach from the opening of the mouth to the back angle of the jaw.	Correct size ensures correct insertion and fit, allowing for conformation of the airway to the curvature of the palate.
8. **Check mouth for any loose teeth, dentures, or other foreign material. Remove dentures or material if present.**	Prevents aspiration or swallowing of objects. During insertion, the airway may push any foreign objects in the mouth to the back of the throat.
9. Position patient in semi-Fowler's position.	This position facilitates airway insertion and helps prevent the tongue from moving back against the posterior pharynx.
10. Suction the patient, if necessary.	This removes excess secretions and helps maintain a patent airway.

ACTION

RATIONALE

11. Open the patient's mouth by using your thumb and index finger to gently pry teeth apart. **Insert the airway with the curved tip pointing up toward the roof of the mouth (Figure 2).**

This is done to advance the tip of the airway past the tongue, toward the back of the throat.

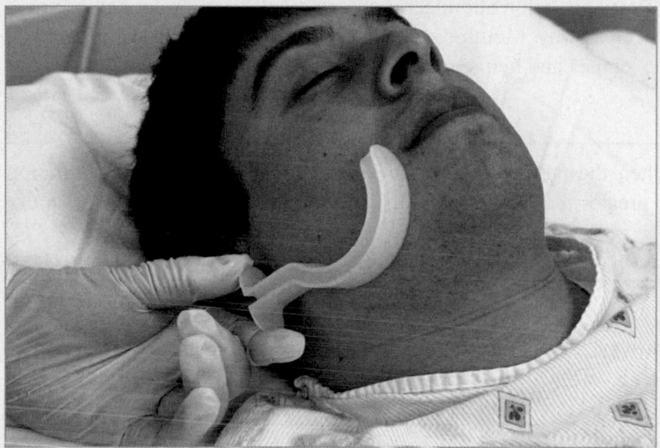

FIGURE 1 Measuring for oropharyngeal airway.

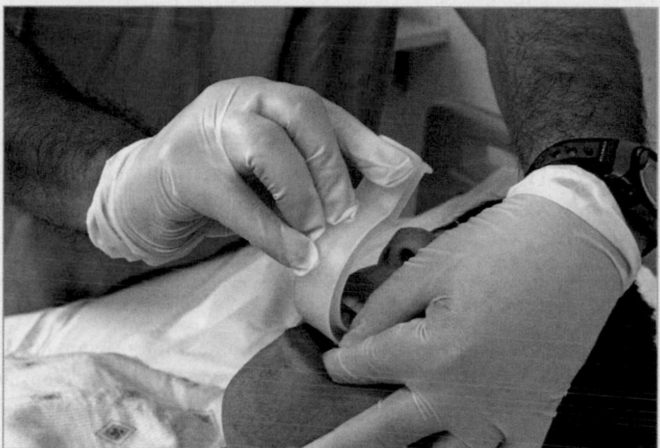

FIGURE 2 Inserting airway.

12. Slide the airway across the tongue to the back of the mouth. Rotate the airway 180 degrees as it passes the uvula (Figure 3). The tip should point down and the curvature should follow the contour of the roof of the mouth. Use a flashlight to confirm the position of the airway with the curve fitting over the tongue.

This is done to shift the tongue anteriorly, thereby allowing the patient to breathe through and around the airway.

13. Ensure accurate placement and adequate ventilation by auscultating breath sounds (Figure 4).

If the airway is placed correctly, lung sounds should be audible and equal in all lobes.

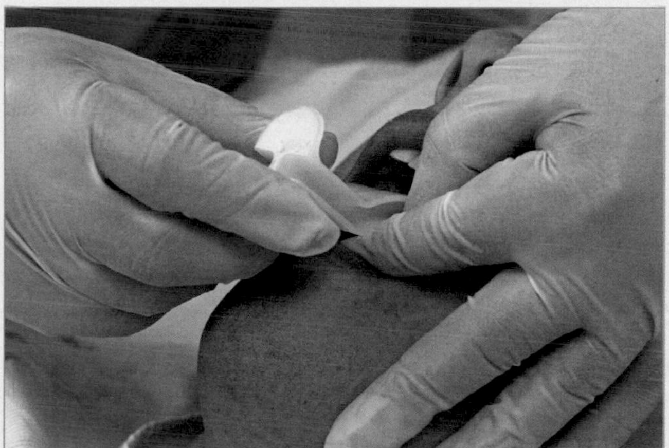

FIGURE 3 Rotating airway.

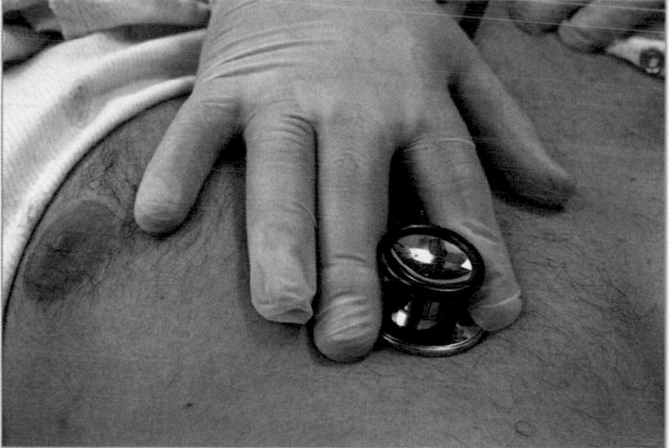

FIGURE 4 Auscultating breath sounds.

14. Position the patient on his or her side when the airway is in place.

This position helps keep the tongue out of the posterior pharynx area and helps to prevent aspiration if the unconscious patient should vomit.

(continued)

SKILL 14-7 INSERTING AN OROPHARYNGEAL AIRWAY continued

ACTION	RATIONALE
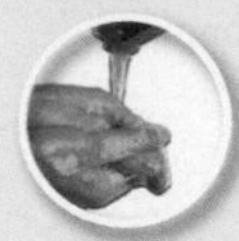 15. Remove gloves and additional PPE, if used. Perform hand hygiene.	Removing PPE properly reduces the risk for infection transmission and contamination of other items. Hand hygiene prevents the spread of microorganisms.
16. Remove the airway for a brief period every 4 hours, or according to facility policy. Assess mouth; provide mouth care and clean the airway according to facility policy before reinserting it.	Tissue irritation and ulceration can result from prolonged use of an airway. Mouth care provides moisture to mucous membranes and helps maintain tissue integrity.

EVALUATION

The expected outcome is met when the patient exhibits a patent airway with oxygen saturation within acceptable parameters, or greater than 95%. In addition, the patient remains free of injury and aspiration.

DOCUMENTATION

Guidelines

Document the placement of the airway, airway size, removal/cleaning, assessment before and after intervention, and oxygen saturation level.

Sample Documentation

9/22/15 1210 Patient noted to have gurgling with respirations, tongue back in posterior pharynx. Difficult to suction oropharynx. Size 4 oropharyngeal airway inserted. Patient placed on left side. Lung sounds clear and equal in all lobes. Pulse oximeter 98% on room air.

—*C. Bausler, RN*

UNEXPECTED SITUATIONS AND ASSOCIATED INTERVENTIONS

- *The patient awakens:* Remove the oral airway once the patient is awake because it may be uncomfortable and cause vomiting. Conscious patients can usually protect their airway.
- *The tongue is sliding back into the posterior pharynx, causing respiratory difficulties:* Put on disposable gloves and remove the airway. Make sure the airway is the appropriate size for the patient.
- *Patient vomits as oropharyngeal airway is inserted:* Quickly position patient onto his or her side to prevent aspiration. Remove oral airway. Suction mouth if needed.

SPECIAL CONSIDERATIONS

General Considerations

- Wearing gloves, remove the airway briefly every 4 hours to provide mouth care. Assess the mouth and tongue for tissue irritation, tooth damage, bleeding, and ulceration. Ensure that the lips and tongue are not between the teeth and the airway to prevent injury.
- When reinserting the oropharyngeal airway, attempt to insert it on the other side of the mouth. This helps to prevent irritation to the tongue and mouth.
- Suction secretions, as needed, by manipulating around and through the oropharyngeal airway.

SKILL VARIATION Inserting a Nasopharyngeal Airway

Nasopharyngeal airways (nasal trumpet) are curved, uncuffed, soft plastic tubes inserted into the back of the pharynx through the nose in patients who are breathing spontaneously. The nasal trumpet provides a route from the nares to the pharynx to help maintain a patent airway. These airways may be indicated if the teeth are clenched, the tongue is enlarged, or the patient needs frequent nasopharyngeal suctioning. The appropriate size range for a nasal trumpet for adolescents to adults is 24F to 36F. Additional assessments include assessing for the presence of nasal conditions, such as a deviated septum or recent nasal or oral surgery, traumatic brain injury, central facial fractures, basilar skull or cribriform fractures, and increased risk for bleeding, such as anticoagulant therapy, which would contraindicate the use of a nasopharyngeal airway.

1. Bring necessary equipment to the bedside stand or overbed table.

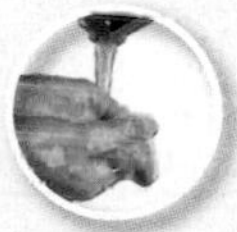

2. Perform hand hygiene and put on PPE, if indicated.

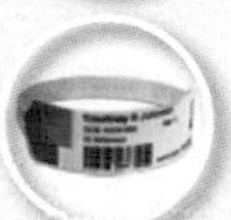

3. Identify the patient.
4. Close the curtains around the bed and close the door to the room, if possible.
5. Explain what you are going to do and the reason you are doing it to the patient, even if the patient does not appear to be alert.
6. Put on disposable gloves. If the patient is coughing or has copious secretions, also wear a mask and goggles.
7. Measure the nasopharyngeal airway for correct size (Figure A). Measure the nasopharyngeal airway length by holding the airway on the side of the patient's face. The airway should reach from the tragus of the ear to the nostril plus 1 inch. The diameter should be slightly smaller than the diameter of the nostril.

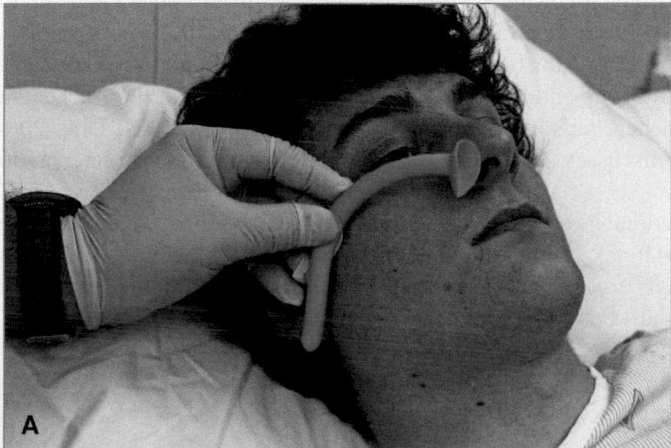

FIGURE A Measuring nasopharyngeal airway.

8. Adjust the bed to a comfortable working level, usually elbow height of the caregiver (VISN 8 Patient Safety Center, 2009). Lower side rail closest to you. **If the patient is awake and alert, position in semi-Fowler's position. If the patient is not conscious or alert, position in a side-lying position.**
9. Suction patient, if necessary.
10. Lubricate the nasopharyngeal airway generously with the water-soluble lubricant, covering the airway from the tip to the guard rim (Figure B).

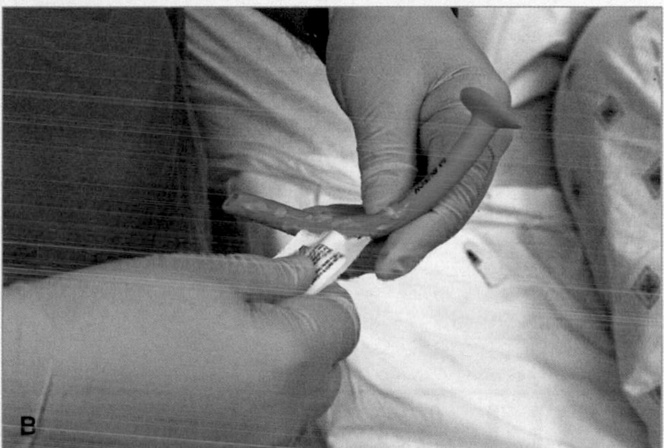

FIGURE B Lubricating nasopharyngeal airway.

11. **Gently insert the airway into the naris (Figure C), narrow end first, until the rim is touching the naris (Figure D). If resistance is met, stop and try the other naris.**

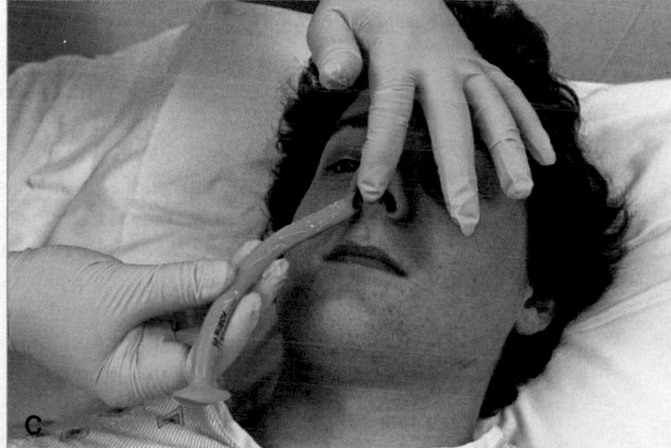

FIGURE C Inserting nasopharyngeal airway.

(continued)

SKILL 14-7 INSERTING AN OROPHARYNGEAL AIRWAY continued

SKILL VARIATION Inserting a Nasopharyngeal Airway continued

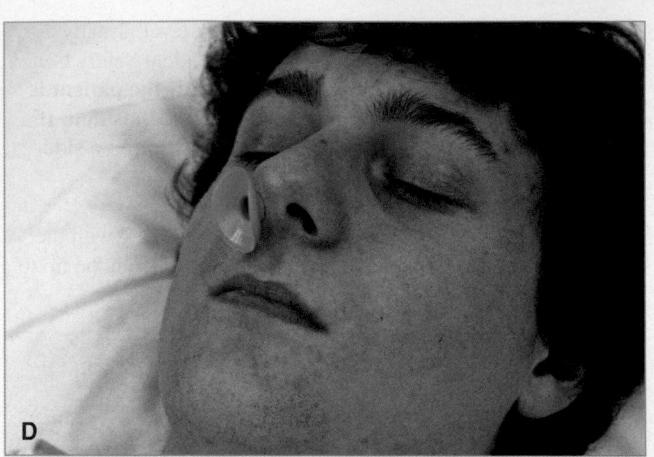

FIGURE D Nasopharyngeal airway inserted.

12. Check placement by closing the patient's mouth and placing your fingers in front of the tube opening to check for air movement. Assess the pharynx to visualize the tip of the airway behind the uvula. Assess the nose for blanching or skin stretching.
13. Remove gloves and raise the bed rail. Place bed in the lowest position. Remove additional PPE, if used. Perform hand hygiene.
14. Remove the airway, clean in warm soapy water, and place in other naris at least every 8 hours, or according to facility policy. If the patient coughs or gags on insertion, the nasal trumpet may be too long. Assess the pharynx. You should be able to visualize the tip of the airway behind the uvula.

SKILL 14-8 SUCTIONING AN ENDOTRACHEAL TUBE: OPEN SYSTEM

The purpose of suctioning is to maintain a patent airway and remove pulmonary secretions, blood, vomitus, or foreign material from the airway. When suctioning via an **endotracheal tube**, the goal is to remove secretions that are not accessible to **cilia** bypassed by the tube itself. Remember, tracheal suctioning can lead to hypoxemia, cardiac dysrhythmias, trauma, atelectasis, infection, bleeding, and pain. Therefore, it is imperative to be diligent in maintaining aseptic technique and in following facility guidelines and procedures to prevent potential hazards. Frequency of suctioning is based on clinical assessment.

Because suctioning removes secretions not accessible to bypassed cilia, the recommendation is to insert the catheter only as far as the end of the endotracheal tube. Catheter contact and suction can cause tracheal mucosal damage, loss of cilia, edema, and fibrosis, and increase the risk of infection and bleeding for the patient. Insertion of the suction catheter to a predetermined distance, no more than 1 cm past the length of the endotracheal tube, avoids contact with the trachea and carina, reducing the effects of tracheal mucosal damage (Hahn, 2010; Ireton, 2007; Pate, 2004; Pate & Zapata, 2002). Box 14-1 discusses several methods for determining appropriate suction catheter depth.

Some consider open system suctioning to be the most efficient way to suction the endotracheal tube, arguing that there are no limitations to the movement of the suction catheter while suctioning. However, the nurse may unknowingly contaminate an open system during the procedure. In addition, with the open system, the patient must be removed from the ventilator during suctioning.

Box 14-1 METHODS TO DETERMINE SUCTION CATHETER DEPTH

Open Suction System

Method 1 (Endotracheal Tubes)

- Using a suction catheter with centimeter increments on it, insert the suction catheter into the endotracheal tube until the centimeter markings on both the endotracheal tube and catheter align.
- Insert the suction catheter no further than an additional 1 cm.

Method 2 (Endotracheal Tubes)

- Combine the length of the endotracheal tube and any adapter being used, and add an additional 1 cm.
- Document the determined length at the bedside or on the plan of care, according to facility policy.

Method 3 (Endotracheal and Tracheostomy Tubes)

- Using a spare endotracheal or tracheostomy tube of the same size as being used for the patient, insert the suction catheter to the end of the tube.
- Note the length of catheter used to reach the end of the tube.
- Document the determined length at the bedside or on the plan of care. Alternately, mark the distance on the suction catheter with permanent ink or tape and place the catheter at the bedside for reference. Refer to facility policy.

Closed Suction System (Endotracheal and Tracheostomy Tubes)

- Combine the length of the endotracheal or tracheostomy tube and any adapter being used, and add an additional 1 cm.
- Advance the catheter until the appropriate length can be seen through the catheter sheath or window.
- Document the depth of the catheter at the bedside or on the plan of care.

(Adapted from Hahn, M. [2010]. 10 considerations for endotracheal suctioning. *The Journal for Respiratory Care Practitioners, 23*(7), 32–33. Republished with permission of American Association of Critical Care Nurses, from Pate, M., & Zapata, T. [2002]. Ask the experts: How deeply should I go when I suction an endotracheal tube or tracheostomy tube? *Critical Care Nurse,* 22[2], 130–131, permission conveyed through Copyright Clearance Center, Inc.)

DELEGATION CONSIDERATIONS

Suctioning an endotracheal tube is not delegated to nursing assistive personnel (NAP) or to unlicensed assistive personnel (UAP). Depending on the state's nurse practice act and the organization's policies and procedures, suctioning of an endotracheal tube in a stable situation, such as long-term care and other community-based care settings, may be delegated to licensed practical/vocational nurses (LPN/LVNs). The decision to delegate must be based on careful analysis of the patient's needs and circumstances, as well as the qualifications of the person to whom the task is being delegated. Refer to the Delegation Guidelines in Appendix A.

EQUIPMENT

- Portable or wall suction unit with tubing
- A commercially prepared suction kit with an appropriate size catheter (see General Considerations) or
- Sterile suction catheter with Y-port in the appropriate size
- Sterile, disposable container
- Sterile gloves
- Towel or waterproof pad
- Goggles and mask or face shield
- Additional PPE, as indicated
- Disposable, clean gloves
- Resuscitation bag connected to 100% oxygen
- Assistant (optional)

ASSESSMENT

Assess lung sounds. Patients who need to be suctioned may have wheezes, crackles, or gurgling present. Assess oxygen saturation level. Oxygen saturation usually decreases when a patient needs to be suctioned. Assess respiratory status, including respiratory rate and depth. Patients may become tachypneic when they need to be suctioned. Assess the patient for signs of respiratory distress, such as nasal flaring, retractions, or grunting. Additional indications for suctioning via an endotracheal tube include secretions in the tube, acute respiratory distress, and frequent or sustained coughing. Also assess for pain and the potential to cause pain during the intervention. Perform individualized pain management in response to the patient's needs (Arroyo-Novoa et al., 2008). Administer pain medication, as prescribed, before suctioning. Assess appropriate suction catheter depth. Refer to Box 14-1. Assess the characteristics and amount of secretions while suctioning.

SKILL 14-8 SUCTIONING AN ENDOTRACHEAL TUBE: OPEN SYSTEM continued

NURSING DIAGNOSIS

Determine the related factors for the nursing diagnoses based on the patient's current status. Appropriate nursing diagnoses may include:

- Ineffective Airway Clearance
- Risk for Aspiration
- Risk for Infection
- Impaired Gas Exchange

OUTCOME IDENTIFICATION AND PLANNING

The expected outcome is that the patient will exhibit improved breath sounds and a clear, patent airway. Other outcomes that may be appropriate include the following: the patient will exhibit an oxygen saturation level within acceptable parameters; the patient will demonstrate a respiratory rate and depth within age-acceptable range; and the patient will remain free of any signs of respiratory distress.

IMPLEMENTATION

ACTION	RATIONALE
1. Bring necessary equipment to the bedside stand or overbed table.	Bringing everything to the bedside conserves time and energy. Arranging items nearby is convenient, saves time, and avoids unnecessary stretching and twisting of muscles on the part of the nurse.
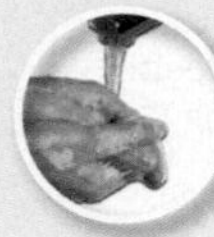 2. Perform hand hygiene and put on PPE, if indicated.	Hand hygiene and PPE prevent the spread of microorganisms. PPE is required based on transmission precautions.
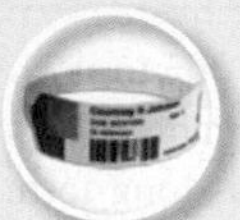 3. Identify the patient.	Identifying the patient ensures the right patient receives the intervention and helps prevent errors.
4. Close the curtains around the bed and close the door to the room, if possible.	This ensures the patient's privacy.
5. Determine the need for suctioning. Verify the suction order in the patient's medical record. **Assess for pain or the potential to cause pain. Administer pain medication, as prescribed, before suctioning.**	To minimize trauma to airway mucosa, suctioning should be done only when secretions have accumulated or adventitious breath sounds are audible. Suctioning can cause moderate to severe pain for patients. Individualized pain management is imperative (Arroyo-Novoa et al., 2008). Suctioning stimulates coughing, which is painful for patients with surgical incisions.
6. Explain what you are going to do and the reason for doing it to the patient, even if the patient does not appear to be alert. Reassure the patient you will interrupt the procedure if he or she indicates respiratory difficulty.	Explanation alleviates fears. Even if the patient appears unconscious, the nurse should explain what is happening. Any procedure that compromises respiration is frightening for the patient.
7. Adjust the bed to a comfortable working position, usually elbow height of the caregiver (VISN 8 Patient Safety Center, 2009). Lower side rail closest to you. **If conscious, place in a semi-Fowler's position. If unconscious, place the patient in the lateral position, facing you.** Move the overbed table close to your work area and raise it to waist height.	Having the bed at the proper height prevents back and muscle strain. A sitting position helps the patient to cough and makes breathing easier. Gravity also facilitates catheter insertion. The lateral position prevents the airway from becoming obstructed and promotes drainage of secretions. The overbed table provides a work surface and maintains sterility of objects on work surface.
8. Place towel or waterproof pad across the patient's chest.	This protects bed linens and the patient.

ACTION	RATIONALE
9. Turn suction to appropriate pressure (Figure 1): • For a wall unit for an adult: 100–150 mm Hg; neonates: 60–80 mm Hg; infants: 80–125 mm Hg; children: 80–125 mm Hg; adolescents: 80–150 mm Hg (Hess et al., 2012). • For a portable unit for an adult: 10–15 cm Hg; neonates: 6–8 cm Hg; infants: 8–10 cm Hg; children: 8–10 cm Hg; adolescents: 8–15 cm Hg.	Higher pressures can cause excessive trauma, hypoxemia, and atelectasis.

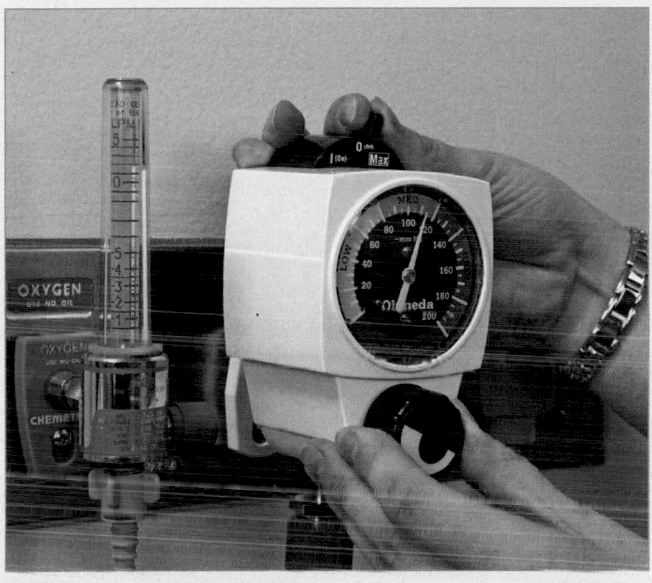

FIGURE 1 Turning suction device to appropriate pressure.

ACTION	RATIONALE
10. Put on a disposable, clean glove and occlude the end of the connecting tubing to check suction pressure. Place the connecting tubing in a convenient location. Place the resuscitation bag connected to oxygen within convenient reach, if using.	Glove prevents contact with blood and body fluids. Checking pressure ensures equipment is working properly. Allows for an organized approach to the procedure.
11. Open sterile suction package using aseptic technique. The open wrapper becomes a sterile field to hold other supplies. Carefully remove the sterile container, touching only the outside surface. Set it up on the work surface and pour sterile saline into it.	Sterile normal saline or water is used to lubricate the outside of the catheter, minimizing irritation of mucosa during introduction. It is also used to clear the catheter between suction attempts.
12. Put on face shield or goggles and mask. Put on sterile gloves. **The dominant hand will manipulate the catheter and must remain sterile. The nondominant hand is considered clean rather than sterile and will control the suction valve (Y-port) on the catheter.**	Handling the sterile catheter using a sterile glove helps prevent introducing organisms into the respiratory tract; the clean glove protects the nurse from microorganisms.
13. With dominant gloved hand, pick up sterile catheter. Pick up the connecting tubing with the nondominant hand and connect the tubing and suction catheter.	Sterility of the suction catheter is maintained.
14. Moisten the catheter by dipping it into the container of sterile saline, unless it is a silicone catheter. Occlude Y-tube to check suction.	Lubricating the inside of the catheter with saline helps move secretions in the catheter. Silicone catheters do not require lubrication. Checking suction ensures equipment is working properly.

SKILL 14-8 SUCTIONING AN ENDOTRACHEAL TUBE: OPEN SYSTEM continued

ACTION	RATIONALE
15. Hyperventilate the patient using your nondominant hand and a manual resuscitation bag and delivering three to six breaths (Figure 2) or use the sigh mechanism on a mechanical ventilator.	Hyperventilation and hyperoxygenation aids in preventing hypoxemia during suctioning.

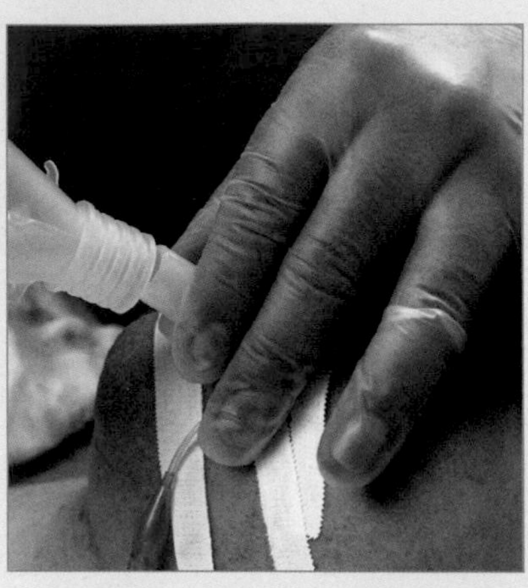

FIGURE 2 Removing ventilator tubing from endotracheal tube to hyperventilate the patient using a manual resuscitation bag.

ACTION	RATIONALE
16. Open the adapter on the mechanical ventilator tubing or remove the manual resuscitation bag with your nondominant hand.	This exposes the endotracheal tube without contaminating sterile gloved hand.
17. Using your dominant hand, gently and quickly insert the catheter into the trachea (Figure 3). **Advance the catheter to the predetermined length. Do not occlude Y-port when inserting the catheter.**	Catheter contact and suction cause tracheal mucosal damage, loss of cilia, edema, and fibrosis, and increase the risk of infection and bleeding for the patient. Insertion of the suction catheter to a predetermined distance, no more than 1 cm past the length of the endotracheal tube, avoids contact with the trachea and carina, reducing the effects of tracheal mucosal damage (Hahn, 2010; Ireton, 2007; Pate, 2004; Pate & Zapata, 2002). If resistance is met, the carina or tracheal mucosa has been hit. Withdraw the catheter at least 0.5 inch before applying suction. Occluding the Y-port (i.e., suctioning) when inserting the catheter increases the risk for trauma to the airway mucosa and increases the risk of hypoxemia.
18. Apply suction by intermittently occluding the Y-port on the catheter with the thumb of your nondominant hand, and gently rotate the catheter as it is being withdrawn (Figure 4). **Do not suction for more than 10 to 15 seconds at a time.**	Turning the catheter as it is withdrawn minimizes trauma to the mucosa. Suctioning for longer than 10 to 15 seconds robs the respiratory tract of oxygen, which may result in hypoxemia. Suctioning too quickly may be ineffective at clearing all secretions.

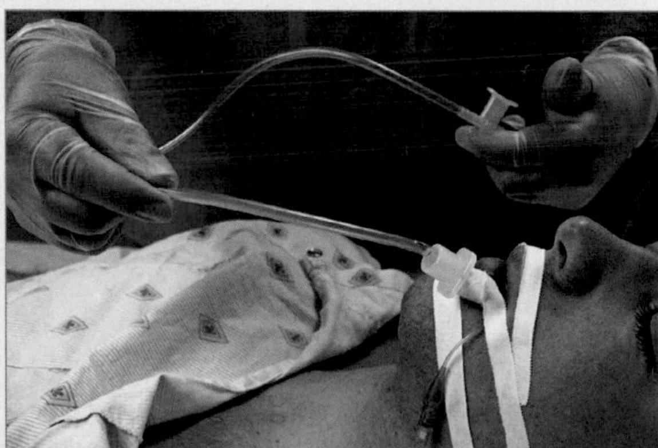

FIGURE 3 Inserting suction catheter into endotracheal tube.

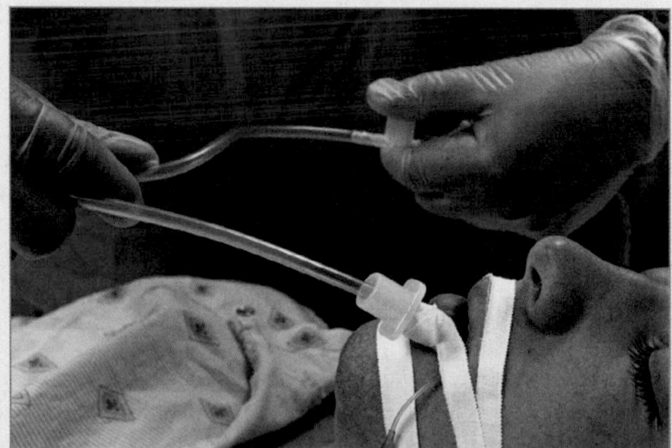

FIGURE 4 Withdrawing suction catheter and intermittently occluding Y-port with thumb to apply suction.

ACTION	RATIONALE
19. Hyperventilate the patient using your nondominant hand and a manual resuscitation bag and delivering three to six breaths. Replace the oxygen delivery device, if applicable, using your nondominant hand and have the patient take several deep breaths. If the patient is mechanically ventilated, close the adapter on the mechanical ventilator tubing or replace the ventilator tubing and use the sigh mechanism on a mechanical ventilator.	Suctioning removes air from the patient's airway and can cause hypoxemia. Hyperventilation and hyperoxygenation can help prevent suction-induced hypoxemia.
20. Flush catheter with saline. Assess the effectiveness of suctioning and repeat, as needed, and according to patient's tolerance.	Flushing clears the catheter and lubricates it for next insertion. Reassessment determines need for additional suctioning.
Wrap the suction catheter around your dominant hand between attempts.	Wrapping the catheter prevents inadvertent contamination of the catheter.
21. **Allow at least a 30-second to 1-minute interval if additional suctioning is needed. Do not make more than three suction passes per suctioning episode.** Suction the oropharynx after suctioning the trachea. Do not reinsert in the endotracheal tube after suctioning the mouth.	The interval allows for reventilation and reoxygenation of airways. Excessive suction passes contribute to complications. Suctioning the oropharynx clears the mouth of secretions. More microorganisms are usually present in the mouth, so it is suctioned last to prevent transmission of contaminants.
22. When suctioning is completed, remove gloves from dominant hand over the coiled catheter, pulling off inside-out. Remove glove from nondominant hand and dispose of gloves, catheter, and container with solution in the appropriate receptacle. Assist patient to a comfortable position. Raise bed rail and place bed in the lowest position.	This technique of glove removal and disposal of equipment reduces transmission of microorganisms. Proper positioning with raised side rails and proper bed height provide for patient comfort and safety.
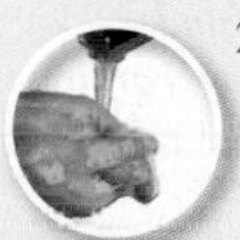 23. Turn off suction. Remove face shield or goggles and mask. Perform hand hygiene.	Removing face shield or goggles and mask properly reduces the risk for infection transmission and contamination of other items. Hand hygiene prevents transmission of microorganisms.
24. Perform oral hygiene after suctioning.	Respiratory secretions that are allowed to accumulate in the mouth are irritating to mucous membranes and unpleasant for the patient.
25. Reassess the patient's respiratory status, including respiratory rate, effort, oxygen saturation, and lung sounds.	These assess effectiveness of suctioning and the presence of complications.
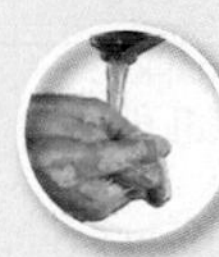 26. Remove additional PPE, if used. Perform hand hygiene.	Removing PPE properly reduces the risk for infection transmission and contamination of other items. Hand hygiene prevents the spread of microorganisms.

EVALUATION

The expected outcome is met when the patient exhibits improved breath sounds and a clear and patent airway. In addition, the oxygen saturation level is within acceptable parameters, and the patient does not exhibit signs or symptoms of respiratory distress or complications.

DOCUMENTATION

Guidelines

Document the time of suctioning, your assessments before and after interventions, reason for suctioning, oxygen saturation levels, and the characteristics and amount of secretions.

(continued)

SKILL 14-8 SUCTIONING AN ENDOTRACHEAL TUBE: OPEN SYSTEM continued

Sample Documentation

9/1/15 1850 Lung sounds coarse in lower lobes, wheezes in upper lobes bilaterally. Respirations 24 breaths per minute, regular rhythm. Intercostal retractions noted. Endotracheal tube suctioning completed with 12F catheter. Small amount of thin, white secretions obtained. Specimen for culture collected and sent. After suctioning, lung sounds clear in all lobes, respirations 18 breaths per minute, no intercostal retractions noted.

—*C. Bausler, RN*

UNEXPECTED SITUATIONS AND ASSOCIATED INTERVENTIONS

- *Catheter or sterile glove is contaminated:* Reconnect patient to ventilator. Discard gloves and suction catheter. Gather supplies and begin procedure again.
- *When suctioning, your eye becomes contaminated with respiratory secretions:* After attending to the patient, perform hand hygiene and flush your eye with large amount of sterile water. Contact employee health or house supervisor immediately for further treatment. Wear goggles or a face shield when suctioning to prevent exposure to body fluids.
- *Patient is extubated during suctioning:* Remain with patient. Call for help to notify the primary care provider. Assess patient's vital signs, ability to breathe without assistance, and oxygen saturation. Be ready to deliver assisted breaths with a bag-valve mask (see Skill 14-15) or administer oxygen. Anticipate the need for reintubation.
- *Oxygen saturation level decreases after suctioning:* Hyperoxygenate patient. Auscultate lung sounds. If lung sounds are absent over one lobe, alert staff to notify primary care provider. Remain with patient. Patient may have **pneumothorax**. Anticipate an order for a stat chest x-ray and chest tube placement.
- *When suctioning, you notice small yellow plugs in the secretions:* Assess the patient's hydration status as well as the humidification on the ventilator. These mucous plugs may cause a ventilation-perfusion mismatch if not resolved. Patient may need more humidification.
- *Patient develops signs of intolerance to suctioning; oxygen saturation level decreases and remains low after hyperoxygenation; patient becomes cyanotic or patient becomes bradycardic:* Stop suctioning. Auscultate lung sounds. Consider hyperventilating patient with manual resuscitation device. Remain with patient. Alert staff to notify primary care provider.

SPECIAL CONSIDERATIONS

General Considerations

- Determine the size of catheter to use by the size of the endotracheal tube. The external diameter of the suction catheter should not exceed half of the internal diameter of the endotracheal tube. Larger catheters can contribute to trauma and hypoxemia.
- Make sure emergency equipment is easily accessible at the bedside. Keep a bag-valve mask, oxygen, and suction equipment at the bedside of a patient with an endotracheal tube at all times.

Infant and Child Considerations

- Maximal time for application of negative pressure (suction) for neonates should be less than 5 seconds (Ireton, 2007).
- Maximal time for application of negative pressure (suction) for children and adolescents should be less than 10 seconds (Ireton, 2007).

SKILL 14-9 SUCTIONING AN ENDOTRACHEAL TUBE: CLOSED SYSTEM

The purpose of suctioning is to maintain a patent airway and remove pulmonary secretions, blood, vomitus, or foreign material from the airway. When suctioning via an endotracheal tube, the goal is to remove secretions that are not accessible to cilia bypassed by the tube itself. Tracheal suctioning can lead to hypoxemia, cardiac dysrhythmias, trauma, atelectasis, infection, bleeding, and pain. It is imperative to be diligent in maintaining aseptic technique and following facility guidelines and procedures to prevent potential hazards. Suctioning frequency is based on clinical assessment to determine the need for suctioning.

Suctioning removes secretions not accessible to bypassed cilia, so recommendation is to insert the catheter only as far as the end of the endotracheal tube. Catheter contact and suction cause tracheal mucosal damage, loss of cilia, edema, and fibrosis, and increase the risk of infection and bleeding for the patient. Insertion of the suction catheter to a predetermined distance, no more than 1 cm past the length of the endotracheal tube, avoids contact with the trachea and carina, reducing the effects of tracheal mucosal damage (Hahn, 2010; Ireton, 2007; Pate, 2004; Pate & Zapata, 2002). Box 14-1 (in Skill 14-8) discusses several methods for nurses to use to determine appropriate suction catheter depth.

Closed system suction (Figure 1) may be used routinely or when a patient must be suctioned frequently and quickly due to an excess of secretions, depending on the policies of the facility. One drawback of closed suctioning is thought to be the hindrance of the sheath when rotating the suction catheter upon removal.

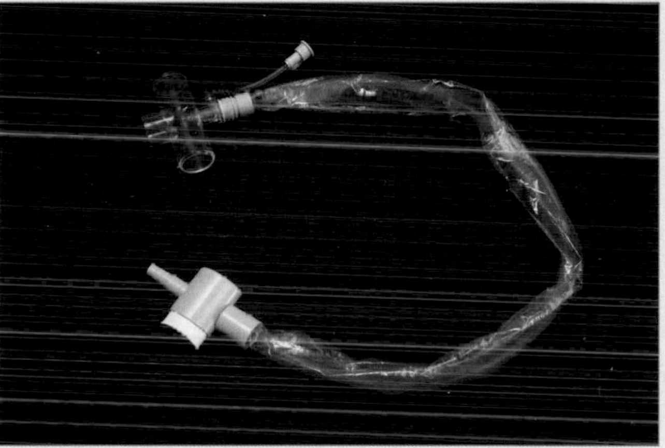

FIGURE 1 Closed suction device.

DELEGATION CONSIDERATIONS

Suctioning an endotracheal tube is not delegated to nursing assistive personnel (NAP) or to unlicensed assistive personnel (UAP). Depending on the state's nurse practice act and the organization's policies and procedures, suctioning of an endotracheal tube in a stable situation, such as long-term care and other community-based care settings, may be delegated to licensed practical/vocational nurses (LPN/LVNs). The decision to delegate must be based on careful analysis of the patient's needs and circumstances, as well as the qualifications of the person to whom the task is being delegated. Refer to the Delegation Guidelines in Appendix A.

EQUIPMENT

- Portable or wall suction unit with tubing
- Closed suction device of appropriate size for patient
- 3 mL or 5 mL normal saline solution in dosette or syringe
- Sterile gloves
- Additional PPE, as indicated

ASSESSMENT

Assess lung sounds. Patients who need to be suctioned may have wheezes, crackles, or gurgling present. Assess oxygen saturation level. Oxygen saturation usually decreases when a patient needs to be suctioned. Assess respiratory status, including respiratory rate and depth. Patients may become tachypneic when they need to be suctioned. Assess the patient for signs of respiratory distress, such as nasal flaring, retractions, or grunting. Additional indications for suctioning via an endotracheal

(continued)

SKILL 14-9 SUCTIONING AN ENDOTRACHEAL TUBE: CLOSED SYSTEM continued

tube include secretions in the tube, acute respiratory distress, and frequent or sustained coughing. Also assess for pain and the potential to cause pain during the intervention. Perform individualized pain management in response to the patient's needs (Arroyo-Novoa et al., 2008). Administer pain medication, as prescribed, before suctioning. Assess appropriate suction catheter depth. Refer to Box 14-1 (in Skill 14-8). Assess the characteristics and amount of secretions while suctioning.

NURSING DIAGNOSIS

Determine the related factors for the nursing diagnoses based on the patient's current status. Appropriate nursing diagnoses may include:

- Ineffective Airway Clearance
- Risk for Aspiration
- Risk for Infection
- Impaired Gas Exchange

OUTCOME IDENTIFICATION AND PLANNING

The expected outcome is that the patient will exhibit improved breath sounds and a clear, patent airway. Other outcomes that may be appropriate include the following: the patient will exhibit an oxygen saturation level within acceptable parameters; the patient will demonstrate a respiratory rate and depth within age-acceptable range; and the patient will remain free of any signs of respiratory distress.

IMPLEMENTATION

ACTION	RATIONALE
1. Bring necessary equipment to the bedside stand or overbed table.	Bringing everything to the bedside conserves time and energy. Arranging items nearby is convenient, saves time, and avoids unnecessary stretching and twisting of muscles on the part of the nurse.
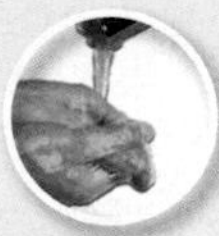 2. Perform hand hygiene and put on PPE, if indicated.	Hand hygiene and PPE prevent the spread of microorganisms. PPE is required based on transmission precautions.
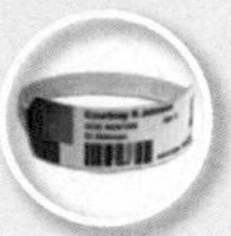 3. Identify the patient.	Identifying the patient ensures the right patient receives the intervention and helps prevent errors.
4. Close the curtains around the bed and close the door to the room, if possible.	This ensures the patient's privacy.
5. Determine the need for suctioning. Verify the suction order in the patient's medical record. **Assess for pain or the potential to cause pain. Administer pain medication, as prescribed, before suctioning.**	To minimize trauma to airway mucosa, suctioning should be done only when secretions have accumulated or adventitious breath sounds are audible. Suctioning can cause moderate to severe pain for patients. Individualized pain management is imperative (Arroyo-Novoa et al., 2008). Suctioning stimulates coughing, which is painful for patients with surgical incisions.
6. Explain what you are going to do and the reason for doing it to the patient, even if the patient does not appear to be alert. Reassure the patient you will interrupt the procedure if he or she indicates respiratory difficulty.	Explanation alleviates fears. Even if the patient appears unconscious, the nurse should explain what is happening. Any procedure that compromises respiration is frightening for the patient.
7. Adjust the bed to a comfortable working position, usually elbow height of the caregiver (VISN 8 Patient Safety Center, 2009). Lower side rail closest to you. **If conscious, place the patient in a semi-Fowler's position. If unconscious, place the patient in the lateral position, facing you.** Move the overbed table close to your work area and raise to waist height.	Having the bed at the proper height prevents back and muscle strain. A sitting position helps the patient to cough and makes breathing easier. Gravity also facilitates catheter insertion. The lateral position prevents the airway from becoming obstructed and promotes drainage of secretions. The overbed table provides work surface and maintains sterility of objects on work surface.

ACTION	RATIONALE
8. Turn suction to appropriate pressure (Figure 2). • For a wall unit for an adult: 100–150 mm Hg; neonates: 60–80 mm Hg; infants: 80–125 mm Hg; children: 80–125 mm Hg; adolescents: 80–150 mm Hg (Hess et al., 2012). • For a portable unit for an adult: 10–15 cm Hg; neonates: 6–8 cm Hg; infants: 8–10 cm Hg; children: 8–10 cm Hg; adolescents: 8–15 cm Hg.	Higher pressures can cause excessive trauma, hypoxemia, and atelectasis.

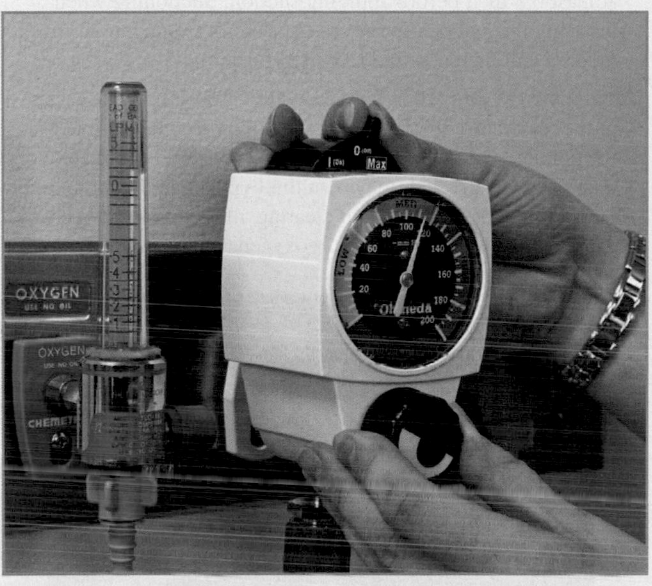

FIGURE 2 Turning suction device to appropriate pressure.

ACTION	RATIONALE
9. Open the package of the closed suction device using aseptic technique. Make sure that the device remains sterile.	The device must remain sterile to prevent a nosocomial infection.
10. Put on sterile gloves.	Gloves deter the spread of microorganisms.
11. Using nondominant hand, disconnect ventilator from endotracheal tube. Place ventilator tubing in a convenient location so that the inside of the tubing remains sterile or continue to hold the tubing in your nondominant hand.	This provides access to the endotracheal tube while keeping one hand sterile. The inside of the ventilator tubing should remain sterile to prevent a nosocomial infection.
12. **Using dominant hand and keeping device sterile, connect the closed suctioning device so that the suctioning catheter is in line with the endotracheal tube.**	Keeping the device sterile decreases the risk for a nosocomial infection.
13. **Keeping the inside of the ventilator tubing sterile, attach ventilator tubing to port perpendicular to the endotracheal tube.** Attach suction tubing to suction catheter.	The inside of the ventilator tubing must remain sterile to prevent a nosocomial infection. By connecting the ventilator tubing to the port, the patient does not need to be disconnected from the ventilator to be suctioned.
14. Pop top off sterile normal saline dosette. Open plug to port by suction catheter and insert saline dosette or syringe.	The saline will help to clean the catheter between suctioning.
15. Hyperventilate the patient by using the sigh button on the ventilator before suctioning. Turn safety cap on suction button of catheter so that button is depressed easily.	Hyperoxygenating and hyperventilating before suctioning helps to decrease the effects of oxygen removal during suctioning. The safety button keeps the patient from accidentally depressing the button and decreasing the oxygen saturation.

(continued)

SKILL 14-9 SUCTIONING AN ENDOTRACHEAL TUBE: CLOSED SYSTEM continued

ACTION	RATIONALE
16. Grasp suction catheter through protective sheath, about 6 inches (15 cm) from the endotracheal tube. Gently insert the catheter into the endotracheal tube (Figure 3). Release the catheter while holding on to the protective sheath. Move hand farther back on catheter. **Grasp catheter through sheath and repeat movement, advancing the catheter to the predetermined length. Do not occlude Y-port when inserting the catheter.**	The sheath keeps the suction catheter sterile. Catheter contact and suction cause tracheal mucosal damage, loss of cilia, edema, and fibrosis, and increase the risk of infection and bleeding for the patient. Insertion of the suction catheter to a predetermined distance, no more than 1 cm past the length of the endotracheal tube, avoids contact with the trachea and carina, reducing the effects of tracheal mucosal damage (Hahn, 2011; Ireton, 2007; Pate, 2004; Pate & Zapata, 2002). If resistance is met, the carina or tracheal mucosa has been hit. Withdraw the catheter at least 0.5 inch before applying suction. Suctioning when inserting the catheter increases the risk for trauma to airway mucosa and increases the risk of hypoxemia.
17. Apply intermittent suction by depressing the suction button with thumb of nondominant hand (Figure 4). Gently rotate the catheter with thumb and index finger of dominant hand as catheter is being withdrawn. **Do not suction for more than 10 to 15 seconds at a time.** Hyperoxygenate or hyperventilate with sigh button on ventilator, as ordered.	Turning the catheter while withdrawing it helps clean surfaces of the respiratory tract and prevents injury to tracheal mucosa. Suctioning for longer than 10 to 15 seconds robs the respiratory tract of oxygen, which may result in hypoxemia. Suctioning too quickly may be ineffective at clearing all secretions. Hyperoxygenation and hyperventilation reoxygenates the lungs.

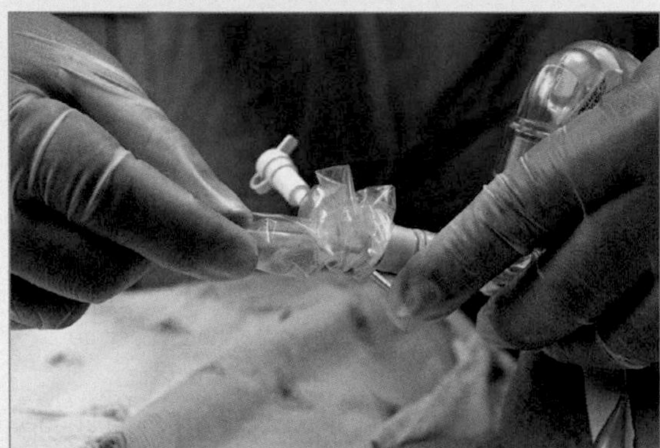

FIGURE 3 Inserting catheter through sheath and into endotracheal tube.

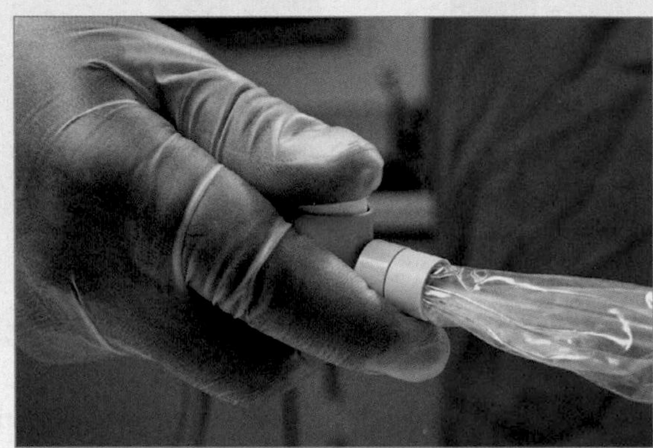

FIGURE 4 Pushing on suction button.

ACTION	RATIONALE
18. Once the catheter is withdrawn back into the sheath (Figure 5), depress the suction button while gently squeezing the normal saline dosette until the catheter is clean. **Allow at least a 30-second to 1-minute interval if additional suctioning is needed. No more than three suction passes should be made per suctioning episode.**	Flushing cleans and clears the catheter and lubricates it for next insertion. Allowing time interval and replacing oxygen delivery setup help compensate for hypoxia induced by the suctioning. Excessive suction passes contribute to complications.

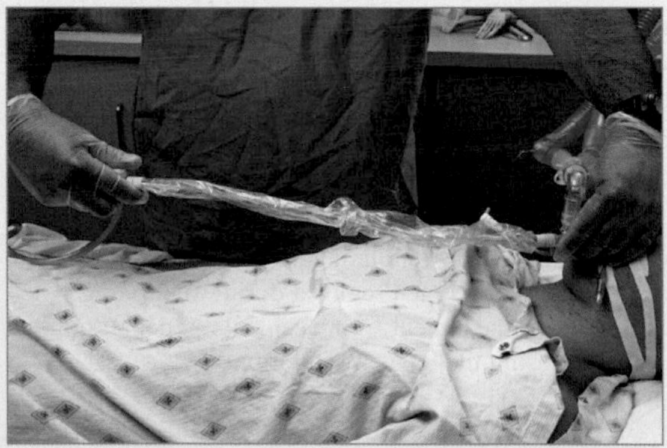

FIGURE 5 Removing suction catheter by pulling back into sheath.

ACTION	RATIONALE
19. When the procedure is completed, **ensure that the catheter is withdrawn into the sheath,** and turn the safety button. Remove normal saline dosette and apply cap to port.	By turning the safety button, the suction is blocked at the catheter so the suction cannot remove oxygen from the endotracheal tube.
20. Suction the oral cavity with a separate single-use, disposable catheter and perform oral hygiene. Remove gloves. Turn off suction.	Suctioning of the oral cavity removes secretions that may be stagnant in the mouth and pharynx, reducing the risk for infection. Oral hygiene offers comfort to the patient. Removing PPE properly reduces the risk for infection transmission and contamination of other items.
21. Assist the patient to a comfortable position. Raise the bed rail and place the bed in the lowest position.	Ensures patient comfort. Proper positioning with raised side rails and proper bed height provide for patient comfort and safety.
22. Reassess the patient's respiratory status, including respiratory rate, effort, oxygen saturation, and lung sounds.	These assess effectiveness of suctioning and the presence of complications.
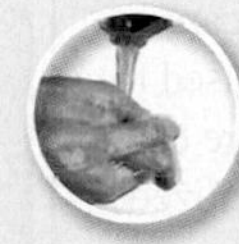 23. Remove additional PPE, if used. Perform hand hygiene.	Removing PPE properly reduces the risk for infection transmission and contamination of other items. Hand hygiene prevents the spread of microorganisms.

EVALUATION

The expected outcome is met when the patient exhibits improved breath sounds and a clear and patent airway. In addition, the oxygen saturation level is within acceptable parameters, and the patient does not exhibit signs or symptoms of respiratory distress or complications.

DOCUMENTATION

Guidelines

Document the time of suctioning, your assessments before and after intervention, reason for suctioning, oxygen saturation levels, and the characteristics and amount of secretions.

Sample Documentation

9/1/15 1850 Lung sounds coarse in lower lobes, wheezes in upper lobes bilaterally. Respirations 24 breaths per minute, irregular rhythm. Intercostal retractions noted. Endotracheal tube suctioning completed with 12F catheter. Small amount of thin, white secretions obtained. After suctioning, lung sounds clear in all lobes, respirations 18 breaths per minute, regular rhythm, no intercostal retractions noted.

—C. Bausler, RN

UNEXPECTED SITUATIONS AND ASSOCIATED INTERVENTIONS

- *Patient is extubated during suctioning:* Remain with patient. Call for help to notify the primary care provider. Assess patient's vital signs, ability to breathe without assistance, and oxygen saturation. Be ready to deliver assisted breaths with a bag-valve mask (see Skill 14-15) or administer oxygen. Anticipate the need for reintubation.
- *Oxygen saturation level decreases after suctioning:* Hyperoxygenate patient. Auscultate lung sounds. If lung sounds are absent over one lobe, alert staff to notify primary care provider. Remain with patient. Patient may have pneumothorax. Anticipate an order for a stat chest x-ray and chest tube placement.
- *When suctioning, you notice small yellow plugs in the secretions:* Assess patient's hydration status as well as the humidification on the ventilator. These mucous plugs may cause a ventilation-perfusion mismatch if not resolved. Patient may need more humidification.
- *Patient develops signs of intolerance to suctioning; oxygen saturation level decreases and remains low after hyperoxygenation; patient becomes cyanotic or patient becomes bradycardic:* Stop suctioning. Auscultate lung sounds. Consider hyperventilating patient with manual resuscitation device. Remain with patient. Alert staff to notify primary care provider.

(continued)

SKILL 14-9 SUCTIONING AN ENDOTRACHEAL TUBE: CLOSED SYSTEM continued

SPECIAL CONSIDERATIONS

General Considerations

- Determine the size catheter to use by the size of the endotracheal tube. The external diameter of the suction catheter should not exceed half of the internal diameter of the endotracheal tube. Larger catheters can contribute to trauma and hypoxemia.
- Make sure emergency equipment is easily accessible at the bedside. Keep bag-valve mask, oxygen, and suction equipment at the bedside of a patient with an endotracheal tube at all times.

Infant and Child Considerations

- Maximal time for application of negative pressure (suction) for neonates should be less than 5 seconds (Ireton, 2007).
- Maximal time for application of negative pressure (suction) for children and adolescents should be less than 10 seconds (Ireton, 2007).

EVIDENCE FOR PRACTICE ▶

ENDOTRACHEAL SUCTIONING

Suctioning of endotracheal tubes is one of the most frequent nursing interventions in the care of patients with these tubes. Two methods of suctioning, open system and closed system, are used to keep the airway open and clean by removing secretions, allowing the patient to breathe more efficiently and comfortably. Serious complications can occur if the correct technique is not utilized.

Related Research

Özden, D., & Gövgülü, R.S. (2012). Development of standard practice guidelines for open and closed system suctioning. *Journal of Clinical Nursing, 21*(9–10), 1327–1338.

This study was carried out to determine the knowledge and practice of nurses related to best practice guidelines for open and closed system suctioning in patients with endotracheal tubes. A standard practice guideline was developed using information from published studies and evidence-based information. A total of 48 nurses working in a cardiovascular surgery intensive care unit were evaluated related to level of knowledge and compliance with standard practice guidelines before and after instruction. There was a significant difference between scores on evaluations related to knowledge of these suctioning systems before and after instruction. Observed compliance with the standard practice guidelines for open and closed suctioning also significantly increased after instruction.

Relevance for Nursing Practice

Nurses are in an important position to influence patient care practices. It is imperative to keep skills up to date and based on current best practice evidence, to ensure use of correct technique and reduce risk of patient complications related to care. Nurses should advocate for examination of current practice and research to clarify issues related to endotracheal suction, as well as to advocate for appropriate instructional activities to keep individual nursing practice current.

Refer to thePoint for additional research on related nursing topics.

SKILL 14-10 SECURING AN ENDOTRACHEAL TUBE

Endotracheal tubes provide an airway for patients who cannot maintain a sufficient airway on their own. A tube is passed through the mouth or nose into the trachea. Patients who have an endotracheal tube have a high risk for skin breakdown related to the securing of the endotracheal tube, compounded by the risk of increased secretions. The endotracheal tube should be retaped every 24 hours to prevent skin breakdown and to ensure that the tube is secured properly. Retaping an endotracheal tube requires two people. There are other ways of securing an endotracheal tube besides using tape. Figure 1 shows an example of a commercially available endotracheal tube holder. To secure with another device, follow the manufacturer's recommendations. However, the literature suggests using tape to secure an endotracheal tube may be the best method (Shimizu et al., 2011; Carlson et al., 2007). One example of taping an endotracheal tube is provided below, but this skill might be performed differently in your facility. Always refer to specific agency policy.

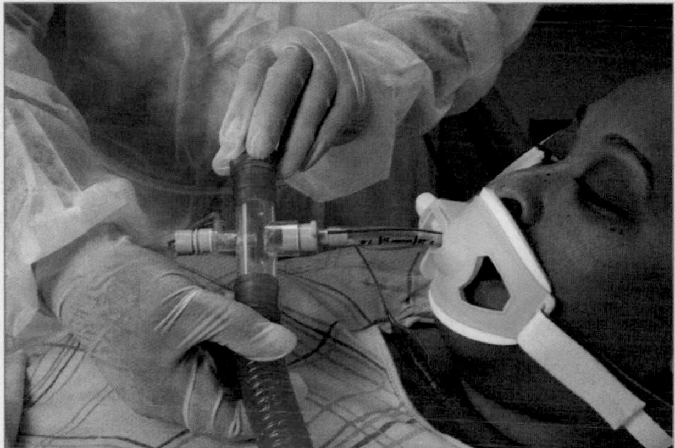

FIGURE 1 Commercially available endotracheal tube holder.

DELEGATION CONSIDERATIONS

Securing an endotracheal tube is not delegated to nursing assistive personnel (NAP) or to unlicensed assistive personnel (UAP). Depending on the state's nurse practice act and the organization's policies and procedures, securing of an endotracheal tube in a stable situation, such as long-term care and other community-based care settings, may be delegated to licensed practical/vocational nurses (LPN/LVNs). The decision to delegate must be based on careful analysis of the patient's needs and circumstances, as well as the qualifications of the person to whom the task is being delegated. Refer to the Delegation Guidelines in Appendix A.

EQUIPMENT

- Assistant (nurse or respiratory therapist)
- Portable or wall suction unit with tubing
- Sterile suction catheter with Y-port
- 1-inch tape (adhesive or waterproof tape)
- Disposable gloves
- Mask and goggles or face shield
- Additional PPE, as indicated
- Sterile suctioning kit
- Oral suction catheter
- Two 3-mL syringes or tongue blade
- Scissors
- Washcloth and cleaning agent
- Skin barrier (e.g., 3M or SkinPrep)
- Adhesive remover swab
- Towel
- Razor (optional)
- Shaving cream (optional)
- Sterile saline or water
- Handheld pressure gauge

ASSESSMENT

Assess for the need for retaping, which may include loose or soiled tape, pressure on mucous membranes, or repositioning of tube. Assess endotracheal tube length. The tube has markings on the side to ensure it is not moved during the retaping. Note the centimeter (cm) marking at the patient's lip or naris. Assess lung sounds to obtain a baseline. Ensure that the lung sounds are still heard throughout the lobes. Assess oxygen saturation level. If the tube is dislodged, the oxygen saturation level may change. Assess the chest for symmetric rise and fall during respiration. If the tube is dislodged, the rise and fall of the chest will change. Assess the patient's need for pain medication or sedation. Assess pain. The patient should be calm, free of pain, and relaxed during the retaping so as not to move and cause an accidental **extubation**. Inspect the area on the posterior portion of the neck for any skin breakdown that may result from irritation or pressure from tape or endotracheal tube holder.

NURSING DIAGNOSIS

Determine the related factors for the nursing diagnoses based on the patient's current status. Appropriate nursing diagnoses may include:

- Risk for Impaired Skin Integrity
- Impaired Oral Mucous Membrane
- Risk for Infection
- Risk for Injury

(continued)

SKILL 14-10 SECURING AN ENDOTRACHEAL TUBE continued

OUTCOME IDENTIFICATION AND PLANNING

The expected outcome to achieve is that the tube remains in place, and the patient maintains bilaterally equal and clear lung sounds. Other outcomes may include the following: the patient demonstrates understanding about the reason for the endotracheal tube; skin remains intact; oxygen saturation remains within acceptable parameters, or greater than 95%; chest rises symmetrically; and airway remains clear.

IMPLEMENTATION

ACTION	RATIONALE
1. Bring necessary equipment to the bedside stand or overbed table.	Bringing everything to the bedside conserves time and energy. Arranging items nearby is convenient, saves time, and avoids unnecessary stretching and twisting of muscles on the part of the nurse.
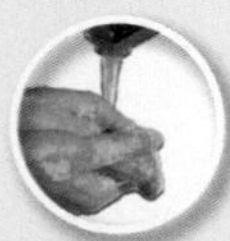 2. Perform hand hygiene and put on PPE, if indicated.	Hand hygiene and PPE prevent the spread of microorganisms. PPE is required based on transmission precautions.
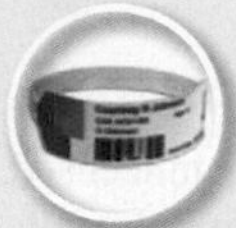 3. Identify the patient.	Identifying the patient ensures the right patient receives the intervention and helps prevent errors.
4. Close the curtains around the bed and close the door to the room, if possible.	This ensures the patient's privacy.
5. Assess the need for endotracheal tube retaping. **Administer pain medication or sedation, as prescribed, before attempting to retape endotracheal tube.** Explain what you are going to do and the reason for doing it to the patient, even if the patient does not appear to be alert.	Retaping the endotracheal tube can stimulate coughing, which may be painful for patients, particularly those with surgical incisions. Explanation alleviates fears, facilitates cooperation, and provides reassurance for the patient. Any procedure that may compromise respiration is frightening for the patient. Even if the patient appears unconscious, the nurse should explain what is happening.
6. Obtain the assistance of a second person to hold the endotracheal tube in place while the old tape is removed and the new tape is placed.	This prevents accidental extubation.
7. Adjust the bed to a comfortable working position, usually elbow height of the caregiver (VISN 8 Patient Safety Center, 2009). Lower side rail closest to you. **If conscious, place the patient in a semi-Fowler's position. If unconscious, place the patient in the lateral position, facing you.** Move the overbed table close to your work area and raise to waist height. Place a trash receptacle within easy reach of the work area.	Having the bed at the proper height prevents back and muscle strain. A sitting position helps the patient to cough and makes breathing easier. Gravity also facilitates catheter insertion. The lateral position prevents the airway from becoming obstructed and promotes drainage of secretions. The overbed table provides work surface and maintains sterility of objects on the work surface. Placing the trash receptacle within reach allows for an organized approach to care.
8. Put on face shield or goggles and mask. Suction patient as described in Skill 14-8 or 14-9.	PPE prevents exposure to contaminants. Suctioning decreases the likelihood of the patient coughing during the retaping of the endotracheal tube. If the patient coughs, the tube may become dislodged.
9. Measure a piece of tape for the length needed to reach around the patient's neck to the mouth plus 8 inches. Cut tape. Lay it adhesive-side up on the table.	Extra length is needed so that tape can be wrapped around the endotracheal tube.

ACTION	RATIONALE
10. Cut another piece of tape long enough to reach from one jaw around the back of the neck to the other jaw. Lay this piece on the center of the longer piece on the table, matching the tapes' adhesive sides together.	This prevents the tape from sticking to the patient's hair and the back of the neck.
11. Take one 3-mL syringe or tongue blade and wrap the sticky tape around the syringe until the nonsticky area is reached. Do this for the other side as well.	This helps the nurse or respiratory therapist to manage the tape without it sticking to the sheets or the patient's hair.
12. Take one of the 3-mL syringes or tongue blades and pass it under the patient's neck so that there is a 3-mL syringe on either side of the patient's head.	This makes the tape easy to access when retaping the tube.
13. Put on disposable gloves. Have the assistant put on gloves as well.	Gloves protect hands from exposure to contaminants.
14. Provide oral care, including suctioning the oral cavity.	This helps to decrease secretions in the oral cavity and pharynx region.
15. Take note of the 'cm' position markings on the tube. Begin to unwrap old tape from around the endotracheal tube. After one side is unwrapped, have assistant hold the endotracheal tube as close to the lips or nares as possible to offer stabilization.	Assistant should hold the tube to prevent accidental extubation. Holding the tube as close to lips or nares as possible prevents accidental dislodgement of tube.
16. Carefully remove the remaining tape from the endotracheal tube (Figure 2). **After tape is removed, have assistant gently and slowly move endotracheal tube (if orally intubated) to the other side of the mouth (Figure 3). Assess mouth for any skin breakdown. Before applying new tape, make sure that markings on endotracheal tube are at same spot as when retaping began.**	The endotracheal tube may cause pressure ulcers if left in the same place over time. By moving the tube, the risk for pressure ulcers is reduced.

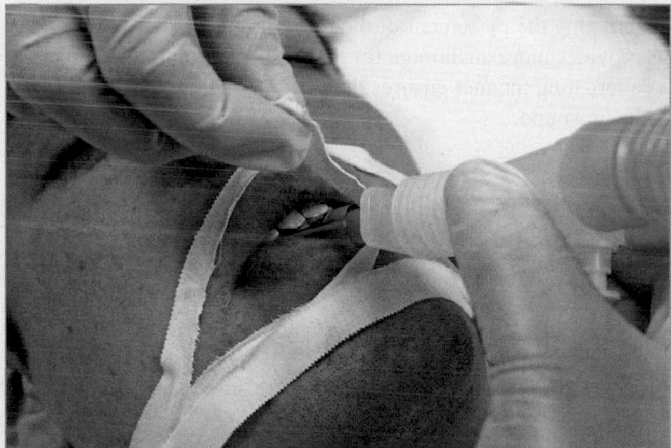

FIGURE 2 Ensuring endotracheal tube is stabilized and removing old tape.

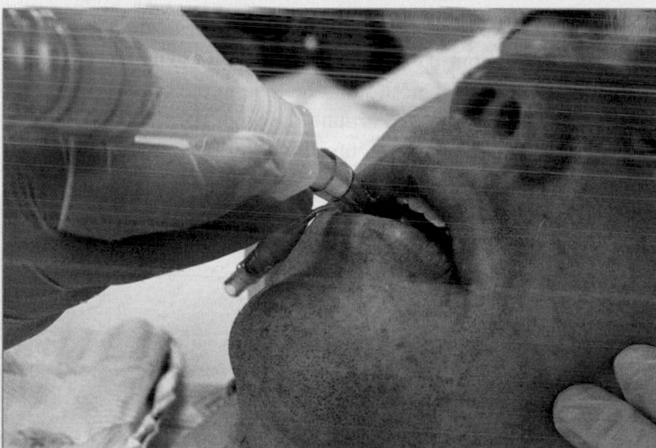

FIGURE 3 Moving endotracheal tube to other side of mouth.

ACTION	RATIONALE
17. Remove old tape from cheeks and side of face. Use adhesive remover to remove excess adhesive from tape (Figure 4). Clean the face and neck with washcloth and cleanser. If patient has facial hair, consider shaving cheeks. Pat cheeks dry with the towel.	To prevent skin breakdown, remove old adhesive. Shaving helps to decrease pain when tape is removed. Cheeks must be dry before new tape is applied to ensure that it sticks.

(continued)

SKILL 14-10 SECURING AN ENDOTRACHEAL TUBE continued

ACTION	RATIONALE
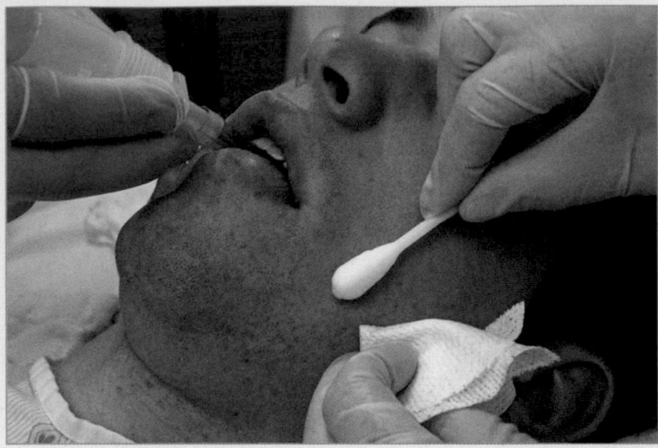	FIGURE 4 Cleaning cheeks at site of tape.
18. Apply the skin barrier to the patient's face (under nose, on cheeks, and lower lip) where the tape will sit. Unroll one side of the tape. Ensure that nonstick part of tape remains behind the patient's neck while pulling firmly on the tape. Place adhesive portion of tape snugly against the patient's cheek. Keep track of the pilot balloon from the endotracheal tube, to avoid taping it to the patient's face. Split the tape in half from the end to the corner of the mouth.	Skin barrier protects the skin from injury with subsequent tape removal and helps the tape adhere better to the skin. The tape should be snug to the side of the patient's face to prevent accidental extubation.
19. Place the top-half piece of tape under the patient's nose (Figure 5). Wrap the lower half around the tube in one direction, such as over and around the tube. Fold over tab on end of tape.	By placing one piece of tape on the lip and the other piece of tape on the tube, the tube remains secure. Tab makes tape removal easier.
20. Unwrap second side of tape. Split to corner of the mouth. Place the bottom-half piece of tape along the patient's lower lip. Wrap the top half around the tube in the opposite direction, such as below and around the tube. Fold over tab on end of tape. Ensure tape is secure (Figure 6). Remove gloves.	Alternating the placement of the top and bottom pieces of tape provides more anchorage for the tube. Wrapping the tape in an alternating manner ensures that the tape will not accidentally be unwound.
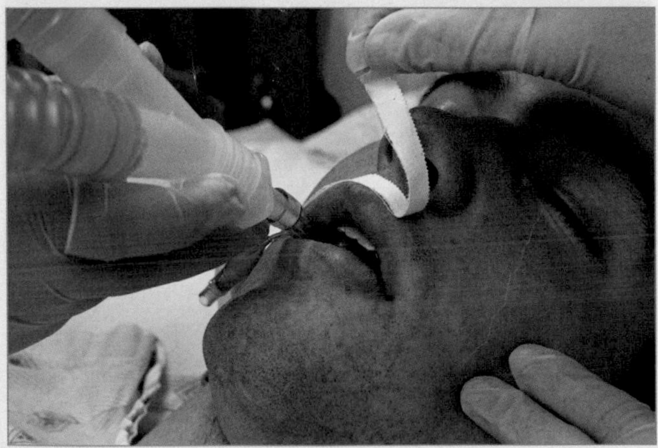 FIGURE 5 Putting new tape in place.	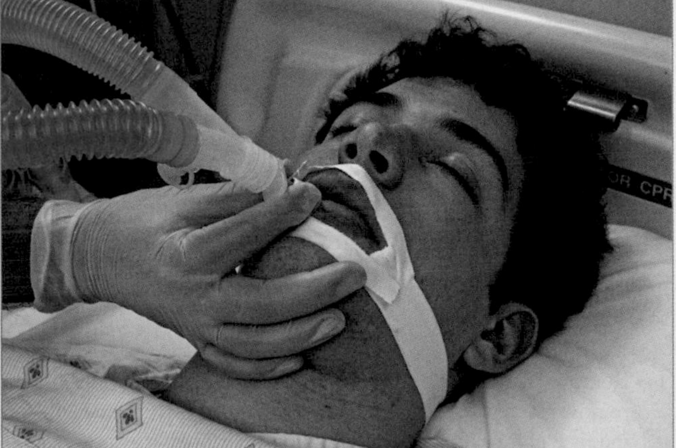 FIGURE 6 Ensuring tape is securely stabilizing the tube.
21. **Auscultate lung sounds. Assess for cyanosis, oxygen saturation, chest symmetry, and endotracheal tube stability. Again check to ensure that the tube is at the correct depth.**	If the tube has been moved from original place, the lung sounds may change, as well as oxygen saturation and chest symmetry. The tube should be stable and should not move with each respiration cycle.

ACTION	RATIONALE
22. **If the endotracheal tube is cuffed, check pressure of the balloon by attaching a handheld pressure gauge to the pilot balloon of the endotracheal tube.**	It is thought cuff pressure should be maintained at less than 25 cm H_2O to prevent excessive pressure on tracheal mucosal wall and surrounding structures (Sultan et al., 2011). Maximal cuff pressures should not exceed 24 to 30 cm H_2O to prevent tracheal ischemia and necrosis.
23. Assist the patient to a comfortable position. Raise the bed rail and place the bed in the lowest position.	Ensures patient comfort. Proper positioning with raised side rails and proper bed height provide for patient comfort and safety.
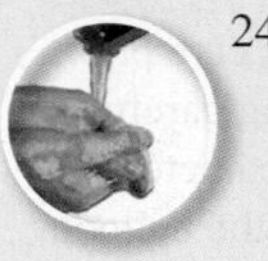 24. Remove face shield or goggles and mask. Remove additional PPE, if used. Perform hand hygiene.	Removing PPE properly reduces the risk for infection transmission and contamination of other items. Hand hygiene prevents the spread of microorganisms.

EVALUATION

The expected outcome is met when the endotracheal tube tape is changed without dislodgement or a depth change of the tube; lung sounds remain equal; no pressure ulcers are noted; airway remains clear; oxygen saturation remains within acceptable parameters, or greater than 95%; chest rises symmetrically; skin remains acyanotic; and cuff pressure is maintained at 20 to 25 cm H_2O.

DOCUMENTATION

Guidelines

Document the procedure, including the depth of the endotracheal tube from teeth or lips; the amount, consistency, and color of secretions suctioned; presence of any skin or mucous membrane changes or pressure ulcers; and your before and after assessments, including lung sounds, oxygen saturation, skin color, cuff pressure, and chest symmetry.

Sample Documentation

9/27/15 1305 Endotracheal tube tape changed; tube remains 12 cm at lips; suctioned for tenacious, yellow secretions, copious in amount; 2-cm pressure ulcer noted on left side of tongue. Tube moved to right side of mouth; lung sounds clear and equal after retaping; pulse oximeter remains 98% on 35% FiO_2 skin pink; cuff pressure 22 cm H_2O; chest rises symmetrically.

—C. Bausler, RN

UNEXPECTED SITUATIONS AND ASSOCIATED INTERVENTIONS

- *Patient is accidentally extubated during tape change:* Stay with patient. Instruct assistant to notify primary care provider. Assess patient's vital signs, ability to breathe without assistance, and oxygen saturation. Be ready to deliver assisted breaths with a bag-valve mask (Skill 14-15) or administer oxygen. Anticipate the need for reintubation.
- *Tube depth changes during retaping:* Tube depth should be maintained at the same level unless otherwise ordered by the primary care provider. Remove tape around tube, adjust tube to ordered depth, and reapply tape.
- *Air leak (air escaping around the balloon) is heard on inspiration cycle of ventilator:* Auscultate lung sounds and check depth of endotracheal tube to ensure that it has not dislodged. Obtain handheld pressure gauge and check pressure. Air may need to be added to the balloon to prevent air leak. If pressure is already 25 cm H_2O, you may need to contact the primary care provider before adding more air to balloon. Sometimes, a change in the patient's position will resolve air leaks.
- *Patient is biting on endotracheal tube:* Obtain a bite block. With the help of an assistant, place the bite block around the endotracheal tube or in patient's mouth. If ordered, consider sedating the patient.
- *Depth of endotracheal tube changes with respiratory cycle:* Remove old tape. Repeat taping of the endotracheal tube, ensuring that tape is snug against the patient's face.
- *Patient has trauma to face that prevents the use of tape when securing the endotracheal tube:* You may need to obtain a commercially prepared endotracheal tube holder. There are various types on the market; check with your facility for availability.

(continued)

SKILL 14-10 SECURING AN ENDOTRACHEAL TUBE continued

- *Lung sounds are greater on one side:* Check the depth of the endotracheal tube. If the tube has been advanced, the lung sounds will appear greater on the side on which the tube is further down. Remove tape and move tube so that it is placed properly. If the depth has not changed, assess patient's oxygen saturation, skin color, and respiratory rate. Notify primary care provider. Anticipate the need for a chest x-ray.
- *Pressure ulcer is noted in the mouth or nares (if patient is intubated via nares):* If the ulcer is painful, you may obtain an order for a topical numbing medication, such as lidocaine viscous jelly. Apply topically with cotton-tipped applicator. Keep area clean by performing more frequent oral or nasal care. Ensure that ventilator or oxygen tubing is not pulling on the endotracheal tube, thus applying pressure on the patient's skin.
- *Pilot balloon is accidentally cut while caring for endotracheal tube:* Notify primary care provider. Obtain a 22-gauge IV catheter and thread it into the pilot balloon tubing, being careful not to puncture the tubing with the needle, below the cut. Remove the needle from the catheter and apply a stopcock or needleless Luer-Lok to the catheter. If air is needed to reinflate the balloon, a syringe can be attached to the stopcock or Luer-Lok so that air may be added. Anticipate the need for an endotracheal tube change.

SPECIAL CONSIDERATIONS

- Make sure emergency equipment is easily accessible at the bedside. Keep bag-valve mask, oxygen, and suction equipment at the bedside of a patient with an endotracheal tube at all times.

EVIDENCE FOR PRACTICE ▶

SECURING ENDOTRACHEAL TUBES

Maintenance of the airway is imperative for patients who are intubated. Oral tracheal intubation is a commonly performed intervention for critically ill patients who need ventilatory support. Unplanned removal or displacement of the tube can be a life-threatening event. Various methods, including tape and commercially marketed devices, are available to prevent accidental removal or displacement.

Related Research

Shimizu, T., Mizutani, T., Yamahita, S., Hagiya, K., & Tanaka, M. (2011). Endotracheal tube extubation force: Adhesive tape versus endotracheal tube holder. *Respiratory Care, 56*(11), 1825–1829.

This study examined the force required to extubate endotracheal tubes from a simulation manikin. Conventional adhesive tape methods, with several tape widths and lengths, and two commercially available endotracheal tube holders were tested. The manikin was intubated with standard tracheal intubation techniques. The endotracheal tube was secured with either tape or one of the commercially available endotracheal tube holders. The endotracheal tube was then connected to a digital push-pull force gauge and manually extubated by pulling perpendicular to the oral cavity, until the entire endotracheal tube cuff was removed from the trachea. Extubation force was defined as the maximal force during each extubation procedure. When tape was used to secure the endotracheal tube, it required a significantly greater force to extubate compared with commercial tube holders. The examiners concluded tape outperformed the commercially available devices.

Relevance for Nursing Practice

Nurses are in an important position to influence patient care practices. It is also important to provide cost-efficient care, because this is becoming an increasingly important issue in health care. The standard use of tape to secure endotracheal tubes may be the best and least expensive method to secure them and to prevent accidental dislodgement or removal of the tube.

Refer to thePoint for additional research on related nursing topics.

SKILL 14-11 SUCTIONING A TRACHEOSTOMY: OPEN SYSTEM

Suctioning through a tracheostomy is indicated to maintain a patent airway. However, tracheal suctioning can lead to hypoxemia, cardiac dysrhythmias, trauma, atelectasis, infection, bleeding, and pain. Therefore, it is imperative to be diligent in maintaining aseptic technique and following facility guidelines and procedures to prevent potential hazards. In the home setting and other community-based settings, clean technique is used, as the patient is not exposed to disease-causing organisms that may be found in health care settings, such as hospitals. Suctioning frequency is based on clinical assessment to determine the need for suctioning.

The purpose of suctioning is to remove secretions that are not accessible to bypassed cilia, so the recommendation is to insert the catheter only as far as the end of the tracheostomy tube. Catheter contact and suction cause tracheal mucosal damage, loss of cilia, edema, and fibrosis, and increase the risk of infection and bleeding for the patient. Insertion of the suction catheter to a predetermined distance, no more than 1 cm past the length of the tracheostomy tube, avoids contact with the trachea and carina, reducing the effects of tracheal mucosal damage (Hahn, 2011; Ireton, 2007; Pate, 2004; Pate & Zapata, 2002). Box 14-1 in Skill 14-8 shows several methods for nurses to use to determine appropriate suction catheter depth.

Note: In-line, closed suction systems are available to suction mechanically ventilated patients. The use of closed suction catheter systems may avoid some of the infection control issues and other complications associated with open suction techniques. The closed suctioning procedure is the same for patients with tracheostomy tubes and endotracheal tubes connected to mechanical ventilation. See Skill 14-9.

DELEGATION CONSIDERATIONS

Suctioning a tracheostomy is not delegated to nursing assistive personnel (NAP) or to unlicensed assistive personnel (UAP). Depending on the state's nurse practice act and the organization's policies and procedures, suctioning of a tracheostomy in a stable situation, such as long-term care and other community-based care settings, may be delegated to licensed practical/vocational nurses (LPN/LVNs). The decision to delegate must be based on careful analysis of the patient's needs and circumstances, as well as the qualifications of the person to whom the task is being delegated. Refer to the Delegation Guidelines in Appendix A.

EQUIPMENT

- Portable or wall suction unit with tubing
- A commercially prepared suction kit with an appropriate-size catheter (see General Considerations) or
- Sterile suction catheter with Y-port in the appropriate size
- Sterile, disposable container
- Sterile gloves
- Towel or waterproof pad
- Goggles and mask or face shield
- Additional PPE, as indicated
- Disposable, clean gloves
- Resuscitation bag connected to 100% oxygen

ASSESSMENT

Assess lung sounds. Patients who need to be suctioned may have wheezes, crackles, or gurgling present. Assess oxygen saturation level. Oxygen saturation usually decreases when a patient needs to be suctioned. Assess respiratory status, including respiratory rate and depth. Patients may become tachypneic when they need to be suctioned. Additional indications for suctioning via a tracheostomy tube include secretions in the tube, acute respiratory distress, and frequent or sustained coughing. Also assess for pain and the potential to cause pain during the intervention. Perform individualized pain management in response to the patient's needs (Arroyo-Novoa et al., 2008). Administer pain medication, as prescribed, before suctioning. Assess appropriate suction catheter depth. (Refer to Box 14-1 in Skill 14-8.) Assess the characteristics and amount of secretions while suctioning.

NURSING DIAGNOSIS

Determine the related factors for the nursing diagnoses based on the patient's current status. Appropriate nursing diagnoses may include:

- Ineffective Airway Clearance
- Risk for Aspiration
- Impaired Gas Exchange

(*continued*)

SKILL 14-11 SUCTIONING A TRACHEOSTOMY: OPEN SYSTEM continued

OUTCOME IDENTIFICATION AND PLANNING

The expected outcome is that the patient will exhibit improved breath sounds and a clear, patent airway. Other outcomes that may be appropriate include the following: the patient will exhibit an oxygen saturation level within acceptable parameters; the patient will demonstrate a respiratory rate and depth within age-acceptable range; and the patient will remain free of any signs of respiratory distress.

IMPLEMENTATION

ACTION	RATIONALE
1. Bring necessary equipment to the bedside stand or overbed table.	Bringing everything to the bedside conserves time and energy. Arranging items nearby is convenient, saves time, and avoids unnecessary stretching and twisting of muscles on the part of the nurse.
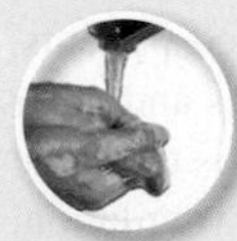 2. Perform hand hygiene and put on PPE, if indicated.	Hand hygiene and PPE prevent the spread of microorganisms. PPE is required based on transmission precautions.
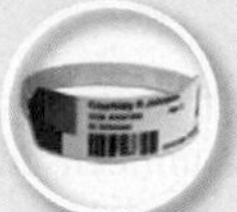 3. Identify the patient.	Identifying the patient ensures the right patient receives the intervention and helps prevent errors.
4. Close the curtains around the bed and close the door to the room, if possible.	This ensures the patient's privacy.
5. Determine the need for suctioning. Verify the suction order in the patient's medical record. **Assess for pain or the potential to cause pain. Administer pain medication, as prescribed, before suctioning.**	To minimize trauma to airway mucosa, suctioning should be done only when secretions have accumulated or adventitious breath sounds are audible. Suctioning can cause moderate to severe pain for patients. Individualized pain management is imperative (Arroyo-Novoa et al., 2008). Suctioning stimulates coughing, which is painful for patients with surgical incisions.
6. Explain to the patient what you are going to do and the reason for doing it, even if the patient does not appear to be alert. Reassure the patient you will interrupt the procedure if he or she indicates respiratory difficulty.	Explanation alleviates fears. Even if the patient appears unconscious, the nurse should explain what is happening. Any procedure that compromises respiration is frightening for the patient.
7. Adjust the bed to a comfortable working position, usually elbow height of the caregiver (VISN 8 Patient Safety Center, 2009). Lower side rail closest to you. **If conscious, place the patient in a semi-Fowler's position (Figure 1). If unconscious, place the patient in the lateral position, facing you.** Move the overbed table close to your work area and raise to waist height.	Having the bed at the proper height prevents back and muscle strain. A sitting position helps the patient to cough and makes breathing easier. Gravity also facilitates catheter insertion. The lateral position prevents the airway from becoming obstructed and promotes drainage of secretions. The overbed table provides a work surface and maintains sterility of objects on the work surface.
8. Place towel or waterproof pad across patient's chest.	This protects bed linens and the patient.
9. Turn suction to appropriate pressure (Figure 2). • For a wall unit for an adult: 100–150 mm Hg; neonates: 60–80 mm Hg; infants: 80–125 mm Hg; children: 80–125 mm Hg; adolescents: 80–150 mm Hg (Hess et al., 2012). • For a portable unit for an adult: 10–15 cm Hg; neonates: 6–8 cm Hg; infants: 8–10 cm Hg; children: 8–10 cm Hg; adolescents: 8–15 cm Hg. Put on a disposable, clean glove and occlude the end of the connecting tubing to check suction pressure. Place the connecting tubing in a convenient location. If using, place resuscitation bag connected to oxygen within convenient reach.	Higher pressures can cause excessive trauma, hypoxemia, and atelectasis. Glove prevents contact with blood and body fluids. Checking pressure ensures equipment is working properly. Allows for an organized approach to the procedure.

ACTION

RATIONALE

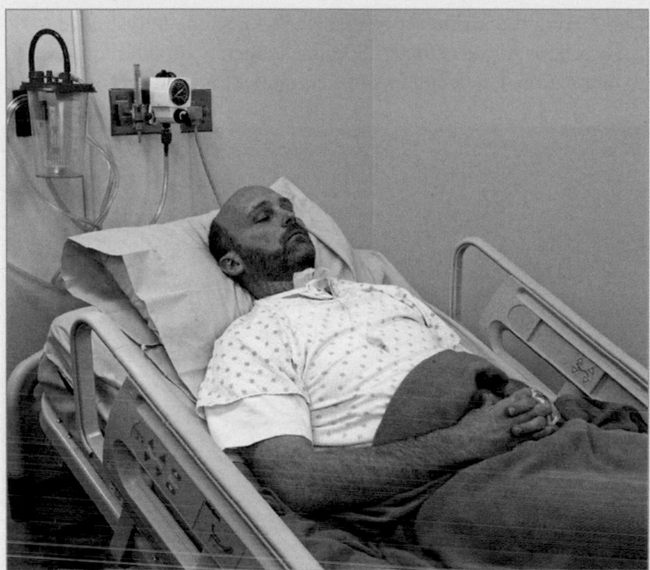

FIGURE 1 Patient in semi-Fowler's position.

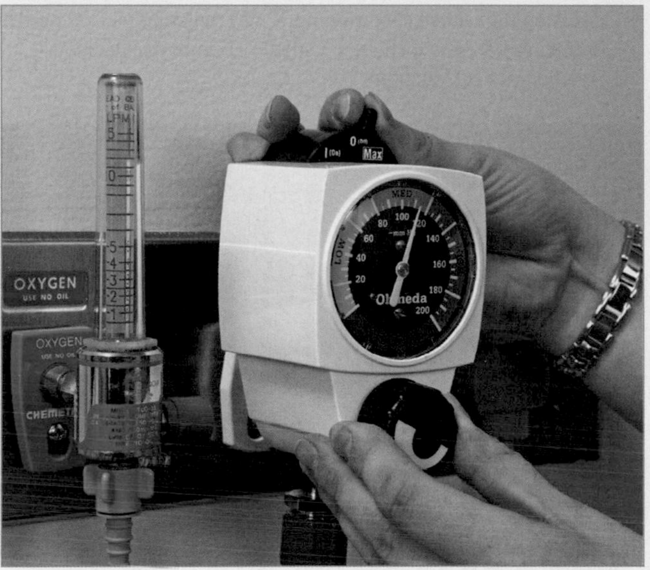

FIGURE 2 Turning suction device to appropriate pressure.

10. Open sterile suction package using aseptic technique. The open wrapper or container becomes a sterile field to hold other supplies. Carefully remove the sterile container, touching only the outside surface. Set it up on the work surface and pour sterile saline into it.

Sterile normal saline or water is used to lubricate the outside of the catheter, minimizing irritation of mucosa during introduction. It is also used to clear the catheter between suction attempts.

11. Put on face shield or goggles and mask (Figure 3). Put on sterile gloves. **The dominant hand will manipulate the catheter and must remain sterile. The nondominant hand is considered clean rather than sterile and will control the suction valve (Y-port) on the catheter.**

Handling the sterile catheter using a sterile glove helps prevent introducing organisms into the respiratory tract; the clean glove protects the nurse from microorganisms.

12. With dominant gloved hand, pick up sterile catheter. Pick up the connecting tubing with the nondominant hand and connect the tubing and suction catheter (Figure 4).

Suction catheter sterility is maintained.

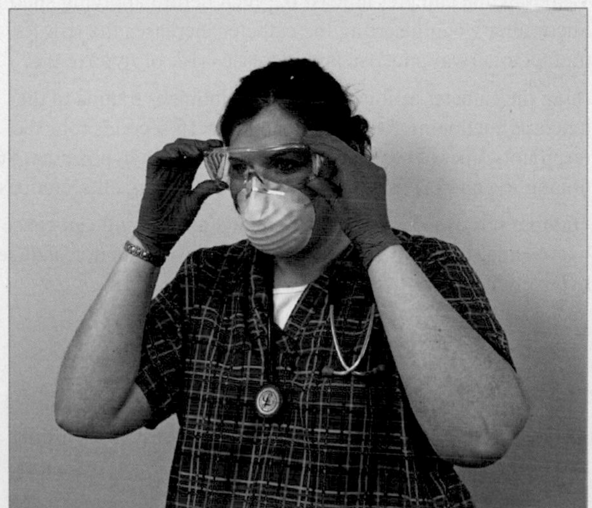

FIGURE 3 Putting on goggles and mask.

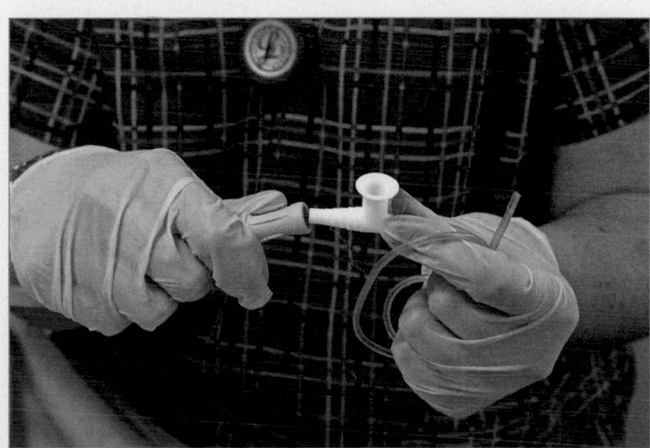

FIGURE 4 Connecting suction catheter to suction tubing.

(continued)

SKILL 14-11 SUCTIONING A TRACHEOSTOMY: OPEN SYSTEM continued

ACTION	RATIONALE
13. Moisten the catheter by dipping it into the container of sterile saline, unless it is a silicone catheter (Figure 5). Occlude Y-tube to check suction (Figure 6).	Lubricating the inside of the catheter with saline helps move secretions in the catheter. Silicone catheters do not require lubrication. Checking ensures equipment is working properly.

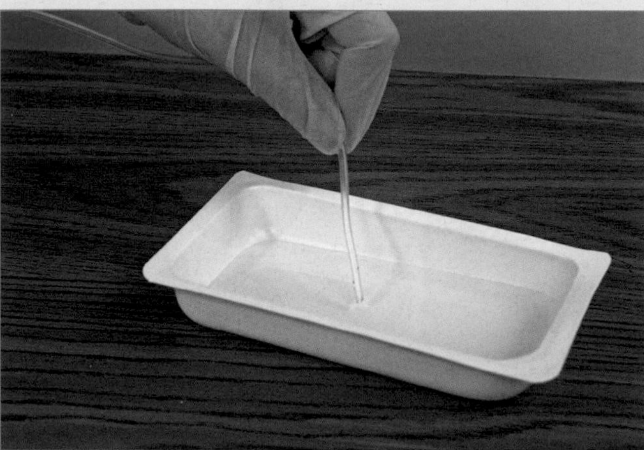

FIGURE 5 Moistening catheter in saline solution.

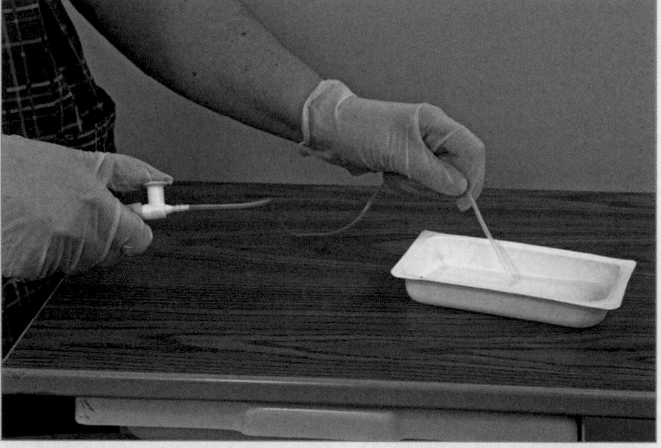

FIGURE 6 Occluding Y-port to check for proper suction.

ACTION	RATIONALE
14. Using your nondominant hand and a manual resuscitation bag, hyperventilate the patient, delivering three to six breaths or use the sigh mechanism on a mechanical ventilator.	Hyperoxygenation and hyperventilation aid in preventing hypoxemia during suctioning.
15. Open the adapter on the mechanical ventilator tubing or remove oxygen delivery setup with your nondominant hand.	This exposes the tracheostomy tube without contaminating sterile gloved hand.
16. Using your dominant hand, gently and quickly insert catheter into trachea. **Advance the catheter to the predetermined length. Do not occlude Y-port when inserting the catheter.**	Catheter contact and suction cause tracheal mucosal damage, loss of cilia, edema, and fibrosis, and increase the risk of infection and bleeding for the patient. Insertion of the suction catheter to a predetermined distance, no more than 1 cm past the length of the endotracheal tube, avoids contact with the trachea and carina, reducing the effects of tracheal mucosal damage (Hahn, 2010; Ireton, 2007; Pate, 2004; Pate & Zapata, 2002). If resistance is met, the carina or tracheal mucosa has been hit. Withdraw the catheter at least 0.5 inch before applying suction. Suctioning when inserting the catheter increases the risk for trauma to airway mucosa and increases risk of hypoxemia.
17. Apply suction by intermittently occluding the Y-port on the catheter with the thumb of your nondominant hand, and gently rotate the catheter as it is being withdrawn (Figure 7). **Do not suction for more than 10 to 15 seconds at a time.**	Turning the catheter as it is withdrawn minimizes trauma to the mucosa. Suctioning for longer than 10 to 15 seconds robs the respiratory tract of oxygen, which may result in hypoxemia. Suctioning too quickly may be ineffective at clearing all secretions.
18. Hyperventilate the patient using your nondominant hand and a manual resuscitation bag, delivering three to six breaths. Replace the oxygen delivery device, if applicable, using your nondominant hand and have the patient take several deep breaths. If the patient is mechanically ventilated, close the adapter on the mechanical ventilator tubing and use the sigh mechanism on a mechanical ventilator.	Suctioning removes air from the patient's airway and can cause hypoxemia. Hyperventilation can help prevent suction-induced hypoxemia.
19. Flush catheter with saline. Assess the effectiveness of suctioning and repeat, as needed, and according to patient's tolerance. Wrap the suction catheter around your dominant hand between attempts.	Flushing clears the catheter and lubricates it for next insertion. Reassessment determines the need for additional suctioning. Prevents inadvertent contamination of the catheter.

ACTION	RATIONALE
20. **Allow at least a 30-second to 1-minute interval if additional suctioning is needed. Do not make more than three suction passes per suctioning episode. Encourage the patient to cough and deep breathe between suctioning attempts.** Suction the oropharynx after suctioning the trachea. Do not reinsert in the tracheostomy after suctioning the mouth.	The interval allows for reventilation and reoxygenation of airways. Excessive suction passes contribute to complications. Clears the mouth of secretions. More microorganisms are usually present in the mouth, so it is suctioned last to prevent transmission of contaminants.
21. When suctioning is completed, remove gloves from dominant hand over the coiled catheter, pulling it off inside-out (Figure 8). Remove glove from nondominant hand and dispose of gloves, catheter, and container with solution in the appropriate receptacle. Assist the patient to a comfortable position. Raise bed rail and place bed in the lowest position.	This technique reduces transmission of microorganisms. Ensures patient comfort. Proper positioning with raised side rails and proper bed height provide for patient comfort and safety.

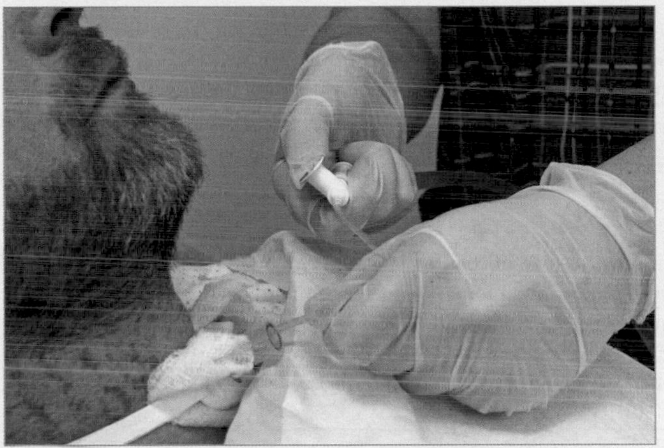

FIGURE 7 Applying intermittent suction while withdrawing catheter.

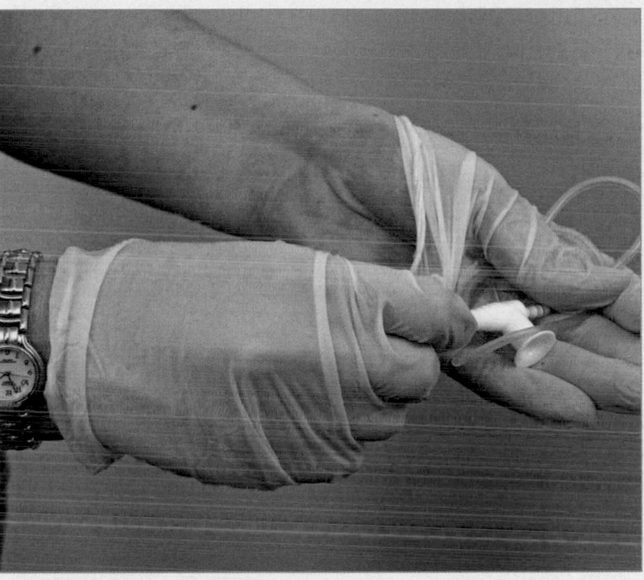

FIGURE 8 Removing gloves while keeping catheter inside.

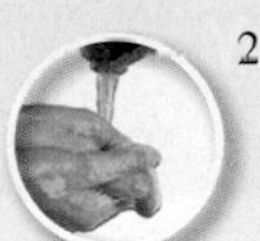

ACTION	RATIONALE
22. Turn off suction. Remove supplemental oxygen placed for suctioning, if appropriate. Remove face shield or goggles and mask. Perform hand hygiene.	Removing PPE properly reduces the risk for infection transmission and contamination of other items. Hand hygiene prevents transmission of microorganisms.
23. Offer oral hygiene after suctioning.	Respiratory secretions that are allowed to accumulate in the mouth are irritating to mucous membranes and unpleasant for the patient.
24. Reassess the patient's respiratory status, including respiratory rate, effort, oxygen saturation, and lung sounds.	Assesses the effectiveness of suctioning and the presence of complications.
25. Remove additional PPE, if used. Perform hand hygiene.	Removing PPE properly reduces the risk for infection transmission and contamination of other items. Hand hygiene prevents the spread of microorganisms.

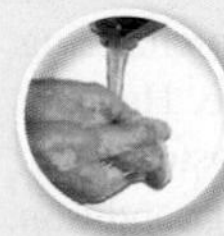

EVALUATION

The expected outcome is met when the patient exhibits improved breath sounds and a clear and patent airway. In addition, the oxygen saturation level is within acceptable parameters, and the patient does not exhibit signs or symptoms of respiratory distress or complications.

(*continued*)

SKILL 14-11 SUCTIONING A TRACHEOSTOMY: OPEN SYSTEM continued

DOCUMENTATION

Guidelines

Document the time of suctioning, your assessments before and after intervention, reason for suctioning, and the characteristics and amount of secretions.

Sample Documentation

9/1/15 1515 Lungs auscultated for wheezes in upper and lower lobes bilaterally. Respirations at 24 breaths per minute. Weak, ineffective cough noted. Tracheal suction completed with 12F catheter. Large amount of thick, yellow secretions obtained. Specimen for culture collected and sent, as ordered. After suctioning, lung sounds clear in all lobes, oxygen saturation at 97%, respirations 18 breaths per minute.

—C. Bausler, RN

UNEXPECTED SITUATIONS AND ASSOCIATED INTERVENTIONS

- *Patient coughs hard enough to dislodge tracheostomy:* Keep a spare tracheostomy and obturator at the bedside. Insert obturator into tracheostomy tube and reinsert tracheostomy into stoma. Remove obturator. Secure ties and auscultate lung sounds. Palpate for any **subcutaneous emphysema**.
- *Tracheostomy becomes dislodged and is not easily replaced:* Notify the primary care provider immediately. This is an emergency situation. Cover the tracheostomy stoma. Assess the patient's respiratory status. Anticipate the possible need for maintaining ventilation using a manual resuscitation device.
- *Lung sounds do not improve greatly and oxygen saturation remains low after three suctioning attempts:* Allow the patient time to recover from previous suctioning. If needed, hyperoxygenate again. Suction the patient again and assess whether the oxygen saturation increases, lung sounds improve, and secretion amount decreases.

SPECIAL CONSIDERATIONS

General Considerations

- Determine the size catheter to use by the size of the tracheostomy. The external diameter of the suction catheter should not exceed half of the internal diameter of the tracheostomy. Larger catheters can contribute to trauma and hypoxemia.
- Make sure emergency equipment is easily accessible at the bedside. Keep bag-valve mask, oxygen, and suction equipment at the bedside of a patient with a tracheostomy tube at all times.

WATCH & LEARN SKILL 14-12 PROVIDING CARE OF A TRACHEOSTOMY TUBE

The nurse is responsible for either replacing a disposable inner cannula or cleaning a nondisposable inner cannula. The inner cannula requires replacement or cleaning to prevent accumulation of secretions that can interfere with respiration and occlude the airway. Because soiled tracheostomy dressings place the patient at risk for the development of skin breakdown and infection, regularly change dressings and tracheostomy collar or ties. Use gauze dressings that are not filled with cotton to prevent aspiration of foreign bodies (e.g., lint or cotton fibers) into the trachea. Clean the skin around a tracheostomy to prevent buildup of dried secretions and skin breakdown. Exercise care when changing the tracheostomy collar or ties to prevent accidental decannulation or expulsion of the tube. Have an assistant hold the tube in place during the changing of a collar. When changing a tracheostomy tie, keep the soiled tie in place until a clean one is securely attached. Agency policy and patient condition determine specific procedures and schedules, but a newly inserted tracheostomy may require attention every 1 to 2 hours. Because the respiratory tract is sterile and the tracheostomy provides a direct opening, meticulous care is necessary when using aseptic technique. Once the tracheostomy site is healed, in the home setting and other community-based settings, clean technique is used, as the patient is not exposed to disease-causing organisms that may be found in health care settings, such as hospitals.

DELEGATION CONSIDERATIONS

Care of a tracheostomy tube is not delegated to nursing assistive personnel (NAP) or to unlicensed assistive personnel (UAP). Depending on the state's nurse practice act and the organization's policies and procedures, care of a tracheostomy tube in a stable situation, such as long-term care and other community-based care settings, may be delegated to licensed practical/vocational nurses (LPN/LVNs). The decision to delegate must be based on careful analysis of the patient's needs and circumstances, as well as the qualifications of the person to whom the task is being delegated. Refer to the Delegation Guidelines in Appendix A.

EQUIPMENT

- Disposable gloves
- Sterile gloves
- Goggles and mask or face shield
- Additional PPE, as indicated
- Sterile normal saline
- Sterile cup or basin
- Sterile cotton-tipped applicators
- Sterile gauze sponges
- Disposable inner tracheostomy cannula, appropriate size for patient
- Sterile suction catheter and glove set
- Commercially prepared tracheostomy or drain dressing
- Commercially prepared tracheostomy holder
- Plastic disposal bag
- Additional nurse

ASSESSMENT

Assess for signs and symptoms of the need to perform tracheostomy care, which include soiled dressings and holder or ties, secretions in the tracheostomy tube, and diminished airflow through the tracheostomy, or in accordance with facility policy. Assess insertion site for any redness or purulent drainage; if present, these may signify an infection. Assess patient for pain. If the tracheostomy is new, pain medication may be needed before performing tracheostomy care. Assess lung sounds and oxygen saturation levels. Lung sounds should be equal in all lobes, with an oxygen saturation level above 93%. If tracheostomy is dislodged, lung sounds and oxygen saturation level will diminish. Inspect the area on the posterior portion of the neck for any skin breakdown that may result from irritation or pressure from tracheostomy holder or ties.

NURSING DIAGNOSIS

Determine the related factors for the nursing diagnoses based on the patient's current status. Appropriate nursing diagnoses may include:

- Impaired Skin Integrity
- Risk for Infection
- Ineffective Airway Clearance
- Risk for Aspiration

OUTCOME IDENTIFICATION AND PLANNING

The expected outcome to achieve when performing tracheostomy care is that the patient will exhibit a tracheostomy tube and site free from drainage, secretions, and skin irritation or breakdown. Other outcomes that may be appropriate include the following: oxygen saturation levels will be within acceptable parameters, and the patient will have no evidence of respiratory distress.

IMPLEMENTATION

ACTION	RATIONALE
1. Bring necessary equipment to the bedside stand or overbed table.	Bringing everything to the bedside conserves time and energy. Arranging items nearby is convenient, saves time, and avoids unnecessary stretching and twisting of muscles on the part of the nurse.
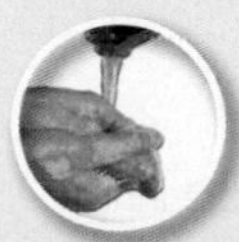 2. Perform hand hygiene and put on PPE, if indicated.	Hand hygiene and PPE prevent the spread of microorganisms. PPE is required based on transmission precautions.
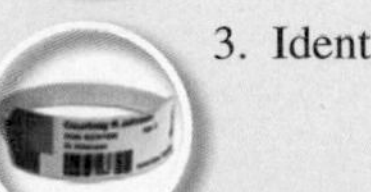 3. Identify the patient.	Identifying the patient ensures the right patient receives the intervention and helps prevent errors.

(continued)

SKILL 14-12 PROVIDING CARE OF A TRACHEOSTOMY TUBE continued

ACTION	RATIONALE
4. Close the curtains around the bed and close the door to the room, if possible.	This ensures the patient's privacy.
5. Determine the need for tracheostomy care. **Assess patient's pain and administer pain medication, if indicated.**	If tracheostomy is new, pain medication may be needed before performing tracheostomy care.
6. Explain what you are going to do and the reason for doing it to the patient, even if the patient does not appear to be alert. Reassure the patient you will interrupt the procedure if he or she indicates respiratory difficulty.	Explanation alleviates fears. Even if the patient appears unconscious, the nurse should explain what is happening. Any procedure that compromises respiration is frightening for the patient.
7. Adjust the bed to a comfortable working position, usually elbow height of the caregiver (VISN 8 Patient Safety Center, 2009). Lower side rail closest to you. **If conscious, place the patient in a semi-Fowler's position. If unconscious, place the patient in the lateral position, facing you.** Move the overbed table close to your work area and raise it to waist height. Place a trash receptacle within easy reach of the work area.	Having the bed at the proper height prevents back and muscle strain. A sitting position helps the patient to cough and makes breathing easier. Gravity also facilitates catheter insertion. The lateral position prevents the airway from becoming obstructed and promotes drainage of secretions. The overbed table provides a work surface and maintains sterility of objects on the work surface. Trash receptacle within reach prevents reaching over the sterile field or turning back to the field to dispose of trash.
8. Put on face shield or goggles and mask. Suction tracheostomy, if necessary. If tracheostomy has just been suctioned, remove soiled site dressing and discard before removal of gloves used to perform suctioning.	PPE prevents contact with contaminants. Suctioning removes secretions to prevent occluding the outer cannula while the inner cannula is removed.

Cleaning the Tracheostomy: Disposable Inner Cannula

(See the accompanying Skill Variation for steps for cleaning a nondisposable inner cannula.)

ACTION	RATIONALE
9. Carefully open the package with the new disposable inner cannula, taking care not to contaminate the cannula or the inside of the package (Figure 1). Carefully open the package with the sterile cotton-tipped applicators, taking care not to contaminate them. Open sterile cup or basin and fill 0.5 inch deep with saline. Open the plastic disposable bag and place within reach on work surface.	Inner cannula must remain sterile. Saline and applicators will be used to clean the tracheostomy site. Plastic disposable bag will be used to discard removed inner cannula.

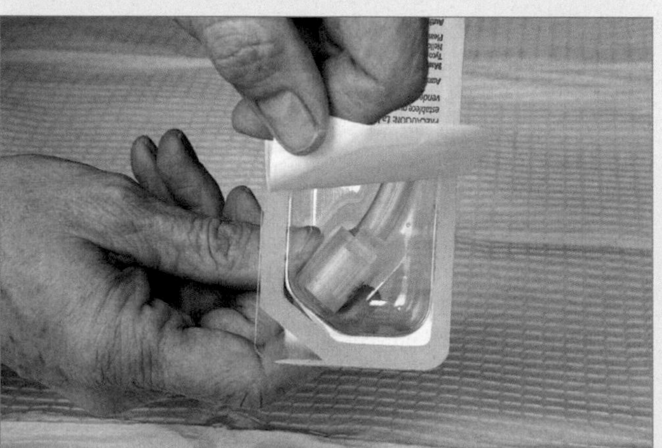

FIGURE 1 Carefully opening package with new disposable inner cannula. *(Photo by B. Proud.)*

ACTION	RATIONALE
10. Put on disposable gloves.	Gloves protect against exposure to blood and body fluids.
11. Remove the oxygen source if one is present. Stabilize the outer cannula and faceplate of the tracheostomy with your nondominant hand. Grasp the locking mechanism of the inner cannula with your dominant hand. Press the tabs and release the lock (Figure 2). Gently remove inner cannula and place in disposal bag. If not already removed, remove site dressing and dispose of it in the trash.	Stabilizing the faceplate prevents trauma to, and pain from, the stoma. Releasing the lock permits removal of the inner cannula.
12. Discard gloves and put on sterile gloves. Pick up the new inner cannula with your dominant hand; stabilize the faceplate with your nondominant hand and gently insert the new inner cannula into the outer cannula. Press the tabs to allow the lock to grab the outer cannula (Figure 3). Reapply oxygen source, if needed.	Sterile gloves are necessary to prevent contamination of the new inner cannula. Locking to outer cannula secures the inner cannula in place. Maintains oxygen supply to the patient.

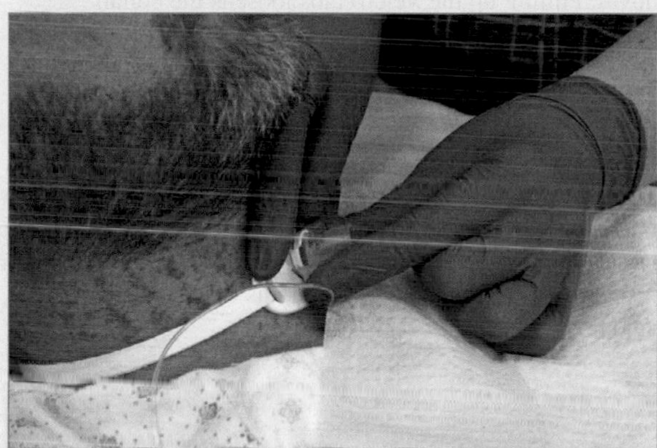

FIGURE 2 Releasing lock on inner cannula.

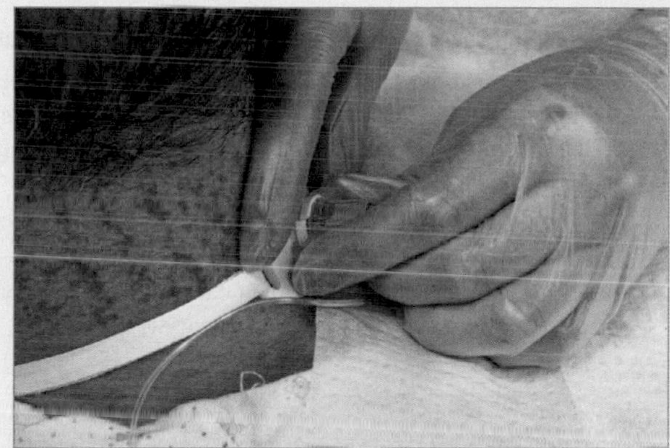

FIGURE 3 Locking new inner cannula in place.

Applying Clean Dressing and Holder

(See accompanying Skill Variations for steps for an alternate site dressing if a commercially prepared sponge is not available and to secure a tracheostomy with tracheostomy ties/tape instead of a collar.)

ACTION	RATIONALE
13. Remove oxygen source, if necessary. Dip cotton-tipped applicator or gauze sponge in cup or basin with sterile saline and clean stoma under faceplate. Use each applicator or sponge only once, moving from stoma site outward (Figure 4).	Saline is nonirritating to tissue. Cleansing from stoma outward and using each applicator only once promotes aseptic technique.

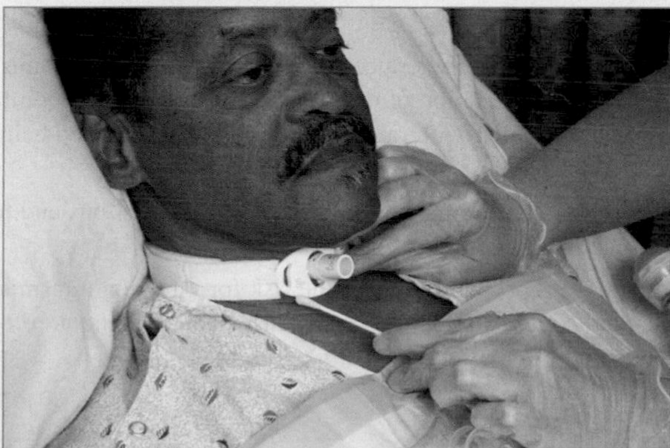

FIGURE 4 Cleaning from stoma site, outward.

(*continued*)

SKILL 14-12 PROVIDING CARE OF A TRACHEOSTOMY TUBE continued

ACTION	RATIONALE
14. Pat skin gently with dry 4 × 4 gauze sponge.	Gauze removes excess moisture.
15. Slide commercially prepared tracheostomy dressing or prefolded non–cotton-filled 4 × 4-inch dressing under the faceplate.	Lint or fiber from a cut cotton-filled gauze pad can be aspirated into the trachea, causing respiratory distress, or can embed in the stoma and cause irritation or infection.
16. Change the tracheostomy holder:	
a. **Obtain the assistance of a second person to hold the tracheostomy tube in place while the old collar is removed and the new collar is placed.**	Holding the tracheostomy tube in place ensures that the tracheostomy will not inadvertently be expelled if the patient coughs or moves.
	Doing so provides attachment for one side of the faceplate.
b. Open the package for the new tracheostomy collar.	Allows access to the new collar.
c. Both nurses should put on clean gloves.	Gloves prevent contact with blood, body fluids, and contaminants.
d. One nurse holds the faceplate while the other pulls up the Velcro tabs. Gently remove the collar.	Holding the tracheostomy tube in place ensures that the tracheostomy will not inadvertently be expelled if the patient coughs or moves. Pulling up the Velcro tabs loosens the collar.
e. The first nurse continues to hold the tracheostomy faceplate.	Prevents accidental extubation.
f. The other nurse places the collar around the patient's neck and inserts first one tab, then the other, into the openings on the faceplate and secures the Velcro tabs on the tracheostomy holder (Figure 5).	Securing the Velcro tabs holds the tracheostomy in place and prevents accidental expulsion of the tracheostomy tube.
g. Check the fit of the tracheostomy collar. You should be able to fit one finger between the neck and the collar. Check to make sure that the patient can flex neck comfortably. Reapply oxygen source, if necessary (Figure 6).	Allowing one fingerbreadth under the collar permits neck flexion that is comfortable and ensures that the collar will not compromise circulation to the area. Maintains oxygen supply to the patient.

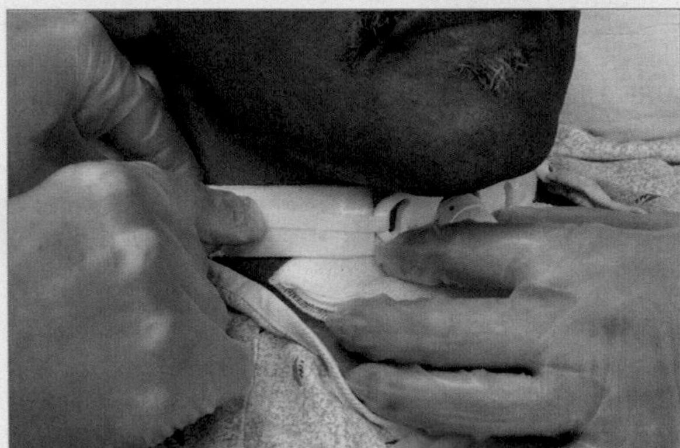

FIGURE 5 Securing tabs on tracheostomy holder.

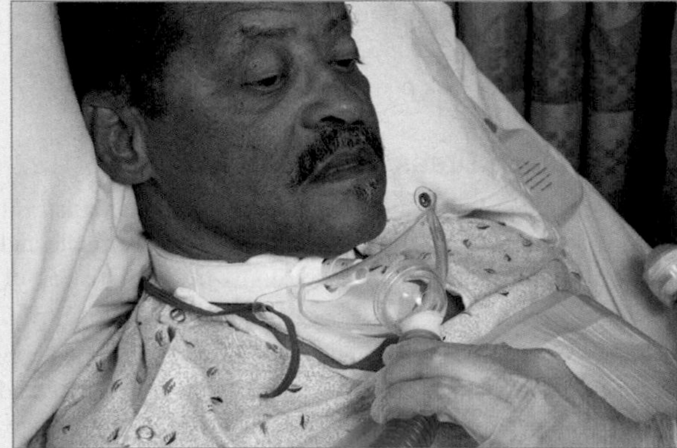

FIGURE 6 Reapplying oxygen source.

ACTION	RATIONALE
17. Remove gloves. Remove face shield or goggles and mask. Assist the patient to a comfortable position. Raise the bed rail and place the bed in the lowest position.	Removing PPE properly reduces the risk for infection transmission and contamination of other items. Ensures patient comfort. Proper positioning with raised side rails and proper bed height provide for patient comfort and safety.
18. Reassess the patient's respiratory status, including respiratory rate, effort, oxygen saturation, and lung sounds.	Assessments determine the effectiveness of interventions and for the presence of complications.
19. Remove additional PPE, if used. Perform hand hygiene.	Removing PPE properly reduces the risk for infection transmission and contamination of other items. Hand hygiene prevents the spread of microorganisms.

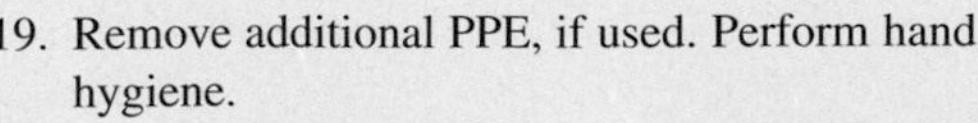

EVALUATION

The expected outcome is met when the patient exhibits a tracheostomy tube and site that are free from drainage, secretions, and skin irritation or breakdown; oxygen saturation level is within acceptable parameters; and the patient is without evidence of respiratory distress. In addition, the patient verbalizes that the site is free of pain and exhibits no evidence of skin breakdown on the posterior portion of the neck.

DOCUMENTATION

Guidelines

Document your assessments before and after interventions, including site assessment, presence of pain, lung sounds, and oxygen saturation levels. Document presence of skin breakdown that may result from irritation or pressure from the tracheostomy collar. Document care given.

Sample Documentation

9/26/15 1300 Tracheostomy care completed; lung sounds clear in all lobes; respirations even/unlabored; site without erythema or edema; small amount of thick, yellow secretions noted at site.

—*C. Bausler, RN*

UNEXPECTED SITUATIONS AND ASSOCIATED INTERVENTIONS

- *Patient coughs hard enough to dislodge tracheostomy:* Keep a spare tracheostomy and obturator at bedside. Insert obturator into the new tracheostomy and insert tracheostomy into stoma. Remove obturator. Secure ties and auscultate lung sounds. Palpate for any subcutaneous emphysema.
- *Tracheostomy becomes dislodged and is not easily replaced:* Notify the primary care provider immediately. This is an emergency situation. Cover the tracheostomy stoma. Assess the patient's respiratory status. Anticipate the possible need for maintaining ventilation using a manual resuscitation device.
- *On palpating around the insertion site, you note a moderate amount of subcutaneous emphysema in tissue:* Assess for dislodgement of the tracheostomy tube. If the tube has become displaced, a buildup of air in the subcutaneous portion of the skin is likely. Notify primary care provider if the subcutaneous emphysema is a change in the status of the tracheostomy.

SPECIAL CONSIDERATIONS

General Considerations

- One nurse working alone should always place new tracheostomy ties before removing old ties to prevent accidental extubation of the tracheostomy. If it is necessary to remove old ties first, obtain the assistance of a second person to hold the tracheostomy tube in place while the old tie is removed and the new tie is replaced.
- Make sure emergency equipment is easily accessible at the bedside. Keep a bag-valve mask, oxygen, the obturator from the current tracheostomy, spare tracheostomy of the same size, spare tracheostomy one size smaller, and suction equipment at the bedside of a patient with a tracheostomy tube at all times.
- If the patient is currently using a tracheostomy without a cuff, keep a spare tracheostomy of the same size with a cuff at the bedside for emergency use.

Home Care Considerations

- Instruct the patient and home caregiver on how to perform tracheostomy care. Observe a return demonstration and provide feedback.
- Clean, rather than sterile, technique can be used in the home setting.
- Sterile saline can be made by mixing 1 teaspoon of table salt in 1 quart of water and boiling for 15 minutes. The solution is cooled and stored in a clean, dry container. Discard saline at the end of each day to prevent growth of bacteria.
- Instruct the patient who is performing self-care to use a mirror to view the steps in the procedure.

(continued)

SKILL 14-12 PROVIDING CARE OF A TRACHEOSTOMY TUBE continued

SKILL VARIATION Cleaning a Nondisposable Inner Cannula

Some tracheostomies use nondisposable inner cannulas, requiring the nurse to clean the inner cannula. Aseptic technique is maintained during the procedure. Clean, rather than sterile, technique can be used in the home setting. Additional equipment includes the following: sterile tracheostomy cleaning kit, if available, or three sterile basins; sterile brush/pipe cleaners; and sterile cleaning solutions (hydrogen peroxide and normal saline solution).

1. Bring necessary equipment to the bedside stand or overbed table.

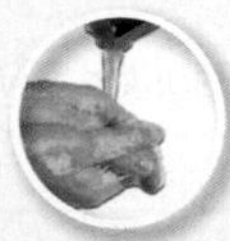

2. Perform hand hygiene and put on PPE, if indicated.

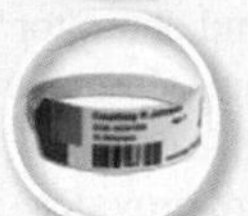

3. Identify the patient.
4. Close the curtains around the bed and close the door to the room, if possible.
5. Determine the need for tracheostomy care. **Assess the patient's pain and administer pain medication, if indicated.** Explain what you are going to do and the reason for doing it to the patient, even if the patient does not appear to be alert. Reassure the patient that you will interrupt the procedure if he or she indicates respiratory difficulty.
6. Adjust the bed to a comfortable working position, usually elbow height of the caregiver (VISN 8 Patient Safety Center, 2009). Lower the side rail closest to you. **If conscious, place the patient in a semi-Fowler's position. If unconscious, place thee patient in the lateral position, facing you.** Move the overbed table close to your work area and raise it to waist height. Place a trash receptacle within easy reach of the work area.
7. Put on face shield or goggles and mask. Suction tracheostomy, if necessary. If tracheostomy has just been suctioned, remove soiled site dressing and discard before removal of gloves used to perform suctioning.
8. Prepare supplies: Open the tracheostomy care kit and separate basins, touching only the edges. If kit is not available, open three sterile basins. Fill one basin 0.5 inch deep with hydrogen peroxide or half hydrogen peroxide and half saline, based on facility policy. Fill other two basins 0.5 inch with saline. Open sterile brush or pipe cleaners, cotton-tipped applicators, and gauze pads, if they are not already available in the cleaning kit.
9. Put on disposable gloves.
10. Remove the oxygen source if one is present. If not already removed, remove site dressing and dispose of it in the trash can. Stabilize the outer cannula and faceplate of the tracheostomy with your nondominant hand. Rotate the inner cannula in a counterclockwise motion with your dominant hand to release the lock (Figure A).

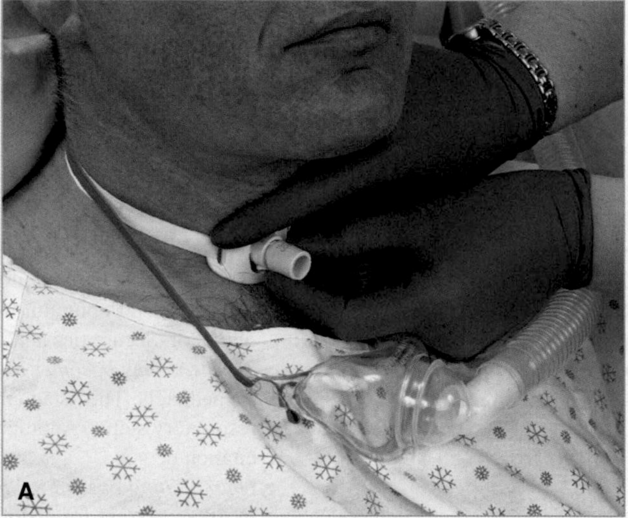

FIGURE A Rotating inner cannula while stabilizing outer cannula.

11. Continue to hold the faceplate. Gently remove the inner cannula (Figure B) and carefully drop it in the basin with the hydrogen peroxide. Replace the oxygen source over the outer cannula.

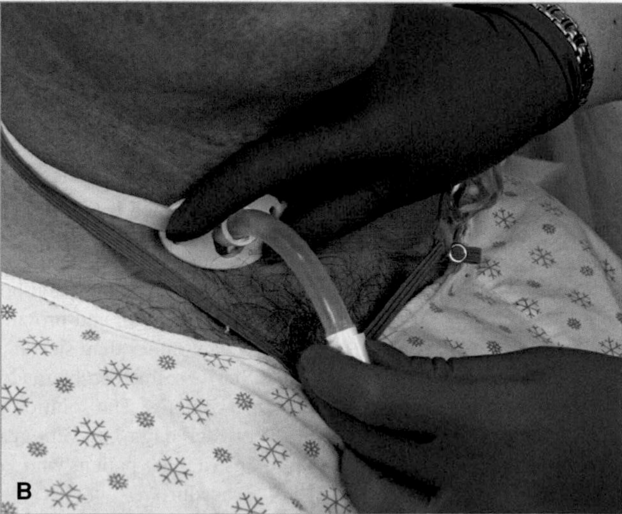

FIGURE B Removing inner cannula for cleaning.

SKILL VARIATION Cleaning a Nondisposable Inner Cannula continued

12. Discard gloves and put on sterile gloves. Remove the inner cannula from the soaking solution. Moisten the brush or pipe cleaner in saline and insert into tube, using a back-and-forth motion to clean (Figure C).
13. Agitate the cannula in saline solution. Remove and tap against the inner surface of the basin. Place on sterile gauze pad. If secretions have accumulated in outer cannula during cleaning of inner cannula, suction outer cannula using sterile technique.
14. Stabilize the outer cannula and faceplate with nondominant hand. Replace inner cannula into outer cannula with dominant hand. Turn clockwise and check that the inner cannula is secure (Figure D). Reapply oxygen source, if needed.
15. Continue with site care as detailed above.

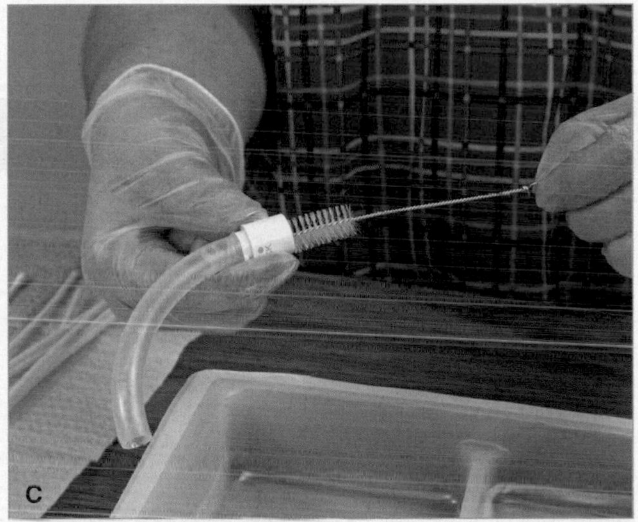

FIGURE C Using brush to clean inner cannula.

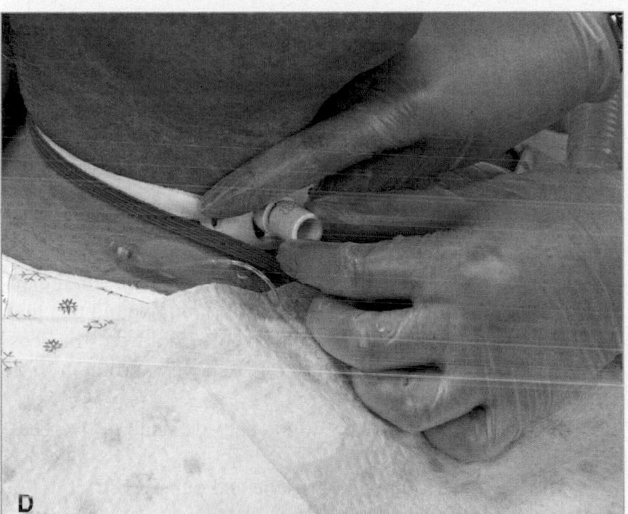

FIGURE D Replacing inner cannula.

SKILL VARIATION Using Alternate Site Dressing if Commercially Prepared Sponge is Not Available

If a commercially prepared site dressing or drain sponge is not available, do not cut a gauze sponge to use at the tracheostomy site. Cutting the gauze can cause loose fibers, which can become lodged in the stoma, causing irritation or infection. Loose fibers could also be inhaled into the trachea, causing respiratory distress.

1. Bring necessary equipment to the bedside stand or overbed table.
2. Perform hand hygiene and put on PPE, if indicated.
3. Identify the patient.
4. Close the curtains around the bed and close the door to the room, if possible.
5. Determine the need for tracheostomy care. **Assess the patient's pain and administer pain medication, if indicated.**
6. Explain what you are going to do and the reason for doing it to the patient, even if the patient does not appear to be alert. Reassure the patient that you will interrupt the procedure if he or she indicates respiratory difficulty.
7. Adjust the bed to a comfortable working position, usually elbow height of the caregiver (VISN 8 Patient Safety Center, 2009). Lower side rail closest to you. **If conscious, place the patient in a semi-Fowler's position. If unconscious, place the patient in the lateral position, facing you.** Move the overbed table close to your work area and raise it to waist height. Place a trash receptacle within easy reach of the work area.

(continued)

SKILL 14-12 PROVIDING CARE OF A TRACHEOSTOMY TUBE continued

SKILL VARIATION Using Alternate Site Dressing if Commercially Prepared Sponge is Not Available continued

8. Remove oxygen source. Dip cotton-tipped applicator or gauze sponge in second basin with sterile saline and clean stoma under faceplate. Use each applicator or sponge only once, moving from stoma site outward.
9. Pat skin gently with dry 4 × 4 gauze sponge.
10. Fold two gauze sponges on the diagonal, to form triangles. Slide one triangle under the faceplate on each side of the stoma, with the longest side of the triangle against the tracheostomy tube.

SKILL VARIATION Securing a Tracheostomy With Ties/Tape

A tracheostomy may be secured in place using twill ties or tape. One nurse working alone should always place new tracheostomy ties in place before removing old ties to prevent accidental extubation of tracheostomy. If it is necessary to remove old ties first, obtain the assistance of a second person to hold the tracheostomy tube in place while the old tie is removed and the new tie is replaced.

1. Bring necessary equipment to the bedside stand or overbed table.
2. Perform hand hygiene and put on PPE, if indicated.
3. Identify the patient.

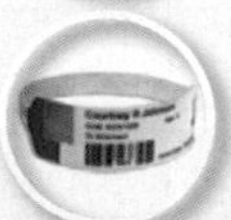

4. Close the curtains around the bed and close the door to the room, if possible.
5. Determine the need for tracheostomy care. **Assess the patient's pain and administer pain medication, if indicated.** Explain what you are going to do and the reason for doing it to the patient, even if the patient does not appear to be alert. Reassure the patient that you will interrupt the procedure if he or she indicates respiratory difficulty.
6. Adjust the bed to a comfortable working position, usually elbow height of the caregiver (VISN 8 Patient Safety Center, 2009). Lower side rail closest to you. **If conscious, place the patient in a semi-Fowler's position. If unconscious, place the patient in the lateral position, facing you.** Move the overbed table close to your work area and raise to waist height. Place a trash receptacle within easy reach of the work area.
7. Put on clean gloves. If another nurse is assisting, both nurses should put on clean gloves.
8. Cut a piece of the tape twice the length of the neck circumference plus 4 inches. Trim ends of tape on the diagonal.
9. Insert one end of the tape through the faceplate opening alongside the old tie. Pull through until both ends are even length (Figure E).

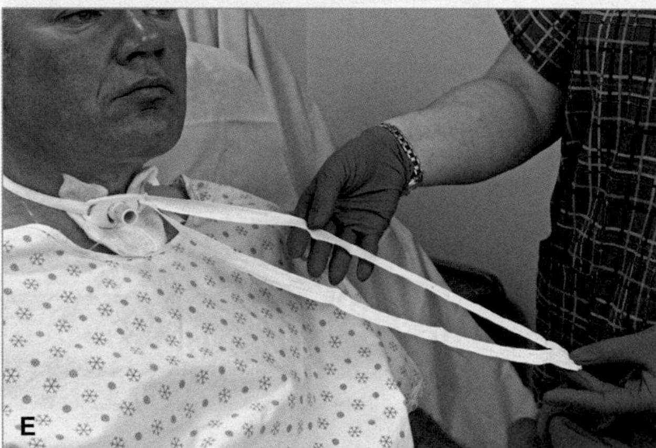

FIGURE E Pulling tape through faceplate opening alongside old tie.

10. Slide both ends of the tape under the patient's neck and insert one end through the remaining opening on other side of the faceplate. Pull snugly and tie ends in double square knot to the side of the patient's neck. You should be able to fit one finger between the neck and the ties. Avoid tying knot at the back of patient's neck, as this can cause excess pressure and skin breakdown. In addition, the ties could be confused with the patient's gown and mistakenly untied. Check to make sure the patient can flex his or her neck comfortably.
11. Carefully cut and remove old ties. Reapply oxygen supply, if necessary.
12. Continue with care as detailed above.

SKILL 14-13 PROVIDING CARE OF A CHEST DRAINAGE SYSTEM

Chest tubes may be inserted to drain fluid (pleural effusion), blood (hemothorax), or air (pneumothorax) from the pleural space. A chest tube is a firm plastic tube with drainage holes in the proximal end that is inserted in the pleural space. Once inserted, the tube is secured with a suture and tape, covered with an airtight dressing, and attached to a drainage system that may or may not be attached to suction. Other components of the system may include a closed water-seal drainage system that prevents air from reentering the chest once it has escaped and a suction control chamber that prevents excess suction pressure from being applied to the pleural cavity. The suction chamber may be a water-filled or a dry chamber. A water-filled suction chamber is regulated by the amount of water in the chamber, whereas dry suction is automatically regulated to changes in the patient's pleural pressure. Many health care agencies use a molded plastic, three-compartment disposable chest drainage unit for management of chest tubes. There are also portable drainage systems that use gravity for drainage. Table 14-2 compares different types of chest drainage systems. The following procedure is based on the use of a traditional water seal, three-compartment chest drainage system. Figure 1 is an example of this system. The Skill Variation following the procedure describes a technique for caring for a chest drainage system using dry seal or suction.

Table 14-2 COMPARISON OF CHEST DRAINAGE SYSTEMS

TYPE	DESCRIPTION	COMMENTS
Traditional water-seal (also referred to as wet-suction) chamber	Has three chambers: a collection chamber, water-seal chamber (middle chamber), and wet suction-control chamber	• Requires that sterile fluid be instilled into water seal and suction chambers. • Has positive and negative pressure–release valves. • Intermittent bubbling indicates that system is functioning properly. • Additional suction can be added by connecting system to a suction source.
Dry-suction water seal (also referred to as dry suction)	Has three chambers: a collection chamber, water-seal chamber (middle chamber), and wet-suction control	• Requires that sterile fluid be instilled in water-seal chamber at 2-cm level. • No need to fill suction chamber with fluid • Suction pressure is set with a regulator. • Has positive and negative pressure–release valves. • Has an indicator to signify that the suction pressure is adequate. • Quieter than traditional water-seal systems.
Dry-suction (also referred to as one-way valve system)	Has a one-way mechanical valve that allows air to leave the chest and prevents air from moving back into the chest	• No need to fill suction chamber with fluid; can be set up quickly in an emergency. • Works even if knocked over, making it ideal for patients who are ambulatory.

From Hinkle J.L., & Cheever, K.H. (2014). *Brunner & Suddarth's textbook of medical-surgical nursing* (13th ed.). Philadelphia: Wolters Kluwer Health/Lippincott Williams & Wilkins.

DELEGATION CONSIDERATIONS

Care of a chest tube is not delegated to nursing assistive personnel (NAP) or to unlicensed assistive personnel (UAP). Depending on the state's nurse practice act and the organization's policies and procedures, care of a chest tube may be delegated to licensed practical/vocational nurses (LPN/LVNs). The decision to delegate must be based on careful analysis of the patient's needs and circumstances, as well as the qualifications of the person to whom the task is being delegated. Refer to the Delegation Guidelines in Appendix A.

(continued)

SKILL 14-13 PROVIDING CARE OF A CHEST DRAINAGE SYSTEM continued

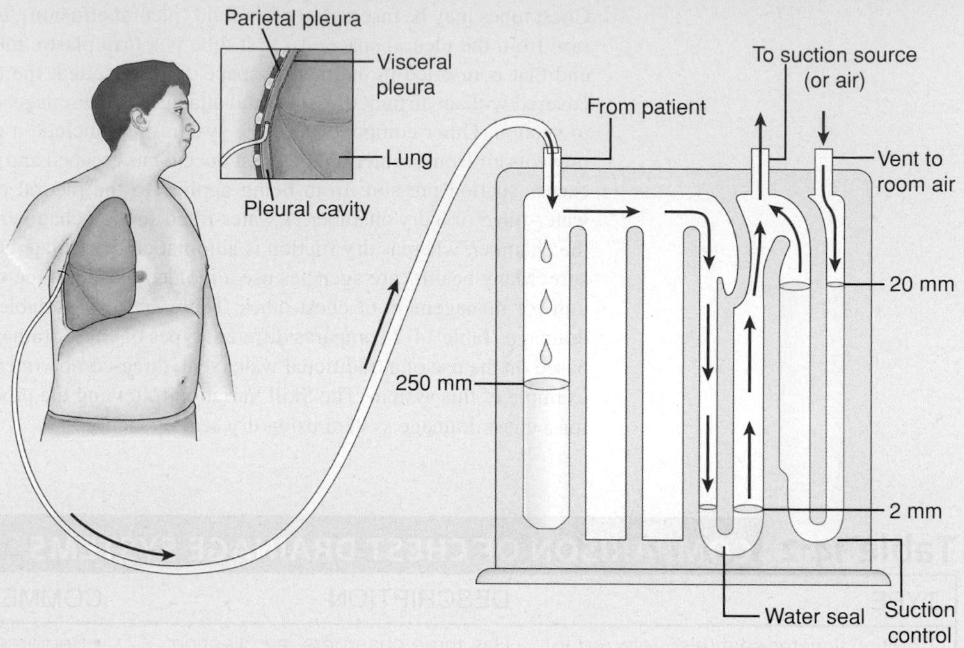

FIGURE 1 Chest drainage system.

EQUIPMENT

- Bottle of sterile normal saline or water
- Two pairs of padded or rubber-tipped Kelly clamps
- Pair of clean scissors
- Disposable gloves
- Additional PPE, as indicated
- Foam tape
- Prescribed drainage system, if changing is required

ASSESSMENT

Assess the patient's vital signs. Significant changes from baseline may indicate complications. Assess for restlessness and shortness of breath. Assess the patient's respiratory status, including oxygen saturation level. If the chest tube is not functioning appropriately, the patient may become tachypneic and hypoxic. Assess the patient's lung sounds. The lung sounds over the chest tube site may be diminished due to the presence of fluid, blood, or air. Also assess the patient for pain. Sudden pressure or increased pain indicates potential complications. In addition, many patients report pain at the chest tube insertion site and request medication for the pain. Assess the patient's knowledge of the chest tube to ensure that he or she understands the rationale for the chest tube.

NURSING DIAGNOSIS

Determine the related factors for the nursing diagnoses based on the patient's current status. Appropriate nursing diagnoses may include:

- Impaired Gas Exchange
- Deficient Knowledge
- Acute Pain

OUTCOME IDENTIFICATION AND PLANNING

The expected outcome to achieve is that the patient will not experience any complications related to the chest drainage system or respiratory distress. Other outcomes that may be appropriate include the following: the patient understands the need for the chest tube; the patient will have adequate pain control at the chest tube insertion site; lung sounds will be clear and equal bilaterally; and the patient will be able to increase activity tolerance gradually.

IMPLEMENTATION

ACTION	RATIONALE
1. Bring necessary equipment to the bedside stand or overbed table.	Bringing everything to the bedside conserves time and energy. Arranging items nearby is convenient, saves time, and avoids unnecessary stretching and twisting of muscles on the part of the nurse.
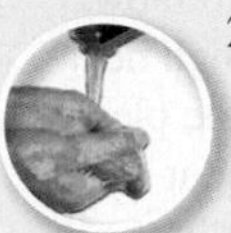 2. Perform hand hygiene and put on PPE, if indicated.	Hand hygiene and PPE prevent the spread of microorganisms. PPE is required based on transmission precautions.
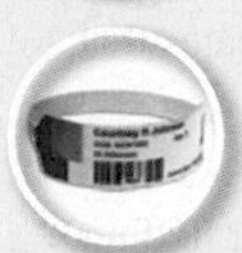 3. Identify the patient.	Identifying the patient ensures the right patient receives the intervention and helps prevent errors.
4. Close the curtains around the bed and close the door to the room, if possible.	This ensures the patient's privacy.
5. Explain what you are going to do and the reason for doing it to the patient.	Explanation relieves anxiety and facilitates cooperation.
6. **Assess the patient's level of pain. Administer prescribed medication, as needed.**	Regular pain assessments are required to maintain adequate analgesic relief from the discomfort and pain caused by chest drains (Crawford, 2011; Sullivan, 2008).
7. Put on clean gloves.	Gloves prevent contact with contaminants and body fluids.

Assessing the Drainage System

ACTION	RATIONALE
8. Move the patient's gown to expose the chest tube insertion site. Keep the patient covered as much as possible, using a bath blanket to drape the patient, if necessary. Observe the dressing around the chest tube insertion site and ensure that it is dry, intact, and occlusive (Figure 2).	Keeping the patient as covered as possible maintains the patient's privacy and limits unnecessary exposure of the patient. If the dressing is not intact and occlusive, air can leak into the space, causing displacement of the lung tissue, and the site could be contaminated. Some patients experience significant drainage or bleeding at the insertion site. If this occurs, the dressing needs to be replaced to maintain occlusion of the site.

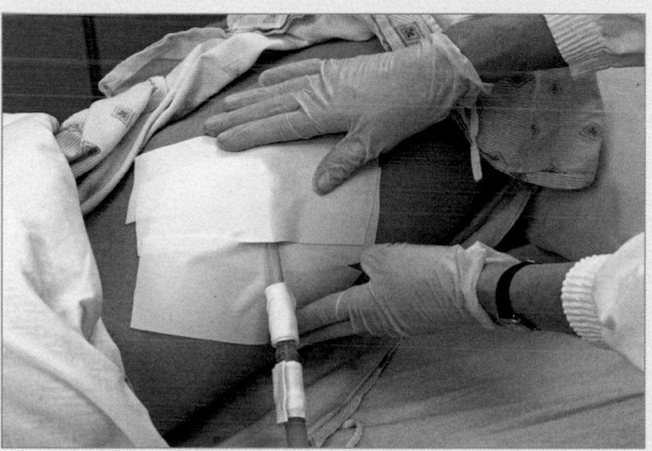

FIGURE 2 Assessing chest tube insertion site.

ACTION	RATIONALE
9. Check that all connections are securely taped. Gently palpate around the insertion site, feeling for crepitus, a result of air or gas collecting under the skin (subcutaneous emphysema). This may feel crunchy or spongy, or like "popping" under your fingers.	The body will absorb small amounts of subcutaneous emphysema after the chest tube is removed. If larger amounts or increasing amounts are present, it could indicate improper placement of the tube or an air leak and can cause discomfort to the patient.

(continued)

SKILL 14-13 PROVIDING CARE OF A CHEST DRAINAGE SYSTEM continued

ACTION	RATIONALE
10. Check drainage tubing to ensure that there are no dependent loops or kinks. Position the drainage collection device below the tube insertion site.	Dependent loops or kinks in the tubing can prevent the tube from draining appropriately (Bauman & Handley, 2011; Sullivan, 2008). The drainage collection device must be positioned below the tube insertion site so that drainage can move out of the tubing and into the collection device.
11. If the chest tube is ordered to be connected to suction, note the fluid level in the suction chamber and check it with the amount of ordered suction. Look for bubbling in the suction chamber. Temporarily disconnect the suction to check the level of water in the chamber. Add sterile water or saline, if necessary, to maintain correct amount of suction.	Some fluid is lost due to evaporation. If suction is set too low, the amount needs to be increased to ensure that enough negative pressure is placed in the pleural space to drain the pleural space sufficiently. If suction is set too high, the amount needs to be decreased to prevent any damage to the fragile lung tissue. Gentle bubbling in the suction chamber indicates that suction is being applied to assist drainage.
12. Observe the water-seal chamber for fluctuations of the water level with the patient's inspiration and expiration (tidaling). If suction is used, temporarily disconnect the suction to observe for fluctuation. Assess for the presence of bubbling in the water-seal chamber. Add water, if necessary, to maintain the level at the 2-cm mark, or the mark recommended by the manufacturer.	Fluctuation of the water level in the water-seal chamber with inspiration and expiration is an expected and normal finding. Bubbles in the water-seal chamber after the initial insertion of the tube or when air is being removed are a normal finding. Constant bubbles in the water-seal chamber after initial insertion period indicate an air leak in the system. Leaks can occur within the drainage unit, or at the insertion site.
13. Assess the amount and type of fluid drainage. Measure drainage output at the end of each shift by marking the level on the container or placing a small piece of tape at the drainage level to indicate date and time (Figure 3). The amount should be a running total, because the drainage system is never emptied. If the drainage system fills, remove and replace it. (See Guidelines below.)	Measurement allows for accurate intake and output measurement and assessment of the effectiveness of therapy, and it contributes to the decision to remove the tube. The drainage system would lose its negative pressure if it were opened.

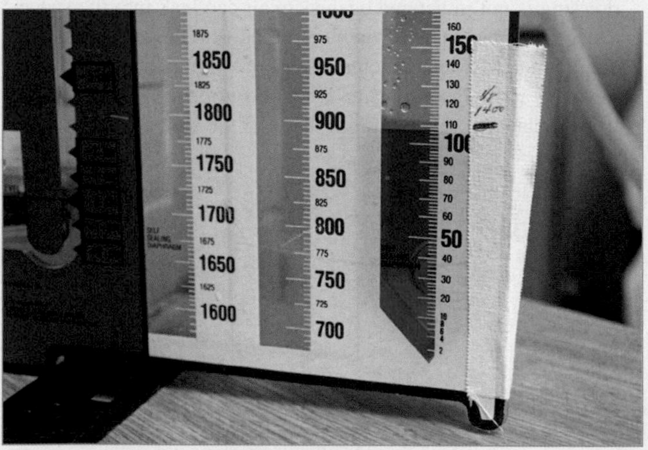

FIGURE 3 Drainage marked on device.

ACTION	RATIONALE
14. Remove gloves. Assist the patient to a comfortable position. Raise the bed rail and place the bed in the lowest position, as necessary.	Removing PPE properly reduces the risk for infection transmission and contamination of other items. Placing the patient in a comfortable position ensures patient comfort. Proper positioning with raised side rails and proper bed height provide for patient comfort and safety.
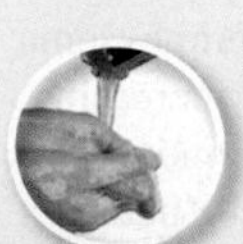 15. Remove additional PPE, if used. Perform hand hygiene.	Removing PPE properly reduces the risk for infection transmission and contamination of other items. Hand hygiene prevents the spread of microorganisms.

ACTION | RATIONALE

Changing the Drainage System

16. Obtain two padded Kelly clamps, a new drainage system, and a bottle of sterile water. Add water to the water-seal chamber in the new system until it reaches the 2-cm mark or the mark recommended by the manufacturer. Follow manufacturer's directions to add water to the suction system if suction is ordered.

Gathering equipment provides for an organized approach. Appropriate level of water in the water-seal chamber is necessary to prevent air from entering the chest. Appropriate level of water in the suction chamber provides the ordered suction.

17. Put on clean gloves and additional PPE, as indicated.

Gloves prevent contact with contaminants and body fluids.

18. **Apply Kelly clamps 1.5 to 2.5 inches from insertion site and 1 inch apart, going in opposite directions (Figure 4).**

Clamps provide a more complete seal and prevent air from entering the pleural space through the chest tube.

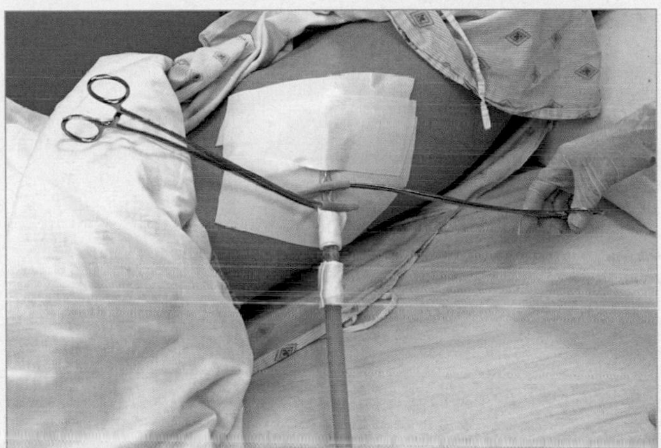

FIGURE 4 Using padded clamps on chest tube.

19. Remove the suction from the current drainage system. Unroll (Figure 5) or use scissors to carefully cut away (Figure 6) any foam tape on the connection of the chest tube and drainage system. Using a slight twisting motion, remove the drainage system. **Do not pull on the chest tube.**

Removing suction permits application of new system. In many facilities, bands or foam tape are placed where the chest tube meets the drainage system to ensure that the chest tube and the drainage system remain connected. Due to the negative pressure, a slight twisting motion may be needed to separate the tubes. The chest tube is sutured in place; do not tug on the chest tube and dislodge it.

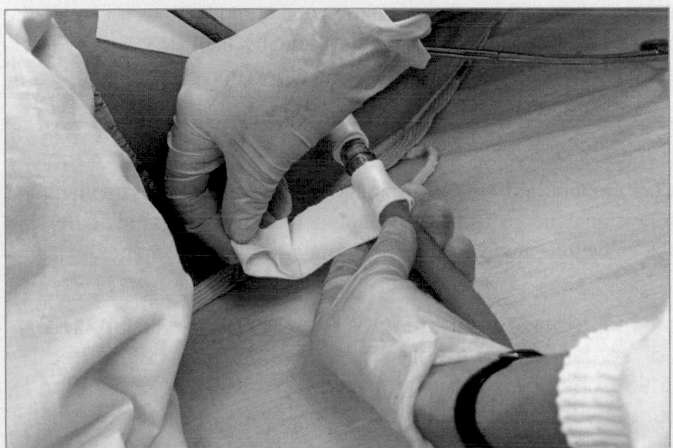

FIGURE 5 Unrolling foam tape.

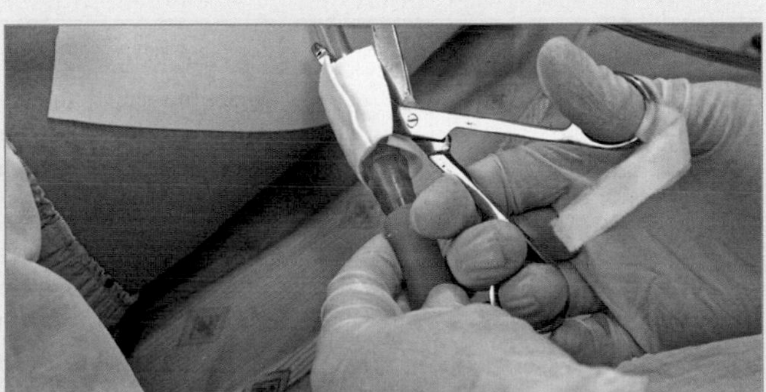

FIGURE 6 Cutting foam tape.

(*continued*)

SKILL 14-13 PROVIDING CARE OF A CHEST DRAINAGE SYSTEM continued

ACTION	RATIONALE
20. Keeping the end of the chest tube sterile, insert the end of the new drainage system into the chest tube (Figure 7). **Remove Kelly clamps.** Reconnect suction, if ordered. Apply foam tape to chest tube/drainage system connection site.	Chest tube is sterile. Tube must be reconnected to suction to form a negative pressure and allow for re-expansion of lung or drainage of fluid. Prolonged clamping can result in a pneumothorax. Bands or foam tape help prevent the separation of the chest tube from the drainage system.

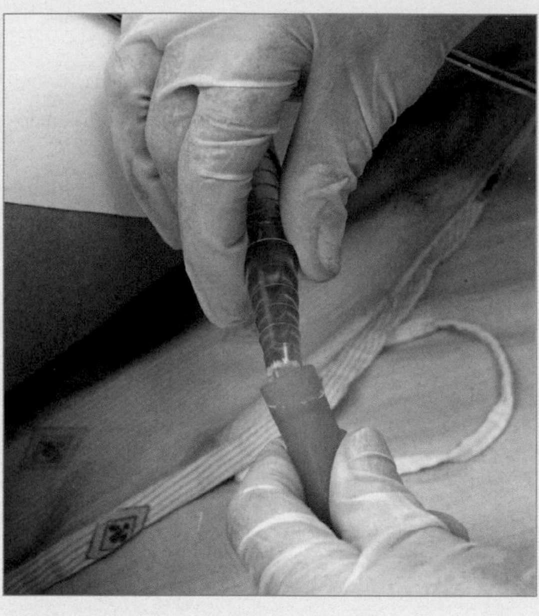

FIGURE 7 Attaching new drainage tube.

ACTION	RATIONALE
21. Assess the patient and the drainage system as outlined (Steps 5–15).	Assess for changes related to the manipulation of the system and placement of a new drainage system.
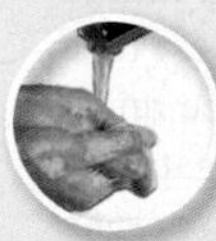 22. Remove additional PPE, if used. Perform hand hygiene.	Removing PPE properly reduces the risk for infection transmission and contamination of other items. Hand hygiene prevents the spread of microorganisms.

EVALUATION

The expected outcome is met when the chest drainage system is patent and functioning. In addition, the patient remains free of signs and symptoms of respiratory distress and complications related to the chest drainage system; the patient verbalizes adequate pain relief, gradually increases activity tolerance, and demonstrates an understanding of the need for the chest tube.

DOCUMENTATION

Guidelines

Document the site of the chest tube, amount and type of drainage, amount of suction applied, and presence of any bubbling, tidaling, or subcutaneous emphysema noted. Document the type of dressing in place and the patient's pain level, as well as any measures performed to relieve the patient's pain.

Sample Documentation

9/10/15 1805 Chest tube present in right lower portion of rib cage at the axillary line. Draining moderate amount of serosanguinous fluid. Suction at 20 cm H_2O noted; gentle bubbling noted in suction chamber. Tidaling present in water-seal chamber, no air leak noted. Small amount of subcutaneous emphysema noted around insertion site, unchanged from previous assessment; patient denies any pain; occlusive dressing remains intact.

—C. Bausler, RN

UNEXPECTED SITUATIONS AND ASSOCIATED INTERVENTIONS

- *The chest tube becomes separated from the drainage device:* Put on gloves. Open the normal saline solution or sterile water and submerge the chest tube into the bottle 1 to 2 inches below the surface of the solution, taking care to avoid contaminating the chest tube. This creates a water seal until a new drainage unit can be attached. Assess the patient for any signs of respiratory distress. Notify the primary care provider. Do not leave the patient. Anticipate the need for a new drainage system and a chest x-ray.
- *The chest tube becomes dislodged:* Put on gloves. Immediately apply an occlusive dressing to the site. There is a controversy in the literature over whether the occlusive dressing should be a sterile Vaseline-impregnated gauze covered with an occlusive tape or a sterile 4 × 4 gauze folded and covered with an occlusive tape. (An example of an occlusive tape would be foam tape or the clear dressing used to cover IV insertion sites.) Assess the patient for any signs of respiratory distress. Notify the primary care provider. Anticipate the need for a chest x-ray. The primary care provider will determine whether the chest tube needs to be replaced.
- *While assessing the chest tube, you notice a lack of drainage when there had been drainage previously:* Check for kinked tubing or a clot in the tubing. Note the amount of suction on which the chest tube is set. Do not perform "milking" of the tubing (squeezing and releasing small segments of tubing between the fingers) and "stripping" of the tubing (squeezing the length of the tube without releasing it) (Bauman & Handley, 2011; Crawford, 2011). Bruising and trauma of lung tissue can occur as a result, as well as dangerously increased negative pressure in the pleural space. If the suction is not set appropriately, adjust until the ordered amount is achieved. Keeping the tubing horizontal across the bed or chair before dropping vertically into the drain device, and avoiding dependent loops optimize drainage. Notify the primary care provider if the lack of drainage persists.
- *Drainage dramatically increases or becomes bright red:* Notify the primary care provider immediately. This can indicate fresh bleeding.
- *Chest tube drainage suddenly decreases and the water-seal chamber is not tidaling:* Notify the primary care provider immediately. This could signal that the tube is blocked.

SPECIAL CONSIDERATIONS

General Considerations

- Ensure that a bottle of sterile water or normal saline is at the bedside at all times. Never clamp chest tubes except to change the drainage system, or when there is a medical order, such as for a trial before chest tube removal. If the chest tube becomes accidentally disconnected from the drainage system, place the end of the chest tube into the sterile solution (see Unexpected Situations above). This prevents more air from entering the pleural space through the chest tube, but allows for any air that does enter the pleural space, through respirations, to escape once pressure builds up.
- Keep two rubber-tipped clamps and additional dressing material at the bedside for quick access, if needed.
- If the patient has a small pneumothorax with little or no drainage and suction is not used, the tube may be connected to a Heimlich valve. A Heimlich valve is a water-seal chamber that allows air to exit from, but not enter, the chest tube. Check to assure that the valve is pointing in the correct direction. The blue end should be connected to the chest tube and the clear end is open as the vent. The arrow on the casing points away from the patient.
- Maintain the chest drainage system in an upright position and lower than the level of the tube insertion site. This is necessary for proper function of the system and to aid drainage.
- Encourage the use of an incentive spirometer if ordered and/or frequent deep breathing and coughing by the patient. This helps drain the lungs, promotes lung expansion, and prevents atelectasis.

Infant and Child Considerations

- Illness and hospitalization alone can be a source of overwhelming distress and anxiety for children and their families. The presence and discomfort related to strand equipment that prevents children from freely moving and invades their body may add to the situation. Provide age-appropriate activities and distraction to help decrease discomfort and promote the child's coping abilities (Crawford, 2011).

(continued)

SKILL 14-13 PROVIDING CARE OF A CHEST DRAINAGE SYSTEM continued

SKILL VARIATION Caring for a Chest Drainage System Using Dry Seal or Suction

1. Bring necessary equipment to the bedside stand or overbed table.

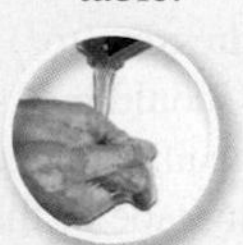

2. Perform hand hygiene and put on PPE, if indicated.

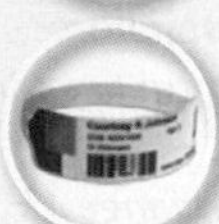

3. Identify the patient.
4. Close the curtains around the bed and close the door to the room, if possible.
5. Explain what you are going to do and the reason for doing it to the patient.
6. **Assess the patient's level of pain. Administer prescribed medication, as needed.**
7. Put on clean gloves. Move the patient's gown to expose the chest-tube insertion site. Keep the patient covered as much as possible, using a bath blanket to drape the patient, if necessary. Observe the dressing around the chest tube insertion site and ensure that it is dry, intact, and occlusive.
8. Check that all connections are taped securely. Gently palpate around the insertion site, feeling for subcutaneous emphysema, a collection of air or gas under the skin. This may feel crunchy or spongy, or like "popping" under your fingers.
9. Check drainage tubing to ensure that there are no dependent loops or kinks. The drainage collection device must be positioned below the tube insertion site.
10. If the chest tube is ordered to be to suctioned, assess the amount of suction set on the chest tube against the amount of suction ordered. Assess for the presence of the suction control indicator, which is a bellows or float device, when adjusting the regulator to the desired level of suction, if prescribed.
11. Assess for fluctuations in the diagnostic indicator with the patient's inspiration and expiration.
12. Check the air-leak indicator for leaks in dry systems with a one-way valve.
13. Assess the amount and type of fluid drainage. Measure drainage output at the end of each shift by marking the level on the container or placing a small piece of tape at the drainage level to indicate date and time. The amount should be a running total, because the drainage system is never emptied. If the drainage system fills, it is removed and replaced.
14. Some portable chest drainage systems require manual emptying of the collection chamber. Follow the manufacturer's recommendations for timing of emptying. Typically, the unit should not be allowed to fill completely because drainage could spill out. Wear gloves, clean the syringe port with an alcohol wipe, use a 60-mL Luer-Lok syringe, screw the syringe into the port, and aspirate to withdraw fluid. Repeat, as necessary, to empty the chamber. Dispose of the fluid according to facility policy.

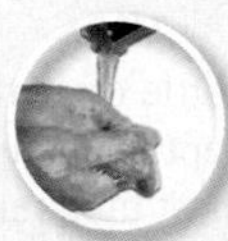

15. Remove gloves, and additional PPE, if used. Perform hand hygiene.

SKILL 14-14 ASSISTING WITH REMOVAL OF A CHEST TUBE

Chest tubes are removed after the lung is re-expanded and drainage is minimal. An advanced-practice professional usually performs chest tube removal. The practitioner will determine when the chest tube is ready for removal by evaluating the chest x-ray and assessing the patient and the amount of drainage from the tube.

DELEGATION CONSIDERATIONS

Assisting with the removal of a chest tube is not delegated to nursing assistive personnel (NAP) or to unlicensed assistive personnel (UAP). Depending on the state's nurse practice act and the organization's policies and procedures, assisting with the removal of a chest tube may be delegated to licensed practical/vocational nurses (LPN/LVNs). The decision to delegate must be based on careful analysis of the patient's needs and circumstances, as well as the qualifications of the person to whom the task is being delegated. Refer to the Delegation Guidelines in Appendix A.

EQUIPMENT

- Disposable gloves
- Additional PPE, as indicated
- Suture removal kit (tweezers and scissors)
- Sterile Vaseline-impregnated gauze and 4 × 4 gauze dressings or other occlusive dressings, based on facility policy
- Occlusive tape, such as foam tape

ASSESSMENT

Assess the patient's respiratory status, including respiratory rate and oxygen saturation level. This provides a baseline for comparison after the tube is removed. If the patient begins to have respiratory distress, he or she will usually become tachypneic and hypoxic. Assess the patient's lung sounds. The lung sounds over the chest tube site may be diminished due to the tube. Assess the patient for pain. Many patients report pain at the chest tube insertion site and request medication for the pain. If the patient has not recently received pain medication, give it before the chest tube removal to decrease the pain felt with the procedure and ease anxiety (Bauman & Handley, 2011).

NURSING DIAGNOSIS

Determine the related factors for the nursing diagnoses based on the patient's current status. Appropriate nursing diagnoses may include:

- Deficient Knowledge
- Acute Pain
- Risk for Injury

OUTCOME IDENTIFICATION AND PLANNING

The expected outcome to achieve when caring for a patient after removal of a chest tube is that the patient will remain free of respiratory distress. Other outcomes that may be appropriate include the following: the insertion site will remain clean and dry without evidence of infection; the patient will experience adequate pain control during the chest tube removal; lung sounds will be clear and equal bilaterally; and the patient will be able to increase activity tolerance gradually.

IMPLEMENTATION

ACTION	RATIONALE
1. Bring necessary equipment to the bedside stand or overbed table.	Bringing everything to the bedside conserves time and energy. Arranging items nearby is convenient, saves time, and avoids unnecessary stretching and twisting of muscles on the part of the nurse.
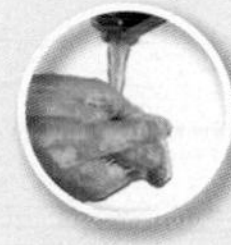 2. Perform hand hygiene and put on PPE, if indicated.	Hand hygiene and PPE prevent the spread of microorganisms. PPE is required based on transmission precautions.
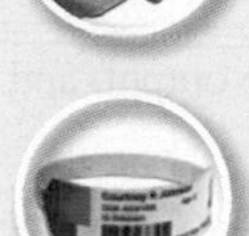 3. Identify the patient.	Identifying the patient ensures the right patient receives the intervention and helps prevent errors.
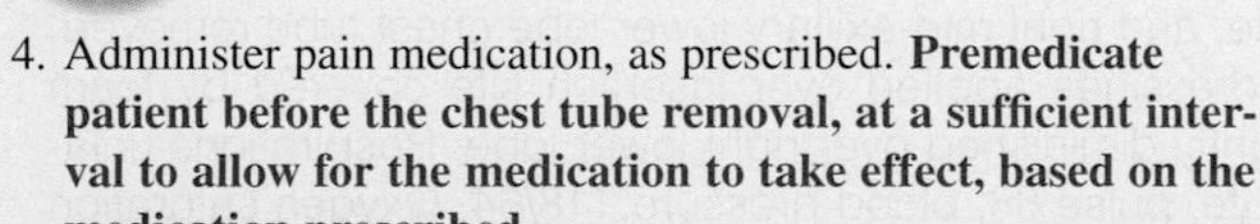 4. Administer pain medication, as prescribed. **Premedicate patient before the chest tube removal, at a sufficient interval to allow for the medication to take effect, based on the medication prescribed.**	Most patients report discomfort during chest tube removal.
5. Close the curtains around the bed and close the door to the room, if possible.	This ensures the patient's privacy.
6. Explain what you are going to do and the reason for doing it to the patient. Explain any nonpharmacologic pain interventions the patient may use to decrease discomfort during tube removal.	Explanation relieves anxiety and facilitates cooperation. Nonpharmacologic pain management interventions, such as relaxation exercises, have been shown to help decrease pain during chest tube removal (Ertuğ & Ülker, 2011; Friesner et al., 2006).

(continued)

SKILL 14-14 ASSISTING WITH REMOVAL OF A CHEST TUBE continued

ACTION	RATIONALE
7. Teach the patient how to do the Valsalva maneuver. Instruct the patient to take a deep breath, keep the mouth closed, and attempt to exhale forcibly while keeping the mouth and nose closed. Bearing down with abdominal muscles can assist with the process.	The chest tube must be removed during breath holding or expiration to prevent air from reentering the pleural space (Bauman & Handley, 2011; Crawford, 2011). The Valsalva maneuver may be contraindicated in people with cardiovascular problems and other illnesses.
8. Put on clean gloves.	Gloves prevent contact with contaminants and body fluids.
9. Provide reassurance to the patient while the practitioner removes the dressing and then the tube.	The removal of the dressing and the tube can increase the patient's anxiety level. Offering reassurance will help the patient feel more secure and help decrease anxiety.
10. **After the practitioner has removed the chest tube and secured the occlusive dressing, assess patient's lung sounds, vital signs, oxygen saturation, and pain level.**	In most facilities, advanced practice professionals remove chest tubes, but some facilities train nurses to remove them. Once the tube is removed, the patient's respiratory status will need to be assessed to ensure that no distress is present.
11. Anticipate an order for a chest x-ray.	A chest x-ray is performed to evaluate the status of the lungs after chest tube removal, to ensure that the lung is still fully inflated.
12. Dispose of equipment appropriately.	This reduces the risk for transmission of microorganisms and contamination of other items.
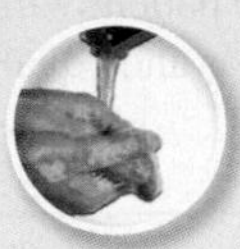 13. Remove gloves and additional PPE, if used. Perform hand hygiene.	Removing PPE properly reduces the risk for infection transmission and contamination of other items. Hand hygiene prevents the spread of microorganisms.
14. Continue to monitor the patient's cardiopulmonary status and comfort level. Monitor the site for drainage.	Continued monitoring allows for assessment of possible respiratory distress if lung does not remain inflated. Checking dressing ensures the assessment of changes in patient condition and enables timely intervention to prevent complications.

EVALUATION

The expected outcome is met when the patient exhibits no signs and symptoms of respiratory distress after the chest tube is removed. In addition, the patient verbalizes adequate pain control; lung sounds are clear and equal; and the patient's activity level gradually increases.

DOCUMENTATION

Guidelines

Document the patient's respiratory rate, oxygen saturation, lung sounds, total chest tube output, and status of the insertion site and dressing.

Sample Documentation

9/16/15 1950 Procedure explained to patient. Morphine sulfate 2 mg IV given, as ordered. Physician at bedside, and right mid-axillary lower lobe chest tube removed. Vaseline gauze and gauze dressings applied over insertion site covered by foam tape. Lung sounds clear, slightly diminished over right lower lobe. Respirations unlabored at 16 breaths per minute, pulse 88, blood pressure 118/64. Oxygen saturation 97% on room air; 322 mL of serosanguinous drainage noted in drainage device. Patient denies pain or respiratory distress.

—C. Bausler, RN

UNEXPECTED SITUATIONS AND ASSOCIATED INTERVENTIONS

- *Patient experiences respiratory distress after chest tube removal:* Auscultate lung sounds. Diminished or absent lung sounds could be a sign that the lung has not fully reinflated or that the fluid has returned. Notify the primary care provider immediately. Anticipate an order for a chest x-ray and possible reinsertion of a chest tube.
- *Chest tube dressing becomes loosened:* Change the chest tube dressing at least every 24 hours or per agency policy in order to assess the site for erythema and drainage. Replace the occlusive dressing using a sterile technique. The dressing should remain occlusive for at least 3 days.

SPECIAL CONSIDERATIONS

Infant and Child Considerations

- It may be difficult to gain the cooperation of the child when performing the Valsalva maneuver. Distraction may be helpful. Ask child to blow up a balloon or blow bubbles (Crawford, 2011).

EVIDENCE FOR PRACTICE ▶

PAIN AND CHEST TUBE REMOVAL

Chest tube removal is a painful procedure for many, if not most, patients. Pharmacologic and nonpharmacologic interventions have been used to decrease patients' discomfort during this procedure.

Related Research

Ertuğ, N., & Ülker, S. (2011). The effect of cold application on pain due to chest tube removal. *Journal of Clinical Nursing, 21*(5/6), 784–790.

The objective of this study was to determine if the effect of application of cold to the chest wall on the pain related to chest tube removal. The study was conducted with 140 patients, divided evenly between an experimental group and a control group. Data were collected regarding the patient's demographic and health history. Skin temperature and pain intensity, using a Visual Analogue Scale, was measured at various points before and after tube removal. There were significant differences related to pain between the two groups. Age, gender, and the number of days the chest tube was inserted had no effect on the pain related to chest tube removal. This study concluded that the application of cold is effective in reducing the pain related to removal of a chest tube.

Relevance for Nursing Practice

Nursing interventions related to decreasing pain and increasing patient comfort are an important nursing responsibility. Interventions should include the use of nonpharmacologic interventions, in addition to the administration of analgesics. The application of cold to the chest wall could significantly decrease the pain and discomfort experienced by a patient during removal of a chest tube. Nurses could easily incorporate this simple intervention as part of nursing care for these patients.

Refer to thePoint for additional research on related nursing topics.

SKILL 14-15 USING A MANUAL RESUSCITATION BAG AND MASK

If the patient is not breathing with an adequate rate and depth, or if the patient has lost the respiratory drive, a bag and mask may be used to deliver oxygen until the patient is resuscitated or can be intubated with an endotracheal tube. Bag and mask devices are frequently referred to as Ambu bags ("air mask bag unit") or BVM ("bag-valve-mask" device). The bags come in infant, pediatric, and adult sizes. The bag consists of an oxygen reservoir (commonly referred to as the tail), oxygen tubing, the bag itself, a one-way valve to prevent secretions from entering the bag, an exhalation port, an elbow so that the bag can lie across the patient's chest, and a mask.

(*continued*)

SKILL 14-15 USING A MANUAL RESUSCITATION BAG AND MASK continued

DELEGATION CONSIDERATIONS

The use of a BVM may be delegated to nursing assistive personnel (NAP) or to unlicensed assistive personnel (UAP) in an emergency situation. The use of a BVM may be delegated to licensed practical/vocational nurses (LPN/LVNs). The decision to delegate must be based on careful analysis of the patient's needs and circumstances, as well as the qualifications of the person to whom the task is being delegated. Refer to the Delegation Guidelines in Appendix A.

EQUIPMENT

- Handheld resuscitation device with a mask
- Oxygen source
- Disposable gloves
- Face shield or goggles and mask
- Additional PPE, as indicated

ASSESSMENT

Assess the patient's respiratory effort and drive. If the patient is breathing less than 10 breaths per minute, is breathing too shallowly, or is not breathing at all, assistance with a BVM may be needed. Assess the oxygen saturation level. Patients who have decreased respiratory effort and drive may also have a decreased oxygen saturation level. Assess heart rate and rhythm. Bradycardia may occur with a decreased oxygen saturation level, leading to a cardiac dysrhythmia. Many times, a BVM is used in a crisis situation. Manual ventilation is also used during airway suctioning.

NURSING DIAGNOSIS

Determine the related factors for the nursing diagnoses based on the patient's current status. Appropriate nursing diagnoses may include:

- Ineffective Breathing Pattern
- Impaired Gas Exchange

OUTCOME IDENTIFICATION AND PLANNING

The expected outcome is that the patient will exhibit signs and symptoms of adequate oxygen saturation. Other outcomes that may be appropriate include the following: the patient will receive adequate volume of respirations with the BVM; and the patient will maintain normal sinus rhythm.

IMPLEMENTATION

ACTION	RATIONALE
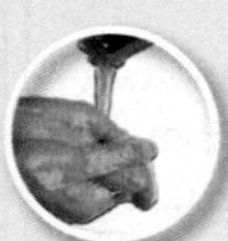 1. If not a crisis situation, perform hand hygiene.	Hand hygiene prevents the spread of microorganisms.
2. Put on PPE, as indicated.	PPE prevents the spread of microorganisms. PPE is required based on transmission precautions.
3. If not a crisis situation, identify the patient.	Identifying the patient ensures the right patient receives the intervention and helps prevent errors.
4. Explain what you are going to do and the reason for doing it to the patient, even if the patient does not appear to be alert.	Explanation alleviates fears. Even if the patient appears unconscious, the nurse should explain what is happening.
5. Put on disposable gloves. Put on face shield or goggles and mask.	Using gloves deters the spread of microorganisms. PPE protects the nurse from pathogens.
6. **Ensure that the mask is connected to the bag device (Figure 1), the oxygen tubing is connected to the oxygen source, and the oxygen is turned on, at a flow rate of 10 to 15 L per minute (Figure 2).** This may be done by visualizing or by listening to the open end of the reservoir or tail: if air is heard flowing, the oxygen tubing is attached and on.	Expected results might **not** be accomplished if the oxygen tubing is not attached and on.

ACTION

RATIONALE

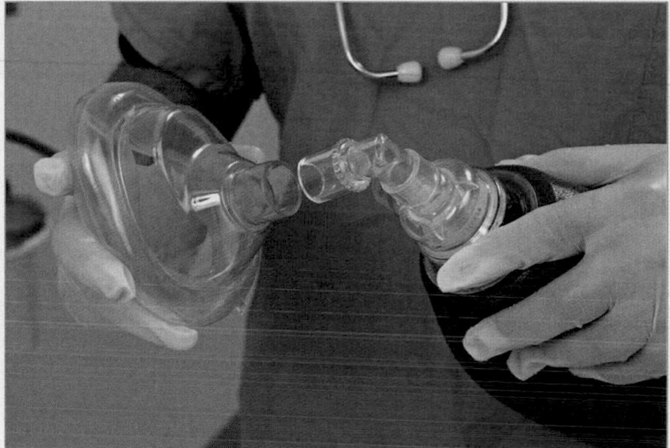

FIGURE 1 Connecting mask to bag-valve device.

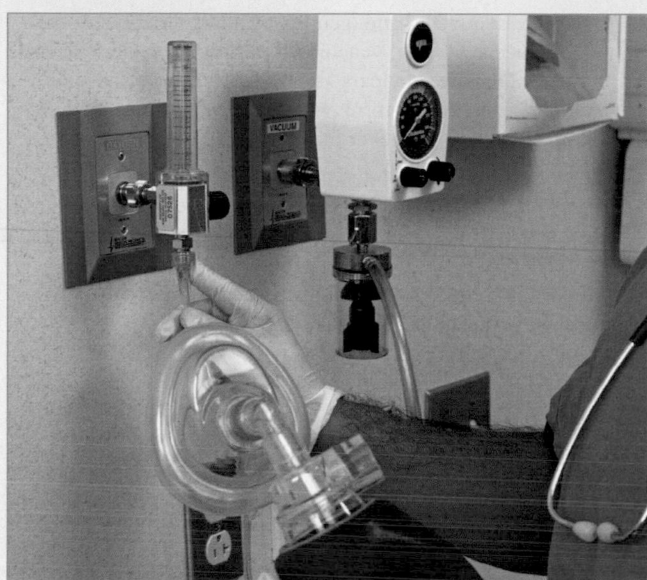

FIGURE 2 Connecting oxygen tubing on bag to oxygen source.

7. Initiate CPR, if indicated.

Start CPR in any situation in which either breathing alone or breathing and a heartbeat are absent. The brain is sensitive to hypoxia and will sustain irreversible damage after 4 to 6 minutes of no oxygen. The faster CPR is initiated, the greater the chance of survival.

8. If possible, get behind head of bed and remove headboard. **Slightly hyperextend the patient's neck (unless contraindicated). If unable to hyperextend, use jaw thrust maneuver to open airway.**

Standing at head of bed makes positioning easier when obtaining seal of mask to face. Hyperextending the neck opens the airway.

9. Place mask over the patient's face with opening over oral cavity. If mask is teardrop-shaped, the narrow portion should be placed over the bridge of the nose.

This helps ensure an adequate seal so that oxygen can be forced into the lungs.

10. **With dominant hand, place three fingers on the mandible, keeping head slightly hyperextended. Place thumb and one finger in C position around the mask, pressing hard enough to form a seal around the patient's face (Figure 3).**

This helps ensure that an adequate seal is formed so that oxygen can be forced into the lungs.

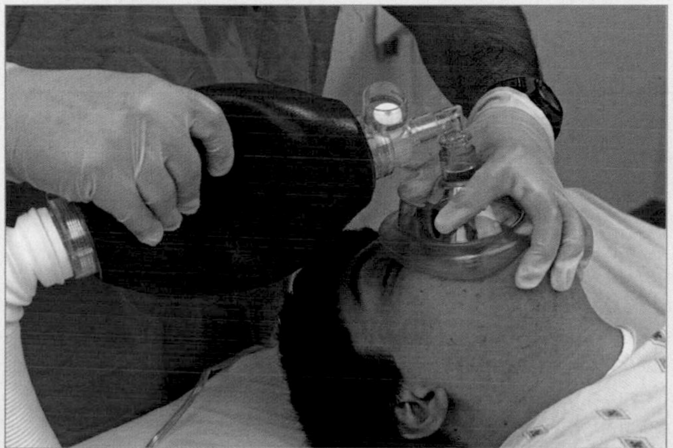

FIGURE 3 Creating a seal between mask and patient's face.

(continued)

SKILL 14-15 USING A MANUAL RESUSCITATION BAG AND MASK continued

ACTION	RATIONALE
11. Using nondominant hand, gently and slowly (over 2 to 3 seconds) squeeze the bag, watching the chest for symmetric rise. If two health care providers are available, one person should maintain a seal on the mask with two hands while the other squeezes the bag to deliver the ventilation and oxygenation.	Volume of air needed is based on patient's size. Enough has been delivered if the chest is rising. If air is introduced rapidly, it may enter the stomach.
12. Deliver the breaths with the patient's own inspiratory effort, if present. Avoid delivering breaths when the patient exhales. Deliver one breath every 5 seconds, if patient's own respiratory drive is absent. Continue delivering breaths until the patient's drive returns or until the patient is intubated and attached to mechanical ventilation.	Once patient's airway has been stabilized or patient is breathing on own, bag-mask delivery can be stopped.
13. Dispose of equipment appropriately.	Reduces the risk for transmission of microorganisms and contamination of other items.
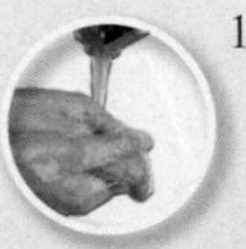 14. Remove face shield or goggles and mask. Remove gloves and additional PPE, if used. Perform hand hygiene.	Removing PPE properly reduces the risk for infection transmission and contamination of other items. Hand hygiene prevents the spread of microorganisms.

EVALUATION

The expected outcome is met when the patient demonstrates improved skin color and nail beds without evidence of cyanosis, the oxygen saturation level is within acceptable parameters, and normal sinus rhythm is evident. In addition, the patient maintains a patent airway and exhibits spontaneous respirations.

DOCUMENTATION

Guidelines

Document the incident, including the patient's respiratory effort before initiation of bag-mask breaths, lung sounds, oxygen saturation, chest symmetry, and resolution of incident (i.e., intubation or patient's respiratory drive returns).

Sample Documentation

9/1/15 2015 Patient arrived to emergency department with respiratory rate of four breaths per minute; respirations shallow; manual breaths delivered using adult bag with mask and 100% oxygen, oxygen saturation increased from 78% to 100% after eight breaths delivered; Dr. Alsup at bedside; patient sedated with 5 mg midazolam before intubation with 7.5-mm oral endotracheal tube, taped 10 cm at lips; lung sounds clear and equal in all lobes; see graphics for ventilator settings. Nasogastric tube placed via R naris to low intermittent suction, small amount of dark green drainage noted, chest x-ray obtained.

—*C. Bausler, RN*

UNEXPECTED SITUATIONS AND ASSOCIATED INTERVENTIONS

- *Breaths become increasingly difficult to deliver due to resistance:* Obtain order for placement of naso- or orogastric tube to remove air from the stomach (many facilities have policies that allow placement of a gastric tube during resuscitation). If air is delivered too fast, it may be introduced into the stomach. When the stomach fills with air, it decreases the space available for the lungs to inflate.
- *Chest is not rising when breaths are delivered, and resistance is felt:* Reposition the head or perform the jaw thrust maneuver. If the chest is not rising at all and resistance is being met, the tongue or another object is most likely obstructing the airway. If repositioning does not resolve the effort, consider performing the Heimlich maneuver.
- *Chest is rising asymmetrically:* Instruct assistant to listen to lung sounds bilaterally. Patient may need a chest tube placed due to pneumothorax. Anticipate the need for chest tube placement.

- *Oxygen saturation decreases from 100% to 80%:* Assess whether the chest is rising. If the chest is rising asymmetrically, the patient may have a pneumothorax. Anticipate the need for a chest tube. Check oxygen tubing. Someone may have stepped on the tubing, either kinking the tubing or pulling the tubing from the oxygen device.
- *A seal cannot be formed around the patient's face, and a large amount of air is escaping around mask:* Assess face and mask. Is the mask the correct size for the patient? If the mask size is correct, reposition fingers, or have a second person hold the mask while you compress the bag.

SPECIAL CONSIDERATIONS

- Have equipment to suction airway readily available when using a BVM. Air can be forced into the stomach during manual ventilation with a mask, causing abdominal distention. This distention can cause vomiting and possible aspiration. Be alert for vomiting; watch through the mask. If the patient starts to vomit, stop ventilating immediately, remove the mask, wipe and suction vomitus as needed, then resume ventilation.

ENHANCE YOUR UNDERSTANDING

FOCUSING ON PATIENT CARE: DEVELOPING CLINICAL REASONING

Consider the case scenarios at the beginning of the chapter as you answer the following questions to enhance your understanding and apply what you have learned.

QUESTIONS

1. Scott Mingus has a chest drain in place after thoracic surgery. The chest tube has been draining 20 to 30 mL of serosanguinous fluid every hour. Suddenly, the chest tube output is 110 mL/hour and the drainage is bright red. What should the nurse do?
2. Saranam Srivastava has a history of smoking and is scheduled for abdominal surgery. She needs to learn how to use an incentive spirometer. What should the nurse include in patient education regarding the use of an incentive spirometer?
3. Paula Cunningham needs to be suctioned via her endotracheal tube. What assessment findings would lead to this conclusion? How would the nurse determine if the suctioning of Ms. Cunningham's airway was effective?

You can find suggested answers after the Bibliography at the end of this chapter.

INTEGRATED CASE STUDY CONNECTION

The case studies in the back of the book are designed to focus on integrating concepts. Refer to the following case studies to enhance your understanding of the concepts related to the skills in this chapter.

- Basic Case Studies: Kate Townsend, page 1073.
- Intermediate Case Studies: Olivia Greenbaum, page 1077; George Patel, page 1091.
- Advanced Case Studies: Cole McKean, page 1093; Dewayne Wallace, page 1095; Jason Brown, Gwen Galloway, Claudia Tran, and James White, page 1099.

TAYLOR SUITE RESOURCES

Explore these additional resources to enhance learning for this chapter:

- NCLEX-Style Questions and other resources on thePoint, http://thePoint.lww.com/Lynn4e
- *Skill Checklists for Taylor's Clinical Nursing Skills,* 4e
- *Taylor's Video Guide to Clinical Nursing Skills:* Oxygenation and Tracheostomy Care
- *Fundamentals of Nursing:* Chapter 38, Oxygenation and Perfusion
- *Lippincott DocuCare* Fundamentals cases

Bibliography

Ackley, B.J., & Ladwig, G.B. (2011). *Nursing diagnosis handbook* (9th ed.). St. Louis: Mosby/Elsevier.

American Association for Respiratory Care (AARC). (2004). Clinical practice guideline: Nasotracheal suctioning—2004 revision & update. *Respiratory Care, 49*(9), 1080–1084.

American Association for Respiratory Care (AARC) Clinical Practice Guideline. (1999). Suctioning of the patient in the home. *Respiratory Care, 44*(1), 99–104.

American Heart Association (AHA). (2011). *BLS for healthcare providers. Student manual. Professional.* Author.

American Heart Association (AHA). (2012). CPR & ECC. *Two steps to staying alive with hands-only CPR.* Available http://www.heart.org/HEARTORG/CPRAndECC/HandsOnlyCPR/Hands-Only-CPR_UCM_440559_SubHomePage.jsp. Accessed June 19, 2012.

Arroyo-Novoa, C., Figueroa-Ramos, M., Puntillo, K., et al. (2008). Pain related to tracheal suctioning in awake acutely and critically ill adults: A descriptive study. *Intensive & Critical Care Nursing, 24*(1), 20–27.

Bauman, M., & Handley, C. (2011). Chest-tube care: The more you know, the easier it gets. *American Nurse Today, 6*(9), 27–32. Available http://www.americannursetoday.com/Article.aspx?id = 8256&fid = 8172. Accessed June 27, 2012.

Bullard, D., Brothers, K., Davis, C., Kingsley, E., & Waters III, J. (2012). Contraindications to nasopharyngeal airway insertion. *Nursing, 42*(10), 9–12.

Carlson, J., Mayrose, J., Krause, R., & Jehle, D. (2007). Extubation force: Tape versus endotracheal tube holders. *Annals of Emergency Medicine, 50*(6), 686–691.

Centers for Disease Control and Prevention (CDC). (2010). *Smoking and tobacco use. Health effects. Heart disease and stroke.* Available http://www.cdc.gov/tobacco/basic_information/health_effects/index.htm. Accessed June 11, 2012.

Collins, C., & Anderson, C. (2007). Deceptive simplicity: systemic oxygen delivery and pulse oximetry. *Journal of Paediatrics & Child Health, 43*(7–8), 510–512.

Crawford, D. (*2011*). Care and nursing management of a child with a chest drain. *Nursing Children and Young People, 23*(10), 27–33.

Davis, M., & Johnston, J. (2008). Maintaining supplemental oxygen during transport. *American Journal of Nursing, 108*(1), 35–36.

Day, W. (2011). On alert for iatrogenic pneumothorax. *Nursing, 41*, 66–67.

DeMeulenaere, S. (2007). Pulse oximetry: uses and limitations. *The Journal for Nurse Practitioners, 3*(5), 312–317.

Eastwood, G., Gardner, A., & O'Connell, B. (2007). Low-flow oxygen therapy: Selecting the right device. *Australian Nursing Journal, 15*(4), 27–30.

Ertuğ, N., & Ülker, S. (2011). The effect of cold application on pain due to chest tube removal. *Journal of Clinical Nursing, 21*(5/6), 784–790.

Fernandez, M., Burns, K., Calhoun, B., et al. (2007). Evaluation of a new pulse oximeter sensor. *American Journal of Critical Care, 16*(2), 146–152.

Field, J.M., Hazinski, M.F., Sayre, M.R., Chameides, L., Schexnayder, S.M., Hemphill, R., et al. (2010). 2010 American Heart Association Guidelines for cardiopulmonary resuscitation and emergency cardiovascular care. Part 1: Executive summary. *Circulation, 122*(Suppl 3), S640–S656.

Freeman, S. (2011). Care of adult patients with a temporary tracheostomy. *Nursing Standard, 26*(2), 49–56.

Friesner, S., Curry, D., & Moddeman, G. (2006). Comparison of two pain-management strategies during chest tube removal: Relaxation exercise with opioids and opioids alone. *Issues in Pain Management, 35*(4), 269–276.

Grossman, S., & Porth, C.M. (2014). Porth's pathophysiology: concepts of altered health states. (9th ed.). Philadelphia: Wolters Kluwer Health/Lippincott Williams & Wilkins.

Hahn, M. (2010). 10 considerations for endotracheal suctioning. *The Journal for Respiratory Care Practitioners, 23*(7), 32–33.

Hess, D.R., MacIntyre, N.R., Mishoe, S.C., Galvin, W.F., & Adams, A.B. (2012). *Respiratory care. Principles and practice* (2nd ed.). Sudbury, MA: Jones & Bartlett Learning.

Higginson, R., Jones, B, & Davies, K. (2010). Airway management for nurses: Emergency assessment and care. *British Journal of Nursing, 19*(16), 1006–1014.

Hinkle, J.L., & Cheever, K.H. (2014). *Brunner & Suddarth's textbook of medical-surgical nursing* (13th ed.). Philadelphia: Wolters Kluwer Health/Lippincott Williams & Wilkins.

Hogan-Quigley, B., Palm, M.L., & Bickley, L. (2012). *Bates' nursing guide to physical examination and history taking.* Philadelphia: Wolters Kluwer Health/Lippincott Williams & Wilkins.

Ireton, J. (2007). Tracheostomy suction: A protocol for practice. *Paediatric Nursing, 19*(10), 14–18.

Jarvis, C. (2012). *Physical examination & health assessment.* (6th ed.). St. Louis: Saunders/Elsevier.

Jensen, S. (2011). *Nursing health assessment. A best practice approach.* Philadelphia: Wolters Kluwer Health/Lippincott Williams & Wilkins.

The Joanna Briggs Institute. (2000). Tracheal suctioning of adults with an artificial airway. *Best Practice, 4*(4), 1–6.

Johnson, A., Schweitzer, D., & Ahrens, T. (2011). Time to throw away your stethoscope? Capnography: Evidence-based patient monitoring technology. *Journal of Radiological Nursing, 30*(1), 25–34.

Johnson, C.L., Anderson, M.A., & Hill, P.D. (2012). Comparison of pulse oximetry measures in a healthy population. *MEDSURG Nursing, 21*(2), 70–76.

Jongerden, I., Rovers, M., Grypdonck, M., et al. (2007). Open and closed endotracheal suction systems in mechanically ventilated intensive care patients: A meta-analysis. *Critical Care Medicine, 35*(1), 260–270.

Kee, J.L., Hayes, E.R., McCuistion, L.E. (2012). *Pharmacology. A nursing process approach* (7th ed.). St. Louis: Elsevier/Saunders.

Kyle, T., & Carman, S. (2013). *Essentials of pediatric nursing* (2nd ed.). Philadelphia: Wolters Kluwer Health/Lippincott Williams & Wilkins.

Lamar, J. (2012). Relationship of respiratory care bundle with incentive spirometry to reduce pulmonary complications in a medical general practice unit. *MEDSURGNursing, 21*(1), 33–36.

Macnee, W. (2007). Pathogenesis of chronic obstructive pulmonary disease. *Clinics in Chest Medicine, 28*(3), 479–513.

Maliakal, M. (2011). Chest tubes. *Nursing, 41*(7), 33.

Massey, D. (2010). Respiratory assessment 1: Why do it and how to do it? *British Journal of Cardiac Nursing, 6*(11), 537–541.

McCool, F., & Rosen, M. (2006). Nonpharmacologic airway clearance therapies: ACCP evidence-based clinical practice guidelines. *Chest, 129*(1), (Suppl): 250S–259S.

Meredith, T., & Massey, D. (2011). Respiratory assessment 2: More key skills to improve care. *British Journal of Cardiac Nursing, 6*(2), 63–68.

NANDA International. (2012). *Nursing diagnoses: Definitions & classification 2012–2014.* West Sussex, UK: Wiley-Blackwell.

Özden, D., & Gövgülü, R.S. (2012). Development of standard practice guidelines for open and closed system suctioning. *Journal of Clinical Nursing, 21*(9–10), 1327–1338.

Parkes, R. (2011). Rate of respiration: The forgotten vital sign. *Emergency Nurse, 19*(2), 12–17.

Pate, M. (2004). Placement of endotracheal and tracheostomy tubes. *Critical Care Nurse, 24*(3), 13.

Pate, M., & Zapata, T. (2002). Ask the experts: How deeply should I go when I suction an endotracheal or tracheostomy tube? *Critical Care Nurse, 22*(2), 130–131.

Pease, P. (2006). Oxygen administration: Is practice based on evidence? *Paediatric Nursing, 18*(8), 14–18.

Perry, S.E., Hockenberry, M.J., Lowdermilk, D.L., & Wilson, D. (2010). *Maternal child nursing care* (4th ed.). Maryland Heights, MO: Mosby/Elsevier.

Pruitt, B. (2007a). Latest advances in respiratory care. *Nursing, 37*(7), 56cc1, 56cc3.

Pruitt, B. (2007b). Take an evidence-based approach to treating acute lung injury. *Nursing, 37*(Suppl): 14–18.

Pullen, R.L. (2010). Using pulse oximetry accurately. *Nursing, 40*(4), 63.

Roman, M. (2005). Tracheostomy tubes. *MEDSURGNursing, 14*(2), 143–144.

Rubin, B.K. (2010). Air and soul: The science and application of aerosol therapy. *Respiratory Care, 55*(7), 911–921.

Rushing, J. (2007). Clinical do's and don'ts: Managing a water-seal chest drainage unit. *Nursing, 37*(12), 12.

Shimizu, T., Mizutani, T., Yamahita, S., Hagiya, K., & Tanaka, M. (2011). Endotracheal tube extubation force: Adhesive tape versus endotracheal tube holder. *Respiratory Care, 56*(11), 1825–1829.

Sole, M.L., Penoyer, D.A., Bennett, M., Bertrand, J., & Talbert, S. (2011). Oropharyngeal secretion volume in intubated patients: The importance of oral suctioning. *American Journal of Critical Care, 20*(6), e141–e145. Available ajcconline.org. Accessed June 26, 2012.

Stoller, J.K. (2011). An overview of home oxygen delivery devices and prescribing practices. *Canadian Journal of Respiratory Therapy, 47*(4), 22–27.

Subirana, M., Solà, I., & Benito, S. (2007). Closed tracheal suction systems versus open tracheal suction systems for mechanically ventilated adult patients. *Cochrane Database of Systematic Reviews*, Issue 4. Art. No.: CD004581.DOI: 10.1002/14651858.CD004581.pub2.

Sullivan, B. (2008). Nursing management of patients with a chest drain. *British Journal of Nursing, 17*(6), 388–393.

Sultan, P., Carvalho, B., Rose, B.O., & Cregg, R. (2011). Endotracheal tube cuff pressure monitoring: A review of the evidence. *Journal of Perioperative Practice, 21*(11), 379–386.

Tabloski, P. (2010). *Gerontological nursing* (2nd ed.). Upper Saddle River, NJ: Pearson.

Taylor, C.R, Lillis, C., & Lynn, P. (2015). *Fundamentals of nursing.* (8th ed.). Philadelphia: Wolters Kluwer Health/Lippincott Williams & Wilkins.

Taylor, J.J., & Cohen, B.J. (2013). *Memmler's structure and function of the human body* (10th ed.). Philadelphia: Wolters Kluwer Health/Lippincott Williams & Wilkins.

Van Leeuwen, A.M., Poelhuis-Leth, D., & Bladh, M.L. (2011). *Davis's comprehensive handbook of laboratory & diagnostic tests with nursing implications* (4th ed.). Philadelphia: F.A. Davis.

Vates, S. (2011). Delivering oxygen therapy in acute care: Part 2. *Nursing Times, 107*(22), 21–23.

VISN 8 Patient Safety Center. (2009). *Safe patient handling and movement algorithms.* Tampa, FL: Author. Available at http://www.visn8.va.gov/patientsafetycenter/safePtHandling. Accessed June 28, 2012.

Yönt, G.H., Korhan, E.A., & Khorshid, L. (2011). Comparison of oxygen saturation values and measurement times by pulse oximetry in various parts of the body. *Applied Nursing Research, 24*(4), e39–e43.

SUGGESTED ANSWERS FOR FOCUSING ON PATIENT CARE: DEVELOPING CLINICAL REASONING

1. Notify the primary care provider immediately. This can indicate fresh bleeding. Assess the patient's vital signs and level of consciousness. Significant changes from baseline may indicate complications. Assess the patient's respiratory status, including oxygen saturation level. The patient may become tachypneic and hypoxic. Assess the patient's lung sounds. The lung sounds over the chest tube site may be diminished due to the presence of increased blood. Also assess the patient for pain. Sudden

pressure or increased pain indicates potential complications. Reassure the patient, as necessary, to decrease anxiety. Maintain the patient on bed rest and monitor closely. Anticipate the need for additional IV fluids or blood transfusions, as well as the potential for surgery to control the bleeding.

2. Assess the patient's level of knowledge regarding the use of an incentive spirometer. Assess the patient's level of pain. Administer pain medication, as prescribed, if needed. Wait the appropriate amount of time for the medication to take effect. Explain the rationale for use of an incentive spirometer and the goal of the activity. If the patient has recently undergone abdominal or chest surgery, place a pillow or folded blanket over a chest or abdominal incision for splinting. Demonstrate how to steady the device with one hand and hold the mouthpiece with the other hand. If the patient cannot use hands, assist the patient with the incentive spirometer. Instruct the patient to exhale normally and then place lips securely around the mouthpiece. Instruct the patient to inhale slowly and as deeply as possible through the mouthpiece without using the nose (if desired, a nose clip may be used). When the patient cannot inhale anymore, the patient should hold her breath and count to three. Check the position of gauge to determine progress and level attained. If the patient begins to cough, splint an abdominal or chest incision. Instruct the patient to remove lips from mouthpiece and exhale normally. If the patient becomes light-headed during the process, tell her to stop and take a few normal breaths before resuming incentive spirometry. Encourage the patient to perform incentive spirometry 5 to 10 times every 1 to 2 hours, if possible. Clean the mouthpiece with water and shake to dry. Patient should verbalize an understanding of the rationale, procedure, and cleaning of equipment and be able to give a return demonstration of the use of the incentive spirometer.

3. Assess lung sounds. Patients who need to be suctioned may have wheezes, crackles, or gurgling present. Assess oxygen saturation level. Oxygen saturation usually decreases when a patient needs to be suctioned. Assess respiratory status, including respiratory rate and depth. Patients may become tachypneic when they need to be suctioned. Assess patient for signs of respiratory distress, such as nasal flaring, retractions, or grunting. Additional indications for suctioning via an endotracheal tube include secretions in the tube, acute respiratory distress, and frequent or sustained coughing. Also assess for pain and the potential to cause pain during the intervention. Perform individualized pain management in response to the patient's needs (Arroyo-Novoa et al., 2008). If the patient has had abdominal surgery or other procedures, administer pain medication before suctioning. Assess appropriate suction catheter depth. (Refer to Box 14-1.) Determine if suctioning the patient's airway was effective by reassessing the patient. The symptoms that indicated the need for airway suctioning should be absent or greatly diminished. The patient should not exhibit signs of respiratory distress, and should have an oxygen saturation level within normal limits.

15 Fluid, Electrolyte, and Acid–Base Balance

FOCUSING ON PATIENT CARE

This chapter will help you develop some of the skills related to fluid, electrolyte, acid–base balance necessary to care for the following patients:

SIMON LAWRENCE, age 3 years, has been admitted to the pediatric floor with dehydration after vomiting for 2 days. He needs intravenous fluids to become rehydrated.

MELISSA COHEN, age 32, was just involved in a motor vehicle crash. She has lost a large amount of blood and needs a blood transfusion.

JACK TRACY, age 67, is undergoing chemotherapy. He is to be discharged and needs his port deaccessed.

Refer to Focusing on Patient Care: Developing Clinical Reasoning at the end of the chapter to apply what you learn.

LEARNING OBJECTIVES

After studying this chapter, you will be able to:

1. Initiate a peripheral venous access IV infusion.
2. Change an IV solution container and administration set.
3. Monitor an IV site and infusion.
4. Change a peripheral venous access dressing.
5. Cap for intermittent use and flush a peripheral venous access device.
6. Administer a blood transfusion.
7. Change the dressing and flush a central venous access device.
8. Access an implanted port.
9. Deaccess an implanted port.
10. Remove a peripherally inserted central catheter (PICC).

KEY TERMS

autologous transfusion: a blood transfusion donated by the patient in anticipation that he or she may need the transfusion during a hospital stay

blood typing: determining a person's blood type (A, B, AB, or O)

central venous access device (CVAD): a venous access device in which the tip of the catheter terminates in the central venous circulation, usually in the superior vena cava just above the right atrium

crossmatching: determining the compatibility of two blood specimens

dehydration: the loss or deprivation of water from the body or tissues

edema: accumulation of fluid in body tissues

hypertonic: having a greater concentration of solutes than the solution with which it is being compared

hypervolemia (fluid volume excess): excess of isotonic fluid (water and sodium) in the extracellular space

hypotonic: having a lesser concentration than the solution with which it is being compared

hypovolemia (fluid volume deficit): deficiency of isotonic fluid (water and sodium) from the extracellular space

implanted port: a type of CVAD; subcutaneous injection port attached to a catheter; distal catheter tip dwells in the lower one third of the superior vena cava to the junction of the superior vena cava and the right atrium (Infusion Nurses Society [INS], 2006), and the proximal end or port is usually implanted in a subcutaneous pocket of the upper chest wall. Implanted ports placed in the antecubital area of the arm are referred to as *peripheral access system ports*.

isotonic: having about the same solute concentration as the solution with which it is being compared

nontunneled percutaneous central venous catheter: a type of CVAD that has a short dwell time (3 to 10 days); may have double, triple, or quadruple lumens; are more than 8 cm, depending on patient size; introduced through the skin into the internal jugular, subclavian, or femoral veins and sutured into place; and are mainly used in critical care and emergency settings (Gabriel, 2008)

peripherally inserted central catheter (PICC): a type of CVAD, more than 20 cm, depending on patient size, that can be introduced into a peripheral vein (usually the basilic, brachial, or cephalic vein), and advanced so the distal tip dwells in the lower one third of the superior vena cava to the junction of the superior vena cava and the right atrium (INS, 2006)

peripheral venous access device: a short (less than 3 inches) peripheral catheter placed in a peripheral vein for short-term therapy. This device is not appropriate for certain therapies, such as vesicant chemotherapy, drugs that are classified as irritants, or TPN.

tunneled central venous catheter: a type of CVAD; intended for long-term use; implanted into the internal or external jugular or subclavian vein; length of this catheter is more than 8 cm (approximately 90 cm on average), depending on patient size; tunneled in subcutaneous tissue under the skin (usually the midchest area) for 3 to 6 inches to its exit site

This chapter discusses the skills needed to care for patients with fluid, electrolyte, and acid–base balance needs. Because fluid is the main constituent of the body, the body's fluid balance is very important. The balance, or homeostasis, of water and dissolved substances (electrolytes) is maintained through the functions of almost every organ of the body. In a healthy person, fluid intake and fluid losses are about equal. Fundamentals Review 15-1 lists the average adult daily fluid sources and losses.

A common form of therapy for handling fluid and electrolyte disturbances is the use of various solutions infused intravenously (IV). The primary care provider is responsible for prescribing the kind and amount of solution to be used. The nurse is responsible for critically evaluating all patient orders prior to administration. Any concerns regarding the type or amount of therapy prescribed should be immediately and clearly communicated to the prescribing practitioner. The contents of selected IV solutions are listed, along with comments about their use, in Fundamentals Review 15-2. The nurse is responsible for initiating, monitoring, and discontinuing the therapy. As with other therapeutic agents, the nurse must understand the patient's need for intravenous therapy, the type of solution being used, its desired effect, and potential adverse reactions and effects (Fundamentals Review 15-3).

FUNDAMENTALS REVIEW 15-1

AVERAGE ADULT DAILY FLUID SOURCES AND LOSSES

Fluid Intake (mL)		Fluid Output (mL)	
Ingested water	1,650	Kidneys	1,500
Ingested food	650	Skin	600
Metabolic oxidation	300	Lungs	300
Total	*2,600*	Gastrointestinal	200
		Total	*2,600*

FUNDAMENTALS REVIEW 15-2

SELECTED INTRAVENOUS SOLUTIONS

Solution	Comments
Isotonic	
5% dextrose in water (D_5W)	Supplies about 170 cal/L and free water (contains 50 g of glucose) Used in fluid loss, dehydration, hypernatremia Should not be used in excessive volumes because it does not contain any sodium; thus, the fluid dilutes the amount of sodium in the serum. Brain swelling, or *hyponatremic encephalopathy,* can develop rapidly and cause death unless it is recognized and treated promptly.
0.9% NaCl (normal saline)	Not desirable as a routine maintenance solution because it provides only Na^+ and Cl^-, which are provided in excessive amounts. May be used to expand temporarily the extracellular compartment if circulatory insufficiency is a problem; also used to treat hypovolemia, metabolic alkalosis, hyponatremia, and hypochloremia. Used with administration of blood transfusions.
Lactated Ringer's solution	Contains multiple electrolytes in about the same concentrations as found in plasma (note that this solution is lacking in Mg^{2+} and PO_4^{3-}). Used in the treatment of hypovolemia, burns, and fluid lost from gastrointestinal sources. Useful in treating metabolic acidosis.
Hypotonic	
0.33% NaCl (⅓-strength normal saline)	Provides Na^+, Cl^-, and free water. Na^+ and Cl^- allow kidneys to select and retain needed amounts. Free water is desirable as aid to kidneys in elimination of solutes. Used in treating hypernatremia.
0.45% NaCl (½-strength normal saline)	A hypotonic solution that provides Na^+, Cl^-, and free water. Used as a basic fluid for maintenance needs. Often used to treat hypernatremia (because this solution contains a small amount of Na^+, it dilutes the plasma sodium while not allowing it to drop too rapidly).

FUNDAMENTALS REVIEW 15-2 continued

SELECTED INTRAVENOUS SOLUTIONS

Solution	Comments
Hypertonic	
5% dextrose in 0.45% NaCl	Used to maintain fluid intake.
10% dextrose in water ($D_{10}W$)	Supplies 340 cal/L. Used in peripheral parenteral nutrition (PPN).
5% dextrose in 0.9% NaCl (normal saline)	Used to treat SIADH (Syndrome of Inappropriate Antidiuretic Hormone). Can temporarily be used to treat hypovolemia if plasma expander is not available.

Adapted from Hinkle, J.L., & Cheever, K.H. (2014). *Brunner & Suddarth's textbook of medical-surgical nursing* (13th ed.). Philadelphia: Wolters Kluwer Health/Lippincott Williams & Wilkins.; Metheny, N.M. (2012). *Fluid and electrolyte balance. Nursing Considerations* (5th ed.). Sudbury, MA: Jones& Bartlett Learning; and *Fluids & electrolytes made incredibly easy!* (5th ed.). (2011). Philadelphia: Wolters Kluwer Health/Lippincott Williams & Wilkins.

FUNDAMENTALS REVIEW 15-3

COMPLICATIONS ASSOCIATED WITH INTRAVENOUS INFUSIONS

Complication/Cause	Signs and Symptoms	Nursing Considerations
Infiltration: the escape of fluid into the subcutaneous tissue Dislodged needle Penetrated vessel wall	Swelling, pallor, coldness, or pain around the infusion site; significant decrease in the flow rate	Check the infusion site every hour for signs/symptoms. Discontinue the infusion if symptoms occur. Restart the infusion at a different site. Use site-stabilization device.
Venous access device-related infection: Improper hand decontamination/hand hygiene Frequent disconnection of tubing, access ports, and/or access caps Poor insertion technique, multiple insertion attempts Multilumen catheters Long-term catheter insertion Frequent dressing changes Inadequate/improper decontamination of hub prior to use An IV solution that becomes contaminated when solutions are changed, a medication is added, or the solution is allowed to infuse for too long a period Inappropriate administration set changes	Erythema, edema, induration, drainage at the insertion site Fever, malaise, chills, other vital sign changes	Perform hand hygiene before and after palpating catheter insertion sites; before and after inserting, replacing, accessing, and dressing a venous access device. Assess catheter site at least daily. Notify primary care provider immediately if any signs of infection. Use scrupulous aseptic technique when starting an infusion. Follow best-practice guidelines for site care, changing of administration tubing sets, connectors, caps and other administration equipment. Follow facility protocol for culture of drainage. Consider use of 2% chlorhexidine wash for daily skin cleansing.

(continued)

FUNDAMENTALS REVIEW 15-3 continued

COMPLICATIONS ASSOCIATED WITH INTRAVENOUS INFUSIONS

Complication/Cause	Signs and Symptoms	Nursing Considerations
Phlebitis: an inflammation of a vein Mechanical trauma from needle or catheter Chemical trauma from solution	Local, acute tenderness; redness, warmth, and slight edema of the vein above the insertion site	Discontinue the infusion immediately. Apply warm, moist compresses to the affected site. Avoid further use of the vein. Restart the infusion in another vein.
Thrombus: a blood clot Tissue trauma from needle or catheter	Symptoms similar to phlebitis IV fluid flow may cease if clot obstructs needle	Stop the infusion immediately. Apply warm compresses as ordered by the primary care provider. Restart the IV at another site. *Do not rub or massage the affected area.*
Speed shock: the body's reaction to a substance that is injected into the circulatory system too rapidly Too rapid a rate of fluid infusion into circulation	Pounding headache, fainting, rapid pulse rate, apprehension, chills, back pains, and dyspnea	Use the proper IV tubing. Carefully monitor the rate of fluid flow. Check the rate frequently for accuracy. A time tape is useful for this purpose.
Fluid overload: the condition caused when too large a volume of fluid infuses into the circulatory system Too large a volume of fluid infused into circulation	Engorged neck veins, increased blood pressure, and difficulty in breathing (dyspnea)	If symptoms develop, slow the rate of infusion. Notify the primary care provider immediately. Monitor vital signs. Carefully monitor the rate of fluid flow. Check the rate frequently for accuracy.
Air embolus: air in the circulatory system Break in the IV system above the heart level allowing air in the circulatory system as a bolus	Respiratory distress Increased heart rate Cyanosis Decreased blood pressure Change in level of consciousness	Pinch off catheter or secure system to prevent entry of air. Place patient on left side in Trendelenburg position. Call for immediate assistance. Monitor vital signs and pulse oximetry.

SKILL 15-1 INITIATING A PERIPHERAL VENOUS ACCESS IV INFUSION

Administering and monitoring IV fluids is an essential part of routine patient care. The primary care provider often orders IV therapy to prevent or correct problems in fluid and electrolyte balance. For IV fluid and other therapies to be administered, an intravenous access must be established. Please review Figure 1, which illustrates potential infusion sites for peripheral venous catheters.

The nurse must also verify the amount and type of solution to be administered, as well as the prescribed infusion rate. The nurse is responsible for critically evaluating all patient orders prior to administration. Any concerns regarding the type or amount of therapy prescribed should be immediately and clearly communicated to the prescribing practitioner. The nurse must understand the patient's need for IV therapy, the type of solution being used, its desired effect, and potential adverse reactions and effects. Follow the facility's policies and guidelines to determine if the infusion should be administered by electronic infusion device or by gravity. Refer to Box 15-1 for guidelines to calculate flow rate for gravity infusion.

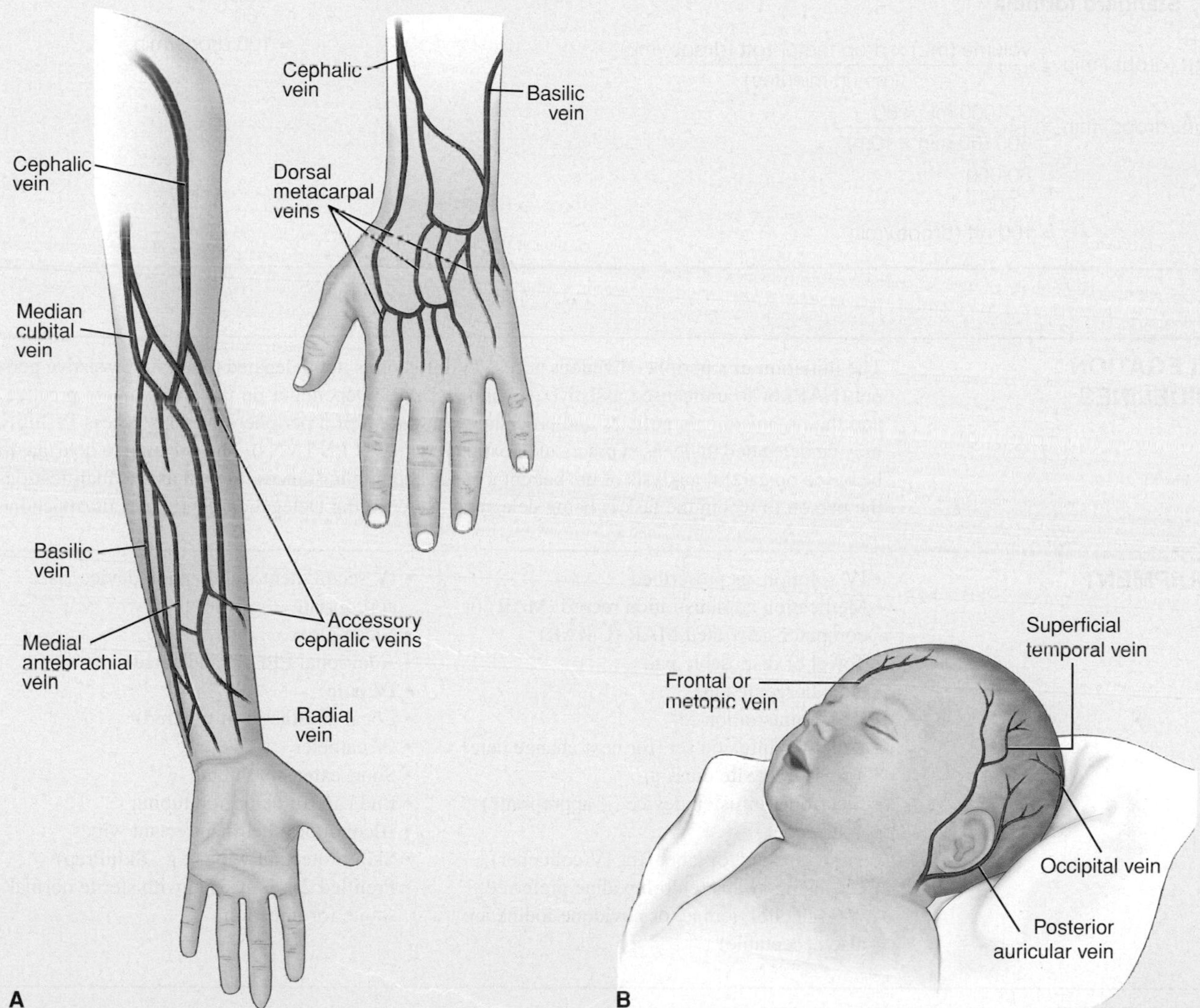

FIGURE 1 Infusion sites. (**A**) Ventral and dorsal aspects of lower arm and hand. (**B**) Scalp.

(continued)

SKILL 15-1 INITIATING A PERIPHERAL VENOUS ACCESS IV INFUSION continued

BOX 15-1 REGULATING IV FLOW RATE

Follow agency's guidelines to determine if infusion should be administered by electronic infusion device or by gravity.

- Check medical order for IV solution.
- Check patency of IV access.

If the infusion is to be administered by gravity infusion:

- Verify drop factor (number of gtt [drops] in 1 mL) of the equipment in use.
- Calculate the flow rate:

EXAMPLE—Administer 1000 mL D_5W over 10 hours (set delivers 60 gtt drops/1 mL).

a. Standard formula

$$\text{gtt (drops)/min} = \frac{\text{volume (mL)} \times \text{drop factor (gtt (drops)/mL)}}{\text{time (in minutes)}}$$

$$\text{gtt (drops)/min} = \frac{1000\text{ mL} \times 60}{600\ (60\text{ min} \times 10\text{ h})}$$

$$= \frac{60{,}000}{600}$$

$$= 100\text{ gtt (drops)/min}$$

b. Short formula using milliliters per hour

$$\text{gtt (drops)/min} = \frac{\text{milliliters per hour} \times \text{drop factor (gtt (drops)/mL)}}{\text{time (60 min)}}$$

Find milliliters per hour by dividing 1000 mL by 10 hours:

$$\frac{1000}{10} = 100\text{ mL/60}$$

$$\text{gtt (drops)/min} = \frac{100\text{ mL} \times 60}{60\text{ min}}$$

$$= \frac{6000}{60}$$

$$= 100\text{ drops/min}$$

DELEGATION GUIDELINES

The initiation of a peripheral venous access IV infusion is not delegated to nursing assistive personnel (NAP) or to unlicensed assistive personnel (UAP). Depending on the state's nurse practice act and the organization's policies and procedures, initiation of a peripheral venous access IV infusion may be delegated to licensed practical/vocational nurses (LPN/LVNs). The decision to delegate must be based on careful analysis of the patient's needs and circumstances, as well as the qualifications of the person to whom the task is being delegated. Refer to the Delegation Guidelines in Appendix A.

EQUIPMENT

- IV solution, as prescribed
- Medication administration record (MAR) or computer-generated MAR (CMAR)
- Towel or disposable pad
- Nonallergenic tape
- IV administration set
- Label for infusion set (for next change date)
- Transparent site dressing
- Electronic infusion device (if appropriate)
- Tourniquet
- Time tape and/or label (for IV container)
- Cleansing swabs (chlorhexidine preferred; 70% alcohol, iodine, or povidone-iodine are also acceptable)
- IV securement/stabilization device, as appropriate
- Clean gloves
- Additional PPE, as indicated
- IV pole
- Local anesthetic (if ordered)
- IV catheter
- Short extension tubing
- End cap for extension tubing
- Alcohol or other disinfectant wipes
- Skin protectant wipe (e.g., SkinPrep)
- Prefilled 2-mL syringe with sterile normal saline for injection

ASSESSMENT

Review the patient's record for baseline data, such as vital signs, intake and output balance, and pertinent laboratory values, such as serum electrolytes. Assess the appropriateness of the solution for the patient. Review assessment and laboratory data that may influence solution administration. Assess arms and hands for potential sites for initiating the IV. Keep in mind the following guidelines related to peripheral venous catheters and access sites:

- Determine the most desirable accessible vein. The dorsal and ventral surfaces of the upper extremities are appropriate sites for infusion (INS, 2011). The superficial veins on the dorsal aspect of the hand can also be used successfully for some people, but can be more painful (I.V. Rounds, 2008). Avoid the ventral surface of the wrist and the lateral surface of the wrist for approximately 4 to 5 inches because of the potential risk for nerve damage. Initiate venous access in the distal areas of the upper extremities, as this allows for future sites proximal to the previous insertion site (INS, 2011).

- Generally, either arm may be used for IV therapy. Usually the nondominant arm is selected for patient comfort and to limit movement in the impacted extremity. For example, if the patient is right-handed, the IV is preferably placed on the left extremity to improve the patient's ability to complete activities of daily living. This is particularly important if the duration of infusion is expected to be prolonged.
- Determine accessibility based on the patient's condition. The use of an extremity for IV therapy may be contraindicated in some circumstances. For example, patients with a history of breast cancer with same side surgical axillary lymph node removal; patients with burns, infections or traumatic injury to the extremity; and patients with upper extremity arterial-venous fistulas or catheters for dialysis treatment will not be able to have an IV catheter placed on the impacted extremity.
- Do not use the antecubital veins if another vein is available. They are not a good choice for infusion because flexion of the patient's arm can displace the IV catheter over time. By avoiding the antecubital veins for peripheral venous catheters, a PICC line may be inserted at a later time, if needed.
- Do not use veins in the leg of an adult, unless other sites are inaccessible, because of the danger of stagnation of peripheral circulation and possible serious complications. The cannulation of the lower extremities is associated with risk of tissue damage, thrombophlebitis, and ulceration (INS, 2011). Some facilities require a medical order to insert an IV catheter in an adult patient's lower extremity.

NURSING DIAGNOSIS

Determine the related factors for the nursing diagnoses based on the patient's current status. Appropriate nursing diagnoses may include:

- Deficient Fluid Volume
- Risk for Shock
- Risk for Deficient Fluid Volume

OUTCOME IDENTIFICATION AND PLANNING

The expected outcome to achieve when initiating a peripheral venous access IV infusion is that the access device is inserted using sterile technique on the first attempt. Also, the patient experiences minimal trauma, and the IV solution infuses without difficulty.

IMPLEMENTATION

ACTION	RATIONALE
1. Verify the IV solution order on the MAR/CMAR with the medical order. Consider the appropriateness of the prescribed therapy in relation to the patient. Clarify any inconsistencies. Check the patient's chart for allergies. Check for color, leaking, and expiration date. Know techniques for IV insertion, precautions, purpose of the IV administration, and medications if ordered. Gather necessary supplies.	This ensures that the correct IV solution and rate of infusion, and/or medication will be administered. The nurse is responsible for critically evaluating all patient orders prior to administration. Any concerns regarding the type or amount of therapy prescribed should be immediately and clearly communicated to the prescribing practitioner. This knowledge and skill is essential for safe and accurate IV and medication administration. Preparation promotes efficient time management and an organized approach to the task.
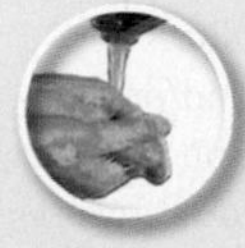 2. Perform hand hygiene and put on PPE, if indicated.	Hand hygiene and PPE prevent the spread of microorganisms. PPE is required based on transmission precautions.

(continued)

SKILL 15-1 INITIATING A PERIPHERAL VENOUS ACCESS IV INFUSION continued

ACTION	RATIONALE
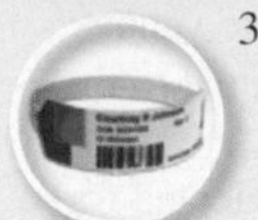 3. Identify the patient.	Identifying the patient ensures the right patient receives the intervention and helps prevent errors.
4. Close the curtains around the bed and close the door to the room, if possible. Explain what you are going to do and why you are going to do it to the patient. Ask the patient about allergies to medications, tape, or skin antiseptics, as appropriate. If considering using a local anesthetic, inquire about allergies for these substances as well.	This ensures the patient's privacy. Explanation relieves anxiety and facilitates cooperation. Possible allergies may exist related to medications, tape, or local anesthetic. Injectable anesthetic can result in allergic reactions and tissue damage.
5. If using a local anesthetic, explain the rationale and procedure to the patient. Apply the anesthetic to a few potential insertion sites. Allow sufficient time for the anesthetic to take effect.	Explanations provide reassurance and facilitate the patient's cooperation. Local anesthetic decreases the degree of pain felt at the insertion site. Some of the anesthetics take up to an hour to become effective.
Prepare the IV Solution and Administration Set	
6. Compare the IV container label with the MAR/CMAR. Remove IV bag from outer wrapper, if indicated. Check expiration dates. Scan bar code on container, if necessary. Compare on patient identification band with the MAR/CMAR. Alternately, label the solution container with the patient's name, solution type, additives, date, and time. Complete a time strip for the infusion and apply to IV container.	Checking the label with MAR/CMAR ensures the correct IV solution will be administered. Identifying the patient ensures the right patient receives the medications and helps prevent errors. Time strip allows for quick visual reference by the nurse to monitor infusion accuracy.
7. Maintain aseptic technique when opening sterile packages and IV solution. Remove administration set from package (Figure 2). Apply label to tubing reflecting the day/date for next set change, per facility guidelines.	Asepsis is essential for preventing the spread of microorganisms. Labeling tubing ensures adherence to facility policy regarding administration set changes and reduces the risk of spread of microorganisms. Refer to Box 15-2 in Skill 15-2 for recommended administration set change guidelines.

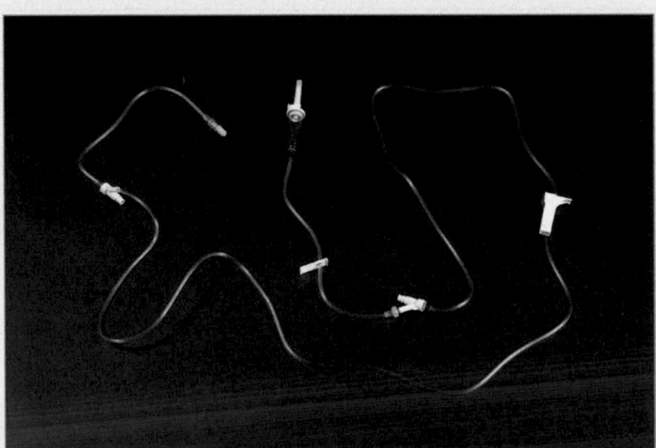

FIGURE 2 Basic administration set for gravity infusion. *(Photo by B. Proud.)*

ACTION	RATIONALE
8. Close the roller clamp or slide the clamp on the IV administration set (Figure 3). Invert the IV solution container and remove the cap on the entry site, taking care not to touch the exposed entry site. Remove the cap from the spike on the administration set. Using a twisting and pushing motion, insert the administration set spike into the entry site of the IV container (Figure 4). Alternately, follow the manufacturer's directions for insertion.	Clamping the IV tubing prevents air and fluid from entering the IV tubing at this time. Inverting the container allows easy access to the entry site. Touching the opened entry site on the IV container and/or the spike on the administration set results in contamination and the container/administration set would have to be discarded. Inserting the spike punctures the seal in the IV container and allows access to the contents.

ACTION	RATIONALE

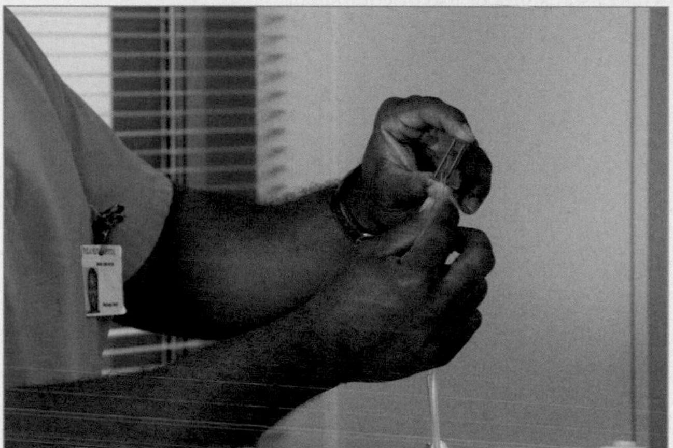

FIGURE 3 Closing clamp on administration set.

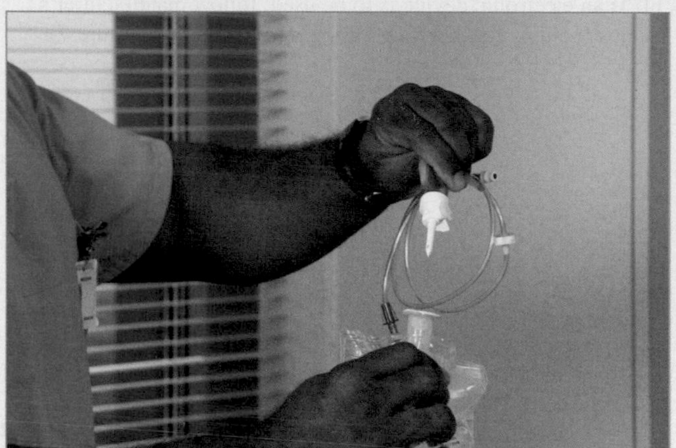

FIGURE 4 Inserting administration set spike into entry site of IV fluid container.

ACTION	RATIONALE
9. Hang the IV container on the IV pole. Squeeze the drip chamber and fill at least halfway (Figure 5).	Suction causes fluid to move into drip chamber. Fluid prevents air from moving down the tubing.
10. Open the IV tubing clamp, and allow fluid to move through tubing. Follow additional manufacturer's instructions for specific electronic infusion pump, as indicated. **Allow fluid to flow until all air bubbles have disappeared and the entire length of the tubing is primed (filled) with IV solution** (Figure 6). Close the clamp. Alternately, some brands of tubing may require removal of the cap at the end of the IV tubing to allow fluid to flow. Maintain its sterility. After fluid has filled the tubing, recap the end of the tubing.	This technique prepares for IV fluid administration and removes air from the tubing. If not removed from the tubing, large amounts of air can act as an embolus. Touching the open end of the tubing results in contamination and the administration set would have to be discarded.

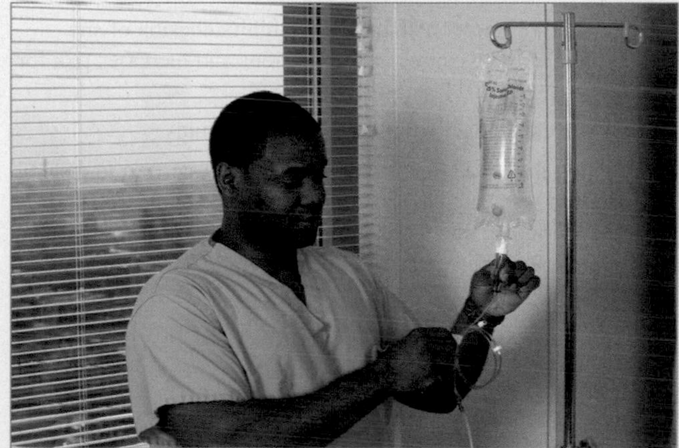

FIGURE 5 Squeezing drip chamber to fill at least halfway.

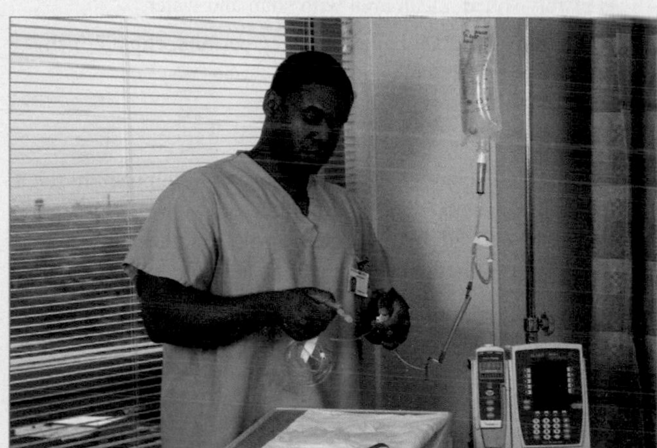

FIGURE 6 Priming administration set.

(continued)

SKILL 15-1 INITIATING A PERIPHERAL VENOUS ACCESS IV INFUSION continued

ACTION	RATIONALE
11. If an electronic device is to be used, follow manufacturer's instructions for inserting tubing into the device (Figure 7).	This ensures proper use of equipment.

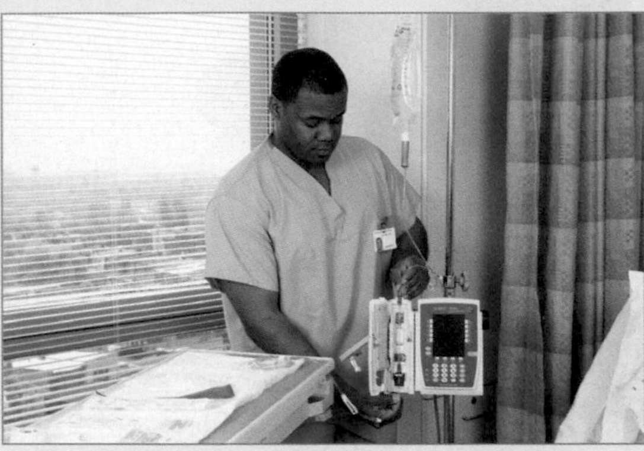

FIGURE 7 Inserting administration set into electronic infusion device.

Initiate Peripheral Venous Access

ACTION	RATIONALE
12. Place patient in low-Fowler's position in bed. Place protective towel or pad under patient's arm.	The supine position permits either arm to be used and allows for good body alignment. Towel protects underlying surface from blood contamination.
13. Provide emotional support, as needed.	Patient may experience anxiety because he/she may, in general, fear needlestick or IV infusion.
14. Open the short extension tubing package. Attach end cap, if not in place. Clean end cap with alcohol wipe. Insert syringe with normal saline into extension tubing. Fill extension tubing with normal saline and apply slide clamp. Remove the syringe and place extension tubing and syringe back on package, within easy reach.	Priming the extension tubing removes air from the tubing and prevents administration of air when connected to venous access. Having tubing within easy reach facilitates accomplishment of procedure.
15. Select and palpate for an appropriate vein. Refer to guidelines in previous Assessment section. If the intended insertion site is visibly soiled, clean area with soap and water.	The use of an appropriate vein decreases discomfort for the patient and reduces the risk for damage to body tissues.
16. If the site is hairy and agency policy permits, clip a 2-inch area around the intended entry site.	Hair can harbor microorganisms and inhibit adhesion of site dressing. Shaving causes microabrasions and increases risk for infection (INS, 2011, p. S44).
17. Put on gloves.	Gloves prevent contact with blood and body fluids.
18. Apply a tourniquet 3 to 4 inches above the venipuncture site to obstruct venous blood flow and distend the vein (Figure 8). Direct the ends of the tourniquet away from the entry site. Make sure the radial pulse is still present.	Interrupting the blood flow to the heart causes the vein to distend. Distended veins are easy to see, palpate, and enter. The end of the tourniquet could contaminate the area of injection if directed toward the entry site.

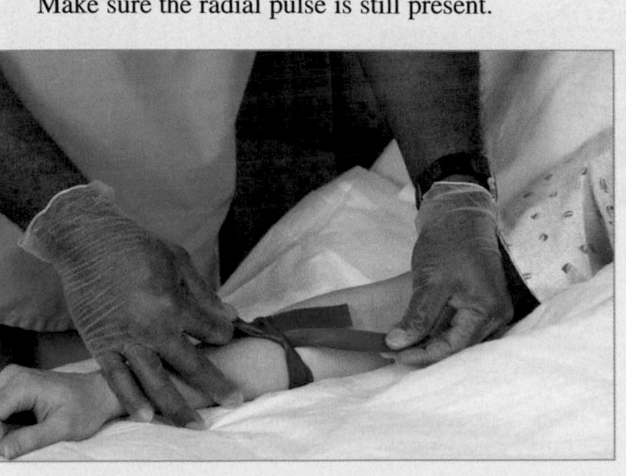

FIGURE 8 Applying tourniquet.

ACTION	RATIONALE
	Tourniquet may be applied too tightly so assessment for radial pulse is important.
	Checking radial pulse ensures arterial supply is not compromised.
19. Instruct the patient to hold the arm lower than the heart.	Lowering the arm below the heart level helps distend the veins by filling them.
20. Ask the patient to open and close the fist. Observe and palpate for a suitable vein. Try the following techniques if a vein cannot be felt:	Contracting the muscles of the forearm forces blood into the veins, thereby distending them further.
a. Lightly stroke the vein downward.	Massaging and tapping the vein help distend veins by filling them with blood.
b. Remove tourniquet and place warm, dry compresses over intended vein for 10 to 15 minutes.	Warm compresses help dilate veins. The use of dry heat increases the likelihood of successful peripheral catheter insertion (INS, 2011).
21. **Cleanse site with an antiseptic solution, such as chlorhexidine, or according to facility policy. Press applicator against the skin and apply chlorhexidine using a gentle back and forth motion. Do not wipe or blot. Allow to dry completely.**	Cleansing is necessary because organisms on the skin can be introduced into the tissues or the bloodstream with the needle. Chlorhexidine is the preferred antiseptic solution, but iodine, povidone-iodine, and 70% alcohol are considered acceptable alternatives (INS, 2011). Scrubbing motion creates friction and lets the solution more effectively penetrate the epidermal layers (Hadaway, 2006).
22. Alternately, for patients who bruise easily, are at risk for bleeding, or have fragile skin, **apply the chlorhexidine without scrubbing for at least 30 seconds. Allow to dry completely. Do not wipe or blot.**	Cleansing is necessary because organisms on the skin can be introduced into the tissues or the bloodstream with the needle. Avoiding use of scrubbing decreases risk of injury. A minimum of 30 seconds is the length of time that is necessary for chlorhexidine to be effective (Hadaway, 2006).
23. Using the nondominant hand placed about 1 or 2 inches below the entry site, hold the skin taut against the vein. **Avoid touching the prepared site.** Ask the patient to remain still while performing the venipuncture.	Pressure on the vein and surrounding tissues helps prevent movement of the vein as the needle or catheter is being inserted. The planned IV insertion site is not palpated after skin cleansing unless sterile gloves are worn to prevent contamination (INS, 2011). Patient movement may prevent proper technique for IV insertion.
24. Enter the skin gently, holding the catheter by the hub in your dominant hand, bevel side up, at a 10- to 15-degree angle (Figure 9). Insert the catheter from directly over the vein or from the side of the vein. While following the course of the vein, advance the needle or catheter into the vein. A sensation of "give" can be felt when the needle enters the vein.	This allows the needle or catheter to enter the vein with minimal trauma and deters passage of the needle through the vein.

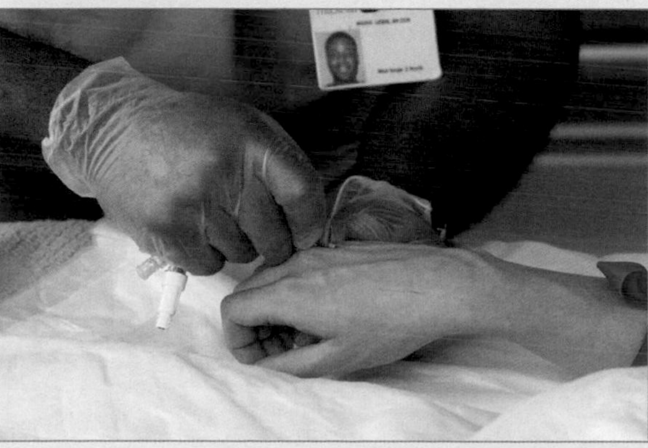

FIGURE 9 Stretching skin taut and inserting needle.

(continued)

SKILL 15-1 INITIATING A PERIPHERAL VENOUS ACCESS IV INFUSION continued

ACTION	RATIONALE
25. When blood returns through the lumen of the needle or the flashback chamber of the catheter, advance either device into the vein until the hub is at the venipuncture site. The exact technique depends on the type of device used.	The tourniquet causes increased venous pressure, resulting in automatic backflow. Placing the access device well into the vein helps to prevent dislodgement.
26. Release the tourniquet. Quickly remove the protective cap from the extension tubing and attach it to the catheter or needle. Stabilize the catheter or needle with your nondominant hand.	Bleeding is minimized and the patency of the vein is maintained if the connection is made smoothly between the catheter and tubing.
27. Continue to stabilize the catheter or needle and flush gently with the saline, observing the site for infiltration and leaking.	Infiltration and/or leaking and patient reports of pain and/or discomfort indicate that the insertion into the vein is not successful and should be discontinued.
28. Open the skin protectant wipe. Apply the skin protectant to the site, making sure to apply—at minimum—the area to be covered with the dressing. Place sterile transparent dressing or catheter securing/stabilization device over venipuncture site. Loop the tubing near the entry site, and anchor with tape (nonallergenic) close to the site.	Skin protectant aids in adhesion of the dressing and decreases the risk for skin trauma when the dressing is removed. Transparent dressing allows easy visualization and protects the site. Stabilization/securing devices preserve the integrity of the access device, minimize catheter movement at the hub, and prevent catheter dislodgement and loss of access (INS, 2011, p. S46). Some stabilization devices act as a site dressing also. The weight of the tubing is sufficient to pull it out of the vein if it is not well anchored. Nonallergenic tape is less likely to tear fragile skin.
29. Label the IV dressing with the date, time, site, and type and size of catheter or needle used for the infusion (Figure 10).	Other personnel working with the infusion will know the site, type of device is being used, and when it was inserted. Peripheral venous catheter IV insertion sites are changed every 72 to 96 hours for an adult (O'Grady et al., 2011).
30. Using an antimicrobial swab, cleanse the access cap on the extension tubing. Remove the end cap from the administration set. Insert the end of the administration set into the end cap (Figure 11). Loop the administration set tubing near the entry site, and anchor with tape (nonallergenic) close to the site. Remove gloves.	Inserting the administration set allows initiation of the fluid infusion. The weight of the tubing is sufficient to pull it out of the vein if it is not well anchored. Nonallergenic tape is less likely to tear fragile skin. Removing gloves properly reduces the risk for infection transmission and contamination of other items.

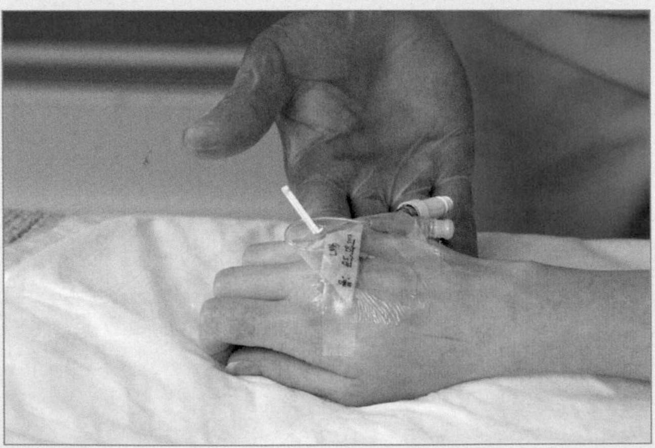

FIGURE 10 Venous access site with labeled dressing.

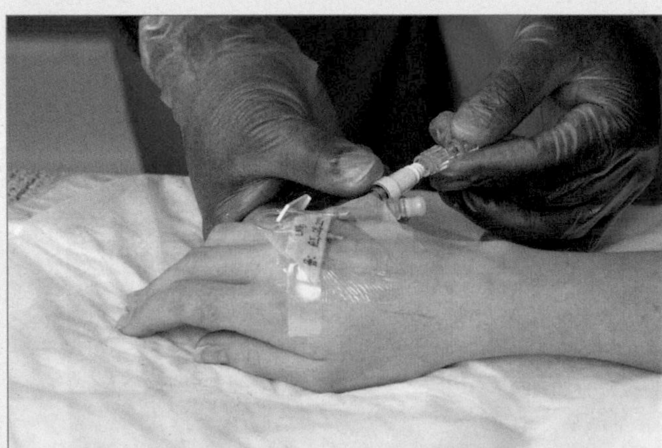

FIGURE 11 Inserting administration set into the end cap of venous access device.

ACTION	RATIONALE
31. Open the clamp on the administration set. Set the flow rate and begin the fluid infusion (Figure 12). Alternately, start the flow of solution by releasing the clamp on the tubing and counting the drops. Adjust until the correct drop rate is achieved. Assess the flow of the solution and function of the infusion device. Inspect the insertion site for signs of infiltration (Figure 13).	Verifying the rate and device settings ensures the patient receives the correct volume of solution. If the catheter slips out of the vein, the solution will accumulate (infiltrate) into the surrounding tissue.

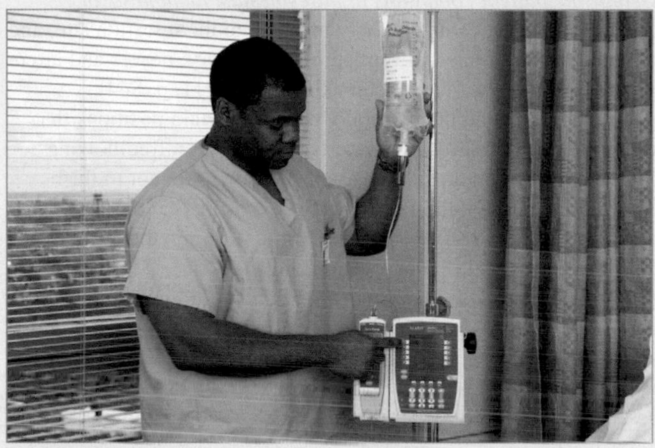

FIGURE 12 Initiating IV fluid infusion.

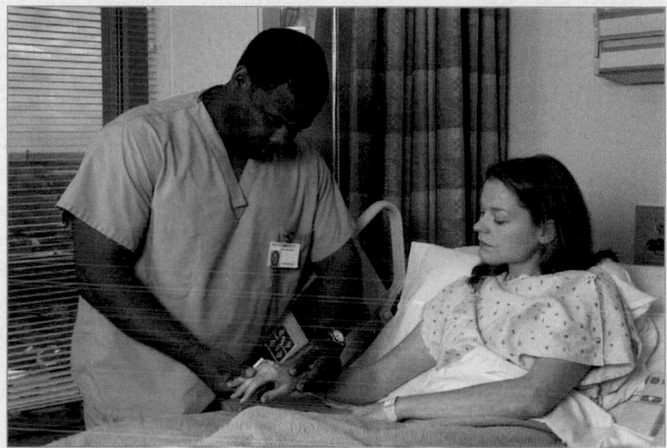

FIGURE 13 Inspecting insertion site.

ACTION	RATIONALE
32. Apply an IV securement/stabilization device if not already in place as part of the dressing, as indicated, based on facility policy. Explain to the patient the purpose of the device and the importance of safeguarding the site when using the extremity.	These systems are recommended for use on all venous access sites, and particularly central venous access sites, to preserve the integrity of the access device, minimize catheter movement at the hub, and prevent catheter dislodgement and loss of access (INS, 2011, p. S46). Some devices act as a site dressing also and may already have been applied.
33. Remove equipment and return the patient to a position of comfort. Lower bed, if not in lowest position.	Promotes patient comfort and safety.
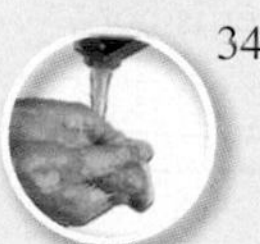 34. Remove additional PPE, if used. Perform hand hygiene.	Removing PPE properly reduces the risk for infection transmission and contamination of other items. Hand hygiene prevents transmission of microorganisms.
35. Return to check flow rate and observe IV site for infiltration and/or other complications 30 minutes after starting infusion, and at least hourly thereafter. Ask the patient if he/she is experiencing any pain or discomfort related to the IV infusion.	Continued monitoring is important to maintain correct flow rate. Early detection of problems ensures prompt intervention.

EVALUATION

The expected outcome is met when the IV access is initiated on the first attempt; fluid flows easily into the vein without any sign of infiltration; and the patient verbalizes minimal discomfort related to insertion and demonstrates an understanding of the reasons for the IV.

DOCUMENTATION

Guidelines

Document the location where the IV access was placed, as well as the size of the IV catheter or needle, the type of IV solution, and the rate of the IV infusion, as well as the use of a securing or stabilization device. Additionally, document the condition of the site. Record the patient's reaction to the procedure and pertinent patient teaching, such as alerting the nurse if the patient experiences any pain from the IV or notices any swelling at the site. Document the IV fluid solution on the intake and output record.

(*continued*)

SKILL 15-1 INITIATING A PERIPHERAL VENOUS ACCESS IV INFUSION continued

Sample Documentation

DocuCare Practice documenting peripheral venous access infusion in *Lippincott DocuCare.*

11/02/15 0830 20G IV started in L hand via the dorsal metacarpal vein. Transparent dressing and peripheral stabilization device applied. Site without redness, drainage, or edema. $D_5$1/2 NS with 20 mEq KCl begun at 110 mL/hour. Patient instructed to call with any pain, discomfort, or swelling.

—S. Barnes, RN

UNEXPECTED SITUATIONS AND ASSOCIATED INTERVENTIONS

- *An artery is inadvertently accessed or the patient complains of paresthesias, numbness, or tingling upon insertion:* Immediately remove the catheter, apply pressure to the insertion site, and notify the primary care provider. Rapid attention may prevent permanent injury; nerves and arteries are often located in very close proximity to the venipuncture site (INS, 2011, p. S44).
- *Fluid does not easily flow into the vein:* Reposition the extremity because certain positions that the patient may assume may prevent the IV from infusing properly. If the IV is a free-flowing IV, raise the height of the IV pole. This may promote an increase in IV flow. Attempt to flush the IV with 2 to 3 mL of saline in a syringe. Check the IV connector to ensure that the clamp is fully open. If fluid still does not flow easily, or if resistance is met while flushing, the IV may be against a valve and may need to be restarted in a different location.
- *Fluid does not flow easily into the vein and the skin around the insertion site is edematous and cool to the touch:* IV has infiltrated. Put on gloves and remove the catheter. Apply pressure with a sterile gauze pad. Secure gauze with tape over the insertion site and restart the IV in a new location. Estimate the volume of fluid that escaped into the tissue based on the rate of infusion and length of time since last assessment. Large volumes (greater than 25 to 50 mL) increase the risk of tissue damage (INS, 2011).
- *A small hematoma is forming at the site while you are inserting the catheter:* The vein is "blowing," which means a small hole has been made in the vein and blood is leaking out into the tissues. Remove and discard the catheter and choose an alternate insertion site.
- *Fluids are leaking around the insertion site:* Change dressing on IV. If site continues to leak, remove IV and restart it in a new location.
- *IV infusion set becomes disconnected from IV:* Discard IV tubing to prevent infection. Attempt to flush IV with 3 mL of normal saline. If the IV is still patent, the site may still be used, as long as the catheter hub has not been contaminated.
- *IV catheter is partially pulled out of insertion site (migrates externally):* Do not reinsert the catheter. Whether the IV is salvageable depends on how much of the catheter remains in the vein. Assess for proper placement in the vein before further use (INS, 2011). If this catheter is not removed, monitor it closely for signs of infiltration.

SPECIAL CONSIDERATIONS

General Considerations

- No more than two attempts at vascular access placement should be made by any one nurse when initiating venous access for a patient. If unsuccessful after two attempts, a colleague with advanced skills, such as a member of the nurse IV team, should attempt to initiate the venous access (Arbique & Arbique, 2007).
- Factors that may interfere with successful placement of a peripheral catheter include increased patient age, obesity, hypovolemia, injection drug use, and the presence of multiple, chronic diseases. These patients lack easy access using the traditional techniques of direct visualization, anatomic landmarks, and palpation (Houston, 2013; White et al., 2010). Ultrasound guided peripheral IV placement is a safe, efficient intervention for patients who are difficult to access (Maiocco & Coole, 2012; White et al., 2010). Consider the use of ultrasound to guide placement of a peripheral IV catheter by a specially trained nurse.
- Closed IV catheter systems are available. These systems have the short extension tubing integrated into the catheter, eliminating the need to attach extension tubing to the IV catheter before insertion, which reduces potential contamination.

Infant and Child Considerations

- Do not choose hand insertion sites as the first choice for children because their nerve endings are very close to the surface of the skin, and such an insertion is more painful. Once the child can walk, do not use the feet as insertion sites.
- Additional potential sites for neonates and children include veins of the scalp, foot, and fingers in infants and toddlers (INS, 2011). Scalp arteries in infants are visible (see Figure 1). Carefully palpate the site before insertion. If the site is pulsating, do not use.
- Do not replace peripheral catheters in children unless a complication develops (Centers for Disease Control and Prevention, 2011).
- Chlorhexidine is not recommended for infants under 2 months of age (INS, 2011). Use of chlorhexidine (in infants and children older than 2 months), 70% alcohol, iodine, or povidone-iodine is recommended for skin antisepsis for peripheral venous catheters (INS, 2011; O'Grady et al., 2011).
- For infants under 2 months of age or pediatric patients with compromised skin integrity, remove dried povidone-iodine with normal saline wipes or sterile water (INS, 2011).

Older Adult Considerations

- Avoid using vigorous friction at the insertion site, which can traumatize fragile skin and veins in older adults.
- To decrease the risk for trauma to the vessel, experienced nurses may omit use of a tourniquet if the patient has prominent but especially fragile veins.

EVIDENCE FOR PRACTICE ▶

INFUSION NURSING STANDARDS OF PRACTICE

Infusion Nurses Society. (2011). Infusion nursing standards of practice. *Journal of Infusion Nursing, 34*(1S), S1–S96.

The Infusion Nurses Society is recognized as the global authority in infusion therapy. The *Infusion Nursing Standards of Practice* is an evidence-based document, providing guidelines for nurses related to infusion therapy for use in all patient settings and addressing all patient populations.

Refer to thePoint for additional research on related nursing topics.

EVIDENCE FOR PRACTICE ▶

INTRAVENOUS ACCESS INSERTION AND USE OF LOCAL ANESTHETICS

Health care providers have an obligation to minimize patient discomfort and anxiety related to procedures. Fear and anxiety related to initiation of an intravenous access can be a source of stress for patients. Intradermal agents can provide effective local anesthesia for venipuncture. What is the effectiveness on pain and cost-effectiveness of these agents?

Related Research

Ganter-Ritz, V., Speroni, K.G., & Atherton, M. (2012). A randomized double-blind study comparing intradermal anesthetic tolerability, efficacy, and cost-effectiveness of lidocaine, buffered lidocaine, and bacteriostatic normal saline for peripheral intravenous insertion. *Journal of Infusion Nursing, 35*(2), 93–99.

The purpose of this randomized, double-blind study was to determine the tolerability, efficacy, and cost-effectiveness of three intradermal anesthetics for IV site preparation. Surgical patients (256) were randomized into one of three groups prior to insertion of a peripheral venous access device. Group 1 received intradermal anesthetic with 1% lidocaine. Group 2 received intradermal anesthetic using 1% buffered lidocaine. Group 3 received intradermal anesthetic using bacteriostatic normal saline with a benzyl alcohol preservative. Data were collected on patient demographics, type of surgery, dominant hand, insertion site, and number of venipunctures for successful IV placement. Patient evaluations were completed before the intradermal anesthetic IV site preparation/needlestick, after the intradermal anesthetic IV site preparation/needlestick, and after IV cannulation/catheter needlestick. Results demonstrated significant variations in patient pain perceptions for tolerability (average level of pain from intradermal insertion) and

(continued)

SKILL 15-1 INITIATING A PERIPHERAL VENOUS ACCESS IV INFUSION continued

efficacy (average level of pain at IV cannulation). The most tolerable solution was buffered lidocaine (Group 2). The most efficacious were Groups 1 and 2. Group 3 was the most cost-effective.

Relevance for Nursing Practice

Nurses are often responsible for initiating peripheral venous access for their patients. Many adult patients experience pain and stress related to initiation of venous access. Using the most efficient techniques can result in decreased pain and anxiety. Nurses and patients may be resistant to the use of intradermal anesthetics because of the need for a second needlestick. However, the use of these agents can significantly reduce the pain associated with initiation of IV access, possibly leading to increased patient satisfaction. Nurses should consider interventions to provide the best care for patients. This information can be used to assist in developing policies for nursing interventions and standards of practice related to insertion of peripheral IV access devices.

Refer to thePoint for additional research on related nursing topics.

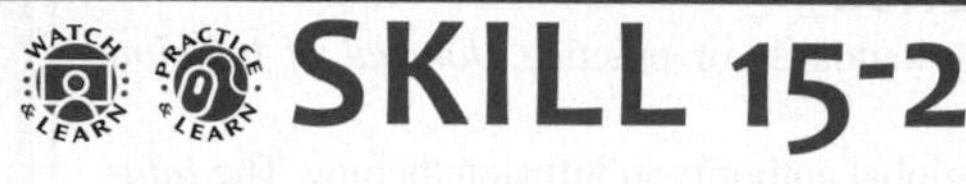

SKILL 15-2 CHANGING AN IV SOLUTION CONTAINER AND ADMINISTRATION SET

Intravenous fluid administration frequently involves multiple bags or bottles of fluid infusion. Verify the amount and type of solution to be administered, as well as the prescribed infusion rate. The nurse is responsible for critically evaluating all patient orders prior to administration. Any concerns regarding the type or amount of therapy prescribed should be immediately and clearly communicated to the prescribing practitioner. The nurse must understand the patient's need for IV therapy, the type of solution to be used, its desired effect, and potential adverse reactions and effects. Follow the facility's policies and guidelines to determine if the infusion should be administered by electronic infusion device or by gravity. Refer to Box 15-1 in Skill 15-1 for guidelines to calculate flow rate for gravity infusion. In addition, monitor these fluid infusions and replace the fluid containers, as needed. Focus on the following points:

- If more than one IV solution or medication is ordered, check facility policy and appropriate literature to make sure that the additional IV solution can be attached to the existing tubing.
- As one bag is infusing, prepare the next bag so it is ready for a change when less than 50 mL of fluid remains in the original container.
- Ongoing assessments related to the desired outcomes of the IV therapy, as well as assessing for both local and systemic IV infusion complications, are required. Refer to Fundamentals Review 15-3.
- Before switching the IV solution containers, check the date and time of the infusion administration set to ensure it does not also need to be replaced. Check facility policy for guidelines for changing IV administration sets. Refer to Box 15-2 for recommended administration set change guidelines.

Box 15-2 RECOMMENDED ADMINISTRATION SET CHANGE SCHEDULE

Type of Infusion/Type of Device	Recommended Frequency
• Primary and secondary continuous administration sets used to administer fluids other than lipid, blood, or blood products	• Change no more frequently than every 96 hours
• Anti-infective CVAD	• Change every 7 days
• Primary intermittent administration sets	• Change every 24 hours
• Secondary intermittent administration sets detached from the primary administration set	• Change every 24 hours
• Administration sets used to administer nonlipid-containing parenteral nutrition	• Change no more frequently than every 96 hours
• Administration sets used to administer parenteral nutrition containing fat emulsions	• Change every 24 hours
• Administration sets used to administer blood and blood components	• Change after the completion of each unit or every 4 hours

(Adapted from Infusion Nurses Society (INS). (2011). Infusion nursing standards of practice. *Journal of Infusion Nursing, 34* (Suppl1S); and O'Grady, N.P., Alexander, M., Burns, L.A., Dellinger, E.P., Garland, J., Heard, S.O., et al., & the Healthcare Infection Control Practices Advisory Committee (HICPAC). (2011). Guidelines for the prevention of intravascular catheter-related infections. *American Journal of Infection Control, 39* (4 Suppl.), S1–S34.)

DELEGATION CONSIDERATIONS

The changing of an IV solution container and administration set is not delegated to nursing assistive personnel (NAP) or to unlicensed assistive personnel (UAP). Depending on the state's nurse practice act and the organization's policies and procedures, these procedures may be delegated to licensed practical/vocational nurses (LPN/LVNs). The decision to delegate must be based on careful analysis of the patient's needs and circumstances, as well as the qualifications of the person to whom the task is being delegated. Refer to the Delegation Guidelines in Appendix A.

EQUIPMENT

For solution container change:
- IV solution, as prescribed
- MAR/CMAR
- Time tape and/or label (for IV container)
- PPE, as indicated

For tubing change:
- Administration set
- Label for administration set (for next change date)
- Sterile gauze
- Nonallergenic tape
- IV securement/stabilization device, as appropriate
- Clean gloves
- Additional PPE, as indicated
- Alcohol or other disinfectant wipes

ASSESSMENT

Review the patient's record for baseline data, such as vital signs, intake and output balance, and pertinent laboratory values, such as serum electrolytes. Assess the appropriateness of the solution for the patient. Review assessment and laboratory data that may influence solution administration.

Inspect the IV site. The dressing should be intact, adhering to the skin on all edges. Check for any leaks or fluid under or around the dressing. Inspect the tissue around the IV entry site for swelling, coolness, or pallor. These are signs of fluid infiltration into the tissue around the IV catheter. Also inspect the site for redness, swelling, and warmth. These signs might indicate the development of phlebitis or an inflammation of the blood vessel at the site. Ask the patient if he/she is experiencing any pain or discomfort related to the IV line. Pain or discomfort can be a sign of infiltration, extravasation, phlebitis, thrombophlebitis, and infection related to IV therapy. Refer to Fundamentals Review 15-3.

NURSING DIAGNOSIS

Determine the related factors for the nursing diagnoses based on the patient's current status. Appropriate nursing diagnoses may include:

- Deficient Fluid Volume
- Risk for Infection
- Impaired Skin Integrity

(continued)

SKILL 15-2 CHANGING AN IV SOLUTION CONTAINER AND ADMINISTRATION SET continued

OUTCOME IDENTIFICATION AND PLANNING

The expected outcome to achieve when changing an IV solution container and tubing is that the prescribed IV infusion continues without interruption and no infusion complications are identified.

IMPLEMENTATION

ACTION	RATIONALE
1. Verify the IV solution order on the MAR/CMAR with the medical order. Consider the appropriateness of the prescribed therapy in relation to the patient. Clarify any inconsistencies. Check the patient's chart for allergies. Check for color, leaking, and expiration date. Know the purpose of the IV administration, and medications if ordered. Gather necessary supplies.	This ensures that the correct IV solution and rate of infusion, and/or medication will be administered. The nurse is responsible for critically evaluating all patient orders prior to administration. Any concerns regarding the type or amount of therapy prescribed should be immediately and clearly communicated to the prescribing practitioner. This knowledge and skill is essential for safe and accurate IV and medication administration. Preparation promotes efficient time management and an organized approach to the task.
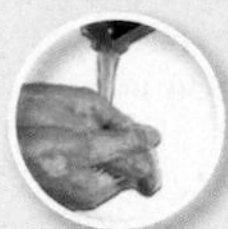 2. Perform hand hygiene and put on PPE, if indicated.	Hand hygiene and PPE prevent the spread of microorganisms. PPE is required based on transmission precautions.
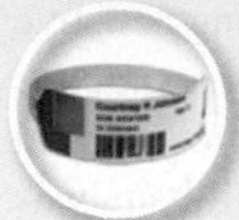 3. Identify the patient.	Identifying the patient ensures the right patient receives the intervention and helps prevent errors.
4. Close the curtains around the bed and close the door to the room, if possible. Explain what you are going to do and why you are going to do it to the patient. Ask the patient about allergies to medications or tape, as appropriate.	This ensures the patient's privacy. Explanation relieves anxiety and facilitates cooperation. Possible allergies may exist related to the IV solution additive or tape.
5. Compare IV container label with the MAR/CMAR (Figure 1). Remove IV bag from outer wrapper, if indicated. Check expiration dates. Scan bar code on container, if necessary. Compare patient identification band with the MAR/CMAR. Alternately, label solution container with the patient's name, solution type, additives, date, and time. Complete a time strip for the infusion and apply to IV container.	Checking label with MAR/CMAR ensures the correct IV solution will be administered. Identifying the patient ensures the right patient receives the medications and helps prevent errors. Time strip allows for quick visual reference by the nurse to monitor infusion accuracy.

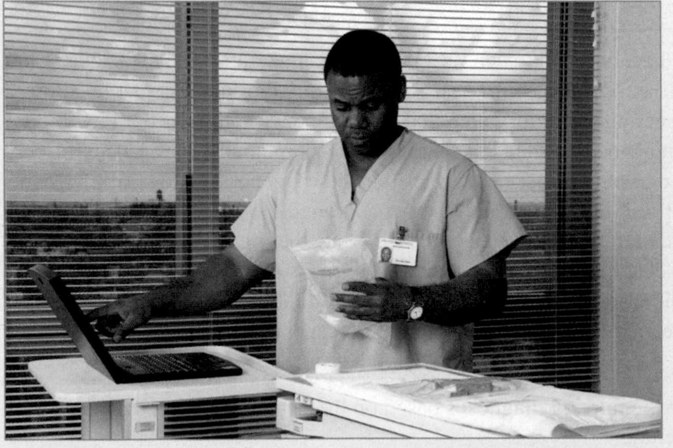

FIGURE 1 Comparing IV fluid container label with MAR/CMAR.

ACTION	RATIONALE
6. Maintain aseptic technique when opening sterile packages and IV solution. Remove administration set from package. Apply label to tubing reflecting the day/date for next set change, per facility guidelines.	Asepsis is essential for preventing the spread of microorganisms. Labeling tubing ensures adherence to facility policy regarding administration set changes and reduces risk of spread of microorganisms. Refer to Box 15-2 for recommended administration set change guidelines.
To Change IV Solution Container	
7. If using an electronic infusion device, pause the device or put on “hold.” Close the slide clamp on the administration set closest to the drip chamber. If using gravity infusion, close the roller clamp on the administration set.	The action of the infusion device needs to be paused while the solution container is changed. Closing the clamp prevents the fluid in the drip chamber from emptying and air from entering the tubing during the procedure.
8. Carefully remove the cap on the entry site of the new IV solution container and expose the entry site, **taking care not to touch the exposed entry site.**	Touching the opened entry site on the IV container results in contamination and the container would have to be discarded.
9. Lift empty container off IV pole and invert it. Quickly remove the spike from the old IV container, **being careful not to contaminate it**. Discard old IV container.	Touching the spike on the administration set results in contamination and the tubing would have to be discarded.
10. Using a twisting and pushing motion, insert the administration set spike into the entry site of the IV container. Alternately, follow the manufacturer’s directions for insertion. Hang the container on the IV pole.	Inserting the spike punctures the seal in the IV container and allows access to contents.
11. Alternately, hang the new IV fluid container on an open hook on the IV pole. Carefully remove the cap on the entry site of the new IV solution container and expose the entry site, **taking care not to touch the exposed entry site**. Lift empty container off the IV pole and invert it. Quickly remove the spike from the old IV container, **being careful not to contaminate it (Figure 2)**. Discard old IV container. Using a twisting and pushing motion, insert the administration set spike into the entry port of the new IV container as it hangs on the IV pole (Figure 3).	Touching the opened entry site on the IV container or the administration set spike results in contamination and both would have to be discarded. Inserting the spike punctures the seal in the IV container and allows access to contents.

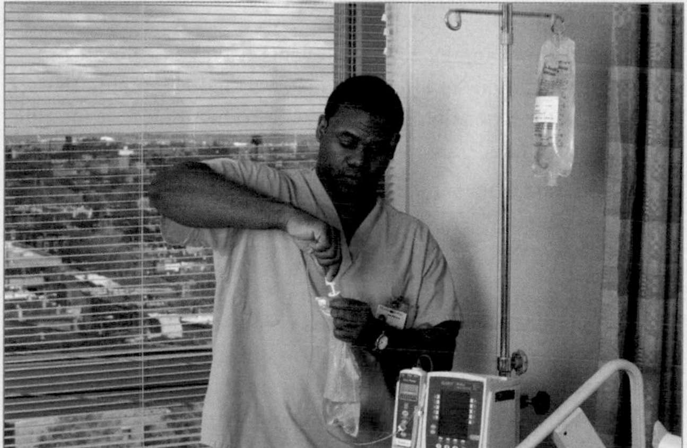

FIGURE 2 Removing administration spike from old IV fluid container.

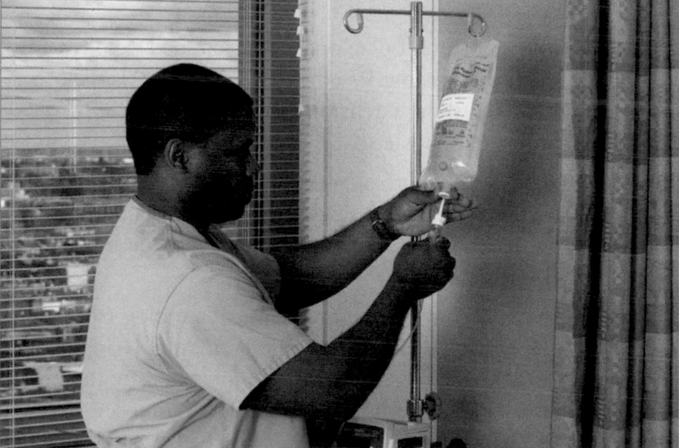

FIGURE 3 Inserting administration set spike into entry port of new IV fluid container.

(continued)

SKILL 15-2 CHANGING AN IV SOLUTION CONTAINER AND ADMINISTRATION SET continued

ACTION	RATIONALE
12. If using an electronic infusion device, open the slide clamp, check the drip chamber of the administration set, verify the flow rate programmed in the infusion device, and turn the device to "run" or "infuse."	Verifying the rate and device settings ensures the patient receives the correct volume of the solution.
13. If using gravity infusion, slowly open the roller clamp on the administration set and count the drops. Adjust until the correct drop rate is achieved (Figure 4).	Opening the clamp regulates the flow rate into the drip chamber. Verifying the rate ensures that the patient receives the correct volume of solution.

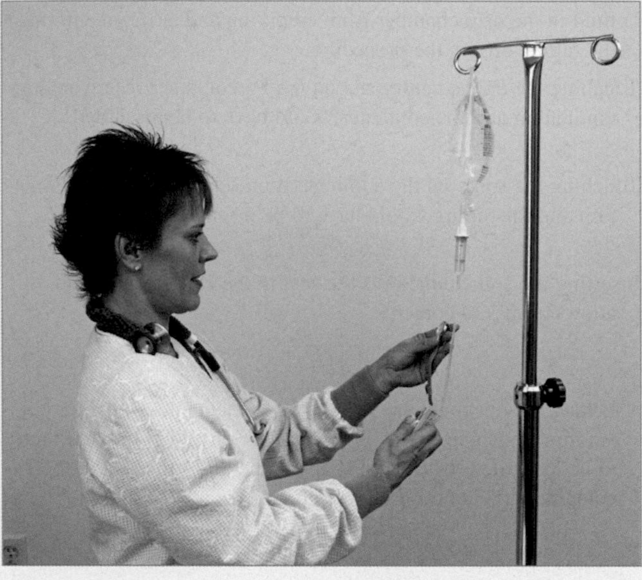

FIGURE 4 Reopening clamp and adjusting flow rate.

To Change IV Solution Container and Administration Set

ACTION	RATIONALE
14. Prepare the IV solution and administration set. Refer to Skill 15-1, Steps 6–10.	
15. Hang the IV container on an open hook on the IV pole. Close the clamp on the existing IV administration set. Also, close the clamp on the short extension tubing connected to the IV catheter in the patient's arm.	Clamping the existing IV tubing prevents leakage of fluid from the administration set after it is disconnected. Clamping the tubing on the extension set prevents introduction of air into the extension tubing.
16. If using an electronic infusion device, remove the current administration set from the device. Following manufacturer's directions, insert a new administration set into the infusion device.	Administration set has to be removed in order to insert new tubing into device.
17. Put on gloves. Remove the current infusion tubing from the access cap on the short extension IV tubing. Using an antimicrobial swab, cleanse access cap on extension tubing. Remove the end cap from the new administration set. Insert the end of the administration set into the access cap. Loop the administration set tubing near the entry site, and anchor with tape (nonallergenic) close to the site (Figure 5).	Cleansing the cap or port reduces the risk of contamination. Inserting the administration set allows initiation of the fluid infusion. The weight of the tubing is sufficient to pull it out of the vein if it is not well anchored. Nonallergenic tape is less likely to tear fragile skin.
18. Open the clamp on the extension tubing. Open the clamp on the administration set.	Opening clamps allows solution to flow to patient.

ACTION	RATIONALE

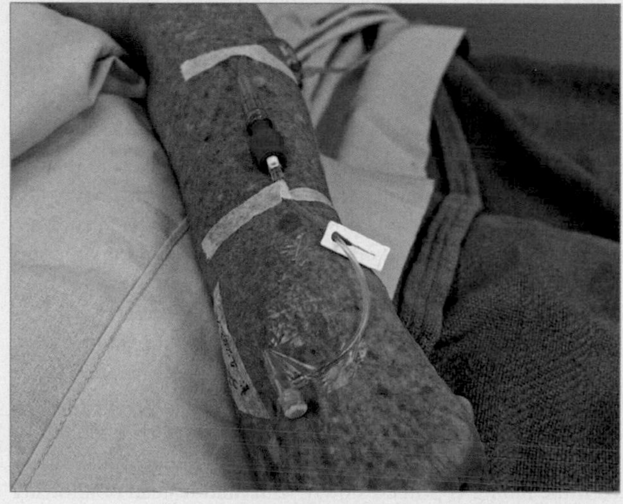

FIGURE 5 Making sure clamp is open on new tubing, with short extension tubing taped in place.

ACTION	RATIONALE
19. If using an electronic infusion device, open the slide clamp, check the drip chamber of the administration set, verify the flow rate programmed in the infusion device, and turn the device to "run" or "infuse."	Verifying the rate and device settings ensures the patient receives the correct volume of solution.
20. If using gravity infusion, slowly open the roller clamp on the administration set and count the drops. Adjust until the correct drop rate is achieved.	Opening the clamp regulates flow rate into the drip chamber. Verifying the rate ensures the patient receives the correct volume of solution.
21. Remove equipment. Ensure patient's comfort. Remove gloves. Lower bed, if not in lowest position.	Promotes patient comfort and safety. Removing gloves properly reduces the risk for infection transmission and contamination of other items.
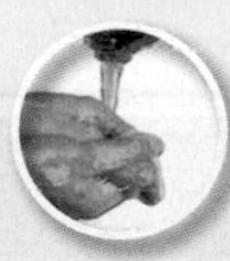 22. Remove additional PPE, if used. Perform hand hygiene.	Removing PPE properly reduces the risk for infection transmission and contamination of other items. Hand hygiene prevents transmission of microorganisms.
23. Return to check flow rate and observe IV site for infiltration and/or other complications 30 minutes after starting infusion, and at least hourly thereafter. Ask the patient if he/she is experiencing any pain or discomfort related to the IV infusion.	Continued monitoring is important to maintain the correct flow rate. Early detection of problems ensures prompt intervention.

EVALUATION

The expected outcome is achieved when the IV solution container and administration set are changed; the IV infusion continues without interruption; and no infusion complications are identified.

DOCUMENTATION

Guidelines

Document the type of IV solution and the rate of infusion (often done in the CMAR/MAR); and the assessment of the access site. Record the patient's reaction to the procedure and pertinent patient teaching, such as alerting the nurse if the patient experiences any pain from the IV or notices any swelling at the site. Document the IV fluid solution on the intake and output record.

(continued)

SKILL 15-2 CHANGING AN IV SOLUTION CONTAINER AND ADMINISTRATION SET continued

Sample Documentation

11/3/15 1015 IV fluid changed from $D_5$1/2 NS with 20 mEq KCl/L at 125 mL/hour to D_5 0.9% NS with 20 mEq KCl/L at 80 mL/hour. IV site intact; no swelling, redness, or drainage noted.

—*S. Barnes, RN*

UNEXPECTED SITUATIONS AND ASSOCIATED INTERVENTIONS

- *Infusion does not flow or flow rate changes after bag and tubing are changed:* Make sure that the flow clamp is open and the drip chamber is approximately half full. Check the electronic device for proper functioning. Check the IV site for possible problems with the catheter, such as bending of the catheter or position of the patient's extremity, and inspect the IV site for signs and symptoms of complications. Readjust the flow rate.
- *After attaching new IV tubing, you note air bubbles in the tubing:* If the bubbles are above the roller clamp, you can easily remove them by closing the roller clamp, stretching the tubing downward, and tapping the tubing with your finger so the bubbles rise to the drip chamber. If there is a larger amount of air in the tubing, swab the medication port on the tubing below the air with an antimicrobial solution and attach a syringe to the port below the air. Clamp the tubing below the access port. Aspirate the air from the tubing via the syringe. Remember that air bubbles in the tubing can be reduced if the tubing is primed slowly with fluid instead of allowing a wide-open flow of the solution.

EVIDENCE FOR PRACTICE ▶

INFUSION NURSING STANDARDS OF PRACTICE

Infusion Nurses Society. (2011). Infusion nursing standards of practice. *Journal of Infusion Nursing, 34*(1S), S1–S96.

Refer to details in Skill 15-1, Evidence for Practice, and refer to thePoint for additional research on related nursing topics.

SKILL 15-3 MONITORING AN IV SITE AND INFUSION

The nurse is responsible for monitoring the infusion rate and the IV site. This is routinely done as part of the initial patient assessment and at the beginning of a work shift. In addition, IV sites are checked at specific intervals and each time an IV medication is given, as dictated by the facility's policies. It is common to check IV sites every hour, but it is important to be familiar with the requirements of your facility. Monitoring the infusion rate is a very important part of the patient's overall management. If the patient does not receive the prescribed rate, he/she may experience a fluid volume deficit. In contrast, if the patient is administered too much fluid over a period of time, he/she may experience fluid volume overload. Other responsibilities involve checking the IV site for possible complications and assessing for both the desired effects of an IV infusion as well as potential adverse reactions to IV therapy.

DELEGATION CONSIDERATIONS

The monitoring of an IV site and infusion is not delegated to nursing assistive personnel (NAP) or to unlicensed assistive personnel (UAP). Depending on the state's nurse practice act and the organization's policies and procedures, these procedures may be delegated to licensed practical/vocational nurses (LPN/LVNs). The decision to delegate must be based on careful analysis of the patient's needs and circumstances, as well as the qualifications of the person to whom the task is being delegated. Refer to the Delegation Guidelines in Appendix A.

EQUIPMENT

- PPE, as indicated

ASSESSMENT

Inspect the IV infusion solution for any particulates and check the IV label. Confirm it is the solution ordered. Assess the current rate of flow by verifying the settings on the electronic infusion device or timing the drops if it is a gravity infusion. Check the tubing for kinks or anything that might clamp or interfere with the flow of the solution. Inspect the IV site. The dressing should be intact, adhering to the skin on all edges. Check for any leaks or fluid under or around the dressing. Inspect the tissue around the IV entry site for swelling, coolness, or pallor. These are signs of fluid infiltration into the tissue around the IV catheter. Also inspect the site for redness, swelling, and warmth. These signs might indicate the development of phlebitis or an inflammation of the blood vessel at the site. Ask the patient if he/she is experiencing any pain or discomfort related to the IV line. Pain or discomfort can be a sign of infiltration, extravasation, phlebitis, thrombophlebitis, and infection related to IV therapy. Refer to Fundamentals Review 15-3. Assess fluid intake and output. Assess the patient's knowledge of IV therapy.

NURSING DIAGNOSIS

Determine the related factors for the nursing diagnoses based on the patient's current status. Appropriate nursing diagnoses may include:

- Excess Fluid Volume
- Deficient Fluid Volume
- Risk for Infection

OUTCOME IDENTIFICATION AND PLANNING

The expected outcome to be met when monitoring the IV infusion and site is that the patient remains free from complications and demonstrates signs and symptoms of fluid balance.

IMPLEMENTATION

ACTION	RATIONALE
1. Verify IV solution order on the MAR/CMAR with the medical order. Consider the appropriateness of the prescribed therapy in relation to the patient. Clarify any inconsistencies. Check the patient's chart for allergies. Check for color, leaking, and expiration date. Know the purpose of the IV administration and medications, if ordered.	This ensures that the correct IV solution and rate of infusion, and/or medication will be administered. The nurse is responsible for critically evaluating all patient orders. Any concerns regarding the type or amount of therapy prescribed should be immediately and clearly communicated to the prescribing practitioner. This knowledge and skill is essential for safe and accurate IV and medication administration.
2. **Monitor IV infusion every hour or per facility policy. More frequent checks may be necessary if medication is being infused.**	Promotes safe administration of IV fluids and medication.
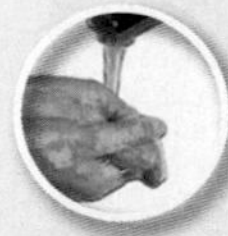 3. Perform hand hygiene and put on PPE, if indicated.	Hand hygiene and PPE prevent the spread of microorganisms. PPE is required based on transmission precautions.
4. Identify the patient.	Identifying the patient ensures the right patient receives the intervention and helps prevent errors.
5. Close the curtains around the bed and close the door to the room, if possible. Explain what you are going to do and why you are doing it to the patient.	This ensures the patient's privacy. Explanation relieves anxiety and facilitates cooperation.

(continued)

SKILL 15-3 MONITORING AN IV SITE AND INFUSION continued

ACTION	RATIONALE
6. If an electronic infusion device is being used, check settings, alarm, and indicator lights. Check set infusion rate (Figure 1). Note position of fluid in IV container in relation to time tape. Teach patient about the alarm features on the electronic infusion device.	Observation ensures that the infusion control device and the alarm are functioning. Lack of knowledge about "alarms" may create anxiety for the patient.

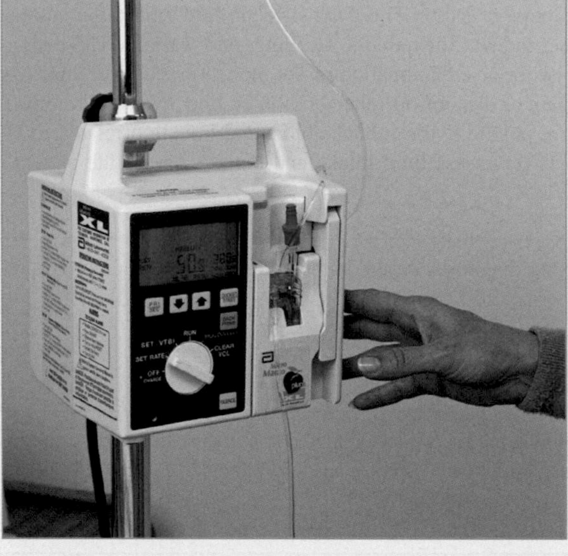

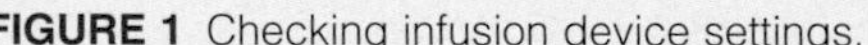

FIGURE 1 Checking infusion device settings.

ACTION	RATIONALE
7. If IV is infusing via gravity, check the drip chamber and time the drops (Figure 2). Refer to Box 15-1 in Skill 15-1 to review calculation of IV flow rates for gravity infusion.	This ensures that the flow rate is correct. Use a watch with a second hand for counting the drops in regulating a gravity drip IV infusion.
8. Check tubing for anything that might interfere with the flow (Figure 3). Be sure clamps are in the open position.	Any kink or pressure on tubing may interfere with the flow.

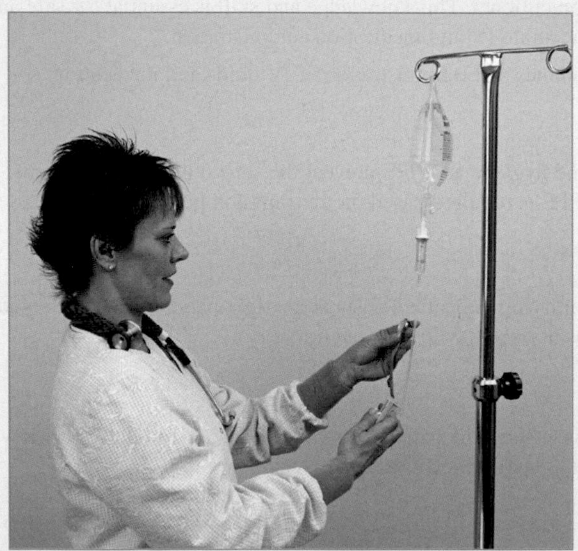

FIGURE 2 Checking drip chamber and timing drops.

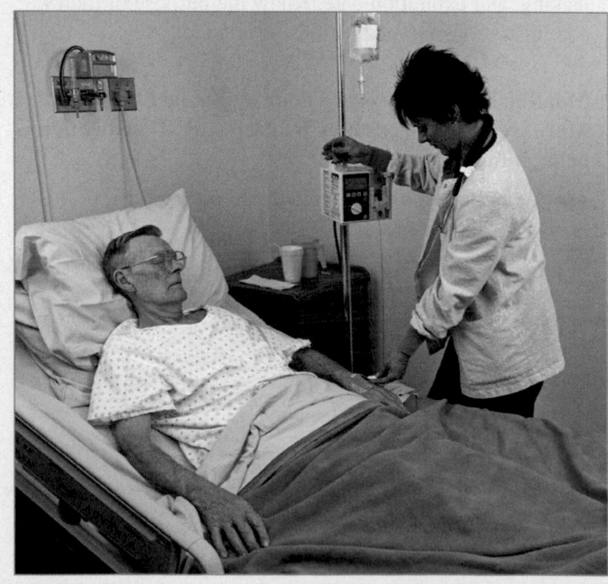

FIGURE 3 Checking tubing for anything that might interfere with flow rate.

ACTION	RATIONALE
9. Observe dressing for leakage of IV solution.	Leakage may occur at the connection of the tubing with the hub of the needle or the catheter and allow for loss of IV solution.
10. Inspect the site for swelling, leakage at the site, coolness, or pallor, which may indicate infiltration (Figure 4). Ask if patient is experiencing any pain or discomfort. If any of these symptoms are present, the IV will need to be removed and restarted at another site. Check facility policy for treating infiltration. See Fundamentals Review 15-3 and Box 15-3.	Catheter may become dislodged from the vein, and IV solution may flow into subcutaneous tissue.

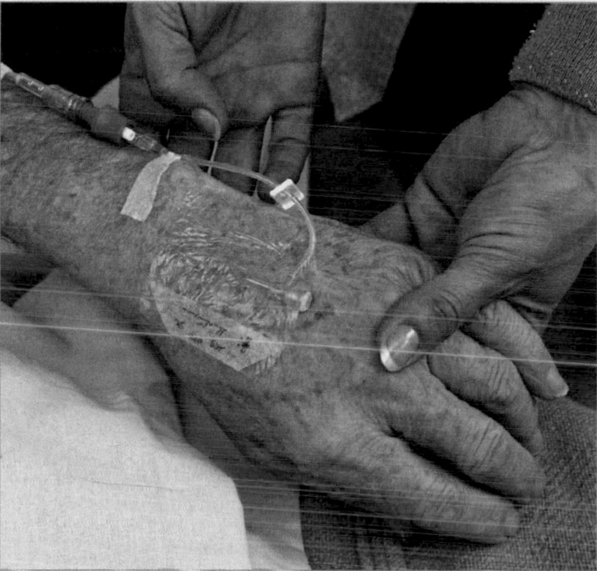

FIGURE 4 Inspecting IV site.

BOX 15-3 INFILTRATION SCALE

Grade and document infiltration according to the most severe presenting indicator.

Grade	Clinical Criteria
0	No symptoms
1	Skin blanched Edema <1 inch in any direction Cool to touch With or without pain
2	Skin blanched Edema 1 to 6 inches in any direction Cool to touch With or without pain
3	Skin blanched, translucent Gross edema >6 inches in any direction Cool to touch Mild to moderate pain Possible numbness
4	Skin blanched, translucent Skin tight, leaking Skin discolored, bruised, swollen Gross edema >6 inches in any direction Deep pitting tissue edema Circulatory impairment Moderate to severe pain Infiltration of any amount of blood product, irritant, or vesicant

(From Infusion Nurses Society. [2006]. Infusion nursing standards of practice. *Journal of Infusion Nursing, 29*(1S), p. S60, with permission.)

(*continued*)

SKILL 15-3 MONITORING AN IV SITE AND INFUSION continued

ACTION	RATIONALE
11. Inspect site for redness, swelling, and heat. Palpate for induration. Ask if patient is experiencing pain. These findings may indicate phlebitis. Notify the primary care provider if phlebitis is suspected. IV will need to be discontinued and restarted at another site. Check facility policy for treatment of phlebitis. Refer to Fundamentals Review 15-3 and Box 15-4.	Chemical irritation or mechanical trauma causes injury to the vein and can lead to phlebitis. Phlebitis is the most common complication related to IV therapy (Ingram & Lavery, 2005).

Box 15-4 PHLEBITIS SCALE

Grade and document phlebitis according to the most severe presenting indicator.

Grade	Clinical Criteria	Grade	Clinical Criteria
0	No symptoms	4	Pain at access site with erythema and/or edema Streak formation Palpable venous cord >1 inch in length Purulent drainage
1	Erythema at access site with or without pain		
2	Pain at access site with erythema and/or edema		
3	Pain at access site with erythema and/or edema Streak formation Palpable venous cord		

(From Infusion Nurses Society. [2011]. Infusion nursing standards of practice. *Journal of Infusion Nursing, 34*(1S), p. S65, with permission.)

ACTION	RATIONALE
12. Check for local manifestations (redness, pus, warmth, induration, and pain) that may indicate an infection is present at the site. Also check for systemic manifestations (chills, fever, tachycardia, hypotension) that may accompany local infection at the site. If signs of infection are present, discontinue the IV and notify the primary care provider. Be careful not to disconnect IV tubing when putting on patient's hospital gown or assisting the patient with movement.	Poor aseptic technique may allow bacteria to enter the needle, catheter insertion site, or tubing connection and may occur with manipulation of equipment.
13. Be alert for additional complications of IV therapy, such as fluid overload bleeding. Refer to Fundamentals Review 15-3.	Infusing too much IV solution results in an increased volume of circulating fluid volume.
a. Fluid overload can result in signs of cardiac and/or respiratory failure. Monitor intake and output and vital signs. Assess for edema and auscultate lung sounds. Ask if patient is experiencing any shortness of breath.	Older patients are most at risk for this complication due to possible decrease in cardiac and/or renal functions.
b. Check for bleeding at the site.	Bleeding may be caused by anticoagulant medication. Bleeding at the site is most likely to occur when the IV is discontinued.
14. If appropriate, instruct patient to call for assistance if any discomfort is noted at site, solution container is nearly empty, flow has changed in any way, or if the electronic pump alarm sounds.	This facilitates patient cooperation and safe administration of IV solution.
15. Remove PPE, if used. Perform hand hygiene.	Removing PPE properly reduces the risk for infection transmission and contamination of other items. Hand hygiene prevents transmission of microorganisms.

EVALUATION

The expected outcome is achieved when the patient remains free of complications related to IV therapy, exhibits patent IV site, and the IV solution infuses at the prescribed flow rate.

DOCUMENTATION

Guidelines

Document the type of IV solution as well as the infusion rate. Note the insertion site location and site assessment. Document the patient's reaction to the IV therapy as well as the absence of subjective reports that he/she is not experiencing any pain or other discomfort, such as coolness or heat associated with the infusion. Additionally, record that the patient is not demonstrating any other IV complications, such as signs or symptoms of fluid overload. Document the IV fluid solution on the intake and output record.

Sample Documentation

11/6/15 1020 IV site right forearm/cephalic vein intact without swelling, redness, or drainage. D_5 0.9% NS with 20 mEq KCl continues to infuse at 110 mL/hour. Patient instructed to call nurse with any swelling or pain.

—*S. Barnes, RN*

UNEXPECTED SITUATIONS AND ASSOCIATED INTERVENTIONS

- *Patient's lung sounds were previously clear, but now some crackles in the bases are auscultated:* Notify the primary care provider immediately. The patient may be exhibiting signs of fluid overload. Be prepared to tell the health care provider what the past intake and output totals were, as well as the vital signs and pulse oximetry findings of the patient.
- *IV is not flowing as easily as it previously had been:* Check all clamps on the tubing and check tubing for any kinking. Check that the patient is not lying on the tubing. If the IV is over a joint, reposition the extremity and see if this helps the flow. You may need to apply an arm board. Attempt to flush the IV with 2 to 3 mL of normal saline. If the IV is painful or you meet resistance when attempting to flush, discontinue the IV and restart in another place.

EVIDENCE FOR PRACTICE ▶

INFUSION NURSING STANDARDS OF PRACTICE

Infusion Nurses Society. (2011). Infusion nursing standards of practice. *Journal of Infusion Nursing, 34*(1S), S1–S96.

Refer to details in Skill 15-1, Evidence for Practice, and refer to thePoint for additional research on related nursing topics.

SKILL 15-4 CHANGING A PERIPHERAL VENOUS ACCESS DRESSING

The IV site is a potential entry point for microorganisms into the bloodstream. To prevent this, sealed IV dressings are used to occlude the site and prevent complications. Transparent semipermeable membrane (TSM) dressings are used most commonly to protect the insertion site. TSM dressings (e.g., Tegaderm or OpSite IV) allow easy inspection of the IV site and permit evaporation of moisture that accumulates under the dressing. Sterile gauze may also be used to cover the catheter site. A gauze dressing is recommended if the patient is diaphoretic or if the site is bleeding or oozing. However, the gauze dressing should be replaced with a TSM once this is resolved (O'Grady et al., 2011). The particular facility's policies determine the type of dressing used and when these dressings are changed. Routine site care and dressing changes are not performed on peripheral catheters unless the dressing is soiled or no longer intact (INS, 2011). However, dressing

(continued)

SKILL 15-4 CHANGING A PERIPHERAL VENOUS ACCESS DRESSING continued

changes might be required more often, based on nursing assessment and judgment. Any access site dressing that is damp, loosened, or soiled should be changed immediately. Whenever these dressings need to be changed, it is important to observe meticulous aseptic technique to minimize the possibility of contamination.

DELEGATION CONSIDERATIONS

The changing of a peripheral venous access dressing is not delegated to nursing assistive personnel (NAP) or to unlicensed assistive personnel (UAP). Depending on the state's nurse practice act and the organization's policies and procedures, the changing of a peripheral venous access dressing may be delegated to licensed practical/vocational nurses (LPN/LVNs). The decision to delegate must be based on careful analysis of the patient's needs and circumstances, as well as the qualifications of the person to whom the task is being delegated. Refer to the Delegation Guidelines in Appendix A.

EQUIPMENT

- Transparent occlusive dressing
- Cleansing swabs (chlorhexidine preferred; 70% alcohol, iodine, or povidone-iodine are also acceptable)
- Adhesive remover (optional)
- Alcohol or other disinfectant wipes
- Skin protectant wipe (e.g., SkinPrep)
- IV securement/stabilization device, as appropriate
- Tape
- Clean gloves
- Towel or disposable pad
- Additional PPE, as indicated

ASSESSMENT

Assess the IV site. The dressing should be intact, adhering to the skin on all edges. Check for any leaks or fluid under or around the dressing, or other indications that the dressing needs to be changed. Inspect the tissue around the IV entry site for swelling, coolness, or pallor. These are signs of fluid infiltration into the tissue around the IV catheter. Also inspect the site for redness, swelling, and warmth. These signs might indicate the development of phlebitis or an inflammation of the blood vessel at the site. Ask the patient if he/she is experiencing any pain or discomfort related to the IV line. Pain or discomfort can be a sign of infiltration, extravasation, phlebitis, thrombophlebitis, and infection related to IV therapy. Refer to Fundamentals Review 15-3. Note the insertion date and date of last dressing change, if different from insertion date. Also assess the patient's need to maintain venous access. If patient does not need the access, discuss the possibility of discontinuation with the primary care provider. Ask the patient about any allergies.

NURSING DIAGNOSIS

Determine the related factors for the nursing diagnoses based on the patient's current status. Appropriate nursing diagnoses may include:

- Risk for Infection
- Risk for Injury
- Risk for Impaired Skin Integrity

OUTCOME IDENTIFICATION AND PLANNING

The expected outcome to achieve when changing a peripheral venous access dressing is that the patient will exhibit an access site that is clean, dry, and without evidence of any signs and symptoms of infection, infiltration, or phlebitis. In addition, the dressing will be clean, dry, and intact and the patient will not experience injury.

IMPLEMENTATION

ACTION	RATIONALE
1. Determine the need for a dressing change. Check facility policy. Gather equipment.	The particular facility's policies determine the type of dressing used and when these dressings are changed. Dressing changes might be required more often, based on nursing assessment and judgment. Immediately change any access site dressing that is damp, loosened, or soiled. Preparation promotes efficient time management and an organized approach to the task.

ACTION	RATIONALE
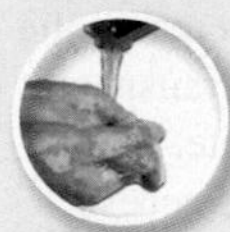 2. Perform hand hygiene and put on PPE, if indicated.	Hand hygiene and PPE prevent the spread of microorganisms. PPE is required based on transmission precautions.
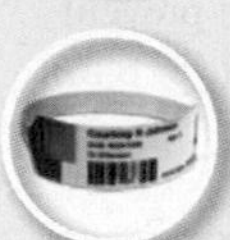 3. Identify the patient.	Identifying the patient ensures the right patient receives the intervention and helps prevent errors.
4. Close the curtains around the bed and close the door to the room, if possible. Explain what you are going to do and why you are going to do it to the patient. Ask the patient about allergies to tape and skin antiseptics.	This ensures the patient's privacy. Explanation relieves anxiety and facilitates cooperation. Possible allergies may exist related to tape or antiseptics.
5. Put on gloves. Place towel or disposable pad under the arm with the venous access. If solution is currently infusing, temporarily stop the infusion. Hold the catheter in place with your nondominant hand and **carefully remove old dressing and/or stabilization/securing device** (Figure 1). Use adhesive remover as necessary. Discard dressing.	Gloves prevent contact with blood and body fluids. Pad protects underlying surface. Proper disposal of dressing prevents transmission of microorganisms.

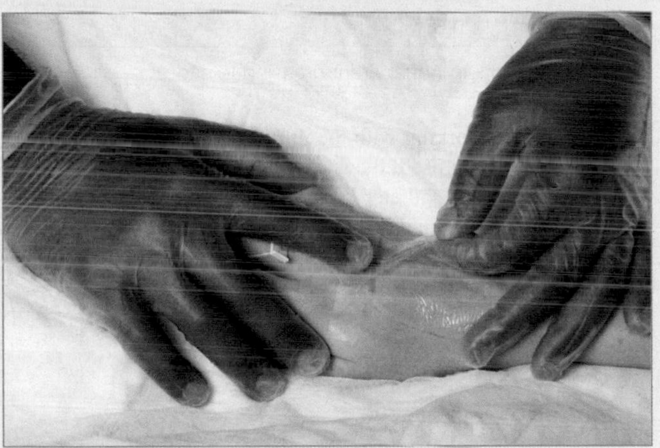

FIGURE 1 Carefully removing old dressing.

ACTION	RATIONALE
6. **Inspect IV site for presence of phlebitis (inflammation), infection, or infiltration.** Discontinue and relocate IV, if noted. Refer to Fundamentals Review 15-3 and Boxes 15-3 and 15-4 (in Skill 15-3).	Inflammation (phlebitis), infection, or infiltration causes trauma to tissues and necessitates removal of the venous access device.
7. **Cleanse the site with an antiseptic solution, such as chlorhexidine, or according to facility policy. Press applicator against the skin and apply chlorhexidine using a gentle back and forth motion. Do not wipe or blot. Allow to dry completely.**	Cleansing the skin is necessary because organisms on the skin can be introduced into the tissues or the bloodstream with the venous access. Chlorhexidine is the preferred antiseptic solution, but iodine, povidone-iodine, and 70% alcohol are considered acceptable alternatives (INS, 2011). A scrubbing motion creates friction and lets the solution more effectively penetrate the epidermal layers (Hadaway, 2006).

(continued)

SKILL 15-4 CHANGING A PERIPHERAL VENOUS ACCESS DRESSING continued

ACTION	RATIONALE
8. Open the skin protectant wipe. Apply it to the site, making sure to cover at minimum the area to be covered with the dressing (Figure 2). Allow to dry. Place sterile transparent dressing or catheter securing/stabilization device over the venipuncture site (Figure 3).	Skin protectant aids in adhesion of the dressing and decreases the risk for skin trauma when the dressing is removed. Transparent dressing allows easy visualization and protects the site. Stabilization/securing devices preserve the integrity of the access device, minimize catheter movement at the hub, and prevent catheter dislodgement and loss of access (INS, 2011, p. S46). Some stabilization devices act as a site dressing also.

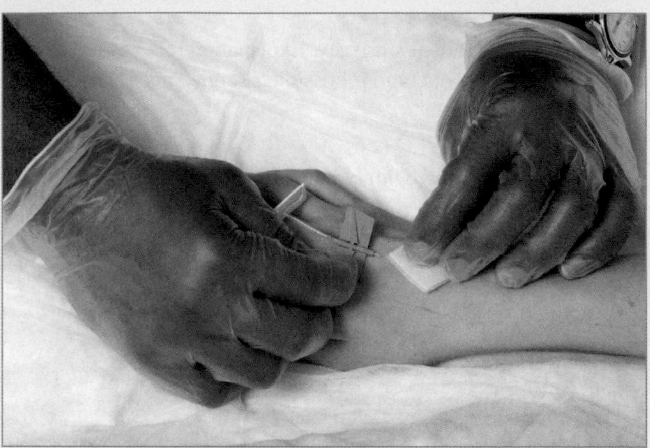

FIGURE 2 Applying skin protectant to site.

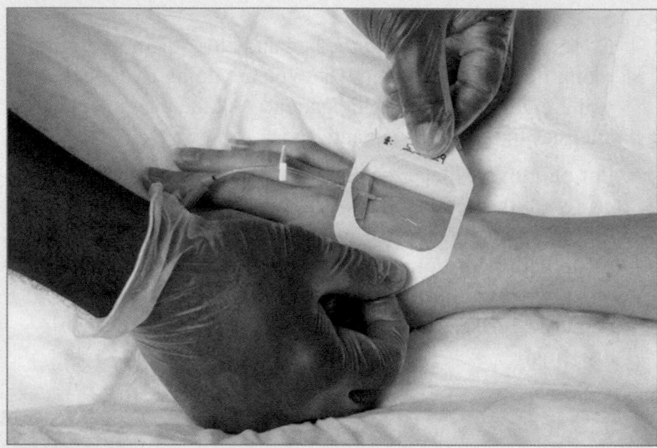

FIGURE 3 Applying transparent dressing to site.

ACTION	RATIONALE
9. Label dressing with date, time of change, and initials. Loop the tubing near the entry site, and anchor with tape (nonallergenic) close to site (Figure 4). Resume fluid infusion, if indicated. Check that IV flow is accurate and system is patent. Refer to Skill 15-3.	Other personnel working with the infusion will know what type of device is being used, the site, and when it was inserted. Peripheral venous catheter IV insertion sites are changed every 72 to 96 hours for an adult (O'Grady et al., 2011).

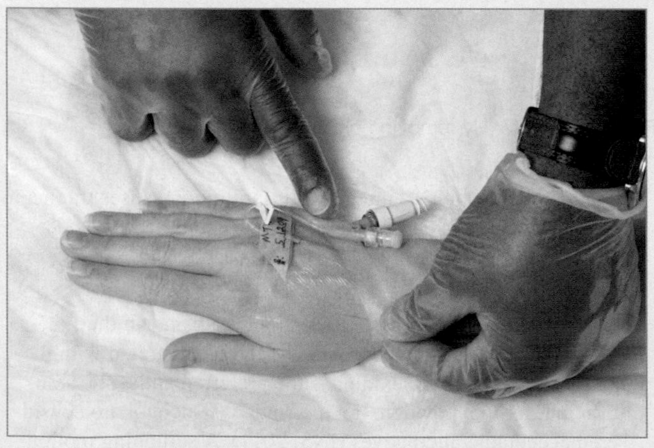

FIGURE 4 Site dressing with label and anchored tubing.

ACTION	RATIONALE
10. Apply an IV securement/stabilization device if not already in place as part of the dressing, as indicated, based on facility policy. Explain to the patient the purpose of the device and the importance of safeguarding the site when using the extremity.	These systems are recommended for use on all venous access sites, and particularly central venous access sites, to preserve the integrity of the access device, minimize catheter movement at the hub, and prevent catheter dislodgement and loss of access (INS, 2011, p. S46). Some devices also act as a site dressing and may already have been applied.

ACTION	RATIONALE
11. Remove equipment. Ensure patient's comfort. Remove gloves. Lower bed, if not in lowest position.	Promotes patient comfort and safety. Removing gloves properly reduces the risk for infection transmission and contamination of other items.
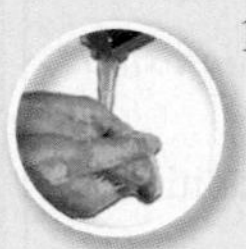 12. Remove additional PPE, if used. Perform hand hygiene.	Removing PPE properly reduces the risk for infection transmission and contamination of other items. Hand hygiene prevents transmission of microorganisms.

EVALUATION

The expected outcome is met when the patient remains free of any signs and symptoms of infection, phlebitis, or infiltration at the venous access site. In addition, the access site dressing is clean, dry, and intact; and the patient has not experienced injury.

DOCUMENTATION

Guidelines

Document the location of the venous access as well as the condition of the site. Include the presence or absence of signs of erythema, redness, swelling, or drainage. Document the clinical criteria for site complications. Refer to Fundamentals Review 15-3 and Boxes 15-3 and 15-4 (in Skill 15-3). Record the subjective comments of the patient regarding the absence or presence of pain at the site. Record the patient's reaction to the procedure and pertinent patient teaching, such as alerting the nurse if the patient experiences any pain from the IV or notices any swelling at the site.

Sample Documentation

11/15/15 1120 Dressing change to IV site in L hand (dorsal metacarpal) complete. Transparent dressing and peripheral stabilization device applied. Site without erythema, redness, edema, or drainage. D_5 NS infusing at 75 mL/hour. Patient instructed to call nurse with any pain, discomfort, swelling, or questions.

—S. Barnes, RN

UNEXPECTED SITUATIONS AND ASSOCIATED INTERVENTIONS

- *Patient complains that IV site feels "funny" and hurts:* Observe venous access site for redness, edema, and warmth. If present, clamp the tubing to stop the IV solution flow, remove the catheter, and apply a gauze dressing. Initiate a new venous access in a different site. Record site assessment and interventions, as well as site for new venous access.
- *IV catheter is partially pulled out of insertion site (migrates externally):* Do not reinsert the catheter. Whether the IV is salvageable depends on how much of the catheter remains in the vein. Assess for proper placement in the vein before further use (INS, 2011). If this catheter is not removed, monitor it closely for signs of infiltration.

SPECIAL CONSIDERATIONS

General Considerations

- Use of chlorhexidine, 70% alcohol, iodine, or povidone-iodine is recommended for skin antisepsis for peripheral venous catheters (INS, 2011; O'Grady et al., 2011).
- Use of topical antibiotic ointments or creams on insertion sites is not recommended because of their potential to promote fungal infections and antimicrobial resistance (O'Grady et al., 2011).
- Do not submerge venous catheters and catheter sites in water; showering is permitted with use of impermeable coverings to protect the catheter and connecting device (O'Grady et al., 2011).

Infant and Child Considerations

- Chlorhexidine is not recommended for infants under 2 months of age (INS, 2011).
- For infants under 2 months of age or pediatric patients with compromised skin integrity, remove dried povidone-iodine with normal saline wipes or sterile water (INS, 2011).

(continued)

SKILL 15-4 CHANGING A PERIPHERAL VENOUS ACCESS DRESSING continued

Older Adult Considerations

- Avoid using vigorous friction at the insertion site, which can traumatize fragile skin and veins in elderly adults.

EVIDENCE FOR PRACTICE ▶

INFUSION NURSING STANDARDS OF PRACTICE

Infusion Nurses Society. (2011). Infusion nursing standards of practice. *Journal of Infusion Nursing, 34*(1S), S1–S96.

Refer to details in Skill 15-1, Evidence for Practice, and refer to thePoint for additional research on related nursing topics.

SKILL 15-5 CAPPING FOR INTERMITTENT USE AND FLUSHING A PERIPHERAL VENOUS ACCESS DEVICE

When a continuous IV is no longer necessary, the primary IV line (short peripheral venous catheter or CVAD) can be capped and converted to an intermittent infusion device. A capped line consists of the IV catheter connected to a short length of extension tubing sealed with a cap. Capping of a short peripheral venous catheter is commonly referred to as a medication or saline lock. Capping of a vascular access device provides venous access for intermittent infusions or emergency medications. This can be accomplished in different ways. Refer to facility policy for the procedure to convert an access for intermittent use. Vascular access devices used for intermittent infusions should be flushed with normal saline solution prior to each infusion as part of the assessment of catheter function. Flushing of the device is also required after each infusion to clear the infused medication or other solution from the catheter lumen. Vascular access devices should also be 'locked' after completion of the flush solution at each use to decrease the risk of occlusion. According to the guidelines from the INS (2011), short **peripheral venous access devices** are locked with normal saline solution after each intermittent use. If the device is not in use, periodic flushing according to facility policy is required to keep the catheter patent. Refer to facility policy for specific guidelines.

The following skill describes converting a primary line when extension tubing is present; the accompanying skill variation describes converting a primary line when the administration set is connected directly to the hub of the IV catheter, without extension tubing.

DELEGATION CONSIDERATIONS

Capping and flushing of a peripheral venous access device is not delegated to nursing assistive personnel (NAP) or to unlicensed assistive personnel (UAP). Depending on the state's nurse practice act and the organization's policies and procedures, these procedures may be delegated to licensed practical/vocational nurses (LPN/LVNs). The decision to delegate must be based on careful analysis of the patient's needs and circumstances, as well as the qualifications of the person to whom the task is being delegated. Refer to the Delegation Guidelines in Appendix A.

EQUIPMENT

- End cap device
- Clean gloves
- Additional PPE, as indicated
- 4 × 4 gauze pad
- Normal saline flush prepared in a syringe (1 to 3 mL) according to facility policy
- Alcohol or other disinfectant wipes
- Tape

ASSESSMENT

Assess the insertion site for signs of any complications. Refer to Fundamentals Review 15-3 and Boxes 15-3 and 15-4 (in Skill 15-3). Verify the medical order for discontinuation of IV fluid infusion.

NURSING DIAGNOSIS

Determine the related factors for the nursing diagnoses based on the patient's current status. Appropriate nursing diagnoses may include:

- Risk for Infection
- Risk for Injury

OUTCOME IDENTIFICATION AND PLANNING

The expected outcome to achieve when converting a primary peripheral IV line is that the patient will remain free of injury and any signs and symptoms of IV complications. In addition, the capped venous access device will remain patent.

IMPLEMENTATION

ACTION	RATIONALE
1. Determine the need for conversion to an intermittent access. Verify medical order. Check facility policy. Gather equipment.	Ensures correct intervention for correct patient. Preparation promotes efficient time management and an organized approach to the task.
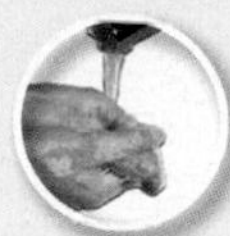 2. Perform hand hygiene and put on PPE, if indicated.	Hand hygiene and PPE prevent the spread of microorganisms. PPE is required based on transmission precautions.
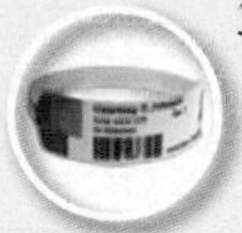 3. Identify the patient.	Identifying the patient ensures the right patient receives the intervention and helps prevent errors.
4. Close the curtains around the bed and close the door to the room, if possible. Explain what you are going to do and why you are going to do it to the patient. Ask the patient about allergies to tape and skin antiseptics.	This ensures the patient's privacy. Explanation relieves anxiety and facilitates cooperation. Possible allergies may exist related to tape or antiseptics.
5. Assess the IV site. Refer to Skill 15-3.	Complications, such as infiltration, phlebitis, or infection, necessitate discontinuation of the IV infusion at that site.
6. If using an electronic infusion device, stop the device (Figure 1). Close the roller clamp on the administration set. If using gravity infusion, close the roller clamp on the administration set.	The action of the infusion device needs to be stopped and clamp closed to prevent leaking of fluid when tubing is disconnected.
7. Put on gloves. Close the clamp on the short extension tubing connected to the IV catheter in the patient's arm.	Clamping the tubing on the extension set prevents introduction of air into the extension tubing.

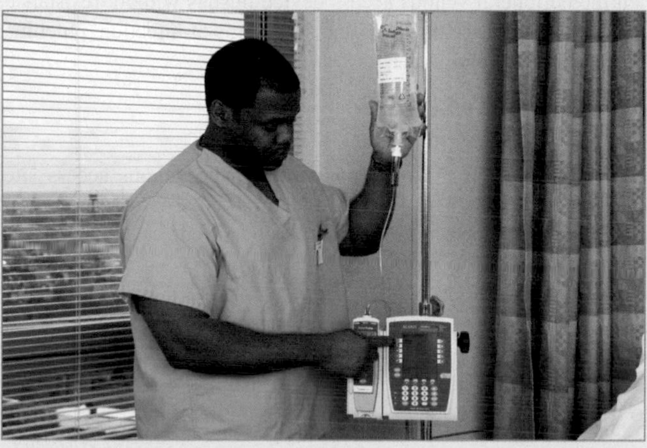

FIGURE 1 Stopping IV fluid infusion.

(continued)

SKILL 15-5 CAPPING FOR INTERMITTENT USE AND FLUSHING A PERIPHERAL VENOUS ACCESS DEVICE continued

ACTION	RATIONALE
8. Remove the administration set tubing from the extension set. Cleanse the end cap with an antimicrobial swab.	Removing the infusion tubing discontinues the infusion. Cleaning the cap reduces the risk for contamination.
9. Insert the saline flush syringe into the cap on the extension tubing. Pull back on the syringe to aspirate the catheter for positive blood return. If positive, instill the solution over 1 minute or flush the line according to facility policy (Figure 2). Remove syringe and reclamp the extension tubing.	Positive blood return confirms patency before administration of medications and solutions (INS, 2011, p. S60). Flushing maintains patency of the IV line. Action of positive pressure end cap is maintained with removal of syringe before clamp is engaged. Clamping prevents air from entering the extension set.

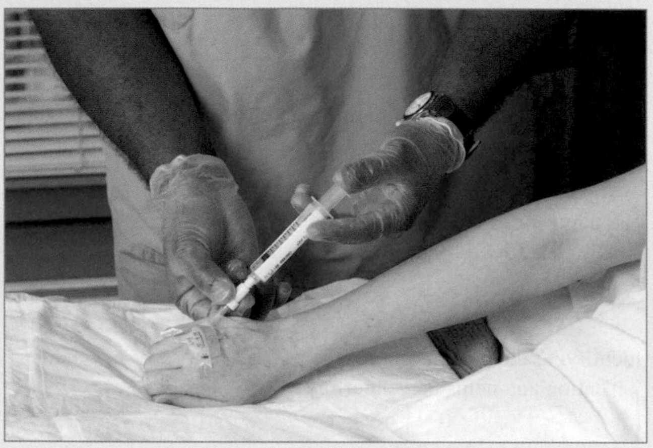

FIGURE 2 Flushing venous access device.

ACTION	RATIONALE
10. If necessary, loop the extension tubing near the entry site and anchor it with tape (nonallergenic) close to the site.	The weight of the tubing is sufficient to pull it out of the vein if it is not well anchored. Nonallergenic tape is less likely to tear fragile skin.
11. Remove equipment. Ensure patient's comfort. Remove gloves. Lower bed, if not in lowest position.	Promotes patient comfort and safety. Removing gloves properly reduces the risk for infection transmission and contamination of other items.
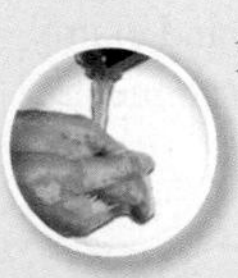 12. Remove additional PPE, if used. Perform hand hygiene.	Removing PPE properly reduces the risk for infection transmission and contamination of other items. Hand hygiene prevents transmission of microorganisms.

EVALUATION

The expected outcome is met when the peripheral venous access device flushes without resistance; the patient exhibits an access site that is intact, free of the signs and symptoms of infection, phlebitis, or infiltration; and the site dressing is clean, dry, and intact.

DOCUMENTATION

Guidelines

Document discontinuation of IV fluid infusion. Record the condition of the venous access site. Document the flushing of the venous access device. This is often done in the CMAR/MAR. Record the patient's reaction to the procedure and any patient teaching that has occurred.

Sample Documentation

12/13/15 1720 IV infusion capped per order. Peripheral site right forearm (cephalic) flushed without resistance using 3 mL of saline. Dressing remains intact. Site without redness, swelling, drainage, or heat. Patient denies discomfort. Patient verbalized an understanding of the need to maintain IV access.

—A. Lynn, RN

UNEXPECTED SITUATIONS AND ASSOCIATED INTERVENTIONS

- *Peripheral venous access site leaks fluid when flushed:* To prevent infection and other complications, remove from site and restart in another location.
- *IV does not flush easily:* Assess insertion site. Infiltration and/or phlebitis may be present. If present, remove and restart in another location. In addition, the catheter may be blocked or clotted due to a kinked catheter at the insertion site. Aspirate and attempt to flush again. If resistance remains, do not force. Forceful flushing can dislodge a clot at the end of the catheter. Remove and restart in another location.
- *IV catheter is partially pulled out of insertion site (migrates externally):* Do not reinsert the catheter. Whether the IV is salvageable depends on how much of the catheter remains in the vein. Assess for proper placement in the vein before further use (INS, 2011). If this catheter is not removed, monitor it closely for signs of infiltration.

SPECIAL CONSIDERATIONS

- Some facilities may use end caps for venous access devices that are not positive pressure devices. In this case, flush with the recommended volume of saline, ending with 0.5 mL of solution remaining in the syringe. While maintaining pressure on the syringe, clamp the extension tubing. This provides positive pressure, preventing backflow of blood into the catheter, decreasing risk for occlusion.

SKILL VARIATION Capping a Primary Line When No Extension Tube is in Place

It is good practice to add a short extension tubing to decrease the risk of contact with blood, and for infection-control purposes if one was not placed during initiation of the peripheral venous access. After checking the medical order to convert the peripheral venous access, the nurse brings the end cap and the extension tubing to the bedside, as well as other required equipment.

1. Gather equipment and verify medical order.

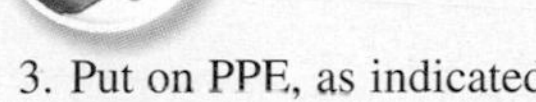

2. Perform hand hygiene.
3. Put on PPE, as indicated.

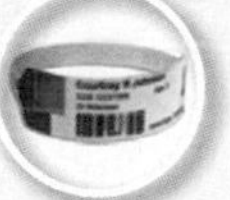

4. Identify the patient.
5. Explain the procedure to the patient.
6. Fill the cap and extension tubing with normal saline.
7. Assess IV site.
8. Put on gloves.
9. Remove site dressing as outlined in Skill 15-4.
10. Put on sterile gloves. Place gauze 4 × 4-inch sponge underneath IV connection hub, between IV catheter and tubing.
11. **Stabilize hub of IV catheter with nondominant hand. Use dominant hand to quickly twist and disconnect IV tubing from the catheter. Discard it. Attach the primed extension tubing to the IV catheter hub using aseptic technique.**
12. Cleanse cap with an antimicrobial solution.
13. Insert the syringe into the cap and gently flush with saline per facility policy. Remove syringe. Engage slide clamp on extension tubing.
14. Redress site as outlined in Skill 15-4.
15. Remove gloves.
16. Loop the extension tubing near the entry site and anchor with tape (nonallergenic) close to the site.
17. Apply an IV securement/stabilization device if not already in place as part of the dressing, as indicated, based on facility policy. Explain to the patient the purpose of the device and the importance of safeguarding the site when using the extremity.
18. Ensure that the patient is comfortable. Perform hand hygiene.
19. Chart on IV administration record, MAR, or CMAR, per facility policy.

EVIDENCE FOR PRACTICE ▶

INFUSION NURSING STANDARDS OF PRACTICE

Infusion Nurses Society. (2011). Infusion nursing standards of practice. *Journal of Infusion Nursing, 34*(1S), S1–S96.

Refer to details in Skill 15-1, Evidence for Practice, and refer to thePoint for additional research on related nursing topics.

SKILL 15-6 ADMINISTERING A BLOOD TRANSFUSION

A blood transfusion is the infusion of whole blood or a blood component, such as plasma, red blood cells, cryoprecipitate, or platelets, into the patient's venous circulation (Table 15-1). A blood product transfusion is given when a patient's red blood cells, platelets, or coagulation factors decrease to levels that compromise a patient's health. Before a patient can receive a blood product, his/her blood must be typed to ensure that he/she receives compatible blood. Otherwise, a serious and life-threatening transfusion reaction may occur involving clumping and hemolysis of the red blood cells and, possibly, death (Table 15-2). The nurse must also verify the infusion rate, based on facility policy or medical order. Follow the facility's policies and guidelines to determine if the transfusion should be administered by an electronic infusion device or by gravity. Refer to Box 15-1 in Skill 15-1 for guidelines to calculate flow rate for gravity infusion.

Table 15-1 BLOOD PRODUCTS

BLOOD PRODUCT	FILTER	RATE OF ADMINISTRATION	ABO COMPATIBILITY	DOUBLE-CHECKED BY TWO LICENSED PRACTITIONERS (e.g., registered nurse, physician)
Packed red blood cells	Yes	1 unit over 2–3 hours; no longer than 4 hours	Yes	Yes
Platelets	Yes (in tubing provided)	As fast as patient can tolerate	No	Yes
Cryoprecipitate	No	IV push over 3 minutes	Recommended	Yes
Fresh-frozen plasma	No	200 mL/hr	Yes	Yes
Albumin	In tubing provided	1–10 mL/min (5%) 0.2–0.4 mL/min (25%)	No	No

Table 15-2 TRANSFUSION REACTIONS

REACTION	SIGNS AND SYMPTOMS	NURSING ACTIVITY
Allergic reaction: allergy to transfused blood	Hives, itching Anaphylaxis	• Stop transfusion immediately and keep vein open with normal saline. • Notify primary care provider stat. • Administer antihistamine parenterally, as necessary.
Febrile reaction: fever develops during infusion	Fever and chills Headache Malaise	• Stop transfusion immediately and keep vein open with normal saline. • Notify primary care provider. • Treat symptoms.
Hemolytic transfusion reaction: incompatibility of blood product	Immediate onset Facial flushing Fever, chills Headache Low back pain Shock	• Stop infusion immediately and keep vein open with normal saline. • Notify primary care provider stat. • Obtain blood samples from site. • Obtain first voided urine. • Treat shock if present. • Send unit, tubing, and filter to laboratory. • Draw blood sample for serologic testing and send urine specimen to the laboratory.
Circulatory overload: too much blood administered	Dyspnea Dry cough Pulmonary edema	• Slow or stop infusion. • Monitor vital signs. • Notify primary care provider. • Place in upright position with feet dependent.
Bacterial reaction: bacteria present in blood	Fever Hypertension Dry, flushed skin Abdominal pain	• Stop infusion immediately. • Obtain culture of patient's blood and return blood bag to laboratory. • Monitor vital signs. • Notify primary care provider. • Administer antibiotics stat.

DELEGATION CONSIDERATIONS

The administration of a blood transfusion is not delegated to nursing assistive personnel (NAP), to unlicensed assistive personnel (UAP), or to licensed practical/vocational nurses (LPN/LVNs).

EQUIPMENT

- Blood product
- Blood administration set (tubing with in-line filter, or add-on filter, and Y for saline administration)
- 0.9% normal saline for IV infusion
- IV pole
- Venous access; if peripheral site, preferably initiated with a 20-gauge catheter or larger
- Alcohol or other disinfectant wipes
- Clean gloves
- Additional PPE, as indicated
- Tape (hypoallergenic)
- Second registered nurse (or other licensed practitioner; e.g., a physician) to verify blood product and patient information

ASSESSMENT

Obtain a baseline assessment of the patient, including vital signs, heart and lung sounds, and urinary output. Review the most recent laboratory values, in particular, the complete blood count (CBC). Ask the patient about any previous transfusions, including the number he/she has had and any reactions experienced during a transfusion. Inspect the IV insertion site, noting the gauge of the IV catheter. Blood or blood components may be transfused via a 14- to 24-gauge peripheral venous access device. Transfusion for neonate or pediatric patients is usually given using a 22- to 24-gauge peripheral venous access device (INS, 2011).

NURSING DIAGNOSIS

Determine the related factors for the nursing diagnoses based on the patient's current status. Appropriate nursing diagnoses may include:

- Risk for Injury
- Excess Fluid Volume
- Ineffective Peripheral Tissue Perfusion

OUTCOME IDENTIFICATION AND PLANNING

The expected outcome to achieve when administering a blood transfusion is that the patient will remain free of injury and any signs and symptoms of IV complications. In addition, the capped venous access device will remain patent.

IMPLEMENTATION

ACTION	RATIONALE
1. Verify the medical order for transfusion of a blood product. Verify the completion of informed consent documentation in the medical record. Verify any medical order for pretransfusion medication. If ordered, administer medication at least 30 minutes before initiating transfusion.	Verification of order ensures the right patient receives the correct intervention. Premedication is sometimes administered to decrease the risk for allergic and febrile reactions for patients who have received multiple previous transfusions.
2. Gather all equipment.	Preparation promotes efficient time management and an organized approach to the task.
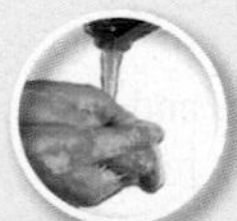 3. Perform hand hygiene and put on PPE, if indicated.	Hand hygiene and PPE prevent the spread of microorganisms. PPE is required based on transmission precautions.
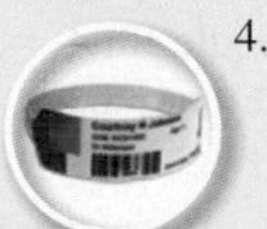 4. Identify the patient.	Identifying the patient ensures the right patient receives the intervention and helps prevent errors.
5. Close the curtains around the bed and close the door to the room, if possible. Explain what you are going to do and why you are going to do it to the patient. Ask the patient about previous experience with a transfusion and any reactions. Advise the patient to report any chills, itching, rash, or unusual symptoms.	This ensures the patient's privacy. Explanation relieves anxiety and facilitates cooperation. Previous reactions may increase the risk for reaction to this transfusion. Any reaction to the transfusion necessitates stopping the transfusion immediately and evaluating the situation.

(continued)

SKILL 15-6 ADMINISTERING A BLOOD TRANSFUSION continued

ACTION	RATIONALE
6. Prime blood administration set with the normal saline IV fluid. Refer to Skill 15-2.	Normal saline is the solution of choice for blood product administration. Solutions with dextrose may lead to clumping of red blood cells and hemolysis.
7. Put on gloves. If patient does not have a venous access in place, initiate peripheral venous access. (Refer to Skill 15-1.) Connect the administration set to the venous access device via the extension tubing. (Refer to Skill 15-1.) Infuse the normal saline per facility policy.	Gloves prevent contact with blood and body fluids. Infusion of fluid via venous access maintains patency until the blood product is administered. Start an IV before obtaining the blood product in case the initiation takes longer than 30 minutes. Blood must be stored at a carefully controlled temperature (4°C) and transfusion must begin within 30 minutes of release from the blood bank.
8. Obtain blood product from blood bank according to agency policy. Scan for bar codes on blood products if required.	Bar codes on blood products are currently being implemented in some agencies to identify, track, and assign data to transfusions as an additional safety measure.
9. Two nurses compare and validate the following information with the medical record, patient identification band, and the label of the blood product: • Medical order for transfusion of blood product • Informed consent • Patient identification number • Patient name • Blood group and type • Expiration date • Inspection of blood product for clots, clumping, gas bubbles	Most states/agencies require two registered nurses to verify the following information: unit numbers match; ABO group and Rh type are the same; expiration date (after 35 days, red blood cells begin to deteriorate). Blood is never administered to a patient without an identification band. If clots or signs of contamination (clumping, gas bubbles) are present, return blood to the blood bank.
10. **Obtain baseline set of vital signs before beginning the transfusion.**	Any change in vital signs during the transfusion may indicate a reaction.
11. Put on gloves. If using an electronic infusion device, put the device on "hold." Close the roller clamp closest to the drip chamber on the saline side of the administration set. Close the roller clamp on the administration set below the infusion device. Alternately, if infusing via gravity, close the roller clamp on the administration set.	Gloves prevent contact with blood and body fluids. Stopping the infusion prevents blood from infusing to the patient before completion of preparations. Closing the clamp to saline allows blood product to be infused via electronic infusion device.
12. Close the roller clamp closest to the drip chamber on the blood product side of the administration set. Remove the protective cap from the access port on the blood container. Remove the cap from the access spike on the administration set. Using a pushing and twisting motion, insert the spike into the access port on the blood container, taking care not to contaminate the spike. Hang the blood container on the IV pole. Open the roller clamp on the blood side of the administration set. Squeeze drip chamber until the in-line filter is saturated (Figure 1). Remove gloves.	Filling the drip chamber prevents air from entering the administration set. The filter in the blood administration set removes particulate material formed during storage of blood. If the administration set becomes contaminated, the entire set would have to be discarded and replaced.
13. **Start administration slowly (no more than 25 to 50 mL for the first 15 minutes). Stay with the patient for the first 5 to 15 minutes of transfusion.** Open the roller clamp on the administration set below the infusion device. Set the flow rate and begin the transfusion. Alternately, start the flow of solution by releasing the clamp on the tubing and counting the drops. Adjust until the correct drop rate is achieved. Assess the flow of the blood and function of the infusion device. Inspect the insertion site for signs of infiltration.	Transfusion reactions typically occur during this period, and a slow rate will minimize the volume of red blood cells infused. Verifying the rate and device settings ensures the patient receives the correct volume of solution. If the catheter or needle slips out of the vein, the blood will accumulate (infiltrate) into the surrounding tissue.

ACTION	RATIONALE

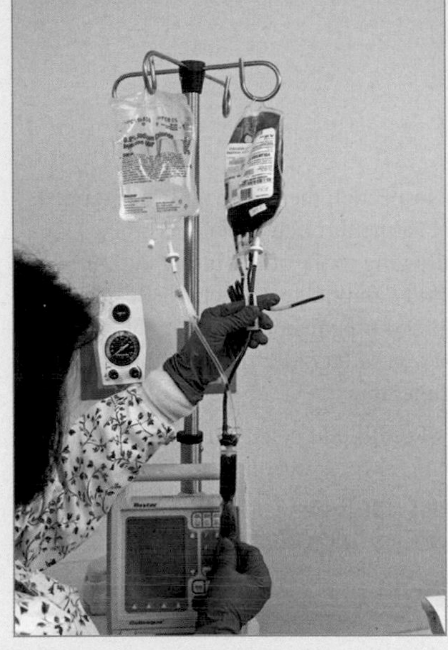

FIGURE 1 Squeezing the drip chamber to saturate the filter.

ACTION	RATIONALE
14. Observe the patient for flushing, dyspnea, itching, hives or rash, or any unusual comments.	These signs and symptoms may be an early indication of a transfusion reaction.
15. After the observation period (5 to 15 minutes) increase the infusion rate to the calculated rate to complete the infusion within the prescribed time frame, no more than 4 hours.	If no adverse effects occurred during this time, the infusion rate is increased. If complications occur, they can be observed and the transfusion can be stopped immediately. Verifying the rate and device settings ensures the patient receives the correct volume of solution. Transfusion must be completed within 4 hours due to potential for bacterial growth in blood product at room temperature.
16. Reassess vital signs after 15 minutes (Figure 2). Obtain vital signs thereafter according to facility policy and nursing assessment.	Vital signs must be assessed as part of monitoring for possible adverse reaction. Facility policy and nursing judgment will dictate frequency.

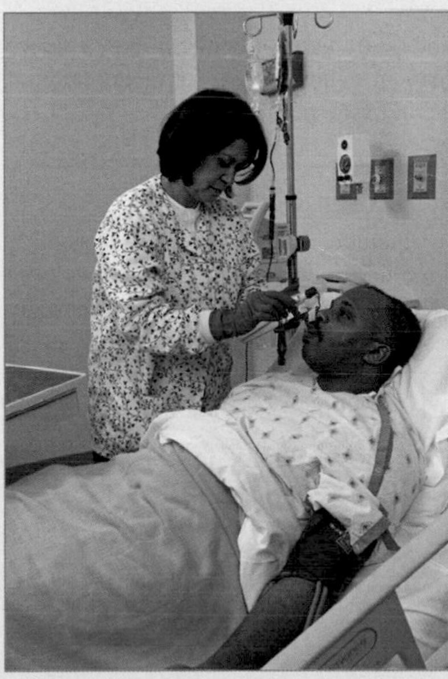

FIGURE 2 Assessing vital signs after 15 minutes.

(continued)

SKILL 15-6 ADMINISTERING A BLOOD TRANSFUSION continued

ACTION	RATIONALE
17. Maintain the prescribed flow rate as ordered or as deemed appropriate based on the patient's overall condition, keeping in mind the outer limits for safe administration. Ongoing monitoring is crucial throughout the entire duration of the blood transfusion for early identification of any adverse reactions.	Rate must be carefully controlled, and the patient's reaction must be monitored frequently.
18. **During transfusion, assess frequently for transfusion reaction. Stop blood transfusion if you suspect a reaction. Quickly replace the blood tubing with a new administration set primed with normal saline for IV infusion. Initiate an infusion of normal saline for IV at an open rate, usually 40 mL/hour. Obtain vital signs. Notify primary care provider and blood bank.**	If a transfusion reaction is suspected, the blood must be stopped. Do not infuse the normal saline through the blood tubing because you would be allowing more of the blood into the patient's body, which could complicate a reaction. Besides a serious life-threatening blood transfusion reaction, the potential for fluid–volume overload exists in older patients and patients with decreased cardiac function.
19. When transfusion is complete, close the roller clamp on blood side of the administration set and open the roller clamp on the normal saline side of the administration set. Initiate infusion of normal saline. When all of blood has infused into the patient, clamp the administration set. Obtain vital signs. Put on gloves. Cap access site or resume previous IV infusion. (Refer to Skill 15-1 and Skill 15-5.) Dispose of blood-transfusion equipment or return to blood bank, according to facility policy.	Saline prevents hemolysis of red blood cells and clears remainder of blood in IV line. Proper disposal of equipment reduces transmission of microorganisms and potential contact with blood and body fluids.
20. Remove equipment. Ensure patient's comfort. Remove gloves. Lower bed, if not in lowest position.	Promotes patient comfort and safety. Removing gloves properly reduces the risk for infection transmission and contamination of other items.
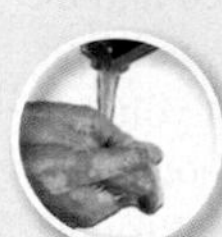 21. Remove additional PPE, if used. Perform hand hygiene.	Removing PPE properly reduces the risk for infection transmission and contamination of other items. Hand hygiene prevents transmission of microorganisms.
22. Monitor and assess the patient for one hour after the transfusion for signs and symptoms of delayed transfusion reaction. Provide patient education about signs and symptoms of delayed transfusion reactions.	Ensures early detection and prompt intervention. Delayed transfusion reactions can occur one to several days after transfusion.

EVALUATION

The expected outcome is met when the patient receives the blood transfusion without any evidence of a transfusion reaction or complication. In addition, the patient exhibits signs and symptoms of fluid balance, improved cardiac output, and enhanced peripheral tissue perfusion.

DOCUMENTATION

Guidelines

Document that the patient received the blood transfusion; include the type of blood product. Record the patient's condition throughout the transfusion, including pertinent data, such as vital signs, lung sounds, and the subjective response of the patient to the transfusion. Document any complications or reactions and whether the patient had received the transfusion without any complications or reactions. Document the assessment of the IV site, and any other fluids infused during the procedure. Document transfusion volume and other IV fluid intake on the patient's intake and output record.

Sample Documentation

11/2/15 1100 T 97.6°F P 82 R 14 B/P 116/74. 1 unit of packed blood red cells initiated via left forearm (basilic) 18-gauge venous access without difficulty. Patient states "no discomfort." IV site intact, no swelling, redness, or pain.

—*S. Barnes, RN*

11/2/15 1115 T 97.6°F P 78 R 16 B/P 118/68. 1 unit of packed blood red cells infusing via left forearm (basilic) 18-gauge venous access without difficulty. Patient states "no discomfort." IV site intact, no swelling, redness, or pain.

—*S. Barnes, RN*

11/2/15 1445 T 97.6°F P 82 R 14 B/P 120/74. 1 unit of packed blood red cells completed via left forearm (basilic) 18-gauge venous access without difficulty. Patient denies symptoms of complications. IV site intact, no swelling, redness, or pain.

—*S. Barnes, RN*

UNEXPECTED SITUATIONS AND ASSOCIATED INTERVENTIONS

- *Patient is becoming febrile, but is exhibiting no other signs of a transfusion reaction:* Notify the primary care provider. The primary care provider may order acetaminophen and an antihistamine for the patient.
- *Patient reports shortness of breath; on auscultation you note crackles bilaterally in the bases:* Compare vital signs with normal vital sounds for this patient. Obtain a pulse oximetry reading. Notify the primary care provider. The primary care provider may order a dose of a diuretic or may decrease the rate of the transfusion. Continue to assess the patient for signs and symptoms of fluid overload.
- *Patient is febrile, tachycardic, and complaining of back pain:* Patient is having a transfusion reaction. Stop the transfusion immediately. Obtain new IV tubing with 0.9% sodium chloride. Notify the primary care provider and blood bank. Send blood unit, tubing, and filter to the laboratory. Obtain additional diagnostic tests, such as blood and urine tests, based on facility policy.

SPECIAL CONSIDERATIONS

General Considerations

- If an electronic infusion device is used to maintain the prescribed rate, ensure it is designed for use with blood transfusions before initiating transfusion.
- Never warm blood in a microwave. Use a blood-warming device, if indicated or ordered, especially with rapid transfusions through a CVAD. Blood warmers should also be used for large-volume transfusions, exchange transfusions, patients with clinically significant conditions, and the neonate/pediatric population (INS, 2011, p. S93). Rapid administration of cold blood can result in cardiac arrhythmias.
- External compression devices, if used for rapid transfusions, should be equipped with a pressure gauge, should totally encase the blood bag, and should apply uniform pressure against all parts of the blood container. Do not use blood pressure cuffs (INS, 2011, p. S93).

Home Care Considerations

- Home care agencies evaluate patients who are candidates for a blood transfusion at home.
- Home transfusion is not appropriate for patients who are actively bleeding or who recently had a reaction to a blood transfusion.
- The nurse transports the blood product to the patient's home in a special cooler. The nurse and competent adult check the serial number and other identification information together (INS, 2011).

EVIDENCE FOR PRACTICE ▶

INFUSION NURSING STANDARDS OF PRACTICE

Infusion Nurses Society. (2011). Infusion nursing standards of practice. *Journal of Infusion Nursing, 34*(1S), S1–S96.

Refer to details in Skill 15-1, Evidence for Practice, and refer to thePoint for additional research on related nursing topics.

SKILL 15-7 CHANGING THE DRESSING AND FLUSHING CENTRAL VENOUS ACCESS DEVICES

Central venous access devices (CVAD) are venous access devices where the tip of the catheter terminates in the central venous circulation, usually in the superior vena cava near its junction with the right atrium (INS, 2011). Types of CVAD include **peripherally inserted central catheters (PICC)** (Figure 1), **nontunneled percutaneous central venous catheters** (Figure 2), tunneled percutaneous central venous catheters (Figure 3), and **implanted ports**. (Refer to Skill 15-8, Figure 1.) They provide access for a variety of IV fluids, medications, blood products, and TPN solutions and provide a means for hemodynamic monitoring and blood sampling. The patient's diagnosis, the type of care that is required, and other factors (e.g., limited venous access, irritating drugs, patient request, or the need for long-term intermittent infusions) determine the type of CVAD used.

Dressings are placed at the insertion site to occlude the site and prevent the introduction of microorganisms into the bloodstream. Scrupulous care of the site is required to control contamination. Facility policy generally determines the type of dressing used and the intervals for dressing change. TSM dressings (e.g., Tegaderm or OpSite IV) allow easy inspection of the IV site and permit evaporation of moisture that accumulates under the dressing. Sterile gauze may also be used to cover the catheter site. A gauze dressing is recommended if the patient is diaphoretic or if the site is bleeding or oozing, but this should be replaced with a TSM dressing once this is resolved (O'Grady et al., 2011). Perform site care and replace TSM dressings on CVADs every 5 to 7 days and every 2 days for CVAD sites with gauze dressings (INS, 2011; O'Grady et al., 2011). Change any dressing that is damp, loosened, or soiled immediately. Whenever these dressings need to be changed, it is important to observe meticulous aseptic technique to minimize the possibility of contamination.

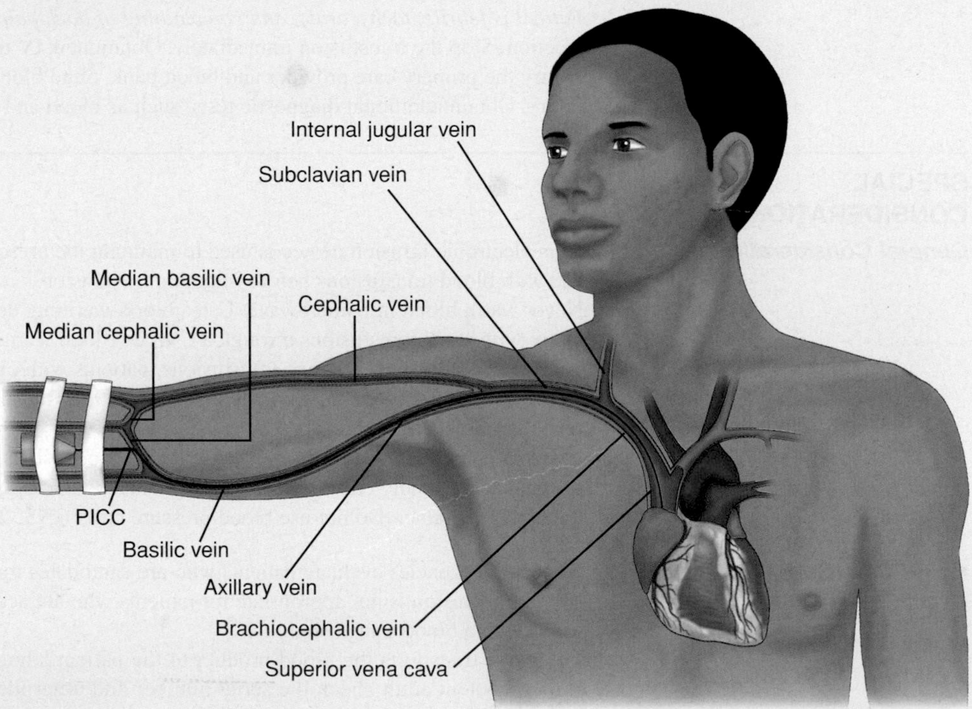

FIGURE 1 Placement of peripherally inserted central catheter (PICC).

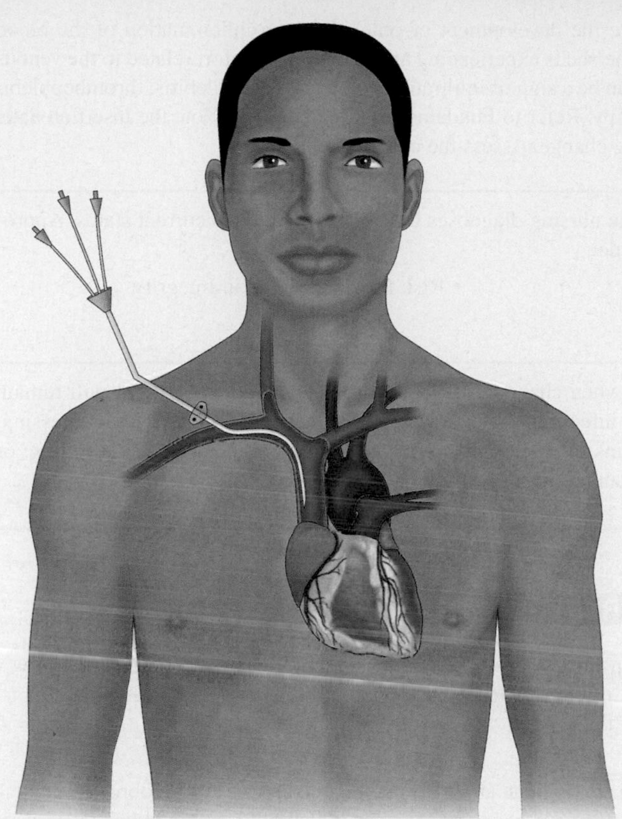

FIGURE 2 Placement of triple-lumen, nontunneled percutaneous central venous catheter.

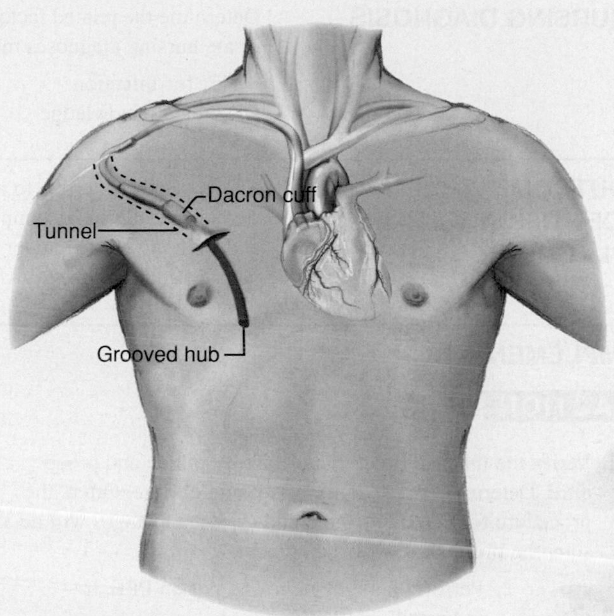

FIGURE 3 Tunneled percutaneous central venous catheter.

DELEGATION CONSIDERATIONS

The changing of a CVAD dressing is not delegated to nursing assistive personnel (NAP) or to unlicensed assistive personnel (UAP). Depending on the state's nurse practice act and the organization's policies and procedures, the changing of a CVAD dressing may be delegated to licensed practical/vocational nurses (LPN/LVNs). The decision to delegate must be based on careful analysis of the patient's needs and circumstances, as well as the qualifications of the person to whom the task is being delegated. Refer to the Delegation Guidelines in Appendix A.

EQUIPMENT

- Sterile tape or Steri-Strips
- Sterile semipermeable transparent dressing
- Several 2 × 2 gauzes
- Sterile towel or drape
- Cleansing swabs (>0.5% chlorhexidine preparation with alcohol)
- NSS vial and 10-mL syringe or prefilled 10-mL NSS syringe; one for each lumen of the CVAD
- Heparin 10 U/mL in 10-mL syringe; one for each lumen of the CVAD
- Masks (2), depending on facility policy
- Clean gloves
- Sterile gloves
- Additional PPE, as indicated
- Skin protectant wipe (e.g., SkinPrep)
- Alcohol or other disinfectant wipes
- Positive pressure end caps; one for each lumen of the CVAD
- IV securement/stabilization device, as appropriate
- Measuring tape
- Bath blanket

ASSESSMENT

Assess the IV site. The dressing should be intact, adhering to the skin on all edges. Check for any leaks or fluid under or around the dressing, or other indications that the dressing needs to be changed. Inspect the tissue around the IV entry site for swelling, coolness, or pallor. These are signs of fluid infiltration into the tissue around the IV catheter. Also inspect the site for redness, swelling, and

(continued)

SKILL 15-7 CHANGING THE DRESSING AND FLUSHING CENTRAL VENOUS ACCESS DEVICES continued

warmth. These signs might indicate the development of phlebitis or an inflammation of the blood vessel at the site. Ask the patient if he/she is experiencing any pain or discomfort related to the venous access device. Pain or discomfort can be a sign of infiltration, extravasation, phlebitis, thrombophlebitis, and infection related to IV therapy. Refer to Fundamentals Review 15-3. Note the insertion date/access date and date of last dressing change. Assess the catheter condition.

NURSING DIAGNOSIS

Determine the related factors for the nursing diagnoses based on the patient's current status. Appropriate nursing diagnoses may include:

- Risk for Infection
- Deficient Knowledge
- Risk for Impaired Skin Integrity

OUTCOME IDENTIFICATION AND PLANNING

The expected outcome to achieve when changing a CVAD dressing is that the patient will remain free of any signs and symptoms of infection. The site will be clean and dry, with an intact dressing, and will show no signs or symptoms of IV complications, such as redness, drainage, swelling, or pain. In addition, the CVAD will remain patent.

IMPLEMENTATION

ACTION	RATIONALE
1. Verify the medical order and/or facility policy and procedure. Determine the need for a dressing change. Often, the procedure for CVAD flushing and dressing changes will be a standing protocol. Gather equipment.	Ensures correct intervention for correct patient. Preparation promotes efficient time management and an organized approach to the task.
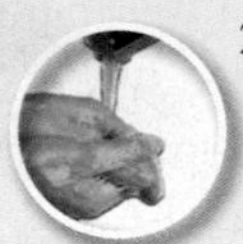 2. Perform hand hygiene and put on PPE, if indicated.	Hand hygiene and PPE prevent the spread of microorganisms. Unclean hands and improper technique are potential sources for infecting a CVAD. PPE is required based on transmission precautions.
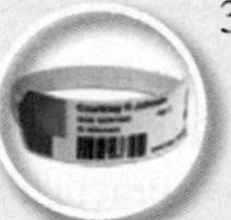 3. Identify the patient.	Identifying the patient ensures the right patient receives the intervention and helps prevent errors.
4. Close the curtains around the bed and close the door to the room, if possible. Explain what you are going to do and why you are going to do it to the patient. Ask the patient about allergies to tape and skin antiseptics.	This ensures the patient's privacy. Explanation relieves anxiety and facilitates cooperation. Possible allergies may exist related to tape or antiseptics.
5. Place a waste receptacle or bag at a convenient location for use during the procedure.	Having a waste container handy means the soiled dressing can be discarded easily, without the spread of microorganisms.
6. Adjust the bed to a comfortable working height, usually elbow height of the caregiver (VISN 8 Patient Safety Center, 2009).	Having the bed at the proper height prevents back and muscle strain.
7. Assist the patient to a comfortable position that provides easy access to the CVAD insertion site and dressing. If the patient has a PICC, position the patient with the arm extended from the body below heart level. Use the bath blanket to cover any exposed area other than the site.	Patient positioning and use of a bath blanket provide for comfort and warmth. This position is recommended to reduce the risk of air embolism.
8. Apply a mask, depending on facility policy. Ask the patient to turn his/her head away from the access site. Alternately, have the patient put on a mask, depending on facility policy. Move the overbed table to a convenient location within easy reach. Set up a sterile field on the table. Open dressing supplies and add to sterile field. If IV solution is infusing via CVAD, interrupt and place on hold during dressing change. Apply slide clamp on each lumen of the CVAD.	Masks are recommended to help to deter the spread of microorganisms (INS, 2011, p. S64). Patient should wear a mask if unable to turn the head away from the site or if based on facility policy. Many facilities have all sterile dressing supplies gathered in a single package. Stopping infusion and clamping each lumen prevents air from entering CVAD.

ACTION

9. Put on clean gloves. Assess CVAD insertion site through old dressing (Figure 4). (Refer to Assessment discussion above.) Note the status of any sutures that may be present. Palpate the site, noting pain, tenderness, or discomfort. Remove old dressing by lifting it distally and then working proximally, making sure to stabilize the catheter (Figure 5). Discard dressing in trash receptacle. Remove gloves and discard.

RATIONALE

Some CVADs may be sutured in place. Note how the CVAD is secured. Care should be taken to avoid dislodgement when changing dressings. Pain, tenderness, or discomfort on palpation may be a sign of infection. Proper disposal of dressing prevents transmission of microorganisms. Removing gloves properly reduces the risk for infection transmission and contamination of other items.

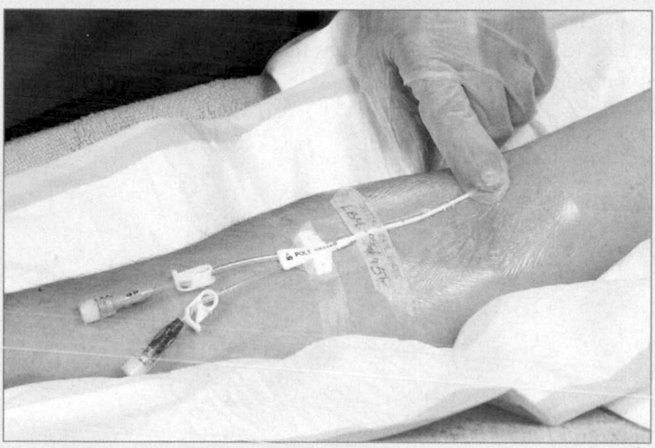

FIGURE 4 Inspecting CVAD insertion site.

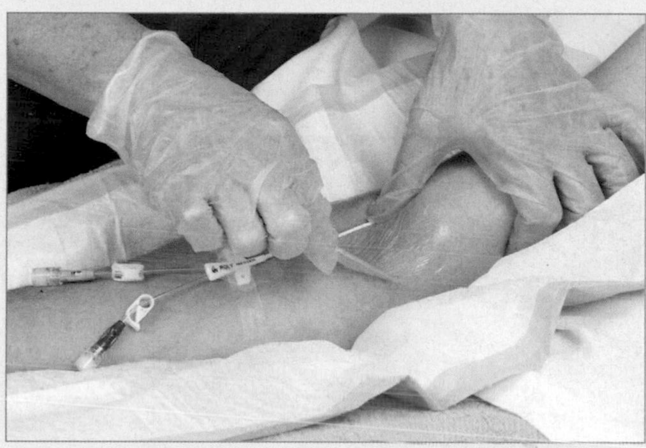

FIGURE 5 Removing dressing.

10. Put on sterile gloves. Starting at the insertion site and continuing in a circle, wipe off any old blood or drainage with a sterile antimicrobial wipe. Using the chlorhexidine swab, cleanse the site. Cleanse directly over the insertion site by pressing the applicator against the skin. **Apply chlorhexidine using a gentle back and forth motion (Figure 6).** Moving outward from the site, use a scrubbing motion to continue to clean, covering at least a 2- to 3-inch area. **Do not wipe or blot. Allow to dry completely.** Apply the skin protectant to the same area, avoiding direct application to the insertion site, and allow to dry.

Site care and replacement of dressing are accomplished using sterile technique. Cleansing is necessary because organisms on the skin can be introduced into the tissues or the bloodstream with venous access. Chlorhexidine is recommended for CVAD site care. Chlorhexidine is the preferred antiseptic solution, but iodine, povidone-iodine, and 70% alcohol are considered acceptable alternatives in patients who are allergic to chlorhexidine (INS, 2011). Scrubbing motion creates friction and lets the solution more effectively penetrate the epidermal layers (Hadaway, 2006). Skin protectant improves adhesion of dressing and protects the skin from damage and irritation when the dressing is removed.

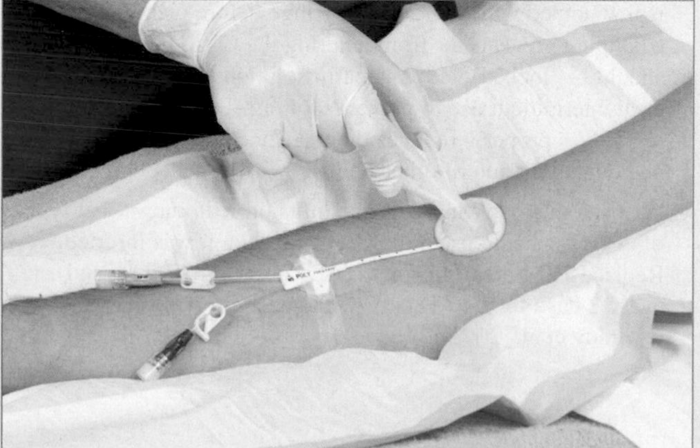

FIGURE 6 Cleansing with a gentle back and forth motion.

(*continued*)

SKILL 15-7 CHANGING THE DRESSING AND FLUSHING CENTRAL VENOUS ACCESS DEVICES continued

ACTION	RATIONALE
11. Stabilize catheter hub by holding it in place with nondominant hand. Use an alcohol wipe to clean each lumen of the catheter, starting at the insertion site and moving outward.	Cleansing is necessary because organisms on the skin can be introduced into the tissues or the bloodstream with the device.
12. Apply transparent site dressing or securement/stabilization device, centering over insertion site (Figure 7). Measure the length of the catheter that extends out from the insertion site.	Dressing prevents contamination of the IV catheter and protects the insertion site. Stabilization/securing devices preserve the integrity of the access device, minimize catheter movement at the hub, and prevent catheter dislodgement and loss of access (INS, 2011, p. S46). Measurement of the extending catheter can be compared with the documented length at time of insertion to assess if the catheter has migrated inward or moved outward.

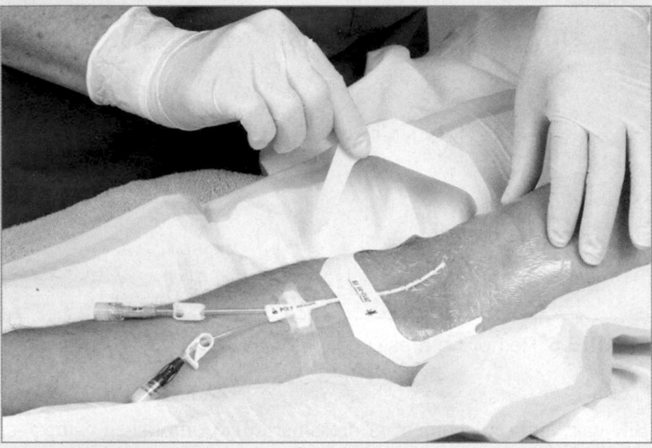

FIGURE 7 Applying site dressing

ACTION	RATIONALE
13. Working with one lumen at a time, remove end cap. Cleanse the end of the lumen with an alcohol swab and apply new end cap. Repeat for each lumen. Secure catheter lumens and/or tubing that extend outside dressing with tape.	The catheter ends should be cleansed and injection caps changed to prevent infection. Weight of tubing and/or tugging on tubing could cause catheter dislodgment.
14. If required, flush each lumen of the CVAD. Amount of saline and heparin flushes varies depending on specific CVAD and facility policy.	Cleaning the cap reduces the risk for contamination.
15. Cleanse end cap with an antimicrobial swab. Insert the saline flush syringe into the cap on the extension tubing. Pull back on the syringe to aspirate the catheter for positive blood return. If positive, instill the solution over 1 minute or flush the line according to facility policy. Remove syringe. Insert heparin syringe and instill the volume of solution designated by facility policy over 1 minute or according to facility policy. Remove syringe and reclamp the lumen. Remove gloves.	Positive blood return confirms patency before administration of medications and solutions (INS, 2011, p. S60). Flushing maintains patency of the IV line. Action of positive pressure end cap is maintained with removal of syringe before clamp is engaged. Clamping prevents air from entering the CVAD. CVADs should be 'locked' with a heparin solution (10 U/mL) after each intermittent use to prevent clotting (INS, 2011). Removing gloves properly reduces the risk for infection transmission and contamination of other items.
16. Label dressing with date, time of change, and initials. Resume fluid infusion, if indicated. Check that IV flow is accurate and system is patent. (Refer to Skill 15-3.)	Other personnel working with the infusion will know what type of device is being used, the site, and when it was inserted. Replace TSM dressings on CVADs every 5 to 7 days and every 2 days for CVAD sites with gauze dressings (INS, 2011; O'Grady et al., 2011).

ACTION	RATIONALE
17. Apply an IV securement/stabilization device if not already in place as part of the dressing, as indicated, based on facility policy. Explain to patient the purpose of the device and the importance of safeguarding the site when using the extremity.	These systems are recommended for use on all venous access sites, and particularly central venous access sites, to preserve the integrity of the access device, minimize catheter movement at the hub, and prevent catheter dislodgement and loss of access (INS, 2011, p. S46). Some devices act as a site dressing also and may already have been applied.
18. Remove equipment. Ensure patient's comfort. Lower bed, if not in lowest position.	Promotes patient comfort and safety.
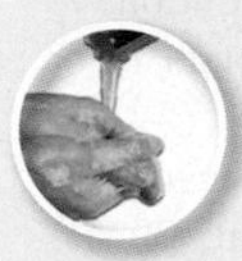 19. Remove additional PPE, if used. Perform hand hygiene.	Removing PPE properly reduces the risk for infection transmission and contamination of other items. Hand hygiene prevents transmission of microorganisms.

EVALUATION

The expected outcome is met when the dressing is changed without any complications, including dislodgement of the CVAD; the patient exhibits an insertion site that is clean and dry without redness or swelling; the dressing is clean, dry, and intact; and the CVAD remains patent.

DOCUMENTATION

Guidelines

Document the location, appearance and condition of the CVAD site. Include the presence or absence of signs of erythema, redness, swelling, or drainage. Record if the patient is experiencing any pain or discomfort related to the CVAD. Document the clinical criteria for site complications. Refer to Fundamentals Review 15-3 and Boxes 15-3 and 15-4 (in Skill 15-3). Record the subjective comments of the patient regarding the absence or presence of pain at the site. Record the patient's reaction to the procedure and pertinent patient teaching, such as alerting the nurse if the patient experiences any pain from the IV or notices any swelling at the site. The CVAD lumens should flush without difficulty. Report any abnormal findings, such as dislodgement of the CVAD, abnormal insertion assessment findings, or inability to flush the CVAD, to the primary care provider.

Sample Documentation

11/12/15 0400 PICC line located in the right basilic vein. Old dressing removed, no drainage, redness, or swelling noted at site. Site care performed; transparent dressing applied and end caps changed. Extending catheter length 5 cm. NSS flush followed by heparin flush per protocol without difficulty. Patient denies pain or discomfort. Patient instructed to inform nurse of any pain, swelling, or leakage related to PICC line.

—S. Barnes, RN

UNEXPECTED SITUATIONS AND ASSOCIATED INTERVENTIONS

- *While dressing is being changed, PICC is inadvertently dislodged:* If PICC is not all the way out, notify primary care provider. The primary care provider will most likely want a chest x-ray to determine the location of the end of the PICC line. Before the chest x-ray, reapply a dressing so that the PICC is not further dislodged.
- *When the dressing is removed, purulent drainage is noted at the insertion site:* Obtain a culture of the site; clean the area; reapply a dressing; and then notify the primary care provider. This prevents the PICC line from being open to air and unprotected while you are notifying the primary care provider. In addition, the culture is obtained without having to remove the dressing a second time. If the primary care provider does not want the culture, discard it in the appropriate receptacle.
- *When flushing the catheter, you are unable to withdraw blood, there is a sluggish flow, and/or you are unable to flush or infuse through the CVAD:* These signs may indicate CVAD occlusion. Consult with the nurse IV team and the primary care provider for appropriate catheter clearance procedure to preserve the function of the CVAD.

(continued)

SKILL 15-7 CHANGING THE DRESSING AND FLUSHING CENTRAL VENOUS ACCESS DEVICES continued

SPECIAL CONSIDERATIONS

- Flushing of PICC devices requires the use of syringes no smaller than 10-mL volume to avoid excessive pressure. Syringes smaller than 10 mL may provide pressures great enough to damage the PICC.
- Implanted ports require larger flush volumes due to volume required to fill the device.
- Groshong devices do not require the use of heparin for flushing.
- Some facilities call for a power flush (rapidly pushing the flush in small amounts).
- Heparin-induced thrombocytopenia (HIT) has been reported with the use of heparin flush solutions. Monitor all patients closely for signs and symptoms of HIT. If present or suspected, discontinue heparin (INS, 2011, p. S60).
- Monitor platelet counts for patients receiving heparin flush solution when there is an increased risk of HIT. For postoperative patients receiving heparin lock solutions of any concentration, monitoring platelet counts for HIT is recommended every 2 to 3 days from day 4 through 14 or until heparin is stopped (INS, 2011, p. S60).
- Use of topical antibiotic ointments or creams on insertion sites is not recommended because of their potential to promote fungal infections and antimicrobial resistance (O'Grady et al., 2011).
- Do not submerge venous catheters and catheter sites in water; showering is permitted with use of impermeable coverings to protect the catheter and connecting device (O'Grady et al., 2011).

Infant and Child Considerations

- Chlorhexidine is not recommended for infants under 2 months of age (INS, 2011).
- For infants under 2 months of age or pediatric patients with compromised skin integrity, remove dried povidone-iodine with normal saline wipes or sterile water (INS, 2011).

Older Adult Considerations

- Avoid using vigorous friction at the insertion site, which can traumatize fragile skin and veins in older adults.

EVIDENCE FOR PRACTICE ▶

INFUSION NURSING STANDARDS OF PRACTICE

Infusion Nurses Society. (2011). Infusion nursing standards of practice. *Journal of Infusion Nursing, 34*(1S), S1–S96.

Refer to details in Skill 15-1, Evidence for Practice, and refer to thePoint for additional research on related nursing topics.

EVIDENCE FOR PRACTICE ▶

PREVENTION OF INTRAVASCULAR CATHETER-RELATED INFECTIONS

O'Grady, N.P., Alexander, M., Burns, L.A., Dellinger, E.P., Garland, J., Heard, S.O., et al., & the Healthcare Infection Control Practices Advisory Committee (HICPAC). (2011). Guidelines for the prevention of intravascular catheter-related infections. *American Journal of Infection Control, 39*(4 Suppl.), S1–S34.

These guidelines were prepared by a working group composed of members from professional organizations representing the disciplines of critical care medicine, infectious diseases, health care infection control, surgery, anesthesiology, interventional radiology, pulmonary medicine, pediatric medicine, and nursing. These guidelines are intended to provide evidence-based recommendations for preventing intravascular catheter-related infections.

Refer to thePoint for additional research on related nursing topics.

SKILL 15-8 ACCESSING AN IMPLANTED PORT

An implanted port consists of a subcutaneous injection port attached to a catheter. The distal catheter tip dwells in the lower one third of the superior vena cava to the junction of the superior vena cava and the right atrium (INS, 2011), and the proximal end or port is usually implanted in a subcutaneous pocket of the upper chest wall (Figure 1). Implanted ports placed in the antecubital area of the arm are referred to as peripheral access system ports. When not in use, no external parts of the system are visible. When venous access is desired, the location of the injection port must be palpated. A special angled, noncoring needle is inserted through the skin and septum and into the port reservoir to access the system. Once accessed, patency is maintained by periodic flushing. The length and gauge of the needle used to access the port should be selected based on the patient's anatomy, amount of subcutaneous tissue at the site, and anticipated infusion requirements. In general, a 0.75-inch 20-gauge needle is frequently used. If the patient has a significant amount of subcutaneous tissue, a longer length (1 or 1.5 inch) may be selected. Site dressings are maintained and changed as outlined in Skill 15-7.

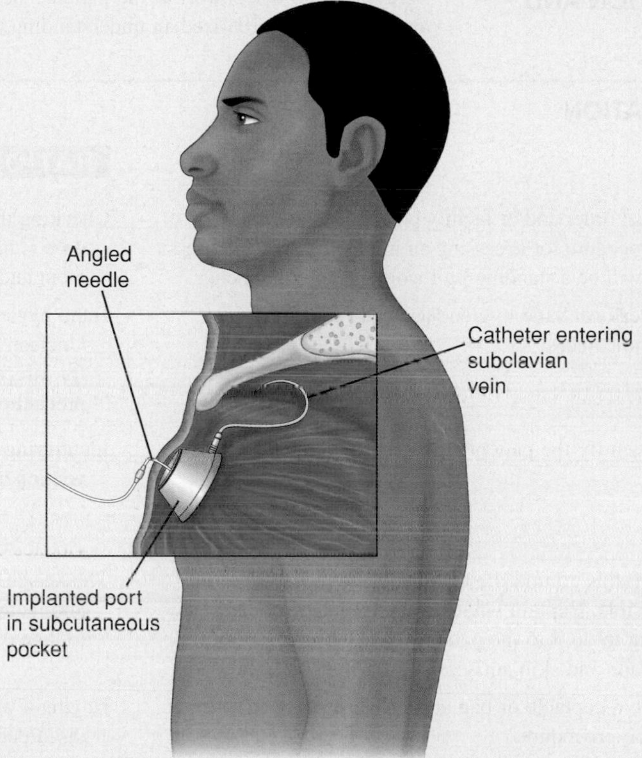

FIGURE 1 An implanted port with catheter inserted in subclavian vein and noncoring needle inserted into port.

DELEGATION CONSIDERATIONS

Accessing an implanted port is not delegated to nursing assistive personnel (NAP), to unlicensed assistive personnel (UAP), or to licensed practical/vocational nurses (LPN/LVNs).

EQUIPMENT

- Sterile tape or Steri-Strips
- Sterile semipermeable transparent dressing
- Several 2 × 2 gauzes
- Sterile towel or drape
- Cleansing swabs (>0.5% chlorhexidine preparation with alcohol)
- NSS vial and 10-mL syringe or prefilled 10-mL NSS syringe
- Heparin 100 U/mL in 10-mL syringe
- Noncoring needle (Huber needle) of appropriate length and gauge
- Masks (2), depending on facility policy
- Clean gloves
- Sterile gloves
- Additional PPE, as indicated
- Skin protectant wipe (e.g., SkinPrep)
- Alcohol or other disinfectant wipes
- Positive pressure end cap
- IV securement/stabilization device, as appropriate
- Bath blanket

(continued)

SKILL 15-8 ACCESSING AN IMPLANTED PORT continued

ASSESSMENT

Inspect the skin over the port, looking for any swelling, redness, or drainage. Also assess the site over the port for any pain or tenderness. Review the patient's history for the length of time the port has been in place. If the port has been placed recently, assess surgical incision. Note presence of Steri-Strips, approximation, ecchymosis, redness, edema, and/or drainage.

NURSING DIAGNOSIS

Determine the related factors for the nursing diagnoses based on the patient's current status. Appropriate nursing diagnoses may include:

- Risk for Infection
- Deficient Knowledge
- Risk for Impaired Skin Integrity

OUTCOME IDENTIFICATION AND PLANNING

The expected outcome to achieve when accessing an implanted port is that the port is accessed with minimal to no discomfort to the patient; the patient experiences no trauma to the site or infection; and the patient verbalized an understanding of care associated with the port.

IMPLEMENTATION

ACTION	RATIONALE
1. Verify medical order and/or facility policy and procedure. Often, the procedure for accessing an implanted port and dressing changes will be a standing protocol. Gather equipment.	Checking the order and/or policy ensures that the proper procedure is initiated. Preparation promotes efficient time management and an organized approach to the task.
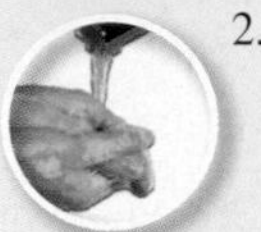 2. Perform hand hygiene and put on PPE, if indicated.	Hand hygiene and PPE prevent the spread of microorganisms. Unclean hands and improper technique are potential sources for infecting a CVAD. PPE is required based on transmission precautions.
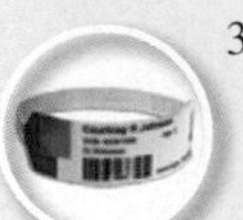 3. Identify the patient.	Identifying the patient ensures the right patient receives the intervention and helps prevent errors.
4. Close the curtains around the bed and close the door to the room, if possible. Explain what you are going to do, and why you are going to do it to the patient. Ask the patient about allergies to tape and skin antiseptics.	This ensures the patient's privacy. Explanation relieves anxiety and facilitates cooperation. Possible allergies may exist related to tape or antiseptics.
5. Place a waste receptacle or bag at a convenient location for use during the procedure.	Having a waste container handy means the soiled dressing can be discarded easily, without the spread of microorganisms.
6. Adjust the bed to a comfortable working height, usually elbow height of the caregiver (VISN 8 Patient Safety Center, 2009).	Having the bed at the proper height prevents back and muscle strain.
7. Assist the patient to a comfortable position that provides easy access to the port site. Use the bath blanket to cover any exposed area other than the site.	Patient positioning and use of a bath blanket provide for comfort and warmth.
8. Apply a mask, depending on facility policy. Ask the patient to turn his/her head away from the access site. Alternately, have the patient put on a mask, depending on facility policy. Move the overbed table to a convenient location within easy reach. Set up a sterile field on the table. Open dressing supplies and add to the sterile field. If IV solution is infusing via CVAD, interrupt and place on hold during dressing change. Apply slide clamp on each lumen of the CVAD.	Masks are recommended to help to deter the spread of microorganisms (INS, 2011, p. S64). Patient should wear mask if unable to turn the head away from the site or if based on facility policy. Many facilities have all sterile dressing supplies gathered in a single package. Stopping infusion and clamping each lumen prevent air from entering the CVAD.
9. Put on clean gloves. Palpate the location of the port. Assess site. Note the status of any surgical incisions that may be present. Remove gloves and discard.	Knowledge of location and boundaries of port are necessary to access the site safely.

ACTION	RATIONALE
10. Put on sterile gloves. Connect the end cap to the extension tubing on the noncoring needle. Clean end cap with alcohol wipe. Insert syringe with normal saline into end cap. Fill extension tubing with normal saline and apply clamp. Place on sterile field.	Priming extension tubing removes air from tubing and prevents administration of air when connected to the port.
11. Using the chlorhexidine swab, cleanse the port site. Press the applicator against the skin. **Apply chlorhexidine using a gentle back and forth motion.** Moving outward from the site, use a circular, scrubbing motion to continue to clean, covering at least a 2- to 3-inch area. **Do not wipe or blot. Allow to dry completely.**	Site care and replacement of dressing are accomplished using sterile technique. Organisms on the skin can be introduced into the tissues or the bloodstream with the needle. Chlorhexidine is the preferred antiseptic solution, but iodine, povidone-iodine, and 70% alcohol are considered acceptable alternatives in patients who are allergic to chlorhexidine (INS, 2011). Scrubbing motion creates friction and lets the solution more effectively penetrate the epidermal layers (Hadaway, 2006).
12. Using the nondominant hand, locate the port. Hold the port stable, keeping the skin taut (Figure 2).	The edges of the port must be palpated so that the needle can be inserted into the center of the port. Hold the port with your nondominant hand so that the needle is inserted into the port with the dominant hand.
13. Visualize the center of the port. Pick up the needle. Coil extension tubing into the palm of your hand. Holding needle at a 90-degree angle to the skin, insert **through the skin into the port septum (Figure 3) until the needle hits the back of the port (Figure 4).**	To function properly, the needle must be located in the middle of the port and inserted to the back of the port.

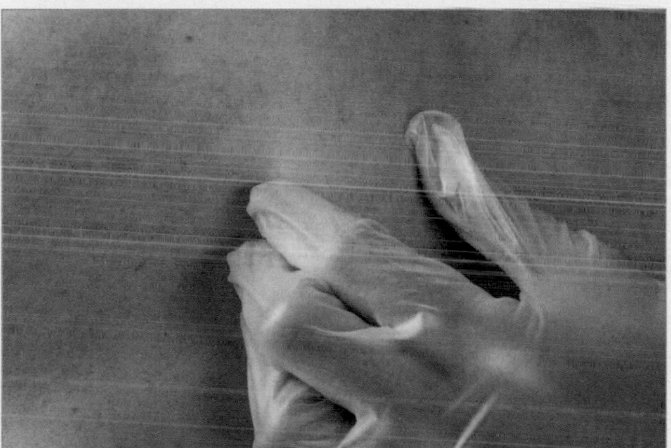

FIGURE 2 Stabilizing port with nondominant hand. *(Photo by B. Proud.)*

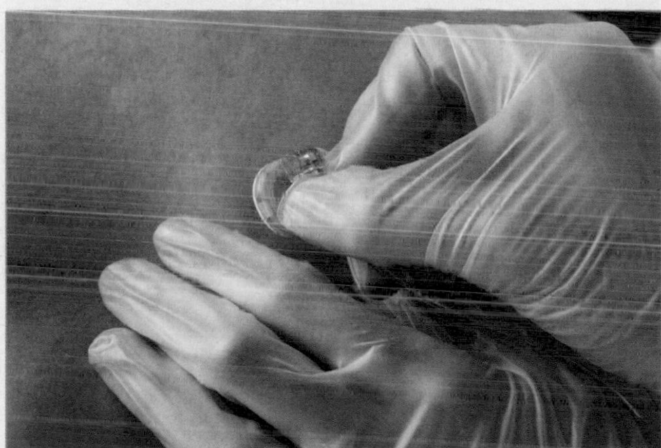

FIGURE 3 Inserting needle through skin into port. *(Photo by B. Proud.)*

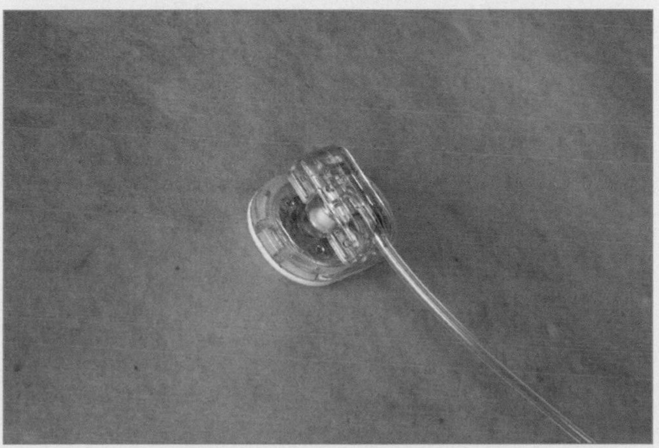

FIGURE 4 Noncoring (Huber) needle in place. *(Photo by B. Proud.)*

(continued)

SKILL 15-8 ACCESSING AN IMPLANTED PORT continued

ACTION	RATIONALE
14. Cleanse the end cap on the extension tubing with an antimicrobial swab and insert the syringe with normal saline. **Open the clamp on extension tubing and flush with 3 to 5 mL of saline, while observing the site for fluid leak or infiltration. It should flush easily, without resistance.**	If needle is not inserted correctly, fluid will leak into tissue, causing the tissue to swell and producing signs of infiltration. Flushing without resistance is also a sign that the needle is inserted correctly.
15. Pull back on the syringe plunger to aspirate for blood return (Figure 5). Do not allow blood to enter the syringe. If positive, instill the solution over 1 minute or flush the line according to facility policy. Remove syringe. Insert heparin syringe and instill the solution over 1 minute or according to facility policy. Remove syringe and clamp the extension tubing. Alternately, if IV fluid infusion is to be started, do not flush with heparin.	Positive blood return indicates the port is patent. Positive blood return confirms patency before administration of medications and solutions (INS, 2011, p. S60). Not allowing blood to enter the syringe ensures that the needle will be flushed with pure saline. Flushing maintains patency of the IV line. **Amount and number of saline and heparin flushes varies depending on specific CVAD and facility policy.** Action of positive pressure end cap is maintained with removal of syringe before clamp is engaged. Clamping prevents air from entering the CVAD. CVADs should be 'locked' with a heparin solution (10 U/mL) after each intermittent use to prevent clotting.

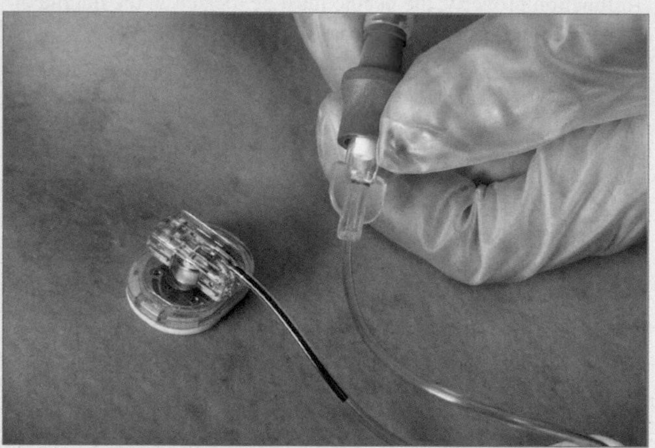

FIGURE 5 Aspirating for blood return. *(Photo by B. Proud.)*

ACTION	RATIONALE
16. If using a "Gripper" needle, remove the gripper portion from the needle by squeezing the sides together and lifting off the needle while holding the needle securely to the port with the other hand.	Gripper facilitates needle insertion and needs to be removed before application of dressing.
17. Apply the skin protectant to the site, avoiding direct application to needle insertion site. Allow to dry.	Skin protectant improves adhesion of dressing and protects skin from damage and irritation when dressing is removed.
18. Apply tape or Steri-Strips in a star-like pattern over the needle to secure it.	Secures needle to help prevent the needle from accidentally pulling out.
19. Apply transparent site dressing or securement/stabilization device, centering over insertion site.	Dressing prevents contamination of the IV catheter and protects the insertion site. Stabilization/securing devices preserve the integrity of the access device, minimize catheter movement at the hub, and prevent catheter dislodgement and loss of access (INS, 2011, p. S46).
20. Label dressing with date, time of change, and initials. If IV fluid infusion is ordered, attach administration set to extension tubing and begin administration. Refer to Skill 15-1.	Other personnel working with the infusion will know what type of device is being used, the site, and when it was inserted. Replace TSM dressings on CVADs every 5 to 7 days and every 2 days for CVAD sites with gauze dressings (INS, 2011; O'Grady et al., 2011).

ACTION	RATIONALE
21. Apply an IV securement/stabilization device if not already in place as part of dressing, as indicated, based on facility policy. Explain to the patient the purpose of the device and the importance of safeguarding the site when using the extremity.	These systems are recommended for use on all venous access sites, and particularly central venous access sites, to preserve the integrity of the access device, minimize catheter movement at the hub, and prevent catheter dislodgement and loss of access (INS, 2011, p. S46). Some devices act as a site dressing also and may already have been applied.
22. Remove equipment. Ensure patient's comfort. Lower bed, if not in lowest position.	Promotes patient comfort and safety.
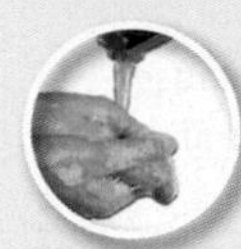 23. Remove additional PPE, if used. Perform hand hygiene.	Removing PPE properly reduces the risk for infection transmission and contamination of other items. Hand hygiene prevents transmission of microorganisms.

EVALUATION

The expected outcome is met when the port can be accessed without difficulty or pain; the patient remains free of signs and symptoms of infection or trauma; and the patient verbalizes an understanding of care related to the port.

DOCUMENTATION

Document the location of the port and the size of needle used to access the port. Document the presence of a blood return and the ease of ability to flush the port. Record the patient's reaction to the procedure and if the patient is experiencing any pain or discomfort related to the port. Document the assessment of the site. Record any appropriate patient teaching.

Sample Documentation

11/22/15 1245 Implanted port R chest wall. Site without drainage, swelling, or redness. 20-G 0.75-inch Huber needle used to access port. Flushes easily with good blood return. Steri-Strips and transparent dressing applied. Patient denies pain or discomfort. Patient instructed to call nurse with any swelling, pain, or leaking.

—S. Barnes, RN

UNEXPECTED SITUATIONS AND ASSOCIATED INTERVENTIONS

- *Port insertion site begins to swell when flushing with saline:* Stop flushing. Verify that needle is against the back of the port septum. Attempt to flush. If swelling persists, stop flush. Remove needle. Obtain additional supplies and reaccess port with new needle. Check blood return and flush. If swelling persists, stop flush. Depending on facility policy, leave access needle in place. Cover with transparent dressing. Notify the primary care provider. Anticipate diagnostic tests to determine patency of port.
- *Port does not flush:* Check clamp to make sure it is open. Gently push down on needle and again try to flush. Ask the patient to perform a Valsalva maneuver. Try having the patient change position or place the affected arm over the head, or try raising or lowering the head of the bed. If the port still does not flush, remove needle. Obtain additional supplies and reaccess with new needle. Check blood return and flush. If still unable to flush, notify the primary care provider. Depending on facility policy, leave access needle in place. Cover with transparent dressing. Anticipate diagnostic tests to determine patency of port.
- *Port flushes, but does not have a blood return:* Ask the patient to perform a Valsalva maneuver. Try having the patient change position or place the affected arm over the head, or try raising or lowering the head of the bed. If the port still does not have a blood return, remove needle. Obtain additional supplies and reaccess with new needle. Check blood return and flush. If it still does not have a blood return, notify the primary care provider. Depending on facility policy, leave access needle in place. Cover with transparent dressing. Anticipate diagnostic tests to determine patency of the port and/or instillation of thrombolytic.

(continued)

SKILL 15-8 ACCESSING AN IMPLANTED PORT continued

SPECIAL CONSIDERATIONS

General Considerations

- Implanted ports require larger flush volumes due to volume required to fill device.
- Groshong devices do not require the use of heparin for flushing.
- Some institutions call for a power flush (rapidly pushing the flush in small amounts).
- The most common practice is to replace the needle every 7 days when using a port for continuous infusions (INS, 2011).
- Monitor platelet counts for patient receiving heparin flush solution when there is an increased risk of HIT. For postoperative patients receiving heparin lock solutions of any concentration, monitoring platelet counts for HIT is recommended every 2 to 3 days from day 4 through 14 or until heparin is stopped (INS, 2011, p. S60).
- Use of topical antibiotic ointments or creams on insertion sites is not recommended because of their potential to promote fungal infections and antimicrobial resistance (O'Grady et al., 2011).
- Do not submerge venous catheters and catheter sites in water; showering is permitted with use of impermeable coverings to protect the catheter and connecting device (O'Grady et al., 2011).

Infant and Child Considerations

- Chlorhexidine is not recommended for infants under 2 months of age (INS, 2011).
- For infants under 2 months of age or pediatric patients with compromised skin integrity, remove dried povidone-iodine with normal saline wipes or sterile water (INS, 2011).

Older Adult Considerations

- Avoid using vigorous friction at the insertion site, which can traumatize fragile skin and veins in older adults.

Home Care Considerations

- Patients often are discharged with a CVAD. The patient and family or significant other requires teaching to care for CVAD in the home.
- Implanted ports need to be accessed every 4 to 6 weeks (according to agency policy) to be flushed.

EVIDENCE FOR PRACTICE ▶

INFUSION NURSING STANDARDS OF PRACTICE

Infusion Nurses Society. (2011). Infusion nursing standards of practice. *Journal of Infusion Nursing, 34*(1S), S1–S96.

Refer to details in Skill 15-1, Evidence for Practice, and refer to thePoint for additional research on related nursing topics.

EVIDENCE FOR PRACTICE ▶

PREVENTION OF INTRAVASCULAR CATHETER-RELATED INFECTIONS

O'Grady, N.P., Alexander, M., Burns, L.A., Dellinger, E.P., Garland, J., Heard, S.O., et al., & the Healthcare Infection Control Practices Advisory Committee (HICPAC). (2011). Guidelines for the prevention of intravascular catheter-related infections. *American Journal of Infection Control, 39*(4 Suppl.), S1–S34.

Refer to details in Skill 15-7, Evidence for Practice, and refer to thePoint for additional research on related nursing topics.

SKILL 15-9 DEACCESSING AN IMPLANTED PORT

When an implanted port will not be used for a period of time, such as when a patient is being discharged, the port is deaccessed. Deaccessing a port involves flushing the port and removing the needle from the port.

DELEGATION CONSIDERATIONS

Deaccessing an implanted port is not delegated to nursing assistive personnel (NAP), to unlicensed assistive personnel (UAP), or to licensed practical/vocational nurses (LPN/LVNs).

EQUIPMENT

- Clean gloves
- Additional PPE, as indicated
- Syringe filled with 10 mL saline
- Syringe filled with 5 mL heparin (100 U/mL or facility's recommendations)
- Sterile gauze sponge
- Alcohol or other disinfectant wipes
- Band-Aid

ASSESSMENT

Inspect the insertion site, looking for any swelling, redness, or drainage. Also assess site over port for any pain or tenderness. Review the patient's history for the length of time the port and needle have been in place.

NURSING DIAGNOSIS

Determine the related factors for the nursing diagnoses based on the patient's current status. Appropriate nursing diagnoses may include:

- Risk for Infection
- Deficient Knowledge
- Risk for Injury

OUTCOME IDENTIFICATION AND PLANNING

The expected outcome to achieve when deaccessing an implanted port is that the needle is removed with minimal to no discomfort to the patient; the patient experiences no trauma or infection; and the patient verbalizes an understanding of port care.

IMPLEMENTATION

ACTION	RATIONALE
1. Verify medical order and/or facility policy and procedure. Often, the procedure for deaccessing an implanted port will be a standing protocol. Gather equipment.	Checking the order and/or policy ensures that the proper procedure is initiated. Preparation promotes efficient time management and an organized approach to the task.
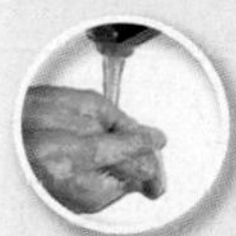 2. Perform hand hygiene and put on PPE, if indicated.	Hand hygiene and PPE prevent the spread of microorganisms. Unclean hands and improper technique are potential sources for infecting a CVAD. PPE is required based on transmission precautions.
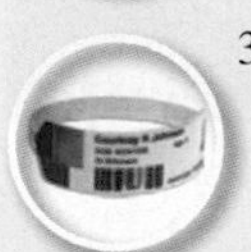 3. Identify the patient.	Identifying the patient ensures the right patient receives the intervention and helps prevent errors.
4. Close the curtains around the bed and close the door to the room, if possible. Explain what you are going to do and why you are going to do it to the patient.	This ensures the patient's privacy. Explanation relieves anxiety and facilitates cooperation.
5. Adjust the bed to a comfortable working height, usually elbow height of the caregiver (VISN 8 Patient Safety Center, 2009).	Having the bed at the proper height prevents back and muscle strain.
6. Assist the patient to a comfortable position that provides easy access to the port site. Use the bath blanket to cover any exposed area other than the site.	Patient positioning and use of a bath blanket provide for comfort and warmth.

(continued)

SKILL 15-9 DEACCESSING AN IMPLANTED PORT continued

ACTION	RATIONALE
7. Put on gloves. Stabilize port needle with nondominant hand. Remove any IV securement/stabilization device that may be in place. Gently pull back transparent dressing, beginning with edges and proceeding around the edge of the dressing. Carefully remove all the tape that is securing the needle in place.	Gloves prevent contact with blood and body fluids. Removal of stabilization device and dressing is necessary to remove access needle. Gently pulling the edges of the dressing is less traumatic to the patient.
8. Clean the end cap on the extension tubing and insert the saline-filled syringe. Unclamp the extension tubing and flush with a minimum of 10 mL of normal saline (Figure 1).	It is important to flush all substances out of the well of the implanted port, because it may be inactive for an extended period of time. **Amount and number of saline and heparin flushes varies depending on specific CVAD and facility policy.**
9. Remove the syringe and insert the heparin-filled syringe, flushing with 5 mL heparin (100 U/mL or per facility policy). Remove syringe and clamp the extension tubing.	**Amount of saline and heparin flushes varies depending on specific CVAD and facility policy.** Action of positive pressure end cap is maintained with removal of syringe before clamp is engaged. Clamping prevents air from entering the CVAD. Implanted ports should be 'locked' with a heparin solution (100 U/mL) before removal on an access needle and/or for periodic access and flushing to prevent clotting (INS, 2011, p. S61).
10. Secure the port on either side with the fingers of your nondominant hand. Grasp the needle/wings with the fingers of dominant hand. Firmly and smoothly, pull the needle straight up at a 90-degree angle from the skin to remove it from the port septum (Figure 2). Engage needle guard, if not automatic on removal.	The port is held in place while the needle is removed.

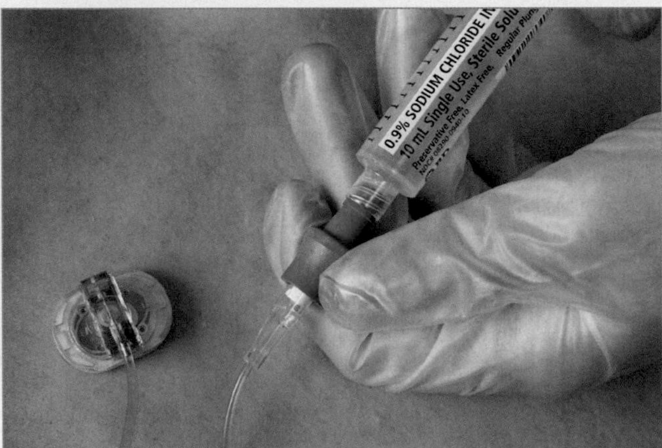

FIGURE 1 Flushing port with saline. *(Photo by B. Proud.)*

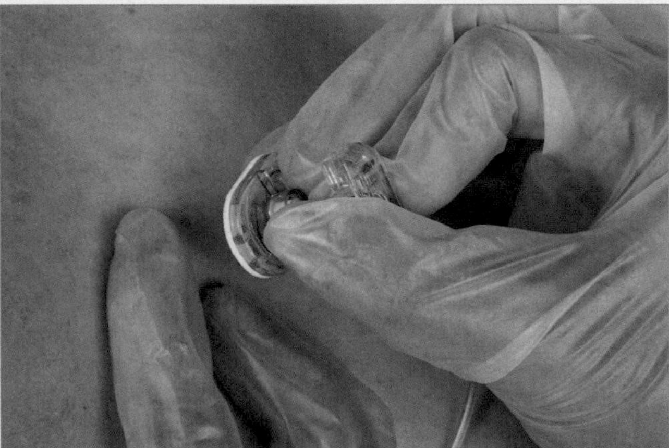

FIGURE 2 Pulling needle from port with auto-engagement of needle guard. *(Photo by B. Proud.)*

ACTION	RATIONALE
11. Apply gentle pressure with the gauze to the insertion site. Apply a Band-Aid over the port if any oozing occurs. Otherwise, a dressing is not necessary. Remove gloves.	A small amount of blood may form from the needlestick. Intact skin provides a barrier to infection.
12. Ensure patient's comfort. Lower bed, if not in lowest position. Put on one glove to handle needle. Dispose of needle with extension tubing in sharps container.	Promotes patient comfort and safety. Proper disposal of needle prevents accidental injury.
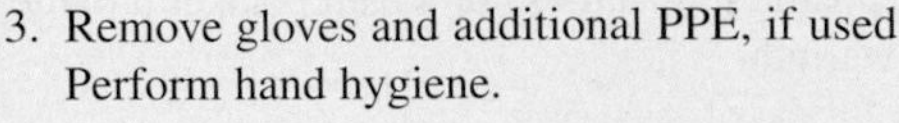 13. Remove gloves and additional PPE, if used. Perform hand hygiene.	Removing PPE properly reduces the risk for infection transmission and contamination of other items. Hand hygiene prevents transmission of microorganisms.

EVALUATION

The expected outcome is met when the port flushes easily; the needle is removed without difficulty; the site is clean, dry, without evidence of redness, irritation, or warmth; and the patient verbalizes an understanding of port care.

DOCUMENTATION

Guidelines

Document the location of the port and the ease or difficulty of flushing the port. Record the locking of the port with heparin (100 U/mL). This may be done on the CMAR/MAR. Document removal of the access needle. Record the appearance of the site, including if there is any drainage, swelling, or redness. Record any appropriate patient teaching.

Sample Documentation

11/13/15 1020 Implanted port L chest wall flushed without resistance using 10 mL of saline and 5 mL of heparin/100 U/mL. No hematoma noted. Access needle removed without difficulty. Site without redness, swelling, drainage, or heat. Patient denies discomfort. Patient verbalized an understanding of site care.

—S. Barnes, RN

UNEXPECTED SITUATIONS AND ASSOCIATED INTERVENTIONS

- *Port does not flush:* Check clamp to make sure tubing is open. Gently push down on needle and again try to flush. Ask patient to perform a Valsalva maneuver. Have patient change position or place the affected arm over the head and raise or lower the head of the bed. If the port still does not flush, notify the primary care provider.
- *Site does not stop bleeding:* Continue to hold pressure. If the patient has some clotting disturbances, pressure may need to be applied for a longer duration.

SPECIAL CONSIDERATIONS

General Considerations

- Groshong devices do not require heparin.
- Some institutions call for a power flush (rapidly pushing the flush in small amounts).
- Monitor platelet counts for patient receiving heparin flush solution when there is an increased risk of HIT. For postoperative patients receiving heparin lock solutions of any concentration, monitoring platelet counts for HIT is recommended every 2 to 3 days from day 4 through 14 or until heparin is stopped (INS, 2011, p. S60).
- Patients often are discharged with a CVAD. The patient and family or significant other requires teaching to care for CVAD in the home.
- Implanted ports need to be accessed every 4 to 6 weeks (according to agency policy) to be flushed. Implanted ports should be 'locked' with a heparin solution (100 U/mL) before removal on an access needle and/or for periodic access and flushing to prevent clotting (INS, 2011, p. S61).

EVIDENCE FOR PRACTICE ▶

INFUSION NURSING STANDARDS OF PRACTICE

Infusion Nurses Society. (2011). Infusion nursing standards of practice. *Journal of Infusion Nursing, 34*(1S), S1–S96.

Refer to details in Skill 15-1, Evidence for Practice, and refer to thePoint for additional research on related nursing topics.

EVIDENCE FOR PRACTICE ▶

PREVENTION OF INTRAVASCULAR CATHETER-RELATED INFECTIONS

O'Grady, N.P., Alexander, M., Burns, L.A., Dellinger, E.P., Garland, J., Heard, S.O., et al., & the Healthcare Infection Control Practices Advisory Committee (HICPAC). (2011). Guidelines for the prevention of intravascular catheter-related infections. *American Journal of Infection Control, 39*(4 Suppl.), S1–S34.

Refer to details in Skill 15-7, Evidence for Practice, and refer to thePoint for additional research on related nursing topics.

SKILL 15-10 REMOVING A PERIPHERALLY INSERTED CENTRAL CATHETER (PICC)

When PICC is no longer required or when the patient has developed complications, it will be discontinued. Nurses or specialized IV team nurses may be responsible for removing a PICC line. Specific protocols must be followed to prevent breakage or fracture of the catheter.

DELEGATION CONSIDERATIONS

The removal of a PICC is not delegated to nursing assistive personnel (NAP), to unlicensed assistive personnel (UAP), or to licensed practical/vocational nurses (LPN/LVNs).

EQUIPMENT

- Clean gloves
- Additional PPE, as indicated
- Sterile gauze sponges
- Tape
- Disposable measuring tape

ASSESSMENT

Inspect the insertion site, looking for any swelling, redness, or drainage. Check pertinent laboratory values, particularly coagulation times and platelet counts. Patients with alterations in coagulation require that pressure be applied for a longer period of time after catheter removal. Measure the length of the PICC after removal.

NURSING DIAGNOSIS

Determine the related factors for the nursing diagnoses based on the patient's current status. Appropriate nursing diagnoses may include:

- Risk for Infection
- Risk for Injury
- Deficient Knowledge

OUTCOME IDENTIFICATION AND PLANNING

The expected outcome to achieve when removing a PICC is that the PICC is removed with minimal to no discomfort to the patient and the patient experiences no trauma or infection.

IMPLEMENTATION

ACTION	RATIONALE
1. Verify medical order for PICC removal and facility policy and procedure. Gather equipment.	Checking the order and/or policy ensures that the proper procedure is initiated. Preparation promotes efficient time management and an organized approach to the task.
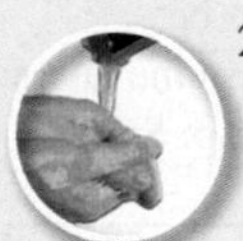 2. Perform hand hygiene and put on PPE, if indicated.	Hand hygiene and PPE prevent the spread of microorganisms. Unclean hands and improper technique are potential sources for infecting a CVAD. PPE is required based on transmission precautions.
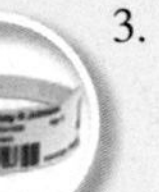 3. Identify the patient.	Identifying the patient ensures the right patient receives the intervention and helps prevent errors.
4. Close the curtains around the bed and close the door to the room, if possible. Explain what you are going to do and why you are going to do it to the patient.	This ensures the patient's privacy. Explanation relieves anxiety and facilitates cooperation.
5. Adjust the bed to a comfortable working height, usually elbow height of the caregiver (VISN 8 Patient Safety Center, 2009).	Having the bed at the proper height prevents back and muscle strain.
6. Assist the patient to a supine position with the arm straight and the catheter insertion site at or below heart level. Use the bath blanket to cover any exposed area other than the site.	This position is recommended to reduce the risk of air embolism. Use of a bath blanket provides for comfort and warmth.

ACTION	RATIONALE
7. Put on gloves. Stabilize catheter hub with your nondominant hand. Gently pull back transparent dressing, beginning with edges and proceeding around the edge of the dressing. Carefully remove all the tape that is securing the catheter in place.	Gloves prevent contact with blood and body fluids. Gently pulling the edges of the dressing is less traumatic to the patient.
8. Instruct the patient to hold his/her breath, and perform a Valsalva maneuver as the last portion of the catheter is removed; if unable to do so, time the removal during patient expiration.	Use of Valsalva maneuver or removal during expiration reduces risk for air embolism (Feil, 2012).
9. Using dominant hand, remove the catheter slowly. Grasp the catheter close to the insertion site and slowly ease it out, keeping it parallel to the skin. Continue removing in small increments, using a smooth and constant motion (Figure 1).	Gentle pressure reduces risk of breakage. Catheter should come out easily.

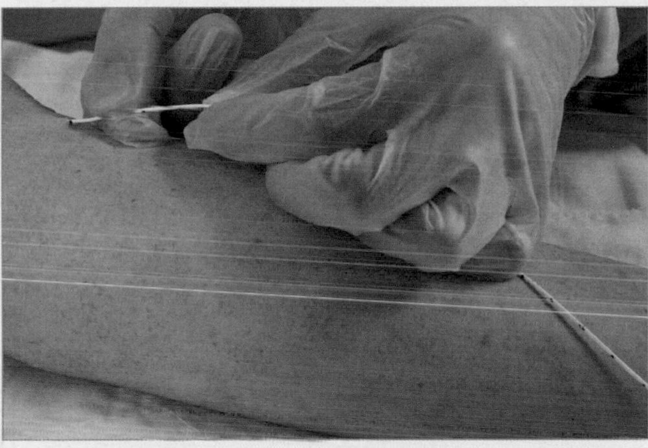

FIGURE 1 Removing PICC in small increments, using a smooth and constant motion. *(Photo by B. Proud.)*

ACTION	RATIONALE
10. After removal, apply pressure to the site with sterile gauze until hemostasis is achieved (minimum 1 minute). Then apply petroleum-based ointment and a sterile dressing to the access site.	Adequate pressure prevents hematoma formation. Use of a petroleum-based ointment and a sterile dressing at the access site seals the skin-to-vein tract and decreases the risk of air embolus (INS, 2011).
11. Measure the catheter and compare it with the length listed in the chart when it was inserted. Inspect the catheter for patency. Dispose of PICC according to facility policy.	Measurement and inspection ensures entire catheter was removed. Proper disposal reduces transmission of microorganisms and prevents contact with blood and body fluids.
12. Remove gloves. Ensure patient's comfort. Lower bed, if not in lowest position.	Promotes patient comfort and safety.
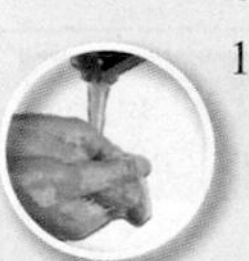 13. Remove additional PPE, if used. Perform hand hygiene.	Removing PPE properly reduces the risk for infection transmission and contamination of other items. Hand hygiene prevents transmission of microorganisms.

EVALUATION

The expected outcome is met when the PICC is removed with minimal to no discomfort to the patient and the patient experiences no trauma or infection.

DOCUMENTATION

Guidelines

Document the location of the PICC and its removal. Record the catheter length and patency. Record the appearance of the site, including if there is any drainage, swelling, or redness. Record any appropriate patient teaching.

(continued)

SKILL 15-10 REMOVING A PERIPHERALLY INSERTED CENTRAL CATHETER (PICC) continued

Sample Documentation

4/1/15 1230 PICC removed from L brachial. Length of catheter 37.5 cm; entire length intact. Pressure applied to insertion site for 2 minutes; site without bleeding, ecchymosis, redness, drainage. Dry dressing applied. Patient instructed to notify nurse if pain or bleeding noted.

—S. Stone, RN

UNEXPECTED SITUATIONS AND ASSOCIATED INTERVENTIONS

- *You encounter resistance while attempting to remove the PICC.* If resistance is felt when removing a catheter, stop removal. Resistance typically is caused by smooth muscle spasm inside the vein wall. Encourage the patient to relax and take deep breaths. Wait a few minutes and then try again (Hadaway, 2009). Do not forcibly remove the catheter (INS, 2011). Replace the sterile dressing and notify the patient's primary care provider.
- *You are removing the PICC and a portion of the catheter breaks:* Immediately apply a tourniquet to the upper arm, close to the axilla, to prevent advancement of the piece of catheter into the right atrium. Check the patient's radial pulse. If unable to detect a pulse, the tourniquet is too tight. Notify the primary care provider immediately. Anticipate the need for an x-ray study to locate the piece of catheter and possible surgery to retrieve the catheter.
- *You measure the catheter after removal and it is shorter than the documented length at insertion:* Notify the primary care provider. Monitor the patient for signs of distress. The piece of catheter could be lodged in the venous system or have migrated to the right atrium. Anticipate the need for an x-ray study to locate the piece of catheter and possible surgery to retrieve the catheter.

EVIDENCE FOR PRACTICE ▶

INFUSION NURSING STANDARDS OF PRACTICE

Infusion Nurses Society. (2011). Infusion nursing standards of practice. *Journal of Infusion Nursing, 34*(1S), S1–S96.

Refer to details in Skill 15-1, Evidence for Practice, and refer to thePoint for additional research on related nursing topics.

ENHANCE YOUR UNDERSTANDING

FOCUSING ON PATIENT CARE: DEVELOPING CLINICAL REASONING

Consider the case scenarios at the beginning of the chapter as you answer the following questions to enhance your understanding and apply what you have learned.

QUESTIONS

1. Simon Lawrence's mother is asking about the risks associated with IV placement. What would you tell her about the risks associated with IV placement and rehydration?
2. During the first 5 minutes of Melissa Cohen's transfusion of packed red blood cells, she reports a headache and low back pain. When you assess her, you find that she has a temperature of 101°F and she is shivering. What actions would be most appropriate at this time?
3. Mr. Tracy asks about care of his new implanted port. What are some topics you should discuss with him before he is discharged?

You can find suggested answers after the Bibliography at the end of this chapter.

INTEGRATED CASE STUDY CONNECTION

The case studies in Unit 3 are designed to focus on integrating concepts. Refer to the following case studies to enhance your understanding of the concepts related to the skills in this chapter.

- Intermediate Case Studies: Olivia Greenbaum, page 1077; Jason Brown, page 1083; Kent Clark, page 1085; Janice Romero, page 1088; Gwen Galloway, page 1089.
- Advanced Case Studies: Robert Espinoza, page 1097.

TAYLOR SUITE RESOURCES

Explore these additional resources to enhance learning for this chapter:

- NCLEX-Style Questions and other resources on thePoint, http://thePoint.lww.com/Lynn4e
- *Skill Checklists for Taylor's Clinical Nursing Skills*, 4e
- *Taylor's Video Guide to Clinical Nursing Skills:* Intravenous Therapy and Central Venous Access Devices
- *Lippincott DocuCare* Fundamentals cases

Bibliography

Ackley, B.J., & Ladwig, G.B. (2011). *Nursing diagnosis handbook* (9th ed.). St. Louis: Mosby/Elsevier.

American Red Cross. (2013). *Donating blood. Eligibility requirements.* Available at http://www.redcrossblood.org/donating-blood/eligibility-requirements.

Arbique, J., & Arbique, D. (2007). I.V. rounds. Reducing the risk of nerve injuries. *Nursing, 37*(11), 20–21.

Baxter, A.L., Ewing, P.H., Young, G.B., Ware, A., Evans, N., & Manworren, R.C.B. (2013). EMLA application exceeding two hours improves pediatric emergency department venipuncture success. *Advanced Emergency Nursing Journal, 35*(1), 67–75.

Bulechek, G.M, Butcher, H.K., Dochterman, J.M., & Wagner, C.M. (Eds.). (2013). *Nursing interventions classification (NIC)* (6th ed.). St. Louis: Mosby Elsevier.

Casey, A.L., Elliott, T.S.J. (2010). Prevention of central venous catheter-related infection: Update. *British Journal of Nursing, 19*(2), 78, 80, 82, 84, 86–87.

Centers for Disease Control and Prevention (CDC). (2011). *Guidelines for the prevention of intravascular catheter-related infections.* Available at www.cdc.gov/hicpac/pdf/guidelines/bsi-guidelines 2011.pdf.

Charron, K. (2012). Decreasing central line infections and needlestick injury rates. *Journal of Infusion Nursing, 35*(6), 370–375.

Cook, L.S. (2013). Infusion-related air embolism. *Journal of Infusion Nursing, 36*(1), 26–36.

Dudek, S. (2014). *Nutrition essentials for nursing practice* (7th ed.). Philadelphia: Wolters Kluwer Health/Lippincott Williams & Wilkins.

Dychter, S., Gold, D., Carson, D., & Haller, M. (2012). Intravenous therapy: A review of complications and economic considerations of peripheral access. *Journal of Infusion Nursing, 35*(2), 84–91.

Ead, H. (2011). Blood products and the phases of perianesthesia care—Reviewing the implications. *Journal of PeriAnesthesia Nursing, 26*(4), 262–276.

Eastwood, G.M., Peck, L., Young, H., Prowle, J., Vasudevan, V., Jones, D., et al. (2012). Intravenous fluid administration and monitoring for adult ward patients in a teaching hospital. *Nursing and Health Sciences, 14*(2), 265–271.

Feil, M. (2012). Pennsylvania Patient Safety Authority. *Pennsylvania patient safety advisory. Reducing risk if air embolism associated with central venous access devices.* Available at http://patientsafetyauthority.org/ADVISORIES/AdvisoryLibrary/2012/Jun;9(2)/Pages/58.aspx.

Fluids & electrolytes made incredibly easy! (5th ed.). (2011). Philadelphia: Wolters Kluwer Health/Lippincott Williams & Wilkins.

Gabriel, J. (2012). Venipuncture and cannulation: Considering the ageing vein. *British Journal of Nursing (Intravenous Supplement), 21*(2), S22–S28.

Gabriel, J. (2008). Infusion therapy part one: Minimising the risks. *Nursing Standard, 22*(31), 51–56.

Ganter-Ritz, V., Speroni, K.G., & Atherton, M. (2012). A randomized double-blind study comparing intradermal anesthetic tolerability, efficacy, and cost-effectiveness of lidocaine, buffered lidocaine, and bacteriostatic normal saline for peripheral intravenous insertion. *Journal of Infusion Nursing, 35*(2), 93–99.

Grossman, S., & Porth, C.M. (2014). Porth's pathophysiology: concepts of altered health states. (9th ed.). Philadelphia: Wolters Kluwer Health/Lippincott Williams & Wilkins.

Hadaway, L. (2006). 5 steps to preventing catheter-related bloodstream infections. *LPN2009, 2*(5), 50–55.

Hadaway, L.C. (2010). Extra! Extra! Preventing extravasation. *Nursing Made Incredibly Easy, 8*(2), 13–14.

Hadaway, L.C. (2009). Central venous access devices. *Nursing2009 Critical Care, 3*(5), 26–33.

Hammond, T. (2004). Choice and use of peripherally inserted central catheters by nurses. *Professional Nurse, 19*(9), 493–497.

Higginson, R. (2011). IV therapy and infection control in patients in the community. *British Journal of Nursing, 20*(3), 152–155.

Hinkle, J.L., & Cheever, K.H. (2014). *Brunner & Suddarth's textbook of medical-surgical nursing* (13th ed.). Philadelphia: Wolters Kluwer Health/Lippincott Williams & Wilkins.

Hogan-Quigley, B., Palm, M.L., & Bickley, L. (2012). *Bates' nursing guide to physical examination and history taking.* Philadelphia: Wolters Kluwer Health/Lippincott Williams & Wilkins.

Houston, P.A. (2013). Obtaining vascular access in the obese patient population. *Journal of Infusion Nursing, 36*(1), 52–56.

Huether, S.E., & McCance, K.L. (2012.) *Understanding pathophysiology* (5th ed.). St. Louis: Elsevier.

Hughes, T. (2012). Providing information to children before and during venipuncture. *Nursing Children and Young People, 24*(5), 23–28.

Infusion Nurses Society (INS). (2011). Infusion nursing standards of practice. *Journal of Infusion Nursing, 34*(Suppl 1S).

Infusion Nurses Society (INS). (2006). Infusion nursing standards of practice. *Journal of Infusion Nursing, 29*(1S), S60.

Ingram, P., & Lavery, I. (2005). Peripheral intravenous therapy: key risks and implications for practice. *Nursing Standard, 19*(46), 55–64.

Institute for Safe Medication Practices (ISMP). (2013). *ISMP summit on the use of smart infusion pumps: Guidelines for safe implementation and use.* Available at http://www.ismp.org/tools/guidelines/smartpumps/default.asp#benefits.

I.V. Rounds. Comparing short peripheral cannula insertion sites. (2008). *Nursing, 38*(5), 60.

Jarvis, C. (2012). *Physical examination & health assessment* (6th ed.). St. Louis: Saunders/Elsevier.

The Joint Commission (TJC). (2014). *National patient safety goals.* Available at http://www.jointcommission.org/standards_information/npsgs.aspx.

Julian, M.K. (2013). Caring for your patient receiving TPN. *Nursing Made Incredibly Easy!, 11*(1), 8–11.

Kassab, M.I., Roydhouse, J.K., Fowler, C., & Foureur, M. (2012). The effectiveness of glucose in reducing needle-related procedural pain in infants. *Journal of Pediatric Nursing, 27*(1), 3–17.

Kee, J.L., Hayes, E.R., & McCuistion, L.E. (2012). *Pharmacology. A nursing process approach* (7th ed.). St. Louis: Elsevier/Saunders.

Koshy, R. (2011). Vascular access device selection for intravenous therapy. *Journal of Illinois Nursing, 109*(3), 24–28.

Kyle, T., & Carman, S. (2013). *Essentials of pediatric nursing* (2nd ed.). Philadelphia: Wolters Kluwer Health/Lippincott Williams & Wilkins.

Lopez, A.C. (2011). A quality improvement program combining maximal barrier precaution compliance monitoring and daily chlorhexidine gluconate baths resulting in decreased central line bloodstream infections. *Dimensions of Critical Care Nursing, 30*(5), 293–298.

Maiocco, G., & Coole, C. (2012). Use of ultrasound guidance for peripheral intravenous placement in difficult-to-access patients. Advancing practice with evidence. *Journal of Nursing Care Quality, 27*(1), 51–55.

Malarkey, L.M., & McMorrow, M.E. (2012). *Saunders nursing guide to laboratory and diagnostic tests* (2nd ed.). St. Louis: Elsevier Saunders.

Mathers, D. (2011). Evidence-based practice: Improving outcomes for patients with a central venous access device. *Journal of the Association for Vascular Access, 16*(2), 64–72.

Moorhead, S., Johnson, M., Maas, M.L., & Swanson, E. (Eds.). (2013). *Nursing outcomes classification (NOC)* (5th ed.). St. Louis: Mosby Elsevier.

Moureau, N. (2013). Safe patient care when using vascular access devices. *British Journal of Nursing, 22*(2), S14–S21.

Moureau, N.L. (2008). Tips for inserting an I.V. device in an older adult. *Nursing, 38*(12), 12.

NANDA-I International. (2012). *Nursing diagnoses: Definitions & classification 2012–2014.* West Sussex, UK: Wiley-Blackwell.

O'Grady, N.P., Alexander, M., Burns, L.A., Dellinger, E.P., Garland, J., Heard, S.O., et al., & the Healthcare Infection Control Practices Advisory Committee (HICPAC). (2011). Guidelines for the prevention of intravascular catheter-related infections. *American Journal of Infection Control, 39*(4 Suppl.), S1–S34.

Ogston-Tuck, S. (2012). Intravenous therapy: Guidance on devices, management and care. *British Journal of Community Nursing, 17*(10), 474–484.

Perry, S.E., Hockenberry, M.J., Lowdermilk, D.L., & Wilson, D. (2010). *Maternal child nursing care* (4th ed.). Maryland Heights, MO: Mosby/Elsevier.

Scales, K. (2008). Intravenous therapy: A guide to good practice. *British Journal of Nursing, 17*(19) (Suppl.): S4–S12.

Smith, B., & Hannum, F. (2008). Optimizing IV therapy in the elderly. *Advance for Nurses, 10*(18), 27–28.

Tabloski, P. (2010). *Gerontological nursing* (2nd ed.). Upper Saddle River, NJ: Pearson.

Taylor, C., Lillis, C., & Lynn P. (2015). *Fundamentals of nursing.* (8th ed.). Philadelphia: Wolters Kluwer Health/Lippincott Williams & Wilkins.

Taylor, J.J., & Cohen, B.J. (2013). *Memmler's structure and function of the human body* (10th ed.). Philadelphia: Wolters Kluwer Health/Lippincott Williams & Wilkins.

Thayer, D. (2012). Skin damage associated with intravenous therapy. *Journal of Infusion Nursing, 35*(6), 390–401.

VISN 8 Patient Safety Center. (2009). *Safe patient handling and movement algorithms.* Tampa, FL: Author. Available at http://www.visn8.va.gov/visn8/patientsafetycenter/safePtHandling/default.asp.

White, A., Lopez, F., & Stone, P. (2010). Developing and sustaining an ultrasound-guided peripheral intravenous access program for emergency nurses. *Advanced Emergency Nursing Journal, 32*(2), 173–188.

Wilkins, R.G., & Unverdorben, M. (2012). Accidental intravenous infusion of air. A concise review. *Journal of Infusion Nursing, 35*(6), 404–408.

SUGGESTED ANSWERS FOR FOCUSING ON PATIENT CARE: DEVELOPING CLINICAL REASONING

1. Explain the reason the IV access is necessary and the rationale for IV fluid replacement. Discuss the potential complications related to peripheral venous access and IV fluid infusion, including infiltration, phlebitis, and infection. Explain the steps the nurses will take to prevent these complications; discuss the steps Ms. Lawrence can take to help prevent complications, as well as the signs and symptoms of which she should be aware. Encourage her to continue to ask questions and report any signs or symptoms she feels her son exhibits. Discuss the advantages related to using a topical anesthetic before peripheral venous access insertion. Explain any securement/stabilization devices that will be used with Simon to prevent accidental dislodgement or removal of the venous access device.
2. Ms. Cohen is exhibiting signs and symptoms consistent with a hemolytic transfusion reaction. This type of reaction typically occurs immediately and is the result of incompatibility of the donor blood with the recipient's blood. Stop the blood immediately. Disconnect the blood and begin infusing normal saline via a different, new administration set. Notify the primary care provider immediately. Monitor vital signs and symptoms. Anticipate the administration of medications to treat the reaction, including hypotension. Prepare to obtain required blood samples for serologic testing and a urine specimen. Return blood product and administration tubing to laboratory.
3. Provide Mr. Tracy with information regarding skin care and assessment related to his port site. Inform him about how to care for his port if it is accessed. It is important that he is aware of signs and symptoms that he should report to his primary care provider. He also needs to be aware of the time interval for surgical follow-up and the interval for appointments to reheparinize the port, if not used.

16 Cardiovascular Care

FOCUSING ON PATIENT CARE

This chapter will help you develop some of the skills related to cardiovascular care necessary to care for the following patients:

COBY PRUDER, age 40, is to undergo an electrocardiogram as part of his physical examination. Although he considers himself healthy, he is nervous.

HARRY STEBBINGS, age 67, is admitted to the emergency department for chest pain and cardiac monitoring.

ANN KRIBELL, age 54, is a patient in the cardiac care unit. She has been diagnosed with heart failure and is receiving cardiac monitoring. She needs to have arterial blood samples drawn from her arterial catheter.

Refer to Focusing on Patient Care: Developing Clinical Reasoning at the end of the chapter to apply what you learn.

LEARNING OBJECTIVES

After studying this chapter, you will be able to:

1. Perform cardiopulmonary resuscitation (CPR).
2. Perform emergency automated external defibrillation.
3. Perform emergency manual external defibrillation (asynchronous).
4. Obtain a 12-lead ECG.
5. Apply a cardiac monitor.
6. Apply and monitor an external pacemaker.
7. Obtain an arterial blood sample from an arterial catheter.
8. Remove a peripheral arterial catheter.

KEY TERMS

cardiac arrest: sudden cessation of functional circulation of the heart (pulse), such as asystole or defibrillation, typically caused by the occlusion of one or more of the coronary arteries or cardiomyopathy

cardiac monitoring: visualization and monitoring of the cardiac electrical activity stimulating the heartbeat

cardiopulmonary resuscitation (CPR): also known as basic life support: revival in the absence of spontaneous respirations and heartbeat to preserve heart and brain function while waiting for defibrillation and advanced cardiac life support care. Achieved by manually pumping the heart by compressing the sternum and forcing oxygen into the lungs using mouth-to-mouth or rescue breathing.

cardioversion: conversion of a pathologic cardiac rhythm to normal sinus rhythm through low doses of electricity, using a device that applies synchronized counter shocks to the heart

circulation: the continuous one-way circuit of blood through the heart and blood vessels, with the heart as the pump (Taylor & Cohen, 2013)

defibrillation: the use of a large amount of electric current to the heart through the chest wall over a brief period of time to treat chaotic cardiac rhythms; temporarily depolarizes the myocardium, producing a momentary asytole (absence of ventricular activity), providing an opportunity for the heart's normal pacemaker to restore a normal rhythm

dysrhythmia: group of conditions in which the electrical activity of the heart is irregular or is faster or slower than normal

electrocardiogram (ECG/EKG): graphic record of the electrical activity of the heart

electrocardiography: the making and study of records of the electrical activity of the heart

fibrillation: small, local, involuntary contraction of muscle, resulting from spontaneous activation of a single muscle fiber or of an isolated bundle of nerve fibers (Grossman & Porth, 2014)

The cardiovascular system is composed of the heart and the blood vessels. The heart is the main organ of **circulation**, which is the continuous one-way circuit of blood through the blood vessels (Taylor & Cohen, 2013). The heart is the circulatory pump, squeezing through the heart and out into the body. This is accomplished by contractions starting in the atria, followed by contraction of the ventricles, with a subsequent resting of the heart. Figure 16-1 provides an overview of cardiac anatomy. Deoxygenated blood (low in oxygen; high in carbon dioxide) is carried from the right side of the heart to the lungs, where oxygen is picked up and carbon dioxide is released, and then returned to the left side of the heart. This oxygenated blood (high in oxygen; low in carbon dioxide) is pumped out to all other parts of the body and back again (refer to Figure 14-2 in Chapter 14). The contraction of the muscles of the heart is controlled by electrical impulses produced in and carried over specialized tissue within the heart. These tissues make up the heart's conduction system. Figure 16-2 provides a review of the cardiac conduction system.

Assessment of cardiovascular function commonly involves noninvasive techniques such as inspection, auscultation, and palpation. Additional basic and important indicators of the heart's effectiveness are pulse rate, strength, and rhythm; blood pressure; skin color and temperature; and level of consciousness. Refer to Chapters 2 and 3 for additional information related to these assessments. Chapter 14 provides additional information related to oxygenation and cardiopulmonary function.

This chapter covers selected skills to assist the nurse in providing cardiovascular care. Should the heart stop pumping, it can be manually pumped via **cardiopulmonary resuscitation (CPR)** until electrical **defibrillation** and additional medical support arrives. These interventions are discussed in Skills 16-1 through 16-3. Noninvasive heart monitoring involves **electrocardiography** and **cardiac monitoring**, discussed in Skills 16-4 and 16-5. The application and use of an external pacemaker is discussed in Skill 16-6. Figure 16-3 highlights cardiac landmark reference lines that are used in assessment and also for placing devices related to these interventions. Other electrical therapy devices are discussed in Fundamentals Review 16-1. The last two skills in the chapter focus on obtaining an arterial blood sample from an arterial catheter and removing a peripheral arterial catheter.

Invasive techniques, such as pulmonary artery monitoring, Swan-Ganz catheterization, cardiac output determination, and cardiac support via an intra-aortic balloon pump (IABP), typically are used by trained critical care personnel to provide additional monitoring and support. These techniques are beyond the scope of this text.

FUNDAMENTALS REVIEW 16-1

ELECTRICAL THERAPY DEVICES

In addition to defibrillation, electrical therapy may be delivered via the following devices:

- **Implantable cardioverter-defibrillator** (ICD) is a sophisticated device that automatically discharges an electric current to provide bradycardia and antitachycardia pacing, synchronized cardioversion, and defibrillation (convert abnormal cardiac rhythms to normal sinus rhythm) when it senses ventricular bradycardia and tachyarrhythmias. Patients with a history of ventricular fibrillation, with poor ejection fraction (<35%), or with heart failure (New York Heart Association [NYHA] class III or IV) may be candidates for this type of device.
- **Synchronized cardioversion** is the treatment of choice for arrhythmias that do not respond to vagal maneuvers or to drug therapy, such as atrial tachycardia, atrial flutter, atrial fibrillation, and symptomatic ventricular tachycardia. Cardioversion is performed similarly to defibrillation but is synchronized with the heart rhythm and uses fewer joules. Cardioversion works by delivering an electrical charge to the myocardium at the peak of the R wave. This causes immediate depolarization, interrupting reentry circuits and allowing the sinoatrial node to resume control. Synchronizing the electrical charge with the R wave ensures that the current will not be delivered on the vulnerable T wave and thus disrupts repolarization. It is usually performed in a critical care area, in the presence of a physician, an anesthesiologist, and emergency equipment. The patient is premedicated with pain medicine.
- **Pacemakers** are electronic devices that can be used to initiate the heartbeat when the heart's intrinsic electrical system cannot effectively generate a rate adequate to support cardiac output. Pacemakers help control abnormal heart rhythms (NHLBI, 2012). Pacemakers can be temporary: placed on the skin (transcutaneous); via temporary epicardial pacing wires inserted during surgery; or transvenous, via a pacing electrode wire passed through a vein (the brachial, internal, or external jugular, subclavian, or femoral) and into the right atrium or right ventricle. Pacemakers can also be permanent surgically implanted devices.
- **Biventricular pacemakers** (cardiac resynchronization therapy pacing device) use electrical current to improve synchronization of left ventricular contraction. Biventricular pacemakers are used in patients with heart failure (NYHA class III or IV), with an intraventricular conduction delay (QRS >120 ms), and in patients with left-ventricular ejection fraction ≤35%. These devices improve right and left ventricle contraction, resulting in improved cardiac function, with improved ejection fraction (Cleveland Clinic, 2013).

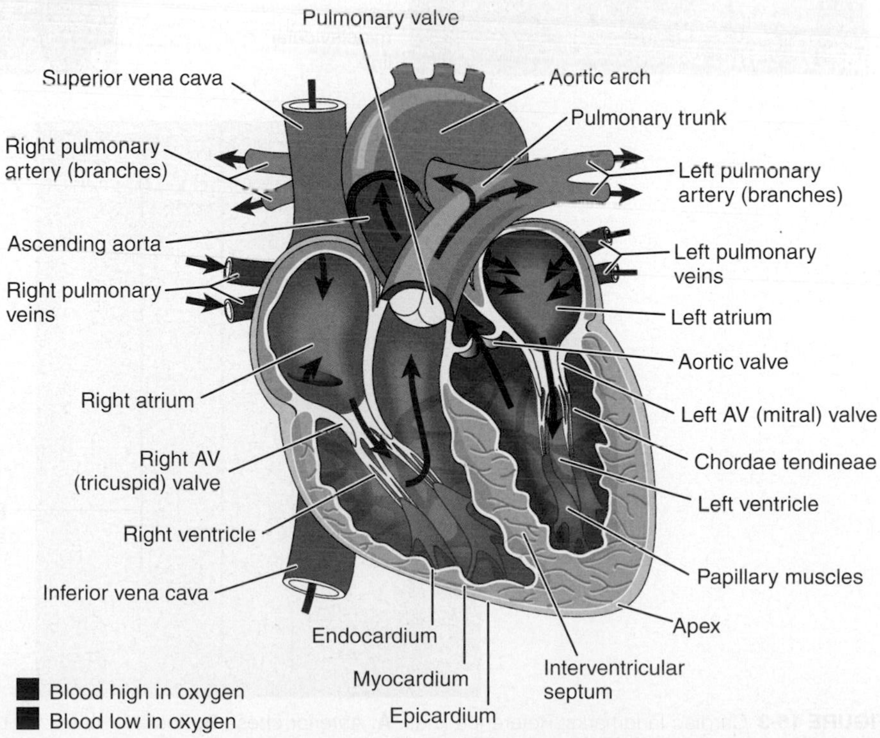

FIGURE 16-1 Cardiac anatomy. (Adapted from Taylor, J.J., & Cohen, B.J. (2013). *Memmler's structure and function of the human body* (10th ed.). Philadelphia: Wolters Kluwer Health/Lippincott Williams & Wilkins.)

Sinoatrial node
Left atrium
Internodal pathways
Right atrium
Atrioventricular node
Atrioventricular bundle (bundle of His)
Right and left bundle branches
Purkinje fibers

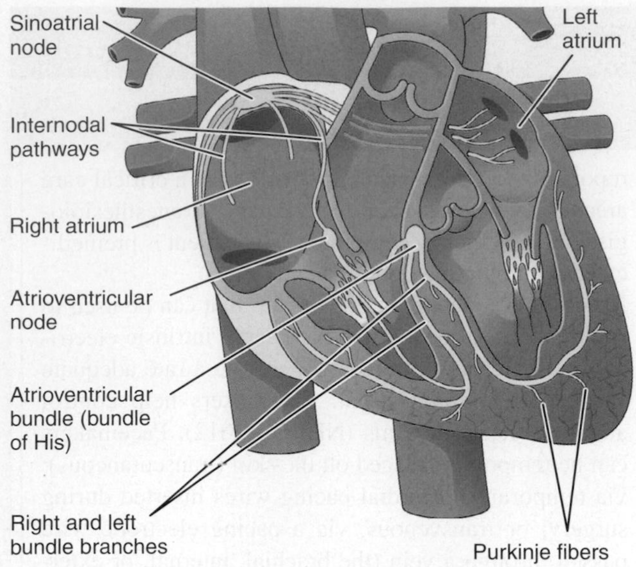

FIGURE 16-2 Cardiac conduction system. (From Taylor, J.J., Cohen, B.J. (2013). *Memmler's structure and function of the human body* (10th ed.). Philadelphia: Wolters Kluwer Health/ Lippincott Williams & Wilkins. Figure 13-9, page 256.)

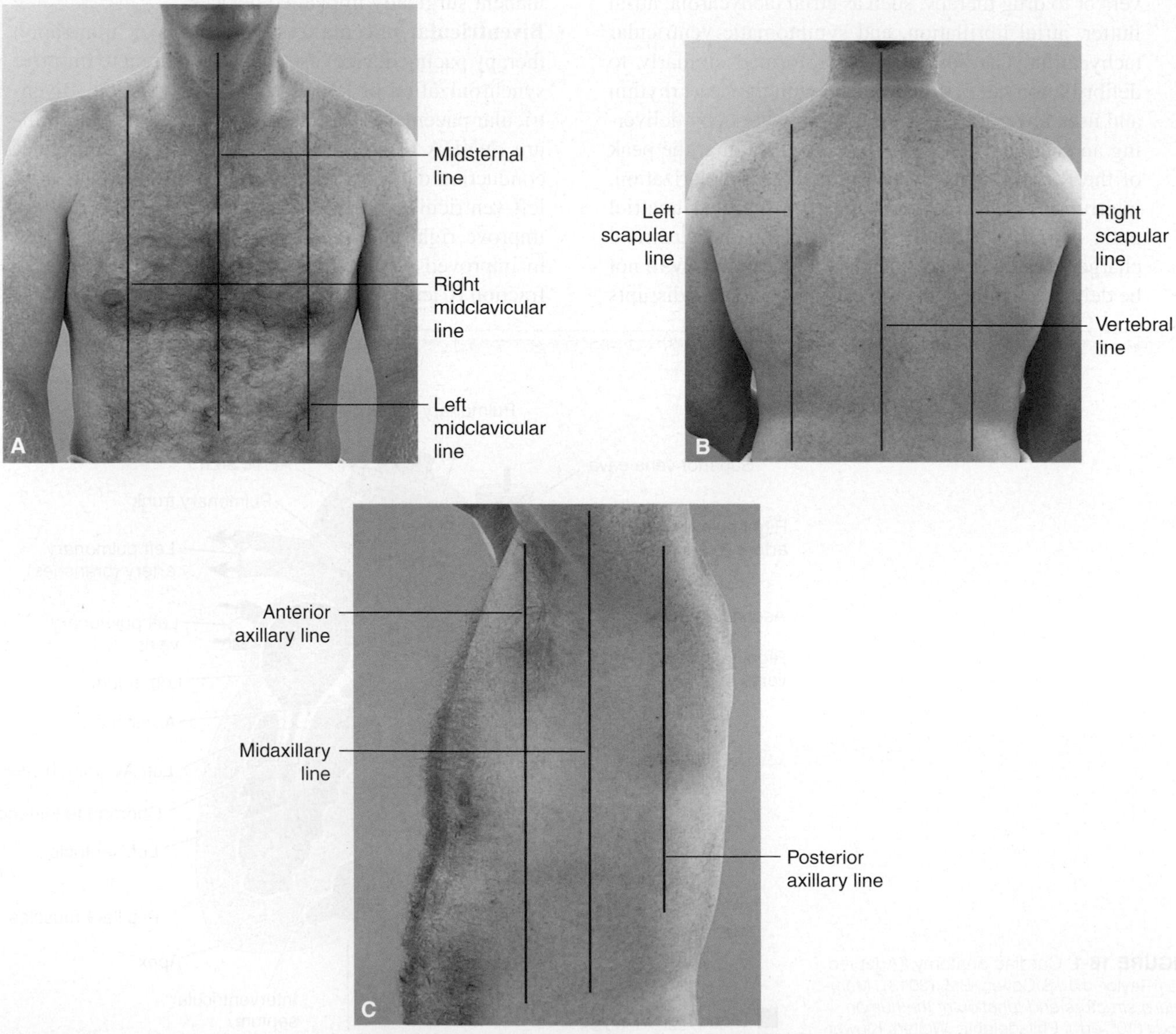

Midsternal line
Right midclavicular line
Left midclavicular line
A
Left scapular line
Right scapular line
Vertebral line
B
Anterior axillary line
Midaxillary line
Posterior axillary line
C

FIGURE 16-3 Cardiac landmarks: Reference lines. **A.** Anterior chest. **B.** Posterior chest. **C.** Lateral chest.

SKILL 16-1 PERFORMING CARDIOPULMONARY RESUSCITATION (CPR)

Cardiopulmonary resuscitation (CPR), also known as basic life support, is used in any situation in which either breathing alone or breathing and a heartbeat are absent. It is a combination of chest compressions, which circulate blood, and mouth-to-mouth breathing, which supplies oxygen to the lungs. The brain is sensitive to hypoxia and will sustain irreversible damage after 4 to 6 minutes of no oxygen. The faster CPR is initiated, the greater the chance of survival.

If breathing alone or breathing and a heartbeat are absent, assess the victim for a response, activate the emergency response system, get an automated external defibrillator (AED) or defibrillator, and begin CPR with the CAB sequence (chest compressions, airway, breathing) and defibrillation (American Heart Association [AHA], 2011).

In the hospital setting, it is imperative that personnel be aware of the patient's stated instructions regarding any wish not to be resuscitated. This should be clearly expressed and documented in the patient's medical record.

Learning conventional CPR is still recommended for emergency interventions outside of health care facilities. However, the AHA alternately recommends that when a teen or an adult suddenly collapses, people near the victim should call 911 (to activate the emergency response system), and push hard and fast in the center of the victim's chest. Studies of real emergencies that have occurred in homes, at work, or in public locations, show that these two steps, called Hands-Only CPR, can be as effective as conventional CPR. Providing Hands-Only CPR to an adult who has collapsed from a sudden **cardiac arrest** can more than double that person's chance of survival (AHA, 2012).

DELEGATION CONSIDERATIONS

The initiation and provision of cardiopulmonary resuscitation is appropriate for all health care providers.

EQUIPMENT

- Personal protective equipment, such as a face shield or one-way valve mask and gloves, if available
- Ambu-bag and oxygen, if available

ASSESSMENT

Assess the patient's vital parameters and determine the patient's level of responsiveness. Check for partial or complete airway obstruction. Assess for the absence or ineffectiveness of respirations. Assess for the absence of signs of circulation and pulses.

NURSING DIAGNOSIS

Determine the related factors for the nursing diagnoses based on the patient's current status. Appropriate nursing diagnoses may include:

- Decreased Cardiac Output
- Impaired Gas Exchange
- Impaired Spontaneous Ventilation

OUTCOME IDENTIFICATION AND PLANNING

The expected outcome to achieve when performing CPR is that CPR is performed effectively without adverse effect to the patient. Additional outcomes include the following: the patient regains a pulse and respirations; the patient's heart and lungs maintain adequate function to sustain life; and advanced cardiac life support is initiated. Another appropriate outcome may be that the patient does not experience injury.

IMPLEMENTATION

ACTION	RATIONALE
1. Assess responsiveness. Look for breathing. If the patient is not responsive and is not breathing or not breathing normally, call for help, pull call bell, and call the facility emergency response number. Call for the automated external defibrillator (AED) or defibrillator, if available.	Assessing responsiveness prevents starting CPR on a conscious patient. Activating the emergency response system initiates a rapid response.

(continued)

SKILL 16-1 PERFORMING CARDIOPULMONARY RESUSCITATION (CPR) continued

ACTION	RATIONALE
2. Put on gloves, if available. Position the patient supine on his or her back on a firm, flat surface, with arms alongside the body. If the patient is in bed, place a backboard or other rigid surface under the patient (often the footboard of the patient's bed). Position yourself at the patient's side.	Gloves prevent contact with blood and body fluids. The supine position is required for resuscitative efforts and evaluation to be effective. Backboard provides a firm surface on which to apply compressions. If the patient must be rolled, move as a unit so the head, shoulders, and torso move simultaneously without twisting.
3. **Provide defibrillation at the earliest possible moment, as soon as an AED becomes available.** Refer to Skill 16-2: Automated External Defibrillation and Skill 16-3: Manual External Defibrillation.	The interval from collapse to defibrillation is one of the most important determinants of survival from sudden cardiac arrest (AHA, 2011).
4. Check for a pulse, palpating the carotid pulse. This assessment should take at least 5 seconds and no more than 10 seconds. If you do not definitely feel a pulse within 10 seconds, begin CPR using the compression:ventilation ratio of 30 compressions to 2 breaths, starting with chest compressions (CAB sequence).	Pulse assessment evaluates cardiac function. Delays in chest compressions should be minimized, so the health care provider should take no more than 10 seconds to check for a pulse. If it is not felt within that time period, chest compressions should be started (Neumar et al., 2010)
5. Position the heel of one hand in the center of the chest between the nipples, directly over the lower half of the sternum. Place the heel of the other hand directly on top of the first hand. Extend or interlace fingers to keep fingers above the chest. Straighten arms and position shoulders directly over hands.	Proper hand positioning ensures that the force of compressions is on the sternum, thereby reducing the risk of rib fracture, lung puncture, or liver laceration.
6. Push hard and fast. Chest compressions should depress the sternum 2 inches. Push straight down on the patient's sternum. Perform 30 chest compressions at a rate of 100 per minute, counting "one, two, etc." up to 30, keeping elbows locked, arms straight, and shoulders directly over the hands. Allow full chest recoil (re-expand) after each compression (Figure 1). Chest compression and chest recoil/relaxation times should be approximately equal.	Direct cardiac compression and manipulation of intrathoracic pressure supply blood flow during CPR. Compressing the chest 2 inches ensures that compressions are not too shallow and provides adequate blood flow. Full chest recoil allows adequate venous return to the heart.
7. Give two breaths (as described below) after each set of 30 compressions. Do five complete cycles of 30 compressions and two ventilations.	Breathing and compressions simulate lung and heart function, providing oxygen and circulation.

FIGURE 1 Using correct body alignment for chest compressions. Depress the sternum 2 inches.

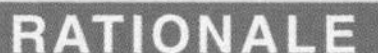

ACTION

RATIONALE

8. Use the head tilt–chin lift maneuver to open the airway (Figure 2). Place one hand on the patient's forehead and apply firm, backward pressure with the palm to tilt the head back. Place the fingers of the other hand under the bony part of the lower jaw near the chin and lift the jaw upward to bring the chin forward and the teeth almost to occlusion.

The head tilt-chin lift maneuver lifts the tongue, relieving airway obstruction by the tongue in an unresponsive person.

9. If trauma to the head or neck is present or suspected, use the jaw-thrust maneuver to open the airway (Figure 3). Place one hand on each side of the patient's head. Rest elbows on the flat surface under the patient, grasp the angle of the patient's lower jaw, and lift with both hands.

The jaw-thrust maneuver may reduce neck and spine movement.

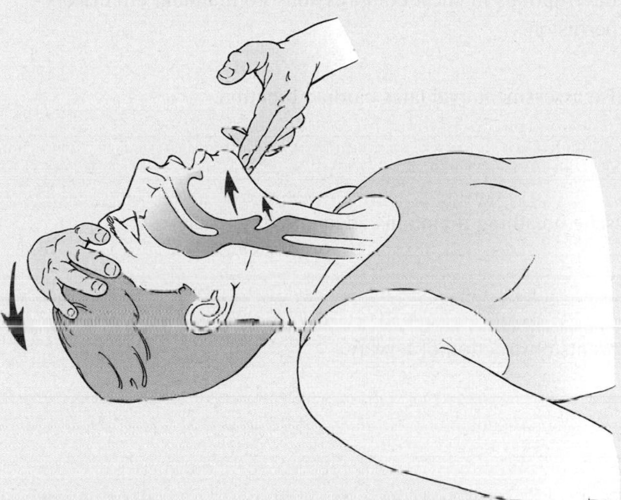

FIGURE 2 Using the head tilt–chin lift method to open the airway.

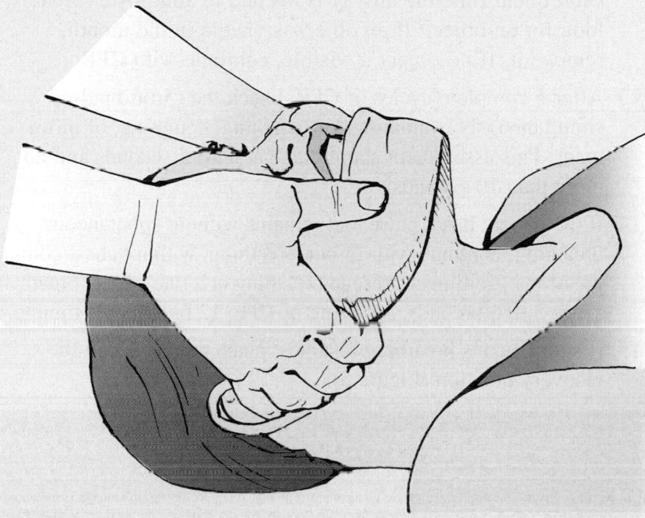

FIGURE 3 Using the jaw-thrust maneuver to open the airway.

10. Seal the patient's mouth and nose with the face shield, one-way valve mask (Figure 4A), or Ambu-bag (handheld resuscitation bag), if available (Figure 4B). If not available, seal the patient's mouth with your mouth.

Sealing the patient's mouth and nose prevents air from escaping. Devices such as masks reduce the risk for transmission of infections.

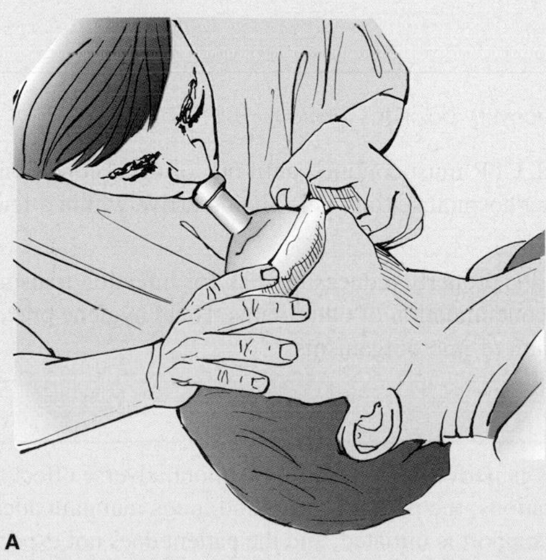

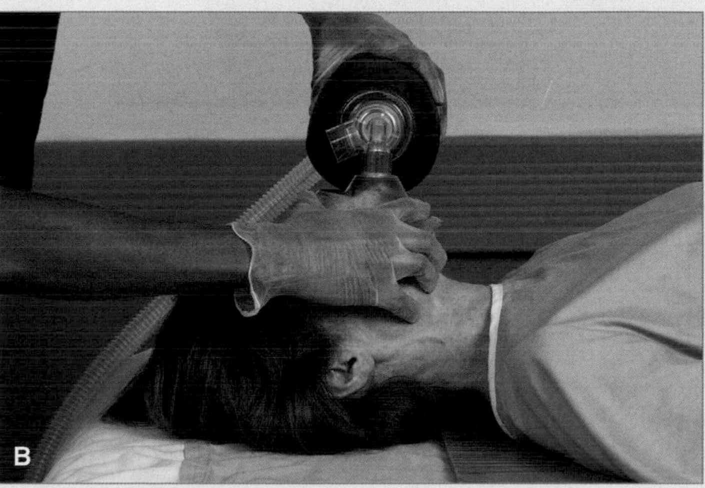

FIGURE 4 A. Using a one-way valve mask. **B.** Using a handheld resuscitation bag. (*Photo by B. Proud.*)

(continued)

SKILL 16-1 PERFORMING CARDIOPULMONARY RESUSCITATION (CPR) continued

ACTION	RATIONALE
11. Instill two breaths, each lasting 1 second, making the chest rise.	Breathing into the patient provides oxygen to the patient's lungs. Hyperventilation results in increased positive chest pressure and decreased venous return. Blood flow to the lungs during CPR is only about 25% to 33% normal; patient requires less ventilation to provide oxygen and remove carbon dioxide. Longer breaths reduce the amount of blood that refills the heart, reducing blood flow generated by compressions. Delivery of large, forceful breaths may cause gastric inflation and distension.
12. If you are unable to ventilate or the chest does not rise during ventilation, reposition the patient's head and reattempt to ventilate. If still unable to ventilate, resume CPR. Each subsequent time the airway is opened to administer breaths, look for an object. If an object is visible in the mouth, remove it. If no object is visible, continue with CPR.	Inability to ventilate indicates that the airway may be obstructed. Repositioning maneuvers may be sufficient to open the airway and promote spontaneous respirations. It is critical to minimize interruptions in chest compressions, to maintain circulatory perfusion.
13. After 5 complete cycles of CPR, check the carotid pulse, simultaneously evaluating for breathing, coughing, or movement. This assessment should take at least 5 seconds and no more than 10 seconds.	Pulse assessment evaluates cardiac function.
14. If the patient has a pulse, but remains without spontaneous breathing, continue with rescue breathing, without chest compressions. Administer rescue breathing at a rate of one breath every 5 to 6 seconds, for a rate of 10 to 12 breaths per minute.	Rescue breathing maintains adequate oxygenation.
15. If spontaneous breathing resumes, place the patient in the recovery position (Figure 5).	Prevents obstruction of airway.

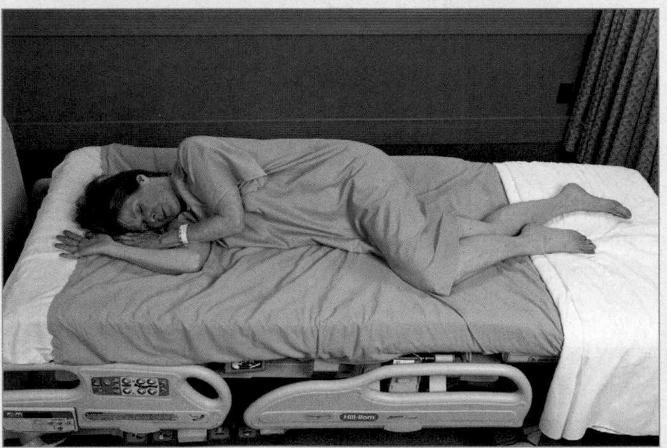

FIGURE 5 Recovery position. (*Photo by B. Proud.*)

ACTION	RATIONALE
16. Otherwise, continue CPR until advanced care providers take over, the patient starts to move, you are too exhausted to continue, or a physician discontinues CPR.	Once started, CPR must continue until one of these conditions is met. In a hospital setting, help should arrive within a few minutes.
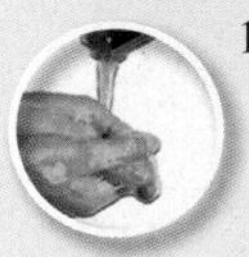 17. Remove gloves, if used. Perform hand hygiene.	Removing PPE properly reduces the risk for infection transmission and contamination of other items. Hand hygiene prevents transmission of microorganisms.

EVALUATION

The expected outcome is achieved when CPR is performed effectively without adverse effect to the patient; the patient regains a pulse and respirations; the patient's heart and lungs maintain adequate function to sustain life; advanced cardiac life support is initiated; and the patient does not experience serious injury.

DOCUMENTATION

Guidelines

Document the time you discovered the patient unresponsive and started CPR. Continued intervention, such as by the code team, is typically documented on a code form, which identifies the actions and drugs provided during the code. Provide a summary of these events in the patient's medical record.

Sample Documentation

> 07/06/15 2230 Called to patient's room by wife. Patient noted to be without evidence of respirations or circulation. Emergency response system activated, CPR initiated. See code sheet.
>
> —*B. Clapp, RN*

UNEXPECTED SITUATIONS AND ASSOCIATED INTERVENTIONS

- *When performing chest compression, there is an audible crack:* Be aware that this sound most commonly indicates cracking of the ribs. Recheck hand position. Then continue compressions.
- *You find a patient lying on the floor:* Determine the patient's level of responsiveness. If the patient is unresponsive, quickly clear an area, call for assistance and AED, and begin CPR.

SPECIAL CONSIDERATIONS

General Considerations

- If unsure whether the patient has a pulse, initiate CPR. Unnecessary CPR is less harmful than not performing CPR when it is truly needed (AHA, 2010).
- **Every effort should be taken to minimize interruptions in chest compressions. Causes for not providing compressions may include prolonged pulse checks, taking too long to give breaths, moving the patient, and using the AED. Try to limit interruptions to less than 10 seconds (AHA, 2011).**
- Perform CPR in the same manner if the patient is obese.
- Perform CPR for pregnant patients using the same guidelines, with a few additional measures. Manual left uterine displacement in the supine position should be performed to reduce aortic and vena cava compression and optimize the quality of compressions. If uterine displacement does not result in adequate chest compressions and a wedge is available, consider placing the patient in a 30-degree left lateral tilt position (Vanden Hoek et al., 2010; Castle, 2007). The left lateral tilt position is accomplished by using a wedge or other firm device behind the patient's back. The rescuer's hands are placed slightly above the center of the patient's chest and compressions are directed to move the sternum toward the spine, not vertically downward. Use additional pressure with chest compressions; greater force is required to generate measurable cardiac output (Puck et al., 2012). Pregnancy-related decreased chest-wall compliance decreases the efficiency of chest compressions. Anteroposterior placement of electrode pads can avoid difficulties associated with increased breast size (Castle, 2007). If the gestational age of the pregnancy is beyond 20 weeks and the mother is not responding to initial attempts at resuscitation, anticipate emergency cesarean delivery within 4 to 5 minutes (Puck et al., 2012).
- If it is not possible to seal the patient's mouth completely for reasons such as oral trauma, perform mouth-to-nose breathing. If the patient has a tracheostomy, provide ventilation through the tracheostomy instead of the mouth.
- The American Heart Association instituted changes in their suggestions regarding emergency interventions by people untrained in CPR outside of health care facilities. Learning conventional CPR is still recommended. However, the AHA alternately recommends when a teen or adult suddenly collapses, persons near the victim should call 911 (to activate the emergency response system), and push hard and fast in the center of the victim's chest. Studies of real emergencies that have occurred in homes, at work, or in public locations, show that these two steps, called Hands-Only CPR, can be as effective as conventional CPR. Providing Hands-Only CPR to a teen or adult who has collapsed from a sudden cardiac arrest can more than double or triple that person's chance of survival (AHA, 2012).
- Know that Hands-Only CPR is not recommended for victims of drowning, drug overdose, airway obstruction, and acute respiratory distress (AHA, 2012).

(*continued*)

SKILL 16-1 PERFORMING CARDIOPULMONARY RESUSCITATION (CPR) continued

- Be familiar with facility guidelines and/or standards of care related to family presence during resuscitation, and advocate for the presence of a family facilitator and support for family needs. The presence of people who are relatives or significant others with whom the patient shares an established relationship during resuscitation or invasive procedures is controversial. Research suggests multiple benefits (Pankop et al., 2013; AACN, 2010; ENA, 2009). The American Association of Critical Care Nurses (AACN) and the Emergency Nurses Association (ENA) recommend family members of all patients undergoing resuscitation and invasive procedures should be given the option of presence at the bedside, as well as recommending the development of related policies or standards of practice in all patient care areas (AACN; ENA). The American Heart Association (AHA) supports offering family members the opportunity to be present during resuscitation, assuming the patient has not indicated this is undesirable. In addition, current guidelines from the AHA indicate resuscitation team members should be sensitive to the presence of family members, assign a team member to remain with the patient, answer questions, clarify information, and offer comfort (Morrison et al., 2010, p. S670).

Infant and Child Considerations

- Once a child reaches puberty (breast development on the female; underarm, chest, and facial hair on the male), use adult CPR guidelines for resuscitation (Berg et al., 2010).
- As soon as it is determined that an infant or child is unresponsive, shout for help. If you did not witness the arrest and are alone, initiate CPR immediately for approximately 2 minutes (about five cycles of CPR) at the rate of 100 compressions per minute (compression-to-ventilation ratio 30 to 2), before leaving the infant/child to activate the emergency response system and getting the AED or defibrillator. If the child is small and it is safe to do so, consider carrying the child with you to activate the emergency response system.
- If the child suddenly collapses, first activate the emergency response system and get an AED or defibrillator, if available, then begin CPR.
- If the victim is age 1 to puberty, palpate a carotid or femoral pulse to perform a pulse check. Use the heel of one or two hands to provide chest compressions, based on the child's body size. Depth of compressions is at least one-third the depth of the chest, approximately 2 inches.
- For an infant under 1 year of age, palpate a brachial pulse to perform a pulse check. Use two fingers placed in the midline one fingerbreadth just below the nipple line and compress one-third the depth of the chest, approximately 1.5 inches.
- To open the airway of a child, place one hand on the child's forehead and gently lift the chin with the other hand (called the sniffing position in infants). If head or neck injury is suspected, use the jaw-thrust method.
- If available, use a one-way valve mask over the child's nose and mouth when performing CPR.
- Perform rescue breathing for infants and children with a pulse at a rate of one breath every 3 to 5 seconds, to deliver 12 to 20 breaths per minute.
- Be aware that Hands-Only CPR is not recommended for unresponsive infants and children (Berg et al., 2010).

Older Adult Considerations

- Nurses can help promote informed decision-making about CPR to older adults and their families (Cadogan, 2010). Educate, support, and advocate for patients as they face this critical choice. Provide evidence-based information, supportive listening, and a willingness to respect their choices (Buck, 2012).

EVIDENCE FOR PRACTICE ▶

CARDIOPULMONARY RESUSCITATION AND EMERGENCY CARDIAC CARE

The American Heart Association provides guidelines for cardiopulmonary resuscitation and emergency cardiac care and has incorporated these guidelines into the Basic Life Support and Advanced Life Support education for health care providers who respond to cardiovascular and respiratory emergencies.

- Field, J.M., Hazinski, M.F., Sayre, M.R., Chameides, L., Schexnayder, S.M., Hemphill, R., et al. (2010). 2010 American Heart Association guidelines for cardiopulmonary resuscitation and emergency cardiovascular care. Part 1: Executive summary. *Circulation, 122*(18 Suppl. 3), S640–S656.
- American Heart Association (AHA). (2011). *BLS for healthcare providers.* Dallas, TX: Author.

Refer to thePoint for additional research on related nursing topics.

EVIDENCE FOR PRACTICE ▶

CARDIOPULMONARY RESUSCITATION AND EMERGENCY CARDIAC CARE

The option for family presence during resuscitation or invasive procedures is recommended by multiple professional organizations. What information is available related to the actual implementation of this intervention?

Related Research

Pankop, R., Chang, K., Thorlton, J., & Spitzer, T. (2013). Implemented family presence protocols. An integrative review. *Journal of Nursing Care Quality, 28*(3), 281–288.

This integrative literature review examined research evidence regarding the use of protocols related to family presence during resuscitation or invasive procedures and providers' feedback related to family presence protocols for adults in the hospital setting. Studies included for review described the use of a family presence protocol for adult patients, implemented the protocol in the hospital setting, and included nurses in the study. Four key findings were identified by the authors. The reviewed literature identified a (1) positive trend in the practice of family presence at the bedside. Problems (2) related to the identification and availability of a family facilitator, which is a critical part of successful family presence protocols, were recognized. Factors that facilitate or inhibit the implementation of family presence protocols (3) were identified, including provider and staff education, enabling family facilitators to fulfill the role, and providing ongoing support and feedback about the practice. Finally, providers' differing attitudes about family presence during CPR and invasive procedures (4) were identified. Nurses continue to practice family presence despite lack of protocols to guide practice. Reviewed studies showed about 50% of nurses practice family presence in facilities with low adoption rate of protocols, covering geographic areas including the United States, Canada, and Europe. Nurses practicing family presence without a protocol and training could experience many issues as a result, such as interruption of care, misinterpretation of team activities, litigation, family distress, and staff distress.

The authors concluded that to ensure safe patient- and family-centered care, a continuous quality improvement process should be used. They propose that each hospital should integrate available resources and guidelines to develop family presence protocols to avoid potential problems associated with practicing family presence without protocols. Hospitals should provide sufficient resources (e.g., space and staff) to support the practice of family presence. Hospitals should offer in-service and continuing education to staff, including simulated scenarios, to prepare health care providers, alleviate concerns, and ensure protocols are implemented as recommended. In addition, hospitals should collect data on the implementation of family presence and perspectives of all stakeholders. Data should be used to reexamine the protocols, revise them as necessary, and improve the practice of family presence.

Relevance for Nursing Practice

Nurses are important patient advocates. Evidence supports the development, implementation, and evaluation of family presence protocols to ensure that patient- and family-centered care is provided. Protocols can reduce harm caused in the delivery of care, engage patients and family members as partners in care, and promote effective communication and coordination of care among health care providers, patients, and family members. Nurses can and should be active participants in this process.

See additional Evidence for Practice related to cardiopulmonary resuscitation at the end of Skill 16-2, and refer to thePoint for additional research on related nursing topics.

SKILL 16-2 PERFORMING EMERGENCY AUTOMATED EXTERNAL DEFIBRILLATION

Early defibrillation, as part of cardiopulmonary resuscitation (CPR) (see Skill 16-1), is critical to survival from sudden cardiac arrest (Link et al., 2010). The interval from collapse to defibrillation is one of the most important determinants of survival from sudden cardiac arrest with ventricular **fibrillation** or pulseless ventricular tachycardia (AHA, 2011). The most frequent initial cardiac rhythm in out-of-hospital witnessed sudden cardiac arrest is ventricular fibrillation (Link et al., 2010). Electrical therapy can be administered by defibrillation, **cardioversion**, or a pacemaker. (See Fundamentals Review 16-1 at the beginning of the chapter.) Early defibrillation is critical to increase patient survival (AHA, 2011; Link et al., 2012).

Defibrillation delivers large amounts of electric current to a patient over brief periods of time. It is the standard treatment for ventricular fibrillation (VF) and is also used to treat pulseless ventricular tachycardia (VT). The goal is to depolarize the irregularly beating heart temporarily and allow more coordinated contractile activity to resume. It does so by completely depolarizing the myocardium, producing a momentary asystole. This provides an opportunity for the natural pacemaker centers of the heart to resume normal activity.

The automated external defibrillator (AED) is a portable external defibrillator that automatically detects and interprets the heart's rhythm and informs the operator if a shock is indicated (Figure 1). AEDs are appropriate for use in situations where the patient is unresponsive, not breathing, and has no pulse (AHA, 2011). The defibrillator responds to the patient information by advising 'shock' or 'no shock.' Fully automatic models automatically perform rhythm analysis and shock, if indicated. These are usually found in out-of-hospital settings. Semiautomatic models require the operator to press an 'Analyze' button to initiate rhythm analysis and then press a 'Shock' button to deliver the shock, if indicated. Semiautomatic models are usually found in the hospital setting. An AED will not deliver a shock unless the electrode pads are correctly attached and a shockable rhythm is detected. Some AEDs have motion-detection devices that ensure the defibrillator will not discharge if there is motion, such as motion from personnel in contact with the patient. The strength of the charge is preset. Once the pads are in place and the device is turned on, follow the prompts given by the device. The following guidelines are based on the American Heart Association (AHA, 2011) guidelines. AHA guidelines state that these recommendations may be modified for the in-hospital setting, where continuous electrocardiographic or hemodynamic monitoring may be in place. CPR should be immediately initiated (see Skill 16-1) and the AED/defibrillator should be used as soon as it is available (Link et al., 2010).

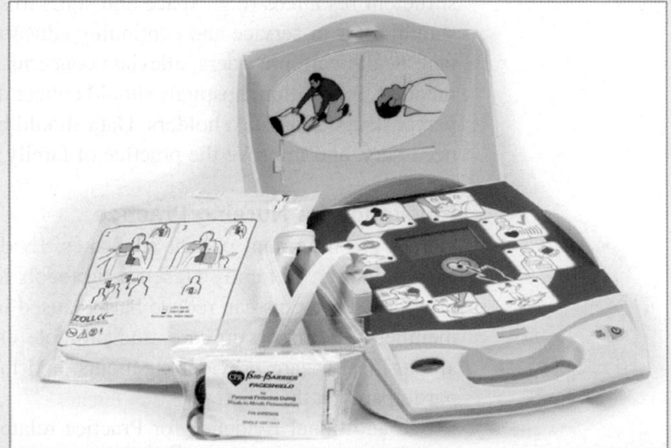

FIGURE 1 Automated external defibrillator (AED).

Current recommendations call for the application of the AED as soon as it is available, allowing for analysis of cardiac status and delivery of an initial shock, if indicated, for adults and children. After an initial shock, deliver five cycles of chest compressions/ventilations (30/2), and then reanalyze cardiac rhythm. Provide sets of one shock alternating with 2 minutes of CPR until the AED indicates a 'no shock indicated' message or until advanced cardiac life support (ACLS) is available (AHA, 2011).

In the hospital setting, it is imperative that personnel be aware of the patient's stated instructions regarding a wish not to be resuscitated. This should be clearly expressed and documented in the patient's medical record.

DELEGATION CONSIDERATIONS	The initiation and provision of cardiopulmonary resuscitation, including use of an AED, is appropriate for all health care providers.
EQUIPMENT	• Automated external defibrillator (AED) (some models have the pads, cables, and AED pre-connected) • Self-adhesive, pregelled monitor-defibrillator pads (6) • Cables to connect the pads and AED • Razor • Towel
ASSESSMENT	Assess the patient for unresponsiveness, effective breathing, and signs of circulation. Assess the patient's vital parameters and determine the patient's level of responsiveness. Check for partial or complete airway obstruction. Assess for the absence or ineffectiveness of respirations. Assess for the absence of signs of circulation and pulses. An AED should be used only when a patient is unresponsive, not breathing, or not breathing normally, and without signs of circulation (pulseless, lack of effective respirations, coughing, movement). Determine the age of the patient; some AED systems are designed to deliver both adult and child shock doses. Choose correct electrode pad for size/age of patient. If available, use child pads or a child system for children less than 8 years of age. Determine whether special situations exist that require additional actions before the AED is used or that contraindicate its use. (Refer to Box 16-1, Special Situations Related to AED, for details of these situations and appropriate actions.)
NURSING DIAGNOSIS	Determine the related factors for the nursing diagnoses based on the patient's current status. Appropriate nursing diagnoses may include: • Decreased Cardiac Output • Impaired Spontaneous Ventilation • Risk for Ineffective Cerebral Tissue Perfusion
OUTCOME IDENTIFICATION AND PLANNING	The expected outcome to achieve when performing AED is that it is performed correctly without adverse effect to the patient, and the patient regains signs of circulation, with organized electrical rhythm and pulse. Additional outcomes include the following: the patient regains respirations; the patient's heart and lungs maintain adequate function to sustain life; the patient does not experience serious injury; and advanced cardiac life support is initiated.

BOX 16-1 SPECIAL SITUATIONS RELATED TO AUTOMATED EXTERNAL DEFIBRILLATION (AED)

- ***The patient is in water.*** Water is a good conductor of electricity. Do not use an AED in water. Defibrillation administered to a patient in water could result in shocking the AED operator and bystanders. Another possible effect is that water on the patient's skin will provide a direct path for the electrical current from one electrode to the other. The arcing of the electrical current between the electrodes bypasses the heart, resulting in the delivery of inadequate current to the heart. If the patient is in water, pull the patient out of the water. If water is covering the patient's chest, quickly dry the chest before attaching the AED pads. If the patient is lying on snow or in a small puddle, the AED may be used (AHA, 2011).
- ***The patient has an implanted pacemaker or defibrillator.*** If possible, avoid placing the AED pad directly over the implanted device, which will appear as a hard lump (half the size of a deck of cards) beneath the skin of the upper chest or abdomen with an overlying scar (AHA, 2011, p. 22). If an AED electrode pad is placed directly over an implanted device, the device may block delivery of the shock to the heart. If the implanted device is delivering shocks to the patient (observed external chest muscle contractions), wait 30 to 60 seconds for the device to complete the treatment cycle before delivering a shock from the AED.
- ***A transdermal medication patch or other object is located on the patient's skin where the electrode pads are to be placed.*** Do not place AED pads directly on top of a medication patch. The patch may block the delivery of energy to the heart and cause small burns to the skin. If it will not delay shock delivery, remove the patch and wipe the area clean before attaching the electrode pads (AHA, 2011, p. 23).

(Adapted from American Heart Association. [2011]. *BLS for healthcare providers.* Dallas, TX: Author.)

(*continued*)

SKILL 16-2 PERFORMING EMERGENCY AUTOMATED EXTERNAL DEFIBRILLATION continued

IMPLEMENTATION

ACTION	RATIONALE
1. Assess responsiveness. Look for breathing. If the patient is not responsive and is not breathing or not breathing normally, call for help, pull call bell, and call the facility emergency response number. Call for the AED. Put on gloves, if available. Begin cardiopulmonary resuscitation (CPR) (see Skill 16-1).	Assessing responsiveness prevents starting CPR on a conscious patient. Activating the emergency response system initiates a rapid response. Gloves prevent contact with blood and body fluids. Initiating CPR preserves heart and brain function while awaiting defibrillation.
2. **Provide defibrillation at the earliest possible moment, as soon as AED becomes available.**	The interval from collapse to defibrillation is one of the most important determinants of survival from sudden cardiac arrest (AHA, 2011).
3. Prepare the AED. Power on the AED. Push the power button. Some devices will turn on automatically when the lid or case is opened.	Proper setup ensures proper functioning.
4. Attach AED cables to the adhesive electrode pads (may be preconnected).	Proper setup ensures proper functioning.
5. Stop chest compressions. Peel away the covering from the electrode pads to expose the adhesive surface. Attach the electrode pads to the patient's chest. Place one pad on the upper right sternal border, directly below the clavicle. Place the second pad lateral to the left nipple, with the top margin of the pad a few inches below the axilla (anterolateral positioning) (Figure 2). Alternately, if two or more rescuers are present, one rescuer should continue chest compressions while another rescuer attaches the AED pads. Attach the AED connecting cables to the AED box, if not preconnected.	Proper setup ensures proper functioning. AHA (2011) specifies anterolateral placement. See note below in *Special Considerations* for alternate electrode placement. Application by second rescuer minimizes interruptions in chest compressions.

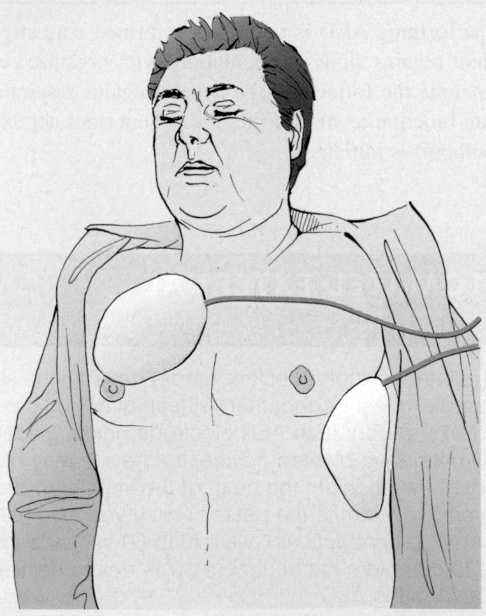

FIGURE 2 AED electrode pad placement.

ACTION	RATIONALE
6. Once the pads are in place and the device is turned on, follow the prompts given by the device. Clear the patient and analyze the rhythm. Ensure no one is touching the patient. Loudly state a "Clear the patient" message. Press 'Analyze' button to initiate analysis, if necessary. Some devices automatically begin analysis when the pads are attached. Avoid all movement affecting the patient during analysis.	Movement and electrical impulses cause artifact during analysis. Avoidance of artifact ensures accurate rhythm analysis. Avoidance of contact with the patient avoids accidental shock to personnel.

ACTION	RATIONALE
7. If a shockable rhythm is present, the device will announce that a shock is indicated and begin charging. Once the AED is charged, a message will be delivered to shock the patient.	Shock message is delivered through a written or visual message on the AED screen, an auditory alarm, or a voice-synthesized statement.
8. **Before pressing the 'Shock' button, loudly state a "Clear the patient" message. Visually check that no one is in contact with the patient (Figure 3).** Press the 'Shock' button. If the AED is fully automatic, a shock will be delivered automatically.	Ensuring a clear patient avoids accidental shocking of personnel.

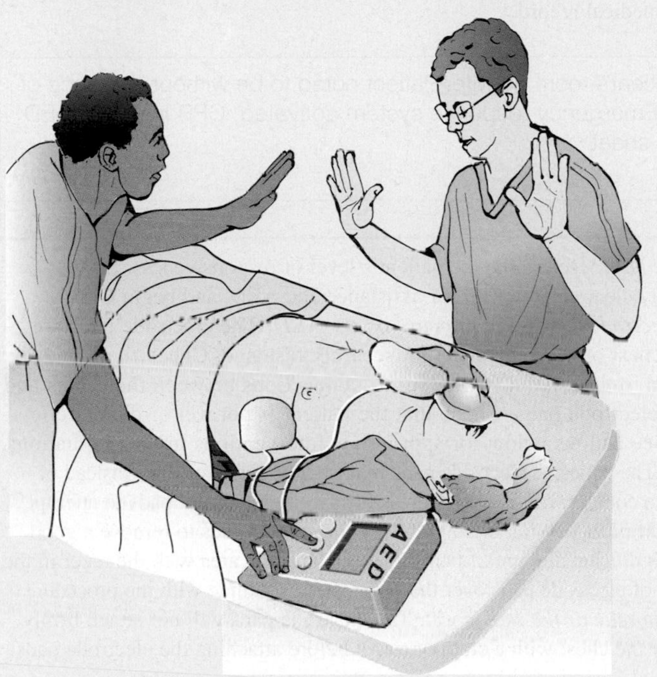

FIGURE 3 Clearing the patient.

ACTION	RATIONALE
9. Immediately resume CPR, beginning with chest compressions. After five cycles (about 2 minutes), allow the AED to analyze the heart rhythm. If a shock is not advised, resume CPR, beginning with chest compressions. Do not recheck to see if there is a pulse. Follow the AED voice prompts.	Resuming CPR provides optimal treatment. CPR preserves heart and neurologic function (based on AHA, 2011 recommended guidelines). Even when a shock eliminates the **dysrhythmia**, it may take several minutes for a heart rhythm to establish and even longer to achieve perfusion. Chest compressions can provide coronary and cerebral perfusion during this period. Some AEDs in the community for use by lay persons are automatically programmed to cycle through three analysis/shock cycles in one set. This would necessitate turning off the AED after the first shock and turning it back on for future analysis and defibrillation. Be familiar with the type of AED available for use.
10. Continue CPR until advanced care providers take over, the patient starts to move, you are too exhausted to continue, or a physician discontinues CPR.	Once started, CPR must continue until one of these conditions is met. In a hospital setting, help should arrive within a few minutes.
11. Remove gloves, if used. Perform hand hygiene.	Removing PPE properly reduces the risk for infection transmission and contamination of other items. Hand hygiene prevents transmission of microorganisms.

(*continued*)

SKILL 16-2 PERFORMING EMERGENCY AUTOMATED EXTERNAL DEFIBRILLATION continued

EVALUATION

The expected outcome is achieved when automatic external defibrillation is applied correctly without adverse effect to the patient and the patient regains signs of circulation. Additional outcomes may include the following: the patient regains respirations; the patient's heart and lungs maintain adequate function to sustain life; the patient does not experience injury; and advanced cardiac life support is initiated.

DOCUMENTATION

Guidelines

Document the time you discovered the patient unresponsive and started CPR. Document the time(s) AED shocks are initiated. Continued intervention, such as by the code team, is typically documented on a code form, which identifies the actions and drugs provided during the code. Provide a summary of these events in the patient's medical record.

Sample Documentation

07/06/15 2230 Called to patient's room by wife. Patient noted to be without evidence of respirations or circulation. Emergency response system activated, CPR initiated. AED applied at 2232. See code sheet.

—*B. Clapp, RN*

UNEXPECTED SITUATIONS AND ASSOCIATED INTERVENTIONS

- *You find a patient lying on the floor:* Determine the patient's level of responsiveness. If the patient is unresponsive, quickly clear an area, call for assistance and AED, and begin CPR.
- *A 'Check pads' or 'Check electrodes' message appears on the AED:* The electrode pads are not securely attached to the chest or the cables are not securely fastened. Check that the pads are firmly and evenly adhered to the patient's skin. Verify connections between the cables and the AED and the cables and electrode pads. Check that the patient is not wet or diaphoretic, or has excessive chest hair. See actions below for appropriate interventions in these situations.
- *The patient has a hairy chest:* The adhesive electrode pads may stick to the chest hair instead of to the skin, preventing adequate contact with the skin. Press firmly on the current pads to attempt to provide sufficient adhesion. If unsuccessful, briskly remove the current pads to remove a good portion of the chest hair. If a significant amount of hair remains, shave the area with the razor in the AED case. Apply a second set of electrode pads over the same sites. Continue with the procedure.
- *The patient is noticeably diaphoretic or the skin is wet:* The electrode pads will not attach firmly to wet or diaphoretic skin. Dry the chest with a cloth or towel before attaching the electrode pads.

SPECIAL CONSIDERATIONS

General Considerations

- **Every effort should be taken to minimize interruptions in chest compressions. Causes for not providing compressions may include prolonged pulse checks, taking too long to give breaths, moving the patient, and using the AED. Try to limit interruptions to less than 10 seconds to maximize effectiveness (AHA, 2011).**
- Additional options for placement of electrodes include anteroposterior, anterior-left infrascapular, and anterior-right infrascapular. These electrode placement positions are equally acceptable for use and equally effective (Link et al., 2010).
- Anteroposterior placement of electrode pads can avoid difficulties associated with increased breast size in patients who are pregnant (Castle, 2007).
- Appropriate maintenance of the AED is critical for proper operation. Check the AED for any visible signs of damage. Check the 'ready for use' indicator on the AED daily. Perform maintenance according to the manufacturer's recommendations and facility policy.
- When hospitals deploy AEDs, the goal of providing the first shock for any sudden cardiac arrest is within 3 minutes of collapse. The objective is to make goals for in-hospital use of AEDs consistent with goals established in the out-of-hospital setting (Link et al., 2010).

Infant and Child Considerations

- For infants less than 1 year of age, a manual defibrillator is preferred. If a manual defibrillator is not available, an AED with pediatric settings is desirable. If neither is available, use an AED with adult pads and deliver the adult shock dose (Link et al., 2010).

- Patients who are 8 years of age and older should be defibrillated with adult pads and adult shock dose.
- If child pads are available and the AED has a key or switch that will deliver a child shock dose, use both for patients 1 to 8 years of age (AHA, 2011).
- If the AED does not have child pads or a child key or switch, use the adult pads and deliver the adult shock dose. Ensure the standard pads do not touch or overlap (AHA, 2011).

Older Adult Considerations

- Nurses can help promote informed decision-making about CPR to older adults and their families (Cadogan, 2010). Educate, support, and advocate for patients as they face this critical choice. Provide evidence-based information, supportive listening, and a willingness to respect their choices (Buck, 2012).

EVIDENCE FOR PRACTICE ▶

CARDIOPULMONARY RESUSCITATION AND EMERGENCY CARDIAC CARE

The American Heart Association provides guidelines for cardiopulmonary resuscitation and emergency cardiac care and has incorporated these guidelines into the Basic Life Support and Advanced Life Support education for health care providers who respond to cardiovascular and respiratory emergencies.

Refer to the Evidence for Practice in Skill 16-1 for details, and refer to thePoint for additional research on related nursing topics.

EVIDENCE FOR PRACTICE ▶

CARDIOPULMONARY RESUSCITATION AND EMERGENCY CARDIAC CARE

During patient cardiac arrest, the health care team members must perform according to established guidelines and function effectively to optimize the outcome from emergency interventions. Can simulation for repeated practice improve performance of skills related to CPR and defibrillation?

Related Research

Delac, K., Blazier, D., Daniel, L., & N-Wilfong, D. (2013). Five alive. Using mock code simulation to improve responder performance during the first 5 minutes of a code. *Critical Care Nursing Quarterly, 36*(2), 244–250.

The purpose of this study was to evaluate the effectiveness of simulation for mock code training to improve skills related to CPR and defibrillation. Monthly in-situ mock code simulations on telemetry and medical surgical units were implemented and video recorded. Participants responded to two different scenarios during each simulation. Data were collected in pre- and post- surveys and evaluation tools, including pre- and post- confidence levels, and recorded time to initiation of CPR and defibrillation, and compared with data collected from several years of emergency code data, including time to CPR and defibrillation. Video debriefing was utilized for reflective learning, to review and correct technical skills, and to identify and modify critical behaviors. Results indicated a significant decrease in the responders' time to both CPR and defibrillation between the first and second scenarios. The data revealed 65% improvement in the participants' response time of 1 minute to CPR and a 67% improvement in the goal of 3 minutes to defibrillation. In addition, the surveys demonstrated an improvement in the nurses' confidence in initiating first responder interventions and their ability to utilize and operate emergency equipment prior to arrival of a rapid response team or code team. Furthermore, the percentage of nurses who expressed the belief that they were confident in their hand-off communication when the rapid response team or code team arrived increased from 60.2% before the training to 80.6% afterward. The authors concluded that an in-situ mock code simulation improves the performance of responders to code situations.

Relevance for Nursing Practice

Nurses are responsible for the initiation of CPR and defibrillation. Skills learned in basic or advance life support may deteriorate without practice and reinforcement. Skills related to these interventions must be maintained to ensure effective interventions to optimize patient outcomes. Nurses need to be prepared at any moment to utilize emergency skills and should advocate for the use of interventions to maintain these skills.

See additional Evidence for Practice related to cardiopulmonary resuscitation at the end of Skill 16-1, and refer to thePoint for additional research on related nursing topics.

SKILL 16-3 PERFORMING EMERGENCY MANUAL EXTERNAL DEFIBRILLATION (ASYNCHRONOUS)

Electrical therapy is used to terminate or control potentially lethal dysrhythmias quickly. Electrical therapy can be administered by defibrillation, cardioversion, or a pacemaker. (See Fundamentals Review 16-1 at the beginning of the chapter.) Early defibrillation is critical to increase patient survival (AHA, 2011; Link et al., 2010). Defibrillation delivers large amounts of electric current to a patient over brief periods of time. It is the standard treatment for ventricular fibrillation (VF) and is also used to treat ventricular tachycardia (VT), in which the patient has no pulse. The goal is temporarily to depolarize the irregularly beating heart and allow more coordinated contractile activity to resume. It does so by completely depolarizing the myocardium, producing a momentary asystole. This provides an opportunity for the natural pacemaker centers of the heart to resume normal activity. The electrode paddles delivering the current may be placed on the patient's chest or, during cardiac surgery, directly on the myocardium.

Manual defibrillation is accomplished with an external defibrillator (Figure 1) and it depends on the operator for analysis of rhythm, charging, proper application of the paddles to the patient's thorax, and delivery of counter shock. It requires the user to have immediate and accurate dysrhythmia recognition skills. The following guidelines are based on the American Heart Association 2011 guidelines.

In the hospital setting, it is imperative that personnel be aware of the patient's stated instructions regarding a wish not to be resuscitated. This should be clearly expressed and documented in the patient's medical record.

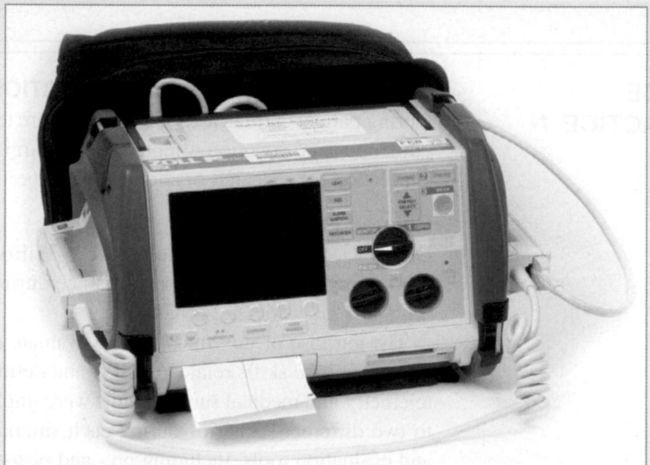

FIGURE 1 External defibrillator.

DELEGATION CONSIDERATIONS

The initiation and provision of manual external defibrillation should be performed by health care providers who are certified in Advanced Cardiac Life Support measures.

EQUIPMENT

- Defibrillator (monophasic or biphasic)
- External paddles (or internal paddles sterilized for cardiac surgery)
- Conductive medium pads
- Electrocardiogram (ECG) monitor with recorder (often part of the defibrillator)
- Oxygen therapy equipment
- Handheld resuscitation bag
- Airway equipment
- Emergency pacing equipment
- Emergency cardiac medications

ASSESSMENT

Assess the patient for unresponsiveness, effective breathing, and signs of circulation. Assess the patient's vital parameters and determine the patient's level of responsiveness. Check for partial or complete airway obstruction. Assess for the absence or ineffectiveness of respirations. Assess for the absence of signs of circulation and pulses. Call for help and perform cardiopulmonary resuscitation (CPR) until the defibrillator and other emergency equipment arrive.

NURSING DIAGNOSIS

Determine the related factors for the nursing diagnoses based on the patient's current status. Appropriate nursing diagnoses may include:

- Decreased Cardiac Output
- Risk for Injury
- Impaired Spontaneous Ventilation

OUTCOME IDENTIFICATION AND PLANNING

The expected outcome to achieve when performing manual external defibrillation is that it is performed correctly without adverse effect to the patient, and the patient regains signs of circulation. Additional outcomes may include the following: the patient regains respirations; the patient's heart and lungs maintain adequate function to sustain life; the patient does not experience serious injury; and advanced cardiac life support is initiated.

IMPLEMENTATION

ACTION	RATIONALE
1. Assess responsiveness. If the patient is not responsive, call for help, pull call bell, and call the facility emergency response number. Call for the AED. Put on gloves, if available. Begin cardiopulmonary resuscitation (CPR).	Assessing responsiveness prevents starting CPR on a conscious victim. Activating the emergency response system initiates a rapid response. Gloves prevent contact with blood and body fluids. Initiating CPR preserves heart and brain function while awaiting defibrillation.
2. Turn on the defibrillator.	Charging and placement prepare for defibrillation.
3. If the defibrillator has "quick-look" capability, place the paddles on the patient's chest. Otherwise, connect the monitoring leads of the defibrillator to the patient and assess the cardiac rhythm.	Connecting the monitor leads to the patient allows for a quick view of the cardiac rhythm.
4. Expose the patient's chest, and apply conductive pads at the paddle placement positions. For anterolateral placement, place one pad to the right of the upper sternum, just below the right clavicle, and the other over the fifth or sixth intercostal space at the left anterior axillary line (Figure 2). For anteroposterior placement, place the anterior pad/paddle directly over the heart at the precordium, to the left of the lower sternal border. Place the flat posterior pad/paddle under the patient's body beneath the heart and immediately below the scapulae (but not on the vertebral column) (Figure 3). 'Hands-free' defibrillator pads can be used with the same placement positions, if available.	This placement ensures that the electrical stimulus needs to travel only a short distance to the heart.

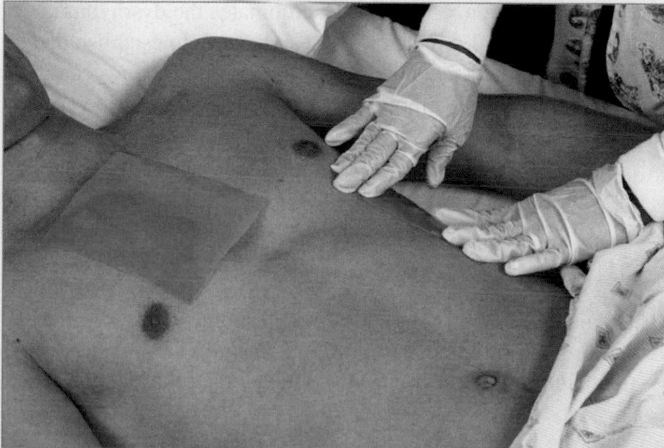

FIGURE 2 Anterolateral placement of conductive pads and defibrillator paddles.

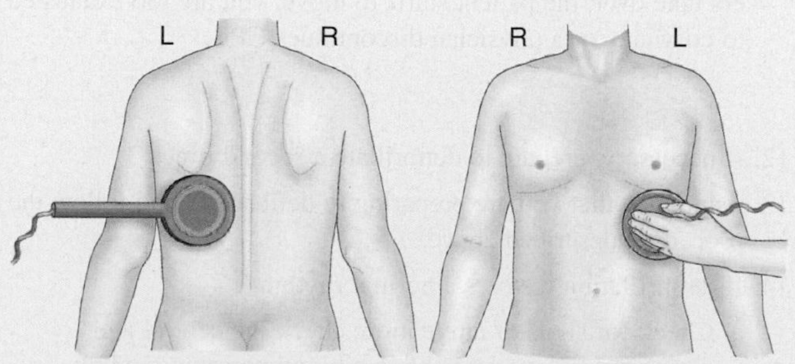

FIGURE 3 Anteroposterior placement of conductive pads and defibrillator paddles. (From Hinkle, J.L., & Cheever, K.H. (2014). *Brunner and Suddarth's textbook of medical-surgical nursing* (13th ed.). Philadelphia: Wolters Kluwer Health/Lippincott Williams & Wilkins, with permission, Figure 26-25.)

(continued)

SKILL 16-3 PERFORMING EMERGENCY MANUAL EXTERNAL DEFIBRILLATION (ASYNCHRONOUS) continued

ACTION	RATIONALE
5. Set the energy level for 360 J (joules) for an adult patient when using a monophasic defibrillator. Use clinically appropriate energy levels for biphasic defibrillators, beginning with 120 to 200 J, depending on device (Morton & Fontaine, 2013).	Proper setup ensures proper functioning.
6. Charge the paddles by pressing the charge buttons, which are located either on the machine or on the paddles themselves.	Proper setup ensures proper functioning.
7. **Place the paddles over the conductive pads (Figure 4) and press firmly against the patient's chest, using 25 pounds (11 kg) of pressure. If using hands-off pads, do not touch the paddles.**	Proper setup ensures proper functioning. Solid adhesion is necessary for conduction.

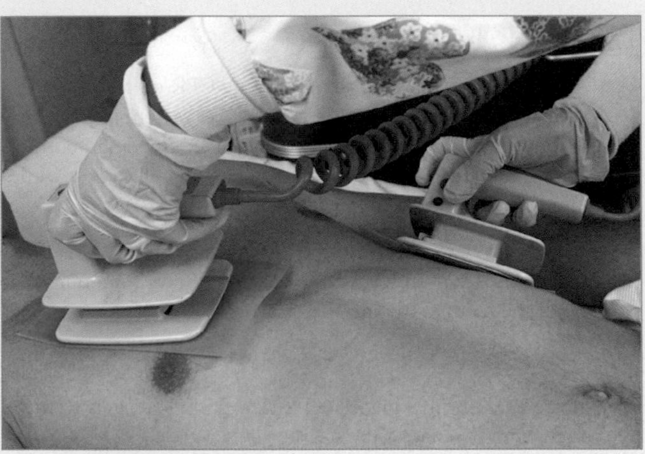

FIGURE 4 Placing paddles on patient's chest.

ACTION	RATIONALE
8. Reassess the cardiac rhythm.	The rhythm may have changed during preparation.
9. **If the patient remains in VF or pulseless VT, instruct all personnel to stand clear of the patient and the bed, including the operator.**	Standing clear of the bed and patient helps prevent electrical shocks to personnel.
10. Discharge the current by pressing both paddle charge buttons simultaneously. If using remote defibrillator pads, press the discharge or shock button on the machine.	Pressing the charge buttons discharges the electric current for defibrillation.
11. After the shock, immediately resume CPR, beginning with chest compressions. After five cycles (about 2 minutes), reassess the cardiac rhythm. Continue until advanced care providers take over, the patient starts to move, you are too exhausted to continue, or a physician discontinues CPR.	Resuming CPR provides optimal treatment. CPR preserves heart, and neurologic function (based on AHA 2006 recommended guidelines). Even when a shock eliminates the dysrhythmia, it may take several minutes for a heart rhythm to establish and even longer to achieve perfusion. Chest compressions can provide coronary and cerebral perfusion during this period (Zed et al., 2008).
12. If necessary, prepare to defibrillate a second time.	Additional shocking may be needed to stimulate the heart.
13. Announce that you are preparing to defibrillate and follow the procedure described above.	Additional shocking may be needed to stimulate the heart.
14. If defibrillation restores a normal rhythm:	
a. Check for signs of circulation; check the central and peripheral pulses, and obtain a blood pressure reading, heart rate, and respiratory rate.	The patient will need continuous monitoring to prevent further problems. Continuous monitoring helps provide for early detection and prompt intervention should additional problems arise.
b. If signs of circulation are present, check breathing. If breathing is inadequate, assist breathing. Start rescue breathing (one breath every 5 seconds).	

ACTION	RATIONALE
c. If breathing is adequate, place the patient in the recovery position. Continue to assess the patient.	
d. Assess the patient's level of consciousness, cardiac rhythm, blood pressure, breath sounds, skin color, and temperature.	Reassessment determines the need for continued intervention. Provides optimal treatment.
e. Obtain baseline ABG levels (Skill 18-11) and a 12-lead ECG (Skill 16-5), if ordered.	
f. Provide supplemental oxygen, ventilation, and medications, as needed.	
g. Anticipate the possible use of induced therapeutic hypothermia.	Cooling the patient after cardiac arrest protects the brain and may preserve neurologic function by reducing the cerebral metabolic rate of oxygen (Morton & Fontaine, 2013; Bucher et al., 2012).
15. Check the chest for electrical burns and treat them, as ordered, with corticosteroid- or lanolin-based creams. If using 'hands-free' pads, keep pads on in case of recurrent ventricular tachycardia or ventricular fibrillation.	Skin inspection identifies injury. Keeping pads in place provides preparation for future use.
16. Remove gloves, if used. Perform hand hygiene.	Removing PPE properly reduces the risk for infection transmission and contamination of other items. Hand hygiene prevents transmission of microorganisms.
17. Prepare the defibrillator for immediate reuse.	A patient may remain unstable and could require further intervention.

EVALUATION

The expected outcome is achieved when manual external defibrillation is performed correctly without adverse effect to the patient and the patient regains signs of circulation. Additional outcomes may include the following: the patient regains respirations; the patient's heart and lungs maintain adequate function to sustain life; the patient does not experience serious injury; and advanced cardiac life support is initiated.

DOCUMENTATION

Guidelines

Document the time you discovered the patient unresponsive and started CPR. Document the procedure, including the patient's ECG rhythms both before and after defibrillation; the number of times defibrillation was performed; the voltage used during each attempt; whether a pulse returned; the dosage, route, and time of drug administration; whether CPR was used; how the airway was maintained; and the patient's outcome. Continued intervention, such as by the code team, is typically documented on a code form, which identifies the actions and drugs provided during the code. Provide a summary of these events in the patient's medical record.

Sample Documentation

07/06/15 2230 Called to patient's room by wife. Patient noted to be without evidence of respirations or circulation. Emergency response system activated, CPR initiated. Manual defibrillation initiated at 2232. See code sheet.

—B. Clapp, RN

UNEXPECTED SITUATIONS AND ASSOCIATED INTERVENTIONS

- *The defibrillator fails to fire:* Check that the power is turned on. If the defibrillator is not plugged in, check if the battery is low. Check that it is fully charged.
- *The patient develops a skin burn at the site of the pad placement:* Prepare to treat the burn area as ordered, such as with corticosteroid- or lanolin-based creams. In most cases, an insufficient amount of conductive medium is the cause.

(*continued*)

SKILL 16-3 PERFORMING EMERGENCY MANUAL EXTERNAL DEFIBRILLATION (ASYNCHRONOUS) continued

SPECIAL CONSIDERATIONS

General Considerations

- **Every effort should be taken to minimize interruptions in chest compressions. Causes for not providing compressions may include prolonged pulse checks, taking too long to give breaths, moving the patient, and using the AED. Try to limit interruptions to less than 10 seconds (AHA, 2011).**
- Defibrillation can cause accidental electric shock to those providing care.
- Defibrillators vary from one manufacturer to another, so familiarize yourself with your facility's equipment. Defibrillator operation should be checked at least every 8 hours, or per facility policy, and after each use.
- Defibrillation can be affected by several factors, including paddle size and placement, condition of the patient's myocardium, duration of the arrhythmia, chest resistance, and the number of counter shocks.

Infant and Child Considerations

- If using a manual defibrillator, use adult paddles for children older than 1 year of age (>10 kg) and infant size paddles for infants <10 kg in weight. Weight-based dosing is recommended for children under 8 years of age or 55 pounds (25 kg). First shock: 2 J/kg; second: 4 J/kg; third and subsequent: ≥4 J/kg with maximum dose not to exceed 10 J/kg or the adult dose, whichever is lower (Kleinman et al., 2010).
- A manual defibrillator is preferred for infants under the age of 1 year.

Older Adult Considerations

Nurses can help promote informed decision making about CPR to older adults and their families (Cadogan, 2010). Educate, support, and advocate for patients as they face this critical choice. Provide evidence-based information, supportive listening, and a willingness to respect their choices (Buck, 2012).

EVIDENCE FOR PRACTICE ▶

CARDIOPULMONARY RESUSCITATION AND EMERGENCY CARDIAC CARE

The American Heart Association provides guidelines for cardiopulmonary resuscitation and emergency cardiac care and has incorporated these guidelines into the Basic Life Support and Advanced Life Support education for health care providers who respond to cardiovascular and respiratory emergencies.

Refer to the Evidence for Practice in Skills 16-1 and 16-2 for details, and refer to thePoint for additional research on related nursing topics.

SKILL 16-4 OBTAINING AN ELECTROCARDIOGRAM (ECG)

Electrocardiography (ECG [also abbreviated as EKG in some references]) is one of the most valuable and frequently used diagnostic tools. ECG measures the heart's electrical activity. Impulses moving through the heart's conduction system create electric currents that can be monitored on the body's surface. Electrodes attached to the skin can detect these electric currents and transmit them to an instrument that produces a record, the **electrocardiogram,** of cardiac activity. The data are graphed as waveforms (Figure 1). ECG can be used to identify myocardial ischemia and infarction, rhythm and conduction disturbances, chamber enlargement, electrolyte imbalances, and drug toxicity.

The standard 12-lead ECG uses a series of electrodes placed on the extremities and the chest wall to assess the heart from 12 different viewpoints (leads) by attaching ten cables with electrodes to the patient's limbs and chest: four limb electrodes and six chest electrodes (Figure 2). Each lead provides

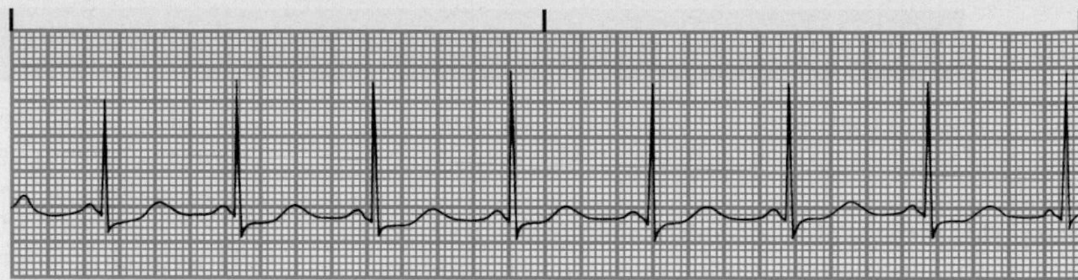

FIGURE 1 Electrocardiogram (waveform) strip.

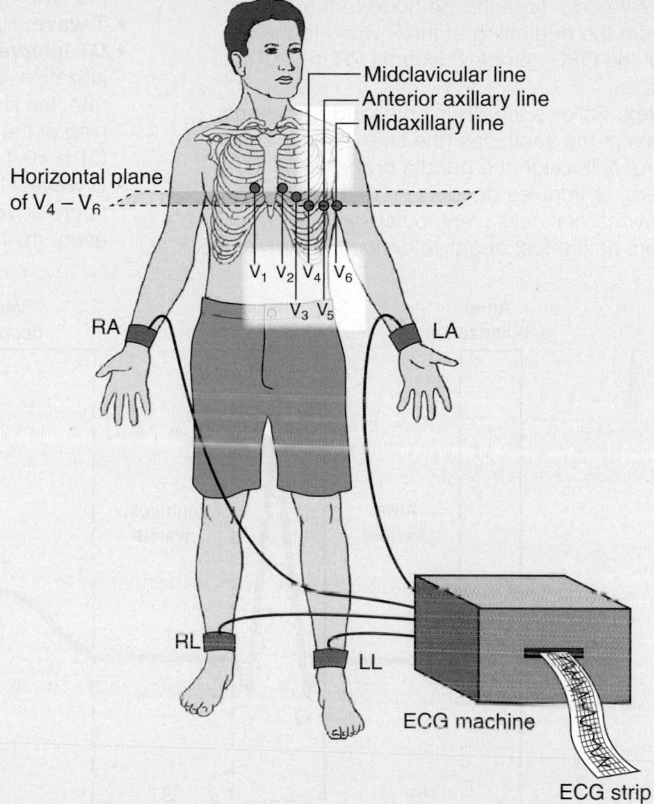

FIGURE 2 12-lead ECG lead placement. (From Morton, P.G., & Fontaine, D.K. (2013). *Essentials of critical care nursing. A holistic approach.* Philadelphia: Wolters Kluwer Health/Lippincott Williams & Wilkins, with permission.)

an electrographic snapshot of electrochemical activity of the myocardial cell membrane. The ECG device measures and averages the differences between the electrical potential of the electrode sites for each lead and graphs them over time, creating the standard ECG complex, called PQRST (Box 16-2). These electrodes provide views of the heart from the frontal plane as well as the horizontal plane. It is essential that connection or placement of the ECG electrodes/leads is accurate to prevent misdiagnosis. The ECG tracing needs to be clear to enable accurate and reliable interpretation (Jevon, 2010).

An ECG is typically accomplished using a multichannel method. All electrodes are attached to the patient at once and the machine prints a simultaneous view of all leads. It is important to reassure the patient that the leads just sense and record and do not transmit any electricity. The patient must be able to lie still and refrain from speaking to prevent body movement from creating artifact in the ECG. Variations of standard ECG include exercise ECG (stress ECG) and ambulatory ECG (Holter monitoring).

Interpreting the ECG requires the following actions:

- Determine the rhythm.
- Determine the rate.
- Evaluate the P wave.
- Determine the duration of the PR interval.
- Determine the duration of the QRS complex.
- Evaluate the T waves.
- Determine the duration of the QT interval.
- Evaluate any other components.

(continued)

SKILL 16-4 OBTAINING AN ELECTROCARDIOGRAM (ECG) continued

BOX 16-2 ECG COMPLEX

The ECG complex consists of five waveforms labeled with the letters P, Q, R, S, and T. In addition, sometimes a U wave appears.

- **P wave:** Represents atrial depolarization (conduction of the electrical impulse through the atria); the first component of ECG waveform.
- **PR interval:** Tracks the atrial impulse from the atria through the AV node, from the SA node to the AV node. Measures from the beginning of the P wave to the beginning of the QRS complex. Normal PR is 0.12 to 0.2 seconds.
- **QRS complex:** Follows the PR interval and represents depolarization of the ventricles (the time it takes for the impulse to travel through the bundle branches to the Purkinje fibers) or impulse conduction and contraction of the myocardial cells (ventricular systole). The Q wave appears as the first negative deflection in the QRS complex, the R wave as the first positive deflection. The S wave appears as the second negative deflection or the first negative deflection after the R wave. Normal QRS is 0.06 to 0.1 seconds.
- **ST segment:** Represents the end of ventricular conduction or depolarization and the beginning of ventricular recovery or repolarization; the J point marks the end of the QRS complex and the beginning of the ST segment.
- **T wave:** Represents ventricular recovery or repolarization.
- **QT interval:** Measures ventricular depolarization and repolarization; varies with the heart rate (i.e., the faster the heart rate, the shorter the QT interval); extends from the beginning of the QRS complex to the end of the T wave. Normal QT is <0.4 seconds, but can vary with heart rate.
- **U wave:** Represents the recovery period of the Purkinje fibers or ventricular conduction fibers; not present on every rhythm strip.

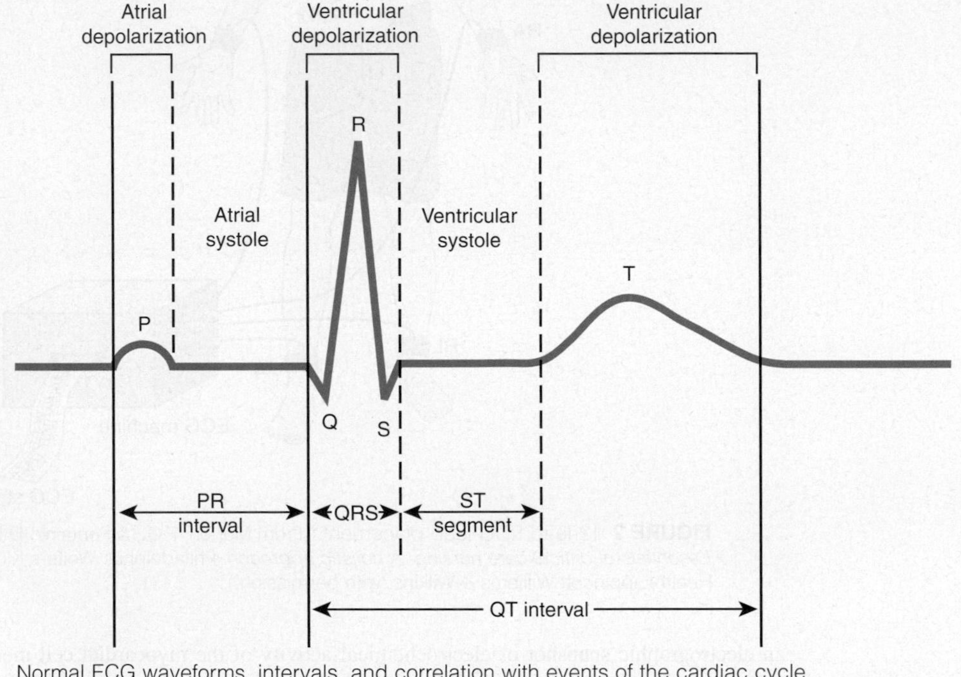

Normal ECG waveforms, intervals, and correlation with events of the cardiac cycle.

DELEGATION CONSIDERATIONS

Obtaining an electrocardiogram is not delegated to nursing assistive personnel (NAP) or to unlicensed assistive personnel (UAP). Depending on the state's nurse practice act and the organization's policies and procedures, this procedure may be delegated to licensed practical/vocational nurses (LPN/LVNs). The decision to delegate must be based on careful analysis of the patient's needs and circumstances, as well as the qualifications of the person to whom the task is being delegated. Refer to the Delegation Guidelines in Appendix A.

EQUIPMENT

- ECG machine
- Recording paper
- Disposable pregelled electrodes
- Adhesive remover swabs
- 4 × 4 gauze pads
- Skin cleanser and water, if necessary
- Additional PPE, as indicated
- Bath blanket

ASSESSMENT

Review the patient's medical record and plan of care for information about the patient's need for an ECG. Assess the patient's cardiac status, including heart rate, blood pressure, and auscultation of heart sounds. If the patient is already connected to a cardiac monitor, remove the electrodes to accommodate the precordial leads and minimize electrical interference on the ECG tracing. Keep the patient away from objects that might cause electrical interference, such as equipment, fixtures, and power cords. Inspect the patient's chest for areas of irritation, breakdown, or excessive hair that might interfere with electrode placement.

NURSING DIAGNOSIS

Determine the related factors for the nursing diagnoses based on the patient's current status. Appropriate nursing diagnoses may include:

- Decreased Cardiac Output
- Acute Pain
- Activity Intolerance

OUTCOME IDENTIFICATION AND PLANNING

The expected outcome to achieve is that a cardiac electrical tracing is obtained without any complications. Other appropriate outcomes may include the following: the patient displays an increased understanding about the ECG, and the patient has reduced anxiety.

IMPLEMENTATION

ACTION	RATIONALE
1. Verify the order for an ECG in the patient's medical record.	This ensures that the correct intervention is performed on the correct patient.
2. Gather all equipment.	Assembling equipment provides for an organized approach to the task.
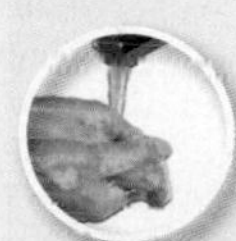 3. Perform hand hygiene and put on PPE, if indicated.	Hand hygiene and PPE prevent the spread of microorganisms. PPE is required based on Transmission Precautions.
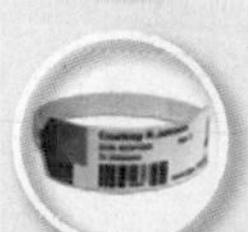 4. Identify the patient.	Identifying the patient ensures the right patient receives the intervention and helps prevent errors.
5. Close curtains around the bed and close the door to the room, if possible. As you set up the machine to record a 12-lead ECG, explain the procedure to the patient. Tell the patient that the test records the heart's electrical activity, and it may be repeated at certain intervals. Emphasize that no electrical current will enter his or her body. Tell the patient the test typically takes about 5 minutes. Ask the patient about allergies to adhesive, as appropriate.	This ensures the patient's privacy. Explanation relieves anxiety and facilitates cooperation. Possible allergies may exist related to adhesive on ECG leads.
6. Place the ECG machine close to the patient's bed, and plug the power cord into the wall outlet.	Having equipment available saves time and facilitates accomplishment of the task.
7. If the bed is adjustable, raise it to a comfortable working height, usually elbow height of the caregiver (VISN 8 Patient Safety Center, 2009).	Having the bed at the proper height prevents back and muscle strain.
8. Have the patient lie supine in the center of the bed with the arms at the sides. Raise the head of the bed if necessary to promote comfort. Expose the patient's arms and legs, and drape appropriately. Encourage the patient to relax the arms and legs. Ensure the wrists do not touch the waist. Make sure the feet do not touch the bed's footboard.	Proper positioning helps increase patient comfort and will produce a better tracing. Proper positioning and relaxation of the arms and legs minimizes muscle tension and trembling and electrical interference.

(continued)

SKILL 16-4 OBTAINING AN ELECTROCARDIOGRAM (ECG) continued

ACTION	RATIONALE
9. If necessary, prepare the skin for electrode placement. If an area is excessively hairy, clip the hair. **Do not shave hair.** Clean excess oil or other substances from the skin with skin cleanser and water and dry it completely. If wet gel electrodes are used, shaving and abrading skin is not necessary. If solid gel electrodes are used, clean, degrease, and debride the skin (gently rub with gauze pad) and clip hair, if necessary.	Shaving causes microabrasions on the chest skin. Oils and excess hair interfere with electrode contact and function. Alcohol, benzoin, and antiperspirant are not recommended to prepare skin.
10. Apply the limb electrodes (Figure 3), then connect the limb lead wires to the electrodes. The tip of each lead wire is lettered and color coded for easy identification. The white or RA lead goes to the right arm, just above the wrist bone; the green or RL lead to the right leg, just above the ankle bone; the red or LL lead to the left leg, just above the ankle bone; the black or LA lead to the left arm, just above the wrist bone. Peel the contact paper off the self-sticking disposable electrode and apply directly to the prepared site, as recommended by the manufacturer. Refer to Figure 2 for electrode placement.	Use of recommended standard sites for limb electrodes is essential to obtain accurate recording (Crawford & Doherty, 2010; SCST, 2010).
11. Expose the patient's chest. Apply the chest electrodes (Figure 4A), and then connect the chest lead wires to the electrodes (Figure 4B). The tip of each lead wire is lettered and color coded for easy identification. The V_1 to V_6 leads are applied to the chest. Peel the contact paper off the self-sticking, disposable electrode and apply directly to the prepared site, as recommended by the manufacturer. Position chest electrodes as follows (refer to Figure 2): • V_1: (Red) Fourth intercostal space at right sternal border • V_2: (Yellow) Fourth intercostal space at left sternal border • V_3: (Green) Exactly midway between V_2 and V_4 • V_4: (Blue) Fifth intercostal space at the left midclavicular line • V_5: (Orange) Left anterior axillary line, same horizontal plane as V_4 and V_6 • V_6: (Purple) Left midaxillary line, same horizontal plane as V_4 and V_5	Proper lead placement is necessary for accurate test results (SCST, 2010; Kligfield et al., 2007).

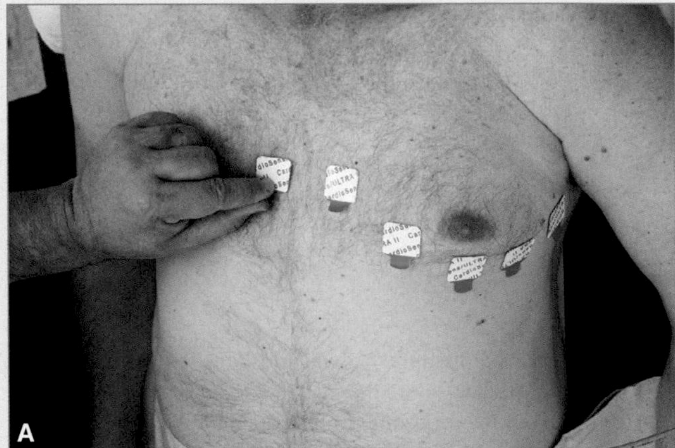

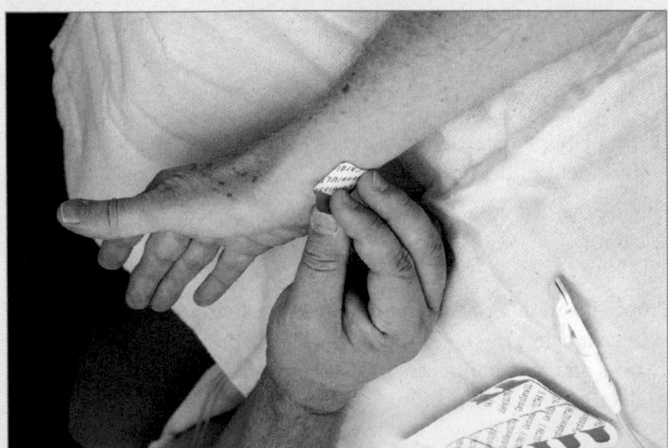

FIGURE 3 Applying limb electrode.

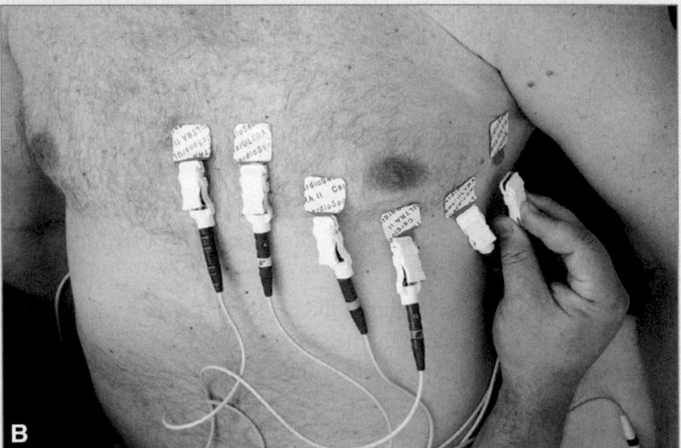

FIGURE 4 **A.** Applying chest electrode. **B.** Applying chest lead.

ACTION	RATIONALE
12. After the application of all the leads (Figure 5), ensure that the cables are not pulling on the electrodes or lying over each other. Make sure the paper-speed selector is set to the standard 25 m/second and that the machine is set to full voltage.	Minimizes electrical artifact and improves quality and accuracy of the ECG (Roberts, 2002, in Jevon, 2010). The machine will record a normal standardization mark—a square that is the height of 2 large squares or 10 small squares on the recording paper.
13. If necessary, enter the appropriate patient identification data into the machine.	This allows for proper identification of the ECG strip.
14. Ask the patient to relax and breathe normally. **Instruct the patient to lie still and not to talk while you record the ECG.**	Lying still and not talking produce a better tracing.
15. Press the AUTO button. Observe the tracing quality (Figure 6). The machine will record all 12 leads automatically, recording 3 consecutive leads simultaneously. Some machines have a display screen so you can preview waveforms before the machine records them on paper. Adjust waveform, if necessary. If any part of the waveform extends beyond the paper when you record the ECG, adjust the normal standardization to half-standardization and repeat. Note this adjustment on the ECG strip, because this will need to be considered in interpreting the results.	Observation of tracing quality allows for adjustments to be made, if necessary. Notation of adjustments ensures accurate interpretation of results.
16. When the machine finishes recording the 12-lead ECG (Figure 7), remove the electrodes and clean the patient's skin, if necessary, with adhesive remover for sticky residue.	Removal and cleaning promote patient comfort.

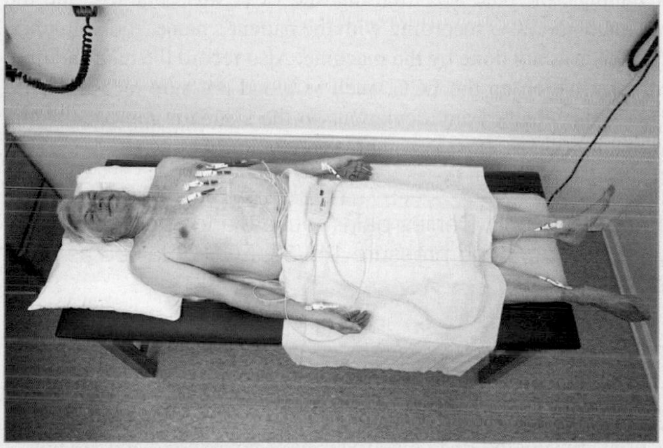

FIGURE 5 Completed application of 12-lead ECG.

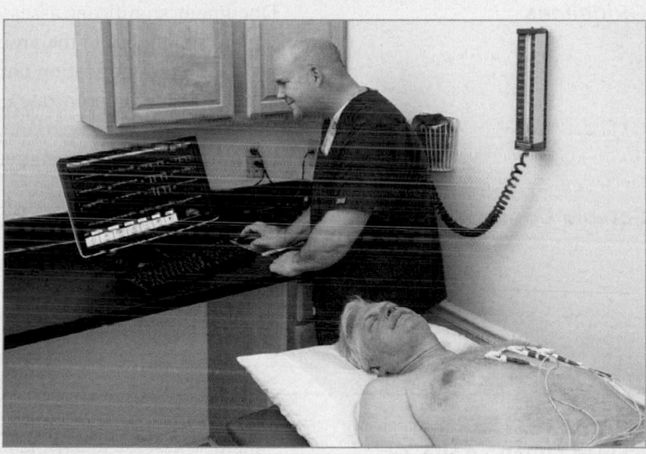

FIGURE 6 Observing tracing quality.

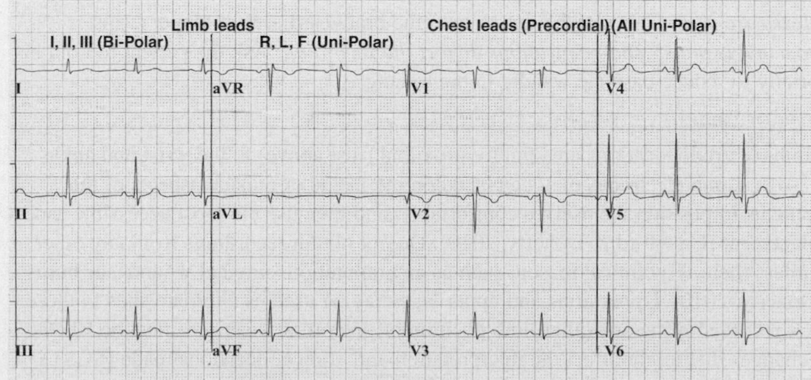

FIGURE 7 Normal 12-lead ECG configuration. (From Diepenbrock, N. (2011). *Quick reference to critical care.* (4th ed.). Philadelphia: Wolters Kluwer Health/Lippincott Williams & Wilkins, with permission, p. 102.)

(continued)

SKILL 16-4 OBTAINING AN ELECTROCARDIOGRAM (ECG) continued

ACTION	RATIONALE
17. After disconnecting the lead wires from the electrodes, dispose of the electrodes. Return the patient to a comfortable position. Lower bed height and adjust the head of bed to a comfortable position.	Proper disposal deters the spread of microorganisms. Positioning with head adjustment promotes patient comfort. Lowering the bed height promotes patient safety.
18. Clean the ECG machine per facility policy. If not done electronically from data entered into the machine, label the ECG with the patient's name, date of birth, location, date and time of recording, and other relevant information, such as symptoms that occurred during the recording (Jevon, 2010). Note any deviations to the standard approach to the recording, such as alternative placement of leads. (See Special Considerations below.)	Cleaning equipment between patient uses decreases the risk for transmission of microorganisms. Accurate labeling ensures the ECG is recorded for the correct patient and accurate and reliable interpretation.
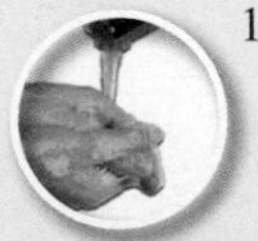 19. Remove additional PPE, if used. Perform hand hygiene.	Removing PPE properly reduces the risk for infection transmission and contamination of other items. Hand hygiene prevents transmission of microorganisms.

EVALUATION

The expected outcome is achieved when a quality ECG reading is obtained without any undue patient anxiety or complications or injury. In addition, the patient verbalizes an understanding of the reason for the ECG.

DOCUMENTATION

Guidelines

Document significant assessment findings, the date and time that the ECG was obtained, and the patient's response to the procedure. Label the ECG recording with the patient's name, room number, and facility identification number, if this was not done by the machine. Also record the date and time as well as any appropriate clinical information on the ECG, such as blood pressure measurement, if the patient was experiencing chest pain. Record any deviations to the standard approach to the recording, such as alternative placement of leads. (See Special Considerations below.)

Sample Documentation

11/10/15 1745 Patient admitted to room 663. Denies pain, nausea, and shortness of breath. Apical heart rate 82 and regular. Blood pressure 146/88. ECG obtained as per admission orders. Copy faxed to Dr. Martin.

—B. Clapp, RN

UNEXPECTED SITUATIONS AND ASSOCIATED INTERVENTIONS

- *An artifact appears on the tracing:* An artifact may be due to loose electrodes or patient movement. Reassess electrode connections. Ensure the ECG electrodes have not expired and are not dry; change electrodes, if necessary (Jevon, 2010). Ask the patient to lie extremely still. Redo the ECG, if necessary.
- *Minimal complexes are seen:* This may be due to extreme bradycardia. Run longer strips.
- *A wandering baseline is noted, and respirations distort the recording:* Ask the patient to hold his or her breath briefly to reduce baseline wander in the tracing.

SPECIAL CONSIDERATIONS

- The standard limb electrode locations are slightly proximal (just above) to the wrist and ankle bones (SCST, 2010). Limb electrodes may be placed on the inside or outside aspects of the limbs. Allow patients to position themselves comfortably, and then use the most accessible aspect for electrode placement (Crawford & Doherty, 2010). Do not obtain recordings from any other limb position unless there is a clinical reason, such as an amputation, surgical wounds, or burns (Crawford & Doherty, 2010). Upper arms and upper legs may be used as alternate sites in these situations. ECGs recorded using any other limb position or precordial positions must be labeled to account for changes that might affect the interpretation and clinical decisions made (SCST).

- To position the chest leads (V_1–V_6) correctly, it is important to be able to accurately locate the relevant intercostal spaces (Jevon, 2010).
- For female patients, place the V_4 electrode, as well as V_5 and V_6 as necessary, under the breast tissue (Kligfield et al., 2007). In a large-breasted woman, you may need to displace the breast tissue laterally and/or superiorly.
- Alternative placement for the chest leads may be indicated. Right-sided chest leads may be ordered for inferior or posterior myocardial infarction, using right-sided electrode positions that mirror the standard V_3–V_6. Posterior chest leads may be ordered for suspected posterior myocardial infarction, with application of chest leads to the patient's back below the left scapula at the level of the fifth intercostal space (Jevon, 2010). ECGs recorded using any other limb position or precordial positions must be labeled to account for changes that might affect the interpretation and clinical decisions made (SCST, 2010).
- If the patient's skin is exceptionally oily, scaly, or diaphoretic, rub the electrode site with a dry 4 × 4 gauze and clean with skin cleanser and water before applying the electrode to help reduce interference in the tracing. Alcohol, benzoin, and antiperspirant are not recommended to prepare the skin.
- If the patient has a pacemaker, perform an ECG with or without a magnet, according to the primary care provider's orders. Note the presence of a pacemaker and the use of the magnet on the strip.
- If self-sticking, disposable electrodes are not used, apply electrode paste or gel to the patient's skin at the appropriate sites. Rub the gel or paste into the skin. The paste or gel facilitates electrode contact and enhances tracing. Secure electrodes promptly after applying the paste or gel. This prevents drying of the medium, which could impair ECG quality.
- Never use alcohol or acetone pads in place of the electrode paste or gel. Acetone and alcohol impair electrode contact with the skin and diminish the transmission of electrical impulses. The use of alcohol as a conducting material can result in burns. After disconnecting the lead wires from the electrodes, dispose of (or clean) the electrodes, as indicated. Proper cleaning after use ensures that the machine will be ready for next use.
- Be aware that a new 80-lead ECG system (body surface mapping) is available, which looks at a patient's heart from 80 views. It can detect more cases of myocardial infarction in patients than a standard 12-lead ECG. Additional education regarding use of this technology is required. An ECG obtained with body surface mapping can be interpreted in about 5 minutes, using the same skills as the standard 12-lead ECG (O'Neil et al., 2010; Self et al., 2006).

SKILL 16-5 APPLYING A CARDIAC MONITOR

Bedside cardiac monitoring provides continuous observation of the heart's electrical activity. It focuses on the detection of clinically significant dysrhythmias (Larson & Brady, 2008). Cardiac monitoring is used for patients with conduction disturbances and for those at risk for life-threatening arrhythmias, such as postoperative patients and patients who are sedated. As with other forms of electrocardiography (ECG), cardiac monitoring uses electrodes placed on the patient's chest to transmit electrical signals that are converted into a tracing of cardiac rhythm on an oscilloscope. Three-lead or five-lead systems may be used (Figure 1). The three-lead–wire monitoring system facilitates monitoring of the patient in any of the limb leads, as well as a modified version of any of the six chest leads (Morton & Fontaine, 2013). The five-lead–wire monitoring system facilitates monitoring of the patient in any one of the standard 12 leads.

(continued)

SKILL 16-5 APPLYING A CARDIAC MONITOR continued

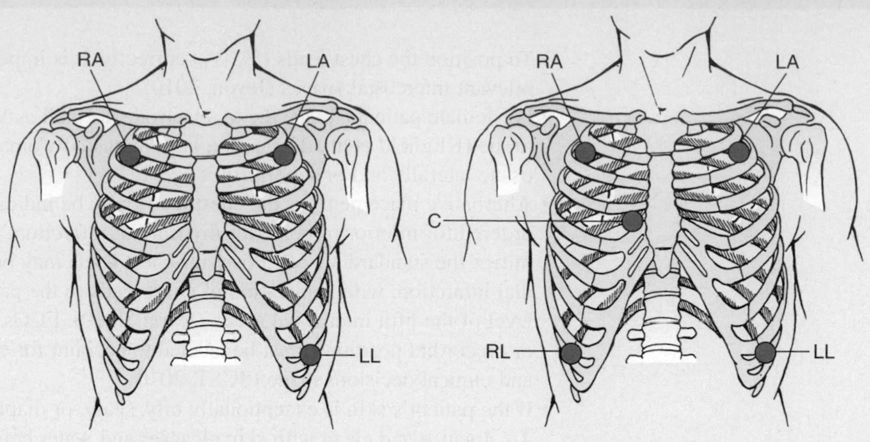

FIGURE 1 Electrode positions for three-lead (*left*) and five-lead (*right*) systems.

Positions for the three-lead system:
RA (white electrode) below right clavicle, second ICS, right midclavicular line
LA (black electrode) below left clavicle, second ICS, left midclavicular line
LL (red electrode) left lower ribcage, eighth ICS, left midclavicular line

Positions for five-lead system:
RA (white electrode) below right clavicle, second ICS, right midclavicular line
RL (green electrode) right lower ribcage, eighth ICS, right midclavicular line
LA (black electrode) below left clavicle, second ICS, left midclavicular line
LL (red electrode) left lower ribcage, eighth ICS, left midclavicular line
Chest (brown electrode) any V lead position, usually V_1 (fourth ICS, right sternal border)

Two types of monitoring may be performed: hardwire or telemetry. In hardwire monitoring, the patient is connected to a monitor at the bedside. The rhythm display appears at the bedside, but may also be transmitted to a console at a remote location. Telemetry uses a small transmitter connected to an ambulatory patient to send electrical signals to another location, where they are displayed on a monitor screen. Battery-powered and portable, telemetry frees patients from cumbersome wires and cables and lets them be comfortably mobile. Telemetry is especially useful for monitoring arrhythmias that occur during sleep, rest, exercise, or stressful situations. Wireless telemetry devices are also being introduced, using microchips to record patient data, eliminating the need for new leads each time the patient is moved to a different location (Goulette, 2008).

Regardless of the type, cardiac monitors can display the patient's heart rate and rhythm, produce a printed record of cardiac rhythm, and sound an alarm if the heart rate exceeds or falls below specified limits. Monitors also recognize and count abnormal heartbeats as well as changes. Cardiac monitoring systems may incorporate computer systems that store, analyze, and trend monitored data, automatic chart documentation, and wireless communication devices that provide data and alarms that can be carried by the nurse (Morton & Fontaine, 2013).

Gel foam electrodes are commonly used. Electrodes should be changed every 24 hours, or according to facility policy, to prevent skin irritation and maintain quality of data. Hypoallergenic electrodes are available for patients with hypersensitivity to tape or adhesive. Any loose or nonadhering electrode should be replaced immediately to prevent inaccurate or missing data.

DELEGATION CONSIDERATIONS

The application of a cardiac monitor is not delegated to nursing assistive personnel (NAP) or to unlicensed assistive personnel (UAP). Depending on the state's nurse practice act and the organization's policies and procedures, application of a cardiac monitor may be delegated to licensed practical/vocational nurses (LPN/LVNs).The decision to delegate must be based on careful analysis of the patient's needs and circumstances, as well as the qualifications of the person to whom the task is being delegated. Refer to the Delegation Guidelines in Appendix A.

EQUIPMENT

- Lead wires
- Pregelled (gel foam) electrodes (number varies from 3 to 5)
- Gauze pads
- Skin cleanser
- Patient cable for hardwire cardiac monitoring
- Transmitter, transmitter pouch, and telemetry battery pack for telemetry
- PPE, as indicated

ASSESSMENT

Review the patient's medical record and plan of care for information about the patient's need for cardiac monitoring. Assess the patient's cardiac status, including heart rate, blood pressure, and auscultation of heart sounds. Inspect the patient's chest for areas of irritation, breakdown, or excessive hair that might interfere with electrode placement. Electrode sites must be dry, with minimal hair. The patient may be sitting or supine, in a bed or chair.

NURSING DIAGNOSIS

Determine the related factors for the nursing diagnoses based on the patient's current status. Appropriate nursing diagnoses may include:

- Decreased Cardiac Output
- Excess Fluid Volume
- Deficient Knowledge

OUTCOME IDENTIFICATION AND PLANNING

The expected outcome to achieve when performing cardiac monitoring is that a clear waveform, free from artifact, is displayed on the cardiac monitor. Other appropriate outcomes may include the following: the patient displays an understanding of the reason for monitoring, and the patient experiences reduced anxiety.

IMPLEMENTATION

ACTION	RATIONALE
1. Verify the order for cardiac monitoring on the patient's medical record.	This ensures that the correct intervention is performed on the correct patient.
2. Gather equipment.	Assembling equipment provides for an organized approach to the task.
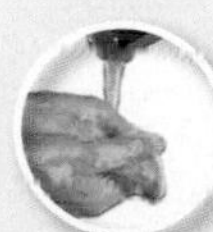 3. Perform hand hygiene and put on PPE, if indicated.	Hand hygiene and PPE prevent the spread of microorganisms. PPE is required based on transmission precautions.
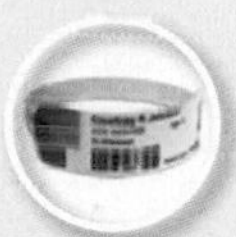 4. Identify the patient.	Identifying the patient ensures the right patient receives the intervention and helps prevent errors.
5. Close curtains around the bed and close the door to the room, if possible. Explain the procedure to the patient. Tell the patient that the monitoring records the heart's electrical activity. Emphasize that no electrical current will enter his or her body. Ask the patient about allergies to adhesive, as appropriate.	This ensures the patient's privacy. Explanation relieves anxiety and facilitates cooperation. Possible allergies may exist related to adhesive on ECG leads.
6. For hardwire monitoring, plug the cardiac monitor into an electrical outlet and turn it on to warm up the unit while preparing the equipment and the patient. For telemetry monitoring, insert a new battery into the transmitter. Match the poles on the battery with the polar markings on the transmitter case. Press the button at the top of the unit, test the battery's charge, and test the unit to ensure that the battery is operational.	Proper setup ensures proper functioning. Not all models have a test button. Test according to manufacturer's directions.
7. Insert the cable into the appropriate socket in the monitor.	Proper setup ensures proper functioning.
8. Connect the lead wires to the cable. In some systems, the lead wires are permanently secured to the cable. For telemetry, if the lead wires are not permanently affixed to the telemetry unit, attach them securely. If they must be attached individually, connect each one to the correct outlet.	Proper setup ensures proper functioning.
9. Connect an electrode to each of the lead wires, carefully checking that each lead wire is in its correct outlet.	Proper setup ensures proper functioning.

(continued)

SKILL 16-5 APPLYING A CARDIAC MONITOR continued

ACTION	RATIONALE
10. If the bed is adjustable, raise it to a comfortable working height, usually elbow height of the caregiver (VISN 8, 2009).	Having the bed at the proper height prevents back and muscle strain.
11. Expose the patient's chest and determine electrode positions, based on which system and leads are being used. (Refer to Figure 1.) If necessary, clip the hair from an area about 10 cm in diameter around each electrode site. Abrade the skin by gently rubbing the area with a gauze pad. Clean the area with skin cleanser and water and dry it completely.	These actions allow for better adhesion of the electrode and thus better conduction. Gentle abrasion removes dead skin cells. Cleaning skin removes oily residues. Alcohol, benzoin, and antiperspirant are not recommended to prepare the skin.
12. Remove the backing from the pregelled electrode. Check the gel for moistness. If the gel is dry, discard it and replace it with a fresh electrode. **Apply the electrode to the site and press firmly to ensure a tight seal.** Repeat with the remaining electrodes to complete the three-lead or five-lead system (Figure 2).	Gel acts as a conduit and must be moist and secured tightly.

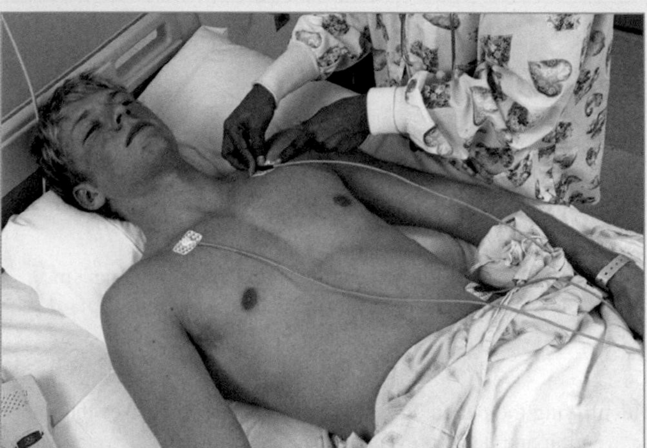

FIGURE 2 Applying the electrodes.

ACTION	RATIONALE
13. When all the electrodes are in place, connect the appropriate lead wire to each electrode. Check waveform for clarity, position, and size. **To verify that the monitor is detecting each beat, compare the digital heart rate display with an auscultated count of the patient's heart rate.** If necessary, use the gain control to adjust the size of the rhythm tracing, and use the position control to adjust the waveform position on the monitor.	This ensures accuracy of reading.
14. Set the upper and lower limits of the heart rate alarm, based on the patient's condition or unit policy.	Setting the alarm allows for audible notification if the heart rate is beyond limits. The default setting for the monitor automatically turns on all alarms; limits should be set for each patient.
15. For telemetry, place the transmitter in the pouch in the hospital gown. If no pouch is available in the gown, use a portable pouch. Tie the pouch strings around the patient's neck and waist, making sure that the pouch fits snugly without causing discomfort. If no pouch is available, place the transmitter in the patient's bathrobe pocket.	Patient comfort leads to compliance.
16. To obtain a rhythm strip, press the RECORD key, either at the bedside for monitoring or at the central station for telemetry. Label the strip with the patient's name and room number, date, time, and rhythm identification. Analyze the strip, as appropriate. Place the rhythm strip in the appropriate location in the patient's chart.	A rhythm strip provides a baseline for future comparison.

ACTION	RATIONALE
17. Return the patient to a comfortable position. Lower the bed height and adjust the head of bed to a comfortable position.	Repositioning promotes patient comfort. Lowering the bed promotes patient safety.
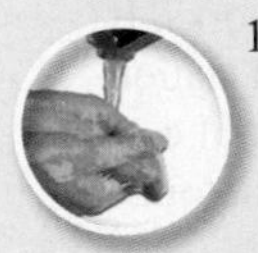 18. Remove additional PPE, if used. Perform hand hygiene.	Removing PPE properly reduces the risk for infection transmission and contamination of other items. Hand hygiene prevents transmission of microorganisms.

EVALUATION

The expected outcome is achieved when the cardiac monitoring waveform displays the patient's cardiac rhythm, with a waveform that is detecting each beat, and is appropriate for clarity, position, and size. In addition, the patient demonstrates no undue anxiety and remains free of complications or injury.

DOCUMENTATION

Guidelines

Record the date and time that monitoring begins and the monitoring lead used in the medical record. Document a rhythm strip at least every 8 hours and with any changes in the patient's condition (or as stated by facility's policy). Label the rhythm strip with the patient's name and room number, date, and time.

Sample Documentation

12/16/15 1615 Patient admitted to room. Cardiac telemetry monitor in place; monitoring in lead II. See flow sheet for assessment data and initial rhythm strip.

— T. Shah, RN

UNEXPECTED SITUATIONS AND ASSOCIATED INTERVENTIONS

- *False high-rate alarm sounds:* Assess for monitor that is interpreting large T waves as QRS complexes, thus doubling the rate, or for skeletal muscle activity. Reposition electrodes to a lead where the QRS complexes are taller than the T waves, and place electrodes away from major muscle masses. Change lead view on monitor. Use "relearn" feature, if available, to identify where the normal complexes are.
- *False low-rate alarm sounds:* Assess for a shift in the electrical axis due to patient movement, making QRS complexes too small to register; low amplitude of QRS; or poor contact between skin and electrode. Reapply electrodes. Set gain so that the height of complex is greater than 1 mV.
- *Low amplitude:* Assess if the size control is adjusted properly; poor contact between skin and electrodes; dried gel; broken or loose lead wires; poor connection between patient and monitor; or malfunctioning monitor. Check connections on all lead wires and monitoring cable. Replace electrodes, as necessary. Reapply electrodes, if required.
- *Wandering baseline:* Assess for poor position or contact between electrodes and skin, or thoracic movement with respirations. Reposition or replace electrodes.
- *Artifact (waveform interference):* Assess for patient movement, improperly applied electrodes, or static electricity. Attach all electrical equipment to a common ground. Check plugs to make sure prongs are not loose.
- *Skin excoriation under electrodes:* Assess for allergic reaction to electrode adhesive or electrodes being left on the skin too long. Remove electrodes and apply hypoallergenic electrodes and hypoallergenic tape, or remove electrode, clean site, and reapply electrode at new site.

SPECIAL CONSIDERATIONS

General Considerations

- Make sure all electrical equipment and outlets are grounded to avoid electric shock and interference (artifacts).
- Avoid opening the electrode package until just before using to prevent the gel from drying out.
- Avoid placing the electrodes on bony prominences, hairy locations, areas where defibrillator pads will be placed, or areas for chest compression.

(continued)

SKILL 16-5 APPLYING A CARDIAC MONITOR continued

- If the patient's skin is very oily, scaly, or diaphoretic, rub the electrode site with a dry 4 × 4 gauze pad before applying the electrode to help reduce interference in the tracing.
- Assess skin integrity and examine the leads every 8 hours. Replace and reposition the electrodes, as necessary.
- If the patient is being monitored by telemetry, show him or her how the transmitter works. If applicable, identify the button that will produce a recording of the ECG at the central station. Instruct the patient to push the button whenever symptoms occur; this causes the central console to print a rhythm strip. Also, advise the patient to notify the nurse immediately if symptoms occur.
- If a medical order is in place, tell the patient to remove the transmitter during showering or bathing, if appropriate, but stress that he or she should let the nurse know the unit is being removed.

Infant and Child Considerations

- Having the infant or child wear a snug undershirt over the leads helps to keep the leads in place (Kyle & Carman, 2013).

EVIDENCE FOR PRACTICE ▶

CARDIAC MONITORING

Many patients admitted to the hospital with cardiac, respiratory, and other acute health problems are placed on electrocardiographic monitoring. This monitoring allows the health care providers, including nurses, to monitor the patient for the development of cardiac dysrhythmias. Frequent monitor alarms are distracting and interfere with the ability to perform critical tasks. Does the changing of monitor electrodes daily impact cardiac monitor alarms?

Related Research

Cvach, M.M., Biggs, M., Rothwell, K.J., & Charles-Hudson, C. (2013). Daily electrode change and effect on cardiac monitor alarms. An evidence-based practice approach. *Journal of Nursing Care Quality, 28*(3), 265–271.

Large numbers of technical alarms distract patient care providers and interfere with patient care. Frequent alarms may lead to errors of omission, inattention, and missed patient status alarms. This study examined the effects of daily electrode change on the number of cardiac monitor alarms, specifically technical alarms. Technical monitor alarms are a result of poor signal quality generated by monitoring equipment, as opposed to patient status alarms related to potentially life-threatening situations or to specific arrhythmias. Eight days of baseline and intervention data were compared for two adult acute care units. Electrodes were changed daily during the hours of 8 a.m. and 12 p.m. Overall average alarms per bed per day were reduced by 47% on one unit and 46% on the other. Technical alarms decreased by 34% on one unit and 45% on the other. The authors concluded daily electrocardiogram electrode change reduces the number of cardiac monitor alarms.

Relevance for Nursing Practice

As primary care providers, nurses have the responsibility to include interventions to provide for the best patient care outcomes possible. Daily changing of monitor electrodes is a simple intervention that can be implemented by nurses. This intervention can lead to fewer technical alarms and decrease the risk for errors related to delayed alarm response.

Refer to thePoint for additional research on related nursing topics.

SKILL 16-6 USING AN EXTERNAL (TRANSCUTANEOUS) PACEMAKER

Temporary cardiac pacing is used to correct life-threatening cardiac dysrhythmias and as an elective procedure, such as to evaluate the need for permanent pacing or after cardiac surgery. A temporary pacemaker consists of an external, battery-powered pulse generator and a lead or electrode system to electrically stimulate heartbeat. Transcutaneous pacing can temporarily supply an electrical current in the heart when electrical conduction is abnormal. This device works by sending an electrical impulse from the pulse generator to the patient's heart by way of two electrodes, which are placed on the front and back of the patient's chest. This stimulates the contraction of cardiac muscle fibers through electrical stimulation (depolarization) of the myocardium. Transcutaneous pacing is quick and effective, but is usually used as short-term therapy until the situation resolves or transvenous or permanent pacing can be initiated.

Transcutaneous pacing can cause significant discomfort. Patient should be made aware of this and adequate sedation is necessary (Morton & Fontaine, 2013).

DELEGATION CONSIDERATIONS

The use of a transcutaneous pacemaker is not delegated to nursing assistive personnel (NAP) or to unlicensed assistive personnel (UAP). Depending on the state's nurse practice act and the organization's policies and procedures, this procedure may be delegated to licensed practical/vocational nurses (LPN/LVNs). The decision to delegate must be based on careful analysis of the patient's needs and circumstances, as well as the qualifications of the person to whom the task is being delegated. Refer to the Delegation Guidelines in Appendix A.

EQUIPMENT

- Transcutaneous noninvasive pacemaker
- Transcutaneous pacing electrodes and cables
- ECG electrodes and cables
- Cardiac monitor
- Medication for analgesia and/or sedation, as prescribed

ASSESSMENT

Review the patient's medical record and plan of care for information about the patient's need for pacing. Transcutaneous pacing is generally an emergency measure. Assess the patient's initial cardiac rhythm, including a rhythm strip and 12-lead ECG. Monitor heart rate, respiratory rate, level of consciousness, and skin color. If the patient is pulseless, initiate CPR.

NURSING DIAGNOSIS

Determine the related factors for the nursing diagnoses based on the patient's current status. Appropriate nursing diagnoses include:

- Decreased Cardiac Output
- Deficient Knowledge
- Anxiety
- Risk for Injury

OUTCOME IDENTIFICATION AND PLANNING

The expected outcome to achieve when using an external transcutaneous pacemaker is that it is applied correctly without adverse effect to the patient, and the patient regains signs of circulation, including the capture of at least the minimal set heart rate. Additional outcomes may include the following: the patient's heart and lungs maintain adequate function to sustain life; and the patient does not experience injury.

IMPLEMENTATION

ACTION	RATIONALE
1. Verify the order for a transcutaneous pacemaker in the patient's medical record.	This ensures that the correct intervention is performed on the correct patient.
2. Gather all equipment.	Assembling equipment provides for an organized approach to the task.
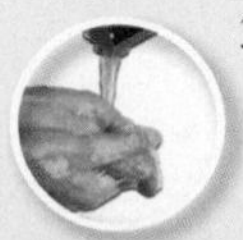 3. Perform hand hygiene and put on PPE, if indicated.	Hand hygiene and PPE prevent the transmission of microorganisms. PPE is required based on transmission precautions.

(continued)

SKILL 16-6 USING AN EXTERNAL (TRANSCUTANEOUS) PACEMAKER continued

ACTION	RATIONALE
4. Identify the patient. 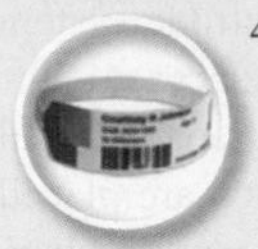	Verifying the patient's identity validates that the correct procedure is being done on the correct patient.
5. If the patient is responsive, explain the procedure to the patient. Explain that it involves some discomfort and that you will administer medication to keep him or her comfortable and help him or her to relax. Administer analgesia and sedation, as ordered, if not an emergency situation.	External pacemakers are typically used with unconscious patients because most alert patients cannot tolerate the uncomfortable sensations produced by the high energy levels needed to pace externally. If responsive, the patient will most likely be sedated.
6. Close curtains around the bed and close the door to the room, if possible. Obtain vital signs.	This provides for patient privacy. Vital signs provide baseline for assessing pacing effectiveness (Del Monte, 2009).
7. If necessary, clip the hair over the areas of electrode placement. **Do not shave the area.**	Shaving can cause tiny nicks in the skin, causing skin irritation. Also, the current from the pulse generator could cause discomfort.
8. Attach cardiac monitoring electrodes to the patient in the lead I, II, and III position. Do this even if the patient is already on telemetry monitoring. If you select the lead II position, adjust the LL (left leg) electrode placement to accommodate the anterior pacing electrode and the patient's anatomy.	Connecting the telemetry electrodes to the pacemaker is required.
9. Attach the patient monitoring electrodes to the ECG cable and into the ECG input connection on the front of the pacing generator. Set the selector switch to the 'Monitor on' position.	These actions ensure that the equipment is functioning properly.
10. Note the ECG waveform on the monitor. Adjust the R-wave beeper volume to a suitable level and activate the alarm by pressing the 'Alarm on' button. Set the alarm for 10 to 20 beats lower and 20 to 30 beats higher than the intrinsic rate.	These actions ensure that the equipment is functioning properly.
11. Press the 'Start/Stop' button for a printout of the waveform.	A printout provides objective data.
12. Apply the two pacing electrodes. Make sure the patient's skin is clean and dry to ensure good skin contact. Pull the protective strip from the posterior electrode (marked 'Back') and apply the electrode on the left side of the thoracic spinal column, just below the scapula (Figure 1).	This placement ensures that the electrical stimulus will travel only a short distance to the heart.

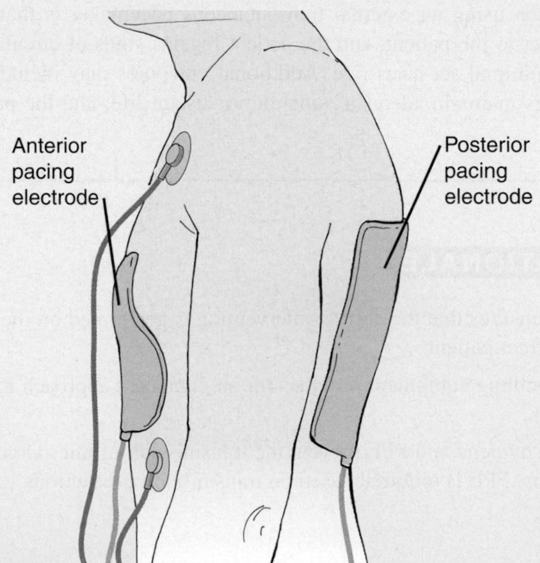

FIGURE 1 Transcutaneous pacemaker pads in place.

ACTION	RATIONALE
13. Apply the anterior pacing electrode (marked 'Front'), which has two protective strips—one covering the gelled area and one covering the outer rim. Expose the gelled area and apply it to the skin in the anterior position, to the left of the precordium in the V_2 to the V_5 position (see Figure 1). Move this electrode around to get the best waveform. Then expose the electrode's outer rim and firmly press it to the skin.	This placement ensures that the electrical stimulus will travel only a short distance to the heart.
14. Prepare to pace the heart. After making sure the energy output in milliamperes (mA) is on 0, connect the electrode cable to the monitor output cable.	This sets the pacing threshold.
15. Check the waveform, looking for a tall QRS complex in lead II.	
16. Check the selector switch to "Pacer on." Select synchronous (demand) or asynchronous (fixed-rate or nondemand) mode, per medical orders. **Tell the patient he or she may feel a thumping or twitching sensation. Reassure the patient you will provide medication if the discomfort is intolerable.**	Asynchronous pacing delivers a stimulus at a set (fixed) rate regardless of the occurrence of spontaneous myocardial depolarizations. Synchronous pacing delivers a stimulus only when the heart's intrinsic pacemaker fails to function at a predetermined rate. Analgesia and/or sedation may be administered, as ordered, for discomfort associated with pacing.
17. Set the pacing rate dial to 60 to 70 beats per minute. Look for pacer artifact or spikes, which will appear as you increase the rate.	Setting the pacing rate dial higher than the intrinsic rhythm ensures adequate cardiac output.
18. Set the pacing current output (in milliamperes [mA]), if not automatically done by the pacemaker. For patients with bradycardia, start with the minimal setting and **slowly increase the amount of energy delivered to the heart by adjusting the 'Output' mA dial. Do this until electrical capture is achieved: you will see a pacer spike followed by a widened QRS complex and a tall broad T wave that resembles a premature ventricular contraction.**	Setting the pacing current output ensures adequate cardiac output.
19. Increase output by 2 mA or 10%. **Do not go higher because of the increased risk of discomfort to the patient.**	Increasing the output ensures consistent capture. With full capture, the patient's heart rate should be approximately the same as the pacemaker rate set on the machine. The usual pacing threshold is 40 to 80 mA. Thresholds may vary due to recent cardiothoracic surgery, pericardial effusions, cardiac tamponade, acidosis, and hypoxia. These conditions may require higher thresholds.
20. Assess for effectiveness of pacing and mechanical capture: observe for pacemaker spike with subsequent capture; assess heart rate and rhythm (using right carotid, brachial or femoral artery); assess blood pressure (using right arm); assess for signs of improved cardiac output (increased blood pressure, improved level of consciousness, improved body temperature).	Both electrical and mechanical capture must occur to benefit the patient (Del Monte, 2009). Use of patient's right side for pulse assessment avoids inaccuracy related to strong contractions from the pacemaker. Use of right arm for blood pressure measurement avoids interference from the pacemaker (Morton & Fontaine, 2013).
21. For patients with asystole, in certain circumstances in hospitalized patients, start with the full output. If capture occurs, slowly decrease the output until capture is lost, then add 2 mA or 10% more.	Although transcutaneous pacing is not recommended for all patients in asystole, there are circumstances when it should be used in hospitalized patients with sudden asystole (Link et al., 2010). Increasing the output ensures consistent capture. With full capture, the patient's heart rate should be approximately the same as the pacemaker rate set on the machine. The usual pacing threshold is 40 to 80 mA.

(continued)

SKILL 16-6 USING AN EXTERNAL (TRANSCUTANEOUS) PACEMAKER continued

ACTION	RATIONALE
22. Secure the pacing leads and cable to the patient's body.	This prevents accidental displacement of the electrode, resulting in failure to pace or sense.
23. Monitor the patient's heart rate and rhythm to assess ventricular response to pacing. Assess the patient's vital signs, skin color, level of consciousness, and peripheral pulses. Take blood pressure in both arms.	Assessment helps determine the effectiveness of the paced rhythm. If the blood pressure reading is significantly higher in one arm, use that arm for measurements.
24. Assess the patient's pain and administer analgesia/sedation, as ordered, to ease the discomfort of chest wall muscle contractions (Craig, 2005).	Analgesia and sedation promote patient comfort.
25. Perform a 12-lead ECG and additional ECG daily or with clinical changes.	ECG monitoring provides a baseline for further evaluation.
26. Continually monitor the ECG readings, noting capture, sensing, rate, intrinsic beats, and competition of paced and intrinsic rhythms. If the pacemaker is sensing correctly, the sense indicator on the pulse generator should flash with each beat.	Continuous monitoring helps evaluate the patient's condition and determine the effectiveness of therapy.
27. Remove PPE, if used. Perform hand hygiene. 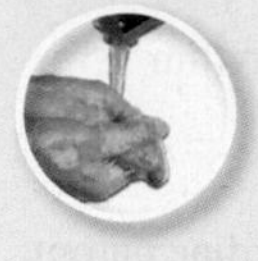	Removing PPE properly reduces the risk for infection transmission and contamination of other items. Hand hygiene and proper disposal of equipment reduce the transmission of microorganisms.

EVALUATION

The expected outcome is achieved when using an external transcutaneous pacemaker when it is applied correctly without adverse effect to the patient; the patient regains signs of circulation, including the capture of at least the minimal set heart rate; the patient's heart and lungs maintain adequate function to sustain life; and the patient does not experience injury.

DOCUMENTATION

Guidelines

Document the reason for pacemaker use, time that pacing began, electrode locations, pacemaker settings, patient's response to the procedure and to temporary pacing, complications, and nursing actions taken. Document the patient's pain-intensity rating, analgesia or sedation administered, and the patient's response. If possible, obtain a rhythm strip before, during, and after pacemaker placement; anytime that pacemaker settings are changed; and whenever the patient receives treatment because of a complication due to the pacemaker.

Sample Documentation

1/2/15 1218 Baseline rhythm strip obtained, sinus bradycardia at 43 bpm; see flow sheet. External temporary pacemaker placed by Dr. Goodman. Cardiac monitoring electrodes placed in the lead I, II, and III positions. Pacer set in synchronous mode at rate of 80 bpm; pacing current output 72 mA. Patient with strong femoral pulses; see flow sheet for vital signs. Patient reports chest discomfort of 4/10. Medicated with morphine 2 mg IV, per order. Pacer alarms set at 50 and 90 bpm, per order.

—*R. Robinson, RN*

1/2/15 1250 Patient reports decreased pain, 1/10.

—*R. Robinson, RN*

UNEXPECTED SITUATIONS AND ASSOCIATED INTERVENTIONS

- *Failure to pace:* This happens when the pacemaker either does not fire or fires too often. The pulse generator may not be working properly, or it may not be conducting the impulse to the patient. If the pacing or sensing indicator flashes, check the connections to the cable and the position/contact of the pacing electrodes on the patient. The cable may have come loose, or the electrode may not be making contact. If the pulse generator is turned on but the indicators still are not flashing, change the battery. If that does not help, use a different pulse generator. Check the settings if the pacemaker is firing too rapidly. If they are correct, or if altering them (according to your facility's policy or the medical order) does not help, change the pulse generator.

- *Failure to capture:* Here, pacemaker spikes are seen but the heart is not responding. The most common reason is failure to increase the current sufficiently. It may also be caused by changes in the pacing threshold from ischemia, an electrolyte imbalance (high or low potassium or magnesium levels), acidosis, an adverse reaction to a medication, or fibrosis. If the patient's condition has changed, notify the primary care provider and ask for new settings. Carefully check all connections, making sure they are placed properly and securely. Increase the milliamperes slowly (according to your facility's policy or the medical order).
- *Failure to sense intrinsic beats:* This could cause ventricular tachycardia or ventricular fibrillation if the pacemaker fires on the vulnerable T wave. This could be caused by the pacemaker sensing an external stimulus as a QRS complex, which could lead to asystole, or by the pacemaker not being sufficiently sensitive, which means it could fire anywhere within the cardiac cycle. If the pacing is undersensing, turn the sensitivity control completely to the right. If it is oversensing, turn it slightly to the left. If the pacemaker is not functioning correctly, change the battery or the pulse generator. Remove items in the room causing electromechanical interference (e.g., razors, radios, cautery devices). Check the ground wires on the bed and other equipment for obvious damage. Unplug each piece and see if the interference stops. When you locate the cause, notify the staff engineer and ask him or her to check it. If the pacemaker is still firing on the T wave and all else has failed, turn off the pacemaker and notify the primary care provider. Make sure atropine is available in case the patient's heart rate drops. Be prepared to call a code and institute cardiopulmonary resuscitation, if necessary.

SPECIAL CONSIDERATIONS

- If possible, avoid placement of anterior electrode over the patient's nipple, diaphragm, or sternum. Avoid placement of the posterior electrode over bony prominences of the spine or scapula (Del Monte, 2009).
- Do not use antiperspirant to prepare the skin for electrode placement; this could hinder conduction of electrical impulses and interfere with therapy, as well as cause skin burns (Del Monte, 2009).
- Do not leave patients unattended during noninvasive pacing. It is safe to touch the patient and perform procedures during pacing (e.g., CPR). Gloves should be worn. Do not touch the conductive surface of the electrodes.
- Monitor for changes in the patient's underlying rhythm. Ventricular fibrillation requires immediate defibrillation. Do not place defibrillation electrodes on the pacing electrodes. Most modern pacemakers are integrated devices with a monitor, defibrillator, and pacemaker in one unit (Del Monte, 2009, p. 22).
- Check the skin where the electrodes are placed for skin burns or tissue damage. Reposition, as needed.
- If the patient needs emergency defibrillation, make sure the pacemaker can withstand the procedure. If you are unsure, disconnect the pulse generator to avoid damage.
- With a female patient, place the anterior electrodes under the patient's breast, but not over her diaphragm.
- Do not use electrical equipment that is not grounded (e.g., telephones, electric shaver, television, or lamps); otherwise, the patient may experience microshock.

SKILL 16-7 OBTAINING AN ARTERIAL BLOOD SAMPLE FROM AN ARTERIAL CATHETER

Obtaining an arterial blood sample requires percutaneous puncture of the brachial, radial, or femoral artery (see Chapter 18: Laboratory Specimen Collection). However, an arterial blood sample can also be obtained from an arterial catheter. Arterial catheters are used for hemodynamic monitoring, blood gas analysis, and obtaining blood samples. A pressure monitoring system (Figure 1) transmits pressures from the intravascular space or cardiac chambers through a catheter and fluid-filled tubing to a pressure transducer, which converts the physiologic signal from the patient to a pressure tracing and digital value. Patency of the system and prevention of backflow of blood through the catheter and tubing is maintained by using a continuous flush solution under pressure (Morton & Fontaine, 2013). ***The procedure below describes obtaining a sample from an open, stopcock system. For information on obtaining an arterial blood sample from a closed reservoir system, please see the Skill Variation at the end of this skill.***

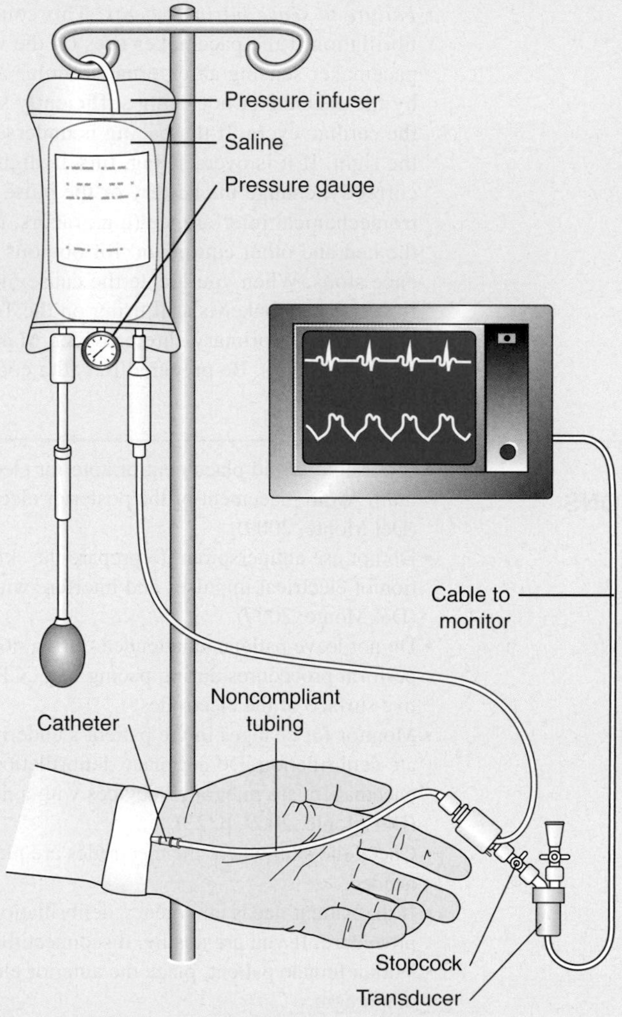

FIGURE 1 Pressure monitoring system. (From Morton, P.G., & Fontaine, D.K. (2013). *Essentials of critical care nursing. A holistic approach.* Philadelphia: Wolters Kluwer Health/Lippincott Williams & Wilkins.)

DELEGATION CONSIDERATIONS

Obtaining an arterial blood sample from an arterial catheter is not delegated to nursing assistive personnel (NAP), unlicensed assistive personnel (UAP), or licensed practical/vocational nurses (LPN/LVNs).

EQUIPMENT

- Arterial blood gas (ABG) syringe with needleless cannula, rubber cap for ABG syringe hub, and ice-filled plastic bag or cup, if ABG is ordered
- Gloves
- Goggles
- Additional PPE, as indicated
- Vacutainer with needleless luer adapter and appropriate blood collection tubes for ordered tests
- Two additional blood collection tubes, for discard blood volume
- Alcohol swabs or chlorhexidine, per facility policy
- Waterproof protective pad
- Sterile cap for arterial catheter stopcock
- Label with patient identification information
- Blank labels (2)
- Biohazard bag
- Bath blanket

ASSESSMENT

Review the patient's medical record and plan of care for information about the patient's need for an arterial blood sample. Assess the patient's cardiac status, including heart rate, blood pressure, and auscultation of heart sounds. Also assess the patient's respiratory status, including respiratory rate, excursion, lung sounds, and use of oxygen, if ordered. Check the patency and functioning of the arterial catheter. Assess the patient's understanding about the need for specimen collection.

NURSING DIAGNOSIS

Determine the related factors for the nursing diagnoses based on the patient's current status. Appropriate nursing diagnoses may include:

- Impaired Gas Exchange
- Decreased Cardiac Output
- Excess Fluid Volume

OUTCOME IDENTIFICATION AND PLANNING

The expected outcome to achieve when obtaining an arterial blood sample is that a specimen is obtained without compromise to the patency of the arterial catheter. In addition, the patient experiences minimal discomfort and anxiety, remains free from infection, and demonstrates an understanding about the need for the specimen collection.

IMPLEMENTATION

ACTION	RATIONALE
1. Verify the order for laboratory testing in the patient's medical record.	This ensures that the correct intervention is performed on the correct patient.
2. Gather all equipment.	Assembling equipment provides for an organized approach to the task.
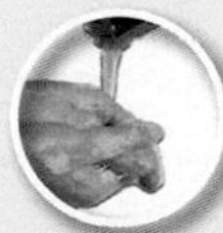 3. Perform hand hygiene and put on PPE, if indicated.	Hand hygiene and PPE prevent the spread of microorganisms. PPE is required based on transmission precautions.
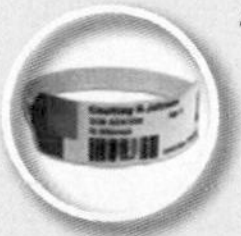 4. Identify the patient.	Identifying the patient ensures the right patient receives the intervention and helps prevent errors.
5. Close curtains around the bed and close the door to the room, if possible. Explain the procedure to the patient.	This ensures the patient's privacy. Explanation relieves anxiety and facilitates cooperation.
6. Assemble equipment on overbed table within reach.	Arranging items nearby is convenient, saves time, and avoids unnecessary stretching and twisting of muscles on the part of the nurse.
7. Compare specimen label with patient identification bracelet. Label should include patient's name and identification number, time specimen was collected, route of collection, identification of the person obtaining the sample, and any other information required by facility policy.	Verifying the patient's identity validates that the correct procedure is being done on the correct patient, and the specimen is accurately labeled.

(continued)

SKILL 16-7 OBTAINING AN ARTERIAL BLOOD SAMPLE FROM AN ARTERIAL CATHETER continued

ACTION	RATIONALE
8. Use blank labels to label the two blood sample collection tubes to be used for discard blood sample and discard flush.	Labeling of discard tubes prevents accidental confusion with blood specimen tubes.
9. Assist the patient to a comfortable position that provides easy access to the sampling site. Use the bath blanket to cover any exposed area other than the sampling site. Place a waterproof pad under the site.	Patient positioning and use of a bath blanket provide for comfort and warmth. Waterproof pad protects underlying surfaces.
10. Put on gloves and goggles or face shield.	Gloves and goggles (or face shield) prevent contact with blood and body fluids.
11. Temporarily silence the arterial pressure monitor alarms.	The integrity of the system is being altered, which will cause the system to sound an alarm. Facility policy may require the alarm be left on.
12. Locate the stopcock nearest the arterial line insertion site (see Figure 1). Remove the nonvented cap from the stopcock. Use the alcohol swab or chlorhexidine to scrub the sampling port on the stopcock. Allow to air dry.	Removal of stopcock cap allows access for blood sampling. Cleansing sampling port reduces the risk of contamination.
13. Attach the needleless luer adapter to the Vacutainer (Figure 2). Connect the needleless adapter of the Vacutainer to the sampling port of the stopcock. Turn off the stopcock to the flush solution. Insert the labeled blood sample tube for the discard sample into the Vacutainer (Figure 3). Follow facility policy for the volume of discard blood to collect (usually 5 to 10 mL).	A sufficient amount of discard volume needs to be withdrawn before obtaining the blood sample to be tested in the laboratory. This sample is discarded because it is diluted with flush solution, possibly leading to inaccurate test results. If an insufficient amount of discard volume is withdrawn, the specimen may be diluted and contaminated with flush solution. If an excessive amount of discard volume is withdrawn, the patient may experience an iatrogenic (treatment-induced) blood loss.
14. Remove the discard syringe and dispose of appropriately, according to facility policy.	Proper disposal reduces the risk of accidental blood exposure and transmission of microorganisms.

FIGURE 2 Blood sample tube holder with Monoject™ needleless luer lock adapter. (Monoject is a trademark of a Covidien company. Copyright © Covidien. Used with permission.)

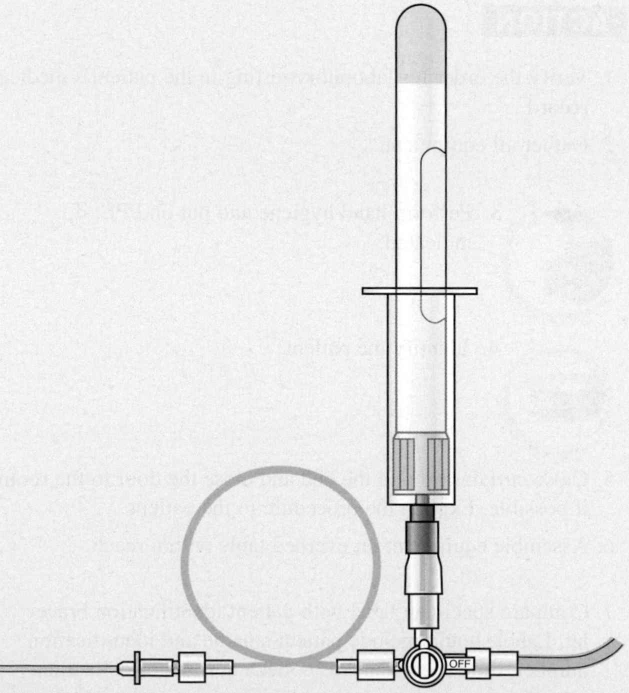

FIGURE 3 Blood sample tube inserted in tube holder connected to the sampling port of stopcock.

ACTION	RATIONALE
15. Insert each blood sample collection tube into the Vacutainer, keeping the stopcock turned off to the flush solution. For each additional sample required, repeat this procedure. If coagulation tests are included in the required tests, obtain blood for this from the final sample. Apply the rubber cap to the ABG syringe hub, if necessary.	Turning the stopcock off to the flush solution allows for sampling and prevents dilution from the flush device. The Vacutainer is a nonvented system, preventing backflow of blood from the patient. Obtaining coagulation samples last prevents dilution from the flush device. The rubber cap on the ABG syringe hub prevents entry of air into the blood sample.
16. After obtaining the final blood sample, turn off the stopcock to the Vacutainer. Activate the in-line flushing device.	Turning the stopcock off and in-line flushing clears the tubing to maintain the integrity of the system and prevent clotting and infection.
17. Turn off the stopcock to the patient. Attach a labeled discard blood sample tube to the Vacutainer. Activate the in-line flushing device.	Turning the stopcock off and in-line flushing clears the stopcock sampling port to maintain the integrity of the system and prevent clotting and infection.
18. Turn off the stopcock to the sampling port. Remove the Vacutainer. Place a new sterile nonvented cap on the blood sampling port of the stopcock.	Capping the port maintains system integrity and reduces the risk for contamination and infection.
19. Remove gloves. Reactivate the monitor alarms. Record date and time the samples were obtained on the labels, as well as the required information to identify the person obtaining the samples. If ABG was collected, record oxygen flow rate (or room air) on label. Apply labels to the specimens, according to facility policy. Place in biohazard bags, place ABG sample in bag with ice.	Removing gloves properly reduces the risk for infection transmission and contamination of other items. Reactivating the system ensures proper functioning. Proper labeling prevents error. Recording oxygen flow rate ensures accurate interpretation of results of ABG. Use of a biohazard bag prevents contact with blood and body fluids. Ice maintains integrity of the sample.
20. Check the monitor for return of the arterial waveform and pressure reading.	This ensures proper functioning and integrity of the system.
21. Return the patient to a comfortable position. Lower bed height, if necessary, and adjust head of bed to a comfortable position.	Repositioning promotes patient comfort. Lowering the bed promotes patient safety.
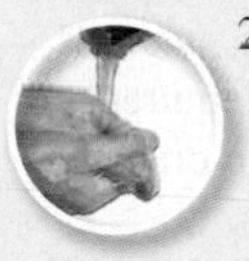 22. Remove goggles and additional PPE, if used. Perform hand hygiene. Send specimens to the laboratory immediately.	Removing PPE properly reduces the risk for infection transmission and contamination of other items. Hand hygiene prevents transmission of microorganisms. Specimens must be processed in a timely manner to ensure accuracy.

EVALUATION

The expected outcome to achieve when obtaining an arterial blood sample is that a specimen is obtained without compromise to the patency of the arterial catheter. In addition, the patient experiences minimal discomfort and anxiety, remains free from infection, and demonstrates an understanding about the need for the specimen collection.

DOCUMENTATION

Guidelines

Document any pertinent assessments, the laboratory specimens obtained, date and time specimens were obtained, and disposition of specimens.

Sample Documentation

10/20/15 0230 Continuous heparin IV infusion at 900 U via left subclavian central catheter. Blood specimens for repeat PT/PTT, CBC, and BMP obtained via right radial arterial catheter, per order. Catheter flushed, per policy; specimens sent to the laboratory.

—R. Chin, RN

UNEXPECTED SITUATIONS AND ASSOCIATED INTERVENTIONS

- *The specimen obtained is dark:* Dark blood means a vein may have been accessed, or the blood may be poorly oxygenated. Ensure that the line from which you are obtaining the specimen is indeed an arterial catheter. Also, check the patient's oxygen saturation level to evaluate for possible hypoxemia.

(continued)

SKILL 16-7 OBTAINING AN ARTERIAL BLOOD SAMPLE FROM AN ARTERIAL CATHETER continued

- *When retracting the syringe for the discarded sample, you feel resistance:* Reposition the affected extremity and check the insertion site for obvious problems (e.g., catheter kinking). Then attempt to obtain the sample to be discarded. If resistance is still felt, notify the primary care provider.
- *After obtaining the specimen and reactivating the arterial pressure monitoring system, no waveform is noted:* Check the stopcock to make sure that it is open to the patient and recheck all connections and components of the system to ensure proper setup. If necessary, rebalance the transducer or replace the system, as necessary. If problem persists, suspect a clotted catheter tip. Follow facility policy to troubleshoot a potentially clotted arterial catheter and notify the primary care provider.

SPECIAL CONSIDERATIONS

- If the patient is receiving oxygen, make sure that this therapy has been underway for at least 15 minutes before collecting an arterial blood sample for ABG analysis. Indicate on the laboratory request slip the amount and type of oxygen therapy the patient is receiving. Also note the patient's current temperature, most recent hemoglobin level, and current respiratory rate. If the patient is receiving mechanical ventilation, note the fraction of inspired oxygen and tidal volume.
- If the patient is not receiving oxygen, indicate that he or she is breathing room air.
- If the patient has just received a nebulizer treatment, wait about 20 minutes before collecting the sample for ABG analysis.

SKILL VARIATION Obtaining an Arterial Blood Sample From a Closed Reservoir System

1. Verify the order for laboratory testing in the patient's medical record. Gather all equipment (including additional syringes to collect blood samples, based on samples ordered).

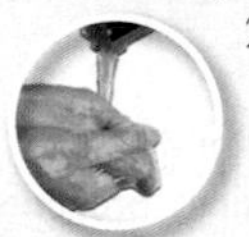

2. Perform hand hygiene. Put on PPE, as indicated.

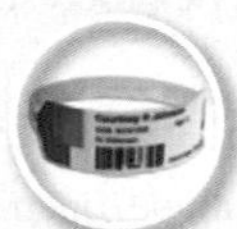

3. Check the patient's identification. Assemble equipment on overbed table within reach. Compare the specimen label with the patient's identification.
4. Explain the procedure to the patient. Close curtains around the bed and close the door to the room, if possible.
5. If the bed is adjustable, raise it to a comfortable working height.
6. Assist the patient to a comfortable position that provides easy access to the sampling site. Use the bath blanket to cover any exposed area other than the sampling site. Place a waterproof pad under the site.
7. Put on gloves and goggles or face shield.
8. Locate the closed-system reservoir and blood-sampling site. Temporarily silence monitor alarms.
9. Clean the sampling site with an alcohol swab or chlorhexidine.
10. Holding the reservoir upright, grasp the flexures, and slowly fill the reservoir with blood over a 3- to 5-second period. If you feel resistance, reposition the extremity and check the catheter site for obvious problems (e.g., kinking of the tubing). Then continue with blood withdrawal.
11. Turn off the one-way valve to the reservoir by turning the handle perpendicular to the tubing. Using a syringe with attached cannula, insert the cannula into the sampling site. Slowly fill the syringe. Then grasp the cannula near the sampling site and remove the syringe and cannula as one unit. Repeat the procedure, as needed, to fill the required number of syringes. If coagulation tests have been ordered, obtain blood for those tests from the final syringe.
12. After filling the syringes, turn the one-way valve to its original position, parallel to the tubing. Push down evenly on the plunger until the flexures lock in place in the fully closed position and all fluid has been re-infused. The fluid should be re-infused over a 3- to 5-second period. Activate the fast-flush release.
13. Clean the sampling site with an alcohol swab or chlorhexidine. Reactivate the monitor alarms. Transfer blood samples to the appropriate specimen tubes, if necessary. Record on the labels the date and time the samples were obtained, as well as the required information to identify the person obtaining the samples. Apply labels to the specimens according to facility policy. Place in biohazard bags; place ABG sample in bag with ice. Remove gloves.
14. Check the monitor for return of the arterial waveform and pressure reading.

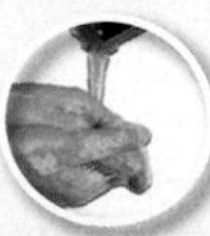

15. Remove any remaining equipment. Remove goggles and additional PPE, if used. Perform hand hygiene. Send specimens to the laboratory immediately.

SKILL 16-8 REMOVING PERIPHERAL ARTERIAL CATHETERS

Arterial catheters, which are used for intensive and continuous cardiac monitoring and intra-arterial access, are ideally placed in the radial, brachial or dorsalis pedis sites in adults to reduce the risk of infection (O'Grady et al., 2011), although the femoral site can be used as well. As soon as the arterial catheter is no longer needed or has become ineffective, it should be removed (O'Grady et al.). Consult facility policy to determine whether nurses are permitted to perform this procedure. Two nurses should be at the bedside until bleeding is controlled, and are available to give emergency medications, if necessary. The patient should be kept NPO until the catheter is removed in case of nausea with a vasovagal response.

DELEGATION CONSIDERATIONS

Removal of an arterial catheter is not delegated to nursing assistive personnel (NAP), unlicensed assistive personnel (UAP), or licensed practical/vocational nurses (LPN/LVNs).

EQUIPMENT

- Sterile gloves
- Clean gloves
- Goggles or face shield
- Sterile gauze pads
- Waterproof protective pad
- Sterile suture removal set
- Transparent dressing
- Hypoallergenic tape
- For femoral catheter: small sandbag (5 to 10 pounds), wrapped in a towel or pillowcase, based on facility policy
- Emergency medications (e.g., atropine, for a vasovagal response with femoral catheter removal) for emergency response, per facility policy and guidelines
- Indelible pen

ASSESSMENT

Review the patient's medical record and plan of care for information about discontinuation of the arterial catheter. Assess the patient's coagulation status, including laboratory studies, to reduce the risk of complications secondary to impaired clotting ability. Assess the patient's understanding of the procedure. Inspect the site for leakage, bleeding, or hematoma. Assess skin color and temperature and assess distal pulses for strength and quality. Mark distal pulses with an 'X' for easy identification after the procedure. Assess the patient's blood pressure; systolic blood pressure should be less than 180 mm Hg before the catheter is removed.

NURSING DIAGNOSIS

Determine the related factors for the nursing diagnoses based on the patient's current status. Appropriate nursing diagnoses may include:

- Risk for Injury
- Impaired Skin Integrity
- Risk for Infection
- Anxiety

OUTCOME IDENTIFICATION AND PLANNING

The expected outcome to achieve when removing an arterial catheter is that the catheter is removed intact and without injury to the patient. In addition, the site remains clean and dry, without evidence of infection, bleeding, or hematoma.

IMPLEMENTATION

ACTION	RATIONALE
1. Verify the order for removal of the arterial catheter in the patient's medical record.	This ensures that the correct intervention is performed on the correct patient.
2. Gather all equipment.	Assembling equipment provides for an organized approach to the task.
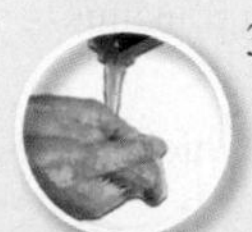 3. Perform hand hygiene and put on PPE, if indicated.	Hand hygiene and PPE prevent the spread of microorganisms. PPE is required based on transmission precautions.

(continued)

SKILL 16-8 REMOVING PERIPHERAL ARTERIAL CATHETERS continued

ACTION	RATIONALE
4. Identify the patient. 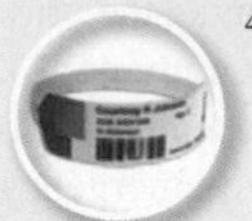	Identifying the patient ensures the right patient receives the intervention and helps prevent errors.
5. Close curtains around the bed and close the door to the room, if possible. Explain the procedure to the patient.	This ensures the patient's privacy. Explanation relieves anxiety and facilitates cooperation.
6. Maintain an IV infusion of normal saline via another venous access during the procedure, as per medical orders or facility guidelines.	IV access may be needed in case of hypotension or bradycardia.
7. If the bed is adjustable, raise it to a comfortable working height, usually elbow height of the caregiver (VISN 8 Patient Safety Center, 2009).	Having the bed at the proper height prevents back and muscle strain.
8. Put on clean gloves, goggles, and gown.	These prevent contact with blood and body fluids.
9. If the catheter being removed is in a femoral site, use Doppler ultrasound to locate the femoral artery 1 to 2 inches above the entrance site of the femoral catheter. Mark with 'X' using an indelible pen.	This ensures accurate location of the femoral artery.
10. Turn off the monitor alarms and then turn off the flow clamp to the flush solution. Carefully remove the dressing over the insertion site. Remove any sutures using the suture removal kit; make sure all sutures have been removed.	These measures help prepare for withdrawal of the catheter.
11. **Withdraw the catheter using a gentle, steady motion. Keep the catheter parallel to the blood vessel during withdrawal. Watch for hematoma formation during catheter removal by gently palpating surrounding tissue. If hematoma starts to form, reposition your hands until optimal pressure is obtained to prevent further leakage of blood.**	Using a gentle, steady motion parallel to the blood vessel reduces the risk for traumatic injury.
12. **Immediately after withdrawing the catheter, apply pressure 1 or 2 inches above the site at the previously marked spot with a sterile 4 × 4 gauze pad. Maintain pressure for at least 10 minutes, or per facility policy (longer if bleeding or oozing persists).** Apply additional pressure to a femoral site or if the patient has a coagulation abnormality or is receiving anticoagulants (INS, 2011).	If sufficient pressure is not applied, a large, painful hematoma may form.
13. **Assess distal pulses every 3 to 5 minutes while pressure is being applied.** Note: Dorsalis pedis and posterior tibial pulses should be markedly weaker from baseline if sufficient pressure is applied to the femoral artery.	Assessment of distal pulses determines blood flow to the extremity. Pulses should return to baseline after pressure is released.
14. Cover the site with an appropriate dressing and secure the dressing with tape. If stipulated by facility policy, make a pressure dressing for a femoral site by folding four sterile 4 × 4 gauze pads in half, and then applying the dressing.	Sufficient pressure is needed to prevent continued bleeding and hematoma formation.
15. Cover the dressing with a tight adhesive bandage, per facility policy. Remove goggles and gloves. If the catheter was in a femoral site, use these additional interventions: Cover the bandage with a sandbag, depending on facility policy. Maintain the patient on bed rest, with the head of the bed elevated less than 30 degrees, for 6 hours with the sandbag in place. Instruct the patient not to lift his or her head while on bed rest. Use logrolling to assist the patient in using the bedpan, if needed.	Sufficient pressure is needed to prevent continued bleeding and hematoma formation. Removing PPE properly reduces the risk for infection transmission and contamination of other items. Raising the head increases intra-abdominal pressure, which could lead to bleeding from the site.

ACTION	RATIONALE
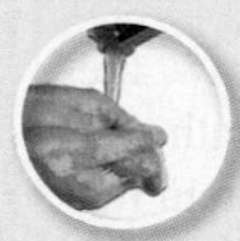 16. Lower the bed height. Remove additional PPE. Perform hand hygiene. Send specimens to the laboratory immediately.	Lowering the bed promotes patient safety. Removing PPE properly reduces the risk for infection transmission and contamination of other items. Hand hygiene prevents transmission of microorganisms. Specimens must be processed in a timely manner to ensure accuracy.
17. Observe the site for bleeding. Assess circulation in the extremity distal to the site by evaluating color, pulses, and sensation. Repeat this assessment every 15 minutes for the first 1 hour, every 30 minutes for the next 2 hours, hourly for the next 2 hours, then every 4 hours, or according to facility policy.	Continued assessment allows for early detection and prompt intervention should problems arise.

EVALUATION

The expected outcome is met when the patient exhibits an arterial catheter site that is clean and dry without evidence of injury, infection, bleeding, or hematoma. In addition, the patient demonstrates intact peripheral circulation and verbalizes a reduction in anxiety.

DOCUMENTATION

Guidelines

Document the time the catheter was removed and how long pressure was applied. Document site assessment every 5 minutes while pressure is being applied (second nurse can do this). Document assessment of peripheral circulation, appearance of site, type of dressing applied, the timed assessments, patient's response, and any medications given.

Sample Documentation

12/20/15 1830 Right radial arterial catheter removed per order. Pressure applied to site for 10 minutes. Site intact without signs of hematoma; radial pulse present, +2 and regular. Hand warm and dry; hand skin tone consistent with left hand. Pressure dressing applied to site. Patient denies pain, nausea, shortness of breath. Vital signs stable before, during, and after procedure. See flow sheet.

—B. Clapp, RN

UNEXPECTED SITUATIONS AND ASSOCIATED INTERVENTIONS

- *Assessment reveals fresh blood on the site dressing:* Apply pressure. If bleeding continues, notify the primary care provider.
- *The patient has a history of peripheral vascular disease:* Assess the peripheral circulation for changes; if necessary, apply slightly decreased pressure at the insertion site.
- *Affected extremity is cold and/or pulseless:* Immediately notify primary care provider.
- *Patient complains of severe back pain or is noted to be hypotensive:* Symptoms may be due to retroperitoneal bleeding. Notify primary care provider immediately.

SPECIAL CONSIDERATIONS

- Sometimes, a culture of the catheter tip is ordered to aid in identifying the source of infection. If ordered, place the catheter tip on a 4 × 4 sterile gauze pad. After the bleeding is under control and the dressing is secure, hold the catheter over the sterile container. Cut the tip of the catheter with sterile scissors and allow it to fall into the sterile container. Label the specimen and send it to the laboratory.

ENHANCE YOUR UNDERSTANDING

FOCUSING ON PATIENT CARE: DEVELOPING CLINICAL REASONING

Consider the case scenarios at the beginning of the chapter as you answer the following questions to enhance your understanding and apply what you have learned.

QUESTIONS

1. Coby Pruder becomes visibly anxious when you bring in the ECG machine and begin to open the supplies. What could you do to help alleviate his anxiety?
2. You go in to assess Harry Stebbings and find him unresponsive. How should you respond?
3. You meet resistance while attempting to draw the discard sample from Ann Kribell's arterial catheter. Should you use excessive pressure to try to obtain the discard sample? Discuss the appropriate actions to problem solve this unexpected situation.

You can find suggested answers after the Bibliography at the end of this chapter.

INTEGRATED CASE STUDY CONNECTION

The case studies in the back of the book are designed to focus on integrating concepts. Refer to the following case studies to enhance your understanding of the concepts related to the skills in this chapter.

- Advanced Case Studies: Cole McKean, page 1093.

TAYLOR SUITE RESOURCES

Explore these additional resources to enhance your learning of this chapter:

- NCLEX-Style Questions and other resources on thePoint, http://thePoint.lww.com/Lynn4e
- *Skill Checklists for Taylor's Clinical Nursing Skills,* 4e

Bibliography

Ackley, B.J., & Ladwig, G.B. (2011). *Nursing diagnosis handbook* (9th ed.). St. Louis: Mosby/Elsevier.

ACLS review made incredibly easy (2nd ed.). (2012). Philadelphia: Wolters Kluwer Health/Lippincott Williams & Wilkins.

American Association of Critical Care Nurses (AACN). (2010). *Family presence during resuscitation and invasive procedures.* Available http://www.aacn.org/wd/practice/docs/practicealerts/family%20presence%2004-2010%20final.pdf.

American Heart Association (AHA). (2011). *BLS for healthcare providers. Student manual. Professional.* Author.

American Heart Association (AHA). (2012). *CPR & ECC. Two steps to staying alive with hands-only CPR.* Available http://www.heart.org/HEARTORG/CPRAndECC/HandsOnlyCPR/Hands-Only-CPR_UCM_440559_SubHomePage.jsp.

Berg, M.D., Schexnayder, S.M., Chameides, L., Terry, M., Donoghue, A., Hickey, R.W., et al. (2010). American Heart Association guidelines for cardiopulmonary resuscitation and emergency cardiovascular care. Part 13: Pediatric basic life support. *Circulation, 122*(18 Suppl. 3), S862–S875.

Bishop, J.P., Brothers, K.B., Perry, J.E., & Ahmad, A. (2010). Reviving the conversation around CPR/DNR. *The American Journal of Bioethics, 10*(1), 61–67.

Bucher, L., Buruschkink, R., Kenyon, D.M., Stenton, K., & Treseder, S. (2012). Improving outcomes with therapeutic hypothermia. *Nursing2012CriticalCare, 7*(5), 22–27.

Buck, H.G. (2012). CPR in older adults: What's the evidence? *Nursing, 42*(5), 14–15.

Bulechek, G.M, Butcher, H.K., Dochterman, J.M., & Wagner, C.M. (Eds.). (2013). *Nursing interventions classification (NIC)* (6th ed.). St. Louis: Mosby Elsevier.

Cadogan, M.P. (2010). CPR decision making and older adults. Clinical implications. *Journal of Gerontological Nursing, 36*(12), 10–15.

Cardiovascular care made incredibly visual (2nd ed.). (2010). Philadelphia: Wolters Kluwer Health/Lippincott Williams & Wilkins.

Castle, N. (2007). Resuscitation of patients during pregnancy. *Emergency Nurse, 15*(2), 20–22.

Centers for Disease Control and Prevention (CDC). (2011). *Guidelines for the prevention of intravascular catheter-related infections.* Available www.cdc.gov/hicpac/pdf/guidelines/bsi-guidelines-2011.pdf.

Cleveland Clinic. (2013). *Biventricular pacemaker.* Available http://my.clevelandclinic.org/heart/services/tests/procedures/biventricular_pm.aspx.

Cottle, E., & James, J. (2008). Role of the family support person during resuscitation. *Nursing Standard, 23*(9), 43–47.

Craig, K.J., & Day, M.P. (2011). Update your knowledge of the latest PALS. *Nursing, 41*(6), 44–47.

Craig, K. (2005). How to provide transcutaneous pacing. *Nursing, 35*(10), 52–53.

Crawford, J., & Doherty, L. (2010). Ten steps to recording a standard 12-lead ECG. *Practice Nurse, 21*(12), 622–630.

Cvach, M.M., Biggs, M., Rothwell, K.J., & Charles-Hudson, C. (2013). Daily electrode change and effect on cardiac monitor alarms. An evidence-based practice approach. *Journal of Nursing Care Quality, 28*(3), 265–271.

Delac, K., Blazier, D., Daniel, L., & N-Wilfong, D. (2013). Five alive. Using mock code simulation to improve responder performance during the first 5 minutes of a code. *Critical Care Nursing Quarterly, 36*(2), 244–250.

Del Monte, L. (2009). *Noninvasive pacing: What you should know.* Educational Series. Redmond, WA: Physio-Control, Inc.

Diaz, M.C.G. (2013). Early use of AEDs can save kids' lives. *Contemporary Pediatrics, 30*(3), 12–20.

Drager, K.K. (2012). Improving patient outcomes with compression-only CPR: Will bystander CPR rates improve? *Journal of Emergency Nursing, 38*(3), 234–238.

Emergency Nurses Association (ENA). Agency for Healthcare Research and Quality. National Guideline Clearinghouse (2009). *Family presence during invasive procedures and resuscitation in the emergency department.* Available http://www.guideline.gov/content.aspx?id = 32594.

Field, J.M., Hazinski, M.F., Sayre, M.R., Chameides, L., Schexnayder, S.M., Hemphill, R., et al. (2010). 2010 American Heart Association guidelines for cardiopulmonary resuscitation and emergency cardiovascular care. Part 1: Executive summary. *Circulation, 122* (18 Suppl. 3), S640–S656.

Goulette, C. (2008). Follow your heart. Wireless telemetry.

Grossman, S., & Porth, C.M. (2014). Porth's pathophysiology: concepts of altered health states. (9th ed.). Philadelphia: Wolters Kluwer Health/Lippincott Williams & Wilkins.

Hazinski, M.F., Nolan, J.P., Billi, J.E., Böttiger, B.W., Bossaert, L., de Caen, A.R., et al. (2010). 2010 International consensus on cardiopulmonary resuscitation and emergency cardiovascular care science with treatment recommendations. Part 1: Executive summary. *Circulation, 122*(16 Suppl. 2), S250–S275.

Hinkle, J.L., & Cheever, K.H. (2014). *Brunner & Suddarth's textbook of medical-surgical nursing* (13th ed.). Philadelphia: Wolters Kluwer Health/Lippincott Williams & Wilkins.

Hogan-Quigley, B., Palm, M.L., & Bickley, L. (2012). *Bates' nursing guide to physical examination and history taking.* Philadelphia: Wolters Kluwer Health/Lippincott Williams & Wilkins.

Huether, S.E., & McCance, K.L. (2012). *Understanding pathophysiology* (5th ed.). St. Louis: Elsevier.

Huseman, K.F. (2012). Improving Code Blue response through the use of simulation. *Journal for Nurses in Staff Development, 28*(3), 120–124.

Infusion Nurses Society (INS). (2011). Infusion nursing standards of practice. *Journal of Infusion Nursing, 34*(Suppl. 1S).

Jarvis, C. (2012). *Physical examination & health assessment* (6th ed.). St. Louis: Saunders/Elsevier.

Jevon, P. (2010). Procedure for recording a standard 12-lead electrocardiogram. *British Journal of Nursing, 19*(10), 649–651.

The Joint Commission (TJC). (2014). *National patient safety goals.* Available http://www.jointcommission.org/standards_information/npsgs.aspx.

Kleinman, M.E., Chameides, L., Schexnayder, S.M., Samson, R.A., Hazinski, M.R., Atkins, D.L., et al. (2010). 2010 American Heart Association guidelines for cardiopulmonary resuscitation and emergency cardiovascular care. Part 14: Pediatric advanced life support. *Circulation, 122*(18 Suppl. 3), S876–S908.

Kligfield, P., Gettes, L.S., Bailey, J.J., Childers, R., Deal, B.J., Hancock, E.W., et al. (2007). Recommendations for the standardization and interpretation of the electrocardiogram. Part 1: The electrocardiogram and its technology. *Journal of the American College of Cardiology, 49*(10), 1109–1127.

Kyle, T., & Carman, S. (2013). *Essentials of pediatric nursing* (2nd ed.). Philadelphia: Wolters Kluwer Health/Lippincott Williams & Wilkins.

Larson, T., & Brady, W. (2008). Electrocardiographic monitoring in the hospitalized patient: A diagnostic intervention of uncertain clinical impact. *American Journal of Emergency Medicine, 26*(9), 1047–1055.

Link, M.S., Atkins, D.L., Passman, R.S., Halperin, H.R., Samson, R.A., White, R.D., et al. (2010). 2010 American Heart Association guidelines for cardiopulmonary resuscitation and emergency cardiovascular care. Part 6: Electrical therapies: Automated external defibrillators, defibrillation, cardioversion, and pacing. *Circulation, 122*(18 Suppl. 3), S706–S719.

Lippincott's nursing procedures (6th ed.). (2013). Philadelphia: Wolters Kluwer Health/Lippincott Williams & Wilkins.

Moorhead, S., Johnson, M., Maas, M.L., & Swanson, E. (Eds.). (2013). *Nursing outcomes classification (NOC)* (5th ed.). St. Louis: Mosby Elsevier.

Morrison, L.J., Kierzek, G., Diekema, D.S., Sayre, M.R., Silvers, S.M., Idris, A.H., & Mancini, M.E. (2010). 2010 American Heart Association guidelines for cardiopulmonary resuscitation and emergency cardiovascular care. Part 3: Ethics. *Circulation, 122*(18 Suppl. 3), S665–S675.

Morton, P.G., & Fontaine, D.K. (2013). *Essentials of critical care nursing. A holistic approach.* Philadelphia: Wolters Kluwer Health/Lippincott Williams & Wilkins.

NANDA-I International. (2012). *Nursing diagnoses: Definitions & classification 2012–2014.* West Sussex, UK: Wiley-Blackwell.

National Heart, Lung, and Blood Institute (NHLBI). (2012). *What is a pacemaker?* Available http://www.nhlbi.nih.gov/health/health-topics/topics/pace/.

Neumar, R.W., Otto, C.W., Link, M.S., Kronick, S.L., Shuster, M., Callaway, C.W., et al. (2010). 2010 American Heart Association guidelines for cardiopulmonary resuscitation and emergency cardiovascular care. Part 8: Adult advanced cardiovascular life support. *Circulation, 122*(18 Suppl. 3), S729–S767.

Oermann, M.H., Kardong-Edgren, S.E., & Odom-Maryon, T. (2012). Competence in CPR. *American Journal of Nursing, 112*(5), 43–46.

O'Grady, N.P., Alexander, M., Burns, L.A., Dellinger, E.P., Garland, J., Heard, S.O., et al., & the Healthcare Infection Control Practices Advisory Committee (HICPAC). (2011). Guidelines for the prevention of intravascular catheter-related infections. *American Journal of Infection Control, 39*(4 Suppl.), S1–S34.

O'Neil, B.J., Hoekstra, J., Pride, Y.B., Lefebvre, C., Diercks, D., Peacock, W.F., et al. (2010). Incremental benefit of 80-lead electrocardiogram body surface mapping over the 12-lead electrocardiogram in the detection of acute coronary syndromes in patients without ST-elevation myocardial infarction: Results from the optimal cardiovascular diagnostic evaluation enabling faster treatment of myocardial infarction (OCCULT MI) trial. *Academic Emergency Medicine, 17*(9), 932–939.

Pankop, R., Chang, K., Thorlton, J., & Spitzer, T. (2013). Implemented family presence protocols. An integrative review. *Journal of Nursing Care Quality, 28*(3), 281–288.

Perry, S.E., Hockenberry, M.J., Lowdermilk, D.L., & Wilson, D. (2010). *Maternal child nursing care* (4th ed.). Maryland Heights, MO: Mosby/Elsevier.

Puck, A.L., Oakeson, A.M., Morales-Clark, A., & Durzin, M. (2012). Obstetric life support. *Journal of Perinatal & Neonatal Nursing, 26*(2), 126–135.

Rijnders, B. (2005). Catheter-related infection can be prevented. .. If we take the arterial line seriously too! *Critical Care Medicine, 33*(6), 1437–1439.

Self, W., Mattu, A., Jartin, M., et al. (2006). Body surface mapping in the ED evaluation of the patient with chest pain: Use of the 80-lead electrocardiogram system. *American Journal of Emergency Medicine, 24*(1), 87–112.

The Society for Cardiological Science & Technology (SCST). (2010). *Clinical guidelines by consensus. Recording a standard 12-lead electrocardiogram.* Available http://www.scst.org.uk/pages/page_box_contents.asp?pageid = 808.

Taylor, C., Lillis, C., & Lynn P. (2015). *Fundamentals of nursing* (8th ed.). Philadelphia: Wolters Kluwer Health/Lippincott Williams & Wilkins.

Taylor, J.J., & Cohen, B.J. (2013). *Memmler's structure and function of the human body* (10th ed.). Philadelphia: Wolters Kluwer Health/Lippincott Williams & Wilkins.

Tough, J. (2008). Elective and emergency defibrillation. *Nursing Standard, 22*(38), 49–56.

Vanden Hoek, T.L., Morrison, L.J., Shuster, M., Donnino, M., Sinz, E., Lavonas, E.J., et al. (2010). 2010 American Heart Association guidelines for cardiopulmonary resuscitation and emergency cardiovascular care. Part 12: Cardiac arrest in special situations. *Circulation, 122*(18 Suppl. 3), S829–S861.

VISN 8 Patient Safety Center. (2009). *Safe patient handling and movement algorithms.* Tampa, FL: Author. Available http://www.visn8.va.gov/visn8/patientsafetycenter/safePtHandling/default.asp.

Zed, P.J., Abu-Laban, R.B., Shuster, M., Green, R.S., Slavik, R.S., & Travers, A.H. (2008). Update on cardiopulmonary resuscitation and emergency cardiovascular care guidelines. *American Journal of Health-System Pharmacy, 65*(24), 2337–2346.

SUGGESTED ANSWERS FOR FOCUSING ON PATIENT CARE: DEVELOPING CLINICAL REASONING

1. Explain the steps involved in obtaining an ECG. Tell Mr. Pruder that the test records the heart's electrical activity, and it may be repeated at certain intervals. Emphasize that no electrical current will enter his body and that the ECG will provide important information to help guide his health care. Tell him the test typically takes about 5 minutes.
2. Call for help, pull call bell, and call the facility emergency response number. Call for the automated external defibrillator (AED). Put on gloves, if available. Position Mr. Stebbings supine on his back on a firm, flat surface, with arms alongside the body. If he is in bed, place a backboard or other rigid surface under him (often the footboard of the patient's bed). Initiate CPR. Provide defibrillation as soon as an AED becomes available.
3. Do not use excessive pressure. Ask Ms. Kribell to reposition the affected extremity. Check the insertion site for obvious problems (e.g., catheter kinking). Attempt to obtain the sample to be discarded. If resistance is still felt, notify the primary care provider.

17

Neurologic Care

FOCUSING ON PATIENT CARE

This chapter will help you develop some of the skills related to neurologic care necessary for the following patients:

ALETA JACKSON, age 68, was involved in a head-on collision. She has been prescribed a cervical collar to stabilize her neck.

YUKA CHONG, age 16, has received spinal rods to resolve her scoliosis. The nurse must logroll Ms. Chong to change her position.

NIKKI GLADSTONE, age 19, is in your intensive care unit following surgery related to a cranial malignancy. She has an external ventriculostomy device in place to monitor intracranial pressure.

Refer to Focusing on Patient Care: Developing Clinical Reasoning at the end of the chapter to apply what you learn.

LEARNING OBJECTIVES

After studying this chapter, you will be able to:

1. Logroll a patient.
2. Apply a two-piece cervical collar.
3. Implement seizure precautions and seizure management.
4. Care for patient in halo traction.
5. Care for a patient with an external ventriculostomy device.
6. Care for a patient with a fiberoptic intracranial catheter.

KEY TERMS

aura: a premonitory or warning sensation of a seizure that can be visual, auditory, or olfactory

cerebral perfusion pressure (CPP): a way of calculating cerebral blood flow; the formula is MAP (mean arterial pressure) minus ICP (intracranial pressure) equals CPP; normal CPP for an adult is 60 to 90 mm Hg (Hickey, 2014)

coma: a pathologic state of unconsciousness characterized by an unarousable sleeplike state; eyes closed at all times; no speech or sound noted; no spontaneous movement of extremities (Hickey, 2014)

consciousness: the degree of wakefulness or ability to be aroused

decerebrate: abnormal body posture associated with severe brain injury; involves muscle tightening and rigidity; the arms and legs are held straight out, the toes are pointed downward, and the head and neck are arched backward

decorticate: abnormal body posture associated with severe brain injury; involves stiffness of the extremities; the arms are bent in toward the body, fists clenched, wrists are bent and held on the chest, and legs held out straight

intracranial compliance: the potential expandability of the brain; the ability of the brain to tolerate stimulation or an increase in intracranial volume without corresponding increase in pressure (Barker, 2008)

intracranial pressure (ICP): pressure within the cranial vault; normal ICP is less than 15 mm Hg (Hickey, 2014; Barker, 2008)

seizure: temporary alteration in brain function due to excessive and abnormal electrical discharges of neurons in the brain that may result in uncontrolled body movements or a convulsion and alteration of consciousness (Bhanushali & Helmers, 2008)

ventriculostomy: a catheter inserted through a hole made in the skull into the ventricular system of the brain; can be used to monitor ICP and/or drain cerebrospinal fluid

Many patients experience injury to the head, neck, or spinal column. In addition, numerous disorders, such as infections and tumors, can affect the brain and spinal cord, interfering with neurologic function. Specialized devices may be used to monitor and control **intracranial pressure**. Meticulous care is needed after injury or trauma to ensure that further injury does not occur. This chapter covers skills to assist the nurse in providing neurologic care. Behavioral scales are used to standardize observations for the objective and accurate assessment of level of **consciousness** (LOC) and monitor changes related to neurologic injury and **coma** (Hickey, 2014). The Glasgow Coma Scale (GCS) and the Full Outline of UnResponsiveness (FOUR) score are examples of two tools used to evaluate LOC. The FOUR score addresses many limitations that have been identified with the GCS, allowing more precise assessment of the extent of brainstem function, through eye response, motor response, brainstem reflexes, and respiratory pattern and drive (Cohen, 2009; Iyer et al., 2009; Palmieri, 2009; Kocak et al., 2012). The FOUR score scale is very useful in evaluating patients who are endotracheally intubated (Iyher et al.; Palmieri; Mink, 2012). Fundamentals Review 17-1 reviews a simple neurologic exam. Refer to Fundamentals Review 17-2 and Fundamentals Review 17-3 for the GCS and the FOUR Score assessment tools. Refer to Chapter 3, Health Assessment, for a review of other components of a neurologic assessment.

FUNDAMENTALS REVIEW 17-1

NEUROLOGIC EXAM

By assessing the patient's appearance and verbal and physical responses, you can obtain important information about the patient's neurologic status, including:

- Is it unchanged from baseline?
- Has the patient developed changes that may indicate a problem with the nervous system?
- Are there symptoms that need further investigation (Vacca, 2010)?

This basic examination can be used during every patient encounter. Refer to Chapter 3, Health Assessment, for details related to other components of a neurologic assessment.

What?	How?	Why?
• Assess level of consciousness, cognition, position, posture, facial symmetry, respiratory pattern. • Assess ability to speak at normal conversational volume. • Identify external forces (e.g., medications, other injuries, or altered laboratory values) that may affect the patient's responses during the assessment. • Identify abnormalities that existed before the patient's current health problem (Mink, 2012).	Does the patient: • Wake up easily? • Hear introduction and question? • Open both eyes and keep them open? • Pay attention to you and remain awake and alert? • Demonstrate behavior appropriate for situation? • Track you with head and eye movements as you move around room? • Speak clearly? • Provide appropriate responses? • Demonstrate symmetry of movement in extremities?	• Alertness, attention, arousal: Assesses reticular activating system, hypothalamus, and thalamus • Interpretation of what is heard and respond appropriately: Assesses cerebral cortex • Motor function: Assesses corticospinal motor pathway and basal ganglia system • Clear, organized, and appropriate speech: Assesses motor speech and language centers in left cerebral hemisphere

Adapted from Vacca, V.M. (2010). How to perform a 60-second neurologic exam. *Nursing, 40*(6), 58–59; Mink, J. (2012). The neurologic assessment toolbox: Key assessments at critical times. *Nursing2012CriticalCare, 7*(3), 12–17; and Barker, E. (2008). *Neuroscience nursing. A spectrum of care* (3rd ed.). St. Louis: Mosby Elsevier.

FUNDAMENTALS REVIEW 17-2

GLASGOW COMA SCALE

The Glasgow Coma Scale (GCS) evaluates three key categories of behavior that most closely reflect activity in the higher centers of the brain: eye opening, verbal response, and motor response. Within each category, each level of response is given a numerical value. The maximal score is 15, indicating a fully awake, alert, and oriented patient; the lowest score is 3, indicating deep coma (Hickey, 2014). The GCS is used in conjunction with other neurologic assessments, including pupillary reaction and vital sign measurement, to evaluate a patient's status.

Component	Score	Response
Eye opening	4	Opens eyes spontaneously when someone approaches
	3	Opens eyes in response to speech (normal tone or shouting)
	2	Opens eyes only to painful stimuli (apply pressure with a pen to the lateral outer aspect of the second or third finger, up to 10 seconds, then release)
	1	No response to painful stimuli
Best motor response	6	Accurately responds to instructions; obeys a simple command, such as "Lift your left hand off the bed"
	5	Localizes (moves hand to point of stimulation) to painful stimuli and attempts to remove source
	4	Flexion reflex action, but unable to locate the source of pain; purposeless movement in response to pain
	3	Flexes elbows and wrists while extending lower legs to pain; decorticate posturing
	2	Extends upper and lower extremities to pain; decerebrate posturing
	1	No motor response to pain on any limb
Best verbal response	5	Converses; oriented to time, place, and person
	4	Converses; disoriented to time, place, or person; any one or all indicators
	3	Converses only in words or phrases that make little sense in the context of the questions
	2	Responds with incomprehensible sounds; no understandable words and/or moaning, groaning, or crying in response to painful stimuli
	1	No response

(Adapted from Hickey, J. V. (2014). *The clinical practice of neurological and neurosurgical nursing* (7th ed.). Philadelphia: Wolters Kluwer Health/Lippincott Williams & Wilkins; Caton-Richards, M. (2010). Assessing the neurological status of patients with head injuries. *Emergency Nurse, 17*(10), 28–31; and Teasdale, G., & Jennett, B. (1974). Assessment of coma and impaired consciousness. A practical scale. *Lancet, 2*(7872), 81–84.)

FUNDAMENTALS REVIEW 17-3

THE FULL OUTLINE OF UNRESPONSIVENESS (FOUR)

Researchers at the Mayo Clinic designed the FOUR score coma scale, which has been proposed as an alternative to the Glasgow Coma Scale (GCS). The FOUR score assigns a value of 0 to 4 to each of four functional categories: eye response, motor response, brainstem reflexes, and respiration. In each of these categories, a score of 0 indicates nonfunctioning status, and a score of 4 represents normal functioning. The FOUR score may provide greater neurologic detail than the GCS due to its ability to evaluate brainstem reflexes and to recognize changes in breathing patterns and stages of brain herniation (Wijdicks et al., 2005, in Cohen, 2009; Kocak et al., 2012). The FOUR score is used in conjunction with other neurologic assessments and vital sign measurement to evaluate a patient's status.

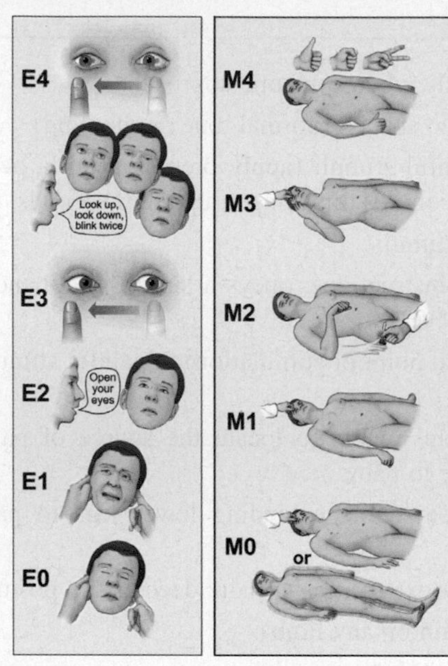

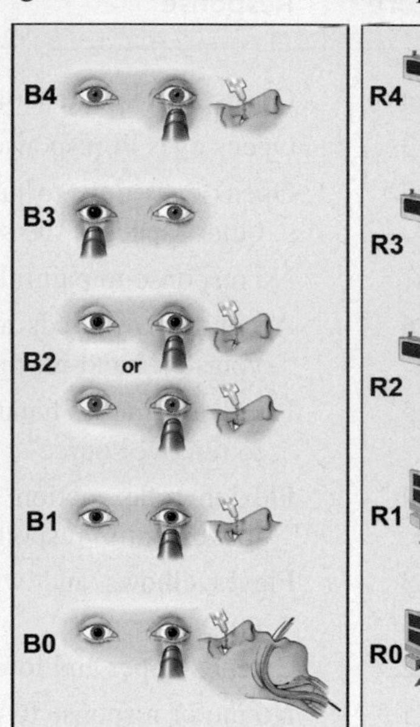

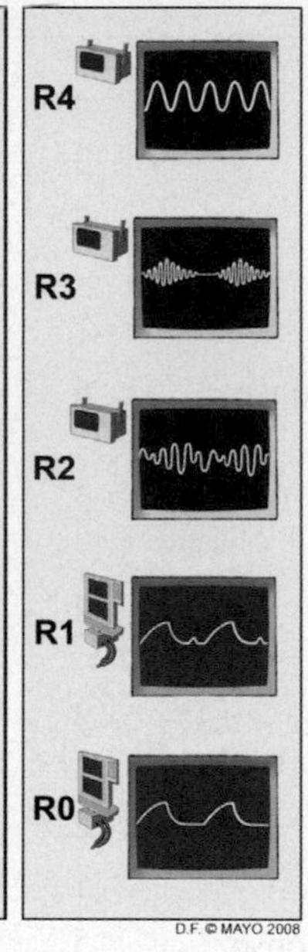

Eye response (E): E4 = eyelids open or opened, tracking or blinking to command
E3 = eyelids open, but not tracking
E2 = eyelids closed, but open to loud voice
E1 = eyelids closed, but open to pain

Motor response (M): M4 = demonstrated thumbs-up, fist, or peach sign to command
M3 = localizing to pain
M2 = flexion response to pain
M1 = extensor posturing
M0 = no response to pain or generalized myoclonus status epilepticus (prolonged repetitive epileptic myoclonic [involuntary twitching of a muscle] activity)

Brainstem reflexes (B): B4 = pupil and corneal reflexes present
B3 = one pupil wide and fixed
B2 = pupil or corneal reflexes absent
B1 = pupil and corneal reflexes absent
B0 = absent pupil, corneal, and cough reflex

Respiration (R): R4 = not intubated, regular breathing
R3 = not intubated, Cheyne-Stokes breathing pattern
R2 = not intubated, irregular breathing pattern
R1 = breathes above ventilator rate
R0 = breathes at ventilator rate or apnea

(Wijdicks, E.F.M., Bamlet, W.R., Maramattom, B.V., Manno, E.M., & McClelland, R.L. (2005). Validation of a new Coma Scale: The FOUR score. *Annals of Neurology, 58*(4), 585–593. By permission of Mayo Foundation for Medical Education and Research.

SKILL 17-1 LOGROLLING A PATIENT

The "logrolling" technique is a maneuver that involves moving the patient's body as one unit so that the spine is kept in alignment, without twisting or bending. This technique is commonly used to reposition patients who have had spinal or back surgery or who have suffered back or neck injuries. The use of logrolling when repositioning the patient helps to maintain neck and spine alignment. If the patient is being logrolled due to a neck injury, do not use a fluffy pillow under the patient's head. However, the patient may need a cervical collar in place for the move (see Skill 17-2). A bath blanket or small pillow under the head may be used to keep the spinal column straight. The patient's neck should remain straight during the procedure and after positioning. Do not twist the patient's head, spine, shoulders, knees, or hips while logrolling. Three caregivers, or more as appropriate, are needed to accomplish the maneuver safely. Do not try to logroll the patient without sufficient help.

DELEGATION CONSIDERATIONS

The use of the logrolling technique may be delegated to nursing assistive personnel (NAP) or to unlicensed assistive personnel (UAP), as well as to licensed practical/vocational nurses (LPN/LVNs). The decision to delegate must be based on careful analysis of the patient's needs and circumstances, as well as the qualifications of the person to whom the task is being delegated. Refer to the Delegation Guidelines in Appendix A.

EQUIPMENT

- At least two additional people to help
- Friction-reducing sheet to facilitate smooth movement, if not already in place; a draw sheet may be substituted if a friction-reducing sheet is not available
- Bath blanket or small pillow for under the head, if indicated
- Small pillow for placement between the legs
- Wedge pillow or two pillows for behind the patient's back
- PPE, as indicated

ASSESSMENT

Assess for conditions that would contraindicate logrolling, such as unstable neurologic status or severe pain. Assess the patient's baseline neurologic status. (See Fundamentals Review 17-1 and Chapter 3, Health Assessment.) Assess for paresthesias and pain. Assess for the need to use a cervical collar (see Skill 17-2). If the patient is complaining of pain, consider medicating the patient before repositioning.

NURSING DIAGNOSIS

Determine the related factors for the nursing diagnoses based on the patient's current status. Appropriate nursing diagnoses may include:

- Risk for Injury
- Impaired Physical Mobility
- Risk for Impaired Skin Integrity
- Impaired Skin Integrity

OUTCOME IDENTIFICATION AND PLANNING

The expected outcome when the patient is moved via logrolling is that the patient's spine remains in proper alignment, thereby reducing the risk for injury. Other outcomes may include the following: patient verbalizes relief of pain, patient maintains joint mobility, and patient remains free of alterations in skin and tissue integrity.

IMPLEMENTATION

ACTION	RATIONALE
1. Review the medical record and nursing plan of care for activity orders and conditions that may influence the patient's ability to move or to be positioned. Assess for tubes, IV lines, incisions, or equipment that may alter the positioning procedure. Identify any movement limitations.	Reviewing the medical record and care plan validates the correct patient and correct procedure. Checking for equipment and limitations reduces the risk for injury during the transfer.

(continued)

SKILL 17-1 LOGROLLING A PATIENT continued

ACTION	RATIONALE
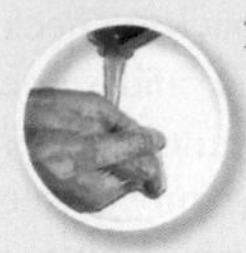 2. Perform hand hygiene and put on PPE, if indicated.	Hand hygiene and PPE prevent the spread of microorganisms. PPE is required based on transmission precautions.
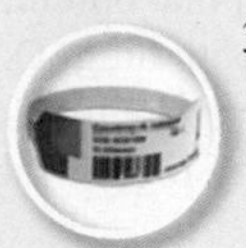 3. Identify the patient.	Identifying the patient ensures the right patient receives the intervention and helps prevent errors.
4. Close curtains around the bed and close the door to the room, if possible. Explain the purpose of the logrolling technique and what you are going to do to the patient, even if the patient is not conscious. Answer any questions.	This ensures the patient's privacy. Explanation relieves anxiety and facilitates cooperation.
5. Place the bed at an appropriate and comfortable working height, usually elbow height of the caregiver (VISN 8 Patient Safety Center, 2009).	Having the bed at the proper height prevents back and muscle strain.
6. Position at least one caregiver on one side of the bed and the two other caregivers on the opposite side of the bed. Position one caregiver at the top of the bed, at the patient's head. Place the bed in flat position. Lower the side rails. Place a small pillow between the patient's knees.	Using three or more people to turn the patient helps ensure that the spinal column will remain in straight alignment. A pillow placed between the knees helps keep the spinal column aligned.
7. If a friction-reducing sheet is not in place under the patient, take the time to place one now, to facilitate future movement of the patient. (See the Unexpected Situations below for information on placing a friction-reducing sheet.)	Use of a friction-reducing sheet facilitates smooth movement in unison and minimizes pulling on the patient's body. A draw sheet may be used if friction-reducing sheets are not available.
8. If the patient can move the arms, ask the patient to cross the arms on the chest. Roll or fanfold the friction-reducing sheet close to the patient's sides and grasp it. In unison, gently slide the patient to the side of the bed opposite to that which the patient will be turned.	Crossing arms across the chest keeps the arms out of the way while rolling the patient. This also encourages the patient not to help by pulling on the side rails. Moving the patient to the side opposite to that which the patient will be turned prevents the patient from being uncomfortably close to the side rail. If the patient is large, more assistants may be needed to prevent injury to the patient.
9. Make sure the friction-reducing sheet under the patient is straight and wrinkle free.	Friction-reducing sheet should be wrinkle free to prevent skin breakdown. Rolling it strengthens the sheet and helps the nurse hold on to the sheet.
10. If necessary, reposition personnel to ensure two stand on the side of the bed to which the patient is turning. The third helper stands on the other side. **Grasp the friction-reducing sheet at hip and shoulder level.**	Proper positioning of personnel provides even division of support and pulling forces on the patient to maintain alignment.
11. Have everyone face the patient. On a predetermined signal, turn the patient by holding the friction-reducing sheet taut to support the body. The caregiver at the patient's head should firmly hold the patient's head on either side, directly above the ears, as appropriate. **Turn the patient as a unit in one smooth motion toward the side of the bed with the two nurses. The patient's head, shoulders, spine, hips, and knees should turn simultaneously (Figure 1).**	Holding the patient's head stabilizes the cervical spine. The patient's spine should not twist during the turn. The spine should move as one unit.

ACTION	RATIONALE

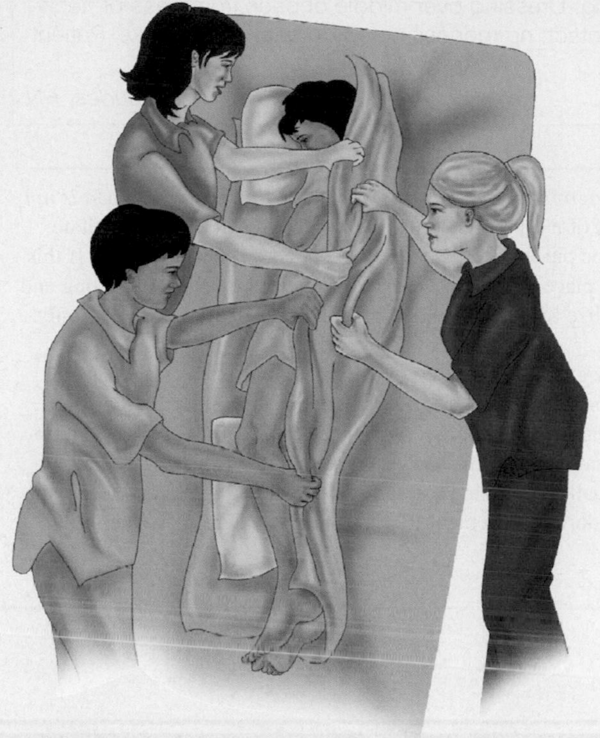

FIGURE 1 Turning patient as one unit.

ACTION	RATIONALE
12. **Once the patient has been turned, use pillows to support the patient's neck, back, buttocks, and legs in straight alignment in a side-lying position.** Raise the side rails, as appropriate.	The pillows or wedge provides support and ensures continued spinal alignment after turning.
13. **Stand at the foot of the bed and assess the spinal column. It should be straight, without any twisting or bending.** Place the bed in the lowest position. Ensure that the call bell and telephone are within reach. Replace covers. Lower bed height.	Inspection of the spinal column ensures that the patient's back is not twisted or bent. Lowering the bed ensures patient safety.
14. Reassess the patient's neurologic status (Fundamentals Review 17-1 and Chapter 3) and comfort level.	Reassessment helps to evaluate the effects of movement on the patient.
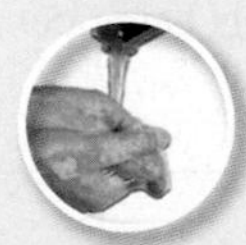 15. Remove PPE, if used. Perform hand hygiene.	Removing PPE properly reduces the risk for infection transmission and contamination of other items. Hand hygiene prevents transmission of microorganisms.

EVALUATION

The expected outcome is met when the patient remains free of injury during and after turning and exhibits proper spinal alignment in the side-lying position. Other expected outcomes are met when the patient states that pain was minimal on turning, the patient demonstrates adequate joint mobility, and the patient exhibits no signs or symptoms of skin breakdown.

DOCUMENTATION

General Guidelines

Document the time of the patient's change of position, use of supports, and any pertinent observations, including neurologic and skin assessments. Document the patient's tolerance of the position change. Many facilities provide areas on bedside flow sheets to document repositioning.

(*continued*)

SKILL 17-1 LOGROLLING A PATIENT continued

Sample Documentation

11/15/15 1120 Patient logrolled with four-person assist. Placed on left side. Patient pushed PCA button prior to turning. Dressing over middle of back from base of neck to lumbar region clean, dry, and intact; no redness noted on back or buttocks. Patient denies pain and discomfort.

—*B. Traudes, RN*

UNEXPECTED SITUATIONS AND ASSOCIATED INTERVENTIONS

- *Patient requires repositioning using logrolling, but a draw sheet or friction-reducing sheet is not in place under the patient:* Placement of a draw sheet or friction-reducing sheet will facilitate future patient movement and should be put into place before the patient occupies the bed. If this was not done, take time to put one in place. This requires careful movement using logrolling and a minimum of three caregivers. Stabilize the cervical spine by holding the patient's head firmly on either side directly above the ears.
- *Patient requires repositioning using logrolling, but you are working alone:* If assistance is not available, wait for at least two additional caregivers for assistance. Do not attempt to reposition the patient alone. At least three caregivers are necessary to perform logrolling to reposition a patient; four or more caregivers for a patient with a cervical spine injury or a large patient. Having one person dedicated to manually stabilizing the spine for a patient with a cervical spine injury is important to restrict motion during movement to prevent further damage to the spinal cord (Strever, 2010).

SKILL 17-2 APPLYING A TWO-PIECE CERVICAL COLLAR

Patients suspected of having injuries to the cervical spine must be immobilized with a cervical collar to stabilize the neck and prevent further damage to the spinal cord. A cervical collar maintains the neck in a straight line, with the chin slightly elevated and tucked inward. Care must be taken when applying the collar not to hyperflex or hyperextend the patient's neck.

DELEGATION CONSIDERATIONS

Application of a cervical collar is not delegated to nursing assistive personnel (NAP) or to unlicensed assistive personnel (UAP). Depending on the state's nurse practice act and the organization's policies and procedures, application of a cervical collar may be delegated to licensed practical/vocational nurses (LPN/LVNs). The decision to delegate must be based on careful analysis of the patient's needs and circumstances, as well as the qualifications of the person to whom the task is being delegated. Refer to the Delegation Guidelines in Appendix A.

EQUIPMENT

- Nonsterile gloves
- Additional PPE, as indicated
- Tape measure
- Cervical collar of appropriate size
- Washcloth
- Skin cleanser and water
- Towel

ASSESSMENT

Assess for a patent airway. If airway is occluded, try repositioning using the jaw-thrust–chin lift method, which helps open the airway without moving the patient's neck. Inspect and palpate the cervical spine area for tenderness, swelling, deformities, or crepitus. Do not ask the patient to move the neck if a cervical spinal cord injury is suspected. Perform a neurologic assessment. (See Fundamentals Review 1 and Chapter 3.) Assess the patient's level of consciousness and ability to follow commands to determine any neurologic dysfunction. If the patient is able to follow commands, instruct him or her not to move the head or neck. Have a second person stabilize the cervical spine by holding the patient's head firmly on either side directly above the ears.

NURSING DIAGNOSIS

Determine the related factors for the nursing diagnoses based on the patient's current status. Appropriate nursing diagnoses may include:

- Risk for Injury
- Acute Pain

OUTCOME IDENTIFICATION AND PLANNING

The expected outcome is that the patient's cervical spine is immobilized, preventing further injury to the spinal cord. Other outcomes that may be acceptable include the following: the patient maintains head and neck without movement; the patient experiences minimal to no pain; and the patient demonstrates an understanding about the need for immobilization.

IMPLEMENTATION

ACTION	RATIONALE
1. Review the medical record and nursing plan of care to determine the need for placement of a cervical collar. Identify any movement limitations. Gather the necessary supplies.	Reviewing the record and care plan validates the correct patient and correct procedure. Identification of limitations prevents injury. Assembling equipment provides for an organized approach to the task.
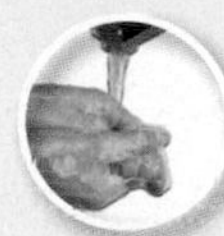 2. Perform hand hygiene and put on PPE, if indicated.	Hand hygiene and PPE prevent the spread of microorganisms. PPE is required based on transmission precautions.
3. Identify the patient.	Identifying the patient ensures the right patient receives the intervention and helps prevent errors.
4. Close curtains around the bed and close the door to the room, if possible. Explain what you are going to do and why you are going to do it to the patient.	This ensures the patient's privacy. Explanation relieves anxiety and facilitates cooperation.
5. Assemble equipment on overbed table within reach.	Arranging items nearby is convenient, saves time, and avoids unnecessary stretching and twisting of muscles on the part of the nurse.
6. Assess the patient for any changes in neurologic status. (See Fundamentals Review 17-1 and Chapter 3 for assessment details.)	Patients with cervical spine injuries are at risk for problems with the neurologic system.
7. Place the bed at an appropriate and comfortable working height, usually elbow height of the caregiver (VISN 8 Patient Safety Center, 2009). Lower the side rails as necessary.	Having the bed at the proper height and lowering the rails prevent back and muscle strain.
8. Gently clean the patient's face and neck with a skin cleanser and water. If the patient has experienced trauma, inspect the area for broken glass or other material that could cut the patient or the nurse. Pat the area dry.	Blood, glass, leaves, and twigs may be present on the patient's neck. The area should be clean before applying the cervical collar to prevent skin breakdown.
9. Have a second caregiver in position to hold the patient's head firmly on either side above the ears. Measure from the bottom of the chin to the top of the sternum, and measure around the neck. Match these height and circumference measurements to the manufacturer's recommended size chart.	This action stabilizes the cervical spine by holding the head firmly on either side above the ears. To immobilize the cervical spine and to prevent skin breakdown under the collar, the correct collar size must be used (Apold & Rydrych, 2012).
10. Slide the flattened back portion of the collar under the patient's head. **The center of the collar should line up with the center of the patient's neck. Do not allow the patient's head to move when passing the collar under the head.**	Stabilizing the cervical spine is crucial to prevent the head from moving, which could cause further damage to the cervical spine. Placing the collar in the center ensures that the neck is aligned properly.

(continued)

SKILL 17-2 APPLYING A TWO-PIECE CERVICAL COLLAR continued

ACTION	RATIONALE
11. Place the front of the collar centered over the chin, while ensuring that the chin area fits snugly in the recess. Be sure that the front half of the collar overlaps the back half. Secure Velcro straps on both sides (Figure 1). Check to see that at least one finger can be inserted between collar and patient's neck.	The collar should fit snugly to prevent the patient from moving the neck and causing further damage to the cervical spine. Velcro will help hold the collar securely in place. Collar should not be too tight to cause discomfort.

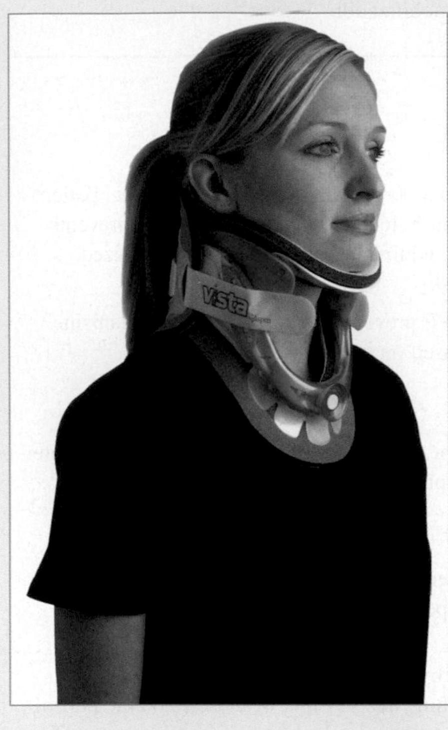

FIGURE 1 Cervical collar in place. (Photo courtesy of Aspen Medical Products, Irvine, California.)

ACTION	RATIONALE
12. Raise the side rails. Place the bed in lowest position. Make sure the call bell is in reach.	Bed in lowest position and access to call bell contribute to patient safety.
13. Reassess the patient's neurologic status and comfort level.	Reassessment helps to evaluate the effects of movement on the patient.
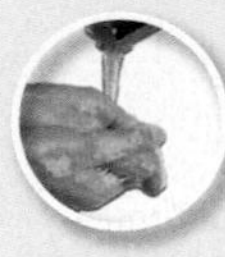 14. Remove PPE, if used. Perform hand hygiene.	Removing PPE properly reduces the risk for infection transmission and contamination of other items. Hand hygiene prevents transmission of microorganisms.
15. **Check the skin under the cervical collar at least every 4 hours for any signs of skin breakdown. Remove the collar every 8 to 12 hours and inspect and cleanse the skin under the collar. When the collar is removed, have a second person immobilize the cervical spine.**	Skin breakdown may occur under the cervical collar if the skin is not inspected and cleansed (Apold & Rydrych, 2012).

EVALUATION

The expected outcomes are met when the cervical collar is placed without adverse effect; the patient's cervical spine is immobilized without further injury; the patient verbalizes minimal to no pain; and the patient demonstrates an understanding of the rationale for cervical spine immobilization.

DOCUMENTATION

Guidelines

Document the application of the collar, including size and any skin care necessary before the application, condition of skin under the cervical collar, and patient's pain level, and neurologic and any other assessment findings.

Sample Documentation

> 11/22/15 0900 Patient arrived on unit; cervical spine immobilized; medium cervical collar applied. Patient awake, alert, and oriented. Admits to right neck pain; denies other pain. See flow sheet for neurologic assessment. Skin pink, warm, and dry. A 3-cm laceration noted on R anterior side of neck. Wound cleansed and antibiotic ointment applied. Patient instructed to refrain from moving without assistance; call bell placed in right hand.
>
> —B. Clapp, RN

UNEXPECTED SITUATIONS AND ASSOCIATED INTERVENTIONS

- *The height and neck circumference measurements are between two sizes:* Start with the smaller size. If the collar is too large, the neck may not be immobilized.
- *Skin breakdown is noted on the shoulder, neck, or ear:* Apply a protective dressing over the area and continue to assess for further skin breakdown.
- *Patient complains that the collar is "choking" him:* If not contraindicated, place the patient in the reverse Trendelenburg position to see if this helps. Elevation of the upper body lessens pressure on the head and neck from the collar. Assess the tightness of the cervical collar; at least one finger should slide under the collar.
- *Patient is able to move head from side to side with cervical collar on:* Tighten the cervical collar, if possible. If the collar is as tight as possible, apply a collar one size smaller and evaluate for a better fit.

SPECIAL CONSIDERATIONS

- Cervical collar-related pressure ulcers may develop on the occiput, chin, ears, mandible, suprascapular area, and over the larynx. The occipital area has very little subcutaneous tissue overlying the bone, making it a particularly vulnerable area (Jacobson et al., 2008). Proper sizing and skin care are an integral part of managing care for these patients.
- If collar has removable inner pads, change and wash the pads every 24 hours and as needed (Apold & Rydrych, 2012).

SKILL 17-3 EMPLOYING SEIZURE PRECAUTIONS AND SEIZURE MANAGEMENT

Seizures occur when the electrical system of the brain malfunctions. Sudden abnormal and excessive discharge from cerebral neurons results in episodes of abnormal motor, sensory, autonomic, or psychic activity, or a combination of these (Hickey, 2014; Hinkle & Cheever, 2014). A seizure manifests as an alteration in sensation, behavior, movement, perception, or consciousness (Barker, 2008). During a seizure, patients are at risk for hypoxia, vomiting, and pulmonary aspiration. Patients who are at risk for seizures and those who have had a seizure(s) are often placed under seizure precautions to minimize the risk of physical injury. Causes of seizures include cerebrovascular disease, hypoxemia, head injury, hypertension, central nervous system infections, metabolic and toxic conditions, brain tumor, drug and alcohol withdrawal, allergies, and a history of epilepsy (seizure disorder) (Hinkle & Cheever, 2014). Seizure management includes interventions by the nurse to prevent aspiration, protect the patient from injury, provide care after the seizure, and observe and document the details of the event (Hinkle & Cheever, 2014; Hickey, 2014). Figure 1 illustrates nursing measures to protect the patient from injury.

(continued)

SKILL 17-3 EMPLOYING SEIZURE PRECAUTIONS AND SEIZURE MANAGEMENT continued

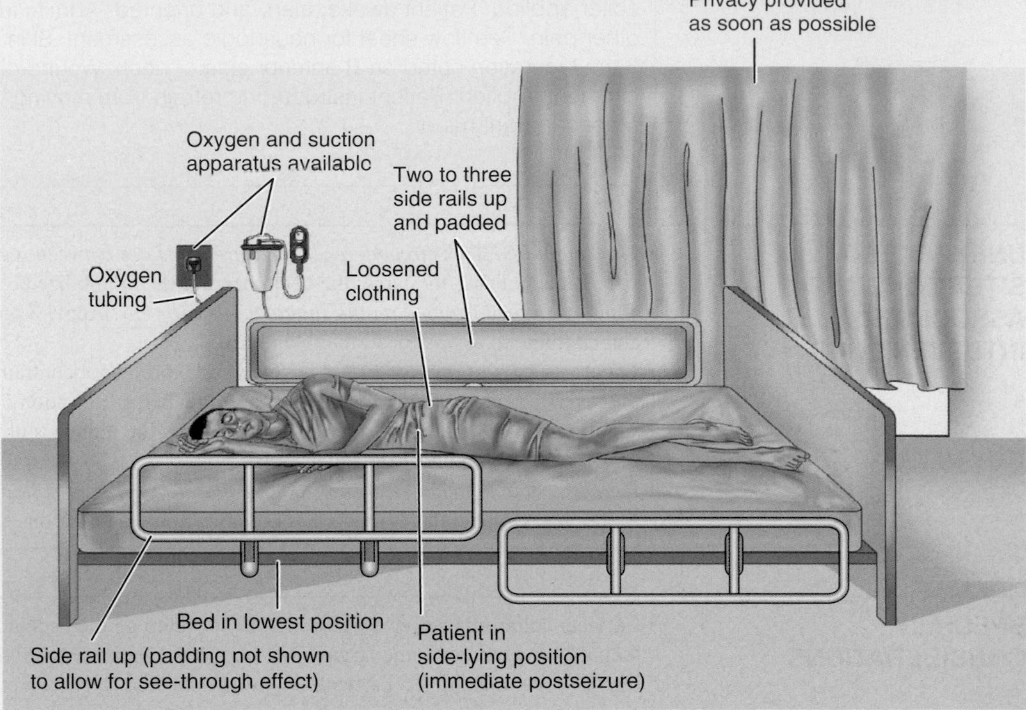

FIGURE 1 Protecting patient from injury. (Adapted from Hinkle, J.L., & Cheever, K.H. (2014). *Brunner & Suddarth's textbook of medical-surgical nursing* (13th ed.). Philadelphia: Wolters Kluwer Health/Lippincott Williams & Wilkins, p. 1961.)

DELEGATION CONSIDERATIONS

The implementation of seizure precautions may be delegated to nursing assistive personnel (NAP) or to unlicensed assistive personnel (UAP). The implementation of seizure management may not be delegated to nursing assistive personnel (NAP) or to unlicensed assistive personnel (UAP). Implementation of seizure precautions as well as seizure management may be delegated to licensed practical/vocational nurses (LPN/LVNs). The decision to delegate must be based on careful analysis of the patient's needs and circumstances, as well as the qualifications of the person to whom the task is being delegated. Refer to the Delegation Guidelines in Appendix A.

EQUIPMENT

- PPE, as indicated
- Portable or wall suction unit with tubing
- A commercially prepared suction kit with an appropriate size catheter or:
  - Sterile suction catheter with Y-port in the appropriate size (adult: 10F to 16F)
  - Sterile disposable container
  - Sterile gloves
- Oral airway
- Bed rail padding
- Oxygen apparatus
- Nasal cannula or mask to deliver oxygen
- Handheld bag valve/resuscitation bag

ASSESSMENT

Assess for preexisting conditions that increase the patient's risk for seizure activity. For example, assess for a history of seizure disorder or epilepsy, cerebrovascular disease, hypoxemia, head injury, hypertension, central nervous system infections, metabolic conditions (e.g., renal failure, hypocalcemia, hypoglycemia), brain tumor, drug/alcohol withdrawal, or allergies. Assess circumstances before the seizure, such as visual, auditory, or olfactory stimuli, tactile stimuli, emotional or psychological disturbances, sleep, or hyperventilation. Assess for the occurrence of an **aura**. Note where the movements or stiffness begin; and the gaze position and position of the head when the seizure begins. Assess the body part(s) and the type of movement(s) involved in the seizure. Assess pupil sizes; if eyes remained open during seizure; and whether eyes or head turned to one side. Assess for the presence or absence of repeated involuntary motor activity (e.g., repeated swallowing); incontinence of urine or stool; duration of seizure; presence of unconsciousness and duration; obvious paralysis or weakness of arms or legs after seizure; and inability to speak, movements, sleeping, and/or confusion after seizure. Assess the patient's neurologic status (refer to Fundamentals Review 17-1 and Chapter 3) and for injury after the seizure is over.

NURSING DIAGNOSIS

Determine the related factors for the nursing diagnoses based on the patient's current health status. An appropriate nursing diagnosis is Risk for Injury. Other nursing diagnoses may include:

- Risk for Aspiration
- Deficient Knowledge

OUTCOME IDENTIFICATION AND PLANNING

The expected outcome to achieve when implementing seizure precautions and seizure management is that the patient remains free from injury. Other specific outcomes will be formulated depending on the identified nursing diagnosis.

IMPLEMENTATION

ACTION	RATIONALE
1. Review the medical record and nursing plan of care for conditions that would place the patient at risk for seizures. Review the medical orders and the nursing plan of care for orders for seizure precautions.	Reviewing the order and plan of care validates the correct patient and correct procedure.
Seizure Precautions	
2. Gather the necessary supplies.	Preparation promotes efficient time management and an organized approach to the task.
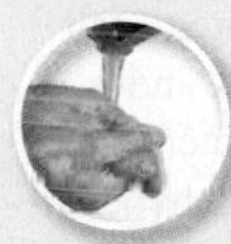 3. Perform hand hygiene and put on PPE, if indicated.	Hand hygiene and PPE prevent the spread of microorganisms. PPE is required based on transmission precautions.
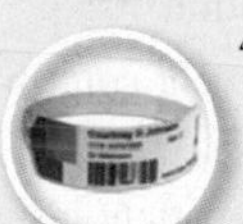 4. Identify the patient.	Identifying the patient ensures the right patient receives the intervention and helps prevent errors.
5. Close curtains around the bed and close the door to the room, if possible. Explain what you are going to do and why you are going to do it to the patient.	This ensures the patient's privacy. Explanation relieves anxiety and facilitates cooperation.
6. Assemble equipment on overbed table within reach.	Arranging items nearby is convenient, saves time, and avoids unnecessary stretching and twisting of muscles on the part of the nurse.
7. Place the bed in the lowest position with two to three side rails elevated. Apply padding to the side rails.	Bed in lowest position promotes safety and decreases risk of injury. Rail padding decreases the risk of injury.
8. Attach oxygen apparatus to oxygen access in the wall at the head of the bed. Place nasal cannula or mask equipment in a location where it can be easily reached if needed.	During a seizure, patients are at risk for hypoxia, vomiting, and pulmonary aspiration. Ready access ensures availability of oxygen in the event of a seizure.
9. Attach suction apparatus to vacuum access in the wall at the head of the bed. Place suction catheter, oral airway, and resuscitation bag in a location where they are easily reached if needed.	During a seizure, patients are at risk for hypoxia, vomiting, and pulmonary aspiration. Ready access ensures availability of suction in the event of a seizure. Oral airway and resuscitation bag ensure availability of emergency ventilation in the event of respiratory arrest.

(continued)

SKILL 17-3 EMPLOYING SEIZURE PRECAUTIONS AND SEIZURE MANAGEMENT continued

ACTION	RATIONALE
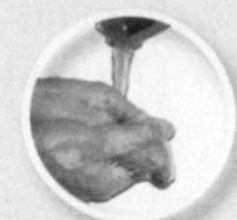 10. Remove PPE, if used. Perform hand hygiene.	Removing PPE properly reduces the risk for infection transmission and contamination of other items. Hand hygiene prevents the spread of microorganisms.
Seizure Management	
11. For patients with known seizures, be alert for the occurrence of an aura, if known. If the patient reports experiencing an aura, have the patient lie down.	Some patients report a warning or premonition before seizures occur; an aura can be a visual, auditory, or olfactory sensation that indicates a seizure is going to occur. Lying down prevents injury that might occur if the patient falls to the floor.
12. Once a seizure begins, close the curtains around the bed and close the door to the room, if possible.	Closing the door or curtain provides for patient privacy.
13. If the patient is seated, ease the patient to the floor.	Getting the patient to the floor prevents injury that might occur if the patient falls to the floor.
14. Remove patient's eyeglasses. Loosen any constricting clothing. Place something flat and soft, such as a folded blanket, under the head. Push aside furniture or other objects in area.	Removing objects and loosening clothing prevents possible injury. Blanket prevents injury from striking a hard surface (floor).
15. If the patient is in bed, remove the pillow, place bed in lowest position, and raise side rails.	Prevents injury.
16. Do not restrain patient. Guide movements, if necessary. Do not try to insert anything in the patient's mouth or open jaws.	Guiding movements prevents injury. Restraint can injure the patient. Attempting to open the mouth and/or insert anything into the mouth can result in broken teeth, and injury to mouth, lips, or tongue.
17. If possible, place patient on the side with the head flexed forward, head of bed elevated 30 degrees. Begin administration of oxygen, based on facility policy. Clear airway using suction, as appropriate. (Refer to Skill 14-6, Suctioning the nasopharyngeal and oropharyngeal airways, Chapter 14, Oxygenation.)	During a seizure, patients are at risk for hypoxia, vomiting, and pulmonary aspiration. This position allows the tongue to fall forward, and facilitates drainage of saliva and mucus and minimizes risk for aspiration. Oxygen supports the increased metabolism associated with neurologic and muscular hyperactivity. Patent airway is necessary to support ventilation.
18. Provide supervision throughout the seizure and time the length of the seizure.	Supervision of the patient ensures safety. Timing of event contributes to accurate information and documentation.
19. Establish/maintain intravenous access, as necessary. Administer medications, as appropriate, based on medical order and facility policy.	Pharmacologic therapy may be appropriate, based on patient history and medical diagnoses. Intravenous access is necessary to administer emergency medications.
20. After the seizure, place the patient in a side-lying position. Clear airway using suction, as appropriate.	Side-lying position facilitates drainage of secretions. Patent airway is necessary to support ventilation.
21. Monitor vital signs, oxygen saturation, response to medications administered, and capillary glucose, as appropriate.	Monitoring of parameters provides information for accurate assessment of patient status.
22. Place the bed in the lowest position. Make sure the call bell is in reach.	Bed in lowest position and access to call bell contribute to patient safety.
23. Reassess the patient's neurologic status and comfort level.	Reassessment helps to evaluate the effects of the event on the patient.
24. Allow the patient to sleep after the seizure. On awakening, orient and reassure the patient. Reassess, as indicated.	The patient will probably experience an inability to recall the seizure; patients may also experience confusion, anxiety, embarrassment, and/or fatigue after a seizure. Reassessment helps to evaluate the effects of the event on the patient.
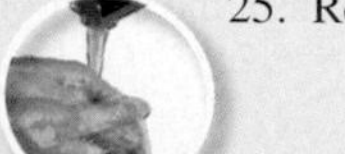 25. Remove PPE, if used. Perform hand hygiene.	Removing PPE properly reduces the risk for infection transmission and contamination of other items. Hand hygiene prevents the spread of microorganisms.

EVALUATION

The expected outcome when implementing seizure precautions and seizure management is met when the patient remains free from injury.

DOCUMENTATION

Guidelines

Document initiation of seizure precautions, including specific interventions put in place. Document if the beginning of the seizure was witnessed. If so, record noted circumstances before the seizure, such as visual, auditory, or olfactory stimuli, tactile stimuli, emotional or psychological disturbances, sleep, or hyperventilation. Note the occurrence of an aura; where the movements or stiffness began; gaze position and position of the head when the seizure began. Record the body part(s) and the type of movement(s) involved in the seizure. Document pupil sizes; if eyes remained open during seizure; whether eyes or head turned to one side; presence or absence of repeated involuntary motor activity (e.g., repeated swallowing); incontinence of urine or stool; duration of seizure; presence of unconsciousness and duration; obvious paralysis or weakness of arms or legs after seizure; and inability to speak, movements, sleeping, and/or confusion after seizure. Document oxygen administration, airway suction, safety measures, and medication administration, if used. If the patient was injured during the seizure, document assessment of injury.

Sample Documentation

1/22/15 0745 Patient bathing with assistance. Stated "I don't feel right." Patient suddenly verbally unresponsive, stiff contractions of legs and arms, with arms extended, lasting approximately 15 seconds; 5-second period of apnea; and bladder incontinence. Continued with approximately 30 seconds of muscle contraction of extremities; eyes closed, facial grimacing. Patient then appeared to sleep; BP 102/68; P 88, R 16; oxygen saturation 94%. Patient awakened after 20 minutes, complaining of headache and fatigue and returned to sleep. Dr. Mason notified of events and assessment. Seizure precautions implemented.

—*D. Tyne, RN*

UNEXPECTED SITUATIONS AND ASSOCIATED INTERVENTIONS

- *You enter room and find patient in the midst of a seizure:* Initiate seizure management interventions outlined above. Note in documentation that the seizure onset was not initially witnessed.

SPECIAL CONSIDERATIONS

Infant and Child Considerations

- Most seizures in children are caused by disorders that originate outside of the brain, such as high fever, infection, head trauma, toxins, or cardiac arrhythmias. Febrile seizures are the most common type during childhood and are usually benign (Kyle & Carman, 2013).
- Seizures in newborns are associated with underlying conditions, such as hypoxic ischemic encephalopathy, hypoglycemia, hypocalcemia, meningitis, encephalitis, and intracranial hemorrhage. The prognosis depends on the underlying cause and severity of the seizure (Kyle & Carman, 2013).
- Children with recurrent seizures should wear a medical alert bracelet.

Home Care Considerations

- Include patient and family/significant other teaching for patients with documented seizures, as well as those at risk for seizures. Teaching should include basic first aid management and the following tips:
  - Help person to lie down.
  - Remove eyeglasses and loosen constrictive clothing.
  - Clear the area around the person of anything hard or sharp.
  - Place something flat and soft (e.g., a folded jacket) under the head. Turn the person gently on the side, if possible.
  - Do not try to force anything into the patient's mouth.

(*continued*)

SKILL 17-3 EMPLOYING SEIZURE PRECAUTIONS AND SEIZURE MANAGEMENT continued

- Stay with the person during the seizure.
- Remain calm.
- After the seizure, stay with the patient until consciousness is regained; reorient as necessary.

- Patients with recurrent seizures should wear a medical alert bracelet.
- Teach the patient and family/significant other guidelines about when to seek emergency medical assistance. Instruct patients' families and significant others to call for emergency assistance if the seizure occurs in water; the person does not begin breathing after the seizure; if the seizure lasts more than 5 minutes without signs of slowing; if the person has trouble breathing afterward, appears to be in pain, or recovery is unusual in some way; the person has one seizure right after another without regaining consciousness; if the patient is injured during the seizure; or if the person has a health condition such as diabetes or heart disease or is pregnant (CDC, 2011).

SKILL 17-4 CARING FOR A PATIENT IN HALO TRACTION

Halo traction provides immobilization to patients with spinal cord injury. Halo traction consists of a metal ring that fits over the patient's head, connected with skull pins into the skull, and metal bars that connect the ring to a vest that distributes the weight of the device around the chest. It immobilizes the head and neck after traumatic injury to the cervical vertebrae and allows early mobility. It is also used to apply spinal traction.

Nursing responsibilities include reassuring the patient, maintaining the device, monitoring neurovascular status, monitoring respiratory status, promoting exercise, preventing complications from the therapy, preventing infection by providing pin-site care, and providing teaching to ensure compliance and self-care. A growing evidence base supports effective management of pin sites, but there is no clear consensus (Walker, 2012; Lagerquist et al., 2012; Sarro et al., 2010). Pin-site care often varies based on primary care provider and facility policy. Dressings are often applied for the first 48 to 72 hours, and then sites may be left open to air. Pin-site care may be performed frequently in the first 48 to 72 hours after application, when drainage may be heavy; other evidence suggests pin care should begin after the first 48 to 72 hours. Routine pin-site care may then be done on a daily or weekly basis (Timms & Pugh, 2012; Lagerquist et al., 2012). Refer to specific patient medical orders and facility guidelines.

DELEGATION CONSIDERATIONS

The care of a patient with halo traction may not be delegated to nursing assistive personnel (NAP) or to unlicensed assistive personnel (UAP). Depending on the state's nurse practice act and the organization's policies and procedures, care for these patients may be delegated to licensed practical/vocational nurses (LPN/LVNs). The decision to delegate must be based on careful analysis of the patient's needs and circumstances, as well as the qualifications of the person to whom the task is being delegated. Refer to the Delegation Guidelines in Appendix A.

EQUIPMENT

- Basin of warm water
- Bath towels
- Skin cleanser, based on facility policy
- Antimicrobial ointment, per primary care provider order or facility policy
- Sterile applicators
- Cleansing solution, usually sterile normal saline or chlorhexidine, per primary care provider order or facility policy
- Sterile gauze or dressing per primary care provider order or facility policy
- Analgesic, per physician's order
- Clean gloves, if appropriate, for bathing under the vest
- Sterile gloves for performing pin care, depending on facility policy
- Additional PPE, as indicated

ASSESSMENT

Review the patient's medical record, medical orders, and nursing plan of care to determine the type of device being used and the prescribed care. Assess the halo traction device to ensure proper function and position. Perform respiratory, neurologic, and skin assessments. Inspect the pin-insertion sites for inflammation and infection, including swelling, cloudy or offensive drainage, pain, or redness. Assess the patient's knowledge regarding the device and self-care activities and responsibilities, and his or her feelings related to treatment.

NURSING DIAGNOSIS

Determine the related factors for the nursing diagnoses based on the patient's current status. Appropriate nursing diagnoses may include:

- Disturbed Body Image
- Self-Care Deficit (toileting, bathing, dressing)
- Disturbed Sleep Pattern
- Risk for Infection

OUTCOME IDENTIFICATION AND PLANNING

The expected outcome to achieve when caring for a patient with halo traction is that the patient maintains cervical alignment. Additional outcomes that may be appropriate include that the patient shows no evidence of infection; the patient is free from complications, such as respiratory impairment, orthostatic hypotension, and skin breakdown; the patient experiences relief from pain; and the patient is free from injury.

IMPLEMENTATION

ACTION	RATIONALE
1. Review the medical record and the nursing plan of care to determine the type of device being used and prescribed care.	Reviewing the medical record and care plan validates the correct patient and correct procedure.
2. Gather the necessary equipment.	Preparation promotes efficient time management and an organized approach to the task.
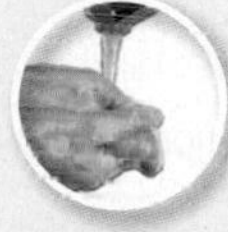 3. Perform hand hygiene and put on PPE, if indicated.	Hand hygiene and PPE prevent the spread of microorganisms. PPE is required based on transmission precautions.
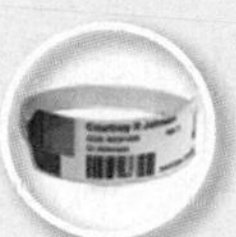 4. Identify the patient.	Identifying the patient ensures the right patient receives the intervention and helps prevent errors.
5. Close curtains around the bed and close the door to the room, if possible. Explain what you are going to do and why you are going to do it to the patient.	This ensures the patient's privacy. Explanation relieves anxiety and facilitates cooperation.
6. Assemble equipment on overbed table within reach.	Arranging items nearby is convenient, saves time, and avoids unnecessary stretching and twisting of muscles on the part of the nurse.
7. Assess the patient for possible need for nonpharmacologic, pain reducing interventions or analgesic medication before beginning. Administer appropriate prescribed analgesic. Allow sufficient time for analgesic to achieve its effectiveness before beginning the procedure.	Pain is a subjective experience influenced by past experience. Pin care may cause pain for some patients.
8. Place a waste receptacle at a convenient location for use during the procedure.	Having a waste container handy means that the soiled dressing may be discarded easily, without the spread of microorganisms.
9. Adjust bed to comfortable working height, usually elbow height of the caregiver if the patient will remain in bed (VISN 8 Patient Safety Center, 2009). Alternatively, have the patient sit up, if appropriate.	Having the bed at the proper height prevents back and muscle strain.

(continued)

SKILL 17-4 CARING FOR A PATIENT IN HALO TRACTION continued

ACTION	RATIONALE
10. Assist the patient to a comfortable position that provides easy access to the head. Place a waterproof pad under the head if the patient is lying down.	Patient positioning provides for comfort. Waterproof pad protects underlying surfaces.
11. Monitor vital signs and perform a neurologic assessment, including level of consciousness, motor function, and sensation, per facility policy. (See Fundamentals Review 17-1 and Chapter 3.) This is usually at least every 2 hours for 24 hours, or possibly every hour for 48 hours.	Changes in the neurologic assessment could indicate spinal cord trauma, which would require immediate intervention.
12. Examine the halo vest unit every 8 hours for stability, secure connections, and positioning (Figure 1). Make sure the patient's head is centered in the halo without neck flexion or extension. Check each bolt for loosening.	Assessment ensures correct function of the device and patient safety. Loose bolts require attention from an appropriate advanced practice professional to maintain correct positioning, proper alignment, and unit stability.

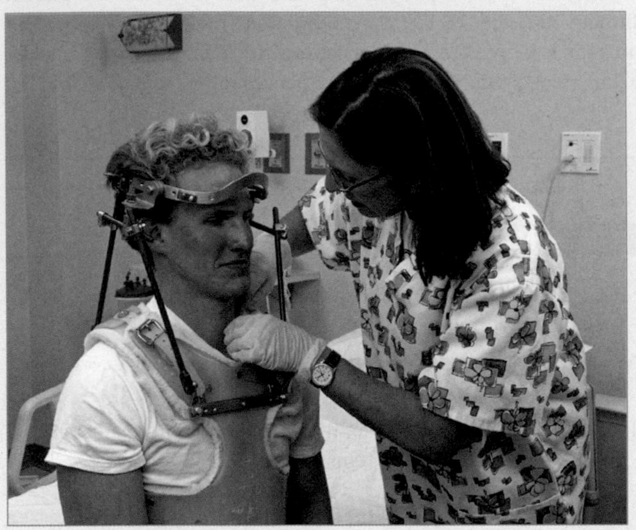

FIGURE 1 Examining halo vest for stability, secure connections, and positioning.

ACTION	RATIONALE
13. Check the fit of the vest. With the patient in a supine position, you should be able to insert one or two fingers under the jacket at the shoulder and chest.	Checking the fit prevents compression on the chest, which could interfere with respiratory status.
14. Put on nonsterile gloves, if appropriate. Remove patient's shirt or gown. Wash the patient's chest and back daily. Loosen the bottom Velcro straps. Protect the vest liner with a waterproof pad.	Gloves prevent contact with blood and body fluids. Removal of clothing from torso allows visualization of, and access to, appropriate areas. Daily cleaning prevents skin breakdown and allows assessment. Loosening the straps allows access to the chest and back. Waterproof pad keeps the vest liner dry and prevents skin irritation and breakdown.
15. Wring out a bath towel soaked in warm water (and skin cleanser, depending of facility policy). Pull the towel back and forth in a drying motion beneath the front.	Using an overly wet towel could lead to skin maceration and breakdown.
16. Thoroughly dry the skin in the same manner with a dry towel. Inspect the skin for tender, reddened areas or pressure spots. Do not use powder or lotion under the vest.	Drying prevents skin irritation and breakdown. Powders and lotions can cause skin irritation.
17. Turn the patient on his or her side, less than 45 degrees if lying supine, and repeat the process on the back. Remove waterproof pad from the vest liner. Close the Velcro straps. Assist the patient with putting on a new shirt, if desired.	Doing so prevents skin breakdown. Cleansers and lotions can cause skin irritation.
18. Perform a respiratory assessment. Check for respiratory impairment, such as absence of breath sounds, the presence of adventitious sounds, reduced inspiratory effort, or shortness of breath.	The halo vest limits chest expansion, which could lead to alterations in respiratory function. Pulmonary embolus is a common complication associated with spinal cord injury.

ACTION	RATIONALE
19. Assess the pin sites for redness, tenting of the skin; prolonged or purulent drainage; swelling; and bowing, bending, or loosening of the pins. Monitor body temperature.	Pin sites provide an entry for microorganisms. Assessment allows for early detection and prompt intervention should problems arise.
20. Perform pin-site care (Figure 2). (See Skills 9-19 and 9-20.)	Pin-site care reduces the risk of infection and subsequent osteomyelitis.
21. Depending on medical order and facility policy, apply antimicrobial ointment to pin sites and a dressing.	Antimicrobial ointment helps prevent infection. Dressing provides protection and helps contain any drainage.

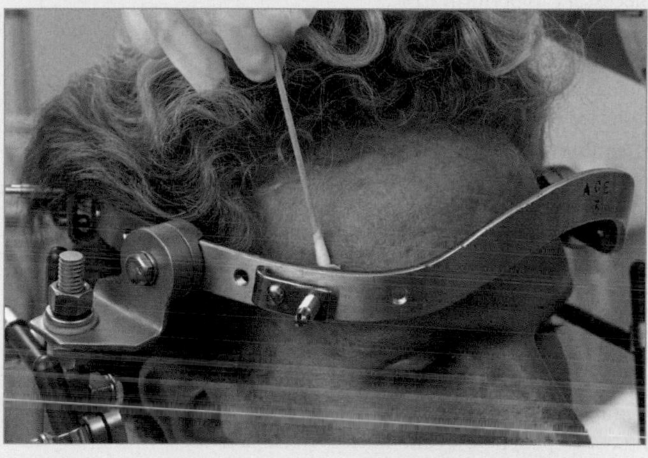

FIGURE 2 Cleansing pin sites.

ACTION	RATIONALE
22. Remove gloves and dispose of them appropriately. Raise rails, as appropriate, and place the bed in the lowest position. Assist the patient to a comfortable position.	Disposing of gloves reduces the risk of microorganism transmission. Rails assist with patient positioning. Proper bed height ensures patient safety.
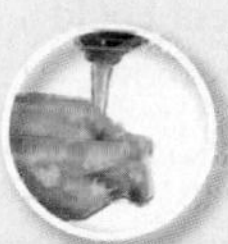 23. Remove additional PPE, if used. Perform hand hygiene.	Removing PPE properly reduces the risk for infection transmission and contamination of other items. Hand hygiene prevents the spread of microorganisms.

EVALUATION

The expected outcome is met when the patient maintains cervical alignment. Additional outcomes are met when the patient shows no evidence of infection; the patient is free from complications, such as respiratory impairment, orthostatic hypotension, and skin breakdown; the patient experiences relief from pain; and the patient is free from injury.

DOCUMENTATION

Guidelines

Document the time, date, and type of device in place. Include the skin assessment, pin-site assessment, personal hygiene, and pin-site care. Document the patient's response to the device and the neurologic assessment and respiratory assessment.

Sample Documentation

11/10/15 2030 Halo traction in place. Skin care provided under jacket; two fingers fit at shoulders and chest. Skin intact without redness or irritation. Pin-site care performed. Pin sites cleaned with normal saline and open to the air. Sites without redness, swelling, and drainage. Neurovascular status intact. Patient reports pain at pin sites 4/10. Medicated with ibuprofen 600 mg per order. Will reevaluate pain in 1 hour.

—*M. Leroux, RN*

(continued)

SKILL 17-4 CARING FOR A PATIENT IN HALO TRACTION continued

UNEXPECTED SITUATIONS AND ASSOCIATED INTERVENTIONS

- *A patient being treated with halo traction complains of a headache after the physician or advanced practice professional has tightened the skull pins:* This is a common complaint; obtain an order for and administer an analgesic. However, if the pain is associated with jaw movement, notify the primary health care provider immediately, because the pins may have slipped onto the temporal plate.

SPECIAL CONSIDERATIONS

General Considerations

- Always keep wrenches specific for the vest at the bedside for emergency removal of the anterior portion of the vest should it be necessary to perform CPR.
- Patient teaching to prevent injury is very important. Patients need to learn to turn slowly and refrain from bending forward to avoid falls.
- Stress to the frame could cause misalignment of the spine and straining or tearing of the skin. Do not use the frame as handles to transfer or position the patient.
- If a pin site becomes unusually painful or tender, or if you notice any fluid discharge, it may be a signal that the pin has loosened or become infected. In the event of unusual pain or irritation, notify the primary care provider (AANN, 2012). Pin loosening may also be indicated by a "tight" feeling or a "clicking" sound (Lagerquist et al., 2012; Patchen et al., 2010).

Home Care Considerations

- Patients and families require information and guidance about the care of their halo in the community. Written information, as well as specific discharge teaching, is crucial in helping to prevent complications (Sarro et al., 2010). Teaching should include the importance of vigilant skin care and signs and symptoms of pin site infection.
- Encourage exercise from walking; teach patient to avoid other exercise activities.
- Keeping hair clean is important. Hair should be shampooed regularly. This can be accomplished by having the patient lie supine in bed, with the head out over foot of the mattress so it is suspended beyond the mattress; shoulders should remain on the mattress with a towel or plastic bag along the back and shoulders of the vest to keep it from getting wet. A garbage can under the patient's head can be used to catch the water (Sarro et al., 2010). Alternately, the patient could rest on the edge of a bathtub, with a towel on the edge of the tub for padding, resting elbows on edge for support. Use a spray attachment or pitcher of water to wash hair.

EVIDENCE FOR PRACTICE ▶

EXTERNAL FIXATOR PIN SITES—CLINICAL EVIDENCE REVIEW

Lagerquist, D., Dabrowski, M., Dock, C., et al. (2012). Clinical evidence review. Care of external fixator pin sites. *American Journal of Critical Care, 21*(4), 288–292.

This clinical evidence review was conducted in CINAHL and MEDLINE, using the search terms *external fixator pin sites, pin sites, and pin site infections,* and included articles from 2003 to 2011. Ten studies were retrieved and included two prospective observational studies, seven randomized controlled trials, and one systematic review. Studies demonstrated mixed approaches to pin-site care. Recommendations for practice based on the evidence reviewed and considerations for practice in the absence of stronger conclusive evidence are provided. The studies addressed solutions for pin-site care, frequency of pin-site management, site dressings, and showering by patients.

Refer to thePoint for additional research on related nursing topics.

SKILL 17-5 CARING FOR A PATIENT WITH AN EXTERNAL VENTRICULOSTOMY (INTRAVENTRICULAR CATHETER–CLOSED FLUID-FILLED SYSTEM)

Intracranial pressure (ICP), the pressure inside the cranium, is the result of blood, tissue, and cerebrospinal fluid circulating in the ventricles and subarachnoid space (Moreda et al., 2009). ICP monitoring is used to assess cerebral perfusion. When ICP increases, as a result of conditions such as a mass (e.g., a tumor), bleeding into the brain or fluid around the brain, or swelling within the brain matter itself, neurologic consequences may range from minor to severe, including death (Hill et al., 2012). Normal ICP is less than 15 mm Hg. Elevated ICP, intracranial hypertension, is a sustained ICP of 20 mm Hg or more (Schimpf, 2012; Barker, 2008). Box 17-1 discusses signs and symptoms of increased intracranial pressure in adults.

Box 17-1 SIGNS AND SYMPTOMS OF INCREASED INTRACRANIAL PRESSURE IN ADULTS

- Decreased level of consciousness
- Changes in mental status
- Lethargy
- Coma
- Headache
- Confusion
- Restlessness, agitation
- Irritability
- Hypoactive reflexes
- Slowed response time
- Ataxia
- Aphasia
- Slowed speech
- Progressively severe headache
- Nausea and vomiting (usually projectile vomiting)
- Seizures
- Changes in pupil size; unequal pupils
- Slowed or lack of pupillary response to light
- Widening of pulse pressure
- Respiratory pattern changes
- Leakage of clear yellow or pinkish fluid from ear or nose

An external **ventriculostomy** is one method used to monitor ICP. It is part of a system that includes an external drainage system and an external transducer. This device is inserted into a ventricle of the brain, most commonly the nondominant lateral ventricle, through a hole drilled into the skull. The catheter is connected by a fluid-filled system to a transducer, which records the pressure in the form on an electrical impulse (Hinkle & Cheever, 2014). The ventriculostomy can be used to measure the ICP, to drain cerebrospinal fluid (CSF), such as removing excess fluid associated with hydrocephalus, or to decrease the volume in the cranial vault, thereby decreasing the ICP, and to instill medications. ICP and blood pressure measurements are used to calculate **cerebral perfusion pressure (CPP)**, the pressure needed to perfuse the blood upward to the brain against gravity (Barker, 2008). ICP monitoring also provides information about intracranial compliance, the ability of the brain to tolerate stimulation or increase in intracranial volume without an increase in pressure through waveform assessment (Box 17-2) (AANN, 2011; Barker, 2008; Hinkle & Cheever, 2014).

DELEGATION CONSIDERATIONS

The care of a patient with an external ventriculostomy may not be delegated to nursing assistive personnel (NAP) or to unlicensed assistive personnel (UAP). Depending on the state's nurse practice act and the organization's policies and procedures, care for these patients may be delegated to licensed practical/vocational nurses (LPN/LVNs). The decision to delegate must be based on careful analysis of the patient's needs and circumstances, as well as the qualifications of the person to whom the task is being delegated. Refer to the Delegation Guidelines in Appendix A.

(continued)

SKILL 17-5 CARING FOR A PATIENT WITH AN EXTERNAL VENTRICULOSTOMY (INTRAVENTRICULAR CATHETER–CLOSED FLUID-FILLED SYSTEM) continued

BOX 17-2 INTERPRETING ICP WAVEFORMS

Sustained periods (>5 minutes) of ICPs greater than 20 mm Hg are considered significant and can be extremely dangerous. Sustained periods of ICPs greater than 60 mm Hg are usually fatal (Morton & Fontaine, 2013, p. 309). A normal waveform correlates with hemodynamic changes. Plotting extended periods of increased ICP measurements over time provides patterns known as A, B, and C waves (waveform trends).

Normal Intracranial Waveform

A normal ICP waveform typically shows a steep upward slope followed by a downward slope with three descending peaks that correlate with hemodynamic changes (forces related to the circulation of blood). P1 correlates with systole; P2 most directly reflects the state of intracranial compliance, so as ICP rises, P2 elevates; P3 tapers down to correlate with diastole (Morton & Fontaine, 2013). In normal circumstances, this waveform occurs continuously and indicates an ICP between 0 and 15 mm Hg—normal pressure. The amplitude of P2 may exceed P1 with increased ICP or decreased intracranial compliance (AACN, 2011).

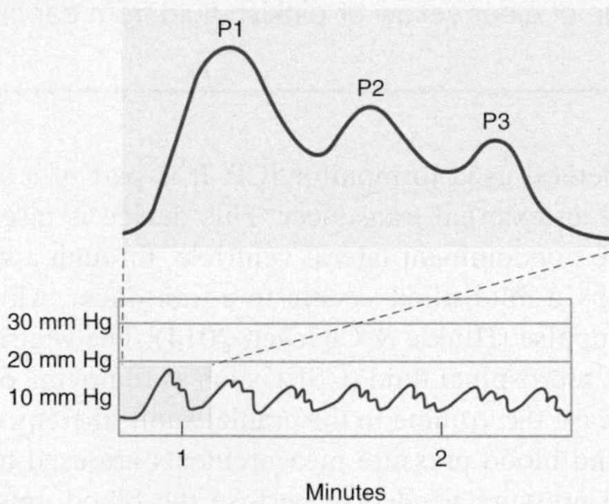

A Waves

A waves are produced by spontaneous, transient, rapid increases of pressure over a period of time (ICP values of 50 to 100 mm Hg, lasting 5 to 20 minutes) and are associated with compromised cerebral perfusion and deteriorating neurologic status.

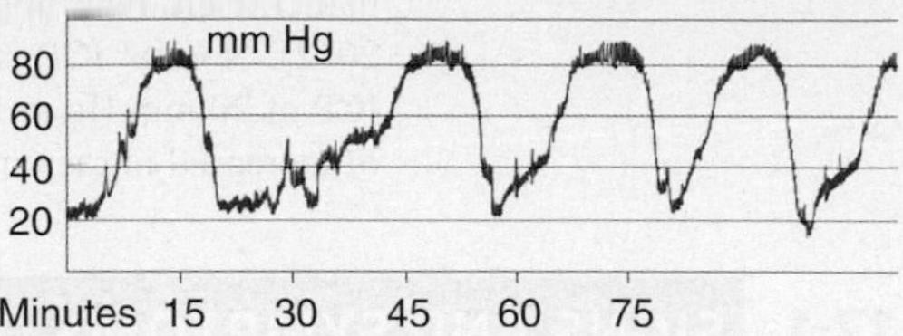

B Waves

B waves, which appear sharp and rhythmic with a saw tooth pattern, are shorter (30 seconds to 2 minutes) with ICP values of 20 to 50 mm Hg. They are seen in patients with intracranial hypertension and decreased intracranial compliance. B waves are an early indication of deteriorating neurologic status and may precede A waves.

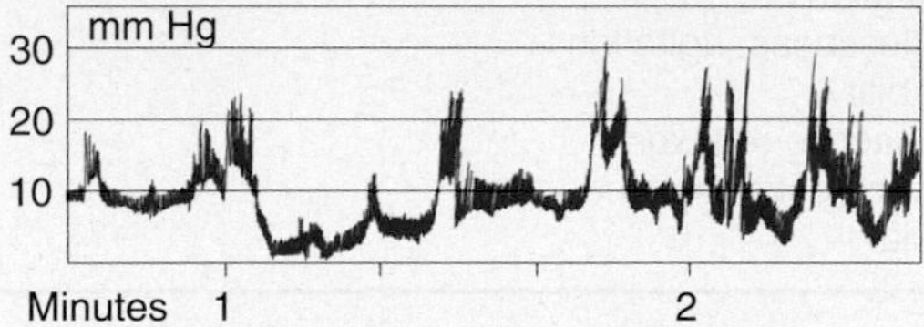

C Waves

C waves are rapid and rhythmic, but they are not as sharp as B waves. C waves are associated with ICPs as high as 20 to 25 mm Hg that persist for less than 5 minutes. They may fluctuate with respirations or systemic blood pressure changes and are considered normal responses to changes in ICP.

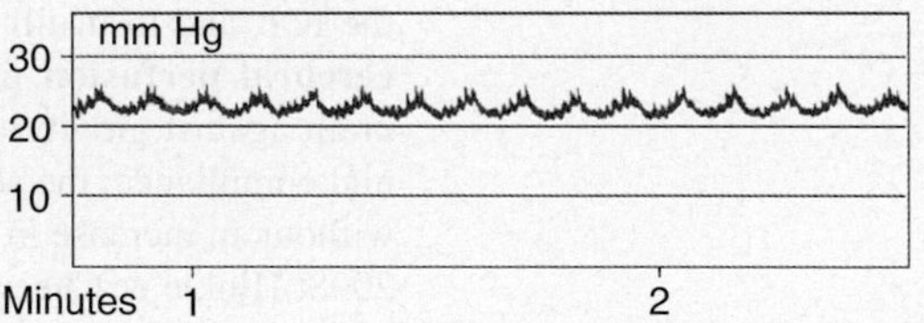

Adapted from Morton, P.G., & Fontaine, D.K. (2013). *Essentials of critical care nursing. A holistic approach.* Philadelphia: Wolters Kluwer Health/Lippincott Williams & Wilkins; Hinkle, J.L., & Cheever, K.H. (2014). *Brunner & Suddarth's textbook of medical-surgical nursing* (13th ed.). Philadelphia: Wolters Kluwer Health/Lippincott Williams & Wilkins; American Association of Critical Care Nurses (AACN). (2011). Lynn-McHale Wiegand, D.J. (Ed.). *AACN procedure manual for critical care* (6th ed.). Philadelphia: Elsevier Saunders; and Barker, E. (2008). *Neuroscience nursing. A spectrum of care* (3rd ed.). St. Louis, MO: Mosby Elsevier.

EQUIPMENT

- Ventriculostomy setup
- Carpenter level, bubble-line level, or laser level, according to facility policy
- PPE, as indicated

ASSESSMENT

Assess the color of the fluid draining from the ventriculostomy. Normal CSF is clear or straw colored. Cloudy CSF may suggest an infection. Red or pink CSF may indicate bleeding. Assess vital signs, because changes in vital signs can reflect a neurologic problem. Assess the patient's pain level. The patient may be experiencing pain at the ventriculostomy insertion site.

Perform a neurologic assessment (see Fundamentals Review 17-1 and Chapter 3). Assess the patient's level of consciousness. If the patient is awake, assess for his or her orientation to person, place, and time. If the patient's level of consciousness is decreased, note the patient's ability to respond and to be aroused. Inspect pupil size and response to light. Pupils should be equal and round and should react to light bilaterally. Any changes in level of consciousness or pupillary response may suggest a neurologic problem. If the patient can move the extremities, assess strength of hands and feet. (See Chapter 3, Health Assessment, for detailed instructions on assessing muscle strength.) A change in strength or a difference in strength on one side compared with the other may indicate a neurologic problem.

NURSING DIAGNOSIS

Determine the related factors for the nursing diagnoses based on the patient's current status. Appropriate nursing diagnoses may include:

- Risk for Injury
- Risk for Ineffective Cerebral Tissue Perfusion
- Pain
- Risk for Infection

OUTCOME IDENTIFICATION AND PLANNING

The expected outcome to achieve is that the patient maintains intracranial pressure at less than 15 mm Hg and cerebral perfusion pressure at 60 to 90 mm Hg (Hickey, 2014). Other outcomes that may be appropriate include the following: patient is free from infection; the patient is free from pain; and the patient/significant others understand the need for the ventriculostomy.

IMPLEMENTATION

ACTION	RATIONALE
1. Review the medical orders for specific information about ventriculostomy parameters.	The nurse needs to know the most recent order for the height of the ventriculostomy. For example, if the health care practitioner has ordered that the ventriculostomy is to be at 10 cm, this means the patient's ICP must rise above 10 cm before the ventriculostomy will drain CSF.
2. Gather the necessary supplies.	Preparation promotes efficient time management and an organized approach to the task.
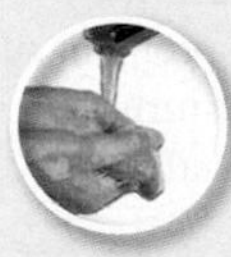 3. Perform hand hygiene and put on PPE, if indicated.	Hand hygiene and PPE prevent the spread of microorganisms. PPE is required based on transmission precautions.
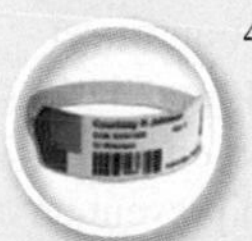 4. Identify the patient.	Identifying the patient ensures the right patient receives the intervention and helps prevent errors.
5. Close curtains around the bed and close the door to the room, if possible. Explain what you are going to do and why you are going to do it to the patient.	This ensures the patient's privacy. Explanation relieves anxiety and facilitates cooperation.
6. Assemble equipment on overbed table within reach.	Arranging items nearby is convenient, saves time, and avoids unnecessary stretching and twisting of muscles on the part of the nurse.
7. Assess patient for any changes in neurologic status. (See Fundamentals Review 17-1 and Chapter 3, Health Assessment, for details of assessment.)	Patients with ventriculostomies are at risk for problems with the neurologic system.

(continued)

SKILL 17-5 CARING FOR A PATIENT WITH AN EXTERNAL VENTRICULOSTOMY (INTRAVENTRICULAR CATHETER–CLOSED FLUID-FILLED SYSTEM) continued

ACTION	RATIONALE
8. Set the zero reference level. **Assess the height of the ventriculostomy system to ensure that the stopcock is at the appropriate reference point: the tragus of the ear (Figure 1), the outer canthus of the patient's eye or the patient's external auditory canal (AANN, 2011; Moreda et al., 2009), using carpenter level, bubble-line level, or laser level, according to facility policy.** Adjust the height of the system if needed.	For measurements to be accurate, the stopcock must be at a reference point to approximate the catheter tip at the level of the foramen of Monro. Use of the same reference point for all readings is critical to ensure accuracy (Moreda et al., 2009). Use of a carpenter level, bubble line level, or laser level, ensures accuracy (Moreda et al., 2009). If the ventriculostomy is used just to measure the ICP and not to drain the CSF, the stopcock will be turned off to the drip chamber.

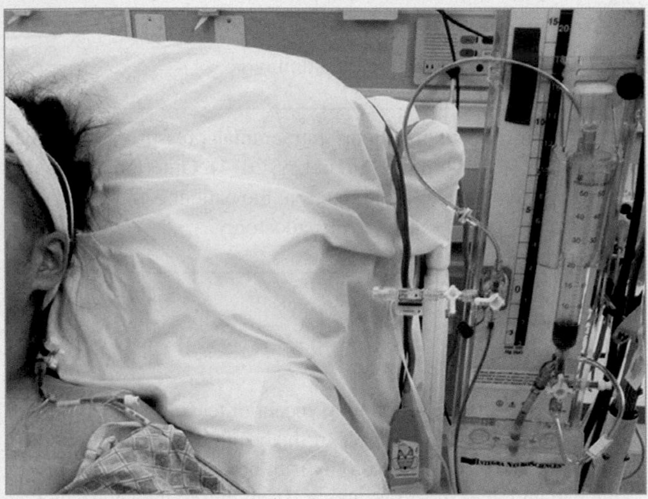

FIGURE 1 Transducer leveled with tragus. (© Copyright 2011 by AANN. All rights reserved.)

ACTION	RATIONALE
9. Set the pressure level, based on prescribed pressure. Move the drip chamber to the ordered height. Assess the amount of CSF in the drip chamber if the ventriculostomy is draining.	When the ICP is higher than the prescribed pressure level, cerebrospinal fluid will drain into the drip chamber. If the ventriculostomy is to drain CSF, the nurse must turn the stopcock off to the drip chamber to obtain a measurement of ICP. After the ICP value is obtained, remember to turn the stopcock back off to the transducer so that CSF is allowed to drain.
10. **Zero the transducer.** Turn the stopcock off to the patient. Remove the cap from the transducer, being careful not to touch the end of the cap. Press and hold the calibration button on the monitor until the monitor beeps. Return the cap to the transducer. **Turn the stopcock off to the drip chamber to obtain an ICP reading and waveform tracing. After obtaining a reading, turn the stopcock off to the transducer.**	The readings would not be considered accurate if the transducer had not been recently zeroed. If the stopcock is not turned off to the patient, when opened to room air, CSF will flow out of the stopcock. The end of the cap must remain sterile to prevent an infection. The stopcock must be off to the drip chamber (open to the transducer) to obtain an ICP. If the ventriculostomy is to drain CSF, the nurse must turn the stopcock off to the drip chamber. After the ICP value is obtained, remember to turn the stopcock back off to the transducer so that CSF is allowed to drain into the drip chamber.
11. **Adjust the ventriculostomy height to prevent too much drainage, too little drainage, or inaccurate ICP readings.**	If the patient's head is lower than the ventriculostomy, the drainage of CSF will slow or stop. If the patient's head is higher than the ventriculostomy, the drainage of CSF will increase. Any ICP readings taken when the ventriculostomy is not level with the outer canthus of the eye would be inaccurate.

ACTION	RATIONALE
12. Care for the insertion site according to the facility's policy. Maintain the system using strict sterile technique. Assess the site for any signs of infection, such as purulent drainage, redness, or warmth. Ensure the catheter is secured at site per facility policy. If the catheter is sutured to the scalp, assess integrity of the sutures (Figure 2).	Site care varies, possibly ranging from leaving the site open to air to applying antibiotic ointment and gauze. Sterile technique helps to prevent infection (Barker, 2008). Securing the catheters after insertion prevents dislodgement and breakage of the device.

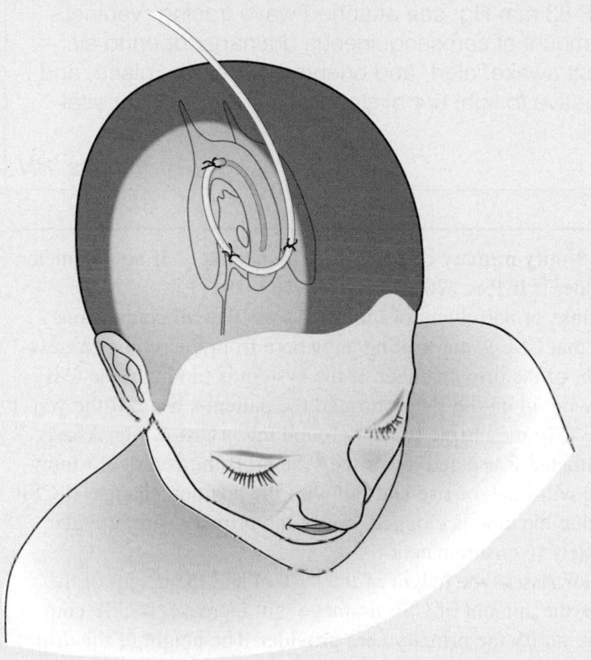

FIGURE 2 Sutured external ventriculostomy catheter.

ACTION	RATIONALE
13. Calculate the CPP, if necessary. Calculate the difference between the systemic MAP and the ICP.	CPP is an estimate of the adequacy of the blood supply to the brain.
14. Remove PPE, if used. Perform hand hygiene.	Removing PPE properly reduces the risk for infection transmission and contamination of other items. Hand hygiene prevents the spread of microorganisms.
15. Assess ICP, MAP, and CPP at least hourly. Note drainage amount, color, clarity. If there is an increase in the ICP, the value should be obtained more often, as often as every 15 minutes (AANN, 2011).	Frequent assessment provides valuable indicators for identifying subtle trends that may suggest developing problems.
16. Assess ICP drainage system at least every 4 hours, checking the insertion site, all drainage system tubing and parts, for cracks in the system or leakage from insertion site or system. Label external ventriculostomy tubing and access ports clearly.	Frequent monitoring allows for early identification of problems and prompt intervention. Clear labeling prevents accidental use as an intravenous access (AANN, 2011).

EVALUATION

The expected outcome is met when the patient demonstrates a CPP and an ICP within identified parameters; remains free from infection; understands the need for the ventriculostomy; and reports no pain.

(continued)

SKILL 17-5 CARING FOR A PATIENT WITH AN EXTERNAL VENTRICULOSTOMY (INTRAVENTRICULAR CATHETER–CLOSED FLUID-FILLED SYSTEM) continued

DOCUMENTATION

Guidelines

Document the following information: amount and color of CSF, ICP, and CPP; pupil status; motor strength bilaterally; orientation to time, person, and place; level of consciousness; vital signs; pain; appearance of insertion site; and height of ventriculostomy.

Sample Documentation

11/2/15 1410 External ventriculostomy zeroed; transducer level with outer canthus of eye, drip chamber 10 cm; draining cloudy, straw-colored CSF (12 mL), physician notified of clarity. ICP 10 mm Hg; CPP 83 mm Hg, see attached wave tracing. Ventriculostomy insertion site with small amount of serosanguineous drainage; open to air. Strong equal grip bilaterally. Patient awake, alert, and oriented to person, place, and time. Pupils equal, round, and reactive to light 6/4 bilaterally. See graphics for vital signs. Patient denies pain.

—B. Traudes, RN

UNEXPECTED SITUATIONS AND ASSOCIATED INTERVENTIONS

- *ICP exceeds established parameters:* Notify primary care provider immediately. If no parameter is specified, notify primary care provider if ICP is >20 mm Hg (AANN, 2011).
- *CSF stops draining:* Assess for any kinks or narrowing of tubing. Assess that all connections on the tubing are well connected and that CSF is not leaking anywhere from the tubing. Assess the height of the system and the height of the drip chamber. If the system is too high, the CSF drainage will taper off. Assess for any liquid on the sheets around the patient's head. If the ventriculostomy has become clogged, the CSF may begin to leak around the insertion site. Assess the patency of the ventriculostomy catheter. Raise and lower the system. If the ventriculostomy catheter is patent, the fluid in the tube will tidal, or rise and fall with the position change. If CSF still is not draining or if you believe that the tube is clogged, notify the primary care provider. The tube may need to be flushed sterilely to ensure patency.
- *The amount of CSF drainage increases:* Assess the height of the system and the height of the drip chamber. If the system is too low, the amount of CSF drainage will increase. If CSF continues to drain at an increased amount, notify the primary care provider. The height of the drip chamber may need to be increased.
- *CSF has changed from clear to cloudy:* Notify the primary care provider immediately. This can signify an infection, and antibiotics may need to be started.
- *CSF has changed from straw-colored to pink tinged or serosanguineous:* Notify the primary care provider immediately. This can signify bleeding in the ventricles of the brain.
- *Catheter is accidentally dislodged:* Notify the primary care provider immediately. Put on sterile gloves and cover the insertion site with sterile gauze. Monitor for color and amount of CSF if draining from site.

SPECIAL CONSIDERATIONS

- Secure the catheters according to facility policy after insertion and use care when moving patients to prevent dislodgement and breakage of these devices.
- Repositioning is important to prevent skin alterations and to decrease the risks associated with immobility. Modest, initial increases in ICP experienced with repositioning quickly return to baseline after repositioning is complete (McNett & Olson, 2013). Turn and position the patient in proper body alignment, avoiding angulation of body parts. Extreme hip flexion or flexion of upper legs can increase intra-abdominal pressure, leading to increased ICP. Use logrolling. Maintain the neck in neutral position at all times to avoid neck vein compression, which can interfere with venous return (Wyatt et al., 2009).
- Maintain the head of the bed elevated 15 to 30 degrees to promote venous return from the brain, depending on medical orders and facility procedure (Kyle & Carman, 2013; Wyatt et al., 2009).
- Endotracheal suctioning episodes should be limited to one to two passes of the catheter. The ICP increases associated with suctioning, tracheal stimulation, and coughing are modest and transient (McNett & Olson, 2013).
- Oral care is a safe intervention; ICP increases experienced with oral care are modest, transient, and resolve quickly when oral care is complete (McNett & Olson).

- Auditory stimulation for critically ill neurologically impaired patients does not increase ICP and is considered a safe intervention (McNett & Olson, 2013).
- Plan care to avoid grouping activities and procedures known to increase ICP. Bathing, turning, and other routine care often have a cumulative effect to increase ICP when performed in succession. Allow rest periods between procedures and carefully assess the patient's response to interventions (Hickey, 2014).

EVIDENCE FOR PRACTICE ▶

CLINICAL PRACTICE GUIDELINE: INTRACRANIAL PRESSURE MONITORING/ EXTERNAL VENTRICULAR DRAINAGE OR LUMBAR DRAINAGE

American Association of Neuroscience Nurses (AANN). (2011). Care of the patient undergoing intracranial pressure monitoring/external ventricular drainage or lumbar drainage. Glenview, IL: Author.

The American Association of Neuroscience Nurses (AANN) is a professional nursing organization committed to the advancement of neuroscience nursing as a specialty through the development and support of nurses to promote excellence in patient care. The AANN provides continuing education, information dissemination, standard setting, and advocacy on behalf of neuroscience patients, families, and nurses. This evidence-based practice guideline is a resource for registered nurses (RNs), patient care units, and facilities in providing safe and effective care to patients undergoing intracranial pressure (ICP) monitoring via an external ventricular drainage device (EVD) or those undergoing subarachnoid drainage of cerebrospinal fluid (CSF) with a lumbar drainage device (LDD).

Refer to thePoint for additional research on related nursing topics.

EVIDENCE FOR PRACTICE ▶

INTRACRANIAL PRESSURE AND ENDOTRACHEAL SUCTIONING

Endotracheal is a routing nursing intervention that can lead to an increase in ICP. Can use of a certain suction technique minimize the effect on ICP?

Related Research

Uğras, G.A., & Aksoy, G. (2012). The effects of open and closed endotracheal suctioning on intracranial pressure and cerebral perfusion pressure: A crossover, single-blind clinical trial. *Journal of Neuroscience Nursing, 44*(6), E1–E8.

This crossover, single-blind clinical trial was planned to determine the appropriate suctioning technique to minimize variability of intracranial pressure (ICP) and cerebral perfusion pressure (CPP) in neurologically impaired patients. The two suctioning techniques examined included open system suctioning and closed system suctioning. According to the need for suctioning, each patient in the experimental and control groups underwent suctioning with both closed and open systems. Recordings were composed of the patients' ICP, mean arterial blood pressure, CPP, heart rate, and arterial blood gases during suctioning. Both suctioning techniques significantly increased ICP, mean arterial blood pressure, CPP, and heart rate; ICP was found to be significantly higher in open suctioning compared with closed suctioning. No significant differences were found in CPP and heart rate between the two techniques. Patient suctioned using an open system had significantly lower mean partial pressure arterial oxygen measurements than those suctioned using a closed system. The authors concluded closed suction technique had fewer effects on ICP, MAP, CPP, and oxygen values.

Relevance for Nursing Practice

Nurses should consider interventions to provide the best care for patients. The information from this study can be used to assist in developing policies for nursing interventions and standards of practice related to endotracheal suctioning.

See additional Evidence for Practice related to caring for patients with intracranial pressure monitoring at the end of Skill 17-6, and refer to thePoint for additional research on related nursing topics.

SKILL 17-6 CARING FOR A PATIENT WITH A FIBER OPTIC INTRACRANIAL CATHETER

Intracranial pressure (ICP), the pressure inside the cranium, is the result of blood, tissue, and cerebrospinal fluid circulating in the ventricles and subarachnoid space (Moreda et al., 2009). ICP monitoring is used to assess cerebral perfusion. When ICP increases, as a result of conditions such as a mass (e.g., a tumor), bleeding into the brain or fluid around the brain, or swelling within the brain matter itself, neurologic consequences may range from minor to severe, including death (Hill et al., 2012). Normal ICP is less than 15 mm Hg. Elevated ICP, intracranial hypertension, is a sustained ICP of 20 mm Hg or more (Schimpf, 2012; Barker, 2008). Refer to Box 17-1 in Skill 17-5 for signs and symptoms of increased ICP in adults.

Fiber optic catheters are one method used to monitor intracranial pressure (ICP). Fiber optic catheters directly monitor ICP using an intracranial transducer located in the tip of the catheter. A miniature transducer in the catheter tip is coupled by a long, continuous wire or fiber optic cable to an external electronic module. This device can be inserted into the lateral ventricle, subarachnoid space, subdural space, brain parenchyma, or under a bone flap. The dura is perforated, and the transducer probe is threaded through the cerebral tissue to the desired depth and fixed in position (Hickey, 2009) (Figure 1). These devices are not fluid-filled systems, eliminating the problems associated with an external transducer and pressure tubing, such as an external ventriculostomy (Skill 17-5). The monitor provides continuous information (Cecil et al., 2011). Fiber optic catheters can be used to monitor the ICP and cerebral perfusion pressure (CPP). Some versions of catheters can also be used to drain cerebral spinal fluid (CSF). These devices are calibrated by the manufacturer and zero-balanced only once at the time of insertion.

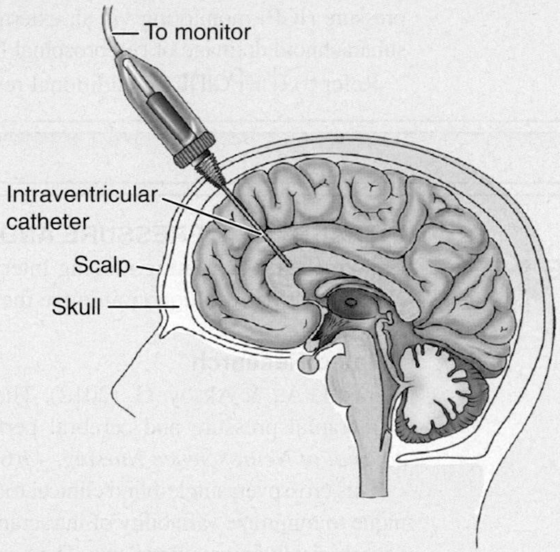

FIGURE 1 Fiber optic catheter in ventricle. (Adapted from Hinkle, J.L. & Cheever, K.H. (2014). *Brunner & Suddarth's textbook of medical-surgical nursing* (13th ed.). Philadelphia: Wolters Kluwer Health/Lippincott Williams & Wilkins, p. 1945.)

ICP and blood pressure measurements are used to calculate CPP, the pressure needed to perfuse the blood upward to the brain against gravity (Barker, 2008). ICP monitoring also provides information about intracranial adaptive capacity, the ability of the brain to tolerate stimulation or increase in intracranial volume without an increase in pressure through waveform assessment (AANN, 2011; Barker, 2008; Hinkle & Cheever, 2014). Box 17-2 in Skill 17-5 reviews ICP waveforms.

DELEGATION CONSIDERATIONS

The care of a patient with a fiber optic intracranial catheter may not be delegated to nursing assistive personnel (NAP) or to unlicensed assistive personnel (UAP). Depending on the state's nurse practice act and the organization's policies and procedures, care for these patients may be delegated to licensed practical/vocational nurses (LPN/LVNs). The decision to delegate must be based on careful analysis of the patient's needs and circumstances, as well as the qualifications of the person to whom the task is being delegated. Refer to the Delegation Guidelines in Appendix A.

EQUIPMENT

- PPE, as indicated

ASSESSMENT

Perform a neurologic assessment (see Fundamentals Review 1 and Chapter 3). Assess the patient's level of consciousness. If the patient is awake, assess the patient's orientation to person, place, and time. If the patient's level of consciousness is decreased, note the patient's ability to respond and to be aroused. Inspect pupil size and response to light. Pupils should be equal and round and should react to light bilaterally. Any changes in level of consciousness or pupillary response may suggest a neurologic problem. If the patient can move the extremities, assess strength of hands and feet. (See Chapter 3, Health Assessment, for detailed instructions on assessing muscle strength.) A change in strength or a difference in strength on one side compared with the other may indicate a neurologic problem. Assess vital signs, because changes in vital signs can reflect a neurologic problem. Assess the patient's pain level. The patient may be experiencing pain at the fiber optic catheter insertion site.

NURSING DIAGNOSIS

Determine the related factors for the nursing diagnoses based on the patient's current status. Appropriate nursing diagnoses may include:

- Risk for Infection
- Risk for Ineffective Cerebral Tissue Perfusion
- Risk for Injury
- Pain

OUTCOME IDENTIFICATION AND PLANNING

The expected outcome to achieve is that the patient maintains intracranial pressure at less than 15 mm Hg and cerebral perfusion pressure at 60 to 90 mm Hg (Hickey, 2014). Other outcomes that may be appropriate include the following: the patient is free from infection; the patient is free from pain; and the patient/significant others understand the need for the ventriculostomy.

IMPLEMENTATION

ACTION	RATIONALE
1. Review the medical orders for specific information about monitoring parameters.	The nurse needs to know the most recent order for acceptable ICP and CPP values.
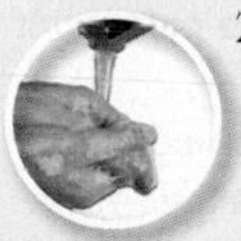 2. Perform hand hygiene and put on PPE, if indicated.	Hand hygiene and PPE prevent the spread of microorganisms. PPE is required based on transmission precautions.
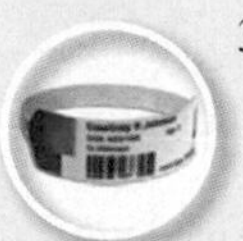 3. Identify the patient.	Identifying the patient ensures the right patient receives the intervention and helps prevent errors.
4. Close curtains around the bed and close the door to the room, if possible. Explain what you are going to do and why you are going to do it to the patient.	This ensures the patient's privacy. Explanation relieves anxiety and facilitates cooperation.
5. Assess the patient for any changes in neurologic status. (See Fundamentals Review 17-1 and Chapter 3, Health Assessment, for details of assessment.)	Patients with ventriculostomies are at risk for problems with the neurologic system.
6. Assess ICP, MAP, and CPP at least hourly. Note ICP value and waveforms as shown on the monitor. If there is an increase in the ICP, the value should be obtained more often, as often as every 15 minutes (AANN, 2011). Note drainage amount, color, clarity, as appropriate.	Frequent assessment provides valuable indicators for identifying subtle trends that may suggest developing problems. Some versions of catheters can also be used to drain cerebral spinal fluid (CSF).

(continued)

SKILL 17-6 CARING FOR A PATIENT WITH A FIBER OPTIC INTRACRANIAL CATHETER continued

ACTION	RATIONALE
7. Care for the insertion site according to the facility's policy. Maintain the system using strict sterile technique. Assess the site for any signs of infection, such as drainage, redness, or warmth. Ensure the catheter is secured at site per facility policy.	Site care varies, possibly ranging from leaving the site open to air to applying antibiotic ointment and gauze. Site care aids in reducing the risk for infection. Sterile technique helps to prevent infection (Barker, 2008). Securing the catheters after insertion prevents dislodgement and breakage of the device.
8. Calculate the CPP, if necessary. Calculate the difference between the systemic MAP and the ICP.	CPP is an estimate of the adequacy of the blood supply to the brain.
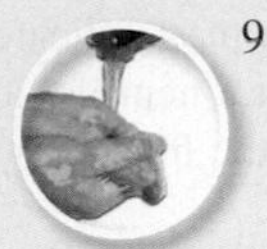 9. Remove PPE, if used. Perform hand hygiene.	Removing PPE properly reduces the risk for infection transmission and contamination of other items. Hand hygiene prevents the spread of microorganisms.

EVALUATION

The expected outcome is met when the patient demonstrates a CPP and an ICP within identified parameters; remains free from infection; understands the need for the catheter and monitoring; and reports no pain.

DOCUMENTATION

General Guidelines

Document the following information: neurologic assessment; ICP and CPP; vital signs; pain; appearance of insertion site.

Sample Documentation

11/2/15 1710 Patient sedated; disoriented and combative when awake. Pupils equal round and reactive to light 6/4 bilaterally. See graphics for vital signs. ICP 22 mm Hg; CPP 61 mm Hg; primary care provider notified. Dopamine drip increased to 8 μg/kg/min. Insertion site with small amount of serosanguineous drainage; site open to air.

—*B. Traudes, RN*

UNEXPECTED SITUATIONS AND ASSOCIATED INTERVENTIONS

- *ICP exceeds established parameters:* Notify primary care provider immediately. If no parameter is specified, notify primary care provider if ICP is >20 mm Hg (AANN, 2011).
- *Fiber optic catheter is accidentally dislodged:* Notify the primary care provider immediately. Put on sterile gloves and cover the site with sterile gauze. Observe for any CSF leakage from the site.
- *Waveforms are not changing with procedures known to cause an increase in the ICP (e.g., suctioning):* Fiber optic catheter may be damaged. Check the manufacturer's instructions for troubleshooting. Notify the primary care provider.
- *CSF is leaking from insertion site:* Notify the primary care provider. CSF is a prime medium for bacteria, and leakage can lead to an infection. Follow the facility's policy. Some facilities may have the nurse apply a sterile dressing around the insertion site; others may have the nurse cleanse the area more frequently.

SPECIAL CONSIDERATIONS

- Secure the catheters according to facility policy after insertion and use care when moving patients to prevent dislodgement and breakage.
- Repositioning is important to prevent skin alterations and to decrease the risks associated with immobility. Modest, initial increases in ICP experienced with repositioning quickly return to baseline after repositioning is complete (McNett & Olson, 2013). Turn and position the patient in proper body alignment, avoiding angulation of body parts. Extreme hip flexion or flexion of upper legs can increase intra-abdominal pressure, leading to increased ICP. Use logrolling. Maintain the neck in neutral position at all times to avoid neck vein compression, which can interfere with venous return (Wyatt et al., 2009).

- Maintain the head of the bed elevated 15 to 30 degrees to promote venous return from the brain, depending on medical orders and facility procedure (Kyle & Carman, 2013; Wyatt et al., 2009).
- Limit endotracheal suctioning episodes to one to two passes of the catheter. The ICP increases associated with suctioning, tracheal stimulation, and coughing are modest and transient (McNett & Olson, 2013).
- Oral care is a safe intervention; ICP increases experienced with oral care are modest, transient, and resolve quickly when oral care is complete (McNett & Olson, 2013).
- Auditory stimulation for critically ill neurologically impaired patients does not increase ICP and is considered a safe intervention (McNett & Olson, 2013).
- Plan care to avoid grouping activities and procedures known to increase ICP. Bathing, turning, and other routine care often have a cumulative effect to increase ICP when performed in succession. Allow rest periods between procedures and carefully assess the patient's response to interventions (Hickey, 2014).

EVIDENCE FOR PRACTICE ▶

NURSING INTERVENTIONS FOR PATIENTS WITH INTRACRANIAL PRESSURE MONITORING

McNett, M.M., & Olson, D.M. (2013). Executive summary. Evidence to guide nursing interventions for critically ill neurologically impaired patients with ICP monitoring. *Journal of Neuroscience Nursing, 45*(3), 120–123.

This Executive Summary addresses the research evidence for common nursing interventions for critically ill neurologically impaired patients with ICP monitoring. The interventions addressed include oral care, endotracheal suctioning, patient repositioning, chest physiotherapy, and auditory stimulation.

See additional Evidence for Practice related to caring for patients with intracranial pressure monitoring at the end of Skill 17-5, and refer to thePoint for additional research on related nursing topics.

ENHANCE YOUR UNDERSTANDING

FOCUSING ON PATIENT CARE: DEVELOPING CLINICAL REASONING

Consider the case scenarios at the beginning of the chapter as you answer the following questions to enhance your understanding and apply what you have learned.

QUESTIONS

1. Aleta Jackson, age 68, was involved in a head-on collision. She has begun to complain that the cervical collar is hurting her neck. How should you address this issue?
2. Yuka Chong had spinal surgery yesterday and is to be logrolled every 2 hours. The nurse caring for Yuka had her push her patient-controlled analgesia button 10 minutes before turning. As you prepare to turn Yuka and change her bed linens, you note that Yuka's dressing has a small saturated spot that has soiled the sheet. How should you address this issue?
3. Mr. and Mrs. Gladstone ask about "the tube coming out of Nikki's head," referring to her ventriculostomy. What should you tell them regarding the ventriculostomy? What should be included in the teaching for her parents? What guidelines regarding positioning and turning Nikki should you keep in mind when caring for her?

You can find suggested answers after the Bibliography at the end of this chapter.

ENHANCE YOUR UNDERSTANDING (continued)

INTEGRATED CASE STUDY CONNECTION

The case studies in Unit 3 are designed to focus on integrating concepts. Refer to the following case studies to enhance your understanding of the concepts related to the skills in this chapter.

- Intermediate Case Studies: Kent Clark, page 1085.

TAYLOR SUITE RESOURCES

Explore these additional resources to enhance learning for this chapter:

- NCLEX-Style Questions and other resources on thePoint, http://thePoint.lww.com/Lynn4e
- *Skill Checklists for Taylor's Clinical Nursing Skills,* 4e

Bibliography

Ackley, B.J., & Ladwig, G.B. (2011). *Nursing diagnosis handbook* (9th ed.). St. Louis: Mosby/Elsevier.

American Association of Critical Care Nurses (AACN). (2011). Lynn-McHale Wiegand, D.J. (Ed.). *AACN procedure manual for critical care* (6th ed.). Philadelphia: Elsevier Saunders.

American Association of Neuroscience Nurses (AANN). (2012). Cervical spine surgery. A guide to preoperative and postoperative patient care. Glenview, IL: Author.

American Association of Neuroscience Nurses (AANN). (2011). Care of the patient undergoing intracranial pressure monitoring/external ventricular drainage or lumbar drainage. Glenview, IL: Author.

Apold, J., & Rydrych, D. (2012). Preventing device-related pressure ulcers. *Journal of Nursing Care Quality, 27*(1), 28–34.

Baird-Holmes, S., & Brown, S. (2005). Skeletal pin site care. National Association of Orthopaedic Nurses: Guidelines for orthopaedic nursing. *Orthopaedic Nursing, 24*(2), 99–106.

Barker, E. (2008). *Neuroscience nursing. A spectrum of care* (3rd ed.). St. Louis: Mosby Elsevier.

Bhanushali, M., & Helmers, S. (2008). Diagnosis and acute management of seizure in adults. *Hospital Physician, 44*(11), 37–42, 48.

Buelow, J.M. (2013). Kathleen Mears Memorial Lecture: An update on patient safety issues in the epilepsy monitoring unit. *Neurodiagnostic Journal, 53*(2), 104–113.

Bulechek, G.M, Butcher, H.K., Dochterman, J.M., & Wagner, C.M. (Eds.). (2013). *Nursing interventions classification (NIC)* (6th ed.). St. Louis: Mosby Elsevier.

Caton-Richards, M. (2010). Assessing the neurological status of patients with head injuries. *Emergency Nurse, 17*(10), 28–31.

Cecil, S., Chen, P.M., Callaway, S.E., Rowland, S.M., Adler, D.E., & Chen, J.W. (2011). Traumatic brain injury: Advance multimodal neuromonitoring from theory to clinical practice. *Critical Care Nurse, 31*(2), 25–37.

Centers for Disease Control and Prevention (CDC). (2011). Epilepsy. First aid for seizures. Available http://www.cdc.gov/epilepsy/basics/first_aid.htm.

Clore, E.T. (2010). Seizure precautions for pediatric bedside nurses. *Pediatric Nursing, 36*(4), 191–194.

Cohen, J. (2009). Interrater reliability and predictive validity of the FOUR score coma scale in a pediatric population. *Journal of Neuroscience Nursing, 41*(5), 261–267.

Cox, B. (2008). The principles of neurological assessment. *Practice Nurse, 36*(7), 45–50.

Epilepsy Foundation. (2012). *About epilepsy. First aid.* Available http://www.epilepsyfoundation.org/aboutepilepsy/firstaid/index.cfm.

Epilepsy Foundation. (2012). *About epilepsy. Seizures.* Available http://www.epilepsyfoundation.org/aboutepilepsy/seizures/index.cfm.

Grossman, S., & Porth, C.M. (2014). Porth's pathophysiology: concepts of altered health states. (9th ed.). Philadelphia: Wolters Kluwer Health/Lippincott Williams & Wilkins.

Hickey, J. (2014). *The clinical practice of neurological and neurosurgical nursing.* (7th ed.). Philadelphia: Wolters Kluwer Health/Lippincott Williams & Wilkins.

Hill, M., Baker, G., Carter, D., Henman, L.J., Marshall, K., Mohn, K., et al. (2012). A multidisciplinary approach to end external ventricular drain infections in the neurocritical care unit. *Journal of Neuroscience Nursing, 44*(4), 188–193.

Hinkle, J.L., & Cheever, K.H. (2014). *Brunner & Suddarth's textbook of medical-surgical nursing* (13th ed.). Philadelphia: Wolters Kluwer Health/Lippincott Williams & Wilkins.

Hogan-Quigley, B., Palm, M.L., & Bickley, L. (2012). *Bates' nursing guide to physical examination and history taking.* Philadelphia: Wolters Kluwer Health/Lippincott Williams & Wilkins.

Iyer, V.N., Mandrekar, J.N., Danielson, R.D., Zubkov, A.Y., Elmer, J.L., & Wijdicks, E.F. (2009). Validity of the FOUR Score Coma Scale in the medical intensive care unit. *Mayo Clinic Proceedings, 84*(8), 694–701.

Jacobson, T., Tescher, A., Miers, A., et al. (2008). Improving practice: Efforts to reduce occipital pressure ulcers. *Journal of Nursing Care Quality, 23*(3), 283–288.

Jarvis, C. (2012). *Physical examination & health assessment* (6th ed.). St. Louis: Saunders/Elsevier.

Johnson, V.D., & Whitcomb, J. (2013). Perception of the use of the Full Outline of Unresponsiveness score versus the Glasgow Coma Scale when assessing the neurological status of intensive care unit patients. *Dimensions of Critical Care Nursing, 32*(4), 180–183.

Kocak, Y., Ozturk, S., Ege, F., & Ekmekci, A.H. (2012). A useful new coma scale in acute stroke patients: FOUR score. *Anaesthesia & Intensive Care, 40*(1), 131–136.

Kyle, T., & Carman, S. (2013). *Essentials of pediatric nursing* (2nd ed.). Philadelphia: Wolters Kluwer Health/Lippincott Williams & Wilkins.

Lagerquist, D., Dabrowski, M., Dock, C., Fox, A., Daymond, M., Sandau, K.E., et al. (2012). Clinical evidence review. Care of external fixator pin sites. *American Journal of Critical Care, 21*(4), 288–292.

Mayo Foundation for Medical Education and Research (MFMER). (2012). *Spinal injury: First aid.* Available http://www.mayoclinic.com/health/first-aid-spinal-injury/FA00010.

McNett, M.M., & Olson, D.M. (2013). Executive summary. Evidence to guide nursing interventions for critically ill neurologically impaired patients with ICP monitoring. *Journal of Neuroscience Nursing, 45*(3), 120–123.

Mink, J. (2012). The neurologic assessment toolbox: Key assessments at critical times. *Nursing2012Critical Care, 7*(3), 12–17.

Moorhead, S., Johnson, M., Maas, M.L., & Swanson, E. (Eds.). (2013). *Nursing outcomes classification (NOC)* (5th ed.). St. Louis: Mosby Elsevier.

Moreda, M.V., Wyatt, A.H., & Olson, D.M. (2009). Keeping the balance. Understanding intracranial pressure monitoring. *Nursing2009Critical Care, 4*(6), 42–47.

Morton, P.G., & Fontaine, D.K. (2013). *Essentials of critical care nursing. A holistic approach.* Philadelphia: Wolters Kluwer Health/Lippincott Williams & Wilkins.

NANDA-I International. (2012). *Nursing diagnoses: Definitions & classification 2012–2014.* West Sussex, UK: Wiley-Blackwell.

National Institute of Neurological Disorders and Stroke. (2013). *Seizures and epilepsy: Hope through research.* Available http://www.ninds.nih.gov/disorders/epilepsy/detail_epilepsy.htm#230383109.

Palmieri, R.L. (2009). Unlocking the secrets of locked-in syndrome. *Nursing, 39*(7), 22–30.

Palmieri, R.L. (2009). Wrapping your head around cranial nerves. *Nursing, 39*(9), 24–31.

Patchen, S.J., Timyam, L., & Atherton, S. (2010). Jerome Medical. *Your life in a halo made easier. Patient information manual.* Available http://assets.ossur.com/lisalib/getfile.aspx?itemid=7127

Perry, S.E., Hockenberry, M.J., Lowdermilk, D.L., & Wilson, D. (2010). *Maternal child nursing care* (4th ed.). Maryland Heights, MO: Mosby/Elsevier.

Puggina, A.C.G., da Silva, M.J.P., Schnakers, C., & Laureys, S. (2012). Nursing care of patients with disorders of consciousness. *Journal of Neuroscience Nursing, 44*(5), 260–270.

Sarro, A., Anthony, T., Magtoto, R., & Mauceri, J. (2010). Developing a standard of care for halo vest and pin site care including patient and family education: A collaborative approach among three greater Toronto area teaching hospitals. *Journal of Neuroscience Nursing, 42*(3), 169–173.

Schimpf, M.M. (2012). Diagnosing increased intracranial pressure. *Journal of Trauma Nursing, 19*(3), 160–167.

Strever, T. (2010). Care of the patient with cervical spine injury. *ORNurse, 4*(4), 26–34.

Taylor, C., Lillis, C., & Lynn, P. (2015). *Fundamentals of nursing.* (8th ed.). Philadelphia: Wolters Kluwer Health/Lippincott Williams & Wilkins.

Timms, A., & Hugh, P. (2012). Pin site care: Guidance and key recommendations. *Nursing Standard, 27*(1), 50–55.

Uğras, G.A., & Aksoy, G. (2012). The effects of open and closed endotracheal suctioning on intracranial pressure and cerebral perfusion pressure: A crossover, single-blind clinical trial. *Journal of Neuroscience Nursing, 44*(6), E1–E8.

Vacca, V.M. (2010). How to perform a 60-second neurologic exam. *Nursing, 40*(6), 58–59.

VISN 8 Patient Safety Center. (2009). *Safe patient handling and movement algorithms.* Tampa, FL: Author. Available http://www.visn8.va.gov/visn8/patientsafetycenter/safePtHandling/default.asp.

Walker, J. (2012). Pin site infection in orthopaedic external fixation devices. *British Journal of Nursing,* 213, 148–151.

Waterhouse, C. (2005). The Glasgow Coma Scale and other neurological observations. *Nursing Standard, 19*(33), 56–64.

Wijdicks, E.F.M., Bamlet, W.R., Maramattom, B.V., Manno, E.M., & McClelland, R.L. (2005) Validation of a new Coma Scale: the FOUR score. *Annals of Neurology, 58*(4), 585–593.

Wyatt, A.H., Moreda, M.V., & Olson, D.M. (2009). Keeping the balance. Understanding intracranial pressure. *Nursing2009CriticalCare, 4*(5), 18–23.

SUGGESTED ANSWERS FOR FOCUSING ON PATIENT CARE: DEVELOPING CLINICAL REASONING

1. Check the fit and placement of the collar. The center of the collar should line up with the center of the patient's neck. Center the front of the collar over the patient's chin, ensuring that the chin area fits snugly in the recess of the collar. Be sure that the front half of the collar overlaps the back half. Check to see that at least one finger can be inserted between collar and patient's neck. Check the skin under the cervical collar for any signs of skin breakdown. Have a second person immobilize the cervical spine. Remove the top half of the collar and cleanse the skin under the collar. Assess the skin for signs of irritation and/or breakdown. If not contraindicated, place the patient in the reverse Trendelenburg position to see if this helps. After replacing the collar, assess the tightness of the cervical collar; at least one finger should slide under the collar.
2. First assess the patient for excessive bleeding from the surgical site. Note the size of the area of drainage on the dressing and the bed linen. Obtain vital signs. Assess the patient for signs/symptoms of excessive bleeding, such as light-headedness, dizziness, and/or pallor. Perform a neurovascular assessment distal to the surgical site. Ensure that at least three other assistants are available to help turn the patient. Gather the linen necessary to change the patient's sheets while they are repositioning her. In addition, plan to place an additional moisture-proof pad under the patient, at the level of the incision and dressing, to protect the linen in case of further drainage. Check the patient's medical record for orders regarding a dressing change or reinforcement of the dressing. Combine changing/reinforcing the dressing, changing the bed linens, and logrolling the patient to prevent having to logroll the patient more times than necessary. Report findings to the primary care provider.
3. Include the following in discussions with the patient and her family: Explain what a ventriculostomy is and the rationale for placing it and the frequency with which it is used and how it helps with the patient's care. Answer any questions they may have regarding the equipment. When positioning and turning the patient, be aware of the location of the ventriculostomy and attached tubing. Ensure that the tubing is not kinked or obstructed by the activity. After positioning the patient, reassess the height of the system to ensure that the location of the stopcock remains at the appropriate reference point: the tragus of the ear, the outer canthus of the patient's eye, or the patient's external auditory canal (AANN, 2011; Moreda et al., 2009). Turn and position the patient in proper body alignment, avoiding angulation of body parts. Avoid extreme hip flexion or flexion of upper legs, which can increase intra-abdominal pressure, leading to increased ICP. Use logrolling and maintain the neck in a neutral position at all times to avoid neck vein compression, which can interfere with venous return. Keep the head of the bed elevated at 15 to 30 degrees to promote venous return from the brain, depending on medical orders and facility procedure (Kyle & Carman, 2013; Wyatt et al., 2009). Bathing, turning, and other routine care often have a cumulative effect to increase ICP when performed in succession. Allow rest periods between procedures and carefully assess the patient's response to interventions (Hickey, 2014).

18 Laboratory Specimen Collection

FOCUSING ON PATIENT CARE

This chapter will help you develop some of the skills related to collecting specimens of body fluids when caring for the following patients:

JOSEPH CONKLIN, age 90, has been admitted to the hospital due to confusion related to a suspected urinary tract infection. You are to obtain a urine specimen for urinalysis and culture.

HUANA YON, age 67, has made an appointment to see her primary physician for a yearly examination. She is to collect a stool specimen for occult blood testing.

CATHERINE YELETSKY, age 54, is a patient in the telemetry unit. She has been diagnosed with congestive heart failure and is receiving cardiac monitoring. She also has diabetes and requires peripheral capillary (fingerstick) blood sampling to monitor her blood glucose levels.

Refer to Focusing on Patient Care: Developing Clinical Reasoning at the end of the chapter to apply what you learn.

LEARNING OBJECTIVES

After studying this chapter, you will be able to:

1. Obtain a nasal swab.
2. Obtain a nasopharyngeal swab.
3. Collect a sputum specimen (expectorated) for culture.
4. Obtain a urine specimen (clean catch, midstream) for urinalysis and culture.
5. Obtain a urine specimen from an indwelling urinary catheter.
6. Test a stool specimen for occult blood.
7. Collect a stool specimen for culture.
8. Obtain a capillary blood sample for glucose testing.
9. Collect a venous blood specimen by venipuncture for routine laboratory testing.
10. Obtain a venous blood specimen for culture and sensitivity.
11. Obtain an arterial blood specimen for blood gas analysis.

KEY TERMS

arterial blood gas (ABG): a laboratory test that evaluates the adequacy of oxygenation, ventilation, and acid–base status

expectorate: expel from the mouth; spit

indole: produced by decomposition of tryptophan in the intestine; contributes to the peculiar odor of feces

lancet: a small, sharp device for piercing the skin
nares: plural for naris
naris: oval openings at the base of the nose
nasopharynx: upper portion of the throat (pharynx) located behind the nasal cavity
occult blood: blood that is hidden in a stool specimen or cannot be seen on gross examination
protocol: written plan that details the nursing activities to be executed in specific situations
skatole: produced by protein decomposition in the intestine; contributes to the peculiar odor of feces
standard: acceptable, expected level of performance established by authority, custom, or consent
Standard Precautions: precautions used in the care of all hospitalized individuals, regardless of their diagnosis or possible infection status; these precautions apply to blood, all body fluids, secretions, and excretions (except sweat), nonintact skin, and mucous membranes
sterile technique: involves practices used to render and keep objects and areas free from microorganisms

Laboratory specimens are collected to aid in the screening and diagnosing of patient health problems, in directing treatment, and in monitoring the treatment effectiveness. The most commonly collected specimens are blood, urine, and stool (Malarkey & McMorrow, 2012). Follow facility **protocol** to collect, handle, and transport specimens. Always observe **Standard Precautions** and use **sterile technique**, where appropriate. It is very important to adhere to protocols and standards, collect the appropriate amount, use appropriate containers and media, and store and transfer the specimen within specified timelines. It is also extremely important to ensure accurate labeling of any specimen collected, according to facility policy. These measures prevent invalid and inaccurate test results.

Patient teaching is an important part of specimen collection. Explain the rationale for the sample collection and the process for obtaining the specimen. Evaluate the patient's ability to follow the specific procedure for collecting the specimen.

When collecting a specimen, take care to prevent the outside of the container from becoming contaminated with any secretions or body fluids. Place all laboratory specimens in plastic bags marked "Biohazard" and seal the bags to prevent leakage during transportation.

This chapter reviews methods to obtain specimens for common laboratory tests. Nurses also must be knowledgeable about normal and abnormal findings associated with these laboratory tests. Fundamentals Review 18-1 and 18-2 highlight the normal findings associated with urine and stool specimens.

FUNDAMENTALS REVIEW 18-1

CHARACTERISTICS OF URINE

Characteristic	Normal Findings	Special Considerations
Color	A freshly voided specimen is pale yellow, straw-colored, or amber, depending on its concentration.	Urine is darker than normal when it is scanty and concentrated. Urine is lighter than normal when it is excessive and diluted. Certain drugs, such as cascara, L-dopa, and sulfonamides, alter the color of urine. Some foods can alter the color; for example, beets can cause urine to appear red in color.
Odor	Normal urine smell is aromatic. As urine stands, it often develops an ammonia odor because of bacterial action.	Some foods cause urine to have a characteristic odor; for example, asparagus causes urine to have a strong, musty odor. Urine high in glucose content has a sweet odor. Urine that is heavily infected has a fetid odor.
Turbidity	Fresh urine should be clear or translucent; as urine stands and cools, it becomes cloudy.	Cloudiness observed in freshly voided urine is abnormal and may be due to the presence of red blood cells, white blood cells, bacteria, vaginal discharge, sperm, or prostatic fluid.
pH	The normal pH is about 6.0, with a range of 4.6 to 8. (Urine alkalinity or acidity may be promoted through diet to inhibit bacterial growth or urinary stone development or to facilitate the therapeutic activity of certain medications.) Urine becomes alkaline on standing when carbon dioxide diffuses into the air.	A high-protein diet causes urine to become excessively acidic. Certain foods tend to produce alkaline urine, such as citrus fruits, dairy products, and vegetables, especially legumes. Certain foods, such as meats, tend to produce acidic urine. Certain drugs influence the acidity or alkalinity of urine; for example, ammonium chloride produces acidic urine, and potassium citrate and sodium bicarbonate produce alkaline urine.
Specific gravity	This is a measure of the concentration of dissolved solids in the urine. The normal range is 1.015 to 1.025.	Concentrated urine will have a higher-than-normal specific gravity, and diluted urine will have a lower-than-normal specific gravity. In the absence of kidney disease, a high specific gravity usually indicates dehydration and a low specific gravity indicates overhydration.
Constituents	*Organic* constituents of urine include urea, uric acid, creatinine, hippuric acid, indican, urene pigments, and undetermined nitrogen. *Inorganic* constituents are ammonia, sodium, chloride, traces of iron, phosphorus, sulfur, potassium, and calcium.	*Abnormal constituents* of urine include blood, pus, albumin, glucose, ketone bodies, casts, gross bacteria, and bile.

FUNDAMENTALS REVIEW 18-2

CHARACTERISTICS OF STOOL

Characteristic	Normal Findings	Special Considerations for Observation
Volume	Variable	Volume of the stool depends on the amount the person eats and the nature of the diet. For example, a diet high in roughage produces more feces than a soft, bland diet. Consistently large diarrheal stools suggest a disorder in the small bowel or proximal colon; small, frequent stools with urgency to pass them suggest a disorder of the left colon or rectum.
Color	Infant: Yellow to brown Adult: Brown	The brown color of the stool is due to stercobilin, a bile pigment derivative. The rapid rate of peristalsis in the breastfed infant causes the stool to be yellow. Stool color is influenced by diet. For example, the stool will be almost black if the person eats red meat and dark green vegetables, such as spinach. The stool will be light brown if the diet is high in milk and milk products and low in meat. The absence of bile may cause the stool to appear white or clay colored. Certain drugs influence the color of the stool. For example, iron salts cause the stool to be black. Antacids cause it to be whitish. Bleeding high in the intestinal tract causes a stool to be black due to the digestion of the blood. Bleeding low in the intestinal tract results in fresh blood in the stool. The stool darkens with standing.
Odor	Pungent; may be affected by foods ingested.	The characteristic odor of the stool is due to **indole** and **skatole**, caused by putrefaction and fermentation in the lower intestinal tract. Stool order is influenced by its pH value, which normally is neutral or slightly alkaline. Excessive putrefaction causes a strong odor. The presence of blood in the stool causes a unique odor.
Consistency	Soft, semisolid, and formed	Stool consistency is influenced by fluid and food intake and gastric motility. The less time stool spends in the intestine (or the shorter the intestine), the more liquid the stool. Many pathologic conditions influence consistency.
Shape	Formed stool is usually about 1 inch (2.5 cm) in diameter and has the tubular shape of the colon, but may be larger or smaller, depending on the condition of the colon.	A gastrointestinal obstruction may result in a narrow, pencil-shaped stool. Rapid peristalsis thins the stool. Increased time spent in the large intestine may result in a hard, marble-like fecal mass.
Constituents	Waste residues of digestion: bile, intestinal secretions, shed epithelial cells, bacteria, and inorganic material (chiefly calcium and phosphates); seeds, meat fibers, and fat may be present in small amounts.	Internal bleeding, infection, inflammation, and other pathologic conditions may result in abnormal constituents. These include blood, pus, excessive fat, parasites, ova, and mucus. Foreign bodies also may be found in the stool.

SKILL 18-1 OBTAINING A NASAL SWAB

A nasal swab provides a sample that can be cultured, which will aid in the diagnosis of infection and detect the carrier state for certain organisms. A nasal swab may be used to diagnose infectious respiratory tract diseases, such as influenza. It is commonly used to detect the presence of organisms, such as *Staphylococcus aureus,* which may colonize on the skin in the nose, skin folds, hairline, perineum, and navel. These organisms often survive in these areas without causing infection, unless the organism invades the skin or deeper tissues (CDC, 2011a). Some strains of *S. aureus* have developed resistance to antibiotics. A nasal swab can be part of the screening process to detect potential infection with drug resistant microorganisms (Higgins, 2008).

DELEGATION CONSIDERATIONS

Obtaining a nasal swab is not delegated to nursing assistive personnel (NAP) or to unlicensed assistive personnel (UAP). Depending on the state's nurse practice act and the organization's policies and procedures, this procedure may be delegated to licensed practical/vocational nurses (LPN/LVNs). The decision to delegate must be based on careful analysis of the patient's needs and circumstances, as well as the qualifications of the person to whom the task is being delegated. Refer to the Delegation Guidelines in Appendix A.

EQUIPMENT

- Nasal swab
- Sterile water (optional)
- Nonsterile gloves
- Goggles and face mask, or face shield
- Additional PPE, as indicated
- Biohazard bag
- Appropriate label for specimen, based on facility policy and procedure

ASSESSMENT

Assess the patient's understanding of the collection procedure, reason for testing, and ability to cooperate. Inspect the patient's **nares** and for the presence of nasal symptoms, such as discharge, erythema, or congestion. Assess for conditions that would contraindicate obtaining a nasal swab, such as injury to the nares or nose, and surgery of nose.

NURSING DIAGNOSIS

Determine the related factors for the nursing diagnoses based on the patient's current status. Appropriate nursing diagnoses may include:

- Risk for Infection
- Acute Pain
- Deficient Knowledge

OUTCOME IDENTIFICATION AND PLANNING

The expected outcome to achieve is that an uncontaminated specimen is obtained without injury to the patient and sent to the laboratory promptly. Additional outcomes that may be appropriate include the following: the patient verbalizes an understanding of the rationale for the procedure; and the patient verbalizes a decrease in anxiety related to specimen collection.

IMPLEMENTATION

ACTION	RATIONALE
1. Verify the order for a nasal swab in the medical record. Gather equipment. Check the expiration date on the swab package.	Verifying the medical order is crucial to ensuring that the proper procedure is administered to the right patient. Assembling equipment provides for an organized approach to the task. Swab package is sterile and should not be used past the expiration date.
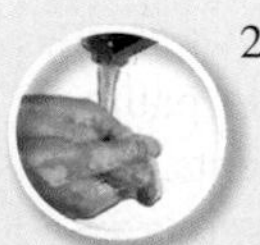 2. Perform hand hygiene and put on PPE, if indicated.	Hand hygiene and PPE prevent the transmission of microorganisms. PPE is required based on transmission precautions.
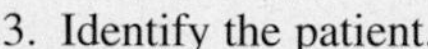  3. Identify the patient.	Identifying the patient ensures the right patient receives the intervention and helps prevent errors.

ACTION	RATIONALE
4. Explain the procedure to the patient. Discuss with the patient the need for a nasal swab. Explain to the patient the process by which the specimen will be collected.	Discussion and explanation help to allay some of the patient's anxiety and prepare the patient for what to expect.
5. Check the specimen label with the patient identification bracelet. Label should include the patient's name and identification number, time specimen was collected, route of collection, identification of the person obtaining the sample, and any other information required by facility policy.	Confirmation of patient identification information ensures the specimen is labeled correctly for the right patient.
6. Assemble equipment on overbed table within reach.	Arranging items nearby is convenient, saves time, and avoids unnecessary stretching and twisting of muscles on the part of the nurse.
7. Close curtains around the bed or close the door to the room, if possible.	Closing the door or curtain provides for patient privacy.
8. Put on goggles and face mask, or face shield and nonsterile gloves.	Goggles, face mask, face shield, and gloves protect the nurse from exposure to blood or body fluids and prevent the transmission of microorganisms.
9. Ask the patient to tip his or her head back slightly. Assist, as necessary.	Tilting the head allows optimal access to the nares, which is where the swab will be inserted.
10. Peel open the swab kit packaging to expose the swab and collection tube. Remove the white plug from the collection tube and discard. Remove the swab from packaging by grasping the exposed end. Take care not to contaminate the swab by touching it to any other surface. Moisten with sterile water, depending on facility policy.	Swab must remain sterile to ensure the specimen is not contaminated. Moistening the end of the swab minimizes discomfort to the patient.
11. Insert swab 2 cm into one **naris** and rotate against the anterior nasal mucosa for 3 seconds or five rotations, depending on facility policy, and then keep it there for 15 seconds (Figure 1).	Contact with the mucosa is necessary to obtain potential pathogens.

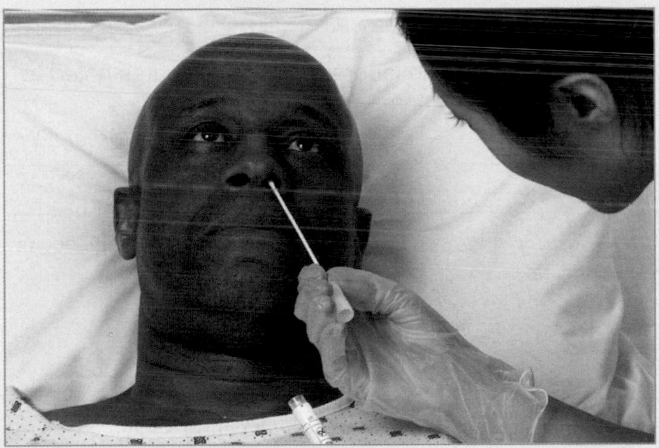

FIGURE 1 Inserting nasal swab into naris. *(Photo by B. Proud.)*

ACTION	RATIONALE
12. Remove the swab and repeat in the second naris, using the same swab.	Repeating in the second naris ensures accurate specimen.
13. Insert the swab fully into the collection tube, taking care not to touch any other surface. The handle end of the swab should fit snugly into the collection tube and the end of swab should be in the culture medium at the distal end of the collection tube. Lightly squeeze the bottom of the collection tube as necessary, depending on type of tube in use in facility, to break the seal on the culture medium.	Swab must remain uncontaminated to ensure accurate results. Full insertion of the swab ensures it will remain in the collection tube. Placement of swab end in culture medium and releasing the liquid transport medium are necessary to ensure accurate specimen processing.

(continued)

SKILL 18-1 OBTAINING A NASAL SWAB continued

ACTION	RATIONALE
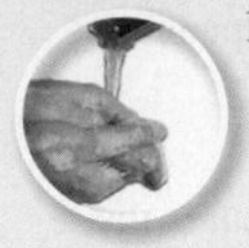 14. Dispose of used equipment per facility policy. Remove gloves. Perform hand hygiene.	Proper disposal of equipment reduces the transmission of microorganisms. Removing gloves properly reduces the risk for infection transmission and contamination of other items. Hand hygiene reduces the transmission of microorganisms.
15. Place label on the collection tube per facility policy. Place container in plastic, sealable biohazard bag.	Ensures specimen is labeled correctly for the right patient and ensures proper processing of the specimen. Packaging the specimen in a biohazard bag prevents the person transporting the container from coming in contact with the specimen.
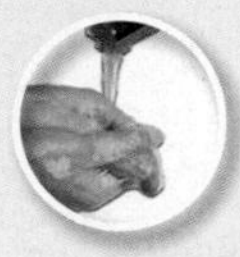 16. Remove other PPE, if used. Perform hand hygiene.	Removing PPE properly reduces the risk for infection transmission and contamination of other items. Hand hygiene reduces the transmission of microorganisms.
17. Transport specimen to the laboratory immediately. If immediate transport is not possible, check with laboratory personnel or policy manual whether refrigeration is contraindicated.	Timely transport ensures accurate results.

EVALUATION

The expected outcome is met when the nasal swab is collected without contamination and is sent to the laboratory as soon as possible. In addition, the patient does not experience injury, verbalizes an understanding of the rationale for the specimen collection, and verbalizes a decrease in anxiety related to the procedure.

DOCUMENTATION

Guidelines

Record the time the specimen was collected and sent to the laboratory. Document any pertinent assessments of the patient's nares and the presence of nasal symptoms, such as discharge, erythema, or congestion.

Sample Documentation

8/21/15 1545 Nasal swab collected and sent to the laboratory. Patient's nares noted to be patent without drainage, congestion, and erythema.

—*S. Turner, RN*

UNEXPECTED SITUATIONS AND ASSOCIATED INTERVENTIONS

- *Swab touches surface other than inner aspect of nares on entry or exit:* Discard the swab, obtain a new culture swab, and recollect the specimen.

SPECIAL CONSIDERATIONS

- If the patient has injury to the nares or nose or has had nose surgery the nurse should contact the primary care provider to discuss the specimen collection. These conditions may prohibit collection.
- If possible, ensure the specimen is obtained before antibiotics are started (Malarkey & McMorrow, 2012).

EVIDENCE FOR PRACTICE ▶

PATIENT-COLLECTED NASAL SWABS AND INFLUENZA TESTING

Influenza viruses, which are transmitted by coughing, sneezing, and contact with contaminated surfaces, are highly contagious. Could self-collected swabs be used to prevent close contact in the health care setting and reduce the spread of influenza? Can self-collected swabs be obtained accurately and efficiently by patients when compared with those collected by a trained health care worker?

Related Research

Dhiman, N., Miller, R.M., Finley, J.L., Sztajnkrycer, M.D., Nestler, D.M., Boggust, A.J., et al. (2012). Effectiveness of patient-collected swabs for influenza testing. *Mayo Clinic Proceedings, 87*(6), 548–554.

The objective of this study was to compare the effectiveness of self-collected and health care worker-collected nasal swabs for detection of influenza viruses and determine the patients' preference for type of collection. Adult patients presenting with influenza-like illness to the emergency department were included in the study. Patients self-collected a midturbinate nasal flocked swab from their right nostril following written instructions. All patients were observed during self-collection by the health care worker for adherence to instructions, but no collection guidance was provided. A second swab was then collected by a health care worker from the left nostril. Swabs were tested for influenza A and B viruses and percent of agreement between collection methods was determined. Of the 72 paired specimens, 25 specimens were positive for influenza A or B by at least one of the collection methods. After patients who had prior health care training were excluded, the agreement between collection methods was 94.8% (55 of 58). Two of the 58 specimens (3.4%) from patients without health care training were positive only by health care worker collection and 1 of 58 (1.7%) was positive only by patient self-collection. A total of 31 of 58 patients (53.4%) preferred the self-collection method over the health care worker collection. Fifteen (15) of 58 patients (25.9%) had no collection preference. The authors concluded self-collected nasal swabs provide a reliable alternative to health care worker collection for influenza testing.

Relevance for Nursing Practice

Self-collected nasal swabs for influenza could be a simple intervention to prevent close contact in the health care setting and decrease unnecessary utilization of health care services during influenza season. Patients could collect their own nasal swab and deliver it to a drop-off location for testing. This would reduce the potential for transmission by infected persons to others in health care settings, such as offices and emergency rooms, where the viruses could be spread rapidly between health care workers and high-risk patient populations. In addition, this intervention could reduce or eliminate unnecessary wait times for patients, decrease the financial burden and workload on emergency departments and outpatient clinics, and decrease costs to patients. Nurses have a role in these settings and are in a position to advocate for alternatives to the provision of health care to improve the care that patients receive and their health status.

Refer to thePoint for additional research on related nursing topics.

SKILL 18-2 OBTAINING A NASOPHARYNGEAL SWAB

A nasopharyngeal swab provides a sample that can be cultured to aid in the diagnosis of infection and to detect the carrier state for certain organisms. A swab on a flexible wire collects a specimen from the posterior **nasopharynx**. It is primarily used to detect viral infections. A nasopharyngeal swab is used for detection of *Bordetella pertussis* and *Corynebacterium diphtheriae,* as well as respiratory syncytial virus, *Neisseria meningitis,* methicillin-resistant *Staphylococcus aureus, Haemophilus influenza,* and viruses causing rhinitis (Azubike et al., 2012).

(continued)

SKILL 18-2 OBTAINING A NASOPHARYNGEAL SWAB continued

DELEGATION CONSIDERATIONS

Obtaining a nasopharyngeal swab is not delegated to nursing assistive personnel (NAP) or to unlicensed assistive personnel (UAP). Depending on the state's nurse practice act and the organization's policies and procedures, this procedure may be delegated to licensed practical/vocational nurses (LPN/LVNs). The decision to delegate must be based on careful analysis of the patient's needs and circumstances, as well as the qualifications of the person to whom the task is being delegated. Refer to the Delegation Guidelines in Appendix A.

EQUIPMENT

- Nasopharyngeal swab (flexible wire)
- Penlight
- Tongue depressor
- Facial tissue
- Nonsterile gloves
- Additional PPE, as indicated
- Biohazard bag
- Appropriate label for specimen, based on facility policy and procedure

ASSESSMENT

Assess the patient's understanding of the collection procedure, reason for testing, and ability to cooperate. Assess the patient's nares and for the presence of nasal symptoms, such as discharge, erythema, or congestion. Inspect the patient's nasopharynx. Assess for conditions that would contraindicate obtaining a nasopharyngeal swab, such as injury to the nares or nose, and surgery of the nose or throat.

NURSING DIAGNOSIS

Determine the related factors for the nursing diagnoses based on the patient's current status. Appropriate nursing diagnoses may include:

- Risk for Infection
- Acute Pain
- Deficient Knowledge

OUTCOME IDENTIFICATION AND PLANNING

The expected outcome to achieve is that an uncontaminated specimen is obtained without injury to the patient and sent to the laboratory promptly. Additional outcomes that may be appropriate include the following: the patient verbalizes an understanding of the rationale for the procedure; and the patient verbalizes a decrease in anxiety related to specimen collection.

IMPLEMENTATION

ACTION	RATIONALE
1. Verify the order for a nasopharyngeal swab in the medical record. Gather equipment. Check the expiration date on the swab package.	Verifying the medical order is crucial to ensuring that the proper procedure is administered to the right patient. Assembling equipment provides for an organized approach to task. Swab package is sterile and should not be used past the expiration date.
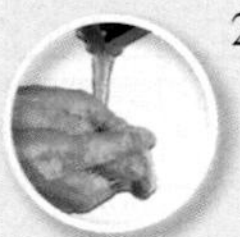 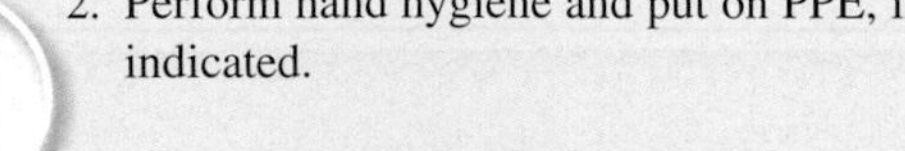 2. Perform hand hygiene and put on PPE, if indicated.	Hand hygiene and PPE prevent the transmission of microorganisms. PPE is required based on transmission precautions.
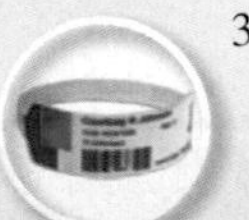 3. Identify the patient.	Identifying the patient ensures the right patient receives the intervention and helps prevent errors.
4. Discuss with patient the need for a nasal swab. Explain to patient the process by which the specimen will be collected. Inform the patient that he or she may experience slight discomfort and may gag.	Discussion and explanation help to allay some of the patient's anxiety and prepare the patient for what to expect.

ACTION	RATIONALE
5. Check the specimen label with the patient's identification bracelet. Label should include the patient's name and identification number, time specimen was collected, route of collection, identification of person obtaining the sample, and any other information required by facility policy.	Confirmation of patient identification information ensures the specimen is labeled correctly for the right patient.
6. Assemble equipment on overbed table within reach.	Arranging items nearby is convenient, saves time, and avoids unnecessary stretching and twisting of muscles on the part of the nurse.
7. Close curtains around the bed or close the door to the room, if possible.	Closing the door or curtain provides for patient privacy.
8. Put on goggles and face mask, or face shield and nonsterile gloves.	Goggles, face mask, face shield, and gloves protect the nurse from exposure to blood or body fluids and prevent the transmission of microorganisms.
9. Ask the patient to blow his or her nose into facial tissue. Ask the patient to cough into facial tissue, and then to tip back his or her head. Assist, as necessary.	Blowing of nose clears nasal passages and coughing clears the nasopharynx of material that may interfere with accurate sampling. Tilting the head allows optimal access to the nares, where the swab will be inserted.
10. Peel open the swab packaging to expose the swab and collection tube. Remove the cap from the collection tube and discard. Remove the swab from packaging by grasping the exposed end. Take care not to contaminate the swab by touching it to any other surface.	Swab must remain sterile to ensure specimen is not contaminated.
11. Ask the patient to open the mouth. Inspect the back of the patient's throat using the tongue depressor.	The swab must make contact with mucosa to ensure collection of potential pathogens.
12. Continue to observe the nasopharynx and gently insert the swab straight back into the nostril, aiming posteriorly along the floor of the nasal cavity (Figure 1A). Insert approximately 6 inches (adult) (approximately the distance from the nose to the ear) to the posterior wall of the nasopharynx (Figure 1B). **Do not insert the swab upward. Do not force the swab.** Rotate the swab. Leave the swab in the nasopharynx for 15 to 30 seconds and remove. Take care not to touch the swab to the patient's tongue or sides of the nostrils.	Observation of the nasopharynx during collection ensures an accurate specimen is collected. Swab must remain uncontaminated to ensure accurate results.

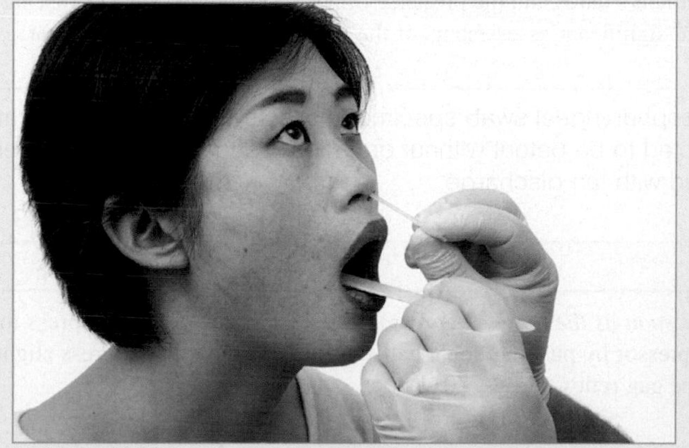

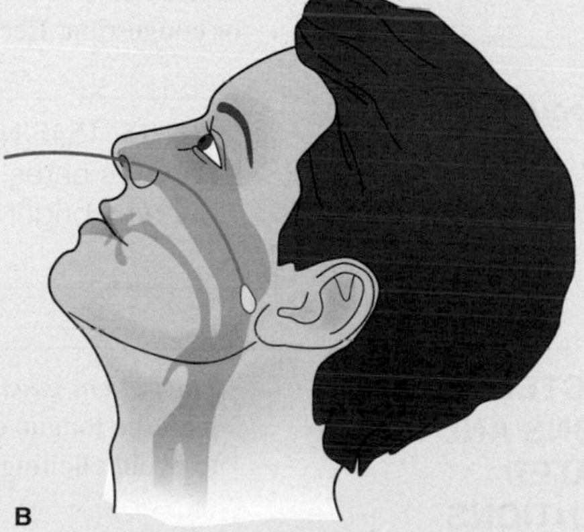

FIGURE 1 A. Observing the nasopharynx and inserting swab. **B.** Nasopharyngeal swab inserted to the posterior wall of the nasopharynx.

(continued)

SKILL 18-2 OBTAINING A NASOPHARYNGEAL SWAB continued

ACTION	RATIONALE
13. Insert the swab fully into the collection tube, taking care not to touch any other surface. The handle end of the swab should fit snugly into the collection tube and the end of swab should be in the culture medium at the distal end of the collection tube. Lightly squeeze the bottom of the collection tube as necessary, depending on type of tube in use in facility, to break the seal on the culture medium.	Swab must remain uncontaminated to ensure accurate results. Full insertion of the swab ensures it will remain in the collection tube. Placement of the swab end in culture medium and releasing of liquid transport medium is necessary to ensure accurate specimen processing.
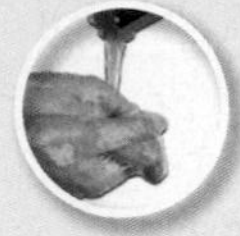 14. Dispose of used equipment per facility policy. Remove gloves. Perform hand hygiene.	Proper disposal of equipment reduces the transmission of microorganisms. Removing gloves properly reduces the risk for infection transmission and contamination of other items. Hand hygiene reduces the transmission of microorganisms.
15. Place label on the collection tube per facility policy. Place container in plastic, sealable biohazard bag.	Ensures specimen is labeled correctly for the right patient and ensures proper processing of specimen. Packaging the specimen in a biohazard bag prevents the person transporting the container from coming in contact with the specimen.
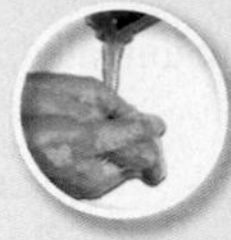 16. Remove other PPE, if used. Perform hand hygiene.	Removing PPE properly reduces the risk for infection transmission and contamination of other items. Hand hygiene reduces the transmission of microorganisms.
17. Transport the specimen to the laboratory immediately. If immediate transport is not possible, check with laboratory personnel or policy manual whether refrigeration is contraindicated.	Timely transport ensures accurate results.

EVALUATION

The expected outcome is met when the nasopharyngeal swab is collected without contamination and sent to the laboratory as soon as possible. In addition, the patient does not experience injury, verbalizes an understanding of the rationale for the specimen collection, and verbalizes a decrease in anxiety related to the procedure.

DOCUMENTATION

Guidelines

Record the time the specimen was collected and sent to the laboratory. Document any pertinent assessments of the patient's nares and the presence of nasal symptoms, such as discharge, erythema, or congestion. Record significant assessments of the patient's oral cavity and throat.

Sample Documentation

8/21/15 1545 Nasopharyngeal swab specimen collected and sent to laboratory. Patient's nares noted to be patent without drainage, congestion, and erythema; nasopharynx bright red with tan discharge.

—*S. Turner, RN*

UNEXPECTED SITUATIONS AND ASSOCIATED INTERVENTIONS

- *The patient gags as soon as the tongue depressor is placed in the mouth:* Depress the tongue with the tongue depressor by pushing down halfway back on the tongue. Press slightly off center to avoid eliciting the gag reflex (Jarvis, 2012).

SPECIAL CONSIDERATIONS

General Considerations

- Warn the patient that the procedure may cause slight discomfort.
- Caution the patient that the procedure may cause gagging.
- If possible, ensure the specimen is obtained before antibiotics are started (Malarkey & McMorrow, 2012).
- Do not force the swab. Forcing could cause injury. If an obstruction is encountered, try the other nostril (CDC, 2011b).

Infant and Child Considerations

- A young child will require restraint so the nurse can depress the tongue and visualize the back of the mouth without injuring the child (Kyle & Carman, 2013).

SKILL 18-3 COLLECTING A SPUTUM SPECIMEN FOR CULTURE

Sputum production is the result of the reaction of the lungs to any constant recurring irritant (Hinkle & Cheever, 2014). A sputum specimen comes from deep within the bronchi, not from the postnasal region. Sputum analysis is used to diagnose disease, test for drug sensitivity, and guide patient treatment. Sputum may be obtained to identify pathogenic organisms, determine if malignant cells are present, and assess for hypersensitivity states. A sputum specimen may be ordered if a bacterial, viral, or fungal infection of the pulmonary system is suspected. A sputum specimen can be collected by patient expectoration into a sterile container, by endotracheal suctioning, during bronchoscopy, and via transtracheal aspiration. Because secretions have accumulated during the night, it is desirable to collect an expectorated sputum specimen first thing in the morning when the patient rises, which aids in the collection process (Hinkle & Cheever, 2014). Characteristics of sputum and potential causes are outlined in Box 18-1. The following procedure describes collecting an expectorated sample. Collecting a sputum specimen by suctioning via an endotracheal tube is discussed in the Skill Variation at the end of this skill.

BOX 18-1 CHARACTERISTICS OF SPUTUM AND POTENTIAL CAUSES

Sputum Characteristic	Potential Cause
• Thick and yellow or green (purulent)	Bacterial infection
• Thin, white, or clear, mucoid (mucous)	Colds, viral infections, bronchitis
• Rust colored	Tuberculosis, pneumococcal pneumonia
• Gradual increase of sputum over time	Chronic bronchitis
• Pink-tinged, mucoid (mucous) sputum	Lung tumor, tuberculosis
• Profuse, frothy, pink sputum	Pulmonary edema
• Foul-smelling sputum and bad breath	Lung abscess, bronchiectasis, anaerobic infection

Adapted from Hinkle, J.L., & Cheever, K.H. (2014). *Brunner & Suddarth's textbook of medical-surgical nursing* (13th ed.). Philadelphia: Wolters Kluwer Health/Lippincott Williams & Wilkins; Jarvis, C. (2012). *Physical examination & health assessment* (6th ed.). St. Louis: Saunders/Elsevier; and Jensen, S. (2011). *Nursing health assessment.* Philadelphia: Wolters Kluwer Health/Lippincott Williams & Wilkins.

(continued)

SKILL 18-3 COLLECTING A SPUTUM SPECIMEN FOR CULTURE continued

DELEGATION CONSIDERATIONS

Obtaining a sputum specimen is not delegated to nursing assistive personnel (NAP) or to unlicensed assistive personnel (UAP). Obtaining a sputum specimen may be delegated to licensed practical/vocational nurses (LPN/LVNs). The decision to delegate must be based on careful analysis of the patient's needs and circumstances, as well as the qualifications of the person to whom the task is being delegated. Refer to the Delegation Guidelines in Appendix A.

EQUIPMENT

- Sterile sputum specimen container
- Nonsterile gloves
- Goggles or safety glasses
- Additional PPE, as indicated
- Biohazard bag
- Appropriate label for specimen, based on facility policy and procedure

ASSESSMENT

Assess the patient's lung sounds. Patients with a productive cough may have crackles, rhonchi, wheezing, or diminished lung sounds. Monitor oxygen saturation levels, because patients with excessive pulmonary secretions may have decreased oxygen saturation. Assess the patient's level of pain. Consider administering pain medication before obtaining the sample, because the patient will have to cough. Assess the characteristics of the sputum: color, quantity, presence of blood, and viscosity.

NURSING DIAGNOSIS

Determine the related factors for the nursing diagnoses based on the patient's current status. Appropriate nursing diagnoses may include:

- Acute Pain
- Ineffective Airway Clearance
- Impaired Gas Exchange

OUTCOME IDENTIFICATION AND PLANNING

The expected outcome to achieve when collecting a sputum specimen is that the patient produces an adequate sample (based on facility policy) from the lungs. Other outcomes that may be appropriate include the following: airway patency is maintained; oxygen saturation increases; the patient demonstrates an understanding about the need for specimen collection; and the patient demonstrates improved respiratory status.

IMPLEMENTATION

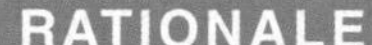

ACTION	RATIONALE
1. Verify the order for a sputum specimen collection in the medical record. Gather equipment.	Verifying the medical order is crucial to ensuring that the proper procedure is administered to the right patient. Assembling equipment provides for an organized approach to the task.
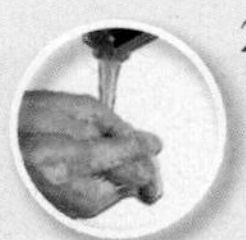 2. Perform hand hygiene and put on PPE, if indicated.	Hand hygiene and PPE prevent the transmission of microorganisms. PPE is required based on transmission precautions.
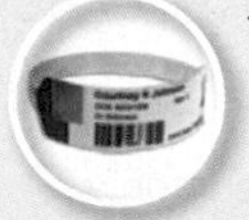 3. Identify the patient.	Identifying the patient ensures the right patient receives the intervention and helps prevent errors.
4. Explain the procedure to the patient. Administer pain medication (if ordered) if the patient might have pain with coughing. If the patient can perform the task without assistance after instruction, leave the container at bedside with instructions to call the nurse as soon as a specimen is produced.	Explanation provides reassurance and promotes cooperation. Pain relief facilitates compliance.
5. Check specimen label with the patient's identification bracelet. Label should include the patient's name and identification number, time specimen was collected, route of collection, identification of the person obtaining the sample, and any other information required by facility policy.	Confirmation of patient identification information ensures the specimen is labeled correctly for the right patient.

ACTION	RATIONALE
6. Assemble equipment on overbed table within reach.	Arranging items nearby is convenient, saves time, and avoids unnecessary stretching and twisting of muscles on the part of the nurse.
7. Close curtains around the bed and close the door to the room, if possible.	Closing the curtain or door provides for patient privacy.
8. Put on disposable gloves and goggles.	The gloves and goggles prevent contact with blood and body fluids.
9. Adjust the bed to a comfortable working height, usually elbow height of the caregiver (VISN 8 Patient Safety Center, 2009). Lower side rail closest to you. Place patient in semi-Fowler's position. **Have patient clear nose and throat and rinse mouth with water before beginning procedure.**	Having the bed at the proper height prevents back and muscle strain. The semi-Fowler's position will help the patient to cough and expectorate the sputum specimen. Water will rinse the oral cavity of saliva and any food particles.
10. Caution the patient to avoid spitting saliva secretion into the sterile container. **Instruct the patient to inhale deeply two or three times and cough with exhalation.** If the patient has had abdominal surgery, assist the patient to splint the abdomen.	Saliva can contaminate the sputum specimen. The specimen will need to come from the lungs; saliva is not acceptable. Splinting helps to reduce the pain in the abdominal incision.
11. If the patient produces sputum, open the lid to the container and have the patient **expectorate** the specimen into the container (Figure 1). Caution the patient to avoid touching the edge or the inside of the collection container.	The specimen needs to come from the lungs; saliva is not acceptable. Touching the edge or inside of the sterile collection container contaminates the specimen.

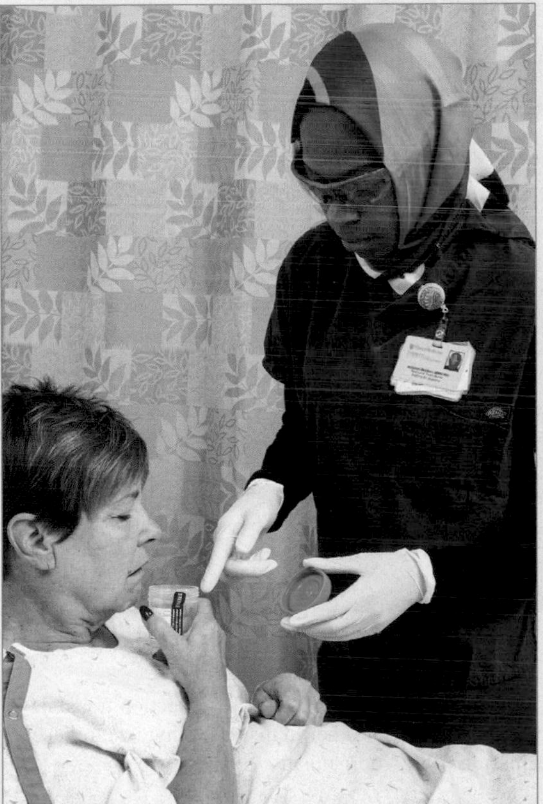

FIGURE 1 Instructing patient to expectorate into the collection container.

(continued)

SKILL 18-3 COLLECTING A SPUTUM SPECIMEN FOR CULTURE continued

ACTION	RATIONALE
12. If patient believes he or she can produce more sputum for the specimen, have the patient repeat the procedure. Collect a volume of sputum based on facility policy.	This ensures an adequate amount of sputum specimen is obtained for analysis.
13. Close the container lid. Offer oral hygiene to the patient.	Closing the container prevents contamination of the specimen and possible infection transmission. Oral hygiene helps to remove pathogens from the oral cavity.
14. Remove equipment and return the patient to a position of comfort. Raise side rail and lower bed.	Repositioning promotes patient comfort. Raising rails promotes safety.
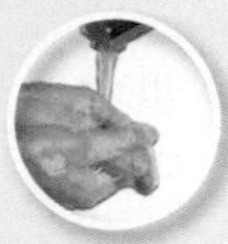 15. Remove gloves and goggles. Perform hand hygiene.	Removing gloves and goggles properly reduces the risk for infection transmission and contamination of other items. Hand hygiene reduces the transmission of microorganisms.
16. Place label on the container per facility policy (Figure 2). Place container in plastic, sealable biohazard bag (Figure 3).	Proper labeling of the specimen ensures the specimen is for the right patient. Packaging the specimen in a biohazard bag prevents the person transporting the container from coming in contact with the specimen.

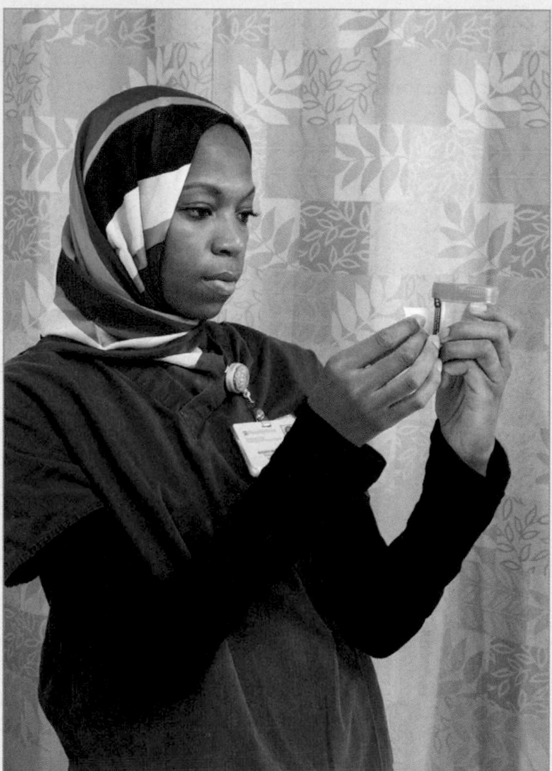

FIGURE 2 Labeling specimen container.

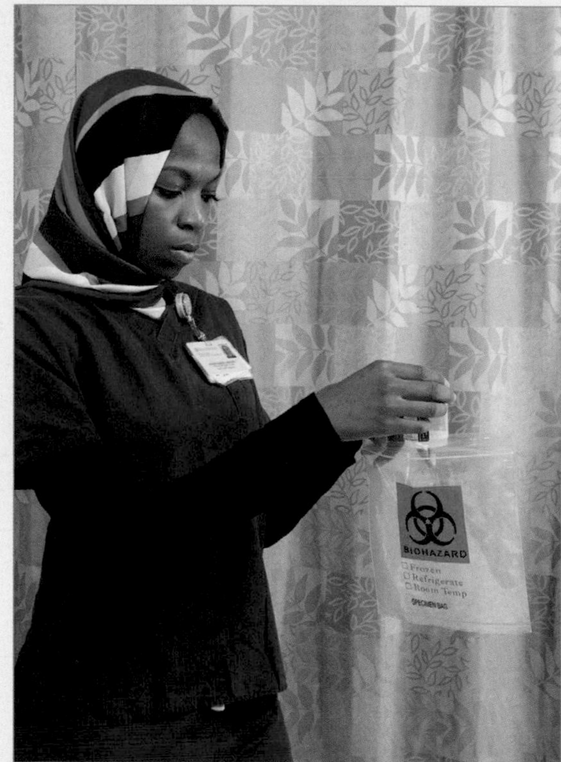

FIGURE 3 Placing specimen container in biohazard bag.

ACTION	RATIONALE
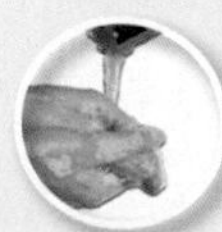 17. Remove other PPE, if used. Perform hand hygiene.	Removing PPE properly reduces the risk for infection transmission and contamination of other items. Hand hygiene reduces the transmission of microorganisms.
18. Transport the specimen to the laboratory immediately. If immediate transport is not possible, check with laboratory personnel or policy manual whether refrigeration is contraindicated.	Timely transport ensures accurate results.

EVALUATION

The expected outcome is met when the patient expectorates sputum, and it is collected in a sterile container and sent to the laboratory as soon as possible. In addition, the patient maintains a patent airway, oxygen saturation level is within expected parameters, and the patient demonstrates understanding about the rationale for the specimen collection.

DOCUMENTATION

Guidelines

Record the time the sputum specimen was collected and sent to the laboratory, and the characteristics and amount of secretions. Document the tests for which the specimen was collected. Note the respiratory assessment pre- and post-collection. Note antibiotics administered in the past 24 hours on the laboratory request form, if required by the facility.

Sample Documentation

9/13/15 0615 Respirations unlabored; lungs with decreased breath sounds at posterior bases. Sputum specimen obtained; patient has moderate amount of thick, yellow sputum; specimen sent to laboratory for culture and sensitivity.

—C. Bausler, RN

UNEXPECTED SITUATIONS AND ASSOCIATED INTERVENTIONS

- *Patient produced a specimen but did not tell you, so you do not know how long the specimen has been sitting at the bedside:* Unless the patient is able to tell you when the specimen was produced, discard the sample and recollect. Most specimens should be sent to the laboratory as soon as possible to ensure valid results.
- *Patient spits saliva into container, without specimen from lungs:* Instruct the patient that the specimen needs to come from the lungs. Review the procedure for collection. Discard the contaminated container and place a new container at the bedside.

SPECIAL CONSIDERATIONS

General Considerations

- If possible, collect sputum sample when patient arises in the morning, to improve chances of obtaining an adequate amount of sputum. Specimens from deep in the lungs are obtained in the early morning after secretions have accumulated overnight (Hinkle & Cheever, 2014).
- If possible, ensure the specimen is obtained before antibiotics are started (Malarkey & McMorrow, 2012).
- Unless contraindicated, assist in providing, and encourage the patient to consume, extra fluids the night before testing; increased fluid intake aids in liquefying secretions and may make it easier to expectorate sputum in the morning (Van Leeuwen et al., 2011).
- Sputum specimens for acid-fast bacilli (AFB; to test for tuberculosis) should be collected at least 8 to 24 hours apart, with at least one specimen produced in the morning (CDC, 2012).
- If the patient understands directions and is able to cooperate, the specimen-collection container may be left at bedside for the patient to collect sputum when available. Container lid should remain in place until the patient is ready to expectorate sputum. Instruct the patient to call to inform staff as soon as sputum is produced, so it can be transported to laboratory in a timely manner.

Home Care Considerations

- If the patient is to collect specimen at home, ensure that he or she has a clear understanding of the collection procedure and that the specimen needs to be transported immediately to the laboratory. Reinforce to the patient that it is important not to touch the inside of the collection container.

(continued)

SKILL 18-3 COLLECTING A SPUTUM SPECIMEN FOR CULTURE continued

SKILL VARIATION Collecting Sputum Specimen via Endotracheal Suctioning

1. Sputum specimens can be collected by suctioning an endotracheal tube or tracheostomy tube. A sterile collection receptacle is attached between the suction catheter and the suction tubing to trap sputum as it is removed from the patient's airway, before reaching the suction collection canister.
2. Refer to Skills 14-8, 14-9, and 14-11 for the procedure for endotracheal suctioning.
3. After checking suction pressure (Step 9, Skill 14-8; Step 8, Skill 14-9; Step 9, Skill 14-11), attach a sterile specimen trap to the suction tubing, taking care to avoid contaminating the open ends (Figure A).
4. Continue with Step 10, Skill 14-8; Step 9, Skill 14-9; Step 10, Skill 14-11, taking care to handle the suction tubing and sputum trap with your nondominant hand. Proceed with suction procedure.
5. After first suction pass, if 5 to 10 mL of sputum has been obtained, disconnect the specimen container, and set aside (LeFever Kee, 2013). If less than this amount has been collected, re-suction the patient, after waiting the appropriate amount of time for the patient to recover.
6. If secretions are extremely thick or tenacious, flush the catheter with a small amount (1 to 2 mL) of sterile normal saline to aid in moving the secretions into the trap.
7. Once the sputum trap is removed, connect suction tubing to the suction catheter. The catheter may then be flushed with normal saline before suctioning again. Continue with the suctioning procedure, if necessary, based on remaining steps in Skill 14-8, Skill 14-9, or Skill 14-11.

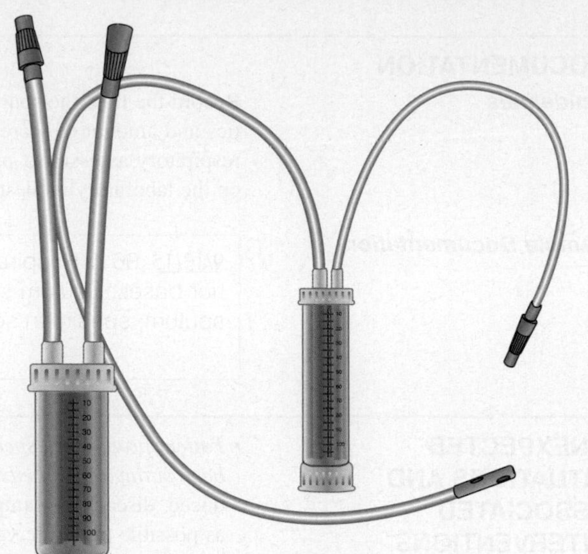

FIGURE A Suction trap for sputum collection.

8. When suctioning is completed, check the specimen label with the patient's identification bracelet. Label should include the patient's name and identification number, time specimen was collected, route of collection, identification of person obtaining the sample, and any other information required by facility policy. Place label on the container per facility policy. Place container in plastic, sealable biohazard bag and send to the laboratory immediately.

SKILL 18-4 COLLECTING A URINE SPECIMEN (CLEAN CATCH, MIDSTREAM) FOR URINALYSIS AND CULTURE

Collecting a urine specimen for urinalysis and culture is an assessment measure to determine the characteristics of a patient's urine. A voided urine specimen for culture is collected midstream to provide a specimen that most closely reflects the characteristics of the urine being produced by the body. If the patient is able to understand and follow the procedure, the patient may collect the sample on his or her own, after explanation and instruction.

DELEGATION CONSIDERATIONS

Obtaining a urine specimen by midstream collection may be delegated to nursing assistive personnel (NAP) or to unlicensed assistive personnel (UAP), as well as to licensed practical/vocational nurses (LPN/LVNs). The decision to delegate must be based on careful analysis of the patient's needs and circumstances, as well as the qualifications of the person to whom the task is being delegated. Refer to the Delegation Guidelines in Appendix A.

EQUIPMENT

- Moist cleansing towelettes or skin cleanser, water, and washcloth
- Nonsterile gloves
- Additional PPE, as indicated
- Sterile specimen container; urine collection tubes, based on facility policy
- Biohazard bag
- Appropriate label for specimen, based on facility policy and procedure

ASSESSMENT

Ask the patient about any medications that he or she is taking, because medications may affect the results of the test. Assess for any signs and symptoms of a urinary tract infection, such as burning, pain (dysuria), or frequency. Assess the patient's ability to cooperate with the collection process. Determine the need for assistance to obtain specimen correctly.

NURSING DIAGNOSIS

Determine the related factors for the nursing diagnoses based on the patient's current status. Possible nursing diagnoses may include:

- Impaired Urinary Elimination
- Anxiety
- Deficient Knowledge

OUTCOME IDENTIFICATION AND PLANNING

The expected outcome to achieve is that an adequate amount of urine is obtained from the patient without contamination. Other outcomes include the following: the patient exhibits minimal anxiety during specimen collection and demonstrates an ability to collect a clean urine specimen.

IMPLEMENTATION

ACTION	RATIONALE
1. Verify the order for a urine specimen collection in the medical record. Gather equipment.	Verifying the medical order is crucial to ensuring that the proper procedure is administered to the right patient. Assembling equipment provides for an organized approach to the task.
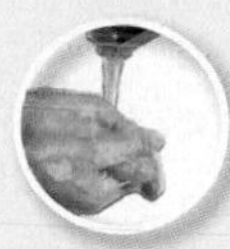 2. Perform hand hygiene and put on PPE, if indicated.	Hand hygiene and PPE prevent the transmission of microorganisms. PPE is required based on transmission precautions.
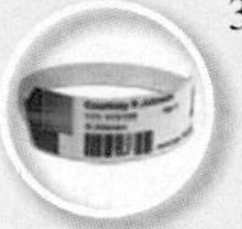 3. Identify the patient.	Identifying the patient ensures the right patient receives the intervention and helps prevent errors.
4. Explain the procedure to the patient. If the patient can perform the task without assistance after instruction, leave the container at bedside with instructions to call the nurse as soon as a specimen is produced.	Explanation provides reassurance and promotes cooperation.
5. Check the specimen label with the patient's identification bracelet. Label should include the patient's name and identification number, time specimen was collected, route of collection, identification of the person obtaining the sample, and any other information required by facility policy.	Confirmation of patient identification information ensures the specimen is labeled correctly for the right patient.
6. Assemble equipment on overbed table within reach.	Arranging items nearby is convenient, saves time, and avoids unnecessary stretching and twisting of muscles on the part of the nurse.
7. Have the patient perform hand hygiene, if performing self-collection.	Hand hygiene prevents the transmission of microorganisms.
8. Close curtains around the bed and close the door to the room, if possible.	Closing the door or curtain provides for patient privacy.

(continued)

SKILL 18-4 COLLECTING A URINE SPECIMEN (CLEAN CATCH, MIDSTREAM) FOR URINALYSIS AND CULTURE continued

ACTION	RATIONALE
9. Put on nonsterile gloves. Assist the patient to the bathroom, or onto the bedside commode or bedpan. Instruct the patient not to defecate or discard toilet paper into the urine (Figure 1).	Gloves reduce the transmission of microorganisms. Stool and/or toilet paper may contaminate the specimen.
10. Instruct the female patient to separate the labia for cleaning of the area and during collection of urine. Female patients should use the towelettes or wet washcloth to clean each side of the urinary meatus, then the center over the meatus, from front to back, using a new wipe or a clean area of the washcloth for each stroke. Instruct the female patient to **keep the labia separated after cleaning and during collection** (Figure 2). Male patients should use a towelette to clean the tip of the penis, wiping in a circular motion away from the urethra. Instruct the uncircumcised male patient to retract the foreskin before cleaning and during collection (Figure 3).	Cleaning the perineal area or penis reduces the risk for contamination of the specimen. Separation of labia avoids contamination by perineal skin and hair. Retraction of foreskin avoids contamination by skin.

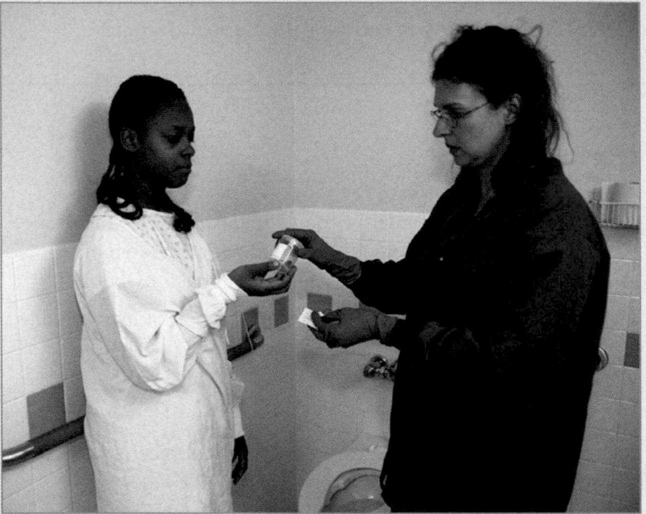

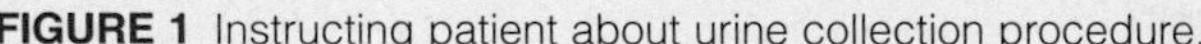

FIGURE 1 Instructing patient about urine collection procedure.

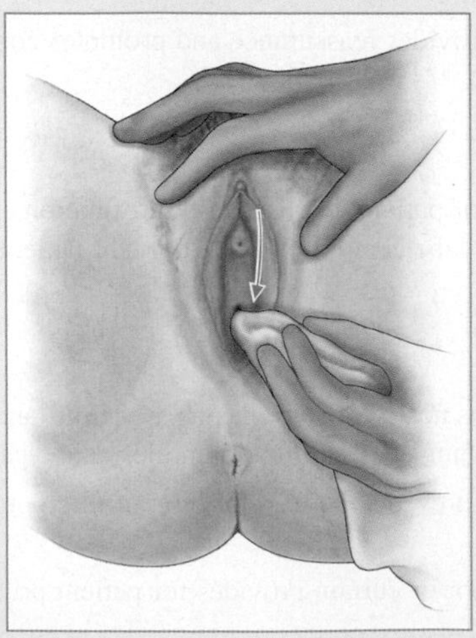

FIGURE 2 Cleaning female perineum. Separating labia and cleansing from front to back.

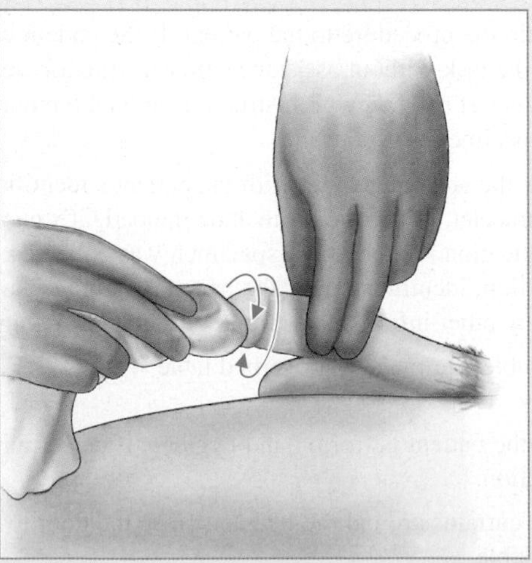

FIGURE 3 Cleaning male perineum. Wiping in a circular motion away from urethra.

ACTION	RATIONALE
11. **Do not let the container touch the perineal skin or hair during collection. Do not touch the inside of the container or the lid. Have patient void a small amount (approx. 30 mL/1 oz.) of urine into the toilet, bedpan, or commode. The patient should then stop urinating briefly, and then continue voiding into the collection container.** Collect the urine specimen (10 to 20 mL is sufficient), and then instruct the patient to finish voiding in the toilet, bedpan, or commode. Instruct the uncircumcised male patient to replace the foreskin after collection.	Collecting a midstream specimen ensures that fresh urine is analyzed. Some urine may have collected in the urethra from the last void. By voiding a little before collecting the specimen, the specimen will contain only fresh urine.
12. Place lid on container. If necessary, transfer the specimen to appropriate containers/tubes for specific test ordered, according to facility policy.	Placing the lid on the container helps to keep the specimen clean and prevents spills.
13. Assist the patient from the bathroom, off the commode, or off the bedpan. Provide perineal care, if necessary.	Perineal care promotes patient comfort and hygiene.
14. Remove gloves and perform hand hygiene.	Removing gloves properly reduces the risk for infection transmission and contamination of other items. Hand hygiene reduces the transmission of microorganisms.
15. Place label on the container per facility policy. Note specimen collection method, according to facility policy. Place container in plastic, sealable biohazard bag.	Proper labeling ensures accurate reporting of results. Packaging the specimen in a biohazard bag prevents the person transporting the container from coming in contact with urine.
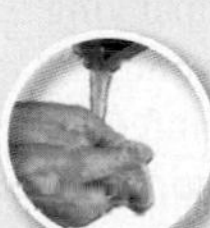 16. Remove other PPE, if used. Perform hand hygiene.	Removing PPE properly reduces the risk for infection transmission and contamination of other items. Hand hygiene reduces the transmission of microorganisms.
17. Transport the specimen to the laboratory as soon as possible. If unable to take the specimen to the laboratory immediately, refrigerate it.	If not refrigerated immediately, urine may act as a culture medium, allowing bacteria to multiply and skewing the results of testing. Refrigeration prevents the bacteria from multiplying.

EVALUATION

The expected outcome is met when an uncontaminated urine specimen is collected and sent to the laboratory promptly. Other outcomes may include the following: the patient demonstrated the proper technique for specimen collection and stated that anxiety is lessened.

DOCUMENTATION

Guidelines

Document that the specimen was sent to the laboratory. Note the specimen collection method. Note the characteristics of the urine, including odor, amount (if known), color, and clarity. Include any significant patient assessments, such as patient complaints of burning or pain on urination.

Sample Documentation

7/10/15 2200 Patient instructed to collect midstream urine sample. Verbalized understanding of directions; 70 mL of cloudy, odorless, yellow urine sent to the laboratory. Patient denies pain or discomfort on urination.

—*A. Blitz, RN*

UNEXPECTED SITUATIONS AND ASSOCIATED INTERVENTIONS

- *Patient cannot provide a sufficient urine sample:* Offer the patient fluids to drink, although drinking too much fluid may dilute the urine, invalidating the test. Patient may return later in day to supply sample. Offer patient assistance with the next void.
- *Patient missed voiding into the specimen container but did void into the collection receptacle in the toilet:* Do not use this urine as a sample for a culture; it could be heavily contaminated with bacteria and give a misleading result. Attempt to collect urine with next void. Offer patient assistance when trying to collect sample.

(*continued*)

SKILL 18-4 COLLECTING A URINE SPECIMEN (CLEAN CATCH, MIDSTREAM) FOR URINALYSIS AND CULTURE continued

SPECIAL CONSIDERATIONS

General Considerations

- For many urine tests, such as a urinalysis, drug testing, or diabetes testing, the specimen does not need to be sterile and does not need to be collected as a midstream specimen. However, in the case of urinalysis, if the specimen shows nitrates and white blood cells, a culture of a urine specimen may be ordered.
- Because the first voiding of the day contains the highest bacterial counts, collect this sample whenever possible.
- If possible, ensure the specimen is obtained before antibiotics are started (Malarkey & McMorrow, 2012).
- Urine specimens may also be obtained by direct urethral catheterization. Refer to Skills 12-5 and 12-6 for catheterization procedure.
- Urine specimens may also be obtained from urinary diversions. See the accompanying Skill Variation below.

Infant and Child Considerations

- The most reliable method to obtain a urine specimen (associated with lower contamination rates) in children less than 2 years of age is to perform a suprapubic aspiration or transurethral catheterization (Tosif et al., 2012). Discuss sampling options with the primary care provider and the patient's parents. Suprapubic aspiration is painful; pain management during the procedure is important (Perry et al., 2010).
- Midstream collection can be accomplished with children older than 2 years of age, provided the child is able to follow direction and will cooperate with the nurse. Try having the child sit facing the back of the toilet, straddling the toilet seat. The nurse or parent can position themself behind the child, holding the sterile container for urine collection (Dulczak, 2005).
- A bagged specimen can be used for urinalysis, but not for urine culture. See the accompanying Skill Variation for the steps used to obtain a bagged urine specimen from an infant or young child. If the urinalysis of the bagged specimen suggests the presence of a urinary tract infection, a second specimen must be obtained for culture, either by urethral catheterization or suprapubic aspiration, to verify the diagnosis and identify the causative microorganism.
- Familiar terms, such as "pee-pee" or "tinkle," may be used with young children to ensure they understand what is being explained (Perry et al., 2010). Enlist the assistance of the patient's parents or significant others to identify appropriate terms.

Home Care Considerations

- If the patient is to collect a specimen at home, ensure that the patient has a clear understanding of collection procedure, understands the need to transport the specimen immediately to the laboratory, and has obtained the necessary equipment from his or her health care provider or laboratory. Reinforce that the patient cannot touch the inside of the collection container. Urine specimens must be refrigerated until they can be brought to the laboratory.

SKILL VARIATION Obtaining a Bagged Urine Specimen for Urinalysis from an Infant or Young Child

1. Verify the order for a urine specimen collection in the medical record. Gather equipment

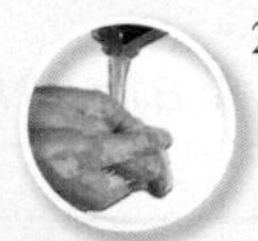

2. Perform hand hygiene and put on PPE, if indicated.

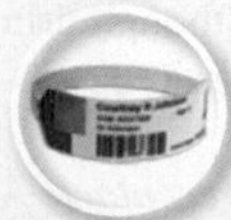

3. Identify the patient. Explain the steps to a young child, if old enough, and to the parents. Talk to the child at the child's level, stressing that no pain will be involved.
4. Check specimen label with the patient's identification bracelet. Label should include the patient's name and identification number, time specimen was collected, route of collection, identification of the person obtaining sample, and any other information required by facility policy.
5. Remove the diaper or underwear. Perform thorough perineal care with skin cleanser and water: for girls, spread labia and cleanse area; for boys, retract foreskin if intact and cleanse glans of penis. Pat skin dry.

SKILL VARIATION Obtaining a Bagged Urine Specimen for Urinalysis from an Infant or Young Child continued

6. Remove paper backing from adhesive faceplate. Apply faceplate over labia or over penis. Gently push faceplate so that seal forms on skin (Figure A).

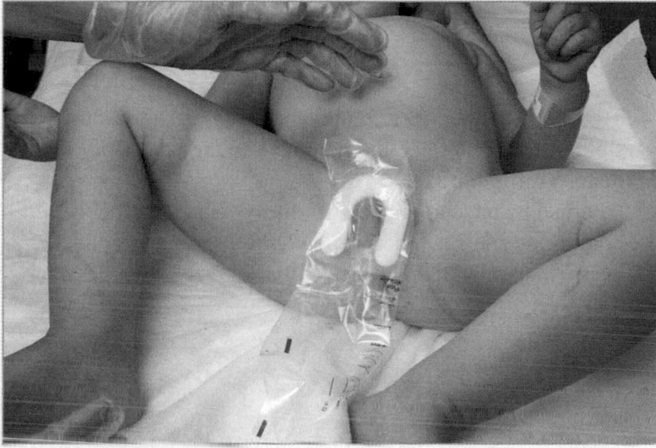

FIGURE A Applying infant urine collection bag.

7. Apply clean diaper or underwear over bag to help prevent dislodgement. Remove gloves and perform hand hygiene. **Check bag every 15 minutes to see whether the child has voided.**
8. As soon as the patient has voided, perform hand hygiene and put on nonsterile gloves. Gently remove bag by pushing skin away from bag. Transfer urine to appropriate containers/tubes for specific test ordered, according to facility policy.
9. Perform perineal care and reapply diaper or clothing.
10. Remove gloves. Perform hand hygiene.
11. Place label on the container per facility policy. Place container in plastic, sealable biohazard bag.

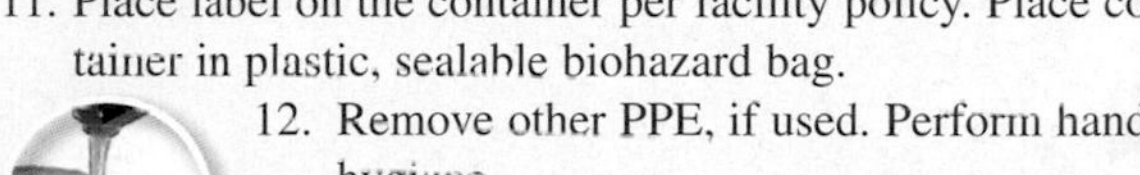

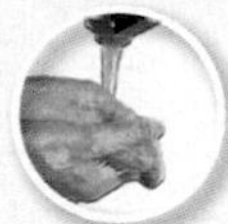

12. Remove other PPE, if used. Perform hand hygiene.
13. Transport the specimen to the laboratory as soon as possible. If unable to take the specimen to the laboratory immediately, refrigerate it.
14. If the collection bag falls off or does not adhere completely, remove the bag, perform perineal care, and apply a new collection bag.

SKILL VARIATION Obtaining a Urine Specimen from a Urinary Diversion

Equipment: Cleansing solution, based on facility policy; sterile gauze; sterile water or saline, or cleansing solution for stoma site (povidone-iodine, chlorhexidine), based on facility policy; double lumen or straight catheter (8 16Fr); sterile water-based lubricant if catheter not self-lubricated; sterile specimen container and urine collection tubes, based on facility policy; sterile and nonsterile gloves; new ostomy appliance; skin cleanser; disposable washcloth or washcloth and towel

1. Verify the order for a urine specimen collection in the medical record. Gather equipment.
2. Perform hand hygiene and put on PPE, if indicated.

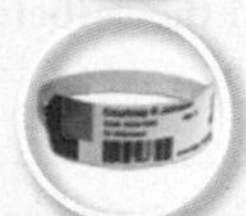

3. Identify the patient. Explain the procedure to the patient.
4. Check specimen label with the patient's identification bracelet. Label should include the patient's name and identification number, time specimen was collected, route of collection, identification of the person obtaining the sample, and any other information required by facility policy.
5. Assemble equipment on overbed table within reach. Open supplies, maintaining sterility of sterile items.
6. Put on nonsterile gloves. Remove ostomy appliance. If one-piece system is in place, remove entire appliance. If two-piece system is in place, remove collection pouch only, leaving appliance pouch only, leaving faceplate wafer intact on skin.
7. Using a circular motion from stoma opening outward, clean the stoma site with the sterile water, sterile saline, or other cleansing solution, based on facility policy.
8. Remove gloves and put on sterile gloves. Blot stoma with sterile gauze.
9. Place open end of urinary catheter into specimen container. Lubricate the catheter with lubricant. If using straight catheter, gently insert the urinary catheter into the stoma site and advance 2 to 3 inches. If using a double-lumen catheter, gently insert catheter tip into stoma and advance the inner catheter approximately 1 to 2 inches. Hold the catheter in position until urine begins to drip. **If you meet resistance, rotate the catheter gently until it slides**

(continued)

SKILL 18-4 COLLECTING A URINE SPECIMEN (CLEAN CATCH, MIDSTREAM) FOR URINALYSIS AND CULTURE continued

SKILL VARIATION Obtaining a Urine Specimen from a Urinary Diversion continued

forward. Do not force the catheter. If you continue to meet resistance, do not force it any further. If urine does not flow into the catheter, ask the patient to shift position and/or cough to mobilize urine (Williams, 2012).

10. Collect approximately 5 to 10 mL of urine before removing catheter. This may take 5 to 15 minutes. Once catheter is removed, cap the specimen container. Clean and dry the stoma and peristomal skin. Replace ostomy appliance. Refer to Skill 12-11. If necessary, transfer the specimen to appropriate containers/tubes for specific test ordered, according to facility policy.
11. Remove gloves and perform hand hygiene.
12. Place label on the container per facility policy. Note specimen collection method, according to facility policy. Place container in plastic, sealable biohazard bag. Dispose of equipment according to facility policy.

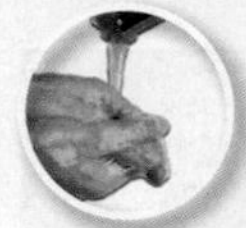

13. Remove other PPE, if used. Perform hand hygiene.
14. Transport the specimen to the laboratory as soon as possible. If unable to take the specimen to the laboratory immediately, refrigerate it.
15. Alternately, once appliance is removed and stoma cleansed, hold the sterile specimen cup under the stoma to collect urine (Mahoney et al., 2013; Williams, 2012).

EVIDENCE FOR PRACTICE ▶

PRACTICE GUIDELINES: URINE SAMPLES AND URINARY DIVERSIONS

Mahoney, M., Baxter, K., Burgess, J., Bauer, C., Downey, C., Mantel, J., et al. (2013). Procedure for obtaining a urine sample from a urostomy, ileal conduit, and colon conduit. A best practice guideline for clinicians. *Journal of Wound, Ostomy & continence Nursing, 40*(3), 277–279.

This best practice guideline was developed by a panel of certified ostomy nurses serving on the Wound, Ostomy and Continence Nurses (WOCN) Society's Clinical Practice Ostomy Committee. This guideline has been validated by the WOCN Society.

Refer to thePoint for additional research on related nursing topics.

SKILL 18-5 OBTAINING A URINE SPECIMEN FROM AN INDWELLING URINARY CATHETER

Indwelling catheter drainage tubes have special sampling ports in the tubing for removal of urine for testing. Most sampling ports are needleless systems. However, some ports require the use of a needle or blunt cannula to access the sampling port. The drainage tubing below the access port may be bent back on itself or clamped so that urine collects near the port, unless contraindicated, based on the patient's condition. **Do not open the drainage system to obtain urine specimens to avoid contamination of the system and bladder infection. Never take urine specimens from the catheter drainage bag because the urine is not fresh and bacteria may be present on the bag.**

DELEGATION CONSIDERATIONS

Obtaining a urine specimen from an indwelling catheter may be delegated to nursing assistive personnel (NAP) or to unlicensed assistive personnel (UAP), as well as licensed practical/vocational nurses (LPN/LVNs). The decision to delegate must be based on careful analysis of the patient's needs and circumstances, as well as the qualifications of the person to whom the task is being delegated. Refer to the Delegation Guidelines in Appendix A.

EQUIPMENT

- 10-mL sterile syringe
- Blunt cannula or 18-gauge needle, if needed, based on specific catheter in use
- Alcohol or other disinfectant wipes
- Nonsterile gloves
- Additional PPE, as indicated
- Sterile specimen container; urine collection tubes, based on facility policy
- Biohazard bag
- Appropriate label for specimen, based on facility policy and procedure

ASSESSMENT

After verifying the medical order for specimen collection, review the medical record for information about any medications that the patient is taking, because medications may affect the results of the test. Assess the characteristics of the urine draining from the catheter. Inspect the catheter tubing to identify the type of sampling port.

NURSING DIAGNOSIS

Determine the related factors for the nursing diagnoses based on the patient's current status. Possible nursing diagnoses may include:

- Impaired Urinary Elimination
- Anxiety
- Deficient Knowledge

OUTCOME IDENTIFICATION AND PLANNING

The expected outcome to achieve is that an adequate amount of urine is obtained from the patient without contamination or adverse effect; the patient experiences minimal anxiety during the collection process; and the patient demonstrates an understanding of the reason for the specimen collection.

IMPLEMENTATION

ACTION	RATIONALE
1. Verify the order for a urine specimen collection in the medical record. Gather equipment.	Verifying the medical order is crucial to ensuring that the proper procedure is administered to the right patient. Assembling equipment provides for an organized approach to the task.
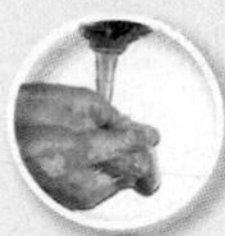 2. Perform hand hygiene and put on PPE, if indicated.	Hand hygiene and PPE prevent the transmission of microorganisms. PPE is required based on transmission precautions.
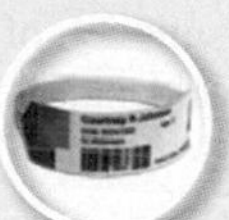 3. Identify the patient.	Identifying the patient ensures the right patient receives the intervention and helps prevent errors.
4. Explain the procedure to the patient.	Explanation provides reassurance and promotes cooperation.
5. Check the specimen label with the patient's identification bracelet. Label should include the patient's name and identification number, time specimen was collected, route of collection, identification of person obtaining the sample, and any other information required by facility policy.	Confirmation of patient identification information ensures the specimen is labeled correctly for the right patient.
6. Assemble equipment on overbed table within reach.	Arranging items nearby is convenient, saves time, and avoids unnecessary stretching and twisting of muscles on the part of the nurse.
7. Close curtains around the bed and close the door to the room, if possible.	Closing curtain or door provides for patient privacy.
8. Put on nonsterile gloves.	Gloves reduce the transmission of microorganisms.
9. Clamp the catheter drainage tubing or bend it back on itself distal to the port. If an insufficient amount of urine is present in the tubing, allow the tubing to remain clamped up to 30 minutes, to collect a sufficient amount of urine, unless contraindicated. Remove lid from specimen container, keeping the inside of the container and lid free from contamination.	Clamping the tubing ensures the collection of an adequate amount of fresh urine. Clamping for an extended period of time leads to overdistention of the bladder. Clamping may be contraindicated based on the patient's condition (e.g., after bladder surgery). The container needs to remain sterile so as not to contaminate the urine.

(continued)

SKILL 18-5 OBTAINING A URINE SPECIMEN FROM AN INDWELLING URINARY CATHETER continued

ACTION	RATIONALE
10. **Cleanse aspiration port vigorously with alcohol or other disinfectant wipe and allow port to air dry.**	Cleaning with alcohol deters entry of microorganisms when the needle punctures the port.
11. Attach the syringe to the needleless port or insert the needle or blunt-tipped cannula into the port. Slowly aspirate enough urine for specimen (usually 10 mL is adequate, check facility requirements) (Figure 1). Remove the syringe from the port. Engage the needle guard, if needle was used. **Unclamp the drainage tubing.**	Using a leur-lock syringe or blunt-tipped needle prevents a needlestick. Collecting urine from the port ensures that the specimen will contain fresh urine. Unclamping catheter drainage tubing prevents overdistention of and injury to the patient's bladder.

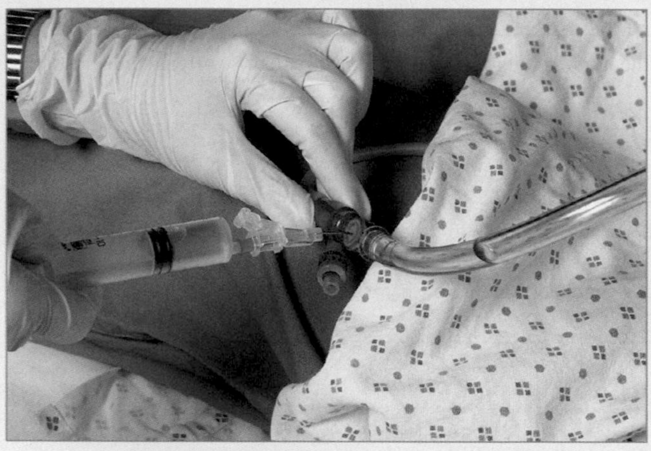

FIGURE 1 Inserting the needle in aspiration port and slowly withdrawing urine specimen.

ACTION	RATIONALE
12. If a needle or blunt-tipped cannula was used on the syringe, remove from the syringe before emptying the urine from the syringe into the specimen cup. Place the needle into a sharps collection container. **Slowly inject urine into the specimen container. Take care to avoid touching the syringe tip to any surface. Do not touch the edge or inside of the collection container.**	Forcing urine through the needle breaks up cells and impedes accurate results of microscopic urinalysis. If the urine is injected quickly into the container, it may splash out of the container or into the nurse's eyes. Avoid touching edge or inside of container to avoid contamination.
13. Replace lid on container. If necessary, transfer the specimen to appropriate containers/tubes for specific test ordered, according to facility policy. Dispose of syringe in a sharps collection container.	Proper disposal of equipment prevents injury and transmission of microorganisms. Safe disposal of sharps prevents accidental injury.
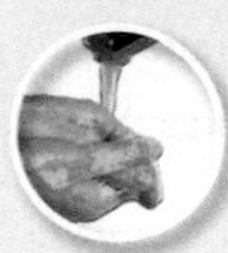 14. Remove gloves and perform hand hygiene.	Removing gloves properly reduces the risk for infection transmission and contamination of other items. Hand hygiene reduces the transmission of microorganisms.
15. Place label on the container per facility policy. Note specimen collection method, according to facility policy. Place container in plastic sealable biohazard bag.	Proper labeling ensures accurate reporting of results. Packaging the specimen in a biohazard bag prevents the person transporting the container from coming in contact with the specimen.
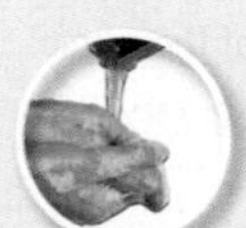 16. Remove other PPE, if used. Perform hand hygiene.	Removing PPE properly reduces the risk for infection transmission and contamination of other items. Hand hygiene reduces the transmission of microorganisms.
17. Transport the specimen to the laboratory as soon as possible. If unable to take the specimen to the laboratory immediately, refrigerate it.	If not refrigerated immediately, urine may act as a culture medium, allowing bacteria to multiply and skewing the results of testing. Refrigeration prevents the bacteria from multiplying.

EVALUATION

The expected outcome is met when an uncontaminated urine specimen is collected and sent to the laboratory without adverse effect. Additionally, the patient does not experience increased anxiety during the collection process.

DOCUMENTATION

Guidelines

Document the method used to obtain the specimen, type of specimen sent, and characteristics of urine. Note any significant patient assessments. Record urine volume on intake and output record, if appropriate.

Sample Documentation

10/20/15 1515 Patient with indwelling urinary catheter in place. Urine noted to be dark yellow and cloudy. Patient's temperature 103°F, pulse 96, respirations 18, BP 118/64. Dr. Burning notified. Specimen for urine culture obtained from indwelling catheter and catheter removed per order. Patient due to void by 2115.

—*B. Clapp, RN*

UNEXPECTED SITUATIONS AND ASSOCIATED INTERVENTIONS

- *No urine or insufficient amount noted in catheter tubing:* Clamp tubing below access port for up to 30 minutes, according to facility policy, unless contraindicated by patient condition.

SPECIAL CONSIDERATIONS

- If possible, collect urine specimens for culture and sensitivity from a newly inserted catheter (SUNA, 2010; Hooten et al., 2010).
- It is very important to remove the clamp from the drainage tubing as soon as the specimen is collected, unless there is a specific order to leave the tubing clamped, to prevent overdistention of the patient's bladder and injury.
- If possible, ensure the specimen is obtained before antibiotics are started (Malarkey & McMorrow, 2012).

EVIDENCE FOR PRACTICE ▶

PRACTICE GUIDELINES AND CATHETER-ASSOCIATED INFECTIONS

Society of Urologic Nurses and Associates (SUNA). (2010). *Prevention & control of catheter-associated urinary tract infection (CAUTI). Clinical practice guideline.* Available https://www.suna.org/sites/default/files/download/cautiGuideline.pdf.

These guidelines provide evidence-based recommendations to guide care for patients requiring catheterization of the urinary bladder to prevent catheter-associated urinary tract infection.

Refer to thePoint for additional research on related nursing topics.

EVIDENCE FOR PRACTICE ▶

PRACTICE GUIDELINES AND CATHETER-ASSOCIATED INFECTIONS

Hooton, T.M., Bradley, S.F., Cardenas, D.D., Colgan, R., Geerlings, S.E., Rice, J.C., et al. (2010). Diagnosis, prevention, and treatment of catheter-associated urinary tract infection in adults: 2009 international clinical practice guidelines from the Infectious Diseases Society of America. *Clinical Infectious Diseases, 50*(5), 625–663. Available http://www.idsociety.org/uploadedFiles/IDSA/Guidelines-Patient_Care/PDF_Library/Comp%20UTI.pdf

These evidence-based practice guidelines include strategies to reduce the risk of catheter-associated urinary tract infections, strategies that have not been found to reduce these infections, and management strategies for patients with catheter-associated urinary tract infection.

Refer to thePoint for additional research on related nursing topics.

SKILL 18-6 TESTING STOOL FOR OCCULT BLOOD

Fecal occult blood testing (FOBT) is used to detect **occult blood** in the stool. It is used for initial screening for disorders such as cancer and for gastrointestinal bleeding in conditions such as ulcer disease, inflammatory bowel disorders, and intestinal polyps. Three consecutive stool samples should be collected over several days to provide the most effective screening for colon cancer (AACC, 2013). FOBT may be performed within an institution, collected at the bedside and sent to the laboratory for analysis. They may also be collected by the patient at home and delivered or mailed to the health care provider's office or to the laboratory for analysis.

The *guaiac fecal occult blood test* (gFOBT) is a chemical test that detects the enzyme peroxidasc in hemoglobin molecules when blood is present in the stool sample. A positive gFOBT result indicates that abnormal bleeding is occurring somewhere in the digestive tract. Ingestion of certain substances before the specimen collection can result in false–positive results. These substances include red meat, salmon, tuna, mackerel, sardines, tomatoes, broccoli, turnips, cauliflower, horseradish, apples, oranges, mushrooms, melon, bananas, and soybeans. Certain medications, such as a salicylate intake of more than 325 mg daily, other nonsteroidal anti-inflammatory drugs, steroids, iron preparations, and anticoagulants, also may lead to false–positive readings (AACC, 2013; Fischbach & Dunning, 2009). Vitamin C ingestion can produce false–negative results even if bleeding is present. The following are recommendations for the patient preparing for a fecal occult blood test:

- Before stool testing, avoid the foods (for 3 days) and drugs (for 7 days) that may alter test results (if clinically possible).
- In a woman who is menstruating, postpone the test until 3 days after her period has ended.
- Postpone the test if hematuria or bleeding hemorrhoids are present.
- Postpone the test if the patient has had a recent nose or throat bleed.

In clinical settings, these restrictions are usually not practical. Be sure to note the presence of any of the previously mentioned conditions in the clinical setting.

The *immunochemical fecal occult blood test* (iFOBT or FIT) uses antibodies directed against human hemoglobin to detect blood in the stool. A positive iFOBT test indicates abnormal bleeding in the lower digestive tract. It cannot detect hemoglobin that came from bleeding sites in the upper gastrointestinal tract or small intestine. Because this test detects only human hemoglobin, other sources of blood, such as from the diet, do not cause a positive result. No dietary or drug restrictions are related to the iFOBT.

A positive result from either the gFOBT or the iFOBT requires follow-up testing, such as a sigmoidoscopy or colonoscopy (AACC, 2013; Malarkey &McMorrow, 2012).

DELEGATION CONSIDERATIONS

Obtaining a stool specimen for FOBT may be delegated to nursing assistive personnel (NAP) or to unlicensed assistive personnel (UAP), as well as to licensed practical/vocational nurses (LPN/LVNs). Developing the FOBT at the point-of-care is not delegated to nursing assistive personnel (NAP) or to unlicensed assistive personnel (UAP). Developing the FOBT at the point-of-care may be delegated to LPN/LVNs. The decision to delegate must be based on careful analysis of the patient's needs and circumstances, as well as the qualifications of the person to whom the task is being delegated. Refer to the Delegation Guidelines in Appendix A.

EQUIPMENT

- Nonsterile gloves; other PPE as indicated
- Wooden applicator
- gFOBT: Wooden applicator, testing card, and developer (if processing is being done at point-of-care)
- iFOBT: Applicator stick or brush, depending on collection kit in use
- Bedpan, or plastic collection receptacle for commode or toilet
- Biohazard bag
- Appropriate label for specimen, based on facility policy and procedure

ASSESSMENT

Assess the patient's understanding of the collection procedure and ability to cooperate. Assess the patient for a history of gastrointestinal bleeding. Review prescribed restrictions for medications and diet, and evaluate patient compliance with required restrictions. Assess patient for any blood in the perineal area, including hemorrhoids, menstruation, urinary tract infection, or vaginal or rectal tears. Blood may be from a source other than the gastrointestinal tract.

NURSING DIAGNOSIS

Determine the related factors for the nursing diagnoses based on the patient's current status. Appropriate nursing diagnoses may include:

- Deficient Knowledge
- Anxiety

OUTCOME IDENTIFICATION AND PLANNING

The expected outcome to achieve is that an uncontaminated stool sample is obtained, following collection guidelines, and then transported to the laboratory within the recommended time frame, without adverse effect. Other outcomes may include the following: the patient demonstrates accurate understanding of testing instructions; the patient verbalizes a decrease in anxiety; and the specimen is obtained with minimal discomfort or embarrassment.

IMPLEMENTATION

ACTION	RATIONALE
1. Verify the order for a stool specimen collection in the medical record. Gather equipment.	Verifying the medical order is crucial to ensuring that the proper procedure is administered to the right patient. Assembling equipment provides for an organized approach to the task.
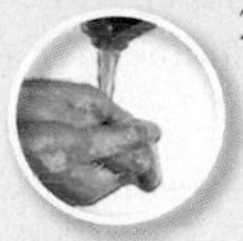 2. Perform hand hygiene and put on PPE, if indicated.	Hand hygiene and PPE prevent the transmission of microorganisms. PPE is required based on transmission precautions.
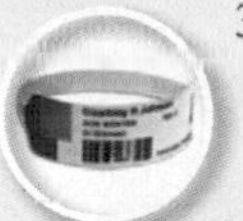 3. Identify the patient.	Identifying the patient ensures the right patient receives the intervention and helps prevent errors.
4. Discuss with the patient the need for a stool sample. Explain to the patient the process by which the stool will be collected, either from a bedpan, commode, or plastic receptacle in the toilet.	Discussion and explanation help to allay some of the patient's anxiety and prepare the patient for what to expect.
5. If sending the specimen to the laboratory, check specimen label with patient identification bracelet. Label should include the patient's name and identification number, time specimen was collected, route of collection, identification of the person obtaining the sample, and any other information required by facility policy.	Facilities may allow point-of-service testing (at bedside or on unit) or the specimen may have to be sent to the laboratory for testing. Confirmation of patient identification information ensures the specimen is labeled correctly for the right patient.
6. Assemble equipment on overbed table within reach.	Arranging items nearby is convenient, saves time, and avoids unnecessary stretching and twisting of muscles on the part of the nurse.
7. Close curtains around the bed or close the door to the room, if possible.	Closing the door or curtain provides for patient privacy.
8. Place the plastic collection receptacle in the toilet, if applicable. Assist the patient to the bathroom or onto the bedside commode, or onto the bedpan. Instruct the patient not to urinate or discard toilet paper with the stool.	Proper collection into an appropriate receptacle for stool prevents inaccurate results. Urine or toilet paper can contaminate the specimen, interfering with accurate results.
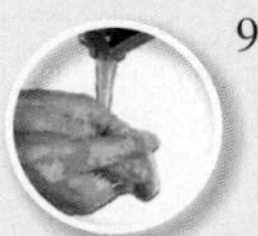 9. After the patient defecates, assist the patient out of the bathroom, off the commode, or remove the bedpan. Perform hand hygiene and put on disposable gloves.	Hand hygiene deters the spread of microorganisms. Gloves protect the nurse from microorganisms in feces.

(continued)

SKILL 18-6 TESTING STOOL FOR OCCULT BLOOD continued

ACTION	RATIONALE
If using gFOBT: 10. Open flap on sample side of card. **With wooden applicator, apply a small amount of stool from the center of the bowel movement onto one window of the testing card. With the opposite end of the wooden applicator, obtain another sample of stool from another area and apply a small amount of stool onto second window of testing card (Figure 1).**	Two separate areas of the same stool sample are tested to ensure accuracy. By using opposite ends of the wooden applicator, cross-contamination is avoided.
11. Close flap over stool samples.	Closing the flap prevents contamination of the samples.
12. If sending stool to the laboratory, label the specimen card per facility policy. Place in a sealable plastic biohazard bag and send to the laboratory immediately.	Facilities may allow point-of-service testing (at bedside or on unit) or the specimen may have to be sent to the laboratory for testing. Correct labeling is necessary to ensure accurate results. Packaging the specimen in a biohazard bag prevents the person transporting the container from coming in contact with the specimen.
13. If testing at the point-of-care, wait 3 to 5 minutes before developing. Open flap on opposite side of card and **place two drops of developer over each window and wait the time stated in the manufacturer's instructions (Figure 2).**	If immediate testing is required, waiting 3 to 5 minutes before developing allows adequate time for the sample to penetrate the test paper (Beckman Coulter, 2009a). The developer will react with any blood in the stool. Following the manufacturer's instructions promotes accuracy of results.
14. Observe card for any blue areas (Figure 3).	Any blue coloring on the card indicates a positive test result for blood.

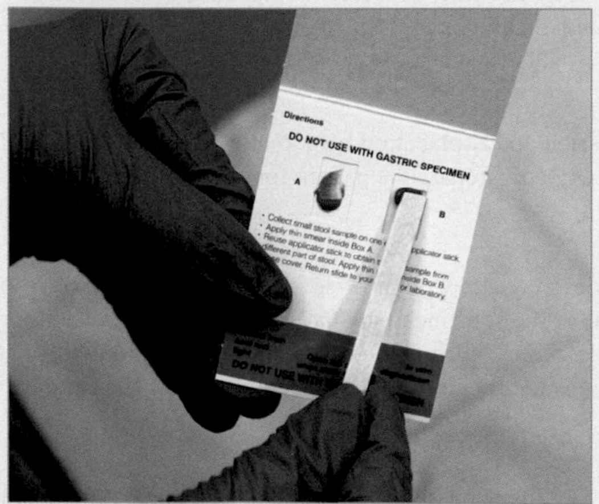

FIGURE 1 Using a wooden applicator to transfer stool specimen to window of testing card.

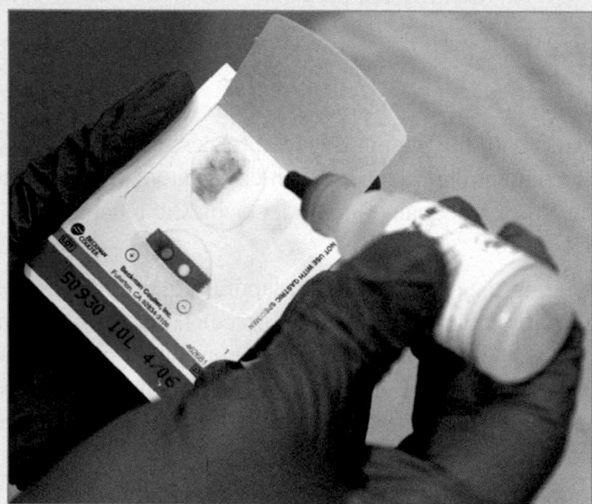

FIGURE 2 Applying developer to card windows.

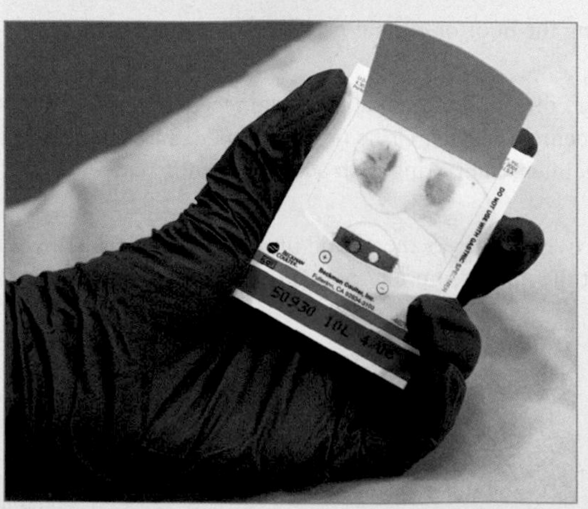

FIGURE 3 Observing windows on card for blue areas.

ACTION	RATIONALE
If using iFOBT:	
15. Open flap on sample side of card. **With applicator, brush, or sampling probe, apply a small amount of stool from the center of the bowel movement onto the top half of window of the testing card. With the opposite end of the device, obtain another sample of stool from another area and apply a small amount of stool onto the bottom half of window of testing card.**	Two separate areas of the same stool sample are tested to ensure accuracy. By using opposite ends of the wooden applicator, cross-contamination is avoided.
16. Spread samples over entire window by pressing gently with device while mixing thoroughly. Close flap over sample (Beckman Coulter, 2009c). Allow card to dry.	Drying of sample stabilizes hemoglobin, if present.
17. If sending to the laboratory, label the specimen card per facility policy. Place in a sealable plastic biohazard bag and send to the laboratory immediately.	Facilities may allow point-of-service testing (at bedside or on unit) or the specimen may have to be sent to the laboratory for testing. Correct labeling is necessary to ensure accurate results. Packaging the specimen in a biohazard bag prevents the person transporting the container from coming in contact with the specimen.
18. If testing at the point-of-care, open collection card according to manufacturer's instructions. Add three drops of developer to center of sample on Sample Pad. Developer should flow through the test (T) line and through the control (C) line. Snap Test Device closed (Beckman Coulter, 2009b).	The developer will react with any blood in the stool. Following the manufacturer's instructions promotes accuracy of results.
19. Wait 5 minutes, or time specified by manufacturer. Observe card for pink color on the test (T) line. The control (C) line must also turn pink within 5 minutes (Figure 4). If the control (C) line turns pink, read and report the result.	The developer will react with any blood in the stool. Following the manufacturer's instructions promotes accuracy of results. Any pink color on the test (T) line indicates a positive result.

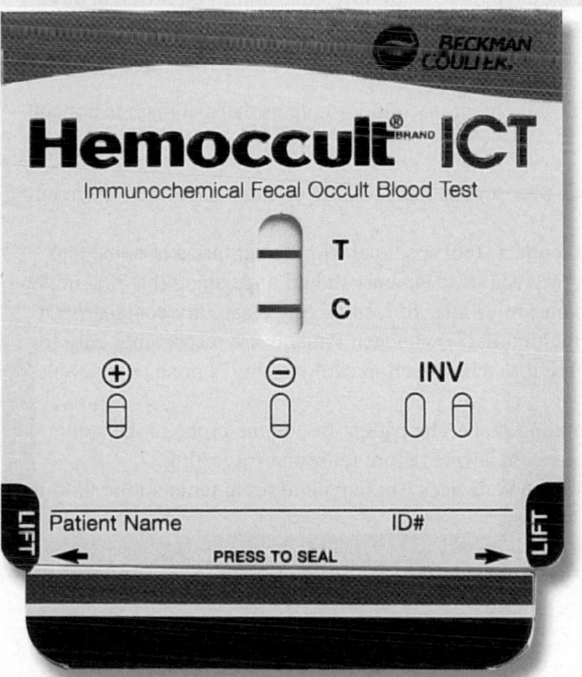

FIGURE 4 Observing for pink color on test (T) line and the control (C) line. (Image courtesy of Beckman Coulter, Inc.)

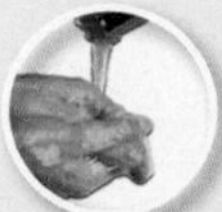

ACTION	RATIONALE
20. After reading results, discard testing slide appropriately, according to facility policy. Remove gloves and any other PPE, if used. Perform hand hygiene.	Removing PPE properly reduces the risk for infection transmission and contamination of other items. Hand hygiene and proper disposal of equipment reduces the transmission of microorganisms.

(continued)

SKILL 18-6 TESTING STOOL FOR OCCULT BLOOD continued

EVALUATION

The expected outcome is met when a stool sample is obtained following collection guidelines and transported to the laboratory within the recommended time frame, without adverse effect; the patient demonstrates accurate understanding of testing instructions; the patient verbalizes decreased anxiety; and the specimen is obtained with minimal discomfort and embarrassment. If the patient is to obtain the stool sample on his or her own, another outcome is met when the patient is able to collect the stool, place it correctly on the collection device, and deliver it to the testing site.

DOCUMENTATION

Guidelines

Document the method used to obtain the specimen and transport it to the laboratory. If testing is done by the nurse, document results and communication of results to the health care provider. Document significant assessment findings and stool characteristics.

Sample Documentation

07/12/15 1040 Stool sample obtained from bowel movement. Labeled and sent to laboratory for occult blood testing. Stool noted to be semi-formed, dark brown, without signs of gross blood.

—K. Sanders, RN

UNEXPECTED SITUATIONS AND ASSOCIATED INTERVENTIONS

- *When developing a gFOBT, one window tests positive, whereas the second window tests negative:* This could indicate that the blood is from a source other than the gastrointestinal tract. Document these results and notify the primary care provider.
- *When developing an iFOBT test, the control (C) line does not turn pink:* Do not report result. Repeat the test with a new collection card and test device (Beckman Coulter, 2009b).

SPECIAL CONSIDERATIONS

General Considerations

- To ensure validity, repeat the test at least three times with different samples on different days.
- Specimen can be collected from an ostomy appliance. Apply a clean ostomy appliance and obtain a sample as soon as patient passes stool into the appliance.

Infant and Child Considerations

- Stool can be collected from the diaper of an infant or child, as long as the specimen is not contaminated with urine.

Home Care Considerations

- Collect three consecutive stool samples over several days to provide the most effective screening for colon cancer (AACC, 2013).
- Patients are often instructed on how to collect stool specimens for occult blood at home and bring the samples to the office, clinic, or laboratory. Patients should understand that it is important to follow instructions carefully to ensure validity of results. Any clean, dry container can be used to collect stool before contact with toilet bowl water. Patients are responsible only for obtaining a sample of stool and applying it to the collection card. Testing is done at the clinic, office, or laboratory.
- Some iFOBT collection kits use a sampling probe; the patient inserts the probe in the stool sample and inserts the probe in the collection device before returning for testing.
- Once the samples are collected, the collection devices can remain at room temperature until they are mailed or delivered to the testing location.

SKILL 18-7 COLLECTING A STOOL SPECIMEN FOR CULTURE

A stool specimen may be ordered to screen for pathogenic organisms, such as *Clostridium difficile* or ova and parasites, electrolytes, fat, and leukocytes. The nurse is responsible for obtaining the specimen according to facility procedure, labeling the specimen, and ensuring that the specimen is transported to the laboratory in a timely manner. The facility's policy and procedure manual or laboratory manual identifies specific information about the amount of stool needed, the time frame during which stool is to be collected, and the type of specimen container to use.

Usually, 1 inch (2.5 cm) of formed stool or 15 to 30 mL of liquid stool is sufficient. If portions of the stool include visible blood, mucus, or pus, include these with the specimen. Also be sure that the specimen is free of any barium or enema solution. Because a fresh specimen produces the most accurate results, send the specimen to the laboratory immediately. If this is not possible, refrigerate it unless contraindicated, such as when testing for ova and parasites. Refrigeration will affect parasites. Ova and parasites are best detected in warm stool. Some institutions require ova and parasite specimens to be placed in a container filled with preservatives; consult facility policy.

DELEGATION CONSIDERATIONS

Obtaining a stool specimen may be delegated to nursing assistive personnel (NAP) or to unlicensed assistive personnel (UAP), as well as to licensed practical/vocational nurses (LPN/LVNs). The decision to delegate must be based on careful analysis of the patient's needs and circumstances, as well as the qualifications of the person to whom the task is being delegated. Refer to the Delegation Guidelines in Appendix A.

EQUIPMENT

- Tongue blade (2)
- Clean specimen container (or container with preservatives for ova and parasites)
- Biohazard bag
- Nonsterile gloves
- Additional PPE, as indicated
- Appropriate label for specimen, based on facility policy and procedure

ASSESSMENT

Assess the patient's understanding of the need for the test and the requirements of the test. Assess the patient's understanding of the collection procedure and ability to cooperate. Ask the patient when his or her last bowel movement was, and check the patient's medical record for this information.

NURSING DIAGNOSIS

Determine the related factors for the nursing diagnoses based on the patient's current status. Appropriate nursing diagnoses include:

- Deficient Knowledge
- Diarrhea
- Anxiety

OUTCOME IDENTIFICATION AND PLANNING

The expected outcome to achieve is that an uncontaminated specimen is obtained and sent to the laboratory promptly. Additional outcomes that may be appropriate include the following: the patient demonstrates the ability to collect a stool specimen and verbalizes a decrease in anxiety related to stool collection.

IMPLEMENTATION

ACTION	RATIONALE
1. Verify the order for a stool specimen collection in the medical record. Gather equipment.	Verifying the medical order is crucial to ensuring that the proper procedure is administered to the right patient. Assembling equipment provides for an organized approach to the task.

(continued)

SKILL 18-7 COLLECTING A STOOL SPECIMEN FOR CULTURE continued

ACTION	RATIONALE
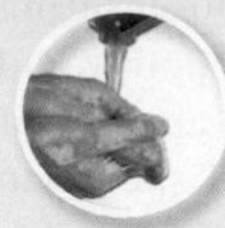 2. Perform hand hygiene and put on PPE, if indicated.	Hand hygiene and PPE prevent the transmission of microorganisms. PPE is required based on transmission precautions.
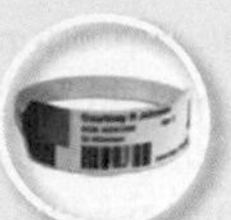 3. Identify the patient.	Identifying the patient ensures the right patient receives the intervention and helps prevent errors.
4. Discuss with the patient the need for a stool sample. Explain to the patient the process by which the stool will be collected, either from a bedpan, commode, or plastic receptacle in the toilet to catch stool without urine. Instruct the patient to void first and not to discard toilet paper with stool. Tell the patient to call you as soon as a bowel movement is completed.	Discussion and explanation help to allay some of the patient's anxiety and prepare the patient for what to expect. The patient should void first because the laboratory study may be inaccurate if the stool contains urine. Placing a container in the toilet or bedside commode aids in obtaining a clean stool specimen uncontaminated by urine.
5. Check specimen label with the patient's identification bracelet. Label should include the patient's name and identification number, time specimen was collected, route of collection, identification of the person obtaining the sample, and any other information required by facility policy.	Confirmation of patient identification information ensures the specimen is labeled correctly for the right patient.
6. Assemble equipment on overbed table within reach.	Arranging items nearby is convenient, saves time, and avoids unnecessary stretching and twisting of muscles on the part of the nurse.
7. After the patient has passed a stool, put on gloves. Use the tongue blades to obtain a sample, free of blood or urine, and place it in the designated clean container.	The container does not have to be sterile, because stool is not sterile. To ensure accurate results, the stool should be free of urine or menstrual blood.
8. Collect as much of the stool as possible to send to the laboratory.	Different tests and laboratories require different amounts of stool. Collecting as much as possible helps to ensure that the laboratory has an adequate amount of specimen for testing.
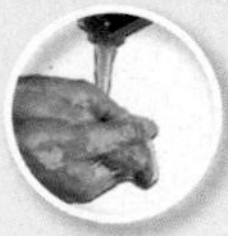 9. Place lid on container. Dispose of used equipment per facility policy. Remove gloves and perform hand hygiene.	Proper disposal of equipment reduces the transmission of microorganisms. Removing gloves properly reduces the risk for infection transmission and contamination of other items. Hand hygiene deters the spread of microorganisms.
10. Place label on the container per facility policy. Place container in plastic, sealable biohazard bag.	Correct labeling is necessary to ensure accurate results. Packaging the specimen in a biohazard bag prevents the person transporting the container from coming in contact with stool.
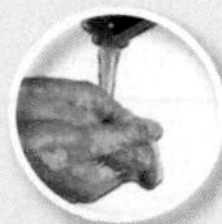 11. Remove other PPE, if used. Perform hand hygiene.	Removing PPE properly reduces the risk for infection transmission and contamination of other items. Hand hygiene reduces the transmission of microorganisms.
12. Transport the specimen to the laboratory while stool is still warm. If immediate transport is impossible, check with laboratory personnel or policy manual whether refrigeration is contraindicated.	Most tests have better results with fresh stool. Different tests may require different preparation if the test is not immediately completed. Some tests will be compromised if the stool is refrigerated.

EVALUATION

The expected outcome is met when the patient passes a stool that is not contaminated by urine or menstrual blood and is placed in a clean container. The specimen is transported appropriately to the laboratory. The patient participates in stool collection and verbalizes feelings of diminished anxiety related to the procedure.

DOCUMENTATION

Guidelines

Document amount, color, and consistency of stool obtained, time of collection, specific test for which the specimen was collected, and transport to laboratory.

Sample Documentation

7/12/15 2045 Large amount of pasty, green stool sent to laboratory for ova and parasite testing.

—K. Sanders, RN

UNEXPECTED SITUATIONS AND ASSOCIATED INTERVENTIONS

- *Patient is menstruating or has discarded toilet paper into commode with stool:* Call laboratory to discuss possible effects on test results. Not all tests will be affected by contaminants. The laboratory may accept the specimen even with the contaminant. Make notation on order card that goes to laboratory with specimen.
- *Specimen is inadvertently left on counter instead of being sent to laboratory:* Call laboratory to discuss possible effects on test results. Not all tests will be affected by leaving the specimen on the counter for a period of time. The laboratory may accept the specimen even though it has been sitting out. Make sure that the time on the card is the actual time the specimen was obtained.

SPECIAL CONSIDERATIONS

General Considerations

- If patient is wearing an adult incontinence brief, the stool may be collected from the brief, as long as it is not contaminated with urine.
- Barium procedures and laxatives should be avoided for 1 week before specimen collection to ensure valid results.
- If bacterial infection is suspected, collect one specimen each day for three days to ensure accuracy.
- Specimen can be collected from ostomy appliance. Apply a clean ostomy appliance and obtain sample as soon as patient passes stool into the appliance.
- If a timed stool test is ordered, such as fecal fat, the entire amount of stool produced for 24 to 72 hours is sent to the laboratory. Be sure to follow instructions for storage while collection is ongoing.

Infant and Child Considerations

- Stool can be collected from the diaper of an infant or child, as long as the specimen is uncontaminated with urine.

Home Care Considerations

- Patients are often instructed on how to collect stool specimens at home and bring the samples to the office, clinic, or laboratory. Patients should understand that it is important to follow instructions carefully to ensure validity of results. Ensure the patient understands the proper procedure for sample storage before bringing it to the laboratory or office.

SKILL 18-8 OBTAINING A CAPILLARY BLOOD SAMPLE FOR GLUCOSE TESTING

Blood glucose monitoring provides information about how the body is controlling glucose metabolism. Controlling the patient's blood glucose levels is an important part of care for patients with many conditions, including diabetes, seizures, enteral and parenteral feeding, liver disease, pancreatitis, head injury, stroke, alcohol and drug intoxication, sepsis, and in patients prescribed corticosteroids (American Diabetes Association [ADA], 2013). Point-of-care testing (testing done at the bedside, where samples are not sent to the laboratory) provides a convenient, rapid, and accurate measurement of blood glucose (ADA, 2013). Patients with diabetes use this type of testing as an important part of disease management to monitor blood glucose and adjust lifestyle interventions and treatment (U.S. FDA, 2013). Blood samples are commonly obtained from the edges of the fingers for adults, but samples can be obtained from the palm of the hand, forearm, upper arm, calf, and anterior thigh, depending on the time of testing and monitor used (U.S. FDA, 2013). Avoid fingertips, because they are more sensitive. Rotate sites to prevent skin damage. **It is important to be familiar with and follow the manufacturer's guidelines and facility policy and procedure to ensure accurate results.** Normal fasting glucose for adults is less than 110 mg/dL (LeFever Kee, 2013).

DELEGATION CONSIDERATIONS

Obtaining a capillary blood sample for glucose testing may be delegated to nursing assistive personnel (NAP) or to unlicensed assistive personnel (UAP), as well as to licensed practical/vocational nurses (LPN/LVNs). The decision to delegate must be based on careful analysis of the patient's needs and circumstances, as well as the qualifications of the person to whom the task is being delegated. Refer to the Delegation Guidelines in Appendix A.

EQUIPMENT

- Blood glucose meter
- Sterile **lancet**
- Cotton balls or gauze squares
- Testing strips for meter
- Nonsterile gloves
- Additional PPE, as indicated
- Skin cleanser and water or alcohol swab

ASSESSMENT

Assess the patient's history for indications necessitating the monitoring of blood glucose levels, such as high-carbohydrate feedings, history of diabetes mellitus, or corticosteroid therapy. Assess for signs and symptoms of hypoglycemia and hyperglycemia. In addition, assess the patient's knowledge about monitoring blood glucose. Inspect the area of the skin to be used for testing. Avoid bruised and open areas.

NURSING DIAGNOSIS

Determine the related factors for the nursing diagnoses based on the patient's current status. Possible nursing diagnoses may include:

- Risk for Unstable Blood Glucose Level
- Deficient Knowledge
- Anxiety

OUTCOME IDENTIFICATION AND PLANNING

The expected outcome to achieve is that the blood glucose level is measured accurately without adverse effect. In addition, the patient remains free of injury; the patient demonstrates a blood glucose level within acceptable parameters; the patient demonstrates the ability to participate in monitoring; and the patient verbalizes increased comfort with the procedure.

IMPLEMENTATION

ACTION	RATIONALE
1. Check the patient's medical record or nursing plan of care for monitoring schedule. You may decide that additional testing is indicated based on nursing judgment and the patient's condition.	This confirms scheduled times for checking blood glucose. Independent nursing judgment may lead to the decision to test more frequently, based on the patient's condition.
2. Gather equipment. Check expiration date on blood test strips.	This provides an organized approach to the task. Blood test strips that are past expiration date could cause inaccurate results and should not be used.

ACTION	RATIONALE
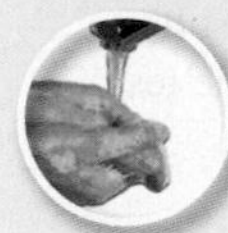 3. Perform hand hygiene and put on PPE, if indicated.	Hand hygiene and PPE prevent the transmission of microorganisms. PPE is required based on transmission precautions.
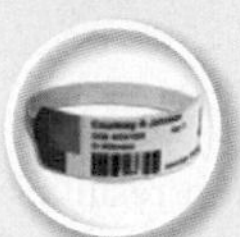 4. Identify the patient. Explain the procedure to the patient and instruct the patient about the need for monitoring blood glucose.	Identifying the patient ensures the right patient receives the intervention and helps prevent errors. Explanation helps to alleviate anxiety and facilitate cooperation.
5. Close curtains around the bed and close the door to the room, if possible.	Closing the curtain or door provides for patient privacy.
6. Turn on the monitor.	The monitor must be on for use.
7. Enter the patient's identification number or scan his or her identification bracelet, if required, according to facility policy.	Use of identification number allows for electronic storage and accurate identification of patient data.
8. Put on nonsterile gloves.	Gloves protect the nurse from exposure to blood or body fluids.
9. Prepare lancet using aseptic technique.	Aseptic technique maintains sterility.
10. Remove test strip from the vial. **Recap container immediately.** Test strips also come individually wrapped. **Check that the code number for the strip matches the code number on the monitor screen.**	Immediate recapping protects strips from exposure to humidity, light, and discoloration. Matching code numbers on the strip and glucose monitor ensures that the machine is calibrated correctly.
11. Insert the strip into the meter according to directions for that specific device. Alternately, strip may be placed in meter after collection of sample on test strip, depending on meter in use.	Correctly inserted strip allows meter to read blood glucose level accurately.
12. **Have the patient wash hands with skin cleanser and warm water and dry thoroughly. Alternately, cleanse the skin with an alcohol swab. Allow skin to dry completely.**	Washing with skin cleanser and water or alcohol cleanses the puncture site. Warm water also helps to cause vasodilation. Alcohol can interfere with accuracy of results if not completely dried.
13. Choose a skin site free of lesions and calluses. Make sure there is no edema, and that the site is warm (Van Leeuwen et al., 2011).	Areas with lesions are not suitable for capillary sampling. Calluses, edema, and vasoconstriction (cool to palpation) interfere with the ability to obtain a blood sample.
14. Hold lancet perpendicular to skin and pierce site with lancet (Figure 1).	Holding lancet in proper position facilitates proper skin penetration.

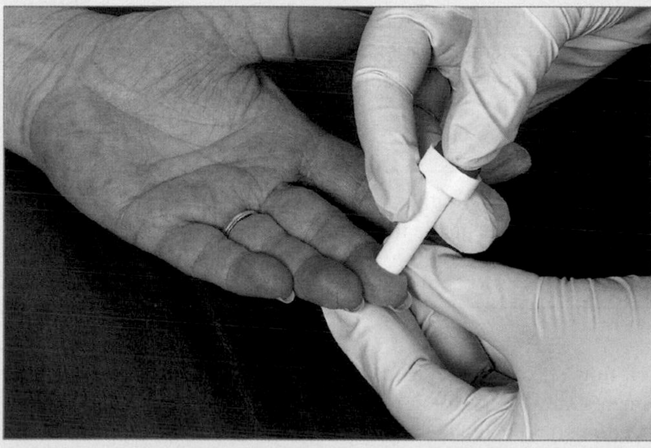

FIGURE 1 Piercing patient's finger with lancet.

ACTION	RATIONALE
15. Wipe away first drop of blood with gauze square or cotton ball if recommended by manufacturer of monitor.	Manufacturers recommend discarding the first drop of blood, which may be contaminated by serum or cleansing product, producing an inaccurate reading.

(*continued*)

SKILL 18-8 OBTAINING A CAPILLARY BLOOD SAMPLE FOR GLUCOSE TESTING continued

ACTION	RATIONALE
16. Encourage bleeding by lowering the hand, making use of gravity. Lightly stroke the finger, if necessary, until a sufficient amount of blood has formed to cover the sample area on the strip, based on monitor requirements (check instructions for monitor). Take care not to squeeze the finger, not to squeeze at puncture site, or not to touch puncture site or blood.	An appropriate-sized droplet facilitates accurate test results. Squeezing can cause injury to the patient and alter the test result (Ferguson, 2005).
17. Gently touch a drop of blood to the test strip without smearing it (Figure 2). Depending on meter in use, insert strip into meter after collection of sample on test strip.	Smearing blood on the strip may result in inaccurate test results.

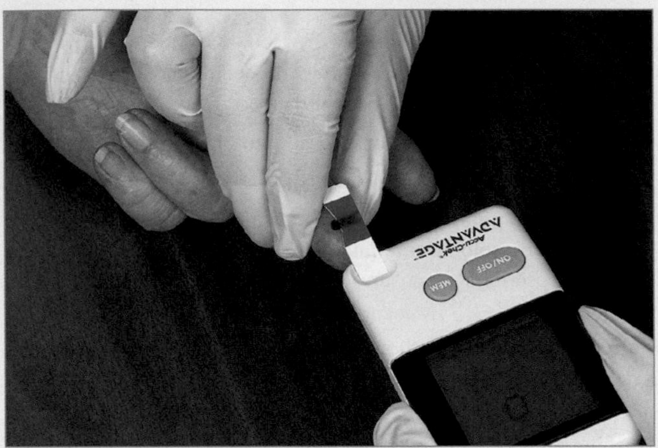

FIGURE 2 Applying blood to test strip.

ACTION	RATIONALE
18. Press time button if directed by manufacturer.	Correct timing produces accurate results.
19. Apply pressure to puncture site with a cotton ball or dry gauze. **Do not use alcohol wipe.**	Pressure causes hemostasis. Alcohol stings and may prolong bleeding.
20. Read blood glucose results and document appropriately at bedside. Inform patient of test result.	Timing depends on type of meter.
21. Turn off meter, remove test strip, and dispose of supplies appropriately. Place lancet in sharps container.	Proper disposal prevents exposure to blood and accidental needlestick.
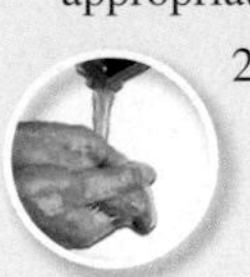 22. Remove gloves and any other PPE, if used. Perform hand hygiene.	Removing PPE properly reduces the risk for infection transmission and contamination of other items. Hand hygiene reduces the transmission of microorganisms.

EVALUATION

The expected outcome is met when the patient's blood glucose level is measured accurately without adverse effect; the blood glucose level is within acceptable limits; the patient participates in monitoring; and the patient verbalizes comfort with the procedure.

DOCUMENTATION

Guidelines

Document blood glucose level on a flow sheet in the medical record, according to facility policy. Document pertinent patient assessments, any intervention related to glucose level, and any patient teaching. Report abnormal results and/or significant assessments to primary health care provider.

Sample Documentation

DocuCare Practice documenting blood glucose testing in *Lippincott DocuCare*.

11/1/15 0800 Patient performed own fingerstick blood glucose test with minimal guidance. Verbalized rationale for fasting measurement and able to state symptoms of hypoglycemia. Patient's fingerstick blood glucose level 168. Four units regular Humulin insulin given per sliding scale, in addition to 10 units NPH Humulin insulin scheduled for 0800. Patient encouraged to review written guidelines for subcutaneous insulin administration; will review procedure and plan to have patient administer insulin at dinnertime. Patient verbalized an understanding.

—B. Clapp, RN

UNEXPECTED SITUATIONS AND ASSOCIATED INTERVENTIONS

- *Extremity is pale and cool to the touch:* Begin by warming the extremity. Have adult patients warm their hands by rubbing them together. Warm, moist compresses also may be used.
- *Blood glucose level results are above or below normal parameters:* Assess the patient for signs of hyperglycemia or hypoglycemia, respectively. Check medical record for ordered interventions, such as insulin dosage or carbohydrate administration. Notify health care provider of results and assessment.

SPECIAL CONSIDERATIONS

General Considerations

- In adults, the middle or ring finger is the preferred site for capillary blood sample (Malarkey & McMorrow, 2012; Van Leeuwen et al., 2011).
- If the selected site feels cool or appears pale, warm compresses can be applied for 3 to 5 minutes to dilate the capillaries
- Sampling of blood from an alternative site other than fingertips may have limitations. Blood in the fingertips shows changes in glucose levels more quickly than blood in other parts of the body. This means that alternative site test results may differ from fingertip test results when glucose levels are changing rapidly (e.g., after a meal, taking insulin, or during or after exercise) because the results may be inaccurate. Caution patients to use a fingertip sample if it is less than 2 hours after eating, less than 2 hours after injecting rapid-acting insulin, during exercise or within 2 hours of exercise, when sick or under stress, when having symptoms of hypoglycemia, if unable to recognize symptoms of hypoglycemia, or if site results do not agree with the way the patient feels (U.S. FDA, 2013).
- Meters require calibration at least monthly or according to the manufacturer's recommendation, and when a new bottle of test strips is opened. Manufacturer's directions for calibration should be followed. After calibration, the meter is checked for accuracy by testing a control solution containing a known amount of glucose.
- Inadequate sampling can cause errors in the results. It is very important to be aware of requirements for the specific monitor used.
- Continuous glucose monitoring systems have become available. These devices use sensors placed just below the skin in the subcutaneous tissue and electrical stimulation to draw interstitial fluid through intact skin into the sensor. A transmitter sends information about glucose levels from the sensor to a pager-like wireless monitor. These devices provide real-time measurements of glucose levels at 1-minute or 5-minute intervals (NDIC, 2012). These systems supplement standard fingerstick meters and provide a way to see glucose trends and track patterns.

Infant and Child Considerations

- Heel sticks, using the outer aspect of the heel, may be used for infants. Warming the heel before the sample is taken dilates the blood vessels in the area and aids in sampling (Perry et al., 2010). This technique is not without controversy, as it is painful and can lead to fibrosis, scarring, and necrotizing osteochondritis (from puncture of the heel bone) (Shah & Ohlsson, 2012; Perry et al., 2010).

Older Adult Considerations

- Meters are available with large digital readouts or audio components for patients with visual impairments.

(continued)

SKILL 18-8 OBTAINING A CAPILLARY BLOOD SAMPLE FOR GLUCOSE TESTING continued

Home Care Considerations

- Patients monitor blood glucose levels routinely at home. Provide education focusing on important elements of diabetes education to assist patients in managing their diabetes, including the signs, symptoms, and management of hypoglycemia and hyperglycemia; correct administration of oral hypoglycemic agents and/or insulin; fingerstick blood glucose monitoring; and the accurate use of fingerstick blood glucose monitoring equipment (Hughes, 2012).
- Many different types of monitors are available. Assist patients to identify desirable features for individual use.

EVIDENCE FOR PRACTICE ▶

BLOOD SAMPLING AND THE USE OF A HEEL LANCE

Heel lance has been traditionally used for blood sampling in neonates for screening tests, including capillary blood glucose sampling. This procedure causes pain for the infants. However, is it less painful when compared with traditional venipuncture? Does use of this technique provide the best care for these infants?

Related Research

Shah, V., & Ohlsson, A. (2012). Venepuncture versus heel lance for blood sampling in term neonates. *Cochrane Database of Systematic Reviews.* Available http://summaries.cochrane.org/CD001452/venepuncture-versus-heel-lance-for-blood-sampling-in-term-neonates.

The objective of this review was to determine whether venipuncture or heel lance is less painful and more effective for blood sampling in newborns. Trials comparing pain response to venipuncture versus heel lance with or without the use of glucose solution as a co-intervention were reviewed. The studies suggested that venipuncture, when done by a trained practitioner, causes less pain than a heel lance. The authors concluded venipuncture, when performed by a skilled phlebotomist, is the method of choice for blood sampling in newborns. In addition, the use of glucose solution given to the infant prior to the venipuncture further lessens the pain associated with venipuncture.

Relevance for Nursing Practice

Nurses are often responsible for obtaining blood samples from their patients, including newborns. Using the most efficient techniques can result in decreased pain and anxiety for both the infant and their parents. Nurses should consider limiting the number and/or frequency of the use of heel lances in infants. This study supports the use of traditional venipuncture to obtain blood samples in term neonates and should be taken into consideration when caring for these young patients.

Refer to thePoint for additional research on related nursing topics.

EVIDENCE FOR PRACTICE ▶

STANDARDS OF MEDICAL CARE IN DIABETES—2013

American Diabetes Association (ADA). (2013). Standards of medical care in diabetes—2013. *Diabetes Care, 36*(Suppl. 1): S11–S66.

These standards of care provide clinicians, patients, researchers, payers, and other interested individuals with the components of diabetes care, general treatment goals, and tools to evaluate the quality of care. The recommendations included are screening, diagnostic, and therapeutic actions that are known or believed to favorably affect health outcomes of patients with diabetes.

Refer to thePoint for additional research on related nursing topics.

SKILL 18-9 USING VENIPUNCTURE TO COLLECT A VENOUS BLOOD SAMPLE FOR ROUTINE TESTING

Venipuncture involves piercing a vein with a needle to obtain a venous blood sample, which is collected in a syringe or tube. The superficial veins of the arm in the antecubital fossa are typically used for venipuncture (Malarkey & McMorrow, 2012), which include the basilic, median cubital, and cephalic veins (Figure 1). However, venipuncture can be performed on a vein in the dorsal forearm, the dorsum of the hand, or another accessible location. When performing a venipuncture, remember the following:

- Do not use the inner wrist because of the high risk for damage to underlying structures.
- Avoid areas that are edematous, paralyzed, burned, scarred, have a tattoo, or are on the same side as a mastectomy, arteriovenous shunt, or graft.
- Avoid an extremity affected by a cerebrovascular accident, areas of infection, or areas with abnormal skin conditions.
- Do not draw blood from the same extremity being used for administration of intravenous medications, fluids, or blood transfusions. Some facilities will allow use of such sites as a 'last resort,' after the infusion has been held for a period of time. If necessary, choose a site distal to the intravenous access site. Check facility policy and procedure (Infusion Nurses Society [INS], 2011; Van Leeuwen et al., 2011).

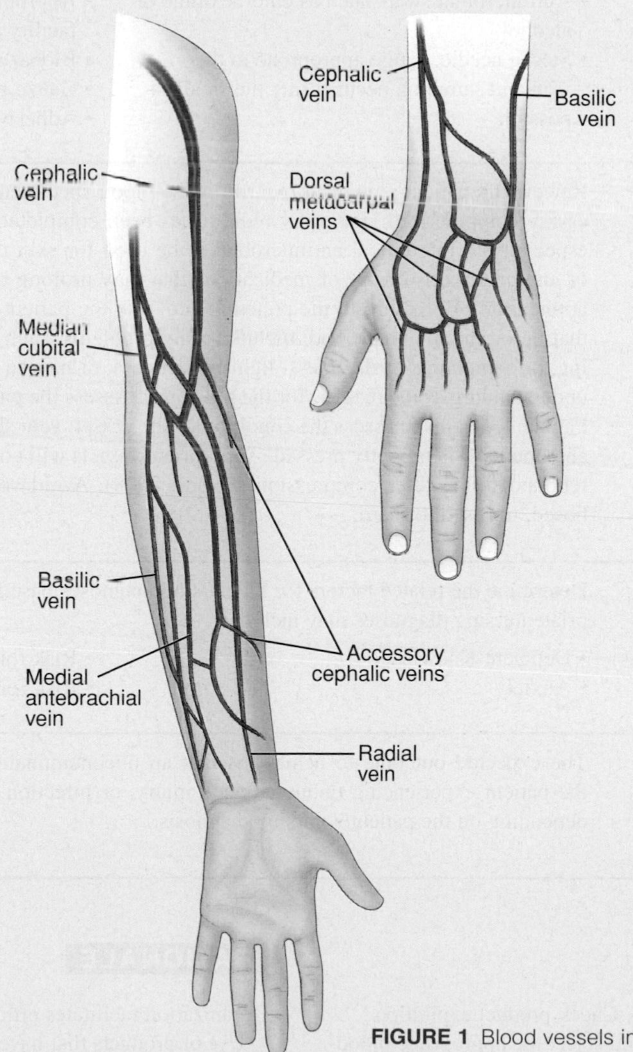

FIGURE 1 Blood vessels in the arm typically used for venipuncture.

(continued)

SKILL 18-9 USING VENIPUNCTURE TO COLLECT A VENOUS BLOOD SAMPLE FOR ROUTINE TESTING continued

Explanation and communication with patients about the need for venipuncture can reduce anxiety. It is important to explain carefully the information about the need for blood tests to ensure patient understanding.

Measures to reduce the risk of infection are an important part of venipuncture. Hand hygiene, aseptic technique, the use of personal protective equipment, and safe disposal of sharps are key to providing safe venipuncture (Adams, 2012; Lavery & Ingram, 2005).

DELEGATION GUIDELINES

The use of venipuncture to obtain a blood sample may be delegated to nursing assistive personnel (NAP) or to unlicensed assistive personnel (UAP) in some settings, as well as to licensed practical/vocational nurses (LPN/LVNs). The decision to delegate must be based on careful analysis of the patient's needs and circumstances, as well as the qualifications of the person to whom the task is being delegated. Refer to the Delegation Guidelines in Appendix A.

EQUIPMENT

- Tourniquet
- Nonsterile gloves
- Additional PPE, as indicated
- Antimicrobial swab, such as chlorhexidine or alcohol
- Sterile needle, gauge appropriate to the vein and sampling needs, using the smallest possible
- Vacutainer needle adaptor
- Blood-collection tubes appropriate for ordered tests
- Appropriate label for specimen, based on facility policy and procedure
- Biohazard bag
- Gauze pads (2 × 2)
- Adhesive bandage

ASSESSMENT

Review the patient's medical record for the blood specimens to be obtained. Ensure that the necessary computerized laboratory request has been completed. Assess the patient for any allergies, especially to the topical antimicrobial to be used for skin cleansing. Investigate for the presence of any conditions or use of medications that may prolong bleeding time, necessitating additional application of pressure to the puncture site. Ask the patient about any previous laboratory testing that he or she may have had, including any problems, such as difficulty with venipuncture, fainting, or complaints of dizziness, light-headedness, or nausea. Assess the patient's anxiety level and understanding of the reasons for the blood test. Assess the patency of the veins in both upper limbs. Palpate the veins to assess the condition of the vessel; vein should be straight, feel soft, cylindrical, and bounce when lightly pressed. Appropriate vessels will compress without rolling, and have rapid rebound filling after compression (Scales, 2008). Avoid veins that are tender, sclerosed, thrombosed, fibrosed, or hard.

NURSING DIAGNOSIS

Determine the related factors for the nursing diagnoses based on the patient's current status. Appropriate nursing diagnoses may include:

- Deficient Knowledge
- Anxiety
- Risk for Injury
- Risk for Infection

OUTCOME IDENTIFICATION AND PLANNING

The expected outcome to achieve is that an uncontaminated specimen will be obtained without the patient experiencing undue anxiety, injury, or infection. Other outcomes may be appropriate, depending on the patient's nursing diagnosis.

IMPLEMENTATION

ACTION	RATIONALE
1. Gather the necessary supplies. Check product expiration dates. Identify ordered tests and select the appropriate blood-collection tubes.	Organization facilitates efficient performance of the procedure. Use of products that have not expired ensures proper functioning of equipment. Using correct bottles ensures accurate blood sampling.

ACTION	RATIONALE
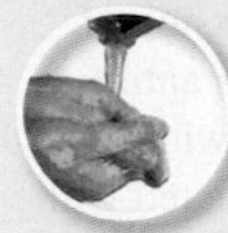 2. Perform hand hygiene and put on PPE, if indicated.	Hand hygiene and PPE prevent the transmission of microorganisms. PPE is required based on transmission precautions.
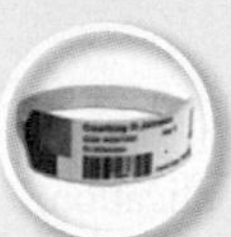 3. Identify the patient.	Identifying the patient ensures the right patient receives the intervention and helps prevent errors.
4. Explain the procedure to the patient. Allow the patient time to ask questions and verbalize concerns about the venipuncture procedure.	Explanation provides reassurance and promotes cooperation.
5. Check the specimen label with the patient's identification bracelet. Label should include the patient's name and identification number, time specimen was collected, route of collection, identification of the person obtaining the sample, and any other information required by facility policy.	Confirmation of patient identification information ensures the specimen is labeled correctly for the right patient.
6. Assemble equipment on overbed table within reach.	Arranging items nearby is convenient, saves time, and avoids unnecessary stretching and twisting of muscles on the part of the nurse.
7. Close curtains around the bed and close the door to the room, if possible.	Closing the door or curtain provides for patient privacy.
8. Provide for good light. Artificial light is recommended. Place a trash receptacle within easy reach.	Good lighting is necessary to perform the procedure properly. Having the trash receptacle within easy reach allows for safe disposal of contaminated materials.
9. Assist the patient to a comfortable position, either sitting or lying. If the patient is lying in bed, raise the bed to a comfortable working height, usually elbow height of the caregiver (VISN 8 Patient Safety Center, 2009).	Proper positioning allows easy access to the site and promotes patient comfort and safety. Proper bed height helps reduce back strain while performing the procedure.
10. Determine the patient's preferred site for the procedure based on his or her previous experience. Expose the arm, supporting it in an extended position on a firm surface, such as a tabletop. Position self on the same side of the patient as the site selected. Apply a tourniquet to the upper arm on the chosen side approximately 3 to 4 inches above the potential puncture site. Apply sufficient pressure to impede venous circulation but not arterial blood flow.	Patient preference promotes patient participation in treatment and gives the nurse information that may aid in site selection (Lavery & Ingram, 2005). Positioning close to the chosen site reduces back strain. Use of a tourniquet increases venous pressure to aid in vein identification. Tourniquet should remain in place no more than 60 seconds to prevent injury (Fischbach & Dunning, 2009).
11. Put on gloves. Assess the veins using inspection and palpation to determine the best puncture site. Refer to the Assessment section above.	Gloves reduce transmission of microorganisms. Using the best site reduces the risk of injury to the patient. Observation and palpation allow for making distinction between other structures, such as tendons and arteries, in the area to avoid injury.
12. **Release the tourniquet. Check that the vein has decompressed.**	Releasing the tourniquet reduces the length of time the tourniquet is applied (Lavery & Ingram, 2005). Tourniquet should remain in place no more than 60 seconds to prevent injury, stasis, and hemoconcentration, which may alter results (Fischbach & Dunning, 2009). Thrombosed veins will remain firm and palpable and should not be used for venipuncture (Lavery & Ingram, 2005).
13. Attach the needle to the Vacutainer device. Place first blood-collection tube into the Vacutainer, but not engaged in the puncture device in the Vacutainer.	Device is prepared for use to ensure efficiency with the task.

(*continued*)

SKILL 18-9 USING VENIPUNCTURE TO COLLECT A VENOUS BLOOD SAMPLE FOR ROUTINE TESTING continued

ACTION	RATIONALE
14. **Clean the patient's skin at the selected puncture site with the antimicrobial swab (Figure 2). If using chlorhexidine, use a gentle back and forth motion or use the procedure recommended by the manufacturer. If using alcohol, wipe in a circular motion spiraling outward. Allow the skin to dry before performing the venipuncture. Do not wipe or blot. Allow to dry completely.**	Cleaning the patient's skin reduces the risk for transmission of microorganisms. Allowing the skin to dry maximizes antimicrobial action and prevents contact of the substance with the needle on insertion, thereby reducing the sting associated with insertion.
15. Alternately, for patients who bruise easily, are at risk for bleeding, or have fragile skin, **apply the chlorhexidine without scrubbing for at least 30 seconds. Allow to dry completely. Do not wipe or blot.**	Avoiding use of scrubbing decreases risk of injury. Application for a minimum 30 seconds is necessary for chlorhexidine to be effective (Hadaway, 2006). Organisms on the skin can be introduced into the tissues or the bloodstream with the needle.
16. Reapply the tourniquet approximately 3 to 4 inches above the identified puncture site (Figure 3). Apply sufficient pressure to impede venous circulation but not arterial blood flow. **After disinfection, do not palpate the venipuncture site unless sterile gloves are worn.**	Use of a tourniquet increases venous pressure to aid in vein identification. Tourniquet should remain in place no more than 60 seconds to prevent injury, stasis, and hemoconcentration, which may alter results (Fischbach & Dunning, 2009).

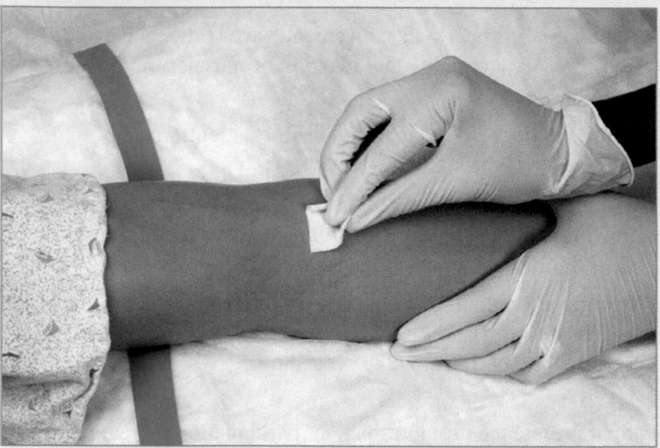

FIGURE 2 Cleaning the patient's skin at the venipuncture site.

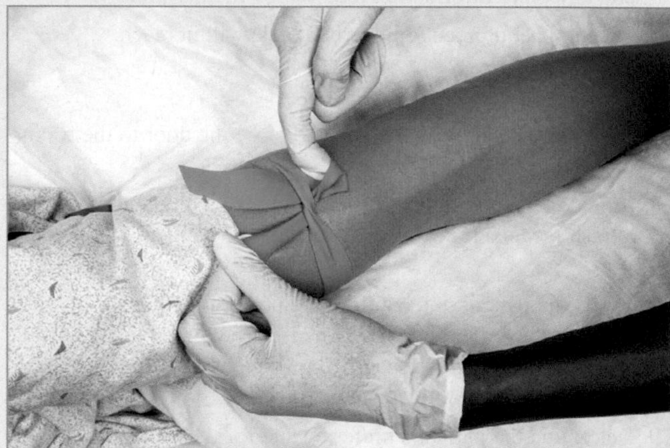

FIGURE 3 Reapplying the tourniquet.

ACTION	RATIONALE
17. Hold the patient's arm in a downward position with your nondominant hand. Align the needle and Vacutainer device with the chosen vein, holding the Vacutainer and needle in your dominant hand. Use the thumb or first finger of your nondominant hand to apply pressure and traction to the skin just below the identified puncture site.	Applying pressure helps immobilize and anchor the vein. Taut skin at entry site aids smooth needle entry.
18. **Inform the patient that he or she is going to feel a pinch.** With the bevel of the needle up, insert the needle into the vein at a 15-degree angle to the skin (Malarkey & McMorrow, 2012) (Figure 4).	Warning the patient prevents reaction related to surprise. Positioning the needle at the proper angle reduces the risk of puncturing through the vein.
19. Grasp the Vacutainer securely to stabilize it in the vein with your nondominant hand, and push the first collection tube into the puncture device in the Vacutainer, until the rubber stopper on the collection tube is punctured. You will feel the tube push into place on the puncture device. Blood will flow into the tube automatically (Figure 5).	The collection tube is a vacuum; negative pressure within the tube pulls blood into the tube.
20. **Remove the tourniquet as soon as blood flows adequately into the tube.**	Tourniquet removal reduces venous pressure and restores venous return to help prevent bleeding and bruising (Van Leeuwen et al., 2011; Scales, 2008).

ACTION	RATIONALE
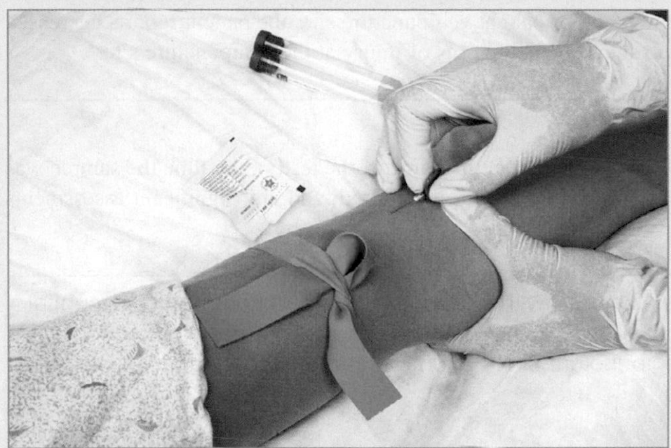 FIGURE 4 Inserting the needle at a 15-degree angle, with the bevel up.	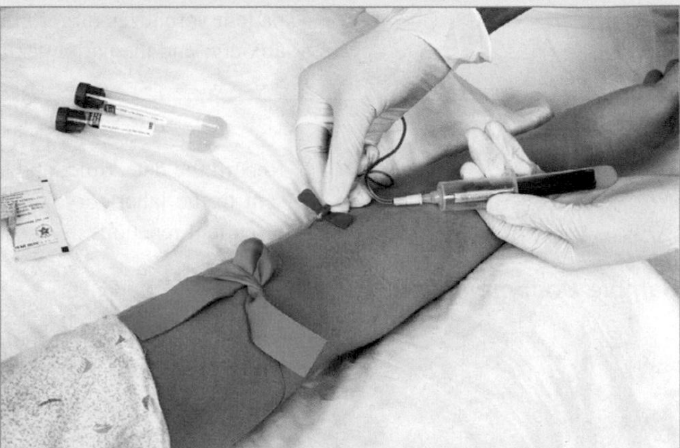 FIGURE 5 Observing blood flowing into the collection tube.
21. Continue to hold the Vacutainer in place in the vein and continue to fill the required tubes, removing one and inserting another. Gently rotate each tube as you remove it.	Filling the required tubes ensures that the sample is accurate. Gentle rotation helps to mix any additive in the tube with the blood sample.
22. After you have drawn all required blood samples, remove the last collection tube from the Vacutainer. **Place a gauze pad over the puncture site and slowly and gently remove the needle from the vein. Engage needle guard. Do not apply pressure to the site until the needle has been fully removed.**	Slow, gentle needle removal prevents injury to the vein. Releasing the vacuum before withdrawing the needle prevents injury to the vein and hematoma formation. Use of a needle guard prevents accidental needlestick injuries.
23. Apply gentle pressure to the puncture site for 2 to 3 minutes or until bleeding stops.	Applying pressure to the site after needle removal prevents injury, bleeding, and extravasation into the surrounding tissue, which can cause a hematoma.
24. After bleeding stops, apply an adhesive bandage.	The bandage protects the site and aids in applying pressure.
25. Remove equipment and return the patient to a position of comfort. Raise side rail and lower bed.	Repositioning promotes patient comfort. Raising rails promotes safety.
26. Discard Vacutainer and needle in sharps container.	Proper disposal of equipment reduces transmission of microorganisms.
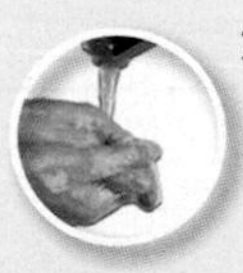 27. Remove gloves and perform hand hygiene.	Removing gloves properly reduces the risk for infection transmission and contamination of other items.
28. Place label on the container per facility policy. Place container in plastic, sealable biohazard bag.	Proper labeling ensures accurate reporting of results. Packaging the specimen in a biohazard bag prevents the person transporting the container from coming in contact with blood and body fluids.
29. Check the venipuncture site to see if a hematoma has developed.	Development of a hematoma requires further intervention.
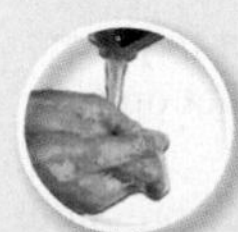 30. Remove other PPE, if used. Perform hand hygiene.	Removing PPE properly reduces the risk for infection transmission and contamination of other items. Hand hygiene reduces the transmission of microorganisms.
31. Transport the specimen to the laboratory immediately. If immediate transport is not possible, check with laboratory personnel or policy manual whether refrigeration is contraindicated.	Timely transport ensures accurate results.

(continued)

SKILL 18-9 USING VENIPUNCTURE TO COLLECT A VENOUS BLOOD SAMPLE FOR ROUTINE TESTING continued

EVALUATION

The expected outcome is achieved when an uncontaminated blood specimen is obtained without adverse event. Other outcomes may include the following: the patient states reason for blood test; the patient verbalizes minor, if any, complaint of pain at venipuncture site; the patient reports decreased anxiety; and the patient exhibits no signs and symptoms of injury at the venipuncture site.

DOCUMENTATION

Guidelines

Record the date, time, and site of the venipuncture; the name of the test(s); the time the sample was sent to the laboratory; the amount of blood collected, if required; and any significant assessments or patient reactions.

Sample Documentation

<u>6/10/15</u> 0945 Blood specimen for CBC with differential obtained from right antecubital space. Approximately 8 mL of blood collected and sent to laboratory. No evidence of bleeding or hematoma at venipuncture site. Patient denied any complaints of pain or feelings of light-headedness.

—*C. Lewis, RN*

UNEXPECTED SITUATIONS AND ASSOCIATED INTERVENTIONS

- *After applying the tourniquet, you have trouble finding a distended vein:* Have the patient make a fist, or try tapping the skin over the vein lightly several times. If unsuccessful, remove the tourniquet and try lowering the patient's arm to allow blood to pool in the veins. If necessary, apply warm compresses for about 10 minutes before reapplying the tourniquet.
- *Patient has large, distended, highly visible veins:* Perform venipuncture without a tourniquet to minimize the risk for hematoma.
- *Patient has a clotting disorder or is receiving anticoagulant therapy:* Maintain firm pressure on the venipuncture site for at least 5 minutes after withdrawing the needle to prevent hematoma formation.
- *Oozing or bleeding continues from the puncture site for more than a few minutes:* Elevate the area and apply a pressure dressing. If bleeding is excessive or persists for longer than 10 minutes, notify the primary health care provider.
- *A hematoma develops at the venipuncture site:* Apply pressure until you are sure bleeding has stopped (about 5 minutes). Notify the primary health care provider. Document size and appearance of hematoma, notification of primary health care provider, and any ordered interventions.
- *Patient reports feeling light-headed and says she is going to faint:* Stop the venipuncture. If the patient is in bed, have the patient lie flat and elevate the feet. If the patient is in a chair, have the patient put her head between her knees. Encourage the patient to take slow, deep breaths. Call for assistance and stay with the patient. Obtain vital signs, if possible.

SPECIAL CONSIDERATIONS

General Considerations

- **Obtain only the volume of blood needed for accurate testing.** Phlebotomy (drawing blood) contributes to iron deficiency and blood loss in newborns and critically ill patients. Consider interventions to conserve blood, including the use of low-volume blood collection tubes, recording the volume of blood obtained for laboratory testing, avoidance of routine testing and consolidation of all daily tests with one blood draw (INS 2011, p. S78).
- Be aware of the facility's policy regarding order of collection of multiple tubes of blood to ensure accurate results.
- If the flow of blood into the collection tube or syringe is sluggish, leave the tourniquet in place longer, but always remove it before withdrawing the needle. Do not leave the tourniquet on for more than 60 seconds.
- If necessary, use a blood pressure cuff inflated to a point between systolic and diastolic pressure values as an alternative to a tourniquet (Fischbach & Dunning, 2009).
- Avoid collecting blood from edematous areas, arteriovenous shunts, an upper extremity on the same side as a previous lymph node dissection or mastectomy, infected sites, same extremity as an intravenous infusion, and sites of previous hematomas or vascular injury.

- Do not use veins in the lower extremities for venipuncture, because of an increased risk of thrombophlebitis. Some facilities allow collection from lower extremities with a physician's order to collect blood from a leg or foot vein. Check your facility's policies.
- Apply warm compresses to the selected site 15 to 20 minutes before venipuncture to aid in distending veins that are difficult to locate.
- Consider the use of topical anesthetic creams to minimize discomfort and pain for the patient, based on facility policy. Be familiar with requirements and specifications for a particular product available for use. Application needs to occur sufficiently in advance to allow enough time to become effective.
- Use distraction, if appropriate. Distraction has been shown to be of benefit in reducing anxiety related to venipuncture, especially with children. Asking the patient to concentrate on relaxing and performing deep breathing may help. Asking the patient to cough at the time of venipuncture is another technique that has been shown to be effective in reducing pain with venipuncture (Usichenko et al., 2004).

Infant and Child Considerations

- Use smaller-gauge needles with infants and children because their veins are smaller and more fragile.
- Consider automatically applying warm compresses to distend the small veins of infants and young children before attempting any venipuncture.
- Use butterfly needles, as appropriate, for obtaining blood from infants and small children.
- Venipuncture by a skilled phlebotomist is the method of choice over a heel lance in infants (Shah & Ohlsson, 2012).
- Administer oral sucrose beginning 1 to 2 minutes before the venipuncture procedure for young infants to decrease the incidence of procedure-related pain (Kassab et al., 2012; Liu et al., 2010).
- Consider using topical anesthetic creams or gels, refrigerant spray, or iontophoresis (application of electric current to carry ionized lidocaine through the skin) with infants and children to decrease the incidence of procedure-related pain (Baxter et al., 2013; İnal & Kelleci, 2012a). Apply the product for sufficient time to reach maximal effectiveness.
- Consider the use of distraction to decrease the incidence of procedure related pain (İnal & Kelleci, 2012b).

Older Adult Considerations

- Keep in mind that the veins of an older adult are fragile and may collapse easily. In addition, the skin is less elastic and may be more difficult to pull taut.
- The superficial veins of the hands of older adults are fragile and venipuncture can cause a hematoma to form. Additionally, these veins move due to the age-related loss of supportive muscle and connective tissue, making it difficult to enter the lumen of the vein (Malarkey & McMorrow, 2012).
- Consider performing venipuncture without a tourniquet for older patients to prevent rupture of capillaries. Instruct the patient to make a tight fist before needle insertion. Do not have the patient pump the fist, because this may increase plasma potassium levels (Fischbach & Dunning, 2009).

EVIDENCE FOR PRACTICE ▶

BLOOD SAMPLING AND THE USE OF A HEEL LANCE

Heel lance has been traditionally used for blood sampling in neonates for screening tests, including capillary blood glucose sampling. This procedure causes pain for the infants. However, is it less painful when compared with traditional venipuncture? Does use of this technique provide the best care for these infants?

Shah, V., & Ohlsson, A. (2012). Venepuncture versus heel lance for blood sampling in term neonates. *Cochrane Database of Systematic Reviews.* Available http://summaries.cochrane.org/CD001452/venepuncture-versus-heel-lance-for-blood-sampling-in-term-neonates.

Refer to Skill 18-8 for details, and refer to thePoint for additional research on related nursing topics.

(*continued*)

SKILL 18-9 USING VENIPUNCTURE TO COLLECT A VENOUS BLOOD SAMPLE FOR ROUTINE TESTING continued

EVIDENCE FOR PRACTICE ▶

RELIEF OF PAIN DURING BLOOD SPECIMEN COLLECTION IN PEDIATRIC PATIENTS

Needle insertion for venipuncture is painful, frightening, and distressful for children. What interventions can assist nurses to reduce the emotional and physical effects of painful procedures, such as venipuncture, in children?

Related Research

İnal, S., & Kelleci, M. (2012). Relief of pain during blood specimen collection in pediatric patients. *The American Journal of Maternal Child Nursing, 37*(5), 339–345.

The purpose of this randomized, controlled study was to investigate the effect of external cold and vibration stimulation on pain and anxiety levels of children during blood specimen collection. Children aged 6 to 12 years who required blood tests were randomly assigned to a control group (no intervention) or an experimental group that received external cold and vibration via a device called Buzzy®. External cold and vibration were applied 5 cm above the venipuncture site, just before the blood specimen collection procedure, and continued until the end of the procedure. Pre-procedural and procedural anxiety were assessed with an objective tool, as well as parent and observer reports. Procedural pain was assessed with an objective tool, as well as self-report of the children, and parents' and observers' reports. The experimental group showed significantly lower pain and anxiety levels compared with the control group during the blood specimen collection procedure. The use of the interventions did not cause a significant difference in the success of the blood specimen collection procedure. The authors concluded the use of external cold and vibration decreased perceived pain and reduced children's anxiety during blood specimen collection.

Relevance for Nursing Practice

Nurses are often responsible for obtaining blood samples from their patients, including children. Using the most efficient techniques can result in decreased pain and anxiety for both the children and their parents. This study suggests a method of reducing pain and anxiety associated with venipuncture and should be taken into consideration when caring for these young patients.

Refer to thePoint for additional research on related nursing topics.

SKILL 18-10 OBTAINING A VENOUS BLOOD SPECIMEN FOR CULTURE AND SENSITIVITY

Normally bacteria-free, blood is susceptible to infection through infusion lines as well as from thrombophlebitis, surgical drains, infected shunts, and bacterial endocarditis due to prosthetic heart-valve replacements. Bacteria may also move into the bloodstream through the lymphatic system from an infection of a specific body site when the person's immune system cannot contain the infection at its source, such as the bladder or kidneys from a urinary tract infection. Patients with a compromised immune system are at higher risk for septicemia.

Blood cultures are performed to detect bacterial invasion (bacteremia) or fungi (fungemia) and the systemic spread of such an infection (septicemia) through the bloodstream. In this procedure, a venous blood sample is collected by venipuncture into two bottles (one set), one containing an anaerobic medium and the other an aerobic medium. The bottles are incubated, encouraging any organisms present in the sample to grow in the media. Ideally, two sets of cultures from two different venipuncture sites should be obtained. In the past, multiple sets of cultures were obtained at different time intervals. Currently, best practice is to draw blood one time, obtaining at least 30 mL of blood (for adults) from two different venipuncture sites. In general, no more than two to three sets of blood specimens over a 24-hour period should be collected (Malarkey & McMorrow, 2012; Myers III & Reyes, 2011).

The main problem encountered with blood-culture testing is that the specimen is easily contaminated with bacteria from the environment. Care must be taken to clean the skin at the venipuncture site properly to prevent contamination with skin flora, and aseptic technique must be used during the procedure. In addition, the access ports on the blood-culture bottles must be properly cleaned before use.

Refer to Skill 18-9 for additional considerations related to venipuncture and blood sample collection.

DELEGATION GUIDELINES

The use of venipuncture to obtain a blood sample for blood culture may be delegated to nursing assistive personnel (NAP) or to unlicensed assistive personnel (UAP) in some settings, as well as to licensed practical/vocational nurses (LPN/LVNs). The decision to delegate must be based on careful analysis of the patient's needs and circumstances, as well as the qualifications of the person to whom the task is being delegated. Refer to the Delegation Guidelines in Appendix A.

EQUIPMENT

- Tourniquet
- Nonsterile gloves
- Additional PPE, as indicated
- Antimicrobial swabs, such as chlorhexidine, per facility policy, for cleaning skin and culture bottle tops
- Vacutainer needle adaptor
- Sterile butterfly needle, gauge appropriate to the vein and sampling needs, using the smallest possible, with extension tubing
- Two blood-culture collection bottles for each set being obtained: one anaerobic bottle and one aerobic bottle
- Appropriate label for specimen, based on facility policy and procedure
- Biohazard bag
- Nonsterile gauze pads (2 × 2)
- Sterile gauze pads (2 × 2)
- Adhesive bandage

ASSESSMENT

Review the patient's medical record and the medical orders for the number and type of blood cultures to be obtained. Ensure that the appropriate computer laboratory request has been completed. Assess the patient for signs and symptoms of infection, including vital signs, and note any antibiotic therapy being administered. Inspect any invasive monitoring insertion sites or incisions for indications of infection. Assess the patient for any allergies, especially related to the topical antimicrobial used for skin cleansing. Assess for presence of any conditions or use of medications that may prolong bleeding time, necessitating additional application of pressure to the puncture site. Ask the patient about any previous laboratory testing that he or she may have had, including any problems, such as difficulty with venipuncture, fainting, or complaints of dizziness, light-headedness, or nausea. Assess the patient's anxiety level and understanding about the reasons for the blood test. Assess the patency of the veins in both upper limbs. Palpate the veins to assess the condition of the vessel; the vein should be straight, feel soft, cylindrical, and bounce when lightly pressed. Appropriate vessels will compress without rolling, and have rapid rebound filling after compression (Scales, 2008). Avoid veins that are tender, sclerosed, thrombosed, fibrosed, or hard.

NURSING DIAGNOSIS

Determine the related factors for the nursing diagnoses based on the patient's current status. Appropriate nursing diagnoses may include:

- Deficient Knowledge
- Anxiety
- Risk for Injury
- Risk for Infection

OUTCOME IDENTIFICATION AND PLANNING

The expected outcome to achieve is that an uncontaminated specimen will be obtained without the patient experiencing undue anxiety and injury. Other outcomes may be appropriate, depending on the patient's nursing diagnosis.

IMPLEMENTATION

ACTION	RATIONALE
1. Gather the necessary supplies. Check product expiration dates. Identify ordered number of blood culture sets and select the appropriate blood-collection bottles (at least one anaerobic and one aerobic bottle). **If tests are ordered in addition to the blood cultures, collect the blood-culture specimens before other specimens.**	Organization facilitates efficient performance of the procedure. Use of products that have not expired ensures proper functioning of equipment. Using correct tubes ensures accurate blood sampling.

(continued)

SKILL 18-10 OBTAINING A VENOUS BLOOD SPECIMEN FOR CULTURE AND SENSITIVITY continued

ACTION	RATIONALE
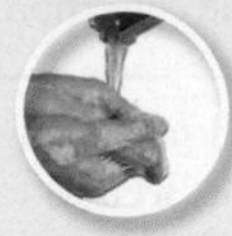 2. Perform hand hygiene and put on PPE, if indicated.	Hand hygiene and PPE prevent the transmission of microorganisms. PPE is required based on transmission precautions.
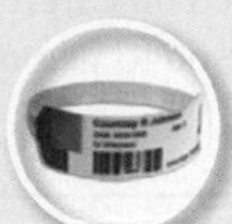 3. Identify the patient.	Identifying the patient ensures the right patient receives the intervention and helps prevent errors.
4. Explain the procedure. Allow the patient time to ask questions and verbalize concerns about the venipuncture procedure.	Explanation provides reassurance and promotes cooperation.
5. Check specimen label with the patient's identification bracelet. Label should include the patient's name and identification number, time specimen was collected, route of collection, identification of person obtaining the sample, and any other information required by facility policy.	Confirmation of patient identification information ensures the specimen is labeled correctly for the right patient.
6. Assemble equipment on overbed table within reach.	Arranging items nearby is convenient, saves time, and avoids unnecessary stretching and twisting of muscles on the part of the nurse.
7. Close curtains around the bed and close the door to the room, if possible.	Closing the door or curtain provides for patient privacy.
8. Provide for good light. Artificial light is recommended. Place a trash receptacle within easy reach.	Good lighting is necessary to perform the procedure properly. Having the trash receptacle within easy reach allows for safe disposal of contaminated materials.
9. Assist the patient to a comfortable position, either sitting or lying. If the patient is lying in bed, raise the bed to a comfortable working height, usually elbow height of the caregiver (VISN 8 Patient Safety Center, 2009).	Proper positioning allows easy access to the site and promotes patient comfort and safety. Proper bed height helps reduce back strain while performing the procedure.
10. Determine the patient's preferred site for the procedure based on his or her previous experience. Expose the arm, supporting it in an extended position on a firm surface, such as a tabletop. Position self on the same side of the patient as the site selected. Apply a tourniquet to the upper arm on the chosen side approximately 3 to 4 inches above the potential puncture site (Figure 1). Apply sufficient pressure to impede venous circulation, but not arterial blood flow.	Patient preference allows the patient to be involved in treatment and gives the nurse information that may aid in site selection (Lavery & Ingram, 2005). Positioning close to the chosen site reduces back strain. Use of a tourniquet increases venous pressure and distention to aid in vein identification. Tourniquet should remain in place no more than 60 seconds to prevent injury, stasis, and hemoconcentration, which may alter results (Fischbach & Dunning, 2009).

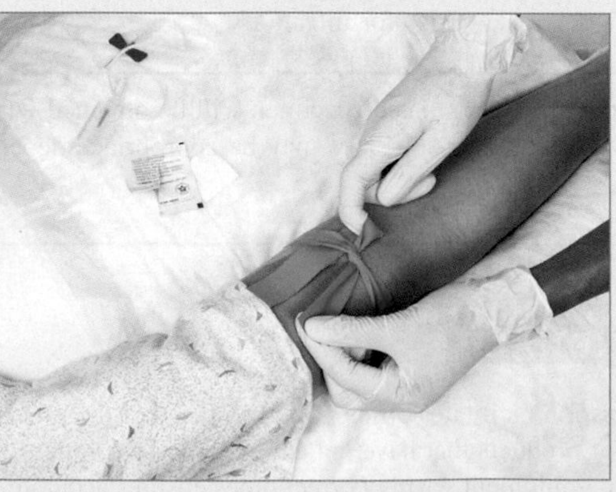

FIGURE 1 Applying the tourniquet.

ACTION	RATIONALE
11. Put on nonsterile gloves. Assess the veins using inspection and palpation to determine the best puncture site. Refer to the Assessment section above.	Gloves reduce transmission of microorganisms. Using the best site reduces the risk of injury to the patient. Palpation allows for making a distinction between other structures, such as tendons and arteries, in the area to avoid injury.
12. **Release the tourniquet. Check that the vein has decompressed.**	Releasing the tourniquet reduces the length of time the tourniquet is applied. Tourniquet should remain in place no more than 60 seconds to prevent injury, stasis, and hemoconcentration, which may alter results (Fischbach & Dunning, 2009). Thrombosed veins will remain firm and palpable and should not be used for venipuncture (Lavery & Ingram, 2005).
13. Attach the butterfly needle extension tubing to the Vacutainer device.	Connection prepares device for use.
14. Move collection bottles to a location close to the arm, with bottles sitting upright on tabletop.	Bottles must be close enough to reach with extension tubing on butterfly needle to fill after venipuncture is completed. Bottles should remain upright to prevent backflow of contents to patient.
15. **Clean the patient's skin at the selected puncture site with the antimicrobial swab, according to facility policy. If using chlorhexidine, use a gentle back and forth motion or use the procedure recommended by the manufacturer. Do not wipe or blot. Allow to dry completely.**	Cleaning the patient's skin reduces the risk for transmission of microorganisms. Allowing the skin to dry maximizes antimicrobial action and prevents contact of the substance with the needle on insertion, thereby reducing the sting associated with insertion.
16. Alternately, for patients who bruise easily, are at risk for bleeding, or have fragile skin, **apply the chlorhexidine without scrubbing for at least 30 seconds. Allow to dry completely. Do not wipe or blot.**	Avoiding use of scrubbing decreases risk of injury. Application for minimum of 30 seconds is necessary for chlorhexidine to be effective (Hadaway, 2006). Organisms on the skin can be introduced into the tissues or the bloodstream with the needle.
17. Using a new antimicrobial swab, clean the stoppers of the culture bottles with the appropriate antimicrobial, per facility policy. Cover bottle top with sterile gauze square, based on facility policy.	Cleaning the bottle top reduces the risk for transmission of microorganisms into the bottle. Covering the top reduces risk of contamination.
18. Reapply the tourniquet approximately 3 to 4 inches above the identified puncture site. Apply sufficient pressure to impede venous circulation, but not arterial blood flow. **After disinfection, do not palpate the venipuncture site unless sterile gloves are worn.**	Use of tourniquet increases venous pressure to aid in vein identification. Tourniquet should remain in place no more than 60 seconds to prevent injury, stasis, and hemoconcentration, which may alter results. Palpation is the greatest potential cause of blood culture contamination (Fischbach & Dunning, 2009).
19. Hold the patient's arm in a downward position with your nondominant hand. Align the butterfly needle with the chosen vein, holding the needle in your dominant hand. Use the thumb or first finger of your nondominant hand to apply pressure and traction to the skin just below the identified puncture site (Figure 2). **Do not touch the insertion site.**	Applying pressure helps immobilize and anchor the vein. Taut skin at the entry site aids smooth needle entry. Not touching the insertion site helps to prevent contamination. Palpation is the greatest potential cause of blood culture contamination (Myers III & Reyes, 2011; Fischbach & Dunning, 2009).

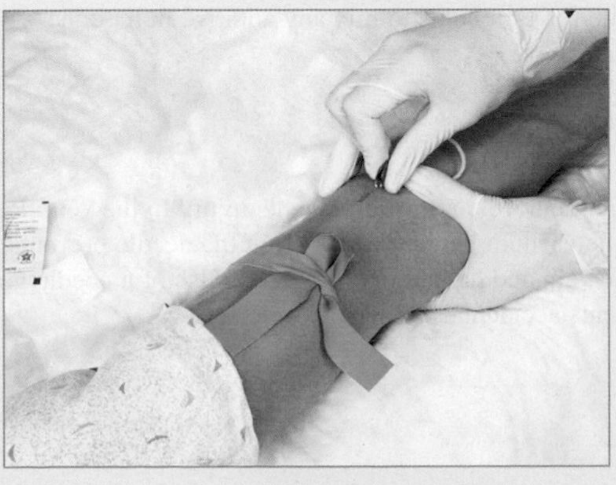

FIGURE 2 Aligning the butterfly needle with the chosen vein.

(continued)

SKILL 18-10 OBTAINING A VENOUS BLOOD SPECIMEN FOR CULTURE AND SENSITIVITY continued

ACTION	RATIONALE
20. **Inform the patient that he or she is going to feel a pinch.** With the bevel of the needle up, insert the needle into the vein at a 15-degree angle to the skin (Malarkey & McMorrow, 2012). You should see a flash of blood in the extension tubing close to the needle when the vein is entered (Figure 3).	Warning the patient prevents reaction related to surprise. Positioning the needle at the proper angle reduces the risk of puncturing through the vein. Flash of blood indicates entrance into the vein.
21. Grasp the butterfly needle securely to stabilize it in the vein with your nondominant hand, and push the Vacutainer onto the first collection bottle (anaerobic bottle), until the rubber stopper on the collection bottle is punctured (Figure 4). You will feel the bottle push into place on the puncture device. Blood will flow into the bottle automatically.	The collection bottle is a vacuum; negative pressure within the bottle pulls blood into the bottle.

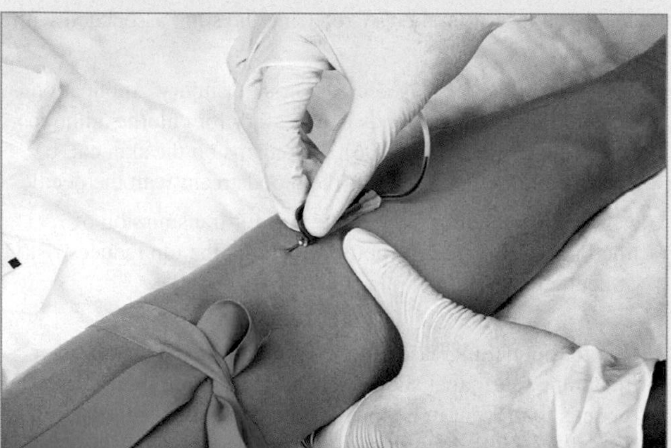
FIGURE 3 Inserting the needle with the bevel up at a 15-degree angle.

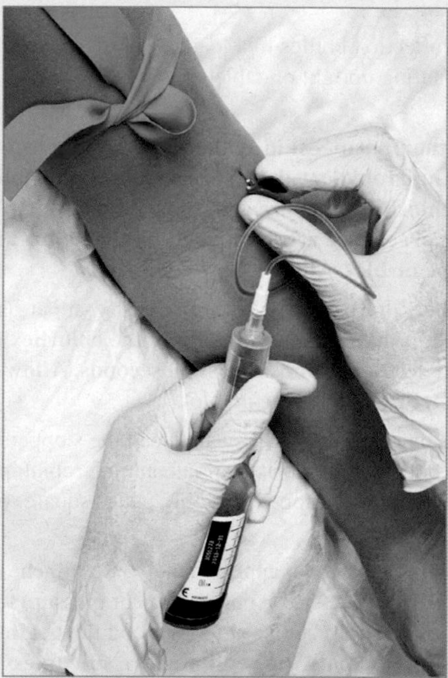
FIGURE 4 Stabilizing the butterfly needle and pushing the Vacutainer onto the anaerobic collection bottle.

ACTION	RATIONALE
22. **Remove the tourniquet as soon as blood flows adequately into the bottle.**	Tourniquet removal reduces venous pressure and restores venous return to help prevent bleeding and bruising (Van Leeuwen et al., 2011; Scales, 2008).
23. Continue to hold the butterfly needle in place in the vein. Once the first bottle is filled, remove it from the Vacutainer and insert the second bottle. After the blood culture specimens are obtained, continue to fill any additional required tubes, removing one and inserting another. Gently rotate each bottle and tube as you remove it.	Filling the required bottles ensures that the sample is accurate. Gentle rotation helps to mix any additive in the tube with the blood sample.
24. After you have drawn all required blood samples, remove the last collection tube from the Vacutainer. **Place a gauze pad over the puncture site and slowly and gently remove the needle from the vein. Engage needle guard. Do not apply pressure to the site until the needle has been fully removed.**	Slow, gentle needle removal prevents injury to the vein. Releasing the vacuum before withdrawing the needle prevents injury to the vein and hematoma formation. Use of a needle guard prevents accidental needlestick injuries.

ACTION	RATIONALE
25. Apply gentle pressure to the puncture site for 2 to 3 minutes or until bleeding stops.	Applying pressure to the site after needle removal prevents injury, bleeding, and extravasation into the surrounding tissue, which can cause a hematoma.
26. After bleeding stops, apply an adhesive bandage.	The bandage protects the site and aids in applying pressure.
27. Remove equipment and return patient to a position of comfort. Raise side rails and lower bed.	Repositioning promotes patient comfort. Raising rails promotes safety.
28. Discard Vacutainer and butterfly needle in sharps container.	Proper disposal of equipment reduces transmission of microorganisms.
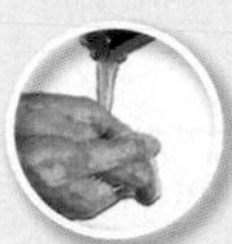 29. Remove gloves and perform hand hygiene.	Removing gloves properly reduces the risk for infection transmission and contamination of other items. Hand hygiene reduces the transmission of microorganisms.
30. Place label on the container, per facility policy (Figure 5). Place containers in plastic, sealable biohazard bag (Figure 6). Refer to facility policy regarding the need for separate biohazard bags for blood culture specimens and other blood specimens.	Proper labeling ensures accurate reporting of results. Packaging the specimen in a biohazard bag prevents the person transporting the container from coming in contact with blood or body fluids. Some facility policies call for individual bagging.
31. Collect blood for second set of cultures from a second site, using the same technique.	Best practice involves drawing blood one time, obtaining at least 30 mL of blood (for adults) from two different venipuncture sites (Malarkey & McMorrow, 2012; Myers III & Reyes, 2011).
32. Check the venipuncture sites to see if a hematoma has developed.	Development of a hematoma requires further intervention.
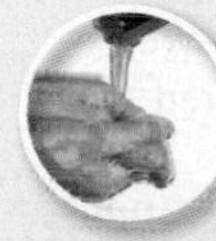 33. Remove other PPE, if used. Perform hand hygiene.	Removing PPE properly reduces the risk for infection transmission and contamination of other items. Hand hygiene reduces the transmission of microorganisms.

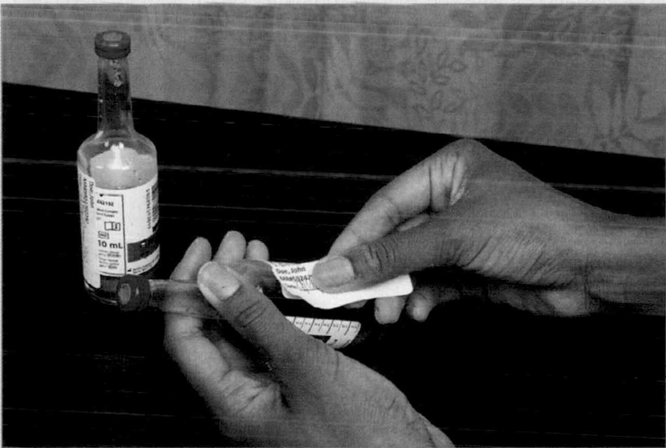

FIGURE 5 Placing a label on specimen container.

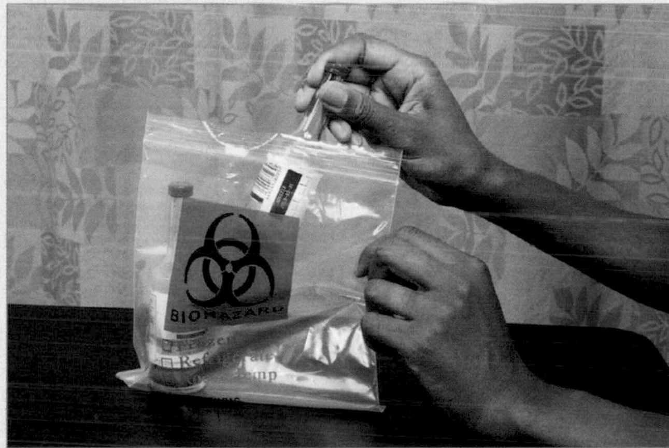

FIGURE 6 Placing specimen containers in biohazard bag.

ACTION	RATIONALE
34. Transport the specimen to the laboratory immediately. If immediate transport is not possible, check with laboratory personnel or policy manual as to appropriate handling.	Timely transport ensures accurate results.

EVALUATION

The expected outcome is achieved when uncontaminated blood culture specimens are obtained without adverse event. Other outcomes may include the following: the patient states reason for blood cultures; the patient verbalizes minor, if any, complaint of pain at venipuncture site; the patient reports decreased anxiety; and the patient exhibits no signs and symptoms of injury at the venipuncture site.

(*continued*)

SKILL 18-10 OBTAINING A VENOUS BLOOD SPECIMEN FOR CULTURE AND SENSITIVITY continued

DOCUMENTATION

Guidelines

Record the date, time, and site of the venipunctures; the name of the test(s); the time the sample was sent to the laboratory; the amount of blood collected, if required; and any significant assessments or patient reactions.

Sample Documentation

6/6/15 1710 Patient's temperature increased to 104.2°F. Patient very lethargic, pale, diaphoretic, with cool, clammy skin. Bradycardic with pulse rate of 56 beats per minute and hypotensive with blood pressure of 90/50 mm Hg. Physician notified. Blood cultures ×2 ordered and obtained from two different sites: left and right antecubital veins. No evidence of bleeding or hematoma at venipuncture site.

—B. Pearson, RN

UNEXPECTED SITUATIONS AND ASSOCIATED INTERVENTIONS

- *After applying the tourniquet, you have trouble finding a distended vein:* Have the patient make a fist, or try tapping the skin over the vein lightly several times. If unsuccessful, remove the tourniquet and try lowering the patient's arm to allow blood to pool in the veins. If necessary, apply warm compresses for about 10 minutes before reapplying the tourniquet.
- *Patient has large, distended, highly visible veins:* Perform venipuncture without a tourniquet to minimize the risk for hematoma.
- *Patient has a clotting disorder or is receiving anticoagulant therapy:* Maintain firm pressure on the venipuncture site for at least 5 minutes after withdrawing the needle to prevent hematoma formation.
- *Oozing or bleeding continues from the puncture site for more than a few minutes:* Elevate the area and apply a pressure dressing. If bleeding is excessive or persists for longer than 10 minutes, notify the primary health care provider.
- *A hematoma develops at the venipuncture site:* Apply pressure until you are sure bleeding has stopped (about 5 minutes). Notify the patient's primary health care provider. Document size and appearance of hematoma, notification of primary health care provider, and any ordered interventions.
- *Patient reports feeling light-headed and says she is going to faint:* Stop the venipuncture. If the patient is in bed, have the patient lie flat and elevate the feet. If the patient is in a chair, have the patient put her head between her knees. Encourage the patient to take slow, deep breaths. Call for assistance and stay with the patient. Obtain vital signs, if possible.

SPECIAL CONSIDERATIONS

General Considerations

- Be aware that the size of the culture bottles may vary according to facility policy, but the sample dilution should always be 1:10.
- If possible, ensure the specimen is obtained before antibiotics are started (Malarkey & McMorrow, 2012).
- Draw blood from two different peripheral venipuncture sites if possible and document each site. This increases the likelihood of detecting a bloodstream infection and helps differentiate true bacteremia from a false–positive finding due to skin contamination. The second specimen may be drawn from a central venous catheter if catheter-related bloodstream infection (CRBSI) is suspected or peripheral access sites are unavailable. If you obtain a blood culture specimen from an intravascular catheter, clearly document it in the patient's medical record. Peripheral sites are preferred (Myers III & Reyes, 2011, p. 62).
- When patients have a central venous access device, clinicians may be tempted to draw blood culture specimens from the central venous catheter upon insertion. Drawing blood culture specimens upon line insertion can result in more false–positive results and should be performed on a separate venous draw from a different site (Myers III & Reyes, 2011, p. 63).
- Avoid collecting blood from edematous areas, arteriovenous shunts, an upper extremity on the same side as a previous lymph node dissection or mastectomy, infected sites, same extremity as an intravenous infusion, and sites of previous hematomas or vascular injury.

- Do not use veins in the lower extremities for venipuncture, because of an increased risk of thrombophlebitis. However, some facilities do allow collection from lower extremities with a physician's order to collect blood from a leg or foot vein. Check your facility's policies.
- Apply warm compresses to the selected site 15 to 20 minutes before venipuncture to aid in distending veins that are difficult to locate.
- Consider the use of topical anesthetic creams to minimize discomfort and pain for the patient, based on facility policy. Be familiar with requirements and specifications for particular products available for use. Application needs to occur sufficiently in advance to allow enough time to become effective.
- Use distraction, which has been shown to be of benefit in reducing anxiety related to venipuncture, especially with children. Asking the patient to concentrate on relaxing and performing deep breathing may help. Asking the patient to cough at the time of venipuncture is another technique that has been shown to be effective in reducing pain with venipuncture (Usichenko et al., 2004).

Infant and Child Considerations

- Consider automatically applying warm compresses to distend the small veins of infants and young children before attempting any venipuncture.
- For pediatric patients, the decision to obtain a sample from a second site is at the discretion of the health care provider.
- The specimen blood volume for children older than 10 years is 20 mL; for children under 10 years of age, the volume is 1 mL for each year of life (Malarkey & McMorrow, 2012).
- Keep in mind that only 1 to 5 mL of blood can safely be drawn for culture from infants and small children. Quantities less than 1 mL may be insufficient to detect bacterial organisms (Fischbach & Dunning, 2009).
- Venipuncture by a skilled phlebotomist is the method of choice over a heel lance in infants (Shah & Ohlsson, 2012).
- Administer oral sucrose beginning 1 to 2 minutes before the venipuncture procedure for young infants to decrease the incidence of procedure-related pain (Kassab et al., 2012; Liu et al., 2010).
- Consider using topical anesthetic creams or gels, refrigerant spray, or iontophoresis (application of electric current to carry ionized lidocaine through the skin) with infants and children to decrease the incidence of procedure-related pain (Baxter et al., 2013; İnal & Kelleci, 2012a). Be sure to apply the product to allow sufficient time to reach maximal effectiveness.
- Consider the use of distraction to decrease the incidence of procedure-related pain (Inal & Kelleci, 2012b).

Older Adult Considerations

- Keep in mind that the veins of an older adult are fragile and may collapse easily. In addition, the skin is less elastic and may be more difficult to pull taut.
- The superficial veins of the hands of older adults are fragile and venipuncture can cause a hematoma to form. Additionally, these veins move due to the age-related loss of supportive muscle and connective tissue, making it difficult to enter the lumen of the vein (Malarkey & McMorrow, 2012)
- Consider performing venipuncture without a tourniquet for older patients to prevent rupture of capillaries. Instruct the patient to make a tight fist before needle insertion. Do not have the patient pump the fist, because this may increase plasma potassium levels (Fischbach & Dunning, 2009).

SKILL 18-11 OBTAINING AN ARTERIAL BLOOD SPECIMEN FOR BLOOD GAS ANALYSIS

Arterial blood gases (ABG) are obtained to determine the adequacy of oxygenation and ventilation, to assess acid–base status, and to monitor the effectiveness of treatment. The most common site for sampling arterial blood is the radial artery. Other arteries may be used, but an advanced health care provider's order may be required to obtain the sample from another artery.

Analysis of ABG evaluates ventilation by measuring blood pH and the partial pressures of arterial oxygen (Pao_2) and partial pressure of arterial carbon dioxide ($Paco_2$). Blood pH measurement reveals the blood's acid–base balance. Pao_2 indicates the amount of oxygen that the lungs deliver to the blood, and $Paco_2$ indicates the lungs' capacity to eliminate carbon dioxide. ABG samples can also be analyzed for oxygen content and saturation, and for bicarbonate values. Table 18-1 highlights the normal values for ABG. A respiratory technician or specially trained nurse can collect most ABG samples, but an advanced practice professional usually performs collection from the femoral artery, depending on facility policy. An Allen's test should always be performed before using the radial artery to determine whether the ulnar artery delivers sufficient blood to the hand and fingers, in case there is damage to the radial artery during the blood sampling. Refer to the guidelines in this skill for performing an Allen's test.

Table 18-1 ARTERIAL BLOOD GAS: NORMAL VALUES

PARAMETER	NORMAL VALUE
pH	7.35–7.45
$PaCO_2$	35–45 mm Hg
HCO_3	22–26 mEq/L
SaO_2	Oxygen saturation >95%
PaO_2	>80–100 mm Hg
Base excess or deficit	±2 mEq/L

DELEGATION CONSIDERATIONS

Obtaining an arterial blood specimen for blood gas analysis is not delegated to nursing assistive personnel (NAP) or to unlicensed assistive personnel (UAP). Depending on the state's nurse practice act and the organization's policies and procedures, obtaining an arterial blood specimen for blood gas analysis may be delegated to licensed practical/vocational nurses (LPN/LVNs). The decision to delegate must be based on careful analysis of the patient's needs and circumstances, as well as the qualifications of the person to whom the task is being delegated. Refer to the Delegation Guidelines in Appendix A.

EQUIPMENT

- ABG kit, *or* heparinized self-filling 10-mL syringe with 22-G, 1-inch needle attached
- Airtight cap for hub of syringe
- 2 × 2 gauze pad
- Band-Aid
- Antimicrobial swab, such as chlorhexidine
- Biohazard bag
- Appropriate label for specimen, based on facility policy and procedure
- Cup or bag of ice and water
- Nonsterile gloves
- Additional PPE, as indicated
- Rolled towel

ASSESSMENT

Review the patient's medical record and plan of care for information about the need for an ABG specimen. Assess the patient's cardiac status, including heart rate, blood pressure, and auscultation of heart sounds. Also assess the patient's respiratory status, including respiratory rate, excursion, lung sounds, and use of oxygen, including the amount being used, if ordered. Determine the adequacy of peripheral blood flow to the extremity to be used by performing the Allen's test (detailed below). If Allen's test reveals no or little collateral circulation to the hand, do not perform an arterial stick to that artery. Assess the patient's radial pulse. If unable to palpate the radial pulse, consider using the other wrist. Assess the patient's understanding about the need for specimen collection. Ask the patient if he or she has ever felt faint, sweaty, or nauseated when having blood drawn.

NURSING DIAGNOSIS

Determine the related factors for the nursing diagnoses based on the patient's current status. Appropriate nursing diagnoses may include:

- Impaired Gas Exchange
- Risk for Injury
- Ineffective Airway Clearance
- Anxiety
- Decreased Cardiac Output

OUTCOME IDENTIFICATION AND PLANNING

The expected outcome to achieve is that the blood sample is obtained from the artery without damage to the artery. Other outcomes that may be appropriate include the following: the patient experiences minimal pain and anxiety during the procedure, and the patient demonstrates an understanding of the need for the ABG specimen.

IMPLEMENTATION

ACTION	RATIONALE
1. Gather the necessary supplies. Check product expiration dates. Identify ordered arterial blood gas analysis. Check the chart to make sure the patient has not been suctioned within the past 20 to 30 minutes. Check facility policy and/or procedure for guidelines on administering local anesthesia for arterial punctures. Administer anesthetic and allow sufficient time for full effect before beginning procedure.	Organization facilitates efficient performance of the procedure. Use of products that have not expired ensures proper functioning of equipment. Suctioning may change the oxygen saturation and is a temporary change not to be confused with baseline for the patient. Arterial puncture is a source of pain and discomfort. Intradermal injection of lidocaine around the puncture site has been shown to decrease the incidence and severity of localized pain when used before arterial puncture (AACN, 2011).
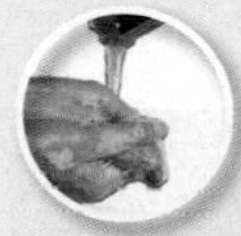 2. Perform hand hygiene and put on PPE, if indicated.	Hand hygiene and PPE prevent the transmission of microorganisms. PPE is required based on transmission precautions.
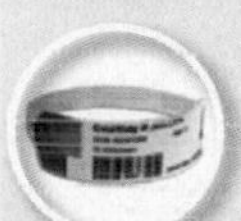 3. Identify the patient.	Identifying the patient ensures the right patient receives the intervention and helps prevent errors.
4. Explain the procedure to the patient. Tell the patient you need to collect an arterial blood sample and the needlestick will cause some discomfort but that he or she must remain still during the procedure.	Explanation facilitates cooperation and provides reassurance for the patient.
5. Check specimen label with the patient's identification bracelet. Label should include patient's name and identification number, time specimen was collected, route of collection, identification of person obtaining the sample, amount of oxygen the patient is receiving, type of oxygen administration device, patient's body temperature, and any other information required by facility policy.	Confirmation of patient identification information ensures the specimen is labeled correctly for the right patient. Oxygen information and patient's body temperature are required for accurate analysis.
6. Assemble equipment on overbed table within reach.	Arranging items nearby is convenient, saves time, and avoids unnecessary stretching and twisting of muscles on the part of the nurse.
7. Close curtains around the bed and close the door to the room, if possible.	Closing the door or curtain provides for patient privacy.
8. Provide for good light. Artificial light is recommended. Place a trash receptacle within easy reach.	Good lighting is necessary to perform the procedure properly. Having the trash receptacle in easy reach allows for safe disposal of contaminated materials.

(continued)

SKILL 18-11 OBTAINING AN ARTERIAL BLOOD SPECIMEN FOR BLOOD GAS ANALYSIS continued

ACTION	RATIONALE
9. If the patient is on bed rest, ask him or her to lie in a supine position, with the head slightly elevated and the arms at the sides. Ask an ambulatory patient to sit in a chair and support the arm securely on an armrest or a table. Place a waterproof pad under the site and a rolled towel under the wrist.	Positioning the patient comfortably helps minimize anxiety. Using a rolled towel under the wrist provides for easy access to the insertion site.
10. **Perform Allen's test (Figure 1) before obtaining a specimen from the radial artery.**	Allen's testing assesses patency of the ulnar and radial arteries.

a. Have the patient clench the wrist to minimize blood flow into the hand.

b. Using your index and middle fingers, press on the radial and ulnar arteries (Figure 1A). Hold this position for a few seconds.

c. Without removing your fingers from the arteries, ask the patient to unclench the fist and hold the hand in a relaxed position (Figure 1B). The palm will be blanched because pressure from your fingers has impaired the normal blood flow.

d. Release pressure on the ulnar artery (Figure 1C). If the hand becomes flushed, which indicates that blood is filling the vessels, it is safe to proceed with the radial artery puncture. This is considered a positive test. If the hand does not flush, perform the test on the other arm.

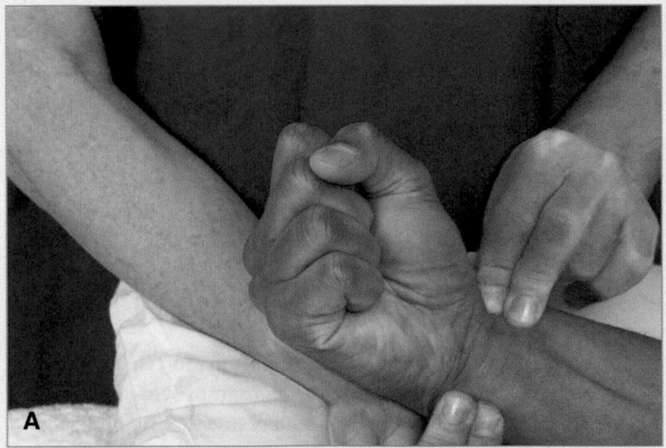

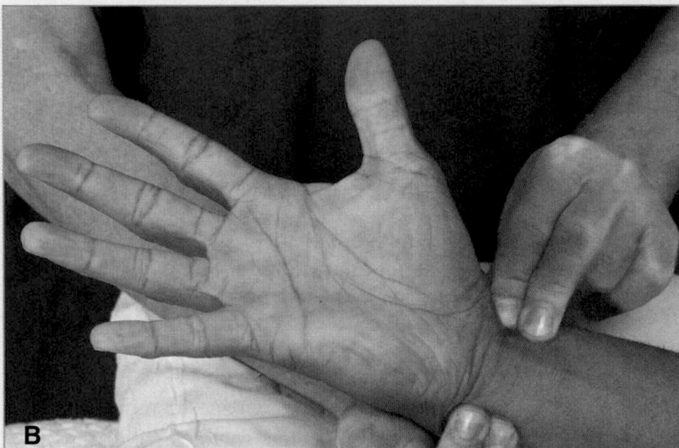

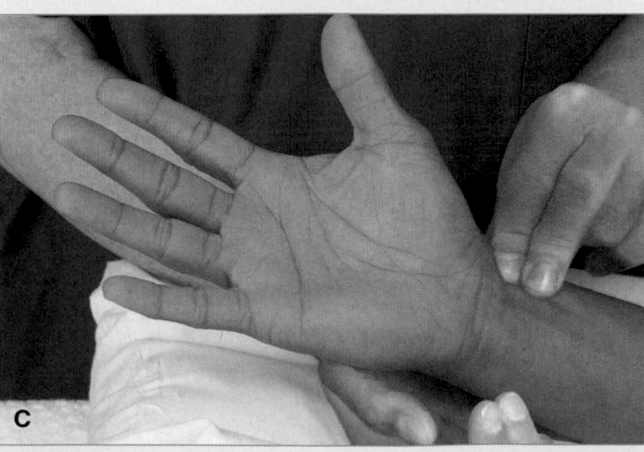

FIGURE 1 Performing Allen's test. (**A**) Compressing the arteries with the patient's fist closed. (**B**) Maintaining compression as patient unclenches fist. (**C**) Compressing only the radial artery.

ACTION	RATIONALE
11. Put on nonsterile gloves. Locate the radial artery and lightly palpate it for a strong pulse.	Gloves reduce transmission of microorganisms. If you push too hard during palpation, the radial artery will be obliterated and hard to palpate.
12. **Clean the patient's skin at the puncture site with the antimicrobial swab, according to facility policy. If using chlorhexidine, use a gentle back and forth motion or use the procedure recommended by the manufacturer. Do not wipe or blot. Allow to dry completely. After disinfection, do not palpate the site unless sterile gloves are worn.**	Site cleansing prevents potentially infectious skin flora from being introduced into the vessel during the procedure. Palpation after cleansing contaminates the area.
13. Alternately, for patients who bruise easily, are at risk for bleeding, or have fragile skin, **apply the chlorhexidine without scrubbing for at least 30 seconds. Allow to dry completely. Do not wipe or blot.**	Avoiding scrubbing decreases the risk of injury. Application for a minimum of 30 seconds is necessary for chlorhexidine to be effective (Hadaway, 2006). Organisms on the skin can be introduced into the tissues or the bloodstream with the needle.
14. Stabilize the hand with the wrist extended over the rolled towel, palm up. Palpate the artery above the puncture site with the index and middle fingers of your nondominant hand while holding the syringe over the puncture site with your dominant hand. **Do not directly touch the area to be punctured.**	Stabilizing the hand and palpating the artery with one hand while holding the syringe in the other provides better access to the artery. Palpating the area to be punctured would contaminate the clean area.
15. Hold the needle bevel up at a 45- to 60-degree angle at the site of maximal pulse impulse, with the shaft parallel to the path of the artery.	The proper angle of insertion ensures correct access to the artery. The artery is shallow and does not require a deeper angle to penetrate.
16. Puncture the skin and arterial wall in one motion. Watch for blood backflow in the syringe (Figure 2). Pulsating blood will flow into the syringe. Do not pull back on the plunger. Fill the syringe to the 5-mL mark.	The blood should enter the syringe automatically due to arterial pressure.

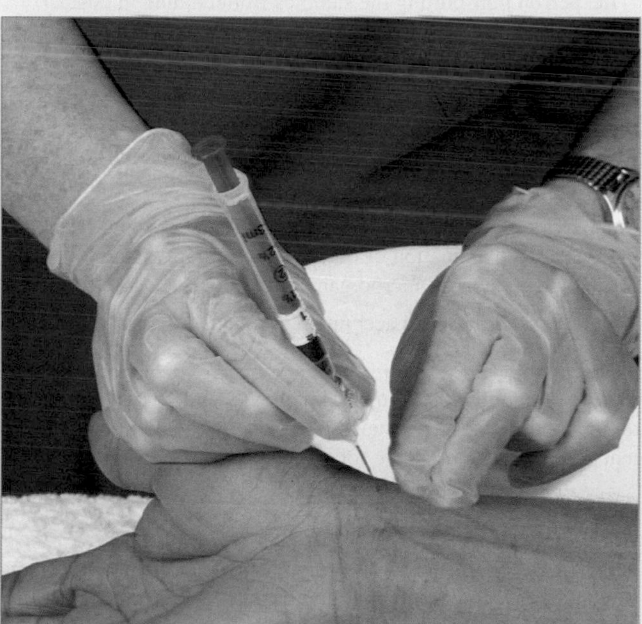

FIGURE 2 Observing blood backflow into syringe. *(Photo by B. Proud.)*

(continued)

SKILL 18-11 OBTAINING AN ARTERIAL BLOOD SPECIMEN FOR BLOOD GAS ANALYSIS continued

ACTION	RATIONALE
17. After collecting the sample, withdraw the syringe while your nondominant hand is beginning to place pressure proximal to the insertion site with the 2 × 2 gauze. **Press a gauze pad firmly over the puncture site until the bleeding stops—at least 5 minutes. If the patient is receiving anticoagulant therapy or has a blood dyscrasia, apply pressure for 10 to 15 minutes; if necessary, ask a coworker to hold the gauze pad in place while you prepare the sample for transport to the laboratory, but do not ask the patient to hold the pad.**	If insufficient pressure is applied, a large, painful hematoma may form, hindering future arterial puncture at the site.
18. When the bleeding stops and the appropriate time has lapsed, apply a small adhesive bandage or small pressure dressing (fold a 2 × 2 gauze into fourths and firmly apply tape, stretching the skin tight).	Applying a dressing also prevents arterial hemorrhage and extravasation into the surrounding tissue, which can cause a hematoma.
19. Once the sample is obtained, check the syringe for air bubbles. If any appear, remove them by holding the syringe upright and slowly ejecting some of the blood onto a 2 × 2 gauze pad.	Air bubbles can affect the laboratory values.
20. Engage the needle guard and remove the needle. Place the airtight cap on the syringe. Gently rotate the syringe. Do not shake.	Engaging the needle guard prevents accidental needlestick injury. Using an airtight cap prevents the sample from leaking and keeps air out of the syringe, because blood will continue to absorb oxygen and will give a false reading if allowed to have contact with air. Rotating the syringe ensures proper mixing of heparin in syringe with the sample; heparin prevents blood from clotting. Vigorous shaking may cause hemolysis.
21. Place label on the syringe per facility policy. Place syringe in plastic, sealable biohazard bag. Insert the syringe into a cup or bag of ice water.	Labeling ensures the specimen is the correct one for the right patient. Packaging the specimen in a biohazard bag prevents the person transporting the samples from coming in contact with blood. Ice prevents the blood from degrading.
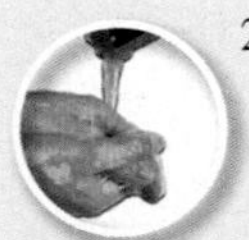 22. Discard the needle in sharps container. Remove gloves and perform hand hygiene.	Proper disposal of equipment prevents accidental injury and reduces transmission of microorganisms. Removing gloves properly reduces the risk for infection transmission and contamination of other items. Hand hygiene reduces transmission of microorganisms.
23. Remove other PPE, if used. Perform hand hygiene.	Removing PPE properly reduces the risk for infection transmission and contamination of other items. Hand hygiene reduces the transmission of microorganisms.
24. Transport the specimen to the laboratory immediately.	Timely transport ensures accurate results.

EVALUATION

The expected outcome is met when an arterial blood specimen is obtained, and the patient reports minimal pain during the procedure. In addition, the site remains free of injury, without evidence of hematoma formation, and the patient verbalizes the rationale for the specimen collection.

DOCUMENTATION

Guidelines

Document results of Allen's test, time the sample was drawn, arterial puncture site, amount of time pressure was applied to the site to control bleeding, type and amount of oxygen therapy that the patient was receiving, pulse oximetry values, respiratory rate, respiratory effort, patient's body temperature, and any other significant assessments.

Sample Documentation

> 9/22/15 1245 Allen's test positive at R radial artery. ABG obtained using R radial artery. Pressure applied to site for 5 minutes. Patient receiving 3 L/NC oxygen, pulse oximetry 94%, respirations even/unlabored, respiratory rate 18 breaths per minute, oral temperature 98.9°F, patient denies dyspnea.
>
> —*C. Bausler, RN*

UNEXPECTED SITUATIONS AND ASSOCIATED INTERVENTIONS

- *While you are attempting to puncture the artery, the patient complains of severe pain:* Using too much force may cause the needle to touch bone, causing the patient pain. Too much force may also result in advancing the needle through the opposite wall of the artery. If this happens, slowly pull the needle back a short distance and check to see if blood returns. If blood still fails to enter the syringe, withdraw the needle completely and restart the procedure.
- *You cannot obtain a specimen from the same site after two attempts:* Stop. Do not make more than two attempts from the same site. Probing the artery may injure it and the radial nerve.
- *Blood will not flow into the syringe:* Typically, this occurs as a result of arterial spasm. Replace the needle with a smaller one and try the puncture again. A smaller-bore needle is less likely to cause arterial spasm.
- *After inserting the needle, you note that the syringe is filling sluggishly with dark red/purple blood:* If the patient is in critical condition, this may be arterial blood. But if the patient is awake and alert with a pulse oximeter reading within normal parameters, you have most likely obtained a venous sample. Discard the sample and redraw.
- *Patient is on anticoagulant therapy:* Expect to hold pressure on the puncture site for at least 10 minutes. If pressure is not held sufficiently long, a hematoma may form, place pressure on the artery, and decrease the flow of blood.
- *Patient cannot keep the wrist extended or lying flat:* Obtain a small arm board, as used for securing an IV, and a roll of gauze. Place the roll of gauze under the patient's wrist. Tape the fingers and forearm to the arm board. This will keep the wrist in an extended position during the blood specimen collection.
- *Blood was drawn without incident, but now, 2 hours later, the patient is complaining of tingling in the fingers and the hand is cool and pale:* Notify the primary health care provider. An arterial thrombosis may have formed. If not treated, the thrombosis can lead to tissue necrosis on the extremity.
- *Puncture site continues to ooze:* If the site is not actively bleeding, consider placing a small pressure bandage on the insertion site. This will prevent the artery from continuing to ooze. Continually check the site for bleeding and assess the extremity to ensure that blood flow is adequate.
- *The Allen's test is negative:* Try the other extremity. If the other extremity has a positive result (collateral circulation), use that extremity. If the Allen's test is negative in both extremities, notify the primary health care provider.

SPECIAL CONSIDERATIONS

General Considerations

- Be aware that use of a particular arterial site is contraindicated for the following reasons: absence of a palpable radial artery pulse; Allen's test showing only one artery supplying blood to the hand; Allen's test showing obstruction in the ulnar artery; cellulitis or infection at the site; presence of arteriovenous fistula or shunt; severe thrombocytopenia (platelet count 20,000/mm^3 or less, or based on facility policy), and a prolonged prothrombin time or partial thromboplastin time.
- If the patient is receiving oxygen, make sure that this therapy has been underway for at least 20 minutes before collecting an arterial blood sample. Also be sure to indicate on the laboratory request and the specimen label the amount and type of oxygen therapy the patient is receiving. If the patient is receiving mechanical ventilation, note the fraction of inspired oxygen and tidal volume.
- If the patient is not receiving oxygen, indicate that he or she is breathing room air.
- Specimens collected within 20 to 30 minutes of respiratory passage suctioning or other respiratory therapy, such as a nebulizer treatment, will not be accurate (Van Leeuwen et al., 2011).
- Consider obtaining an order for the use of a local anesthetic (1% lidocaine solution) to minimize discomfort and pain for the patient, based on facility policy. The use of 1% lidocaine without

(*continued*)

SKILL 18-11 OBTAINING AN ARTERIAL BLOOD SPECIMEN FOR BLOOD GAS ANALYSIS continued

epinephrine injected intradermally around the artery puncture site has been shown to decrease the incidence of localized pain (AACN, 2011). Be familiar with requirements and specifications for particular products available for use. Application needs to occur sufficiently far in advance to allow enough time to become effective, which may be contraindicated by the patient's condition. Consider such use of lidocaine carefully because it can delay the procedure. The patient may be allergic to the drug, or the resulting vasoconstriction may prevent successful puncture.

- If the femoral site is used for the procedure, apply pressure for a minimum of 10 minutes.
- Arterial lines may be used to obtain blood samples. (Refer to Chapter 16, Cardiovascular Care.) When sampling from arterial lines, record the amount of blood drawn for each sampling. Frequent sampling can result in significant amount of blood being removed.

Infant and Child Considerations

- Administer oral sucrose to young infants beginning 1 to 2 minutes before the procedure to decrease the incidence of procedure-related pain (Kassab et al., 2012; Liu et al., 2010).
- Consider using topical anesthetic creams or gels, refrigerant spray, or iontophoresis (application of electric current to carry ionized lidocaine through the skin) with infants and children to decrease the incidence of procedure-related pain (Baxter et al., 2013; İnal & Kelleci, 2012a). Be sure to apply the product to allow for sufficient time to reach maximal effectiveness.
- Consider the use of distraction to decrease the incidence of procedure-related pain (İnal & Kelleci, 2012b).

ENHANCE YOUR UNDERSTANDING

FOCUSING ON PATIENT CARE: DEVELOPING CLINICAL REASONING

Consider the case scenarios at the beginning of the chapter as you answer the following questions to enhance your understanding and apply what you have learned.

QUESTIONS

1. The nurse explained to Mr. Conklin the procedure for obtaining the required urine specimens. Unfortunately, it becomes clear that the patient is too confused at this time to follow the directions and obtain the specimen by himself. How would you handle this situation? How would you successfully obtain an uncontaminated specimen from a patient who is unable to cooperate?
2. Huana Yon's primary care provider provides pre- and postappointment education and information for the patients in the practice. Part of the nurse's responsibilities when contacting patients before their scheduled visit is to provide information related to anticipated laboratory tests and any necessary patient preparation. What information would you include if you were calling this patient before her visit in relation to collecting a stool specimen for occult blood? What medications, dietary habits, or other habits would you question her about? What information would you give her to prepare for the test?
3. The nurse assigned to Mrs. Yeletsky questions her about her blood glucose testing at home. Mrs. Yeletsky states, "I never really figured out how to work the machine they gave me the last time I saw the doctor. The buttons are too small, and I can't see the writing on the screen very well. Besides, I'm only a little diabetic." What additional information would you want to obtain from this patient? How would you address her possible lack of understanding regarding diabetes? What interventions could you attempt to aid her in managing her blood glucose levels? What other aspects of her health habits would you want to assess?

You can find suggested answers after the Bibliography at the end of this chapter.

INTEGRATED CASE STUDY CONNECTION

The case studies in Unit 3 are designed to focus on integrating concepts. Refer to the following case studies to enhance your understanding of the concepts related to the skills in this chapter.

- Basic Case Studies: Joe LeRoy, page 1072; Tula Stillwater, page 1075.
- Intermediate Case Studies: Victoria Holly, page 1079.
- Advanced Case Studies: Cole McKean, page 1093.

TAYLOR SUITE RESOURCES

Explore these additional resources to enhance learning for this chapter:

- NCLEX-Style Questions and other resources on thePoint, http://thePoint.lww.com/Lynn4e
- *Skill Checklists for Taylor's Clinical Nursing Skills,* 4e
- *Lippincott DocuCare* Fundamentals cases

Bibliography

Ackley, B.J., & Ladwig, G.B. (2011). *Nursing diagnosis handbook* (9th ed.). St. Louis: Mosby/Elsevier.

Adams, D. (2012). Needlestick and sharps injuries: Practice update. *Nursing Standard, 26*(37), 49–57.

Allison, J.E. (2007). The role of fecal occult blood testing in screening for colorectal cancer. *Practical Gastroenterology, 31*(6), 20–32.

American Association for Clinical Chemistry (AACC). (2013). *Lab tests online. Fecal occult blood test and fecal immunochemical test.* Available http://labtestsonline.org/understanding/analytes/fecal-occult-blood/tab/glance.

American Association of Critical Care Nurses (AACN). (2011). Lynn-McHale Wiegand, D. (Ed.). *AACN procedure manual for critical care* (6th ed.). Philadelphia: Elsevier Saunders.

American Diabetes Association (ADA). (2013). Standards of medical care in diabetes—2013. *Diabetes Care, 36*(Suppl. 1): S11 S66.

Azubike, N., Bullard, D., Chrisman, J., Davis, C., & Waters III, J. (2012). Navigating the nasopharyngeal culture. *Nursing Made Incredibly Easy, 10*(6), 9–12.

Baxter, A.L., Ewing, P.H., Young, G.B., Ware, A., Evans, N., & Manworren, R.C.B. (2013). EMLA application exceeding two hours improves pediatric emergency department venipuncture success. *Advanced Emergency Nursing Journal, 35*(1), 67–75.

Beckman Coulter. (2009a). *Hemoccult®. Product instructions.* Available https://www.beckmancoulter.com/wsrportal/bibliography?docname=HOII%20-%20462478.EA%20.pdf.

Beckman Coulter. (2009b). *Developing and interpreting Hemoccult® ICT Tests.* Available http://www.hemoccultfobt.com/healthcare/health_hemo_ICT_tests.htm.

Beckman Coulter. (2009c). *Hemoccult® ICT. Patient instructions.* Available http://www.hemoccultfobt.com/patients/patients_Hemo_ICT_Pt_Instr.htm.

Bulechek, G.M, Butcher, H.K., Dochterman, J.M., & Wagner, C.M. (Eds.). (2013). *Nursing interventions classification (NIC)* (6th ed.). St. Louis: Mosby Elsevier.

Centers for Disease Control and Prevention (CDC). (2013). *Colorectal (colon) cancer. Colorectal cancer screening guidelines.* Available http://www.cdc.gov/cancer/colorectal/basic_info/screening/guidelines.htm.

Centers for Disease Control and Prevention (CDC). (2012). *Tuberculosis (TB). Core curriculum on tuberculosis: What the clinician should know. Chapter 4. Diagnosis of tuberculosis disease.* Available http://www.cdc.gov/tb/education/corecurr/index.htm.

Centers for Disease Control and Prevention (CDC). (2011a). *Healthcare-associated infections (HAIs). Staphylococcus aureus in healthcare settings.* Available http://www.cdc.gov/HAI/organisms/staph.html.

Centers for Disease Control and Prevention (CDC). (2011b). *Pertussis (whooping cough). Specimen collection. Pertussis testing video: Collecting a nasopharyngeal swab clinical specimen.* Available http://www.cdc.gov/pertussis/clinical/diagnostic-testing/specimen-collection.html.

Dhiman, N., Miller, R.M., Finley, J.L., Sztajnkrycer, M.D., Nestler, D.M., Boggust, A.J., et al. (2012). Effectiveness of patient-collected swabs for influenza testing. *Mayo Clinic Proceedings, 87*(6), 548–554.

Dulczak, S. (2005). Overview of the evaluation, diagnosis, and management of urinary tract infections in infants and children. *Urologic Nursing, 25*(3), 185–192.

Edden, A., & Hawthorne, G. (2012). A review of insulin delivery devices and glucose meters. *Nursing & Residential Care, 14*(6), 278–281.

Ferguson, A. (2005). Blood glucose monitoring. *Nursing Times, 101*(38), 28–29.

Fischbach, F., & Dunning, M. (2009). *A manual of laboratory and diagnostic tests.* (8th ed.). Philadelphia: Wolters Kluwer Health/Lippincott Williams & Wilkins.

Flitcroft, K.L., Irwig, L.M., Carter, S.M., Saldeld, G.P., & Gillespie, J.A. (2012). *Colorectal cancer screening: Why immunochemical fecal occult blood tests may be the best option. BMC Gastroenterology, 12:* 183. Available http://www.biomedcentral.com/1471-230X/12/183.

Gabriel, J. (2012). Venepuncture and cannulation: Considering the ageing vein. *British Journal of Nursing, 21*(2), S22–S28.

Hadaway, L. (2006). 5 steps to preventing catheter-related bloodstream infections. *LPN2009, 2*(5), 50–55.

Hewison, C.J., Heath, C.H., & Ingram, P.R. (2012). Stool culture. *Australian Family Physician, 41*(10), 775–779.

Higgins, D. (2008). Specimen collection. Part 4: Obtaining a nasal swab. *Nursing Times, 104*(20), 26–27.

Hinkle, J.L., & Cheever, K.H. (2014). *Brunner & Suddarth's textbook of medical-surgical nursing* (13th ed.). Philadelphia: Wolters Kluwer Health/Lippincott Williams & Wilkins.

Hooton, T.M., Bradley, S.F., Cardenas, D.D., Colgan, R., Geerlings, S.E., Rice, J.C., et al. (2010). *Diagnosis, prevention, and treatment of catheter-associated urinary tract infection in adults: 2009 international clinical practice guidelines from the Infectious Diseases Society of America. Clinical Infectious Diseases, 50*(5), 625–663. Available http://www.idsociety.org/uploadedFiles/IDSA/Guidelines-Patient_Care/PDF_Library/Comp%20UTI.pdf.

Huether, S.E., & McCance, K.L. (2012.) *Understanding pathophysiology* (5th ed.). St. Louis: Elsevier.

Hughes, L. (2012). Think "SAFE". Four crucial elements for diabetes education. *Nursing, 42*(1), 58–61.

Hughes, T. (2012). Providing information to children before and during venepuncture. *Nursing Children and Young People, 24*(5), 23–28.

İnal, S., & Kelleci, M. (2012a). Relief of pain during blood specimen collection in pediatric patients. *The American Journal of Maternal Child Nursing, 37*(5), 339–345.

İnal, S., & Kelleci, M. (2012b). Distracting children during blood draw: Looking through distracting cards if effective in pain relief of children during blood draw. *International Journal of Nursing Practice, 18*(2), 210–219.

Infusion Nurses Society (INS). (2011). Infusion nursing standards of practice. *Journal of Infusion Nursing, 34*(Suppl: 1S).

Jarvis, C. (2012). *Physical examination & health assessment* (6th ed.). St. Louis: Saunders/Elsevier.

The Joint Commission (TJC). (2014). *National patient safety goals.* Available http://www.jointcommission.org/standards_information/npsgs.aspx.

Karacan, C., Erkek, N., Senel, S. Gunduz, S.A., Catli, G., & Tavil, B. (2010). Evaluation of urine collection methods for the diagnosis of urinary tract infection in children. *Medical Principles and Practice, 19*(3), 188–191.

Kassab, M.I., Roydhouse, J.K., Fowler, C., & Foureur, M. (2012). The effectiveness of glucose in reducing needle related procedural pain in infants. *Journal of Pediatric Nursing, 27*(1), 3–17.

Kim, N-H., Kim, M., Lee, S., Yun, N.R., Kim, K-H., Park, S.W., et al. (2011). Effect of routine sterile gloving on contamination rates in blood culture. *Annals of Internal Medicine, 154*(3), 145–151.

Kyle, T., & Carman, S. (2013). *Essentials of pediatric nursing* (2nd ed.). Philadelphia: Wolters Kluwer Health/Lippincott Williams & Wilkins.

Lavery, I., & Ingram, P. (2005). Venipuncture: Best practice. *Nursing Standard, 19*(49), 55–66, 68.

LeFever Kee, J. (2013). *Pearson handbook of laboratory and diagnostic tests with nursing implications* (7th ed.). Upper Saddle River, NJ: Pearson.

Liu, M-F., Lin, K-C., Chou, Y-H., & Lee, T-Y. (2010). Using non-nutritive sucking and oral glucose solution with neonates to relieve pain: A randomized controlled trial. *Journal of Clinical Nursing, 19*(11–12), 1604–1611.

Mahoney, M., Baxter, K., Burgess, J., Bauer, C., Downey, C., Mantel, J., et al. (2013). Procedure for obtaining a urine sample from a urostomy, ileal conduit, and colon conduit. A best practice guideline for clinicians. *Journal of Wound, Ostomy & continence Nursing, 40*(3), 277–279.

Malarkey, L.M., & McMorrow, M.E. (2012). *Saunders nursing guide to laboratory and diagnostic tests* (2nd ed.). St. Louis: Elsevier Saunders.

Matheson, A., Christie, P., Stari, T., Kavanagh, K., Gould, I.M., Masterton, R., et al. (2012). Nasal swab screening for methicillin-resistant *Staphylococcus aureus* – How well does it perform? A cross-sectional study. *Infection Control and Hospital Epidemiology, 33*(8), 803–808.

MedlinePlus. (2011). *Nasopharyngeal culture.* Available at www.nlm.nih.gov/medlineplus/ency/article/003747.htm.

Meetoo, D., McAllister, G., & West, A. (2012). Diabetes. Evidence-based management 45. Assessing glycaemic control with self-monitoring of blood glucose. *Practice Nursing, 23*(7), 352–360.

Micheletti, L. (2010). Arterial blood gas: Regulation of acid–base balance rests on the respiratory and renal systems. *Advance for Nurses, 7*(1), 16–19.

Mompoint-Williams, D., Watts, P.I., & Appel, S.J. (2012). Detecting and treating hypoglycemia in patients with diabetes. *Nursing, 42*(8), 50–52.

Moorhead, S., Johnson, M., Maas, M.L., & Swanson, E. (Eds.). (2013). *Nursing outcomes classification (NOC)* (5th ed.). St. Louis: Mosby Elsevier.

Myers III, F.E., & Reyes, C. (2011). Combating infection. Blood cultures: 5 steps to doing it right. *Nursing, 41*(3), 62–63.

NANDA-I International. (2012). *Nursing diagnoses: Definitions & classification 2012–2014.* West Sussex, UK: Wiley-Blackwell.

National Diabetes Information Clearinghouse (NDIC). (2012). *Continuous glucose monitoring.* Available http://diabetes.niddk.nih.gov/dm/pubs/glucosemonitor/index.aspx#continue.

Novotne, T.A., & Kaseb, H.O. (2013). The changing face of *Clostridium difficile* in critical care. *Nursing 2013CriticalCare, 8*(3), 26–34.

Perry, S.E., Hockenberry, M.J., Lowdermilk, D.L., & Wilson, D. (2010). *Maternal child nursing care* (4th ed.). Maryland Heights, MO: Mosby/Elsevier.

Qaseem, A., Denberg, T.D., Hopkins Jr., R.H., Humphrey, L., Levine, J., Sweet, D.E., et al. (2012). Screening for colorectal cancer: A guidance statement from the American College of Physicians. *Annals of Internal Medicine, 156*(5), 378–386.

Rowley, S., & Clare, S. (2011). ANTT: An essential tool for effective blood culture collection. *British Journal of Nursing, 20*(14), S9–S14.

Scales, K. (2008). A practical guide to venepuncture and blood sampling. *Nursing Standard, 22*(29), 29–36.

Shah, V., & Ohlsson, A. (2012). *Venepuncture versus heel lance for blood sampling in term neonates. Cochrane Database of Systematic Reviews.* Available http://summaries.cochrane.org/CD001452/venepuncture-versus-heel-lance-for-blood-sampling-in-term-neonates.

Society of Urologic Nurses and Associates (SUNA). (2010). *Prevention & control of catheter-associated urinary tract infection (CAUTI). Clinical practice guideline.* Available https://www.suna.org/sites/default/files/download/cautiGuideline.pdf.

Tabloski, P. (2010). *Gerontological nursing* (2nd ed.). Upper Saddle River, NJ: Pearson.

Taylor, C., Lillis, C., & Lynn P. (2015). *Fundamentals of nursing.* (8th ed.). Philadelphia: Wolters Kluwer Health/Lippincott Williams & Wilkins.

Taylor, J.J., & Cohen, B.J. (2013). *Memmler's structure and function of the human body* (10th ed.). Philadelphia: Wolters Kluwer Health/Lippincott Williams & Wilkins.

Tosif, S., Baker, A., Oakley, E., Donath, S., & Babl, F.E. (2012). Contamination rates of different urine collection methods for the diagnosis of urinary tract infections in young children: An observational cohort study. *Journal of Paediatrics and Child Health, 48*(8), 659–664.

U.S. Food and Drug Administration (FDA). (2013). *Medical devices. Blood glucose monitoring devices.* Available http://www.fda.gov/%20medicaldevices/productsandmedicalprocedures/invitrodiagnostics/glucosetestingdevices/default.htm.

U.S. National Library of Medicine and the National Institutes of Health. MedlinePlus. (2011). *Nasopharyngeal culture.* Available http://www.nlm.nih.gov/medlineplus/ency/article/003747.htm.

Usichenko, T., Pavlovic, D., Foellner, S., et al. (2004). Reducing venipuncture pain by a cough trick: A randomized crossover volunteer study. *Anesthesia & Analgesia, 98*(2), 343–345.

Van Leeuwen, A.M., Poelhuis-Leth, D., & Bladh, M.L. (2011). *Davis's comprehensive handbook of laboratory & diagnostic tests with nursing implications* (4th ed.). Philadelphia: F.A. Davis Company.

VISN 8 Patient Safety Center. (2009). *Safe patient handling and movement algorithms.* Tampa, FL: Author. Available http://www.visn8.va.gov/visn8/patientsafetycenter/safePtHandling/default.asp.

Washer, L.L., Chenoweth, C., Kim, H-W., Rogers, M.A.M., Malani, A.N., Riddell, J., et al. (2013). Blood culture contamination: A randomized trial evaluating the comparative effectiveness of 3 skin antiseptic interventions. *Infection Control and Hospital Epidemiology, 34*(1), 15–21.

Whitmore, C. (2012). Blood glucose monitoring: An overview. *British Journal of Nursing, 21*(10), 583–587.

Williams, J. (2012). Stoma care: Obtaining a urine specimen from a urostomy. *Gastrointestinal Nursing, 10*(5), 11–12.

SUGGESTED ANSWERS FOR FOCUSING ON PATIENT CARE: DEVELOPING CLINICAL REASONING

1. Obtaining a urine specimen is a priority in Mr. Conklin's care. Results will help determine the underlying cause of his symptoms and direct treatment. As a result, you will have to take a more involved role in the collection. You will have to obtain the specimen. Continue to reinforce the need for the urine specimen. Gather the necessary supplies and place them in the patient's room or bathroom. Plan to obtain the specimen the next time Mr. Conklin has to void. Share the plan with other caregivers. When the patient communicates his need to void, put on nonsterile gloves. Assist him to the bathroom. Explain again the need and rationale for the urine specimen. Explain that you are going to clean his penis to get the specimen. Clean his penis according to the guidelines in the procedure. Ask Mr. Conklin to void into the toilet; be ready to place the specimen cup in the stream of urine to obtain a sample. Put the lid on the specimen container. After assisting the patient with the rest of his toileting needs, clean the outside of the container, if urine contacted the outside during sampling. Label the sample and transport it to the laboratory.

2. Explain the reason for the test and the procedure for stool collection. You should also include information about foods and drugs that need to be avoided, informing Ms. Yon to avoid those foods for 3 days and the drugs for 7 days (if clinically possible). In addition, ask about any hematuria, bleeding hemorrhoids, or recent nose or throat bleeding. These situations would require the test to be postponed. Question Ms. Yon regarding medications she uses, including certain medications, such as a salicylate intake of more than 325 mg daily, steroids, iron preparations, and anticoagulants, that may lead to false–positive readings. Ms. Yon should understand that she should collect the specimen the morning of her appointment and know how to handle the specimen once she has obtained it.

3. Assess Mrs. Yeletsky's knowledge regarding her understanding of what diabetes is, its effects on the body, possible complications, dietary guidelines, medications she is prescribed to treat her diabetes, activity level/habits, and personal hygiene, particularly foot care. You should incorporate education regarding diabetes, including simple explanations of the definition of diabetes, normal blood glucose ranges, effect of insulin and exercise, effect of food and stress, and basic treatment approaches. A referral to the diabetic clinical specialist, if available, would be appropriate, as well as a referral for outpatient follow-up. Review her understanding of blood glucose monitoring and the use of the blood glucose monitor. Investigate alternate blood glucose monitors; models are available to aid people with impaired vision. Explore the support she has available and the possibility of a significant other assisting with her diabetes management, if appropriate.

UNIT

III

Integrated Case Studies

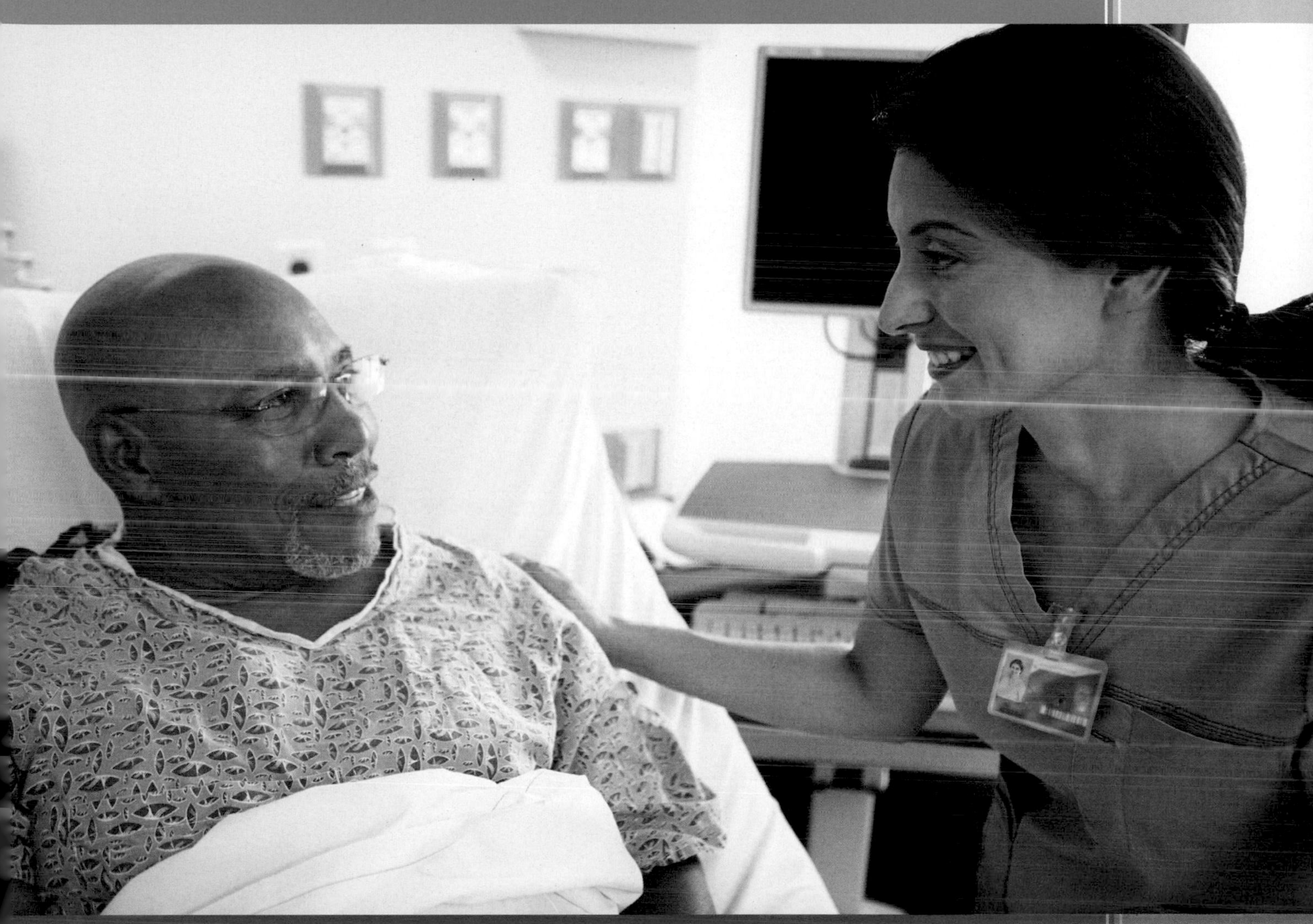

These case studies are designed to focus on integrating concepts. They are not meant to be all-inclusive. The critical thinking questions should guide your discussions of related issues. The discussion within the integrated nursing care section represents possible nursing care solutions to problems; you may find other solutions that are equally acceptable.

1 Basic Case Studies

CASE STUDY

ABIGAIL CANTONELLI

Abigail Cantonelli, age 80, injured her left knee and wrist when she fell on an icy sidewalk. She has been on your orthopedic and neurologic unit for several days. She has an extended history of cardiomyopathy, for which she receives furosemide (Lasix). Her vital signs are stable and she rates her pain as a 2 on a scale of 1 to 10 (10 = worst pain). Because Mrs. Cantonelli has an increased risk of falling, her primary care provider has ordered physical therapy and cane-walking instructions before discharge. Although the physical therapy staff has already initiated the cane-walking instructions, you will need to ambulate Mrs. Cantonelli with her cane during your shift. While you are ambulating down the hall, she says, "Oh, dear! I feel dizzy." She begins to lose her balance and falls toward you.

MEDICAL ORDERS

Physical therapy for cane-walking instruction
Ambulate every shift with cane assistance
Lasix 20 mg PO every morning
Potassium chloride 10 mEq PO every day
Lortab 5 one tab PO q 4–6 hours prn pain

DEVELOPING CLINICAL REASONING

- Identify Mrs. Cantonelli's risk factors for falling.
- Considering these risk factors, what special assessments and precautions should you implement before assisting her to ambulate or while assisting her with ambulation?
- Describe the actions you would implement when Mrs. Cantonelli begins to fall.

continued

SUGGESTED RESPONSES FOR INTEGRATED NURSING CARE

- Falls are the leading cause of accidental death in people over age 79. Because of Mrs. Cantonelli's age, history of falls, and impaired mobility, she continues to be at risk for falls. Her weakness and pain from her injuries also contribute to this risk. In addition, she is taking Lortab for pain and Lasix, which is a diuretic. These medications contribute to an increased risk for falling and subsequent injury (Taylor et al., 2015).
- Before ambulating Mrs. Cantonelli, it is a good idea to implement several assessments and precautions to prevent orthostatic hypotension. Have her sit on the side of the bed for a few minutes and make sure she does not feel dizzy, weak, or light-headed (see Chapter 9). Because she has a history of cardiomyopathy, assess for shortness of breath and chest pain. If she cannot tolerate sitting up on the side of the bed without having these symptoms, then she will not tolerate standing up or ambulating. Assess her pain level immediately before ambulation. If you have to medicate her for pain, then wait until the pain medicine has had time to take effect before ambulating. Because she is weaker on her left side, assess strength on her right side to ensure she will be able to support her weight with the cane (see Chapter 9). If she has difficulty maintaining her balance, apply a special safety belt (gait belt) before she begins to ambulate with the cane (some institutions require the use of a safety belt).
- While Mrs. Cantonelli is ambulating with her cane, observe her closely. Assess her technique with the cane. Observe for symptoms such as dizziness, chest pain, and shortness of breath. As she continues ambulating, evaluate how she tolerates this activity. Before she is discharged from the hospital, assess her self-confidence as well as her overall ability to use the cane.
- If Mrs. Cantonelli begins to fall, it is important to protect her while also protecting yourself. If you feel her start to fall, maintain a wide base of support, grasp the safety belt firmly, and place her weight against your body. You can then gently and slowly guide her down toward the floor (see Chapter 9). Assess her orientation and stay with her while waiting for help from another nurse. Take her vital signs to determine if there is a change from baseline. Thoroughly explore other factors that may have contributed to her fall, and plan interventions that will prevent future falls. If Mrs. Cantonelli continues to have problems with falling, consider having her use a walker.

CASE STUDY

TIFFANY JONES

Tiffany Jones, age 17, is scheduled to undergo an ovarian cyst biopsy under local anesthesia. She has been NPO since midnight. Her ID bracelet is on and her consent form is signed. Her mother is in the waiting room. You are to provide her immediate preoperative care. You place an IV in her left hand without difficulty. The next procedure is to insert an indwelling urinary (Foley) catheter. You set up the sterile field between her legs. As you clean the urinary meatus, Tiffany keeps drawing her legs closer together. When you remind her, she opens her legs and says, "Sorry, I didn't mean to move." As you insert the catheter into the urethra, Tiffany is startled and slams her knees together. When she opens her knees, the catheter appears to be inserted, but no urine is flowing.

MEDICAL ORDERS

Intravenous fluids: D5 ½ NSS at 50 mL/hr

Foley catheter to straight drainage

continued

DEVELOPING CLINICAL REASONING

- Where is the urinary catheter, and should you advance the catheter further?
- How do you determine whether the catheter and the sterile field are still sterile?
- How could you have set up a more stable sterile field?
- Identify issues of concern to patients before surgery.
- Describe methods of responding to Tiffany's nervousness.

SUGGESTED RESPONSES FOR INTEGRATED NURSING CARE

- The female urethra is short, only about 1.5 to 2.5 inches long. If the catheter is advanced that far and no urine is flowing, the catheter may be in the vagina. Do not remove the catheter; it will serve as a guide to locate the urethral opening, which is just above the vagina (see Chapter 12). You would not advance the catheter further even if it were in the urethra, because when Tiffany closed her legs, the catheter probably came into contact with her skin and is no longer sterile. Advancing a nonsterile catheter into the urethra would increase her risk for developing a urinary tract infection. Because you are not certain whether her legs touched the sterile field, the sterile field is also no longer considered sterile (see Chapters 1 and 12).
- You will need to obtain another complete catheter insertion kit. Cover Tiffany and verify that she understands your plans. As you set up the new kit, place it on the bedside table, not between her legs, to prevent accidental contamination (see Chapter 12).
- Teenagers are generally uncomfortable with urinary catheterization because in this procedure, the nurse must look at and touch a very private area. Such an invasion of privacy is traumatic at an age when girls are easily embarrassed. Teenage girls may have "nervous legs:" As you touch their inner thighs or labia, the knees slam shut almost involuntarily. Have a second nurse or a relative attend to the teenager. The nurse or relative can distract and soothe the teen, minimizing the unpleasantness of the experience, and can also keep a "reminder" hand on Tiffany's open knee to help you maintain sterility.
- As with most preoperative patients, Tiffany has several reasons to feel nervous. She is facing surgery, an unknown and anxiety-producing experience. The preoperative procedures, such as IV insertion and urinary catheterization, are unpleasant and uncomfortable. You can implement several strategies to reduce preoperative patients' anxiety. Have a familiar person stay with the patient. Tell the patient your name. Clearly explain procedures, and provide instructions to the patient before you begin. Instructions should include the rationale and the length of time the procedure will take. For urinary catheterization, the patient may also want to know how long he or she will have the catheter in place. Emphasize to the patient that it is all right to ask questions. Describe how the procedure will feel to the patient—for example, "when I clean you, it will feel cold and wet." Keep your voice calm and very matter-of-fact throughout the procedure (see Chapter 6 and Chapter 12).

CASE STUDY

JAMES WHITE

James White, a patient with an exacerbation of COPD, is on your medical–surgical unit. You need to obtain his vital signs and give him a bath. His vital signs at 8 AM were as follows: temperature, 98.4°F; pulse, 86 beats/minute and regular; respirations, 18/minute; blood pressure, 130/68 mm Hg. The physical therapist who is working with this patient on conditioning therapy has just brought him back from his exercises. You notice that his breathing is labored, with audible expiratory wheezes. While you are obtaining his oral temperature and vital signs, you continue to hear audible expiratory wheezing. His vital signs now are as follows: temperature, 96.8°F; pulse, 106 beats/minute and irregular; respirations, 26/minute; blood pressure, 140/74 mm Hg.

MEDICAL ORDERS

Daily physical therapy for conditioning

Oxygen at 2 L via nasal prongs prn for pulse oximetry <90%

Vital signs q 4 hr

Oxygen saturation levels via pulse oximeter every shift and prn

DEVELOPING CLINICAL REASONING

- Did you take the second set of vital signs at the most appropriate time? Why or why not?
- Describe the timing and type of bath you think Mr. White requires and the degree of assistance he will need. Explain your rationale.
- How have Mr. White's exercises affected the accuracy of his vital signs?
- What would be your course of action in response to his labored breathing?

SUGGESTED RESPONSES FOR INTEGRATED NURSING CARE

- Always compare vital signs with the baseline before making further clinical decisions (see Chapter 2). As you compare the previous vital signs with the ones you just obtained, you notice that Mr. White's pulse rate, respiratory rate, and blood pressure are elevated. Your assessment of his pulse also indicates that his pulse is now irregular. Mr. White has just experienced a significant increase in activity; waiting until he has recovered from the exertion would be more appropriate in order to obtain a resting set of vital signs.
- What does the very low temperature indicate? Remember, you continued to hear Mr. White's heavy breathing while obtaining the remainder of the vital signs. Mr. White could not keep his lips pursed in a seal around the thermometer, and this often gives an inaccurate temperature. Mouth breathing and respiratory distress are contraindications for obtaining an oral temperature. As a nurse, you are responsible for determining the most appropriate site to obtain the temperature (see Skill 2-1).

continued

- Does Mr. White's elevated respiratory rate and noisy breathing indicate respiratory distress or a need for oxygen? Obtain an oxygen saturation level via pulse oximetry. If the oxygen saturation level is satisfactory for Mr. White, then you can be confident his body is compensating for the increased oxygen demand. Allow him to rest, with the head of his bed elevated, and retake his vital signs in 15 to 30 minutes. Take vital signs as often as the patient's condition warrants. If Mr. White's oxygen saturation and vital signs continue to deviate from baseline after a rest period, notify the primary care provider (see Chapter 2).
- A bath represents another increase in activity. Mr. White needs time to recover from the exercises before attempting the bath. He should be able to sit in a chair and, in fact, will breathe more comfortably sitting up than lying down. Having him lie flat could make him decompensate, so you should not perform occupied bed-making. If encouraged to sit up, he will probably be able to complete much of his bath by himself.

CASE STUDY

NAOMI BELL

Naomi Bell, age 90, was admitted to the hospital yesterday after experiencing chest pain. She wears a hearing aid in her left ear. In the report you were told that she is "confused" and "doesn't answer questions appropriately." Her night vital signs were as follows: temperature, 98.0°F; pulse, 62 beats/minute; respirations, 18/minute; blood pressure, 132/86 mm Hg. She is due for her AM medications. As you give Mrs. Bell her medications and state their purpose, she points to the digoxin and says, "Honey, I don't take that pill."

MEDICAL ORDERS

Digoxin 0.125 mg PO every morning
Enteric-coated aspirin 81 mg PO every day
Furosemide 20 mg PO every morning
Famotidine 20 mg PO BID
Potassium chloride 10 mEq PO every morning
Captopril 50 mg PO TID

DEVELOPING CLINICAL REASONING

- How would you respond to Mrs. Bell's statement, "Honey, I don't take that pill"?
- Suggest ways in which you can confirm you are giving Mrs. Bell the correct medications.
- Identify the medications that require assessment before administration.
- Describe factors that can contribute to inappropriate answers, and identify nursing actions to diminish these factors.
- How would you determine Mrs. Bell's level of confusion?

continued

SUGGESTED RESPONSES FOR INTEGRATED NURSING CARE

- When patients question you regarding their medications, listen to them. Questions like this should send a "red flag" to the nurse. Often, patients are familiar with what they normally take and can alert you that this may not be the right medication. Do not insist that Mrs. Bell take the digoxin until you confirm the accuracy of the order. In this case, it could be that Mrs. Bell just did not hear what you said. Always confirm what patients say to you by restating it back to them. It could also be that she is more familiar with the trade name for this drug or the medication may look different from the medication she uses at home.
- You can use many safety checks to give medications safely. Some measures include researching the drug before giving it and double-checking all of the "rights." Compare the Medication Administration Record with the original order in the medical record. If the order still remains unclear to you, call the prescriber to clarify it (see Chapter 5).
- Some medications require assessment before you administer them to the patient. In this case, Mrs. Bell takes four medications that will require assessment before administration. Digoxin, furosemide, and captopril will affect pulse and blood pressure. In addition, laboratory test results should be available on potassium and digoxin levels. If Mrs. Bell has a low pulse rate, low blood pressure, or a toxic laboratory value, you will not administer these medications and will notify the primary care provider (see Chapter 5).
- Sometimes, older patients become confused in the hospital. However, do not assume this is always the case. The nurse who gave you the report may have assumed that Mrs. Bell's inappropriate answers were due to confusion, when in fact they may be related to Mrs. Bell's hearing problem. When patients with hearing impairment are admitted to the hospital, encourage them to wear their hearing aids and help them check their batteries to ensure they are working. If you are still unclear whether Mrs. Bell is confused, perform a standard mental status examination used by your institution. This will establish a baseline assessment of her mental status that you can use to individualize her nursing plan of care.
- If you determine she is confused, assess the source of confusion. Given Mrs. Bell's cardiac condition, assess her respiratory status and oxygen saturation level via pulse oximetry to determine whether she is experiencing hypoxia or ischemia. If the cause is physiologic, notify the primary care provider immediately. Another source contributing to confusion could be isolation caused by hearing loss. One way to reduce possible confusion for Mrs. Bell is to improve communication. Ensure that her hearing aid battery is operating and that the unit is placed correctly. Other ways to improve communication include talking to her at eye level, facing her directly when speaking, or even speaking into her unaffected ear. If Mrs. Bell's vision is better than her hearing, you can also give her pertinent information in writing.

CASE STUDY

JOHN WILLIS

You are a nursing student in your first semester of nursing school. Your assigned patient has been discharged before your arrival. Your instructor provides you with the name of another patient to care for, based on the recommendation of the staff. Before you can review the information about the patient with your instructor, she is called to consult with another student and a physician about an emergent patient situation. You read the clinical pathway for John Willis and find that he has methicilllin-resistant *Staphylococcus aureus* (MRSA) in his sputum and suspected pulmonary tuberculosis (TB). You remember reviewing these topics in class and in the learning resource center. Because your instructor is still occupied with the patient emergency, you decide to begin caring for your new patient, instead of wasting time waiting to review the information with her. When

continued

you go to your patient's room, you see the isolation cart containing the infection-control–precaution supplies outside the room, with the hospital's policy and procedure posted for precautions to use for TB and MRSA. You see there are individual masks in plastic bags with different people's names on them, as well as masks with protective eye shields. You recall something from class about wearing a specially fitted mask when implementing these precautions, but realize you do not remember as much as you thought you did. You are unsure of exactly what you need to do. You find the staff nurse assigned to the patient in another patient's room, interrupt his conversation, and say, "I don't have a mask to care for my patient." The nurse sharply responds, "Just go get started. I'm in the middle of something." You consider just going in and introducing yourself and checking on the patient's status. Should you "borrow" a mask from one of the bags? You think it is your duty to care for this patient, but think you may need more information to be safe.

MEDICAL ORDERS

Airborne precautions
Contact precautions
Sputum specimen for culture and sensitivity
Vital signs every shift

DEVELOPING CLINICAL REASONING

- Compare the mode of transmission for TB and MRSA.
- What may have led to the nurse's abrupt and sharp response?
- Identify the appropriate protective equipment needed to care for a patient with TB and a patient with MRSA.
- Describe another way in which you could have approached this situation.
- What can occur if you do not take the appropriate transmission-based precautions and enter other patient rooms?

continued

SUGGESTED RESPONSES FOR INTEGRATED NURSING CARE

- Pulmonary TB transmission occurs through airborne respiratory droplets. MRSA transmission can occur through contact with contaminated blood or body fluids. MRSA can be spread by direct or indirect contact. In this case, MRSA could be transmitted indirectly by coming into contact with items used to care for the patient, such as blood pressure cuffs or linens.
- Agencies will require the use of gowns, gloves, and masks when caring for patients with TB and MRSA. Unique to the Airborne Precautions needed for TB is the use of specially fitted masks called high-efficiency particulate air (HEPA) masks that prevent the inspiration of airborne microorganisms (see Chapter 1). Disposable masks are also available, but they usually require fit-testing as well. If a fit-tested mask is required by your agency, you would either need to be fit-tested for a mask (often done by Employee Health) or reassigned to another patient. In addition, to protect yourself whenever there is the potential for contamination to your eyes, such as coughing, you should wear goggles or a mask with a face shield. Institutions vary greatly in their supplies. If you do not take the appropriate transmission-based precautions, you put yourself at risk for exposure to disease; in this case, TB and MRSA. In addition, entering other patients' rooms results in the potential for transmission of a nosocomial infection. It is always your responsibility, even as a student, to follow the policy and procedure of the facility where you are placed for clinical experiences.
- Hospitals are stressful places. Understanding when and how to communicate with others is an invaluable set of skills. Waiting for the nurse to complete a conversation and task before asking for guidance would have been the ideal situation. Nurses have to prioritize the care they provide. Asking, "Do you have a moment to review something with me?" is a good way to ensure getting the time and attention you need. Because there was no emergency to obtain the vital signs and sputum specimen, they can wait until you are sure you can provide safe care.
- You were right to question the appropriateness of caring for this patient in thinking you may need more information to be safe. In this situation, waiting to review the patient information with your instructor is the ideal solution. Your instructor did not have all the information about the patient before being called away to an emergency. She would not have assigned this patient to you after reviewing his diagnosis, realizing that you would need a specially fitted mask to care for the patient. While waiting for your instructor, you should obtain as much information as possible. Background research and knowledge are powerful tools. Examples of resources you can access include the hospital policy-and-procedure manual, the infection-control manual, the infection-control nurse, and experienced staff members, provided they are able to take time out from their patient care responsibilities. Then, when your instructor is available, you can share this information with him or her to plan your care for that day.

CASE STUDY

CLAUDIA TRAN

Claudia Tran, age 84, has been on your skilled nursing floor for several weeks following a cerebral vascular accident (CVA). She had previously been a resident of a long-term care facility. Her neurologic checks and vital signs are unchanged from her baseline admission. Her CVA has impaired her ability to chew and swallow. She has left-sided weakness, with flaccidity of her left hand. She is emaciated and her skin is very fragile. She has reddened areas on her coccyx, heels, and elbows. She is receiving weekly vitamin B_{12} injections for pernicious anemia. Over the past week, Mrs. Tran has become increasingly confused and incontinent. She constantly pulls at her feeding tube and has had to have it reinserted after pulling it out. Because of this, soft wrist restraints have been ordered. She has a nasogastric tube for tube feedings, which she receives every 8 hours. During your shift, Mrs. Tran is due for a tube feeding. You check the residual and it is 380 mL.

continued

MEDICAL ORDERS

Soft wrist restraints for safety

Nasogastric tube feedings

Vitamin B_{12} injection 1,000 mcg IM weekly

Fiber source 320 mL q 8 hr

Hold feeding for gastric residual ≥200 mL and notify primary care provider.

Physical therapy daily, passive and active range of motion (ROM) as tolerated

DEVELOPING CLINICAL REASONING

- Considering Mrs. Tran's condition, what special safety measures should be implemented with her restraints?
- What are the risks of falling for this patient?
- Identify the risks associated with tube feeding for this patient.
- Identify risk factors and preventive measures for Mrs. Tran's skin breakdown.
- Identify appropriate sites for the vitamin B_{12} injections in Mrs. Tran. Develop a schedule of rotating sites for this injection.

SUGGESTED RESPONSES FOR INTEGRATED NURSING CARE

- Only use restraints as a last resort after all other measures have failed. Other measures could include placing her bed in a low position, having a family member sit with her, and placing her in a room near the nurses' station. Only use restraints with an order from the primary care provider, and follow strict guidelines to protect the patient. Because Mrs. Tran already has skin breakdown, pad the restraints and make sure they are the correct size. An additional safety measure would be performing frequent neurovascular checks, such as checking warmth, sensation, and capillary refill. Restraints are released at specified frequencies. This will improve the circulation to her extremities, reduce the chance of skin breakdown, and give you an opportunity to assess the site. Mrs. Tran has left-sided weakness; therefore, applying a restraint on her flaccid arm could cause harm and is not needed (see Chapter 4).
- Mrs. Tran has many risk factors for skin breakdown, including immobilization, malnutrition, altered mental status, age, incontinence, and positioning for tube feedings. A multifaceted approach is necessary to reduce these risk factors and prevent further skin breakdown. It is essential to develop a schedule for repositioning. Mrs. Tran could benefit from a special type of mattress, such as one with a pressure-reducing surface. Implementing a physical therapy program of active and passive ROM exercises would be helpful. Arrange for a nutritional consult to ensure she will receive adequate protein, as well as other vitamins and minerals essential for skin integrity.
- What skin breakdown complications could result from immobilization and incontinence? A noninvasive way to reduce the chance of recurrent incontinence is to offer Mrs. Tran a bedpan at regular intervals. Frequent skin care and use of skin barriers to prevent damage from excessive moisture is an important part of her nursing care.
- Because Mrs. Tran is confused and in a restraint, her risk for falling is high. Keep her bed in a low position at all times and make sure her call light is within reach. Frequently check on patients such as Mrs. Tran to decrease isolation and provide orientation.
- Mrs. Tran is receiving tube feedings and has an excessive residual. She is at increased risk for aspiration of tube feedings into her lungs if positioned supine. To decrease the risk for aspiration, check the residual amount before every feeding. Additional assessments should include auscultating for the presence of bowel sounds, abdominal distension, and abdominal tenderness. In this situation, Mrs. Tran's gastric residual was greater than 200 mL. Therefore, keep her head elevated, hold her tube feeding, and contact her primary care provider as soon as possible (see Chapter 11).
- When giving Mrs. Tran vitamin B_{12} injections, use larger muscles and rotate sites. Implement the rotation schedule for this injection in her plan of care. This is particularly important because Mrs. Tran is emaciated and does not have good muscle mass. Avoid areas that are reddened or have palpable nodules and scars. Because vitamin B_{12} injections can be irritating, inject the medication slowly to minimize pain, trauma, and discomfort (see Chapter 5).

CASE STUDY

JOE LEROY

Joe LeRoy, age 60, was brought in by his daughter and admitted to your small rural hospital. He has had the stomach flu at home for several days and is suffering from dehydration. He has right-sided hemiplegia due to a cerebral vascular accident (CVA) 3 years ago. Mr. LeRoy has remained in bed during his hospital stay due to extreme weakness and fatigue.

You received the report on your seven patients. From the report, you note that Mr. LeRoy continues to have frequent liquid stools (averaging about three or four times/shift). The doctor has ordered a stool sample for culture and sensitivity. When entering your patient's room, you notice his sheets are very dirty and he has a strong body odor.

MEDICAL ORDERS

Intravenous fluids: D5 ½ NSS IV at 125 mL/hr

Stool sample for culture and sensitivity

Vital signs every shift

DEVELOPING CLINICAL REASONING

- Develop your priorities and rationales for the following nursing care for Mr. LeRoy:
- What considerations should be taken into account when collecting the stool sample?
  - Changing his sheets
  - Completing the AM assessment
- Are there any assessments that you would want to pay particular attention to during your nursing care?
  - Obtaining vital signs
  - Collecting the sample
  - Giving a bath
- Describe how your attitude and nonverbal behavior could affect Mr. LeRoy's hospital experience.

SUGGESTED RESPONSES FOR INTEGRATED NURSING CARE

- Prioritizing care is a difficult, but important skill for all nurses. Determine whether Mr. LeRoy can provide his own morning care, although this is unlikely due to his hemiplegia and weakness. If you need to assist him with his personal care, determine the needs of your other patients before beginning this task. Before leaving Mr. LeRoy, let him know your plan and the time he can expect to have assistance with his bath. Another alternative is asking a nursing assistant (if you have one on your unit) to give Mr. LeRoy a bath and change his bed linens. On your initial assessment of Mr. LeRoy, cover any very obviously dirty areas of his sheets with a blue waterproof pad or a clean sheet. You could also offer him a

continued

wet, warm washcloth and a dry towel for initial cleaning while you are completing his assessment. You should also inform him of the need for a stool specimen.

- If your floor has no nursing aide, return to his room after completing your other patient assessments. First, obtain the warm stool sample, give the bath, and then change his linens. This sequence saves time and energy for both the nurse and the patient, because when providing a bed bath or assisting a patient on a bedpan, you can easily soil the linens.
- While wearing gloves, collect and send the stool specimen promptly to the laboratory. Specimens should be sent while still warm, because the microorganisms present at body temperature may die when the specimen temperature changes, and this would produce a false–negative result (see Chapter 18).
- During your assessment, pay particular attention to his skin. Mr. LeRoy is at risk for pressure ulcers due to his age, diarrhea, altered nutrition, and immobility. Assist Mr. LeRoy to turn over so that you can inspect his back and bony prominences, the most likely areas for skin breakdown. If you notice any skin breakdown, notify the primary care provider so that treatment can begin promptly.
- A nurse's nonverbal behavior can have a dramatic impact on a patient's hospital experience. Projecting a positive attitude and providing nonjudgmental care help a patient cope with hospitalization. You may be offended by Mr. LeRoy's body odor and the smell of his stool, but as a nurse you need to learn strategies to manage strong odors and make sure that your facial expressions or body language do not convey discomfort or disgust.

CASE STUDY

KATE TOWNSEND

Kate Townsend, a 70-year-old patient with chronic obstructive pulmonary disease (COPD), has just returned to your medical–surgical unit from surgery for excision of a nonmalignant intestinal polyp. She has a midline abdominal transverse incision secured with sutures and covered with a dry sterile dressing. She has a right peripheral IV with D5 ½ NSS at 75 mL/hr. She has a history of long-term steroid use for her COPD. She has a nasogastric tube in her right naris, which is clamped at this time. The primary care provider orders oxygen 2 L/minute via nasal cannula. The patient's primary nurse asks you to place the patient on oxygen. When you attempt to place the cannula in the patient's naris with the nasogastric (NG) tube, you think it is uncomfortable and a little odd. For comfort, you decide to place a simple oxygen mask on Mrs. Townsend instead. Her vital signs are as follows: temperature, 99.6°F; pulse, 76 beats/minute; respirations, 24 breaths/minute; blood pressure, 110/70 mm Hg; oxygen saturation, 92%.

MEDICAL ORDERS

Nasogastric tube clamped
Incentive spirometry prn
Morphine sulfate 2 to 4 mg IV q 4 hr prn pain
Oxygen 2 L/minute via nasal cannula
Intravenous fluid: D5 ½ NSS at 75 mL/hr

continued

DEVELOPING CLINICAL REASONING

- What is the difference between oxygen given by nasal cannula and that given via a simple oxygen mask?
- What comfort measures would you want to provide for Mrs. Townsend?
- What complication could occur with Mrs. Townsend when changing her to a simple oxygen mask?
- Develop a discharge plan for Mrs. Townsend.
- Considering Mrs. Townsend's chronic lung disease, what complications can occur, and what nursing interventions could decrease these complications?

SUGGESTED RESPONSES FOR INTEGRATED NURSING CARE

- Several delivery systems exist to provide oxygen to patients, and they deliver varying amounts of oxygen. Oxygen delivered via a nasal cannula set at 2 L/minute would deliver about 28% oxygen, whereas oxygen delivered in a simple mask could deliver 40% to 60% oxygen, depending on the flow meter setting (see Chapter 14). Oxygen is considered a medicine, so it is not a nursing order but a medical order. The oxygen concentration and delivery system are adjusted according to orders or parameters from a physician or other advanced practice professional.
- For people without chronic lung disease, breathing is driven by the buildup of carbon dioxide levels in the blood (hypercapnia). The drive to breathe for patients with COPD is often a lack of oxygen (hypoxia). Because of this, increasing oxygen levels in patients with COPD may decrease their respiratory drive. Therefore, when changing Mrs. Townsend for comfort reasons from the nasal cannula to the mask, you could have increased her oxygen anywhere from 12% to 32%, and even a small increase in oxygen has the potential to stop her breathing. Although it is not entirely comfortable to have an NG tube, much less another tube in the naris, it is not unusual for this to occur. Both will fit with some manipulation by the nurse.
- Patients with chronic lung disease are at increased risk after surgery for pulmonary complications, including atelectasis and pneumonia. General anesthesia alters all of the muscles involved in breathing and clearing the airway. COPD is a restrictive lung disease, meaning that the patient's lungs lose their elasticity and become less compliant. For Mrs. Townsend, this combination of underlying disease and the effects of surgery results in a decreased ability to mobilize secretions, which could lead to atelectasis and possibly pneumonia. Mrs. Townsend may be experiencing atelectasis, indicated by her temperature of 99.6°F. Other signs of atelectasis would be decreased breath sounds and/or crackles in the lung bases, shortness of breath, increased respiratory rate, and decreased oxygen saturation of pulse oximetry. Without nursing intervention, atelectasis could lead to pneumonia. Measures to facilitate lung expansion and mobilization of secretions will minimize atelectasis. These nursing measures include elevation of the head of her bed, deep-breathing exercises, incentive spirometry, adequate pain control, and early ambulation.
- Long-term steroid use can make the skin very fragile, increase the potential for skin breakdown, and delay wound healing. To prevent this, observe the skin under her NG tube and oxygen cannula tubing. The pressure of the tubes on her face and behind her ears could cause a break in skin integrity. Repositioning the tape that is holding the NG tube may make it more comfortable. You may need to protect the skin under the cannula tubing with a hydrocolloid dressing (see Chapter 8), especially if the skin becomes reddened. There are many commercial products to hold oxygen nasal cannulas, as well as NG tubes, which may also increase her comfort.
- Discharge plans for Mrs. Townsend would need to address both her underlying lung disease as well as her recent intestinal surgery. Patient education should focus on measures that enable Mrs. Townsend to improve her lung compliance and increase her oxygenation. Incentive spirometry and a daily activity schedule are imperative. Due to her prolonged use of steroids, she may also have delayed wound healing at her incision site. Patient education should address optimal nutrition and prevention of infection. Before discharge, validate Mrs. Townsend's knowledge of measures to prevent pulmonary and wound complications.

CASE STUDY

TULA STILLWATER

Tula Stillwater is a 36-year-old Native American who has had diabetes since age 26. She weighs 218 lb. She is gravida 1 para 1 and delivered a 9 lb, 6 oz boy via cesarean section 3 days ago. She has a transverse abdominal incision with staples. She reports tenderness on the right side of the incision, but acute pain on the left side of the incision. Her 8 AM vital signs are as follows: temperature, 101.6°F; pulse, 76 beats/minute; respirations, 18/minute; blood pressure, 134/78 mm Hg. Her blood glucose before breakfast is 185 mg/dL; her blood glucose on previous days had ranged from 90 to 124 mg/dL.

On your assessment, you find her incision is open to air and the staples are intact. The incision is well approximated and without erythema on the right side. However, the left side of the incision is pulling apart and is edematous and warm to the touch, with a scant amount of purulent drainage.

MEDICAL ORDERS

Vital signs q 4 hr
Standing order: Remove staples before discharge.
Fingerstick blood glucose before meals and at bedtime
Standing order: Discharge on third day if stable.
Regular insulin per sliding scale

DEVELOPING CLINICAL REASONING

- What is your interpretation of her vital signs? Who should be notified and when?
- How would you determine whether Mrs. Stillwater meets the criteria for discharge?
- What is the relationship between Mrs. Stillwater's diabetes and her postsurgical condition?
- What factors affect her staple removal?
- How should you respond to her fingerstick blood glucose level?
- What nursing interventions do you foresee performing?
- Describe the timing and the technique for administering her insulin.

continued

SUGGESTED RESPONSES FOR INTEGRATED NURSING CARE

- Mrs. Stillwater's vital signs should alert you to a potential complication. She may have an infection related to her incision, as evidenced by her increased temperature and her subjective report of acute pain at the incision. Her blood pressure could be a result of her pain, but you should compare it with her baseline and continue to monitor it. You inspected the incision carefully for signs of infection. Notify her primary care provider immediately of this potential complication.
- Wound healing may be impaired in people with diabetes, so any patient with diabetes requires vigilant wound assessment. Additionally, the stress of surgery usually results in increased blood glucose levels. Mrs. Stillwater's fingerstick blood sugar is elevated from her baseline, another symptom of a possible infection. When you see a dramatic increase in blood sugar in a patient with diabetes, consider the possible causes.
- Despite the urgency of this new complication of wound infection, Mrs. Stillwater should receive her insulin and breakfast as she usually would. Administer her insulin in a subcutaneous site; she can help you identify the site where she should receive her insulin. Patients who are accustomed to managing their diabetes at home will have preferences when in the hospital, and you should honor these preferences when possible (see Chapter 5).
- Many women who have had cesarean sections are discharged on the third day. One of the expected outcomes for discharge would include being free of infection. Mrs. Stillwater is not free of infection; she has pain at her incision site, a fever, and an elevated fingerstick blood sugar. When you notify the primary care provider of these symptoms, blood count, a wound culture, incision site care, and cancellation of the discharge are ordered.
- Given the delayed discharge and impaired wound healing, you would not want to remove the staples from this incision because removing the staples at this time could place Mrs. Stillwater at risk for dehiscence. Another factor affecting the risk for dehiscence and impaired wound healing is Mrs. Stillwater's increased subcutaneous fat.
- Did you foresee obtaining a complete blood count and a wound culture and performing incision site care? Did you also anticipate that this patient should not be discharged nor have her staples removed? In addition, although her physiologic care is very important, you will also need to relieve anxiety related to this infection and acknowledge her disappointment that she cannot go home today.

2

Intermediate Case Studies

CASE STUDY

OLIVIA GREENBAUM

Olivia Greenbaum is a 9-month-old infant admitted with respiratory syncytial virus (RSV). She was born prematurely at 30 weeks' gestation. Her complications at birth included respiratory distress syndrome (RDS), suspected sepsis, and formula intolerance. She was discharged home after 5 weeks on soy-based formula. This is her first hospitalization since her birth. Olivia is Mr. and Mrs. Greenbaum's only child, and they are very anxious. Mrs. Greenbaum is her primary caregiver.

Olivia is receiving supplemental humidified oxygen administered via oxygen tent at 40%. She is very fussy and is not tolerating separation from her mother well. She has a peripheral IV inserted in her right hand with D5 ¼ NSS infusing at 20 mL/hr. It is covered with a sock puppet. She is wearing a T-shirt and a disposable diaper. She is quite active within the crib. Her previous vital signs were as follows: temperature, 36.4°C (97.5°F); pulse, 84 beats/minute; respirations, 38/minute; blood pressure, 94/58 mm Hg.

Mrs. Greenbaum spent the night and is currently sleeping in the recliner in Olivia's room. You enter the room and observe Olivia sleeping. She is pale with circumoral cyanosis. Her respiratory rate is 40/minute with an audible expiratory wheeze. Her heart rate on the monitor is 86 bpm; her pulse rate on the pulse oximeter is 62 bpm. The pulse oximeter is currently showing an oxygen saturation level of 68%.

MEDICAL ORDERS

Vital signs q 4 hr
Encourage coughing.
Oxygen via tent at 40%
Continuous pulse oximetry when quiet; may obtain q hr intermittent pulse oximeter readings when active
Maintain O_2 saturation 93% to 97%. Adjust O_2 in increments of 2% up to a max of 50%.
Isomil 6–8 oz q 4 hr when awake
Intravenous fluids: D5 ¼ NSS at 20 mL/hr
Heart rate/resp. monitor

continued

DEVELOPING CLINICAL REASONING

- What is your first priority after observing Olivia sleeping?
- Should you increase the oxygen being administered?
- What is your interpretation of her vital signs and oxygen saturation?
- Give examples of how to manage thermoregulation within an oxygen tent.
- Identify factors that affect the accuracy of the oxygen saturation reading.
- How frequently should Olivia's IV site be assessed? What is the function of the sock puppet?
- How do you encourage coughing in a 9-month-old baby?

SUGGESTED RESPONSES FOR INTEGRATED NURSING CARE

- Your first priority is to establish whether Olivia is hypoxic. You noted a rapid respiratory rate and circumoral cyanosis, both potential symptoms of hypoxia. The pulse oximeter heart rate does not match the cardiac monitor heart rate. Gently, without disturbing Olivia, you remove and replace the pulse oximeter.
- Your preliminary assessment is that the pulse oximeter is not accurately assessing her oxygenation. You are able to hold the probe to her toe and get a reading of 95%. Olivia begins to wake up. Take her apical heart rate, which is the most reliable site for infants and small children (see Chapter 2). Compare her apical pulse rate with the heart rate on the pulse oximeter as well as the heart rate on the cardiac monitor. Nurses must always verify that the equipment is accurately reflecting the patient's status. Next, you take her temperature, which is 36.2°C (97.1°F). The humidified oxygen is also cooling Olivia, making her hands, feet, and lips appear cold, blue, and dusky (see Chapter 14).
- Once Olivia is awake, she will not tolerate having the pulse oximeter probe on her toe and will keep pulling it off. You will need to check the oxygen saturation intermittently. Your next priority is to warm her up. When children become chilled, they have

continued

increased energy expenditure. When infants are stressed beyond aerobic metabolism, they use anaerobic metabolism. This produces lactic acid, which increases the acidity of the blood, exacerbating respiratory distress. Urge her mother to bring in more clothes and to layer her clothes to keep Olivia thermoregulated within the humidified tent. You do not need to increase the oxygen level; what at first looked like hypoxia is in fact hypothermia!

- The accuracy of a pulse oximetry reading is affected by several factors, including patient perfusion and peripheral vasoconstriction. Other factors that prevent the detection of oxygen saturation may be as simple as nail polish or artificial nails (see Chapter 14).
- Encouraging coughing in an infant is accomplished either through crying or laughing. Crying and laughing require deep breaths and will cause a patient to cough, thus promoting airway clearance. If the infant is periodically crying vigorously, that is sufficient. You can try tickling or playing peek-a-boo to get a 9-month-old to laugh.
- Check this patient's IV site every hour to ensure there are no signs of infiltration. The sock puppet is one way to disguise the IV site dressing while leaving it accessible for examination. If a young child can see the IV site dressing, he or she will often persist in trying to remove the tape and dressing despite all your efforts. If you cover the site, the child will not remember it is there. Piaget's theory of cognitive development includes the concept of object permanence. At 9 months old, a child cannot imagine what he or she cannot see—in other words, what is out of sight is out of mind.

CASE STUDY

VICTORIA HOLLY

Victoria Holly, age 68, is newly admitted to the hospital due to anemia and severe dehydration. To treat the dehydration she has an IV of D5 ½ NSS infusing into the right hand. To treat the anemia, she has a medication or IV lock in her left arm to be used for blood administration only. She recently received 2 units of packed red blood cells. You have medical orders to draw a complete blood count and a complete metabolic profile. Mrs. Holly also has an ileostomy, which she has managed for several years on her own. Upon your initial physical assessment of Mrs. Holly, you find her vital signs are as follows: temperature, 97.2°F; pulse, 96 beats/minute; respirations, 18/minute; blood pressure, 88/50 mm Hg. Her skin is "tenting" and you are having difficulty palpating her peripheral pulses. Her lips are dry and cracked. The skin around her stoma site is bright red and open in areas. You notice that her ostomy pouch was cut much larger than the stoma site. She reports she is very tired and "lacks energy." Her family informs you that she has always been a very independent person but in the last couple of months she just "hasn't been herself."

MEDICAL ORDERS

Intravenous fluids: D5 ½ NSS IV at 125 mL/hr
Strict I&O
Daily weights

Complete blood count (CBC) and complete metabolic profile (CMP) stat.

continued

DEVELOPING CLINICAL REASONING

- Identify appropriate sites and equipment needed to draw the blood.
- Describe how you would assess Mrs. Holly's peripheral circulation.
- What concerns you about Mrs. Holly's present condition in relationship to performing her activities of daily living (ADLs) independently?
- What is alarming about her ileostomy? Identify possible explanations for the stoma's condition.
- What are measurable physical parameters you can use to determine whether fluid replacement therapy and blood administration are sufficient?
- Develop a discharge teaching plan for Mrs. Holly related to her ostomy care.

SUGGESTED RESPONSES FOR INTEGRATED NURSING CARE

- You cannot draw blood specimens from a dedicated line such as the one Mrs. Holly has for blood administration. You also cannot obtain the specimen from above the IV in her right hand because the specimen will be diluted with the D5 ½ NSS solution and, thus, will be inaccurate. It is not considered best practice to draw laboratory specimens from an IV site unless absolutely necessary, according to facility policy. Collect Mrs. Holly's laboratory work from her left arm via venipuncture, avoiding the right arm due to the IV infusion.
- Mrs. Holly's vital signs are disconcerting because her blood pressure is low. Because of her hypotension, ADLs may unduly tax her. Until you see a positive change in her vital signs, provide assistance with her ADLs (see Chapter 7). In addition, Mrs. Holly has an IV in each arm. It may be difficult for her to care for the ostomy while attempting to keep the IV sites free from infection.
- One outcome to anticipate with Mrs. Holly would be an increase in blood pressure. Other outcomes include palpable peripheral pulses and normal skin turgor. Subjectively, Mrs. Holly should report that her energy has increased. Her family may also comment that she is becoming more "like herself." Sometimes health care workers make judgments about older adults, thinking that they are always tired. Since health care workers are often unfamiliar with their patients' normal conditions, comments made by family members can often be very helpful in determining progress. This is especially true if your patient cannot communicate. Objectively, one outcome would be that Mrs. Holly becomes more active in her own care.
- When a patient has no peripheral pulses, you must investigate further. Never ignore the absence of pulses, as this could signal a life-threatening condition. Have another nurse check the pulses, or use a Doppler. Upon checking Mrs. Holly's pulses with a Doppler device, you were able to hear them and marked them with an "x" to facilitate future assessments. In your initial assessment, you were not surprised that

continued

Mrs. Holly's pulses were nonpalpable, as she has a very low circulating volume (see Chapter 2).

- Mrs. Holly's ileostomy site is very red and excoriated. You are alarmed, as this could place her at risk for infection. Do not assume that a primary care provider has seen the excoriation around the ostomy site. If the patient came into the hospital with more pressing matters, such as decreased blood pressure, the primary care provider may not have observed the ileostomy. Notify the primary care provider. Mrs. Holly may lack knowledge about the appropriate method for sizing and cutting her ostomy appliance. You suspect that she may be cutting the faceplate in such a way as to leave her skin exposed to the liquid stool, which is then causing the excoriation (see Chapter 13).
- One area you should investigate is Mrs. Holly's ability to care for the ostomy before she came to the hospital. It is possible that her skin around the stoma site has looked like this for some time. Before her hospital discharge, evaluate her knowledge through return demonstration to ensure that she can care for the stoma and can identify possible family resources. She may benefit from a home health referral to ensure she is caring for her stoma properly.

CASE STUDY

TULA STILLWATER

It is now day 5 in the hospital for Mrs. Stillwater. She has developed a staphylococcal infection in her cesarean section incision. This is the second time you have cared for this patient. You are familiar with her diabetic status, baseline vital signs, and routine postpartum care. She is currently receiving an IV antibiotic. Her vital signs are as follows: temperature, 99.2°F; pulse, 74 beats/minute; respirations, 18/minute; blood pressure, 130/80 mm Hg. Her fingerstick blood glucose before breakfast is 120 mg/dL.

You learned in report that her incision is intact and healing on the right side, but the far left side of her incision is being treated with a calcium alginate wound dressing. The open part of the incision is approximately 1″ long, 0.5″ wide, and 1″ deep. This part of her incision is draining copious amounts of foul-smelling, yellow to green purulent drainage. The incision is very painful. Mrs. Stillwater reports her pain at a 6 on a scale of 1 to 10 (10 = worst) before her pain medication is administered.

Mrs. Stillwater's 5-day-old boy is now bottle-feeding regularly. He is taking 3 oz of Similac with Iron every 4 hours. Mrs. Stillwater is eager to assume the majority of his care.

MEDICAL ORDERS

Medication or IV lock; flush every shift and prn

Vancomycin 1.0 g IV q 12 hr

Sterile dressing change with calcium alginate wound dressing; pack loosely, change when outer dressing is saturated with drainage. Irrigate wound with normal saline before removing dressing.

Irrigate wound with NSS with dressing change

Fingerstick blood glucose before meals and at bedtime

Humalog insulin per sliding scale

Vital signs q 4 hr

Lortab 7.5 mg, 2 tabs q 4 to 6 hr prn pain

continued

DEVELOPING CLINICAL REASONING

- How will you plan her dressing change, and what equipment will you need?
- How will you organize your nursing care to provide uninterrupted time for Mrs. Stillwater to care for her 5-day-old son?
- Describe your assessment and interventions for this wound.
- What techniques can you show Mrs. Stillwater to improve her mobility and ability to hold and care for her infant?
- Identify factors that will promote wound healing in Mrs. Stillwater.
- Describe the procedure you will use to administer the IV antibiotic.

SUGGESTED RESPONSES FOR INTEGRATED NURSING CARE

- Mrs. Stillwater's dressing change will be stressful and uncomfortable. To manage the pain, perform the dressing change after she has taken her pain medication and you have allowed enough time for it to be effective. Given her diabetic status, allow her to eat her breakfast and receive her insulin before you begin her dressing change. Mrs. Stillwater's focus is probably on her son. Encourage her to give him his morning bottle and to be satisfied that he is comfortable before you begin the dressing change.
- Review Chapter 8 to develop the list of equipment you will need for the dressing change. You will need to set up a sterile field and maintain the sterility during the dressing change. Mrs. Stillwater can be positioned supine and rotated slightly to her left to promote drainage of the wound during irrigation.
- Make sure your assessment of the wound includes the size, the presence of granulation tissue, a description of the drainage, wound color, the presence of edema and erythema, and temperature (see Chapter 8). Note the condition of the skin at the wound edges as well as the skin where the wound dressing is taped. Look for changes in the condition of the wound and note how Mrs. Stillwater is tolerating the dressing change. If she will be taught to care for this wound and perform the dressing changes at home, instruction and return demonstration would become part of her discharge planning.
- For Mrs. Stillwater's wound to heal, the infection must be resolved and the wound edges will need to become approximated. To optimize wound healing, Mrs. Stillwater will need a diet high in protein and minerals. Obtain a nutritional consultation.
- The care of her infant son is a priority for Mrs. Stillwater. Cluster your nursing care, such as wound dressings, vital signs, and medication administration, to allow her sufficient time to provide care for her son.
- Make sure Mrs. Stillwater knows how to use a splint, such as a pillow, across her abdomen to give support to her abdominal musculature when moving

continued

or coughing. Spending time in a comfortable chair may be preferable to getting in and out of bed. Assess that Mrs. Stillwater is using the "football hold" to feed and comfort her son. The advantage of this position is that the infant does not rest on the mother's abdomen. Mrs. Stillwater should have several pillows available to provide support for her arms when holding her infant.

- To give the IV antibiotic, assess the IV site for patency, flush the IV per facility policy prior to administration, administer the antibiotics according to the pharmacy or manufacturer's guidelines, and then flush the medication or IV lock after the antibiotic is infused (see Chapter 5).

CASE STUDY

JASON BROWN

Jason Brown is a 21-year-old college football player. It is the second post-op day following surgical repair of a fracture of his right tibia and fibula. He has sutures over the anterior knee and lateral malleolus and a posterior splint on the right leg. He continues to report considerable pain. His vital signs at midnight were as follows 98.3°F; pulse, 58 beats/minute; respirations, 12/minute; blood pressure 118/70 mm Hg. He reported his pain as a 3 on a scale of 1 of 10 (10 = worst) at about 10 pm. He has a peripheral IV in his left forearm infusing D5 ½ NSS at a rate of 20 mL/hr. He is using a PCA pump for pain relief. The nursing care for the morning includes routine AM care, cast care, and a trip to physical therapy. Shortly after morning report, the unit secretary catches you and says, "Jason says he needs a nurse. He is in terrible pain."

You enter the room. Jason is pale and diaphoretic. His sheets are damp with some wet spots. He says, "My leg hurts. It really hurts." You ask him to rate his pain, and he answers, "At least an 8. I've been pushing my pain pump but I'm still in pain." His IV site looks okay. You say, "I'm going to find out why it is hurting. I need to get your vital signs first." His vital signs now are as follows: temperature, 98.9°F; pulse, 72 beats/minute; respirations, 20/minute; blood pressure, 124/78 mm Hg.

MEDICAL ORDERS

Vital signs q 4 hr
Intravenous fluids: D5 ½ NSS at 40 mL/hr
PCA—Morphine sulfate 1 mg/mL, 1 mg q 6 min; lock-out max 10 mg in 1 hr
Ambien 5 mg prn at bedtime for sleep
Physical therapy for weight-bearing, as tolerated

continued

DEVELOPING CLINICAL REASONING

- What is the significance of the changes in Jason's vital signs?
- How do you assess the following:
  - Infection versus inflammation?
  - Neurovascular compromise?
  - IV patency?
- What interventions for Jason's pain must occur immediately before administering nursing care and PT?

SUGGESTED RESPONSES FOR INTEGRATED NURSING CARE

- Always compare vital signs with a comparable baseline and the previous vital signs (see Chapter 2). While Jason's temperature is elevated slightly, it has not increased dramatically, as it would be with an infection. His respiratory rate and pulse rate were quite low at midnight. Since he is a young, healthy athlete, his resting pulse rate may be lower than what is often considered as the norm. You notice that his resting pulse rates on the night shift have been running from 56 to 60 beats/minute. Another factor contributing to his decreased pulse rate is the effect of the Ambien that he took at 9 PM to help him sleep. Therefore, while his morning respiratory rate and pulse rate are still within normal range, they represent a significant increase from his resting baseline. These are objective assessments supporting his assertion of increased pain.
- One reason for an increase in pain with any postsurgical patient is the possibility of infection. Quickly assess all surgical incision sites and observe for redness, swelling, or a foul odor (Chapter 8). Due to short hospital stays, signs and symptoms of infection do not usually appear until after the patient is discharged. The assessment of the surgical site should also include checking for bleeding. Hemorrhage in the postoperative period is always a potential complication (see Chapter 6).
- In addition to infection, Jason is at risk for neurovascular compromise because of the trauma to his right leg as well as from the splint and dressing. Assess for neurovascular compromise and perform cast care (see Chapter 9). Jason's fracture has been placed in a splint rather than a cast, which is a more current surgical practice, but nurses still refer to the care of the affected extremity as "cast care." Determine whether there are any signs of compartment syndrome (see Chapter 9). You need no additional equipment for this assessment, and it should take very little time; do this immediately.
- Upon assessment, you find that Jason's foot and leg are pink and warm with 2+ pulses, no edema, full sensation, motion, and capillary refill measuring less than 3 seconds. The incision sites show no redness, swelling, drainage, or foul odor, and no bleeding is evident.
- Another possible reason for his pain is that his IV may no longer be patent and, therefore, he would not be receiving any pain medication. You remember the wet spots on the bed as you begin systematically checking each of the IV administration-set connections. Your assessment of the IV site shows no swelling, and he reports no pain at the site. Your next check should be from the IV site to the IV tubing. You find that the connection of the IV tubing to the IV insertion catheter is loose and leaking. Determine whether the IV site is still patent (see Chapter 15). If the IV is still patent, replace the IV tubing (see Chapter 15). Check the medication in the PCA pump to ensure it is the correct medication. You will be required to check the PCA history to determine the amount of medication used as well as the amount remaining every 4 hours or according to facility policy (see Chapter 10).
- Contact the primary care provider to explain that the PCA pain medication was infusing onto the sheets, and obtain an order for an appropriate bolus dose so that Jason can obtain immediate pain relief. After 30 minutes, obtain another set of vital signs and perform a pain assessment. Document the evaluation of your interventions. Jason's pain will need to be controlled before initiating additional nursing care. Coordinating with physical therapy to reschedule his therapy until his pain is resolved is a nursing responsibility.

CASE STUDY

KENT CLARK

Kent Clark, age 29, was admitted 24 hours ago for observation related to a suspected closed head injury following a motor vehicle accident (MVA). Mr. Clark's baseline vital signs are stable. He has a cervical collar and is scheduled to undergo an MRI to determine if he has a cervical spine injury. The primary care provider has asked you to reduce his activity until cervical spinal injuries are ruled out.

Currently, Mr. Clark is awake, alert, and oriented (to person, place, and time); his pupils are equally round and reactive to light and accommodation (PERRLA). He moves all four extremities bilaterally. His head is elevated 30 degrees to minimize increased intracranial pressure (ICP) and edema. A peripheral IV in his right arm is infusing D5 ½ NSS at 40 mL/hr.

Just before you are scheduled to take him to Special Procedures, Mr. Clark becomes restless and anxious. During the neuro check you notice that his right pupil is sluggish. Although he denies pain, he says, "I don't care what the doctors say. I am not going to stay in this bed any longer!" When you call the primary care provider, he orders lorazepam 0.5 mg IV push. However, as you give the IV push medication to Mr. Clark, you notice a cloudy substance forming in the IV line and he reports a slight burning at his IV insertion site.

MEDICAL ORDERS

Bed rest
Intravenous fluids: D5 ½ NSS at 20 mL/hr
HOB elevated 30 degrees
Neurologic checks q 2 hr
Cervical collar

DEVELOPING CLINICAL REASONING

- What clinical symptoms alert you that Mr. Clark's condition is changing? What additional assessments will you do?
- Identify the source of the pain at the IV insertion site and the cloudy substance in the IV tubing.
- Describe special positioning and transfer techniques to be followed for Mr. Clark.
- What could you have done to prevent these complications, and how will you intervene now?
- How will you handle Mr. Clark's anger and prevent him from getting out of bed?

continued

SUGGESTED RESPONSES FOR INTEGRATED NURSING CARE

- In a patient with a closed head injury, bleeding or swelling may occur within the confines of the skull, leading to increased intracranial pressure (ICP). This increased ICP could cause extensive brain damage. Mr. Clark became increasingly restless and anxious, which could be a subtle sign of increased ICP. Even slow bleeding inside the cranium can cause changes. When you observe a change, immediately complete a neurologic assessment to determine if there are further neurologic alterations. When Mr. Clark became restless, you found that his right pupil was more sluggish to light than the left, which is another sign of increased ICP. Complete neurologic checks as often as his condition warrants, and immediately report subtle changes in neurologic checks to the physician. Meticulous documentation of baseline neurologic checks and subsequent assessments is important to detect subtle neurologic changes (see Chapter 17).
- Cervical spinal injuries can vary in severity, and even hairline fractures can become unstable if the patient is not positioned and transferred correctly. Mr. Clark has a cervical collar and the primary care provider has asked you to minimize his movement. If you need to turn Mr. Clark, keep his head lowered and then logroll him as a unit without flexing or turning his neck. Obtain help from additional staff so that you can stabilize his head, neck, and torso in straight alignment while he is being turned. When Mr. Clark is transferred from the bed to a stretcher, use a friction-reducing sheet or lateral transfer device to move him gently and carefully as a unit. Even though he has a cervical collar, do not assume that it is safe for him to sit up further in the bed or get up and move around.
- Mr. Clark is angry and wants to get out of bed. For Mr. Clark, careful pharmacologic sedation may be a better option. The physician has ordered lorazepam to reduce his agitation and anxiety. Another possible intervention is to help Mr. Clark feel more in control of his environment. This could be as simple as having a family member stay with him, and frequently checking his needs. Restraints would be the least desirable option for him. At this time, placing restraints on him could increase his agitation and make him feel more trapped, and this could increase his ICP (see Chapter 4).
- Pain at the IV site could mean that the IV is not patent. Carefully observe the IV site for any signs of phlebitis or infiltration before and while giving the IV push. If you determine that Mr. Clark's IV has a good blood return and is not infiltrated, the burning sensation at his IV site may be from the medication administration. Medications given by intravenous bolus can be irritating. Give the medication and the flush that follows at a slower rate. If not contraindicated, some medications can also be diluted if ordered.
- The most probable cause for the cloudy appearance in Mr. Clark's IV line is precipitation of the drug due to chemical incompatibility of the lorazepam and the IV fluid of D5 ½ NSS. When giving any medication through an IV line, you must know whether the drug and IV solution are chemically compatible (see Chapter 5). When IV drugs are not compatible, a reaction immediately occurs that may not be visible to the eye, but nevertheless can be dangerous. To prevent this, flush the IV line before and after medication administration per institution policy. Since a precipitate has already formed, clamp the tubing off closest to Mr. Clark and make sure that the cloudy substance does not reach him (see Chapter 5). Some facilities require discontinuing the IV and restarting another IV with new IV tubing; other hospitals require changing only the IV tubing. If signs of incompatibility occur, notify the primary care provider and continue to assess Mr. Clark's need for further medication.

CASE STUDY

LUCILLE HOWARD

Lucille Howard, age 78, is in the hospital for a severe urinary tract infection (UTI). She has a history of urinary retention and UTIs. She is overweight, has a history of heart failure, and is allergic to many medications, including several antibiotics. Twenty-four hours ago she had severe nausea and vomiting and was ordered nothing by mouth (NPO). She has

continued

an IV catheter inserted in her left arm, infusing D5 ½ NSS at 75 mL/hr. Mrs. Howard just had a triple-lumen urinary retention catheter inserted for continuous bladder irrigation with amphotericin B. The catheter was inserted at 6:30 AM and your shift started at 6:45 AM. During your shift, you notice that she begins to have some coarse audible breath sounds and difficulty breathing. She reports pain in her abdomen.

MEDICAL ORDERS

Amphotericin B 50 mg in 1,000-mL sterile H_2O irrigating in bladder at 40 mL/hr for 5 days

Intravenous fluids: D5 ½ NSS at 75 mL/hr

NPO

Strict I&O

DEVELOPING CLINICAL REASONING

- What are possible causes of Mrs. Howard's current symptoms?
- How would you identify the source of her current symptoms?
- What actions will you take?

SUGGESTED RESPONSES FOR INTEGRATED NURSING CARE

- There are several potential causes for Mrs. Howard's symptoms. In light of her drug sensitivities, she may be allergic to the amphotericin B. Allergic responses can include difficulty breathing as well as itching and a rash. Another source of her symptoms could be related to her heart problems. People with heart problems can easily become overloaded with fluid. Symptoms of fluid overload, a common problem for patients with heart failure, include crackles in the lungs, abnormal heart sounds, and possibly edema. A final possibility is that her catheter is placed incorrectly in the vagina rather than the bladder.
- To determine the cause of Mrs. Howard's symptoms, you need to perform several assessments. First, auscultate her heart and lung sounds and palpate her abdomen. Also assess for a rash on her skin, and ask her if she has any itching. If her heart and lung sounds are normal but her lower abdomen is hard, check for the position of the catheter. Sometimes it is difficult to tell if the catheter is in the right position just by looking, especially if the area around the catheter is swollen or if your patient is overweight. You can also check inputs to see if they match outputs. Currently, Mrs. Howard is getting 75 mL/hr of IV fluid and 40 mL/hr of the amphotericin B irrigant. She should be putting out in her urine at least 70 mL/hr: the hourly output of the urinary irrigant (40 mL) plus the least amount of urine you would expect to see in an hour (30 mL). If the catheter is in the correct place and her overall input is higher than her output, you are placing Mrs. Howard at risk for overload. If the catheter is

continued

not in the correct place, then you are giving her a vaginal irrigation and not the bladder irrigation that is ordered (see Chapter 12).

- If Mrs. Howard is having an allergic reaction, stop the irrigant immediately, follow anaphylactic protocol, and notify the primary care provider. If she is beginning to have problems with fluid overload due to her heart problems, reduce the IV rate to a keep open rate (20 to 40 mL/hr), stop the irrigant, and contact the primary care provider for further orders. If you discover that the catheter was not placed correctly, stop the irrigant, leave the catheter in place, and obtain another catheter kit. Insert the new triple-lumen urinary retention catheter into the urinary meatus and then remove the other catheter. Begin your irrigations once the new catheter is in place, and notify the primary care provider. Continue to monitor Mrs. Howard until you are certain she is stabilized and her symptoms have resolved.

CASE STUDY

JANICE ROMERO

Janice Romero, age 24, has recently been diagnosed with acute lymphocytic leukemia (ALL). To provide long-term venous access, she was admitted to have an implanted port placed. She had a 21-gauge peripheral IV inserted in her right arm prior to surgery. After her port was placed, Mrs. Romero's primary care provider ordered 2 units of packed red blood cells (PRBCs). You note an order for the use of a blood warmer for the transfusions. When you talk to Mrs. Romero about the blood transfusion, she tells you that the last time she received blood she had chills and fever during the transfusion.

MEDICAL ORDERS

2 units packed RBCs via blood warmer stat.

Intravenous fluids: D5 ½ NSS at 50 mL/hr

DEVELOPING CLINICAL REASONING

- Identify the site you will use to administer blood to Mrs. Romero. Why did you choose this site?
- Describe the technique you will use to administer blood to Mrs. Romero.
- Identify the purposes for warming blood, and describe the safest way to warm blood.
- Considering Mrs. Romero's history and diagnosis, describe the precautions you will implement before giving her blood.

continued

SUGGESTED RESPONSES FOR INTEGRATED NURSING CARE

- Before Mrs. Romero can receive blood, you must select an appropriate site (see Chapter 15). Site selection depends on the gauge of the IV and the fluid infusing in the IV. Blood must be given through a large-bore catheter to prevent red blood cell damage. Since dextrose will cause hemolysis, blood can be administered only with normal saline. For these two reasons, the optimal site for blood administration is her implanted port. Before you give her blood through the port, be certain that the port is not dedicated for other infusions, such as chemo.
- Since the implanted port is new, ensure that it is working properly prior to use. Check the medical record for a medical order allowing use of the port. Depending on your hospital policy, wear a mask and sterile gloves when accessing the port, particularly since she has leukemia and may be immunocompromised. In addition, a larger-gauge Huber needle is recommended for administering blood (see Chapter 15). Check the port for patency and blood return per facility policy. Infuse the normal saline slowly while you observe the implanted port site for signs of swelling and pain. If the port shows any sign of infiltration, notify the primary care provider, and choose another site to give her blood.
- Some patients may need to have their blood warmed before it is administered. This includes patients who are at risk for cardiac arrhythmias, patients with unusual immune responses, as well as neonatal and pediatric patients. A medical order is required for the warming of blood products during transfusion. Various devices exist to warm blood. Do not use the microwave to warm any blood product: It coagulates the proteins of the blood and causes severe hemolysis in the patient, which could be fatal. Whenever you need to warm blood, always use a blood warmer that your facility has approved.
- Mrs. Romero's history of chills and fever are signs of a possible transfusion reaction; thus, she is at increased risk for a transfusion reaction. Ensure that she has a signed consent form and that she fully understands her need for the blood. The primary care provider needs to be aware of this history of a transfusion reaction. The primary care provider may order premedication with diphenhydramine (Benadryl), acetaminophen (Tylenol), or steroids prior to blood administration to reduce the risk for developing another reaction. Stay with her for at least 15 minutes at the beginning of the transfusion. Continue to monitor her vital signs frequently per hospital policy. When you leave her room, make sure her call light is available, and instruct her to contact you if she has any unusual symptoms.

CASE STUDY

GWEN GALLOWAY

Mrs. Galloway, age 64, had a left-sided mastectomy and is now receiving follow-up chemotherapy for recurrent breast cancer with axillary node involvement. She has been hospitalized for 48 hours. She reports pain on her left side and under her left arm. She has a right double-lumen Hickman catheter inserted. Recent laboratory work shows a low white blood cell count of 1,800/mm^3 and a low platelet count of 39,000/mm^3. She also bleeds and bruises very easily. You have to obtain vital signs and provide AM care. You also need to draw a complete blood count and change the dressing on her central line.

MEDICAL ORDERS

Vital signs q 4 hr
Complete blood count (CBC) now and every AM
Morphine sulfate IV 6–8 mg q 2 hr prn pain
Cefazolin sodium (Ancef) 1 g IV q 8 hr
Change central line dressing q week

continued

DEVELOPING CLINICAL REASONING

- What special precautions should you take while obtaining Mrs. Galloway's vital signs?
- Identify your interventions when changing Mrs. Galloway's central line dressing and the rationale for these interventions.
- Explain why some sites would be contraindicated when taking Mrs. Galloway's temperature.
- Discuss the equipment used, restrictions, and concerns regarding Mrs. Galloway's personal care.
- Describe the special precautions you would take when drawing blood from Mrs. Galloway. Identify the site where you would draw the blood.

SUGGESTED RESPONSES FOR INTEGRATED NURSING CARE

- To individualize care, always assess your patient's condition and special needs. When a patient undergoes a mastectomy, she will often have lymph nodes removed from the affected side. Taking a blood pressure reading in the affected arm could interfere with circulation and harm the extremity (see Chapter 2). In Mrs. Galloway's case, her affected side is on the left, so take her blood pressure on the right side.
- Mrs. Galloway has a low platelet count, which places her at risk for bleeding. In addition, her low white blood cell count places her at risk for infection and other complications. Therefore, taking a rectal temperature would be contraindicated for Mrs. Galloway. It would also be contraindicated to take a left-sided axillary temperature on Mrs. Galloway because she is still having some discomfort due to her recent mastectomy (see Chapter 2).
- Given Mrs. Galloway's risk for bleeding, would a peripheral venipuncture be the best choice to obtain her CBC? Due to the risk for prolonged bleeding, her central line may provide the best access for a blood specimen. Determine whether her primary care provider has restricted her central line for chemotherapy. If her central line is dedicated to chemotherapy only, obtain a blood specimen by doing a venipuncture. If you needed to do a venipuncture, using Mrs. Galloway's left side would be contraindicated due to the mastectomy. You will need to apply pressure to the site for a longer period of time because of her increased risk for bleeding.
- When changing Mrs. Galloway's central line dressing, use sterile technique due to her increased risk for infection. Depending on facility policy, you may also need to place a mask on yourself and Mrs. Galloway. To prevent bleeding and bruising at the central line site, do not move or pull on the catheter as you are manipulating the central line dressing.
- Several restrictions could apply when performing Mrs. Galloway's personal care. Patients at risk for bleeding should avoid shaving. Another concern is the potential for bleeding from the mucous membranes when using a hard-bristled toothbrush and dental floss. Use mouth rinses and very soft toothettes to minimize trauma (see Chapter 7).

CASE STUDY

GEORGE PATEL

George Patel, age 64, was admitted to your floor 3 days ago following surgical insertion of a tracheostomy tube. His diagnosis prior to surgery was acute upper airway obstruction. He has a left IV or medication lock. Currently, he is receiving oxygen via his tracheostomy at 40%. His pulse oximetry readings have been consistently running in the low 90s. He quickly becomes short of breath when his oxygen is interrupted during suctioning. During your shift, you will have to suction Mr. Patel as needed and provide routine tracheostomy care. You will also need to transport him with portable oxygen to radiology for his AP and lateral chest x-ray.

MEDICAL ORDERS

Morphine sulfate 2 to 6 mg IV q 2 hr prn for pain
AP and lateral chest x-ray
Pulse oximetry every shift and prn
Oxygen via trach Venturi mask at 40%
Tracheostomy care every shift and prn
Medication or IV lock flush every shift
Tracheal suctioning prn

DEVELOPING CLINICAL REASONING

- How would you determine when Mr. Patel needs to be suctioned?
- How would you determine when Mr. Patel needs to have tracheostomy care?
- Describe expected outcomes when suctioning and providing tracheostomy care.
- When transporting Mr. Patel to the radiology department, what precautions should you implement to ensure his safety?

continued

SUGGESTED RESPONSES FOR INTEGRATED NURSING CARE

- To evaluate the need for suctioning, first assess Mr. Patel's respiratory status. Examine his oxygen saturation and compare it with his baseline. If his oxygen saturation is decreased from his baseline, this may be an indication that he needs to be suctioned. Observe his respirations to determine if they are more labored than usual. Listen to his lung sounds for crackles or wheezes. Also, listen around his tracheostomy for gurgling. Does he have a productive cough? All of these signs and symptoms are indications that he needs to be suctioned.
- To assess the need for tracheostomy care (see Chapter 14), closely examine his tracheostomy as well as the tracheostomy holder/ties and precut gauze dressing. If it appears wet or moist, tracheostomy care would be indicated. If his tracheostomy dressing appears dry and intact, you may want to wait until later in your shift to do tracheostomy care. Suctioning and subsequent coughing will often soil the tracheostomy dressings, so wait until after suctioning to change the tracheostomy dressing.
- Your expected outcomes when suctioning a tracheostomy include minimizing hypoxia, discomfort, and fatigue. Hypoxia may be reduced by hyperoxygenating the patient before suctioning according to facility policy. When you suction Mr. Patel, limit the length of suction time to 10 to 15 seconds and allow him to rest before suctioning him again (see Skill 14-11). During tracheostomy care or repeat suctioning, quickly replace his oxygen source and limit the time his oxygen is interrupted. Since Mr. Patel has a new tracheostomy, it is very likely he will need to be premedicated with morphine for pain. Morphine depresses respirations, so continually assess Mr. Patel's respiratory status after administering the pain medication. In addition, adequate rest periods are needed to minimize fatigue from suctioning. Mr. Patel may require a rest period between suctioning the tracheostomy and his tracheostomy care.
- The precautions you would take when transporting Mr. Patel focus on providing adequate oxygenation. First, assess Mr. Patel's oxygen saturation and respiratory status prior to transport. If indicated, suction Mr. Patel before he leaves his room. You must also check that the portable oxygen tank is full and the label says "oxygen." Before turning off his wall oxygen, make sure the portable oxygen tank is working properly and that the equipment is ready. This avoids interruption of his oxygenation while placing him on the portable oxygen.

3 Advanced Case Studies

CASE STUDY

COLE MCKEAN

Cole McKean is a 4-year-old boy in the pediatric intensive care unit (PICU). He weighs 22 kg. He was admitted 3 days ago after nearly drowning in a neighbor's pool. He was submerged for 5 to 10 minutes. The neighbor initiated CPR and the rescue team had a heart rate established within 10 minutes of their arrival. The aspirated pool water caused a severe inflammatory response resulting in pulmonary edema. Cole is intubated with an endotracheal tube (ETT) and is on a mechanical ventilator. Throughout the past 2 days he has been producing copious bronchial secretions and has required suctioning about every 2 hours. Today, his breath sounds are clearer and he requires less frequent suctioning. He is being weaned off oxygen. The care plan for today includes possible extubation. An arterial line is in place in his left radial artery, infusing NSS at 2 to 3 mL/hr. A PICC line with an infusion of D5 ½ NSS at 75 mL/hr is inserted into his right arm. His heart rate, respiratory rate, and arterial waveform are being monitored. The pulse oximeter sensor is applied to his right toe. He has an indwelling urinary (Foley) catheter to gravity drainage and a nasogastric tube in place and set to low intermittent suction. Cole is receiving sedation, but is opening his eyes at times and moving his extremities. He is becoming more active.

Suddenly, the alarm goes off on the ventilator. You look at Cole. His eyes are open and he is making crying sounds. You know when a child is properly intubated he or she cannot make sounds. You notice that his oxygen saturation level has dropped to 81% and his color is dusky. He is breathing on his own around the tube and his abdomen is rounded. You are assessing Cole's respiratory status and oxygenation when the primary care provider comes to the bedside. The primary care provider tells you to remove the ET tube and begin oxygen at 40% via face mask. When you place Cole on the face mask, his oxygen saturation returns to the mid-90s. The primary care provider says, "This little fellow was ready to get rid of his tube." She orders a follow-up arterial blood gas (ABG) to be drawn in 15 minutes.

continued

MEDICAL ORDERS

Continuous pulse oximetry
Foley to gravity
Maintain O_2 saturation 92% to 98%
I&O
Vent settings: 36% O_2, IMV 36, pressures 26/6
Nasogastric tube to low intermittent suction
Vital signs q 1 hr
Arterial blood gases q 2 hr
Neurologic checks q 1 hr
Intravenous fluids: D5 ½ NS at 75 mL/hr
Endotracheal suctioning prn
Arterial line: NS 2 to 3 mL/hr

DEVELOPING CLINICAL REASONING

- Describe your initial actions in response to a possible extubation.
- How can the technique of drawing ABGs be adapted for a pediatric patient?
- How will Cole's response be evaluated now that he is on an oxygen mask?
- Develop a plan of care that will allow Cole rest and sleep periods, but also allow hourly assessments.
- Identify the nursing skills involved in monitoring Cole's respiratory status.

SUGGESTED RESPONSES FOR INTEGRATED NURSING CARE

- When a patient is intubated, the patency of this airway is a critical priority. When you hear Cole cry, you must determine if his ETT is in the proper place. Listen with your stethoscope over the lung fields and abdomen. If you do not hear ventilator-induced breath sounds over the lung fields, then the ETT is not in place. Because a child's neck is so short, it is not difficult to displace a tracheal tube into the esophagus. If this occurs, you may hear ventilator-cycled sounds in the abdomen. Signs that an ETT is not in the correct position include unstable oxygen saturation levels, cyanosis, and abdominal distention. In Cole's situation, you determine that the ETT is no longer in the lungs. All patients on mechanical ventilation must have an Ambu bag and a mask of the correct size at the bedside. Cole did not require mask-bag respirations at this time, but he has the potential for this need.
- When you are evaluating Cole's response, the ABG results will guide clinical decision-making regarding oxygen delivery. In Cole's case, 10 to 15 minutes after changing to the 40% oxygen mask, you draw an ABG (see Chapter 18). The results come back as follows: $Pa{O_2}$, 82 mm Hg; $Pa{CO_2}$, 46 mm Hg; pH, 7.34; HCO_3, 20 mEq/L. This ABG shows that Cole's oxygen level is acceptable and there is no indication for immediate reintubation. Continue to draw

continued

ABGs periodically, as ordered, to evaluate Cole's response to treatment.

- To monitor his respiratory status, observe his work of breathing, count his respiratory rate, observe his color, and auscultate breath sounds. If he shows no significant respiratory distress and has a stable respiratory rate and clear breath sounds, he is responding well to the change in his oxygen source. In addition, continuously monitor the oxygen saturation level via pulse oximetry. Immediately report any increases or decreases in oxygen saturation to the primary care provider.
- Because children have a small total blood volume, the blood drawn back in the arterial line is usually not discarded but returned to the patient after the laboratory sample is drawn. Smaller volumes of blood are sent to the laboratory in pediatric specimen tubes. The setup for a pediatric arterial line delivers a smaller volume of fluid when the fast-flush release is activated (i.e., the pigtail is pulled).
- When a patient, especially a child, is critically ill, cluster your hands-on care so that the patient will have a significant amount of time to sleep and rest between hourly interventions. One of the initial assessments a nurse makes in an intensive care setting is to determine that each of the monitoring devices is accurately displaying the patient's status (see Chapters 14 and 16). After you determine that the monitors accurately reflect the patient's vital signs, obtaining alternating sets of vital signs from the patient and from the monitor may be permitted, according to hospital policy. Maintain a quiet environment. Because of the noise and activity of the intensive care unit, many infant and child intensive care units dim the lights at night to create day/night cycles for the children.

CASE STUDY

DEWAYNE WALLACE

Dewayne Wallace, age 19, was admitted to the emergency department approximately 4 hours ago with a stab wound to the chest that he received in a knife fight while intoxicated. You are asked to care for Dewayne while his nurse attends to a new emergency. She gives you the following report: He was admitted in respiratory distress and bleeding from the stab wound. His wound is on the right side at the sixth intercostal space and is approximately 1 inch in length, sutured and intact. The chest x-ray confirmed a right hemothorax and, as a result, the physician inserted a chest tube. The chest tube is connected to a disposable drainage system and placed to suction at –20 cm H_2O. The chest tube is draining a small amount of dark-red blood. There has not been any new drainage for the past 2 hours.

Dewayne's most recent vital signs were as follows: temperature, 98.4°F; pulse, 88 beats/minute; respirations, 24/minute; blood pressure, 112/74 mm Hg. He is receiving oxygen via face mask at 30% and is on continuous pulse oximetry. The oxygen saturation level is currently 96%. He says he feels short of breath. He does not have labored breathing and is not using accessory muscles. He reports pain at the chest tube insertion site and stab wound site. He has a patent IV infusing in his left forearm. His laboratory work reported a blood alcohol level of 0.12. The nurse giving report says, "Good luck with that delinquent. He says he's in pain, but I think he already drank his pain medication from a bottle."

continued

Dewayne turns on his call light. When you approach him, you notice his breathing is labored with subclavicular retractions. The pulse oximeter reads 95%. Dewayne says, "This thing in my side really hurts."

You take another set of vital signs: temperature, 98.6°F; pulse, 90 beats/minute; respirations, 37/minute; blood pressure, 118/78 mm Hg. You find the breath sounds are diminished on the right. The chest drainage tubing is in the bed without a dependent loop, and Dewayne has been lying on a segment of the tubing. You ask him to rate his pain on a scale of 1 to 10 (10 = worst), and he says, "About a 5." You ask if the medicine he got earlier helped with the pain, and he answers that he didn't get any pain medicine. When you check the chart you find that an order for hydrocodone bitartrate 5 mg/acetaminophen 500 mg (Lortab 5/500) was written about 3 hours ago, but when you look over the medication administration record, you do not see that any has been administered. You find his nurse and ask if the Lortab was given. The response you get is, "Are you kidding? If he's tough enough to drink and fight, he's tough enough for a little chest tube. He made his bed; he can just lie in it."

MEDICAL ORDERS

Chest tube with drainage system to suction at –20 cm H_2O

Intravenous fluids: NSS at 100 mL/hr

Oxygen at 30% via face mask

Lortab 5/500, 1 or 2 tabs q 4 hr PO prn for pain

Continuous pulse oximetry

DEVELOPING CLINICAL REASONING

- Which of Dewayne's needs is your first priority? Describe your assessments related to your first priority.
- How would you troubleshoot his chest tube drainage system? What could be the source of his respiratory distress?
- Describe the purpose of a chest tube drainage system for a hemothorax.
- Discuss valid reasons a nurse might not give a pain medication when there is a prn order.
- Discuss prejudices nurses may have that may prohibit adequate pain management.

continued

SUGGESTED RESPONSES FOR INTEGRATED NURSING CARE

- Your first priority is Dewayne's increased respiratory distress. Although the change in oxygen saturation levels is very small, this is only because Dewayne's body is compensating for it now. Dewayne's work of breathing has dramatically changed, signaling a change in his respiratory status. Your preliminary assessment showed a respiratory rate of 37 breaths/minute, up significantly from his earlier respiratory rate of 24. When you inspected the chest you found subclavicular retractions; this indicates that Dewayne is using his intercostal muscles to breathe. When you auscultated breath sounds, you found decreased air movement on the right, indicating a hemothorax.
- In a hemothorax, blood collects in the pleural space and compresses a lung. The purpose of the chest tube is to evacuate the blood and allow the lung to expand fully. In Dewayne's case, the stab wound created a puncture in the pleura, allowing blood to accumulate within the pleural space. It is important to evaluate the right lung on a routine basis to make sure the blood in the pleural space has been removed so that the lung can re-expand. Any change in respiratory status may indicate a problem with the chest tube drainage system.
- As you noted in this case, Dewayne has had a change in his respiratory status. Since you have completed his physical assessment, now begin inspecting the equipment. As with any equipment check, begin inspection at the patient and move to the equipment. Start your inspection at the insertion site of the chest tube. Observe the dressing to ensure it is occlusive and inspect the tubing for leaks, kinks, and dependent loops. Compare the amount of recent drainage in the drainage system with the volume of old drainage, and check the amount of suction (see Chapter 14). In this case, Dewayne has been lying on his tubing, which would prevent it from draining properly. When you reposition Dewayne's tubing, approximately 60 mL of dark old blood flows into the drainage set. His respiratory status improves quickly. Thus, this accumulated blood in the pleural space was the source of his respiratory distress.
- There are several situations in which giving a narcotic analgesic is contraindicated. During a life-saving procedure, pain is not always a priority. In this case, Dewayne did not receive pain medication before the insertion of his chest tube because he was at risk for respiratory arrest. Narcotics are also contraindicated when it is critical to assess alertness, because the narcotic might mask neurologic changes. Narcotic analgesics also are associated with the side effects of respiratory depression and vital sign changes. Patients sometimes do not receive the pain medication ordered because the nurse is worried about these side effects. Because of this, controversy exists to whether the benefit of pain control outweighs the risk of side effects. Many hospitals have committees that can assist with these ethical decisions. A dialog among nurses, doctors, and pharmacists can result in optimal pain control with minimal side effects. Speak with the primary care provider before independently deciding to withhold pain medication to prevent side effects.
- Another reason nurses may withhold medication is their own preconception of the patient's pain and their own prejudices. Some nurses are not even aware that they have these feelings. As a nursing student, you need to understand how you will respond to patients, and you need to explore your own beliefs and prejudices. The accepted standard in nursing is that a patient defines his or her own pain and that it is the nurse's responsibility to manage it properly. Guidelines for pain management have been written by state Boards of Nursing, the U.S. Department of Health and Human Services, the World Health Organization, as well as other professional organizations.

CASE STUDY

ROBERT ESPINOZA

Robert Espinoza, age 44, has just had exploratory abdominal surgery. The postanesthesia recovery room (PACU) nurse calls at 2:10 PM to report on Mr. Espinoza and tells you he has a peripheral IV inserted in his right arm, infusing NSS at 50 mL/hr. He has a midline abdominal dressing that is dry and intact with two Jackson-Pratt (JP) drains in place. He also

continued

has a nasogastric (NG) tube and an indwelling urinary catheter (Foley) to gravity drainage. She reports that his NG tube has been checked for placement and has been draining moderate amounts of yellow-green contents. His vital signs in the PACU are as follows: temperature, 98.0°F; pulse, 86 beats/minute; respirations, 16/minute; blood pressure, 134/80 mm Hg. At 2 PM, he received 6 mg morphine sulfate IV for a pain rating of 6 on a scale of 1 to 10 (10 = worst).

At 3 PM, you receive Mr. Espinoza on your medical–surgical unit via stretcher by a hospital transporter. The NG tube tape that secured the NG to his nose is no longer in place. You also notice that the urinary drainage bag lying on top of his legs has a small amount of amber urine in the reservoir. While you are in his room, Mr. Espinoza says, "Hey, it feels like there's something wet under my back." His vital signs on arrival are as follows: temperature, 98.0°F; pulse, 130 beats/minute; respirations, 18/minute; and blood pressure, 100/68 mm Hg. His respirations are regular and unlabored and his skin color is pink. He now rates his pain as a 2 on a scale of 1 to 10 (10 = worst). Mr. Espinoza's family is anxiously waiting in the waiting room on your floor.

MEDICAL ORDERS

Indwelling urinary catheter (Foley) to gravity
Routine JP drain care
Strict I&O
Routine postoperative vital signs
Nasogastric tube to intermittent suction
Intravenous fluids: NSS at 50 mL/hr
Morphine sulfate 4 to 10 mg IV q 2 hr prn for pain

DEVELOPING CLINICAL REASONING

- Considering Mr. Espinoza's immediate postoperative status, describe how you would transfer him from the stretcher to his bed.
- Prioritize, with rationales, your assessments and nursing care for Mr. Espinoza in the following areas:
  - Immediate physical assessments and interventions
  - Assessment and management of tubes
  - Pain management and comfort level
  - Care of his family

SUGGESTED RESPONSES FOR INTEGRATED NURSING CARE

- When transferring Mr. Espinoza to his bed, consider the following factors: minimizing his pain level, protecting his incision, and protecting the patency of his tubes. Excessive strain from moving can cause disruption and bleeding to his abdominal incision. Per hospital policy, carefully transfer him with the assistance of others. During transfer, be careful not to disrupt his tubes or dressings. Once Mr. Espinoza is in his bed, place his urinary drainage bag on the bed frame so that it hangs below the level of his bladder. This position will allow the urine to drain by gravity and decrease the possibility of a urinary tract infection (see Chapter 12).

continued

- Because Mr. Espinoza is a new postoperative patient, your first priority is to perform an assessment based on the ABC criteria (airway, breathing, and circulation). Compare his vital signs on arrival with his baseline vital signs. Mr. Espinoza's respiratory rate has not changed significantly from his baseline. If not contraindicated, elevate his head to facilitate deep breathing and continue to assess his airway and respiratory status (see Chapter 6).
- Circulation is the next immediate priority. In Mr. Espinoza's case, his blood pressure has decreased and his heart rate has increased from his baseline in the PACU. Both of these changes could indicate decreased blood volume related to bleeding. Therefore, assess Mr. Espinoza's abdominal dressing to evaluate if it is dry and intact. Never assume that an incision is dry just because you cannot see any blood on top of the dressing. If the abdominal dressing is covered by foam tape, blood underneath the tape may not be easily visualized. Look under the patient to see if blood has trickled underneath the dressing. Mr. Espinoza said that he felt something "wet" under his back, and when turning him, you discover that there is a large puddle of bright-red blood underneath him that is caused by acute bleeding from his abdominal incision. Do not remove the abdominal dressing. You may, however, reinforce the dressing if you have an order.
- Identify all other possible sources of bleeding. When you assess the JP drains, note the color, amount, and consistency of blood. Assess his abdomen for signs of internal bleeding, such as abdominal distention. Also check for decreased urine output, another sign indicating a possible decrease in blood volume. A urine output of less than 30 mL/hr may be a sign of hypovolemic shock. Although Mr. Espinoza is bleeding and has signs of decreased blood volume, he is not yet in hypovolemic shock. If Mr. Espinoza's blood pressure continues to drop, elevate his feet to increase venous return. Report all indications of internal and/or external bleeding to the physician. Acute postoperative bleeding requires surgical repair.
- Your next priority is to ensure that all of his tubes are intact and working properly. One of the first tubes you want to assess for patency is his IV, particularly because he may be returning to surgery. The next tubes you want to examine are the JP drains. To maintain suction, a JP drain must be less than half full. Assess the color and other characteristics of the JP drainage (see Chapter 8). Next, assess his NG tube. Mr. Espinoza's NG tube tape is not secure, so you cannot assume that the tube is still in his stomach. Check the NG for placement; assess the color, pH, and amount of the return; and then place the NG to intermittent suction (see Chapter 13). Measure the length of the exposed tube and compare it with the length documented at the time of insertion. Next, evaluate his urinary catheter to determine if it is draining properly (see Chapter 12).
- The next priority is to monitor Mr. Espinoza's pain level. If he is in acute pain, immediately consider incisional disruption. Because Mr. Espinoza is bleeding, you may need to give small increments as opposed to large amounts of morphine to prevent a further drop in his blood pressure. In addition to his physical comfort, attend to potential anxiety about returning to the operating room. Maintain a calm voice and demeanor when caring for Mr. Espinoza.
- Notify the primary care provider of all assessment findings.
- Do not forget Mr. Espinoza's family, who are anxious to see him. It is helpful to send another staff nurse to keep them updated while you are busy in his room. When his condition stabilizes and before the family visits him, tell them about the tubes that they will see, including the reason for and function of each of the tubes. Be flexible when allowing the family to come in and visit Mr. Espinoza.

CASE STUDY

JASON BROWN, GWEN GALLOWAY, CLAUDIA TRAN, AND JAMES WHITE

This is your first week as an RN in a small rural hospital. You work the night shift on a medical–surgical unit. Tonight your only aide and a staff nurse have called in sick, which makes the unit short-staffed. You have notified the night supervisor that you need help, and she sends an aide from another floor to assist you. She tells you she can get someone on

continued

the floor to help you in about an hour, and instructs you to take care of the priority cases until that time.

You have six relatively uncomplicated patients; caring for them involves checking their vital signs and giving medications. You instruct the aide to obtain their vital signs and report the results back to you. A quick review of the medications reveals nothing that is urgent; you can wait and have the second nurse administer the medications when he or she arrives. You have four other patients with more complicated issues, who require additional assessments and urgent care:

- Jason Brown, a 64-year-old patient with a tracheostomy, has gurgling sounds coming from his tracheostomy and a frequent, nonproductive cough. His oxygen saturation level via pulse oximetry is 88%. You have orders to suction his tracheostomy prn.
- Gwen Galloway had been receiving chemotherapy and has now come back to the hospital with gastroenteritis. When you arrive on your shift, she is experiencing bouts of nausea and vomiting.
- Claudia Tran, an 84-year-old patient from a nursing home, is post-CVA. She has a stage III pressure ulcer on her coccyx and a stage I ulcer on her left hip. She needs to be turned every 15 minutes because of rapidly developing erythema on bony prominences. She is confused and has fallen the past 2 nights when left unattended, even when restrained. Her family is visiting her now but plans to leave in 30 minutes.
- James White has COPD. The aide reports that the blood pressure from the automatic cuff is 168/100 mm Hg; his baseline is usually 130/70 mm Hg. The aide also reports that he is complaining of a severe headache, but has no other complaints.

DEVELOPING CLINICAL REASONING

- Identify the order in which you would provide care to these patients. Explain your rationales as well as your interventions.

SUGGESTED RESPONSES FOR INTEGRATED NURSING CARE

- Mr. Brown is having difficulty with airway clearance and oxygenation, so he will be your first priority. Nursing priorities always follow the ABCs: airway, breathing, and circulation. He will require prompt tracheal suctioning and further evaluation of his respiratory status (see Chapter 14). When his oxygen saturation levels have stabilized, you can then attend to the other patients.
- Next, address the dramatic change in vital signs that Mr. White is experiencing. Mr. White is at risk for a stroke if his blood pressure continues to stay elevated and is not controlled immediately. Before planning any other interventions, verify the blood pressure by taking it yourself with a manual cuff (see Chapter 2). Initial nursing assessment includes assessing the accuracy of the equipment as well as the accuracy of the information reported to you by assistive personnel. The blood pressure you obtain is 190/110 mm Hg. Check for the primary care provider's orders regarding

continued

possible prn blood pressure medications. Call the primary care provider right away and notify him or her of the change in Mr. White's status.

- You know that Mrs. Tran is at high risk for falls if left unattended, and she may injure herself seriously if this occurs. Reducing her risk for injury is your next priority (see Chapter 4). In Mrs. Tran's case, you could ask a family member to stay the night, or at least until you get more help on the unit. Many families are willing to help if you make them aware of such situations. If the family leaves, ask the aide to remove the restraint, place the bed in a low position, and stay with Mrs. Tran until you get further help. You can delegate Mrs. Tran's positioning schedule to the aide.
- Despite the obvious distress of vomiting, this is not a life-threatening situation for Mrs. Galloway. Therefore, her condition is a lower priority than that of the other three patients. Mrs. Galloway requires comfort. Check if an antiemetic medication has been ordered; if not, call the primary care provider and obtain an order. Other interventions you can perform until her medication takes effect are lowering the lights, applying a cool cloth to the neck, decreasing noises, removing substances that may have a strong odor (e.g., food and vomitus), and keeping her head elevated.
- When prioritizing and delegating care, here are some questions that might help guide your decision-making process:
  - Is the situation life threatening?
  - How rapidly could this patient's condition deteriorate?
  - How quickly can you remedy the problem?
  - Who can provide assistance?
- Whenever a patient's airway, breathing, or circulation is jeopardized, this is a life-threatening emergency. Base your priorities on the ABC criteria. Mr. Brown is your first priority because his airway and oxygenation are a problem. When a patient's condition has the potential to deteriorate rapidly, this is also a priority. In Mr. White's case, because of the spike in his blood pressure, he has the potential for a stroke. Preventing this life-threatening event requires immediate action. When two patients have problems of similar urgency, such as oxygenation, respond to the problem that you can remedy the quickest. Sometimes when you have many activities to accomplish in a short period of time, it is difficult to take time to seek additional help. Many hospitals will have night supervisors to assist you with problem solving. Additionally, physicians are available by phone or in the hospital. Nonlicensed personnel, such as aides, are sometimes available to assist with noncritical tasks. A nursing skill to develop is prioritization of nursing care and delegation of noncritical tasks.

Case Study References

Centers for Disease Control and Prevention (CDC). (2013). Methicillin-resistant *Staphylococcus aureus* (MRSA) infections. Available http://www.cdc.gov/mrsa/index.html.

Centers for Disease Control and Prevention. (2004). *Guidance for the selection and use of personal protective equipment (PPE) in healthcare settings.* (Slide presentation). Available http://www.cdc.gov/HAI/pdfs/ppe/PPEslides6-29-04.pdf.

Centers for Disease Control and Prevention (CDC). (2007a). (Updated 2012). *Airborne infection isolation precautions. Excerpted from guideline for isolation precautions: Preventing transmission of infectious agents in healthcare settings.* Available www.cdc.gov/hicpac/pdf/isolation/Isolation2007.pdf.

Centers for Disease Control and Prevention (CDC). (2007b). (Updated 2012). *Standard precautions. Excerpted from guideline for isolation precautions: Preventing transmission of infectious agents in healthcare settings.* Available www.cdc.gov/hicpac/pdf/isolation/Isolation2007.pdf.

The Institute for Safe Medication Practices (ISMP). (2013). ISMP and FDA campaign to eliminate use of error-prone abbreviations. Available http://search.ismp.org/cgi-bin/hits.pl?in–517791&fh=80&ph–1&tk–hTuuku%20TuukuOw%20PukqT%20PukqTOw%20SzzuT%3A%26Sp%26kqw%20SzzuT%3A%26Sp%26kqOw%20Tuukuw%20SzzuT%3A%26Sp%26kq&su=swXX_I%3F%3Ffff.LvQ_.FJu%3FgFF%3Av%3FVEEJPaLVXLFrv%3FkPeVx%3AX.Vv_&qy=hTuuku%20PukqT%20SzzuT%3A%26Sp%26kqw&pd=1.

The Joint Commission (TJC). (2014). *National patient safety goals. Hospital: 2014 National patient safety goals.* Available http://www.jointcommission.org/standards_information/npsgs.aspx.

Taylor, C., Lillis, C., & Lynn, P. (2015). *Fundamentals of nursing.* (8th ed.). Philadelphia: Wolters Kluwer Health/Lippincott Williams & Wilkins.

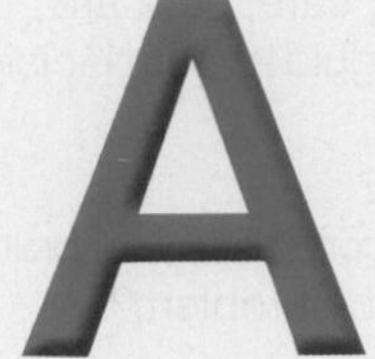

Appendix A Guidelines for Delegation Decision Making

Delegation involves the transfer of responsibility for the performance of an activity to another individual while retaining accountability for the outcome. Used appropriately, delegation can result in safe and effective nursing care. Delegation can free the registered nurse (RN) to focus on assessment and development or revision of the nursing plan of care (Trossman, 2012). Delegation allows the RN to attend to more complex patient care needs, develops the skills of nursing assistive personnel, and promotes cost containment for the healtlh care organization. The RN determines appropriate nursing practice by using nursing knowledge, professional judgment, and the legal authority to practice nursing (American Nurses Association [ANA], 2007).

In delegating, the registered nurse must ensure appropriate assessment, planning, implementation, and evaluation. Decision making about delegation is a continuous process. These guidelines provide a quick reference for the delegation decision-making information found in each skill.

DELEGATION CRITERIA

Three criteria to be considered by the registered nurse when deciding to delegate care activities (National Council of State Boards of Nursing [NCSBN], 2005) are:

1. The State Nursing Practice Act must permit delegation and outline the authorized task(s) to be delegated or authorize the RN to decide delegation;
2. The person delegating has the appropriate qualifications: appropriate education, skills and experience, as well as current competency.
3. The person receiving the delegation must have the appropriate qualifications: appropriate education, training, skills and experience, as well as evidence of current competency.

In addition, according to the ANA and NCSBN (2006), the delegated task(s) must not require critical thinking or professional judgment.

DELEGATION PROCESS

Delegation is a multistep, continuous process.

1. The registered nurse must assess the situation, identifying the needs of the patient, considering the circumstances and setting, as well as the competence of the person to whom the task is being delegated. The RN may proceed with delegation if patient needs, circumstances, and available resources indicate patient safety will be maintained with delegated care.
2. The registered nurse plans for and communicates clearly the specific task(s) to be delegated. The RN may proceed with delegation if the nature of the task, competence of the person receiving the delegation, and patient implications indicate patient safety will be maintained with delegated care.
3. The registered nurse assures appropriate accountability. The RN may proceed with delegation if the RN and person receiving the delegation accept the accountability for their respective roles in the delegated patient care.
4. The registered nurse supervises performance of the delegated task(s), providing directions and clear expectations of how the task(s) is to be performed. The RN monitors performance, intervenes if necessary, and ensures the appropriate documentation.

5. The registered nurse must evaluate the entire delegation process, evaluating the patient, the performance of the task(s), and obtain and provide feedback.
6. The registered nurse must reassess and adjust the overall plan of care, as needed.

FIVE RIGHTS OF DELEGATION

The Five Rights of Delegation provide a resource to facilitate decisions about delegation. The NCSBN (1995) identifies the Five Rights of Delegation as follows:

- **Right Task:** One that is delegable for a specific patient.
- **Right Circumstances:** Appropriate patient setting, available resources, and other relevant factors considered.
- **Right Person:** Right person is delegating the right task to the right person to be performed on the right person.
- **Right Direction/Communication:** Clear, concise description of the task, including its objective, limits, and expectations.
- **Right Supervision:** Appropriate monitoring, evaluation, intervention, as needed, and feedback.

"DO-NOT-DELEGATE" CARE

Nursing care or tasks that should never be delegated except to another RN include:

- Initial and ongoing nursing assessment of the patient and his or her nursing care needs
- Determination of the nursing diagnosis, nursing care plan, evaluation of the patient's progress in relation to the care plan, and evaluation of the nursing care delivered to the patient
- Supervision and education of nursing personnel; patient teaching that requires an assessment of the patient and his or her education needs
- Any other nursing interventions that requires professional nursing knowledge, judgment, and/or skill

DELEGATION DECISION TREE

Using skills, knowledge, and professional judgment, the registered nurse determines appropriate nursing practice based on the state practice act and professional scope of practice, the standards and code of ethics, and the organization's policies and procedures related to delegation (ANA & NCSBN, 2006).

The Decision Tree for Delegation by Registered Nurses distributed by the American Nurses Association and the National Council of State Boards of Nursing can assist nurses with delegation decisions. The Decision Tree for Delegation can be found at https://www.ncsbn.org/Delegation_joint_statement_NCSBN-ANA.pdf.

Taylor Suite Resources

Explore these additional resources for more information on delegation:

- thePoint online resource, http://thepoint.lww.com/Lynn4E
- Fundamentals of Nursing: *Chapter 14, Implementing; Chapter 22, Nurse Leader, Manager, and Care Coordinator*

References and Resources

American Nurses Association (ANA). (2012). Principles for delegation by registered nurses to unlicensed assistive personnel. Silver Spring, MD: Author.

American Nurses Association (ANA). (2007). Unlicensed assistive personnel. Position statement. Available at http://www.nursingworld.org/MainMenuCategories/Policy-Advocacy/Positions-and-Resolutions/ANAPositionStatements/Position-Statements-Alphabetically/Registered-Nurses-Utilization-of-Nursing-Assistive-Personnel-in-All-Settings.html.

American Nurses Association (ANA) and National Council of State Boards of Nursing (NCSBN). (2006) Joint statement on delegation. Available https://www.ncsbn.org/Delegation_joint_statement_NCSBN-ANA.pdf.

Ayers, D. M. & Montgomery, M. (2008). Hospital nursing. Delegating the "right" way: Learn five tips for delegating effectively and safely. *Nursing, 38*(4), 56hn1-2.

Daley, K. (2013). Helping nurses strengthen their delegation skills. *American Nurse Today, 8*(3), 18.

National Council of State Boards of Nursing (NCSBN). (2005). Working with others: A position paper. Available https://www.ncsbn.org/Working_with_Others.pdf

Trossman, S. (2012). Is it OK to delegate?: Revised principles, resources aim to help RNs answer the question. *The American Nurse,* 44(6), 1, 6.

Weydt, A. (2010). Developing delegation skills. *Online Journal of Issues in Nursing, 15*(2), Manuscript 1.

Index

Page numbers followed by t indicate table; those followed by b indicate box.

C

D

E

F

J

Q

R

U

V

CCS0814